Eighteenth Edition

Williams
Obstetrics

F. Gary Cunningham, M.D.
Professor and Chairman, Department of Obstetrics & Gynecology
University of Texas Southwestern Medical Center
Chief of Obstetrics & Gynecology, Parkland Memorial Hospital
Dallas, Texas

Paul C. MacDonald, M.D.
Professor, Departments of Obstetrics & Gynecology and Biochemistry
Director of the Cecil H. and Ida Green Center for Reproductive Biology Sciences
University of Texas Southwestern Medical Center
Senior Attending Staff, Parkland Memorial Hospital
Dallas, Texas

Norman F. Gant, M.D.
Professor, Department of Obstetrics & Gynecology
University of Texas Southwestern Medical Center
Senior Attending Staff, Parkland Memorial Hospital
Dallas, Texas

APPLETON & LANGE
Norwalk, Connecticut/San Mateo, California

ISBN 0-8385-9736-X

Notice: Our knowledge in clinical sciences is constantly changing. As new information becomes available, changes in treatment and in the use of drugs become necessary. The authors and the publisher of this volume have taken care to make certain that the doses of drugs and schedules of treatment are correct and compatible with the standards generally accepted at the time of publication. The reader is advised to consult carefully the instruction and information material included in the package insert of each drug or therapeutic agent before administration. This advice is especially important when using new or infrequently used drugs.

Copyright © 1989 by Appleton & Lange
A Publishing Division of Prentice Hall
Copyright © 1985 by Appleton-Century-Crofts
Copyright © 1971 by Meredith Corporation
Copyright © 1966 by Meredith Publishing Company
Copyright © 1950, 1956, 1961 by Appleton-Century-Crofts, Inc.
Copyright © 1936, 1941, 1945 by D. Appleton-Century Co., Inc.
Copyright © 1902, 1903, 1904, 1907, 1909, 1912, 1917, 1923, 1930 by D. Appleton and Company
Copyright © renewed 1964 by Florence C. Stander
Copyright © renewed 1951 by Anne W. Niles
Copyright © renewed 1935, 1940 by Caroline W. Williams
Copyright © renewed 1930, 1931, 1932 by J. Whitridge Williams

89 90 91 92 93 / 10 9 8 7 6 5 4 3 2 1

Prentice Hall International (UK) Limited, *London*
Prentice Hall of Australia Pty. Limited, *Sydney*
Prentice Hall Canada, Inc., *Toronto*
Prentice Hall Hispanoamericana, S. A., *Mexico*
Prentice Hall of India Private Limited, *New Delhi*
Prentice Hall of Japan, Inc., *Tokyo*
Simon & Schuster Asia Pte. Ltd., *Singapore*
Editora Prentice Hall do Brasil Ltda., *Rio de Janeiro*
Prentice Hall, *Englewood Cliffs, New Jersey*

Library of Congress Cataloging-in-Publication Data
Williams, J. Whitridge (John Whitridge), 1866–1931.
    Williams obstetrics.

    Includes bibliographies and index.
    1. Obstetrics. I. Cunningham, F. Gary.
II. MacDonald, Paul C., 1930–   . III. Gant, Norman F. IV. Title. V. Title: Obstetrics.
[DNLM: 1. Obstetrics. WQ 100 W724w]
RG524.W7 1989   618.2   88–34287
ISBN 0-8385-9736-X

Listed here are some recently translated editions of this book and the publishers:

Italian (*15th edition*), Piccin
Japanese (*15th edition*), Hirokawa
Persian, Franklin
Portuguese (*16th edition*), Ed. Gunabara Koogan
Spanish (*17th edition*), Salvat

Editor: Lin Paterson
Designer: M. Chandler Martylewski, Steven Byrum
Production Editor: John Williams
Production Assistance: Lisa Jenio and Harkavy Publishing Service
Indexer: Maria Coughlin

Printed in the United States of America

Dedication

The eighteenth edition of *Williams Obstetrics* is dedicated, with affection, pride, and honor, to Dr. Jack A. Pritchard. The three authors of this edition each know Jack in an unusual way. First, he was the mentor of all three. Second, all three served as the chairman of this department when Jack was a faculty member. In consequence, each of us has his own special view of Jack as teacher, boss, employee, colleague, and friend.

Jack Pritchard became the second chairman of this department in 1955, at age 33, and he retired as chairman in 1969, at age 47. The three authors of the eighteenth edition followed him as chairman. Based on his beliefs and experiences, he admonished each of us: "Don't become a chairman before you are 40 and don't continue after you are 50." So far, we have pretty well kept to that schedule. But this admonishment was clearly characteristic of the man. He brought to the specialty of obstetrics and gynecology a well-defined discipline. Indeed, one clear view of Jack which each of us shares is that of disciplinarian in the finest sense of the word. He believed in and adopted the scientific approach to the practice of obstetrics; he believed in and created a disciplined training program for students, house officers, and fellows alike; and he believed in and participated in the creation of a disciplined system for the communication of new knowledge and ideas and experiences. In bad times and good times, he stuck doggedly to the principle of providing the optimal in obstetrical care. He was the first to accept proven methods and to embrace new and innovative approaches that

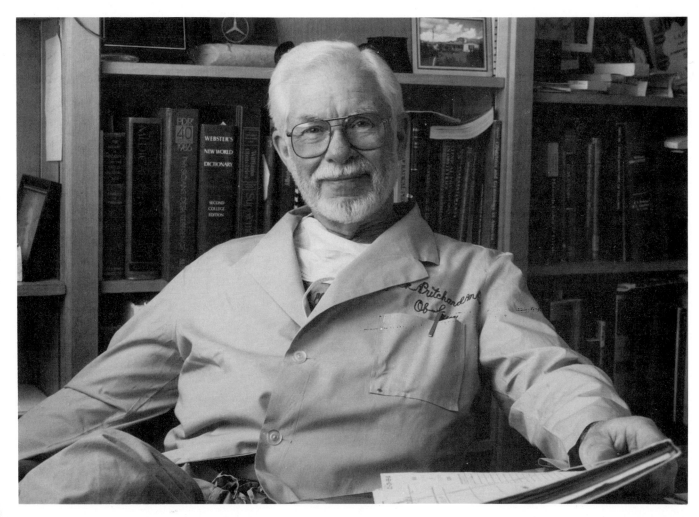

were based on sufficient data and rigorous testing, but he also was the first to reject the unproven and the first to disavow the likely utility of the fad of the day. He is a clinical scientist who recognized and supported the development of the basic sciences and scientists with whom he is associated. He believes in communication among all disciplines of science and medicine and promoted joint appointments of faculty in pediatrics and the basic sciences. He is involved. He has that uniquely difficult-to-define "feel" for the proper approach to a given clinical problem; he is intuitive; he is thorough; and he is always a part of the action. Jack Pritchard has never been disembodied from the mainstream of the obstetrical service, often to the chagrin of social workers, nursing staff, hospital administration, faculty, housestaff, and students. As chairman and chief of obstetrics, he was ever-present. And he never waivered from the disciplined approach to the successful promotion of progress. He is a giant in the field of obstetrics, and our lives and those of countless thousands of obstetricians to follow and countless millions of women, some not yet born, will be enriched because of his disciplined contributions to this art and science, obstetrics. With profound respect, we dedicate this eighteenth edition to him.

Contents

Preface

Obstetrics is an unusual specialty of medicine. Practitioners of this art and science must be concerned simultaneously with the lives and well-being of two persons; indeed, the lives of two who are interwoven. Ordinarily, the expectation for continued good health for these two persons collectively is more than 120 years, and the quality of that life is our most important concern. Hence, the obligation of the obstetrician is clear, the responsibility is enormous, but the rewards of success are monumental.

In this, the eighteenth edition of *Williams Obstetrics,* as in the ones that came before, we emphasize the basic principles of sound obstetrical practice. We have incorporated exciting new findings relevant to the recently distinguished science of maternal–fetal medicine, and to do so, extensive revisions and additions were necessary. The format of the book has been changed to reflect better the narrow margin that too often separates normal pregnancy from those conditions and circumstances in which the life of the mother or the fetus or both is placed suddenly in jeopardy.

Whereas the practice of obstetrics is a clinical science, the principles on which it is based are developed from discoveries made through research conducted by both clinical and basic scientists. In recognition of the importance of knowledge of basic physiology of pregnancy to the practice of obstetrics, Sections I and II are devoted to descriptions of fundamental biomolecular processes involved in the organization of pregnancy, of fetal development and maturation, and of the physiological and biomolecular processes of parturition. These chapters were revised extensively to present clinically relevant vistas of the dynamic role of the fetus and fetal contributions to the maintenance of pregnancy and the initiation of parturition. Sections III and IV are dedicated to descriptions of time-honored practices and proven management plans for the pregnant woman and her fetus. Included are extensive descriptions of useful methods for fetal evaluation by way of biochemical, biomolecular, ultrasonic, and electronic techniques. Section V includes a presentation of obstetrical management strategies for abnormalities encountered during labor and delivery. Section VI is devoted to considerations important in operative obstetrics, and abnormalities of the puerperium are addressed in Section VII. Sections VIII and IX include extensively revised chapters in which the management of pregnancy complications as well as medical and surgical disorders that may develop during pregnancy are addressed in detail. Section X of the new text is devoted to reproductive function in women. It includes chapters on the anatomy of the female reproductive tract, reproductive success and failure, and family planning.

To accomplish these sometimes extensive revisions, the voluminous literature relevant to all aspects of maternal–fetal medicine published since the completion of the seventeenth edition was reviewed. More than 1700 references have been added, along with more than 200 new figures and tables. Continuing the tradition of the past four editions, we cite frequently our cumulative clinical experience gained from the large obstetrical service at Parkland Memorial Hospital. We did so to develop unambiguous recommendations for the management of a variety of obstetrical problems and complications. We emphasize, as was done in the seventeenth edition, that these should not be interpreted as the only acceptable management schemes that would result in a favorable outcome of a given pregnancy. Indeed, the "Parkland Way"—as it is referred to frequently by our faculty and housestaff—is recognized to be but one established approach, but it is one that has served us well. Indeed, this approach has been our cornerstone in the development of obstetrical care plans that have proved useful for the successful medical and surgical management of more than a quarter of a million women and their fetuses.

An incredible amount of research and time in writing is necessary for a textbook revision of this magnitude. The contributions and participation of many persons of the Department of Obstetrics & Gynecology of this university were essential to ensure the timely birth of the eighteenth edition. To these individuals, we are truly grateful. In addition to critical editorial input, Dr. Alvin "Bud" Brekken provided strong leadership for the department when the writing chores took the heaviest toll on the authors' time. The clinical expertness and valuable suggestions of Drs. Kenneth Leveno and Larry Gilstrap were enlightening and served to enrich the entire text. Dr. Linette Casey toiled countless hours to facilitate the incorporation of important basic science principles that underlay clinical obstetrics. Providing expert advice from their specialized fields were Dr. Barry Schwarz for family planning, Dr. Victor Klein for clinical genetics, Dr. Rigoberto Santos for ultrasonography, Dr. Donald Wallace for obstetrical anesthesia, Dr. David Hemsell for ectopic pregnancy, and Drs. Roberto Yazigi and Alan Munoz for trophoblastic disease. Importantly, numerous unmentioned faculty and fellows readily and graciously assumed our duties at particularly busy times. Finally, the inquiring minds of the housestaff and maternal–fetal medicine fellows of Parkland Memorial Hospital served as a constant stimulus. In these respects, we are pleased to acknowledge that this eighteenth edition is the product of the entire department.

From the beginning of this revision, editorial planning, assistance, and encouragement were provided ably and amiably by Lin Paterson of Appleton & Lange. Production efforts were made almost enjoyable because of the technical expertise and cooperation of John Williams of Appleton & Lange. Rosemary Bell, Sarah Aycock, Janice Walton, and Kay Stanley of this department spent innumerable overtime hours preparing manuscript to assure that deadlines were met. Pat Ladd, Scott Bodel, and Renice Crosby provided excellent graphics and artwork. Most importantly, no undertaking of this size would be successful without a project director, and Marsha Congleton served with expertness at the computer keyboard, as production coordinator, as severe taskmaster, and not infrequently, as mother confessor. To all of these people, and to many more who are unnamed, we are grateful.

After working tirelessly to improve the care of the pregnant woman and her fetus by improving and editing the fourteenth through seventeenth editions, Dr. Jack Pritchard elected to make a "clean break" from *Williams Obstetrics*. This eighteenth edition is dedicated to him, but personally, we thank him for being our mentor and for his inspiration in the development of this entire manuscript. Importantly, although Signe Pritchard gave perpetual words of encouragement, her expert editorial assistance that was invaluable for past editions was missed.

During the thousands of hours spent over the 18 months in which the manuscript was produced, we neglected our wives even more so than usual. Despite this neglect, Rebekah Cunningham, Sue MacDonald, and Deann Gant have been not only understanding but have been supportive—at times, unbelievably so. And clearly, the eighteenth edition is also their book. To them, as well as to our neglected families and friends, and to our colleagues, we offer our sincerest thanks and deepest affection.

Part I
HUMAN PREGNANCY

Obstetrics in Broad Perspective

Obstetrics is the branch of medicine that deals with parturition, its antecedents, and its sequels (*Oxford English Dictionary*, 1933). It is concerned principally, therefore, with the phenomena and management of pregnancy, labor, and the puerperium, in both normal and abnormal circumstances. In a broader sense, obstetrics is concerned with the reproduction of a society. Obstetrical care, when appropriately practiced, should promote health and well-being, both physical and mental, among couples and their offspring and help them develop healthy attitudes toward sex, family life, and the place of the family in society. Obstetrics is concerned with all the physiological, psychological, and social factors that profoundly influence both the quantity and the quality of human reproduction. The problems of population growth are the natural heritage of obstetrics. The vital statistics of the nation, published monthly by the National Center for Health Statistics, attest to society's concern with the charge of this specialty.

The word *obstetrics* is derived from the Latin term *obstetrix*, meaning *midwife*. The etymology of *obstetrix*, however, is obscure. In most dictionaries, it is connected with the verb *obstare*, which means to *stand by* or *in front of*. The rationale of this derivation is that the midwife stood by or in front of the parturient. This has long been attacked by some etymologists who believed that the word was originally *adstetrix* and that the *ad* had been changed to *ob*. In that case, *obstetrix* would mean *the woman assisting the parturient*. The fact that on certain inscriptions *obstetrix* is also spelled *opstetrix* has led to the conjecture that it was derived from *ops* (aid) and *stare*, meaning *the woman rendering aid*. According to Temkin,* the most likely interpretation is that *obstetrix* meant *the woman who stood by the parturient*. Whether it alluded merely to the midwife's standing in front of or near the parturient or whether it carried the additional connotation of rendering aid is not clear.

The term *obstetrics* is of relatively recent usage. The *Oxford English Dictionary* gives the earliest example from a book published in 1819, indicating that in 1828 it was necessary to apologize for the use of the word *obstetrician*. Kindred terms, however, are much older. For example, *obstetricate* is found in English works published as early as 1623; *obstetricatory*, in 1640; *obstetricious*, in 1645; and *obstetrical*, in 1775. These terms were often used figuratively. As an example of such usage, the ad-

jective *obstetric* appears in Pope's *Dunciad* (1742) in the famous couplet:

> There all the Learn'd shall at the labour stand,
> and Douglas lend his soft, obstetric hand.

The much older term *midwifery* was used instead of *obstetrics* until the latter part of the 19th century in both the United States and Great Britain. It is derived from the Middle English *mid*, meaning *with*, and *wif*, meaning *wife* in the sense of a woman. The term *midwife* was used as early as 1303, and *midwifery*, in 1483. In England today, the term *midwifery* carries the same connotation as obstetrics, and the two words occasionally may be used synonymously.

AIMS OF OBSTETRICS

The transcendent objective of obstetrics is that every pregnancy be wanted and that it culminate in a healthy mother and a healthy baby. Obstetrics strives to minimize the number of women and infants who die as a result of the reproductive process or who are left physically, intellectually, or emotionally injured therefrom. Obstetrics is concerned further with the number and spacing of children so that both mother and offspring, indeed all the family, may enjoy optimal physical and emotional well-being. Finally, obstetrics strives to analyze and influence the social factors that impinge on reproductive efficiency.

VITAL STATISTICS

To aid in the reduction of the number of mothers and infants who die as the result of pregnancy and labor, it is important to know how many such deaths there are in this country each year and in what circumstances. To evaluate these data correctly, a variety of events concerned with pregnancy outcomes have been defined by various agencies:

> *Birth.* This is the complete expulsion or extraction from the mother of a fetus irrespective of whether the umbilical cord has been cut or the placenta is attached. Fetuses weighing less than 500 g usually are not considered as births, but rather as *abortuses*, for purposes of perinatal statistics. In the absence of a birthweight, a body length of 25 cm, crown to heel, is usually equated with 500 g.

---

*Previous communication. Dr. Owsei Temkin, Associate Professor of the History of Medicine, Johns Hopkins University School of Medicine, graciously devoted time to a study of the etymology of the word *obstetrics*, and the comments cited are entirely his.

Approximately 20 weeks gestational age is commonly considered to be equivalent to 500 g fetal weight, however, a 500 g fetus is more likely to be 22 (menstrual) weeks gestational age.

Birth Rate. The number of births per 1,000 population is the birth rate, or crude birth rate. The birth rate in the United States for the year ending February 1988 was 15.7 (National Center for Health Statistics, 1988).

Fertility Rate. This term refers to the number of live births per 1,000 female population aged 15 through 44 years. In 1987 this was 65.9.

Live Birth. Whenever the infant at or sometime after birth breathes spontaneously or shows any other sign of life such as heart beat or definite spontaneous movement of voluntary muscles, a live birth is recorded.

Stillbirth. None of the signs of life are present at or after birth.

Neonatal Death. Early neonatal death refers to death of a liveborn infant during the first 7 days after birth. Late neonatal death refers to death after 7 but before 29 days.

Stillbirth Rate. The number of stillborn infants per 1,000 infants born.

Fetal Death Rate. This term is synonymous with stillbirth rate.

Neonatal Mortality Rate. The number of neonatal deaths per 1,000 live births.

Perinatal Mortality Rate. This rate is defined as the number of stillbirths plus neonatal deaths per 1,000 total births.

Low Birthweight. If the first newborn weight obtained after birth is less than 2500 g, the infant is termed low birthweight.

Term Infant. An infant born anytime after 37 completed (menstrual) weeks of gestation through 42 completed weeks of gestation (260 to 294 days) is considered by most to be a term infant. Such a definition implies that birth at any time within this period is optimal whereas birth before or afterward is not. Such an implication is not warranted. Some infants born between 37 and 38 weeks are at risk of functional prematurity, for example, the development of respiratory distress in the newborn infant of a diabetic mother (see Chap. 39, p. 816). In the past, some considered gestation extending past 41 weeks to be postterm; however, any risk to the fetus that might be imposed by remaining in utero until 42 weeks rather than 41 weeks does not appear to be appreciable (Chap. 38, p. 758). Consequently, there is no good reason for distorting the range for term birth to 3 weeks below the mean of 40 weeks but only 1 week beyond the mean.

Preterm or Premature Infant. An infant born before 37 completed weeks has been so classified, although born before 38 completed weeks would seem more appropriate for reasons stated above.

Postterm Infant. An infant born anytime after completion of the 42nd week has been classified by some as being postterm.

Abortus. A fetus or embryo removed or expelled from the uterus during the first half of gestation (20 weeks or less), or weighing less than 500 g, or measuring less than 25 cm is also referred to as an abortus.

Direct Maternal Death. Death of the mother resulting from obstetrical complications of the pregnancy state, labor, or puerperium, and from interventions, omissions, incorrect treatment, or a chain of events resulting from any of the above is considered a direct maternal death. An example is maternal death from exsanguination resulting from rupture of the uterus.

Indirect Maternal Death. An obstetrical death not directly due to obstetrical causes but resulting from previously existing disease, or a disease that developed during pregnancy, labor, or the puerperium, but which was aggravated by the maternal physiological adaptation to pregnancy, is classified as an indirect maternal death. An example is maternal death from complications of mitral stenosis.

Nonmaternal Death. Death of the mother resulting from accidental or incidental causes in no way related to the pregnancy may be classified as a nonmaternal death. An example is death from an automobile accident.

Maternal Death Rate or Maternal Mortality. The number of maternal deaths that result from the reproductive process per 100,000 live births.

The Birth Rate and Fertility Rate

One index of the need for obstetrical personnel and facilities is the number of births each year. Additional indices are the birth rate and the fertility rate. From these data, particularly the fertility rate, the expected number of births in future years can be estimated.

According to the National Center for Health Statistics (1988), there were 3.82 million live births in the United States for the year ending February 1988. This was the largest number of births recorded since 1964. The fertility rate was 65.9 in 1987, while it was 64.9 in 1986. There also was an increase of 1 percent in the number of women in the childbearing years, and thus, the reason for more births in 1987 was an increase in the number of women between 15 and 44 years of age as well as a slight increase in their fertility. According to the center, women born during the post–World War II "baby-boom" accounted for much of this increase.

MATERNAL MORTALITY

The number of maternal deaths per 100,000 live births has decreased remarkably in the past half century. There were only 295 maternal deaths in the United States reported in 1985, or 7.8 per 100,000 live births. By way of comparison, there were 12,544 maternal deaths, or 582.1 per 100,000 live births in 1935! Values for intervening years are presented in Table 1–1.

In 1985, the maternal mortality rate for black women was 20.4 per 100,000. The fourfold difference in maternal mortality rate that exists between white and black women appears to result primarily from social and economic factors, such as a relative lack of skilled personnel and appropriate facilities at delivery, lack of antepartum care, lack of family planning services, faulty health education, and dietary deficiencies. Other conditions commonly cited are higher mortality rates due to induced abortion and ectopic pregnancy. As these unfavorable social and economic conditions are improved, the racial difference in the maternal death rates will doubtless decrease.

The maternal mortality rate also varies with the age of the mother. In all races, the remarkable increase in mortality with advancing age can be explained only on the basis of an intrinsic maternal factor(s). The increasing frequency of hypertension with advancing years and the greater tendency to uterine hem-

TABLE 1–1. MATERNAL MORTALITY IN THE UNITED STATES, 1935–1985

	Maternal Deaths	Rate Per 100,000 Live Births		
Year	Number	Total	White	Other
1935	12,544	582.1	530.6	945.7
1940	8,876	376.0	319.8	773.5
1945	5,668	107.2	172.1	454.8
1950	2,960	83.3	61.1	221.6
1955	1,901	47.0	32.8	130.3
1960	1,579	37.1	26.0	97.9
1965	1,189	31.6	21.0	83.7
1970	803	21.5	14.4	55.9
1975	403	12.8	9.1	29.0
1980	334	9.2	6.7	19.8
1985	295	7.8	5.2	18.1

orrhage contribute significantly to the increase of the mortality rate. Advanced age and high parity act independently to increase the risk of childbearing, but their effects are usually additive. In the actual analysis of cases, it is difficult to dissociate these two factors.

Common Causes of Maternal Mortality

Hemorrhage, hypertension that is either induced or aggravated by pregnancy, and infection still account for half the maternal deaths in the United States (Fig. 1–1). The causes of obstetrical hemorrhage are multiple and include postpartum hemorrhage, bleeding in association with abortion, bleeding from ectopic pregnancy, bleeding as the result of abnormal placental location or separation (placenta previa and abruptio placentae), and bleeding from ruptured uteri. Hypertension, induced or aggravated by pregnancy, complicates about 6 or 7 percent of pregnancies and is accompanied commonly by edema and proteinuria (preeclampsia), and in some severe cases by convulsions and coma (eclampsia). Puerperal infection, or postpartum pelvic infection, usually begins as uterine and parametrial in-

fection, but sometimes it undergoes extension to cause peritonitis, thrombophlebitis, and bacteremia. Details of the origin, prevention, and treatment of these conditions form a considerable portion of the subject matter of obstetrics.

Unfortunately, maternal deaths are underreported and causes frequently are derived from birth certificates and thus are erroneous. The Centers for Disease Control, in conjunction with the American College of Obstetricians and Gynecologists, established the Maternal Mortality Collaborative to determine the accuracy of voluntary reporting (Rochat and colleagues, 1988). Over the 5-year period, 1980 through 1984, 19 reporting areas, including 16 states, reported a total of 510 maternal deaths. This number was 37 percent more than the 373 deaths reported for these areas by the National Center for Health Statistics. Still, the causes of death in this smaller sample were remarkably similar to the causes of 2,475 maternal deaths shown in Figure 1–1.

Reasons for Decline in Maternal Mortality Rate

Many factors and agencies are responsible for the dramatic fall in the maternal death rate in this country over the past 50 years. Obviously, there has been a general improvement in medical practice. The widespread use of blood transfusion and antimicrobial drugs and the maintenance of fluid, electrolyte, and acid-base balance in the serious complications of pregnancy and labor have materially changed obstetrical practice. Equally important is the development of widespread obstetrical training and continuing educational programs, which have provided more and better qualified specialists. Similarly, training programs in anesthesia, as well as the recognition that obstetrical anesthesia requires special personnel and equipment, have substantially lowered the maternal death rate from its use.

Obstetrics is unique in that no other branch of medicine is subject to such careful public scrutiny. Not only are births a matter of public record, but maternal and perinatal deaths are examined by municipal, state, and national health authorities. In many areas, local medical or obstetrical and gynecological societies also examine such deaths, and mortality conferences are frequently conducted as part of the continuing medical education of the obstetrician. Unfortunately, the threat that these

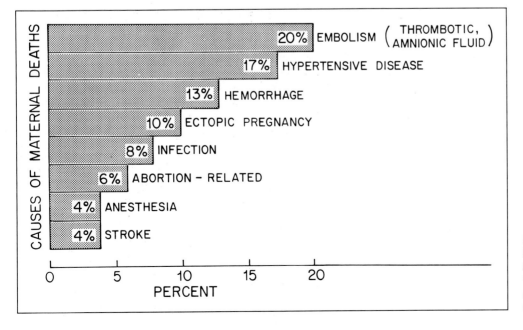

Figure 1–1. Selected distribution of 2,475 maternal deaths from direct causes in the United States from 1974 to 1978. (*Data from Kaunitz and colleagues: Obstet Gynecol 65:605, 1985.*)

proceedings may be subpoenaed to substantiate alleged malpractice claims has greatly detracted from their educational value.

The *sine qua non* of good work in any field is well-trained personnel, but they could not have achieved the excellent results had there not been a great expansion in facilities for good obstetrical care. Despite increased facilities, there remain areas in the United States where obstetrical services are woefully inadequate, particularly in rural areas and in some large inner cities.

From the viewpoint of safer care during labor, the outstanding advance of the past 40 years has been the great increase in the proportion of hospital deliveries. As recently as 1940, only 60 percent of white births took place in hospitals, but this figure now exceeds 99 percent. Hospital births not only mean better facilities but imply care by individuals specially trained in obstetrics and perinatology.

Reproductive Mortality

In more recent years, as the maternal mortality rate decreased markedly, some deaths were occurring as the consequence of a great increase in the use of various contraceptive techniques. The sum of the mortalities from pregnancy and from the use of these techniques to prevent pregnancy has been termed *reproductive mortality*. As shown in Table 1–2, in spite of the innovation and widespread use of oral contraceptives and intrauterine devices accompanied by a marked increase in surgical sterilization, the number of deaths from contraception was slight compared with the decrease in maternal mortality.

PERINATAL MORTALITY

The sum of stillbirths and neonatal deaths is the perinatal mortality. The perinatal death rate has fallen by nearly 50 percent in the past 25 years (Table 1–3). Currently, there are about 180 perinatal deaths for every maternal death. With the current very low incidence of maternal deaths, perinatal loss rates not only are a better index of the level of obstetrical care, but also give a valid indication of an equally important datum, the *infant morbidity*. To some extent, the total perinatal loss is correlated with the age and parity of the mother. The rates tend to be highest for the firstborn of very young women and births of the order of six and over.

Factors Affecting the Stillbirth Rate

Nearly one half of perinatal deaths are stillbirths. Stillbirths tend to decline as the quality of care during and throughout pregnancy improves. With improvement in prenatal care and proper

hospitalization, some of these deaths are preventable. In too large a proportion of fetal deaths, unfortunately, there may be no obvious explanation.

Neonatal Deaths

In 1977, for the first time in the United States, there were fewer neonatal deaths than fetal deaths (stillbirths). Nearly half of the neonatal deaths occur in the first day of life. The number of deaths during those 24 hours exceeds that from the second month to the completion of the first year. The causes of this huge wastage during the neonatal period are numerous, but the most important is low birthweight usually as the consequence of delivery long before term. The proportion of low-birthweight infants differs among ethnic groups, ranging from about 60 per 1,000 for white mothers to approximately 120 per 1,000 for black mothers. The interracial difference in the rates of low birthweight accounts for the major difference in neonatal mortality between these two groups. However, social and environmental factors probably impact more heavily than race in the cause of this difference. As well as deaths, low birthweight has contributed appreciably to infant morbidity and for a large fraction of the neurological and intellectual deficits that are tragic individually and costly to society. Why some women go into labor before term is one of the greatest unsolved problems of obstetrics.

The second most common cause of neonatal death is injury to the central nervous system. Here the word *injury* is used in its broad sense to indicate both cerebral injury resulting from hypoxia in utero and traumatic injury to the brain during labor and delivery. Another important cause of neonatal death is congenital malformation.

The Birth Certificate

Statutes in all 50 states and the District of Columbia require that a birth certificate be submitted promptly to the local registrar. An extensively revised document was implemented in January 1989. After the birth has been duly registered, notification is sent to the parents of the child and a complete report is forwarded to the National Center for Health Statistics in Washington.

There are many reasons why the complete and accurate registration of births is essential. Certification of the facts of birth is needed as evidence of age, citizenship, and family relationships. Moreover, the data provided are of immeasurable importance to all agencies (social, public health, demographic, or obstetrical) dealing with human reproduction. For instance, the data presented in the foregoing paragraphs were culled almost entirely from information published by the National Center for Health Statistics on the basis of birth certificates, and

TABLE 1–2. REPRODUCTIVE MORTALITY IN THE UNITED STATES BY CAUSE—1955, 1975, AND 1982

| | Estimated Number of Deaths | | | | | | | |
| | Pregnancy Related | | | Contraception Related | | | | Reproductive Mortality Rate[b] |
Year	Ectopic Pregnancy	Abortion	Other Deaths	OC[a]	IUD[a]	Sterilization	Total Deaths	
1955	139	485	2,065	—	—	14	2,703	7.8
1975	50	49	428	452	6	14	999	2.1
1982	—	7	369	327	25	23	751	1.4

[a] OC indicates oral contraceptives; IUD, intrauterine device (neither used in 1955).
[b] Rate per 100,000 women aged 15 to 44.
Data from Rosenberg and Rosenthal: Am J Public Health, 77:833, 1987; Sachs and Associates: JAMA 247:2789, 1982.

TABLE 1–3. PERINATAL MORTALITY IN THE UNITED STATES, 1950 THROUGH 1985

Year	Perinatal[a]		Fetal[b]		Neonatal[c]	
	Number	Rate[d]	Number	Rate[d]	Number	Rate[e]
1950	141,117	39.0	68,262	18.8	72,855	20.5
1960	148,213	34.3	68,480	15.8	79,733	18.7
1970	109,240	28.9	52,961	14.0	56,279	15.1
1975	70,212	22.1	33,796	10.6	36,416	11.6
1980	63,971	17.5	33,353	9.1	30,618	8.5
1983	57,259	15.6	30,752	8.4	26,507	7.3
1985	55,840	14.7	29,661	7.8	26,179	7.0
1987	—	—	—	—	—	6.5[f]

[a] Perinatal Definition II is used, which includes fetal deaths of 20 weeks gestation or greater and infant deaths of less than 28 days.
[b] Fetal deaths of 20 weeks gestation or more.
[c] Infant deaths of less than 29 days.
[d] Rate per 1,000 live births and fetal deaths.
[e] Rate per 1,000 live births.
[f] Provisional data based upon a 10 percent sample of U.S. death certificates.
From the National Center for Health Statistics, Vital Statistics of the United States, Volume II, Mortality, 1985, and unpublished data courtesy of Drs. Harry Rosenberg and Marian MacDorman of the National Center for Health Statistics.

this represents only a small fraction of the information obtainable from that source. A birth certificate provides even more data of direct obstetrical importance. **Hence, the prompt and accurate completion of this certificate after each birth is not only a legal duty but a contribution to the broad field of obstetrical knowledge.**

OBSTETRICS AND OTHER BRANCHES OF MEDICINE

Obstetrics is a multifaceted discipline with close and numerous relations to other branches of medicine. It is related so intimately to the kindred subject of gynecology that obstetrics and gynecology are generally regarded as one specialty. Gynecology deals with the physiology and the pathology of the female reproductive organs in the nonpregnant state, whereas obstetrics deals with the pregnant state and its sequels. Correct differential diagnosis in either obstetrics or gynecology entails an intimate acquaintance with the clinical syndromes met in both, and the methods of examination and many operative techniques are common to both disciplines. It is obligatory, therefore, that every obstetrician have extensive experience in gynecology, and vice versa.

The scope of fetal diagnosis and treatment has broadened remarkably, as discussed especially in Chapter 15. This, as well as the concern of obstetrics with the newborn infant, has brought the subject into close relation with pediatrics and given rise to the concept of perinatology. The boundaries between obstetrics and neonatology are not sharp, but rather overlap to the benefit of the fetus and infant. Even in metropolitan centers, inconvenient hours of birth often impose on the obstetrician the management of the newborn during the most critical hour of life. The obstetrician must be knowledgeable, therefore, in the management of the infant at this time as well as before birth.

Because pregnant and nonpregnant women are subject to the same diseases, the obstetrician commonly encounters and therefore must be knowledgeable about a variety of diseases in pregnant women. As emphasized in Chapter 39, the clinical picture presented by some of these disorders may be altered remarkably during pregnancy and the immediate puerperium; conversely, these diseases may affect the course of gestation.

Obstetrics is intimately related to most clinical and preclinical sciences. The study of spontaneous abortion, for example,

depends on knowledge of anomalies in the development of the early embryo and trophoblast. Abortion may also involve hormonal defects, a condition which would link the subjects of obstetrics and endocrinology; or abortion may result from chromosomal defects, and such a condition would forge a link to cytogenetics. The concept of erythrocyte antigen isoimmunization has shown how immunological factors may interfere with the successful outcome of pregnancy, but in turn, by appropriate immunotherapy, be prevented successfully. Obstetrics and general pathology meet closely in the rapidly developing field of perinatal pathology. In studies of fetal malformation, clinical genetics is of prime importance. Other important relations of obstetrics to preclinical sciences include: microbiology, in the study of maternal and fetal infections; biochemistry and physiology, in relation to myriad events including labor; pharmacology, in the action and metabolism of drugs in the mother and in the fetus and newborn infant; and molecular genetics, from which techniques of an ever-increasing number of inherited disease are used to identify affected fetuses. The numerous applications of the preclinical sciences to problems of human reproduction are evident in the relatively short but remarkable history of the National Institute of Child Health and Human Development.

Obstetrics is related also to certain fields that are not strictly medical. Because nutritional requirements are altered by pregnancy, obstetrics requires knowledge of the science of nutrition. Whereas the mother–child relationship is the basis of the family unit, the obstetrician is continually dealing with psychological and sociological problems. Economics play a prominent role in obstetrics because health care may be quite expensive, and especially so when some who provide it have little concern for costs. In addition, obstetrics has important legal aspects, especially in regard to the increasing number of malpractice suits.

OBSTETRICS, THE MOTHER, AND HER FAMILY

In spite of the remarkable record of safety for the hospitalized expectant mother and her fetus-infant that has been achieved in recent years, there has evolved a small but quite vocal group of dissidents made up of former parturients, their partners, and those who would attempt to provide care during home delivery. Hopefully, those complaints about hospitalization for which there are real bases can be resolved short of sacrificing the safety that hospitalization for delivery can provide the mother and especially her fetus-infant.

There is no question but that some individuals who collaborate in the effort to provide optimal in-hospital care for the mother and the fetus-infant have not necessarily been as considerate of the pregnant mother and her family as they should have been. The expectant mother has been commonly treated as if she were seriously ill, even when she was quite healthy. All too often she has been forced to conform to a common pathway of care that stripped her of most of her individuality and much of her dignity. Pleasant surroundings have not always been provided; instead, hospital austerity has prevailed. Hospital administrators have tended not to seek her business claiming they lost money on obstetrics. In recent years, obstetricians, for many good reasons, have worked mostly in groups and as a consequence, about the time of delivery, the ultimate event in the minds of the mother and her family, there may have been either a "changing of the obstetrical guard" or the obstetrician created the appearance of wanting to hurry the labor and delivery since he or she would soon be "going off." The same picture has been presented by the nurses and other personnel intimately involved in providing care for the mother and fetus-infant. Too often the expectant mother has felt that her fate and the fate of her baby were dependent not so much on skilled personnel but upon an electronic cabinet that appeared to possess some great power that prevailed above all others. Fortunately, appropriate applications of medical science do not require that excellent care be a dehumanizing ordeal. Excellent obstetrical care and the many benefits that accrue can be provided in a hospital setting that, at the same time, is enjoyed by the mother and family, and is acceptable economically to all parties involved.

THE FUTURE

Although the recent decline in maternal mortality rate has been enormous, continuous improvements in maternal health care are needed. If the nonwhite mortality rate were reduced to the level of that of white women by providing equal care, and if the deaths in white women considered preventable by many mortality studies were averted, approximately two-thirds of current maternal deaths could be prevented. Maternal mortality affects most seriously the socially and economically deprived. Many of these deaths result from sheer lack of adequate facilities, including lack of properly distributed units for antepartum care, lack of suitable hospital arrangements, and lack of readily available blood for transfusion. Others are caused by errors of management by the obstetrical personnel. Errors of omission include failure to provide antepartum care, failure to follow the woman and fetus carefully throughout labor and the early puerperium, and failure to obtain appropriate consultation. Among errors of commission, traumatic delivery is probably foremost.

These several deficiencies in maternity care obviously must be corrected first if maternal and perinatal mortality rates are to be brought to the irreducible minimum. They can and doubtless will be lowered to that level by the same methods that have proved efficacious in the past: more and better trained personnel and equipped facilities available to all pregnant women and their fetuses.

Along with these improvements to better insure pregnancy outcome is the realization that costs for obstetrical care are rising in an unprecedented fashion. Simply put, technology is expensive and the addition to routine prenatal care of various screening tests to detect relatively uncommon diseases will continue to increase the costs of prenatal care. For example, maternal serum screening is widely used to detect high or low alpha-fetoprotein concentration that may suggest a neural tube defect or chromosomally abnormal fetus. While the yield of such screening techniques is low, the technological and counseling services needed to support such programs are expensive. Along with the availability of easily performed and widely accessible techniques of molecular genetics to diagnose inherited diseases during early pregnancy comes the formidable price tag for the use of such technology.

Commonly used methods of fetal health assessment include ultrasound to visualize the fetus for anatomical aberrations as well as to measure fetal growth. Electronic assessment of fetal heart rate and its reaction to a variety of stimuli is used to predict fetal well-being. Many times, a combination of fetal heart rate reactivity and ultrasonic evaluation is conducted simultaneously. Such innovations also are expensive, both from the technological as well as personnel standpoints. Thus, obstetrical care has become expensive for consumers, who typically are young couples getting started in life, and who can least afford to bear escalating and sometimes overwhelming medical costs.

Finally, the impact of malpractice litigation on obstetrics cannot be ignored. Although the intensive surveillance of perinatal outcome by patients and plaintiff attorneys has served to improve some obstetrical practices, it is unreasonable and unfair to assume automatically that a less than salutary outcome is caused always by neglect or incompetence. An example is cerebral palsy, which, as discussed in Chapter 33, seldom follows recognizable perinatal insults, but whose identification commonly places the health care providers in a defensive posture, forced to prove that medical mismanagement *did not* cause the injury. In these and similar cases with imperfect outcomes, litigation is instituted too frequently by overzealous attorneys in search of huge settlements. In many of these, "expert" witnesses readily provide dogmatic opinions to chronicle alleged obstetrical mismanagement. Such practices also have served to increase the cost of obstetrical care because malpractice insurance premiums are necessarily passed on to patients. Another adverse effect of the so-called malpractice crisis is that a large number of skilled clinicians are voluntarily retiring from the practice of obstetrics.

Nevertheless, the concept of the right of every child to be physically, mentally, and emotionally "well-born" is fundamental to human dignity. If obstetrics is to serve a role in the realization of this goal, the specialty must maintain and even extend its role in the control of population growth. The right to be "well-born" in its broadest sense is simply incompatible with unrestricted fertility. Yet our knowledge of the forces operative in the fluctuation and control of population growth is still rudimentary. This concept of obstetrics as a social as well as a biological science impels us to accept a responsibility unprecedented in American medicine.

REFERENCES

Kaunitz AM, Hughes JM, Grimes DA, Smith JC, Rochat RW, Kafrissen ME: Causes of maternal mortality in the United States. Obstet Gynecol 65:605, 1985
National Center for Health Statistics: Births, marriages, divorces, and deaths for February, 1988. Monthly Vital Stat Rep 37:3, 1988
Rochat RW, Koonin LM, Atrash HK, Jewett JJ, and the Maternal Mortality Collaborative: Maternal mortality in the United States: Report from the Maternal Mortality Collaborative. Obstet Gynecol 72:91, 1988
Rosenberg MJ, Rosenthal SM: Reproductive mortality in the United States: Recent trends and methodologic considerations. Am J Public Health 77:833, 1987
Sachs BP, Layde PM, Rubin GL, Rochat RW: Reproductive mortality in the United States. JAMA 247:2789, 1982

Human Pregnancy: Overview, Organization, and Diagnosis

OVERVIEW OF REPRODUCTIVE FUNCTION IN WOMEN

The physiological investments made by women, indeed all female organisms, in the achievement of pregnancy are astounding. Consider the following: in populations of women in whom early marriage was the rule and in whom contraception was not practiced, menstruation was relatively uncommon. Pregnancy occurred with ovulation in early adolescence; and after delivery, anovulation and amenorrhea persisted during lactation; and, breast feeding was continued for 2 or 3 years. Thereafter, pregnancy occurred again and again, and by the time that 10 or 11 pregnancy-lactation episodes were completed, ovarian function and ovulation had ceased, i.e., the time of menopause. A thought-provoking analysis of the *"evolution of human reproduction"* has been presented by Roger Short (1976).

The development of safe and effective contraceptive agents, according to David Baird (1985), who also referred to the writings of his father, Sir Dugald Baird, *"has relieved [women] from the tyranny of excessive fertility—'the fifth freedom.' Because the social and physical demands of continuous [pregnancy and] breast-feeding are unlikely to be acceptable to women of the 20th century . . ."* they have chosen menstruation as an alternative, *"in the absence of a simple, safe means of inducing amenorrhea pharmacologically."* This predicament was prophesied by Whitehouse, in 1914, who stated: *"Periodic uterine hemorrhage is, in fact, one of the sacrifices which women must offer at the altar of evolution and civilization."*

Accordingly, menstruation must be viewed, in a physiological sense, as the end-result of fertility failure, whether chosen or naturally occurring. This perspective of reproductive function in women is appropriate at the outset of a treatise on obstetrics. It is important that we recognize the incredible endocrinological and physiological expenditures that are obliged, involuntarily, in reproductive-age women, at least in the absence of pharmacological intervention, to ensure the opportunity for the achievement of pregnancy. There can be no doubt that the physiological animus of the ovarian cycle, as well as the accompanying morphological accommodations of the reproductive tract, is ovulation, fertilization, and implantation, namely, the establishment of pregnancy. To be sure, there are fail-safe systems that become operative if there is failure of fertilization of the ovum or failure of implantation of the blastocyst; and these culminate in menstruation.

OVULATION IS THE CARDINAL FUNCTION OF THE OVARY

Ordinarily one egg is released by way of ovulation each month; this process is repeated faithfully every 24 to 35 days from menarche to menopause, or for about 35 years, so long as pregnancy is not achieved and so long as sufficient numbers of follicles remain in the ovary. The endocrine events of the ovarian cycle are optimized to create a hormonal environment that promotes ovulation. The endocrine milieu created during the ovarian cycle also is optimal for endometrial regeneration after a failed fertility cycle (menstruation) in preparation of the uterus for the next pregnancy opportunity. But the somatic effects of estrogen, for example, on bone density, must be viewed as added benefits of follicular estrogen that is produced to regulate ovarian-brain-pituitary function and follicular maturation, which eventuate in ovulation. Namely, there is no mechanism in place by which somatic tissues can act to regulate the rate of ovarian estrogen secretion. Except for ovary and brain-pituitary, this is true of all estrogen-responsive tissues, including breast, uterus, bone, skin, vagina, and liver.

THE OVARY AS AN ENDOCRINE ORGAN

The function and functional regulation of the human ovary is unlike that known for any other endocrine gland. Generally, endocrine glands respond to the appropriate trophic stimulus by producing the major hormone(s) characteristic of that gland: for example, cortisol in response to corticotropin (ACTH) in the adrenal; thyroxine in response to the action of TSH (thyroid-stimulating hormone) in the thyroid; testosterone in response to LH (luteinizing hormone) in the testes; but not the ovary. In the ovary, estrogen formation is confined largely to one ovary at a time, and to the granulosa cells of a single follicle—the chosen follicle, the follicle destined for ovulation during that ovarian cycle. And the rate of formation and secretion of estradiol-17β by the granulosa cells of that chosen follicle corresponds to the maturation and development of that follicle. Indeed, when the follicular apparatus of the ovaries is depleted, ovarian endocrine function also ceases and menopause occurs. Thereafter, gonadotropins do not act on the ovary to effect an increase in estrogen secretion.

During the first and last few days of each ovarian cycle, there is very little estradiol-17β formed in the ovarian follicle(s). Most of the estrogen (estrone) produced at the extremes of the ovarian cycles of women arises by way of the extraglandular formation of estrogen from circulating C_{19}-steroids (androstenedione) through aromatization (principally in adipose tissue). This is the mechanism by which most estrogen is produced in men, children, and postmenopausal women. Thus, the ovary is not an endocrine organ of the same type as the adrenal cortex or the thyroid or even the testis; the formation of estrogen and thence progesterone in the ovary is linked irrevocably to the ovulatory process. At the commencement of each ovarian cycle, there is a gradual and thence a sudden increase in the rate of follicular formation and secretion of estradiol-17β. These momentous endocrine events are parallel to and essential for the development and maturation of the follicle and for the regulation of gonadotropin secretion, including the sudden release or *surge* in LH secretion that brings about ovulation.

After ovulation, the corpus luteum produces prodigious amounts of progesterone. Apart from pregnancy and pregnancy-related phenomena, there is no known metabolic utility of progesterone. But progesterone is believed to be the "pro gestation steroid"; indeed, it is generally accepted that progesterone is essential to the maintenance of pregnancy in most mammalian species. The formation of progesterone by the corpus luteum is important in the early maintenance of pregnancy; and the persistence of corpus luteum function during a fertile cycle is essential to the success of early pregnancy. Progesterone withdrawal, by way of removal of the corpus luteum, before 8 weeks of human pregnancy results in abortion.

Teleologically, therefore, it is easy to accept the proposition that the endocrine events of the ovarian cycle are an investment made almost singularly toward the achievement of pregnancy; the nonreproductive physiological benefits of estrogen in women are achieved as a fortuitous advantage of this process. This, no doubt, serves as an explanation for the success of estrogen treatment of ovariectomized and postmenopausal women by use of a host of different regimens using a variety of estrogenic compounds administered by any of several routes.

REPRODUCTIVE FUNCTION OF WOMEN IN PHYSIOLOGICAL PERSPECTIVE

Another way of envisioning the reproductive function of women is as follows: the most intricate and complex function of the ovary is the extrusion of an egg at cyclic intervals, and if this is accomplished, all other aspects of ovarian function, including the hypothalamic-pituitary participation in this event, are normal. The function of the fallopian tube evolves about sperm and egg transport and the provision of the optimal environment for fertilization of the ovum and cleavage of the zygote. The endometrium may be the optimal (but not the only) site for implantation; but the decidua (endometrium of pregnancy) is the likely site of origin of uterotropins (agents that serve to prepare the uterus for parturition) and uterotonins (agents that cause the contractions of the uterus with labor). Thus, reproductive function in women is focused in a highly directed manner on the achievement of pregnancy and delivery of the mature fetus.

PREGNANCY ORGANIZATION: THE FETAL–MATERNAL COMMUNICATION SYSTEM

DEVELOPMENT OF THE COMMUNICATION SYSTEM

There is no doubt that ovulation is dependent upon brain-pituitary-ovarian interactions in women before pregnancy; but after conception, the establishment and maintenance of pregnancy is highly dependent upon contributions made by the blastocyst, the embryo, and thence the fetus. A biomolecular communication system is established between the zygote/blastocyst/embryo/fetus and mother that is operative from before the time of nidation and persists through the time of parturition. This fetal–maternal communication system is essential to the success of processes involved in blastocyst implantation, maternal recognition of pregnancy, fetal contributions to the maintenance of pregnancy, maternal adaptation to pregnancy, and fetal participation in the initiation of parturition. These physiological processes involve fetal-directed modifications of maternal responses.

Heretofore, we have envisioned the communication system as operative primarily in nutritive supplies from the mother to the fetus. By way of this communication system, the mother serves up nutrients that are effectively taken up by fetal trophoblasts and transferred to the embryo/fetus. But the completeness of the contributions of the fetus to this communication system is evidenced by the fact that the blastocyst is the dynamic force in implantation and the fetus/newborn is even responsible for creating the hormonal milieu that culminates in lactation and thence in milk let-down during suckling.

Today, we recognize that there are two major anatomical and functional arms of the fetal–maternal communication system: One is the **placental arm,** in which a variety of functional components are encompassed, for example, nutritive and endocrine. The other is the **paracrine arm,** the functional components of which include pregnancy maintenance, acceptance of the semiallogeneic fetal graft, physical protection of the fetus, and parturition.

The placental arm of the fetal–maternal communication system is in place by way of blood-borne conduits that involve (1) maternal blood in the intervillous space, which bathes the fetal villous trophoblasts, and (2) fetal blood, which is confined within fetal capillaries in the intravillous space. The paracrine arm of the communication system is in place by way of direct cell-to-cell biomolecular trafficking between fetal membranes (chorion laeve) and maternal decidua. In turn, the amnion, the innermost fetal membrane, is contiguous with amnionic fluid, which is rich in fetal excretions and secretions.

ORGANIZATION OF THE COMMUNICATION SYSTEM

At the very commencement of pregnancy, i.e., at the time of blastocyst implantation, there is, anatomically, only one distinguishable communication system between fetus and mother. This is established between developing trophoblasts and uterine decidua and maternal blood. But even then, the functional progenitors of the two mature arms of the communication system are in place (Fig. 2–1).

1. Placental Arm of the Fetal–Maternal Communication System (Nutrient Transfer and Endocrine System). The placenta (villous trophoblasts) becomes the principal site of nutrient transfer between mother and fetus and the principal site of endocrine function of pregnancy, albeit one that is highly dependent upon the provision of blood-borne, preformed precursors, especially for placental steroid hormone formation. **Ultimately, the proximal anatomical parts of the placental arm (nutrient transfer and endocrine function) of the fetal–maternal communication system are fetal blood, the placenta, and maternal blood.** The human placenta is a hemochorioendothelial type. As stated already, this means that fetal villous trophoblasts are bathed directly by maternal blood, but the fetal blood in placenta is contained in fetal vessels that traverse the intra-

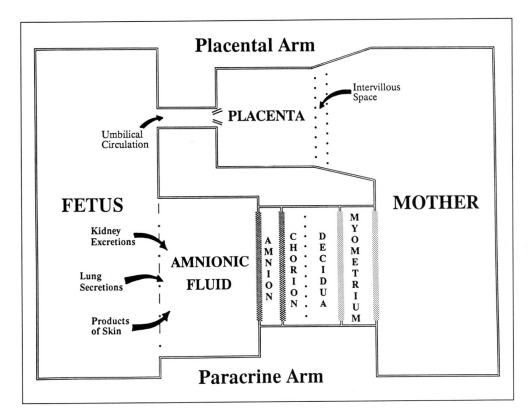

Figure 2–1. The fetal–maternal communication system. The proximal anatomical parts of the two arms of this system, the Placental Arm and the Paracrine Arm, are depicted. Fetal blood perfuses the placenta by way of the fetal villous capillaries. Maternal blood directly bathes the trophoblasts. Amnionic fluid, comprised in large measure by fetal urine, and containing secretions from fetal lung and skin, bathes the avascular amnion, which is contiguous with avascular chorion laeve. The chorion laeve and decidua vera (parietalis) are in direct cell-to-cell contact.

villous space; therefore, fetal blood is separated from trophoblasts by the endothelium of the fetal capillaries and the matrix in the intravillous space (Chap. 4).

2. Paracrine Arm of the Fetal–Maternal Communication System (Fetal Membranes–Decidua). As the embryo grows, the fetal membranes (amnion and chorion laeve) develop as avascular membranous structures that come to lie adjacent to the entire surface of the decidua that is not occupied by the placenta (Chap. 4). This anatomical arrangement gives rise to the fetal-decidual paracrine arm. We refer to this arm as paracrine because there are cell-to-cell interactions of monumental importance that occur between the avascular fetal membranes and the maternal decidua. The amnionic fluid is contained within the space surrounded by the fetal membranes and bathes the innermost, the amnion. The chorion laeve, the outermost fetal membrane, is contiguous with the decidua. **Therefore, the proximal anatomical parts of the paracrine arm of the fetal–maternal communication system are the amnionic fluid, the amnion, the chorion laeve, the decidua vera, and probably the myometrium.** We choose to include myometrium because it is likely that bioactive agents produced in decidua act in a paracrine manner to cause uterine preparedness (uterotropins) that is essential for successful parturition and to cause the myometrial contractions (uterotonins) of labor as well (Chap. 10). Communication between fetus and mother by way of this paracrine arm is possible by way of several mechanisms. After about 20 weeks of gestation, amnionic fluid is comprised largely of fetal urine. Fetal lung secretions also enter amnionic fluid by way of fetal thoracic movements (fetal breathing). Therefore, secretions and excretions of the fetus enter amnionic fluid, which serves as a conduit for the transmission of biomolecular signals in the paracrine arm of the communication system. In the reverse direction, decidual products enter amnionic fluid and these en-

ter the fetus by way of the fetal lung and by way of fetal swallowing. In some cases, there is preferential entry of decidual products into amnionic fluid. For example, large amounts of prolactin are formed in decidua; but little or none of decidual prolactin enters maternal blood. Rather, decidual prolactin enters amnionic fluid almost exclusively (Chaps. 4 and 6).

THE DYNAMIC ROLE OF THE FETUS IN PREGNANCY

Heretofore, the fetus commonly was envisioned as a passive passenger of the pregnancy unit; it is now known that this is not the case. To comprehend the nature and importance of the fetal–maternal communication system of human pregnancy, it is important to acknowledge that the fetus enjoys a position of protection from the external environment that is never to be experienced again in life; but at the same time, it must be recognized that the fetus is the dynamic force in the orchestration of its own destiny.

The fetus and extraembryonic fetal tissues are the source of bioactive agents that serve as the driving force in pregnancy. From the time of conception, a molecular dialogue is established between fetal and maternal tissues; some of the signal transmission systems no doubt are operative even before the time of blastocyst implantation. In several mammalian species, the horse for example, there are clear-cut differences between the transport of fertilized and nonfertilized ova in the fallopian tube.

The impetus for implantation is derived from the blastocyst and blastocyst products; invasion of the maternal decidua and blood vessels in the establishment of the implantation site and subsequent development of the placenta is under the active direction of bioactive products of fetal tissues; the maternal recognition of pregnancy is brought about by way of signals generated by the blastocyst; the maintenance of pregnancy is orchestrated by fetal contributions; the endocrine changes of pregnancy derive from products formed and secreted by fetal placenta; indeed, it is probable that fetal retreat from the maintenance of pregnancy is the penultimate event in the spontaneous initiation of parturition at term. From these interactions, it is established that there is trafficking, at the biomolecular level, that involves intimate signal transmission-responses between tissues of the fetus and its mother.

Therefore, to understand the organization of pregnancy and the functional components that serve to promote the maintenance of pregnancy and the physiological adaptations of the maternal organism to the developing fetus, it is essential that we understand the anatomical and physiological arrangements provided by this communication system in appreciable detail.

OVERVIEW

Fertilization of the human ovum by a spermatozoan nominally occurs in the fallopian tube within a short time (minutes to a few hours) after ovulation; and 6 days after fertilization, the blastocyst begins to implant in the endometrium of the uterus; and pregnancy has begun. Based on the proposition that the fetus is the dynamic force in the orchestration of the physiological events of pregnancy, the concept clearly emerges that the maternal organism is constitutively passive, responding to signals emanating from the fetus or extraembryonic fetal tissues, viz., the placenta and fetal membranes.

The role of the fetus and extraembryonic fetal tissues in pregnancy is not dissimilar to that of a nonmetastasizing, but rapidly growing, neoplasm. The developing embryo and fetus is very demanding; and in general, its demands are met at whatever cost to the maternal organism by way of efficient placental mechanisms for nutrient uptake and transfer. But in other respects, the fetus is a benevolent, albeit self-serving, parasite in that it provides for the development of systems that facilitate maternal adaptation to this rapidly growing, semiallogeneic, tumorlike graft. These systems include those that permit a sizable expansion of the maternal blood volume, an increase in cardiac output, refractoriness to pressor agents, increases in renal blood flow, and efficient utilization of energy sources (Chap. 7).

The fetus also is able to "tap in" to maternal systems that provide for protection, for example, the transplacental passage of antibodies; and in general, the fetus occupies a privileged and protected position during pregnancy. But the fetus is not totally isolated from the maternal environment, being subject to adverse effects of teratogens and some infectious agents and to profound alterations in maternal metabolic function and uteroplacental blood flow.

As specific examples of the active role of the blastocyst/embryo/fetus in guaranteeing its own optimum outcome (Fig. 2–2), consider the following:

IMPLANTATION

Clearly, the endometrium is not essential to implantation; ectopic pregnancies occur in the fallopian tube, ovary, peritoneal cavity, and spleen; and in experimental animals, the blastocyst can be implanted successfully into many tissues, including the testis. Thus, the blastocyst is the driving force in implantation. The capacity for estrogen formation in blastocyst has been documented; and it is speculated that an "estrogen surge" is a fundamental feature of the implantation of the blastocyst. In this regard, it is noteworthy that whereas enzyme deficiencies are known for virtually all steroidogenic enzymes involved in cortisol, mineralocorticosteroid, and androgen formation, a deficiency in aromatase, the pivotal enzyme in estrogen forma-

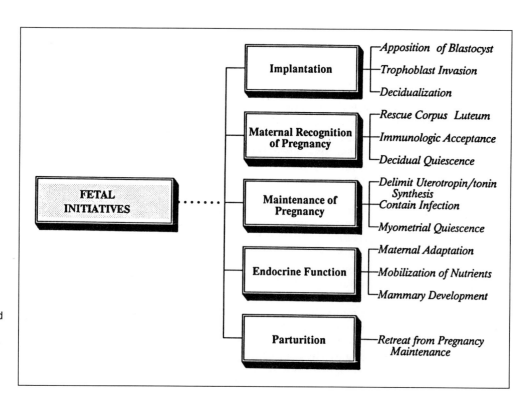

Figure 2–2. Fetal contributions to the maintenance of pregnancy. The fetus and extraembryonic fetal tissues are the dynamic, driving force in the establishment and maintenance of pregnancy. The contributions of the fetus include processes essential to implantation and maternal recognition of pregnancy; but more than this, the physiological and metabolic accommodations in the maternal organism that contribute to successful pregnancy are orchestrated by fetal-directed biomolecular initiatives.

tion, has never been found. Perhaps this enzyme deficiency is incompatible with pregnancy, i.e., blastocyst implantation.

There are components of both the neoplastic and the inflammatory process involved in blastocyst implantation; the blastocyst produces prostaglandins, platelet-activating factor, and plasminogen activator. In fact, complete decidualization of endometrium takes place only after blastocyst implantation. Thus, the blastocyst is an efficient, invasive, aggressive, dynamic force that directs the commencement of successful pregnancy.

MATERNAL RECOGNITION AND FETAL MAINTENANCE OF PREGNANCY

Among the early arrangements provided by the fetal–maternal communication system is one referred to by Short (1969) as the **maternal recognition of pregnancy.** This is an important concept in mammalian pregnancy physiology. But we suggest that the arrangement should be redesignated, for an important reason, namely, the **fetal-induced maternal recognition of pregnancy.** Whereas there is no doubt that there is, physiologically, maternal recognition of pregnancy, it is highly probable that this response is effected by *fetal contributions to the maintenance of pregnancy.* The importance of this distinction is to recognize the fundamental and essential contributions made by fetal tissues to the success of pregnancy. Conceptually, this interpretation also is important in determining the role of the fetus in the initiation of parturition (Chap. 10). The ''maternal recognition'' of pregnancy encompasses a series of processes (Bazer and colleagues, 1986) that include prolongation of the life-span of the corpus luteum to ensure continued progesterone secretion and decidual acceptance of the semiallogeneic fetal graft, which are effected, in part, by the inhibition of decidual prostaglandin formation.

The production of chorionic gonadotropin (hCG) by blastocyst and embryo ensures a continuation of corpus luteum function until the fetal trophoblasts are able to synthesize sufficient amounts of progesterone to maintain pregnancy (Chaps. 5 and 10). In some mammalian species, involution of the corpus luteum during a nonfertile cycle is induced in response to the action of prostaglandin (PG) $F_{2\alpha}$ produced in endometrium. In particular, if there is no implantation of blastocyst, $PGF_{2\alpha}$ is produced in the endometrium; the $PGF_{2\alpha}$ enters the uterine venous circulation and is transported by way of the uterine vein. In sheep and other species, the uterine vein crosses over the ovarian artery. $PGF_{2\alpha}$ is transferred from the uterine vein to the ovarian artery by a transvascular mechanism, and the $PGF_{2\alpha}$ acts on the corpus luteum as a luteolytic agent, bringing an end to the function of the corpus luteum. This event has been referred to as the *murder of the corpus luteum.* There are certain analogies between the regulation of corpus luteum function, i.e., luteolysis, and the initiation of parturition. For example, the formation of $PGF_{2\alpha}$ in endometrium (or decidua), in increased amounts, appears to be critical for both events. In those species in which endometrial $PGF_{2\alpha}$ acts as the luteolytic agent, the blastocyst (after implantation) acts to prevent $PGF_{2\alpha}$ formation and thus prevents luteolysis (Flint and Sheldrick, 1985).

This does not appear to be the case in the human; there is no evidence of endometrial production of a luteolytic agent in women because after hysterectomy, there seems to be normal ovarian function including the development of corpora lutea with normal life-spans. Nonetheless, hCG, produced by embryonic tissues, does function to prolong the life-span of the corpus luteum in women.

There also is appreciable evidence the blastocyst/embryo produces agents that serve to effect directly decidual quiescence early in pregnancy, thus ensuring the maintenance of pregnancy. The most clear-cut example of this process to date is the production of ovine trophoblast protein-1 (oTP-1) in the sheep embryo. OTP-1 (M_r about 18,000) is the major secretory product of the early (13- to 21-day) sheep blastocyst (Godkin and coworkers, 1984) and there is appreciable homology of the amino acid sequence of this protein with interferon-α (Imakawa and associates, 1987). Receptors for oTP-1 are present in sheep endometrium. OTP-1 is produced transiently by sheep blastocyst and serves to prevent luteolysis possibly by inhibiting endometrial prostaglandin $F_{2\alpha}$ formation (Hansen and colleagues, 1985). The infusion of bovine interferon-α into the uterine lumen of the cow prolongs the life-span of the corpus luteum (Plante and co-workers, 1988).

FETAL CONTRIBUTIONS TO THE MATERNAL ACCEPTANCE OF THE ALLOGENEIC FETAL GRAFT

Just after, or at about the time of implantation, there is suppression of HLA antigen formation in extraembryonic fetal tissues (trophoblasts), i.e., in tissues that embrace maternal tissues; this may be a fundamental mechanism by which the developing fetus gains immunological acceptance during blastocyst implantation.

FETAL CONTRIBUTIONS TO THE ENDOCRINOLOGY OF PREGNANCY

The hormonal changes of human pregnancy are monumental and unprecedented in breadth and amount in the annals of mammalian endocrinology (Chap. 5). But almost without exception, the endocrine changes of human pregnancy are the consequence of fetal placental function, either directly or indirectly—thus, the fetus also is the prime contributor to the endocrine alterations of pregnancy. The formation of estrogens during pregnancy occurs by way of the placental aromatization of C_{19}-steroids, which, in turn, are produced primarily in the fetal adrenals. Progesterone also is produced in fetal trophoblasts in massive quantities by way of the utilization of maternal plasma low-density lipoprotein (LDL)-cholesterol; indeed, the rate of utilization of maternal plasma LDL by trophoblasts for progesterone formation is so great in some pregnancies as to be equivalent to the total daily turnover rate of LDL in nonpregnant women (Chap. 5). Placental progesterone is converted in maternal tissues to deoxycorticosterone, a potent mineralocorticosteroid; placental progesterone, secreted into the maternal compartment, serves as the stimulus by way of its natrurietic action for the increase in aldosterone secretion by the maternal adrenal to levels 20 times or more than that found in men and nonpregnant women. All of these changes, and many more, are effected by way of fetal-produced or fetal-induced endocrine contributions to pregnancy (Chaps. 5 and 7).

PLACENTAL SEQUESTRATION OF NUTRIENTS

Fetal villous trophoblasts are remarkably efficient in extracting or sequestering essential nutrients from the maternal circulation. For example, in women with profound iron-deficiency anemia during pregnancy, the iron stores of the fetus are normal; in women with severe folic acid deficiency during pregnancy causing severe anemia, the fetal hematocrit is normal (Chap. 7). The fetus is a demanding and efficient parasite. We have long been fascinated by the fact that the amount of calcium assembled into the shell of the egg of the chicken in a period of 18 hours is equivalent to the amount of calcium contained in the entire bony skeleton of the hen. Thus, even in the avian, a species that arguably is never pregnant, the needs of the embryo are met.

FETAL RETREAT FROM PREGNANCY MAINTENANCE AND THE INITIATION OF PARTURITION

It is probable that the fetus also is in control of his/her own destiny with respect to the timely onset of parturition. Perhaps this comes about by way of fetal retreat from further maintenance of pregnancy. A good example of the importance of the fetus in the maintenance of pregnancy and the initiation of parturition is found in cases of fetal death. Even after fetal death, labor does not immediately ensue. It is common for pregnancies with a dead fetus to proceed for days, weeks, or even months after the time of fetal demise. For example, it has been reported that with fetal death caused by Rh isoimmunization before 35 weeks gestation, 50 percent of such pregnancies remain undelivered, at least in the absence of intervention, for up to 5 weeks after fetal death (Townsend and Shelton, 1964). It is as if there is no built-in mechanism for emptying the uterus by way of processes initiated within the maternal compartment even after the fetus is dead.

LACTATION AND MILK LET-DOWN

During pregnancy, estrogen and progesterone, together with prolactin, act on maternal mammary tissue to induce optimal morphological and biochemical maturation preparatory to lactation, i.e., milk production. Progesterone, however, also acts to prevent lactogenesis; but with progesterone withdrawal after delivery of the placenta, lactogenesis promptly commences. Thereafter, suckling by the newborn induces the secretion of oxytocin in the mother; oxytocin acts on the myoepithelial cells of the breast ducts to cause milk let-down and ensures the success of breast feeding.

These are but a few examples to indicate unambiguously that the fetus, or else extraembryonic fetal tissues, direct the orchestration of the physiological events of pregnancy. The maternal organism passively responds—even to the point of her own detriment. We will refer to this particular arrangement frequently as we consider the physiological adaptations of maternal systems to pregnancy (Chap. 7), acceptance of the fetal semiallogeneic graft (Chap. 4), fetal growth and development (Chap. 6), and the initiation of parturition (Chap. 10).

DIAGNOSIS OF PREGNANCY

By way of molecular communication between fetal and maternal tissues, remarkable physiological and anatomical changes are brought about in pregnant women from very soon after conception. Throughout this book, we will emphasize that ordinarily pregnancy is a normal physiological state; but to be sure, it is one in which there are profound adaptive changes that are monumental and essential to optimal pregnancy outcome. Many of the physiological adaptations of pregnancy are predictable and therefore constitute important milestones that mark the accommodations of the pregnant woman to the development of the fetus. Many of these physiological adaptations constitute important clues that provide for the diagnosis of pregnancy and an evaluation of its progress.

In the life of women, few diagnoses are more important than that of pregnancy. And whereas pregnancy is ordinarily a physiological state, the importance of the correct diagnosis of pregnancy cannot be overstated. For the woman who may be pregnant, there are few diagnoses that can evoke emotions of such absolute joy or else such pains of profound despair. And for all physicians entrusted with the medical management of women of reproductive age, knowledge of the existence of pregnancy is crucial to the proper diagnosis and treatment of all disease processes. For all of these reasons, every physician who assumes the responsibility for the medical care of any woman in the reproductive age range, irrespective of the nature of the physician's practice or special interest, must always raise the question, *Is she pregnant?* Failure to do so often leads to incorrect diagnoses, inappropriate treatment, and, at times, to medicolegal embroilment.

The diagnosis of pregnancy is ordinarily very easy to establish, but unfortunately this is not always the case. On occasion, pharmacological, physiological, or pathophysiological processes may cause endocrine or anatomical changes that mimic pregnancy and cause confusion for the woman or the physician. At times, therefore, the diagnosis of pregnancy is not easy to make, but rarely is it impossible if appropriate clinical and laboratory tests are conducted.

Ordinarily, the woman is aware of the likelihood of pregnancy when she consults a physician, although she may not volunteer this information unless asked specifically. Mistakes in diagnosis are made most frequently in the first several weeks of pregnancy while the uterus is still a pelvic organ. Although it is possible to mistake the enlarged uterus of pregnancy, even at term, for a tumor of some nature, such errors usually are the result of hasty or incomplete examination.

The endocrine, physiological, and anatomical alterations that accompany pregnancy give rise to symptoms and signs that provide presumptive, probable, and even definitive evidence that pregnancy exists. These changes transpire as a consequence of interactions between fetal and maternal tissues, in response to signals that are transmitted between the fetus (and fetal tissues) and the mother (and maternal tissues), and by way of the development of the fetus per se.

The diagnosis of pregnancy is based upon certain symptoms and signs that are elicited by history and found by examination and upon results of laboratory tests. The symptoms and signs of pregnancy are classified into three groups: presumptive evidence, probable signs, and positive signs.

PRESUMPTIVE EVIDENCE OF PREGNANCY

Presumptive evidence of pregnancy is based largely on subjective symptoms and signs that include (1) nausea with or without vomiting, (2) disturbances in urination, (3) fatigue, and (4) the perception of fetal movement. These signs include (1) cessation of menses, (2) anatomical changes in the breasts, (3) discoloration of the vaginal mucosa, (4) increased skin pigmentation and the development of abdominal striae, and (5) especially important, **does she believe that she is pregnant?**

SYMPTOMS OF PREGNANCY

Nausea With or Without Vomiting

Commonly, pregnancy is characterized by disturbances of the digestive system, manifested particularly by nausea and vomiting. This so-called *morning sickness of pregnancy* usually commences during the early part of the day but passes off in a few hours, although occasionally it persists longer and may occur at other times. This disturbing symptom usually appears about 6 weeks after the commencement of the last menstrual period and ordinarily disappears spontaneously 6 to 12 weeks later.

Disturbances in Urination
During the first trimester of pregnancy, the enlarging uterus, by exerting pressure on the urinary bladder, may cause frequent micturition. Gradually, the frequency of urination diminishes as pregnancy progresses and the uterus rises up into the abdomen. This symptom reappears near the end of pregnancy, however, when the fetal head descends into the maternal pelvis.

Fatigue
Easy fatigability is such a frequent characteristic of early pregnancy that it provides a noteworthy diagnostic clue.

Perception of Fetal Movement
Sometime between 16 and 20 weeks after the onset of the last menstrual period, the pregnant woman usually becomes conscious of slight fluttering movements in the abdomen, and these movements gradually increase in intensity. These are caused by fetal activity, and the time that these are first recognized by the pregnant woman is designated as *quickening*, or the perception of life. This sign provides only corroborative evidence of pregnancy and in itself is of little diagnostic value. It is, however, a milestone of the progress of pregnancy that, if dated accurately, can provide corroborative evidence in determining the duration of gestation.

SIGNS OF PREGNANCY

Cessation of Menses
In a healthy woman who previously has experienced spontaneous, cyclic, predictable menstruation, the abrupt cessation of menses is highly suggestive of pregnancy. Because there is appreciable variation in the length of the ovarian (and thus menstrual) cycle among women and even in the same woman, it is not until 10 days or more after the time of expected onset of the menstrual period that the absence of menses is a reliable indication of pregnancy. When a second menstrual period is missed, the probability of pregnancy is very much greater.

Although cessation of menstruation is an early and very important indication of pregnancy, gestation may begin without prior menstruation, i.e., in a girl in whom menarche has not occurred. In certain Oriental countries, where girls marry at a very early age, and in sexually promiscuous groups, pregnancy sometimes occurs before menarche. Indeed, we have managed the pregnancies of a girl who had four children without ever having a menstrual period. She delivered her fourth child at age 16, and conceived her first child at age 12 before menarche, presumably with first ovulation.

Nursing mothers, who usually do not menstruate during lactation, sometimes conceive at that time; and more rarely, women who believe they have passed the menopause may become pregnant. Uterine bleeding that is suggestive of menstruation occurs occasionally after conception. For example, during the first half of pregnancy, one or two episodes of bloody discharge, reminiscent of, and sometimes misinterpreted as, menstruation, are not uncommon, but almost without exception, such bleeding is brief and scant. In a series of 225 consecutive pregnant women who did not abort, Speert and Guttmacher (1954) observed that macroscopic vaginal bleeding, which occurred between the time of conception and the 196th day of pregnancy, was reported by 22 percent of these women. In the absence of any cervical lesion, the bleeding began on or before the 40th day of pregnancy in 8 percent. Speert and Guttmacher interpreted such bleeding to be physiological, viz., the consequence of implantation. Bleeding during pregnancy was three times more frequent among multiparas than among primigravidas. Of 83 multiparas, 25 percent experienced bleeding.

Nonetheless, alleged instances in which women are said to have "menstruated" every month throughout pregnancy are of questionable authenticity; true uterine bleeding during pregnancy is undoubtedly the result of some abnormality of the reproductive organs. **Bleeding per vagina at any time during pregnancy must be regarded as abnormal and portends a greater likelihood of profound pregnancy complications.**

Cessation or absence of menstruation can be caused by a number of conditions other than pregnancy. Probably the most common cause of a delay in the time of onset of the menstrual period is anovulation, which in turn may be the consequence of a number of factors that include physiological aberrations induced by emotional disorders, for example, the fear of pregnancy. Environmental changes as well as a variety of chronic disease processes also may suppress ovulation by inducing anestrogenic or estrogenic anovulation. Delays in the onset of menstruation have been attributed to persistent corpus luteum function, e.g., in association with cystic corpora lutea, but the evidence is not convincing. Most, perhaps all, instances of prolonged function of the corpus luteum are related to a pregnancy episode, even though the pregnancy may be unrecognized as in the case of early missed or incomplete abortion.

Changes in the Breasts
Generally, the anatomical changes in the breast that accompany pregnancy are quite characteristic in primiparas, but are less obvious in multiparas, whose breasts may contain a small amount of milky material or colostrum for months or even years after the birth of their last child (Chap. 7). Occasionally, changes in the breasts similar to those caused by pregnancy are found in women with prolactin-secreting pituitary tumors and in women taking drugs that induce hyperprolactinemia. Instances also have been reported of such breast changes occurring in women with spurious or imaginary pregnancy, *pseudocyesis* (see p. 20).

Discoloration of the Vaginal Mucosa
During pregnancy, the vaginal mucosa frequently appears dark bluish or purplish-red and congested, the so-called *Chadwick's sign* (1886). This appearance of the vagina is taken as presumptive evidence of pregnancy; but it is not conclusive. Similar changes in vaginal appearance may be induced by any condition that causes intense congestion of the pelvic organs.

Increased Skin Pigmentation and the Appearance of Abdominal Striae
These cutaneous manifestations are common to, but not diagnostic of, pregnancy. These signs may be absent during pregnancy, and conversely, these changes may be associated with the use of estrogen-progestin contraceptives.

PROBABLE EVIDENCE OF PREGNANCY

The probable signs of pregnancy include (1) enlargement of the abdomen, (2) changes in the shape, size, and consistency of the uterus, (3) anatomical changes in the cervix, (4) Braxton Hicks contractions, (5) ballottement, (6) physical outlining of the fetus, and (7) results of endocrine tests.

ENLARGEMENT OF THE ABDOMEN

By 12 weeks of gestation, the uterus usually can be felt through the abdominal wall just above the symphysis as a tumor; thereafter, the uterus gradually increases in size to the end of pregnancy. In general, any enlargement of the abdomen during the childbearing period of women is strongly suggestive of pregnancy.

The abdominal enlargement usually is less pronounced in primiparous than in multiparous women in whom some of the tone of the abdominal musculature has been lost; indeed, in some multiparous women, the abdominal wall is so flaccid that the uterus sags forward and downward, producing a pendulous abdomen. This difference in abdominal tone between first and subsequent pregnancies sometimes is so obvious that it is not rare for women in the latter part of a second pregnancy to suspect a twin pregnancy because of the increased size of their abdomen, as compared with that in the corresponding month of their previous pregnancy. The abdomen of the pregnant woman also undergoes significant changes in shape depending on her body position. The uterus is, of course, much less prominent when the woman is in the supine position.

CHANGES IN SIZE, SHAPE, AND CONSISTENCY OF THE UTERUS

During the first few weeks of pregnancy, the increase in size of the uterus is limited principally to the anterioposterior diameter, but at a little later time in gestation, the body of the uterus is almost globular; an average uterine diameter of 8 cm is attained by 12 weeks of pregnancy. On bimanual examination, the body of the uterus during pregnancy feels doughy or elastic and sometimes becomes exceedingly soft.

At about 6 to 8 weeks after the onset of the last menstrual period, *Hegar's sign* becomes manifest. With one hand of the examiner on the abdomen and two fingers of the other hand placed in the vagina, the still-firm cervix is felt, with the elastic body of the uterus above the compressible soft isthmus, which is between the two. Occasionally, the softening at the isthmus is so marked that the cervix and the body of the uterus seem to be separate organs. At this time in pregnancy, the inexperienced examiner may mistake the cervix for a small uterus, and the softened body of the fundus for a tumor of the ovaries or oviducts. This sign of Hegar is not, however, positively diagnostic of pregnancy, because occasionally it may be present when the walls of the nonpregnant uterus are excessively soft for reasons other than pregnancy.

CHANGES IN THE CERVIX

By 6 to 8 weeks gestation, the cervix often becomes considerably softened. In primigravidas, the consistency of the cervical tissue that surrounds the external os is more similar to that of the lips of the mouth than to that of the nasal cartilage, as it is in nonpregnant women. Other conditions, however, may bring about softening of the cervix. Estrogen-progestin contracep-tives, for example, commonly act to cause some softening and congestion of the uterine cervix.

As pregnancy advances, the cervical canal may become sufficiently patulous as to admit the tip of the examiner's finger. In certain inflammatory conditions, as well as with carcinoma, the cervix may remain firm during pregnancy, yielding only with the onset of labor, if at all.

BRAXTON HICKS CONTRACTIONS

During pregnancy, the uterus undergoes palpable but ordinarily painless contractions at irregular intervals from early stages of gestation. These contractions may increase in number and amplitude when the uterus is massaged. These Braxton Hicks contractions, however, are not positive signs of pregnancy because similar contractions sometimes are observed in uteri of women with hematometra and occasionally in uteri in which there are soft myomas, especially those of the pedunculated, submucous variety. The detection of Braxton Hicks contractions, however, may be helpful in excluding the existence of an ectopic abdominal pregnancy.

BALLOTTEMENT

Near midpregnancy, the volume of the fetus is small compared with that of the volume of amnionic fluid; and consequently, sudden pressure exerted on the uterus may cause the fetus to sink in the amnionic fluid and then rebound to its original position; the tap produced (ballottement) is felt by the examining fingers.

OUTLINING THE FETUS

In the second half of pregnancy, the outlines of the fetal body may be palpated through the maternal abdominal wall, and the outlining of the fetus becomes easier the nearer that term is approached. Occasionally, subserous myomas may be of such a size and shape as to simulate the fetal head or small parts, or both, thus causing serious diagnostic errors. A positive diagnosis of pregnancy cannot be made, therefore, from this sign alone.

ENDOCRINE TESTS

The presence of human chorionic gonadotropin (hCG) in maternal plasma and its excretion in urine provides the basis for the endocrine tests for pregnancy. This hormone may be identified in body fluids by any one of a variety of immunoassay or bioassay techniques.

CHORIONIC GONADOTROPIN

One component of the **maternal recognition of pregnancy** arrangement in the human that is induced by blastocyst provides for a convenient chemical test of pregnancy, viz., the production by trophoblasts of a glycoprotein hormone, namely, hCG. The production of hCG by fetal trophoblasts is important in the maternal recognition of pregnancy by way of the action of hCG on the ovary to prevent the involution of the corpus luteum, the principal site of progesterone formation in the first 6 to 8 weeks of pregnancy. HCG is a luteinizing hormone (LH)-like agent that acts as an LH surrogate in responsive tissues, for example, the ovary (corpus luteum) and testis. The detection of hCG in biological fluids, either urine or serum of the woman to be tested, is by far the most common test of pregnancy used throughout the world. For this reason, it is imperative that the student of obstetrics become familiar with the chemistry, biological action, and detection of this unique glycoprotein hormone that is produced by the trophoblasts during human pregnancy.

History

The evolution of our understanding of the biological, physiological, and chemical nature of hCG occupies an important niche in the history of obstetrics. It is interesting to recall that the first species in which a chorionic gonadotropin was discovered was the human. Hirose (1919) is credited with the first demonstration of a trophic effect of human placental tissue fragments on the ovaries and uteri of the rabbit; and it was the demonstration of the *pregnancy hormone* in urine of pregnant women by Ascheim and Zondek (1927) that formed the basis for the original consideration of the presence of hCG in urine as a test for pregnancy.

Hertz (1980) relates the story of an interesting conversation that he had with Bernhard Zondek. In that conversation, Zondek recounted with good humor that he once chastised his technician for the reporting of a positive pregnancy test that was obtained with the urine of a man. Hertz recounts that the matter was complicated further because the man's last name was the same as that of one of the pregnant women whose urine was tested in the same assay. Ultimately, it was found that the man in question was one in whom there was a testicular tumor that was producing hCG. Now we know that a number of *neoplasias* in man produce hCG. Zondek made amends and never doubted that technician's findings again.

The discovery of the *pregnancy hormone* led to the development of the first pregnancy test, and even the laity were familiar with the *Ascheim-Zondek,* or *A-Z test* and the *Friedman tests* for pregnancy because, as Hertz points out, these became household terms. These tests were bioassays that took advantage of the biological property of hCG to stimulate the gonads of experimental animals, either sexually immature animals (the rat) or else induced ovulators (the rabbit). Indeed, the A-Z test, or variations on the theme, namely stimulation of the follicles of the ovaries of experimental animals, including the induction of ovulation in induced ovulators (rabbits) by urine of pregnant women, was the standard test for pregnancy in women for more than 40 years.

Zondek believed that there were two pregnancy-related gonadotropin activities because he observed that concentrates of urine of pregnant women evoked both follicular development and ovulation and corpus luteum formation. For these reasons, he believed that there were two separate agents, and he referred to these putative agents as *prolan A* and *prolan B.* Soon there was considerable controversy as to the relationship between the gonadotropin(s) in urine of pregnant women and those extracted from pituitary tissue. Hertz recounts the history of, and the resolution of, this controversy as follows: Zondek (1931) and others emphasized that, by use of the bioassay procedures employed, there was, in the urine of postmenopausal women, follicle-stimulating activity. It also was demonstrated that whereas the avian gonad and the ovary of the immature rhesus monkey are responsive to extracts of the pituitary, there was no such response to concentrates of urine of pregnant women. Convincing evidence that the two preparations, the pituitary extracts and concentrates of urine of pregnant women, were different in gonadotropin properties was obtained by Reichert and co-workers (1932), who demonstrated that the hypophysectomized rat was virtually unresponsive to extracts of urine of pregnant women but readily responsive to extracts of pituitary tissue.

In 1938, the placental source of hCG was established further and verified by Gey, Jones, and Hellman, who demonstrated the production of the hormone by trophoblastic cells maintained in tissue culture. In 1948, the hormone was crystallized by Claesson and co-workers. Based on the work of these pioneering investigators, we since have come to know (1) the nature of as well as the

structure of hCG, (2) in large measure, the molecular events involved in its mechanism of action, (3) the nature of its biosynthesis and processing, (4) the utility of this protein hormone in the evaluation of certain neoplastic processes, and (5) trials have been conducted to ascertain if the hormone could be used as an antigen for the development of antibodies to hCG as a means of immunization against pregnancy in women.

CHEMISTRY

We now know that hCG is a glycoprotein with a high carbohydrate content. The molecule is a heterodimer comprised of two dissimilar subunits, designated α and β, which are noncovalently linked. These subunits have been separated, isolated in pure form, and the primary structure of each has been characterized (Chap. 5).

CELLULAR SITE OF ORIGIN AND BIOLOGICAL ASPECTS OF hCG ACTION

HCG is produced in placenta almost exclusively by syncytiotrophoblast rather than cytotrophoblasts (Chap. 5).

hCG IN BLOOD AND URINE: PLACENTAL PRODUCTION OF hCG

The production of hCG in blastocyst begins very early and indeed may even precede the time of nidation. After implantation, the levels of hCG in maternal plasma and urine rise very rapidly. Certainly with a sensitive test, for example, a radioimmunoassay employing antibodies directed against the β-subunit of hCG (which is specific for hCG and does not cross-react significantly with LH), the pregnancy hormone can be demonstrated by 8 to 9 days after ovulation, probably on the day of blastocyst implantation. It is estimated that, in early pregnancy, the doubling time of hCG concentrations in plasma is 1.4 to 2.0 days (Chartier and colleagues, 1979). The levels of hCG in blood and urine increase from the day of implantation until about 60 to 70 days of pregnancy. Thereafter; the concentration of hCG declines until a nadir is reached at about 100 to 130 days of pregnancy. The rate of excretion of chorionic gonadotropin into the urine of pregnant women closely parallels the levels in serum; peak levels are attained between 60 and 70 days of gestation. A good rule of thumb is that the concentration of hCG contained in 1 liter of maternal plasma is equivalent to that contained in 24 hours of urine. Thus, if the urine excreted per 24 hours were 1 liter, the concentration of hCG in serum and in urine would be similar.

Although most curves constructed from mean values for hCG in serum or urine are quite similar, these curves are not such as to emphasize the considerable variations in the levels of this hormone in blood or urine among individual women at the same time of gestation.

PREGNANCY TESTS

In this time of wide utilization of the principles of immunoassay for the measurement of thousands of compounds, at a time when radioreceptor assays are common, as are radioenzymatic assays and the use of monoclonal antibodies, it seems strange now that we were obliged to use bioassays for the evaluation of hCG in biological fluids for nearly four decades. On the other hand, it obviously was necessary to establish the general principles of immunoassay before these could be applied to the measurement of hCG as a means of sensitive and accurate testing for pregnancy. Also, in retrospect, it is reasonably impressive to recall that several of the bioassays for hCG, especially those employing the development of ovarian hyperemia in the immature rat as the end-point, were, while insensitive, remarkably accurate by 4 to 5 weeks after ovulation or at least by the time of the second missed menses.

Today, for the vast majority of pregnancy testing conducted, there are inexpensive kits available that can be used for tests that can be completed quickly, i.e., in 3 to 5 minutes, with high accuracy—and with certain precautions—high precision. Almost without exception, chemical detection of pregnancy involves the demonstration of hCG in blood or urine of the woman to be tested. Many different test systems are available in kit form commercially. Each, however, is dependent upon one principle: recognition of hCG (or a subunit thereof) by an antibody to the hCG molecule. Bandi and colleagues (1987) found that there were 39 commercially available urine pregnancy tests in 1986. These included tests involving the principles of agglutination inhibition, radioimmunoassay, and enzyme-linked immunosorbent assay (ELISA) methods.

ANTIBODIES TO hCG

The methods for assaying hCG are of considerable importance because these assays form the basis for the majority of tests for pregnancy in women. Until relatively recently, some of the immunoassays and all of the bioassays commonly employed for pregnancy testing were not absolutely specific for hCG. Antibodies raised against the complete (intact) hCG also recognize LH. The α-subunit of four glycoprotein hormones, namely, follicle-stimulating hormone, thyrotropin, luteinizing hormone, and hCG, are identical (Chap. 5). On the other hand, the β-subunit is distinct for each of these hormones. Antibodies raised against the complete hCG molecule, therefore, will recognize epitopes on the α-subunit of LH and hCG.

The apparent hCG activity in biological fluids at times was found to differ appreciably, depending upon whether immunoassay or bioassay was employed. Wide and Hobson (1967), and also Bridson and associates (1970), demonstrated that hCG synthesized in vitro by cloned choriocarcinoma cells yielded values twice as great by immunoassay as by bioassay. They suggested that the reduction in biologically active material compared with that found employing immunoassays was the result of alterations in the hormone molecule after it was secreted by the trophoblast. We now know, however, that such cells secrete the α-subunit, the β-subunit, and complete hCG; the separate subunits are biologically inactive but are recognized by antibodies in varying reactivities.

With the recognition that LH and hCG were composed of an α- and β-subunit, that the two subunits of each molecular species could be separated and purified, and that the β-subunits of each were structurally distinct, at least at the COOH-terminus (Chap. 5), Vaitukaitis and colleagues (1972) set out to develop antibodies that would specifically recognize epitopes on the β-subunit of hCG. Thereby, an antibody would be available that could discriminate between LH and hCG. The development of such an antibody has become an incredibly useful tool for elucidation of physiological processes, for early detection of pregnancy, and for monitoring hCG production in persons with neoplastic trophoblastic disease, both before and during treatment.

Therefore, antibodies, with high specificity for the β-subunit of hCG, with little cross-reactivity against LH, have been raised by immunization of animals (polyclonal antibodies) or by hybridoma techniques (monoclonal antibodies) against recognition sites on the β-subunit of hCG; and antibodies have been raised against the α-subunit of hCG and LH (which are identical).

IMMUNOASSAYS OF hCG

Agglutination Inhibition
In many immunoassay procedures, the principle of agglutination inhibition, i.e., the prevention of flocculation of hCG-coated particles, for example, latex particles to which hCG is covalently bound, is used. The kits commercially available to offices and laboratories that employ failure of agglutination of latex particles to detect hCG in urine contain two reagents. One is a suspension of latex particles coated with or covalently bound to hCG and the other contains a solution of hCG antibody. To test for hCG, one drop of urine is mixed with one drop of the antibody-containing solution on a black glass slide. If no hCG is present in the urine, antibody will remain available to agglutinate the hCG-coated latex particles, which are added subsequently. Agglutination of the latex particles can be observed easily when a bright light source is illuminated against the dark background of the glass slide. If hCG were present in the urine, it would bind to the antibody and thus prevent antibody-induced agglutination of the hCG-coated latex particles. Therefore, the pregnancy test is positive if no agglutination occurs; the pregnancy test is negative when agglutination occurs.

Recently, commercially available kits have been introduced in which the antibody to hCG is directed specifically to epitopes on the β-subunit, thus avoiding cross-reactivity with LH. This permits greater sensitivity together with greater accuracy in assays of hCG.

Radioimmunoassays
In radioimmunoassays, [^{125}I]iodohCG is used as the radiolabeled ligand for antibodies raised against hCG and is dependent upon displacement of (or competition with) the radiolabeled ligand by nonradiolabeled hCG in the biological sample to be tested. In radioimmunoassays, "free" and "bound" [^{125}I]iodohCG are separated and radioactivity that is unbound is assayed. From a construction of standard curves, hCG is quantified with great accuracy and sensitivity by this method. In this immunoassay, antibodies against the β-subunit of hCG also are used.

Enzyme-Linked Immunosorbent Assay (ELISA)
This technique is useful for the quantification of extremely small amounts of materials in biological samples. In the ELISA for hCG, a monoclonal antibody, bound to a solid phase support (usually plastic), binds the hCG in the test sample; a second antibody is added to "sandwich" the hCG. It is the second antibody to which an enzyme, e.g., alkaline phosphatase, is linked; when substrate for this enzyme is added, a blue color develops, the intensity of which is related directly to the amount of enzyme and, thus, the amount of second antibody bound. This, in turn, is determined by the amount of hCG present in the test sample. The sensitivity of ELISA for hCG in serum is 50 mIU per mL.

Accuracy of Pregnancy Tests
In a multicenter collaborative study sponsored by the National Institutes of Health, Jovanovic and associates (1987) concluded

that laboratories conducting routine clinical tests could measure hCG accurately at the time of "missed" menses, but not necessarily before this time.

"Do It Yourself" Test Kits

Today there are several over-the-counter pregnancy test kits for use at home. In each of the tests, the principle of hemagglutination inhibition using sheep erythrocytes is employed with antibodies to hCG, and the subject's urine. The experience to date has been that women who use the test at home experience a relatively low false-positive rate but a high false-negative result.

Valanis and Perlman (1982) evaluated the prevalence of use of home pregnancy-testing kits among a wide distribution of subjects according to age, race, and socioeconomic status. They also investigated test results. They found that among 144 women interviewed in the settings of a private physician's office, a Planned Parenthood clinic, and a public obstetrics-gynecology clinic, almost one third of the subjects had used a home pregnancy-testing kit. They also found that the false-negative test result incidence was nearly 25 percent, and that only one third of the subjects complied with test kit instructions. They also found a greater use among white women compared with black women and greater use among middle-income women and among women consulting private physicians. These investigators voiced concern about the high false-negative test results even among women who did ultimately seek medical advice. In this study, only women who did initiate medical care were evaluated.

Subsequently, Doshi (1986) found that when women conducted their own in-home pregnancy tests, the predictive value of a negative result was 56 percent and the predictive value of a positive result was 83 percent.

Physician opinion is divided concerning the wisdom of making pregnancy testing available to nonprofessionals. Some argue that such tests will give results that will prompt women to see physicians earlier. We are of the view that the reverse may be more likely in those complicated situations in which early physician consultation is urgently needed.

BIOASSAYS OF hCG

Radioreceptor Assay

Saxena and Landesman (1978) reviewed the development and utilization of a radioreceptor assay for hCC. This assay makes use of the high-affinity receptors on plasma membrane preparations of responsive tissues, for example, bovine corpora lutea. The radioreceptor assay does not distinguish between LH and hCG because these two hormones are operative by way of the same receptor. It requires the utilization of radiolabeled hCG and approximately 2 hours to conduct. The test does offer the advantage of accuracy and applicability to serum testing (Boyko and Russell, 1979).

Pharmacological Endocrine Assay

Progesterone-induced and synthetic progestin-induced withdrawal uterine bleeding was used in the past in attempts to differentiate pregnancy from other causes of amenorrhea. In the absence of pregnancy, withdrawal bleeding usually occurs 3 to 5 days after a test dose of the progestin in estrogen-producing anovulatory women. This response, of course, requires an estrogen-primed endometrium. Withdrawal of the progestin results in uterine bleeding if there is little or no endogenous

progesterone production. If there is sufficient production of endogenous progesterone or if the endometrium is not estrogen-primed, no bleeding occurs.

In general, this method offers little that cannot be accomplished by a careful evaluation of the woman's history and by ascertaining, at the time of pelvic examination, whether there is any cervical mucus and, if so, whether the spread and dried mucus crystallizes to form a fern or a cellular pattern (see Chap. 3, p. 36). If copious thin mucus is present and if a fern pattern develops on drying, early pregnancy is very unlikely and the woman almost certainly will experience uterine bleeding after treatment with and withdrawal from progestin. If little cervical mucus is present and a highly cellular pattern forms, she may or may not be pregnant. If not pregnant, she may or may not sustain uterine bleeding after receiving progestin, depending upon her own supply of endogenous progesterone. Moreover, currently there is the fear that progestins are potential teratogens (see Chap. 32, p. 563). Therefore, progestins should not be used in women who are believed to be pregnant except in unusual circumstances, e.g., after removal of the corpus luteum before completion of the 8th week of pregnancy.

Summary and Critique of Pregnancy Tests for hCG

None of the chemical tests of pregnancy is sufficiently accurate to provide positive proof of pregnancy. Unfortunately, the same or even greater error rate in tests conducted by women at home may give rise to false security or unnecessary alarm if she cannot evaluate the likely validity of the results of such tests in light of other signs or symptoms. If the test employed is so sensitive that it detects very small amounts of hCG (with an antibody that also recognizes LH), the results may give rise to a positive test for pregnancy in nonpregnant women, especially in problem cases, because of the cross-reactivity of circulating or excreted LH. At the time of menopause, for example, amenorrhea not infrequently causes considerable fear of the possibility of pregnancy. At the same time, the levels of pituitary gonadotropins in plasma and urine in the postmenopausal woman usually are elevated and may be the cause of a falsely positive pregnancy test. If, however, the sensitivity of the pregnancy test is reduced so as to exclude a falsely positive result caused by LH cross-reactivity, some early pregnancies will not be identified because the levels of hCG are yet too low to be detected. The falsely negative test is most likely to be encountered during the first few days of pregnancy or after the 4th month, although with abnormal pregnancies, such as a tubal (ectopic) pregnancy, hCG may be present only in small amounts and therefore not identified by the less sensitive methods of testing.

Specific tests for hCG, i.e., those utilizing the antibody directed against recognition sites on the β-subunit of hCG, are currently available commercially. These tests are exquisitely sensitive and have been reviewed by Barnes and colleagues (1985). These tests provide greater specificity because the β-subunit of hCG differs antigenically from the β-subunit of LH.

MEASUREMENT OF hCG IN GYNECOLOGICAL DISORDERS

Ectopic pregnancy (Chap. 30) is a common gynecological disorder that may present a variety of difficulties in diagnosis and management. Frequently, the routinely used clinical tests for pregnancy, when the embryo is implanted outside the endometrial cavity (ectopic pregnancies), are negative for hCG. This may be due to a variety of reasons, likely the most common being reduction in placentation for the stage of gestation because of the ectopic site of implantation, disruption of trophoblasts by hemorrhage, or embryonic death. Nonetheless, hCG is present in plasma and urine of most (probably all) women with ectopic pregnancies, albeit generally in lower concentrations than in women with normal intrauterine pregnancies at comparable stages of gestations (Barnes and associates, 1985).

In many instances of unruptured ectopic pregnancy, the diagnosis may be difficult. For this reason, the detection of hCG in biological fluids of such women or the demonstration of a declining concentration of the levels of hCG may be of considerable assistance in reaching a definitive diagnosis. By use of radioimmunoassay procedures with antibodies directed toward the β-subunit of the molecule, this goal ordinarily is achieved. The same is true of the use of radioreceptor assays; these, however, as pointed out, do not distinguish between LH and hCG. If the case in point is not an emergency situation, the demonstration of a decline in hCG levels early in pregnancy or else a failure of the levels to increase with time is indicative of impending spontaneous abortion or else ectopic pregnancy. Unfortunately, the reverse does not obtain. Namely, normal levels of hCG may be found in women in whom there is an ectopic pregnancy.

Early in pregnancy, the levels of hCG in plasma double about every 2 days. If this doubling time can be demonstrated, a successful pregnancy outcome will be expected in 90 percent of cases (Pelosi and associates, 1983). This same doubling time in the increase in plasma levels of hCG is found in only 20 percent of women with an ectopic pregnancy. Kadar and colleagues (1981) found that the level of hCG in plasma increased by at least 66 percent in 48 hours early in normal pregnancy but by less than this amount in women with an ectopic pregnancy.

By use of sensitive assays for hCG, positive results have been obtained in 80 to 99 percent of proven cases of ectopic pregnancy by various investigators. It is important to remember, however, that low or falling levels of hCG are not such as to distinguish between ectopic pregnancy and impending spontaneous abortion (Barnes and co-workers, 1985).

Lagrew and colleagues (1983) found that the concentration of hCG in plasma of pregnant women increased in an exponential fashion between 30 and 60 days of pregnancy (dated from last menses). By use of a regression line constructed from measurement of hCG in a large population of pregnant women, these investigators found that the level of hCG at this time in pregnancy was an accurate reflection of gestation duration. Thus, in women with infertility and ovulation induction or in other instances in which the last normal menses may not be appropriate for pregnancy dating, the levels of hCG in early pregnancy may be useful.

Sensitive tests for hCG in biological fluids also are of specific utility in the management of persons with neoplastic trophoblastic disease, especially in the evaluation of the results of and effectiveness of treatment (Chap. 31, p. 548).

In some cases of elective abortion, postabortion evaluation of persistence of hCG may be useful in evaluating the possibility of persistent trophoblastic function, which could be indicative of the possibilities that abortion was not accomplished (for example, very early in pregnancy—menstrual extraction), that abortion was incomplete, or that the pregnancy was (and is) ectopically implanted. Yet another explanation could be that a twin pregnancy existed, but only one fetus (placenta) was removed. Given the long half-life of hCG, early postabortal testing for hCG, however, is of little utility. Postabortion follow-up testing for hCG, if indicated, is best conducted 2 to 3 weeks after the procedure (Derman and colleagues, 1981).

POSITIVE SIGNS OF PREGNANCY

The three positive signs of pregnancy are (1) identification of fetal heart action separately and distinctly from that of the woman, (2) perception of active fetal movements by the examiner, and (3) recognition of the embryo and fetus at most any time in pregnancy by sonographic techniques or of the more mature fetus radiographically in the latter half of pregnancy.

IDENTIFICATION OF FETAL HEART ACTION

Hearing or observing the pulsations of the fetal heart assures the diagnosis of pregnancy. Contractions of the fetal heart can be identified by auscultation with a special fetoscope by use of the *Doppler principle* with ultrasound, and by use of sonography.

The heartbeat of the fetus can be detected by auscultation with a stethoscope by 17 weeks gestation, on average, and by 19 weeks in nearly all pregnancies in normal-sized women (Jimenez and co-workers, 1979). Normally, the fetal heart rate ranges from 120 to 160 beats a minute and is heard as a double sound resembling the tick of a watch under a pillow. To establish the diagnosis of pregnancy, it is not sufficient merely to "hear" the "fetal" heart; it must be different from that of the maternal pulse. During much of pregnancy, the fetus moves freely in the amnionic fluid; and consequently, the site on the maternal abdomen where the fetal heart sounds can be heard best will vary as the position of the fetus changes.

Several instruments are available that make use of the *Doppler principle* to detect the action of the fetal heart. By use of these instruments, ultrasound is directed toward the moving blood of the fetus. The sound reflected by the moving blood undergoes a shift in frequency, the echo of which is detected by a receiving crystal immediately adjacent to the transmitting crystal. Because of the difference in heart rates, pulsatile flow in the fetus is differentiated easily from that of the mother unless there is severe fetal bradycardia or else significant maternal tachycardia. Fetal cardiac action can be detected almost always by the 10th week of gestation with appropriate equipment in which the Doppler principle is employed.

Echocardiography can be used to detect fetal heart action as early as 48 days after the first day of the last normal menses (Robinson, 1972). *Real-time sonography* can be used to detect fetal heart action and fetal movement after the second month of pregnancy.

Upon auscultation of the abdomen of the pregnant woman in the later months of pregnancy, the examiner often may hear sounds other than those produced by fetal heart action, the most common of which are (1) the funic (umbilical cord) souffle, (2) the uterine souffle, (3) sounds resulting from movement of the fetus, (4) the maternal pulse, and (5) the gurgling of gas in the intestines of the woman.

The *funic souffle* is caused by the rush of blood through the umbilical arteries. It is a sharp, whistling sound that is synchronous with the fetal pulse and can be heard in perhaps 15 percent of pregnancies. It is inconstant, sometimes being recognizable distinctly at the time of one examination, but not found in the same woman on other occasions.

The *uterine souffle* is heard as a soft, blowing sound that is synchronous with the maternal pulse; it usually is heard most distinctly during auscultation of the lower portion of the uterus. This sound is produced by the passage of blood through the dilated uterine vessels and is characteristic not only of pregnancy but of any condition in which the blood flow to the uterus is greatly increased. Accordingly, a uterine souffle may be heard in nonpregnant women with large uterine myomas or large tumors of the ovaries.

Frequently, the maternal pulse can be heard distinctly by auscultation of the abdomen; and in some women, the pulsation of the aorta is unusually loud. Occasionally during examination, the pulse of the mother may become so rapid as to simulate the fetal heart sounds. In addition to the sounds described, it is not unusual to hear certain other sounds that are produced by the passage of gases or liquids through the intestines of the pregnant woman.

PERCEPTION OF FETAL MOVEMENTS

The second positive sign of pregnancy is the detection by the examiner of movements by the fetus. After about 20 weeks gestation, active fetal movements can be felt, at indeterminate intervals, by placing the examining hand on the woman's abdomen. These fetal movements vary in intensity from a faint flutter early in pregnancy to brisk motions at a later period; the latter are sometimes visible as well as palpable. Occasionally, somewhat similar sensations may be produced by contractions of the intestines or the muscles of the abdominal wall of the pregnant woman, although these should not deceive an experienced examiner.

ULTRASONIC RECOGNITION

A normal intrauterine pregnancy may be demonstrated by pulse-echo sonography after only 4 to 5 weeks of amenorrhea (Fig. 2–3). After 6 weeks of amenorrhea, the small white gestational ring is so characteristic that failure to identify such raises doubts about pregnancy. Thus, there may be ultrasonic confirmation of pregnancy by the time that some of the common tests for hCG in urine become positive. By careful scanning, distinct echoes from the

embryonic poles can be demonstrated within the gestational ring by 7 weeks after commencement of the last normal menstrual period. By 8 weeks, fetal brain is seen and heart action can be detected using Doppler or real-time sonography. By this time, from the length of the embryo, the gestational age can be estimated quite accurately (Fig. 2–4). Up to 12 weeks, the crown–rump length is predictive of gestational age within 4 days (American College of Obstetricians and Gynecologists, 1988).

In addition to the early identification of normal pregnancy, the findings of sonography also may permit the identification of gestations in which there is a blighted ovum, i.e., the embryo is dead and an abortion will occur ultimately. The characteristic features of a blighted ovum are (1) loss of definition of the gestational sac, (2) an unusually small gestational sac, and (3) the absence of echoes emanating from the fetus after 8 weeks gestation.

By 11 weeks of amenorrhea, the pregnancy ring normally is no longer distinctly identifiable in the uterine cavity by sonography. By the 14th week, the fetal head and thorax can be identified; and soon thereafter, the placental site can be visualized by ultrasound techniques. First-trimester fetal ultrasonic findings were reviewed recently by Green and Hobbins (1988).

Subsequently, ultrasonography can be used successfully to identify the number of fetuses, the presenting part(s), various fetal anomalies, and hydramnios, and to assess the rate of fetal growth by measuring, serially, the biparietal diameter of the fetal head and the circumference of the fetal abdomen.

VAGINAL SONOGRAPHY

Ultrasonic scanning, using a vaginal probe, provides a number of methodological advantages for selected diagnostic purposes in obstetrics and gynecology (Bernaschek and colleagues, 1988). By use of this technique, a gestational sac in the uterine cavity as small as 2 mm in diameter was identified. This corresponded to a time about 16 days after ovulation or 10 days after implantation.

The findings of sonography often provide as much, and usually much more, information as do those of radiography

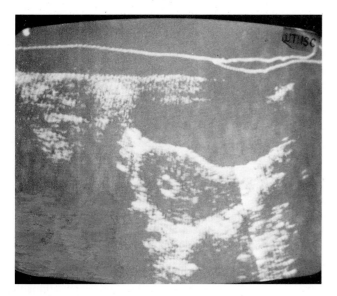

Figure 2–3. Longitudinal sonogram in which a gestation sac at 5 to 6 weeks of gestational (menstrual) age is demonstrated.

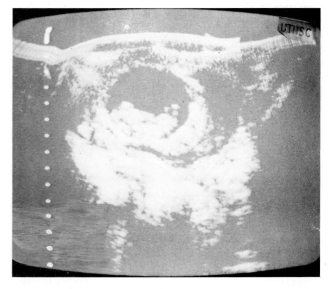

Figure 2–4. Transverse sonographic view of amnionic sac in which there is a fetus of 10 to 12 weeks of gestational age.

without the potential, albeit undefined, risks of irradiation. To date, no adverse effects on the human embryo or fetus have been identified from exposure to energies comparable to those used for clinical sonographic examinations.

FETAL RECOGNITION BY RADIOGRAPHY

Whenever the fetal skeleton is distinguished radiologically, the diagnosis of pregnancy is certain. This method of positive identification of pregnancy usually is not valid until after 16 weeks of gestation, and it is not used today for this purpose. On occasion, however, radiological examination of the abdomen is obliged or is conducted without knowledge of the existence of pregnancy. By x-ray examination, Bartholomew and co-workers (1921) were able to make a positive diagnosis of pregnancy by 20 weeks gestation in only one third of the women examined who were pregnant and in only one half by 24 weeks. Just how early the fetal skeleton is visible in the radiograph depends, in part, upon the thickness of the abdominal wall of the mother and the radiological technique used. Foci of ossification in the fetus have been demonstrated as early as 14 weeks, although ordinarily the gestation must have reached 16 weeks or more before the fetal skeleton can be visualized.

DIFFERENTIAL DIAGNOSIS OF PREGNANCY

The uterus of pregnancy is sometimes mistaken for other tumors occupying the pelvis or abdomen; less frequently, the opposite error is made. The uterine changes of the early weeks of pregnancy may be simulated through enlargement of the uterus caused by myomas, hematometra, adenomyosis, or by apparent enlargement that actually is due to a contiguous but extrauterine mass or masses. As a rule, the enlarged uterus in these circumstances is firmer than it is in pregnancy and is less elastic and boggy. Except in hematometra, moreover, such conditions usually are not attended by cessation of the menses. If uncertainty remains, however, reexamination in a few weeks usually will allow for the correct diagnosis to be established.

SPURIOUS PREGNANCY

Imaginary pregnancy, or *pseudocyesis*, usually occurs in women nearing the menopause or in women who desire intensely to be pregnant. Such women may present all the subjective symptoms of pregnancy in association with a considerable increase in the size of their abdomen, caused either by deposition of fat, by gas in the intestinal tract, or by abdominal fluid. In such women, the menses do not as a rule disappear, but may become unpredictable in time of onset and in amount and duration of bleeding. Changes in the breasts, including enlargement, the appearance of galactorrhea, and increased areolar pigmentation, sometimes occur. In a majority of these women, there is morning sickness, probably of psychogenic origin.

The ingestion of a variety of phenothiazines can lead to amenorrhea, breast enlargement, hyperprolactinemia, and galactorrhea. Obviously, the underlying emotional problem may be compounded by these changes.

The supposed fetal movements that are perceived by women with pseudocyesis usually can be ascribed to intestinal peristalsis or to muscular contractions of her abdominal wall, but occasionally these are so marked as to deceive physicians.

Careful examination of such women usually leads to a correct diagnosis without great difficulty because the small uterus can be palpated on bimanual examination. The greatest difficulty encountered in the care of such women may be that of convincing her of the correct diagnosis. Emotionally distressed women may persist for years in the delusion that they are pregnant.

DISTINCTION BETWEEN FIRST AND SUBSEQUENT PREGNANCIES

Occasionally, it is of practical importance to ascertain whether a woman is pregnant for the first time or has previously borne children. Ordinarily, but not always, there are indelible traces of a former term pregnancy.

In a nullipara, the abdomen usually is tense and firm, and the uterus is felt through it with difficulty. The characteristic old abdominal striae and the distinctive changes in the breasts are absent. The labia majora are usually in close apposition and the frenulum is intact. The vagina is usually narrow and characterized by well-developed rugae. The cervix is softened but usually does not admit the tip of the examiner's finger until the very end of pregnancy.

In multiparas, the abdominal wall usually is lax and, at times, pendulous, and through it the uterus is palpated readily. In addition to the pink abdominal striae associated with the present pregnancy, the silvery cicatrices of past pregnancies also may be present. Usually, the breasts are not so firm as in women during their first pregnancy and frequently there are striae in the skin over the breast tissue similar to those on the abdomen. The vulva of a woman who previously has delivered vaginally usually gapes open to some extent, the frenulum has disappeared, and the hymen is transformed into the myrtiform caruncles. In multiparas who previously have delivered vaginally, the external os of the cervix, even in the early months of pregnancy, may admit the tip of the examiner's finger, which can be carried up to the internal os. Moreover, the sites of healed lacerations of the cervix usually can be identified.

IDENTIFICATION OF FETAL LIFE OR DEATH

A learned review of the problems of diagnosis and management of fetal death was presented by Pitkin (1987). He observes that all too often the occurrence of fetal death comes "utterly without warning in a pregnancy that has previously seemed entirely normal." Regrettably, the cause of this tragic event may go undiscovered; in fact the "unknown" cause group may constitute 50 percent of the total. The scenario that ensues, Pitkin says, all too commonly is as follows: The woman, with anxiety in her voice, reports that she has not felt fetal movement for hours or for 1 or 2 days. The fetal heart is not heard by auscultation or identified by real-time ultrasound examination. Failure to detect heart wall motion after 10 to 12 weeks gestation by real-time ultrasonography is reliable evidence of fetal death. Ancillary findings of sonography in the case of fetal death include scalp edema and sequelae of maceration.

In the early months of pregnancy, the diagnosis of fetal death may present difficulty. Unless ultrasonic techniques are employed, the diagnosis of fetal death can be made with certainty only after it can be shown by repeated examinations that the uterus has remained constant in size or there actually has been a decrease in size of the uterus over a number of weeks.

Because trophoblasts of the placenta may continue to produce hCG for several weeks after death of the embryo or fetus, a positive endocrine test for pregnancy is not necessarily indicative that the fetus is alive.

In the latter half of pregnancy, the cessation of fetal movements usually alerts the woman to the possibility of fetal death, but if fetal cardiac action can still be identified distinct from that of the mother, the fetus certainly is alive. If, by careful auscultation, the fetal heart tones are not heard, however, the fetus probably is dead. There is a possibility of error, of course, especially in pregnancies in which the fetal heart is remote from the examiner, for example, if the woman is obese or if hydramnios exists.

Ultrasonic instruments in which the Doppler shift principle is employed, as described on page 18, are of considerable value in the evaluation of pregnancies in which the fetal heart cannot be heard by auscultation with a stethoscope. The use of Doppler ultrasound is especially valuable when fetal death is suspected but fetal heart action can be identified. If fetal heart action is not demonstrated after careful examination, it can be stated that very likely, but not absolutely, the fetus is dead. Real-time ultrasonic examination when carefully performed will serve to identify accurately the presence or absence of fetal heart motion.

If the fetus has been dead for some time, usually it can be shown by careful examination that the uterus does not correspond in size to the estimated duration of pregnancy or actually that the uterus has become smaller than previously observed. With the death of the fetus, maternal weight gain usually ceases; and not infrequently, there is even a slight decrease in her weight. At the same time, retrogressive changes usually have occurred in the breasts. Ordinarily, the diagnosis of fetal death cannot be made from the findings of a single examination, but fetal death certainly must be considered when the signs just mentioned are identified and fetal cardiac action cannot be detected.

Occasionally, a positive diagnosis of fetal death can be established by palpating the collapsed fetal skull through the partially dilated cervix; in that event, the loose bones of the fetal head feel as though these are contained in a flabby bag.

Radiographic techniques were used in the past but are rarely indicated today to establish fetal death. There are three principal radiological signs of fetal death:

1. Significant overlap of the skull bones (Spalding's sign), caused by liquefaction of the brain, a process that requires several days to develop. A similar sign may develop occasionally with a living fetus, for example, when the fetal head is compressed in the maternal pelvis.
2. Exaggerated curvature of the fetal spine. Because the development of this sign depends on maceration of the spinous ligaments, its development also requires several days; moreover, mild degrees of curvature of the spine in living fetuses may be misleading.
3. Demonstration of gas in the fetus is an uncommon but reliable sign of fetal death (Fig. 2–5).

In instances in which the fetus has been dead for several days to weeks, the amnionic fluid is red to brown and usually turbid rather than nearly colorless and clear. The finding of such amnionic fluid is not absolutely diagnostic of fetal death, however, because prior hemorrhage into the amnionic sac, as rarely occurs during amniocentesis, may lead to similar discoloration of the amnionic fluid even though the fetus is alive.

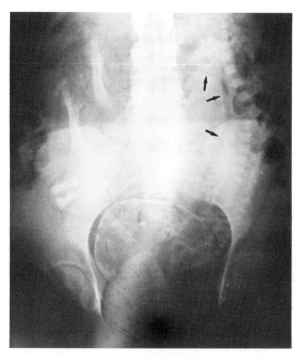

Figure 2–5. Fetal death is established by the presence of gas in a major vessel. The close proximity to the fetal spine implies that the vessel is the aorta.

REFERENCES

American College of Obstetritians and Gynecologists: Ultrasound in pregnancy. Tech Bull No 116, May 1988

Ascheim S, Zondek B: Anterior pituitary hormone and ovarian hormone in the urine of pregnant women. Klin Wochensehr 6:248, 1927

Baird DT: Preface. In Baird DT, Michie EA (eds): Mechanisms of Menstrual Bleeding. New York, Raven Press, 1985, p. v

Bandi ZL, Schoen I, DeLara M: Enzyme-linked immunosorbent urine pregnancy tests: Clinical specificity studies. Am J Clin Pathol 87:236, 1987

Barnes RB, Roy S, Yee B, Duda MJ, Mishell DR: Reliability of urinary pregnancy tests in the diagnosis of ectopic pregnancy. J Reprod Med 30:827, 1985

Bartholomew RA, Sale BE, Calloway JT: Diagnosis of pregnancy by the roentgen ray. JAMA 76:912, 1921

Bazer RW, Vallet JL, Roberts RM, Sharp DC, Thatcher WW: Role of conceptus secretory products in establishment of pregnancy. J Reprod Fert 76:841, 1986

Bernaschek G, Rudelstorfer R, Csaicsich P: Vaginal sonography versus serum human chorionic gonadotropin in early detection of pregnancy. Am J Obstet Gynecol 158:608, 1988

Boyko WL, Russell HT: Evaluation and clinical application of the quantitative radioreceptor assay for serum hCG. Obstet Gynecol 54:737, 1979

Bridson WE, Ross GT, Kohler PO: Immunologic and biologic activity of chorionic gonadotropin synthesized by cloned choriocarcinoma cells in tissue culture. Clin Res 18:356, 1970

Chadwick JR: Value of the bluish coloration of the vaginal entrance as a sign of pregnancy. Trans Am Gynecol Soc 11:399, 1886

Chartier M, Roger M, Barrat J, Michelon B: Measurement of plasma chorionic gonadotropin (hCG) and β-hCG activities in the late luteal phase: Evidence of the occurrence of spontaneous menstrual abortions in infertile women. Fertil Steril 31:134, 1979

Claesson L, Hogberg B, Rosenberg T, Westman A: Crystalline human chorionic gonadotropin and its biological action. Acta Endocrinol 1:1, 1948

Derman R, Corson LS, Horwitz, CA, Lau HD, Solderstrom R: Early diagnosis of pregnancy: A symposium. J Reprod Med 26:149, 1981

Doshi ML: Accuracy of consumer performed in-home tests for early pregnancy detection. Am J Public Health 76:512, 1986

Flint APF, Sheldrick EL: Ovarian peptides and luteolysis. In Edwards RG, Purdy JM, Steptoe PC (eds): Implantation of the Human Embryo. London, Academic Press, 1985, p 235

Gey GO, Jones GES, Hellman LM: The production of a gonadotrophic substance (prolan) by placental cells in tissue culture. Science 88:306, 1938

Godkin JD, Bazer FW, Roberts RM: Ovine trophoblast protein 1, an early secreted blastocyst protein, binds specifically to uterine endometrium and affects protein synthesis. Endocrinology 114:120, 1984

Green JJ, Hobbins JC: Abdominal ultrasound examination of the first-trimester fetus. Am J Obstet Gynecol 159:165, 1988

Hansen PJ, Anthony RV, Bazer RW, Baumbach GA, Roberts RM: In vitro synthesis and secretion of ovine trophoblast protein-1 during the period of maternal recognition of pregnancy. Endocrinology 117:1424, 1985

Hertz R: Early studies of chorionic gonadotropin and antihormones. In Segal SJ (ed): Chorionic Gonadotropin. New York, Plenum, 1980, p 1

Hirose T: Experimentalle histologische studie fur genese corpus luteum. Mitt ad med Fakultd t Univ Z U, Tokyo 23:63, 1919

Imakawa K, Anthony RV, Kazemi M, Marotti KR, Polites HG, Roberts RM: Interferon-like sequence of ovine trophoblast protein secreted by embryonic trophectoderm. Nature 330:377, 1987

Jimenez JM, Tyson JE, Santos-Ramos R, Duenhoelter JH: Comparison of obstetric and pediatric evaluation of gestational age. Pediatr Res 13:498, 1979

Jovanovic L, Singh M, Saxena BB, Mills JL, Tulchinsky D, Holmes LB, Simpson JL, Metzger BE, Labarbera A, Aarons J, Van Allen MI, NICHD-DIEP Study Group: Verification of early pregnancy tests in a multicenter trial. Proc Soc Exp Biol Med 184:201, 1987

Kadar N, Caldwell BV, Romero R: A method of screening for ectopic pregnancy and its indications. Obstet Gynecol 58:162, 1981

Lagrew DC, Wilson EA, Jawad MJ: Determination of gestational age by serum concentrations of human chorionic gonadotropin. Obstet Gynecol 62:37, 1983

Pelosi MC, Apuzzi J, Dwyer JW: Early diagnosis of pregnancy, Part I: Workup and laboratory tests. The Female Patient 8:38, 42, 1983

Pitkin RM: Fetal death: Diagnosis and management. Am J Obstet Gynecol 157:583, 1987

Plante C, Hansen PJ, Thatcher WW: Prolongation of luteal lifespan in cows by intrauterine infusion of recombinant bovine alpha-interferon. Endocrinology 122:2342, 1988

Reichert FL, Pencharz FI, Simpson ME, Meyer K, Evans HM: Relative ineffectiveness of prolan in hypophysectomized animals. Am J Physiol 100:157, 1932

Robinson HP: Detection of fetal heart movement in first trimester of pregnancy using pulsed ultrasound. Br Med J 4:66, 1972

Saxena BB, Landesman R: Diagnosis and management of pregnancy by the radioreceptor assay of human chorionic gonadotropin. Am J Obstet Gynecol 131:97, 1978

Short RV: Maternal recognition of pregnancy. In Wolstenhome GEW, O'Connor M (eds): Foetal Autonomy. London, Churchill, 1969, p 2

Short RV: Definition of the problem: The evolution of human reproduction. In Short RV, Baird DT (eds): Contraceptives of the Future. Cambridge, University Printing House, 1976, p 3

Speert H, Guttmacher AF: Frequency and significance of bleeding in early pregnancy. JAMA 155:172, 1954

Townsend L, Shelton JG: Intrauterine death due to fetal erythroblastosis. Aust NZ J Obstet Gynaecol 4:84, 1964

Vaitukaitis JL, Braunstein GD, Ross GT: A radioimmunoassay which specifically measures chorionic gonadotropin in the presence of human luteinizing hormone. Am J Obstet Gynecol 113:751, 1972

Valanis BG, Perlman CS: Home pregnancy testing kits: Prevalence of use, false-negative rates, and compliance with instructions. Am J Public Health 72:1034, 1982

Whitehouse HB: The physiology and pathology of uterine haemorrhage. Lancet 1:877, 1914

Wide L, Hobson B: Immunological and biological activity of human chorionic gonadotropin in urine and serum of pregnant women and women with a hydatidiform mole. Acta Endocrinol 54:105, 1967

Zondek B: Die hormone des ovariums und des hypophysenvordelappens. Berlin, Springer, 1931

The Endometrium and Uterine Decidua

MATERNAL TISSUES OF THE FETAL–MATERNAL COMMUNICATION SYSTEM

The fetal–maternal communication system is operative even before the time of blastocyst implantation by interchange of secretory products between the developing zygote and those of the maternal fallopian tube and endometrium. The fundamental organization of this system as well as its anatomical parts are described in Chapter 2. Direct contact between fetal and maternal tissues first comes about 6 days after fertilization of the ovum when the blastocyst embraces the endometrium. At the time of *apposition* of blastocyst to the uterine lining, the endometrium is the only maternal tissue in direct contact with fetal trophoblasts; but already, cell-to-cell dialogue between fetal and maternal tissues is established. The fundamental components of implantation, maternal recognition of pregnancy, pregnancy maintenance, and fetal nutrition are then established (Chaps. 2 and 4).

The implanting blastocyst, in some ill-defined manner, incites further decidualization of the secretory endometrium. It is likely that this process involves essential elements of the inflammatory process, including blastocyst generation of prostaglandins, platelet-activating factor, and serine proteases (e.g., plasminogen activator), which are believed to be important in trophoblast invasion of endometrium. In the experimental animal, appropriately primed with estrogen and progesterone, trauma to the endometrium is a potent artificial stimulus to deciduoma formation.

Functionally, there are two maternal tissues involved directly in the fully developed fetal–maternal communication system: (1) maternal uterine decidua and (2) maternal blood. As the trophoblasts of the blastocyst invade the endometrium, the two distinct arms of the fetal–maternal communication system are established. Trophoblasts invade the endometrial blood vessels and thereby the villous trophoblasts become surrounded by "lakes" of maternal blood, the lacunae, which ultimately coalesce to form the intervillous space. At this time, **the placental arm of the fetal–maternal communication system** is established (Chap. 4). And as the embryo and extraembryonic fetal tissues grow, the fetal membranes develop and ultimately come to lie adjacent to all of the uterine decidua, not occupied by placenta, to form **the paracrine arm of the fetal–maternal communication system** (Chap. 4).

THE CARDINAL FUNCTION OF THE UTERUS IS PREGNANCY

To gain greater insights into the function and functional regulation of the uterus (myometrium, endometrium), we believe it to be worthwhile to consider critically the contributions of this unique organ to physiological processes.

Ramsey (1977) has reviewed the history of evolution of knowledge concerning the anatomy of the uterus. She observes that during the Middle Ages, i.e., the "Dark Ages," the popular theory was that the uterus was multicompartmental, the most popular number of compartments being seven. It was commonly believed that male embryos developed in the three right-hand cells, females in the three on the left, and hermaphrodites in the one in the middle. An alternative view was that the female reproductive tract is a mirror image of that of the male, i.e., the vagina being a penis turned inside out and the uterus an inverted scrotum.

In 1315 Mondino dei Luzzi conducted the first public authorized dissection of a human body; and from the findings of Mondino, the uterus, cervix, and vagina were described almost as we know these structures today. Leonardo da Vinci correctly depicted the anatomical relationship between the ovaries, tubes, and ligaments. Clearly, he considered the uterus to consist of a single cavity; and at about the same time, Beringario da Carpi stated that *"it is a pure lie—to say that the uterus has seven cavities."*

The Renaissance in anatomy can be focused on Vesalius, whose epic *De humani corporis fabrica* appeared in 1543. The frontispiece of *Fabrica* shows Vesalius presiding over the dissection of a female cadaver; and the presentation of the gross anatomy of the human female reproductive tract, in this masterpiece, was as we know it today (Chap. 40). The term *uterus* was first used in this treatise; since that time, we have come to understand the morphological and, to some extent, the physiological function of this organ in appreciably greater detail.

We conclude, as have others, that there is but one physiological function of the uterus, namely, pregnancy. There is no known hormonal or other physiological function of the endometrium or myometrium that contributes to the metabolic economy or well-being of women. There is no evidence that removal of the endometrium-myometrium (hysterectomy) serves to affect adversely the lifespan or health of women. On the contrary, blood loss from menstruation, malignant transformation, infections, and benign tumors of this organ may cause significant disability and even death. Indeed, the association between hormonal treatment and an increased incidence of neoplasia in humans is established most clearly in the case of endometrium (estrogen treatment and endometrial carcinoma).

OVERVIEW OF ENDOMETRIAL FUNCTION

The endometrium is the innermost tissue layer of the uterus, forming the lining of the uterine cavity. The growth and functional characteristics of the endometrium are unique. There are relatively few cell types in adult humans that replicate continuously; among these few, those of the endometrium of reproductive-age women are particularly noteworthy. This obtains not only because the superficial epithelial cells of the uterine epithelium grow at a rapid rate, but because the glands and stromal cells of this tissue also are regenerated during each endometrial (menstrual-ovarian) cycle. Indeed, two-thirds of the entire tissue (endometrium) is shed and regenerated more than 400 times in the life of most women. There is no other example in humans of the cyclic shedding and regrowth of an entire tissue. To place menstruation in yet another perspective, the lifetime cumulative menstrual blood loss associated with normal endometrial shedding is 10 to 20 liters or more, an amount of blood that contains at least three times the total body iron content of the average adult woman. And, as we have observed before, in the seventeenth edition of this book, if the doubling time of endometrial growth experienced during the 5th to 20th day of the ovarian cycle were maintained for 1 year, the weight of endometrium would approach 1 ton!

THE CARDINAL FUNCTION OF THE DECIDUA IS PREGNANCY MAINTENANCE AND PARTURITION

The decidua is the specialized endometrium of pregnancy, being comprised largely of decidual cells, which develop from the stromal cells (mesenchyme) of the endometrium. Most of the glandular epithelium and glandular structure of endometrium is lost during pregnancy.

The importance of the uterine endometrium (decidua) in the success of pregnancy cannot be underestimated, but at the same time, it should not be overstated. It is probable that the endometrium is the optimal site for blastocyst implantation and embryo-fetal development; but, it cannot be claimed that this function of endometrium is unique because of the known success, albeit limited, of ectopic pregnancies, i.e., cases in which blastocyst implants and fetus develops outside the uterine cavity. In the same manner, there may be a role for endometrium in sperm capacitation; but, it cannot be argued that this function is unique to endometrium as evidenced by the success of sperm capacitation and fertilization of the ovum in vitro.

Today, there is appreciable evidence that the maintenance of pregnancy and the initiation of parturition are closely aligned in all mammalian species by way of rigid regulation of decidual function. For this reason, we suggest that endometrial (decidual) function is directed to the success of biomolecular processes that forestall the initiation of labor until the achievement of fetal maturity; but thereafter, retreat from pregnancy maintenance is sounded and the decidua becomes the site of formation of uterotropins and uterotonins that direct the parturitional process.

A *uterotropin* is an agent that causes uterine preparedness for labor, including cervical effacement and ripening, the development of gap junctions between myometrial cells, an increase in the number of oxytocin receptors, and increased sensitivity to uterotonins. A *uterotonin* is an agent that serves to effect the myometrial contractions of labor (Chap. 10). There is appreciable evidence today in support of the likelihood that uterine decidua (the endometrium of pregnancy) is one primary source of uterotropins and uterotonins that serve to initiate parturition and maintain labor.

In Chapter 10, the thesis is developed that one of the penultimate events in the initiation of labor is decidual activation. There is no doubt that a number of uterine and extraembryonic fetal tissues are stimulated to new levels of metabolic activity during parturition. And, the generation of uterotropins and uterotonins by these tissues is essential to the success of parturition. During labor, a "set" of bioactive agents is produced in these tissues and these agents accumulate in the amnionic fluid, which is contiguous with the fetal membranes and is an anatomical part of the paracrine arm of the fetal–maternal communication system. Many of the bioactive agents produced during parturition are extremely potent. Therefore, the production of these uterotropins and uterotonins in intrauterine sites permits these agents to act in a paracrine manner on contiguous myometrium without the undesirable side-effects that these substances would produce if delivered by way of the systemic circulation. Some of these bioactive agents of parturition are produced in decidua, which, anatomically, is directly contiguous with the myometrium; therefore, the decidua occupies a key anatomical position in the paracrine arm of the fetal–maternal communication system. It is contiguous on one side with the fetal chorion laeve and on the other side with maternal myometrium.

For these reasons, the functional characteristics of decidua are important in the physiology of pregnancy maintenance, the acceptance of the semiallogeneic fetal graft, and the initiation of parturition and the maintenance of labor. It also is probable that the functional characteristics of the decidua will be profoundly important in devising strategies for the prevention of preterm labor. **Premature perturbation, activation, or stimulation of decidual tissue likely is the cause of a large fraction of preterm births** (Chap. 10).

SPECIALIZED FUNCTIONS OF THE ENDOMETRIUM/DECIDUA

The endometrial cavity is patent, i.e., anatomically open through the cervical canal, which in turn is open to the vagina, which in turn is open to the external environment. The same is true of the decidua during pregnancy—at least at the lower pole of the interface between the chorion laeve (the innermost of the fetal membranes) and decidua vera. To be sure, there is functional closure of the cervical canal by way of a mucus "plug," and there are antimicrobial properties ascribed to the cervical mucus. Nonetheless, because of this anatomical reality, i.e., patency of the female reproductive tract, it is reasonable to presume that endometrium/decidua must be endowed with unique and extraordinary capacities to respond to microbial and immunological challenges. It is highly likely that, normally, decidua functions effectively to contain infectious processes at the lower pole of chorion laeve-decidual interface as a means of preventing the onset of preterm labor (Chap. 10).

In addition, there are other specialized functions of decidua including the production of hormones, unique proteins, and other bioactive agents. Moreover, the functional characteristics of decidual tissue are macrophage-like, an issue of great importance in deciphering selected features of the maternal acceptance of the semiallogeneic fetal graft, the containment of infection, and the induction of parturition, both spontaneously at term and prematurely (p. 35).

THE RELATIONSHIP OF MENSTRUATION TO PARTURITION

In the development of this general concept, i.e., that the cardinal function of endometrium/decidua is as the tissue that serves as the modulator of pregnancy maintenance and the timely initiation of labor, other notable features of endometrium/decidua that are germane to an understanding of the function of this tissue are important. In Chapter 2 we observed that menstruation is the consequence of failed fertility; and, it is probable that the biomolecular processes that eventuate in the initiation of menstruation constellate about the same fundamental processes for which the function of the endometrium is destined, viz., parturition. Indeed, progesterone withdrawal is believed to be the penultimate antecedent endocrinological event that precedes menstruation; and, progesterone withdrawal is the key endocrine event that precedes the initiation of parturition in many mammalian species. Others have referred to the process of parturition as *delayed menstruation* (Gustavii, 1972). We choose another philosophical interpretation: with failed fertility, menstruation is initiated by cellular and biomolecular processes that are characteristic of those involved in parturition (p. 34); therefore, **menstruation is the parturition of fertility failure.**

HORMONAL REGULATION OF ENDOMETRIUM

The endometrium has become a model for investigations directed toward an understanding of the mechanism of action of steroid hormones and other agents, for example, prostaglandins and cytokines. The accessibility of human endometrial tissue, together with the fact that endometrial glandular epithelium can be easily separated from stroma, rightfully has attracted the interest of endocrinologists, molecular biologists, and immunologists who seek to define the molecular nature of hormone action(s) in target tissues as well as the functional relationships between mesenchyme and epithelium of a given tissue, and to solve the riddle of the success of the allogeneic tissue graft of pregnancy.

ESTROGEN ACTION

Estradiol-17β, the potent naturally occurring estrogen secreted by the ovarian follicle, acts to promote responses of the endometrium in a manner that now stands as one model for the mechanism of steroid hormone action. In 1961 Elwood Jensen presented a scintillating lecture, entitled *"Basic Guides to the Mechanism of Estrogen Action,"* to the Laurentian Hormone Conference (Jensen and Jacobson, 1962). By use of radiolabeled estrogens of high specific radioactivity, they were able to show sequestration of nonmetabolized radiolabeled estradiol-17β in estrogen-responsive tissues. This seems to have been the beginning of the contemporary era of the study of steroid mechanism of action. Jensen ended his brilliant lecture with a limerick:

> *To a tissue that's trying to grow*
> *We hope these experiments show:*
> *With steroids phenolic*
> *Don't get metabolic,*
> *Just grab on, and never let go!*

Estradiol-17β enters the endometrial cell, apparently by simple diffusion. In the responsive cell, the hormone, in some manner, is *sequestered* and translocated to the nucleus, where it becomes associated with the estrogen receptor. The receptor is a macromolecule that is characterized by a high affinity, but low capacity, for estradiol-17β and other biologically active estrogens, including synthetic estrogens. The estradiol-17β-receptor complex, probably after transformational changes, becomes associated with chromatin. The result is a gene-transcriptional event that brings about synthesis of messenger RNA and, subsequently, protein synthesis.

Among the many proteins synthesized in response to estrogen action in the endometrium are macromolecules that are characterized by high affinity for progesterone, i.e., *progesterone receptors*, as well as additional receptor molecules for estradiol-17β. Thus, among the actions of estradiol-17β on the endometrium are those that provide both for the perpetuation of the cellular milieu in which estrogen can act and for the initiation of events that provide for responses to the actions of progesterone. Until very recently, we believed that cytosolic receptors became bound to steroid hormones and that the cytosolic receptor-estrogen complex provided for the initiation of steroid hormone action. It was envisioned that steroid hormones became associated with the cytosolic receptor and thereafter the steroid-receptor complex was translocated to the nucleus. It now seems possible that the finding of receptors in cytosolic preparations is, at least in part, an artifact of the tissue preparations and that the receptors for steroid hormones are concentrated principally in the nucleus.

PROGESTERONE ACTION

Progesterone also apparently enters the endometrial cell by diffusion and thence becomes associated with nuclear receptors with high affinity, but low capacity, for progesterone. The concentration of progesterone receptors is dependent, however, on previous estrogen action. The progesterone-receptor complex also is active in promoting gene transcription, but the attendant response is strikingly different from that evoked by the estradiol-17β-receptor complex. The progesterone-receptor complex acts to bring about a decrease in the production of estradiol-17β receptor molecules (Tseng and Gurpide, 1975), an action that serves as one means by which progesterone acts to negate the action of estrogen. Progesterone also acts to cause an increase in the activity of the enzyme *estradiol-17β dehydrogenase*, which catalyzes the interconversion of estradiol-17β and estrone. Tseng and Gurpide (1974) found that the reaction kinetics of estradiol-17β dehydrogenase in endometrium are such that the formation of estrone, a biologically weaker estrogen than estradiol-17β, is favored. Progesterone also acts to increase sulfurylation of estrogen (*estrogen sulfotransferase*), another means of estrogen inactivation (Tseng and Liu, 1981). Thus, progesterone can attenuate estrogen action in endometrium in at least three ways: (1) by reducing the rate of synthesis of estrogen receptors, (2) by bringing about a reduction in the intracellular level of estradiol-17β (through conversion to estrone), and (3) by increasing estrogen inactivation through sulfurylation.

The findings of important studies such as these also have provided tools for investigators to identify markers of estrogen and progesterone action—tools believed to be important in the identification of and thence in the management of hormone-responsive tumors. For example, a marker of estrogen action in a given tissue (or tumor) is the presence of progesterone receptors. Horwitz and colleagues (1975) have pioneered the delineation of estrogen-responsive breast cancers by showing that tumors in which progesterone receptors are demonstrable are likely to be more responsive to endocrine ablation procedures.

The presence of estradiol-17β dehydrogenase activity also is indicative of progesterone action, and the presence of this enzyme activity in endometrial carcinoma tissue may signal responsiveness, therapeutically, of such tumors to progesterone or synthetic progestational agents.

THE ENDOMETRIAL CYCLE

HISTORY

Hitschmann and Adler (1908) were the first to describe cyclic histological changes in the endometrium. And more than 50

years ago, Rock and Bartlett (1937) suggested that the histological features of the endometrium were sufficiently characteristic as to permit the "dating" of the ovarian cycle of the woman from whom the endometrium was obtained. The histological changes that occur in the endometrium during the menstrual cycle are summarized in Figure 3–1; the findings are taken from those of Noyes, Hertig, and Rock (1950). Indeed, this manuscript, in which the day-to-day changes in endometrial histology were described almost 40 years ago, was the first paper published, as noted by Benirschke (1986), in the then-new journal *Fertility and Sterility*.

HORMONE-INDUCED MORPHOLOGICAL CHANGES

In response to the changes that are evoked by hormone actions produced in the ovary during each ovulatory cycle, there are morphological changes in the endometrium that evolve with

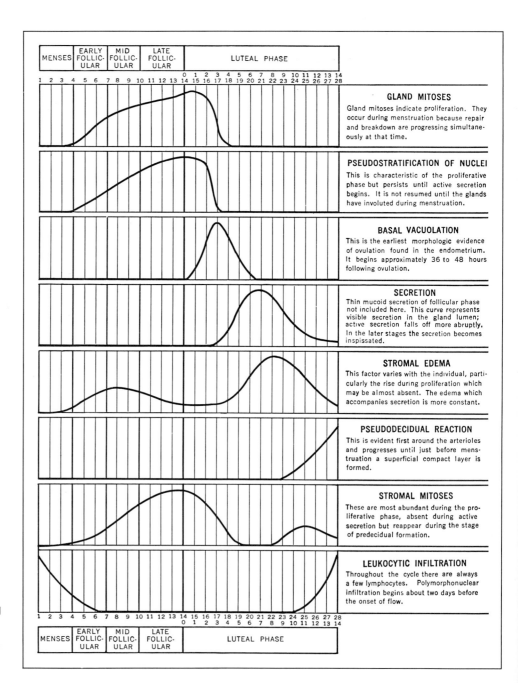

Figure 3–1. Dating of the endometrium according to the day of the menstrual cycle during a hypothetical 28-day ovarian cycle. Correlation of typical morphological findings. (*From Noyes, Hertig, and Rock: Fertil Steril 1:3, 1950.*)

such precise regularity that the histological features of the endometrium can be used by an experienced morphologist to estimate the day of the ovarian cycle on which the endometrium was removed. The endocrine changes during the ovarian cycle can be summarized as follows: (1) During the preovulatory, or follicular, phase of the ovarian cycle, estradiol-17β is secreted principally by the dominant follicle in increasing quantities. (2) During the postovulatory, or luteal, phase of the cycle, progesterone, in addition to estradiol-17β, is secreted by the corpus luteum. (3) During the premenstrual phase, the corpus luteum regresses and the rates of secretion of both estradiol-17β and progesterone diminish.

In response to these changes in sex steroid hormones that are secreted during the ovarian cycle, there are four main stages of the endometrial cycle: (1) postmenstrual reorganization and thence *proliferation* in response to stimulation (directly or indirectly) by estradiol-17β; (2) abundant glandular *secretion*, which results from the combined action of estrogen and progesterone; (3) *premenstrual ischemia* and involution; and, (4) *menstruation*, which is accompanied by collapse and desquamation of all but the deepest layer of the endometrium. Ultimately, menstruation is the consequence of progesterone withdrawal. The follicular, i.e., preovulatory, or proliferative phase, and the postovulatory, i.e., luteal, or secretory phase customarily are divided into early and late stages. The normal secretory phase may be subdivided rather finely (almost day by day), by histological criteria, from shortly after ovulation until the onset of menstruation.

Early Proliferative Phase
During menstruation, about two-thirds of the functional endometrium is destroyed and shed. By the 5th day (day of menses onset equals day 1), the epithelial surface of the endometrium has been restored. The endometrium during the early proliferative phase of the endometrial cycle is thin, usually less than 2 mm in depth. Histologically, the glands are narrow, tubular structures that pursue almost a straight, parallel course from the surface toward the basal layer. The glandular epithelium is low columnar, and the nuclei are round and basal. In the deeper part of the endometrium, the cells of the stroma are packed rather densely and the nuclei of these cells are deep-staining and small. In the superficial, i.e., reorganizing, layer, the stromal cells are packed more loosely and the nuclei are more nearly round, more vesicular, and larger than in the deeper layers.

Mitotic figures, especially in the glands, are present by the 5th day after the onset of menstruation and mitotic activity in both glandular epithelium and stroma is evident until 2 to 3 days after ovulation. Although the blood vessels are numerous and prominent, there is no extravasated blood or lymphocytic infiltration at this stage.

Late Proliferative Phase
The endometrium in the late proliferative phase becomes thicker, as a result of both glandular hyperplasia and an increase in stromal ground substance. The loose stroma is especially prominent superficially, and the glands are separated widely compared with those of the deeper zone, where the glands are crowded and tortuous and the stroma is more dense. Gradually, the glandular epithelium becomes taller and pseudostratified at about the time of ovulation.

Day-by-day "dating" of the endometrium during the proliferative phase is not possible, however, because of the considerable variation among women in the length of the follicular phase of the ovarian cycle. Whereas the luteal or secretory (i.e., postovulatory) phase of the cycle among women is remarkably constant in duration (12 to 14 days), the length of the proliferative or follicular (i.e., preovulatory) phase varies greatly.

Early Secretory Phase
After ovulation, there are changes in endometrial morphology that occur with such regularity as to permit the endometrium to be dated with great precision. During the secretory stage, three zones of the endometrium become well defined: (1) the basal zone, or layer adjacent to the myometrium; (2) the compact zone, or layer immediately beneath the endometrial surface; and, (3) the spongy zone, or layer between the compact and basal layers. Actually, the basal layer undergoes little, if any, histological alteration during the endometrial (menstrual) cycle, but mitoses are found in the glands. The spongy middle layer is comprised of a lacy labyrinth with little stroma between the tortuous, serrated glands, which characterize the luteal phase. In the compact superficial layer, the glands are more nearly straight and are narrower, but the glandular lumens often are filled with secretions. Edema of the abundant stroma is an important factor in the thickening of the endometrium, but there also is an increase in dry weight.

Late Secretory Phase
The endometrium at this time is extremely vascular, succulent, and rich in glycogen; and apparently, it is ideally suited for the implantation and growth of the blastocyst. The stromal cells, and in particular those around the blood vessels, undergo hypertrophic changes similar to, but less extensive than, those of the true decidua of pregnancy (p. 35).

During the late secretory phase of the cycle, there is the commencement of the formation of a pericellular basement membrane that will come to surround completely the stromal, i.e., decidual, cell. This very peculiar pericellular basement membrane and the components thereof are considered in greater detail in the analysis of decidual tissue and the characteristics of this unique tissue in the fetal-decidual paracrine system of human pregnancy.

At the time of the cycle that corresponds to implantation, i.e., about 1 week after ovulation, the endometrium is 5 to 6 mm thick and the secretory changes preparatory to nidation of the blastocyst appear to be maximal.

A further characteristic of the secretory phase endometrium is the striking development of the *spiral*, or *coiled, arteries*, which become much more tortuous. In the compact layer, the arteries branch and the arterioles break up into capillaries within this zone. During the first week of the menstrual cycle, the arterioles extend only about halfway through the endometrium. Because the arterioles lengthen more rapidly than the endometrium thickens, the distal ends of the vessels reach progressively closer to the surface of the endometrium. This unequal growth results in a disproportion between the length of the arterioles and the thickness of the endometrium; and for this reason, the vessels become increasingly coiled.

Premenstrual Phase
This phase of the cycle encompasses the 2 or 3 days before menstruation and corresponds, in time, to the regression of the corpus luteum and, in turn, to the rapid decline in secretion of progesterone and estrogen. The chief histological characteristic of the premenstrual phase is infiltration of the stroma by polymorphonuclear or mononuclear leukocytes, by which is im-

parted a pseudoinflammatory appearance. At the same time, in the superficial zone, the reticular framework of the stroma disintegrates. As a result of the loss of tissue fluid and secretion, the thickness of the endometrium often decreases appreciably during the 2 days before menstruation. In the process of reduction in thickness, the glands and arteries collapse.

Endometrial Ischemia

In a classic study, Markee (1940) described the vascular changes that occur before menstruation, as he observed these alterations in intraocular transplants of endometrium in the rhesus monkey. He found that as the result of the compression of endometrium, the coiling of the arterioles increases markedly. Although the coils are fairly regular earlier in the cycle, just before menstruation these become quite irregular.

Furthermore, Markee observed two entirely different vascular phenomena in endometrial transplants for the few days that precede menstrual bleeding. Beginning 1 to 5 days before the onset of menstruation, there is a period of slowed circulation, or relative stasis, during which vasodilatation may occur. Thereafter, there is a period of vasoconstriction that commences 4 to 24 hours before the extravasation of any blood. The period of stasis is extremely variable, from less than 24 hours to 4 days. It was Markee's opinion that the slowing of the circulation that leads to stasis is caused by the increased resistance to blood flow offered by the coiled arteries. As more coils are added, the blood flow becomes increasingly slower. Another explanation, however, must be invoked for bleeding during anovulatory cycles and for bleeding that follows withdrawal of estrogens, in which circumstances the arteries may be quite simple or relatively uncoiled; in such cases, there may be a more direct mechanism that involves arteriolar vasoconstriction.

Thus, it is envisioned by most authorities that vasoconstriction of the arterioles and coiled arteries precedes the onset of menstrual bleeding by the 4 to 24 hours that correspond to the premenstrual ischemic phase. After the constriction has begun, the superficial half to two-thirds of the endometrium is inadequately supplied with blood during the remainder of that menstrual cycle; the anemic appearance of the functional zone may be striking. When, after a period of constriction, an individual coiled artery relaxes, hemorrhage occurs from that artery or its branches. Then, in sequence, these constricted arteries relax and bleed; the succession of small hemorrhages from individual arterioles or capillaries continues for a variable time. Although this sequence of vasoconstriction, relaxation, and hemorrhage appears to be well established, the mechanism that actually brings about the escape of blood from the vessels remains an enigma. It is entirely possible that the damage to the walls of the vessels during the period of vasoconstriction results in their rupture when the constricted segment relaxes and the blood flow is resumed.

Menstrual Phase

Menstrual bleeding may be of either arterial or venous origin, but the former is predominant. It appears at the outset to result from rhexis of a coiled artery with consequent formation of a hematoma, but occasionally it takes place by leakage through the vessel. When a hematoma forms, the superficial endometrium is distended and then ruptures. Subsequently, fissures develop in the adjacent functional layers, and blood, as well as fragments of tissue of various sizes, becomes detached. Although autolysis occurs, as a rule fragments of tissue can be identified in the menstrual tissue in the vagina. Hemorrhage stops when the coiled artery returns to a state of constriction.

The changes that accompany partial necrosis also serve to seal off the tip of the vessel; and in the superficial portion, often only the endothelium remains. The endometrial surface is restored, according to Markee, by growth of the flanges, or collars, that form the everted free ends of the uterine glands. These flanges increase in diameter very rapidly, and the continuity of the epithelium is effected by the fusion of the edges of these sheets of thin, migrating cells.

Dating of the Endometrium by Histological Criteria

Benirschke (1986), in an excellent review, has summarized the histological features of the endometrium that permit accurate dating of endometrium obtained after ovulation. Immediately after ovulation, i.e., days 14 to 16 of an idealized 28-day cycle, and presumably in response to the action of progesterone secreted by the developing corpus luteum, characteristic subnuclear glycogen-rich vacuoles develop in the glandular epithelium. By day 17 to 18, the vacuoles have displaced the nuclei toward the middle of the cells; mitoses are rare, and by day 18, mitosis has ceased. The migration of vacuoles continues past the nuclei to the luminal surface of the glands and by day 20, near-maximum secretion into the lumen of the glands, has transpired. By this time, there are only a few vacuoles that remain in the glandular epithelium. During the early luteal phase of the cycle, mitosis ceases but the glands become more tortuous as the luteal response continues.

There are, simultaneously, hormonally induced changes in the stroma—indeed, by days 20 to 21, there is considerable interstitial edema. Predecidualization is apparent by days 23 to 24, a process that consists of an increase in the cytoplasm of stromal cells—commencing first in cells around the spiral arterioles. Thereafter, the decidual changes extend throughout the stroma. Granulocytes and lymphocytes infiltrate the predecidual secretory endometrium. The premenstrual phase of the endometrial cycle is characterized by a decrease in thickness of the endometrium, extravasation of blood, and disassociation and thence disintegration of stromal cells. In Benirschke's description of these morphological changes, he points out that "amazingly" at a time when the surface epithelium of the premenstrual endometrium still is intact, there is extensive hemorrhage into and disintegration of the stroma.

THE ROLE OF PROSTAGLANDINS IN MENSTRUATION

The prostaglandins, a unique class of tissue hormones, are synthesized in the cells in which these substances act or else in nearby cells. Thus, this group of substances are tissue hormones rather than humoral hormones. In most tissues, prostaglandins are degraded rapidly in the tissues of origin or in nearby tissues, as well as in more remote sites, such as the lungs. The prostaglandins or prostaglandin-like substances are synthesized from an essential fatty acid, arachidonic acid. Arachidonic acid is present in tissues in an esterified form, usually in the *sn*-2 position of glycerophospholipids. In this esterified form, arachidonic acid *cannot* be converted to prostaglandins. The enzyme *phospholipase A₂* catalyzes the hydrolysis of the *sn*-2 fatty acid ester of certain glycerophospholipids to effect the release of free arachidonic acid. Other lipases, which commonly act in concert in a series of reactions, catalyze the hydrolysis of arachidonic acid from other lipid stores, notably, phosphatidylinositol. Thus, the rate of release of free arachidonic acid commonly is believed to be the rate-limiting step in

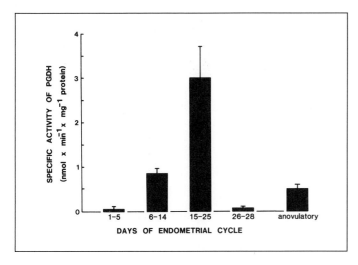

Figure 3–2. Specific activities (mean ± SEM) of NAD⁺-dependent 15-hydroxyprostaglandin dehydrogenase (PGDH) in cytosolic fractions of human endometrial tissues obtained on various days of the menstrual cycle or from anovulatory women. Days of the menstrual cycle were idealized to that of a 28-day ovulatory cycle for postovulatory samples according to menstrual history, histological appearance of the endometrium, and serum estradiol-17β and progesterone concentrations on the day of endometrial sampling. (*From Casey and colleagues: Prostaglandins 19:115, 1980.*)

the formation of prostaglandins in most tissues. Both endometrium and decidua are richly endowed with prostaglandin synthase activity. It has been shown that the decidua also is enriched with arachidonic acid. The role of prostaglandin metabolism in decidua in the initiation of parturition and in the maintenance of labor is discussed in Chapter 10, p. 200.

A role for prostaglandins in the initiation of menstruation also is envisioned. Prostaglandins, administered to nonpregnant women, will bring about menstruation. It has been proposed that this action of prostaglandins is mediated by way of the induction of vasoconstriction of the endometrial arterioles. Large amounts of prostaglandins are found in menstrual blood and prostaglandin administration to women gives rise to symptoms that mimic those of dysmenorrhea, which commonly is associated with normal ovulatory menses, i.e., menses initiated by progesterone withdrawal.

NAD⁺-dependent *15-hydroxyprostaglandin dehydrogenase* (PGDH), the enzyme that catalyzes the first reaction in the degradation of prostaglandins, is found in endometrium, principally in the cells of the glandular epithelium (Casey and coworkers, 1980). The specific activity of this enzyme is highest in endometrial tissue obtained during the luteal phase of the cycle, whereas it is barely detectable or absent on days 26 to 28, just before the onset of menses, and on days 1 to 5 of the menstrual cycle (Fig. 3–2). Thus, the specific activity of PGDH in endometrium appears to follow the levels of progesterone. It has been hypothesized that the fall in activity of PGDH, as the levels of progesterone fall, and, in turn, the reduced rate of degradation of prostaglandins, may serve to increase the levels of prostaglandins in the endometrium. Casey and colleagues (1980) have provided a review of the role of prostaglandins in the menstrual cycle.

Among the more thorough studies of the process of menstruation are those of McLennan and Rydell (1965) who concluded that loss of endometrial tissue may be less extensive than previous investigators had suggested. In their opinion, regeneration of the uterine surface occurs from the residual spongy layer rather than from the most basal elements.

ULTRASTRUCTURE

From the findings of Wynn and associates (1967) and White and Buchsbaum (1973) who studied the ultrastructure of the endo-

metrium, there is secretion of cytoplasmic components of the endometrial cells into the glandular lumens throughout the menstrual cycle (Figs. 3–3 and 3–4). The terms *proliferative* and *secretory*, therefore, are reflective less accurately of the histological pattern of the endometrium than are the terms *preovulatory* (follicular) and *postovulatory* (luteal).

THE ENDOMETRIAL CYCLE IN RETROSPECT

The correlations of the hormonal events of the ovarian cycle and the morphological changes of the endometrial cycle and the action of the pituitary gonadotropic hormones are summarized in Table 3–1 and in Figure 3–5.

Commonly, we presume (incorrectly) that the ovarian cycle and the endometrial or menstrual cycle are coincident in time. And again, somewhat incorrectly, the follicular phase of the ovarian cycle has been presumed to be absolutely coincident with the proliferative phase of the endometrial or menstrual cycle. At the same time, the terms *luteal phase* and *secretory phase* have been regarded, in terms of the cycle, to be coincident if not synonymous.

In fact, the ovarian cycle, as we now understand it, and the menstrual cycle, as we define it, i.e., the endometrial cycle that begins on the 1st day of menses, are not coincident. We now know that follicular recruitment, presumably brought about in part by a modest but significant increase in FSH secretion, commences not with menstruation but a few days before the onset of menses, at a time of maximum regression of the corpus luteum; indeed, the preceding ovarian cycle terminates before the onset of menstruation when the corpus luteum of the succeeding ovarian cycle regresses. Although the cycles are divided into phases for descriptive purposes and for convenience in description, the changes are continuous throughout an ovulatory cycle. Furthermore, there is considerable individual variation in both the activity of the endocrine glands and in the response of the target organ, the uterus. Secretory changes that resemble closely those of the luteal phase may appear occasionally before ovulation. Although the postovulatory phase of the cycle generally is very close to 14 days in length, the normal follicular phase may vary from 1 to 3 weeks. Finally, whereas the bleeding at the end of a typical ovulatory menstrual cycle is preceded by endometrial ischemia, uterine bleeding, on occasion, may appear at the expected time without prior ovulation,

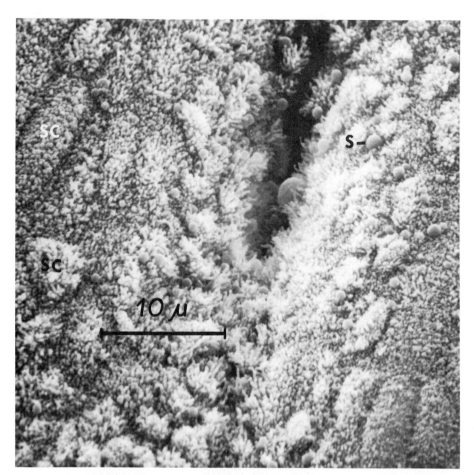

Figure 3–3. Gland ostium and surrounding endometrium in proliferative phase seen by scanning electron microscopy. Many secretory droplets are seen on cell surfaces. Microvilli are prominent on secretory cells (SC) and individual cell margins are identified. (*From White and Buchsbaum: Gynecol Oncol 1:330, 1973.*)

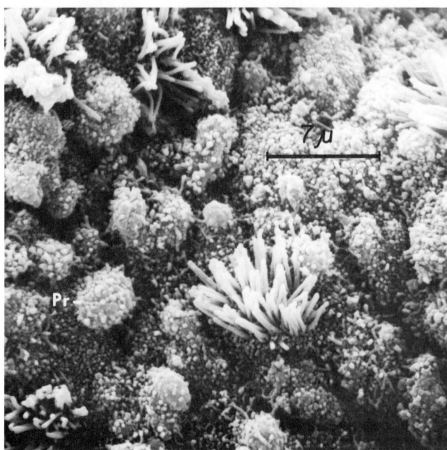

Figure 3–4. Cellular detail for secretory phase endometrium on day 24 of the menstrual cycle, demonstrated by scanning electron microscopy. Microvilli are prominent and cellular protuberances are evident. (*From White and Buchsbaum: Gynecol Oncol 1:330, 1973.*)

TABLE 3–1. IMPORTANT MILESTONES IN THE CORRELATION OF OVARIAN AND ENDOMETRIAL (MENSTRUAL) CYCLES (IDEALIZED 28-DAY CYCLE)

	Phase						
	Menstrual 1–5 Days	Early Follicular 6–8 Days	Advanced Follicular 9–13 Days	Ovulation 14 Days	Early Luteal 15–19 Days	Advanced Luteal 20–25 Days	Premenstrual 26–28 Days
Ovary	Formation of corpus albicans from corpus luteum of preceding cycle. Recruitment of follicles.	Follicular maturation and development of the chosen or dominant follicle.		Ovulation and luteinization of granulosa cells in the ruptured follicle.	Vascularization of granulosa lutein cells and formation of corpus luteum. Follicular atresia.	Mature corpus luteum and continued follicular atresia.	Involution of corpus luteum and initiation of follicular recruitment for the next cycle.
Estrogen	Low; derived principally from extraglandularly produced estrone; little estradiol-17β secretion by the ovary.	Estradiol-17β secretion, principally by granulosa cells of the dominant follicle, increases strikingly, maximal rates being attained just prior to the LH surge.		Immediately after, or coincident with, ovulation, there is an abrupt, indeed, precipitous decline in estradiol-17β secretion.	Gradual and progressive postovulatory rise in estradiol-17β secretion by the corpus luteum.	Maximal rates of postovulatory estradiol-17β secretion are attained; luteal phase estradiol-17β secretion rates, however, are not nearly as great as those observed in the immediate preovulatory phase.	Estradiol-17β secretion declines precipitously and, as during menstruation, the principal estrogen produced is estrone, which is formed in extraglandular sites.
Progesterone	Low secretion; there is little secretion of progesterone by the adrenal cortex and the corpus luteum of the preceding ovarian cycle has regressed.	During the follicular phase of the ovarian cycle, progesterone levels remain low. This is due to the fact that human granulosa cells cannot synthesize cholesterol, the obligate precursor of progesterone, but are dependent upon LDL-cholesterol that can be obtained only from the blood after vascularization of the granulosa cells after ovulation.		Progesterone secretion increases steadily as the consequence of the availability of LDL and LH action to effect cholesterol side-chain cleavage.	Progesterone secretion remains high until the end of the advanced luteal phase.		Precipitous decline in progesterone secretion.
Endometrium	Menstrual desquamation and early reorganization of endometrial glandular epithelium.	Proliferation of glandular epithelium with many mitoses.	Pseudostratification of nuclei—no secretion, early stromal changes.	Appearance of subnuclear vacuoles that are rich in glycogen.	Migration of vacuoles to the luminal surface; cessation of mitosis. The endometrial glands become very tortuous.	Vacuoles have been secreted and decidualization commences. Stromal edema and enlargement of stromal cells is prominent.	Disruption and disintegration of stromal cells. Leukocyte infiltration and interstitial hemorrhage.
Pituitary Secretion: FSH	Continuing decline in FSH levels that had become modestly increased coincident with the decline in steroid secretion by the regressing corpus luteum of the preceding cycle.	FSH secretion is at all times pulsatile in nature but during the proliferative phase of the ovarian cycle, prior to the time of the LH surge at midcycle, FSH levels remain low.		There is a significant surge of FSH secretion, albeit less prominent than that of LH, that heralds the commencement of the ovulatory process.	After the midcycle gonadotropin surge, FSH levels fall abruptly to levels similar to those found during the preovulatory phase of the cycle.		As steroid secretion by the regressing corpus luteum diminishes, there is a modest but significant increase in FSH.
Pituitary Secretion: LH	The levels of LH are low and reasonably constant until just prior to ovulation.			Coincident with, or just after, the striking increase in estradiol-17β secretion by the dominant follicle, there is a striking increase in LH secretion—the LH "surge."	The levels of LH are low and reasonably constant until just prior to ovulation.		

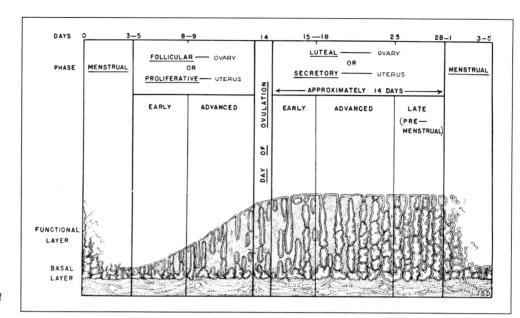

Figure 3–5. Cyclic changes in thickness and in form of glands and arteries of endometrium and the relation of these changes to those of the ovarian cycle.

formation of a corpus luteum, or secretion of progesterone. Anovulatory cycles sometimes occur in otherwise apparently normal women, but the incidence is difficult to ascertain because adequate observations of the ovaries are rarely possible. It appears that in some such cycles a follicle enlarges but then becomes cystic and degenerates. In others, no follicles grow beyond a few millimeters throughout an entire cycle. Withdrawal of progesterone, therefore, is not essential for uterine bleeding. **Nonetheless, in women with persistent anovulation, menstruation is not cyclic unless they are ingesting oral contraceptives.**

At about 27 to 35 days after the first day of the last menstrual period, there may be bleeding around the site of implantation of the fertilized ovum, an event that results in slight vaginal bleeding that is sometimes mistaken for menses. This "placental sign" (Hartman, 1932) of bleeding always occurs during pregnancy in the rhesus monkey.

CLINICAL ASPECTS OF MENSTRUATION

Menstruation is the periodic discharge of blood, mucus, and cellular debris from the uterine mucosa and occurs at more or less regular, cyclic, and predictable intervals from menarche to menopause except during periods of pregnancy and lactation. Physiologically, however, menstruation must be viewed as failed fertility (Chap. 2).

THE MENARCHE AND PUBERTY

Historically, the age at which menstruation begins, *menarche*, has declined steadily until recent years (Fig. 3–6). This decline has ceased in the United States. The average time at which menstruation begins is now between 12 and 13 years of age, but in a small number of apparently normal girls, menarche may occur as early as the 10th or as late as the 16th year. The menarche refers specifically to the first menstruation, whereas puberty is a broader term that refers to the entire transitional stage between childhood and sexual maturity. The menarche, hence, is just one sign of puberty, but if it is the consequence of ovulation (and

attendant hormonal secretion), it is indicative of the completion of the fundamental physiological event of puberty, namely the release of an ovum.

INTERVAL

Although the *modal interval* at which menstruation occurs is considered to be 28 days, there is considerable variation among women, in general, as well as in the cycle lengths of a given woman. Marked variation in the length of menstrual cycles does not necessarily mean infertility.

Arey (1939), who analyzed 12 studies, which comprised about 20,000 calendar records from 1,500 women, reached the conclusion that there is no evidence of perfect menstrual regularity. In a study by Gunn and co-workers (1937) of 479 normal British women, the typical difference between the shortest and longest cycle was 8 or 9 days. In 30 percent of women, it was more than 13 days but in no woman was it fewer than 2 days. Arey found that in an average adult woman, one-third of her cycles departed by more than 2 days from the mean of the lengths of her cycles. Arey's analysis of 5,322 cycles in 485 normal women was indicative of an average interval of 28.4 days; his finding for the average cycle length in pubertal girls was longer, 33.9 days. Chiazze and associates (1968) analyzed the length of 30,655 menstrual cycles of 2,316 women. The mean for all cycles was 29.1 days. For cycles that range from 15 to 45 days, the average length was 28.1 days. The degree of variability was such that only 13 percent of the women experienced cycles that varied in length by less than 6 days. Haman (1942) surveyed 2,460 cycles in 150 housewives who attended a clinic where special attention was directed to recording accurately the length of the menstrual cycles. Arey's data and those of Haman, the distribution curves of which are superimposed and shown in Figure 3–7, are almost identical.

DURATION AND AMOUNT

The duration of menstrual flow also is variable; the usual duration is 4 to 6 days, but lengths between 2 and 8 days may be considered normal. In any individual woman, however, the

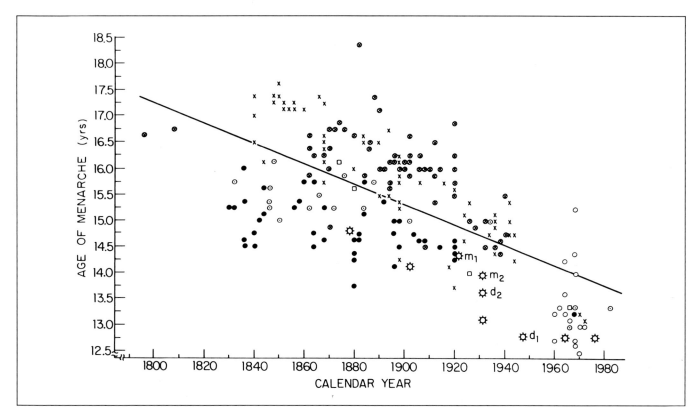

Figure 3–6. Mean or median age of menarche as a function of calendar year from 1790 to 1980. The symbols refer to England (⊙); France (●); Germany (⊗); Holland (□); Scandinavia (Denmark, Finland, Norway, and Sweden) (×); Belgium, Czechoslovakia, Hungary, Italy, Poland (rural), Romania (urban and rural), Russia (15.2 years at an altitude of 2500 m and 14.4 years at 700 m), Spain, and Switzerland (all labeled ✿); and the United States (○, data not included in the regression line). Twenty-seven points for Europe were identical and do not appear on the graph. The regression line cannot, of course, be extended indefinitely. The age of menarche has already leveled off in some European countries, as it has in the United States. (*From Wyshak and Frisch: N Engl J Med 306:1033, 1982.*)

duration of the flow is usually reasonably similar from cycle to cycle.

The menstrual discharge consists of shed fragments of endometrium mixed with a variable quantity of blood. Usually the blood is liquid, but if the rate of blood flow is excessive, clots of various sizes may appear. Considerable attention has been directed to the usual state of incoagulability of menstrual blood. The most logical explanation for its incoagulability is that the blood was coagulated as it was shed, but promptly was liquefied by fibrinolytic activity. In endometrial tissue, there are not only potent thromboplastic properties, which promptly initiate clotting, but also potent fibrinolytic properties (plasmin), which effect prompt lysis of fibrin clots. Plasmin is formed by way of the action of plasminogen activator (produced in endometrium) on blood-borne plasminogen. It is quite likely that hormonal regulation of plasminogen activator and plasminogen activator inhibitor are important cellular features of the biomolecular regulation of menstruation.

The extrusion of clots with uterine bleeding also is indicative of anovulation, i.e., bleeding that occurs without benefit of progesterone action and withdrawal. This issue is further considered below.

At one time, the toxic properties of the menstrual discharge attracted considerable interest. The discharge undoubtedly con-

tains toxic proteins and peptides that arise most likely from proteolytic activity present in the mixture of blood and endometrial tissue fragments, but also from bacterial contamination.

The average amount of blood lost by normal women during a menstrual period has been determined by several groups of

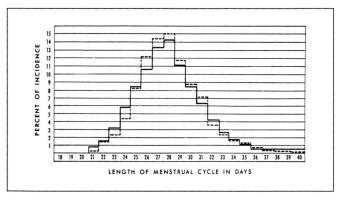

Figure 3–7. Duration of menstrual cycle based on distribution data of Arey (continuous line) and Haman (broken lines). (*Courtesy of Eli Lilly and Co.*)

investigators who found it to range from about 25 to 60 mL (Baldwin and associates, 1961; Barker and Fowler, 1936; Hallberg and co-workers, 1966; Hytten and associates, 1964; Millis, 1951). With a normal hemoglobin concentration of 14 g per dL and a hemoglobin iron content of 3.4 mg per g, these volumes of blood contain from 12 to 29 mg of iron and represent a blood loss equivalent to 0.4 to 1.0 mg of iron for every day of the cycle, or from 150 to 400 mg per year. Finch (1959) determined the rate of decrease in the specific activity of the miscible iron of the body for a period of years after the injection of ^{55}Fe to ascertain the rate of loss of iron from the body. In women who menstruated, the iron loss on average was 0.6 mg per day more than the iron loss in men or postmenopausal women. Because the amount of iron that is absorbed from the diet usually is quite limited, this seemingly "negligible" iron loss is important because it contributes further to the low iron stores that are present in the majority of women (Hallberg and co-workers, 1968; Scott and Pritchard, 1967).

Actually, the blood loss is very small especially considering that the area of the endometrium of normal uteri of nonpregnant women is 10 to 45 cm^2 (Chimbira and colleagues, 1980). Therefore, there must be an effective means of hemostasis in the endometrium during menstruation. The control of blood loss likely is not effected by myometrial contractions to compress uterine vessels, because inhibitors of prostaglandin synthesis usually serve to reduce blood loss during menstruation. On the other hand, excessive blood loss is common in women with coagulation or platelet disorders. It is likely, therefore, that hemostasis in endometrium is effected by hemostatic plug formation as in other tissues (Christiaens and associates, 1985). But lysis of blood clots is accomplished by an active, local fibrinolytic system in endometrium.

CHANGES IN BODY WEIGHT DURING THE OVARIAN CYCLE

It has been reported frequently that about 30 percent of women gain 1 to 3 lb shortly before the onset of menstruation, an amount of weight that is lost promptly as menstruation begins. Although only a minority of women manifest weight gains, there has been a tendency to regard the increase in weight as a normal characteristic of the cycle that is reflective of the influence of steroid hormones. Actually, the average weight gain is insignificant, perhaps a quarter of a pound, as shown in a statistical study of this question by Chesley and Hellman (1957) and by Golub and associates (1965). It would appear, therefore, that the concept of appreciable premenstrual weight gain, as a physiological phenomenon, is not valid. Preece and co-workers (1975) could find no consistent change in total body water during the menstrual cycle.

On the other hand, it is possible that we have not conducted the proper studies to evaluate weight gain due to increases in body water. Most studies have been conducted by carefully weighing women in the morning after first micturition. It is possible that the increased glomerular filtration rate of the supine position during sleep will lead to a water diuresis and thus eliminate from consideration the water loss that occurred during the night.

This is an important consideration in future evaluations of the changes in sodium and water homeostasis during the luteal phase of the ovarian cycle and in deciphering the potential causes of the premenstrual syndrome. During the midluteal phase of the ovarian cycle, there is a sizable increase in the rate

of secretion of aldosterone by the adrenal cortex. Presumably this increase in aldosterone secretion is in response to the natriuretic effect of progesterone produced in large amounts by the corpus luteum. Increased sodium excretion favors the release of renin from the juxtaglomerular apparatus of kidney leading to increased angiotensin II formation; and angiotensin II is the principal stimulus of aldosterone secretion by the adrenal. But in addition, there is a striking increase in the production of another mineralocorticosteroid, deoxycorticosterone (DOC), during the midluteal phase of the ovarian cycle and during pregnancy. This comes about by way of the extraadrenal conversion of plasma progesterone to DOC through the action of steroid 21-hydroxylase activity in nonadrenal tissues, including tissues of mineralocorticosteroid action (Casey and MacDonald, 1982).

The increase in mineralocorticosteroid secretion during the luteal phase of the cycle, which persists and increases as pregnancy progresses, is one of the earliest adaptations of the maternal organism to pregnancy (Chap. 7).

THE MENOPAUSE AND CLIMACTERIC

Menopause is the cessation of menses. There are wide variations in the age at which menopause occurs. About one half of all women cease menstruating between the ages of 45 and 50, about one-quarter stop before the age of 45, and another one quarter continue to menstruate until past 50 years of age. The term *climacteric* is derived from the Greek word that means "rung of a ladder" and bears the same relation to the menopause as the term *puberty* bears to menarche. The climacteric refers to the time in a woman's life known to the laity as the "change of life."

MENSTRUATION AND PARTURITION

There are selected physiological features of menstruation in women that provide important clues as to the biomolecular phenomenon involved in this process. Clearly it is progesterone "withdrawal" that leads to the onset of menstruation in ovulatory women. Treatment of castrated women with estrogen and thence with intermittent progesterone administration causes uterine bleeding after withdrawal of the progesterone, irrespective of the continuation or noncontinuation of the estrogen treatment. Moreover, progesterone withdrawal menses are predictable, i.e., in time of onset, duration of bleeding, and amount of blood loss. Increased prostaglandin production, and in particular PGF$_{2\alpha}$ formation, in endometrium is characteristic of progesterone withdrawal menses, as are contractions of the uterus. And, uterine bleeding in response to progesterone withdrawal is associated with discomfort, varying greatly in intensity among women, but uniformly present.

Another issue is worthy of restatement: normal menstruation, i.e., that which occurs in ovulatory women (progesterone withdrawal), is characterized by the extrusion of incoagulable blood; and there is indirect evidence in favor of the probability that serine proteases (and inhibitors thereof) are produced in endometrium in a cyclic manner that is suggestive of hormonal regulation. Among these, plasminogen activator is recognized as an important enzyme in the fibrinolytic system.

Hahn (1980) quoted John Hunter who described this event more than 200 years ago (1774): *"In healthy menstruation, the blood which is discharged does not coagulate; in the irregular or unhealthy it does.''* Perhaps a remarkably profound insight into the biomolecular regulation of this event was provided as early as 1914 by Whitehouse who observed: *"As the blood escapes into the tissues it is brought into contact with cells rich in thrombokinase, and this induces rapid coagulation. The thrombus is then disintegrated by the enzyme contained in the secretion of the endometrial glands. These two processes are normally balanced, but it will be obvious that abnormalities in either may lead to the production of excessive bleeding.''*

These several physiological correlates are extraordinarily informative and useful in constructing a reasonable hypothesis to explain the hormonal and cellular control of menstruation; in particular, the hormonal regulation of formation of serine proteases and inhibitors thereof in endometrium may be pivotal not only in the fibrinolytic action of endometrium but also in the processing of other proteins.

Interleukin-1 (IL-1) may serve in endometrium and in decidua as the intermediate agent that causes increased prostaglandin formation. The processing of pro-IL-1 to the active, mature form of IL-1 may involve the action of serine proteases. IL-1 is an extraordinarily potent agent that is known to be involved in responses to inflammation and immunological challenge. This immunohormone-immunomodulator is produced primarily by stimulated monocyte-macrophages, but in addition, IL-1 is produced by a number of other cells including the endometrial stromal cells and decidual tissue. Interleukin-1 is known to act in an autocrine manner (e.g., on macrophages), in a paracrine manner (e.g., as lymphocyte-activating factor), and in an endocrine manner (e.g., as *endogenous pyrogen*).

Increased concentrations of interleukin-1 have been demonstrated in blood of women after ovulation, i.e., during the luteal phase of the ovarian cycle (Cannon and Dinarello, 1985). One of the mechanisms of IL-1 action is to promote prostaglandin formation in responsive tissues. The stimulation of PGE_2 formation in the brain by the action of IL-1 is believed to be one mechanism of fever induction during infection. From the perspective of the reproductive biologist, IL-1 acts on amnion, decidua, endometrial stromal cells, and myometrium to induce a striking increase in prostaglandin formation (Word and colleagues, 1989). Therefore, it seems reasonable to suspect that IL-1 serves a crucial role in the induction of prostaglandin synthesis, in particular $PGF_{2\alpha}$, which is fundamental to menstruation and parturition. Clearly, an increase in basal body temperature is characteristic of the luteal phase of the ovarian cycle, and it seems possible that IL-1, the so-called endogenous pyrogen, is involved in this process.

It is interesting, therefore, to speculate as to whether the increased IL-1 in blood of postovulatory women arises from the corpus luteum or from the secretory endometrium or some other tissue site, possibly in response, directly or indirectly, to progesterone action. In support of this possibility, it has been demonstrated that peritoneal macrophages isolated from women during the luteal phase of the ovarian cycle produce IL-1 whereas those obtained from women before ovulation do not (Glover and colleagues, 1987).

IL-1 levels in amnionic fluid increase appreciably during spontaneous parturition (Chap. 10). Therefore, IL-1 produced in decidua may be instrumental in modulating increased prostaglandin formation in fetal membranes and decidua during labor. IL-1 also is produced in endometrial stromal cells; perhaps this IL-1 modulates $PGF_{2\alpha}$ formation in endometrium in the initiation of menstruation; **thereby, menstruation is the parturition of failed fertility.**

THE DECIDUA

The human decidua, the specialized endometrium of pregnancy, is produced by prolonged stimulation of the endometrium by estrogen and progesterone and from stimuli provided by the implanting blastocyst. The special relationship that exists between endometrium-decidua and invading trophoblast seemingly defies the laws of transplantation immunology. The success of this unique autograft not only is a curiosity but an event that many investigators believe may harbor solutions to the future of successful transplantation surgery and perhaps the control of neoplasia as well.

DECIDUAL STRUCTURE

William Hunter, the 19th-century British gynecologist, wrote the first comprehensive treatise on the uterus of pregnant women. In that book, he provided the first scientific description of the *membrana decidua*. According to Damjanov (1985), the term was coined in the best tradition of formal logic applied to scientific writing—*membrana*, denoting its gross appearance, while the qualifier, *decidua*, was added in analogy with deciduous leaves and deciduous teeth to indicate its ephemeral nature and the fact that it is shed from the rest of the uterus at the time of delivery. Wewer and associates (1985) provided evidence that decidua indeed qualifies to be called a membrane, not only because of its gross appearance, but because it contains most, if not all, of the major basement membrane components. But more than that, each mature decidual cell of the decidua at term is surrounded by a basement membrane, one major component of which is *laminin*, a basement membrane protein that is produced in decidual cells.

In the development of this pericellular membrane of decidual cells, there is what appears to be a gradual development of the extracellular matrix. In proliferative endometrium, laminin cannot be identified in association with the stromal cells. In late secretory endometrium, there are punctate areas of laminin identified in extracellular sites. In early pregnancy (8 to 16 weeks), the vast majority of the decidual cells are completely surrounded by the laminin-rich basement membranes (large mature decidual cells). But there also are intermediate-size decidual cells, and these cells are characterized by pericellular or intracellular basement membrane proteins. It has been postulated, and there is some evidence in favor of the postulate, that the small intermediate cells are precursors of the large mature decidual cells.

Thus, in human decidual cells, there is a pericellular basement membrane. These cells clearly build walls around themselves and possibly around the fetus. In addressing this issue, Damjanov was reminded of the verse from Robert Frost, *"Before I build a wall I'd ask to know, what I was walling in or walling out.''* Perhaps a partial answer to this poetic question, in the case of the decidual cell, may serve to answer the unsolved riddle regarding the peculiar properties of decidua in the maintenance of pregnancy and the initiation of parturition.

UNIQUE DECIDUAL FUNCTIONS

The decidual cells develop from transformations of the stromal cells of the endometrium; but the unique nature and histology and endocrine and immunological function of the decidual cell distinguishes it clearly from "fibroblasts." These cells produce prolactin, relaxin, a variety of "pregnancy-specific proteins," prostaglandins, cytokines, and 1,25-dihydroxyvitamin D_3 and are rich in a variety of intriguing enzymes, such as diamine oxidase.

The mysteries of the human decidua continue to increase. Convincing evidence has been presented by Riddick and co-workers (1979) and Golander and associates (1978), for example, that the decidua is the source of prolactin that is found in enormous amounts in the amnionic fluid during human pregnancy. Levels of prolactin of 10,000 ng per mL of amnionic fluid are found during the 20th to 24th week of pregnancy compared with levels of 150 ng per mL in plasma of near-term pregnant women (Tyson and co-workers, 1972). Importantly, prolactin produced in decidua preferentially enters amnionic fluid and little or none enters maternal blood. This is a classic example of the peculiar trafficking of molecules between maternal and fetal tissues of the paracrine arm of the fetal–maternal communication system.

DECIDUAL ORGANIZATION

During pregnancy, the decidua thickens, eventually attaining a depth of 5 to 10 mm. With a magnifying glass, furrows and numerous small openings, representing the mouths of uterine glands, can be detected. The portion of the decidua directly beneath the site of implantation forms the *decidua basalis;* that overlying the developing blastocysts and separating it from the rest of the uterine cavity is the *decidua capsularis.* The remainder of the uterus is lined by *decidua vera* or *decidua parietalis* (Chap. 4).

CERVICAL, VAGINAL, AND TUBAL CYCLES

CERVIX

Cyclic changes occur in the endocervical glands, especially during the follicular phase of the cycle. During the early follicular phase, the glands are only slightly tortuous and the secretory cells are not very tall. Secretion of mucus is meager. The late follicular phase, however, is characterized by pronounced tortuosity of the glands, deep invagination, tumescence of the epithelium, high columnar cells, and abundant secretion. The connective tissue acquires a looser texture and more extensive vascularization. After ovulation, these characteristics regress.

The secretory activity of the endocervical glands is maximal at about the time of ovulation and is the result of estrogenic stimulation. Only at that time, in most women, is the quality of the cervical mucus such as to permit penetration by the spermatozoa. The property of the cervical mucus that permits it to be drawn out in long strands is termed *spinnbarkeit,* a property of mucus that is maximal at the time of ovulation. The synchronization of the height of secretory activity in the cervical and endometrial cycles is precise and purposeful. In the cervix, where the mucus facilitates passage of the spermatozoa, it occurs just before the ovum is to be released (i.e., at ovulation), a period probably of not more than about 36 to 48 hours. In the endometrium, where the purpose of the highly developed secretory activity seems to be to provide a site favorable for nidation of the fertilized ovum, the changes are maximum about 6 to 7 days later, when the fertilized ovum is ready to implant.

CERVICAL MUCUS

If cervical mucus is aspirated, spread on a glass slide, allowed to dry for a few minutes, and examined microscopically, characteristic patterns can be discerned that are dependent on the stage of the ovarian cycle and the presence or absence of pregnancy (i.e., progesterone secretion in large amounts). From about the 7th day of the menstrual cycle to about the 18th day,

a fern-like pattern of dried cervical mucus is seen (Fig. 3–8); it is sometimes called a process of "arborization" or the "palm leaf pattern." After approximately the 21st day, this fern pattern does not develop, but rather there is a quite different pattern that forms, i.e., a beaded or cellular appearance (Fig. 3–9). This beaded pattern usually also is encountered in pregnancy.

The crystallization of the mucus, which is necessary for the production of the fern, or arborized pattern, is dependent upon the concentration of electrolytes, principally sodium chloride, in the secretion. In general, a concentration of sodium chloride of 1 percent is required for the full development of a fern pattern; below that concentration, either a beaded pattern or atypical, incomplete arborization is seen.

The concentration of sodium chloride, and, in turn, the presence or absence of the fern pattern, is determined by the response of the cervix to hormonal action. Whereas the cervical mucus is relatively rich in sodium chloride when estrogen, but not progesterone, is being produced, the secretion of progesterone (even without a reduction in the rate of secretion of estrogen) promptly acts to lower the sodium chloride concentration of the mucus, either cervical or nasal, to levels at which ferning will not occur as the specimen dries. During pregnancy, progesterone usually exerts a similar effect, even though the amount of estrogen produced is enormous compared with that produced during a normal ovarian cycle.

VAGINA

There is constant desquamation of the superficial cells of the vaginal epithelium. Consequently, the nature of maturity of the cells in the vaginal fluid is reflective to some degree of the changes in the epithelium of the surface of the vagina that occur in response to hormone action. Vaginal epithelium, under estrogenic stimulation, is characterized by cyclic changes during which the greatest development is reached at the end of the follicular phase. This stage is characterized by enlargement, flat-

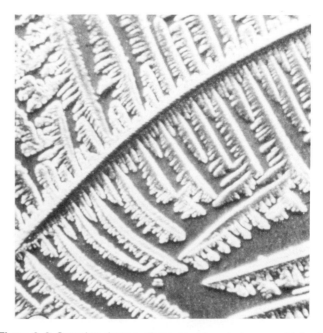

Figure 3–8. Scanning electron microscopy of cervical mucus obtained on day 11 of the menstrual cycle. (*From Zaneveld and colleagues: Obstet Gynecol 46:424, 1975.*)

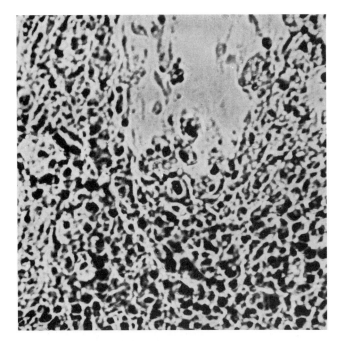

Figure 3–9. Photomicrograph of dried cervical mucus obtained from the cervical canal of a woman pregnant at 32 to 33 weeks. The beaded pattern is characteristic of progesterone action on the endocervical gland mucus composition. (*Courtesy of Dr. J. C. Ullery.*)

tening, and spreading of the superficial cells and by relative leucopenia, whereas in the smear taken in the luteal phase, there is an increase in the number of basophilic cells and leucocytes, as well as irregular grouping of the cells.

FALLOPIAN TUBES

Fertilization of the ovum occurs in the fallopian tube soon after ovulation. Based on considerable experience assembled by investigators around the world, there is evidence that the milieu of the fallopian tube is optimized for early cleavage and development of the zygote. Recapitulation of this environment has been the goal of many investigators seeking to idealize conditions for in vitro fertilization.

REFERENCES

Arey LB: The degree of normal menstrual irregularity: An analysis of 20,000 calendar records from 1,500 individuals. Am J Obstet Gynecol 37:12, 1939

Baldwin RM, Whalley PJ, Pritchard JA: Measurements of menstrual blood loss. Am J Obstet Gynecol 81:739, 1961

Barker AP, Fowler WM: The blood loss during normal menstruation. Am J Obstet Gynecol 31:979, 1936

Benirschke K: The endometrium. In Yen SSC, Jaffe RB (eds): Reproductive Endocrinology: Physiology, Pathophysiology and Clinical Management. Philadelphia, Saunders, 1986, p 385.

Cannon JG, Dinarello CA: Increased plasma interleukin-1 activity in women after ovulation. Science 227:1247, 1985

Casey ML, Hemsell DL, MacDonald PC, Johnston JM: NAD⁺-dependent 15-hydroxyprostaglandin dehydrogenase activity in human endometrium. Prostaglandins 19:115, 1980

Casey ML, MacDonald PC: Extraadrenal formation of a mineralocorticosteroid: Deoxycorticosterone and deoxycorticosterone sulfate biosynthesis and metabolism. Endocr Rev 3:396, 1982

Chesley LC, Hellman LM: Variations in body weight and salivary sodium in the menstrual cycle. Am J Obstet Gynecol 74:582, 1957

Chiazze L, Brayer FT, Macisco JJ, Parker MP, Duffy BJ: The length and variability of the human menstrual cycle. JAMA 203:377, 1968

Chimbira TH, Anderson ABM, Turnbull AC: Relation between measured menstrual blood loss and patient's subjective assessment of loss, duration of bleeding, number of sanitary towels used, uterine weight and endometrial surface area. Br J Obstet Gynaecol 87:603, 1980

Christiaens GCML, Sixma JJ, Haspels AA: Vascular and haemostatic changes in menstrual endometrium. In Baird DT, Michie EA (eds): Mechanism of Menstrual Bleeding. Serono Symposia. New York, Raven Press, 1985, p 27, Vol 25

Damjanov I: Editorial: Vesalius and Hunter were right: Decidua is a membrane. Lab Invest 53:597, 1985

Finch CA: Body iron exchange in man. J Clin Invest 38:392, 1959

Glover DM, Brownstein D, Burchett S, Larsen A, Wilson CB: Expression of HLA class II antigens and secretion of interleukin-1 by monocytes and macrophages from adults and neonates. Immunology 61:195, 1987

Golander A, Hurley T, Barret J, Hizi A, Handwerger S: Prolactin synthesis by human chorion decidual tissue: A possible source of prolactin in the amniotic fluid. Science 202:311, 1978

Golub LJ, Menduke H, Conly SS Jr: Weight changes in college women during the menstrual cycle. Am J Obstet Gynecol 91:89, 1965

Gunn DL, Jenkin PM, Gunn AL: Menstrual periodicity: Statistical observations on a large sample of normal cases. J Obstet Gynaecol Br Emp 44:839, 1937

Gustavii B: Labour: A delayed menstruation? Lancet 2:1149, 1972

Hahn L: Composition of menstrual blood. In Diczfalusy E, Fraser IS, Webb FTG (eds): Endometrial Bleeding and Steroidal Contraception. Proc Symp Steroid Contraception and Mechanism of Menstrual Bleeding. Bath, England, Pitman Press, 1980, p 107

Hallberg L, Hallgren J, Hollender A, Hogdahl AM, Tibblin G: Occurence of iron deficiency anemia in Sweden. Symp Swed Nutri Found 6:19, 1968

Hallberg L, Hogdahl AM, Nilsson L, Rybo G: Menstrual blood loss, a population study: Variation at different ages and attempts to define normality. Acta Obstet Gynecol Scand 45:320, 1966

Haman JO: The length of the menstrual cycle: A study of 150 normal women. Am J Obstet Gynecol 43:870, 1942

Hartman CG: Studies in the reproduction of the monkey Macaca (Pithecus) rhesus with special reference to menstruation and pregnancy. Contrib Embryol 23:1, 1932

Hitschmann F, Adler L: Der Bau der Uterusschleimhaut des geschlechtsreifen Weives mit besonderer Berücksichtigung der Menstruation. Monatsschr Begurtshilfe Gynaekol 27:1, 1908

Horwitz KB, McGuire WL, Pearson OH, Segaloff A: Predicting response to endocrine therapy in human breast cancer: A hypothesis. Science 189:726, 1975

Hytten FE, Cheyne GA, Klopper AI: Iron loss at menstruation. J Obstet Gynaecol Br Commonw 71:255, 1964

Jensen EV, Jacobson HI: Basic guides to the mechanism of estrogen action. Recent Prog Horm Res 18:387 [Pincus G (ed). New York, Academic], 1962

Markee JE: Menstruation in intraocular endometrial transplants in the rhesus monkey. Contrib Embryol 28:219, 1940

McLennan CE, Rydell AH: Extent of endometrial shedding during normal menstruation. Obstet Gynecol 26:605, 1965

Millis J: The iron losses of healthy women during consecutive menstrual cycles. Med J Aust 2:874, 1951

Noyes RW, Hertig AT, Rock J: Dating the endometrial biopsy. Fertil Steril 1:3, 1950

Preece PE, Richards AR, Owen GM, Hughes LE: Mastalgia and total body water. Br Med J 4:498, 1975

Ramsey EM: History. In Wynn RM (ed): Biology of the Uterus. New York, Plenum, 1977, p 1

Riddick DH, Luciano AA, Kusmik WF, Maslar IA: Evidence for a nonpituitary source of amniotic fluid prolactin. Fertil Steril 31:35, 1979

Rock J, Bartlett M: Biopsy studies of human endometrium. JAMA 108:2022, 1937

Scott DE, Pritchard JA: Iron deficiency in healthy young college women. JAMA 199:897, 1967

Tseng L, Gurpide E: Estradiol and 20α-dihydroprogesterone dehydrogenase activities in human endometrium during the menstrual cycle. Endocrinology 94:419, 1974

Tseng L, Gurpide E: Effects of progestins on estradiol receptor levels in human endometrium. J Clin Endocrinol Metab 41:402, 1975

Tseng L, Liu HC: Stimulation of acylsulfotransferase activity by progestins in human endometrium in vitro. J Clin Endocrinol Metab 53:418, 1981

Tyson JE, Hwang P, Guyda H, Friesen HG: Studies of prolactin secretion in human pregnancy. Am J Obstet Gynecol 113:14, 1972

Wewer UM, Faber M, Liotta LA, Albrechtsen R: Immunochemical and ultrastructural assessment of the nature of the pericellular basement membrane of human decidual cells. Lab Invest 53:624, 1985

White AJ, Buchsbaum HJ: Scanning electron microscopy of the human endometrium. Gynecol Oncol 1:330, 1973

Whitehouse HB: Pathological uterine haemorrhage. Lancet 1:951, 1914

Word RA, MacDonald PC, Casey ML: Stimulation of prostaglandin (PG) production in myometrial cells in culture by interleukin-1 (IL-1). Presented at the Society for Gynecological Investigation, San Diego, California, March 1989.

Wynn RM, Harris JA: Ultrastructural cyclic changes in the human endometrium: I. Normal preovulatory phase. Fertil Steril 18:632, 1967

Wynn RM, Woolley RS: Ultrastructural cyclic changes in the human endometrium: II. Normal postovulatory phase. Fertil Steril 18:721, 1967

The Placenta and Fetal Membranes

FETAL TISSUES OF THE FETAL–MATERNAL COMMUNICATION SYSTEM

The basic features of the fetal–maternal communication system of human pregnancy, which is comprised of two arms (placental and paracrine), were described in Chapters 2 and 3 (Fig. 2–1). The villous trophoblasts are the fetal tissue of the anatomical interface of the placental arm; and the fetal membranes, i.e., the amnion-chorion laeve, are the fetal tissues of the anatomical interface of the paracrine arm of this system. Ultimately, a communication link is established by way of the placental arm as follows: maternal blood directly bathes the villous trophoblasts; but the fetal blood is contained in fetal capillaries that traverse the intravillous space. Thus, a *hemochorioendothelial* type of placentation develops in the human pregnancy. The communication link established by the paracrine arm of the fetal–maternal communication system is by way of the anatomical and biomolecular juxtaposition of (fetal) chorion laeve and (maternal) decidua.

Heretofore, interest in the placenta properly has derived primarily from its role in the processes of nidation and in the transfer of nutrients to the developing fetus. Scientific interest in the placenta also evolves from its enormous diversity of form and function and from the unique metabolic, endocrine, and immunological properties of its trophoblasts. Today, we recognize that important metabolic functions of the fetal–maternal communication system also are accomplished by way of the fetal membranes and uterine decidua vera. In this paracrine arm of the communication system, there is direct cell-to-cell molecular trafficking between fetal and maternal tissues. And today, we also know that fundamental contributions, indeed the driving force in pregnancy, are made by fetal tissues through signal transmission responses that affect maternal tissues by way of the two arms of the fetal–maternal communication system.

PLACENTA AND FETAL MEMBRANES: AN OVERVIEW

Kurt Benirschke (1981) observed: *"The placenta is the most accurate record of the infant's prenatal experiences."* Benirschke goes on to suggest: *"Physicians generally are uncomfortable with the task of examining the placenta. Yet, it is a task they should willingly undertake . . . submitting this organ to a reasonably knowledgeable look and touch can provide much insight into prenatal life; the results are often helpful in caring for the neonate; the findings provide a record pediatricians and obstetricians can use to plan the future care for mother and child; and, most important, much of what can be learned cannot be put into the maternal prenatal history if the information is discarded with the organ."*

Evolution of Knowledge of the Placenta

Boyd and Hamilton (1970) presented a marvelous account of the history of placental research. They observe that the term *placenta* is believed to have been introduced by Realdus Columbus in 1559 when he used the Latin word for a *circular cake*. In 1937, Mossman defined *placenta* as that portion of the fetal membranes that was in apposition with or fused to the uterine mucosa. Historically, however, as pointed out by Boyd and Hamilton, man's knowledge of the *afterbirth* can be traced far into human history.

In the Old Testament, the placenta was considered as the External Soul and was sometimes described as being tied up in the so-called Bundle of Life, which probably included the umbilical cord. It is believed that Aristotle (384–322 B.C.) was the first to use the word *chorion*. It was not, however, until the early 16th century, a time of renaissance of anatomy, that opinions were given concerning the function of the placenta. But even then, as pointed out by Boyd and Hamilton, Leonardo da Vinci (1452–1515) and Vesalius (1514–1564) illustrated the human placenta incorrectly. To his credit, however, Vesalius, in 1555, corrected his error in the second edition of his outstanding book.

The concept of the circulation of blood in the placenta apparently was introduced by Harvey in 1628, but it was John Mayow (1643–1679) who more adequately described the nature of the fetal circulation. It can be appreciated that the endocrine function of the placenta was not recognized until much later because the function of hormones in general must necessarily have preceded such an elucidation. It was not until 1564 that Arantius, by way of careful placenta dissections, discounted the concept that there was continuity between the maternal and fetal vascular systems. Harvey, in 1651, set forth clearly that there was a fetal arterial and venous circulation to the placenta, but it was Malpighi, in 1660, who established the concept of a capillary network as the anatomical basis for the regional circulation. By way of the findings of many celebrated anatomists, there was, by the end of the 17th century, a remarkably accurate concept of the structure and functional significance of the human placenta. The basic idea that there was a *placental barrier* already was formulated clearly in the late 17th or early 18th century. John and William Hunter, around 1750, injected liquid wax into the uterine artery; the wax did not appear in the fetal circulation. This finding finally set aside the notion of anastomosis between maternal and fetal vessels (Ramsey, 1985).

William Hunter, in 1774, is credited with the first accurate description of the decidua and, even then, he distinguished a parietal lining (decidua vera) from a capsular one. Later, in 1821, John Hunter described the decidua basalis. It was probably William and John Hunter, although each claimed credit separately, who accurately described what we now know as the intervillous spaces. It was not until the middle of the 19th century that the true nature of the chorionic villi were appreciated; by 1880, however, the basic knowledge of the nature of blood circulation in the intervillous space was established. In 1882, a notable contribution was made by Langhans, who demonstrated clearly that the villi were covered by two layers of cells. Indeed, it is the inner layer of cells, the cytotrophoblasts, that are referred to as the *Langhans cells*. It was in 1889 that the term *trophoblast* was introduced by Hubrecht to distinguish the portion of blastocyst that does not contribute to the cellular portion of the embryo. The superficial layer of the chorionic villi was eventually demonstrated to be syncytial in nature and is now generally referred to as the syncytiotrophoblast.

DEVELOPMENT OF THE HUMAN PLACENTA

FERTILIZATION

Keith Moore (1973) provides a quote by George W. Corner who may have described it best: *"The fertilization of an egg by a sperm is one of the greatest wonders of nature, an event in which magnificently small fragments of animal life are driven by cosmic forces toward their appointed end, the growth of a living being. As a spectacle it can be compared only with an eclipse of the sun or the eruption of a volcano. . . . It is, in fact, the most common and the nearest to us of nature's cataclysms, and yet it is very seldom observed because it occurs in a realm most people never see, the region of microscopic things."*

We also have been captivated by Richard Blandau's pictorial comparison of the ejaculation of seminal fluid with an atomic explosion; and we have contemplated with him the realism that a population explosion in the world is as devastating as an atomic blast. Few, if any, naturally occurring phenomena are of greater importance to man than the union of egg and sperm. Fertilization of the human egg by a spermatozoan occurs in the fallopian tube within minutes or no more than a few hours after ovulation.

DEFINITIONS (MOORE, 1973)

- *Zygote:* the cell that results from the fertilization of the ovum by a spermatozoan.
- *Blastomeres:* mitotic division of the zygote (cleavage) gives rise to daughter cells called blastomeres.
- *Morula:* the solid ball of cells formed by 16 or so blastomeres.
- *Blastocyst:* after the morula reaches the uterus, a fluid-filled cavity is formed, converting the morula to a blastocyst.
- *Embryo:* the embryo-forming cells, which are grouped as an inner cell mass, give rise to the embryo, which usually is designated when the bilaminar embryonic disc forms. The *embryonic period* extends until the end of the 7th week, at which time the major structures are present.
- *Fetus:* after the embryonic period, the developing conceptus is referred to as the fetus.
- *Conceptus:* this term is used to refer to all products of conception, i.e., embryo (fetus), fetal membranes, and placenta. In particular, the conceptus includes all tissues that develop from the zygote, both embryonic and extraembryonic.

HUMAN EMBRYOLOGY

CLEAVAGE OF THE ZYGOTE

The mature ovum, after fertilization in the fallopian tube, becomes a zygote (a diploid cell with 46 chromosomes), which then undergoes segmentation, or cleavage, into blastomeres.

The first typical mitotic division of the segmentation nucleus of the zygote results in the formation of two blastomeres. In a photomicrograph of a living, segmenting zygote of the monkey (Fig. 4–1), the suspension of blastomeres and polar bodies in the perivitelline fluid, which is surrounded by the zona pellucida, is shown. In a fertilized human ovum (Fig. 4–2), there are similar changes.

Within the fallopian tube, the fertilized ovum undergoes slow cleavage for 3 days; indeed, fertilized human ova that are recovered from the uterine cavity may be comprised of only 12 to 16 blastomeres. As the blastomeres continue to divide, a solid mulberry-like ball of cells, the *morula*, is produced. The morula enters the uterine cavity about 3 days after fertilization of the ovum. The gradual accumulation of fluid within the morula between blastomeres results in formation of the blastocyst, at one pole of which there is a compact mass of cells, the *inner cell mass*, which is destined to produce the embryo (Fig. 4–3), and an outer mass of cells, destined to be the *trophoblasts*.

THE EARLY HUMAN ZYGOTE

In a presumably normal 2-cell zygote that was flushed from the oviduct (Fig. 4–2A), Hertig and co-workers (1954) found that the blastomeres (and a polar body, which was free in the perivitelline fluid) were surrounded by a thick zona pellucida (see fertilized ovum of monkey, Fig. 4–1A). In a 58-cell blastocyst (Fig. 4–2B), the outer cells can be distinguished and these presumably are destined to produce the trophoblast from the inner cells (those that form the embryo). The next stage that was obtained was a 107-cell blastocyst (blastodermic vesicle) that was no larger than the earlier cleavage stages, despite the accumulated fluid (Fig. 4–2C). It measured 0.153×0.155 mm in diameter before fixation and after the disappearance of the zona pellucida. The eight formative (embryo-producing) cells were surrounded by 99 trophoblastic cells. The fertilized "ovum," now a blastocyst, was ready for implantation.

IMPLANTATION

Before implantation, the zona pellucida disappears and the blastocyst adheres to the endometrial surface, the time of *apposition*. After erosion of the epithelium of the endometrium, the blastocyst sinks into and becomes totally encased within the endometrium, i.e., **the blastocyst is completely buried in the endometrium.**

At the time of blastocyst implantation, the invading conceptus is very analogous to a locally invasive tumor, but a very unusual one because it is a semiallogeneic graft. At this time, the innermost trophoblasts, i.e., the trophoblasts contiguous with and invading the endometrium coalesce to become an amorphous, multinucleated membrane, the syncytium (made up of the syncytiotrophoblasts). It is important to recognize, however, that these syncytiotrophoblasts are derived from the inner cytotrophoblasts. This is an important concept, so let us restate it. **Cytotrophoblasts (Langhans cells) are the progenitors of the syncytiotrophoblasts.** At this time, there clearly are two distinguishable layers of trophoblasts. Thus, the syncytiotrophoblasts are contiguous with maternal decidua (and later, maternal blood) whereas the cytotrophoblasts are the innermost (embryonic side) layer and ultimately come to be the cell nearest the intravillous space, in which the fetal capillaries traverse as one conduit of the placental arm of the fetal–maternal communication system.

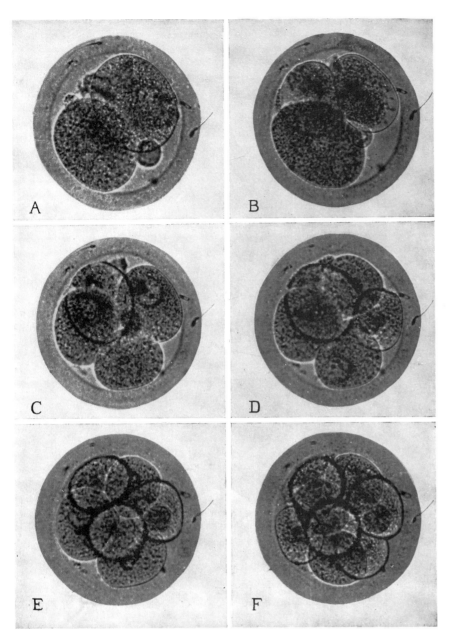

Figure 4–1. Photomicrographs (×300) of living monkey fertilized ovum showing its cleavage divisions. The fertilized ovum was washed out of the tube and cultivated in plasma; its growth changes were recorded cinematographically. The illustrations are enlargements from single frames of the film. **A.** 2-cell stage, 29 hours and 30 minutes after ovulation. **B.** 3-cell stage, 36 hours and 4 minutes after ovulation. **C.** 4-cell stage, 37 hours and 35 minutes after ovulation. **D.** 5-cell stage, 48 hours and 39 minutes after ovulation. **E.** 6-cell stage, 49 hours exactly after ovulation. **F.** 8-cell stage, 48 hours and 48 minutes after ovulation. These cleavages normally occur as the ovum passes down the fallopian tube. Note the spermatozoan in the zona pellucida. (*After Lewis and Hartman: Contrib Embryol 24:187, 1933.*)

Recall again that the entire blastocyst becomes imbedded in the maternal endometrium. Therefore, as the trophoblasts begin to replicate, the entire blastocyst is covered by both trophoblasts and endometrium/decidua. As the developing blastocyst and its surrounding trophoblasts and covering decidua grow, one pole of this mass extends toward the cavity of the uterus and one pole remains buried in the endometrium. The innermost pole ultimately forms the placenta, i.e., the villous trophoblasts, whereas the pole developing toward the endometrial cavity ultimately becomes the *chorion laeve* (the smooth chorion), which is covered by the decidua (capsularis). **In this manner, the fetal tissues of the two arms (placental and paracine) of the fetal–maternal communication system are established.**

With continued growth, the blood supply of the chorion laeve is restricted and the villous nature of this tissue is lost as is the blood supply; ultimately, it becomes the avascular fetal membrane that comes to lie contiguous with the maternal decidua not occupied by the villous trophoblasts—the chorion laeve. The chorion laeve, therefore, is comprised of cytotrophoblasts that survive in a relatively low oxygen atmosphere. The decidua capsularis later comes to be merged with the decidua parietalis—perhaps the decidua capsularis is largely lost by way of pressure and loss of blood supply. This area of the decidua, i.e., where decidua capsularis and decidua parietalis merge is sometimes referred to as the decidua vera.

One of the earliest implantation sites discovered by Hertig and Rock (1944) is shown in Figure 4–4. It measured only 0.36 × 0.31 mm; its discovery was truly a remarkable achievement. The blastocyst shown in Figure 4–4 was believed to be in the process of entering the endometrium, with its thin outer wall still within the uterine cavity. An implanting ovum at a similar stage of development, $7\frac{1}{2}$ days after fertilization is shown

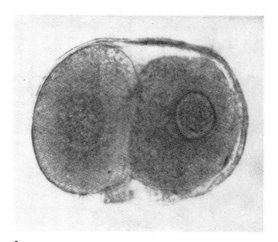

A

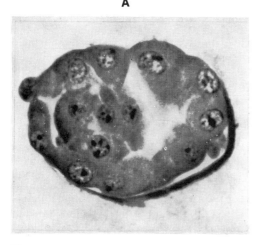

B

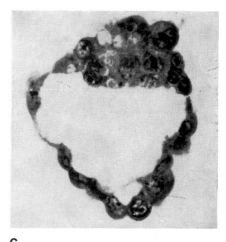

C

Figure 4–2. Human preimplantation stages. **A.** 2-celled stage. Intact fertilized ovum surrounded by zona pellucida, photographed after fixation. Washed from fallopian tube about 1½ days after conception. Nuclei shimmer through granular cytoplasm. Polar body in perivitelline space (Carnegie Collection No. 8698 (×500)). **B.** 58-celled blastula with intact zona pellucida found in uterine cavity 3 to 4 days after conception. Thin section showing outer (probably trophoblastic) and inner (embryo-forming) cells and beginning segmentation cavity (Carnegie Collection No. 8794 (×600)). **C.** 107-celled blastocyst found free in uterine cavity about 5 days after conception. A shell of trophoblastic cells enveloping fluid-filled blastocele and inner mass consisting of embryo-forming cells. (Carnegie Collection No. 8663 (×600)). (*From Hertig and associates: Contrib Embryol 35:199, 1954.*)

in Figure 4–5. It appears to have been flattened in the process of penetrating the uterine epithelium; the enlargement and multiplication of the trophoblastic cells in contact with the endometrium alone are responsible for the increase in size of the implanted blastocyst as compared with the free one. The hole in the uterine epithelium that is created by the fertilized ovum 9 days after fertilization (Fig. 4–6), as it implants, is indicative of the size of the zygote at the time of erosion of the surface. The defect is bounded by a zone of maternal endometrial epithelium that became shriveled as the trophoblast spread out beneath it. When correction was made for the additional artifactual shrinkage, which results from preparation of the histological sections, the diameter of the fertilized ovum at the moment of implantation was estimated to be 0.23 mm.

According to Hertig and Rock, implantation of the human blastocyst takes place 6 days after fertilization of the ovum. Although little is known of the fundamental nature of implantation in the human, some information (based primarily on findings of studies of lower species) is available. As the blasto-

cyst contacts the endometrium, syncytiotrophoblast is differentiated from cytotrophoblast. Development of syncytiotrophoblast undoubtedly is a major factor in the successful invasion of the endometrium, possibly involving trophoblast production of serine proteases, e.g., plasminogen activator. In the human, a full decidual response in endometrium is not elicited until the trophoblast has eroded the superficial uterine epithelium.

Whereas, in the human, the free blastocystic period (fertilization to apposition) is 4 to 6 days, in some species, there is a *developmental diapause,* or delayed implantation, during which time the blastocysts may remain unattached for much longer intervals (6 months or more in the pine marten).

Free blastocysts that were recovered from the uterus of the cow and the sheep and kept frozen in liquid nitrogen for up to 3 weeks have been implanted successfully in recipient animals to produce normal offspring. Human ova have been fertilized in vitro and many successful pregnancies have been reported since the original one in 1978 by Steptoe and Edwards (Chap. 41).

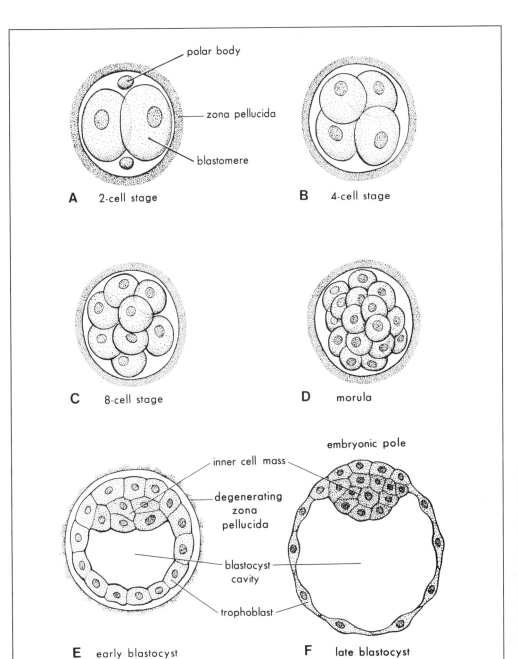

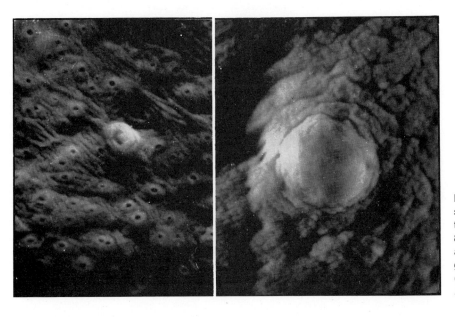

Figure 4–3. Cleavage of the zygote and formation of the blastocyst. **A** to **D** show various stages of cleavage. The period of the morula begins at the 12- to 16-cell stage and ends when the blastocyst forms, which occurs when there are 50 to 60 blastomeres present. **E** and **F** are sections of blastocysts. The zona pellucida has disappeared by the late blastocyst stage (5 days). The polar bodies shown in **A** are small, nonfunctional cells that soon degenerate. (*From Moore: The Developing Human, 3rd ed. Philadelphia, Saunders, 1982.*)

Figure 4–4. Low- and high-power photographs of surface view of an early human implantation obtained on day 22 of the menstrual cycle, less than 8 days after conception. Site was slightly elevated and measured 0.36 × 0.31 mm. Mouths of uterine glands appear as dark spots surrounded by halos. (Carnegie Collection No. 8225.) (*From Hertig and Rock: Am J Obstet Gynecol 47:149, 1944.*)

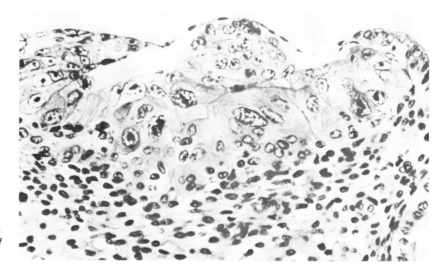

Figure 4–5. An implanting human blastocyst 7½ days after fertilization. (*From Potter and Craig: Pathology of the Fetus and the Infant. Chicago, Year Book, 1975.*)

EARLY TROPHOBLASTS

In the description of the earliest stages of the human blastocyst, the wall of the primitive blastodermic vesicle was defined as consisting of a single layer of ectoderm (Fig. 4–2). As early as 72 hours after fertilization, Hertig (1962) observed that the 58-cell blastula had differentiated into 5 embryo-producing cells and 53 cells destined to form trophoblasts. Although trophoblasts have not been identified before implantation of the blastocyst, both cellular and syncytial trophoblast are identifiable in the earliest implanted blastocyst of the monkey. Indeed, evidence has been presented that the elaboration of human chorionic gonadotropin (hCG) by blastocyst may precede implantation. Soon after implantation, the trophoblasts proliferate rapidly and invade the surrounding decidua. In invasive and cytolytic behavior, in histologically characteristic cytoplasmic vacuolization, and in ultrastructure, the early trophoblasts resemble choriocarcinoma (see Chap. 31, p. 542). And, it seems reasonably clear that the impetus for implantation-invasion is provided by products of the blastocyst.

As invasion of the endometrium by trophoblasts proceeds, maternal blood vessels are tapped to form lacunae, which are soon filled with maternal blood. To understand the nature of human placentation, it is imperative that we recognize the importance of the human type of placentation, i.e., **hemochorioendothelial.** The "hemo" refers to maternal blood, which bathes the syncytiotrophoblasts (chorio), which in turn, are separated from fetal blood by the wall of the capillaries (endothelial) of the fetus in the intravillous space. This is not true of all species, but it is a consideration of signal importance in the human. Maternal blood bathes the syncytiotrophoblasts directly; but, the fetal blood is separated from the trophoblasts by the endothelium of the fetal capillaries in the intravillous space. This arrangement is illustrated in Figures 4–7 and 4–8. As the lacunae join, a complicated labyrinth is formed that is partitioned by solid trophoblastic columns. The trophoblast-lined labyrinthine channels and the solid cellular columns form the intervillous space and primary villous stalks, respectively.

Much of our knowledge of the formation of the intervillous

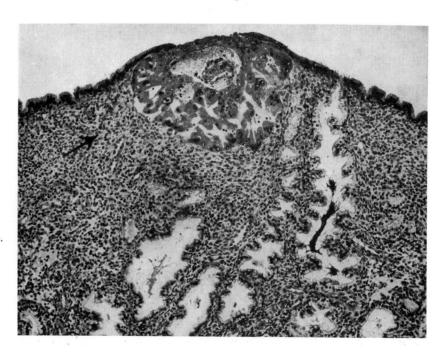

Figure 4–6. A thin section of fertilized ovum obtained on 25th day of cycle, 9½ days or less after fertilization. Area still exposed to uterine lumen as in Figure 4–9. Syncytiotrophoblasts, a complex network fills enlarged implantation site. Within cytotrophoblastic shell, two-layered embryo and amnion-forming cells. Arrow is pointed to zone of enlarged stromal cells. Photomicrograph × 100. (Carnegie Collection No. 8004.) (*From Hertig and Rock: Contrib Embryol 31:65, 1945.*)

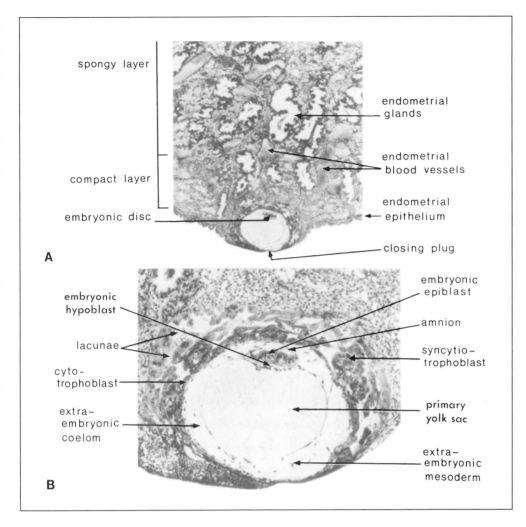

spongy layer

compact layer

embryonic disc

endometrial glands

endometrial blood vessels

endometrial epithelium

closing plug

A

embryonic hypoblast

lacunae

cyto-trophoblast

extra-embryonic coelom

B

embryonic epiblast

amnion

syncytio-trophoblast

primary yolk sac

extra-embryonic mesoderm

Figure 4–7. A. Section through the implantation site of a human embryo 12 days after fertilization. The embryo is embedded in the compact layer of endometrium ($\times 30$). **B.** Higher magnification of the conceptus and surrounding endometrium ($\times 100$). (*From Hertig and Rock: Contrib Embryol 29:127, 1941. Courtesy of Carnegie Institution of Washington, as modified by Moore: The Developing Human, 2nd ed. Philadelphia, Saunders, 1977.*)

space of both the human and the macaque is based on the findings of the classic studies of Wislocki and Streeter (1938). **Maternal blood enters the intervillous space from the spiral arterioles in fountain-like bursts; thus, maternal blood sweeps over and bathes the syncytiotrophoblasts directly.** The maternal surface of these trophoblasts consists of a complex microvillous structure. And during pregnancy, there is continual shedding and reformation of the microvilli.

DEVELOPMENT OF EMBRYO AFTER IMPLANTATION

At 7½ days of development, the stage shown in Figure 4–5, the wall of the blastocyst that faces the uterine lumen consists of a single layer of flattened cells, whereas the thicker opposite wall is comprised of two zones–the trophoblast and the embryo-forming inner cell mass. In maternal tissues that are in contact with trophoblast, signs of injury are apparent; the decidua, immediately adjacent, appears to be condensed, perhaps as a result of withdrawal of water by the invading trophoblast. Among the trophoblast, two subdivisions of cells are distinguishable, the *cytotrophoblast,* which is comprised of individual cells with relatively pale-staining cytoplasm, and the *syncytiotrophoblast,* in which dark-staining nuclei are distributed irregularly within a common basophilic cytoplasm. In the trophoblast, mitotic figures are confined to the cellular (cytotrophoblast) ele-

ments. As early as 7½ days after fertilization, the inner cell mass, now called the *embryonic disc,* already is differentiated into a thick plate of primitive ectoderm and an underlying layer of endoderm. Between the embryonic disc and the trophoblast, some small cells appear that soon enclose a space that will become the amnionic cavity.

To illustrate the next stage of development, a thin section of the 9½-day fertilized ovum (Fig. 4–6) is shown; the increase in size is principally the result of development of the syncytium, which comprises a complex network of protoplasmic strands that enclose irregular fluid-filled spaces, the *lacunae,* which later become confluent. The embryonic disc now consists of a "dorsal" ectoderm, which is made up of tall columnar cells, and a "ventral" endoderm, which is formed of somewhat irregular cells. The remainder of the blastocyst is occupied by a proteinaceous coagulum, which is limited externally by a layer of flattened cells (the *exocelomic,* or *Heuser membrane*), the origin of which is uncertain. The amnionic cavity dorsal to the embryonic disc is now well defined. With regard to the amnion, it seems reasonable that at least the epithelium is delaminated from the trophoblast. There is no convincing evidence that the inner-cell mass produces any of the extraembryonic mesoderm.

As the embryo enlarges, more maternal tissue is destroyed and the walls of the capillaries thereof are eroded; the result is that maternal blood enters the lacunae. With deeper burrowing

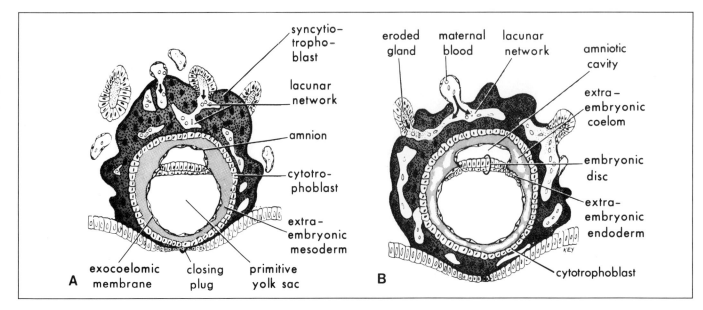

Figure 4–8. Drawings of sections through implanted blastocysts. **A.** 10 days. **B.** 12 days after fertilization. This stage of development is characterized by the intercommunication of the lacunae filled with maternal blood. Note in **B** that large cavities have appeared in the extraembryonic mesoderm, forming the beginning of the extraembryonic coelom. Also note that extraembryonic endodermal cells have begun to form on the inside of the primary yolk sac. (*From Moore: The Developing Human, 2nd ed. Philadelphia, Saunders, 1977.*)

and invasion of the blastocyst into the decidua, the trophoblastic strands branch to form the solid primitive villi that traverse the lacunae. Originally located over the entire surface of the blastocyst, the villi later disappear except over the most deeply implanted portion, i.e., the site destined to form the placenta. The mesenchyme first appears as isolated cells within the cavity of the fertilized ovum. When the cavity is lined completely with mesoderm, it is termed the *chorionic vesicle*, and its membrane, now called the *chorion*, is composed of trophoblasts and mesenchyme.

In the 12-day embryo, as shown in Figure 4–7, the diameter is almost 1 mm. The mesenchymal cells within the cavity are most numerous about the embryo, where these condense, eventually, to form the *body stalk* that serves to join the embryo to the nutrient chorion and later develops into the umbilical cord. Thereafter, the site of entry of the blastocyst into the endometrium is covered by regenerated epithelium. The defect per se is plugged by fibrin and cellular debris.

The syncytiotrophoblast of the chorionic shell is permeated by a system of intercommunicating channels of trophoblastic lacunae that contain maternal blood. At the same time, in the surrounding endometrial stroma, a decidual reaction develops that is characterized by enlargement of the endometrial stromal cells and storage therein of glycogen. The amnionic cavity then is lined by ectoderm, which apparently is contiguous with that of the embryonic disc. At this stage, the endoderm probably delaminates from the inferior surface of the embryonic disc and soon spreads peripherally beyond the disc to line the blastocoele; this process results in the formation of the yolk sac. The remainder of the blastocyst is filled with primary mesoderm, which consists of sparse mesenchymal cells in a loose matrix. It is believed that the mesoderm arises from the trophoblast, but its precise mode of origin in the human remains to be elucidated.

THE GERM LAYERS

In Figures 4–8 and 4–9, the amnion and yolk sac, with both epithelial and mesenchymal components, are illustrated. The body stalk, from which the caudal end of the embryo arises, also can be recognized at this stage. Cellular proliferation in the embryonic disc marks the beginning of a thickening in the midline that clearly is indicative of the embryonic axis and is called the *primitive streak*. Cells spread out laterally from the primitive streak between ectoderm and endoderm to form the mesoderm. These three germ layers give rise to the various organs of the developing embryo. From the *ectoderm* are derived the entire nervous system, central and peripheral, and the epidermis, with such derivatives as the crystalline lens and the hair. The *endoderm* develops into the lining of the gastrointestinal tract, from pharynx to rectum, and such derivative organs as the liver, pancreas, and thyroid. The dermis, the skeleton, the connective tissues, the vascular and urogenital systems, and most skeletal and smooth muscles arise from the *mesoderm*. The cavity that later divides the somatic and visceral sheets of intraembryonic mesoderm is the *coelom*.

FORMATION OF THE SOMITES

During the 3rd week after fertilization (5th week of gestation), the primitive streak becomes a prominent structure and the cephalic and caudal ends of the embryo become distinguishable. As cells proliferate rapidly and spread laterally from the primitive streak, a midline *primitive groove* develops. Simultaneously, the yolk sac enlarges, and hence, the embryonic disc is spread out upon it. In Figure 4–9, there is shown a well-defined body stalk into which a narrow endodermal diverticulum, the allantois, has extended. In many mammals, the allantois develops into a large sac that vascularizes the chorion. A forward extension of the primitive streak, the *notochord* (Fig. 4–10), con-

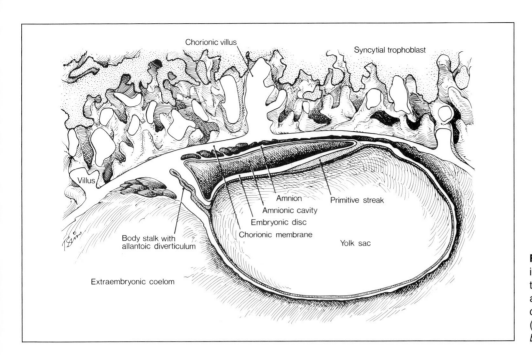

Figure 4–9. Median view of a drawing of a wax reconstruction of Mateer fertilized ovum, showing the amnionic cavity and its relations to chorionic membrane and yolk sac (×50). (*After Streeter: Contrib Embryol 9:389, 1920.*)

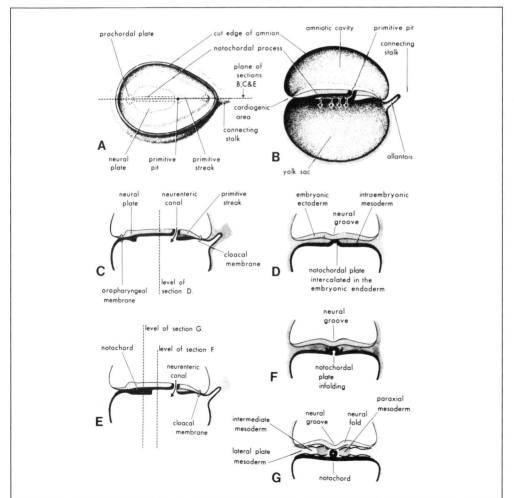

Figure 4–10. Drawings illustrating final stages of notochord development. **A.** Dorsal view of the embryonic disc at about 18 days, exposed by removing the amnion. **B.** Three-dimensional sagittal section of the embryo. **C** and **E.** Sagittal sections of embryos of about 18 to 19 days. **D, F,** and **G.** Transverse sections of the embryonic disc. (*From Moore: The Developing Human, 3rd ed. Philadelphia, Saunders, 1982.*)

stitutes the primordial supporting structure of vertebrates and remains as a continuous column of cells throughout embryonic life. Remnants of the notochord persist in the adult as the nucleus pulposus of the intervertebral discs.

Because differentiation of structures proceeds from cephalic to caudal ends in a sequence characteristic of all vertebrate embryos, most of the substance of the early embryo will enter into formation of the head; the subsequent development of the primitive streak provides material for the rest of the body. Soon, a *neural groove* develops as neural folds arise on either side. The cavity of the future neural tube is connected with the future lumen of the gut by the *neurenteric canal*. As the neural folds develop, the underlying lateral mesoderm is divided into discrete blocks, the *somites* which give rise to the skeletal and connective tissues, the muscles, and the dermis. The first three of four somites enter into formation of the occipital region of the head. The primordium of the heart already has appeared beneath the pharynx and is separated from the yolk sac by a fold that also lifts the cephalic end of the embryo above the level of the yolk sac. In Figure 4–11 (A to E), the elevation of the neural folds is shown as is the closure of these folds to form a tube, which is wider from the outset in the region of the fourth pair of somites. Although the head remains relatively enormous during the embryonic period, the rest of the body takes form after the 4th week, and the head becomes smaller in proportion. By the 7th week after fertilization, the neck can be recognized, the tail filament has disappeared, and the embryo can be identified as human. From the 8th week after fertilization, changes in the shape of the human fetus are less striking. Some of the principal features are presented in Chapter 6.

BIOLOGY OF THE TROPHOBLAST

ORIGIN OF THE SYNCYTIOTROPHOBLAST

Of all placental components, the trophoblast is the most variable in structure, function, and development. Its invasiveness pro-

vides for attachment of the blastocyst to the uterus; its role in nutrition of the conceptus is reflected in its name; and its function as an endocrine organ is essential to the physiological adaptation of the maternal organism to pregnancy. Morphologically, the trophoblast may be cellular or syncytial and it may appear as uninuclear cells or multinuclear giant cells. The true syncytial character of the human syncytiotrophoblast (syncytium) has been confirmed by electron microscopy. The mechanism of growth of the syncytium, however, was a mystery, in view of the discrepancy between an increase in the number of nuclei in the syncytiotrophoblast and only equivocal evidence of intrinsic nuclear replication. Mitotic figures are completely absent from the syncytium, being confined to the cytotrophoblast.

Richart (1961) found early incorporation of triticated thymidine in the cytotrophoblast but not in the syncytium. Midgley and co-workers (1963) subsequently extended the idea that syncytial cells are derived from cytotrophoblasts by demonstrating that although tritiated thymidine appeared at first only in the nuclei of the cytotrophoblast, the label could be detected 22 hours later in the syncytiotrophoblast, indicating that the syncytium is derived from cytotrophoblast and is itself a mitotic end-stage.

Galton (1962) concluded that the rapid accumulation of nuclei in the syncytiotrophoblast is explained by cellular proliferation within the cytotrophoblast, followed by a coalescence of daughter cells in the syncytium. It now seems reasonably clear that the cytotrophoblast is the germinal cell and the syncytium, the secretory cells, are derived from the cytotrophoblasts. Each cytotrophoblast is characterized as a single cell with well-demarcated borders, a single, distinct nucleus, and frequent mitosis. These characteristics are lacking, however, in syncytium, in which the cytoplasm is amorphous, lacking cell borders—nuclei are multiple and diverse in size and shape (Ramsey, 1985).

Strauss and co-workers, in an elegant series of studies, have demonstrated the in vitro conversion of cytotrophoblasts to morphologically and functionally characteristic syncytial cells; and,

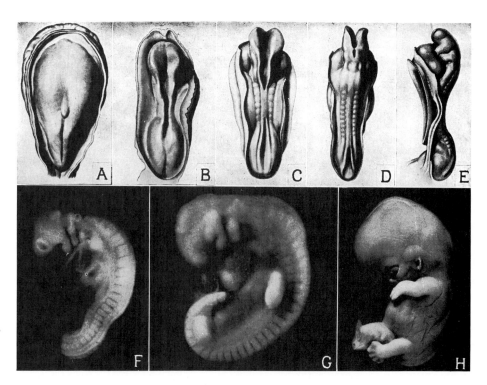

Figure 4–11. Human embryogenesis. **A.** Heuser, ×30, 19 days. **B.** Ingalls, ×28. **C.** Payne, ×23. **D.** Corner, ×23. **E.** Atwell, ×15.5, 21 to 22 days. **F.** ×12, 4th week. **G.** ×8.5, 5th week. **H.** ×2.5, 8th week. (Carnegie Collection) (*From Streeter: Sci Monthly 32:495, 1931.*)

they have shown that at least a part of this differentiation process involves the action of cyclic AMP. They also present a model for the formation of syncytiotrophoblasts in which it is envisioned that isolated cytotrophoblasts migrate toward each other to form aggregates. The aggregates fuse to form syncytiotrophoblasts (Kliman and colleagues, 1986; Ulloa-Aguirre, 1987).

TROPHOBLAST ULTRASTRUCTURE

From the electron microscopic studies of Wislocki and Dempsey (1955), basic data were provided upon which the functional interpretation of the fine structure of the placenta is based. The prominent microvilli of the syncytial surface, corresponding to the so-called brush border of light microscopy, and the associated pinocytotic vacuoles and vesicles are related to the absorptive and secretory functions of the placenta. The cytotrophoblasts, which persist to term although often compressed against the trophoblastic basal lamina, retain their ultrastructural simplicity. There are few specialized organelles in these cells, with abundant free ribosomes but scant ergastoplasm. Desmosomes connect individual cytotrophoblast cells with one another and with the syncytium, from which complete plasma membranes are absent. The syncytium is, ultrastructurally, relatively complex, containing abundant endoplasmic reticulum, Golgi bodies, and mitochondria, as well as numerous secretory droplets, lipid granules, and highly convoluted plasma membranes. As the syncytium matures, the fine structural changes are reflective of functional maturation. Early syncytiotrophoblast often exhibits a microvesicular endoplasmic reticulum; later, at the height of active synthesis of proteins, flattened ergastoplasmic channels assume prominence; and still later, associated with storage and transport of proteins, there appear dilated cisternae of endoplasmic reticulum, the largest of which are visible with the light microscope. Secretory granules, at least those believed to be glycoproteins and osmiophilic lipid granules, correspond to PAS-positive and sudanophilic droplets, respectively (Figs. 4–12 to 4–14).

As the placenta matures, the collagen-rich stromal connective tissue decreases, as do the numbers of fibroblasts and Hofbauer cells. The human placental membrane may be reduced, anatomically, to a thin covering of trophoblast, capillary endothelium, and trophoblastic and endothelial basement membranes separated by mere wisps of connective tissue. Although at term, there is focal villous degeneration, morphological evidence of activity in all layers persists. Because not only the trophoblast but the endothelium and even the basal laminas may show evidence of pinocytosis and other metabolic activity, it is hardly reasonable to equate the number of layers in the histological "barrier" with the functional efficiency of the placenta. Reduction of the number of layers may result in more rapid transplacental passage of substances to which the laws governing simple diffusion apply, but selected substances regulated by "carrier systems" are not proportionally affected. As for pinocytosis, a virtually continuous system of vesicles and vacuoles may be found extending from the syncytial surface to the capillary endothelium. Boyd and co-workers (1968) described a direct connection of some of these vacuoles with the perinuclear space, which receives tubular communications with the endoplasmic reticulum.

The term *barrier* as applied to placental physiology should therefore be replaced by the more accurate term *placental membrane*. The number of layers, furthermore, is a poor index of the true approximation of the circulations; for example, in the 6-layered epitheliochorial placenta of the pig, the indentation of

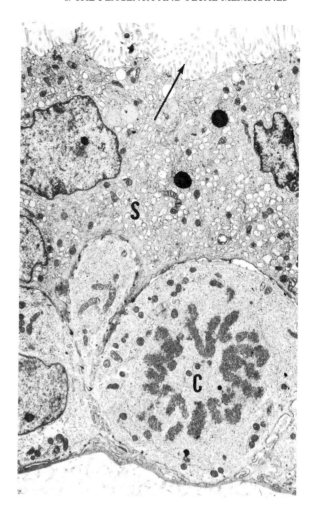

Figure 4–12. Electron micrograph of human placenta at 6 weeks gestation. Note prominent border of microvilli (arrow), syncytium (S), and mitotic figure in cytotrophoblast (C). (*Courtesy of Dr. Ralph M. Wynn.*)

both fetal and maternal epithelium by the respective capillaries results in a rather close vascular relation.

ORGANIZATION OF PLACENTA

CHORIONIC VILLI

Villi can first be distinguished easily in the human placenta on about the 12th day after fertilization. When the solid trophoblast is invaded by a mesenchymal cord, presumably derived from cytotrophoblast, secondary villi are formed. After angiogenesis occurs in situ from the mesenchymal cores, the resulting villi are termed *tertiary*. Maternal venous sinuses are tapped early, but until the 14th or 15th day after fertilization, maternal arterial blood does not enter the intervillous space. By about the 17th day, both fetal and maternal blood vessels are functional and a placental circulation is established. The fetal-placental circulation is completed when the blood vessels of the embryo are connected with chorionic blood vessels, which likely are formed in situ from cytotrophoblast. Some villi, in which absence of angiogenesis results in a lack of circulation, may distend with fluid and form vesicles. A striking exaggeration of this process is present in the development of hydatidiform mole (see Chap. 31, p. 541).

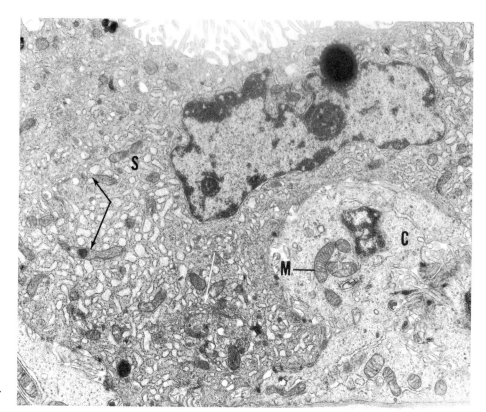

Figure 4–13. First-trimester human placenta, showing well-differentiated syncytiotrophoblast (S) with numerous mitochondria (black arrows) and Golgi complexes (white arrow). Cytotrophoblast (C) has large mitochondria (M) but few other organelles. (*Courtesy of Dr. Ralph M. Wynn.*)

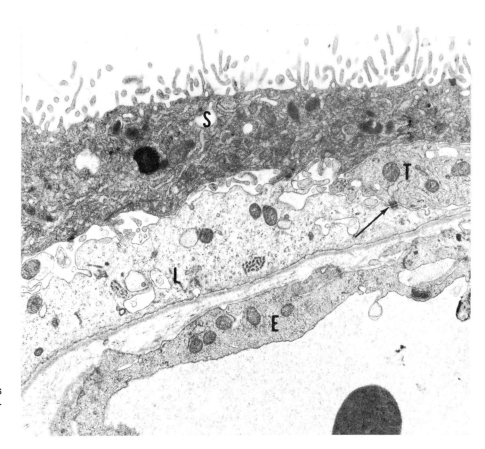

Figure 4–14. Term human placenta showing electron-dense syncytium (S), Langhans cells (L), transitional cytotrophoblast (T), and capillary endothelium (E). Arrow points to desmosome. (*Courtesy of Dr. Ralph M. Wynn.*)

Proliferation of cellular trophoblast at the tips of the villi produces the trophoblastic cell columns, which are not invaded by mesenchyme but are anchored to the decidua at the basal plate. Thus, the floor of the intervillous space (maternal side) consists of cytotrophoblast from the cell columns, peripheral syncytium of the trophoblastic shell, and decidua of the basal plate. The chorionic plate, consisting of the two trophoblasts externally and fibrous mesoderm internally, forms the roof of the intervillous space.

Between the 18th and 19th days of development, the blastocyst (including the chorionic shell) measures 6 × 2.5 mm in diameter. At this time, the embryo is in the primitive-streak stage with a maximal length of 0.6 to 0.7 mm. The trophoblastic shell is thick, with villi formed of cytotrophoblastic projections, a central core of chorionic mesoderm in which blood vessels are developing, and an external covering of syncytiotrophoblast, or syncytium. At this time, the blastocyst lies buried in the decidua and is separated from the myometrium by the decidua basalis and from the uterine epithelium by the decidua capsularis. The embryo itself is trilaminar, and its endoderm is continuous with the lining of the yolk sac. An intermediate layer of intraembryonic mesoderm can be traced and found to be contiguous with the extraembryonic mesoderm, which later forms part of the walls of the amnion and yolk sac and connects the embryonic structures to the chorionic mesoderm by the body stalk, or abdominal pedicle, the forerunner of the umbilical cord. At this stage, the secondary or definitive yolk sac is completely lined by endoderm. External to the yolk sac, the fluid-filled exocelomic cavity is found, the early formation of which prevents approximation of the yolk sac and trophoblasts in man, and hence precludes formation of a choriovitelline placenta.

By about 3 weeks after fertilization, the relations of chorion to decidua are clearly evident in the human embryo. The chorionic membrane consists of an inner connective tissue layer and an outer epithelium from which rudimentary villi project. The connective tissue consists of spindly cells with protoplasmic processes within a loose intercellular matrix. The trophoblast differentiates into cuboidal or nearly round cells with clear cytoplasm and light-staining vesicular nuclei (cytotrophoblast or Langhans cells) and an outer syncytium containing irregularly

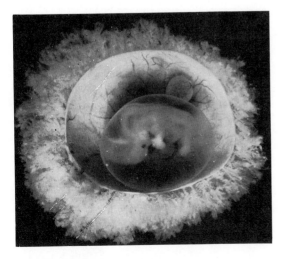

Figure 4–15. Human chorionic vesicle. Ovulatory age, 40 days. (Carnegie Collection No. 8537.)

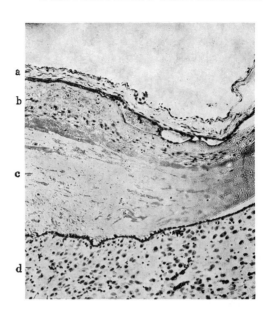

Figure 4–16. Unfused decidua vera and capsularis. Section through uterus at 10 weeks gestation, showing that the decidua vera and capsularis have not yet fused. a = amnion chorionic membrane; b = degenerating decidua capsularis; c = uterine cavity; d = decidua vera.

scattered, dark-staining nuclei within a coarsely granulated cytoplasm (syncytiotrophoblast).

In early pregnancy, the villi are distributed over the entire periphery of the chorionic membrane; grossly, an ovum dislodged from the endometrium at this stage of development appears shaggy (Fig. 4–15). The villi in contact with the decidua basalis proliferate to form the leafy chorion, or *chorion frondosum*, the fetal component of the placenta, whereas those in contact with the decidua capsularis cease to grow and undergo almost complete degeneration, the *chorion laeve*. The greater part of the chorion, thus denuded of villi, is designated the smooth, or bald, chorion or the chorion laeve. It is formed, according to Hertig (1962), as the result of a combination of direct pressure and interference with its vascular supply. The chorion laeve is more nearly opaque generally than the amnion even though rarely exceeding 1 mm in thickness. The chorion laeve contains ghost villi and, clinging to its surface, a few shreds of decidua. Until near the end of the 3rd month, the chorion laeve remains separated from the amnion by the exocelomic cavity. Thereafter the amnion and chorion are in intimate contact (Fig. 4–16). **In the human, the chorion laeve and amnion form an avascular amniochorion which, nevertheless, is an important site of transfer and metabolic activity.** The chorion laeve is the fetal tissue of the interface of the paracrine arm of the fetal–maternal communication system.

PLACENTAL COTYLEDONS

Certain villi of the chorion frondosum extend from the chorionic plate to the decidua and serve as anchoring villi. Most villi, however, arboresce and end freely in the intervillous space without reaching the decidua (Fig. 4–17). As the placenta matures, the short, thick, early stem villi branch repeatedly, forming progressively finer subdivisions and greater numbers of increasingly small villi (Fig. 4–18). Each of the main stem villi and its ramifications constitute a placental cotyledon, the fetal tissue interface of the placental arm of the fetal–maternal communication system.

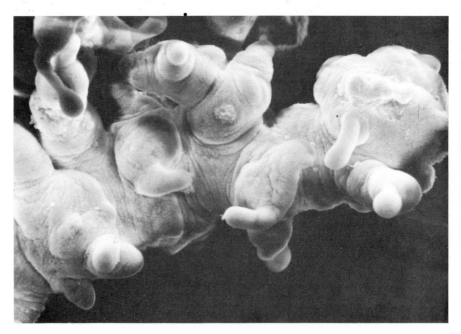

Figure 4–17. Scanning electron micrograph of the placental villi at 10 to 14 weeks gestation. Note the larger stem villi and the small syncytial sprouts at various stages of formation. Furrows or creases on the surface are also evident, especially at the bases of larger villi (× 289). (*From King and Menton: Am J Obstet Gynecol 122:824, 1975.*)

PLACENTAL SEPTA

The origin and exact composition of the placental septa continue to stimulate controversy. These appear to consist of decidual tissue in which trophoblastic elements are encased and thus are very likely of dual origin, i.e., fetal and maternal. Especially recommended for an elegant pictorial description of human placentation is Boyd and Hamilton's extensively illustrated treatise, *The Human Placenta* (1970).

PLACENTAL SIZE AND WEIGHT

The data obtained from weighing the placenta vary considerably, depending upon how the placenta is prepared. If membranes and most of the cord are left attached and adherent maternal blood clot is not removed, the weight is increased by nearly 50 percent (Thomson and co-workers, 1969). Crawford (1959) suggested that the total number of cotyledons remains the same throughout gestation, but individual cotyledons continue to grow until term, although less actively in the final weeks.

PLACENTAL AGING

As the villi continue to branch and the terminal ramifications become more numerous and smaller, the volume and prominence of cytotrophoblast (Langhans cells) in the villi decrease, although cytotrophoblast remains obvious in the placental floor. As the syncytium thins and forms knots, the vessels become more prominent and lie closer to the surface. The stroma of the villi also exhibits changes associated with aging. In placentas of early pregnancy, the branching connective tissue cells are separated by an abundant loose intercellular matrix; later the stroma becomes denser, and the cells more spindly and more closely packed. Another change in the stroma involves the so-called *Hofbauer cells*, still of somewhat uncertain nature, origin, and significance. These are nearly round cells with vesicular, often eccentric nuclei and very granular or vacuolated cytoplasm. These cells are characterized, histochemically, by intracytoplasmic lipid and are readily distinguished from plasma cells.

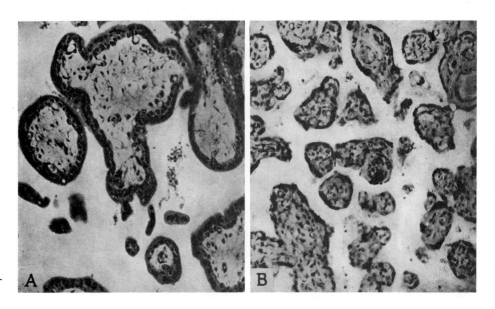

Figure 4–18. Comparison of chorionic villi in early and late pregnancy. **A.** 2-months gestation. Note inner Langhans cells and outer syncytial layer. **B.** Term placenta. Syncytial layer is obvious, but Langhans cells are difficult to recognize at low magnification in light micrographs.

As the placenta grows and ages, certain of the accompanying histological changes are suggestive of an increase in the efficiency of transport to meet the metabolic requirements of the growing fetus. Such changes involve a decrease in thickness of the syncytium, partial disappearance of Langhans cells, decrease in the stroma, and an increase in the number of capillaries and their approximation to the syncytial surface. By 4 months, the apparent continuity of the cytotrophoblast is broken, and the syncytium forms knots on the more numerous, smaller villi. At term, the villous covering may be focally reduced to a thin layer of syncytium with minimal connective tissue with fetal capillaries that apparently abut the trophoblast. The villous stroma, Hofbauer cells, and Langhans cells are markedly reduced, and the villi appear filled with thin-walled capillaries. Other changes, however, appear to decrease the efficiency for placental exchange, as, for example, the thickening of basement membranes of endothelium and trophoblast, obliteration of certain vessels, deposition of fibrin on the surface of the villi, and deposits of fibrin in the basal and chorionic plates and elsewhere in the intervillous space.

THE DECIDUA

DECIDUAL REACTION

The decidua is the endometrium of pregnancy and is so named because much of it is shed after parturition. The decidual reaction encompasses the changes that begin in response to progesterone produced after ovulation and prepare the endometrium for implantation and nutrition of the blastocyst (Chap. 3, p. 35). In human pregnancy, the decidual reaction is not completed until several days after nidation. It commences first around maternal blood vessels, spreading in waves throughout the mucosa of the uterus. During development of the decidua, the endometrial stromal cells enlarge and form polygonal or round *decidual cells.* The nuclei become round and vesicular, and the cytoplasm becomes clear, slightly basophilic, and surrounded by a translucent membrane.

During pregnancy, the decidua thickens, eventually attaining a depth of 5 to 10 mm. With a magnifying glass, furrows and numerous small openings, representing the mouths of uterine glands, can be detected. The portion of the decidua directly beneath the site of implantation forms the *decidua basalis;* that overlying the developing ovum and separating it from the rest of the uterine cavity is the *decidua capsularis* (Figs. 4–19 and 4–20). The remainder of the uterus is lined by *decidua vera,* or *decidua parietalis.*

There is a space between the decidua capsularis and the decidua vera because the gestational sac does not fill the entire uterine cavity during the early months of pregnancy. By the 4th month, the growing sac fills the uterine cavity; and with fusion of the capsularis and vera, the uterine cavity is obliterated. The decidua capsularis is most prominent about the 2nd month of pregnancy, consisting of decidual cells covered by a single layer of flattened epithelial cells without traces of glands; internally, it contacts the chorion laeve.

The decidua vera and the decidua basalis each are composed of three layers: a surface, or compact zone (*zona compacta*); a middle portion, or spongy zone (*zona spongiosa*) with glands and numerous small blood vessels; and a basal zone (*zona basalis*). The compacta and the spongiosa together form the functional zone (*zona functionalis*). The basal zone remains after delivery and gives rise to new endometrium. As pregnancy advances, the glandular epithelium of the decidua vera changes from a cylindrical to a cuboidal or flattened form, at times even resembling endometrium. After the 4th month, because of uterine distension, the decidua vera gradually thins from its maximal height of 1 cm in the first trimester to only 1 or 2 mm at term.

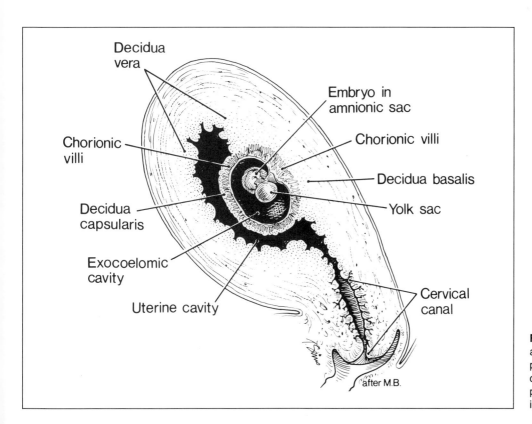

Figure 4–19. Chorion frondosum and chorion laeve of early pregnancy. Three portions of the decidua (basalis, capsularis, and parietalis, or vera) are also illustrated.

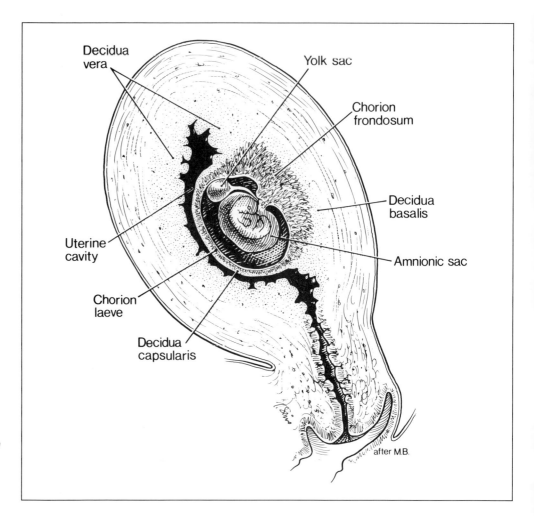

Figure 4–20. More advanced stage of pregnancy, showing atrophic chorion laeve and chorion frondosum (chorionic villi) proliferating into decidua basalis.

HISTOLOGY

The compact layer of the decidua consists of large, closely packed, epithelioid, polygonal, lightly staining cells with round vesicular nuclei (Fig. 4–21). Many stroma cells appear stellate, particularly when the decidua is edematous, with long protoplasmic processes that anastomose with those of adjacent cells. Numerous small round cells, which contain very little cytoplasm, are scattered among typical decidual cells, especially early in pregnancy. Formerly considered to be lymphocytes, these cells are now regarded as precursors of new decidual elements. In the early months of pregnancy, ducts of uterine glands are found in the decidua compacta, but these become less obvious in late pregnancy. Beginning during the late secretory phase of the ovarian cycle, a pericellular basement membrane develops around each large decidual cell. Indeed, each cell is walled-off from the other (Chap. 3, p. 35).

The spongy layer of the decidua consists of large distended glands, often exhibiting marked hyperplasia but separated by minimal stroma. At first, the glands are lined by typical cylindrical uterine epithelium with abundant secretory activity. Presumably the glandular secretion contributes to the nourishment of the ovum during its histotrophic phase, before the establishment of a placental circulation. The epithelium gradually becomes cuboidal or even flattened, later degenerating and sloughing to a greater extent into the lumens of the glands. The stroma of the spongy zone undergoes little change.

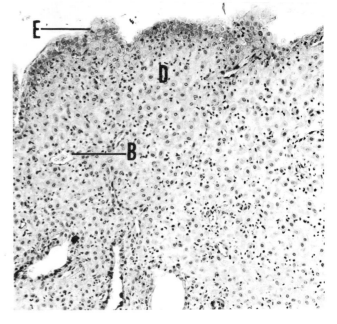

Figure 4–21. Photomicrograph of decidua vera (parietalis) in which epithelium (E), decidualized stromal cells (D), and blood vessels (B) are shown. (*Courtesy of Dr. Ralph M. Wynn.*)

From the basal zone of the decidua vera (not to be confused with decidua basalis) some of the endometrium regenerates during the puerperium. In comparing the decidua vera at 4 months gestation with the early proliferative endometrium of the uterus of nonpregnant women, it is clear that during decidual transformation of the endometrial stroma, there is marked hypertrophy but only slight hyperplasia.

The decidua basalis enters into the formation of the *basal plate* of the placenta and differs, histologically, from the decidua vera in two respects (Fig. 4–22). First, the spongy zone of the decidua basalis consists mainly of arteries and widely dilated veins; by term, the glands have virtually disappeared. Second, the decidua basalis is invaded extensively by trophoblastic giant cells, which first appear as early as the time of implantation. The number and depth of penetration of the giant cells vary greatly. Although generally confined to the decidua, these cells may penetrate the myometrium. In such circumstances, their number and invasiveness may be so extensive as to be suggestive of choriocarcinoma to the inexperienced observer.

AGING OF THE DECIDUA

Where invading trophoblast meets the decidua, there is a zone of fibrinoid degeneration, *Nitabuch's layer*. Whenever the decidua is defective, as in placenta accreta (see Chap. 24, p. 419), Nitabuch's layer is usually absent. There also is an inconstant deposition of fibrin, *Rohr's stria*, at the bottom of the intervillous space and surrounding the fastening villi. McCombs and Craig (1964) found that decidual necrosis is a normal phenomenon in the first and probably the second trimester. The presence of necrotic decidua obtained through curettage after spontaneous abortion in the first trimester should not, therefore, be interpreted necessarily as either a cause or an effect of the abortion.

HISTOCHEMISTRY AND ULTRASTRUCTURE

In their elegant studies of placental histochemistry, Wislocki and Dempsey (1948, 1955) found difficulty in distinguishing, with conventional stains, trophoblast from decidua in the basal plate. They observed differences, however, in the distribution

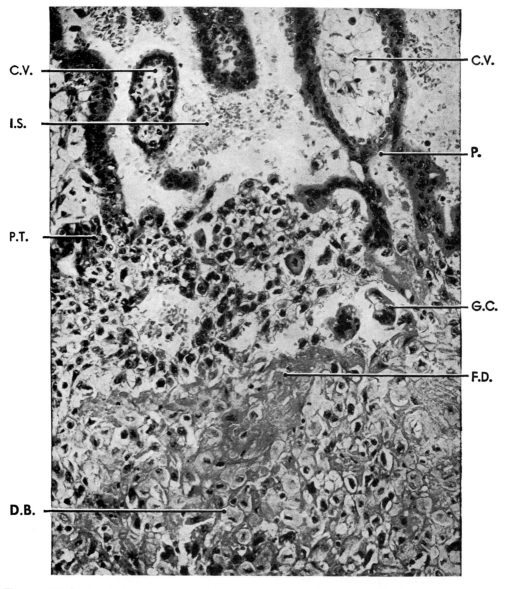

Figure 4–22. Section through junction of chorion and decidua basalis. Fourth month of gestation. C.V. = chorionic villi; D.B. = decidua basalis; F.D. = fibrinoid degeneration; G.C. = giant cell; I.S. = intervillous space containing maternal blood; P. = fastening villus; P.T. = proliferating trophoblast.

of RNA and mitochondria and characteristic "capsules" surrounding individual decidual cells. Wynn's electron microscopic findings (1967) of the human basal plate demonstrated that this complex region of the placenta comprises intimately related fetal and maternal cells. Well-preserved trophoblastic and endometrial cells are rarely in direct contact, however, but remain separated by degenerating tissue and fibrinoid. The giant cells in the region are derived from the syncytium or arise from differentiation of cytotrophoblast in situ. These syncytial masses may be hormonally active late in pregnancy. Moe (1969) confirmed these findings by showing that there is no intimate contact between apparently viable cytotrophoblast and decidua. The immunologic implications of these cellular relations are discussed subsequently.

BIOACTIVE SUBSTANCES IN DECIDUA

As described in Chapter 7, the concentration of prolactin in amnionic fluid is extraordinarily high compared with the levels in fetal or maternal plasma; this prolactin arises in the decidua (Riddick and co-workers, 1983). There are a number of lines of evidence in favor of this conclusion: (1) prolactin concentrations in decidua are extraordinarily high, (2) the synthesis of prolactin

persists in decidual tissue maintained in organ culture, (3) prolactin has been isolated from culture medium of dispersed decidual cells in monolayer culture, (4) pituitary and decidual prolactin are immunologically indistinguishable, as are the biological activities of pituitary and decidual prolactin, (5) cycloheximide treatment of decidual tissue in culture inhibits prolactin secretion, (6) radiolabeled leucine is incorporated into prolactin by decidual tissue, and (7) bromocriptine treatment of pregnant women, while causing a striking reduction in the concentration of prolactin in fetal and maternal plasma, does not affect the concentration of prolactin in amnionic fluid.

The factor(s) that regulates prolactin secretion in decidua is not clearly defined. Those factors known to affect, either negatively or positively, the rate of secretion of prolactin by the anterior pituitary, for example, dopamine and dopamine agonists and thryotropin-releasing hormone, do not act either in vivo or in vitro to alter the rate of decidual prolactin secretion. It has been reported that arachidonic acid, but not prostaglandins E_2 and $F_{2\alpha}$, will attenuate the rate of decidual prolactin secretion. The physiological role of prolactin produced in decidua is not known. Because all or most all of prolactin produced in decidua enters amnionic fluid, it has been speculated that there may be a role for this hormone in solute and water

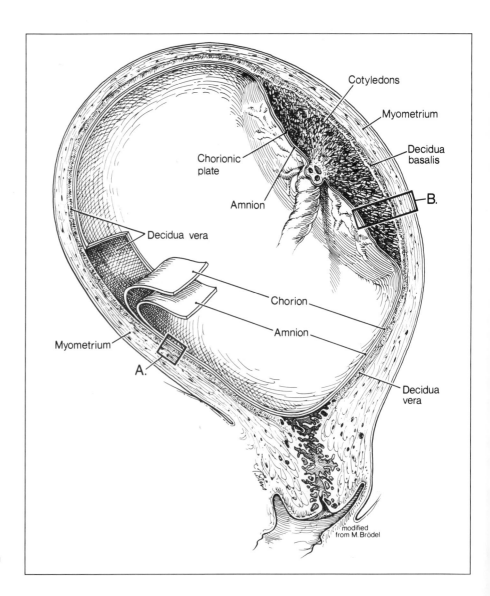

Figure 4–23. Uterus of pregnant woman showing normal placenta in situ. **A.** Location of section shown in Figure 4–24. **B.** Location of section shown in Figure 4–25.

transport across the chorioamnion and, thus, in the maintenance of amnionic fluid volume homeostasis. Various other roles for decidual prolactin have been suggested but, presently, these must be considered as speculative. Excellent reviews of the synthesis of prolactin in decidua have been presented by Tyson and McCoshen (1983) and by Bigazzi (1983).

It now also seems likely that *relaxin, β-endorphin,* and *1,25-dihydroxyvitamin D3* also are produced in human decidua; and, numerous *pregnancy-specific proteins,* and a number of *cytokines* are produced in this macrophage-like tissue (Chap. 10, p. 202).

POLYAMINE SYNTHESIS AND METABOLISM IN DECIDUA

Many investigators have established the probability that the accelerated production of the polyamines, viz., putrescine, spermidine, and spermine, is essential in processes that involve both hypertrophy and hyperplasia. Human pregnancy would seem to be a physiological process in which extraordinary rates of polyamine production exist. Not only is there a rapidly growing fetus and placenta but there is extensive hypertrophy of the uterus and other tissues as well. Yet, as discussed in Chapter 7, increased levels of polyamines are demonstrable in the urine of pregnant women only briefly during pregnancy, at about 12 to 14 weeks gestation. The enzyme that catalyzes the first and rate-limiting step in polyamine formation, *ornithine decarboxylase,* is present in and has been characterized in decidua of women (Garza and coworkers, 1983). Thus, it seems enigmatic and, in view of the growth of the fetus, disappointing that the levels of polyamines in maternal blood and urine are not reflective of the rate of growth of fetus, decidua, and uterine hypertrophy; if this were the case, it could be that the measurement of polyamines would be useful as an index of fetal growth.

An explanation, however, may be offered for this apparent paradox. The activity of the enzyme *diamine oxidase,* also known as *histaminase,* rises dramatically in blood of pregnant women

early in pregnancy at about the time that the levels of polyamines begin to decline, namely, at about 14 weeks gestation. The importance of this observation is that diamine oxidase is the enzyme that catalyzes the metabolism of putrescine. Thus, it may be that the rate of polyamine synthesis is indeed strikingly accelerated and increases throughout pregnancy but the rate of catabolism of these compounds is greater than the rate of synthesis. This is easily envisioned when one considers that diamine oxidase activity in plasma of pregnant women may increase a thousandfold by 20 weeks gestation (Ahlmark, 1944). It is believed that this increased amount of diamine oxidase is principally of decidual origin (Swanberg, 1948).

For this reason and others, many investigators have determined the activity of diamine oxidase in plasma of pregnant women in the hope of using such values as an index of fetal well-being. Although some correlates appear to exist, it now is generally accepted that such measurements are not of specific usefulness in the selection of clinical management plans (Resnik and Levine, 1969).

CIRCULATION IN THE MATURE PLACENTA

Elizabeth Ramsey (1985), the preeminent researcher of the contemporary era of the investigation of placental circulation, states, *"The modern era in the understanding of the placenta could not have commenced while scientists still thought that maternal and fetal vessels were anastomosed end to end."* Because the placenta functionally represents a rather intimate presentation of the fetal capillary bed to maternal blood, its gross anatomy primarily concerns vascular relations. The human placenta at term is a discoid organ measuring approximately 15 to 20 cm in diameter and 2 to 3 cm in thickness. It weighs approximately 500 g and generally is located in the uterus anteriorly or posteriorly near the fundus. The fetal side is covered by transparent amnion beneath which the fetal vessels course, with the arteries passing over the veins. A section through the placenta in situ (Figs. 4–23

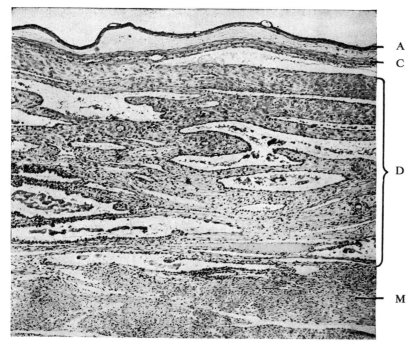

Figure 4–24. Section of fetal membranes and uterus opposite placental site at A in Figure 4–23. A = amnion; C = chorion; D = decidua parietalis; M = myometrium.

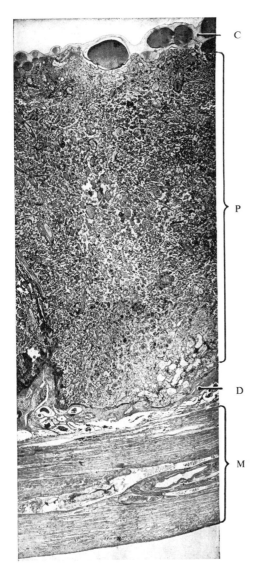

Figure 4–25. Section of placenta and uterus through B in Figure 4–23. C = chorionic plate with fetal blood vessels; P = placental villi; D = decidua basalis; M = myometrium.

to 4–25) includes amnion, chorion, chorionic villi and intervillous spaces, decidual plate, and myometrium.

The maternal surface of the placenta (Fig. 4–26) is divided into irregular lobes by furrows produced by septa, which consist of fibrous tissue with sparse vessels confined mainly to their bases. The broad-based septa ordinarily do not reach the chorionic plate, thus providing only incomplete partitions.

FETAL CIRCULATION

Fetal blood flows to the placenta through the two umbilical arteries, which carry deoxygenated, or "venous-like," blood. The vessels branch repeatedly beneath the amnion and again within the dividing villi, forming capillary networks in the terminal divisions (Figs. 4–27 and 4–28). Blood, with a significantly higher oxygen content, returns to the fetus from the placenta through the single umbilical vein (see Chap. 6, p. 99).

MATERNAL CIRCULATION

Only relatively recently has the mechanism of the maternal placental circulation been explained in physiological terms. Insofar as fetal homeostasis is dependent on efficient placental circulation, the extensive efforts of investigators to define the factors that regulate the flow of blood into and from the intervillous space have led to important practical applications in obstetrics. An adequate theory must explain how blood may actually leave the maternal circulation, flow into an amorphous space lined by trophoblastic syncytium rather than capillary endothelium, and return through maternal veins without producing arteriovenous-like shunts that would prevent the blood from remaining in contact with the villi long enough for adequate exchange.

It was not until the objective studies of Ramsey and her co-workers (1963, 1966) that a "physiological" mechanism of placental circulation, consistent with both experimental and clinical findings, was available (Fig. 4–28). Discarding the crude corrosion technique of her predecessors, Ramsey and colleagues, by careful, slow injections of radiocontrast material under low pressure that avoided disruption of the circulation, proved that the arterial entrances as well as the venous exits are scattered at random over the entire base of the placenta. This arrangement was reviewed by Ramsey and Donner (1980).

The maternal blood entering through the basal plate is driven by the head of maternal arterial pressure high up toward the chorionic plate before lateral dispersion occurs. After bathing the chorionic villi, the blood drains through venous orifices in the basal plate and enters the maternal placental veins. The maternal blood thus traverses the placenta randomly without preformed channels, propelled by the maternal arterial pressure. The spiral arteries are generally perpendicular and the veins parallel to the uterine wall, an arrangement that facilitates closure of the veins during a uterine contraction and prevents squeezing of essential maternal blood from the intervillous space. According to Brosens and Dixon (1963), there are about 120 spiral arterial entries into the intervillous space of the human placenta at term, discharging blood in spurts that displace the adjacent villi, as described by Borell and co-workers (1958).

Ramsey and Harris (1966) compared the uteroplacental vasculature and circulation of the rhesus monkey with those of the human. The most significant morphological variation is the greater dilatation of human uteroplacental arteries. In the human, particularly in early pregnancy, there may be multiple openings from a single arterial stem into the intervillous space. The force of the spurts of blood is eventually dissipated with the creation of a small lake of blood roughly 5 mm in diameter about halfway toward the chorionic plate. The closeness of the villi slows the flow of blood, providing adequate time for exchange.

Ramsey's concept is supported by the findings of numerous arteriographic studies. Clearly, the spiral arterial spurts are associated with the "lakes" and the closure of uteroplacental veins are effected by pressure produced at the beginning of uterine contractions. Corroboration has been provided by results of cine-radioangiography, in which it was shown how, in the macaque, debouching streams from the spiral arteries connect with and develop into the small lakes, which then disperse in a general effusion of blood throughout the intervillous space (Fig. 4–29).

In Ramsey's motion pictures, the effect of myometrial contractions upon placental circulation is shown unequivocally to involve diminution of arterial inflow and cessation of venous drainage. Continued observation of the contrast medium by televised fluoroscopy was indicative that myometrial contractions cause a slight delay in appearance of the contrast medium in the veins of the uterine wall when injection occurs during a strong contraction. The pressure in the intervillous space may be decreased to the point at which blood cannot be expressed

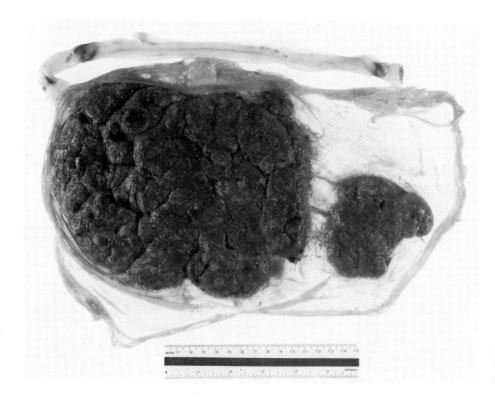

Figure 4–26. Maternal surface of term placenta. Variably discrete, irregularly shaped adjacent lobes are evident plus a large separate (succenturiate) lobe.

against the prevailing myometrial pressure. Ramsey has provided further evidence of independent activity of the spiral arterioles, as indicated by the appearance of spurts in different locations even when injections are performed under conditions of minimal myometrial pressure. Not all endometrial spiral arteries are continuously patent, nor do they all necessarily discharge blood into the intervillous space simultaneously.

In summary, Ramsey's concept holds that the maternal blood enters the intervillous space in spurts produced by the maternal blood pressure. The *vis a tergo* forces blood in discrete streams toward the chorionic plate until the head of pressure is reduced. Lateral spread then occurs. Continuing influx of arterial blood exerts pressure on the contents of the intervillous space, pushing the blood toward exits in the basal plate, from which it

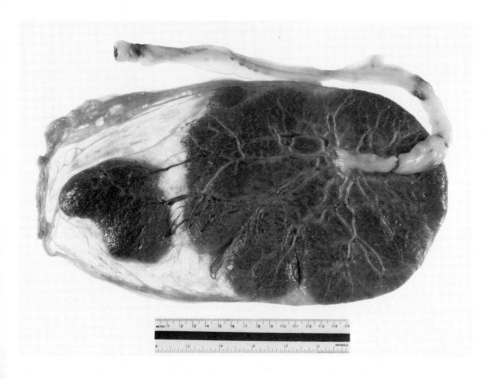

Figure 4–27. Fetal surface of term placenta. Fetal vessels are visible beneath the amnion overlying the placenta. The fetal vessels extend to the adjacent separate (succenturiate) lobe.

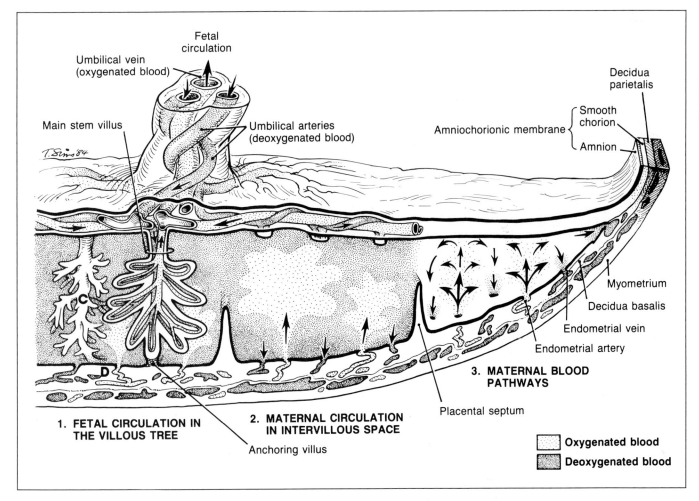

Figure 4–28. Schematic drawing of a section through a full-term placenta: **1.** The relation of the villous chorion (C) to the decidua basalis (D) and the fetal placental circulation. **2.** The maternal placental circulation. Maternal blood flows into the intervillous spaces in funnel-shaped spurts, and exchanges occur with the fetal blood as the maternal blood flows around the villi. **3.** The inflowing arterial blood pushes venous blood into the endometrial veins, which are scattered over the entire surface of the decidua basalis. Note that the umbilical arteries carry deoxygenated fetal blood to the placenta and that the umbilical vein carries oxygenated blood to the fetus. Note that the cotyledons are separated from each other by placental (decidual) septa of the maternal portion of the placenta. Each cotyledon consists of two or more main stem villi and their many branches. (*Based on Moore: The Developing Human, 3rd ed. Philadelphia, Saunders, 1982, p 116.*)

is drained through uterine and other pelvic veins. During uterine contractions, both inflow and outflow are curtailed, although the volume of blood in the intervillous space is maintained, thus providing for continual, though reduced, exchange.

Freese (1968) added support to older anatomical studies in which it was shown that in both the rhesus monkey and man, each placental cotyledon is supplied by one spiral artery, which is located beneath a central empty space. He believed that this relatively hollow central portion of the cotyledon, which he called the intracotyledonary space, is the preferential site of entry of blood. Wigglesworth (1969) suggested that the structure of the fetal cotyledon may determine, in part, the pattern of maternal blood flow through the placenta and that fetal cotyledons develop around the spiral artery. Variations in structure of the villi in this region imply that growth occurs around the center of the cotyledon because villi there are less mature. The intervillous space thus has arterial, capillary, and venous zones.

In this connection, Reynolds and co-workers (1968) showed that the blood pressure was highest around the central cavity of the cotyledon, the gradient diminishing radially and toward the subchorial lake. They postulated that Braxton–Hicks contractions (p. 14) enhance the movement of blood from the center of the cotyledon through the intervillous space.

Bleker and associates (1975) identified by serial sonography in normally laboring women that the length, thickness, and surface of the placenta increased during uterine contractions. They attributed these changes to distension of the intervillous spaces by blood as the consequence of relatively greater impairment of venous outflow compared to arterial inflow. During contractions, therefore, a somewhat larger volume of blood is available for exchange even though the rate of flow is decreased. More recently, by the use of Doppler velocimetry, it was shown that diastolic flow velocity in spiral arterioles is diminished during uterine contractions (see Chap. 15, p. 285).

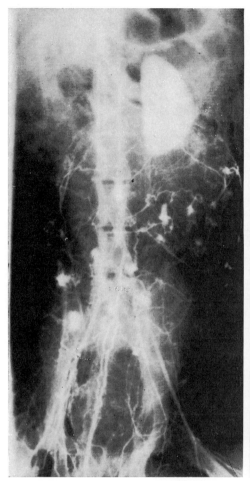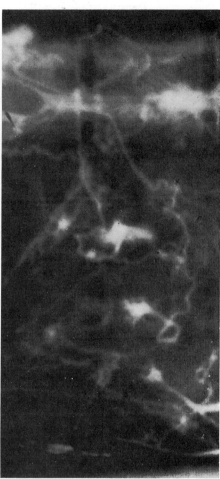

Figure 4–29. *Left:* Radiogram 6 seconds after injection of a radiopaque contrast medium into the right femoral artery of a monkey of day 111 of pregnancy. The primary placenta is below on the left; the secondary placenta is above on the right. *Right:* High magnification of an artery at the center of the secondary placenta in the same monkey. (*Courtesy of Dr. Elizabeth M. Ramsey.*)

The principal factors regulating the flow of blood in the intervillous space are thus shown to include arterial blood pressure, intrauterine pressure, the pattern of uterine contraction, including the contour of the individual contraction wave, and factors acting specifically upon the arteriolar walls. The lack of homogeneity of blood throughout the intervillous space has been emphasized by Fuchs and co-workers (1963), who measured blood samples believed to be from the intervillous space and found considerable variations in the P_{O_2}, P_{CO_2}, and pH. The values of some samples resembled arterial and others uterine venous blood. They stressed, however, the difficulty of ascertaining the precise source of blood obtained by transuterine puncture of the placenta.

Studies of the human placental circulation provide no evidence of countercurrent flow, a system by which fetal blood of low oxygen content as it enters the villous capillaries would flow first close to maternal blood of low oxygen content and then move in close proximity to progressively more oxygenated maternal blood. In the hemochorioendothelial placenta of the human, strict countercurrent flow is precluded by the random distribution of villi, in the capillaries of which the direction of fetal-to-maternal flow can bear no fixed relationship.

Ramsey and Donner (1980) presented a summary of anatomical studies of the uteroplacental vasculature. They noted that cytotrophoblastic elements are confined initially to the terminal portions of the uteroplacental arteries but later extend proximally. By the 16th week, cytotrophoblasts are found in many of the arteries of the inner layer of myometrium. Intraarterial accumulation of trophoblast ultimately may stop circulation through some of these vessels. The number of arterial openings into the intervillous space gradually is reduced by cytotrophoblast and by breaching of the walls of the more proximal parts of the arteries by deeply penetrating trophoblast. Brosens and co-workers (1967) found that the cytotrophoblast not only breaches the maternal spiral vessels but also serves a major role in their progressive conversion to large tortuous channels by replacement of the normal muscular and elastic tissue of the wall by fibrous tissue and fibrinoid. After the 30th week, a prominent venous plexus separates the decidua basalis from the myometrium, thus providing a plane of cleavage for separation of the placenta.

PLACENTAL IMMUNOLOGY

The placenta and extraembryonic fetal membranes appear to defy the laws of transplantation immunology. Today, it still is enigmatic that the mother tolerates the fetal graft.

IMMUNOLOGICAL CONSIDERATIONS

Attempts to explain the survival of the semiallogeneic fetal graft have occupied the attention of several of the world's outstanding biologists. The first explanation based on antigenic immaturity of the fetus must be discarded in light of Billingham's demonstration (1964) that transplantation antigens (in embryonic tissues) appear very early in life. But ordinarily, in the fetal–maternal communication system, only extraembryonic fetal tissues are in direct contact with maternal tissues. Namely, trophoblasts are contiguous with maternal blood and decidua. And except for the abnormal passage of fetal blood cellular elements through "breaks" in the placenta, cells of the embryo do not come into direct contact with maternal tissues. Nonetheless, except in parthenogenesis, or in situations in which both parents are genetically identical, the trophoblasts confront the mother with foreign antigens.

A second explanation, based on diminished immunological reactivity of the mother during pregnancy, provides only an ancillary factor in the prevention of the development of maternal isoimmunization during pregnancy in a few species. If the uterus were an immunologically privileged site, as in a third explanation, advanced ectopic pregnancies could never occur. Because transplantation immunity can be evoked and expressed in the uterus as elsewhere, the survival of the homograft must be related to a peculiarity of the fetus, primarily the trophoblasts, rather than of the uterus. A fourth explanation involves a physiological barrier between fetus and mother. Lanman and colleagues (1962) provided indirect support for the last hypothesis in their experiments in which fertilized rabbit's ova were transferred to a recipient's uterus. Neither prior exposure of the foster mother to skin grafts from the parents nor reexposure to homografts of these donors at the time of egg transfer or at midpregnancy adversely affected the pregnancy.

Kobayashi and co-workers (1979) have reported a dose-dependent suppression of the bidirectional mixed lymphocyte reaction by progesterone in concentrations comparable to those of the placenta. Therefore, they suggest a role for progesterone at its site of production in immunoregulation during pregnancy. Siiteri and co-workers (1977) previously demonstrated that the rejection of grafted hamster skin is delayed by the presence of progesterone.

HLA ANTIGEN EXPRESSION IN FETAL TROPHOBLASTS

Head and co-workers (1987) have provided an excellent review of the most attractive hypothesis for the unique success of fetal acceptance by its immunocompetent maternal host. They point out that as early as 1932, Witebsky and Reisch found that blood group antigens are lacking in human trophoblasts. Subsequently much research has been focused on the expression of the major histocompatibility (MHC) antigens (HLA, by international agreement, is the logo of the human MHC) as a function of trophoblast development. Before blastocyst implantation in the mouse, low levels of MHC class I antigens are expressed on the trophectoderm, but these antigens disappear at the time of implantation, not to reappear except later in selected subpopulations of trophoblasts in the mature placenta. **Class II MHC antigens are absent from trophoblasts at all stages of gestation.**

The same generalities of HLA expression are applicable to human trophoblasts. Whereas there is no doubt that class I antigens are expressed, the precise nature of the antigens that are expressed in trophoblasts is not fully defined. There is appreciable evidence that the class I antigens expressed in human trophoblasts are novel. Moreover, it is possible that expression of these antigens may be modulated, e.g., by the action of interferons. But, the responsiveness of human trophoblast to interferon action may be crucial to trophoblast survival. This latter issue is important because it is clear that increased expression of class I antigens after exposure to interferon leads to better killing of allogeneic and virus-infected targets.

The important question today, therefore, is related to the potential immunogenicity of trophoblasts. Expression of class II HLA antigens is believed to be very important in the immunogenicity of tissue and organ allografts; the complete absence of class II antigens in human (and other mammalian) trophoblasts is no doubt important in maternal acceptance of the fetus. The elimination of class II antigen-presenting macrophages from kidney permits transplantation in experimental animals without immunosuppression (Schreiner and associates, 1988).

The absence of class I antigens from trophoblasts during the perimplantation period and the absence of class II antigens on trophoblasts in contact with maternal blood may provide the "immunological buffer zone" between maternal and fetal tissues (Head and colleagues, 1987).

ROLE OF HLA CLASS I ANTIGENS ON TROPHOBLASTS

The most simplistic answer to maternal acceptance of the semiallogeneic graft would have been the complete absence of MHC (HLA) antigens. This is not the case (except for class II). It seems possible, therefore, that selected expression of class I antigens, both in time and type, are beneficial to pregnancy. As pointed out by Head and co-workers (1987), one possibility is that such antigen expression may elicit the formation of growth-promoting cytokines. Other possibilities include the participation of class I antigens with the binding of peptide hormones to the cell surface. Such a proposal has been made in the case of insulin and epidermal growth factor.

ANCILLARY IMMUNOLOGICAL CONSIDERATIONS

One ancillary explanation for the survival of the homograft appears to be a fairly complete anatomical separation of maternal and fetal circulations. Comparative electron microscopy of the placenta has supported the concept of the prime role of the trophoblast in maintaining the "immunological barrier." In all placentas examined with the electron microscope, at least one layer of trophoblast has been shown to persist essentially throughout gestation.

The suggestion by Kirby and co-workers (1964) that deposition of fibrinoid was a general phenomenon of mammalian placentation rekindled interest in these amorphous deposits. The term *fibrinoid* is used in the restricted conventional sense of the histopathologist to refer to a group of substances recognized with the light microscope. Although fibrinoids are not demonstrable in all mammalian placentas, a submicroscopic glycocalyx may be found with the electron microscope to coat most trophoblastic plasma membranes. It is still not clear whether these polysaccharide barriers serve as mechanical barriers to the passage of transplantation antigens from fetus to mother, or to provide for local shields from maternal lymphocytes.

Maternal lymphocyte function may be altered during pregnancy, as reflected by a reduction in phytohemagglutinin-induced transformation (Finn and colleagues, 1972; Purtilo and associates, 1972). It has been suggested that both trophoblasts and decidua produce agents that suppress lymphocyte immune responses. Sargent and co-workers (1987) recently reviewed these associations.

BREAKS IN THE PLACENTAL "BARRIER"

The failure of the placenta to maintain absolute integrity of the fetal and maternal circulations is documented by numerous findings of the passage of cells between mother and fetus in both directions, and best exemplified clinically by the occurrence of erythroblastosis fetalis (see Chap. 33, p. 599). Typically a few fetal blood cells are found in the mother's blood; and, rarely, the fetus may exsanguinate into the maternal circulation (see Chap. 33, p. 598). Leucocytes from the fetus may replicate in the mother; leucocytes bearing a Y chromosome have been identified in women for up to 5 years after giving birth to a son (Ciaranfi and colleagues, 1977). Desai and Creger (1963) labeled maternal leucocytes and platelets with atabrine and found that they crossed the placenta from mother to fetus. Lymphocytes passing into the fetus create the possibility of chimerism, the subject of a review by Benirschke (1970). If the maternal cells then colonize, a *graft-versus-host* reaction or autoimmune process may result.

Cells of fetal origin other than constituents of the blood have also been identified in the maternal circulation. Cells morphologically identical with trophoblast have been identified in the uterine venous blood (Douglas and associates, 1959) as well as in cord blood (Salvaggio and co-workers, 1960). The immunological significance of continuous release of fetal elements into the maternal circulation remains to be explained.

THE AMNION

The human amnion either develops from the delamination of the cytotrophoblast about the 7th or 8th day of development of the normal ovum or it develops essentially as an extension of the fetal ectoderm. Initially a minute vesicle (see Fig. 4–8), the amnion develops into a small sac that covers the dorsal surface of the embryo. As the amnion enlarges, it gradually engulfs the growing embryo, which prolapses into its cavity. Distension of the amnionic sac eventually brings it into contact with the interior of the chorion; apposition of the mesoblasts of chorion and amnion near the end of the first trimester results in obliteration of the extraembryonic coelom. The amnion and chorion, though slightly adherent, are never intimately connected and usually can be separated easily, even at term.

The normal amnion is 0.02 to 0.5 mm in thickness. The epithelium normally consists of a single layer of nonciliated, cuboid cells. According to Bourne (1962), there are five layers, comprising, from within outward, epithelium, basement membrane, the compact layer, the fibroblastic layer, and the spongy layer. Electron microscopic studies of amnion by Wynn and French (1968) and by Hoyes (1968) have not, however, confirmed such sharply defined layers (Fig. 4–30).

Bourne (1962) was unable to find blood vessels or nerves in the amnion at any stage of development and, despite the occurrence of suggestive spaces in the fibroblastic and spongy layers, could not identify distinct lymphatic channels.

At term, small rounded plaques are often found on the amnion, particularly near the attachment of the umbilical cord. These *amnionic caruncles* consist of stratified squamous epithelium that histologically resembles skin (see Chap. 31, p. 554).

FETAL MEMBRANES AND PARTURITION

Studies directed toward a definition of the role of the fetal membranes in the initiation of parturition were initiated by MacDonald and co-workers (1974). Among the early findings was the clear demonstration that both the amnion and chorion laeve possess extensive enzymatic capabilities for steroid hormone metabolism including 5α-reductase, 3β-hydroxysteroid dehydrogenase, Δ^{5-4}-isomerase, 20α-steroid oxidoreductase, 17β-dehydrogenase, and other enzyme activities.

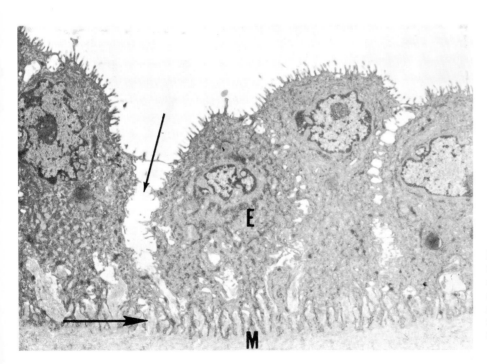

Figure 4–30. Electron micrograph of human amnion at term obtained at time of cesarean section. Epithelium (E) and mesenchyme (M) are shown. Thin arrow indicates intercellular space. Thick arrow points to specializations of basal plasma membranes. (*Courtesy of Dr. Ralph M. Wynn.*)

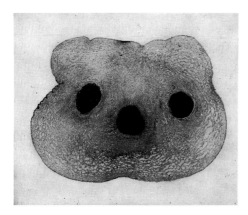

Figure 4–31. Cross section of umbilical cord fixed after blood vessels had been emptied. The umbilical vein, carrying oxygenated blood to the fetus, is in the center; on either side are the two umbilical arteries carrying deoxygenated blood from the fetus to the placenta. (*From Reynolds: Am J Obstet Gynecol 68:69, 1954.*)

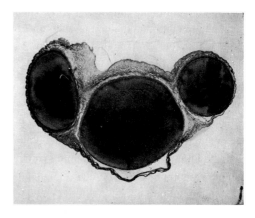

Figure 4–32. Cross section of the same umbilical cord shown in Figure 4–31, but through a segment from which the blood vessels had not been emptied. This photograph probably represents more accurately the conditions in utero. (*From Reynolds: Am J Obstet Gynecol 68:69, 1954.*)

The fetal membranes also are rich in arachidonic acid, the obligate precursor of prostaglandins E_2 and $F_{2\alpha}$. The fetal membranes are endowed with lipases that utilize arachidonoyl-glycerophospholipids preferentially to give free arachidonic acid. The availability of free arachidonic acid is the rate-limiting step in many tissues in prostaglandin biosynthesis (see Chap. 10, p. 199), and there is appreciable evidence in favor of increased PGE_2 formation in amnion during human parturition.

AMNIONIC FLUID

The normally clear fluid that collects within the amnionic cavity increases in quantity as pregnancy advances until near term, when it normally decreases. An average volume of somewhat less than 1,000 mL is found at term, although the volume may vary widely from a few milliliters to many liters in abnormal conditions (oligohydramnios and polyhydramnios, or hydramnios). The origin, composition, and function of the amnionic fluid are discussed further in Chapter 6 (p. 105).

UMBILICAL CORD AND RELATED STRUCTURES

DEVELOPMENT OF THE CORD AND RELATED STRUCTURES

The yolk sac and the umbilical vesicle into which it develops are quite prominent at the beginning of pregnancy. At first the embryo is a flattened disc interposed between amnion and yolk sac. Because the dorsal surface grows faster than the ventral surface, in association with the elongation of the neural tube, the embryo bulges into the amnionic sac and the dorsal part of the yolk sac is incorporated into the body of the embryo to form the gut. The allantois projects into the base of the body stalk from the caudal wall of the yolk sac or, later, from the anterior wall of the hindgut. As pregnancy advances, the yolk sac becomes smaller and its pedicle relatively longer. By about the middle of the 3rd month, the expanding amnion obliterates the exocelom, fuses with the chorion laeve, and covers the bulging placental disc and the lateral surface of the body stalk, which is then called the umbilical cord, or funis. Remnants of the exo-

celom in the anterior portion of the cord may contain loops of intestine, which continue to develop outside the embryo. Although the loops are later withdrawn, the apex of the midgut loop retains its connection with an attenuated vitelline duct that terminates in a crumpled, highly vascular sac 3 to 5 cm in diameter lying on the surface of the placenta between amnion and chorion or in the membranes just beyond the placental margin, where occasionally it may be identified at term.

In an electron microscopic study of the human yolk sac, Hoyes (1969) confirmed that its endoderm is the origin of fetal blood cells. The epithelium of the yolk sac has ultrastructural features that are usually associated with those of a tissue that serves as a site of transfer metabolites.

The three vessels in the cord at term normally are two arteries and one vein. The right umbilical vein usually disappears early during fetal development, leaving only the original left vein. Section of any portion of the cord frequently reveals, near the center, the small duct of the umbilical vesicle, lined by a single layer of flattened or cuboid epithelial cells. In sections just beyond the umbilicus, but never at the maternal end of the cord, another duct representing the allantoic remnant occasionally is found. The intra-abdominal portion of the duct of the umbilical vesicle, which extends from umbilicus to intestine, usually atrophies and disappears, but occasionally it remains patent, forming Meckel's diverticulum. The most common vascular anomaly in man is the absence of one umbilical artery. This subject is discussed further in Chapter 31 (p. 537).

STRUCTURE AND FUNCTION OF THE UMBILICAL CORD

The umbilical cord, or funis, extends from the fetal umbilicus to the fetal surface of the placenta. Its exterior is dull white, moist, and covered by amnion, through which three umbilical vessels may be seen. Its diameter is 1 to 2.5 cm, with an average length of 55 cm and a usual range of 30 to 100 cm. Folding and tortuosity of the vessels, which are longer than the cord itself, frequently create nodulations on the surface, or *false knots*, which are essentially varices. The matrix of the cord consists of Wharton's jelly (Figs. 4–31 and 4–32). After fixation, the umbilical vessels appear empty, but Figure 4–32 is more accurately representative of the situation in vivo, when the vessels are not emptied of blood. The two arteries are smaller in diameter than the vein. When fixed in its normally distended state, the umbilical artery exhibits transverse intimal *folds of Hoboken* across part of its lumen (Chacko and Reynolds, 1954). The mesoderm of the cord, which is of allantoic origin, fuses with that of the amnion.

The egress of blood from the umbilical vein is by way of two routes, the ductus venosus, which empties directly into the inferior vena cava, and numerous smaller openings into the fetal hepatic circulation and thence into the inferior vena cava by the hepatic vein. The blood takes the path of least resistance through these alternate routes. Resistance in the ductus venosus is controlled by a sphincter, which is situated at the origin of the ductus at the umbilical recess and innervated by a branch of the vagus nerve.

Ellison and co-workers (1970) studied the innervation of the umbilical cord of the rat by means of localization of acetylcholinesterase and catecholamines. Cholinesterase-positive nerves were confined to periarterial plexus while adrenergic nerves were entirely absent from the cord. By these techniques, certain nerves could be traced to the placenta but not into it.

REFERENCES

Ahlmark A: Studies on the histaminolytic power of plasma with special reference to pregnancy. Acta Physiol Scand (Suppl 28) 9:1, 1944

Benirschke K: Spontaneous chimerism in mammals: A critical review. In Current Topics in Pathology. Berlin, Springer-Verlag, 1970, p 1

Benirschke K: The placenta: How to examine it and what you can learn. Contemp Ob/Gyn 17:117, 1981

Bigazzi M: Specific endocrine function of human decidua. Semin Reprod Endocrinol 1:343, 1983

Billingham RE: Transplantation immunity and the maternal–fetal relation. N Engl J Med 270:667, 720, 1964

Bleker OP, Kloosterman GJ, Mieras DJ, Oosting J, Salle HJA: Intervillous space during uterine contractions in human subjects: An ultrasonic study. Am J Obstet Gynecol 123:697, 1975

Borell U, Fernstrom I, Westman A: An arteriographic study of the placental circulation. Geburtshilfe Frauenheilkd 18:1, 1958

Bourne GL: The Human Amnion and Chorion. Chicago, Year Book, 1962

Boyd JD, Boyd CAR, Hamilton WJ: Observations on the vacuolar structure of the human syncytiotrophoblast. Z Zellforsch Mikrosk Anat 88:57, 1968

Boyd JD, Hamilton WJ: The Human Placenta. Cambridge, England, Heffer, 1970

Brosens I, Dixon HG: The anatomy of the maternal side of the placenta. Br J Obstet Gynaecol 73:357, 1963

Brosens I, Robertson WB, Dixon HB: The physiological response of the vessels of the placental bed to normal pregnancy. J Pathol Bact 98:569, 1967

Chacko AW, Reynolds SRM: Architecture of distended and nondistended human umbilical cord tissues, with special references to the arteries and veins. Contrib Embryol 35:135, 1954

Ciaranfi A, Curchod A, Odartchenko N: Survie de lymphocytes foetaux dans de sany maternal post-partum. Schweiz Med Wschr 107:134, 1977

Crawford JM: A study of human placental growth with observations on the placenta in erythroblastosis foetalis. Br J Obstet Gynaecol 66:855, 1959

Desai RG, Creger WP: Maternofetal passage of leukocytes and platelets in man. Blood 21:665, 1963

Douglas GW, Thomas L, Carr M, Cullen NM, Morris R: Trophoblast in the circulating blood during pregnancy. Am J Obstet Gynecol 78:960, 1959

Ellison JP, Hibbs RG, Ferguson MA, Mahan M, Blasini EJ: The innervation of the umbilical cord. Anat Rec 166:302, 1970

Finn R, St Hill CA, Govan AJ, Ralfs IG, Gurney FJ, Denye V: Immunological responses in pregnancy and survival of fetal homograft. Br Med J 3:150, 1972

Freese UE: The uteroplacental vascular relationship in the human. Am J Obstet Gynecol 101:8, 1968

Fuchs F, Spackman T, Assali NS: Complexity and nonhomogenicity of the intervillous space. Am J Obstet Gynecol 86:226, 1963

Galton M: DNA content of placental nuclei. J Cell Biol 13:183, 1962

Garza JR, MacDonald PC, Johnston JM, Casey ML: Characterization of ornithine decarboxylase activity in human uterine decidua vera. Am J Obstet Gynecol 145:509, 1983

Harris JWS, Ramsey EM: The morphology of human uteroplacental vasculature. Contrib Embryol 38:43, 1966

Head JR, Drake BL, Zuckermann FA: Major histocompatibility antigens on trophoblast and their regulation: Implications in the maternal-fetal relationship. Am J Reprod Immunol Microbiol 15:12, 1987

Hertig AT: The placenta: Some new knowledge about an old organ. Obstet Gynecol 20:859, 1962

Hertig AT, Rock J, Adams EC, Mulligan WJ: On the preimplantation stages of the human ovum. Contrib Embryol 35:199, 1954

Hoyes AD: Fine structure of human amniotic epithelium in early pregnancy. Br J Obstet Gynecol 75:949, 1968

Hoyes AD: The human foetal yolk sac: An ultrastructural study of four specimens. Z Zellforsch 99:469, 1969

Kirby DRS, Billington WD, Bradbury S, Goldstein DJ: Antigen barrier of the mouse placenta. Nature 204:548, 1964

Kliman HJ, Nestler JE, Sermasi E, Sanger JM, Strauss JF: Purification, characterization, and *in vitro* differentiation of cytotrophoblasts from human term placenta. Endocrinology 118:1567, 1986

Kobayashi H, Mori T, Suzuki A, Nishimura T, Nishimoto H, Harada M: Suppression of mixed lymphocyte reaction by progesterone and estradiol-17β. Am J Obstet Gynecol 134:255, 1979

Lanman JT, Dinerstein J, Fikrig S: Homograft immunity in pregnancy: Lack of harm to fetus from sensitization of mother. Ann NY Acad Sci 99:706, 1962

Lavery JP (ed): The Human Placenta: Clinical Perspectives. Rockville, MD, Aspen, 1987

MacDonald PC, Schultz FM, Duenhoelter JH, Gant NF, Jimenez JM, Pritchard JA, Porter JC, Johnston JM: Initiation of human parturition: I. Mechanism of action of arachidonic acid. Obstet Gynecol 44:629, 1974

McCombs HL, Craig MJ: Decidual necrosis in normal pregnancy. Obstet Gynecol 24:436, 1964

Midgley AR Jr, Pierce GB Jr, Deneau GA, Gosling JRS: Morphogenesis of syncytiotrophoblast *in vivo*: An autoradiographic demonstration. Science 141:349, 1963

Moe N: The deposits of fibrin and fibrin-like materials in the basal plate of the normal human placenta. Acta Pathol Microbiol Immunol Scand 75:1, 1969

Moore KL: The Developing Human: Clinically Oriented Embryology. Philadelphia, Saunders, 1973

Mossman HW: Comparative morphogenesis of the fetal membranes and accessory uterine structures. Contrib Embryol 26:129, 1937

Purtilo DT, Hallgren H, Yunis EJ: Depressed maternal lymphocyte response to phytohaemagglutinin in human pregnancy. Lancet 1:769, 1972

Ramsey EM: What we have learned about placental circulation. J Reprod Med 30:312, 1985

Ramsey EM, Davis RW: A composite drawing of the placenta to show its structure and circulation. Anat Rec 145:366, 1963

Ramsey EM, Donner MW: Placental Vascular and Circulation. Philadelphia, Saunders, 1980

Ramsey EM, Harris JWS: Comparison of uteroplacental vasculature and circulation in the rhesus monkey and man. Contrib Embryol 38:59, 1966

Resnik R, Levine RJ: Plasma diamine oxidase activity in pregnancy: A reappraisal. Am J Obstet Gynecol 104:1061, 1969

Reynolds SRM, Freese UE, Bieniarz J, Caldeyro-Barcia R, Mendez-Bauer C, Escarcena L: Multiple simultaneous intervillous space pressures recorded in several regions of the hemochorial placenta in relation to functional anatomy of the fetal cotyledon. Am J Obstet Gynecol 102:1128, 1968

Richart RM: Studies of placental morphogenesis: I. Radioautographic studies of human placenta utilizing tritiated thymidine. Proc Soc Exp Biol Med 106:829, 1961

Riddick DH, Daly DC, Walters CA: The uterus as an endocrine compartment. Clin Perinatol 10:627, 1983

Salvaggio AT, Nigogosyan G, Mack HC: Detection of trophoblasts in cord blood and fetal circulation. Am J Obstet Gynecol 80:1013, 1960

Sargent IL, Redman CWG: The placenta as a graft. In Lavery JP (ed): The Human Placenta: Clinical Perspectives. Rockville, MD, Aspen, 1987, p 79

Schreiner GF, Flye W, Brunt E, Korber K, Lefkowith JB: Essential fatty acid depletion of renal allografts and prevention of rejection. Science 240:1032, 1988

Siiteri PK, Febres F, Clemens LE, Chang JR, Gondos B, Sites D: Progesterone and maintenance of pregnancy: Is progesterone nature's immunosuppressant? Ann NY Acad Sci 286:384, 1977

Steptoe PC, Edwards RG: Birth after the reimplantation of human embryo. Lancet 2:366, 1978 [letter]

Swanberg H: Source of histaminolytic enzyme in blood of pregnant women. Acta Physiol Scand 16:83, 1948

Thomson AM, Billewicz WZ, Hytten FE: The weight of the placenta in relation to birthweight. Br J Obstet Gynaecol 76:865, 1969

Tyson JE, McCoshen JA: Decidual prolactin: An enigmatic cybernin in human reproduction. Semin Reprod Endocrinol 1:197, 1983

Ulloa-Aguirre A, August AM, Golos TG, Kao L-C, Sakuragi N, Kliman HJ, Strauss JF: 8-Bromo-adenosine 3′,5′-monophosphate regulates expression of chorionic gonadotropin and fibronectin in human cytotrophoblasts. J Clin Endocrinol Metab 64:1002, 1987

Wigglesworth JS: Vascular anatomy of the human placenta and its significance for placental pathology. J Obstet Gynaec Brit Commonw 76:979, 1969

Wislocki GB, Dempsey EW: The chemical histology of human placenta and decidua with reference to mucoproteins, glycogen, lipids and acid phosphatase. Am J Anat 83:1, 1948

Wislocki GB, Dempsey EW: Electron microscopy of the human placenta. Anat Rec 123:133, 1955

Wislocki GB, Streeter GL: On the placentation of the macaque (*Macaca mulatta*), from the time of implantation until the formation of the definitive placenta. Contrib Embryol 27:1, 1938

Witebsky ES, Reich H: Zur gruppenspezifischen differenzierung der placentarorgan. Klin Wochenschr 11:1960, 1932

Wynn RM: Fetomaternal cellular relations in the human basal plate: An ultrastructural study of the placenta. Am J Obstet Gynecol 97:832, 1967

Wynn RM, Davies J: Comparative electron microscopy of the hemochorial villous placenta. Am J Obstet Gynecol 91:533, 1965

The Placental Hormones

ENDOCRINE COMPONENT OF THE PLACENTAL ARM OF THE FETAL–MATERNAL COMMUNICATION SYSTEM

The biomolecular interactions between fetus and mother during human pregnancy are orchestrated by means of a fetal–maternal communication system (Chaps. 2, 3, and 4). The placental arm of this system is the conduit for nutrient transfer to the fetus and it is the principal instrument by which the endocrine milieu, one that is so uniquely characteristic of human pregnancy, is established. The anatomical parts of the endocrine component of the placental arm of this communication system are the fetal adrenal glands and liver, fetal blood, placenta, and maternal blood. Endocrine responsive tissues of both mother and fetus constitute the end-organs of this remarkable system (Fig. 5–1).

In 1905, Halban first suggested that the placenta was an endocrine organ. Since then, many investigators have contributed to a definition of the endocrine functions of the human placenta, including the formation of steroid, protein, and polypeptide hormones. And from the demonstration of a unique relationship between the hyperestrogenic state of human pregnancy and the fetal adrenal secretion of massive quantities of C_{19}-steroids (which are used as precursors for estrogen synthesis in placental trophoblasts), the existence of an interactive fetal–placental communication system was established.

THE PLACENTA AS AN ENDOCRINE ORGAN

The endocrine alterations that accompany human pregnancy are perhaps the most unique and astounding that are recorded in mammalian physiology or pathophysiology. A compendium of steroid hormone production rates in near-term pregnant women and in nonpregant women is presented in Table 5–1. From a perusal of these values, it is evident that the endocrine changes of pregnancy are phenomenal. In addition to these increases in the formation of sex steroid and mineralocorticosteroid hormones, there also are striking increases in the levels of plasma renin, angiotensinogen, and angiotensin II, together with the daily production of 1 g of human placental lactogen (hPL) and massive quantities of human chorionic gonadotropin (hCG). The placenta also produces chorionic adrenocorticotropin (ACTH), as well as other products of pro-opiomelanocortin, human chorionic thyrotropin (hCT), and also hypothalamic-like releasing and inhibiting hormones, e.g., thyrotropin-releasing hormone (TRH), gonadotropin-releasing hormone (GnRH) (or luteinizing hormone-releasing hormone [LHRH]), corticotropin-releasing factor (CRF), and somatostatin, as well as inhibin and a variety of proteins that are unique to pregnancy (pregnancy-specific) or neoplastic processes.

Thus, one of the more remarkable physiological events of pregnancy is the establishment of mechanisms whereby the gravid woman is able to adapt to this unusual endocrine milieu, an issue considered in appreciable detail in Chapter 7.

PROTEIN HORMONES OF THE PLACENTA

CHORIONIC GONADOTROPIN

Overview

The early history of the discovery of hCG is recounted in Chapter 2 (p. 15). HCG is a glycoprotein hormone with LH (luteinizing hormone)-like biological activity that is produced almost exclusively during human pregnancy. HCG acts by way of the LH receptor on responsive cells; but, the half-life of hCG (24 hours) in plasma is much longer than is that of LH (2 hours). The pituitary of normal men and nonpregnant women produces very small quantities of hCG in an episodic fashion (Odell and Griffin, 1987) and a variety of tumors produce this glycoprotein, sometimes in reasonably large amounts. Nonetheless, the detection of hCG in blood or urine of reproductive age women by customary procedures used to identify this glycoprotein is almost always indicative of pregnancy (Chap. 2). Incredible amounts of hCG are produced during human pregnancy; but this is not common to all mammals. Chorionic gonadotropin has been found in a few, but not all, mammals. No other species has been identified in which large amounts of chorionic gonadotropin are produced, comparable to that of the human.

Chemical Characteristics of hCG

HCG is a glycoprotein (M_r about 36,700) with a high carbohydrate (30 percent) content; indeed, this is the highest carbohydrate content of any human hormone. The carbohydrate component, and especially the terminal sialic acid, protects the molecule from catabolism; the enzymatic removal of the terminal sialic acid by use of specific enzymes greatly accelerates the rate of clearance of hCG from the circulation.

The hCG molecule is comprised of two dissimilar subunits, designated α and β, which are noncovalently linked. The α- and β-subunits are held together by electrostatic and hydrophobic forces and can be separated by treatment with acidified urea. The subunits of hCG have been isolated in pure form; and the primary structure of each has been characterized. There is no intrinsic biological activity in either separated subunit (neither subunit binds to receptor); but if the subunits are recombined, near 100 percent of bioactivity is restored. Talamantes and Ogren (1988) have presented an excellent review of this subject.

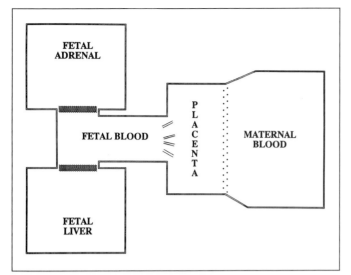

Figure 5–1. The anatomical parts of the endocrine component of the placental arm of the fetal–maternal communication system. Fetal liver is the principal site of production of low-density lipoprotein (LDL)–cholesterol, the principal precursor for fetal adrenal steroidogenesis. Dehydroisoandrosterone sulfate, secreted in prodigious amounts by the fetal adrenal, is converted to 16α-hydroxydehydroisoandrosterone sulfate in fetal liver. These steroids, dehydroisoandrosterone and 16α-hydroxydehydroisoandrosterone, are converted in placenta to estrogens, namely, estradiol-17β and estriol, respectively. Cholesterol, derived from LDL-cholesterol in maternal blood, serves as the precursor for progesterone biosynthesis in placenta. The majority (90 percent) of the steroids formed in placenta (both estrogens and progesterone) enters maternal blood; 10 percent enters fetal blood.

The nature of the purified subunits is of considerable interest to both investigators and clinicians (Chap. 2). HCG is related structurally to three other glycoprotein hormones, viz., LH, FSH (follicle-stimulating hormone), and TSH (thyroid-stimulating hormone). The primary amino acid structure of the α-subunits of all four of these human glycoprotein hormones is identical; but in contrast, while sharing certain similarities, there are distinctive differences among the amino acid sequences of the β-subunits of hFSH, hTSH, as well as those of hCG and hLH. The β-subunits of hCG and hLH, however, are more similar one to the other; there is 80 percent sequence homology of the first 121 amino acids of β-hLH and β-hCG, but there is a 24-amino-acid extension at the carboxy-terminus in the hCG β-subunit not present in β-hLH.

Recombination of an α- and a β-subunit of the four glycoprotein hormones gives rise to a molecule with biological activity characteristic of the hormone from which the β-subunit was derived. The carbohydrate moieties of the molecules apparently are not crucial to receptor binding or antibody recognition, but may be important in coupling of the hormone to adenylate cyclase.

Biosynthesis of hCG

The syntheses of the α- and β-chains of hCG are regulated separately; a single gene codes for the α-subunit of all four glycoprotein hormones; but, there are eight separate genes of the family that codes the β-subunit of β-hCG and β-hLH. Seven of these genes code for β-hCG and one for β-hLH. All eight of the genes for the β-subunit are on chromosome 19. Only two

(possibly three) of the β-hCG genes are expressed. It has been speculated that the seven β-hCG genes evolved from an ancestral gene for β-LH.

The rate of synthesis of the β-subunit is limiting in the formation of the complete hCG molecule. Trophoblasts of normal placenta and those of hydatidiform mole and choriocarcinoma tissues secrete the α- and β-subunits as well as intact hCG; but there is an excess of hCG α-subunits in placenta and in plasma of pregnant women whereas the hCG β-subunit is present in small or undetectable quantities. Interestingly, the same obtains with respect to the synthesis and secretion of the α- and β-subunits of LH by the pituitary.

Both the α- and β-subunits are synthesized as larger molecular weight precursors; the signal sequences are cleaved by microsomal endopeptidases. Once hCG is synthesized, it is rapidly released from the cell; but, the regulation of hCG secretion from the cell is not understood.

Cellular Site of Origin of hCG

The complete hCG molecule is believed to be produced principally in syncytiotrophoblasts rather than cytotrophoblasts. It has been demonstrated, however, that mRNA for α-hCG is present in cytotrophoblasts and syncytiotrophoblasts whereas mRNA for β-hCG is present primarily in syncytiotrophoblasts.

It is somewhat paradoxical, therefore, that the greatest concentration of hCG in plasma of pregnant women is found at a time in gestation when there are the greatest number of cytotrophoblasts in the placenta, viz., in early pregnancy, at 8 to 10 weeks gestation. As the number of cytotrophoblasts in placenta decline, the levels of hCG in maternal blood also decline. Later in gestation, in some complicated pregnancies, there is a reappearance of cytotrophoblasts, e.g., with D-antigen isoimmunization and an affected fetus and in pregnancies complicated by maternal diabetes mellitus. And in such circumstances, there also is an increase in the concentration of hCG. Indeed in some such pregnancies, theca lutein cysts develop late in pregnancy, possibly in response to the increase in the concentration of hCG in maternal plasma. It is possible, as will be addressed subsequently, that GnRH, produced in cytotrophoblasts, acts on syncytiotrophoblast, in a paracrine manner, to stimulate the secretion of hCG in a fashion analogous to the stimulation of pituitary LH release by GnRH of hypothalamic origin.

Concentrations of hCG in Serum and Urine

The intact (complete) hCG molecule is detectable in the plasma of pregnant women within 8 to 10 days after the midcycle surge

TABLE 5–1. STEROID PRODUCTION RATES IN NONPREGNANT AND NEAR-TERM PREGNANT WOMEN

	Production Rate (mg per 24 hr)	
Steroid[a]	Nonpregnant	Pregnant
Estradiol-17β	0.1–0.6	15–20
Estriol	0.02–0.1	50–150
Progesterone	0.1–20	250–600
Aldosterone	0.05–0.1	1–2
Deoxycorticosterone	0.05–0.5	1–12
Cortisol	10–30	10–20

[a] Estrogens and progesterone are produced by placenta. Aldosterone is produced by the maternal adrenal in response to the stimulus of angiotensin II. Deoxycorticosterone is produced in extraglandular tissue sites by way of the 21-hydroxylation of plasma progesterone. Cortisol production during pregnancy is not increased, even though the blood levels are elevated because of decreased clearance caused by increased cortisol-binding globulin (Chap. 7).

of LH secretion that precedes ovulation. Thus, it is likely that hCG begins to enter maternal blood on the day of blastocyst implantation. Thereafter, the levels of hCG in blood increase rapidly, maximal levels being attained at about 10 weeks of pregnancy. There is no discernible, predictable rhythmicity in the secretion of hCG during the day, but appreciable fluctuations in plasma levels are observed in the same pregnant woman (Chap. 2).

The level of hCG in fetal plasma is much less than that in maternal plasma, viz., about 3 percent; but the pattern of appearance of hCG in fetal blood (as a function of gestational age) is similar to that in the mother. HCG is present in amnionic fluid; and early in pregnancy, the concentration of hCG in this biological space is similar to that in maternal plasma. As pregnancy progresses, however, the concentration of hCG in amnionic fluid declines to levels that are about one fifth that in maternal blood.

Beginning at about 10 to 12 weeks of pregnancy, the level of hCG in maternal blood begins to decline, a nadir being reached by about 20 weeks gestation. But, this lower plasma level of hCG persists during the remainder of pregnancy. The level of hCG in the serum is closely parallel to that in the urine, rising rapidly from approximately 1 IU per mL by 6 weeks after the commencement of the last menstrual period to an average value of about 100 IU per mL between the 60th and 80th day after the last menses (Fig. 5–2).

The levels of the α- and β-subunit in plasma of pregnant women are substantially different from those of the intact molecule. As cited, the levels of the β-subunit are low or undetectable throughout human pregnancy (Fig. 5–2). On the other hand, the levels of the α-subunit increase gradually and steadily until about 36 weeks gestation when a plateau is attained that is maintained for the remainder of pregnancy, similar to the pattern of human placental lactogen ([hPL] Fig. 5–2), as discussed subsequently (Ashitaka and co-workers, 1980). Thus, the formation of α-hCG corresponds to placental mass whereas the formation of the complete hCG molecule is maximal at 8 to 10 weeks gestation. The concentration of α-hCG in maternal blood, however, always is much less (10 percent or less) than that of intact hCG.

Significantly higher levels of hCG are likely to be found in pregnancies with multiple fetuses, in pregnancies with a single erythroblastotic fetus resulting from maternal isoimmunization, and especially in women with hydatidiform mole and choriocarcinoma. Interestingly, a variety of nontrophoblastic tumors also produce hCG; and, Yoshimoto and co-workers (1979) have demonstrated that many normal tissues also secrete hCG, albeit in very small amounts. It has been shown that the β-subunit of hCG is produced in fetal kidney (McGregor and co-workers, 1981); but more than that, it now has been shown that a number of fetal tissues produce the intact hCG molecule (McGregor and associates, 1983).

Regulation of hCG Biosynthesis

The complete hCG molecule is synthesized primarily in the syncytiotrophoblasts. And, the amount of total mRNA for both the α- and β-subunits of hCG is greater in placentas from first trimester than from those at term. But, the concentration of α-mRNA in syncytiotrophoblasts increases as pregnancy advances. The finding of mRNA for the α- and β-subunits of hCG in cytotrophoblasts or in intermediate trophoblasts is suggestive that the genes for hCG are expressed before full differentiation of the cells.

This conclusion is supported by the fact that cytotrophoblasts begin to disappear from the placenta at the end of the first trimester; and, when there is a reappearance of cytotrophoblasts, hCG levels rise, e.g., with D-antigen isoimmunization. Alternatively, as stated, GnRH may be produced in cytotrophoblasts and then act on syncytial cells to stimulate hCG formation. There are several lines of evidence in favor of a role for placental GnRH in the regulation of trophoblast formation hCG. Recently, a role for placental inhibin in the regulation of hCG formation also has been proposed (p. 72).

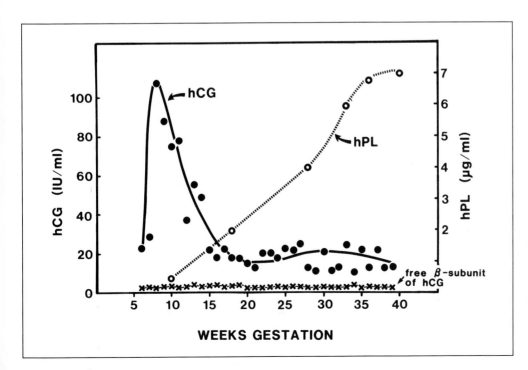

Figure 5–2. Mean concentration of chorionic gonadotropin (hCG) and placental lactogen (hPL) in serum of women throughout normal pregnancy. Free β-subunit of hCG is in low concentration or else is undetectable throughout pregnancy. The concentration of free α-subunit of hCG in serum increases gradually during pregnancy in a manner similar to that of hPL, albeit in much smaller amounts than hPL. (*Data from Ashitaka and colleagues, 1980; Selenkow and co-workers, Diabetes 20:696, 1971.*)

Biomolecular Regulation of hCG Formation

It has been demonstrated that a number of agents act to increase hCG secretion by trophoblasts in vitro. Among these are bu-tyrated derivatives of cyclic AMP, GnRH, and epidermal growth factor; on the other hand, dibutyryl cyclic GMP, AMP, insulin, progesterone, epinephrine, or prostaglandin do not cause an increase in hCG secretion.

Metabolic Disposition of hCG

The metabolic clearance rate (MCR) of hCG is about 3 mL per minute; i.e., about 4 liters of plasma are cleared of hCG each day. The renal clearance of hCG as the native molecule accounts for 30 percent of the total MCR, the remainder being metabo-lized by pathways other than renal excretion, likely in liver and kidney (Nishula and Wehmann, 1980). The MCR of the β-subunit and of the α-subunit are about 10-fold and 30-fold, respectively, greater than that of native hCG. On the other hand, the renal clearance rates of the subunits are considerably less than that of hCG. Thus, renal clearance is not the means by which the subunits are cleared so rapidly from plasma.

Assay of hCG

The methods for detecting hCG are of considerable importance because these assays form the basis for the majority of tests for pregnancy in women (Chap. 2).

Biological Functions of hCG

The most apparent function of hCG in pregnancy is to maintain the function of the corpus luteum during early gestation. Brad-bury and colleagues (1950) demonstrated that the lifespan of the corpus luteum in nonpregnant women could be prolonged by the administration of hCG during the luteal phase of the ovarian cycle. Until recently, however, this action of hCG, while ac-cepted without question from the findings of Bradbury and co-workers, seemed to offer an incomplete explanation for the physiological role of hCG. This obtains because the maximum concentrations of hCG in plasma of pregnant women are at-tained at a time in gestation after the function of the corpus luteum, with respect to progesterone formation, has declined, viz., at 8 to 10 weeks gestation (Fig. 5–2). While not rigorously proven, a tentative explanation for these several observations may be formulated. HCG, which is present in high concentra-tions at 8 to 10 weeks gestation, may serve to "down-regulate" the hCG/LH receptors in corpus luteum; the consequence would be a decrease in the rate of cholesterol side-chain cleavage and, thereby, a reduction in the rate of corpus luteum progesterone secretion at a time in gestation when trophoblasts are capable of producing sufficient progesterone for the maintenance of pregnancy.

Fetal testicular testosterone secretion is maximum at the same time in gestation that the rate of placental secretion of hCG is maximum. Thus, at a critical time in male fetal develop-ment, hCG serves as an LH surrogate on fetal testes to promote testosterone synthesis and secretion and thereby male sexual differentiation.

In the adult human ovary, appropriately primed by FSH, hCG induces ovulation and is sometimes used therapeutically, together with FSH, as an LH surrogate in the treatment of infertility caused by anovulation because of hypogonadotropic hypogonadism. In this context, it is important to reiterate that the half-life of hCG is quite long (24 hours) compared with that of LH (2 hours), which may account for a longer lifespan of the corpus luteum after ovulation induction with hCG compared with that induced by LH in hypophysectomized women.

HUMAN PLACENTAL LACTOGEN

History

Prolactin-like activity in the human placenta was first described by Ehrhardt in 1936. The hormone responsible for this activity was isolated and partially purified by Ito and Higashi (1961) and by Josimovich and MacLaren (1962). They isolated and charac-terized this polypeptide from extracts of human placenta and retroplacental blood. Because of potent lactogenic and growth hormone-like activity (and an immunochemical resemblance to human growth hormone), it first was called *human placental lactogen or chorionic growth hormone*. This hormone also has been referred to as chorionic somatomammotropin. Recently, most authors have used the original terminology, i.e., human pla-cental lactogen (hPL). Grumbach and Kaplan (1964) found, by immunofluorescence studies, that this hormone, like hCG, was concentrated in the syncytiotrophoblast. HPL is detected in the trophoblast as early as the second or third week after ovulation.

Chemical Characteristics

HPL consists of a single polypeptide chain with a molecular weight of 22,279. The gene for hPL has been cloned, and the nucleotide sequence for DNA complementary to the mRNA encoding for hPL has been determined (Shine and colleagues, 1977). Placental lactogen contains 191 amino acid residues, com-pared with 188 in human growth hormone; the amino acid sequence in each hormone is strikingly similar (96 percent ho-mology, including conservative substitutions). HPL also is struc-turally similar to human prolactin (hPRL) with about 67 percent amino-acid-sequence homology. For these reasons, it has been suggested that the genes for hPL, hPRL, and hGH evolved from a common ancestral gene by repeated gene duplication as re-viewed by Talamantes and Ogren (1988). Large molecular weight forms of hPL (dimers and higher oligomers) are found in serum and in extracts of the placenta.

Gene Structure and Expression

There are five genes in the growth hormone–placental lactogen gene family; the genes are linked and located on chromosome 17. Two of these genes, hCS-A and hCS-B, both code for hPL, and the amount of mRNA for each (in term placentas) is similar. On the other hand, the gene for hPRL is located on chromo-some 6 (Owerbach and co-workers, 1980, 1981).

The mRNA for hPL in placenta is localized in the syncy-tiotrophoblasts and is not found in cytotrophoblasts, indicating that the genes for hPL are expressed only in the fully differen-tiated trophoblast. Incredibly, at term, hPL represents 7 to 10 percent of the peptides synthesized by placental ribosomes. In fact, 20 percent of the mRNA of term placenta is hPL mRNA. The synthesis of hPL is stimulated by insulin and cAMP. PGE_2 and $PGF_{2\alpha}$ seem to inhibit the secretion of hPL.

Secretion and Metabolism

The metabolic clearance rate of hPL, about 175 L per day, is considerably greater than that of hCG; and, the production rate near term, 1 g or more per day, is the greatest of any known hormone in the human.

Serum Concentration

HPL is demonstrable in syncytiotrophoblasts within 2 to 3 weeks after conception; and, placental lactogen can be detected in the serum of pregnant women as early as the 5th week of gestation (3 weeks after fertilization). The concentration of hPL rises steadily until about the 34th to 36th week of pregnancy and the concentration in maternal blood is approximately proportional to placental mass. The concentration of hPL in maternal serum, as measured by radioimmunoassay, reaches higher levels in late pregnancy (5 to 15 μg per mL) than those of any other known protein hormone (Fig. 5–2). These high levels, coupled with a very short half-life in the circulation, attest to a rate of production of hPL by the placenta of considerable magnitude. The half-life of hPL in maternal plasma is between 10 and 30 minutes.

Very little hPL is found in the circulation of the human fetus or in the urine of the mother or newborn; the concentration of the hormone in amnionic fluid is somewhat lower than that in maternal plasma. Because hPL is secreted primarily into the maternal circulation, with only very small amounts found in cord blood, it appears that the role of the hormone in pregnancy, if any, is mediated through action in maternal rather than in fetal tissues.

Regulation of hPL Biosynthesis

The concentration of mRNA for hPL in syncytiotrophoblasts remains relatively constant throughout pregnancy. This finding also is supportive of the likelihood that the rate of hPL secretion is proportional to placental mass. As stated, the absence of mRNA for hPL in cytotrophoblasts may be indicative that only the mature, differentiated cell produces hPL; the finding of very high levels of hCG in blood of women with neoplastic trophoblastic disease together with low levels of hPL in plasma of these same women is supportive of this view. Prolonged starvation in the first half of pregnancy leads to an increase in the concentration of hPL in plasma. Short-term changes in plasma glucose or insulin have relatively little effect on plasma levels of hPL.

Metabolic Actions of hPL

It has been postulated that hPL participates, directly or indirectly, in a number of important metabolic processes. These putative actions include (1) lipolysis and an increase in the levels of circulating free fatty acids (thereby providing a source of energy for maternal metabolism and fetal nutrition) and (2) inhibition of both the uptake of glucose and of gluconeogenesis in the mother, thereby sparing both glucose and protein (Chap. 7, p. 138). The latter proposed anti-insulin action of hPL is believed to lead to an increase in maternal levels of insulin, which favors protein synthesis; this, in turn, ensures a mobilizable source of amino acids for transport to the fetus.

The presence of the hormone, however, does not appear to be required for a successful pregnancy outcome. Nielsen and associates (1979) described a pregnancy in which hPL could not be identified in either maternal serum or in the placenta when analyzed by several techniques in a number of laboratories. Since the account of Nielsen and co-workers, other cases of very low or undetectable levels of hPL in otherwise normal pregnancies have been described. It has been estimated that deficiency in hPL production may occur in about 1 of 12,000 pregnancies. Hubert and associates (1983) found that the level of mRNA for hPL in placental tissue of a pregnancy in which hPL in maternal plasma was undetectable, was very low compared with that in a normal placenta. These findings are consistent with the likelihood that hPL functions primarily as a fail-safe mechanism to ensure nutrient supply to the fetus, for example, in times of maternal starvation.

Spellacy and Buhi (1969) could not detect hPL in the early postpartum period and also noted a deficient output of pituitary growth hormone at this time. They suggested that this relative lack of insulin antagonists is associated with low fasting levels of blood glucose during this period.

HPL production is not restricted to the trophoblast. The hormone has been detected by direct radioimmunoassay in sera from men and women with various malignancies, other than those originating in trophoblast or gonad, including bronchogenic carcinoma, hepatoma, lymphoma, and pheochromocytoma (Weintraub and Rosen, 1970).

Possible indications in clinical obstetrics for assaying hPL are considered especially in Chapter 15 (p. 289); however, clear utility for its measurement in high-risk pregnancy has not been established.

CHORIONIC ADRENOCORTICOTROPIN AND THYROTROPIN

An ACTH-like protein has been isolated from placental tissue and considerable evidence has accrued to support the proposition that this compound is of placental origin. There are several lines of evidence that are supportive of the likelihood that ACTH is produced in chorionic tissue. Odagiri and colleagues (1979) found that ACTH, lipotropin, and β-endorphin are all found in placental extracts and presumably are derived from the same or a similar 31K precursor molecule, pro-opiomelanocortin (Fig. 5–3), as are the pituitary peptides. Liotta and colleagues (1977) also found that ACTH is produced by dispersed placental cells.

Dexamethasone treatment does not alter the levels of ACTH in placental tissue whether the ACTH is measured by bioassay or immunoassay. To evaluate the biosynthesis of ACTH and ACTH-like compounds in placental tissue, the incorporation of [35S]methionine and [3H]leucine into ACTH and related peptides by dispersed trophoblastic cells was demonstrated. By use of pulse-chase studies, the radiolabel was first incorporated into a high molecular weight (M_r about 34,000) peptide similar to that of the ACTH, β-lipotropin precursor of the pituitary and

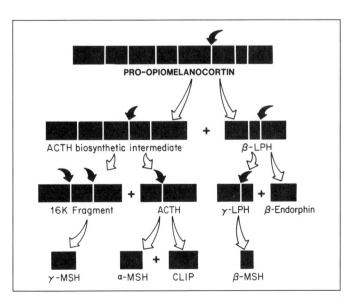

Figure 5–3. Processing of pituitary pro-opiomelanocortin (31K protein).

hypothalamus. With longer incubations, the radiolabel disappeared progressively from the high molecular weight form and began to appear, in increasing amounts, in smaller peptides that corresponded to peptides with antigenic determinants of ACTH and α-MSH, as well as β-lipotropin and β-endorphin. For a review of the placental processing of pro-opiomelanocortin, see Simpson and MacDonald (1981) and Krieger (1982).

Nonetheless, the physiological significance of placental ACTH and related compounds is unclear. In pregnant women, the plasma levels of ACTH at all times in pregnancy (before labor) are lower than those found in men and nonpregnant women; nonetheless, the concentration of immunoreactive ACTH in maternal plasma increases as pregnancy advances (Carr and colleagues, 1981). The placenta may produce ACTH that is secreted into the mother or fetus during pregnancy, but it is likely that ACTH does not cross the placenta. The administration of dexamethasone to pregnant women does not cause suppression of the levels of urinary free cortisol as effectively as it does in men and nonpregnant women.

There also is evidence that the placenta produces a chorionic thyrotropin (hCT), but there is little or no evidence that there is a significant biological role for this substance in normal human pregnancy. The neoplastic trophoblasts of hydatidiform mole and choriocarcinoma may produce a family of chorionic thyrotropins, but the increased thyroid-stimulating activity in women with neoplastic trophoblastic disease may be attributed chiefly to the thyroid-stimulating properties of hCG, which are low; but, enormous quantities of hCG are produced in women with hydatidiform mole (Chap. 31, p. 545).

HYPOTHALAMIC-LIKE–RELEASING HORMONES OF THE PLACENTA

There is an appreciable amount of immunoreactive gonadotropin-releasing hormone (GnRH) in placenta (Siler-Khodr and Khodr, 1978, and Siler-Khodr, 1988). Interestingly, these investigators also demonstrated that immunoreactive GnRH was present in the cytotrophoblast, but not in the syncytiotrophoblast. Siler-Khodr (1983) has referred to this substance as hCG-releasing hormone. Gibbons and co-workers (1975) and Khodr and Siler-Khodr (1980) have demonstrated that the human placenta can synthesize both GnRH and TRH in vitro.

Indeed, for each known hypothalamic-releasing hormone or -inhibiting hormone described, namely GnRH, TRH, corticotropin-releasing hormone (CRF), and somatostatin, there are reports of analogous hormones produced in human placenta, as reviewed by Siler-Khodr (1988). The role of these hypothalamic-like releasing or inhibiting hormones in chorionic tissue, however, cannot be resolved presently. It is interesting to speculate that the finding of these substances in placental tissue is indicative that there may be a hierarchy of control of formation of chorionic trophic agents such as hCG, hCT, and pro-opiomelanocortin-derived peptides of the placenta. CRF is found in umbilical venous blood, indicative of placenta secretion of this peptide into the fetal compartment. Margioris and associates (1988) demonstrated that placental fragments perifused in vitro release immunoreactive corticotropin-releasing hormone.

INHIBIN

Inhibin, a glycoprotein hormone that acts preferentially to inhibit FSH release by the pituitary, is known to be produced by human testis and by the granulosa cells of the human ovary. Inhibin is a heterodimer, i.e., composed of dissimilar α- and β-subunits. Inhibin also is produced in placenta; and in conjunction with the large amounts of sex steroid hormones produced in human pregnancy, may serve to inhibit FSH secretion and thereby preclude ovulation during pregnancy. In placenta, inhibin is produced in cytotrophoblasts and may serve, in a paracrine fashion, to regulate syncytiotrophoblast function, e.g., the regulation of hCG release. HCG and cyclic AMP analogues stimulate inhibin secretion in isolated trophoblast cells; antibodies to the inhibin α-subunit cause an increase in hCG secretion, suggesting that inhibin may act to regulate hCG release/secretion in placenta (Petraglia and associates, 1987).

"Pregnancy-Specific" Proteins

In the past two decades, a host of proteins has been discovered that most investigators refer to as pregnancy specific or pregnancy related. For the most part, these "newly discovered" proteins were identified by use of antibodies developed in animals against the serum of pregnant women. The resulting antibodies in animal serum were treated with serum of men or nonpregnant women to remove antibodies not specific for proteins of human pregnancy; and, those antibodies remaining should be directed toward antigens specific in, or in far greater concentration in, serum of pregnant women. The residual antiserum can then be used to isolate proteins peculiar to the serum of pregnant women. Many investigators have employed this approach; and, in consequence, it is estimated that more than 20 such proteins have been isolated (Klopper, 1981). This estimate, however, is difficult to make with certainty because there is no consistent nomenclature or precise standards for indentification of these pregnancy-related proteins. The precise role(s) or function(s) of these proteins produced in placenta or decidua or both is not defined. Many possibilities exist. Among those proposed are involvements in the immunological acceptance of the fetal semiallogenic graft, binding proteins for other agents and hormones, stimulants of cellular formation of other hormones or bioactive agents, and others.

ESTROGENS

ESTROGEN PRODUCTION IN PREGNANCY

Normal human pregnancy, near term, is a hyperestrogenic state of nearly unbelievable magnitude. The amount of estrogen produced each day during the last few weeks of pregnancy is equivalent to that produced, on average, by no fewer than 1,000 ovulatory premenopausal women each day. By way of another analogy, during the course of one normal human pregnancy, more estrogen is produced by the placenta than is secreted by the ovaries of 150 ovulatory premenopausal women during an entire year. This hyperestrogenic state is one of continually increasing proportions as pregnancy progresses, terminating abruptly immediately after delivery of the fetus and placenta.

The small amount of estrogen produced by the maternal ovaries is limited to the first 2 to 4 postovulatory weeks of pregnancy. Diczfalusy and Borell (1961) found no reduction in the levels of urinary estrogens after bilateral oophorectomy performed as early as the 78th day of pregnancy. Similar results were obtained in several studies of urinary estrogen excretion by pregnant women after surgical removal of the corpus luteum. As early as the 7th week of gestation, more than 50 percent of the estrogens entering the maternal circulation are produced in placenta (MacDonald, 1965; Siiteri and MacDonald, 1963, 1966a).

ESTROGEN BIOSYNTHESIS IN PLACENTA

The biosynthetic mechanisms of estrogen formation in human pregnancy differ from those in men and nonpregnant women. Androstenedione, the immediate precursor of estrone, is produced de novo in the ovary, i.e., from acetate or cholesterol, in theca cells of the developing follicle. Androstenedione is transferred from the theca cells into the follicular fluid and thence utilized by the granulosa cells for estrogen formation. Therefore, it is clear that estradiol-17β synthesized in the granulosa cells is produced from ovarian theca cell precursor produced de novo, i.e., from acetate or cholesterol (Chap. 2).

This is not true of placenta. Acetate or cholesterol, or even progesterone, cannot serve as precursor for estrogen biosynthesis in the human placenta. Steroid 17α-hydroxylase activity is not expressed in the human placenta; and consequently, the conversion of C_{21}-steroids to C_{19}-steroids, the latter being the immediate precursors of estrogen, is not possible in human placenta.

This is an important consideration for reasons that are related to both the endocrinology of human pregnancy and to the endocrine antecedents of parturition as well (p. 191). Steroid 17α-hydroxylase activity is demonstrable in the placenta of most mammalian species, but not in the placentas of primates. In those species in which steroid 17α-hydroxylase is present, the induction of this enzyme is usually possible by treatment with glucocorticosteroids (e.g., cortisol of fetal adrenal origin); and, increased placental 17α-hydroxylase activity leads to a fall in progesterone secretion and a "surge" in estrogen formation, endocrine antecedents that herald the onset of parturition in many species, but not the human (Chap. 10).

In classic experiments, Ryan (1959a) demonstrated that there is an exceptionally high capacity of placenta to convert certain C_{19}-steroids to estrone and estradiol-17β. He found that dehydroisoandrosterone, androstenedione, and testosterone were converted efficiently to estrone or estradiol-17β, or both, by preparations of human placental tissue. These findings were important later in the design of investigations to define the role of preformed C_{19}-steroids delivered to placenta in maternal or fetal plasma as precursors for the biosynthesis of estrogen.

PLASMA-BORNE PRECURSORS FOR PLACENTAL ESTROGEN BIOSYNTHESIS

Prophetically, Amoroso (1960) suggested that the placenta might, through its abundant enzymatic activity, bring about the formation of active agents by way of the conversion of inactive materials derived from elsewhere in the body. Support for this deduction was provided by Frandsen and Stakemann (1961) who discovered that the amount of estrogen in the urine of women pregnant with an anencephalic fetus was approximately one-tenth that found in the urine of women pregnant with a normal fetus at the same stage of gestation. Pointing to the characteristic absence of the fetal zone of the adrenal cortex in anencephalic human fetuses, Frandsen and Stakemann deduced that the fetal adrenal may be the site of origin of a substance(s) that serves as the placental estrogen precursor.

The first proof that the placenta uses plasma-borne precursors for estrogen biosynthesis was provided by the demonstration that radiolabeled dehydroisoandrosterone sulfate, intro-

duced into the maternal circulation, was converted extensively to radioactive estrogens by the placenta (Baulieu and Dray, 1963; Siiteri and MacDonald, 1963). It also was shown that other C_{19}-steroids, namely, nonconjugated dehydroisoandrosterone, androstenedione, and testosterone, when introduced into the maternal circulation, also were converted to estrogens.

The abundance of dehydroisoandrosterone sulfate in the plasma, however, and its much longer half-life uniquely qualified this steroid as the principal circulating precursor of placental estrone and estradiol-17β. The presentation of dehydroisoandrosterone as the sulfate ester at the site of conversion does not preclude its use in the synthesis of estrogen; this obtains because the placenta normally is a rich source of sulfatase activity (Pulkkinen, 1961; Warren and Timberlake, 1962). By infusing radiolabeled dehydroisoandrosterone sulfate into pregnant women, it was shown as early as the 7th week of gestation that there is conversion of circulating maternal dehydroisoandrosterone sulfate to estradiol-17β. By the 30th week of pregnancy, 25 percent or more of dehydroisoandrosterone sulfate in the maternal plasma is converted to estradiol-17β by the placenta (Siiteri and MacDonald, 1963, 1966a).

METABOLISM OF MATERNAL PLASMA DEHYDROISOANDROSTERONE SULFATE

The extensive use of maternal plasma dehydroisoandrosterone sulfate for placental estrogen biosynthesis undoubtedly accounts, in part, for the progressive decrease in the concentration of dehydroisoandrosterone sulfate in the plasma of pregnant women as pregnancy progresses, as well as the decrease in the amount of 11-deoxy-17-ketosteroids excreted in the urine of pregnant women (Migeon and associates, 1955; Milewich and colleagues, 1978; Siiteri and MacDonald, 1966b).

In extensive studies of the metabolism of maternal plasma dehydroisoandrosterone sulfate in human pregnancy, Gant and co-workers (1971) found that there is a striking increase in the metabolic clearance rate (MCR) of plasma dehydroisoandrosterone sulfate in normally pregnant women at term compared with its clearance in men and nonpregnant women. The MCR of dehydroisoandrosterone sulfate in men and nonpregnant women is small, viz., 6 to 8 liters per 24 hours; but, the rate of clearance of this substance from plasma of pregnant women at term is increased by 10- to 20-fold. Because the production rate of dehydroisoandrosterone sulfate in maternal adrenals is not changed significantly during the course of human pregnancy, the plasma concentration must decrease as the rate of clearance increases.

The increase in the MCR of dehydroisoandrosterone sulfate from the plasma of pregnant women appears to be attributable principally to two processes: (1) its removal through conversion to estradiol-17β by the trophoblasts; and, (2) an increased rate of metabolism that is accounted for by increased 16α-hydroxylation of dehydroisoandrosterone sulfate in the maternal compartment (probably in maternal liver). Approximately 30 percent of dehydroisoandrosterone sulfate in the plasma of pregnant women is converted to 16α-hydroxydehydroisoandrosterone sulfate (Madden and associates, 1976, 1978). The extent of these conversions is high; nonetheless, the maternal adrenal does not produce significantly increased amounts of dehydroisoandrosterone sulfate during pregnancy; therefore, the fetal adrenal constitutes the quantitatively important source of placental estrogen precursor in the human.

FETAL ADRENAL GLANDS

FETAL ADRENAL AND ESTROGEN FORMATION IN PLACENTA

As pregnancy advances, the placental utilization of maternal plasma dehydroisoandrosterone sulfate accounts for only a small fraction of total placental estrogen production. The observation by Frandsen and Stakemann (1961) of lower excretion of estrogens in women pregnant with an anencephalic fetus, in whom the fetal zone of the adrenal cortex characteristically is absent, together with the finding of high levels of dehydroisoandrosterone sulfate in the cord blood of normal infants (Colas and co-workers, 1964), were suggestive of the likelihood that the fetal adrenal cortex was the principal source of placental estrogen precursors, both for estradiol-17β and estriol.

Confirmation for part of this hypothesis was provided by the experiments of Bolté and co-workers (1964a,b), who demonstrated that dehydroisoandrosterone sulfate, introduced into the umbilical artery and perfused through the placenta in situ, was converted to estrone and estradiol-17β. Ultimately it was established that, near term, about 50 percent of estradiol-17β produced in placenta arises from the utilization of maternal plasma dehydroisoandrosterone sulfate and 50 percent arises from fetal plasma dehydroisoandrosterone sulfate (Siiteri and MacDonald, 1966a).

FETAL ADRENAL CONTRIBUTION TO ESTRIOL FORMATION IN PLACENTA

Therefore, dehydroisoandrosterone sulfate, circulating in both fetal and maternal plasma, is used in the production of estrone and estradiol-17β by the placenta; nonetheless, these findings did not provide an explanation for the inordinately large amount of estriol produced in human pregnancy.

In nonpregnant women, the estrogen secreted by the granulosa cells of the "chosen" follicle is estradiol-17β; the estrogen formed in extraglandular tissues is estrone; and from these two primary estrogens, the multiple estrogenic metabolites (including estriol), which are found in urine of nonpregnant women, are derived. The ratio of the concentration of urinary estriol to that of estrone plus estradiol-17β in nonpregnant women is approximately one. But during pregnancy, this ratio increases to ten or even much more near term (Brown, 1956).

Estriol produced during human pregnancy cannot be accounted for as a metabolite of estrone or estradiol-17β. Brown (1956) and Fishman and associates (1961) demonstrated that the metabolic fate of estradiol-17β in pregnant women was not significantly different from that found in nonpregnant women.

Moreover, it has not been possible to demonstrate the conversion of more than trace amounts of estradiol-17β to estriol in the placenta, indicating that the critical step of 16α-hydroxylation necessary for the conversion of estrone or estradiol-17β to estriol is not efficiently performed by placental tissue.

Consequently, several other explanations were offered to account for the formation of estriol in pregnancy. One of the several hypotheses held that placental estrone and estradiol-17β were circulated to the fetus and therein converted to estriol, which thereafter reentered the maternal circulation (Fishman and associates, 1961; Gurpide and co-workers, 1962). A second explanation, advanced by Bolté and colleagues (1964c), held that placental estrone was converted to 16α-hydroxyestrone by the fetus and that this product circulated back to the placenta where reduction to estriol occurred.

A third explanation was that a 16α-hydroxy-C_{19}-steroid(s) produced in the fetus or mother is a circulating precursor for placental biosynthesis of estriol. Although all three explanations are supported by data, quantitatively, the third mechanism is the most important.

Ryan (1959b) had demonstrated that 16α-hydroxylated C_{19}-steroids such as 16α-hydroxydehydroisoandrosterone, 16α-hydroxy-Δ^4-androstenedione, and 16α-hydroxytestosterone were converted efficiently to estriol by preparations of human placental tissue. In addition, large amounts of 16α-hydroxydehydroisoandrosterone sulfate are found in umbilical cord blood (Colas and associates, 1964). Finally, the conversion of radiolabeled 16α-hydroxydehydroisoandrosterone and 16α-hydroxydehydroisoandrosterone sulfate, introduced into the maternal circulation, to radiolabeled estriol was demonstrated (MacDonald and Siiteri, 1965a; Madden and associates, 1978).

The disproportionate increase in estriol formation during human pregnancy, therefore, results from the direct placental formation of estriol from 16α-hydroxylated C_{19}-steroids, principally 16α-hydroxydehydroisoandrosterone sulfate, rather than from an alteration in the metabolism of estrone or estradiol-17β to estriol in mother or fetus or from 16α-hydroxylation in placenta, which does not occur. 16α-Hydroxydehydroisoandrosterone sulfate, which is present in large concentrations in fetal blood, arises by synthesis in the fetal adrenal and by 16α-hydroxylation of fetal plasma dehydroisoandrosterone sulfate

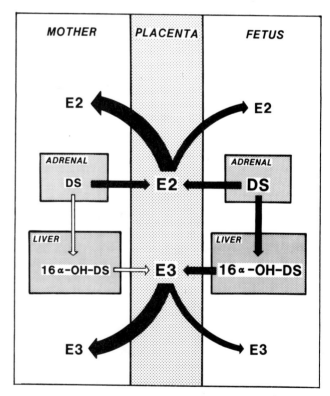

Figure 5–4. Schematic presentation of the biosynthesis of estrogen in human placenta. Near term, 50 percent of estradiol-17β is derived from fetal adrenal dehydroisoandrosterone sulfate (DS) and 50 percent from maternal DS. On the other hand, 90 percent of estriol in placenta arises from fetal 16α-OH-dehydroisoandrosterone sulfate (16α-OH-DS) and only 10 percent from all other sources. Most (80 to 90 percent) of steroids produced in placenta are secreted into the maternal blood.

in the fetal liver (Fig. 5–4). **The fetus is the source of 90 percent of the precursor of estriol formed in placenta in normal near-term human pregnancy** (Siiteri and MacDonald, 1966a).

Maternal plasma dehydroisoandrosterone sulfate also is converted to estriol by way of an estrone/estradiol-17β-independent pathway; namely, plasma dehydroisoandrosterone sulfate is converted in maternal liver to 16α-hydroxydehydrosisandrosterone sulfate, which, in placenta, is converted to estriol (MacDonald and Siiteri, 1965a,b; Madden and colleagues, 1976, 1978).

FETAL ADRENAL FUNCTION: AN OVERVIEW

Based on the importance of the fetal adrenal in the biogenesis of placental estrogen precursors and based on the potential importance of fetal adrenal secretions in fetal lung maturation (Chap. 6), and in the initiation of labor (Chap. 10), considerable interest and investigative efforts have been directed toward an elucidation of the factors that serve to regulate the steroidogenic activity and growth of this remarkable gland.

The fetal adrenal cortex is unique; compared with organs of the adult, it is the largest organ of the fetus; but, it is an unusual structure in other ways. At term, the weight of the fetal adrenals approximates the weight of the adrenals of the adult; but more than 85 percent of the fetal adrenal gland normally is composed of the peculiar fetal zone, which is not found in the adrenals of adults.

Direct measurements of fetal adrenal steroid secretory rates have not been possible; nonetheless, it can be estimated that normally, near term, the fetal adrenals must produce 100 to 200 mg of steroids per day. If one considers that the normal rate of steroid secretion by the adrenals of the nonstressed, resting adult rarely exceeds 20 to 30 mg per day, it is apparent that the fetal adrenal is a truly remarkable endocrine organ.

The fetal adrenal cortex of the neonate undergoes rapid involution immediately after birth; and, the weight of the adrenals decreases strikingly during the first few weeks of life. The size attained by the adrenals of the human fetus just before birth is not achieved again until late in adolescent or early adult life (Fig. 5–5).

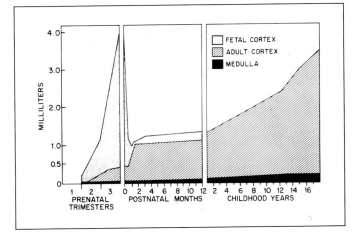

Figure 5–5. Size of the adrenal gland and its component parts in utero, during infancy, and during childhood. (*Adapted from Bethune: The Adrenal Cortex, A Scope Monograph. Kalamazoo, MI, Upjohn, 1974.*)-

EARLY FETAL ADRENAL DEVELOPMENT

Early in embryonic life, the fetal adrenal is composed of cells that resemble those of the fetal zone of the fetal adrenal cortex; these cells rapidly appear and proliferate prior to the time that vascularization of the pituitary by the hypothalamus is complete. This is suggestive that the early development of the fetal adrenal is under trophic influences that may not conform exactly to those of the adult (Mulchahey and colleagues, 1987). Possibly, ACTH is secreted by the fetal pituitary in the absence of hypothalamic corticotropin-releasing factor (CRF), or else ACTH (or CRF) arises from a source(s) other than the fetal pituitary, e.g., from chorionic ACTH (or CRF) that is synthesized by trophoblast. ACTH does not cross the placenta. But there are other possibilities; these include the likelihood that there is an agent(s) other than ACTH that promotes the replication of adrenal cells of the fetal zone.

The adrenal cortex of the normal fetus continues to grow throughout gestation; and during the last 5 to 6 weeks of pregnancy, there is a sharp increase in size of the human fetal adrenal. It is quite clear that the rate of fetal adrenal growth and steroid secretion are not controlled by a single trophic stimulus (ACTH), but rather must be regulated by more than one type of growth-promoting agent. The peculiar development, growth rate, and steroid synthetic pattern that are characteristic of the fetal adrenal can be explained only in this way.

Enzymatic Considerations

There is a relative deficiency in the expression of the microsomal enzyme 3β-hydroxysteroid dehydrogenase $\Delta^{5,4}$-isomerase in the fetal adrenal. The absence of effective expression of this enzyme activity limits the conversion of pregnenolone to progesterone, an obligatory step in cortisol biosynthesis, and it also precludes the conversion of dehydroisoandrosterone to androstenedione. Presently, it is not totally clear whether the absence of expression of 3β-hydroxysteroid dehydrogenase is due to lack of synthesis of this enzyme or else inhibition of enzyme activity, e.g., by steroid hormones produced in placenta and circulated to the fetal adrenal. In any event, the failure of expression of 3β-hydroxysteroid dehydrogenase enzyme activity causes a relative inefficiency in the capacity for cortisol biosynthesis. By contrast, there is very active steroid sulfotransferase activity in the fetal adrenal. In consequence, the principal secretory products of the human fetal adrenal cortex are dehydroisoandrosterone sulfate and pregnenolone sulfate. Comparatively, cortisol is a quantitatively minor secretory product of the human fetal adrenal.

Fetal Adrenal Size and Steroidogenesis

Relative to body weight, the fetal adrenals of the human at term are 25 times larger than those of the adult. Because of the enormous size of the human fetal adrenal and its capacity for steroid production, many investigators have deduced that there must be more than one growth stimulus for this gland. As stated, it is probable that ACTH alone does not bring about the total physiological response observed in fetal adrenal growth and steroid secretion; indeed, there is a continual decrease in the concentration of immunoreactive ACTH in human fetal plasma as pregnancy progresses (Winters and associates, 1974), at a time when the fetal adrenal is growing most rapidly. And, generally, ACTH evokes hypertrophy but not replication of adrenal cells.

For all of these reasons, many investigators have searched

for a second trophic agent that acts cooperatively with ACTH to stimulate the fetal adrenal cortex in its rate of growth and steroid secretion. In this quest, every compound known to be secreted by the pituitary (Fig. 5–3) and each of the peptide hormones of the placenta have been considered to be potential candidates for this role. By way of brief summary, none of these agents acts acutely to cause significant increases in steroid production by human fetal adrenal tissues.

It is likely that the rate of growth of the fetal adrenal is determined, at least in part, by growth factors that may not affect directly the rate of steroidogenesis. There appears to be sufficient ACTH in the fetal circulation at all stages of gestation to ensure optimal cholesterol side-chain cleavage, the rate-limiting step in adrenal steroidogenesis. If this were true, it follows that stimulation of fetal adrenal growth leading to an increased mass of functional cells would cause a striking increase in the capacity of the gland for steroid formation even if the putative growth factor did not act directly to increase steroidogenesis. Therefore, growth of the human fetal adrenal cortex may be determined, in part, by factors that affect cell replication without necessarily altering the rate of synthesis or activities of steroidogenic enzymes.

THE SOURCE OF STEROID PRECURSOR IN THE FETAL ADRENAL

Because of the very high rate of steroid production in the fetal adrenal cortex, yet another consideration becomes pivotal. Namely, **what is the precursor of steroids produced in the fetal adrenals?**

Others had proposed that progesterone and pregnenolone produced by the placenta may serve as precursors for fetal adrenal cortisol and dehydroisoandrosterone sulfate biosynthesis, respectively. The conversion of radiolabeled progesterone, introduced into the fetal circulation, to radiolabeled cortisol has been demonstrated. The relative importance, however, of this pathway of cortisol formation compared with that of the de novo synthesis of fetal cortisol from cholesterol likely is small. And it also is clear that the utilization of pregnenolone in the fetal circulation cannot account for more than a tiny fraction of the enormous quantity of dehydroisoandrosterone sulfate secreted by the fetal adrenals near term.

Therefore, it seemed reasonable that the precursor for fetal adrenal steroidogenesis must be cholesterol. The rate of steroid biosynthesis in the fetal adrenal is so great that fetal adrenal steroid hormone production alone requires the use of an amount of cholesterol equivalent to one fourth to one fifth of the total daily LDL-cholesterol turnover in the adult. If the relative size of the fetus is taken into account, it can be computed that the rate of turnover of the cholesterol pool in the fetus must be six times that of the total cholesterol turnover in the adult just to accommodate the needs of the fetal adrenal for steroidogenesis.

LDL-CHOLESTEROL AND FETAL ADRENAL STEROIDOGENESIS

We come then to another important issue with respect to the regulation of fetal adrenal steroidogenesis; namely, what then is the source of cholesterol that is used for fetal adrenal steroidogenesis? Several investigators have demonstrated that fetal adrenal tissue, in vitro, can synthesize steroid hormones. From these findings, it is clear that the fetal adrenal also can synthesize cholesterol from two carbon fragments, viz., acetate. The rate of cholesterol synthesis by fetal adrenal tissue, how-

ever, is insufficient to account for more than a fraction of the steroids produced by the fetal adrenals at term.

Therefore, the fetal adrenal must assimilate cholesterol from the circulation to meet the demands for optimal steroidogenesis. In plasma, cholesterol and cholesterol esters are present principally in the form of lipoproteins. Lipoproteins are designated according to density as determined by ultracentrifugation, e.g., very low-density lipoprotein (VLDL), low-density lipoprotein (LDL), and high-density lipoprotein (HDL). In studies of human fibroblasts in culture, Goldstein and Brown (1974), demonstrated the presence of specific plasma membrane receptors with high affinity for LDL. After binding of LDL to the plasma membrane receptor, LDL is internalized by an adsorptive endocytotic process. The internalized endocytotic vesicles fuse with lysosomes and the hydrolytic enzymes of the lysosomes catalyze the hydrolysis of the protein component of LDL, which gives rise to amino acids, and the hydrolysis of the cholesterol esters of LDL, which gives rise to cholesterol and fatty acids.

Simpson and co-workers (1979) conducted experiments to ascertain if human fetal adrenals use circulating lipoproteins as a source of cholesterol for steroidogenesis. Using explants of human fetal adrenal tissue maintained in organ culture, they found that when LDL was present in the culture medium, there was a marked stimulation of steroidogenesis by ACTH-treated fetal adrenal tissue. HDL was much less effective than LDL, whereas VLDL was devoid of stimulatory activity.

Carr and associates (reviewed by Carr and Simpson, 1981) also evaluated the relative contribution of cholesterol synthesized de novo and that of cholesterol derived from the uptake of LDL for fetal adrenal steroidogenesis. First, they found that the activity of the rate-limiting enzyme in de novo cholesterol synthesis in the fetal adrenal 3-hydroxy-3-methylglutaryl coenzyme A (HMG CoA) reductase was sufficient to account for only a fraction of the cholesterol required for fetal adrenal steroidogenesis. Second, they demonstrated that if LDL were removed from the medium of fetal adrenal explants in organ culture, the rate of steroidogenesis decreased, even in the presence of ACTH. Thus, the fetal adrenal is highly dependent upon circulating LDL as a source of cholesterol for steroidogenesis. A model of cholesterol metabolism in the fetal adrenal is presented in Figure 5–6.

REGULATION OF CHOLESTEROL LEVELS IN THE HUMAN FETUS

Therefore, an important question to be addressed was the source of circulating cholesterol in the human fetus. Pitkin and co-workers (1972), from the results obtained in studies of subhuman primates, and in the study of one human pregnancy, concluded that no more than 20 percent of cholesterol in fetal plasma could be attributed to transfer from the mother.

More recently, Carr and Simpson (1984) have shown that most of the LDL in fetal plasma arises by de novo synthesis in the fetal liver. The low level of LDL-cholesterol in the plasma of the fetus likely is due to the rapid use of LDL by the fetal adrenal for steroidogenesis. Early in human pregnancy, the levels of LDL-cholesterol are similar to those of the adult. But as pregnancy progresses, the levels of LDL-cholesterol in fetal plasma decline as the fetal adrenal grows. In the normal newborn delivered at term, the concentration of LDL-cholesterol is only about 30 mg per dL (Parker and associates, 1980, 1983a).

The levels of LDL-cholesterol are high in umbilical cord

plasma of the anencephalic newborn in whom the adrenal is atrophic (Parker and co-workers, 1983b). Moreover, there is a higher level of LDL in newborn infants of women with hypertension in whom estriol levels are low; thus, there is an inverse correlation between the cord plasma levels of LDL and dehydroisoandrosterone sulfate (Parker and associates, 1983b, 1986a).

REGULATION OF FETAL ADRENAL GROWTH

The unique pattern of fetal adrenal secretion, i.e., the secretion of large amounts of dehydroisoandrosterone sulfate and small amounts of cortisol, is reminiscent of the adrenal steroid secretory patterns observed with virilizing adrenal adenomas that sometimes affect women.

In yet another pathophysiological state, i.e., hyperprolactinemia with microadenomas of the anterior pituitary, high plasma levels of dehydroisoandrosterone sulfate and normal levels of cortisol are sometimes observed. Importantly, when such women were treated with dopamine agonists, which lower plasma levels of prolactin, dehydroisoandrosterone sulfate levels in plasma decreased appreciably. Thus, a second hormone that may serve a role in fetal adrenal steroidogenesis is fetal pituitary prolactin. In support of this view, it has been demonstrated that whereas the levels of immunoreactive ACTH in fetal plasma decline throughout the course of gestation, increasing concentrations of prolactin are observed. Indeed, the concentrations of prolactin during the last 5 weeks of pregnancy increase and are maintained at a high level during the time of maximum fetal adrenal growth (Winters and associates, 1975).

Most investigators, including ourselves, however, have been unable to show a direct stimulatory effect of prolactin on fetal adrenal tissue. Therefore, it appears that if there is a role for prolactin in fetal adrenal growth and steroidogenesis, it must be indirect, e.g., by way of an effect on the growth of the fetal adrenal without necessarily affecting steroid synthesis directly or else by increasing the availability of LDL.

Indeed, it now seems likely that the third trophic agent for the human fetal adrenal (ACTH and LDL being the first two discovered) will be one that acts as a growth-promoting factor, perhaps a growth factor per se, even one produced in placenta.

SECRETION OF PLACENTAL STEROIDS INTO THE MATERNAL AND FETAL COMPARTMENTS

The estrogens that are synthesized in trophoblast enter the maternal circulation preferentially. Gurpide and co-workers (1966) have shown that more than 90 percent of estradiol-17β and estriol produced in trophoblast enter maternal plasma. The same is true of progesterone that is formed in the trophoblast. Specifically, Gurpide and co-workers (1972) also found that 85 percent or more of progesterone that is formed in trophoblast enters maternal plasma; and, very little of the progesterone in the maternal circulation enters the fetus.

In the case of estradiol-17β and estrone, estradiol-17β is the primary estrogen that enters the maternal compartment; but somewhat surprisingly, the reverse appears to be true for the fetus; namely, there is preferential entry of estrone rather than estradiol-17β into the fetus (Gurpide and co-workers, 1982; Walsh and McCarthy, 1981). This finding, however, as Gurpide and colleagues point out, may be caused by extratrophoblastic conversion of estradiol-17β to estrone in fetal tissues or erythrocytes. Estriol synthesized in trophoblasts enters both fetal and maternal plasma, but most (90 percent) enters the mother.

FETAL ADRENAL FUNCTION AND FETAL "STRESS"

In the past, it was commonly assumed that the fetus would respond, physiologically, to adverse conditions, e.g., hypoxia, as the adult responds to stress. This is not the case. Much of the adult response to stress involves the "fight or flight" phenomenon, which includes fear. So far as we know, the fetus does not experience fear. Fight, flight, and fear in the adult are preludes to increased ACTH secretion and, in consequence, an increase in cortisol secretion by the adrenal.

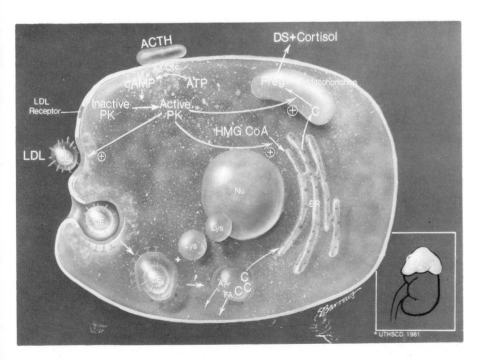

Figure 5–6. A model proposed for the regulation of fetal adrenal steroidogenesis, lipoprotein utilization, and cholesterol metabolism in the human fetal gland. Lys = lysosome; Nu = nucleus; ER = endoplasmic reticulum; Ad. Cyc. = adenylate cyclase; Preg = pregnenolone; CE = cholesterol esters; AA = amino acids; C = cholesterol; FA = fatty acids; PK = protein kinase; + = stimulation. (*From Carr and Simpson, 1981, with permission.*)

The importance of this issue is related to the response of the fetus during times of hypoxia insofar as maturation of key fetal tissues are concerned. For example, it has been observed that "stressed" fetuses may experience more rapid lung maturation than is the case in nonstressed fetuses. It has been assumed commonly that this circumstance may be related to increased secretion of glucocorticosteroids by the adrenal cortex of the "stressed" fetus. There probably is an alternative explanation, however, for these observations.

In instances of decreased uteroplacental blood flow in human pregnancies, e.g., with maternal hypertension, there is a reduction in maternal plasma and urinary estrogen levels. The decrease in estrogen levels is the result of decreased placental estrogen formation because of a decrease in supply of fetal adrenal precursor, viz., dehydroisoandrosterone sulfate (and 16α-hydroxydehydroisoandrosterone sulfate). Thus, in times of fetal "stress," fetal adrenal function, at least with respect to the secretion of dehydroisoandrosterone sulfate, is suppressed. Because of decreased adrenal steroidogenesis, use of fetal plasma LDL-cholesterol by the fetal adrenal is reduced; thereby, cholesterol levels in fetal blood of such fetuses are increased. Indeed, alterations in LDL-cholesterol levels in cord plasma appear to be highly dependent, inversely, upon the rate of fetal adrenal steroid biosynthesis before birth (Parker and colleagues, 1980, 1983a, 1983b).

On the other hand, several groups of investigators have found increased levels of arginine vasopressin (AVP) in blood of newborns that were "stressed" in utero (Chap. 6, p. 117). AVP commonly acts to increase ACTH secretion. Nonetheless, it has been difficult to establish increased cortisol secretion in such fetuses. Higher blood levels of cortisol in these newborns commonly can be accounted for by transfer of cortisol from the mother to the fetus. During labor, for example, the levels of cortisol in maternal plasma are increased markedly.

ALTERATIONS IN TRANSFER OF STEROIDS FROM TROPHOBLASTS

Recall that the placental arm of the fetal–maternal communication system of human pregnancy is established by way of hemochorioendothelial placentation. Accordingly, steroids leaving the trophoblasts enter directly into maternal blood in the intervillous space. There is no evidence of specific estrogen binding within trophoblast; therefore, net transfer between trophoblast and intervillous space favors entry into maternal blood, which rapidly enters the general circulation of the mother.

Steroids that leave trophoblasts toward the fetal compartment, however, do not enter fetal blood directly. First, steroids traversing toward the fetus must enter the intravillous space. Steroids in this space can reenter the trophoblasts. Second, steroids that escape the intravillous space toward the fetus must then traverse the wall of the fetal capillaries to reach fetal blood. And, steroids in the fetal capillaries of the intravillous space can reenter the intravillous space and thence the trophoblasts.

The dynamic result of this arrangement is substantially greater net entry of steroids formed in trophoblasts into the maternal circulation compared with the amount of steroids arising in trophoblast that ultimately enters the fetal blood.

Recently, we have discovered an interesting phenomenon with respect to the distribution of steroids formed in trophoblasts to the maternal and fetal compartments in pregnancies in which decreased uteroplacental blood flow was suspected.

In newborn infants of women with pregnancy-induced hypertension, chronic hypertension, and the more severe forms of diabetes mellitus, the umbilical cord plasma levels of estrogens and progesterone are significantly greater than in newborn infants of normal women. Initially, this was a surprise because we know that with decreased uteroplacental blood flow, estrogen production in placenta is decreased, as are the levels of estrogen in the maternal compartment. We interpret these findings as follows: with a reduction in uteroplacental blood flow, and thereby relative stasis of maternal blood in the intervillous space, there is a redistribution of trophoblastic steroid in favor of the fetal compartment. In particular, there is a decrease in the net exit of steroid from trophoblast into the maternal circulation, undoubtedly this is because of greater reentry of steroids from intervillous space into trophoblasts. This favors a relative increase in the transfer of trophoblast steroids to the fetal compartment. Thereby, there is an increase in the concentration of trophoblast-formed steroids in the umbilical vein. This occurs even in the face of a decrease in total placental estrogen formation and, in consequence, a decrease in estrogen levels in the maternal compartment. This is an important concept that may be useful in evaluations of the role of estrogen in fetal lung maturation, which we know may be accelerated in fetuses of pregnancies in which uteroplacental blood flow is presumed to be reduced (Parker and associates, 1987 and Chap. 6).

ESTROGEN PRODUCTION IN PREGNANCY: CLINICAL CORRELATIONS

A schematic representation of the pathways of estrogen formation in the placenta is presented in Figure 5–4.

Fetal Anencephaly

In the absence of the fetal zone of the adrenal cortex, as in anencephaly, the rate of formation of placental estrogens (especially estriol) is limited severely because of the lack of precursor formation in the fetus. Verification of the diminished levels of precursors in anencephalic fetuses was provided by the finding of low levels of dehydroisoandrosterone sulfate in cord blood of such newborns (Nichols and co-workers, 1958).

In addition, it was shown that almost all of the estrogens produced in women pregnant with an anencephalic fetus at 33 to 40 weeks of gestation can be accounted for by the placental utilization of maternal plasma dehydroisoandrosterone sulfate (MacDonald and Siiteri, 1965a,b). Furthermore, in such pregnancies, the production of estrogens can be increased by the administration (to the mother) of ACTH, which stimulates the rate of dehydroisoandrosterone sulfate secretion by the maternal adrenal. Finally, placental production of estrogens is decreased in women pregnant with an anencephalic fetus during the administration of a potent glucocorticosteroid, which suppresses ACTH secretion and thus decreases the rate of secretion of dehydroisoandrosterone sulfate from the maternal adrenal cortex (MacDonald and Siiteri, 1965a).

Maternal Adrenal Dysfunction

In women with Addison disease, there is decreased excretion of estrogens in urine during pregnancy (Baulieu and co-workers, 1956), although the decrease is principally in the urinary estrone and estradiol-17β fractions, because the fetal contribution to the synthesis of estriol, particularly in the latter part of pregnancy, is of paramount importance.

Maternal Ovarian Androgen-producing Tumors

The extraordinary efficiency of the placenta in the aromatization of C_{19}-steroids may be exemplified by two considerations. First, Edman and associates (1981) found that the placental clearance of maternal plasma androstenedione to estradiol-17β was very similar (when corrected to total blood cleared) to the estimated blood flow to the placenta. This means that all of the androstenedione entering trophoblast was converted to estrogen and therefore none of this C_{19}-steroid escaped into the fetus. Second, it is rare that a female fetus is virilized in a pregnant woman who is known to have an androgen-secreting ovarian tumor. This finding also is indicative that the placenta efficiently converts aromatizable C_{19}-steroids (including bioactive testosterone) to estrogens, thereby precluding transplacental passage of bioactive androgen from the mother to the fetus. Indeed, it may be that the female fetuses who are virilized in women with an androgen-producing tumor are those in whom a nonaromatizable C_{19}-steroid androgen is produced by the tumor, e.g., 5α-dihydrotestosterone.

Placental Sulfatase Deficiency

Generally, estrogen formation in placenta is regulated by the availability of C_{19}-steroid prohormones in fetal and maternal plasma. Specifically, there is no rate-limiting enzymatic reaction in placenta in the sequence leading to estrogen biosynthesis. And aside from minor alterations in placental aromatase induced by xenobiotics, the excess of placental enzymatic machinery for estrogen formation is large. An exception to this generality was found by France and Liggins (1969), who were the first to establish placental sulfatase deficiency as the cause of very low estrogen levels in otherwise normal pregnancies (except possibly for dysfunctional labor). Sulfatase deficiency precludes the hydrolysis of C_{19}-steroid sulfate precursors of estrogen, the first enzymatic step in the placental use of these circulating prehormones for estrogen biosynthesis. This is an X-linked disorder (all affected fetuses are male) that is associated with the development of icthyosis later in life.

Glucocorticosteroid Treatment

The administration of glucocorticosteroids to pregnant women causes a striking reduction in estrogen formation. Glucocorticosteroids act to inhibit ACTH secretion by the maternal and fetal pituitary resulting in decreased maternal and fetal adrenal secretion of placental estrogen precursor.

Neoplastic Trophoblastic Disease

In the case of neoplastic trophoblastic disease, namely, hydatidiform mole or choriocarcinoma, there is no fetal adrenal source of C_{19}-steroid precursor for the trophoblasts. Thereby, estrogen formation is limited to the utilization of maternal plasma C_{19}-steroids, and therefore, the estrogen produced is principally estradiol-17β (MacDonald and Siiteri, 1964, 1966).

Deficiency in Fetal LDL-Cholesterol Biosynthesis

A successful pregnancy in a woman with abetalipoproteinemia was recently described (Parker and colleagues, 1986b). This pregnancy is extraordinarily interesting for many reasons. The absence of LDL in the maternal plasma led to very low progesterone formation in both the corpus luteum and placenta; in addition, the levels of estriol also were lower than normal. Presumably, the depressed levels of estrogen were the result of decreased LDL formation in the fetus who was heterozygous for

LDL deficiency. Decreased fetal LDL-cholesterol formation would lead to decreased fetal adrenal production of dehydroisoandrosterone sulfate and thereby reduced precursor for placental estrogen formation.

Decreased Fetal Adrenal Use of LDL

The most common cause of decreased placental estrogen formation (aside from fetal death) is caused by a reduction in fetal adrenal utilization of plasma LDL. This leads to a reduction in the rate of formation of dehydroisoandrosterone sulfate and thereby a reduction in placental estrogen precursor. As noted before, the final consequence may be as follows: Estrogen formation in placenta is decreased and estrogen levels in maternal blood and urine are decreased. The levels of dehydroisoandrosterone sulfate in umbilical venous blood are decreased, but the levels of LDL-cholesterol are increased. At the same time, because of a redistribution of placental estrogens, the levels of estriol in umbilical venous blood may be increased. This sequence of events is observed most commonly in pregnancies complicated by hypertension or the more severe forms of diabetes mellitus (Parker and associates, 1984, 1987).

ESTRIOL AS A TEST OF FETAL WELL-BEING

RATIONALE

With the discovery that there are large amounts of estrogens in the urine of pregnant women and that these originate in the placenta, measurements of these urinary metabolites have been conducted in an attempt to provide an index of *placental function* or *fetal well-being*. Because the principal estrogen in the urine of pregnant women is estriol, most investigators concentrated on developing reliable methods for the measurement of this metabolite. The discovery that the fetus serves an important role in contributing precursors for the synthesis of estriol added impetus to the possibility that abnormalities in pregnancy may be recognized or monitored by the evaluation of estriol production.

URINARY ESTRIOL

It has been known for many decades that death of the human fetus is accompanied by a striking reduction in the levels of urinary estrogens; moreover, Cassmer (1959) demonstrated that after ligation of the umbilical cord with the fetus and placenta left in situ, there was an abrupt and striking decrease in the production of placental estrogens. The findings of Cassmer's classic study were subject to at least two interpretations. The first explanation was that maintenance of the fetal placental circulation is essential to the functional integrity of the placenta. This explanation was unlikely to be correct, however, because in Cassmer's preparation the placental production of progesterone was maintained at "preligation" levels even after occlusion of the umbilical cord. A second explanation for the marked decrease in urinary estrogens after fetal death was that, after umbilical cord ligation, there is an elimination of an important source of precursors of placental estrogen biosynthesis was eliminated, i.e., the fetus.

The latter explanation was proven to be correct because fetal precursors of placental estrogen in normal pregnancy are derived largely from C_{19}-steroids secreted by fetal adrenals. Levels of estriol in the urine of pregnant women, therefore, are not regulated primarily by the biosynthetic integrity of the placenta (except in rare instances) but by the availability of precursors of placental estrogens, mostly of fetal adrenal origin.

In the past, there was clinical usefulness for the measurements of estriol as corroborative evidence of fetal death. But the critical question has been whether estrogen measurements provide a clinically useful index of placental function or insights into the condition of the living fetus. The clinical value of such tests can be established only by proof of increased infant salvage resulting directly from therapeutic regimens predicated upon the results of estriol measurements.

Twenty-five years ago, the development of this aspect of obstetrical endocrinology was discussed extensively by Frandsen and Stakemann (1963). They reviewed the development of methods for measuring urinary estriol and described reliable procedures for the estimation of urinary estriol throughout normal human pregnancy. The range of variation in the amount of urinary estriol excreted among different normal pregnant women is great, as illustrated in Figure 5–7. With reliable urine collections and accurate chemical methods, however, they found that the day-to-day variation of estriol excretion by the same woman was relatively small; in four fifths of the women in this study, there was less than 20 percent day-to-day variation in estriol levels during the last 30 weeks of pregnancy.

The interpretation of ''abnormal'' levels of urinary or plasma estriol associated with possibly or definitely abnormal pregnancies must be made with caution and with appreciation of several factors as follow:

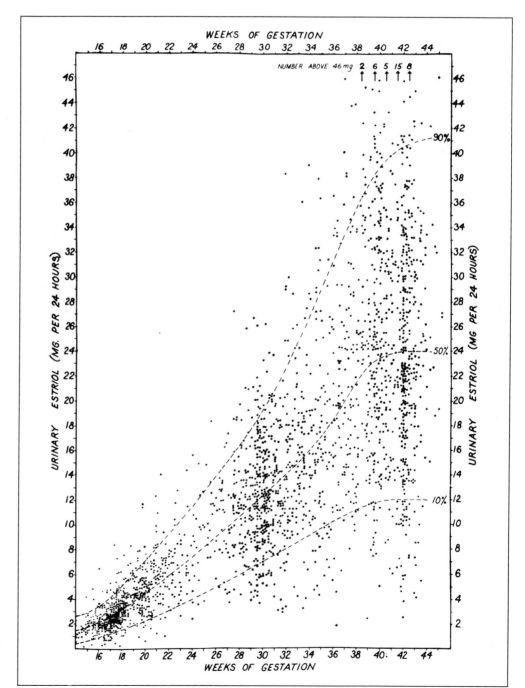

Figure 5–7. Urinary estriol values from 14 weeks of gestation showing 10th, 50th, and 90th percentiles. (*From Beischer and associates: Am J Obstet Gynecol 103:483, 1969.*)

1. The wide range of normal values for estriol in plasma or urine severely restricts the significance of a single measurement that falls in the "normal range" (Fig. 5–7).
2. In view of the difficulties of accurately ascertaining both duration of gestation and completeness of urine collection, and of eliminating technical error, a **single measurement that falls considerably outside the "normal range" must be verified.**
3. Restriction of the supply of placental precursors of estriol, as in anencephaly, isolated fetal pituitary ACTH deficiency, or during the administration of potent glucocorticosteroids to the mother, will result in decreased production of placental estriol, independent of placental function.
4. Factors apparently unrelated to the fetoplacental unit may be associated with decreased urinary estriol levels. For example, Taylor and colleagues (1963) found low levels of urinary estriol in women with acute pyelonephritis who subsequently recovered and delivered a healthy infant. Moreover, low levels of estriol are found during the ingestion of certain drugs, including certain antibiotics, phenobarbital, and even aspirin (Castellanos and associates, 1975).
5. Low levels of urinary and plasma estriol can be caused by placental deficiency of sulfatase activity (France and Liggins, 1969), a situation that precludes the use of the sulfurylated precursors, dehydroisoandrosterone sulfate or 16α-hydroxydehydroisoandrosterone sulfate, for placental estrogen biosynthesis.

High rates of excretion of estriol may occur in women with multiple fetuses and in some sensitized D-negative women who are pregnant with an erythroblastotic fetus (Greene and Touchstone, 1963; Taylor and colleagues, 1963). It also is theoretically possible that women pregnant with a fetus affected by congenital adrenal hyperplasia will have elevated levels of urinary estriol as a result of the increased production of C_{19}-steroids by the affected fetal adrenal cortex.

PLASMA ESTRIOL

In addition to the use of urinary estriol levels to monitor high-risk pregnancies, plasma estriol has been measured for the same purpose. Generally, the results of plasma estriol measurements, by a variety of techniques, as well as total plasma estrogens, have correlated well with the results of urinary estrogen determinations. The advantages of the use of plasma estriol are the ease of collection of blood compared with 24-hour urine collections and the avoidance of technical difficulties both in the collection and in the processing of urine.

ESTETROL

Some interest was focused on the possible merits of the measurement of plasma or urinary estetrol to monitor fetal well-being. Estetrol is 15α-hydroxyestriol; and, there are several features of this metabolite that make it uniquely representative of fetal metabolic function. First, it is derived principally from estriol, the production of which is attributable primarily to the use of fetal precursors; and, second, estetrol is produced almost exclusively in the fetus. The 15α-hydroxylation capability resident in the fetus and requisite for the formation of estetrol is not demonstrable in the maternal compartment. Thus, estetrol represents a compound, the production of which is dependent principally upon fetal precursors and upon fetal metabolism for its finite and final formation. To date, however, the results reported are not supportive of the view that the measurement of estetrol is advantageous over that of estriol determinations in the monitoring of the pregnancies in which the fetus may be at high risk.

CLINICAL UTILITY

One of the greatest problems in obstetrical management today is the proper timing of delivery when complications of a given pregnancy threaten the life or well-being of the fetus. The difficult, but common, problem is to choose between prematurity on the one hand and high risk for the fetus (if intrauterine existence in a deteriorating environment is continued) on the other hand. In such situations, notably diabetes mellitus, pregnancy-induced or chronic hypertension, poor previous obstetrical history, fetal growth retardation, suspected postmaturity, and others, the need for an accurate index of fetal well-being is urgent.

Barnes (1965) emphasized that there is little evidence that therapy based on levels of urinary estriol increased the rate of infant salvage beyond that accomplished by sound clinical judgment alone. Moreover, the results of the only prospective, controlled study reported to date are suggestive that the measurement of estriol has little or no clinical utility in reducing perinatal mortality or morbidity (Duenhoelter and co-workers, 1976). Specifically, the results of this study were supportive of the proposition that expert clinical management offers the greatest potential to date for the reduction of perinatal mortality and morbidity and that the measurement of hormones produced by the placenta offers no unique insight into a complicated pregnancy in which the fetus is at high risk. In a study of pregnancies complicated by mild chronic hypertension, Arias and Zamora (1979) also found that estriol measurements were of no utility in the management of such complicated pregnancies. Similarly, Schneider and associates (1978) concluded that 24-hour urinary estriol excretion measured three times per week was of no value in the management of postterm pregnancies. Finally, Dooley and associates (1984) found such measurements of no value—in fact, misleading—in the management of pregnant women with diabetes.

Regrettably, there still is no evidence of clinical utility for the measurement of urinary or plasma estriol in selection of management options for the pregnancy believed to be at high risk for the fetus.

PROGESTERONE

TISSUE SITE OF PRODUCTION

The biosynthesis of progesterone in human pregnancy is accomplished by the placental utilization of maternal plasma low-density lipoprotein-cholesterol in syncytiotrophoblast. Recall that the capacity for de novo synthesis of steroids in placenta is limited; in part, this is because of low rates of cholesterol formation in trophoblasts. Although much more progesterone than estrogen is produced during normal human pregnancy, relatively much less was known about its biosynthesis until recently.

Very little of the progesterone produced during human pregnancy arises in the ovary after the first few weeks of gestation (Diczfalusy and Troen, 1961). Surgical removal of the corpus luteum or even bilateral oophorectomy conducted during the 7th to 10th weeks of pregnancy does not result in a decrease in the rate of urinary excretion of pregnanediol, the principal metabolite of progesterone. There is a gradual increase in the levels of plasma progesterone as well as those of estradiol-17β and estriol in normal human pregnancy, as shown in Figure 5–8.

PRODUCTION RATE

Isotope dilution techniques for the measurement of endogenous rates of hormone production in the human were first applied to a study of progesterone production in pregnancy. The results of these studies, conducted by Pearlman in 1957, were indicative that the daily production of progesterone in late normal, singleton pregnancies was about 250 mg. The results of studies in which other methods have been employed are in agreement with that value. In some pregnancies with multiple fetuses, however, the daily progesterone production rate may exceed 600 mg per day.

SOURCE OF CHOLESTEROL PRECURSOR FOR PROGESTERONE BIOSYNTHESIS

Progesterone is formed from cholesterol in all steroidogenic tissues in a two-step enzymatic reaction. First, cholesterol is converted, in mitochondria, to the steroid intermediate pregnenolone, in a reaction catalyzed by cytochrome P-450 cholesterol side-chain cleavage enzyme. In turn, pregnenolone is converted to progesterone in microsomes by another P-450 enzyme, 3β-hydroxysteroid dehydrogenase.

Solomon and colleagues (1954) demonstrated that perfusion of the placenta in vitro with radiolabeled cholesterol resulted in the formation of radiolabeled progesterone. In addition, incubation of pregnenolone with placental tissue preparations also resulted in the formation of progesterone; and, an exceedingly great capacity of the placenta to convert pregnenolone to

progesterone has been demonstrated by in situ placental perfusion studies conducted in Diczfalusy's laboratories.

But whereas the placenta produces a prodigious amount of progesterone, there is a very limited capacity for the biosynthesis of cholesterol in this organ. The rate of incorporation of radiolabeled acetate into cholesterol by placental tissue proceeds very slowly and the activity of the rate-limiting enzyme in cholesterol biosynthesis, viz., 3-hydroxy-3 methylglutaryl coenzyme A (HMG CoA) reductase, in placental tissue microsomes is limited. This raised the question as to the source of cholesterol for placental progesterone formation.

By in vivo studies, Bloch (1945) and Werbin and co-workers (1957) demonstrated that after the intravenous administration of radiolabeled cholesterol to pregnant women, the specific activity of urinary pregnanediol was similar to that of plasma cholesterol. Hellig and associates (1970) also demonstrated that maternal plasma cholesterol was the principal precursor (up to 90 percent) of progesterone biosynthesis in human pregnancy.

PLACENTAL USE OF LOW-DENSITY LIPOPROTEIN-CHOLESTEROL

In studies similar to those described by use of fetal adrenal tissue (p. 76), Simpson and associates demonstrated that the placenta preferentially uses lipoprotein-cholesterol for progesterone biosynthesis. Thus, the formation of placental progesterone, like that of placental estrogens, occurs through the use of circulating precursors; but unlike estrogens, which are formed principally from the use of fetal adrenal precursors, placental progesterone biosynthesis proceeds by way of the use of a maternal precursor, which is taken up in the form of LDL-cholesterol. This was reviewed by Casey and colleagues (1985) and Simpson and MacDonald (1981).

These findings not only provide new insights into the biochemical mechanisms of placental progesterone formation, but also may provide insights into other aspects of maternal–placental–fetal physiology. The rate of progesterone biosynthesis is largely dependent on the number of LDL receptors on the plasma membrane of the trophoblasts and, thereby, primarily independent of uteroplacental blood flow. This obtains for several reasons:

1. Cholesterol side-chain cleavage by placental mitochondria is continually in a highly activated state.
2. De novo synthesis of cholesterol by the placenta is limited.
3. The fetus contributes little or no precursors for placental progesterone biosynthesis in normal human pregnancy.
4. Maternal levels of LDL-cholesterol should not be rate-limiting in the placental assimilation of cholesterol from the maternal circulation, except in very unusual circumstances, e.g., homozygous familial abetalipoproteinemia. Reduced placental progesterone formation was observed in a successful pregnancy of a woman with abetalipoproteinemia, i.e., a homozygous deficiency in LDL formation (Parker and co-workers, 1986b, and Chap. 10, p. 194)

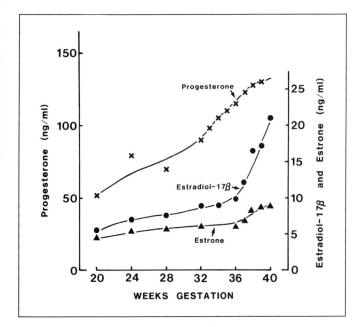

Figure 5–8. Mean plasma levels (± SEM) for progesterone, unconjugated estradiol-17β, and unconjugated estriol in 33 normal women during the last 9 weeks before delivery. (*Adapted from Tungsubutra and France: Aust NZ J Obstet Gynaecol, 18:97, 1978.*)

The metabolism of LDL by the trophoblasts will result in the hydrolysis of the apoprotein and the cholesterol esters of the LDL particle. This is an important consideration because such a prodigious amount of LDL is processed each day by the near-term placenta. In fact, it can be computed that the placenta alone may process an amount of LDL-cholesterol equal to the total daily LDL turnover in nonpregnant women. The hydrolysis of the protein component of LDL gives rise to amino acids, many of which are essential amino acids. The hydrolysis of the cholesterol esters of LDL gives rise to cholesterol, which is used for progesterone biosynthesis, and to fatty acids. The principal fatty acid of LDL-cholesterol esters is linoleic acid, an essential fatty acid. It seems reasonable to speculate, therefore, that the metabolism of LDL by trophoblast constitutes a means of obtaining cholesterol for placental progesterone biosynthesis and a mechanism for sequestering essential fatty acids and amino acids for transport to the fetus.

Simpson and Burkhart (1980) also found that progesterone, in concentrations similar to those found in placental tissue, inhibits the activity of the enzyme that catalyzes the esterification of cholesterol. It can be envisioned that this physiological event will serve to ensure a supply of cholesterol for progesterone biosynthesis by preventing the sequestration of cholesterol into an inappropriate storage form, viz., cholesterol esters, and will protect essential fatty acids from reesterification with cholesterol.

The intimate relationships that exist between fetal well-being and the placental production of estrogen cannot be demonstrated in the case of progesterone. Fetal death, ligation of the umbilical cord with the fetus and placenta remaining in situ, and anencephaly all are conditions associated with very low maternal plasma levels and urinary excretion of estrogens. In these circumstances, there is no concomitant decrease in the plasma levels of progesterone to anywhere near the same extent as those of estrogen until some indeterminate time after fetal death. Thus, placental endocrine function, including the formation of protein hormones, e.g., hCG, and progesterone biosynthesis may persist indefinitely after death of the fetus.

PROGESTERONE METABOLISM DURING PREGNANCY

The metabolic clearance rate of progesterone in pregnant women is similar to that found in men and nonpregnant women. This is an important consideration in evaluating the role of progesterone in the initiation of parturition (Chap. 10, p. 193).

During pregnancy, there is a disproportionate increase in the concentration of 5α-dihydroprogesterone in plasma and thus the ratio of the concentration of this metabolite to the concentration of progesterone is reduced in pregnant women (Milewich and co-workers, 1975). The mechanisms by which this comes about are not defined, but may be relevant to the resistance to pressor agents that develops in normally pregnant women (Everett and associates, 1978 and Chap. 7, p. 145). Progesterone also is converted to the potent mineralocorticosteroid deoxycorticosterone (DOC) in pregnant women and in the fetus. During human pregnancy, the concentration of DOC is increased strikingly in both the maternal and fetal compartments; and, the extraadrenal formation of deoxycorticosterone from circulating progesterone accounts for the vast majority of this mineralocorticosteroid produced in human pregnancy (Casey and MacDonald, 1982a,b).

REFERENCES

Amoroso EC: Comparative aspects of the hormonal functions. In Villee CA (ed): The Placenta and Fetal Membranes. Baltimore, Williams & Wilkins, 1960, p 3
Arias F, Zamora J: Antihypertensive treatment and pregnancy outcome in patients with mild chronic hypertension. Obstet Gynecol 53:489, 1979
Ashitaka Y, Nishimura R, Takemori M, Tojo S: Production and secretion of hCG and hCG subunits by trophoblastic tissue. In Segal S (ed): Chorionic Gonadotropins. New York, Plenum Press, 1980, p 151
Barnes AC: Discussion of paper by JW Greene. Am J Obstet Gynecol 91:688, 1965
Baulieu EE, Bricaire H, Jayle MF: Lack of secretion of 17-hydroxycorticosteroids in a pregnant woman with Addison's disease. J Clin Endocrinol 16:690, 1956
Baulieu EE, Dray F: Conversion of ³H-dehydroisoandrosterone (3β-hydroxy- Δ⁵-androsten-17-one) sulfate to ³H-estrogens in normal pregnant women. J Clin Endocrinol 23:1298, 1963
Bloch K: The biological conversion of cholesterol to pregnanediol. J Biol Chem 157:661, 1945
Bolté E, Mancuso S, Eriksson G, Wiqvist N, Diczfalusy E: Studies on the aromatization of neutral steroids in pregnant women: 1. Aromatization of C-19 steroids by placenta perfused in situ. Acta Endocrinol 35:535, 1964a
Bolté E, Mancuso S, Eriksson G, Wiqvist N, Diczfalusy E: Studies on the aromatization of neutral steroids in pregnant women: 2. Aromatization of dehydroisoandrosterone and of its sulphate administered simultaneously into a uterine artery. Acta Endocrinol 45:560, 1964b
Bolté E, Mancuso S, Eriksson G, Wiqvist N, Diczfalusy E: Studies on the aromatization of neutral steroids in pregnant women: 3. Over-all aromatization of dehydroisoandrosterone sulphate circulating in the foetal and maternal compartments. Acta Endocrinol 45:576, 1964c
Bradbury JT, Brown WE, Guay LA: Maintenance of the corpus luteum and physiologic action of progesterone. Recent Prog Horm Res 5:151, 1950
Brown JB: Urinary excretion of oestrogens during pregnancy, lactation, and the reestablishment of menstruation. Lancet 1:704, 1956
Carr BR, Parker CR Jr, Madden JD, MacDonald PC, Porter JC: Maternal plasma adrenocorticotropin and cortisol relationships throughout human pregnancy. Am J Obstet Gynecol 139:416, 1981
Carr BR, Simpson ER: Lipoprotein utilization and cholesterol synthesis by the human fetal adrenal gland. Endocr Rev 2:306, 1981
Carr BR, Simpson ER: Cholesterol synthesis by human fetal hepatocytes: Effect of lipoproteins. Am J Obstet Gynecol 150:551, 1984
Casey ML, MacDonald PC: Extraadrenal formation of a mineralocorticosteroid: Deoxycorticosterone and deoxycorticosterone sulfate biosynthesis and metabolism. Endocr Rev 3:396, 1982a
Casey ML, MacDonald PC: Metabolism of deoxycorticosterone and deoxycorticosterone sulfate in men and women. J Clin Invest 70:312, 1982b
Casey ML, MacDonald PC, Simpson ER: Endocrinologic changes in pregnancy. In Foster DW, Wilson JD (eds): Williams Textbook of Endocrinology. Philadelphia, Saunders, 1985, p 422
Cassmer O: Hormone production of the isolated human placenta. Acta Endocrinol (Suppl) 32:45, 1959
Castellanos JM, Aranda M, Cararach J, Cararach V: Effect of aspirin on oestriol excretion in pregnancy. Lancet 1:859, 1975
Colas A, Heinrichs WL, Tatum HJ: Pettenkofer chromogens in the maternal and fetal circulations: Detection of 3β,16α-dihydroxyandrost-5-en-17-one in umbilical cord blood. Steroids 3:417, 1964
Diczfalusy E, Borell U: Influence of oophorectomy on steroid excretion in early pregnancy. J Clin Endocrinol 21:1119, 1961
Diczfalusy E, Troen P: Endocrine functions of the human placenta. Vitam Horm 19:229, 1961
Dooley SL, Depp R, Socol ML, Tamura RK, Vaisrub N: Urinary estriols in diabetic pregnancy: A reappraisal. Obstet Gynecol 64:469, 1984
Duenhoelter JH, Whalley PJ, MacDonald PC: An analysis of the utility of plasma immunoreactive estrogen measurements in determining delivery time of gravidas with a fetus considered at high risk. Am J Obstet Gynecol 125:889, 1976
Edman CD, Toofanian A, MacDonald PC, Gant NF: Placental clearance rate of maternal plasma androstenedione through placental estradiol formation: An indirect method of assessing uteroplacental blood flow. Am J Obstet Gynecol 141:1029, 1981
Everett RB, Worley RJ, MacDonald PC, Gant NF: Modification of vascular responsiveness to angiotensin II in pregnant women by intravenously infused 5α-dihydroprogesterone. Am J Obstet Gynecol 131:555, 1978
Fishman J, Brown JB, Hellman L, Zumoff B, Gallagher TF: Estrogen metabolism in normal and pregnant women. J Biol Chem 237:1489, 1961
France JT, Liggins GC: Placental sulfatase deficiency. J Clin Endocrinol 29:138, 1969
Frandsen VA, Stakemann G: The site of production of oestrogenic hormones in human pregnancy: Hormone excretion in pregnancy with anencephalic foetus. Acta Endocrinol 38:383, 1961
Frandsen VA, Stakemann G: The urinary excretion of oestriol during the early months of pregnancy. Acta Endocrinol 44:196, 1963
Gant NF, Hutchinson HT, Siiteri PK, MacDonald PC: Study of the metabolic clearance rate of dehydroisoandrosterone sulfate in pregnancy. Am J Obstet Gynecol 111:555, 1971
Gibbons JM, Mitnick M, Chieffo V: In vitro biosynthesis of TSH- and LH-releasing factors by human placenta. Am J Obstet Gynecol 121:127, 1975

Goldstein JL, Brown MS: Binding and degradation of low density lipoproteins by cultured human fibroblasts. J Biol Chem 249:5153, 1974

Greene JW, Touchstone JC: Urinary estriol as an index of placental function. Am J Obstet Gynecol 85:1, 1963

Grumbach MM, Kaplan SL: On placental origin and purification of chorionic growth hormone–prolactin and its immunoassay in pregnancy. Trans NY Acad Sci 27:167, 1964

Gurpide E, Angers M, VandeWiele R, Lieberman S: Determination of secretory rates of estrogens in pregnant and nonpregnant women from the specific activities of urinary metabolites. J Clin Endocrinol 22:935, 1962

Gurpide E, Marks C, de Ziegler D, Berk PD, and Brandes JM: Asymmetric release of estrone and estradiol derived from labeled precursors in perfused human placentas. Am J Obstet Gynecol 144:551, 1982

Gurpide E, Schwers J, Welch MT, VandeWiele RL, Lieberman S: Fetal and maternal metabolism of estradiol during pregnancy. J Clin Endocrinol Metab 26:1355, 1966

Gurpide E, Tseng J, Escarcena L, Fahning M, Gibson C, Fehr P: Fetomaternal production and transfer of progesterone and uridine in sheep. Am J Obstet Gynecol 113:21, 1972

Halban J: Die innere secretion von ovarium und Placenta und ihre Bedeutung fur die function der milchdrusen. Arch Gynecol 75:343, 1905

Hellig HD, Gattereau D, Lefevre Y, Bolté E: Steroid production from plasma cholesterol: I. Conversion of plasma cholesterol to placental progesterone in humans. J Clin Endocrinol Metab 30:624, 1970

Hubert C, Descombey D, Mondon F, Daffos F: Plasma human chorionic somatomammotropin deficiency in a normal pregnancy is the consequence of low concentration of messenger RNA coding for human chorionic somatomammotropin. Am J Obstet Gynecol 147:676, 1983

Ito Y, Higashi K: Studies on prolactin-like substance in human placenta: II. Endocrinol Jpn 8:279, 1961

Josimovich JB, MacLaren JA: Presence in human placenta and term serum of highly lactogenic substance immunologically related in pituitary growth hormone. Endocrinology 71:209, 1962

Khodr GS, Siler-Khodr TM: Placental luteinizing hormone-releasing factor and its synthesis. Science 207:315, 1980

Klopper A: The new placental proteins: Their role in pregnancy. In Givens JR (ed): Endocrinology of Pregnancy. Chicago, Year Book, 1981, p 203

Krieger DT: Placenta as a source of "brain" and "pituitary hormones." Biol Reprod 26:55, 1982

Liotta A, Osathanondh R, Ryan KJ, Krieger DT: Presence of corticotropin in human placenta: Demonstration of in vitro synthesis. Endocrinology 101:1552, 1977

MacDonald PC: Placental steroidogenesis. In Wynn RM (ed): Fetal Homeostasis. New York, New York Academy of Sciences, 1965, p 265, Vol I

MacDonald PC, Siiteri PK: Study of estrogen production in women with hydatiform mole. J Clin Endocrinol Metab 24:685, 1964

MacDonald PC, Siiteri PK: Origin of estrogen in women pregnant with an anencephalic fetus. J Clin Invest 44:465, 1965a

MacDonald PC, Siiteri PK: The conversion of isotope-labeled dehydroisoandrosterone and dehydroisoandrosterone sulfate to estrogen in normal and abnormal pregnancy. In Paulsen CA (ed): Estrogen Assays in Clinical Medicine. Seattle, University of Washington Press, 1965b, p 251

MacDonald PC, Siiteri PK: The in vivo mechanisms of origin of estrogen in subjects with trophoblastic tumors. Steroids 8:589, 1966

Madden JD, Gant NF, MacDonald PC: Studies of the kinetics of conversion of maternal plasma dehydroisoandrosterone sulfate to 16α-hydroxydehydroisoandrosterone sulfate, estradiol and estriol. Am J Obstet Gynecol 132:392, 1978

Madden JD, Siiteri PK, MacDonald PC, Gant NF: The pattern and rates of metabolism of maternal plasma dehydroisoandrosterone sulfate in human pregnancy. Am J Obstet Gynecol 125:915, 1976

Margioris AN, Grino M, Protos P, Gold PW, Chrousos GP: Corticotropin-releasing hormone and oxytocin stimulate the release of placental proopiomelanocortin peptides. J Clin Endocrinol Metab 66:922, 1988

McGregor WG, Kuhn RW, Jaffe RB: Biologically active chorionic gonadotropin: Synthesis by the human fetus. Science 220:306, 1983

McGregor WG, Raymoure WJ, Kuhn RW, Jaffe RB: Fetal tissue can synthesize a placental hormone: Evidence for chorionic gonadotropin β-subunit synthesis by human fetal kidney. J Clin Invest 68:306,1981

Migeon CJ, Keller AT, Holmstrom EG: Dehydroisoandrosterone, androsterone and 17-hydroxycorticosteroid levels in maternal and cord plasma in cases of vaginal delivery. Bull Johns Hopkins Hosp 97:415, 1955

Milewich L, Gomez-Sanchez CE, Madden JD, Bradfield DJ, Parker PM, Smith SL, Carr BR, Edman CD, MacDonald PC: Dehydroisoandrosterone sulfate in peripheral blood of premenopausal, pregnant, and postmenopausal women and men. J Steroid Biochem 9:1159, 1978

Milewich L, Gomez-Sanchez CE, Madden JD, MacDonald PC: Isolation and characterization of 5α-pregnane-3,20-dione and progesterone in peripheral blood of pregnant women: Measurement throughout pregnancy. Gynecol Invest 6:291, 1975

Mulchahey JJ, DiBlasio AM, Martin MC, Blumenfeld A, Jaffe RB: Hormone production and peptide regulation of the human fetal pituitary gland. Endocr Rev 8:406, 1987

Nichols J, Lescure OL, Migeon CJ: Levels of 17-hydroxycorticosteroids and 17-ketosteroids in maternal and cord plasma in term anencephaly. J Clin Endocrinol 18:444, 1958

Nielsen PV, Pedersen J, Kampmann E-M: Absence of human placental lactogen in an otherwise uneventful pregnancy. Am J Obstet Gynecol 135:322, 1979

Nishula BC, Wehmann R: Distribution, metabolism, and excretion of human chorionic gonadotropin and its subunits in man. In Segal S (ed): Chorionic Gonadotropin. New York, Plenum Press, 1980, p 199

Odagiri E, Sherrill BJ, Mount CD, Nicholson WE, Orth DN: Human placental immunoreactive corticotropin, lipotropin, and β-endorphin: Evidence for a common precursor. Proc Natl Acad Sci USA 16:2027, 1979

Odell WD, Griffin J: Pulsatile secretion of human chorionic gonadotropin in normal adults. N Engl J Med 317:1688, 1987

Owerbach D, Martial JA, Baxter JD, Rutter WJ, Shows TB: Genes for growth hormone, chorionic somatomammotropin, and growth hormone–like gene on chromosome 17 in humans. Science 209:289, 1980

Owerbach D, Rutter WJ, Cooke NE, Martial JA, Shows TB: The prolactin gene is located on chromosome 6 in humans. Science 212:815, 1981

Parker CR Jr, Carr BR, Simpson ER, MacDonald PC: Decline in the concentration of low-density lipoprotein-cholesterol in human fetal plasma near term. Metabolism 32:919, 1983a

Parker CR Jr, Carr BR, Winkel CA, Casey ML, Simpson ER, MacDonald PC: Hypercholesterolemia due to elevated low-density lipoprotein-cholesterol in newborns with anencephaly and adrenal atrophy. J Clin Endocrinol Metab 57:37, 1983b

Parker CR Jr, Hankins GDV, Carr BR, Gant NF, MacDonald PC, Porter JC: Prolactin levels in umbilical cord serum and its relation to fetal adrenal activity in newborns of women with pregnancy-induced hypertension. Pediatr Res 20:876, 1986a

Parker CR Jr, Hankins GDV, Carr BR, Leveno KJ, Gant NF, MacDonald PC: The effect of hypertension in pregnant women on fetal adrenal function and fetal plasma lipoprotein-cholesterol metabolism. Am J Obstet Gynecol 150:263, 1984

Parker CR Jr, Hankins GDV, Guzick DS, Rosenfeld CR, MacDonald PC: Ontogeny of unconjugated estriol in fetal blood and the relation of estriol levels at birth to the development of respiratory distress syndrome. Pediatr Res 21:386, 1987

Parker CR Jr, Illingworth DR, Bissonnette J, Carr BR: Endocrinology of pregnancy in abetalipoproteinemia: Studies in a patient with homozygous familial hypobetalipoproteinemia. N Engl J Med 314:557, 1986b

Parker CR Jr, Simpson ER, Bilheimer DW, Leveno KJ, Carr BR, MacDonald PC: Inverse relation between low-density lipoprotein-cholesterol and dehydroisoandrosterone sulfate in human fetal plasma. Science 208:512, 1980

Pearlman WH: [16-³H]Progesterone metabolism in advanced pregnancy and in oophorectomized-hysterectomized women. Biochem J 67:1, 1957

Petraglia F, Sawchenko P, Lim AT, Rivier J, Vale W: Localization, secretion, and action of inhibin in human placenta. Science 237:187, 1987

Pitkin RM, Connor WE, Lin DS: Cholesterol metabolism and placental transfer in the pregnant rhesus monkey. J Clin Invest 51:2584, 1972

Pulkkinen MO: Arylsulphatase and the hydrolysis of some steroid sulphates in developing organism and placenta. Acta Physiol Scand (Suppl) 180s:52, 1961

Ryan KJ: Biological aromatization of steroids. J Biol Chem 234:268, 1959a

Ryan KJ: Metabolism of C-16-oxygenated steroids by human placenta: The formation of estriol. J Biol Chem 234:2006, 1959b

Schneider JM, Olson RW, Curet LB: Screening for fetal and neonatal risk in the postdate pregnancy. Am J Obstet Gynecol 131:473, 1978

Selenkow HA, Varma K, Younger D, White P, Emerson K Jr: Patterns of serum immunoreactive human placental lactogen (IR-HPL) and chorionic gonadotropin (IR-HCG) in diabetic pregnancy. Diabetes 20:696, 1971

Shine J, Seeburg PH, Marial JA, Baxter JD, Goodman HM: Construction and analysis of recombinant DNA for human chorionic somatomammotropin. Nature 270:494, 1977

Siiteri PK, MacDonald PC: The utilization of circulating dehydroisoandrosterone sulfate for estrogen synthesis during human pregnancy. Steroids 2:713, 1963

Siiteri PK, MacDonald PC: Placental estrogen biosynthesis during human pregnancy. J Clin Endocrinol Metab 26:751, 1966a

Siiteri PK, MacDonald PC: The origin of placental estrogen precursor during human pregnancy. Excerpta Medica Int Cong Series 132:726, 1966b

Siler-Khodr TM: Hypothalamic-like peptides of the placenta. Semin Reprod Endocrinol 1:321, 1983

Siler-Khodr TM: Chorionic peptides. In McNellis D, Challis JRG, MacDonald PC, Nathanielsz P, Roberts J (eds): Cellular and Integrative Mechanisms in the Onset of Labor. An NICHD workshop. Ithaca, NY, Perinatology Press, 1988

Siler-Khodr TM, Khodr GS: Content of luteinizing hormone-releasing factor in the human placenta. Am J Obstet Gynecol 130:216, 1978

Simpson ER, Burkhart M: Acyl CoA: Cholesterol acyl transferase activity in human placental microsomes: Inhibition by progesterone. Arch Biochem Biophys 200:79, 1980

Simpson ER, Carr BR, Parker CR, Milewich L, Porter JC, MacDonald PC: The role of serum lipoproteins in steroidogenesis by the human fetal adrenal cortex. J Clin Endocrinol Metab 49:146, 1979

Simpson ER, MacDonald PC: Endocrine physiology of the placenta. Ann Rev Physiol 43:163, 1981

Solomon S, Lentz AL, VandeWiele RL, Lieberman S: Pregnenolone as intermediate in the biogenesis of progesterone and the adrenal hormones. Proc Am Chem Soc [Abstract 29C], 1954

Spellacy WN, Buhi WC: Pituitary growth hormone and placental lactogen levels measured in normal term pregnancy and at the early and late postpartum periods. Am J Obstet Gynecol 105:888, 1969

Talamantes F, Ogren L: The placenta as an endocrine organ: Polypeptides. In Knobil E, Neill J (eds): The Physiology of Reproduction. New York, Raven Press, 1988, p 2093

Taylor ES, Hassner A, Bruns PD, Drose VE: Urinary estriol excretion of pregnant patients with pyelonephritis and Rh isoimmunization. Am J Obstet Gynecol 85:10, 1963

Walsh SW, McCarthy MS: Selective placental secretion of estrogens into fetal and maternal circulations. Endocrinology 109:2152, 1981

Warren JC, Timberlake CE: Steroid sulfatase in the human placenta. J Clin Endocrinol 22:1148, 1962

Weintraub D, Rosen SW: Ectopic production of human chorionic somatomammotropin (HCS) in patients with cancer. Clin Res 18:375, 1970

Werbin H, Plotz EJ, LeRoy GV, David ME: Cholesterol: A precursor of estrone in vivo. J Am Chem Soc 79:1012, 1957

Winters AJ, Colston C, MacDonald PC, Porter JC: Fetal plasma prolactin levels. J Clin Endocrinol Metab 41:626, 1975

Winters AJ, Oliver C, Colston C, MacDonald PC, Porter JC: Plasma ACTH levels in the human fetus and neonate as related to age and parturition. J Clin Endocrinol Metab 39:269, 1974

Yoshimoto Y, Wolfsen AR, Hirose F, Odell WD: Human chorionic gonadotropin-like material: Presence in normal human tissues. Am J Obstet Gynecol 134:729, 1979

Part II
PHYSIOLOGY OF PREGNANCY

6

The Morphological and Functional Development of the Fetus

FETAL DEVELOPMENT

THE CONTEMPORARY ERA OF OBSTETRICS: THE FETUS

The high purpose of obstetrics is to ensure that every newborn is physically invested, *mens sana in corpore sano;* sound in mind and body, for the lifelong pursuit of the quintessence of earthly existence. To this end, investigations of the nature of human life in utero have been, and will continue to be, among the most fascinating and rewarding in all of biological research. This obtains, in large measure, because the findings of these inquiries are of momentous import to all mankind. It is for this reason that the contemporary era of obstetrics, arbitrarily defined as that period encompassed by the past quarter of a century, has been a time that obstetrical research has been focused on the physiology and pathophysiology of the fetus, its development, and environment. As an important consequence, the status of the fetus has been elevated to that of a patient who, in large measure, can be given the same meticulous care that physicians long have given the pregnant woman.

During this time, we also have come to understand that the conceptus is the dynamic force in the pregnancy unit; the maternal organism, in general, responds passively to signals generated in fetal or extraembryonic fetal tissues (Chaps. 2 to 5). Therefore, research directed toward an understanding of fetal development and maturation must necessarily take cognizance of the fetal contributions to implantation, maternal recognition of pregnancy, immunological acceptance, endocrine function, nutrition, and parturition (Fig. 2–1).

In this chapter, we consider the development of the normal fetus. In Chapter 15, the techniques used currently for identifying fetal well-being, or fetal health, are considered in greater detail; and in Chapters 32 and 33, anomalies, injuries, and diseases that affect the fetus and newborn infant are addressed.

DATING OF PREGNANCY

The several different terms that commonly are used to indicate the duration of pregnancy, and thus fetal age, are somewhat confusing. *Menstrual age or gestational age* is estimated by computing from the 1st day of the last menstrual period, a time that precedes conception; namely, this is about 2 weeks before ovulation and fertilization and nearly 3 weeks before implantation of the fertilized ovum. About 280 days, or 40 weeks, elapse, on average, between the 1st day of the last menstrual period and delivery of the infant; 280 days corresponds to 9⅓ calendar months, or 10 units of 28 days each. The unit of 28 days has been referred to commonly, but imprecisely, as a lunar month of pregnancy; actually, the time from one new moon to the next is 29½ days.

Obstetricians customarily calculate gestational age on the basis of menstrual age of a given pregnancy. Embryologists, however, cite events in days or weeks from the time of ovulation (*ovulation age*) or conception (*postconception age*), these two being nearly identical. Occasionally, it is of some value to divide the period of gestation into three units of three calendar months each, or three *trimesters,* because some important obstetrical milestones may be designated conveniently by trimesters. The possibility of spontaneous abortion, for example, is limited principally to the first trimester of pregnancy, whereas the likelihood of survival of the infant born preterm is increased greatly in pregnancies that reach the third trimester.

A short description of various periods of development of the fertilized ovum and embryo is presented. For a more detailed description, based on Streeter's (1920) timetables of human development, "*Horizons,*" the reader is referred to the text by Hamilton and Mossman (1972).

THE OVUM, ZYGOTE, AND BLASTOCYST

During the first 2 weeks from ovulation, there are several successive phases of development that are identified as follow: (1) ovulation, (2) fertilization of the ovum, (3) formation of free blastocyst (the events of the first week after ovulation are illustrated diagrammatically in Figure 6–1), and (4) implantation of the blastocyst, a process that begins at the end of the 1st week after conception. Primitive chorionic villi begin to form after implantation. It is conventional to refer to the products of conception after the development of chorionic villi not as a fertilized ovum, or zygote, but as an embryo. The early stages of preplacental development, and the formation of the placenta are described in Chapter 4.

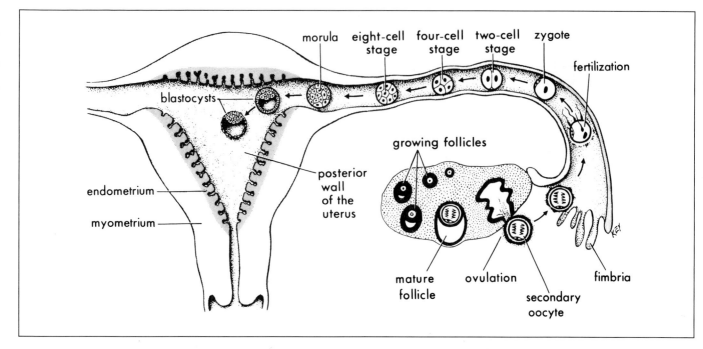

Figure 6–1. Diagrammatic summary of the ovarian cycle, fertilization, and human development during the 1st week. Developmental stage 1 begins with fertilization and ends when the zygote forms. Stage 2 (days 2 to 3) comprises the early stages of cleavage (from 2 to about 16 cells, or the morula). Stage 3 (days 4 to 5) consists of the free unattached blastocyst. Stage 4 (days 5 to 6) is represented by the blastocyst attaching to the center of the posterior wall of the uterus, the usual site of implantation. (*From Moore: The Developing Human, 3rd ed. Philadelphia, Saunders, 1982.*)

THE EMBRYO

The beginning of the embryonic period is taken as the beginning of the 3rd week after ovulation (fertilization), or the 5th week after the 1st day of the last menstrual period, and coincides in time with the expected time of the next menstruation. Most pregnancy tests in clinical use are positive by this time (Chap. 2, p. 15).

At this stage, the embryonic disc is well defined and the body stalk is differentiated; the chorionic sac measures approximately 1 cm in diameter (Figs. 6–2 and 6–3). The chorionic villi are distributed equally around the circumference of the chori-

onic sac. There is a true intervillous space that contains maternal blood and villous cores in which there is angioblastic chorionic mesoderm.

By the end of the 4th week after ovulation, the chorionic sac measures 2 to 3 cm in diameter, and the embryo about 4 to 5 mm in length (Fig. 6–4). The heart and pericardium are very prominent because of the dilatation of the chambers of the heart. Arm and leg buds are present, and the amnion is beginning to ensheath the body stalk, which thereafter becomes the umbilical cord.

At the end of the 6th week after fertilization, or about 8 weeks after the onset of the last menstrual period, the embryo

Figure 6–2. Early human embryos. Only the chorion adjacent to the body stalk is shown. Small outline to right of each embryo gives its actual size. Ovulation ages: **A.** 19 days (presomite). **B.** 21 days (7 somites). **C.** 22 days (17 somites). (*After drawings and models in the Carnegie Institution.*)

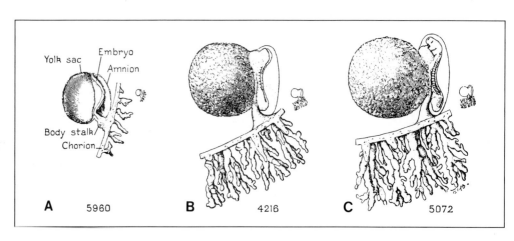

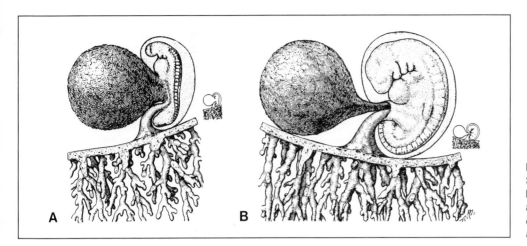

Figure 6–3. Early human embryos. Small outline to right of each embryo gives its actual size. Ovulation ages: **A.** 22 days. **B.** 23 days. (*After drawings and models in the Carnegie Institution.*)

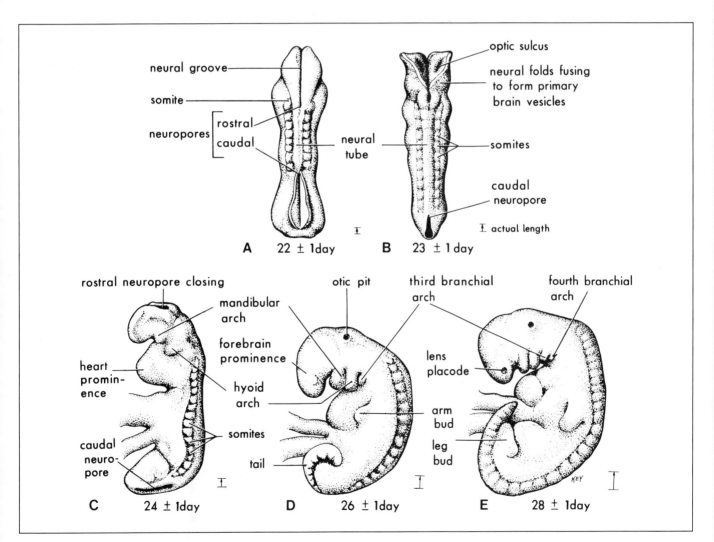

Figure 6–4. Three- to four-week-old embryos. **A** and **B.** Dorsal views of embryos during stage 10 of development (about 22 to 23 days) showing 8 and 12 somites, respectively. **C–E.** Lateral views of embryos during stages 11, 12, and 13 of development (24 to 28 days), showing 16, 27, and 33 somites, respectively. (*From Moore: The Developing Human, 3rd ed. Philadelphia, Saunders, 1982.*)

is 22 to 24 mm in length, and the head is quite large compared with the trunk. Fingers and toes are present, and the external ears form definitive elevations on either side of the head.

THE FETUS

The end of the embryonic period and the beginning of the fetal period are arbitrarily designated by most embryologists to occur 8 weeks after fertilization, or 10 weeks after the onset of the last menstrual period. At this time, the embryo is nearly 4 cm long. Few, if any, new major structures are formed thereafter; development during the fetal period of gestation consists of growth and maturation of structures that were formed during the embryonic period.

Three Lunar Months

By the end of the 12th week of pregnancy, by menstrual age, or 10 weeks after ovulation, the crown-rump length of the fetus is 6 to 7 cm (Figs. 6–5 and 6–6); and by this time, the uterus usually is palpable just above the symphysis pubis. Centers of ossification have appeared in most of the fetal bones; the fingers and toes have become differentiated and are provided with nails; scattered rudiments of hair appear; and the external genitalia are beginning to show definite signs of male or female sex. A fetus delivered at this time may make spontaneous movements if still within the amnionic sac or if immersed in warm saline.

Four Lunar Months

By the end of the 16th week, by menstrual age, the crown-rump length of the fetus is 12 cm, and it weighs about 110 g. By careful examination of the external genital organs, the sex of the fetus can be identified.

Five Lunar Months

The end of the 5th lunar month, or the end of the 20th week, is the midpoint of pregnancy or gestation as estimated from the time of the last normal menstrual period. The fetus now weighs somewhat more than 300 g. The skin has become less transparent, a downy lanugo covers its entire body, and some scalp hair is visible.

Six Lunar Months

By the end of the 24th week, the fetus weighs about 630 g. The skin is characteristically wrinkled, and fat is deposited beneath it. The head is still comparatively quite large; eyebrows and eyelashes usually are recognizable. A fetus born at this period will attempt to breathe, but almost always dies shortly after birth.

Seven Lunar Months

By the end of the 28th week after the onset of the last menstrual period, a crown-rump length of about 25 cm is attained and the fetus weighs about 1,100 g. The thin skin is red and covered with vernix caseosa. The pupillary membrane has just disappeared from the eyes. An infant born at this time in gestation moves his

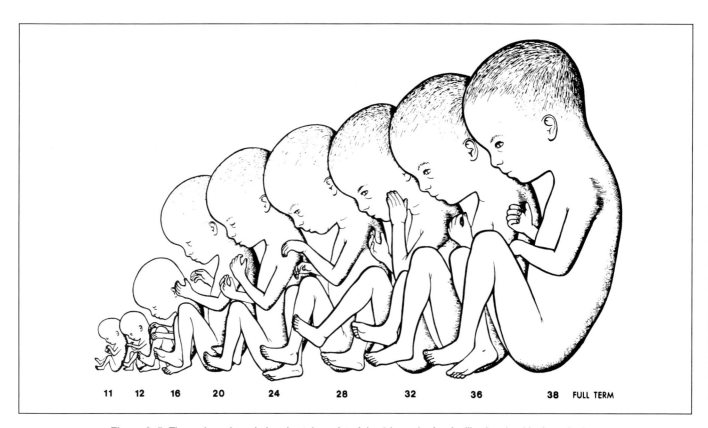

Figure 6–5. The embryonic period ends at the point of the 8th week after fertilization; by this time, the beginnings of all essential structures are present. The fetal period, extending from the 9th week until birth, is characterized by growth and elaboration of structures. Sex is clearly distinguishable by 12 weeks. (*From Moore: The Developing Human, 3rd ed. Philadelphia, Saunders, 1982.*)

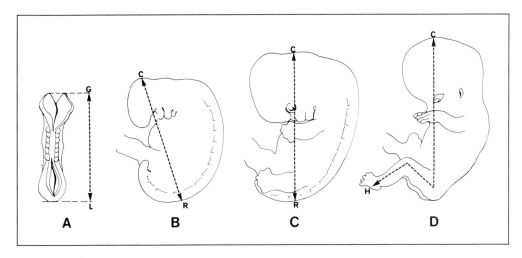

Figure 6–6. Sketches showing methods of measuring the length of embryos. **A.** Greatest length. **B** and **C.** Crown-rump length. **D.** Crown-heel length.(*From Moore: The Developing Human, 3rd ed. Philadelphia, Saunders, 1982.*)

or her limbs quite energetically and cries weakly. The infant of this gestational age, with expert care, most often will survive.

Eight Lunar Months
At the end of the 8th lunar month, or 32 weeks, the fetus has attained a crown-rump length of about 28 cm and a weight of about 1,800 g. The surface of the skin is still red and wrinkled. Infants born at this period, with proper care, usually survive.

Nine Lunar Months
At the end of 36 weeks gestation, the average crown-rump length of the fetus is about 32 cm long and the weight is about 2,500 g. Because of the deposition of subcutaneous fat, the body has become more rotund and the previous wrinkled appearance of the face is lost. Infants born at this time have an excellent chance of survival with proper care.

Ten Lunar Months
Term is reached at 10 lunar months, or 40 weeks after the onset of the last menstrual period. At this time the fetus is fully developed, with the characteristic features of the newborn infant to be described here. The average crown-rump length of the fetus at term is about 36 cm, and the weight is approximately 3,400 g, with variations to be discussed subsequently.

Length of Fetus
Because of the variability in the length of the legs and the difficulty of maintaining them in extension, measurements corresponding to the sitting height (crown to rump) are more accurate than are those corresponding to the standing height (Fig. 6–6). The average sitting height and weight of the fetus at the end of each lunar month were ascertained by Streeter (1920) from 704 specimens and still are similar to those found more recently, as shown in Table 6–1. Such values are approximate, but generally, the length is a more accurate criterion of the age of a fetus than is the weight.

Haase (1875) suggested that, for clinical purposes, the length in centimeters of the fetus measured from crown to heel may be approximated during the first 5 months by squaring the number of the lunar month to which the pregnancy has advanced and, in the second half of pregnancy, by multiplying the month by 5.

Weight of the Newborn
The average term infant at birth weighs about 3,000 to 3,600 g, depending upon race, parental economic status, size of the parents, and parity of the mother, with boys about 100 g (3 oz) heavier than girls. From the observations of Gruenwald (1967) and other investigators, it is established that during the second half of pregnancy the fetal weight increases in a linear manner with time until about the 37th week of gestation, and then it slows in rate variably. Gruenwald emphasized that the principal determinants of the extent to which fetal growth late in pregnancy departs from the previously linear pattern are related, in large part, to the socioeconomic status of the mother. In general, the greater the socioeconomic deprivation, the slower the rate of fetal growth late in pregnancy.

Birthweights over 5,000 g occur occasionally, but most tales of huge babies vastly exceeding this figure are based on hearsay and inaccurate measurements at best. Presumably, the largest baby recorded in the medical literature is that described by Belcher (1916), a stillborn female weighing 11,340 g (25 lb). In spite of these exceptional cases of macrosomia, extreme skepticism is justified in accepting reports concerning phenomenally heavy newborns. Term infants, however, frequently weigh less than 3,200 g and sometimes as little as 2,250 g (5 lb) or even less. In the past, it was customary, when the birth weight was 2,500 g or less, to classify the infant as premature even though in some cases the low birthweight was not the consequence of preterm birth but rather was because of retardation in growth during intrauterine development.

The many factors intimately involved in fetal growth are considered further in this chapter in the sections on placental transfer and fetal nutrition (p. 94, 97), as well as in Chapters 15 and 38.

Fetal Head
Obstetrically, the head of the fetus is a most important body part because an essential feature of labor is the adaptation between the fetal head and the maternal bony pelvis. Only a comparatively small part of the head of the fetus at term is represented by the face; the rest is composed of the firm skull, which is made up of two frontal, two parietal, and two temporal bones, along with the upper portion of the occipital bone and the wings of the sphenoid.

These bones are not united rigidly, but rather are separated by membranous spaces, the *sutures* (Fig. 6–7). The most

TABLE 6–1. CRITERIA FOR ESTIMATING AGE DURING THE FETAL PERIOD

Age (Wk)		CR Length (mm)[a]	Foot Length (mm)[a]	Fetal Weight (g)[b]	Main External Characteristics
Menstrual	Fertilization				
11	9	50	7	8	Eyes closing or closed. Head more rounded. External genitalia still not distinguishable as male or female. Intestines are in the umbilical cord.
12	10	61	9	14	Intestines in abdomen. Early fingernail development.
14	12	87	14	45	Sex distinguishable externally. Well-defined neck.
16	14	120	20	110	Head erect. Lower limbs well developed.
18	16	140	27	200	Ears stand out from head.
20	18	160	33	320	Vernix caseosa present. Early toenail development.
22	20	190	39	460	Head and body (lanugo) hair visible.
24	22	210	45	630	Skin wrinkled and red.
26	24	230	50	820	Fingernails present. Lean body.
28	26	250	55	1000	Eyes partially open. Eyelashes present.
30	28	270	59	1300	Eyes open. Good head of hair. Skin slightly wrinkled.
32	30	280	63	1700	Toenails present. Body filling out. Testes descending.
34	32	300	68	2100	Fingernails reach finger tips. Skin pink and smooth.
38	36	340	79	2900	Body usually plump. Lanugo hairs almost absent. Toenails reach toe tips.
40	38	360	83	3400	Prominent chest; breasts protrude. Testes in scrotum or palpable in inguinal canals. Fingernails extend beyond finger tips.

[a]These measurements are averages and so may not apply to specific cases; dimensional variations increase with age. The method for taking CR (crown-rump) measurements is illustrated in Figure 6–6.
[b]These weights refer to fetuses that have been fixed for about two weeks in 10 percent formalin. Fresh specimens usually weigh about 5 percent less.
From Moore: The Developing Human, 2nd ed. Philadelphia, Saunders, 1977.

important sutures are the *frontal,* between the two frontal bones; the *sagittal,* between the two parietal bones; the two *coronal,* between the frontal and parietal bones; and the two *lambdoid,* between the posterior margins of the parietal bones and upper margin of the occipital bone. With vertex presentation, all of the sutures are palpable during labor, except the *temporal* sutures, which are situated on either side between the inferior margin of the parietal and upper margin of the temporal bones, covered by soft parts, and cannot be felt in the living fetus.

Where several sutures meet, an irregular space forms, which is enclosed by a membrane and designated as a *fontanel* (Fig. 6–7). Three such structures usually are distinguished, namely the greater, the lesser, and the temporal fontanels. The *greater,* or *anterior, fontanel* is a lozenge-shaped space that is situated at the junction of the sagittal and the coronal sutures. The *lesser,* or *posterior, fontanel* is represented by a small triangular area at the intersection of the sagittal and lambdoid sutures. Both can be palpated readily during labor, and the localization of these fontanels gives important information concerning the presentation and position of the fetus. The *temporal,* or *casserian,* fontanels, situated at the junction of the lambdoid and temporal sutures, have no diagnostic significance.

It is customary to measure certain critical *diameters* (Fig.

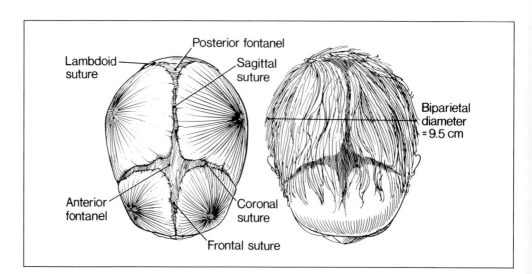

Figure 6–7. Fetal head at term showing various fontanels, sutures, and the biparietal diameter.

6–8), and *circumferences* of the infant's head. The diameters most frequently used and the average lengths thereof are:

1. The *occipitofrontal* (11.5 cm), which follows a line extending from a point just above the root of the nose to the most prominent portion of the occipital bone
2. The *biparietal* (9.5 cm), the greatest transverse diameter of the head, which extends from one parietal boss to the other
3. The *bitemporal* (8.0 cm), the greatest distance between the two temporal sutures
4. The *occipitomental* (12.5 cm), from the chin to the most prominent portion of the occiput
5. The *suboccipitobregmatic* (9.5 cm), which follows a line drawn from the middle of the large fontanel to the undersurface of the occipital bone just where it joins the neck (Figs. 6–7 and 6–8).

The greatest circumference of the head, which corresponds to the plane of the occipitofrontal diameter, averages 34.5 cm, and the smallest circumference, corresponding to the plane of the suboccipitobregmatic diameter, is 32 cm. As a rule, white infants have larger heads than do nonwhite infants; boys, somewhat larger than girls; and the infants of multiparas, larger heads than those of nulliparas.

Because of the widely varying mobility between the bones of the skull at the sutures, fetal heads differ appreciably in adaptation to the maternal pelvis by *molding*. The bones of one fetus may be soft and readily molded, whereas those of another are firmly ossified, only slightly mobile, and therefore incapable of significant reduction in size. This variation undoubtedly contributes to the incidence of fetopelvic disproportion, a leading indication for cesarean delivery (Chaps. 19 and 20).

Fetal Brain

As pregnancy advances, the fetal brain changes remarkably in appearance, as well as in function (Fig. 6–9). Therefore, it is possible to identify fetal age rather precisely from the external appearance of the brain (Dolman, 1977).

THE FETAL–MATERNAL COMMUNICATION SYSTEM: PLACENTAL ARM

The transfer of oxygen and a great variety of nutrients from the mother to the fetus and, conversely, the transfer of carbon dioxide and other metabolic wastes from fetus to mother is accomplished by way of the nutritive component of the placental arm of the fetal–maternal communication system. Thus, the placenta is the organ of transfer between mother and fetus. The placenta, and to a limited extent the attached membranes, supply all material for fetal growth and energy production while removing all products of fetal catabolism.

There are no continuous direct communications between the fetal blood (contained in the fetal capillaries in the intravillous space of the chorionic villi) and the maternal blood (in the intervillous space). The one exception to this generalization regarding the independence of the circulations is the development of occasional breaks in the chorionic villi, permitting the escape of fetal erythrocytes, in various numbers, into the maternal circulation (Chaps. 4 and 7). This leakage is the mechanism by which some D-negative women become sensitized by the erythrocytes of their D-positive fetus (see Chap. 33, p. 599). These occasional leaks, however, do not controvert the basic principle that there is no gross intermingling of the macromolecular constituents of the two circulations. The transfer of substances from mother to fetus and from fetus to mother, therefore, depends primarily on the mechanisms that permit or facilitate the transport of such substances through the intact chorionic villus.

THE INTERVILLOUS SPACE: MATERNAL BLOOD

The intervillous space is the maternal biological compartment of transfer; the maternal blood in this compartment directly bathes the trophoblasts. Transfer of substances from mother to fetus is accomplished first by transfer from the intervillous space into trophoblasts. This also is the biological space into which substances from the fetus are transported by way of the trophoblasts. This process of transfer supplies the fetus with oxygen as

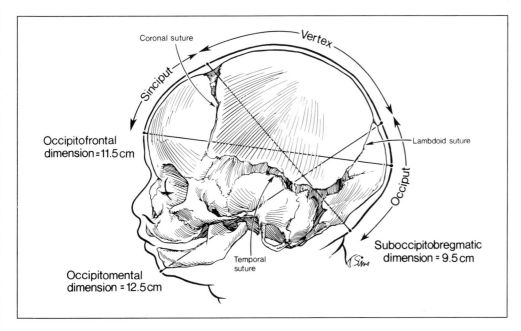

Figure 6–8. Diameters of the fetal head at term.

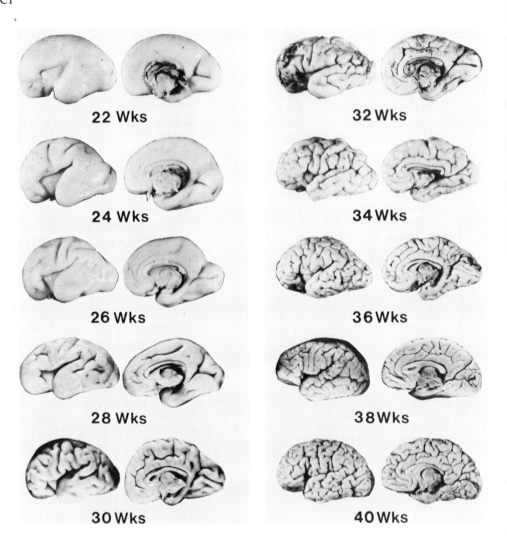

Figure 6–9. Characteristic configuration of fetal brains from 22 to 40 weeks of gestation at 2-week intervals. (*From Dolman: Arch Pathol Lab Med 101:193, 1977.*)

well as nutrients and provides for elimination of metabolic waste products; therefore, the chorionic villi and the intervillous space, together, function for the fetus as lung, gastrointestinal tract, and kidney. Fetal urination does commence early in pregnancy, and the fetal urine enters amnionic fluid. But fetal kidney function develops as pregnancy progresses, as is true of all other fetal organs.

The circulation of maternal blood within the intervillous space is described in detail in Chapter 4. The residual volume of the intervillous space of the delivered term placenta measures about 140 mL; the normal volume of the intervillous space before delivery, however, is probably twice this value (Aherne and Dunnill, 1966). Uteroplacental blood flow near term has been estimated to be about 600 mL per minute, with most of the blood apparently going through the intervillous space.

Uterine contractions cause a reduction in the flow of blood into the intervillous space, the degree of reduction depending, in large measure, upon the intensity of the contraction. Blood pressure within the intervillous space is significantly less than uterine arterial pressure, but somewhat greater than uterine venous pressure. Uterine venous pressure, in turn, varies depending upon several factors, including the body position of the pregnant woman. When she is supine, for example, pressure in the lower part of the inferior vena cava is elevated; consequently, in this position, pressure in the uterine and ovarian veins and, in turn, the intervillous space, is increased. An even greater increase in intervillous pressure is likely when she is standing.

FETAL CAPILLARIES OF THE INTRAVILLOUS SPACE: FETAL BLOOD

The hydrostatic pressure in the fetal capillaries that traverse the chorionic villi is probably not appreciably different from that in the intervillous space. During normal labor, the rise in fetal blood pressure must be parallel to the pressure in the amnionic fluid and the intervillous space. Otherwise, the capillaries in the chorionic villi would collapse and fetal blood flow through the placenta would cease.

PLACENTAL TRANSFER

CHORIONIC VILLUS

Substances that pass from the maternal blood to the fetal blood must traverse (1) trophoblast, (2) stroma of the intravillous space, and (3) fetal capillary wall. These three layers would have a minimal aggregate thickness of 3 to 6 μm, according to Wislocki (1955). Although this histological "barrier" separates the blood in the maternal and fetal circulations, it does not behave uniformly like a simple physical barrier because throughout pregnancy it either actively or passively permits, facilitates, and adjusts the amount and rate of transfer of a wide range of substances to the fetus. After midpregnancy, the number of Langhans cells, or cytotrophoblasts, decreases and the villous epithelium then consists predominantly of syncytiotrophoblast. The walls of the villous capillaries likewise become thinner, and the relative number of fetal vessels increases in relation to the villous connective tissue.

Several attempts have been made to estimate the total surface area of chorionic villi in the human placenta at term. The planimetric measurements made by Aherne and Dunnill (1966) of the villous surface area of the placenta indicate that there is a close correlation with fetal weight. They calculated that the total surface area at term was approximately 10 m^2.

REGULATION OF PLACENTAL TRANSFER

The syncytiotrophoblast is the primary fetal tissue interface of the placental arm of the transport system. The maternal-facing surface of this tissue is characterized by a complex microvillous structure. The fetal-facing, i.e., basal cell membrane of the trophoblast is the site of transfer to the intravillous space in which the fetal capillaries traverse. Because of the syncytial nature of the trophoblasts, there are no lateral or intercellular spaces in this membrane. In the case of transport from the intravillous space into fetal blood, or vice versa, the walls of the fetal capillaries pose an additional transport site.

At least 10 variables are important in determining the effectiveness of the human placenta as an organ of transfer:

1. The concentration of the substance under consideration in the maternal plasma and in some instances the extent to which it is bound to another compound, for example, a carrier protein;
2. The rate of maternal blood flow through the intervillous space;
3. The area available for exchange across the villous trophoblast epithelium;
4. In case the substance is transferred by diffusion, the physical properties of the tissue barrier interposed between blood in the intervillous space and blood in the fetal capillaries;
5. For any substance actively transported, the capacity of the biochemical machinery of the placenta for effecting active transfer, e.g., specific receptors on the plasma membrane of the trophoblasts;
6. The amount of the substance metabolized by the placenta during transfer;
7. The area for exchange across the fetal capillaries in the placenta;
8. The concentration of the substance in the fetal blood, exclusive of any that is bound;
9. Specific binding or carrier proteins in the fetal or maternal circulation; and
10. The rate of fetal blood flow through the villous capillaries.

TRANSFER BY DIFFUSION

Most substances with a molecular mass less than 500 daltons diffuse readily through the placental tissue interposed between the maternal and fetal circulations. Molecular weight clearly is important in determining the rate of transfer by diffusion; all

other things equal, the smaller the molecule, the more rapid is the transfer rate. Simple diffusion, however, is by no means the only mechanism of transfer of low molecular weight compounds. The trophoblasts actually facilitate the transfer of a variety of small compounds, especially those that are in low concentration in maternal plasma but are essential for the normal growth and development of the fetus.

Simple diffusion appears to be the mechanism involved in the transfer of oxygen, carbon dioxide, water, and most (but not all) electrolytes. Anesthetic gases also pass through the placenta rapidly and do so apparently by simple diffusion.

Insulin, steroid hormones, and thyroid hormones cross the placenta but at very slow rates. The hormones synthesized in situ in the trophoblasts enter both the maternal and fetal circulations but not necessarily to the same degree (Chap. 5). For example, the concentrations of chorionic gonadotropin and placental lactogen are very much lower in fetal plasma than in maternal plasma. Substances of very high molecular weight usually do not traverse the placenta, but there are important exceptions, such as immune gamma globulin G [(IgG); M_r is about 160,000], which is transferred by way of a specific trophoblast receptor-mediated mechanism (p. 98).

TRANSFER OF OXYGEN AND CARBON DIOXIDE

Morriss and Boyd (1988), in an excellent account of placental transport, provide an interesting observation. They recall that Mayow, in 1674, suggested that the placenta served as the fetal lung. Moreover, Erasmus Darwin, in 1796, only 22 years after the discovery of oxygen, reasoned that the function of the placenta was comparable with that of lungs and gills. Inasmuch as Darwin observed that the color of blood passing through each organ became bright red, he deduced that *"from the structure as well as the use of the placenta, it appears to be a respiratory organ, like the gills of the fish, by which the fetus becomes oxygenated."*

The transfer of carbon dioxide across the placenta is diffusion-limited; but the transfer of oxygen is blood-flow limited. Normal values for oxygen, carbon dioxide, and pH in maternal and fetal blood, as compiled by Longo (1972), are presented in Table 6–2. Because of the continuous passage of oxygen from the maternal blood in the intervillous space to the fetus, the oxygen saturation of this blood resembles that in the maternal capillaries; namely, it is somewhat less than that of the mother's arterial blood. The average oxygen saturation of intervillous space blood is estimated to be 65 to 75 percent, with a partial pressure (P_{O_2}) of about 30 to 35 mm Hg. The oxygen saturation

TABLE 6–2. NORMAL VALUES FOR OXYGEN, CARBON DIOXIDE, AND pH IN HUMAN MATERNAL AND FETAL BLOOD

	Uterine		Umbilical	
	Artery	*Vein*	*Vein*	*Artery*
P_{O_2} (mm Hg)	95	40	27	15
O_2Hb (percent saturation)	98	76	68	30
O_2 content (mL/dL)	15.8	12.2	14.5	6.4
Hemoglobin (g/dL)	12.0	12.0	16.0	16.0
O_2 capacity (mL O_2/dL)	16.1	16.1	21.4	21.4
P_{CO_2} (mm Hg)	32	40	43	48
CO_2 content (mM/L)	19.6	21.8	25.2	26.3
HCO_3 (mM/L)	18.8	20.7	24.0	25.0
pH	7.40	7.34	7.38	7.35

of umbilical vein blood is similar, but with an oxygen partial pressure somewhat lower.

In the estimations reported for the PO₂ of blood from the intervillous space, inconsistently high or low figures were often encountered, suggesting that if the needle were actually in the intervillous space, the blood is not thoroughly mixed. If the needle or electrode were placed at a point where it is bathed by arterial blood jetting into the intervillous space, the estimate of oxygen saturation would be inordinately high, whereas the reverse would obtain if the needle or electrode were placed at a location where the circulation was relatively sluggish. The collection of umbilical venous or arterial blood at delivery that is truly representative of the oxygenation in utero is fraught with even greater errors.

Despite the relatively low PO₂, the fetus normally does not suffer from lack of oxygen. The human fetus probably behaves like the lamb fetus and, therefore, has a cardiac output considerably greater per unit of body weight than does the adult. The high cardiac output and, late in pregnancy, the increased oxygen-carrying capacity of fetal blood (attributable to fetal hemoglobin), and a higher hemoglobin concentration than in adults, compensate effectively for the low oxygen tension. Both of these mechanisms are considered further in this chapter under "Fetal Circulation" and under "Fetal Blood." Additional evidence that the fetus does not normally experience lack of oxygen is provided by measurements of the lactic acid content of fetal blood, which is only slightly higher than that of the mother.

Assali and co-workers (1968b) and Assali (1974) were able to raise the PO₂ in the umbilical vein of the lamb fetus by 10 mm Hg when the mother breathed 100 percent oxygen at atmospheric pressure. They detected no fall in uteroplacental or umbilical blood flow in response to 100 percent oxygen. When the ewe breathed hyperbaric oxygen that raised the maternal arterial PO₂ to 1,300 mm Hg, uteroplacental blood flow did not change and umbilical flow decreased only slightly, although the PO₂ in umbilical blood rose to nearly 600 mm Hg (Fig. 6–10). With normally functioning maternal and fetal circulations, therefore, oxygen can be delivered across the placenta, at least to the sheep fetus, under increased tension and without remarkably restricting umbilical blood flow. Employing the usual clinical equipment for providing oxygen to the mother, the increase is modest, however.

There are no precise measurements of the ability of the human fetus to withstand severe hypoxia. Myers (1970) measured the tolerance of the brain of the monkey fetus to hypoxia induced by cord compression with complete cessation of flow. The rates at which bradycardia, hypotension, and acidosis developed varied with gestational age, so that the more mature the fetus, the more rapid the rate of deterioration.

In general, the transfer of carbon dioxide from the fetus to the mother is accomplished by diffusion, the placenta being highly permeable to carbon dioxide, which traverses the chorionic villus more rapidly than does oxygen. Near term, the partial pressure of carbon dioxide in the umbilical arteries is estimated to average about 48 mm Hg, or about 5 mm or so more than in the maternal blood in the intervillous space. Fetal blood has somewhat less affinity for carbon dioxide than does the blood of the mother, thereby favoring the transfer of carbon dioxide from the fetus to the mother. Also, mild hyperventilation by the pregnant woman results in a fall in PCO₂ favoring a transfer of CO₂ from the fetal compartment into maternal blood.

SELECTIVE TRANSFER AND FACILITATED DIFFUSION

Although diffusion is an important method of placental transfer, the trophoblasts and the chorionic villus unit exhibit enormous selectivity in transfer, maintaining different concentrations of a variety of metabolites on the two sides of the villus. One example of this process was observed more than 30 years ago when Page and associates (1957) found selectivity in placental transfer of the two isomers of histidine. D-histidine, the unnatural isomer, traversed the placenta more slowly, coming to equilibrium with the fetal blood within 3 or 4 hours. If only passive transfer by simple diffusion were involved, L-histidine, the natural isomer, would have been expected to behave similarly, but in the case of this isomer, equilibrium was attained within a few minutes. As it turns out, we now know that there are specific transport processes by which trophoblast assimilate amino acids from maternal plasma.

The concentrations of a number of substances, which are not synthesized by the fetus, are several times higher in fetal than in maternal blood. Ascorbic acid is a good example of this phenomenon. This relatively low molecular weight substance resembles the pentose and hexose sugars and might be expected to traverse the placenta by simple diffusion. The concentration of ascorbic acid, however, is 2 to 4 times higher in fetal

Figure 6–10. Changes in umbilical vein blood PO₂ during progressively increasing maternal blood PO₂ in the sheep. Note that when the maternal blood PO₂ was raised to about 300 mm Hg by ventilating the maternal lungs with 100 percent oxygen (black dots), umbilical vein blood PO₂ remained below 60 mm Hg. This illustrates the boundary imposed on fetal oxygenation. Only when maternal blood PO₂ was increased by hyperbaric oxygenation (open circles) did the fetal blood PO₂ increase to high levels. (*From Assali: In Gluck (ed): Modern Perinatal Medicine. Chicago, Year Book, 1974.*)

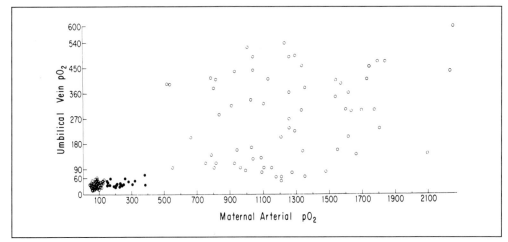

plasma than in maternal plasma (Braestrup, 1937; Manahan and Eastman, 1938; Morriss and Boyd, 1988). The unidirectional transfer of iron across the placenta provides another example of the unique capabilities of the human placenta for transport. Typically, iron is present in the plasma at a lower concentration in the pregnant women than in her fetus; and at the same time, the iron-binding capacity of the plasma is much greater in the pregnant woman than in the fetus. Nonetheless, iron is transported actively from maternal to fetal plasma; and in the human fetus, the amount transferred appears to be independent of maternal iron status.

Fetal infections caused by viruses, bacteria, and protozoa are occasionally encountered (Chap. 33, p. 613). Many viruses, including those responsible for rubella, chickenpox, measles, mumps, smallpox, vaccinia, poliomyelitis, cytomegalic inclusion disease, coxsackie virus disease, and western equine encephalitis, may cross the placenta and infect the fetus. *Treponema pallidum, Toxoplasma, Plasmodium* species, and *Mycobacterium tuberculosis* also may produce fetal infection. With protozoal and bacterial, but not necessarily viral, infections, there is almost always histological evidence of involvement of the placenta.

Rarely, malignant cells arising in neoplasias in the pregnant woman can be transferred to the placenta or fetus or both. According to Read and Platzer (1981), approximately 50 percent of these are malignant melanomas or else they are hematopoietic in origin (see Chap. 31, p. 553).

NUTRITION OF THE FETUS

PLACENTAL ARM OF THE FETAL–MATERNAL COMMUNICATION SYSTEM: NUTRIENT COMPONENT

During the first 2 months of pregnancy, the embryo consists almost entirely of water; in later months, relatively more solids are added. The amounts of water, fat, nitrogen, and certain minerals in the fetus at successive weeks of pregnancy are shown in Table 6–3. Because of the small amount of yolk in the human ovum, growth of the fetus from the very early stage of development depends on nutrients obtained from the mother. During the first few days after implantation, the nutrition of the blastocyst arises directly from the interstitial fluid of the endometrium and from the surrounding maternal tissue, which has undergone proteolysis due to trophoblastic invasion. Within the next week, the forerunners of the intervillous space are formed; in the beginning, there are simply lacunae filled with maternal blood. During the 3rd week after fertilization, fetal blood vessels appear in the chorionic villi. During the 4th week after ovulation, a cardiovascular system has formed, and thereby a true circulation, both within the embryo and between the embryo and the chorionic villi.

Ultimately, the maternal diet is the source of the nutrients supplied to the fetus; but ingested foodstuff is translated into storage forms that are then made available continuously, in an orderly way, to meet the demands for energy, tissue repair, and new growth, including those related to pregnancy. Three major storage depots, namely, the liver, muscle, and adipose tissue, and the storage hormone, insulin, are involved intimately in the metabolism of the nutrients absorbed from the maternal gut. Insulin is released from the maternal islands of Langerhans in response to various materials liberated from food during digestion and absorption. The secretion of insulin is sustained by rising levels of blood glucose and amino acids. The net effect is to store glucose as glycogen primarily in the liver and muscle, to retain some amino acids as protein, and to store the excess as fat. This storage of maternal fat peaks in the second trimester, then declines as fetal demands increase in late pregnancy (Pipe and colleagues, 1979).

During the fasting state, glucose is released from glycogen, but glycogen stores are not large in the mother and these cannot provide an adequate amount of glucose to meet the requirements of the mother and fetus for energy and growth. The cleavage of triacylglycerols, stored in adipose tissue, however, provides the mother with energy in the form of free fatty acids. The process of lipolysis is activated, directly or indirectly, by a number of hormones, including glucagon, norepinephrine, placental lactogen, glucocorticosteroids, and thyroxine.

GLUCOSE

D-glucose transfer across the placenta is accomplished by a carrier-mediated, stereospecific, nonconcentrating process that can be saturated—*facilitated diffusion.* Transporter proteins for D-glucose have been isolated from the plasma membrane of the microvilli of human trophoblasts (Morriss and Boyd, 1988).

Because glucose is a major nutrient for growth and energy in the fetus, it would seem advantageous during pregnancy, as

TABLE 6–3. TOTAL AMOUNTS OF FAT, NITROGEN, AND MINERALS IN THE BODY OF THE DEVELOPING FETUS

Body Weight (g)	Approx. Fetal Age (wk)	Water (g)	Fat (g)	N (g)	Ca (g)	P (g)	Mg (g)	Na (mEq)	K (mEq)	Cl (mEq)	Fe (mg)	Cu (mg)	Zn (mg)
30	13	27	0.2	0.4	0.09	0.09	0.003	3.6	1.4	2.4	—	—	—
100	15	89	0.5	1.0	0.3	0.2	0.01	9	2.6	7	5.1	—	—
200	17	177	1.0	2.8	0.7	0.6	0.03	20	7.9	14	10	0.7	2.6
500	23	440	3.0	7.0	2.2	1.5	0.10	49	22	33	28	2.4	9.4
1000	26	860	10	14	6.0	3.4	0.22	90	41	66	64	3.5	16
1500	31	1270	35	25	10	5.6	0.35	125	60	96	100	5.6	25
2000	33	1620	100	37	15	8.2	0.46	160	84	120	160	8.0	35
2500	35	1940	185	49	20	11	0.58	200	110	130	220	10	43
3000	38	2180	360	55	25	14	0.70	240	130	150	260	12	50
3500	40	2400	560	62	30	17	0.78	280	150	160	280	14	53

From Widdowson: In Assali (ed): Biology of Gestation, Vol. II, The Fetus and Neonate. New York, Academic, 1968.

emphasized by Freinkel (1969), for the operational mechanisms to be those that minimize glucose utilization by the mother and thereby make the limited maternal supply available to the fetus. One metabolic action of placental lactogen, a hormone normally present in abundance in the mother but not the fetus, is believed to be the blocking of the peripheral uptake and utilization of glucose by maternal tissues while promoting the mobilization and utilization of free fatty acids. Placental lactogen does not appear to be absolutely required for a normal pregnancy outcome, however. Nielsen and co-workers (1979) described an otherwise normal pregnancy in which placental lactogen could not be identified by a variety of techniques applied in several laboratories (Chap. 5). The fetus is not exposed to a constant supply of glucose; even in normal pregnant women, the plasma levels may vary by up to 75 percent.

Whereas the fetus is quite dependent on the mother for nutrition, the fetus is not a passive parasite, it actively participates in providing for its own nutrition. At midpregnancy, fetal glucose concentration is independent of and may exceed maternal levels (Bozzetti and colleagues, 1988).

LACTATE

Lactate also is transported across the placenta by facilitated diffusion. By way of co-transport with hydrogen ions, lactate is probably transported as lactic acid.

FREE FATTY ACIDS AND TRIGLYCERIDES

Neutral fat (triacylglycerols) does not cross the placenta but glycerol does. The extent of transport of free fatty acids is not known, although Szabo and associates (1969) found active transfer of palmitic acid from the maternal to the fetal side of the human placenta perfused in vitro. Portman and co-workers (1969), furthermore, demonstrated rapid transfer of palmitic and linoleic acids from mother to fetus in subhuman primates. Lipoprotein lipase is present on the maternal surface but not on the fetal surface of the placenta. This arrangement should favor hydrolysis of triacylglycerols in the maternal intervillous space while preserving these neutral lipids in the fetal blood.

In Chapter 5, we pointed to the likelihood that the placental uptake and use of low-density lipoprotein (LDL) by the placenta may account for an additional mechanism for the assimilation of essential fatty acids and essential amino acids. The LDL particle of maternal plasma becomes bound to specific LDL receptors in the coated-pit region of the microvilli on the maternal-facing side of the trophoblasts. The LDL particle is taken up by a process of endocytosis. The apoprotein and cholesterol esters of LDL are hydrolyzed by lysosomal enzymes in trophoblasts to give (1) cholesterol for progesterone synthesis, (2) free amino acids (including essential amino acids), and (3) an essential fatty acid, linoleic acid, from the hydrolysis of the cholesterol esters of LDL. Indeed, the concentration of arachidonic acid in fetal plasma is greater than that in maternal plasma; most of the arachidonic acid arises from linoleic acid assimilated from the diet.

AMINO ACIDS

In addition to the use of LDL, the placenta is known to concentrate a large number of amino acids intracellularly (Lemons, 1979). Neutral amino acids from maternal plasma are taken up by trophoblasts by at least three specific processes. Presumably, the amino acids, concentrated in trophoblasts, are thence transferred to the fetal side by diffusion.

PROTEINS AND OTHER LARGE MOLECULES

Generally, the transfer of larger proteins across the placenta is very limited. There are important exceptions. A major one is immunoglobulin G (IgG). In the human, IgG crosses the placenta in major amounts.

Near term, IgG is present in approximately the same concentrations in cord and maternal sera but IgA and IgM are considerably lower in cord serum. Although IgA and IgM of maternal origin are effectively excluded from the fetus, IgG crosses the placenta with considerable efficiency (Gitlin and colleagues, 1972). Fc receptors are present on trophoblasts; and the transport of IgG is accomplished by way of these receptors through a classic process of endocytosis. Increased amounts of IgM are found in the fetus only after the fetal immune system has been provoked into antibody response by an infection in the fetus.

IONS AND TRACE METALS

Iodide transport across the placenta clearly is carrier-mediated by an active process; indeed the placenta concentrates iodide. Calcium and phosphorus also are actively transported across the placenta from mother to fetus. A calcium-binding protein is present in placenta. Iron is accumulated in placenta by an active, energy-requiring process. The concentrations of zinc in the fetal plasma also are greater than those in maternal plasma.

VITAMINS

Vitamin A (Retinol)
The concentration of vitamin A is greater in fetal than in maternal plasma. Vitamin A in fetal plasma is bound to retinol-binding protein and to prealbumin.

Vitamin C (Ascorbic Acid)
The transport of vitamin C across the placenta from mother to fetus is accomplished by an energy-dependent carrier-mediated process.

Vitamin D (Cholecalciferol)
The levels of the principal vitamin D metabolites, including 1,25-dihydroxycholecalciferol, are greater in maternal plasma than are those in fetal plasma. The 1α-hydroxylation of 25-hydroxyvitamin D_3 is known to take place in placenta and in decidua.

MATERNAL NUTRITION

For obvious reasons, a great deal of investigative effort continues to be focused on maternal nutrition and its effect on the growth and development of the fetus. Fetal size is not just a function of fetal age. For example, in some forms of maternal diabetes mellitus (i.e., without significant maternal vascular disease), the fetus may be larger than normal; but if severe maternal vascular disease further complicates the diabetes, the fetus may be appreciably smaller than normal (see Chap. 39, p. 820). Fetal macrosomia usually complicates the pregnancy when maternal diabetes is not well controlled.

Page (1970), in an interesting theoretical discussion of fetal growth, analyzed the factors known to control the delivery of a primary nutrient, glucose, to the fetus. Because maternal hyperglycemia leads to increased transfer of glucose across the placenta, he suggested that hyperglycemia and hyperinsulinemia in the fetus function together to accelerate fetal growth. Brinsmead and Liggins (1979) found that insulin levels were higher in cord plasma from large-for-gestational-age infants and lower when infants were small for gestational age.

GROWTH RETARDATION

The cause of growth retardation in the human fetus is not always clearly defined. Theoretically, growth retardation might result from insufficient concentration of a nutrient in the maternal arterial plasma, inadequate uterine blood flow and placental perfusion, reduced functional surface area of the chorionic villi, impairment of placental transport mechanisms, inadequate fetal vascularity of the chorionic villi, or insufficient umbilical blood flow to transfer the nutrient in appropriate amounts from the placenta to the fetus. Among species in which the weight of the fetus is relatively large compared with the mother's weight, and in which the duration of gestation is short, maternal dietary deficiencies commonly cause fetal growth retardation. In humans, however, where fetal size is small compared with that of the mother and the duration of gestation is long, it has been difficult to demonstrate a correlation between maternal nutritional deficiency and fetal growth retardation (see Chap. 38, p. 765). It is possible that subtle but nonetheless deleterious changes in the human fetus may be induced by faulty maternal nutrition, be it either undernutrition or the ingestion of excessive amounts of nutrients, including protein (Stein and colleagues, 1978).

PHYSIOLOGY OF THE FETUS

The fetus does swallow amnionic fluid; and late in gestation, large volumes are ingested. Nonetheless, it is unlikely that this represents a major source of nutrients to the fetus. On the other hand, there may be an important function of amnionic fluid in fetal development other than physical protection of the fetus. Fetal kidney is known to produce an epidermal growth factor-like agent (kidney-derived growth factor [KDGF]) that is excreted into fetal urine and thence into amnionic fluid. This agent acts on amnion to promote amnion cell replication, possibly promoting amnion growth as fetal urine volume and the volume of the amnionic fluid (including the fetus) increase. In fetal conditions in which amnionic fluid is not taken into the lungs by fetal thoracic excursions (fetal breathing), lung hypoplasia invariably results. Heretofore, this phenomenon has been attributed to failure of lung expansion by amnionic fluid. And no doubt this is a partial explanation. But on the other hand, we also know that epidermal growth factor (EGF)-like growth factors, may serve an important role in fetal lung development (p. 116). Thus, the ingestion of amnionic fluid into the lung and gastrointestinal tract of the fetus may promote growth and differentiation by way of growth factors in amnionic fluid.

FETAL CIRCULATION

Because almost all nutrient materials required for fetal growth and maturation are delivered to the fetus from the placenta by the umbilical vein, the fetal circulation must differ fundamentally from that of the adult (Fig. 6–11). The single umbilical vein in the umbilical cord carries oxygenated, nutrient-bearing blood from the placenta to the fetus. The *umbilical vein* enters the fetus through the umbilical ring and ascends along the anterior abdominal wall toward the liver. The vein then divides into the portal sinus and the ductus venosus, the former carrying blood to the hepatic veins primarily of the left side of the liver, the latter or major "branch" of the umbilical vein traversing the liver to enter directly the *inferior vena cava*. The blood flowing to the fetal heart from the inferior vena cava, therefore, consists of an admixture of "arterial-like" blood that passes through the ductus venosus and less well-oxygenated blood that collects from most of the veins below the level of the diaphragm. As a consequence, the oxygen content of blood delivered to the heart from the inferior vena cava is less than that which leaves the placenta, but it is greater than that from the superior vena cava.

As emphasized by Dawes (1962), the *foramen ovale* opens directly off the inferior vena cava so that blood from the inferior vena cava is, for the most part, immediately deflected by the *crista dividens* through the foramen ovale into the left atrium. Little or none of the less-well oxygenated blood from the *superior vena cava* normally passes through the foramen ovale. The preferential flow of blood from the inferior vena cava through the foramen ovale to the left atrium bypasses the right ventricle and pulmonary circulation and permits delivery to the left ventricle of more highly oxygenated blood than if complete admixture had occurred in the right atrium. The more highly oxygenated blood that passes through the foramen ovale and is ejected from the left ventricle perfuses two vital organs, the heart and the brain. The blood that is typically venous in character, coming from the superior vena cava and ejected from the right ventricle into the pulmonary trunk, is, for the most part, shunted through the *ductus arteriosus* into the descending aorta.

The lamb fetus has been studied intensively by several groups of investigators who take the view that the circulatory function of the mature lamb fetus is similar in many respects to that of the mature human fetus. Before birth, in human and in sheep, both ventricles of the fetal heart, as the consequence of the shunts just described, work in parallel rather than in series. Attempts to measure cardiac output in the lamb fetus have yielded somewhat variable results. Assali (1974) and associates (1968a) have ascertained a mean value of about 225 mL per kg per minute, but with considerable individual variation; Paton and co-workers (1973) found very similar values in baboon fetuses. Such a high fetal cardiac output, which per unit of weight is about 3 times that of an adult at rest, would serve to compensate for the low oxygen content of fetal blood. The high cardiac output is accomplished in part by the fast heart rate of the fetus and a low systemic (peripheral) resistance.

Before birth and expansion of the lungs, the high pulmonary vascular resistance accounts for the high pressure and the low blood flow in the fetal pulmonary circuit. At the same time, resistance to flow through the ductus arteriosus and the umbilicoplacental circulation is low, probably accounting for the overall low fetal systemic vascular resistance. It is estimated that in the fetal lamb about one-half the combined output of the two ventricles goes to the placenta. Rudolph and Heymann (1968), by injecting isotopically labeled plastic microspheres into the fetal lamb circulation at various sites, determined the distribution of cardiac output during the last third of gestation to be approximately as follows: placenta, 41 percent; carcass, 35 percent; brain, 5 percent; heart, 5 percent; gastrointestinal tract, 5 percent; lungs, 4 percent; kidneys, 2 percent; spleen, 2 percent; liver (hepatic artery only), 2 percent.

Blood is returned to the placenta through the two *hypogastric arteries*, which distally become the *umbilical arteries*.

After birth, the umbilical vessels, the ductus arteriosus, the foramen ovale, and the ductus venosus normally constrict or collapse and consequently the hemodynamics of the fetal circulation undergo pronounced changes. According to Assali (1974) and Assali and associates (1968), clamping of the umbilical cord and expansion of the fetal lungs, either through spontaneous breathing or artificial respiration, promptly induce a variety of hemodynamic changes in sheep. The systemic arterial pressure initially falls slightly, apparently the result of the reversal in the direction of blood flow in the ductus ateriosus, but it soon recovers and then rises above the control value. They concluded that several factors served to regulate the flow of blood through the ductus arteriosus, including the difference in pressure between the pulmonary artery and aorta and especially the oxygen tension of the blood passing through the ductus arteriosus. They were able to influence flow through the ductus arteriosus by altering the P_{O_2} of the blood. When the lungs were ventilated with oxygen

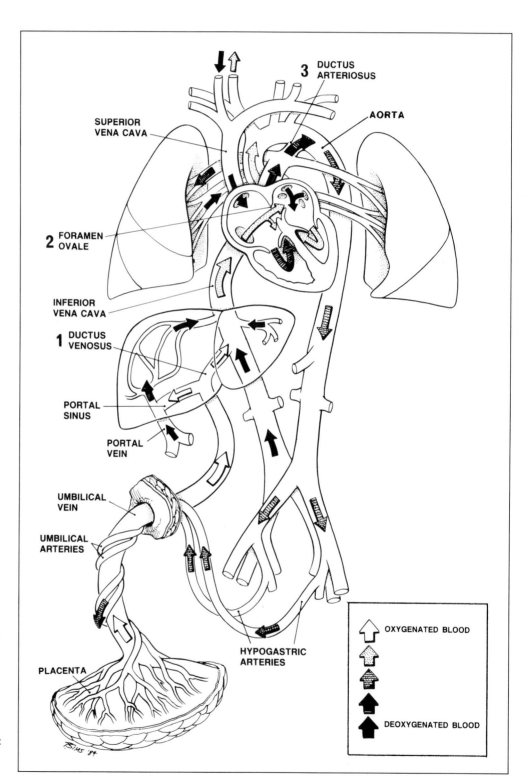

Figure 6–11. The intricate nature of the fetal circulation is evident. The degree of oxygenation of blood in various vessels differs appreciably from that in the postnatal state as the consequences of oxygenation being provided by the placenta rather than the lungs and the presence of three major vascular shunts: **1.** Ductus venosus. **2.** Foramen ovale. **3.** Ductus arteriosus.

and the PO_2 rose above 55 mm Hg, ductus flow dropped, but ventilation with nitrogen, initially at least, returned the ductus flow to the original pattern. The ductus is functionally closed by 10 to 96 hours after birth, and anatomically closed by 2 to 3 weeks (Clymann and Heymann, 1981).

The effects from variations in oxygen tension of blood flowing through the ductus arteriosus are believed to be mediated through the actions of prostaglandins on the ductus. Prostaglandin E_2 (PGE_2) dilates the constricted ductus arteriosus and is intimately involved in maintaining normal patency in utero. Inhibitors of prostaglandin synthase, when given to the mother, may lead to premature closure of the ductus arteriosus (see Chap. 38, p. 757), but can be used pharmacologically to close a symptomatic patent ductus arteriosus postnatally (Brash and associates, 1981).

With expansion of the lungs, pressures in the right ventricle and pulmonary arteries fall because of the marked decrease in pulmonary vascular resistance. Theoretically, at least, an increase in the left arterial pressure above that of the right atrium would cause functional closure of the foramen ovale immediately after birth. There is some disagreement, however, as to when closure actually occurs. The experiments of Barclay and co-workers (1939) are consistent with the view that functional closure of the foramen ovale occurs within several minutes of birth. Arey (1946), however, states that anatomical fusion of the two septa of the foramen ovale is not completed until about 1 year after birth, and that in 25 percent of cases perfect closure is never attained. When the foramen ovale remains functionally patent, circulatory disturbances of variable gravity result.

The more distal portions of the hypogastric arteries, which course from the level of the bladder along the abdominal wall to the umbilical ring and into the cord as the umbilical arteries, undergo atrophy and obliteration within 3 to 4 days after birth, to become the *umbilical ligaments*; intraabdominal remnants of the umbilical vein form the *ligamentum teres*. The ductus venosus constricts and its lumen closes resulting in the formation of the *ligamentum venosum*.

FETAL BLOOD

Hematopoiesis

Hematopoiesis, in the very early embryo, is demonstrable first in the yolk sac. The next major site of erythropoiesis is the liver and finally the bone marrow. The contributions made by each site throughout the growth and development of the embryo and fetus are demonstrated graphically in Figure 6–12.

The first erythrocytes formed in the fetus are nucleated, but as fetal development progresses, more and more of the circulating erythrocytes are nonnucleated. As the fetus grows, not only does the volume of blood in the common circulation of the fetus and placenta increase, but the hemoglobin concentration rises as well. As shown by the studies of Walker and Turnbull (1953), the hemoglobin of fetal blood rises to the adult male level of about 15 g per dL at midpregnancy, and at term it is somewhat higher, about 18 g per dL. Fetal blood at or near term is characterized, therefore, by a high hemoglobin concentration that is high by maternal standards.

The reticulocyte count falls from a very high level in the very young fetus to about 5 percent at term. Pearson (1966), using a variety of techniques, found the life span of erythrocytes from more mature fetuses to be approximately two thirds of erythrocytes of normal adults, but erythrocytes of less mature fetuses have an even shorter life span. This is related undoubt-

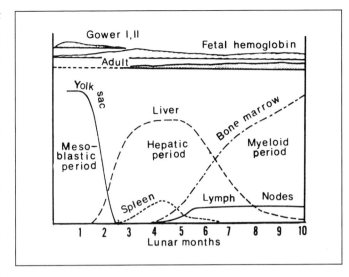

Figure 6–12. Sites of hematopoiesis and kinds of hemoglobin synthesized at various stages of fetus development. (*From Brown: Biology of Gestation, Vol. II. The Fetus and Neonate, New York. Academic, 1968, p 361.*)

edly to their large volume, and these data are supportive of the concept that fetal erythrocytes are "stress erythrocytes." The erythrocytes of the fetus differ structurally and metabolically from those of the adult. Fetal erythrocytes are more deformable, which serves to offset their higher viscosity (Smith and co-workers, 1981), and they contain several enzymes that have appreciably different activities.

Erythropoiesis

The fetus is capable of making erythropoietin in increased amounts when severely anemic and of excreting it into the amnionic fluid (Finne, 1966; Zivny and co-workers, 1982). Evidence of a physiological role for erythropoietin in fetal erythropoiesis has been provided by Zanjani and co-workers (1974). The injection of antierythropoietin into the sheep fetoplacental circulation was followed by a decrease in reticulocytes and decreased incorporation of radioiron into erythrocytes; moreover, induction of anemia in the fetus resulted in elevated levels of erythropoietin-like material. In utero, the fetal liver, rather than the kidney, appears to be an important source of erythropoietin. After birth, erythropoietin normally may not be detectable for up to 3 months.

Fetal Blood Volume

Precise measurements of the volume of blood contained in the human fetoplacental circulation are lacking. Usher and associates (1963), however, have measured the volume of blood of term normal infants very soon after birth and found an average of 78 mL per kg when immediate cord-clamping was conducted. Gruenwald (1967) found the volume of blood of fetal origin contained in the placenta after prompt cord-clamping to average 45 mL per kg of fetus. Thus, fetoplacental blood volume at term is approximately 125 mL per kg of fetus. Pritchard and co-workers (unpublished observations) measured the volumes of blood in infants with erythroblastosis fetalis as well as their placenta and cord immediately after delivery. The "fetoplacental" blood volume in these circumstances was very close to 120 mL per kg of infant weight.

Fetal Hemoglobin

In the embryo and fetus, the globin moiety of much of the hemoglobin differs from that of the normal adult. In the embryo, three major forms of hemoglobin may be found. The most primitive forms are Gower-1 and Gower-2 (Pearson, 1966). The third form is hemoglobin Portland. The globin moiety of Gower-1 consists of two ξ-peptide chains and two γ-chains per molecule of protein, whereas in Gower-2 there are two α- and two ε-chains. All normal hemoglobins elaborated after Gower-1 contain a pair of α-chains, but the other pair of peptide chains differs for each kind of hemoglobin. Hemoglobin F (so-called fetal hemoglobin or alkaline-resistant hemoglobin) contains a pair of α-peptide chains and a pair of γ-chains per molecule of hemoglobin. Actually, two varieties of γ-chains have been identified in hemoglobin F, the ratios changing steadily as the fetus and infant mature (Fadel and Abraham, 1981; Huisman and colleagues, 1970).

Hemoglobin A, the final hemoglobin to be formed by the fetus and the major hemoglobin formed after birth in normal adults, is present after the 11th week of gestation in progressively greater amounts as the fetus matures (Pataryas and Stamatoyannopoulos, 1972).

Evidence has been presented that the switch from hemoglobin F to hemoglobin A that begins at 32 to 34 weeks gestation is associated with methylation of the γ-globin genes. In newborns of women with diabetes mellitus, there is commonly a persistence of the hemoglobin F and there is hypomethylation of the γ-globin genes (Perrine and associates, 1988). The globin of hemoglobin A is made up of a pair of α-chains and a pair of β-chains. Hemoglobin A_2, the globin of which contains a pair of α-chains and a pair of δ-chains, is present in very small concentrations in the mature fetus but increases after birth. Thus, as growth proceeds, there is a shift not only in the amounts but also in the kinds of globin synthesized by the embryo and fetus.

As illustrated in Figure 6–13, at any given oxygen tension and at identical pH, fetal erythrocytes that contain mostly hemoglobin F bind more oxygen than do erythrocytes that contain nearly all hemoglobin A. The major reason for this difference is that hemoglobin A binds 2,3-diphosphoglycerate more avidly than does hemoglobin F (De Verdier and Garby, 1969) and 2,3-diphosphoglycerate so bound lowers the affinity of the hemoglobin molecule for oxygen. The increased oxygen affinity of the fetal erythrocyte results from a lower concentration of 2,3-diphosphoglycerate compared with that of the maternal erythrocyte, in which the 2,3-diphosphoglycerate level is increased compared with the nonpregnant state. Gilbert and associates (1983) found that, at higher temperatures, the affinity of fetal blood for oxygen decreases. They concluded that increases in fetal temperature as a consequence of maternal hyperthermia could significantly compound fetal hypoxia.

Because fetal erythrocytes that are formed late in pregnancy contain less hemoglobin F and more hemoglobin A than do the cells formed earlier, the content of hemoglobin F of the fetal erythrocytes falls somewhat during the latter weeks of pregnancy. At term, about three-fourths of the total hemoglobin normally is hemoglobin F. During the first 6 to 12 months after delivery, the proportion of hemoglobin F continues to decrease, eventually to reach the low level found in erythrocytes of normal adults (Schulman and Smith, 1953).

Coagulation Factors in the Fetus

The concentrations of several coagulation factors at birth are appreciably below the levels that develop within a few weeks after birth (Sell and Corrigan, 1973). The factors that are low in

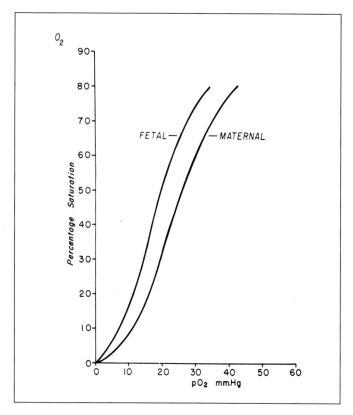

Figure 6–13. Oxygen dissociation curves of fetal and maternal human bloods prepared at pH 7.40. (*Courtesy of the late Dr. Andre Hellergers.*)

cord blood are II, VII, IX, X, XI, XII, XIII, and fibrinogen. Without prophylactic vitamin K, vitamin K–dependent coagulation factors usually decrease even further during the first few days after birth, especially in breast-fed infants, and may lead to hemorrhage in the newborn infant (Shearer and co-workers, 1982) (see Chap. 33, p. 611). Platelet counts in cord blood are in the normal range for nonpregnant adults, while fibrinogen levels are somewhat less than in nonpregnant adults. For reasons unknown, the time for conversion of fibrinogen in plasma to fibrin clot when thrombin is added (thrombin time) is somewhat prolonged compared with that of older children and adults. The measurement of factor VIII coagulant activity in the cord is of value in accurately making or excluding the diagnosis of hemophilia in male infants (Kasper and colleagues, 1964). Functional factor XIII (fibrin-stabilizing factor) levels in plasma are significantly reduced compared with those in normal adults (Henriksson and co-workers, 1974) but the clinical diagnosis of factor XIII deficiency is usually made by observing a continuous "ooze" from the umbilical stump. Nielsen (1969) described the finding of low levels of plasminogen and somewhat increased fibrinolytic activity in cord plasma compared with that in maternal plasma. This may be due to a structurally and functionally different fetal plasminogen (Estelles and co-workers, 1980).

Fetal Plasma Proteins

The mean total plasma protein and plasma albumin concentrations in maternal and cord blood are similar. For example, Foley and associates (1978) identified maternal and cord total plasma proteins to average 6.5 and 5.9 g per dL, respectively, with maternal and cord plasma albumin levels of 3.6 and 3.7 g per dL, respectively.

Fetal Blood Viscosity

The viscosities of maternal and cord bloods are similar (Foley and associates, 1978). The increase in viscosity imposed by the higher hematocrit of cord blood is offset by the lower levels of fibrinogen and IgM in the cord plasma and by the more deformable fetal erythrocytes (Smith and co-workers, 1981).

IMMUNOCOMPETENCE OF THE FETUS

In the absence of a direct antigenic stimulus in the fetus, such as infection, the immunoglobulins in the fetus consist almost totally of immune globulin G (IgG) synthesized by the mother and subsequently transferred across the placenta by receptor-mediated processes in trophoblast as described on page 98 of this chapter. Therefore, the antibodies in the fetus and the newborn infant most often reflect the immunological experiences of the mother.

Immunoglobulin G

IgG transport from mother to fetus begins at about 16 weeks gestation and increases as gestation proceeds. But the bulk of IgG is acquired by the fetus (from the mother) during the last 4 weeks of pregnancy (Gitlin, 1971). Accordingly, preterm infants are endowed relatively poorly with maternal antibodies. Newborns begin to produce IgG, but slowly; adult values are not attained until 3 years of age.

Immunoglobulin M

IgM is not transported from mother to fetus; therefore, any IgM in the fetus or newborn is that which was produced in the fetus. Very little IgM is produced by normal, healthy fetuses; that which is produced may include antibody to maternal T lymphocytes (Hayward, 1983). Increased levels of IgM are found in newborns with congenital infection (rubella, cytomegalovirus, toxoplasmosis). Adult levels of IgM normally are attained by 9 months of age.

Lymphocytes

The immune system begins to mature early in fetal life. B lymphocytes appear in liver by 9 weeks and are present in blood and spleen by 12 weeks gestation. T lymphocytes begin to leave the thymus at about 14 weeks (Hayward, 1983).

Monocytes

Monocytes of newborns are able to process and present antigen when tested with maternal antigen-specific T cells.

Ontogeny of the Immune Response

The transfer of some IgG antibodies from mother to fetus is harmful rather than protective to the fetus. The classic clinical example of antibodies of maternal origin that are dangerous to the fetus is hemolytic disease of the fetus and newborn resulting from D-antigen isoimmunization. In this disease, maternal antibody to fetal erythrocyte antigen crosses the placenta to destroy the fetal erythrocytes (see Chap. 33, p. 602).

Infections in utero have provided an opportunity to examine some of the mechanisms for immune response by the human fetus. The opinion that the fetus is immunologically incompetent is no longer tenable. Indeed, morphological evidence of immunological competence in the human fetus has been reported as early as 13 weeks gestational age by Altshuler (1974), who described infection of the placenta and fetus by cytomegalovirus with characteristic severe inflammatory cell proliferation as well as virus inclusions. Moreover, synthesis of complement late in the first trimester by fetal organs has been demonstrated by Kohler (1973) and confirmed by Stabile and co-workers (1988). All components of human complement are produced at an early stage of fetal development. In cord blood at or near term, the average level for most components of complement are about one half the values for adults (Adinolfi, 1977).

The newborn responds poorly to immunization, and especially poorly to bacterial capsular polysaccharides. This immaturity of response may be due to (1) deficient response of newborn B cells to polyclonal activators or (2) lack of T cells that proliferate in response to specific stimuli (Hayward, 1983).

Differing from many animals, the human newborn infant does not acquire much in the way of passive immunity from the absorption of humoral antibodies ingested in the colostrum. Nevertheless, IgA ingested in colostrum may provide protection against enteric infections, since the antibody resists digestion and is effective on mucosal surfaces. The same is possibly true for IgA ingested with amnionic fluid before delivery.

In the adult, production of immune globulin M (IgM) in response to antigen is superseded in a week or so predominantly by production of IgG. In contrast, the IgM response remains the dominant one for weeks to months in the fetus and newborn. IgM serum levels in umbilical cord blood and identification of specific antibodies may be of aid in the diagnosis of intrauterine infection.

NERVOUS SYSTEM AND SENSORY ORGANS

Synaptic function is developed sufficiently by the 8th week of gestation to demonstrate flexion of neck and trunk (Temiras and co-workers, 1968). If the fetus is removed from the uterus during the 10th week, spontaneous movements may be observed, although movements in utero usually are not felt by the mother until several weeks later. At 10 weeks, local stimuli may evoke squinting, opening the mouth, incomplete finger closure, and plantar flexion of the toes. Complete finger closure is achieved during the 4th lunar month. Swallowing and respiration are also evident during the 4th lunar month but the ability to suck is not present until the 6th month or even later (Lebenthal and associates, 1983).

During the third trimester of pregnancy, integration of nervous and muscular function proceeds rapidly, so that the majority of fetuses delivered after the 32nd week of gestation survive.

By the 7th lunar month, the eye is sensitive to light, but perception of form and color is not complete until long after birth.

The internal, middle, and external components of the ear are well developed by midpregnancy. The fetus apparently hears some sounds in utero as early as the 24th to 26th week of gestation.

Taste buds are evident histologically in the 3rd lunar month; and by the 7th month of gestation, the fetus is responsive to variations in the taste of ingested substances.

DIGESTIVE SYSTEM

GASTROINTESTINAL TRACT

Development

By the 11th week of gestation, the small intestine undergoes peristalsis and is capable of transporting glucose actively (Koldovsky and colleagues, 1965). Gastrointestinal function is sufficiently developed at four months to allow the fetus to swallow amnionic fluid, absorb much of the water from it, and propel unabsorbed matter as far as the lower colon (Fig. 6–14). Hydrochloric acid and some adult digestive enzymes are present in very small amounts in the early fetus; therefore, in the premature infant, transient deficiencies of these enzymes are often present depending upon the gestational age of the infant when born (Lebenthal and Lee, 1983).

Fetal Swallowing

Fetal swallowing at various stages of pregnancy has been measured by introducing a small volume of maternal erythrocytes labeled with isotopic chromium into the amnionic sac and subsequently measuring the chromium that accumulated in the gastrointestinal tract either directly in fetuses that succumbed from immaturity after delivery or in the meconium and feces passed after birth by more mature fetuses (Pritchard, 1965, 1966). Term-size fetuses are believed to swallow relatively large volumes of amnionic fluid; in one study, the amount appeared to average nearly 450 mL per 24 hours. Gitlin and associates (1972) found that the rate of clearing of radiolabeled albumin from amnionic fluid, presumably by swallowing, was very similar to this value. It is likely, however, that the volumes of amnionic fluid swallowed directly by the fetus are less than what has been reported. Probably some of the label in the amnionic fluid was removed by inhalation; and the inspired

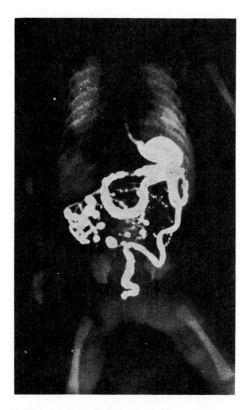

Figure 6–14. X-ray of 115 g fetus in which Thorotrast is present in the lungs, esophagus, stomach, and entire intestinal tract following injection of Thorotrast into the amnionic cavity 26 hours before delivery. This demonstrates not only intrauterine respiration of the fetus but also active swallowing of amnionic fluid. (*From Davis and Potter: JAMA 131:1194, 1946.*)

radiolabeled material, in turn, was either absorbed across the lung or was propelled from the lung by ciliary movement into the pharynx from which it was swallowed.

Fetal swallowing appears to have little effect on the amnionic fluid volume early in pregnancy because the volume swallowed is small compared with the total volume of amnionic fluid present. Late in pregnancy, however, the volume of amnionic fluid appears to be regulated substantially by fetal swallowing, for when swallowing is inhibited, hydramnios is common (see Chap. 31, p. 555).

The act of swallowing may enhance growth and development of the alimentary canal and condition the fetus for alimentation after birth, although anencephalic fetuses, which usually swallow little amnionic fluid, have gastrointestinal tracts that appear normal. In late pregnancy, swallowing serves to remove some of the insoluble debris that is normally shed into the amnionic sac and sometimes abnormally excreted into it. The undigested portions of the swallowed debris can be identified in meconium collected at birth. The amnionic fluid swallowed probably contributes little to the caloric requirements of the fetus but may contribute essential nutrients. Gitlin (1974) demonstrated that late in pregnancy about 0.8 g of soluble protein, approximately one-half albumin, appears to be ingested by the fetus each day.

Meconium

Meconium consists not only of undigested debris from swallowed amnionic fluid, but to a larger degree, of various products of secretion, excretion, and desquamation by the gastrointestinal tract. The dark greenish-black appearance is caused by pigments, especially biliverdin. Hypoxia has been implicated in the evacuation of meconium from the large bowel into the amnionic fluid. This mechanism may result from the release of arginine vasopressin (AVP) from the fetal pituitary secondary to hypoxia. The AVP thus released stimulates the smooth muscle of the colon to contract resulting in intraamnionic defecation (DeVane and co-workers, 1982; Rosenfeld and Porter, 1985).

Small-bowel obstruction may lead to vomiting in utero (Shrand, 1972). Fetuses who suffer from congenital chloride diarrhea may have diarrhea in utero, which leads to hydramnios and preterm delivery (Holmberg and associates, 1977).

LIVER AND PANCREAS

Liver

Hepatic function in the fetus differs, in several ways, from that of the adult. Many enzymes of the fetal liver are present in considerably reduced amounts compared with those in later life. The liver has a very limited capacity for converting free *bilirubin* to bilirubin diglucuronoside (see Chap. 33, p. 608). The more immature the fetus, the more deficient is the system for conjugating bilirubin.

Because the life span of the fetal erythrocyte is shorter than is that of normal adult erythrocytes, relatively more bilirubin is produced. Only a small fraction of the bilirubin is conjugated by the fetal liver and excreted through the biliary tract into the intestine and ultimately oxidized to biliverdin. Bashore and associates (1969) demonstrated that radiolabeled unconjugated bilirubin is cleared promptly from the monkey fetal circulation by the placenta to the maternal liver where it is conjugated and excreted through maternal bile. The transfer of the unconjugated bilirubin across the placenta, however, is bidirectional.

This observation is supported by the rarely encountered case of high levels of unconjugated bilirubin in maternal plasma. Conjugated bilirubin is not exchanged to any significant degree between mother and fetus.

Most of the cholesterol in the fetus is produced in fetal liver. Indeed, the large demand for LDL-cholesterol by the fetal adrenal is met primarily by fetal hepatic synthesis.

Glycogen appears in low concentration in fetal liver during the second trimester of pregnancy, but near term there is a rapid and marked increase in normal fetuses to levels 2 to 3 times those in adult liver. After delivery, the glycogen content falls precipitously.

Pancreas

It is interesting to remember that the discovery of insulin by Banting and Best (1922) came from its extraction from the pancreas of the fetal calf. Insulin-containing granules can be identified in the human fetal pancreas by 9 to 10 weeks gestation, and insulin in fetal plasma is detectable at 12 weeks (Adam and associates, 1969). The fetal pancreas responds to hyperglycemia by increasing plasma insulin (Obsenshain and colleagues, 1970). Although the precise role of insulin of fetal origin is not clear, fetal growth must be determined to a considerable extent by the amounts of basic nutrients from the mother and, through the action of insulin, the anabolism of these materials by the fetus. Insulin levels are high in serum from newborn infants of diabetic mothers and in other large-for-gestational-age infants, but insulin levels are low in infants who are small for gestational age (Brinsmead and Liggins, 1979).

Glucagon has been identified in the fetal pancreas at 8 weeks gestation. Induced hypoglycemia and infused alanine cause an increase in glucagon levels in the rhesus mother, yet similar stimuli to the fetus do not. Within 12 hours of birth, however, the infant is capable of responding (Chez and co-workers, 1975). Moreover, fetal alpha cells of the pancreas are capable of responding to L-dopa (Epstein and associates, 1977). Therefore, alpha cell nonresponsiveness to hypoglycemia and infused alanine likely is the consequence of failure of glucagon release rather than inadequate production of the hormone.

The exocrine function of the fetal pancreas appears to be limited but not necessarily absent. For example, radioiodine-labeled human albumin injected into the amnionic sac and swallowed by the fetus is absorbed from the fetal intestine. It is not absorbed as undigested protein, however, because the iodine is excreted promptly in the maternal urine when pretreatment with iodide has been provided to enhance the clearance of the digested radiolabeled iodine (Pritchard, 1965).

URINARY SYSTEM

Two primitive urinary systems, the pronephros and the mesonephros, precede the development of the metanephros. Embryological failure of either of the first two may result in anomalous development of the definitive urinary system.

By the end of the first trimester, the nephrons have some capacity for excretion through glomerular filtration, although the kidneys are functionally immature throughout fetal life. The ability to concentrate and modify the pH of urine is quite limited even in the mature fetus. Fetal urine is hypotonic with respect to fetal plasma because of low concentrations of electrolytes. In the lamb fetus, and most likely in the human fetus, the fraction of the cardiac output perfusing the kidneys is low and renal vascular resistance is high, compared with these values later in life (Assali and colleagues, 1968a; Rudolph and Heymann, 1968). In the lamb fetus, urine flow varies considerably in response to stress. Transient marked fetal polyuria postoperatively that dissipates apparently with recovery of fetal well-being has been noted by Gresham and co-workers (1972).

Urine is usually found in the bladder even in small fetuses. Wladimiroff and Campbell (1974) estimated urine production for human fetuses using an ultrasonic method to determine bladder volumes. They found a mean production of 10 mL per hour at 30 weeks, with an increase at term to 27 mL, or 650 mL per day. Maternally administered diuretic (furosemide) increases fetal urine formation. Kurjak and associates (1981) confirmed the findings of Wladimiroff and Campbell and measured fetal glomerular filtration rates and fetal tubular water reabsorption. All three measurements were decreased in 33 percent of growth-retarded infants and in 17 percent of infants of diabetic mothers. All values were normal in anencephalic infants and in cases of polyhydramnios.

After obstruction of the urethra, the bladder, ureters, and renal pelves may become quite dilated; the bladder may become sufficiently distended that dystocia results. The kidneys in these circumstances seem capable of excreting urine until back pressure ultimately destroys the renal parenchyma. Kidneys are not essential for survival in utero, but are important in the control of the composition and volume of amnionic fluid (see Chap. 31, p. 555). Abnormalities that cause chronic anuria most often are accompanied by oligohydramnios and hypoplasia of the lungs.

AMNIONIC FLUID

The fluid filling the amnionic sac serves several important functions. It provides a medium in which the fetus can readily move, cushions the fetus against possible injury, helps maintain an even temperature, and provides, when appropriately tested, useful information concerning the health and maturity of the fetus (see Chap. 15). If the presenting part of the fetus is not closely applied to the lower uterine segment during labor, the hydrostatic action of the amnionic fluid also may be important in dilating the cervix.

By the 12th day after fertilization of the ovum, a cleft enclosed by primitive amnion has formed adjacent to the embryonic plate. Rapid enlargment of the cleft and fusion of the surrounding amnion first with the body stalk, and later with the chorion, create the amnionic sac, which fills with an essentially colorless fluid. The amnionic fluid increases rapidly to an average volume of 50 mL at 12 weeks gestation and 400 mL at midpregnancy; it reaches a maximum of about 1,000 mL at 36 to 38 weeks gestation. The volume then decreases as term approaches, and if the pregnancy is prolonged, amnionic fluid may become relatively scant (see Chap. 38, p. 557). There are rather marked individual differences in amnionic fluid volume, however, as reported by Fuchs (1966). Similar data reported by Gillibrand (1969) is shown in Figure 6–15. The physician performing amniocentesis for diagnostic purposes soon appreciates the considerable variability in the volume of amnionic fluid present at the same time in different pregnancies as well as at different times in the same pregnancy.

The composition and volume of amnionic fluid change as pregnancy advances. In the first half of pregnancy, the fluid is the same as the extracellular fluid of the fetus, and it is nearly devoid of particulate matter.

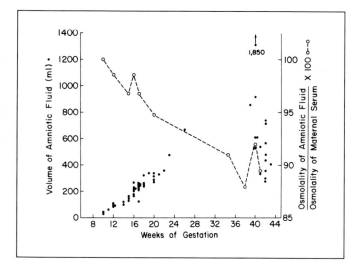

Figure 6–15. Amnionic fluid volume (black dots) and osmolality (open circles). The first and second trimesters are characterized by a rather orderly increase in volume, but at term the volume is quite variable. The osmolality decreases in approximately linear fashion as pregnancy advances. (*From Gillibrand: Br J Obstet Gynaecol 76:893, 1969.*)

Ions and small molecules move rapidly into and out of amnionic fluid but at rates that are specific for each substance. In contradistinction to bulk movement of amnionic fluid, as with swallowing, this process involves simply molecular or ionic trade across a membrane without necessarily inducing changes in volume or concentration (Plentl, 1968).

There is no single mechanism that will account for all the variations in composition and volume of amnionic fluid that have been observed during the course of a normal pregnancy. One relatively simple explanation is that amnionic fluid in early pregnancy is a product primarily of the amnionic membrane covering the placenta and cord. It is likely that fluid also passes across the fetal skin at this time (Lind and colleagues, 1972). As pregnancy advances, the surface of the amnion expands and the volume of fluid increases, but from about the 4th month, the fetus is capable of modifying amnionic fluid composition and volume by urinating and swallowing progressively larger amounts of fluid. At the same time, movement of fluid into and out of the respiratory tract is likely to modify further the volume and composition of amnionic fluid.

As gestation advances, fetal urine makes an increasingly important contribution to the amnionic fluid. Fetal urine is quite hypotonic compared with maternal or fetal plasma, because of the lower electrolyte concentration in the urine, but it contains more urea, creatinine, and uric acid than does plasma. The net effect is that the osmolality of fluid decreases with increasing length of gestation. These observations have been shown to exist in utero as early as the 24th week of pregnancy. Mandelbaum and Evans (1969) examined urine obtained inadvertently from the fetal bladder at the time of attempted transfusion and compared the concentrations of several of the constituents of the urine with those of amnionic fluid. Even at 24 weeks gestation, the urea and creatinine concentrations were 2 to 3 times higher in the urine, whereas the concentrations of sodium, potassium, and chloride were only about one-third to one-fifth as great as those in the amnionic fluid. The admixture of sizable volumes of fetal urine with the amnionic fluid, therefore, would

logically be expected to lower the osmolality, as shown in Figure 6–15, and, at the same time, raise the concentration of urea, creatinine, and uric acid. Indeed, late in pregnancy, amnionic fluid normally differs from plasma in precisely these ways.

As pregnancy progresses, glycerophospholipids, primarily from the lung, accumulate in the fluid (p. 107) and variable amounts of particulate matter in the form of desquamated fetal cells, lanugo and scalp hair, and vernix caseosa are shed into the fluid. The concentrations of various solutes also change significantly and, as a consequence, the osmolality decreases on the average about 20 to 30 mOsm, or about 10 percent, as shown in Figure 6–15.

The fetus swallows amnionic fluid during much of pregnancy. Often, but not always, a great excess of amnionic fluid (hydramnios) develops whenever fetal swallowing is greatly impaired (see Chap. 31, p. 555). A classic example of a lesion in which fetal swallowing cannot take place and thereby leads to hydramnios is fetal esophageal atresia. Conversely, when urination in utero cannot take place, as in instances of renal agnesis or atresia of the urethra, the volume of amnionic fluid surrounding the fetus typically is extremely limited (oligohydramnios).

Although lack of fetal swallowing with continuous production of normal amounts of fluid by the amnion and by the fetal kidneys may lead to hydramnios, this mechanism is certainly not the sole cause of hydramnios. Progressive hydramnios has been observed in instances in which a normal fetus was known to ingest relatively large amounts of amnionic fluid, and in which maternal diseases known to predispose to hydramnios, such as diabetes, were not identified (Pritchard, 1966). Presumably, in these instances, increased production by the amnion or, unlikely, intense fetal polyuria, or even both, cause the increase in amnionic fluid volume. Whether the respiratory tract is involved at times in the development of hydramnios is not clear. What is clear, however, is that if the volume of amnionic fluid is reduced to abnormal levels, as may occur in anephric fetuses or in instances of early and prolonged rupture of the fetal membranes, fetal pulmonary hypoplasia may result to such a severe degree that extrauterine life is impossible (Fliegner and co-workers, 1981; Wigglesworth and Desai, 1982).

RESPIRATORY SYSTEM

FETAL LUNG

The timetable of lung maturation and the identification of biochemical indices of lung functional maturity in the fetus are of considerable importance and concern to the obstetrician. This obtains because functional immaturity of the lung at birth leads to the development of the respiratory distress syndrome.

RESPIRATORY DISTRESS SYNDROME: IMMATURE LUNGS OF THE NEWBORN

History

Kiedel and Gluck (1975), as well as Farrell and Avery (1975), have recounted succinctly the history of the clinical identification of the respiratory distress syndrome. The signs and symptoms of this disorder were described first in 1903 by Hocheim, who observed a nebulous lining in the lungs of two infants who died shortly after birth. His observation led to the use of the descriptive phrase *hyaline membrane disease,* which is used to describe the pathological features of the respiratory distress

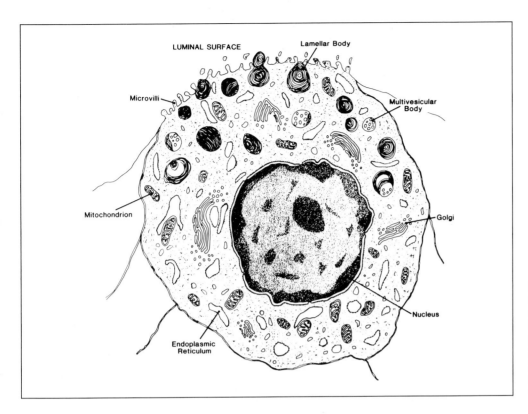

Figure 6–16. Type II pneumonocyte. There are prominent microvilli on the apical surface identifiable. Many multivesicular bodies, the precursor of lamellar bodies, and many lamellar bodies (rich in surfactant) that are migrating toward the luminal surface prior to extrusion into the alveolar space are illustrated.

syndrome. In 1929, von Neergard compared the pressure-volume curves of lungs distended with air with those of lungs distended with a gum arabic solution; and from the results of these studies, he concluded that the forces that promote deflation or collapse of the air-containing lung are those that result principally from surface tension at the air-tissue interface of the alveolus. Clements (1957) found that a surface tension-lowering material was present in saline extracts of lung lavage material. Subsequently, it was demonstrated that the surface-active properties of the alveoli are attributable to the components of a complex lipoprotein, viz., *surfactant*.

Surfactant

Klaus and associates (1961) determined that the principal surface-active component of surfactant was attributable to a specific *lecithin*, i.e., *dipalmitoylphosphatidylcholine*, a unique phosphatidylcholine moiety in which palmitate is present in both the *sn*-1 and *sn*-2 positions of this glycerophospholipid. This is a peculiar species of phosphatidylcholine; this is true because it is rare to find a saturated fatty acid in both the *sn*-1 and -2 positions of a glycerophospholipid. Ordinarily there is a saturated fatty acid in the *sn*-1 position but a polyunsaturated fatty acid in the *sn*-2 position.

Avery and Mead (1959) were the first to point out that the respiratory distress syndrome is caused by a deficiency in surfactant biosynthesis in fetal and neonatal lung. Subsequently, several investigators have shown that augmented surfactant synthesis normally appears in fetal lungs according to a developmental timetable; and, it is known that of the 40 cell types of the lung, surfactant is formed specifically in the type II pneumonocytes that line the alveoli (Fig. 6–16). The type II cells are characterized by multivesicular bodies (Fig. 6–16), the cellular progenitors of the lamellar bodies (Figs. 6–17 and 6–18) in which surfactant is assembled. Ultimately, the lamellar bodies are se-

creted from the lung. During late fetal life, at a time when the alveolus is characterized by a water-to-tissue interface, the intact lamellar bodies are swept into the amnionic fluid during fetal respiratory-like movements, i.e., fetal breathing.

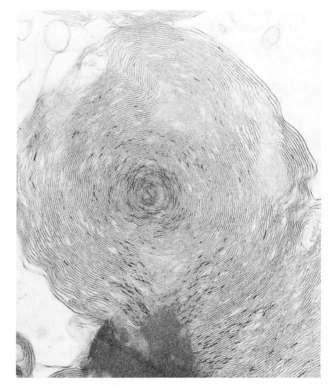

Figure 6–17. Transmission electron micrograph of fused human fetal lung lamellar bodies. (*Courtesy of Dr. J. Snyder and Dr. J. M. Johnston.*)

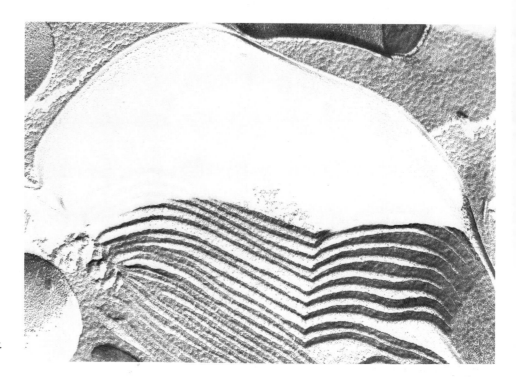

Figure 6–18. Freeze-fracture scanning electron micrograph of a lamellar body. (*Courtesy of Dr. R. C. Reynolds and Dr. J. M. Johnston.*)

This is a particularly important feature of human pregnancy because the appearance of surfactant in amnionic fluid heralds the commencement of functional maturation of the fetal lungs. In other species, lung secretions do not necessarily enter amnionic fluid; for example, in the sheep fetus, the lung secretions are swallowed. After birth, with the first breath, an air-to-tissue interface is produced in the lung alveolus of the newborn. This permits the "uncoiling" of surfactant from the lamellar bodies and this surface tension-lowering material then spreads to line the alveolus and thereby prevent alveolar collapse during expiration. Therefore, it is the capacity for fetal lungs to produce surfactant and not the actual laying down of this material in utero that characterizes lung maturity before birth.

Surfactant Composition

The recognition of the important role of surfactant in the prevention of respiratory distress syndrome prompted many investigators to study the composition of this lipoprotein (Fig. 6–19). About 90 percent of surfactant (dry weight) is lipid; and, approximately 80 percent of the glycerophospholipids are comprised of phosphatidylcholines (lecithins); but, importantly, a single phosphatidylcholine, namely, *dipalmitoylphosphatidylcholine* (*disaturated phosphatidylcholine* or *disaturated lecithin*), accounts for nearly 50 percent of the glycerophospholipids of surfactant. There also is an unusually high content of *phosphatidylglycerol* in surfactant, viz., 9 to 15 percent, an amount that is much greater than that found in any other mammalian tissue (Keidel and Gluck, 1975).

Phosphatidylglycerol is the second most surface-active component of surfactant; but more importantly, phosphatidylglycerol appears to confer a certain unique feature to the surfactant moiety, a surface-active property that is over and above that which can be attributed to its surface tension-lowering properties alone. This as yet ill-defined action of phosphatidylglycerol is believed to be important in the prevention of the respiratory distress syndrome because infants born before the

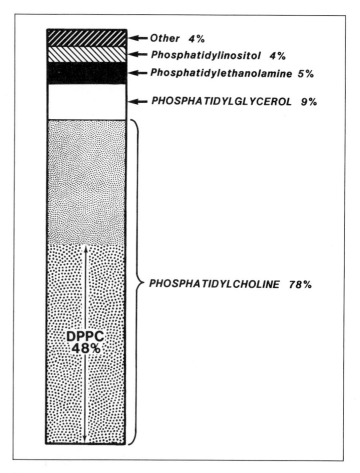

Other 4%
Phosphatidylinositol 4%
Phosphatidylethanolamine 5%
PHOSPHATIDYLGLYCEROL 9%
PHOSPHATIDYLCHOLINE 78%
DPPC 48%

Figure 6–19. Glycerophospholipid composition of "mature" surfactant. Surfactant is especially enriched in lecithin (phosphatidylcholine) and, in particular, the surface-active dipalmitoylphosphatidylcholine (DPPC, 48 percent). The phosphatidylglycerol content of surfactant (8 to 15 percent) is also very high.

appearance of phosphatidylglycerol in surfactant are at increased risk of development of the respiratory distress syndrome even in those newborns in whom the dipalmitoylphosphatidylcholine content of the surfactant is normal for mature lungs.

Regulation of Surfactant Synthesis

In an elegant series of studies, Gluck and associates (1967, 1970, 1971, 1972, 1974) demonstrated that an increasing concentration of dipalmitoylphosphatidylcholine (lecithin) in amnionic fluid, relative to that of sphingomyelin (the lecithin to sphingomyelin, or L/S, ratio), constitutes a marker of fetal lung maturation. These studies were successful because of the ingenious idea of determining the concentration of sphingomyelin as a reference for glycerophospholipid synthesis by the lung in general, whereas the measurement of acetone-precipitable dipalmitoylphosphatidylcholine (disaturated lecithin) is a specific index of surfactant synthesis in type II pneumonocytes. Hallman and co-workers (1976) later demonstrated that the identification of phosphatidylglycerol in amnionic fluid also is an indicator of lung maturation.

From these many and complementary observations, it became apparent that augmented synthesis of surfactant, and specifically that which is enriched with dipalmitoylphosphatidylcholine and phosphatidylglycerol, is essential for the successful preparation of the fetal lung for the transition from a water-alveolar interface to an air-alveolar interface, events that must take place if alveolar collapse on expiration after birth is to be prevented. Thus, the regulation of the rate of synthesis of dipalmitoylphosphatidylcholine and phosphatidylglycerol in fetal lung is of signal importance. The biosynthetic pathways involved in the formation of the glycerophospholipids of surfactant are illustrated in Figures 6–20 through 6–22.

In the past few years, we also have come to appreciate and understand the nature of and the regulation of synthesis of the apoproteins of surfactant. The protein moiety is essential not

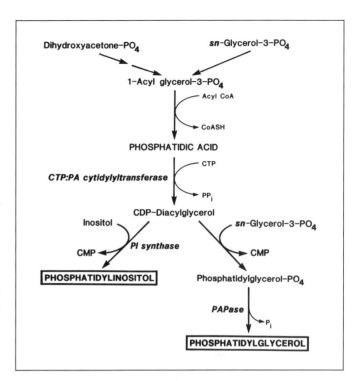

Figure 6–21. Biosynthetic pathway for the synthesis of phosphatidyl-inositol and phosphatidylglycerol in type II pneumonocytes. CTP:PA = cytidine triphosphage: phosphatidic acid. For other abbreviations, see Figure 6–20.

only to the synthesis of surfactant but also to the function and recycling of the lipoprotein in the alveolus of the lung.

Regulation of Surfactant Formation: Glycerophospholipids

Surfactant biosynthesis is confined to the type II cells of the lung. The apoproteins are produced in the endoplasmic reticulum. The surface-active components of surfactant, i.e., the glycerophospholipids, are synthesized by way of cooperative interactions of several cellular organelles. Common reactions are involved in the initial steps in the biosynthesis of phosphatidylcholine and phosphatidylglycerol. The glycerol backbone for phosphatidylcholine, phosphatidylinositol, and phosphatidylglycerol synthesis (phosphatidic acid) is provided by dihydroxyacetone phosphate from one or two reaction sequences (Figs. 6–20 and 6–21). It is unlikely that glycerol from blood is used in the formation of glycerol-3-phosphate in fetal lung (for review: Odom and colleagues, 1986). It is most likely that plasma glucose also is not involved primarily in glycerol synthesis in the type II cells; rather, the ultimate precursor more likely is glycogen, which is stored in these cells prior to the time of accelerated surfactant synthesis. Glycerol-3-phosphate is acylated in a stepwise fashion in a process that gives rise to phosphatidic acid in which there are two of a variety of fatty acids. Phosphatidic acid is the precursor of all the glycerophospholipids of surfactant. The acyl donor to the glycerol backbone is fatty acid–coenzyme A (CoA). Generally, there is a saturated fatty acid in the sn-1 position and an unsaturated fatty acid in the sn-2 position of phosphatidic acid. In lung tissue, however, there is considerable capacity for the de novo synthesis of palmitic acid and thus a greater likelihood of finding palmitate in the sn-2 position of

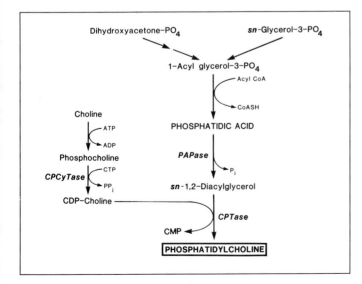

Figure 6–20. Biosynthetic pathway for phosphatidylcholine (lecithin) synthesis in type II pneumonocytes. PAPase = phosphatidate phosphohydrolase; CPTase = choline phosphotransferase; CPCyTase = choline phosphate cytidylyltransferase; CDP = choline diphosphate; CMP = cytidine monophosphate.

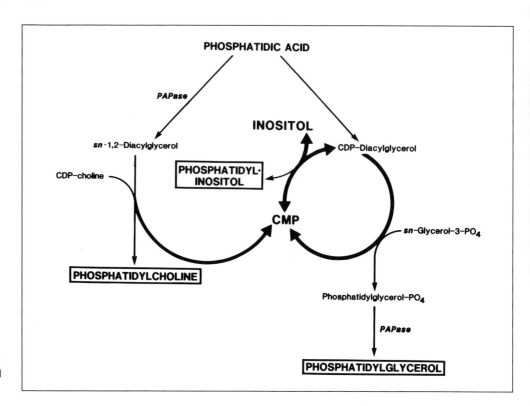

Figure 6–22. The proposed CMP cycle for the regulation of the relative rates of synthesis of phosphatidylcholine, phosphatidylinositol, and phosphatidylglycerol.

glycerolipids in lung tissue compared with that in other tissues. In the biosynthesis of phosphatidic acid by lung tissue, however, there is no evidence for preferential incorporation of palmitoyl-CoA in the *sn*-2 position.

It is important to emphasize that phosphatidic acid is a substrate common to the formation of the two principal surface-active glycerophospholipids, i.e., dipalmitoylphosphatidylcholine and phosphatidylglycerol (Figs. 6–20 through 6–22). Thus, the metabolism of phosphatidic acid constitutes a critical branch point in the regulation of the biosynthesis of the principal surface-active glycerophospholipids of surfactant.

Regulation of Surfactant Formation: Lecithin (Dipalmitoylphosphatidylcholine)

Dipalmitoylphosphatidylcholine, or lecithin, is the major glycerophospholipid of surfactant. In the synthesis of lecithin, phosphatidic acid is hydrolyzed, through the action of the enzyme phosphatidate phosphohydrolase (PAPase), to give *sn*-1,2-diacylglycerols (Fig. 6–20). The *sn*-1,2-diacylglycerols serve as co-substrate with cytidine diphosphate (CDP)-choline in the formation of phosphatidylcholines. This latter reaction is catalyzed by the enzyme choline phosphotransferase (CPTase). The co-substrate, CDP-choline, is formed in a sequence of reactions; through the action of choline kinase, phosphorylcholine is formed. Phosphorylcholine, in turn, is converted to CDP-choline in a reaction that is catalyzed by cytidine triphosphate (CTP)-phosphocholine cytidylyltransferase ([CTP-CyT] Fig. 6–20). In the resultant phosphatidylcholines, there may be a saturated fatty acid, commonly palmitic acid, in the *sn*-1 position, whereas an unsaturated fatty acid may be present in the *sn*-2 position.

Obviously, some molecular rearrangement of such phosphatidylcholines must occur to produce dipalmitoylphosphatidylcholine, the surface-active lecithin. Two separate mech-

anisms have been proposed to account for the enrichment of phosphatidylcholines with palmitic acid in the *sn*-2 position. In both mechanisms, the action of the enzyme phospholipase A$_2$ is required. The action of phospholipase A$_2$ results in the deacylation of glycerophospholipids at the *sn*-2 position. One product of this reaction is *sn*-1-palmitoyllysophosphatidylcholine. This lysophosphatidylcholine product may be acylated with palmitoyl-CoA through the action of acyltransferase, resulting in the product dipalmitoylphosphatidylcholine (Lands, 1958). It is interesting that this pathway was demonstrated first in lung tissue. Alternatively, the remodeling of phosphatidylcholine can come about as the result of the transfer of the acyl moiety from the *sn*-1 position of an *sn*-1-palmitoyllysophosphatidylcholine to the *sn*-2 position of a second *sn*-1-palmitoyllysophosphatidylcholine. Dipalmitoylphosphatidylcholine also can be formed by way of this pathway. This latter mechanism for remodeling phosphatidylcholine was demonstrated originally in liver tissue (Marinetti and colleagues, 1958), but it also has been demonstrated in lung tissue (Van den Bosch and associates, 1965).

Regulation of Surfactant Formation: Phosphatidylglycerol

The regulation of phosphatidylglycerol synthesis is especially important because Hallman and co-workers (1976) have shown that increased concentrations of phosphatidylglycerol, together with decreased concentrations of phosphatidylinositol, in surfactant also herald lung maturation. Some infants who are born of diabetic mothers develop the respiratory distress syndrome despite high concentrations of dipalmitoylphosphatidylcholine in their amnionic fluid. The surfactant in lung and amnionic fluid of affected fetuses and neonates is characterized by low levels of phosphatidylglycerol and high levels of phosphatidylinositol. Furthermore, it has been shown that phosphatidylglycerol also acts to increase the activity of the lung tissue enzyme CTP:phosphocholine cytidylyltransferase, an enzyme necessary for phosphatidylcholine biosynthesis. Thus, an understanding of the regulation of formation of phosphatidylglycerol becomes of crucial importance in a consideration of the final biochemical events in fetal lung maturation.

At presently, the regulation of phosphatidylinositol and phosphatidylglycerol biosynthesis is incompletely understood. It seems likely that the decrease in concentration of phosphatidylinositol that is associated with a concomitant increase in phosphatidylglycerol in surfactant with lung maturation is brought about by a change in the flux of CDP-diacylglycerol through the pathways involved in the synthesis of these acidic glycerophospholipids (Bleasdale and colleagues, 1979 [Figs. 6–21 and 6–22]). In any event, it is known that with fetal lung maturation there is first a "surge" in phosphatidylcholine synthesis that is followed, in time, by an increase in phosphatidylglycerol together with a concomitant decrease in phosphatidylinositol in surfactant (Fig. 6–23).

From an evaluation of the metabolic pathways involved in the biosynthesis of phosphatidylglycerol and phosphatidylinositol, it was difficult to envision a mechanism that could account for (1) the increase in phosphatidylcholine synthesis for surfactant formation with lung maturation, which thereafter is followed in time by (2) an increase in phosphatidylglycerol content, and (3) a concomitant decrease in phosphatidylinositol concentration in surfactant. The difficulty in resolving the mechanisms involved was related to the proposition that each of these glycerophospholipids is derived ultimately from a common precursor, viz., phosphatidic acid; but more than that, phosphatidylinositol and phosphatidylglycerol both are derived from a common precursor that is a product of phosphatidic acid, namely CDP-diacylglycerol. How, then, can there be a reciprocal relationship between the rates of formation of phosphatidylglycerol and phosphatidylinositol when both are biosynthesized from common precursors?

Batenburg and co-workers (1982) reviewed the three mechanisms by which the switchover from phosphatidylinositol to phosphatidylglycerol synthesis for surfactant could come about:

1. An increase in enzymatic activity for glycerolphosphate phosphatidyltransferase;
2. A decrease in fetal plasma inositol; and
3. Increased levels of cytidine monophosphate (CMP), resulting from increased phosphatidylcholine (lecithin) synthesis.

Based on findings of studies conducted in isolated type II cells of the adult rat lung, Batenburg and co-workers concluded that mechanism 2 was most important. Bleasdale and associates presented convincing evidence in favor of mechanism 3. There is little support for mechanism 1. Possibly the solution is to be found through a combination of mechanisms 2 and 3.

Elegant studies were conducted by Johnston, Bleasdale, and associates (Bleasdale and associates, 1979; Bleasdale and Johnston, 1982; Quirk and co-workers, 1980) that are relevant to this issue. First, they demonstrated that the phosphatidylinositol synthetase reaction is *reversible* (Figs. 6–21 and 6–22). Heretofore, this was not generally believed to be physiologically important. Nonetheless, the reaction that catalyzes the conversion of CDP-diacylglycerol and *myo*-inositol to phosphatidylinositol and CMP (cytidine monophosphate) is reversible in the presence of CMP in optimum concentrations; the latter issue is of great importance when the temporal relationships that exist between increased phosphatidylcholine formation and the subsequent decline in phosphatidylinositol synthesis in favor of phosphatidylglycerol in the formation of "mature" surfactant are considered. For the moment, suffice it to say that the reversibility of the reaction(s) catalyzed by phosphatidylinositol synthetase is such as to permit the possibility of a flux of the common precursor, CDP-diacylglycerol, to phosphatidylglycerol at the expense of phosphatidylinositol.

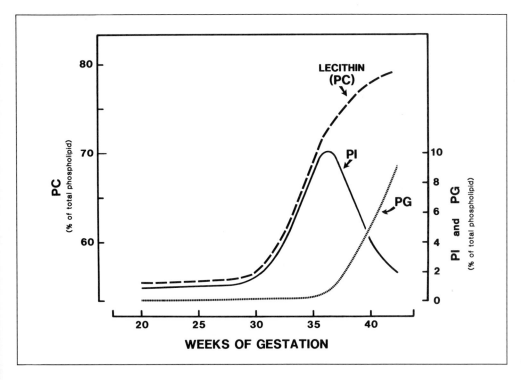

Figure 6–23. Relation between the levels of lecithin (dipalmitoylphosphatidylcholine [PC]), phosphatidylinositol (PI), and phosphatidylglycerol (PG) in amnionic fluid as a function of gestational age.

The first indication of maturation of the fetal lung with respect to accelerated surfactant formation is the increased synthesis and secretion of dipalmitoylphosphatidylcholine. At this time, phosphatidylinositol levels in surfactant are high and those of phosphatidylglycerol are low (Fig. 6–23). And, it is only later in maturation, after a considerable increase in the rate of lecithin synthesis, that there occurs, simultaneously, an increase in phosphatidylglycerol and a decrease in phosphatidylinositol in surfactant. These several observations (together with the demonstration of the reversibility of the reaction catalyzed by phosphatidylinositol synthetase) led to the concept of a CMP cycle, a concept first fostered by Johnston, Bleasdale, and colleagues (Bleasdale and Johnston, 1984).

The first evidence of accelerated surfactant synthesis, i.e., increased synthesis of dipalmitoylphosphatidylcholine may come about as a consequence of a maturational increase in PAPase activity and a resultant increase in diacylglycerol synthesis en route to the formation of phosphatidylcholine. As a by-product of this reaction, there is an increase in the rate of formation of CMP (Fig. 6–20).

Based on the proposition that CMP is a co-substrate for the reverse reaction that is catalyzed by phosphatidylinositol synthetase, i.e., PI + CMP $\leftrightarrows$ CDP-diacylglycerol + *myo*-inositol, it seemed reasonable that accelerated phosphatidylcholine synthesis would promote the flux of phosphatidylinositol through CDP-diacylglycerol and thence to phosphatidylglycerol phosphate and on to phosphatidylglycerol. The latter reaction should not be rate limiting because, as stated, some form of PAPase catalyzes the hydrolysis of phosphatidylglycerophosphate to phosphatidylglycerol; and for practical purposes, the hydrolysis of phosphatidylglycerol phosphate is irreversible.

Let us then take inventory of the role of CMP in these reactions. (1) Increased phosphatidylcholine biosynthesis gives rise to increased CMP. (2) The forward reaction of the phosphatidylinositol synthetase enzyme gives rise to CMP. (3) In the formation of phosphatidylglycerol phosphate from CDP-diacylglycerol, CMP is a product. Thus, a CMP cycle is established with respect to the relative rates of formation of the glycerophospholipids of surfactant (Fig. 6–22). It has been suggested that the activation of this CMP cycle is initiated first by way of an increase in phosphatidylcholine formation. In consequence, CMP levels rise, phosphatidylinositol conversion to CDP-diacylglycerol is favored and the resultant CDP-diacylglycerol can be rerouted toward phosphatidylglycerol. In consequence, the concentration of phosphatidylcholine in surfactant rises first, and thereafter, the levels of phosphatidylinositol decrease and at the same time there is an increase in the concentration of phosphatidylglycerol—features characteristic of "mature" surfactant.

To complement this CMP cycle–mediated set of events, the lowering of *myo*-inositol in fetal plasma as gestation advances would serve to promote phosphatidylglycerol synthesis at the expense of phosphatidylinositol.

In this regard, it is known that early in gestation, the concentration of *myo*-inositol in fetal plasma is much greater than that in maternal plasma. As pregnancy progresses, however, the concentration of *myo*-inositol in fetal plasma declines. This is believed to be an important maturational event because only a limited amount of lung tissue *myo*-inositol arises by de novo synthesis; the remainder is obtained by lung tissue in an energy-dependent uptake of *myo*-inositol from blood (Quirk and Bleasdale, 1983). It has been suggested, therefore, that the developmental decline in *myo*-inositol concentrations in blood

may favor a decrease in phosphatidylinositol synthesis in favor of phosphatidylglycerol by way of an alteration in flux of CDP-diacylglycerol.

Hyperinositolemia in the fetus of a woman with diabetes mellitus could lead to a delay in the developmental change in surfactant composition from one that is rich in phosphatidylinositol to one that is rich in phosphatidylglycerol. Recently, it also was shown that insulin acts on fetal lung tissue in vitro to inhibit the synthesis of the apoprotein, SAP-35 (Snyder and Mendelson, 1987).

REGULATION OF SURFACTANT FORMATION: APOPROTEINS

Surfactant is composed primarily of glycerophospholipids; but in the past 5 to 10 years, the functional importance of the unique apoproteins of surfactant have been investigated. The major apoprotein of surfactant is a glycoprotein (M_r about 35,000) referred to as SAP-35. The SAP-35 is synthesized in the type II cells, and increased synthesis is related temporally to increased surfactant formation in maturing fetal lungs. The amnionic fluid content of SAP-35 also increases as does the L/S ratio as a function of gestational age and fetal lung maturity. Synthesis of SAP-35 is known to be increased by treatment of fetal lung tissue with cyclic AMP (analogues) and by epidermal growth factor and triiodothyronine. On the other hand, glucocorticosteroids may inhibit apoprotein (SAP-35) synthesis (Whitsett and associates, 1987), and insulin definitely inhibits its synthesis (Snyder and Mendelson, 1987).

SAP-35 seems to be important in the structural transformation of the secreted lamellar body into tubular myelin within the lumen of the alveolus. SAP-35 also may be involved in the endocytosis and recycling of secreted surfactant by the type II cells. In addition to SAP-35, there are a number of smaller molecular weight proteins of surfactant (M_r about 5,000 to 18,000). These lower molecular weight surfactant proteins are believed to be important in optimizing the surface-active properties of surfactant. In addition, the surfactant apoproteins, after being taken back into the type II cells by receptor-mediated endocytosis, act to inhibit surfactant synthesis and secretion.

In studies of surfactant replacement therapy, natural surfactants that contain the surfactant proteins are more effective than are synthetic lipid mixtures. And surfactant therapy, using natural surfactants, is meritorious in preventing or treating respiratory distress syndrome in newborns (see Chap. 33, p. 594).

ALTERATIONS IN THE TIMETABLE OF "MATURE" SURFACTANT FORMATION

If this were a correct formulation of the means by which the relative amounts of glycerophospholipids and apoproteins in surfactant are regulated, it can be envisioned that certain physiological or pathophysiological events may cause a delay in the timetable of fetal lung maturation. By way of example, if the levels of plasma *myo*-inositol were elevated, phosphatidylinositol formation, at the expense of phosphatidylglycerol, would be favored (Fig. 6–22). This pattern of surfactant formation, i.e., one rich in phosphatidylcholine and phosphatidylinositol and deficient in phosphatidylglycerol is characteristic of that found in some newborn infants of diabetic mothers. Such infants are at greater risk of respiratory distress syndrome in spite of high levels of lecithin in amnionic fluid. Inositolemia and inositol intolerance are common in persons with diabetes mellitus. Quirk and Bleasdale (1984) and Odom and colleagues (1986) have presented an in-depth review of the maturation of the fetal lung in pregnancies complicated by maternal diabetes mellitus. At the same time, hyperinsulinemia of the fetus may serve to inhibit the synthesis of the apoprotein of surfactant.

HORMONAL REGULATION OF SURFACTANT FORMATION IN HUMAN FETAL LUNG

Although it is of signal importance to define the biochemical events involved in the synthesis and release of surfactant, it is equally important to define the mechanisms involved in the control of the synthesis and release (secretion) of surfactant. Many substances (generally hormones) have been proposed as potentially important modulators of these processes. Ballard (1986) has presented a comprehensive review of this subject. The interest of most investigators who have directed their attention to this question, however, has been centered on only a few agents. Of these, the most intensively investigated compounds are hormones, in particular, cortisol and other glucocorticosteroids.

Cortisol and Fetal Lung Maturation

The basis for suspecting that glucocorticosteroids promote lung maturation was provided first by Liggins (1969). In studies designed to induce preterm labor in the sheep (Chap. 10), he observed that there appeared to be accelerated lung maturation in prematurely delivered lambs that had been treated with glucocorticosteroids prior to birth. Since that time, many investigators have suggested that cortisol produced in the fetal adrenal is the natural stimulus for augmented surfactant synthesis.

Glucocorticosteroid receptors have been demonstrated in cytosolic and nuclear fractions prepared from fetal lung tissues (Ballard and Ballard, 1972; Giannopoulus, 1973). The administration of glucocorticosteroids to the rabbit and rat fetus causes an increase in the rate of incorporation of radiolabeled choline into phosphatidylcholine of lung (Barrett and colleagues, 1975; Farrell and Zachman, 1973; Russell and associates, 1974). The inclusion of glucocorticosteroids in the medium of human fetal lung tissue explants (Ekelund and co-workers, 1975) and mixed rabbit lung cells grown in tissue culture (Smith and Torday, 1974) caused increased incorporation of radiolabeled choline into phosphatidylcholine. The administration of glucocorticosteroids to rabbit fetuses causes an increase in the specific activity of lung CPTase (Farrell and Zachman, 1973), lipoprotein lipase (Hamosh and Hamosh, 1977), and PAPase (Brehier and co-workers, 1978).

On the other hand, Rooney and co-workers (1975) and Brehier and colleagues (1977), could not demonstrate an increase in the specific activity of CPTase or glycerophosphate phosphatidyltransferase after glucocorticosteroid administration in the rabbit.

There is appreciable evidence in support of the view that glucocorticosteroids, when administered in large amounts to the mother at certain critical times during gestation, effect an increase in the rate of maturation of the human fetal lung as indicated by a reduced incidence of respiratory distress syndrome in newborn infants of such glucocorticosteroid-treated mothers compared with that in those whose mothers were not so treated (Liggins and Howie, 1972).

The precise role of glucocorticosteroids in fetal lung maturation has not been fully defined, however; and from the evidence available, it cannot be concluded that cortisol is the single physiological regulator of the activities of enzymes involved in surfactant formation in most species, including man.

There is little doubt that the administration of glucocorticosteroids to pregnant women during the 29th to 33rd week of gestation is associated with a reduced incidence of respiratory distress in their prematurely born infants; but various conclusions have been reached regarding the mechanism(s) by which such treatment is effective. Some investigators have found that the lecithin (phosphatidylcholine)-to-sphingomyelin ratio in amnionic fluid increases after glucocorticosteroid treatment of the mother (Spellacy and colleagues, 1973; Zuspan and associates, 1977); yet, Liggins and Howie found no consistent increase. Some investigators have found a temporal relationship between the levels of cortisol in amnionic fluid and increasing lecithin-to-sphingomyelin ratios (Fencl and colleagues, 1975; Tan and co-workers, 1976); but we (Milewich and associates, 1978) and others (Sivakumaran and associates, 1975) have not found such a relationship. Murphy (1975) found a significant correlation between the level of cortisol in umbilical cord plasma and the lecithin-to-spingomyelin ratio in amnionic fluid; Sybulski and Manghan (1976) did not. Murphy found a relationship between the levels of cortisol in cord plasma and the subsequent development of respiratory distress syndrome in newborn infants; Hauth and associates (1978) did not.

It should be emphasized, however, that the failure to find a correlation between the levels of cortisol in umbilical cord plasma and in amnionic fluid with alterations in the L/S ratio in the amnionic fluid and with the subsequent development of respiratory distress syndrome should be viewed with caution. This obtains because it is likely that the metabolic clearance rate of plasma cortisol in the fetus increases as a function of the size of the fetus and its vascular volume. Thus, the levels of fetal plasma cortisol may remain relatively constant during the latter few weeks of gestation, at a time when the rate of cortisol secretion by the fetal adrenal may be rising appreciably. If this were the case, then static measurements of fetal plasma cortisol at one point in time, i.e., at the time of birth, would not be reflective of the rate of secretion of cortisol by the fetal adrenal cortex. At the same time, the level of cortisol in amnionic fluid may not necessarily be reflective of the rate of cortisol secretion by the fetal adrenal. This obtains because cortisone, arising in the maternal compartment, can be converted to cortisol by the human fetal membranes (Murphy, 1977). Moreover, alterations in the rate of excretion of cortisol sulfate by the developing fetal kidneys, together with increasing clearance of substances in amnionic fluid through increased fetal breathing movements and fetal swallowing as gestation advances, as well as transport from the amnionic fluid to the maternal compartment, are factors likely to give rise to significant alterations in the levels of cortisol in amnionic fluid that are independent of the rate of secretion of cortisol by the fetal adrenal cortex. Nonetheless, Johnson and colleagues (1978) found that the administration of glucocorticosteroids to pregnant subhuman primates was not associated with an increase in surfactant content in the fetal lungs. Rather, they found that the principal alteration in the fetal lungs of corticosteroid-treated pregnant monkeys was a decrease in the content of collagenous tissue.

Thus, in view of the failure to find a consistent relationship between glucocorticosteroid administration and an increase in activity of an enzyme involved in surfactant synthesis, the failure to find consistently a response in phosphatidylcholine formation (as indicated by an increased L/S ratio) after the administration of glucocorticosteroids to pregnant women, the failure to demonstrate consistently a temporal relationship between increased cortisol (as indicated by cortisol levels in amnionic fluid or in umbilical cord plasma) and increased surfactant formation, some investigators have concluded that cortisol may not be the single stimulus for augmented surfactant formation in the maturing human fetal lung (Hauth and co-workers, 1978). This conclusion is strengthened by the well-known clinical observation that the respiratory distress syndrome is not necessarily observed in many human neonates in whom the capacity to secrete cortisol is limited. Such infants include those with anencephaly, adrenal hypoplasia, and congenital adrenal hyperplasia. It may be that cortisol is one of several hormones that act cooperatively to effect fetal lung maturation. For example, cortisol is believed to stabilize the ribosomal-endoplasmic reticulum complex of mammary tissue such that this organ can respond to prolactin and insulin and thereby secrete milk (Oka and Topper, 1971).

Fibroblast Pneumocyte Factor

Smith (1978) observed that a factor produced in stromal cells of lung (fibroblast pneumocyte factor [FPF]) may serve as an intermediate modulator for type II cell maturation. Purified type II cells responded poorly to glucocorticosteroids; but in the presence of fibroblasts or partially purified FPF, the cells do respond. Post and co-workers (1984) demonstrated that antibodies raised against partially purified FPF inhibited cortisol-stimulated surfactant formation.

Prolactin and Fetal Lung Maturation

Winters and colleagues (1974) found that the levels of prolactin in fetal plasma increased strikingly during the last few weeks of human pregnancy. Hauth and co-workers (1978) found that the rise in fetal prolactin levels was temporally related to the increase in the L/S ratio in amnionic fluid (Fig. 6–24). They also suggested that a role for prolactin in fetal lung maturation can be envisioned by recalling that prolactin has a profound effect on the gills of fish, the phylogenetic homologue of lung (Lam, 1969) and that there are certain metabolic similarities between the maturing human lung and the prolactin-stimulated mammary gland. For example, these two tissues share a common

and almost unique lipid biosynthetic capability, i.e., an extraordinary capacity to incorporate palmitic acid into the sn-2 position of the glycerophospholipids of surfactant and into the sn-2 position of triacylglycerols of milk (Breckenridge and associates, 1969). Prolactin acts to increase the capacity of mammary tissue that is maintained in culture to synthesize fatty acids (Hollowes and colleagues, 1973) and other milk constituents such as casein and lactose (Turkington and co-workers, 1973). In type II cell tumors of the lung, and presumably nontumorous type II pneumonocytes, there is a large capacity to synthesize palmitic acid when compared with that of the other cells of the lung (Voelker and associates, 1976).

It has been shown that prolactin administration to fetal rabbits results in an increase in the phosphatidylcholine concentration of the fetal lung (Hamosh and Hamosh, 1977). (Interestingly, the action of prolactin in mammary tissue is dependent upon pretreatment of such tissue with glucocorticosteroids and insulin). On the other hand, it should be pointed out that Ballard and colleagues (1978) were unable to induce increased phosphatidylcholine content in the lung tissue of rabbit fetuses by prolactin treatment. Specifically, after the injection of prolactin into fetal rabbits, they did not find an increase in phosphatidylcholine concentration of similar magnitude to that found by Hamosh and Hamosh (1977). Moreover, Ballard and associates (1978) administered prolactin to sheep fetuses and again were unable to find an increase in the phosphatidylcholine content of the tracheal fluid of these fetuses. It should be noted, however, that the lecithin content of tracheal fluid in the sheep fetus does not rise during glucocorticosteroid treatment. It has been reported that the newborn infant of a woman treated with bromocriptine did not suffer from respiratory distress syndrome (Bigazzi and colleagues, 1979) even though such treatment caused low levels of prolactin in fetal blood. This finding is important, because the levels of prolactin in the mother and in the newborn infant of this bromocriptine-treated woman were quite low. On the other hand, the level of prolactin in amnionic fluid of this pregnancy was not reduced; amnionic fluid prolactin is believed to arise in decidua and is not subject to dopaminergic regulation (Chaps. 4 and 7). Johnson and associates (1979) have proposed that prolactin in amnionic fluid, inspired into the fetal alveoli during fetal thoracic movements, may serve an important role in the maturation of fetal lungs. Thus, as in the case of cortisol, one cannot conclude that prolactin, either of fetal pituitary or amnionic fluid origin, is the sole stimulant for the biochemical maturation of the fetal lung.

Nonetheless, it has been found that the concentration of prolactin in umbilical cord plasma and the incidence of respiratory distress syndrome are correlated inversely (Table 6–4). In the study conducted by Hauth and co-workers, it was found that in those infants in whom the prolactin concentration in cord plasma was equal to or greater than 200 ng per mL, respiratory distress occurred uncommonly, in no infants delivered from 29.5 to 33 weeks of gestation and 5 percent in infants delivered from 33.5 to 36 weeks of gestation. When the prolactin level in cord plasma was less than 200 ng per mL, respiratory distress occurred often, 80 percent in infants delivered from 29.5 to 33 weeks, and 28 percent in those delivered from 33.5 to 36 weeks. All infants delivered from 25 to 29 weeks of gestation had prolactin levels less than 200 ng per mL; and among these infants, the incidence of respiratory distress was 89 percent. Smith and co-workers (1978) also measured cord plasma prolactin levels in 58 newborns ranging from 27 weeks gestation to term. They found that the incidence of respiratory distress was

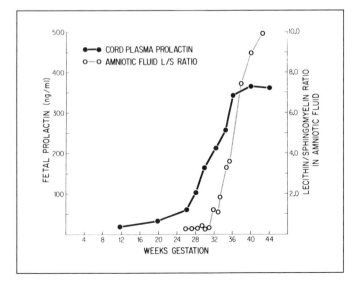

Figure 6–24. Temporal relationship between fetal plasma prolactin concentrations and the amnionic fluid L/S ratio. (*From Hauth and colleagues: Obstet Gynecol 51:81, 1978.*)

TABLE 6–4. THE INCIDENCE OF RESPIRATORY DISTRESS AND CORD PLASMA PROLACTIN LEVELS IN VARIOUS GESTATIONAL AGE GROUPS

| Gestational Age at Delivery (wk) | Newborn Cord Plasma Prolactin | | | | |
| | < 200 ng/mL | | ≥ 200 ng/mL | | |
	Incidence	%	Incidence	%	P[a]
≤ 26	4/4	100	0/0		—
26.5–29	12/14	86	0/0		—
29.5–33	20/26	80	0/10	0	<0.001
33.5–36	7/25	28	2/43	5	<0.01
≥ 36.5	1/20	5	2/50	4	0.64

[a]Computed from the exact probability test of Fisher.
From Hauth and associates: Obstet Gynecol 51:81, 1978.

markedly increased in those infants in whom the cord plasma prolactin levels were less than 140 ng per mL, as compared to those in whom the prolactin levels were greater than 140 ng per mL. Gluckman and associates (1978) also found that infants who develop respiratory distress had lower prolactin plasma concentrations at the time of birth than did those infants who did not develop respiratory distress. Similar findings were reported by Grosso and colleagues (1980).

It can be argued that augmented surfactant biosynthesis and increased prolactin secretion are independent milestones in fetal lung maturation. The presence of prolactin receptors in fetal lung tissue (Josimovich and co-workers, 1977), however, and the demonstrated participation of prolactin in lipid biosynthesis by the fetal lung and by mammary tissue are supportive of the view that there is a role for prolactin in the process of augmented surfactant formation. Additional support for this proposed action of prolactin in the biochemical maturation of the fetal lung is provided by the finding that the incidence of respiratory distress syndrome in preterm infants born of heroin addicts is markedly decreased (Glass and associates, 1971). Opiates, for example morphine, are potent stimuli for prolactin secretion (Tolis and colleauges, 1975). These several lines of evidence taken together have led some investigators to the conclusion that increased prolactin secretion and augmented synthesis of surfactant by the human fetus during the last trimester of gestation may be causally related, and that prolactin and cortisol may act in concert to bring about augmented surfactant synthesis.

Snyder and colleagues (1981) have developed an elegant system for the study of human fetal lung maturation in vivo. They find that there is a striking morphological and biochemical maturation in explants of fetal lung tissue (16 to 20 weeks gestational age abortuses) that are maintained in organ culture. In such tissues, there is a remarkable increase in phosphatidylcholine formation and a rapid (4 to 5 days of culture) appearance of multivesicular bodies and lamellar bodies in type II pneumonocytes in these tissues. In such preparations, Mendelson and co-workers (1981) found that cortisol plus prolactin (but neither hormone alone) caused an acceleration in the rate of increase in phosphatidylcholine synthesis by human fetal lung tissue in organ culture. Thus, cortisol and prolactin, acting in concert, may be the lead hormones in the orchestration of a multihormonal stimulation of surfactant biosynthesis in fetal lung.

If the account presented were an accurate description of the events that transpire in vivo, it easily can be envisioned

that other hormones may serve a supportive role in this orchestration of fetal lung maturation. Estrogens affect phospholipid turnover in many tissues, act to promote prolactin release from the anterior pituitary, and, in many tissues, may be involved in the synthesis of prolactin receptors. Quirk and colleagues (1982) have reviewed the role of prolactin in fetal lung maturation.

Estrogens and Fetal Lung Maturation

It is of interest that in many of the tissues in which there are prolactin receptors, there also are receptors for estrogens. In fact, it appears that estrogens, directly or indirectly, act to regulate the number of prolactin receptors in the liver and mammary gland (Gelato and co-workers, 1975; Kelly and associates, 1975; Posner and Kelly, 1975). Many of the actions of prolactin and estrogens appear to be interrelated, especially with regard to lipid metabolism and growth. Estrogens are anabolic steroids that are known to regulate lipoprotein synthesis in the liver (Luskey and co-workers, 1974) and lipid metabolism in the rat uterus (Chan and colleagues, 1976). Increased lipid synthesis is one of the earliest and most dramatic responses of the rat uterus to estrogenic hormones (Aizawa and Mueller, 1961). Spooner and Gorski (1972) showed that estrogens caused enhanced fatty acid synthesis and an increase in rate of the incorporation of choline into glycerophospholipids of the rat uterus. Dickey and Robertson (1969) found that maternal and neonatal urinary estrogens in infants in whom respiratory distress subsequently developed were decreased. Pasqualini and associates (1976), studying guinea pig fetuses, demonstrated a high concentration of estradiol-17β receptors in lung tissue cytosol as well as nuclear binding of the steroid. The number of estrogen receptors in the lung of the guinea pig fetus increased with gestational age (Sumida and colleagues, 1977). Mendleson and associates (1980) have demonstrated high-affinity estrogen binding in cytosolic fractions prepared from rat and human fetal lung tissues. Moreover, Khosla and Rooney (1979) found that when pregnant rabbits were injected with estradiol-17β, fetal lung surfactant content was increased. Rooney and Brehier (1982) suggested that the estrogen-induced increase in the incorporation of choline into phosphatidylcholine is mediated by changes in CTP:phosphocholine cytidylyltransferase activity.

Nonetheless, the human fetus appears to be relatively estrogen-insensitive, at least in many tissues other than brain. Therefore, a role for estrogen in human fetal lung maturation may be indirect, e.g., by way of the modulation of pituitary prolactin secretion.

Thyroxine and Fetal Lung Maturation

A role for thyroxine in the rate of surfactant synthesis has been proposed by a number of investigators. Thyroxine administration to rabbit fetuses at 24 to 25 days of gestation is associated with accelerated maturation of the fetal lung and an early appearance of osmophilic lamellar inclusions within the type II pneumonocytes (Rooney and colleagues, 1974; Wu and associates, 1971, 1973). Smith and Torday (1974) found that thyroxine treatment was associated with an increased incorporation of choline into phosphatidylcholine in cultured cells prepared from rabbit fetuses of 28 days gestation. On the other hand, Rooney and co-workers (1974) found no effect of thyroxine treatment on the activities of lysophosphatidic acid acyltransferase, CPTase, CDP-diglyceride:inositol phosphatidyltransferase, glycerolphosphate phosphatidyltransferase, acyltransferase, or fatty acid biosynthesis. Mason (1973), in a study of the effect of thyroxine treatment on the concentration of dipalmitoylphosphatidylcholine in lungs of hyperthyroid and in euthyroid rats, found that thyroxine had little effect on the concentration of dipalmitoylphosphatidylcholine. Thus, the role of thyroxine, if any, in the biochemical maturation of the fetal lung type II pneumonocyte is unclear.

Growth Factors and Fetal Lung Maturation

Epidermal growth factor (EGF) acts to promote surfactant secretion and specifically to increase the synthesis of SAP-35, the apoprotein of surfactant (Whitsett and associates, 1987).

Conclusion

At presently, it seems reasonable to conclude that the hormonal stimulation of surfactant synthesis in the type II pneumonocytes of developing fetal lung is brought about by a complex interaction of several hormones. It is well established that pretreatment of breast tissue with estrogens, followed by cortisol, prolactin, and insulin treatment is essential for lactation. Perhaps a similar sequence of events leads to accelerated surfactant formation in maturing fetal lungs.

On the other hand, it now seems most reasonable to conclude that the regulation of fetal lung maturation (1) does not evolve singularly about the maturation of the type II pneumonocyte and (2) does not necessarily involve similar stimuli for the synthesis of both the glycerophospholipids and the apoproteins of surfactant. Moreover, it is clear that lung growth and maturation are not synonymous—perhaps the two events are not even complementary; to wit: lung growth may involve processes that inhibit functional maturation. If this were true, considerable initial confusion would be presented to investigators seeking to define the regulation of fetal lung growth, maturation, and function.

Several curious features of human fetal lung development are supportive of this proposition. For example, glucocorticosteroid treatment of pregnant women to effect fetal lung maturation is generally effective only during one brief window in gestation, viz., 29 to 33 weeks of gestation. This may be indicative that the therapeutic benefits of glucocorticosteroids at this time are derived from processes largely independent of accelerated surfactant formation. Possibly, the benefits are the consequence of alterations in extracellular matrix that facilitate lung expandability, a proposition suggested before from studies of the rhesus fetus (Johnson and associates, 1978).

Yet other facets of our confusion concerning fetal lung maturation may be related to the likelihood that the hormonal stimuli for the synthesis of apoprotein and those for glycerophospholipid synthesis are not identical. This seems to be the case and is especially germane to the delayed lung maturation of fetuses of diabetic women. For example, the hyperinsulinemia of such fetuses may retard apoprotein formation and not affect glycerophospholipid synthesis. On the other hand, dexamethasone may stimulate glycerophospholipid biosynthesis (perhaps indirectly through factors produced in stroma) but inhibit apoprotein formation.

RESPIRATION

Within a very few minutes after birth, the respiratory system must be able to provide oxygen as well as eliminate carbon dioxide if the neonate is to survive. Development of air ducts and alveoli, pulmonary vasculature, muscles of respiration, and coordination of their activities through the central nervous system to a degree that allows fetal survival, at least for a time, can be demonstrated by the end of the second trimester of pregnancy. The majority of fetuses born before this time succumb immediately or during the next few days from respiratory insufficiency, as pointed out in Chapter 38 (p. 746).

Movements of the fetal chest wall have been detected by ultrasonic techniques as early as 11 weeks gestation (Boddy and Dawes, 1975). From the beginning of the 4th month, the fetus is capable of respiratory movement sufficiently intense to move amnionic fluid in and out of the respiratory tract. In the radiograph in Figure 6–14, obtained 26 hours after injection of Thorotrast into the amnionic sac, the contrast medium is present in fetal lung. Davis and Potter (1946) reported that the longer the exposure in utero after a single injection of Thorotrast, the greater the apparent concentration in the lungs.

Duenhoelter and Pritchard (1976, 1977) demonstrated in both the human and the rhesus fetus that chromium-labeled erythrocytes and other labeled particles injected into the amnionic sac accumulated in the lungs as well as the gastrointestinal tract (Fig. 6–25). They concluded that throughout the last two trimesters progressively larger volumes of amnionic fluid are normally inspired and presumably expired by the fetus. The pressure changes with some inspirations are sufficient to account for such movement in the rhesus fetus (Martin and co-workers, 1974).

Boddy and Dawes (1975) identified fetal breathing movements in the normal human fetus that are episodic and irregular, their frequency ranging typically from 30 to 70 per minute. Asphyxia was followed by cessation of normal breathing movements and the initiation of gasping respiratory efforts. Such cessation of normal respiratory movements may be the consequence of increased levels of fetal β-endorphin (Browning and co-workers, 1983).

Vagitus Uteri

Crying in utero is a rare phenomenon. After rupture of the membranes, air may gain access to the amnionic cavity and be inspired by the fetus. Thiery and associates (1973) described three cases in which fetal crying was heard during vaginal examination, amnioscopy, or application of a clip electrode to the fetus. Fetal hiccuping is a more common phenomenon and frequently the movement produced by the fetus is appreciated by the mother.

ENDOCRINE GLANDS

ANTERIOR PITUITARY

Mulchahey and associates (1987), in an elegant review of the ontogenesis of fetal pituitary gland function and regulation, put forward an interesting and plausible view. First, they discounted the validity of the concept that the control of fetal anterior pituitary secretion was dependent upon maturation of the central nervous system. Second, they pointed out that the fetal endocrine system is functional for some time before "*the central nervous system completes its synaptogenesis and other integrative systems have reached a state of maturity competent to perform many of the tasks associated with homeostasis.*" Third, they go on to suggest that the endocrine system of the fetus does not necessarily mimic that of the adult but nonetheless may be one of the first homeostatic systems to develop.

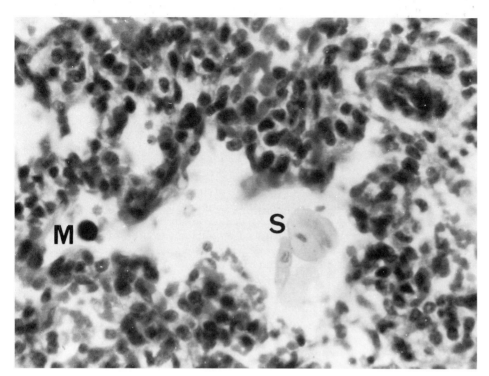

Figure 6–25. Photomicrograph of lung of a near-term rhesus fetus delivered 24 hours after labeling the amnionic fluid with radio-strontium-labeled microspheres as well as chromium-labeled erythrocytes. Contained in the alveolus immediately adjacent to the dense microsphere (M) are labeled erythrocytes that were also inhaled, as were fetal squamous cells, or squames (S). From the amount of chromium within the lungs, it was calculated that at least 62 mL of amnionic fluid was inhaled in 24 hours by a fetus that weighed 281 g. (*From Duenhoelter and Pritchard: Am J Obstet Gynecol 125:306, 1976.*)

Ultimately, the fetal anterior pituitary differentiates into five cell types, which secrete six protein hormones: (1) lactotropes, producing prolactin (PRL); (2) somatotropes, producing growth hormone (GH); (3) corticotropes, producing corticotropin (ACTH); (4) thyrotropes, producing thyroid-stimulating hormone (TSH); and (5) gonadotropes, producing luteinizing hormone (LH) and follicle-stimulating hormone (FSH). ACTH is first detected in the fetal pituitary at 7 weeks gestation; and before the end of the 17th week, the fetal pituitary is able to synthesize and store all pituitary hormones. GH, ACTH, and LH have been identified in the pituitary of the human fetus by 13 weeks gestation. Moreover, the fetal pituitary is responsive to hypophysiotropic hormones and is capable of secreting these hormones from early in gestation (Grumbach and Kaplan, 1974).

The levels of pituitary *growth hormone* are rather high in cord blood, although the role for the hormone in fetal growth and development is not clear. Decapitation in utero does not appreciably impair the growth of the rest of the animal fetus, as shown by Bearn (1967) as well as others. Furthermore, human anencephalic fetuses, with little pituitary tissue, are not remarkably different in weight from normal fetuses.

The fetal pituitary produces and releases β-endorphin in a manner separate from maternal plasma levels (Browning and colleagues, 1983). Furthermore, cord blood levels of β-endorphin and β-lipotrophin were found to decrease with declining fetal pH but correlate in a positive manner with fetal PCO₂ (Browning and co-workers, 1983).

NEUROHYPOPHYSIS

The fetal neurohypophysis is well developed by 10 to 12 weeks gestation and oxytocin and arginine vasopressin (AVP) are demonstrable. In addition, the neurohypophyseal hormone of submammalian vertebrates, arginine vasotocin (AVT), is present in fetal pituitary and pineal glands. AVT is present only in fetal

life in the human (Fisher, 1986). In adult animals, the infusion of AVT promotes sleep and stimulates prolactin release.

It is probable that oxytocin as well as AVP are functional in the fetus to conserve water; but these actions may be largely at the level of lung and placenta rather than kidney. PGE₂ formation in fetal kidney may serve to attenuate AVP action in this organ.

Several investigators have found that the levels of AVP in umbilical cord plasma are increased strikingly compared with the levels found in maternal plasma (Chard and associates, 1971; Polin and co-workers, 1977). Additionally, AVP in cord and fetal blood appears to be elevated by fetal stress (DeVane and Porter, 1980; De Vane and co-workers, 1982).

FETAL INTERMEDIATE PITUITARY

There is a well-developed intermediate lobe of the pituitary in the human fetus. The cells of this structure begin to disappear before term and are absent from the pituitary of adults. The principal secretory products of the intermediate lobe cells are α-melanocyte-stimulating hormone (α-MSH) and β-endorphin. The levels of fetal α-MSH decrease progressively with gestation.

THYROID

The pituitary-thyroid system is capable of function by the end of the first trimester (Table 6–5). Until midpregnancy, however, secretion of thyroid-stimulating hormone and thyroid hormones is low. There is a considerable increase after this time (Fisher, 1975, 1985; Fisher and Klein, 1981). Probably very little *thyrotropin* crosses the placenta from mother to fetus, whereas the long-acting thyroid stimulators LATS and LATS-protector do so when present in high concentrations in the mother (see Chap. 7, p. 154). Also, maternal IgG antibodies against thyroid-stimulating hormone (TSH) also may cross the placenta result-

TABLE 6–5. PHASES OF THYROID MATURATION IN THE HUMAN FETUS AND NEWBORN INFANT

Phase	Events	Gestational Age
I	Embryogenesis of pituitary-thyroid axis	2 to 12 weeks
II	Hypothalamic maturation	10 to 35 weeks
III	Development of neuroendo-crine control	20 weeks to 4 weeks after birth
IV	Maturation of peripheral mon-odeiodination systems	30 weeks to 4 weeks after birth

From Fisher: Ross Conference on Obstetrical Decisions and Neonatal Outcome, San Diego, May 1979.

ing in falsely high TSH levels in the neonate (Lazarus and associates, 1983).

The human placenta actively concentrates iodide on the fetal side; and throughout the second and third trimesters of pregnancy, the fetal thyroid concentrates iodide more avidly than does the maternal thyroid. Therefore, the hazard to the fetus of administering either radioiodide or appreciable amounts of ordinary iodide to the mother is obvious.

Thyroid hormones of maternal origin cross the placenta to a very *limited* degree, with triiodothyronine crossing more readily than thyroxine. There is limited action of thyroid hormones during fetal life. The athyroid human fetus is normally grown at birth. Only selected fetal tissues may be responsive to thyroid hormone, e.g., brain and lung.

Immediately after birth there are major changes in thyroid function and metabolism. Atmospheric cooling evokes sudden and marked increase in thyrotropin secretion which, in turn, causes a progressive increase in serum thyroxine levels maximal 24 to 36 hours after birth. There are nearly simultaneous elevations of serum triiodothyronine levels.

PARATHYROID GLANDS

There is good evidence that the fetal parathyroids elaborate *parathormone* by the end of the first trimester, and the glands appear to respond in utero to regulatory stimuli. Newborn infants of mothers with hyperparathyroidism, for example, may suffer hypocalcemic tetany. Plasma calcium levels in the fetus, 11 to 12 mg per dL, are maintained by active transport from maternal blood. Parathyroid levels in fetal blood are relatively low and those of calcitonin are high. In the sheep, fetal parathyroidectomy causes a fall in fetal plasma calcium concentrations. Fetal nephrectomy also causes a fall in calcium; and, 1α-hydroxylation of 25-OH-cholecalciferol takes place in fetal kidney.

ADRENAL GLANDS

The *adrenal* of the human fetus is very much larger in relation to total body size than is that of the adult; the bulk of the enlargement is made up of the inner or so-called fetal zone of the adrenal cortex. The normally hypertrophied fetal zone involutes rapidly after birth. The fetal zone is scant to absent in rare instances where the fetal pituitary is congenitally absent. The function of the fetal adrenal and the control of fetal adrenal steroidogenesis (dehydroisoandrosterone sulfate and cortisol) are discussed in detail in Chapter 5 (p. 74).

The fetal adrenal also synthesizes *aldosterone.* In one study, aldosterone levels in cord plasma near term exceeded those in maternal plasma, as did renin and renin substrate (Katz and colleagues, 1974). The renal tubules of the newborn, and presumably the fetus, appear relatively insensitive to aldosterone (Kaplan, 1972).

GONADS

Siiteri and Wilson (1974) demonstrated the synthesis of testosterone by the fetal testis from progesterone and pregnenolone by 10 weeks gestation. Moreover, Leinonen and Jaffe (1985) found that fetal testicular Leydig cells escape desensitization characteristic of adult testes subjected to repeated hCG challenges. This phenomenon in fetal testis may be due to (1) absence of estrogen receptors in fetal testes and (2) prolactin stimulation of hCG/LH receptors in fetal testes. Therefore, there is a close relationship between (1) the appearance of development of Leydig cells in fetal testes and levels of hCG, (2) fetal testicular testosterone formation and levels of hCG, (3) receptor concentration for LH/hCG and hCG levels, and (4) the absence of down-regulation of LH/hCG receptors and continued fetal testicular testosterone secretion during the time that hCG levels are high. The formation of estrogen in fetal ovaries has been demonstrated; but, estrogen formation in the ovaries is not required for female phenotypic development.

SEX OF THE FETUS

SEX RATIO

The accepted secondary sex ratio, that is, the sex ratio of human fetuses that reach viability, is approximately 106 males to 100 females. This figure has been obtained by the examination of term and preterm infants. Many attempts have been made to establish a sex ratio for fetuses of earlier gestational age. In general, such studies have been misleading, for as Wilson (1926) showed, the appearance of external genitals are an unreliable index of sex before the 50 mm stage.

Because, theoretically, there should be as many Y-bearing as X-bearing sperm, the primary sex ratio, or the ratio at the time of fertilization, should be one-to-one. If so, the secondary sex ratio of 106 to 100 is suggestive that more females than males are lost during the early months of pregnancy. Establishment of the primary sex ratio in humans is at present impracticable, for it requires the recovery and assignment of zygotes that fail to cleave and blastocysts that fail to implant. The results of Carr's studies (1963), nevertheless, are suggestive that the primary sex ratio in the human may be unity.

SEXUAL DIFFERENTIATION

One of the greatest responsibilities of the obstetrician is the assignment of sex to the newborn. But if the external genitalia of the newborn are ambiguous (with respect to complete male or female development), a profound dilemma is faced.

Griffin and Wilson (1986) have stated that *"it is no exaggeration to say that the detection of sexual ambiguity in the newborn constitutes a true medical emergency."* An incorrect assignment of sex portends grave psychological and social problems for the baby and family. Yet, we are of the view that the proper functional sex assignment for the newborn can be made almost always at the time of delivery even in newborns with ambiguity of the external genitalia. To address this issue, and to address the issue of establishing a definitive diagnosis as to the cause of development of ambiguous external genitalia, the mechanisms of normal and abnormal sexual differentiation must be understood.

It is clear that male phenotypic sexual differentiation is directed by the function of the fetal testis. **In the absence of the testis, female differentiation ensues irrespective of the genetic sex.**

Chromosomal Sex

Genetic sex, XX or XY, is established at the time of fertilization of the ovum. Thereafter, however, for the first 8 weeks, the development of male and female embryos is identical. It is the differentiation of the primordial gonad into testis or ovary that heralds the establishment of gonadal sex (Fig. 6–26).

Gonadal Sex

In the process of gonadal differentiation, it is known that the Y-chromosome is of paramount importance in the direction of gonadal differentiation into testes. It is reasonably clear that the testis-determining gene is located near the centromere on the short arm of the Y-chromosome. This subject was reviewed in an in-depth analysis by George and Wilson (1988). Nonetheless, it still is not clear how the Y-chromosome directs testicular differentiation. It is known that there are male-specific, cell-surface proteins, e.g., the H-Y antigen(s), that are correlated with testicular development in many species. Indeed, evidence has been presented that the H-Y antigen(s) actually induces testicular differentiation (Ohno and associates, 1978). It may be,

however, that the structural gene that specifies the H-Y antigen is located on an autosome with positive regulation caused by a locus on the Y-chromosome and a negative regulatory control caused by a locus on the X-chromosome (Wolf, 1981). As pointed out by Silvers and colleagues (1982), however, there likely are a number of male-specific antigens; and at present, no invariable relation can be defined between the presence of a given antigen and the development of a testis.

The contribution of chromosomal sex to gonadal sex may be deciphered best from an understanding of the apparent paradox presented by the XX male. The incidence of 46,XX phenotypic human males is estimated to be about 1 in 20,000 to 24,000 male births. Most cases in the human seem to result from interchange of a Y-chromosome fragment with the X-chromosome. Translocation of a testis-determining region of the Y-chromosome to the X-chromosome during meiosis of male germ cells gives rise to this possibility (George and Wilson, 1988).

Nonetheless, with establishment of the gonadal sex, there is the very rapid development of the phenotypic sex.

Phenotypic Sex

The urogenital tract of the human fetus is identical in the two sexes before the 8th week of gestation. Thereafter, development of the internal and external genitalia of the male phenotype is dependent upon testicular function.

The fundamental experiments to determine the role of the testis in male sexual differentiation were conducted by a French anatomist, Alfred Jost. Ultimately, he established that the induced-phenotype is male and that secretions from the gonad, including the ovary, are not necessary for female differentiation.

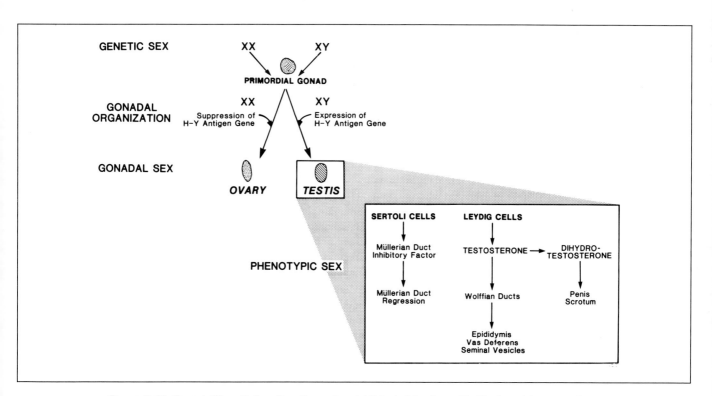

Figure 6–26. Sexual differentiation. Genetic sex is established at the time of fertilization of the ovum. At a time thereafter, the primordial gonad is acted upon by male-specific substances, e.g., H-Y antigen(s), that effect the organization of the gonad as a testis, the secretions of which effect male phenotypic sex differentiation.

Fetal Castration

Jost and associates (1973) found that if castration of the rabbit fetus were conducted before differentiation of the genital anlagen, all newborns were phenotypic females with female external genitalia; and the müllerian ducts had developed into uterus, fallopian tubes, and upper vagina.

Fetal Castration with Testis Implant

If castration of the fetus were conducted before differentiation of the genital anlagen and this was followed by implantation of a testis on one side, the phenotype of all fetuses was male; the external genitalia of such fetuses was masculinized; and on the side of the testicular implant, there was wolffian duct development in that a vas deferen, epididymis, and seminal vesicle were formed. On the side of the testicular implant, müllerian structures, i.e., uterine horn and fallopian tube, were not present. On the other hand, the müllerian duct did develop on the side of castration in which there was no testis graft.

Fetal Castration with Androgen Pellet Implant

Jost also found that if after castration of the fetus, at the sexually indifferent stage, a testosterone pellet were implanted on one side (in the site of a removed gonad), the external genitalia masculinized, as did the wolffian duct; but, the müllerian duct did not regress, i.e., the uterine horn and fallopian tubes did develop in spite of the "androgen" implant.

These fundamental observations, together with those of Wilson and collaborators (Wilson and Gloyna, 1970; Wilson and Lasnitzki, 1977), form the basic framework of our understanding of the mechanisms of sexual differentiation.

Testosterone Conversion to 5α-Dihydrotestosterone

Wilson and Gloyna (1970) demonstrated convincingly that in most androgen-responsive tissues, the androgen testosterone is converted to 5α-dihydrotestosterone in a reaction catalyzed by the enzyme 5α-reductase. In these tissues, androgen action is expressed by way of this 5α-reduced metabolite. The 5α-dihydrotestosterone is bound to an androgen-binding protein and the steroid-receptor protein complex in the nucleus becomes associated with chromatin. Thus, in the genital tubercle and urogenital sinus, testosterone acts only after conversion to 5α-dihydrotestosterone.

There is a notable and important exception, however, to this generalization for testosterone action in genital tissues. Namely, Wilson and Lasnitzki (1977) also demonstrated that testosterone, as testosterone, acts on the wolffian duct of the embryo to cause development of the male ductal system; indeed, this action of testosterone is expressed before 5α-reductase activity is detectable in this tissue.

Physiological and Biomolecular Basis of Sexual Differentiation

Based on these observations, the biochemical basis of sexual differentiation can be formulated as illustrated diagrammatically in Figure 6–26 and summarized as follows:

1. Genetic sex is established at the time of fertilization of the ovum.
2. Gonadal sex is determined by organizing factor(s) that may arise on autosomes, but by way of genic action that is affected positively by factors encoded on loci on the Y-chromosome or negatively by factors encoded on loci on the X-chromosome. By way of these coordinated processes, differentiation of the primitive gonad as a testis is accomplished.
3. The fetal testis secretes a proteinaceous substance called *müllerian-inhibiting substance,* a dimeric glycoprotein (M_r about 140,000) that acts locally (i.e., not as a hormone) to cause regression of the müllerian duct; i.e., it causes failure of development of uterus, fallopian tube, and upper vagina. Müllerian-inhibiting substance is produced by the Sertoli cells of the seminiferous tubules; importantly, the seminiferous tubules appear in fetal gonads before the Leydig cells, the cellular site of origin of testosterone. And, müllerian-inhibiting substance is produced by Sertoli cells even before differentiation of the seminiferous tubules. Therefore, regression of the müllerian ducts is initiated at a time in fetal development before testosterone secretion commences. Müllerian-inhibiting substance acts locally, i.e., near its site of formation; therefore, if a testis were absent on one side, the müllerian duct on that side would persist and the uterus and fallopian tubes would develop therefrom. It also may be that müllerian-inhibiting substance is important in testicular descent because the testes of newborn boys with cryptorchidism contain less müllerian-inhibiting substance than those of normal newborns.
4. The fetal testis, under the influence of the action of chorionic gonadotropin initially and thence fetal pituitary LH, secretes testosterone that acts directly on the wolffian duct to effect the development of the vas deferens, epididymides, and seminal vesicles. Testosterone, of fetal testicular origin, enters the blood, reaches the genital tubercle and urogenital sinus, and, in these tissues, testosterone is converted to 5α-dihydrotestosterone, the active androgen that brings about the virilization of the external genitalia.

GENITAL AMBIGUITY OF THE NEWBORN

The development of ambiguous genitalia is brought about, invariably, by abnormal androgenic representation in utero. This means, simply, too much androgen for an embryo that was destined to be female or too little androgenic representation for an embryo or a fetus that was destined to be male.

In the case of the fetus destined to be male, inadequate androgenic representation may be caused by deficient fetal testicular secretion of testosterone or else by a deficiency in responsiveness to testosterone or 5α-dihydrotestosterone in tissues that nominally respond to androgen.

Based on these premises, we believe that all abnormalities of sexual differentiation can be assigned to one of three general categories:

Category 1. Female pseudohermaphroditism
Category 2. Male pseudohermaphroditism
Category 3. Dysgenetic gonads and true hermaphroditism

Category 1. Female pseudohermaphroditism. In this category, abnormalities are found that conform to several guidelines as follow: (1) müllerian-inhibiting substance is *not* produced; (2) androgen exposure of the embryo and fetus is variable; (3) karyotype is 46,XX; and (4) ovaries are present. Therefore, all subjects in this category were destined to be female by virtue of genetic and gonadal sex.

Thus, the only abnormality that can occur is androgenic excess. Because müllerian-inhibiting substance was not produced (ovaries, not testes, are present), there will be a uterus, fallopian tubes, and upper vagina in each subject of this category. If such embryos were exposed to a small androgenic excess reasonably late in embryonic (early fetal) development, the only abnormality would be slight clitoral hypertrophy, with an otherwise normal female phenotype. With somewhat greater androgenic excess, clitoral hypertrophy and posterior labial fusion may develop. With progressively increasing androgenic excess, somewhat earlier in embryonic development, there is greater virilization. This process of virilization can proceed through the formation of labioscrotal folds, the development of a urogenital sinus (in which the vagina empties into the posterior urethra), and even to the development of a penile urethra with scrotal formation, the "empty scrotum" syndrome.

The cause of female pseudohermaphroditism is excessive androgen for a fetus that is destined to be female. The androgenic excess most commonly arises by secretion from the fetal adrenal because of increased secretion of androgen or androgen prehormones as a result of enzymatic defects in the pathway to cortisol formation in the adrenal cortex, i.e., congenital adrenal hyperplasia. With inadequate cortisol synthesis, it is presumed that ACTH secretion is elevated. Excessive stimulation of the adrenals leads to excessive secretion of precursors of cortisol and metabolites thereof, which include androgens or androgenic prehormones that can be converted, principally by way of androstenedione to testosterone, in extraglandular tissues. The enzyme deficiency may involve any of the five enzymatic reactions in the pathway to cortisol biosynthesis, i.e., cholesterol side-chain cleavage, 3β-hydroxysteroid dehydrogenase, 17α-hydroxylase, 21-hydroxylase, or 11β-hydroxylase.

Another cause of female pseudohermaphroditism is androgen excess in the fetus that is caused by increased androgen formation in the maternal compartment. Excess androgen in the mother may arise by secretion from maternal ovaries, i.e., hyperreactio lutealis, or from tumors of the maternal ovary, e.g., luteomas, arrhenoblastomas, or hilar cell tumors. Most commonly, however, the female fetus of a pregnant woman with an androgen-secreting tumor is not virilized. During most, perhaps all, of pregnancy, the female fetus is protected from androgen excess in the mother because of the extraordinary capacity of the trophoblast to convert aromatizable C_{19}-steroids (androgens) to estrogens (see Chap. 5).

In addition, if certain drugs are given to pregnant women, virilization of their female fetuses may occur. Most commonly, such drugs are synthetic progestins. It is not altogether clear how progestins cause virilization of the female fetus. On the one hand, some of these compounds, especially those of the 19-nortestosterone configuration, may act on fetal tissues as androgens. On the other hand, these agents may act to inhibit aromatization in the placenta and thus allow the transfer to the fetus of androgens that escape aromatization.

Importantly, all subjects of category 1 can be normal, fertile women if the proper diagnosis is made and appropriate therapy is initiated.

Category 2. Male pseudohermaphroditism. In this category, we find abnormalities that conform to several guidelines as follow: (1) müllerian-inhibiting substance is produced; (2) androgenic representation is variable; (3) karyotype is 46,XY; and (4) testes, or else no gonads, are present. All subjects in this category were destined to be male by virtue of genetic sex. Thus, the abnormalities in sexual differentiation are the result of

incomplete virilization, i.e., inadequate androgenic representation.

Incomplete masculinization of the fetus can be caused by inadequate production of testosterone by the fetal testis or else by diminished responsiveness of the genital anlagen to normal quantities of androgen, including failure of in situ formation of 5α-dihydrotestosterone in tissues destined to form the external genitalia.

Because müllerian-inhibiting substance is produced during embryonic life in these subjects (testes present, at least at some time in embryonic life), there is no uterus, fallopian tubes, or upper vagina.

Diminished Fetal Testicular Testosterone Secretion

Deficient fetal testicular testosterone production may occur if there is an enzymatic defect in the testis that involves any one of the four enzymes (which catalyze five enzymatic reactions) in the biosynthetic pathway to testosterone formation (Fig. 6–27). Defects in each of these enzymatic reactions, as a cause of abnor-

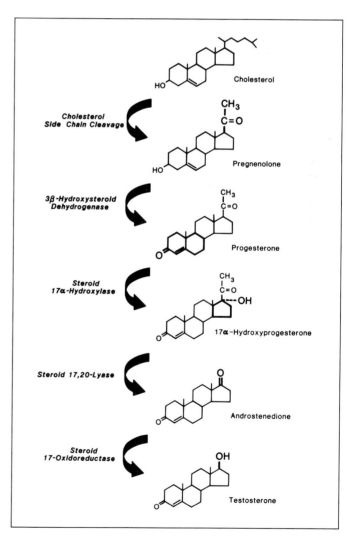

Figure 6–27. Biosynthetic pathway of testosterone formation in the testis. There are five enzymatic reactions involved in the conversion of cholesterol to testosterone. A defect in each of these enzymes has been identified as the cause of inadequate fetal testicular testosterone production.

mal sex differentiation, have been described. Enzymatic defects in testicular testosterone biosynthesis give rise to decreased rates of fetal testosterone secretion; and, incomplete masculinization of the external genitalia is the consequence. The phenotype of such newborns is variable in the degree of ambiguity because the degree of enzyme deficiency varies.

Embryonic Testicular Regression

Embryonic or fetal loss of testes gives rise to a phenotype that is dependent upon the time in embryonic life that the testes regressed. If the testes regress during embryonic or fetal life, there will be, thereafter, deficient testosterone production. Such an occurrence has been referred to as embryonic testicular regression (Edman and associates, 1977).

The time course of gonadal development and sexual differentiation is illustrated in Figure 6–28. Edman and associates (1977) analyzed the phenotypes of reported cases of agonadism in 46,XY persons, and in three cases of their own. They compared these findings with those that would be expected to occur if the testes regressed at various stages of development according to embryological findings of the time course of sexual differentiation in man (Jirasek, 1967, 1970, 1971). They found that a spectrum of phenotypes (cases a to i, Fig. 6–28) had been described, and among affected persons the phenotypes varied from normal female with absent uterus, fallopian tubes, and upper vagina, to that of a normal male, but with anorchia. Because müllerian duct regression commences before virilization is initiated in embryonic life, such a spectrum of phenotypes was to be expected if testicular regression were to occur at various times during the process of sexual differentiation.

Androgen Resistance

Deficiencies in androgen responsiveness are caused by inadequate or abnormal, or both, androgen receptor macromolecules in androgen-responsive tissues or else may be due to failure of conversion of testosterone to 5α-dihydrotestosterone in such tissues because of deficient 5α-reductase enzyme activity (Wilson and MacDonald, 1978).

The most extreme form of the disorders of androgen resistance is that of *testicular feminization*. In this entity, there appears to be little or no tissue responsiveness to androgen. In affected subjects, there is a female phenotype and a short, blind-ending vagina, no uterus or fallopian tubes, and no wolffian duct structures. At the expected time of puberty, testosterone levels in such women rise to values similar to or greater than those found in normal adult men. Nonetheless, virilization does not occur and even sexual hair, i.e., pubic and axillary hair, does not develop because of end-organ resistance to androgen action. Presumably, because of androgen resistance at the level of the brain and pituitary, LH levels are elevated in these women. In response to LH, in high concentrations, there also is increased testicular secretion of estrogen compared with that found in normal men (MacDonald and colleagues, 1979). The increased estrogen, together with the absence of androgen responsiveness, may act in concert to cause feminization, i.e., breast development.

In the disorder referred to as *incomplete testicular feminization*, there appears to be slight androgen responsiveness. In such subjects, there ordinarily is modest clitoral hypertrophy at birth; but at the expected time of puberty, virilization does not occur, pubic and axillary hair do develop. These women also develop feminine breasts, presumably through the same

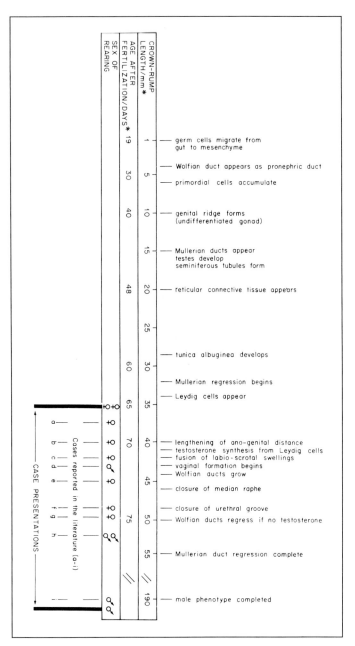

Figure 6–28. The temporal relations of the sequence or morphological changes that occur during male embryogenesis, and a comparison of this sequence to the phenotypes reported in subjects with embryonic testicular regression.

endocrine mechanisms as in women with the complete form of testicular feminization (Madden and co-workers, 1975).

A third syndrome of androgen resistance has been referred to as *familial male pseudohermaphroditism*, type I (Walsh and colleagues, 1974). This entity is also referred to commonly as *Reifenstein syndrome* but constitutes a spectrum of abnormalities of genital virilization varying from a phenotype similar to that of women with incomplete testicular feminization to that of a male phenotype with only a bifid scrotum, infertility, and gynecomastia. In these subjects, androgen resistance also was established by the demonstration of diminished 5α-dihydrotestosterone-binding capacity in fibroblasts grown in culture from genital skin biopsies.

A fourth form of androgen resistance is caused by *5α-reductase deficiency* in androgen-responsive tissues. Because androgen action in the genital tubercle and urogenital sinus is mediated by the action of 5α-dihydrotestosterone, in persons with 5α-reductase deficiency there are female external genitalia (modest clitoral hypertrophy). But because androgen action in the wolffian duct of the embryo is mediated by testosterone per se, in such persons there are well-developed epididymides, seminal vesicles, and vas deferens, and the male ejaculatory ducts empty into the vagina (Walsh and associates, 1974).

A composite photograph of the genitalia of subjects with each of the four types of androgen resistance is shown in Figure 6–29.

Category 3. In this category of our classification, we find subjects with abnormalities of sexual differentiation that conform to several guidelines as follow: (1) müllerian-inhibiting substance was not produced, (2) fetal androgen production among subjects was variable, (3) karyotype varies among subjects and commonly is abnormal, and (4) gonads are not present, neither ovaries or testis (but rarely both). In all of the subjects of this category, there is a uterus, fallopian tubes, and upper vagina.

In the majority of subjects in category 3, dysgenetic gonads are found. With the typical case of gonadal dysgenesis (e.g., those with Turner syndrome) there is a female phenotype; but, at the time of expected puberty, sexual infantilism persists. In some persons with gonadal dysgenesis, there are ambiguous genitalia, a finding that is indicative that an abnormal gonad produced androgen, albeit in small amounts, during embryonic development. Generally, in such subjects, we find mixed gonadal dysgenesis, i.e., a dysgenetic gonad on one side and an abnormal testis or dysontogenetic tumor on the other side. In most subjects with true hermaphroditism, the guidelines for category 3 are met. True hermaphrodites are those persons in whom both ovarian and testicular tissues are present; and, in particular, the germ cells, i.e., ova and sperm, of both sexes are formed.

PRELIMINARY DIAGNOSIS OF THE CAUSE OF GENITAL AMBIGUITY

A preliminary diagnosis of the etiology and pathogenesis of genital ambiguity can be made at the time of birth of an affected child. By physical and ultrasonic examination of the newborn, the experienced examiner can ascertain whether the child has a uterus. If the uterus is present, the diagnosis must be female

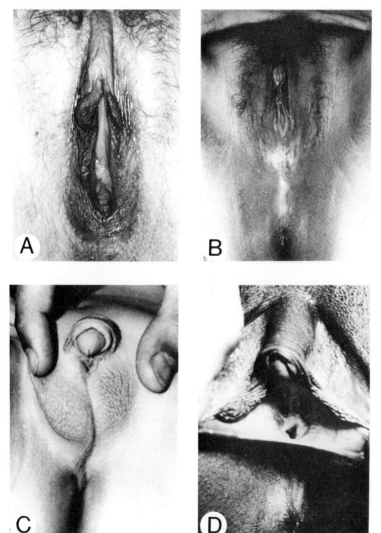

Figure 6–29. External genitalia of representative patients with male pseudohermaphroditism due to androgen resistance. **A.** Testicular feminization. **B.** Incomplete testicular feminization. **C.** Familial male pseudohermaphroditism, type I (Reifenstein syndrome). **D.** 5α-reductase deficiency. (*From Wilson and MacDonald, In Metabolic Basis of Inherited Disease. New York, McGraw-Hill, 1978.*)

pseudohermaphroditism, testicular or gonadal dysgenesis, or true hermaphroditism. A family history of congenital adrenal hyperplasia is helpful. If the uterus is not present, the diagnosis is male pseudohermaphroditism. Androgen resistance and enzymatic defects in testicular testosterone biosynthesis are familial.

SEX ASSIGNMENT

The critical decision of sex assignment by the obstetrician, in our view, is usually easy, although sometimes a painful decision to make. In our judgment, any newborn with ambiguity of the genitalia so severe as to represent more than hypospadius should be designated as female. This conclusion is reached on the basis of several considerations as follow: (1) All persons in category 1 of our classification (i.e., female pseudohermaphroditism) can be normal, fertile women. (2) The subjects of category 2 of this classification either cannot produce testosterone or else are refractory to its action. Moreover, all of the subjects of category 2 will be infertile. (3) Currently, reconstruction of the penis in persons with androgen resistance is possible, but the achievement of male sexual function, let alone fertility, is not.

REFERENCES

Adam PAJ, Teramo K, Raiha N, Gitlin D, Schwartz R: Human fetal insulin metabolism early in gestation: Response to acute elevation of the fetal glucose concentration and placental transfer of human insulin-I-131. Diabetes 18:409, 1969

Adinolfi M: Human complement: Onset and site of synthesis during fetal life. Am J Dis Child 131:1015, 1977

Aherne W, Dunnill MS: Morphometry of the human placenta. Br Med Bull 22:1, 1966

Aizawa Y, Mueller GC: The effect in vivo and in vitro of estrogens on lipid synthesis in the rat uterus. J Biol Chem 236:381, 1961

Altshuler G: Immunologic competence of the immature human fetus. Obstet Gynecol 43:811, 1974

Arey LB: Developmental Anatomy: A Textbook and Laboratory Manual of Embryology, 5th ed. Philadelphia, Saunders, 1946

Assali NS: In Gluck L (ed): Modern Perinatal Medicine. Chicago, Year Book, 1974

Assali NS, Bekey GA, Morrison LW: Fetal and neonatal circulation. In Assali NS (ed): Biology of Gestation, Vol II: The Fetus and Neonate. New York, Academic, 1968a

Assali NS, Kirschbaum TH, Dilts PV: Effects of hyperbaric oxygen on uteroplacental and fetal circulation. Circ Res 22:573, 1968b

Avery ME, Mead J: Surface properties in relation to atelectasis and hyaline membrane disease. Am J Dis Child 97:517, 1959

Ballard PL: Hormones and lung maturation. Monographs in Endocrinology, New York, Springer-Verlag, 1986, Vol 28

Ballard PL, Ballard RA: Glucocorticoid receptors and the role of glucocorticoids in fetal lung development. Proc Natl Acad Sci USA 69:2668, 1972

Ballard PL, Gluckman PD, Brehier A, Kitterman JA, Kaplan SL, Rudolph AM, Grumbach MM: Failure to detect an effect of prolactin on pulmonary surfactant and adrenal steroids in fetal sheep and rabbits. J Clin Invest 62:879, 1978

Banting FG, Best CH: Pancreatic extracts. J Lab Clin Med 1:464, 1922

Barclay AE, Barcroft J, Barron DH, Franklin KJ: Radiographic demonstration of circulation through heart in adult and in foetus, and identification of ductus arteriosus. Br J Radiol 12:505, 1939

Barrett CT, Sevanian A, Kaplan SA: Cyclic AMP (cAMP) and surfactant production: New means for enhancing lung maturation in the fetus. Pediatr Res 9:394, 1975

Bashore RA, Smith F, Schenker S: Placental transfer and disposition of bilirubin in the pregnant monkey. Am J Obstet Gynecol 103:950, 1969

Batenburg JJ, Klazinga W, Van Golde LMG: Regulation of phosphatidylglycerol and phosphatidylinositol synthesis in alveolar type II cells isolated from adult rat lung. FEBS Lett 147:171, 1982

Bearn JG: Role of fetal pituitary and adrenal glands in the development of the fetal thymus of the rabbit. Endocrinology 80:979, 1967

Belcher DP: A child weighing 25 pounds at birth. JAMA 67:950, 1916

Bigazzi M, Ronga R, Lancranjan I, Ferraro S, Branconi F, Buzzoni P, Martorana G, Scarselli GF, Del Pozo E: A pregnancy in an acromegalic woman during bromocriptine treatment: Effects on growth hormone and prolactin in maternal, fetal, and amniotic compartments. J Clin Endocrinol Metab 48:9, 1979

Bleasdale JE, Johnston JM: CMP-dependent incorporation of [¹⁴C] glycerol 3-phosphate into phosphatidylglycerol and phosphatidylglycerol phosphate by rabbit lung microsomes. Biochim Biophys Acta 710:377, 1982

Bleasdale JE, Johnston JM: Developmental biochemistry of lung surfactant. In Nelson GH (ed): Pulmonary Development and Transition to Extrauterine Life. Marcell Dekker (in press), 1984

Bleasdale JE, Wallis P, MacDonald PC, Johnston JM: Characterization of the forward and reverse reactions catalyzed by CDP-diacylglycerol: Inositol transferase in rabbit lung tissue. Biochim Biophys Acta 575:135, 1979

Boddy K, Dawes GS: Fetal breathing. Br Med Bull 31:3, 1975

Bozzetti P, Ferrari MM, Marconi AM, Ferrazzi E, Pardi G, Makowski EL, Battaglia FC: The relationship of maternal and fetal glucose concentrations in the human from midgestation until term. Metabolism 37:358, 1988

Braestrup PW: Studies of latent scurvy in infants: II. Content of ascorbic (cevitamic) acid in the blood serum of women in labor and in children at birth. Acta Paediatr (Suppl 1) 19:328, 1937

Brash AR, Hickey DE, Graham TP, Stahlman MT, Oates JA, Cotton RB: Pharmacokinetics of indomethacin in the neonate: Relation of plasma indomethacin levels to response of the ductus arteriosus. N Engl J Med 305:67, 1981

Breckenridge WC, Makai L, Kuksis A: Triglyceride structure of human milk fat. Can J Biochem 47:761, 1969

Brehier A, Benson BJ, Williams MC, Mason RJ, Ballard PL: Corticosteroid induction of phosphatidic acid phosphatase in fetal rabbit lung. Biochem Biophys Res Commun 77:886, 1977

Brinsmead MW, Liggins GC: Somatomedin-like activity, prolactin, growth hormone and insulin in human cord blood. Aust NZ J Obstet Gynaec 19:129, 1979

Browning AJF, Butt WR, Lynch SS, Shakespear RA: Maternal plasma concentrations of β-lipotropin, β-endorphin and γ-lipotrophin throughout pregnancy. Br J Obstet Gynaecol 90:1147, 1983

Carr D: Chromosome studies in abortuses and stillborn infants. Lancet 2:603, 1963

Chan L, Jackson RL, O'Malley BW: Synthesis of very low density lipoproteins in the cockerel: Effects of estrogen. J Clin Invest 58:368, 1976

Chard T, Hudson CN, Edwards CRW, Boyd NRH: Release of oxytocin and vasopressin by the human foetus during labour. Nature 234:352, 1971

Chez RA, Mintz DH, Reynolds WA, Hutchinson DL: Maternal-fetal plasma glucose relationships in late monkey pregnancy. Am J Obstet Gynecol 121:938, 1975

Clements JA: Surface tension of lung extracts. Proc Soc Exp Biol Med 95:170, 1957

Clymann RI, Heymann MA: Pharmacology of the ductus arteriosus. Pediatr Clin North Am 28:77, 1981

Davis ME, Potter EL: Intrauterine respiration of the human fetus. JAMA 131:1194, 1946

Dawes GS: The umbilical circulation. Am J Obstet Gynecol 84:1634, 1962

DeVane GW, Naden RP, Porter JC, Rosenfeld CR: Mechanism of arginine vasopressin release in the sheep fetus. Peediatr Res 16:504, 1982

DeVane GW, Porter JC: An apparent stress-induced release of arginine vasopressin by human neonates. J Clin Endocrinol Metab 51:1412, 1980

De Verdier CH, Garby L: Low binding of 2,3-diphosphoglycerate to hemoglobin F. Scand J Clin Lab Invest 23:149, 1969

Dickey RP, Robertson AF: Newborn estrogen excretion. Am J Obstet Gynecol 104:551, 1969

Dolman CL: Characteristic configuration of fetal brains from 22 to 40 weeks gestation at two week intervals. Arch Pathol Lab Med 101:193, 1977

Duenhoelter JH, Pritchard JA: Fetal respiration: Quantitative measurements of amnionic fluid inspired near term by human and rhesus fetuses. Am J Obstet Gynecol 125:306, 1976

Duenhoelter JH, Pritchard JA: Fetal respiration. A review. Am J Obstet Gynecol 129:326, 1977

Edman CD, Winters AJ, Porter JC, Wilson J, MacDonald PC: Embryonic testicular regression. A clinical spectrum of XY agonadal individual. Obstet Gynecol 49:208, 1977

Ekelund L, Arvidson G, Astedt B: Cortisol induced accumulation of phospholipids in organ culture of human fetal lung. Scand J Clin Lab Invest 35:419, 1975

Epstein M, Chez RA, Oakes GK, Mintz DH: Fetal pancreatic glucagon responses in glucose-intolerant nonhuman primate pregnancy. Am J Obstet Gynecol 127:268, 1977

Estelles A, Aznar J, Gilabert J, Parrilla JJ: Dysfunctional plasminogen in full-term newborn. Pediatr Res 14:1180, 1980

Fadel HE, Abraham EC: Minor fetal hemoglobins in relation to gestational age. Am J Obstet Gynecol 141:704, 1981

Farrell PM, Avery ME: Hyaline membrane disease. Am Rev Respir Dis 111:657, 1975

Farrell PM, Zachman RD: Induction of choline phosphotransferase and lecithin synthesis in the fetal lung by corticosteroids. Science 179:297, 1973

Fencl MD, Tulchinsky D: Total cortisol in amniotic fluid and fetal lung maturation. N Engl J Med 292:133, 1975

Finne PH: Antenatal diagnosis of the anemia in erythroblastosis. Acta Paediatr Scand 55:609, 1966

Fisher DA: Fetal thyroid hormone metabolism. Contemp Ob/Gyn 3:47, 1975

Fisher DA: Control of thyroid hormone production in the fetus. In Albrecht ED, Pepe GJ (eds): Research in Perinatal Medicine, Vol IV: Perinatal Endocrinology. Ithaca, NY, Perinatology Press, 1985, p 55

Fisher DA: The unique endocrine milieu of the fetus. J Clin Invest 78:603, 1986

Fisher DA, Klein AH: Thyroid development and disorders of thyroid function in the newborn. N Engl J Med 304:702, 1981

Fliegner JR, Fortune DW, Eggers TR: Premature rupture of the membranes, oligohydramnios and pulmonary hypoplasia. Aust NZ J Obstet Gynaec 21:77, 1981

Foley ME, Isherwood DM, McNicol GP: Viscosity, haematocrit, fibrinogen and plasma proteins in maternal and cord blood. Br J Obstet Gynaecol 85:500, 1978

Freinkel N: Homeostatic factors in fetal carbohydrate metabolism. In Wynn RM (ed): Fetal Homeostasis. New York, Appleton, 1969, Vol IV

Fuchs F: Volume of amniotic fluid at various states of pregnancy. Clin Obstet Gynecol 9:449, 1966

Gelato M, Marshall S, Boudreau M, Bruni J, Campbell GA, Meit J: Effects of thyroid and ovaries on prolactin binding activity in rat liver. Endocrinology 96:1292, 1975

George FW, Wilson JD: Embryology of the genital tract. In Walsh PC, Gittes RF, Perlmutter AD, Stamey RA (eds): Campbell's Urology. Philadelphia, Saunders, 1986, p 1804

George FW, Wilson JD: Sex determination and differentiation. In Knobil E, Neill J (eds): The Physiology of Reproduction. New York, Raven, 1988, p 3

Giannopoulus G: Glucocorticoid receptors in lung: I. Specific binding of glucocorticoids to cytoplasmic components of rabbit fetal lung. J Biol Chem 248:3876, 1973

Gilbert RD, Lis L, Longo LD: Temperature effects on O_2 affinity of fetal blood. Presented at the 30th Annual Meeting of the Society for Gynecologic Investigation. Washington, DC, March 17–20, 1983

Gillibrand PN: Changes in amniotic fluid volume with advancing pregnancy. J Obstet Gynaecol Br Commonw 76:527, 1969

Gitlin D: Development and metabolism of the immune globulins. In Kaga BM, Stiehm ER (eds): Immunologic Incompetence. Chicago, Year Book, 1971

Gitlin D: Protein transport across the placenta and protein turnover between amnionic fluid, maternal and fetal circulation. In Moghissi KS and Hafez ESE (eds): The Placenta. Springfield, IL, Thomas, 1974

Gitlin D, Kumate J, Morales C, Noriega L, Arevalo N: The turnover of amniotic fluid protein in the human conceptus. Am J Obstet Gynecol 113:632, 1972

Glass L, Rajegowda BK, Evans HE: Absence of respiratory distress syndrome in premature infants of heroin-addicted mothers. Lancet 2:685, 1971

Gluck L, Kulovich MV, Borer RC: The interpretation and significance of the lecithin-sphingomyelin ratio in amniotic fluid. Am J Obstet Gynecol 120:142, 1974

Gluck L, Kulovich MV, Borer RC, Brenner PH, Anderson GG, Spellacy WN: Diagnosis of the respiratory distress syndrome by amniocentesis. Am J Obstet Gynecol 109:440, 1971

Gluck L, Kulovich MV, Eidelman AI, Cordero L, Khazin AF: Biochemical development of surface activity in mammalian lung: IV. Pulmonary lecithin synthesis in the human fetus and newborn and etiology of the respiratory distress syndrome. Pediatr Res 6:81, 1972

Gluck L, Landowne RA, Kulovich MV: Biochemical development of surface activity in mammalian lung: III. Structural changes in lung lecithin during development of the rabbit fetus and newborn. Pediatr Res 4:352, 1970

Gluck L, Motoyama EK, Smits HL, Kulovich, MV: The biochemical development of surface activity in mammalian lung: I. The surface-active phospholipids; the separation and distribution of surface-active lecithin in the lung of the developing rabbit fetus. Pediatr Res 1:237, 1967

Gluckman PD, Ballard PL, Kaplan SL, Liggins GC, Grumbach MM: Prolactin in umbilical cord blood and the respiratory distress syndrome. J Pediatr 93:1011, 1978

Gresham EL, Rankin JHG, Makowski EL, Meschia G, Battaglia FC: An evaluation of fetal renal function in unstressed pregnancies. J Clin Invest 51:149, 1972

Griffin JE, Wilson JD: Disorders of sexual differentiation. In Walsh PC, Gittes RF, Perlmutter AD, Stamey RA (eds): Campbell's Urology. Philadelphia, Saunders, 1986, p 1819

Grosso DS, MacDonald CP, Thomasson JE, Christian CD: Relationship of newborn serum prolactin to the respiratory distress syndrome and maternal hypertension. Am J Obstet Gynecol 137:569, 1980

Gruenwald P: Growth of the human foetus. In McLaren A (ed): Advances in Reproductive Physiology. New York, Academic, 1967

Grumbach MM, Kaplan SL: Fetal pituitary hormones and the maturation of central nervous system regulation of anterior pituitary function. In Gluck L (ed): Modern Perinatal Medicine. Chicago, Year Book, 1974

Haase W: Maternity annual report for 1875. Charite Annalen 2:669, 1875

Hallman M, Kulovich MV, Kirkpatrick E, Sugarman RG, Gluck L: Phosphatidylinositol and phosphatidylglycerol in amniotic fluid: Indices of lung maturity. Am J Obstet Gynecol 125:613, 1976

Hamilton WJ, Mossman HW: Human Embryology, 4th ed. Baltimore, Williams & Wilkins, 1972

Hamosh M, Hamosh P: The effect of prolactin on the lecithin content of fetal rabbit lung. J Clin Invest 59:1002, 1977

Hauth JC, Parker CR, MacDonald PC, Porter JC, Johnston JM: Role of fetal prolactin in lung maturation. Obstet Gynecol 51:81, 1978

Hayward AR: The human fetus and newborn: Development of the immune response. Birth Defects 19:289, 1983

Henriksson P, Hedner V, Nilsson IM, Boehm J, Robertson B, Lorand L: Fibrin-stabilization factor XIII in the fetus and the newborn infant. Pediatr Res 8:789, 1974

Hocheim H: Cited by Kiedel W and Gluck L in Scarpelli (ed): Pulmonary Physiology of the Fetus, Newborn, and Child. Philadelphia, Lea & Febiger, 1975

Hollowes RC, Wang DY, Lewis DJ: The stimulation by prolactin and growth hormone of fatty acid synthesis in explants from rat mammary glands. J Endocrinol 57:265, 1973

Holmberg C, Perheentupa J, Launiala K, Hallman N: Congenital chloride diarrhoea. Arch Dis Child 52:255, 1977

Huisman THJ, Schroder WA, Brown AK: Changes in the nature of human fetal hemoglobin during the first year of life. Presented before Society for Pediatric Research, Atlantic City, NJ, May 1, 1970

Jirasek JE: The relationship between the structure of the testis and differentiation of the external genitalia and phenotype in man. In Wolstenholme GEW,

O'Connor M (eds): Ciba Foundation Colloquia on Endocrinology: Endocrinology of the Testis. Boston, Little, Brown, 1967

Jirasek JE: The relationship between differentiation of the testicle, genital ducts and external genitalia in fetal and postnatal life. In Rosenberg E, Paulsen CA (eds): The Human Testis: Advances in Experimental Medicine and Biology. New York, Plenum Press, 1970, Vol 10

Jirasek JE: Development of the genital system in human embryos and fetuses. Development of the Genital System and Male Pseudohermaphroditism. Baltimore, Johns Hopkins Press, 1971

Johnson JWC, Mitzner W, Lindon WJ, Palmer AE, Scott R, Kearney K: Glucocorticoids and the rhesus fetal lung. Am J Obstet Gynecol 130:905, 1978

Johnson JWC, Tyson JE, Mitzner W, London W, Palmer A, Andreassen B, Beck J: Prolactin and rhesus fetal lung characteristics. Presented before Society of Gynecologic Investigation, San Diego, CA, March 21, 1979

Josimovich JB, Merisko K, Boccella L: Binding of prolactin by fetal rhesus cell membrane fractions. Endocrinology 100:557, 1977

Jost A, Vigier B, Prepin J: Studies on sex differentiation in mammals. Recent Prog Horm Res 29:1, 1973

Kaplan S: Disorders of the endocrine system. In Assali NS (ed): Pathophysiology of Gestation: III. Fetal and Neonatal Disorders. New York, Academic, 1972

Kasper CK, Hoag MS, Aggeler PM, Stone S: Blood clotting factors in pregnancy: Factor VIII concentrations in normal and AHF-deficient women. Obstet Gynecol 24:242, 1964

Katz FH, Beck P, Makowski EL: The renin-aldosterone system in mother and fetus at term. Am J Obstet Gynecol 118:51, 1974

Keidel WN, Gluck L: Lipid biochemistry and biochemical development of the lung. In Scarpelli E (ed): Pulmonary Physiology of the Fetus, Newborn, and Child. Philadelphia, Lea & Febiger, 1975, p 96

Kelly PA, Posner BI, Friesen HG: Effects of hypophysectomy, ovariectomy, and cycloheximide on specific binding sites for lactogenic hormones in rat liver. Endocrinology 97:1408, 1975

Khosla SS, Rooney SA: Stimulation of fetal lung surfactant production by administration of 17β-estradiol to the maternal rabbit. Am J Obstet Gynecol 133:213, 1979

Klaus MH, Clements JA, Havel RJ: Composition of surface-active material isolated from beef lung. Proc Natl Acad Sci USA 47:185, 1961

Kohler PF: Maturation of the human complement system. J Clin Invest 52:671, 1973

Koldovsky O, Heringova A, Jirsova U, Jirasek JE, Uher J: Transport of glucose against a concentration gradient in everted sacs of jejunum and ileum of human fetuses. Gastroenterology 48:185, 1965

Kurjak A, Kirkinen P, Latin V, Ivankovic D: Ultrasonic assessment of fetal kidney function in normal and complicated pregnancies. Am J Obstet Gynecol 141:266, 1981

Lam TJ: Effect of prolactin on loss of solutes via the head region of the early-winter marine threespine stickleback (Gasterosteus aculeatus L, form tacherus) in fresh water. Can J Zool 47:865, 1969

Lands WE: Metabolism of glycerolipids: A comparison of lecithin and triglyceride synthesis. J Biol Chem 231:883, 1958

Lazarus JH, John R, Ginsberg J, Hughes IA, Shewring G, Smith BR, Woodhead JS, Hall R: Transient neonatal hyperthyrotrophinaemia: A serum abnormality due to transplacentally acquired antibody to thyroid stimulating hormone. Br Med J 286:592, 1983

Lebenthal E, Lee PC: Interactions of determinants of the ontogeny of the gastrointestinal tract: a unified concept. Pediatr Res 1:19, 1983

Leinonen PK, Jaffe RB: Leydig cell desensitization by human chorionic gonadotropin does not occur in the human fetal testis. J Clin Endocrinol Metab 61:234, 1985

Lemons JA: Fetal placental nitrogen metabolism. Semin Perinatol 3:177, 1979

Liggins GC: Premature delivery of foetal lambs infused with glucocorticoids. J Endocrinol 45:515, 1969

Liggins GC, Howie MB: A controlled trial of antepartum glucocorticoid treatment of prevention of the respiratory distress syndrome in premature infants. Pediatrics 50:515, 1972

Lind R, Kendall A, Hytten FE: The role of the fetus in the formation of amniotic fluid. J Obstet Gynaecol Br Commonw 79:289, 1972

Longo L: Disorders of placental transfer. In Assali NS (ed): Pathophysiology of Gestation. New York, Academic, 1972, Vol II

Luskey KL, Brown MS, Goldstein JL: Stimulation of the synthesis of very low density lipoproteins in rooster liver by estradiol. J Biol Chem 249:5939, 1974

MacDonald PC, Madden JD, Brenner PF, Wilson JD, Siiteri PK: Origin of estrogen in normal men and in women with testicular feminization. J Clin Endocrinol Metab 49:905, 1979

Madden JD, Walsh PC, MacDonald PC, Wilson JD: Clinical and endocrinological characterization of a patient with syndrome of incomplete testicular feminization. J Clin Endocrinol 41:751, 1975

Manahan CP, Eastman NJ: The cevitamic acid content of fetal blood. Bull Johns Hopkins Hosp 62:478, 1938

Mandelbaum B, Evans TN: Life in the amniotic fluid. Am J Obstet Gynecol 104:365, 1969

Marinetti GV, Erbland J, Witter RF, Petix J, Stotz E: Metabolic pathways of lipolecithin in a soluble rat-liver system. Biochim Biophys Acta 30:223, 1958

Martin CB, Murata Y, Petrie RH: Respiratory movements in fetal rhesus monkeys. Am J Obstet Gynecol 119:934, 1974

Mason RJ: Disaturated lecithin concentration of rabbit tissues. Am Rev Respir Dis 107:678, 1973

Mendelson CR, Johnston JM, MacDonald PC, Snyder JM: Multihormonal regulation of surfactant synthesis by human fetal lung *in vitro*. J Clin Endocrinol Metab 53:307, 1981

Mendelson CR, MacDonald PC, Johnston JM: Estrogen binding in human fetal lung cytosol. Endocrinology 106:368, 1980

Milewich L, Johnston JM, Bradfield DJ, Herbert WNP, MacDonald PC, Jimenez JM: The relationship of amniotic fluid dehydroisoandrosterone sulfate (DS) and cortisol (F) concentrations with lecithin to sphingomyelin (L/S) ratios during human gestation. Pediatr Res 12:397 [Abstract], 1978

Moore KL: The Developing Human, 2nd ed. Philadelphia, Saunders, 1977

Morriss FH Jr, Boyd RDH: Placental transport. In Knobil E, Neill J (eds): The Physiology of Reproduction. New York, Raven Press, 1988, p 2043

Mulchahey JJ, DiBlasio AM, Martin MC, Blumenfeld Z, Jaffe RB: Hormone production and peptide regulation of the human fetal pituitary gland. Endocr Rev 8:406, 1987

Murphy BEP: Cortisol and cortisone levels in the cord blood at delivery of infants with and without the respiratory distress syndrome. Am J Obstet Gynecol 119:1112, 1975

Murphy BEP: Chorionic membrane as an extra-adrenal source of foetal cortisol in human amniotic fluid. Nature 266:179, 1977

Myers RE: Fetal brain tolerance to umbilical cord compression according to gestational age. Presented at the 17th Annual Meeting of the Society for Gynecologic Investigation, New Orleans, April 2, 1970

Nielsen NC: Coagulation and fibrinolysin in normal women immediately postpartum and in newborn infants. Acta Obstet Gynecol Scand 48:371, 1969

Nielsen PV, Pedersen J, Kampmann E-M: Absence of human placental lactogen in an otherwise uneventful pregnancy. Am J Obstet Gynecol 135:322, 1979

Obenshain SS, Adam PAJ, King KC, Teramo K, Raivio KO, Raiha N, Schwartz R: Human fetal insulin response to sustained maternal hyperglycemia. N Engl J Med 283:566, 1970

Odom MJ, MacDonald PC, Bleasdale JE: Diabetes and fetal lung maturation. Williams Supplement No. 7. Appleton-Century-Crofts, July/August, 1986.

Ohno S, Najai Y, Cicares S: Testicular cells lyso-stripped by H-Y antigen organize ovarian follicle-like aggregates. Cytogenet Cell Genet 20:351, 1978

Oka T, Topper YJ: Hormone-dependent accumulation of rough endoplasmic reticulum in mouse mammary epithelial cells *in vitro*. J Biol Chem 246:7701, 1971

Page EW: Problems of nutrition in the perinatal period. Report of the 60th Ross Conference on Pediatric Research, Columbus, OH, 1970

Page EW, Glendening MB, Margolis A, Harper HA: Transfer of D- and L-histidine across the human placenta. Am J Obstet Gynecol 73:589, 1957

Pasqualini JR, Sumida C, Gelly C: Cytosol and nuclear [³H]oestradiol binding in the foetal tissues of guinea pig. Acta Endocrinol 83:811, 1976

Pataryas HA, Stammatoyannopoulos G: Hemoglobins in human fetuses: Evidence for adult hemoglobin production after the 11th gestational week. Blood 39:688, 1972

Paton JB, Fisher DE, DeLannoy CW, Behram RE: Umbilical blood flow, cardiac output, and organ blood flow in the immature baboon fetus. Am J Obstet Gynecol 117:560, 1973

Pearson HA: Recent advances in hematology. J Pediatr 69:466, 1966

Perrine SP, Greene MF, Cohen RA, Faller DV: A physiological delay in human fetal hemoglobin switching is associated with specific globin DNA hypomethylation. FEBS Lett 228:139, 1988

Pipe NGJ, Smith T, Halliday D, Edmonds CJ, Williams C, Coltart TM: Changes in fat, fat-free mass and body water in human normal pregnancy. Br J Obstet Gynaecol 86:929, 1979

Plentl AA: Physiology of the placenta: III. Dynamics of amniotic fluid. In Assali NS (ed): Biology of Gestation, Vol I: The Maternal Organism. New York, Academic, 1968

Polin RA, Husain MK, James LS, Frantz AG: High vasopressin concentrations in human umbilical cord blood—lack of correlation with stress. J Perinat Med 5:114, 1977

Portman OW, Behrman RE, Soltys P: Transfer of free fatty acids across the primate placenta. Am J Obstet Gynecol 216:143, 1969

Posner BI, Kelly PA: Prolactin receptors in rat liver: Possible induction by prolactin. Science 188:57, 1975

Post M, Foros J, Smith BT: Inhibition of lung maturation by monoclonal antibodies against fibroblast-pneumocyte factor. Nature 308:284, 1984

Pritchard JA: Deglutition by normal and anencephalic fetuses. Obstet Gynecol 25:289, 1965

Pritchard JA: Fetal swallowing and amniotic fluid volume. Obstet Gynecol 28:606, 1966

Quirk JG, Bleasdale JE: Myo-inositol homeostasis in the human fetus. Obstet Gynecol 62:41, 1983

Quirk JG, Bleasdale JE: Fetal lung maturation in the pregnancy complicated by diabetes mellitus. In DiRenzo GC, Hawkins PF (eds): Perinatal Medicine: Updates and Controversies. London, Wiley, 1984

Quirk JG, Bleasdale JE, MacDonald PC, Johnston JM: A role for cytidine monophosphate in the regulation of the glycerophospholipid composition of surfactant in developing lung. Biochem Biophys Res Commun 95:985, 1980

Quirk JG, MacDonald PC, Johnston JM: Role of fetal pituitary prolactin in fetal lung maturation. Semin Perinatol 6:328, 1982

Read EJ Jr, Platzer PB: Placental metastasis from maternal carcinoma of the lung. Obstet Gynecol 58:387, 1981

Rooney SA, Brehier A: The CDP-choline pathway: Cholinephosphate cytidylyltransferase. In Farrell PM (ed): Lung Development: Biological and Clinical Perspectives. New York, Academic, 1982, p 317, Vol 1

Rooney SA, Gross I, Motoyama EK, Warshaw JB: Effects of cortisol and thyroxine on fatty acid and phospholipid biosynthesis in fetal rabbit lung. Physiologist 17:323, 1974

Rooney SA, Gross I, Gassenheimer LN, Motoyama EK: Stimulation of glycerolphosphate phosphatidyltransferase activity in fetal rabbit lung by cortisol administration. Biochim Biophys Acta 398:433, 1975

Rosenfeld CR, Porter JC: Arginine vasopressin in the developing fetus. In Albrecht ED, Pepe GJ (eds): Research in Perinatal Medicine. IV: Perinatal Endocrinology. Ithaca, NY, Perinatology Press, 1985, p 91

Rudolph AM, Heymann MA: The fetal circulation. Ann Rev Med 19:195, 1968

Russell BJ, Nugent L, Chernick V: Effects of steroids on the enzymatic pathways of lecithin production in fetal rabbits. Biol Neonate 24:306, 1974

Schulman I, Smith CH: Fetal and adult hemoglobins in premature infants. Am J Dis Child 86:354, 1953

Sell EJ, Corrigan JJ Jr: Platelet counts, fibrinogen concentrations, and factor V and factor VIII levels in healthy infants according to gestational age. J Pediatr 82:1028, 1973

Shrand II: Vomiting in utero with intestinal atresia. Pediatrics 49:767, 1972

Siiteri PK, Wilson JD: Testosterone formation and metabolism during male sex differentiation in human embryo. J Clin Endocrinol 38:113, 1974

Silvers WK, Glasser DL, Eicher EM: H-Y antigen, serologically detectable male antigen and sex determination. Cell 28:439, 1982

Sivakumaran T, Duncan ML, Effer SB, Younglai EV: Relationship between cortisol and lecithin/sphingomyelin ratios in human amniotic fluid. Am J Obstet Gynecol 122:291, 1975

Smith BT: Fibroblast-pneumocyte factor: Intercellular mediator of glucocorticoid effect on fetal lung. In Stern L (ed): Intensive Care in the Newborn. New York, Masson, 1978, p 25

Smith BT, Torday JS: Factors affecting lecithin synthesis by fetal lung cells in culture. Pediatr Res 8:848, 1974

Smith CM II, Tukey DP, Krivit W, White JG: Fetal red cells (FC) differ in elasticity, viscosity, and adhesion from adult red cells (AC). Pediatr Res 15:588, 1981

Smith YF, Mullan DK, Hamosh M, Scanlon JW, Hamosh P: Prolactin and human lung maturation. Pediatr Res 12:569, 1978

Snyder JM, Johnston JM, Mendelson CR: Differentiation of type II cells of human fetal lung in vitro. Cell Tissue Res 220:17, 1981

Snyder JM, Mendelson CR: Insulin inhibits the accumulation of the major lung surfactant apoprotein in human fetal lung explants maintained *in vitro*. Endocrinology 120:1250, 1987

Spellacy WN, Buhi WC, Riggall FC, Holsinger KL: Human amniotic fluid lecithin/sphingomyelin ratio changes with estrogen or glucocorticoid treatment. Am J Obstet Gynecol 115:216, 1973

Spooner PM, Gorski J: Early estrogen effects on lipid metabolism in the rat uterus. Endocrinology 91:1273, 1972

Stabile I, Nicolaides KH, Bach A, Teisner B, Rodeck C, Westergaard JG, Grudzinskas JG: Complement factors in fetal and maternal blood and amniotic fluid during the second trimester of normal pregnancy. Br J Obstet Gynaecol 95:281, 1988

Stein Z, Susser M, Rush D: Prenatal nutrition and birth weight: Experiments and quasi-experiments in the past decade. J Reprod Med 21:287, 1978

Streeter GL: Weight, sitting height, head size, foot length, and menstrual age of the human embryo. Contrib Embryol 11:143, 1920

Sumida C, Gelly C, Nguyen BL, Pasqualini JR: Cytosol and nuclear ³H-estradiol receptors in fetal guinea pig kidney, lung, and uterus during fetal development. Acta Endocrinol (Suppl 212) 85:36, 1977

Sybulski S, Manghan GB: Relationship between cortisol levels in umbilical cord plasma and development of the respiratory distress syndrome in premature newborn infants. Am J Obstet Gynecol 125:239, 1976

Szabo AJ, Grimaldi RCD, Jung WF: Palmitate transport across perfused human placenta. Metabolism 18:406, 1969

Tan SY, Gewolb IH, Hobbins JC: Unconjugated cortisol in human amniotic fluid: Relationship to lecithin/sphingomyelin ratio. J Clin Endocrinol Metab 43:412, 1976

Temiras PS, Vernadakis A, Sherwood NM: Development and plasticity of the nervous system. In Assali NS (ed): Biology of Gestation: VII. The Fetus and Neonate. New York, Academic, 1968

Thiery M, Yo Le Sian A, Vrijens M, Janssens D: Vagitus uterinus. J Obstet Gynaecol Brit Commonw 80:183, 1973

Tolis G, Hickey J, Guyda H: Effect of morphine on serum growth hormone, cortisol, prolactin, and thyroid stimulating hormone in man. J Clin Endocrinol Metab 41:797, 1975

Turkington RW, Majumderi GC, Kadohama N: Hormone regulation of gene expression in mammary cells. Recent Prog Horm Res 29:417, 1973

Usher R, Shephard M, Lind J: The blood volume of the newborn infant and placental transfusion. Acta Paediatr 52:497, 1963

Van Den Bosch J, Bonte HA, van Deenen LLM: On the anabolism of lipolecithin. Biochim Biophys Acta 98:648, 1965

Voelker DR, Ten-Cheng L, Snyder F: Fatty acid biosynthesis and dietary regulation in pulmonary adenomas. Arch Biochem Biophys 176:753, 1976

Von Neergaad K: Neue Auffassungen über einen Grundbegriff der Atemmechanik Die Retrakionskraft der Lunge Abhangig von der Oberflach enspannung in den Alveolen. Z Ges Expt Med 66:373, 1929

Walker J, Turnbull EPN: Haemoglobin and red cells in the human foetus and their relation to the oxygen content of the blood in the vessels of the umbilical cord. Lancet 2:312, 1953

Walsh PC, Madden JD, Harrod MJ, Goldstein JL, MacDonald PC, Wilson JD: Familial incomplete male pseudohermaphroditism, type 2: Decreased dihydrotestosterone formation in pseudovaginal perineoscrotal hypospades. N Engl J Med 291:944, 1974

Whitsett JA, Weaver TE, Lieberman MA, Clark JC, Daugherty C: Differential effects of epidermal growth factor and transforming growth factor-β on synthesis of M_r = 35,000 surfactant-associated protein in fetal lung. J Biol Chem 262:7908, 1987

Widdowson EM: Growth and composition of the fetus and newborn. In Assali NS (ed): Biology of Gestation, Vol II: The Fetus and Neonate. New York, Academic, 1968

Wigglesworth JS, Desai R: Is fetal respiratory function a major determinant of perinatal survival? Lancet 1:264, 1982

Wilson JD, Gloyna RE: The intranuclear metabolism of testosterone in the accessory organs of reproduction. Recent Prog Horm Res 26:309, 1970

Wilson JD, Lasnitzki I: Dihydrotestosterone formation in fetal tissues of the rabbit and rat. Endocrinology 89:659, 1971

Wilson JD, MacDonald PC: Male pseudohermaphroditism due to androgen resistance: Testicular feminization and related syndromes. In Stanbury JB, Wyngaarden JD, Frederickson DS (eds): The Metabolic Basis of Inherited Disease. New York, McGraw-Hill, 1978

Wilson KM: Correlation of external genitalia and sex-glands in the human embryo. Contrib Embryol 18:23, 1926

Winters AJ, Oliver C, Colston C, MacDonald PC, Porter JC: Plasma ACTH levels in the human fetus and neonate as related to age and parturition. J Clin Endocrinol Metab 39:269, 1974

Wislocki GB: Electron microscopy of the human placenta. Anat Rec 123:133, 1955

Wladimiroff JW, Campbell S: Fetal urine-production rates in normal and complicated pregnancy. Lancet 1:151, 1974

Wolf U: Genetic aspects of H-Y antigen. Hum Genet 58:25, 1981

Wu B, Kikkawa Y, Orzalesi MM, Motoyama EK, Kaibara M, Zigas CJ, Cook CD: Accelerated maturation of fetal rabbit lungs by thyroxine. Physiologist 14:253, 1971

Wu B, Kikkawa Y, Orzalesi MM, Motoyama EK, Kaibara M, Zigas CJ, Cook CD: The effect of thyroxine on the maturation of fetal rabbit lungs. Biol Neonate 22:161, 1973

Zanjani ED, Peterson EN, Gordon AS, Wasserman LR: Erythropoietin production in the fetus: Role of the kidney and maternal anemia. J Lab Clin Med 83:281, 1974

Zivny J, Kobilkova J, Neuwirt J, Andrasova V: Regulation of erythropoiesis in fetus and mother during normal pregnancy. Obstet Gynecol 60:77, 1982

Zuspan FR, Cordero L, Semchyshyn S: Effects of hydrocortisone on lecithin-sphingomyelin ratio. Am J Obstet Gynecol 128:571, 1977

Maternal Adaptations to Pregnancy

The anatomical, physiological, and biochemical adaptations that take place in women during the short span of human pregnancy are profound. Many of these changes begin soon after fertilization and continue throughout gestation, and as noted already (Chaps. 2 through 6), most of these remarkable adaptations occur in response to physiological stimuli provided by the fetus or fetal tissues: the fetal–maternal communications system. Equally astounding is that the woman who was pregnant is returned almost completely to her prepregnancy state after delivery and cessation of lactation. The understanding of these adaptations to pregnancy remains a major goal of obstetrics, and without such knowledge, it is almost impossible to understand the disease processes—pregnancy induced or coincidental—that can threaten women during pregnancy and the puerperium.

UTERUS

HYPERTROPHY AND DILATATION

The capacity of the uterus to increase rapidly in size during pregnancy and then to return almost to its original state within a few weeks is remarkable. In the nonpregnant woman, the uterus is an almost solid structure weighing 70 g or so and with a cavity of 10 mL or less. During pregnancy, the uterus is transformed into a relatively thin-walled muscular organ of sufficient capacity to accommodate the fetus, placenta, and amnionic fluid. The total volume of the contents of the uterus at term averages about 5 L but may be as much as 20 L or more, so that by the end of pregnancy the uterus has achieved a 500 to 1,000 times greater capacity than in the nonpregnant state. There is a corresponding increase in uterine weight and the body of the uterus at term weighs approximately 1,100 g. During pregnancy, uterine enlargement involves stretching and marked hypertrophy of existing muscle cells, whereas the appearance of new muscle cells is limited. At the time of parturition, a single myometrial cell is about 500 μm in length and the nucleus is eccentrically placed in the thickest part of the cell. The myometrial smooth muscle cell is surrounded by an irregular array of collagen fibrils. The force of contraction is transmitted from the contractile proteins of the muscle cell to the surrounding connective tissue through the reticulum of collagen (Carsten, 1968).

Accompanying the increase in size of the uterine muscle cells during pregnancy, there is an accumulation of fibrous tissue, particularly in the external muscular layer, together with a considerable increase in elastic tissue. The network that is formed adds materially to the strength of the uterine wall. Concomitantly, there is a great increase in the size and number of blood vessels and lymphatics. The veins that drain the placental site are transformed into large uterine sinuses and there is hypertrophy of the nerves exemplified by the increase in size of Frankenhäuser's cervical ganglion.

During the first few months of pregnancy, hypertrophy of the uterine wall is probably stimulated chiefly by the action of estrogen and perhaps that of progesterone. It is apparent that the early hypertrophy of the uterus is not entirely in response to mechanical distension by the products of conception because similar uterine changes occur when the embryo is ectopically implanted in the fallopian tube or ovary. But, after the 3rd month, the increase in uterine size is, in large part, related in some manner to the effect of pressure exerted by the expanding products of conception.

Rapid growth of most (perhaps all) tissues is correlated with increased synthesis of *polyamines*, which include *spermidine* and *spermine* and their immediate precursor, *putrescine*. These polyamines are believed to occupy crucial roles in tissue growth and cell hypertrophy. Russell and colleagues (1978) found that polyamine levels in the urine of normally pregnant women are strikingly elevated and that the highest levels are attained at 13 to 14 weeks gestation (Fig. 7–1). It is interesting to speculate that the increased rate of synthesis of polyamines at this time is related to the myometrial hypertrophy that occurs during this stage of pregnancy. But equally important, at 13 to 14 weeks of pregnancy there is a striking increase in diamine oxidase activity in blood. This enzyme probably is produced in decidua but is released into blood in large amounts. Indeed, the activity of diamine oxidase in blood of pregnant women is 1,000 times that found in men or nonpregnant women. This enzyme serves to catalyze the metabolism of polyamines. Thus, it is likely that the rate of polyamine formation is increased strikingly throughout pregnancy, but the rate of metabolism of these growth-promoting agents increases so remarkably, due to the action of diamine oxidase, that the levels of polyamines decline after 12 to 14 weeks of pregnancy. Russell and Durie (1978) have provided a concise review of these interactions.

During the first few months of pregnancy, the uterine walls become considerably thicker than in the nonpregnant state, but as gestation advances the walls gradually thin. At term, the walls of the uterine corpus are for the most part 1.5 cm or less in thickness. Early in pregnancy, the uterus loses the firmness and resistance characteristic of the nonpregnant organ. In the later months, the uterus is changed into a muscular sac with thin, soft, readily indentable walls, demonstrable by the ease with which the fetus usually can be palpated through the abdominal wall and by the readiness with which the uterine walls yield to the movements of the fetal extremities.

The enlargement of the uterus is not symmetrical and it is

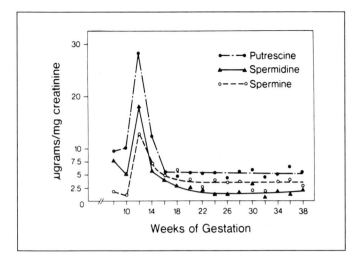

Figure 7–1. Polyamines in the urine of women with normal pregnancies are plotted as a function of weeks of gestation. Each point is the mean value of results obtained in the urine of at least five separate women. (*From Russell and colleagues: Am J Obstet Gynecol 132:649, 1978.*)

most marked in the fundus. The differential growth is readily apparent by observing the relative positions of the attachments of the fallopian tubes and ovarian ligaments. In the early months of pregnancy, these structures insert only slightly below the apex of the fundus, whereas in the later months, they are inserted slightly above the middle of the uterus. The position of the placenta also influences the extent of uterine hypertrophy, since the portion of the uterus surrounding the placental site enlarges more rapidly than does the myometrium distal to the site of placental implantation.

Arrangement of the Muscle Cells

Uterine musculature during pregnancy is arranged in three strata: an external hoodlike layer, which arches over the fundus and extends into the various ligaments; an internal layer, consisting of sphincterlike fibers around the orifices of the tubes and the internal os; and (lying between these two) a dense network of muscle fibers perforated in all directions by blood vessels. The main portion of the uterine wall is formed by the middle layer, which consists of an interlacing network of muscle fibers between which extend the blood vessels. Each cell in this layer has a double curve, so that the interlacing of any two gives approximately the form of the figure 8. As a result of this arrangement, when the cells contract after delivery they constrict the penetrating blood vessels and thus act as ligatures.

The muscle cells composing the uterine wall in pregnancy, especially in its lower portion, overlap one another like shingles on a roof. One end of each fiber arises beneath the serosa of the uterus and extends obliquely downward and inward toward the decidua, forming a large number of muscular lamellae which are interconnected by short muscular processes. When the tissue is slightly spread apart, it appears sievelike and, on closer examination, is found to comprise innumerable rhomboidal spaces.

CHANGES IN UTERINE SIZE, SHAPE, AND POSITION

As the uterus increases in size, it also undergoes important modifications in shape. For the first few weeks, its original pear shape is maintained, but as pregnancy advances the corpus and fundus soon assume a more globular form, becoming almost

spherical by the 3rd lunar month. Subsequently, the organ increases more rapidly in length than in width and assumes an ovoid shape (Fig. 4–23).

By the end of 12 weeks, the uterus has become too large to remain wholly within the pelvis. Thereafter, as the uterus continues to enlarge, it contacts the anterior abdominal wall, displaces the intestines laterally and superiorly, and continues to rise, reaching ultimately almost to the liver. As the uterus rises, tension is exerted upon the broad ligaments, which partly unfold their median and lower portions, and upon the round ligaments.

During pregnancy, the uterus is movable. With the pregnant woman standing, the longitudinal axis of the uterus corresponds to an extension of the axis of the pelvic inlet. The abdominal wall supports the uterus and, unless it is quite relaxed, maintains this relation between the long axis of the uterus and the axis of the pelvic inlet. When the pregnant woman is supine, the uterus falls back to rest upon the vertebral column and the adjacent great vessels, especially the inferior vena cava and the aorta.

With ascent of the uterus from the pelvis, it usually undergoes rotation to the right, resulting in the left margin facing anteriorly. This *dextrorotation* likely results in large measure from the presence of the rectosigmoid on the left side of the pelvis. However, *levorotation* occurs occasionally, especially if there is a pelvic or low abdominal mass on the right side, for example, a transplanted kidney.

CHANGES IN CONTRACTILITY

From the first trimester of pregnancy onward, the uterus undergoes irregular contractions, which normally are painless. In the second trimester, these contractions may be detected by bimanual examination. The relaxed uterus transiently becomes firm and then returns to its original relaxed state. Since attention was first called to this phenomenon by Braxton Hicks, the contractions have been known by his name. Such contractions appear unpredictably and sporadically, are usually nonrhythmic, and their intensity, according to Alvarez and Caldeyro-Barcia (1950), is somewhat more than 8 cm of water. Until the last month of gestation, *Braxton Hicks contractions* are infrequent, but increase in frequency during the last week or two. At this time, the contractions may occur as often as every 10 to 20 minutes and also may assume some degree of rhythmicity. Late in pregnancy, these contractions may cause some discomfort and account for so-called *false labor*.

UTEROPLACENTAL BLOOD FLOW

The delivery of most substances essential for the growth and metabolism of the fetus and placenta, as well as the removal of most metabolic wastes, is dependent upon adequate perfusion of the placental intervillous space. Placental perfusion by maternal blood is dependent in turn upon blood flow to the uterus through the uterine and ovarian arteries. There is no question that there is a progressive increase in uteroplacental blood flow during pregnancy. The reported values, which average about 500 mL per minute late in pregnancy, must be viewed as approximations because of inherent errors in the methods of measurement as well as the undoubtedly appreciable changes in uterine blood flow that likely are induced by changes in body positions (Kauppila and associates, 1980).

Assali and co-workers (1953, 1960), Metcalfe and colleagues (1955), and Blechner and associates (1975), using the nitrous oxide method to estimate uteroplacental blood flow in human pregnancy, found that the total flow averages about 500 mL per minute at term. Browne and Veall (1953) arrived at approximately the same values, calculating the rate of disappearance of [24]Na.

Rekonen and co-workers (1976) attempted measurement of intervillous and myometrial blood flow in pregnant women in the supine position using intravenously injected [133]Xe. They obtained mean values for intervillous flow of 135 mL per minute per dL and myometrial flow of 7.7 mL per minute per 100 g. Thus for a placenta of 500 g and a uterus of 1,000 g, uteroplacental blood flow estimated by this technique averaged 650 mL per minute. There was appreciable variation among individuals, although reproducibility in the same person was good.

Edman and colleagues (1981) calculated minimal placental intervillous blood flow from the placental clearance rate of maternal plasma Δ^4-androstenedione through placental estradiol-17β formation. They reported values of approximately 450 mL per minute for placental intervillous flow at or near term.

Campbell and co-workers (1983) reported on the use of pulsed Doppler techniques to study waveforms in uterine wall arteries in normal and complicated pregnancies. Normally there was appreciable diastolic flow velocity; however, in cases of fetal hypoxia and fetal growth retardation and in hypertensive pregnancies, the systolic pulsatile pattern was high but the diastolic flow was low. The use of Doppler waveform analysis to assess vascular resistance has expanded rapidly. In some fetal and maternal vessels, actual volume flow calculations can be made (see Chap. 15, p. 286).

Assali and co-workers (1968), and others, using electromagnetic flow meters, studied the effects of spontaneous and oxytocin-induced labor on uteroplacental blood flow in sheep and dogs at term. They found that uterine contractions, either spontaneous or induced, caused a decrease in uterine blood flow that was approximately proportional to the intensity of the contraction and that a tetanic contraction caused a precipitous fall in uterine blood flow. Harbert and associates (1969) made similar observations in gravid monkeys, and the same pattern of

change undoubtedly follows the myometrial contractions of human parturition.

Janbu and Nesheim (1987) measured uterine artery velocities during labor using pulsed Doppler spectrum analysis. They studied normal women in labor and correlated these Doppler waveforms with intrauterine pressure readings. They found an almost linear correlation between pressure and decreased velocity (Fig. 7–2), and with contractions generating 50 mm Hg pressure, velocity was decreased by 60 percent. However, Brar and colleagues (1988) reported no adverse effects on umbilical artery flow.

CONTROL OF UTEROPLACENTAL BLOOD FLOW

The factors that serve to regulate uteroplacental perfusion remain largely unknown. By the use of animal models and indirect methods of assessing uteroplacental perfusion in the human, however, a partial understanding is evolving.

Increases in total uterine blood flow occur progressively throughout gestation in both the human and sheep. But, there is a definite redistribution of blood flow within the gravid ovine (sheep) uterus (Makowski and co-workers, 1968). Before pregnancy, uterine blood flow is equally divided between myometrium, endometrium, and future placental implantation sites (caruncles). By the end of the first third of ovine pregnancy, endometrial blood flow is 50 percent of the total. By term, blood flow to the placental cotyledons accounts for approximately 90 percent of total uterine blood flow (Rosenfeld and associates, 1974).

There appear to be at least two distinct stages of placental development associated with the changes in distribution of uterine blood flow just noted. The first is associated with implantation and is completed near the end of the middle third of pregnancy when placental weight is maximal and total uterine blood flow temporarily plateaus at 400 to 500 mL per minute. The second stage occurs during the last third of pregnancy. At this time, there is no further placental growth. Despite this, vessel diameters increase without an increase in the number of endothelial cells (Teasdale, 1976) and placental blood flow doubles to values of approximately 900 to 1,000 mL per minute. These observations imply, at least, that vasodilation is occurring at this time.

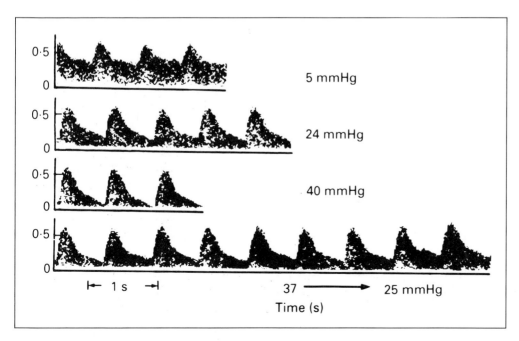

Figure 7–2. Doppler waveforms from a branch of the uterine artery in a normal woman during spontaneous labor. Uterine pressures were measured using an intrauterine catheter. In the top three panels, decreased diastolic blood flow velocity follows increased intrauterine pressures from 5 to 40 mm Hg. In the bottom panel, the spectrum following decreased pressure from 37 to 25 mm Hg is seen. (*From Janbu and Nesheim: Br J Obstet Gynecol 94:1150, 1987, with permission.*)

What actually induces the increase in uterine blood flow during the first two-thirds of ovine pregnancy is not clearly understood. There is, however, no doubt that it is in part the consequence of increasing placental size and number of blood vessels (Teasdale, 1976). An additional factor may be the localized production of Wharton's jelly, a major component of which is glucosamine. Greiss and Wagner (1983) reported that glucosamine can induce significant increases in uteroplacental blood flow and may function locally to redistribute blood flow early in pregnancy from the endometrium and myometrium to the uterine caruncles and placental cotyledons. The role, if any, of prostaglandins at this stage or later in pregnancy remain to be defined.

During the last third of ovine pregnancy, the increase in maternal-placental blood flow occurs principally by means of vasodilation whereas fetal-placental blood flow is increased by a continuing increase in placental vessels (Teasdale, 1976). This appears to result in an optimal match of maternal and fetal placental blood flows such that maternal-fetal transfer should be maximal. It appears likely that this late-pregnancy vasodilation is at least in part the consequence of estrogen stimulation (Rosenfeld and co-workers, 1976). The administration of estradiol-17β to sheep late in pregnancy can cause an increase in placental blood flow by as much as 25 percent without a change in perfusion pressure, further evidence of placental vasodilation (Rosenfeld and co-workers, 1976). Moreover, Naden and Rosenfeld (1985) showed that estradiol-17β administration to nonpregnant sheep induced cardiovascular changes similar to those observed in pregnant animals.

The observation that estrogen-induced increased uterine blood flow by vasodilation could be partially blocked by surgical and/or anesthetic stress (Killam and colleagues, 1973; Rosenfeld and associates, 1973) is consistent with the hypothesis that vascular systems are likely responsive to a number of vasoactive compounds such as catecholamines and angiotensin II. This hypothesis has been confirmed.

Catecholamines

Both epinephrine and norepinephrine cause significant decreases in placental perfusion in sheep even in the absence of any change in arterial blood pressure (Rosenfeld and co-workers, 1976; Rosenfeld and West, 1977). Such a response is likely the consequence of a greater sensitivity to catecholamines of the uteroplacental vascular beds when compared with the systemic vasculature. It is worrisome to speculate that any stressful situation—for example, pain, anesthesia, and/or surgery—that results in an elevation of catecholamines may decrease uteroplacental perfusion even in the absence of an elevation in blood pressure.

Angiotensin II

Vascular refractoriness to the pressor effects of angiotensin II appears to be a normal response of both human (Chesley and associates, 1965; Gant and co-workers, 1973) and ovine pregnancy (Rosenfeld and Gant, 1981; Naden and Rosenfeld, 1981). Despite a marked refractoriness of the systemic vasculature to angiotensin II, the uterine vasculature in sheep is even more refractory. This is clearly illustrated in Figure 7–3, where greater changes in mean arterial blood pressure and systemic vascular resistance are found at lower doses of infused angiotensin II compared with changes in uterine vascular resistance. This observation has been confirmed and expanded by Matsuura and co-workers (1983) who reported that the systemic infusion of hypertonic saline caused a decrease in systemic vascular resistance to angiotensin II but did not affect uterine vascular resistance.

The physiological implications of uterine vascular refractoriness to angiotensin II are not immediately apparent but may be of signal importance. This response may result in a potential advantage to the fetus in cases where there is a decreased refractoriness of the systemic vasculature to pressor agents (increased sensitivity to pressor agents), as occurs in women destined to develop pregnancy-induced hypertension and where uterine vascular refractoriness to pressor agents is maintained at least initially. This would be expected to result in an increased uteroplacental perfusion in such pregnancies prior to the development of actual hypertension. Such a situation is known to occur in women destined to develop pregnancy-induced hypertension (Gant and associates, 1972, 1976). In these women, uteroplacental blood flow, as reflected by the metabolic clearance rate of dehydroisoandrosterone sulfate, is increased initially, then falls as pregnancy advances and hypertension develops or worsens (Fig. 7–4). The initial increase in uteroplacental blood flow likely results as a consequence of a blunted uterine vascular resistance to angiotensin II, and possibly other pressor agents as well, compared with systemic vascular resistance (Fig. 7–3). Uteroplacental perfusion then decreases as uterine vascular resistance increases compared with systemic vascular resistance (Fig. 7–3). This is analogous to the effect observed on the uteroplacental vasculature which occurs at higher doses of infused angiotensin II when uterine vascular resistance exceeds mean arterial pressure, resulting in decreased uterine blood flow.

These observations have additional clinical significance as to whether mild to moderate blood pressure increases, such as in women with chronic hypertension, should be treated with antihypertensive drugs during pregnancy. Antihypertensive drugs may cause a greater decrease in vascular resistance than in uterine vascular resistance, thereby resulting in a greater fall in uterine blood

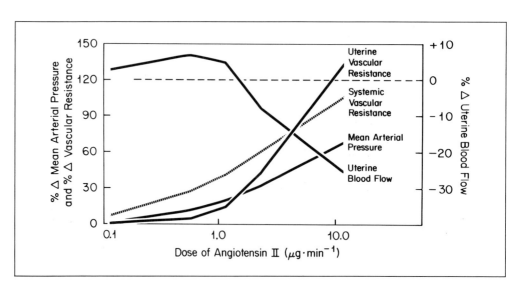

Figure 7–3. The relative changes in uterine blood flow, mean arterial pressure, systemic vascular resistance, and uterine vascular resistance during the systemic infusion of angiotensin II in term pregnant ewes. Responses were recorded after 4 to 5 minutes of stabilization at each dose of angiotensin II. *(From Rosenfeld: Sem Perinatol 8:42, 1984.)*

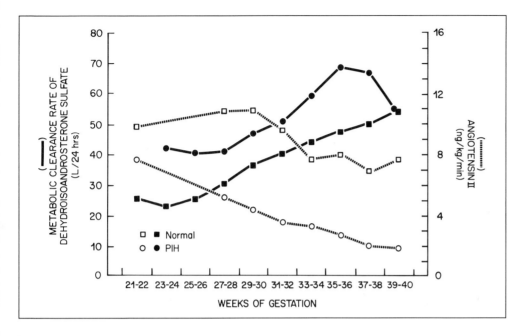

Figure 7–4. Comparison of the metabolic clearance rate of dehydroisoandrosterone sulfate and the amount of angiotensin II required to evoke a standard pressor response in primigravidas who remained normotensive (*squares*) and in primigravidas who subsequently developed pregnancy-induced hypertension (*circles*). (*Adapted from Excerpta Medica Int Congr Series 273:1026, 1972; J Clin Invest 52:2682, 1982; Gant and co-workers: Obstet Gynecol 47:319, 1976.*)

flow. Such a possible risk has been confirmed, not as a consequence of antihypertensive therapy, but as a consequence of the **hypotensive side effect** of tocolytic treatment with calcium channel blocking drugs. Such agents produce significant reductions in peripheral vascular resistance in the pregnant sheep. The reduction in peripheral vascular resistance apparently exceeds that occurring with uterine vascular resistance and this results in a decrease in uteroplacental blood flow. The reduction in uteroplacental blood flow leads to fetal acidemia (Besinger and Niebyl, 1988; Murad and associates, 1985). Similar fetal acidemia has been noted in human neonates after maternal treatment with calcium channel blockers. Gant and colleagues (1976) found that uteroplacental perfusion appeared to be greater in pregnancies complicated by moderate essential hypertension than in normotensive women. This also likely is the consequence of an increased arterial blood pressure (less refractoriness of the systemic vascular tree to pressor agents) and a greater refractoriness of the uterine vasculature to pressor agents resulting in an increased blood flow as described in women destined to develop pregnancy-induced hypertension and in the angiotensin II studies conducted during ovine pregnancy.

Whereas many of the studies described above were conducted in pregnant sheep, thus far these studies are consistent with less extensive and certainly less invasive studies conducted during human pregnancy. The interested reader is referred to the review by Rosenfeld (1984).

CHANGES IN THE CERVIX

During pregnancy, pronounced softening and cyanosis of the cervix occurs, often demonstrable as early as a month after conception. These changes comprise two of the very earliest physical signs of pregnancy (Chap. 2). The factors responsible for these changes are increased vascularity and edema of the entire cervix, together with hypertrophy and hyperplasia of the cervical glands.

As shown in Figure 7–5A and B, the glands of the cervical mucosa undergo such marked proliferation that by the end of pregnancy, they occupy approximately one-half of the entire mass of the cervix, rather than a small fraction, as in the nonpregnant state. Moreover, the septa separating the glandular spaces become progressively thinner, resulting in the formation of a structure resembling a honeycomb, the meshes of which are filled with tenacious mucus. Soon after conception a clot of very thick mucus obstructs the cervical canal. At the onset of labor, if not before, this so-called *mucus plug* is expelled resulting in a *bloody show*. The glands near the external os proliferate beneath the stratified squamous epithelium of the portio vaginalis, giving the cervix the velvety consistency characteristic of pregnancy.

So-called *erosions* of the cervix are common during pregnancy. These lesions are customarily red and velvety in appearance and are covered by columnar epithelium, spreading from the external os to involve the portio vaginalis of the cervix to various degrees. The high frequency of cervical *erosions* in pregnancy is best explained on the basis that these are not abnormal, but rather represent an extension, or *eversion*, of the proliferating endocervical glands and the columnar endocervical epithelium. Although the term *erosion* implies an "eating out" or ulceration, of the covering epithelium, the cause in pregnancy is rarely inflammatory.

During pregnancy, there is a change in the consistency of the cervical mucus. In the great majority of pregnant women, cervical mucus, spread and dried on a glass slide, is characterized by fragmentary crystallization, or *beading*, typical of the effect of progesterone (see Chap. 3, p. 37). Arborization of the crystals, or *ferning*, however, is not necessarily associated with a poor outcome of pregnancy (Salvatore, 1968). Chrétien (1978), employing scanning electron microscopy, has studied the structural variations in cervical mucus during normal pregnancy.

During pregnancy, basal cells near the squamocolumnar junction of the cervix, histologically are likely to be prominent in size, shape, and staining qualities. These changes are considered by most authorities to be estrogen-induced (Hellman and colleagues, 1954). Although the cervix contains a small amount of smooth muscle, its major component is connective tissue. The cervix undergoes profound changes during pregnancy, including a rearrangement of collagen-rich connective tissue to produce a 12-fold reduction in mechanical strength (Rechberger and colleagues, 1988) (see Chap. 10, p. 212).

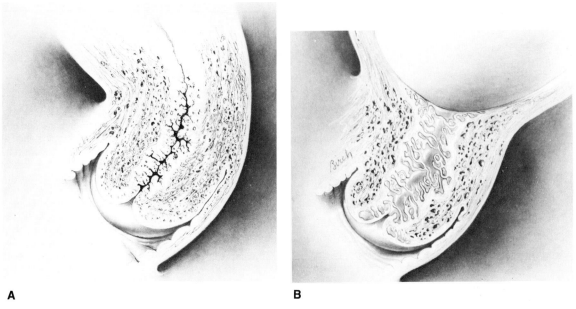

Figure 7–5. Changes in the cervix induced by pregnancy. **A.** Cervix in the nonpregnant woman. **B.** Cervix in pregnancy. Note the elaboration of the mucosa into a honeycomb-like structure, the meshes of which are filled with a tenacious mucus plug.

OVARIES AND FALLOPIAN TUBES

OVARIAN FUNCTION

Ovulation ceases during pregnancy and the maturation of new follicles is suspended. Ordinarily, only a single corpus luteum of pregnancy can be found in the ovaries of pregnant women. In gonadotropin-induced pregnancies, Yoshima and associates (1969) found that the level of plasma progesterone after having risen during the luteal phase of the ovarian cycle reached a nadir by the 8th week of pregnancy (6th week post ovulation) and then rose again. Such a nadir was not observed by Tulchinsky and Hobel (1973) in spontaneous ovulatory cycles, but instead a less rapid increase or plateau in plasma progesterone levels was found. By contrast, maternal plasma 17α-hydroxyprogesterone levels continued to decline in early pregnancy to a level only somewhat greater than those found during the luteal phase. Thus, the corpus luteum of pregnancy most likely functions maximally during the first 6 to 7 weeks of pregnancy (4 to 5 weeks post ovulation), and thereafter, the corpus luteum contributes relatively little to progesterone production during the remainder of human pregnancy. This has been confirmed in vivo by the surgical removal of the corpus luteum before 7 weeks gestation (5 weeks post ovulation), which results in a rapid fall in maternal serum progesterone and abortion (Csapo and co-workers, 1973). After this time in pregnancy, however, corpus luteum removal ordinarily does not cause abortion or labor.

RELAXIN

Human relaxin (M_r about 6,000) is a protein hormone composed of nonidentical A and B chains of similar length. There are structural features of relaxin that are similar to insulin and insulin-like growth factors I and II. As is the case for insulin, relaxin is synthesized initially as a single chain preprohormone that includes the signal peptide: B chain: connecting peptide: A

chain. Although the gene for human insulin is located on the short arm of chromosome 11 and the two genes for relaxin on the short arm of chromosome 9, Crawford and associates (1984) concluded that the insulin and relaxin genes separated during a chromosomal translocation involving a breakpoint between the two genes. They also hypothesized that the two human relaxin genes evolved by a second gene duplication. The reason for the two human relaxin genes is unknown but relaxin gene 2 appears to be the functional member of the two.

The variation in structure of relaxin from species to species is remarkable and likely accounts for the various effects attributed to the use of relaxin from one species to study biological events in a second species. Therefore, studies of the effects of relaxin in the human using nonhuman sources of relaxin must be viewed with suspicion until confirmed with human relaxin. Sources of human relaxin are now available since Hudson and co-workers (1983) cloned a human gene capable of encoding biologically active human relaxin.

Human relaxin is secreted by the corpus luteum of pregnancy and possibly by uterine decidua during pregnancy. The pattern of secretion is similar to human chorionic gonadotropin (Eddie and co-workers, 1986). Therefore, secretion of relaxin differs from that of ovarian steroid hormones. Whereas 17-α-hydroxyprogesterone and likely progesterone secretion by the corpus luteum declines to negligible rates by the 7th to 8th gestational week, appreciable relaxin secretion continues throughout pregnancy (Eddie and associates, 1986).

The decidua has been reported to secrete human relaxin but significant amounts, as yet, have not been obtained from decidual tissue. In fact, the amounts of relaxin present in human decidua appear to be quite low compared with the corpus luteum.

The role of relaxin during human pregnancy is not defined. Although relaxin is a major myometrial inhibitory substance in the pregnant guinea pig uterus (Porter, 1972), the hormone is not essential to the maintenance of human pregnancy (Bryant-Greenwood, 1982). The mechanism of action of relaxin in producing uterine relaxation during rat pregnancy and likely in other animals as well is very similar to the action of β-mimetic drugs. Specifically, relaxin appears to react or combine with a β-adrenergic receptor on the cell membrane to stimulate an increase in adenylate cyclase, which in turn increases cyclic AMP and protein kinase. The protein kinase then disassociates into a regulatory subunit–cyclic AMP complex and an active protein kinase subunit that promotes the phosphorylation of intracellular proteins. Thus, as cyclic AMP and protein kinase activities increase, the affinity of myosin light chain kinase for the calmodulin-calcium complex decreases resulting in a reduction in myosin light chain phosphorylation and actomyosin ATPase. The result is uterine muscle relaxation (Sanborn, 1986). Whether such a mechanism occurs in the human as either a primary or secondary modulating system for maintaining uterine relaxation is not known.

The role of human relaxin in producing softening and effacement of the uterine cervix also is unknown. The topical administration of pharmacological doses of a highly purified porcine relaxin to the human cervix, however, results in cervical softening and effacement, as well as a more successful rate of labor inductions in treated versus untreated women (Evans and colleagues, 1983; Porter, 1980).

A variety of other actions of relaxin have been reported in animals including changes in blood pressure, changes in symphysis mobility, regulation of lactation, and remodeling of connective tissues. Such effects vary from animal species to species, but there is little evidence to support such actions in the human. The origin, production, secretion, and actions of relaxin in a variety of animal species, as well as in man, were presented recently in an excellent review by Sherwood (1988).

PREGNANCY LUTEOMA

In 1963, Sternberg described a solid ovarian tumor that developed during pregnancy that was composed of large acidophilic luteinized cells. The observations of Krause and Stembridge (1966) and Garcia-Bunuel and co-workers (1975) are consistent with the view that a luteoma of pregnancy represents an exaggeration of the luteinization reaction of the ovary of normal pregnancy and is not a true neoplasm. The luteoma regresses after delivery, and normal ovarian function returns even in those instances in which the luteoma is responsible transiently for maternal virilization. In the immediate puerperal state, the luteoma may be responsive to exogenously administered hCG (Cohen and associates, 1982). These lesions may recur in subsequent pregnancies (Shortle and associates, 1987).

Even though maternal virilization may be prominent, the female fetus usually is not affected, presumably because of the protective role of the placenta through its high capacity to convert androgens and androgen-like steroids to estrogens (Edman and co-workers, 1979). There is no question, however, that a female fetus can in some cases be virilized (Cohen and associates, 1982; Hensleigh and Woodruff, 1978; Verkauf and co-workers, 1977).

HYPERREACTIO LUTEINALIS

Hyperreactio luteinalis is a second benign lesion of the ovary that causes maternal virilization during pregnancy. While the cellular pattern is similar to that of a luteoma of pregnancy, the two tumors are different grossly. The luteoma is a solid and the

hyperreactio luteinalis a cystic tumor. Additionally, hyperreactio luteinalis commonly is associated with extremely high human chorionic gonadotropin values (Muechler and colleagues, 1987). An excellent review of the anatomical, microscopic, and clinical characteristics of luteomas of pregnancy and hyperreactio luteinalis was presented by Hensleigh and Woodruff (1978). Virilization of the female fetus may occur with hyperreactio luteinalis, but the incidence is much less than with a luteoma.

> Why one fetus will be virilized and another not remains incompletely understood. Edman and associates (1979) presented evidence that the androgens produced in at least two cases of luteoma of pregnancy are extensively converted into estrogens in the placenta, thus serving to protect the fetus. Cohen and associates (1982) speculated that in some cases, the high androgen levels might in fact suppress testosterone-binding globulin resulting in more free testosterone. Another possibility is that 5α-reductase activity is increased (or not suppressed) resulting in higher concentrations of 5α-dihydrotestosterone. Even more critical is the time at which androgen levels are presented to the fetal compartment. That is, if excessive androgen levels are present early enough in pregnancy, their concentration may exceed the enzymatic capacity of a small placenta to clear the androgens into estrogens.

OTHER CHANGES

A *decidual* reaction on and beneath the surface of the ovaries, similar to that found in the endometrial stroma, is common in pregnancy and may be observed at cesarean section. These elevated patches of tissue bleed easily and may, on first glance, resemble freshly torn adhesions. Similar decidual reactions are occasionally seen on the posterior uterine serosa and upon or within other pelvic or even extrapelvic abdominal organs.

By inspection of the ovarian veins at cesarean section, their enormous caliber is startling. Through actual measurement, Hodgkinson (1953) found that the diameter of the ovarian vascular pedicle increased during pregnancy from 0.9 cm to approximately 2.6 cm at term.

FALLOPIAN TUBES

The musculature of the fallopian tubes undergoes little hypertrophy during pregnancy. The epithelium of the tubal mucosa is flattened during gestation, compared to that of the nonpregnant state. Decidual cells may develop in the stroma of the endosalpinx, but a continuous decidual membrane is not formed.

VAGINA AND PERINEUM

During pregnancy increased vascularity and hyperemia develop in the skin and muscles of the perineum and vulva and there is softening of the normally abundant connective tissue of these structures.

Increased vascularity prominently affects the vagina. The copious secretion and the characteristic violet color of the vagina during pregnancy (*Chadwick's sign*), similar to the changes that occur in the cervix during pregnancy, probably result chiefly from hyperemia. The vaginal walls undergo striking changes seemingly in preparation for the distension that occurs during labor, with a considerable increase in thickness of the mucosa, loosening of the connective tissue, and hypertrophy of the smooth-muscle cells to nearly the same extent as in the uterus. These changes effect such an increase in length of the vaginal walls that sometimes, in parous women, the lower portion of the anterior vaginal wall protrudes slightly through the vulvar opening. The papillae of the vaginal mucosa also undergo considerable hypertrophy, creating a fine hobnailed appearance.

VAGINAL SECRETION

The considerably increased cervical and vaginal secretion during pregnancy consists of a somewhat thick, white discharge. Its pH is acidic, varying from 3.5 to 6, the result of increased production of lactic acid from glycogen in the vaginal epithelium by the action of *Lactobacillus acidophilus*. The acidic pH probably serves to control the rate of multiplication of pathogenic bacteria in the vagina.

VAGINAL CYTOLOGY

Early in pregnancy the vaginal epithelial cells are similar to those found during the luteal phase of the menstrual cycle (see Chap. 3, p. 36), but as pregnancy advances, two patterns of response are seen:

1. Small intermediate cells, called navicular cells by Papanicolaou, are found in abundance in small, dense clusters. The ovoid navicular cell contains a vesicular, somewhat elongated nucleus.
2. Vesicular nuclei without cytoplasm, or so-called naked nuclei, are evident along with an abundance of *Lactobacillus*, a normal organism in the vagina.

ABDOMINAL WALL AND SKIN

STRIAE GRAVIDARUM

In the later months of pregnancy, reddish, slightly depressed streaks commonly develop in the skin of the abdomen and sometimes in the skin over the breasts and thighs. These striae gravidarum occur in about one-half of all pregnant women. In multiparous women, in addition to the reddish striae of the present pregnancy, glistening, silvery lines that represent the cicatrices of previous striae are seen frequently.

DIASTASIS RECTI

Occasionally the muscles of the abdominal walls do not withstand the tension to which they are subjected, and the rectus muscles separate in the midline, creating a diastasis recti of varying extent. If severe, a considerable portion of the anterior uterine wall is covered by only a layer of skin, attenuated fascia, and peritoneum. In extreme instances, herniation of the gravid uterus through the diastasis may be so great that the fundus of the uterus drops below the level of the pelvic inlet when the woman is standing.

PIGMENTATION

In many women, the midline of the abdominal skin becomes markedly pigmented, assuming a brownish-black color to form the *linea nigra*. Occasionally, irregular brownish patches of varying size appear on the face and neck, giving rise to *chloasma* or *melasma gravidarum* (*mask of pregnancy*), which, fortunately, usually disappears, or at least regresses considerably, after delivery. Oral contraceptives may cause similar pigmentation in these same women. There is very little known of the nature of these pigmentary changes, although melanocyte-stimulating

hormone, a polypeptide similar to ACTH, has been shown to be remarkably elevated from the end of the second month of pregnancy until term.

It is known, however, that pro–opinomelanocorticotrophin is metabolized in the intermediate lobe of the pituitary to β-endorphin and to α-melanotrophin (α-MSH). This activity is under the inhibitory influence of dopaminic control, which when blocked results in a marked increase in β-endorphin plasma levels in pregnant *but not in nonpregnant women* (Abou-Samra and co-workers, 1984). The response in the pregnant but not in the nonpregnant women likely is due to hypertrophy of the intermediate lobe of the pituitary gland during pregnancy. Thus, it may be that estrogen and progesterone stimulation during pregnancy results in hypertrophy of the intermediate lobe with an increased release of β-endorphin and *possibly* α-MSH.

Estrogen and progesterone have been reported to exert a melanocyte-stimulating effect (Diczfalusy and Troen, 1961).

CUTANEOUS VASCULAR CHANGES

Angiomas, called *vascular spiders,* develop in about two thirds of white women and approximately 10 percent of black women during pregnancy (Bean and colleagues, 1949). These are minute, red elevations on the skin, particularly common on the face, neck, upper chest, and arms, with radicles branching out from a central body. The condition is often designated as nevus, angioma, or telangiectasis. *Palmar erythema* is also frequently encountered in pregnancy, having been observed by Bean and associates in about two thirds of white women and one third of black women. The two conditions frequently occur together but are of no clinical significance and disappear in most women shortly after the termination of pregnancy. The high incidence of vascular spiders and palmar erythema in pregnancy is most likely the consequence of the hyperestrogenemia of pregnancy.

BREASTS

During pregnancy, striking changes occur in the breasts. In the early weeks, the pregnant woman often experiences tenderness and tingling of the breasts. After the 2nd month, the breasts increase in size and become nodular as a result of hypertrophy of the mammary alveoli. As the breasts increase in size, delicate veins become visible just beneath the skin. The changes in the nipples and areolae are even more characteristic. The nipples become considerably larger, more deeply pigmented, and more erectile. After the first few months, a thick, yellowish fluid, *colostrum*, often can be expressed from the nipples by gentle massage. At that time, the areolae become broader and more deeply pigmented. The depth of pigmentation varies with the woman's complexion. Scattered through the areolae are a number of small elevations, the so-called glands (follicles) of Montgomery, which are hypertrophic sebaceous glands. If the increase in size of the breasts is very extensive, striations similar to those observed in the abdomen may develop. Histological and functional changes of the breasts induced by pregnancy and lactation are discussed further in Chapter 13 (p. 248).

METABOLIC CHANGES

In response to the rapidly growing fetus and placenta and their increasing demands, the pregnant woman undergoes metabolic changes that are numerous and intense. Certainly no other physiological event in postnatal life induces such profound metabolic alterations.

WEIGHT GAIN

Most of the increase in weight during pregnancy is attributable to the uterus and its contents, the breasts, and increases in blood volume and extravascular extracellular fluid. A smaller fraction of the increased weight is the result of metabolic alterations which result in an increase in cellular water and deposition of new fat and protein, so-called maternal reserves. Chesley (1944) reported that the average total weight gain in pregnancy was 24 lb (11 kg). During the first trimester, the average gain was 2 lb (1 kg), compared to about 11 lb (5 kg) during each of the last two trimesters. More recently, Hytten (1981) reported similar but somewhat higher average weights for English women (Table 7–1).

Hytten and Leitch (1971) have calculated the excess energy costs for normal pregnancy to be 80,000 kcal (335 MJ). Illingworth and associates (1987) found that the energetic response to a mixed constituent meal was reduced by 28 percent in midtrimester. They suggested that this was a maternal adaptation to increased energetic efficiency at the time fetal demands were highest. Oxygen consumption with exercise is apparently reduced at 35 weeks gestation compared to 15 and 25 weeks and postpartum (McMurray and colleagues, 1988).

WATER METABOLISM

Increased water retention is a normal physiological alteration of pregnancy. This is mediated, at least in part, by a fall in plasma osmolality of approximately 10 milliosmoles per kg induced by a resetting of osmotic thresholds for thirst and vasopressin secretion (Lindheimer and co-workers, 1987a). This phenomenon was demonstrated by Brown and associates (1988) to be operable by midpregnancy. Marked retention of sodium and water, however, with the development of edema, is commonly present with pregnancy-induced hypertension. An excellent review of the control of sodium excretion in normal and hypertensive pregnancies has been presented by Gallery and Brown (1987).

At term, the water content of the fetus, placenta, and amnionic fluid amounts to about 3.5 L. Approximately 3.0 L more water accumulates as a result of increases in the maternal blood volume and in the size of the uterus and the breasts. Thus, the minimum amount of extra water that the average woman could be expected to retain during normal pregnancy is about 6.5 L. Clearly demonstrable pitting edema of the ankles and legs occurs in a substantial proportion of pregnant women, especially at the end of the day, before retiring. This accumulation of fluid, which may amount to a liter or so, is caused by an increase in venous pressure below the level of the uterus as a consequence of partial occlusion of the vena cava by the gravid uterus (p. 147). A decrease in interstitial colloid osmotic pressure induced by normal pregnancy also favors edema formation late in pregnancy (Øian and co-workers, 1985).

The amount of water to be mobilized and excreted by the mother after delivery will depend upon the amount retained during pregnancy, the degree of hydration or dehydration during labor, and the amount of blood lost at delivery. In normal primiparas without demonstrable edema before vaginal delivery, weight loss during the first 10 days after delivery averaged nearly 5 pounds (2 kg) (Dennis and Bytheway, 1965).

PROTEIN METABOLISM

The products of conception, as well as the uterus and maternal blood, are relatively rich in protein rather than fat or carbohydrate. Nonetheless, their protein content is rather small compared with the total body protein of the mother. At term, the fetus and placenta together weigh about 4 kg and contain approximately 500 g of protein, or about one half of the total increase normally induced by pregnancy (Hytten and Leitch, 1971; Widdowson, 1968). The remaining 500 g of protein is added to the uterus as contractile protein, to the breasts primarily in the glands, and to the maternal blood in the form of hemoglobin and plasma proteins.

The utilization of ingested protein is dependent upon the protein's digestibility and amino acid composition. The *biological value* of ingested protein is defined as the percent of the absorbed nitrogen retained by the body. The product of the biological value and *digestibility* gives the net *protein utilization* (National Research Council, Food and Nutrition Board, 1974). The human appears to utilize high-quality protein such as egg protein at a rate of approximately 70 percent, so this arbitrarily has been assigned a protein utilization value of 100. Using the egg protein value of 100, it is estimated that the protein utilization value of the average American diet is approximately 75.

TABLE 7–1. DISTRIBUTION OF WEIGHT GAIN DURING PREGNANCY

Tissue/Fluid	Increase in Weight in Grams (and Pounds)[a] up to:			
	10 wk	*20 wk*	*30 wk*	*40 wk*
Fetus	5 (0.01)	300 (0.7)	1,500 (3.3)	3,400 (7.5)
Placenta	20 (0.04)	170 (0.4)	430 (0.9)	650 (1.4)
Amnionic fluid	30 (0.07)	350 (0.8)	750 (1.7)	800 (1.8)
Uterus	140 (0.3)	320 (0.7)	600 (1.3)	970 (2.1)
Breasts	45 (0.1)	180 (0.4)	360 (0.8)	405 (0.9)
Blood	100 (0.2)	600 (1.3)	1,300 (2.9)	1,250 (2.8)
Extracellular				
Extravascular fluid (no edema present)	0 (0)	30 (0.06)	80 (0.2)	1,680 (3.7)
Subtotal	340 (0.7)	1,950 (4.3)	5,020 (11.1)	9,155 (20.2)
Maternal reserves	310 (0.7)	2,050 (4.5)	3,480 (7.7)	3,345 (7.4)
Total weight gain	650 (1.4)	4,000 (8.8)	8,500 (18.7)	12,500 (27.5)

[a]Where possible, numbers are rounded to the nearest one-tenth pound.
Modified from Hytten and Chamberlain: Clinical Physiology in Obstetrics, 1981, p 221, Table 7.8.

From nitrogen balance studies in pregnant women, however, it appears that actual nitrogen utilization is only 26 percent (Calloway, 1974). Therefore, daily requirements for protein intake during pregnancy are increased appreciably (Chap. 14, p. 263) to correct for this and to supply the increased protein demands.

Equally important to an increase in protein in pregnancy is the ingestion of adequate sources of energy foods, e.g., carbohydrates and fat. If these are not consumed in adequate amounts, the energy requirements of the mother must be met by catabolism of maternal protein stores. The liberated amino acids used for energy are not available for synthesis of maternal protein (King, 1975). Therefore, with increasing intake of fat and carbohydrates as energy sources, less dietary protein is required to maintain a positive nitrogen balance, a concept proven in a study conducted in Guatemala in which a dietary supplement containing only energy sources was provided. The use of this approach in Guatemala served to reduce infant mortality by one half (Habicht and associates, 1973). This observation is important and is consistent with the view that the concept of "empty calories" or of "nonnutritious calories" is not valid, at least during pregnancy.

Concentrations of several plasma proteins are altered by pregnancy. The albumin concentration decreases significantly (p. 151) while fibrinogen rises (p. 143). The concentrations of IgG, IgA, and IgM fall somewhat (Amino and colleagues, 1978). The plasma concentrations of α_1-antitrypsin, α_2-macroglobulin, ceruloplasmin, and transferrin all increase, but complement C_3 and haptoglobin apparently are not changed (Killingsworth, 1979).

CARBOHYDRATE METABOLISM

Pregnancy is potentially diabetogenic. Diabetes mellitus may be aggravated by pregnancy and clinical diabetes may appear in some women only during pregnancy. Consequently, considerable attention has been focused on the metabolism of carbohydrates and insulin in pregnant women. In healthy women, the fasting plasma glucose concentration falls somewhat during pregnancy, possibly due to increased plasma levels of insulin (Lind, 1979; Spellacy and Goetz, 1963). The increased levels of insulin cannot be explained, however, by a change in the metabolism of insulin because the half-life of insulin during pregnancy is not changed (Lind and associates, 1977). Whereas the exact mechanisms responsible for the beta cell hypertrophy, hyperplasia, and hypersecretion observed in pregnancy are not understood completely, estrogen, progesterone, and human placental lactogen likely are involved.

The peak in human placental lactogen concentrations corresponds to the greatest insulin responses by the beta cell (Freinkel, 1980). Furthermore, it has been reported that human placental lactogen acts to stimulate directly the synthesis and secretion of insulin in mouse islet cells in culture (Nielsen, 1982). Regardless, these changes regress rapidly postpartum (Hubinont and colleagues, 1988).

Progesterone, when administered to nonpregnant adults in amounts similar to that produced during pregnancy, results in increased basal insulin concentrations and similar responses to oral glucose challenges as those found in normal pregnant women (Bender and Chickering, 1985). Additionally, estradiol induces hyperinsulinism in both control and oopherectomized rats (Faure and associates, 1983).

The increased basal level of plasma insulin observed in normal pregnancy is associated with several unique responses

to the ingestion of glucose. For example, after an oral glucose meal, there is both prolonged hyperglycemia and hyperinsulinemia in pregnant women with a greater suppression of glucagon (Lind, 1979; Phelps and associates, 1981). The purpose of such a mechanism likely is to ensure a sustained or maintained postprandial supply of glucose to the fetus. This response is consistent with a pregnancy-induced state of peripheral resistance to insulin (Freinkel and colleagues, 1985; Lind, 1979).

The existence of tissue resistance to insulin during pregnancy is suggested by three observations: (1) increased insulin response to glucose (increased plasma level and duration); (2) reduced peripheral uptake of glucose (increased plasma level and duration); and (3) suppressed glucagon response (Lind, 1979). The mechanism(s) responsible for the tissue resistance to insulin is not understood completely. Progesterone and estrogen may act, directly or indirectly to mediate this resistance to insulin (Bauman and colleagues, 1981; Tsibris and co-workers, 1980). The plasma levels of human placental lactogen increase with gestation and this protein hormone is characterized by growth hormone-like action that may result in increased lipolysis and increased liberation of free fatty acids (Freinkel, 1980). The increased concentration of circulating free fatty acids also may facilitate increased tissue resistance to insulin.

The mechanisms cited ensure that a continuous supply of glucose is available for transfer to the fetus. The pregnant woman, however, changes rapidly from a postprandial state characterized by elevated and sustained glucose levels to a fasting state characterized by decreased plasma glucose and amino acids such as alanine. There also are higher plasma concentrations of free fatty acids, triglycerides, and cholesterol in the pregnant woman during fasting (Fig. 7–6). Freinkel and colleagues (1985) have referred to this pregnancy-induced switch in fuels from glucose to lipids as "accelerated starvation." Certainly, when fasting is prolonged in the pregnant woman, these alterations are exaggerated and ketonemia appears rapidly (Bender and Chickering, 1985).

Insulinase activity has been found in the human placenta. It seems unlikely, however, that accelerated degradation of insulin by placental insulinase contributes appreciably to the diabetogenic state induced by pregnancy, since the rate of degradation of radiolabeled insulin in vivo does not appear to differ among pregnant and nonpregnant women (Burt and Davidson, 1974).

The role of glucagon during pregnancy is not totally defined. Hornnes and Kuhl (1980) measured glucagon and insulin responses to a standard glucose stimulus in the same women late in normal pregnancy and again postpartum. The insulin response to glucose infusion was increased 3.8 times in late pregnancy. The glucagon suppression was similar in late pregnancy and the puerperium. These results are consistent with the view that β-cell sensitivity to a glucose challenge is significantly increased in normal pregnant women, but the α-cell sensitivity to a glucose stimulus is unaltered during pregnancy.

FAT METABOLISM

The concentrations of lipids and lipo- and apolipoproteins in plasma increase appreciably during pregnancy (Figs. 7–6 and 7–7). Plasma levels of lipids increase continuously throughout gestation and Desoye and co-workers (1987) found by time-series analysis that there were positive correlations between the concentrations of lipids (shown in Fig. 7–6) with those of estradiol, progesterone, and human placental lactogen.

Apolipoproteins AI, AII, and B concentrations increase until weeks 25, 28, and 28 respectively, and then usually remain

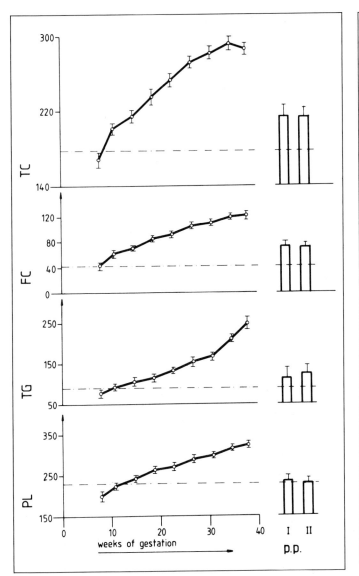

Figure 7–6. Mean (± SEM) plasma lipid concentrations (mg per dL) throughout gestation (N = 42) and during the luteal (I) and follicular (II) phases postpartum (p.p.; N = 23). The *dashed lines* represent the mean values of the control group (N = 24). TC = total cholesterol; FC = free cholesterol; TG = triglycerides; PL = phospholipids. (*From Desoye and associates: J Clin Endocrinol Metab 64:704, 1987, with permission.*)

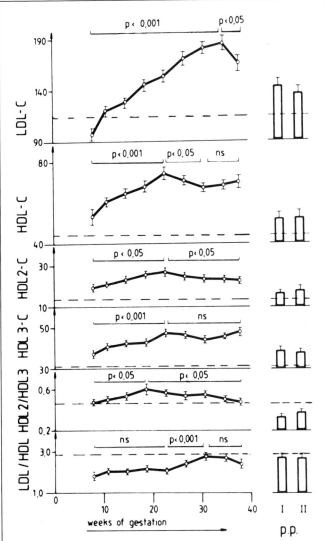

Figure 7–7. Mean (± SEM) plasma lipoprotein cholesterol levels (mg per dL) throughout gestation (N = 42) and during the luteal (I) and follicular (II) phases postpartum (p.p.; N = 23). The *dashed lines* represent the mean values of the control group (100 percent). LDL-C = low-density lipoprotein cholesterol; HDL-C = high-density lipoprotein cholesterol; HDL2-C = high-density lipoprotein-2 cholesterol; HDL3-C = high-density lipoprotein-3 cholesterol. (*From Desoye and associates: J Clin Endocrinol Metab 64:704, 1987, with permission.*)

unchanged until delivery (figure not shown). The concentration changes in apolipoprotein B are similar to those of estradiol after a 2-week time shift and this effect may be causally related (Desoye and associates, 1987).

Plasma lipoprotein cholesterol levels through pregnancy are illustrated in Figure 7–7. Low-density lipoprotein cholesterol (LDL-C) levels peak at approximately week 36. High-density lipoprotein cholesterol (HDL-C) peaks at week 25, decreases until week 32, and remains constant for the remainder of pregnancy. High-density lipoprotein-2 and -3 cholesterol levels peak at approximately 28 weeks and remain unchanged throughout the remainder of pregnancy.

The increase in LDL-C is likely the consequence of the hepatic effects of estradiol and progesterone (Desoye and asso-

ciates, 1987). The decrease in LDL-C before term was paralleled by a fall in the estradiol/progesterone ratio. This, in fact, might be the consequence of increased utilization of LDL-C for placental progesterone production because the estradiol/progesterone ratio change was due principally to an increase in progesterone relative to estradiol.

The increase in HDL-C levels in the first half of gestation is believed to be caused by estrogen action. Interestingly, the decrease after weeks 22 to 24 coincides with the onset of increasing resistance to insulin and the increase in concentration of plasma insulin. Therefore, the HDL-C concentration may be controlled, in part, by insulin.

After approximately 30 weeks, HDL-C levels plateau. One possible explanation for this is that human placental lactogen, through its lipolytic activity, causes an increase in plasma concentrations of free fatty acids. The free fatty acids then may be incorporated into triglycerides and very low-density lipoproteins in the liver. The increased specific activity of hepatic lipase induced by progesterone in turn likely results in increased concentrations of high-density lipoproteins (Desoye and coworkers, 1987). Maternal lipoprotein lipase activity favors hypertriglyceridemia (Herrera and colleagues, 1988).

Handwerger and colleagues (1987) found that high-density lipoproteins stimulate, in a dose-dependent manner, the release of human placental lactogen from placental tissue explants. The stimulation also was observed after delipidation of apolipoproteins AI, AII, and CI. Furthermore, delipidation of high-density lipoprotein did not prevent its activity but tryptic digestion did. It is likely, therefore, that the high-density lipoprotein effect is due to its apoprotein components. Finally, placental cells have specific high-density lipoprotein receptors. These results are consistent with the view that high-density lipoproteins are involved in the regulation of human placental lactogen release during pregnancy in a manner possibly independent from the usual role of this lipoprotein as a plasma lipid carrier.

After delivery, the concentrations of these lipids, lipoproteins, and apolipoproteins decrease at different rates (Desoye and co-workers, 1987). Lactation increases the rate of decrease of many of these compounds (Darmady and Postle, 1982).

In pregnant women, starvation induces a more intense ketonemia (see p. 138) than occurs in nonpregnant women. For example, remarkably increased levels of plasma-free fatty acids, glycerol, and ketones were observed in women at midpregnancy who were starved experimentally for up to four days prior to abortion.

Hytten and Thomson (1968) and Pipe and co-workers (1979) concluded that storage of fat occurs primarily during midpregnancy, the fat being deposited mostly in central rather than peripheral sites. Later in pregnancy, as the nutritional demands of the fetus increase remarkably, storage of fat decreases. Hytten and Thomson cited some evidence that progesterone may act to reset a "lipostat" in the hypothalamus, and at the end of pregnancy the lipostat returns to its previous nonpregnant level and the added fat is lost. Such a mechanism for energy storage, theoretically at least, might protect the mother and fetus during times of prolonged starvation or hard physical exertion.

MINERAL METABOLISM

The requirements for iron during pregnancy are considerable and often exceed the amounts available (p. 142). With respect to most other minerals, pregnancy induces little change in their metabolism other than their retention in amounts equivalent to those used for growth of fetal and, to a lesser extent, maternal tissues (see Chap. 6, p. 97; Chap. 14, p. 264).

Copper and ceruloplasmin in the plasma increase considerably early in pregnancy because of the increases in estrogens, which will produce the same changes when administered to nonpregnant subjects (Russ and Raymunt, 1956). Vir and co-workers (1981) reported that copper levels in hair were similar in nonpregnant and pregnant women, but values in pregnancy decreased from first through third trimester. They added that there was a significant positive correlation between third trimester maternal hair and serum copper levels and neonatal weight but a significant negative correlation with respect to maternal serum copper and neonatal head circumference.

During pregnancy, calcium and magnesium levels are reduced very slightly, the reduction probably reflecting for the most part the lowered plasma protein concentration and, in turn, the consequent decrease in the amount of each electrolyte that is bound to protein. However, Fogh-Anderson and Schultz-Larsen (1981) demonstrated a small but significant increase in free calcium ion concentration in late pregnancy by correcting for blood pH changes. Serum phosphorus levels are within the nonpregnant range. Cole and co-workers (1987) reported that bone turnover was reduced during early pregnancy, returned toward normal during the third trimester and increased in postpartum lactating women. The status of zinc metabolism in pregnancy, as discussed in Chapter 14, p. 265, is currently somewhat confused.

ACID-BASE EQUILIBRIUM AND BLOOD ELECTROLYTES

Normally, the pregnant woman hyperventilates, compared with the nonpregnant subject, and this causes a respiratory alkalosis by lowering the P_{CO_2} of the blood. A moderate reduction in plasma bicarbonate from about 26 to about 22 mmol per L partially compensates for the respiratory alkalosis. As a result, there is only a minimal increase in blood pH (Sjöstedt, 1962). The increase in blood pH shifts the oxygen dissociation curve to the left and increases the affinity of maternal hemoglobin for oxygen (Bohr effect), thereby decreasing the oxygen-releasing capacity of maternal blood. Thus, the hyperventilation which results in a reduced maternal P_{CO_2} facilitates transport of carbon dioxide from the fetus to the mother but appears to impair release of oxygen from the mother's blood to the fetus. The increase in blood pH, however, while minimal, stimulates an increase in 2,3-diphosphoglycerate in maternal erythrocytes (Tsai and co-workers, 1982) which counteracts the Bohr effect by shifting the oxygen dissociation curve back to the right, facilitating oxygen release to the fetus. These subtle but important changes insure that the fetus has every advantage from blood gas exchange.

Despite large accumulations during pregnancy of sodium and potassium, the serum concentration of these electrolytes decreases. During normal pregnancy, nearly 1,000 mEq of sodium and 300 mEq of potassium are retained (Lindheimer and colleagues, 1987b). Brown and colleagues (1986, 1988) showed that sodium and potassium excretion are unchanged during pregnancy despite the fact that their filtration by the glomerulus is increased. Obviously, fractional excretion of these electrolytes is decreased, and it has been postulated that progesterone counteracts the natriuretic and kaliuretic effects of aldosterone (see p. 155).

HEMATOLOGICAL CHANGES OF NORMAL PREGNANCY

BLOOD VOLUME

The maternal blood volume increases markedly during pregnancy. In a study of 50 normal women, the blood volumes at or very near term averaged about 45 percent above their nonpregnant levels (Pritchard, 1965). This increase is similar to that described by Caton and associates (1949), by Dahlström and Ihrman (1960), and by Ueland (1976).

The degree of expansion varies considerably, and in some women there is only a modest increase and in others their blood volume nearly doubles. A fetus is not essential for the development of hypervolemia during pregnancy, for increases in blood volume identical with those found during normal pregnancy have been demonstrated in some women with hydatidiform mole (Pritchard, 1965).

The pregnancy-induced hypervolemia serves to meet the demands of the enlarged uterus with its greatly hypertrophied vascular system, to protect the mother and, in turn, the fetus against the deleterious effects of impaired venous return in the supine and erect positions, and, very importantly, to safeguard the mother against the adverse effects of blood loss associated with parturition.

The maternal blood volume starts to increase during the first trimester, expands most rapidly during the second trimester, and then rises at a much slower rate during the third trimester to attain a plateau during the last several weeks of pregnancy.

The increase in blood volume results from an increase in both plasma and erythrocytes. The usual pattern is that of an initial rise in the plasma volume, followed by an increase in the volume of circulating erythrocytes. Although more plasma than erythrocytes is usually added to the maternal circulation, the increase in the volume of circulating erythrocytes is considerable, averaging, in the 50 women previously mentioned, about 450 mL of erythrocytes, or an increase of about 33 percent. The importance of this increase in creating a demand for iron is discussed below. The increase in the volume of circulating erythrocytes in pregnancy is accomplished by accelerated production rather than by prolongation of the life span of the erythrocyte (Pritchard and Adams, 1960).

The mean age of circulating maternal red cells is lower during the latter half of pregnancy because the rate of red cell production exceeds that of destruction. The *mean cell volume* is increased with the red blood cells becoming more spherical due to a decreased diameter and an increased thickness (Bolton and colleagues, 1982).

Moderate erythroid hyperplasia is present in the bone marrow, and the reticulocyte count is elevated slightly during normal pregnancy. This is almost certainly due to increased levels of erythropoietin, which have been noted in maternal plasma and urine during pregnancy (Cotes and associates, 1983; Zivný and associates, 1982).

Jepson and Friesen (1968) reported that administration of purified human placental lactogen to polycythemic mice accelerated the incorporation of iron into their erythrocytes, an effect that was abolished by its incubation with antibody to placental lactogen but not with antisheep erythropoietin. Cotes and co-workers (1983) reported that serum erythropoietin levels and placental lactogen were significantly related. It should be noted, however, that apparently quite normal pregnancies develop with no detectable levels of placental lactogen.

ATRIAL NATRIURETIC PEPTIDE AND PLASMA VOLUME

Atrial natriuretic peptides are a group of biologically active peptides synthesized and secreted by atrial myocytes. Three separate forms (α, β, γ) of the peptide have been isolated from human atrial cells (Kangawa and Matsu, 1984; Kangawa and co-workers, 1985). The biologically active form of the peptide is not known definitely but indirect evidence has accrued that the 28-amino-acid α-atrial natriuretic peptide is the active form (Sagnella and associates, 1985).

The atrial natriuretic peptide has been reported to produce significant natriuresis and diuresis in mammals, including man.

The peptide induces an increase in renal blood flow and glomerular filtration rate and a decreased renin secretory rate (Burnett, 1984). However, the actual mechanism(s) responsible for the natriuresis remains unclear, with evidence consistent for both a hemodynamically induced natriuresis (Wakitani and colleagues, 1985) and an inhibitory effect upon tubular sodium reabsorption (Borenstein, 1983).

The atrial natriuretic peptides also have been shown to reduce basal release of aldosterone from cultured zona glomerulosa cells and to blunt ACTH and angiotensin II–stimulated release of aldosterone as well (Atarashi and associates, 1984). As mentioned earlier, the rate of renin secretion also is inhibited by this peptide (Burnett, 1984). Finally, the atrial natriuretic peptides also have a direct vasorelaxant action upon angiotensin II– or norepinephrine-stimulated vascular smooth muscle. Thus, the peptide appears to behave as a functional antagonist to endogenous vasoconstrictors (Kleinert and co-workers, 1984).

In the human, increased secretion of atrial natriuretic peptides follows volume expansion and atrial stretch and also in response to a high sodium diet (Sagnella and co-workers, 1985). Conversely, a low sodium diet results in a decrease in peptide concentration.

During normotensive pregnancy, atrial natriuretic peptides were reported by Cusson and associates (1985) and Miyamoto and colleagues (1988) to increase. This observation has not been confirmed by Rutherford (1987), Grace (1987), Hirai (1988), or Steegers (1987) and their co-workers, who found no increase. The reason for this discrepancy is not apparent but may be the result of different assay techniques. Interestingly, Rutherford and Steegers found that the peptide rapidly increased in concentration during the first few days postpartum with a resulting prompt natriuresis likely due to a puerperal shift of fluid from the extravascular space into the vascular compartment.

The actual effect of this peptide on plasma volume in the normally pregnant woman remains to be defined. There is no doubt, however, that the peptide has a rapid and effective action upon plasma volume during the early puerperium. It seems unlikely that such a potent mediator of volume and sodium hemostasis would not have an effect during pregnancy as well.

CHANGES IN HEMATOCRIT

In spite of an augmented erythropoiesis, the concentrations of hemoglobin and erythrocytes, as well as the hematocrit, decrease slightly during normal pregnancy. Consequently, whole blood viscosity decreases (Huisman and colleagues, 1987). In a careful study in which iron was readily available to the mother for erythropoiesis, Pritchard and Hunt (1958) found that the hemoglobin concentration at term averaged 12.5 g, with a level below 11.0 g per dL present in only 6 percent of the pregnant subjects. A hemoglobin concentration below 11.0 g per dL, especially late in pregnancy, should be considered as probably abnormal and usually due to iron deficiency, rather than to hypervolemia of pregnancy (see Chap. 14, p. 264).

IRON METABOLISM

Iron Stores

It has been stated commonly that the total body iron content averages about 4 g, or slightly more, in the adult. This value, however, applies to normal men. In healthy young women of average size, the body iron content is probably not much more than half that amount (Table 7–2). Commonly, iron stores of normal young women are only about 300 mg (Pritchard and Mason, 1964; Scott and Pritchard, 1967). As in men, heme iron in myoglobin and enzymes and tranferrin-bound circulating iron together total only a few hundred milligrams. The total iron content of normal adult women, therefore, is probably in the range of 2.0 to 2.5 g.

Iron Requirements

The iron requirements of normal pregnancy total about 1 g (Fig. 7–8). About 300 mg are actively transferred to the fetus and placenta (Widdowson and Spray, 1951) and about 200 mg are lost through various normal routes of excretion. These are obligatory losses and occur even when the mother is iron deficient. The average increase in the total volume of circulating erythrocytes of about 450 mL during pregnancy, when iron is available, uses another 500 mg of iron since 1 mL of normal erythrocytes contains 1.1 mg of iron. Practically all the iron for these purposes is used during the latter half of pregnancy. Therefore, the iron requirement becomes quite large during the second half of pregnancy, averaging 6 to 7 mg per day (Pritchard and Scott, 1970). Since this amount of iron is not available from body stores in most women, the desired increase in maternal erythrocyte volume and hemoglobin mass will not develop unless exogenous iron is made available in adequate amounts. In the absence of added exogenous iron, the hemoglobin concentration and hematocrit fall appreciably as the maternal blood volume increases. Hemoglobin production in the fetus, however, will not be impaired, because the placenta obtains iron from the mother in amounts sufficient for the fetus to establish normal hemoglobin levels even when the mother has severe iron-deficiency anemia.

The amounts of iron absorbed from diet, together with that mobilized from stores, is usually insufficient to meet the demands imposed by pregnancy, even though iron absorption from the gastrointestinal tract appears to be moderately increased during pregnancy (Hahn and associates, 1951). Supplemental iron, therefore, is valuable during the latter half of pregnancy, and for several weeks after delivery if the infant is to be breast-fed (see Chap. 14, p. 264).

Without supplemental iron, the maternal *plasma iron concentration* often decreases during pregnancy. Undoubtedly, in most instances, iron deficiency contributes significantly to the fall. The *plasma iron-binding capacity* (transferrin) increases during pregnancy even when iron deficiency has been eliminated

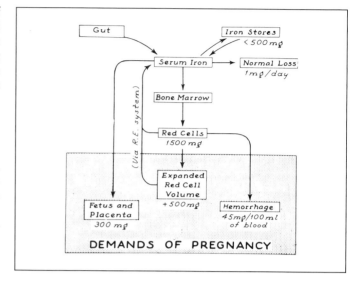

Figure 7–8. The iron requirements of normal pregnancy. The 300 mg of iron transferred to the fetus are permanently lost from the mother. The 500 mg incorporated into maternal hemoglobin usually are not all lost; the amount recovered for storage depends upon the amount of blood lost at and after delivery.

by appropriate treatment (Sturgeon, 1959). Estrogen has been shown when administered to nonpregnant women to produce an increase in plasma transferrin levels comparable to those of pregnancy.

Blood Loss

Not all the iron added to the maternal circulation in the form of hemoglobin is necessarily lost from the mother. During normal vaginal delivery and through the next few days, only about one-half of the erythrocytes added to the maternal circulation during pregnancy are lost from the majority of women by way of the placental implantation site, the placenta itself, the episiotomy wound and lacerations, and in the lochia. On the average, an amount of maternal erythrocytes corresponding to about 600 mL of predelivery blood is lost during and after vaginal delivery of a single fetus (Pritchard, 1965; Ueland, 1976). The average blood loss associated with cesarean section or with the vaginal delivery of twins is about 1 L, or nearly twice that lost with the delivery of a single fetus (Pritchard, 1965; Ueland, 1976). Unfortunately, it is not rare for the quantity of erythrocytes lost to equal or exceed the added volume accumulated during pregnancy.

Generally, the pattern of change in maternal blood volume during labor, vaginal delivery, and puerperium is as follows: (1) there is some hemoconcentration during labor, which varies with the degree of muscular activity and dehydration, (2) during and soon after delivery there is a further reduction in volume which closely parallels the amount of blood lost, (3) during the first few days of the puerperium there is little change or a slight increase in blood volume, especially if hemoconcentration during labor or blood loss at delivery was sizable, and (4) by 1 week after delivery there is a further reduction in plasma volume to the extent that the maternal blood volume is only slightly greater than several months later (Pritchard, 1965).

After delivery, any excess circulating hemoglobin above the amount normally present in the nonpregnant state ultimately

---

TABLE 7–2. MEASUREMENT OF HEMOGLOBIN IRON AND IRON STORES IN HEALTHY NULLIGRAVID WOMEN WHO NEVER EXPERIENCED ABNORMAL BLOOD LOSS

	Average	Range
Age	23	21 – 26
Weight (kg)	60	49 – 72
Height (inches)	65	60 – 68
Hemoglobin (g per dL)	14.1	13 – 15.6
Serum iron (µg per dL)	105	76 – 132
Hemoglobin mass (g)	443	358 – 492
Hemoglobin iron (mg)	1,505	1,210 – 1,670
Iron stores[a] (mg)	347	150 – 629

[a]Iron converted to hemoglobin following repeated phlebotomies.
From Pritchard and Mason: JAMA 190:897, 1964.

yields iron for storage. The mechanism by which this occurs is most likely not accelerated erythrocyte destruction during the late puerperium, but rather normal destruction with reduced production of new erythrocytes. A similar process occurs after a normal nonanemic person receives transfused cells, or when a normal person with polycythemia, induced by high altitude, returns to sea level.

IMMUNOLOGICAL AND LEUCOCYTE FUNCTIONS

Pregnancy has been assumed to be associated with suppression of a variety of humoral and cellularly mediated immunological functions in order to accommodate the "foreign" semiallogeneic fetal graft. In fact, humoral antibody titers against several viruses, for example, herpes simplex, measles, and influenza A, are decreased during pregnancy. The decrease in titers, however, is in proportion to the hemodilutional effect of pregnancy (Baboonnian and Griffiths, 1983). The prevalence of a variety of autoantibodies is unchanged (Patton and colleagues, 1987). Furthermore, α-interferon, which is present in almost all fetal tissues and fluids, most often is absent in normally pregnant women (Chard and coworkers, 1986). There is evidence, as yet unexplained, that polymorphonuclear leucocyte chemotaxis and adherence functions are depressed beginning in the second trimester and continuing throughout pregnancy (Krause and associates, 1987). Therefore, it is possible that these depressed functions in the polymorphonuclear leucocytes of pregnant women account, in part, for the improvement observed in some pregnant women with autoimmune diseases and the possibly increased susceptibility of pregnant women to certain infections. Thus, both function and absolute numbers of leucocytes appear to be important factors when considering the leucocytosis of normal pregnancy.

The blood leucocyte count varies considerably during normal pregnancy (Efrati and co-workers, 1964). Usually it ranges from 5,000 to 12,000 per μL. During labor and the early puerperium it may become markedly elevated, attaining levels of 25,000 or even more; however, the concentration averages 14,000 to 16,000 per μL (Taylor and co-workers, 1981). The cause for the marked increase is not known, but the same response occurs during and after strenuous exercise. It probably represents the reappearance in the circulation of leucocytes previously shunted out of the active circulation.

Beginning quite early in pregnancy, the activity of alkaline phosphatase in the leucocytes is increased. Such elevated activity is not peculiar to pregnancy but occurs in a wide variety of conditions, including most inflammatory states. During pregnancy there is a neutrophilia which consists predominantly of mature forms; however, an occasional myelocyte is found.

BLOOD COAGULATION

The levels of several blood coagulation factors are increased during pregnancy. Plasma fibrinogen (factor I) measured as thrombin-clottable protein in normal pregnant women, averages very close to 300 mg per dL and ranges from about 200 to 400. During normal pregnancy the concentration of fibrinogen increases about 50 percent to average about 450 mg per dL late in pregnancy, with a range from approximately 300 to 600. The increase in the concentration of fibrinogen undoubtedly contributes greatly to the striking increase in the blood *sedimentation rate* in normal pregnancy (Ozanne and co-workers, 1983). The increased sedimentation rate in pregnancy, therefore, has no diagnostic or prognostic value when employed for usual clinical purposes, for example, the assessment of the activity of lupus erythematosus.

Other clotting factors, the activities of which are increased appreciably during normal pregnancy, are factor VII (proconvertin), factor VIII (antihemophiliac globulin), factor IX (plasma thromboplastin component or Christmas factor), and factor X (Stuart factor). Usually the level of factor II (prothrombin) is increased only slightly, whereas those of factors XI (plasma thromboplastin antecedent) and XIII (fibrin-stabilizing factor) are decreased somewhat during pregnancy (Coopland and associates, 1969; Kasper and colleagues, 1964; Talbert and Langdell, 1964). The Quick one-stage prothrombin time and the partial thromboplastin time are both shortened slightly as pregnancy progresses.

Some investigators have described a moderate decrease in the number of platelets per unit volume (Pitkin and Witte, 1980). This may be the consequence of increased platelet consumption throughout normal pregnancy (Fay and co-workers, 1983). The clotting times of whole blood in either plain glass tubes (wettable surface) or silicone-coated or plastic tubes (nonwettable surface) do not differ significantly in normal pregnant and nonpregnant women. Some, but not all, of the pregnancy-induced changes in the levels of coagulation factors can be duplicated by the administration of one of several of the commonly used estrogen plus progestin contraceptive tablets (Fletcher and Alkjaersig, 1969).

High-molecular-weight soluble fibrin-fibrinogen complexes circulate in normal pregnancy. Also, an increased capacity for neutralizing heparin has been described, but plasma antithrombin III does not appear to be reduced during pregnancy (Weiner and Brandt, 1980). Some of these alterations in coagulation factors during normal pregnancy may be equated with continuing low-grade intravascular coagulation (Fletcher and co-workers, 1979). In support of this concept, Tygart and associates (1986) observed a mildly elevated mean platelet volume and a greater and significant increase in platelet distribution width as pregnancy advanced. They interpreted these observations to represent an increased level of thrombocytopoiesis as a consequence of both dilutional and consumptive stimuli of normal pregnancy. Rakoczi and co-workers (1979) reported a shorter half-life for platelets in pregnant compared to nonpregnant women. Beta-thromboglobulin, a platelet-specific release protein, also is increased during the second and third trimesters in normally pregnant women (Douglas and associates, 1982). Finally, Bonnar (1978) used electron microscopy and identified fibrin deposited in the intervillous space of the placenta and in the walls of the spiral arteries that supply blood to the intervillous space.

During normal pregnancy, the level of maternal plasminogen (profibrinolysin) in plasma increases considerably, a phenomenon that can be induced by estrogen treatment. Even so, fibrinolytic, or plasmin, activity, measured either as the time for clotted plasma to dissolve or as the time for the clotted euglobulin fraction from plasma to undergo lysis, is distinctly prolonged compared with that of the normal nonpregnant state. Astedt (1972) implicated the placenta in the reduced fibrinolytic activity that characterizes normal pregnancy, since delivery normally is promptly followed by a prompt increase in plasma fibrinolytic activity (Ratnoff and co-workers, 1954). At the same time, fibrin degradation products usually rise slightly after delivery (Woodfield and associates, 1968).

CARDIOVASCULAR SYSTEM

During pregnancy and the puerperium there are remarkable changes involving the heart and the circulation.

HEART

Typically, the resting pulse rate increases about 10 to 15 beats per minute during pregnancy. As the diaphragm is elevated progressively during pregnancy, the heart is displaced to the left and upward, while at the same time it is rotated somewhat on its long axis. As a result, the apex of the heart is moved somewhat laterally from its position in the normal nonpregnant state, and an increase in the size of the cardiac silhouette is found in radiographs (Fig. 7–9). The extent of these changes is influenced by the size and position of the uterus, the strength of the abdominal muscles, and the configurations of the abdomen and thorax. Furthermore, normally pregnant women apparently have some degree of benign pericardial effusion which may increase the cardiac silhouette on x-ray (Enein and colleagues, 1987). Variability of these factors makes it difficult to precisely identify moderate degrees of cardiomegaly by physical examination or by simple x-ray studies. The physician must, therefore, be cautious in making a diagnosis of pathological cardiomegaly during pregnancy.

In several studies using frontal and sagittal roentgenograms, the cardiac volume was found to increase normally by about 75 mL, or a little more than 10 percent, between early and late pregnancy (Ihrman, 1960). Katz and co-workers (1978) studied left ventricular performance during pregnancy and the puerperium using echocardiography. Both left ventricular wall mass and end-diastolic dimensions were observed to increase during pregnancy, as did heart rate, calculated stroke volume, and cardiac output. The changes in stroke volume were directly proportional to end-diastolic volume, implying, at least, that there is little change in the inotropic state of the myocardium during normal singleton pregnancy and the puerperium. In multifetal pregnancies, however, cardiac output is increased even more than in singleton pregnancies. This occurs predominantly by virtue of an **increased inotropic effect** as measured

by an increased fractional shortening of the ventricular diameters (Veille and co-workers, 1985). The increased heart rate and inotropic contractility imply that cardiovascular reserve is reduced.

During pregnancy some of the cardiac sounds may be altered to the extent that they would be considered abnormal in the absence of pregnancy. Cutforth and MacDonald (1966) obtained phonocardiograms at varying stages of pregnancy in 50 normal women and documented the following changes: (1) an exaggerated splitting of the first heart sound with increased loudness of both components; no definite changes in the aortic and pulmonary elements of the second sound; and a loud, easily heard third sound, and (2) a systolic murmur in 90 percent of pregnant women, intensified during inspiration in some or expiration in others, and disappearing very shortly after delivery; a soft diastolic murmur transiently in 19 percent; and continuous murmurs arising apparently in the breast vasculature in 10 percent.

The physician must be cautious when interpreting the significance of murmurs during pregnancy, especially systolic murmurs. Normal pregnancy induces no characteristic changes in the *electrocardiogram* other than slight deviation of the electrical axis to the left as a result of the altered position of the heart.

CARDIAC OUTPUT

During normal pregnancy, arterial blood pressure and vascular resistance decrease while blood volume, maternal weight, and basal metabolic rate increase. Each of these events would be expected to affect cardiac output with some leading to decreased output but others causing an increase. It is now evident that cardiac output *at rest*, when measured in the lateral recumbent position, increases appreciably during the first trimester and remains elevated during the second and third trimesters (Fig. 7–10). Typically, cardiac output in late pregnancy is appreciably higher when the woman is in the lateral recumbent position than when she is supine, since in the supine position the large uterus and its contents often impede venous return to the heart. Ueland and Hansen (1969), for example, found cardiac output to increase 1,100 mL (22 percent) when the pregnant woman was moved from her back onto her side. When she assumes the standing position after sitting, cardiac output in the pregnant woman falls to the same degree as in the nonpregnant woman (Easterling and associates, 1988).

Cardiac output in response to physical activity by the ambulatory woman must be greater late in pregnancy than it would be if she were not pregnant. Increase in mass alone demands such a response.

During the first stage of labor, maternal cardiac output increases moderately, and during the second stage of labor, with vigorous expulsive efforts, the cardiac output is appreciably greater (Fig. 7–10). Most of the increase in cardiac output induced by pregnancy is lost very soon after delivery (Ueland and Metcalfe, 1975).

Reviews of cardiac function and cardiovascular physiology have been provided by Metcalfe and co-workers (1981) and by Hankins and associates (1983).

FACTORS CONTROLLING VASCULAR REACTIVITY IN PREGNANCY

Gant and associates (1973) conducted a prospective study of vascular reactivity to angiotensin II throughout pregnancy to ascertain when vascular refractoriness to angiotensin II was lost

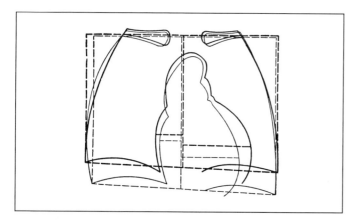

Figure 7–9. Change in cardiac outline that occurs in pregnancy. The light lines represent the relations between the heart and thorax in the nonpregnant woman, and the heavy lines represent the conditions existing in pregnancy. These findings are based on teleoroentgenograms and represent the average findings in 33 women. (*From Klafen and Palugyay: Arch Gynaekol 131:347, 1927.*)

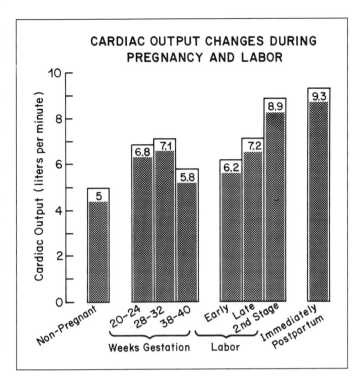

Figure 7–10. Cardiac outputs during three stages of gestation, labor, and immediately postpartum are compared with values of nonpregnant women. All values were determined with women in the lateral recumbent position. (*Adapted from Ueland and Metcalfe: Clin Obstet Gynecol 18:41, 1975.*)

in normal women who later became hypertensive. The results of these studies are given in Figure 35–1 (p. 658). Briefly, the 192 primigravid women in this study were less than 17 years of age and were studied sequentially throughout pregnancy. At each clinic visit, the women were infused with angiotensin II in doses sufficient to increase baseline diastolic blood pressure by 20 mm Hg. The dose of angiotensin II in ng/kg/min required to elevate diastolic blood pressure 20 mm Hg was recorded as the *effective pressor dose.* Women destined to develop pregnancy-induced hypertension became progressively more sensitive to the pressor effects of infused angiotensin II after 18 weeks. In a retrospective analysis of the data obtained between 28 and 32 weeks, it was ascertained that more than 90 percent of women in whom the effective pressor dose of angiotensin II was less than 8 ng/kg/minute developed hypertension 10 to 14 weeks later. Conversely, hypertension did not develop in over 90 percent of those women who remained refractory to angiotensin II infusion at doses greater than 8 ng/kg/minute.

The early and clear divergence in the effective pressor dose of angiotensin II observed in normal and subsequently preeclamptic women likely was the result of significant alterations in a variety of physiological processes that serve to control vascular reactivity to angiotensin II. Gant and associates (1974b) speculated that possible factors included alterations in circulating plasma levels of renin, angiotensin II, aldosterone, and possibly prostaglandins. Certainly in pregnancies complicated by pregnancy-induced hypertension, plasma renin concentration, renin activity, angiotensin II, and aldosterone levels are lower than in normotensive women (Chesley, 1978).

Renin, Angiotensin II, and Plasma Volume

Pressor responsiveness to angiotensin II and the renin-angiotensin-aldosterone system is altered remarkably in pregnant compared to nonpregnant women. In normotensive pregnant women, there are marked increases in the concentrations of plasma renin, renin activity, renin substrate, angiotensin II, and aldosterone, as well as a blunted pressor response to infused angiotensin II (Chesley, 1978). Gant and co-workers (1974b) and Cunningham and associates (1975) found that various volume loads including normal saline (1 L), dextran (500 mL), and packed red blood cells (950 mL) did not alter pressor responsiveness to angiotensin II in normotensive pregnant women despite significant increases in blood volume and decreases in the plasma levels of renin following volume expansion. Therefore, the increased refractoriness to angiotensin II characteristic of normal pregnancy likely is the consequence of individual vessel refractoriness to angiotensin II. That is, in the woman destined to develop preeclampsia, or in the woman already acutely ill with preeclampsia, the increased sensitivity to angiotensin II was the result of an alteration in vessel wall refractoriness *rather* than the consequence of changes in blood volume or circulating renin-angiotensin levels.

Prostaglandins

McGiff and Itskovitz (1973) found that prostaglandins are potent mediators of vascular reactivity in several different organs under a variety of conditions. Moreover, Terragno and colleagues (1974) reported that late in canine pregnancy, uterine blood flow was related to the concentration of prostaglandin E in uterine venous blood. These investigators also observed that the intravenous infusion of angiotensin II into pregnant dogs led to an increase in uterine blood flow and a rise in the level of prostaglandin E in uterine blood.

Everett and co-workers (1978c) evaluated the effect of prostaglandin synthase inhibitors on the effective pressor dose of angiotensin II in normally pregnant women after 28 weeks. They found that indomethacin and aspirin resulted in a significant reduction in the amount of infused angiotensin II required to evoke an increase in diastolic blood pressure of 20 mm Hg. Thus, the refractoriness to angiotensin II usually observed during normal human pregnancy may be mediated, in part, by the action of prostaglandin-related substances that are produced in situ by arteriolar endothelium. Decreases in the rate of prostaglandin synthesis, or increases in the rate of prostaglandin catabolism, therefore might result in increased vascular responsiveness to infused angiotensin II, a characteristic of the pregnant woman who has developed or is destined to develop pregnancy-induced hypertension.

The likelihood of prostaglandin involvement in the regulation of vascular reactivity in pregnancy was confirmed by Broughton-Pipkin and Meirelles (1982). They infused prostaglandin E_2 intravenously into pregnant women and found that the amount of angiotensin II required to increase diastolic blood pressure by 20 mm Hg was increased. The same group also found increased vascular refractoriness to infused angiotensin II in pregnant sheep treated intravenously with prostaglandin E_2.

Progesterone and Progesterone Metabolites

Other factors appear to participate in modulating vascular responsiveness to angiotensin II during pregnancy. Gant and associates (1977) observed that normally pregnant women lose pregnancy-acquired vascular refractoriness to angiotensin II within 15 to 30 minutes after the placenta is delivered and that intramuscular administration of large amounts of progesterone to the mother during the later stages of labor delays this loss (Gant and associates, 1977). On the other hand, intravenously administered progesterone does not restore angiotensin II refractoriness to women with pregnancy-induced hypertension; however, the infusion of a major progesterone metabolite, 5α-pregnane-3, 20-dione (5α-dihydroprogesterone), does. Thus, a progestin mechanism may modulate the expression of prostaglandin-mediated vascular responsiveness in normal pregnancy. The mechanism by which 5α-dihydroprogesterone restores vascular refractoriness to women with pregnancy-induced hypertension is not known, but infusion of this steroid into five normally pregnant women who had been rendered angiotensin II–sensitive by the administration of indomethacin also restored vascular refractoriness (Everett and associates, 1978a).

Thus, a progestin-induced mechanism may modulate the prostaglandin-mediated vascular responsiveness to the pressor effects of angiotensin II that is characteristic of normal human pregnancy. Alternatively, the steroid may act independently of prostaglandin action(s).

Alterations in Cyclic AMP

Administration of theophylline to angiotensin II–sensitive pregnant women with early onset pregnancy-induced hypertension more than doubled the mean effective pressor dose of angiotensin II, restoring the vascular refractoriness characteristic of normal pregnancy (Everett and co-workers, 1978b). This effect of theophylline likely results from its inhibition of the enzyme phosphodiesterase, a known action of theophylline. Phosphodiesterase is a principal regulator of intracellular cyclic nucleotide accumulation. Inhibition of phosphodiesterase activity would promote the accumulation of cyclic adenosine monophosphate (cAMP) within vascular smooth muscle and should lead to the promotion of vascular smooth muscle relaxation.

Alterations in Calcium Entry to Vascular Smooth Muscle

Reductions in vascular refractoriness to infused angiotensin II have been reported in normal women and several different animals after the administration of various agents that act as calcium channel blockers (Anderson, 1987; Pasanisi, 1985; Vierhapper, 1982; and their co-workers; Hof, 1984, 1985). The safety of these compounds in human pregnancy has not been established. Moreover, their use has resulted in significant acidosis in the fetal lamb, likely due to a reduction in uteroplacental blood flow (Parisi, 1986).

Dietary Manipulations

Everett and co-workers (1977) administered 40 g of *linoleic acid* per day to a group of angiotensin II-sensitive women who had been admitted to the hospital prior to 34 weeks for pregnancy-induced hypertension. A similar group of women were given 40 g of palmitic acid per day. In this double-blind study, only the women who received the linoleic acid became refractory to infused angiotensin II. They suggested that because linoleic acid, but not palmitic acid, was a precursor of arachidonic acid, the precursor of prostacyclin, it was possible that linoleic acid served to increase the production of prostacyclin and thereby increase vascular refractoriness to infused angiotensin II. However, they noted that while vascular reactivity in the women given the linoleic acid increased (6 to 12 ng/kg/minute), refrac-

toriness was not restored to characteristically normal late pregnancy values (16 to 20 ng/kg/minute).

Calcium, added to the diet of pregnant women, increases the amount of angiotensin II required to elicit a pressor response (Noriyoshi and co-workers, 1985). Moreover, Belizan and Villar (1971) reported that in populations of women with a high calcium intake, the incidence of eclampsia was decreased. Belizan and co-workers (1983) also reported that blood pressure in pregnant women could be reduced by oral calcium administration.

In summary, it appears likely that vascular reactivity in human pregnancy is controlled, at least in part, by: (1) the action of a prostaglandin(s) or prostaglandin-related substance(s) on vascular smooth muscle, (2) progestin action which may modify the prostaglandin effect, (3) alterations in the cyclic nucleotide system of vascular smooth muscle, and (4) changes in intracellular calcium concentration.

PHARMACOLOGICAL ALTERATIONS OF VASCULAR REACTIVITY IN PREGNANCY

As discussed above, the pressor effects of infused angiotensin II can be altered. If loss of vascular refractoriness has a central role in the pathogenesis of pregnancy-induced hypertension or other pregnancy abnormalities, it may be possible that a simple means for restoring refractoriness, or of preventing its loss, may be used clinically to improve pregnancy outcome. A list of such potentially effective drugs or diet manipulations is presented below.

Theophylline, Calcium Channel Blockers, and Dietary Manipulations

As discussed above, each of these methods has been shown to restore vascular refractoriness to angiotensin II in women with pregnancy-induced hypertension. Whether these methods will be successful to treat or prevent pregnancy-induced hypertension remains to be proven.

Aspirin

Wallenburg and co-workers (1986) administered 60 mg of aspirin, or a placebo, to primigravid women beginning at 28 weeks. These women were identified as high risk by the finding of increased sensitivity to infused angiotensin II. The reduced incidence of preeclampsia in the treated group was attributed to a selective suppression of thromboxane synthesis by platelets, with sparing of endothelial prostacyclin production. In a group of women with prior poor pregnancy outcomes as a result of hypertension and placental insufficiency, Beaufils and colleagues (1985) found that early prophylactic treatment with dipyridamole and low-dose aspirin reduced the recurrence of these conditions. The effectiveness of the treatment was attributed to antiplatelet actions of these drugs.

Despite these encouraging reports of low-dose aspirin efficacy in decreasing the incidence and severity of pregnancy-induced hypertension, more extensive evaluations must be conducted before the safety of this regimen is established. For example, Spitz and associates (1988) found that 81 mg of aspirin per day does not selectively inhibit thromboxane and spare prostacyclin. They reported that thromboxane production was inhibited by 75 percent but prostacyclin and prostaglandin E were also inhibited, 21 and 29 percent, respectively (see also Chap. 35, p. 659).

In summary, as the control of vascular reactivity in pregnancy is better understood, it is reasonable to expect that pharmacological and dietary interventions might be useful to maintain or restore normal pregnancy-induced refractoriness to pressor agents.

CIRCULATION

The posture of the pregnant woman affects *arterial blood pressure.* Typically, blood pressure in the brachial artery is highest when she is sitting, lowest when lying in the lateral recumbent position, and intermediate when supine, except for some women who become quite hypotensive in the supine position. Usually, arterial blood pressure decreases to a nadir during the second trimester or early third trimester and rises thereafter. A sustained rise of 30 mm Hg systolic or 15 mm Hg diastolic under basal conditions may be indicative of an abnormality, most likely pregnancy-induced hypertension (see Chap. 35, p. 654).

The antecubital *venous pressure* remains unchanged during pregnancy, but in the supine position the femoral venous pressure rises steadily from 8 cm H_2O early in pregnancy to 24 cm H_2O at term (Fig. 7–11). Employing radiolabeled tracers, Wright and co-workers (1950) and many others have demonstrated that blood flow in the legs is retarded during pregnancy except when the subjects were in the lateral recumbent position. This tendency toward stagnation of blood in the lower extremities during the latter part of pregnancy is attributable to the occlusion of the pelvic veins and inferior vena cava by pressure of the enlarged uterus. The elevated venous pressure returns to normal if the pregnant woman lies on her side and immediately after delivery of the infant by cesarean section (McLennan, 1943). From a clinical viewpoint, the retarded blood flow and increased lower extremity venous pressure are of great importance. These alterations contribute to the dependent edema frequently experienced by women as they approach term and to the development of varicose veins in the legs and vulva, as well as hemorrhoids.

OTHER CIRCULATORY EFFECTS FROM SUPINE POSITION

In the supine position, the large pregnant uterus rather consistently compresses the venous system that returns blood from the lower half of the body to the extent that cardiac filling may be reduced and cardiac output decreased. Infrequently, this causes significant arterial hypotension, sometimes referred to as the *supine hypotensive syndrome* (Howard and colleagues, 1953). Moreover, Bieniarz and associates (1968) observed that in the supine position the large pregnant uterus may compress the aorta sufficiently to lower arterial blood pressure below the level of compression. They demonstrated that the usual measurement of blood pressure in the brachial artery does not provide a reliable estimate of the pressure in the uterine or other arteries that lie distal to the compression exerted on the aorta by the gravid uterus and its contents. When the pregnant woman is supine, uterine arterial pressure is significantly lower than that in the brachial artery. In the presence of systemic hypotension, as occurs with spinal analgesia, the decrease in uterine arterial pressure is even more marked than in arteries above the level of aortic compression. Gant and associates (1974a) reported that an appreciable number of women destined to develop pregnancy-induced hypertension exhibited more than a 20 mm Hg increase in diastolic blood pressure when they were turned from the lateral to the supine position. They called this a *supine pressor test,* but its exact mechanism remains to be defined.

BLOOD FLOW TO SKIN

Increased cutaneous blood flow in pregnancy serves to dissipate excess heat generated by the increased metabolism imposed by pregnancy (Burt, 1950; Spetz, 1964).

RESPIRATORY TRACT

ANATOMICAL CHANGES

The level of the diaphragm rises about 4 cm during pregnancy. The subcostal angle widens appreciably as the transverse diameter of the thoracic cage increases about 2 cm. The thoracic circumference increases about 6 cm but not sufficiently to prevent a reduction in the residual volume of air in the lungs created by the elevated diaphragm. The idea that the elevated diaphragm was "splinted" during normal pregnancy has been disproved using fluoroscopic studies (Möbius, 1961). Diaphragmatic excursion is actually greater during pregnancy than when nonpregnant. As a result, the tidal volume increases.

PULMONARY FUNCTION

At any stage of normal pregnancy, the amount of oxygen delivered by the increase in tidal volume clearly exceeds the oxygen need imposed by the pregnancy. Moreover, the amount of hemoglobin in the circulation and, in turn, the total oxygen-carrying capacity, increases appreciably during normal pregnancy, as does cardiac output. As the consequence, *maternal arteriovenous oxygen difference* is decreased.

The respiratory rate is changed little during pregnancy but the *tidal volume, minute ventilatory volume,* and *minute oxygen uptake* increase appreciably as pregnancy advances (Table 7–3). The *maximum breathing capacity* and *forced or timed vital capacity* are not altered appreciably. The *functional residual capacity* and the *residual volume* of air are decreased as the consequence of the elevated diaphragm. *Lung compliance* is unaffected by pregnancy while *airway conductance* is increased and *total pulmonary resistance* is reduced. Gee and associates (1967) speculated that in-

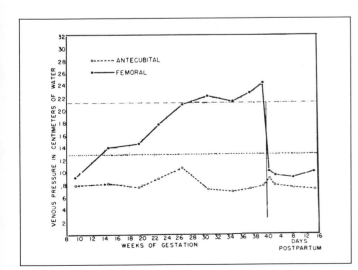

Figure 7–11. Serial changes in antecubital and femoral venous blood pressure throughout normal pregnancy and early puerperium. These measurements were made on women in the supine position. (*From McLennan: Am J Obstet Gynecol 45:568, 1943.*)

TABLE 7–3.   RESTING RESPIRATORY FUNCTION

Function	Not Pregnant	Pregnant	Change (%)
Respiratory rate	15	16	—
Tidal volume (mL)	487	678	+39[a]
Minute ventilation (mL)	7,270	10,340	+42[a]
Minute O_2 uptake	201	266	+32[a]
Vital capacity (mL)	3,260	3,310	+1
Maximum breathing capacity (% of predicted)	102	97	−5
Inspiratory capacity (mL)	2,625	2,745	+5
Residual volume (mL)	965	770	−20[a]

[a]Highly significant differences.
From Cugell and associates: Am Rev Tuberc 67:568, 1953.

creased airway conductance from decreased bronchomotor tone may be effected by progesterone action.

The *closing volume*, or the lung volume at which airways in the dependent parts of the lung begin to close during expiration, has been considered to be higher in pregnancy by some investigators but not by others (Baldwin and associates, 1977).

An increased awareness of a desire to breathe is common even early in pregnancy (Milne and colleagues, 1978) and may be interpreted as dyspnea which, in turn, suggests pulmonary or cardiac abnormalities even though most often none exists. The increased tidal volume normally lowers slightly the blood P_{CO_2} causing mild respiratory alkalosis, which is partially compensated for by a lowering of the bicarbonate concentration.

The increased respiratory effort and, in turn, the reduction in P_{CO_2} during pregnancy most likely is induced in large part by progesterone and to a lesser degree estrogen. Oral medroxyprogesterone has been administered to stimulate an increased respiratory drive in obese nonpregnant subjects who hypoventilate (Sutton and co-workers, 1975). The site of action of the hormones appears to be central through a direct stimulatory effect on the respiratory center.

Although pulmonary function is not impaired by pregnancy, disease of the respiratory tract may be more serious during gestation (see Chap. 39, p. 805). Important factors are undoubtedly the increased oxygen requirements imposed by pregnancy and perhaps an increase in closing volume, especially when supine.

URINARY SYSTEM

Remarkable changes in both structure and function take place in the urinary tract during normal pregnancy.

KIDNEY

The kidney increases slightly in size during pregnancy. Bailey and Rolleston (1971), for example, found that the kidney was 1.5 cm longer during the early puerperium than when measured 6 months later.

The glomerular filtration rate (GFR) and renal plasma flow (RPF) increase early in pregnancy, the former as much as 50 percent by the beginning of the second trimester, and the latter not quite so much (Chesley, 1963; Dunlop, 1981). The precise mechanism by which these are increased in pregnancy has not been identified. Elevated glomerular filtration has been found by most investigators to persist to term (Fig. 7–12),

whereas the renal plasma flow decreases during late pregnancy.

Most studies of renal function conducted during pregnancy have been performed while the subjects were supine, a position that late in pregnancy may produce marked systemic hemodynamic changes (see p. 147) that lead to alterations in several aspects of renal function. Late in pregnancy, for instance, urinary flow and sodium excretion are affected significantly by posture, averaging less than half the rate of excretion in the supine position, compared to the lateral recumbent position.

Whereas posture clearly affects sodium and water excretion in late pregnancy, its impact on glomerular filtration and renal plasma flow seems to be much more variable. Chesley and Sloan (1964), for example, found both to be reduced commonly when the pregnant woman was in the supine position, whereas Dunlop (1976) identified little or no reduction. Pritchard and associates (1955) detected decreases in these while supine compared to lateral recumbent in some, but not most, of the late pregnant women studied. Ezimokhai and associates (1981) presented evidence that the late pregnancy decrease in renal plasma flow is not due simply to a positional effect. Davison and Hytten (1974) rightfully pointed out that an estimate of glomerular filtration rate is only valid for the conditions under which it is measured and that changes with posture represent the real-life situation rather than artifact.

A possible cause of the changes in renal function in the supine position compared to the lateral recumbent is reduced venous return to the heart, which results from obstruction of the inferior vena cava and iliac veins by the large pregnant uterus, which could lead to reduction in cardiac output and, in turn, lowering of renal plasma flow and glomerular filtration. This sequence of events, however, does not appear to be essential to the mechanism that triggers sodium and water retention when supine. In a woman at term with a renal transplant in the right iliac fossa, a change to the supine from the lateral recumbent position had no obvious effect on water and sodium excretion or on glomerular filtration (J. Pritchard, unpublished).

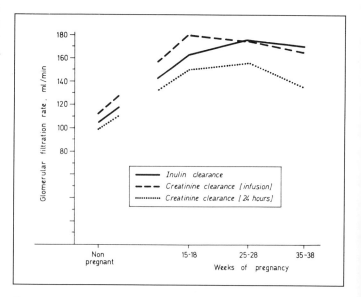

Figure 7–12. Mean glomerular filtration rate in healthy women over a short period with infused inulin (*solid line*), simultaneously as creatinine clearance during the inulin infusion (*broken line*), and over 24 hours as endogenous creatinine clearance (*dotted line*). (*From Davison and Hytten: J Obstet Gynaecol Brit Commonw 81:588, 1974.*)

Another possible mechanism to account for decreased sodium and water excretion in supine pregnant women is elevated ureteral pressure. Fulop and Brazeau (1970) induced increased tubular reabsorption of sodium and water in dogs by elevating ureteral pressure moderately. Pritchard and associates (1955) were not able to prevent such decreases in the supine position following the insertion of ureteral catheters well above the pelvic brim; however, increased intraureteric pressure may not have been completely prevented by this maneuver.

It has been suggested by some that the release of antidiuretic hormone (ADH) plays a role, but ADH probably is not essential, since postural changes have produced similar reductions in a pregnant woman with severe diabetes insipidus (Whalley and co-workers, 1961).

LOSS OF NUTRIENTS

One unusual feature of the pregnancy-induced changes in renal excretion is the remarkably increased amounts of various nutrients in the urine. Amino acids and water-soluble vitamins are lost in the urine of pregnant women in much greater amounts than in the urine of nonpregnant women (Hytten and Leitch, 1971).

TESTS OF RENAL FUNCTION

The results of several of the tests of renal function in general clinical use may be altered during normal pregnancy and therefore may be quite misleading. During pregnancy the concentrations in plasma of creatinine and urea normally decrease as a consequence of their increased glomerular filtration. At times, the urea concentration may be so low as to suggest impaired hepatic synthesis, which sometimes occurs with severe liver disease.

Creatinine clearance is a useful test to estimate renal function in pregnancy provided that complete urine collection is made over an accurately timed period, preferably several hours at least. *Urine concentration tests* may give results that are misleading (Davison and colleagues, 1981). During the day, pregnant women tend to accumulate water in the form of dependent edema (see p. 137), and at night, while recumbent, they mobilize this fluid and excrete it via the kidneys. This reversal of the usual nonpregnant diurnal pattern of urinary flow causes nocturia and the urine is more dilute than in the nonpregnant state. The failure of a pregnant woman to excrete a concentrated urine after withholding fluids for approximately 18 hours does not necessarily mean renal damage. The kidney, in fact, in these circumstances functions perfectly normally by excreting mobilized extracellular fluid of relatively low osmolality.

URINALYSIS

Glucosuria during pregnancy is not necessarily abnormal. The appreciable increase in glomerular filtration, together with impaired tubular reabsorptive capacity for filtered glucose accounts in most cases for the glucosuria (Davison and Hytten, 1975). Chesley (1963) calculated that for these reasons alone about one sixth of all pregnant women should spill glucose in the urine. Even though glucosuria is common during pregnancy, the possibility of diabetes mellitus cannot be ignored. *Proteinuria* does not occur normally during pregnancy except occasionally in slight amounts during or soon after vigorous labor. Lopez-Espinoza and colleagues (1986) measured serial urinary albumin excretion using a sensitive radioimmunoassay in 14 healthy pregnant women. There was a slight but signifi-

cant rise from a median of 7 to 18 mg/24 h from early to late pregnancy, however, albuminuria was not detected using conventional testing methods. If not the result of contamination during collection, blood cells in the urine during pregnancy are compatible with a diagnosis of urinary tract disease. Difficult labor and delivery, of course, can cause hematuria because of trauma to the lower urinary tract.

HYDRONEPHROSIS AND HYDROURETER

In pregnant women, after the uterus rises completely out of the pelvis, it rests upon the ureters, compressing them at the pelvic brim. Increased intraureteral tonus above the level of the pelvic brim compared with that of the pelvic portion of the ureter has been identified (Rubi and Sala, 1968). No such differences were demonstrable in nonpregnant women.

Typically, ureteral dilatation above the pelvic brim is more marked on the right side. Schulman and Herlinger (1975) found ureteral dilatation to be greater on the right side in 86 percent of pregnant women studied (Fig. 7–13). A similar result has been reported by Peake and co-workers (1983) using ultrasonic techniques. The unequal degrees of dilatation may result from a cushioning provided the left ureter by the sigmoid colon and perhaps from greater compression of the right ureter as the consequence of dextrorotation of the uterus. Bellina and co-workers (1970) emphasized that the right ovarian vein complex, which is remarkably dilated during pregnancy, lies obliquely

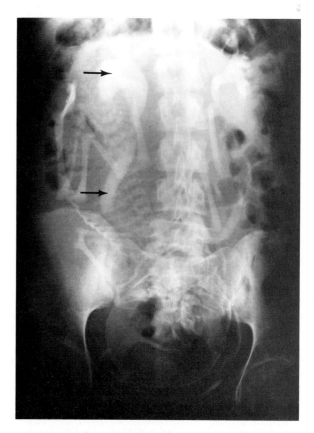

Figure 7–13. Normal intravenous pyelogram at 36 weeks gestation. Pregnancy-induced hydronephrosis (*upper arrow*) and hydroureter (*lower arrow*) are more marked on the mother's right side. Elongation, dilatation, and peristalsis of the ureter create the appearance of discontinuity of the ureter.

over the right ureter and may contribute significantly to right ureteral dilatation.

Another possible mechanism causing hydronephrosis and hydroureter is hormonal, presumably an effect of progesterone. Major support for this concept was provided by Van Wagenen and Jenkins (1939), who described in the monkey further dilatation of the ureters after removal of the fetus if the placenta remained in situ. The relatively abrupt onset of dilatation in women at midpregnancy, described by Schulman and Herlinger (1975), is more consistent with ureteral compression from a translocated enlarging uterus than a hormonal effect.

Elongation accompanies distension of the ureter, which is frequently thrown into curves of varying size, the smaller of which may be sharply angulated, producing, at least theoretically, partial or complete obstruction. These so-called kinks are poorly named, since the term connotes obstruction. They are, usually merely single or double curves, which, when viewed in the radiograph taken in the same plane as the curve, appear as more or less acute angulations of the ureter (Fig. 7–13). Another exposure at right angles nearly always identifies them to be more gentle curves rather than kinks. The ureter, in both its abdominal and pelvic portions, undergoes not only elongation but frequently lateral displacement by the pressure of the enlarged uterus.

Remarkable pregnancy-induced hydronephrosis with some degree of hydroureter has been demonstrated after transplant of a donor kidney to the iliac fossa (Fig. 7–14A,B). In this particular subject, the creatinine clearance increased from 75 mL per minute very early in pregnancy to 120 mL per minute during the third trimester, a normal response for pregnancy.

After delivery, there is resolution so that by 6 to 8 weeks the urinary tract has returned to prepregnancy dimensions. The stretching and dilatation do not continue long enough to impair permanently the elasticity of the ureter unless infection supervenes.

URINARY BLADDER

There are few significant anatomical changes in the bladder before the 4th month of pregnancy. From that time onward, however, the increased size of the uterus, together with the hyperemia which affects all pelvic organs and the hyperplasia of the muscle and connective tissues, elevates the bladder trigone and causes thickening of its posterior, or intraureteric, margin. Continuation of this process to the end of pregnancy produces marked deepening and widening of the trigone. The bladder mucosa undergoes no change other than an increase in the size and tortuosity of its blood vessels.

Using urethrocystometry, Iosif and colleagues (1980) found that bladder pressure doubled from 8 cm H_2O early in primigravid pregnancy to 20 cm H_2O at term. To compensate for reduced bladder capacity, absolute and functional urethral lengths increased by 6.7 and 4.8 mm, respectively. Finally, to preserve continence, maximal intraurethral pressure increased from 70 to 93 cm H_2O.

Toward the end of pregnancy, particularly in nulliparas in whom the presenting part often engages before the onset of labor, the entire base of the bladder is pushed forward and upward, converting the normal convex surface into a concavity. As a result, difficulties in diagnostic and therapeutic procedures are increased greatly. In addition, the pressure of the presenting part impairs the drainage of blood and lymph from the base of the bladder, often rendering the area edematous, easily trau-

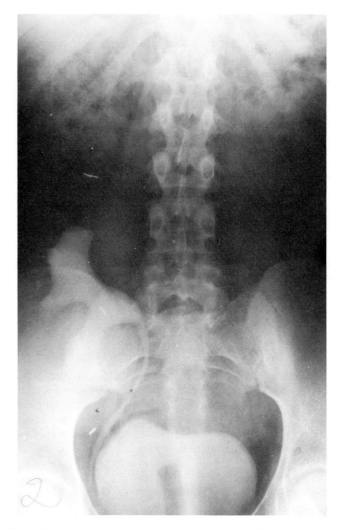

Figure 7–14. A. Intravenous pyelogram of renal transplant: Before pregnancy.

matized, and probably more susceptible to infection. Both urethral pressure and length have been shown to be decreased in women following vaginal but not abdominal delivery (Van Geelen and co-workers, 1982). These investigators suggested that a weakness of the urethral sphincter mechanism due to pregnancy or delivery may play a role in the pathogenesis of urinary stress incontinence.

Normally there is little residual urine in nulliparas, but occasionally it develops in the multipara with relaxed vaginal walls and a cystocele. Incompetence of the ureterovesical valve may supervene, with the consequent probability of vesicoureteral reflux of urine.

GASTROINTESTINAL TRACT

As pregnancy progresses, the stomach and intestines are displaced by the enlarging uterus. As the result of the positional changes in these viscera, the physical findings in certain diseases are altered. The appendix, for instance, is usually displaced upward and somewhat laterally as the uterus enlarges, and at times it may reach the right flank (Chap. 39, p. 833).

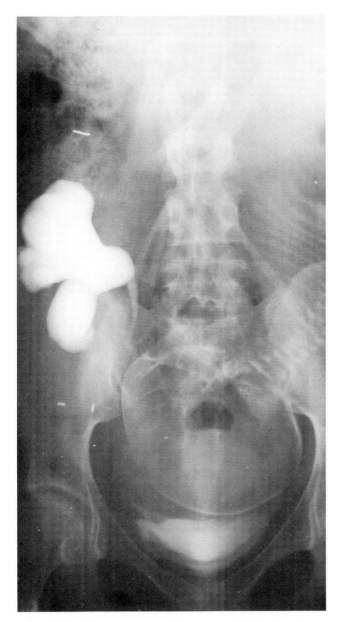

Figure 7–14. B. Intravenous pyelogram of renal transplant: Late in pregnancy. Marked levorotation of the uterus was identified at cesarean section.

There are usually decreased tone and motility of the gastrointestinal tract, which lead to prolongation of the times of gastric emptying and intestinal transit. This may be the result of the large amounts of progesterone which are present during pregnancy, decreased levels of *motalin*, a hormonal peptide known to have smooth muscle stimulating effects (Christofides and associates, 1982), or both. During labor, especially after administration of analgesic agents, *gastric-emptying time* typically is appreciably prolonged. A major danger of general anesthesia for delivery is regurgitation and aspiration of either food-laden or highly acidic gastric contents (see Chap. 17, p. 331).

Pyrosis (*heartburn*), common during pregnancy, is most likely caused by reflux of acidic secretions into the lower esophagus, the altered position of the stomach probably contributing

to its frequent occurrence. Esophageal and gastric tone are altered by pregnancy, with intraesophageal pressures being lower and intragastric pressures higher in pregnant women. At the same time, esophageal peristalsis has lower wave speed and lower amplitude (Ulmsten and Sundström, 1978). These changes favor gastroesophageal reflux.

The gums may become hyperemic and softened during pregnancy and may bleed when mildly traumatized, as with a toothbrush. A focal, highly vascular swelling of the gums, the so-called *epulis* of pregnancy develops occasionally but typically regresses spontaneously after delivery. There is no good evidence that pregnancy per se incites tooth decay.

Hemorrhoids are fairly common during pregnancy. They are caused in large measure by constipation and the elevated pressure in veins below the level of the enlarged uterus.

LIVER AND GALLBLADDER

LIVER

Although the liver in some animals increases remarkably in size during pregnancy, there is no evidence of such an increase in human pregnancy (Combes and Adams, 1971). Moreover, by histological evaluation of liver obtained by biopsy, including examination with the electron microscope, it has been demonstrated that no distinct changes in liver morphology occur in response to normal pregnancy (Ingerslev and Teilum, 1946). The results of the very few measurements of hepatic blood flow during pregnancy are conflicting, and there is perhaps a slight increase.

Some of the laboratory tests commonly used to evaluate hepatic function yield appreciably different results during normal pregnancy. Moreover, the changes induced by pregnancy often occur in the same direction as those found in patients with hepatic disease. Total *alkaline phosphatase* activity in serum almost doubles during normal pregnancy and commonly reaches levels that would be considered abnormal in the nonpregnant woman. Much of the increase is attributable to alkaline phosphatase isozymes from the placenta, which are heat-stable up to 65°C. Whether all of the increase is caused by enzymes of placental origin is not clear, since nonpregnant women given estrogen in amounts comparable with those found in pregnancy frequently have increased serum alkaline phosphatase activity in their blood (Song and Kappas, 1968). Mendenhall (1970) reconfirmed the presence of a decrease in *plasma albumin* concentration, showing it to average 3.0 g per dL late in pregnancy compared with 4.3 g per dL in nonpregnant women. The reduction in serum albumin, combined with a slight increase in globulins in plasma that occur normally during pregnancy, results in a decrease in the albumin to globulin ratio similar to that seen in certain hepatic diseases. Plasma *cholinesterase* activity is reduced during normal pregnancy. The magnitude of the decrease is about the same as the decrease in the concentration of albumin (Pritchard, 1955; Kamban and associates, 1988).

Leucine aminopeptidase activity is markedly elevated in serum from pregnant women and at term it reaches a level approximately three times the nonpregnant value. The increase in total serum leucine aminopeptidase activity during pregnancy results from the appearance of a pregnancy-specific enzyme (or enzymes) with distinct substrate specificities (Song and Kappas, 1968). Pregnancy-induced aminopeptidase has oxytocinase activity.

Combes and associates (1963) demonstrated that the capacity of the liver for excreting sulfobromophthalein into bile is somewhat decreased during normal pregnancy, while, at the same time, the ability of the liver to extract and store sulfobromophthalein is increased. The administration of estrogens to nonpregnant women induces comparable changes (Mueller and Kappas, 1964). *Spider nevi* and *palmer erythema,* both of which occur in patients with liver disease, are commonly found in normal pregnant women, most likely as a result of the increased circulating estrogens during pregnancy, but they disappear soon after delivery.

GALLBLADDER

Gallbladder function is altered during pregnancy. Potter (1936) noted at the time of cesarean section that quite often the gallbladder is distended but hypotonic; moreover, aspirated bile was quite thick. It is commonly accepted that pregnancy predisposes to formation of gallstones (see Chap. 39, p. 827).

ENDOCRINE GLANDS

Some of the most important endocrine changes of pregnancy have been discussed elsewhere, especially in Chapter 5.

PITUITARY

The pituitary enlarges during pregnancy by approximately 136 percent compared to nonpregnant controls (Gonzalez and colleagues, 1988). Although there have been suggestions that it may increase in size sufficiently to compress the optic chiasma and reduce the visual fields, such visual changes during normal pregnancy are either absent or minimal. Striking enlargement of microadenomas of the pituitary can occur, however, during pregnancy (see Chap. 39, p. 826).

The maternal pituitary gland is not essential for the maintenance of pregnancy. A number of women have undergone hypophysectomy, completed pregnancy successfully and have undergone spontaneous labor while receiving glucocorticosteroids along with thyroid hormone and vasopressin. Extensive destruction of both the maternal and the fetal pituitary glands in monkeys during the second trimester does not interrupt gestation (Hutchinson and co-workers, 1962). In these hypophysectomized primates, marked adrenal atrophy did not occur; thus the placenta may be a source of an adrenal corticotropin in this species.

PITUITARY GROWTH HORMONE

Although placental lactogen (hPL) is abundant in the blood of pregnant women, the level of pituitary growth hormone is increased only slightly. During the first trimester, serum and amnionic fluid growth-hormone values are within nonpregnant values of 0.5 to 7.5 ng per mL (Kletzky and associates, 1985). Serum values increase slowly from approximately 3.5 ng per mL at 10 weeks to plateau after 28 weeks at approximately 14 ng per mL. Growth hormone in amnionic fluid peaks at 14 to 15 weeks and slowly declines thereafter (Fig. 7–15) to reach baseline values after 36 weeks. After delivery, placental lactogen rapidly disappears, but growth hormone is elevated for some time but at levels lower than late pregnancy values (Spellacy and Buhi, 1969). The relative lack of these hormones, with the loss of their diabetogenic effect, may account in part for the usually abrupt

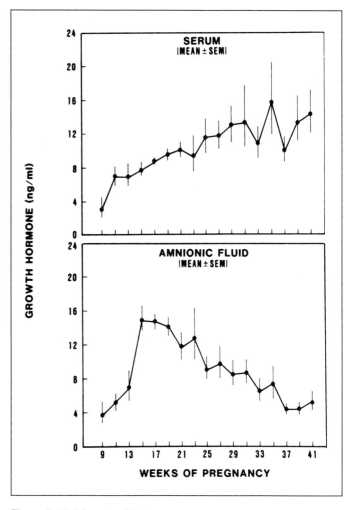

Figure 7–15. Mean (± SEM) concentrations of human growth hormone in maternal serum and in amnionic fluid throughout pregnancy. (*From Kletzky and associates: Am J Obstet Gynecol 151:878, 1985, with permission.*)

and rather marked reduction in insulin requirements of women with diabetes mellitus during the early puerperium.

PROLACTIN

During the course of human pregnancy, there is a marked increase in the levels of prolactin in the maternal plasma. In fact, the levels increase to such an extent that mean concentrations of 150 ng per mL, values 10 times greater than those in normal nonpregnant women, are observed at term (Kletzky and associates, 1985) (Fig. 7–16). Paradoxically, after delivery, there is a decrease in plasma prolactin concentration even in women who are breastfeeding. During early lactation, there are pulsatile bursts of secretion of prolactin apparently in response to suckling. The physiological cause of the marked increase in prolactin prior to parturition is not entirely certain; however, estrogen stimulation increases the number of anterior pituitary lactotrophs (prolactin producing cells) and may stimulate the release of prolactin from these cells (Andersen, 1982). Thyroid-releasing hormone acts to cause an increased level of prolactin in pregnant compared to nonpregnant women but the response decreases in each trimester as pregnancy advances (Andersen,

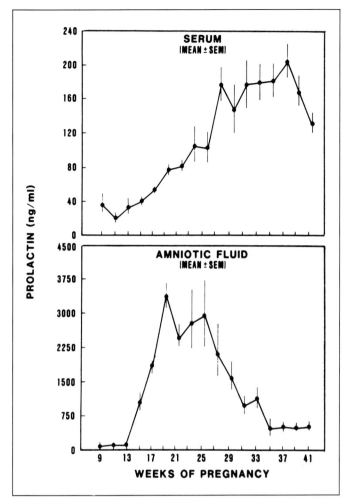

Figure 7–16. Mean (± SEM) concentrations of human prolactin in maternal serum and in amnionic fluid throughout pregnancy. (*From Kletzky and associates: Am J Obstet Gynecol 151:878, 1985, with permission.*)

1982; Miyamoto, 1984). Serotonin also is believed to increase prolactin but prolactin-inhibiting factor (probably identical to dopamine) is believed to inhibit its secretion (Andersen, 1982).

The principal function of maternal serum prolactin is believed to be to ensure lactation. Early in pregnancy, prolactin acts to initiate DNA synthesis and mitosis of glandular epithelial cells and the presecretory alveolar cells of the breast. Prolactin also increases the number of estrogen and prolactin receptors in these same cells. Finally, prolactin promotes mammary alveolar cell RNA synthesis, galactopoiesis, and production of casein and lactalbumin, lactose, and lipids (Andersen, 1982). Kauppila and co-workers (1987) found that a woman with an isolated prolactin deficiency failed to lactate after two pregnancies, establishing the absolute necessity of prolactin for lactation but *not* for successful pregnancy outcome.

Prolactin also is found, throughout the course of gestation, in high concentration in the fetal plasma, attaining highest concentrations during the last 5 weeks of pregnancy (Winters and associates, 1975). Considerable evidence has accrued that is supportive of the view that prolactin in fetal plasma is of fetal pituitary origin and not of maternal pituitary origin.

Prolactin is present in amnionic fluid in high concentrations, and indeed, levels of 10,000 ng per mL can be observed in

the amnionic fluid at 20 to 26 weeks gestation (Fig. 7–16). Several groups of investigators have presented convincing evidence that the uterine decidua is the site of synthesis of the prolactin in amnionic fluid. The levels of prolactin in amnionic fluid decrease after about 26 weeks and plateau after 34 weeks at approximately 500 ng per mL.

The function of amnionic fluid prolactin is not known. Some investigators have suggested that prolactin in amnionic fluid impairs the transfer of water from the fetal into the maternal compartment, thus preserving fetal extracellular fluid and preventing fetal dehydration during the last trimester of pregnancy when amnionic fluid is normally hypotonic (Andersen, 1982).

β-LIPOTROPHIN

The major precursor for a number of pituitary and likely chorionic peptide hormones is proopiomelanocortin, a large peptide chain that is processed at a variety of sites by specific proteolytic enzymes (see Chap. 5, p. 71, and Fig. 5–3). One of the major fragments from this process is a 91-amino-acid chain, β-lipotrophin. This compound may then be cleaved again to give two additional fragments, one a 51-amino-acid peptide called γ-lipotrophin and the other a 31-amino-acid chain called β-endorphin. β-Endorphin is a potent endogenous opioid that is elevated in a variety of stressful situations, including labor, in parallel with pituitary ACTH (Fletcher and associates, 1980; Genazzani and colleagues, 1981; Goland and associates, 1981).

Maternal plasma concentrations of β-lipotrophin, β-endorphin, and γ-lipotrophin are increased steadily throughout pregnancy (Browning and co-workers, 1983a, 1983b; Newnham and associates, 1983). Their levels are lower in women delivering vaginally who have epidural analgesia than in women receiving either a narcotic or no analgesics. The specific physiological function for these opioid agents in maternal plasma during pregnancy and labor has not been established. However, such agents obviously could serve to blunt the pain of childbirth.

Browning and co-workers (1983b) speculated that a flaccid baby with depressed respiratory drive may be the consequence of fetal acidosis, increasing the opioid agent β-endorphin to very high levels which, in turn, depress respiratory drive and result in a depressed neonate.

THYROID

During pregnancy there is moderate enlargement of the thyroid caused by hyperplasia of the glandular tissue and increased vascularity. However, normal pregnancy does not cause significant thyromegaly and any goiter in pregnancy should be considered as pathological (Levy and co-workers, 1980). The basal metabolic rate increases progressively during normal pregnancy by as much as 25 percent. Most of this increase in oxygen consumption is the result of the metabolic activity of the products of conception. If the body surface of the fetus is considered along with that of the mother, the predicted and the measured basal metabolic rates are quite similar.

Thyroxine

Beginning as early as the second month of pregnancy, the concentration of *thyroxine* (T$_4$) rises sharply in the maternal plasma to a plateau, which is maintained until after delivery. The plateau is reached at levels from 9 to 16 μg per dL as compared with 5 to 12 μg per dL in nonpregnant euthyroid women.

This elevation of circulating thyroid hormone is not indicative of hyperthyroidism. During pregnancy, the *thyroxine-binding proteins* of plasma, principally an α-globulin, are increased considerably. Mulaisho and Utiger (1977) provided the following mean values for thyroid-binding globulin levels in plasma: 7.1 mg per dL in the first trimester, 9.0 in the second, and 8.9 in the third trimester, compared to values of 3.6 mg per dL for normal nonpregnant women. Even though the total concentrations of thyroxine and triiodothyronine (T_3) are elevated, the amounts of unbound, or effective, hormone are not appreciably higher (Osathanondh and colleagues, 1976). The increase in circulating estrogens during pregnancy presumably is the major cause of these changes in hormone levels and binding capacity, for they can be reproduced by administering estrogen, including most oral contraceptives, to nonpregnant women. Although the normal early increase in thyroxine and thyroid-binding globulin and the decrease in triiodothyronine resin uptake are sometimes absent in women destined to abort, the abortion almost certainly is not the result of failure of hormones and binding protein to increase, but rather is due to an abnormal conceptus.

Reverse Triiodothyronine (rT_3)

Reverse T_3 is formed from the inner ring (5-deiodinase) monodeiodination of thyroxine. The level of reverse triiodothyronine in maternal blood is 3 to 5 times less than in fetal blood and amnionic fluid (Roti and associates, 1983) likely because the conversion of thyroxine to reverse triiodothyronine occurs in fetal membranes and in the placenta.

There is almost no transfer of thyroxine, triiodothyronine, or reverse triiodothyronine from the maternal into the fetal compartment. Therefore, fetal thyroid function appears to be independent of maternal thyroid status. This protection of the fetus likely is the consequence of the previously mentioned placental inner ring deiodination of thyroxine.

Long-acting Thyroid Stimulator (LATS)

The usually protected status of the fetal thyroid is overcome in some cases of Graves' disease. Long-acting thyroid stimulator (LATS) may cross the placenta in women with Graves' disease and stimulate the fetal thyroid to produce neonatal thyrotoxicosis. The long-acting thyroid stimulator now is recognized to be only one of a variety of thyroid-stimulating immunoglobulins that may be detected in women with Graves' disease (Roti and co-workers, 1983).

Thyroid-releasing Hormone (TRH)

Thyroid-releasing hormone is a neurotransmitter present throughout the brain but in highest concentrations in the hypothalamus. This compound stimulates the synthesis and release of thyroid-stimulating hormone from the anterior pituitary. It is not increased during normal pregnancy but it does cross the placenta and may stimulate the fetal pituitary to increase thyroid-stimulating hormone (Roti and associates, 1983). The role, if any, served by maternal thyroid-releasing hormone in fetal homeostasis is not clear at this time.

Thyroid-stimulating Hormone (TSH)

Thyroid-stimulating hormone is not bound by a carrier protein in the blood but circulates in the free form. Its concentration is not elevated by pregnancy, and it does not cross the placenta. Thus, there is no correlation between maternal and fetal thyroid-stimulating hormone.

During pregnancy, there is increased uptake of ingested radioiodide by the maternal thyroid gland, again suggesting a hyperthyroid state. Some of this is undoubtedly because renal iodide excretion is increased concomitant with increased glomerular filtration. This causes decreased serum iodide concentration and iodide deficiency. Aboul-Khair and associates (1964) claim that although the clearance of inorganic iodine is increased by the thyroid gland during pregnancy, the absolute uptake is not increased. They concluded that the thyroid enlargement of pregnancy simply compensates for the lower concentration of circulating iodide available for synthesis of thyroxine.

Hershman and Starnes (1969), as well as others, identified a thyrotropic substance obtained from human placenta but the role of *chorionic thyrotropin*, if any, in stimulating the thyroid is unclear. In women with hydatidiform moles, increased thyroid activity is likely due primarily to the action of chorionic gonadotropin, which is known to have intrinsic thyroid-stimulating activity. In Table 7–4, the pregnancy-induced changes, those found in hyperthyroidism and those induced by administration of estrogen, are compared.

Thyroxine, thyroxine-binding capacity, and triiodothyronine resin uptake values in cord serum are less than those in maternal serum but greater than levels in nonpregnant adults (Russell and colleagues, 1964).

PARATHYROID AND CALCIUM METABOLISM

The regulation of calcium concentration is closely interrelated to magnesium, phosphate, parathyroid hormone, vitamin D, and

TABLE 7–4. COMPARISON OF EFFECTS OF PREGNANCY AND OF ESTROGEN ADMINISTRATION ON TESTS USED TO EVALUATE THYROID FUNCTION

Tests	Normal Pregnancy	Estrogen Administration	Hyperthyroidism
Basal metabolic rate	Increased	Not increased	Increased
Total thyroxine	Increased	Increased	Increased
Thyroxine-binding globulin	Increased	Increased	Not increased
Free thyroxine	Not increased	Not increased	Increased
Total triiodothyronine	Increased	Increased	Increased
Free triiodothyronine	Not increased	Not increased	Increased
Radioiodine uptake (percent)	Increased	Not increased	Increased
Absolute iodine uptake	Not increased	Not increased	Increased
Triiodothyronine resin uptake	Decreased	Decreased	Increased
Serum cholesterol level	Increased	Variable	Decreased

calcitonin physiology. Any alteration of one of these factors is likely to change the others.

Parathyroid Hormone and Calcium Interrelationships

Acute or chronic decreases in plasma calcium or acute decreases in magnesium stimulate the release of parathyroid hormone whereas increases in calcium and magnesium suppress parathyroid hormone levels. The known actions of parathyroid hormone are presented in Table 7–5. The net effect of the action of this hormone on bone resorption, intestinal absorption, and kidney reabsorption is to increase extracellular fluid calcium and decrease phosphate (Tsang and co-workers, 1976).

Parathyroid hormone concentrations in plasma decrease during the first trimester, then increase progressively throughout the remainder of pregnancy (Pitkin, 1985). Increased parathyroid hormone levels likely result from increased plasma volume, increased glomerular filtration rate, and increased fetal transfer of calcium, all resulting in a chronic suppression of calcium concentration in the pregnant woman. Despite the well-observed decrease in total calcium concentration during pregnancy, ionized calcium, which is the major feedback mechanism regulating secretion of parathyroid hormone, is decreased only slightly during pregnancy (Pitkin, 1985). Reitz and co-workers (1977) suggest that during pregnancy a new "set point" exists between ionized calcium and parathyroid hormone. Estrogens also appear to block the action of parathyroid hormone on bone resorption resulting in another mechanism to increase parathyroid hormone during pregnancy. The net result of these actions is a "physiological hyperparathyroidism" of pregnancy, likely in order to supply the fetus with adequate calcium.

Calcitonin and Calcium Interrelationships

The calcitonin-secreting C-cells are derived embryologically from the neural crest and are located predominantly in the parafollicular areas of the thyroid gland. Calcium and magnesium increase the biosynthesis and secretion of calcitonin. Various gastric hormones (gastrin, pentagastrin, glucagon, and pancreoxymin) and food ingestion also increase calcitonin plasma levels.

The known actions of calcitonin are shown in Table 7–5 and can generally be considered to oppose those of parathyroid hormone and vitamin D to protect the calcification of the skeleton during times of calcium stress. Pregnancy and lactation are two examples of profound calcium stress; and during these times, calcitonin levels are appreciably higher than in nonpregnant women (Whitehead and associates, 1981).

Vitamin D and Calcium Interrelationships

Vitamin D is produced in the skin or ingested and is converted into 25-hydroxyvitamin D_3 in the liver. This product then is converted in the kidney, decidua, and placenta to 1,25-dihydroxyvitamin D_3 (Weisman and co-workers, 1979), which is most likely the biologically active compound, the known actions of which are listed in Table 7–5.

The actual control of 1,25-dihydroxyvitamin D_3 production and release is unknown, but the conversion of 25-hydroxyvitamin D_3 to 1,25-dihydroxyvitamin D_3 is facilitated by parathyroid hormone and by low calcium and phosphate plasma levels and opposed by calcitonin (Tsang and associates, 1976). A possible role of prolactin has been suggested by Robinson and colleagues (1982). They found that in the lactating rat, prolactin increased the plasma levels of 1,25-dihydroxyvitamin D_3 and this in turn increased intestinal absorption of calcium. As yet, this effect has not been reported in the human, but 1,25-dihydroxyvitamin D_3 levels are increased during normal pregnancy (Whitehead and associates, 1981).

ADRENAL GLANDS

In normal pregnancy, there is probably very little morphological change in the maternal adrenal glands.

Cortisol

There is a considerable increase in the concentration of circulating cortisol, but much of it is bound by cortisol-binding globulin, *transcortin*. The rate of cortisol secretion by the maternal adrenal is not increased, and probably it is decreased compared to the nonpregnant state. The metabolic clearance rate of cortisol, however, is lower during pregnancy, as indicated by the fact that in a pregnant woman, the half-life of intravenously injected radiolabeled cortisol is nearly twice as long as it is in nonpregnant women (Migeon and associates, 1957). Administration of estrogen, including most oral contraceptives, causes changes in levels of cortisol and transcortin similar to those of pregnancy.

In early pregnancy, the levels of circulating corticotropin (ACTH) are strikingly reduced. As pregnancy progresses, the levels of ACTH and free cortisol rise. This apparent paradox is not completely understood. Nolten and Rueckert (1981) have presented evidence that the higher free cortisol levels observed in pregnancy are the result of a "resetting" of the maternal feedback mechanisms to higher levels. They further propose that the "resetting" might result from *tissue refractoriness* to cortisol. Thus an elevated free cortisol would be needed during pregnancy to maintain homeostasis.

Aldosterone

As early as the 15th week of normal pregnancy, the maternal adrenal secretes considerably increased amounts of aldosterone. By the third trimester, about 1 mg per day is secreted. If sodium intake is restricted, aldosterone secretion is elevated even further (Watanabe and co-workers, 1963). At the same

TABLE 7–5. RELATIONSHIP BETWEEN PARATHYROID HORMONE (PTH), VITAMIN D, AND CALCITONIN TO CALCIUM (Ca), PHOSPHATE (P), AND MAGNESIUM (Mg)

| | Bone Resorption | | | Intestinal Absorption | | Kidney Reabsorption | | | Extracellular Fluid | |
	Ca	P	Mg	Ca	Mg	Ca	P	Mg	Ca	P
PTH	↑	↑	↑	↑	↑	↑	↓	↑	↑	↓
Vitamin D	↑	↑	—	↑	↑	—	—	—	↑	↑
Calcitonin	↓	↓	↓	—	↓	↓	↓	↓	↓	↓

Modified from Tsang and colleagues: Ped Clin North Am 23:611, 1976.

time, levels of renin and angiotensin II substrate are normally increased, especially during the latter half of pregnancy (Geelhoed and Vander, 1968; Massani and associates, 1967). This gives rise to increased plasma levels of angiotensin II, which, by acting on the zona glomerulosa of the maternal adrenal glands, likely accounts for the markedly elevated secretion of aldosterone. It has been suggested that the increased secretion of aldosterone during normal pregnancy affords protection against the natriuretic effect of progesterone (Landau and Lugibihl, 1961). Progesterone administered to nonpregnant women is associated with a prompt increase in aldosterone excretion (Laidlaw and colleagues, 1962).

Deoxycorticosterone

There is a striking increase in the maternal plasma levels of deoxycorticosterone (DOC) during pregnancy. Brown and co-workers (1972) and Nolten and associates (1978) found that in nonpregnant women and during the first two trimesters of pregnancy, the levels of plasma DOC are less than 100 pg / mL. During the last few weeks of pregnancy, DOC levels rise to 1,500 pg per mL or more (Fig. 7–17). Interestingly, Nolten and associates found that the administration of a potent glucocorticosteroid, dexamethasone, to pregnant women to reduce ACTH secretion is not accompanied by a reduction in plasma DOC levels. Moreover, ACTH administration to pregnant women is not accompanied by an increase in plasma DOC concentration. This was highly suggestive that DOC and DOC-SO_4 in plasma of pregnant women do not arise principally by maternal adrenal secretion. The levels of DOC and DOC-SO_4 in fetal blood are appreciably higher than those in the maternal blood, and this finding led some investigators to suggest that DOC and DOC-SO_4 in the maternal compartment may arise, at least in part, by way of transfer from the fetus. This may be true; nonetheless, transfer of DOC and DOC-SO_4 from fetus to mother must account for no more than a small fraction of the total amount of these compounds in the maternal compartment.

Most of the DOC in maternal plasma arises by way of the extraadrenal 21-hydroxylation of plasma progesterone in maternal tissues (Winkel and associates, 1980). The product of the fractional conversion of plasma progesterone to DOC and the plasma production rate of progesterone is very nearly equal to the total production rate of DOC in the maternal compartment. This is a very interesting and potentially important phenomenon for several reasons. First, the extraadrenal conversion of plasma progesterone to DOC is known to occur in tissue sites of mineralocorticosteroid action, viz., kidney, skin, blood vessels. Thus, there is in situ formation of a potent mineralocorticosteroid in its potential site of action. It is possible that far greater concentrations of DOC can be achieved in a given responsive cell by way of this mechanism than could reasonably be achieved by way of delivery through blood. Second, there is great individual variation in the fractional conversion of plasma progesterone to DOC among persons. This is very unusual for steroid conversions or interconversions. Ordinarily, the fractional conversion of one steroid to another is reasonably similar among persons, but this is not true in the case of the fractional conversion of plasma progesterone to DOC. Indeed, variations in this conversion by 30-fold or more have been observed among normal women. Therefore, the capacity of one woman to produce DOC from extraadrenal utilization of plasma progesterone to DOC may be remarkably greater than that found in another woman. For these two reasons, it is quite possible that much more DOC is produced during pregnancy in one woman compared with another, and the DOC produced may be formed largely in tissues that are mineralocorticosteroid-responsive. The clinical implications of these findings, if any, with respect to sodium homeostasis during pregnancy and with alterations in sodium retention are unknown. In any event, it is startling that the adaptation to pregnancy includes accommodations for marked increases in the formation of both aldosterone and DOC in most normally pregnant women without the development of hypertension. Teleologically, it is probable that the increased formation of mineralocorticosteroids is important in the plasma volume expansion that accompanies pregnancy.

The mechanisms of origin of DOC-SO_4 during pregnancy are equally or more provocative than are those of DOC. It is clearly established that plasma DOC is not converted to plasma DOC-SO_4. Therefore, DOC-SO_4 in plasma must arise by way of some DOC-independent mechanism. Plasma progesterone is not converted to DOC-SO_4. Recently, however, evidence was obtained that DOC-SO_4 in the blood of pregnant women probably arises by way of a fetal-placental interaction. It has been known for some time that the fetal plasma concentration of pregnenolone-3,21-disulfate is elevated strikingly with fetal plasma levels to 1,000 ng per mL. Yet, it is believed that pregnenolone and pregnenolone sulfate are not good substrates for steroid 21-hydroxylase activity in the fetal adrenal. On the other hand, large amounts of pregnenolone sulfate are known to be secreted by the fetal adrenal glands. It is likely that pregnenolone sulfate is converted in fetal liver to pregnenolone-3,21-disulfate and, in the placenta, the latter is converted to DOC-SO_4. This is probably accomplished because "placental sulfatase" readily removes sulfates from the C-3 position of steroids, but the Km of the enzyme for 21-sulfates is much greater than that for 3-sulfates. Thus, in placenta pregnenolone-3,21-disulfate is converted to pregnenolone-21-sulfate, which in turn is converted by way of 3β-hydroxysteroid dehydrogenase to DOC-SO_4. The DOC-SO_4 formed is secreted into the maternal compartment. This set of findings raises again the interesting question that the extraadrenal steroid 21-hydroxylase(s) may be a different enzyme(s) than that primarily expressed in the adrenal cortex.

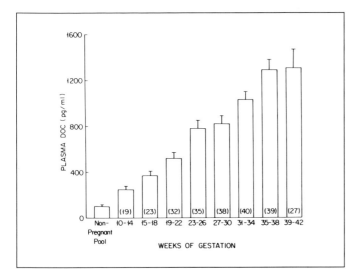

Figure 7–17. Plasma deoxycorticosterone (DOC) in primigravid women (*From Parker and co-workers: Am J Obstet Gynecol 138:626, 1980.*)

In summary, DOC present in maternal plasma arises primarily by way of the 21-hydroxylation of plasma progesterone and this transformation occurs in tissue sites of mineralocorticosteroid action. Great person-to-person variability in this peripheral conversion is known to exist. DOC-SO$_4$ in maternal plasma arises, at least in part, by way of placental formation of DOC-SO$_4$ from the utilization of fetal plasma pregnenolone-3,21-disulfate (Casey and associates, 1987; Casey and MacDonald, 1982; Parker and co-workers, 1983).

DEHYDROISOANDROSTERONE SULFATE

As discussed in Chapter 5 (p. 73), the levels of *dehydroisoandrosterone sulfate* circulating in maternal blood and excreted in the urine are not increased during normal pregnancy, but rather decreased as a consequence of an increased rate of removal, through extensive 16α-hydroxylation in the maternal liver and estrogen formation in the placenta.

ANDROSTENEDIONE AND TESTOSTERONE

Maternal plasma levels of *androstenedione* and *testosterone* are increased during pregnancy. This finding is not totally explained by alterations in the metabolic clearance rates of these steroids. On the one hand, maternal plasma androstenedione and testosterone are converted to estradiol in the placenta, which increases the rate of clearance, but, on the other hand, there is an increased amount of sex hormone–binding globulin in plasma of pregnant women which retards the rate of testosterone clearance. Thus, there is an increased plasma production rate of maternal testosterone and androstenedione during human pregnancy. The source of this increased C$_{19}$-steroid production is unknown but it likely originates in the ovary. Interestingly, little or no testosterone in maternal plasma enters the fetal circulation as testosterone. Even when massive testosterone levels are found in the circulation of pregnant women with androgen-secreting tumors, the testosterone level in umbilical cord venous plasma is likely to be too low to be detected. This finding is the result of the near complete conversion of testosterone to 17β-estradiol by the trophoblast (Edman and associates, 1979).

MUSCULOSKELETAL SYSTEM

Progressive *lordosis* is a characteristic feature of normal pregnancy. Compensating for the anterior position of the enlarging uterus, the lordosis shifts the center of gravity back over the lower extremities. There is increased mobility of the sacroiliac, sacrococcygeal, and the pubic joints during pregnancy, presumably as a result of hormonal changes. Their mobility may contribute to the alteration of maternal posture and, in turn, cause discomfort in the lower portion of the back, especially late in pregnancy. During the last trimester of pregnancy, aching, numbness, and weakness are occasionally experienced in the upper extremities, possibly as a result of the marked lordosis with anterior flexion of the neck and slumping of the shoulder girdle, which, in turn, produces traction on the ulnar and median nerves (Crisp and DeFrancesco, 1964).

PRECOCIOUS AND LATE PREGNANCY

PRECOCIOUS PREGNANCY

The youngest mother whose history is authenticated is Lina Medina, who was delivered by cesarean section in Lima, Peru,

on May 15, 1939. It was claimed that she was 4 years and 8 months old, but a careful review of her birth records indicates that she may have been 5 years and 8 months of age. In either event, it is a record. Ms. Medina related to a reporter (*The National Enquirer*, September 30, 1980) that she always knew that the child, who had been raised as her brother, had come from her own body, but she did not completely comprehend the significance of this until she was about eleven. Gerardo (named for the doctor who performed the cesarean section) was 10 years old before he knew that Lina was his mother. Ms. Medina went on to marry Raul Gonzalez and has had one child in this marriage. Gerardo married at age 18 and had two daughters. He died on September 8, 1979, of an apparent heart attack at the age of 40.

Although true precocious puberty, as suffered by Lina Medina, is still very uncommon, the average age of menarche and ovulation is appreciably lower than it was several decades ago (see Chap. 3, Fig. 3–6). The mean age of menarche in the United States is now estimated to be 12.3 years.

As a consequence of earlier menarche, and perhaps of greater sexual freedom, most obstetrical services have witnessed a marked increase in the number of extremely young pregnant women.

LATE PREGNANCY

The large number of women born during the so-called baby boom after World War II are now centered around 40 years of age. This, coupled with evidence that women are delaying childbearing, has caused a disproportionate increase in older women giving birth in the United States. For example, the Census Bureau estimates that total births to women aged 35 to 49 will increase from 5 percent in 1982 to 8.6 percent in the year 2000 (Spencer, 1984).

Although it was predicted by some that long-term suppression of ovulation by oral contraceptives might result in continued ovulation for years after the usual time of menopause, there is no evidence to support the occurrence of such a phenomenon. Pregnancy after age 47 is uncommon. In a careful review of the literature from 1860 to 1964 on this subject, Wharton (1964) cited 26 women over the age of 50 with normal pregnancy and the oldest was said to be 63. The paucity of reports of pregnancy in women of advanced age is probably an underestimate of the prevalence, but it nevertheless indicates the rarity of pregnancy in the sixth decade of life.

Specific risks related to childbearing in older women have been identified by Hansen (1986), who described the first risk to the older woman as an inability to conceive with advancing age. In this extensive review, he found that during pregnancy in older women, hypertension, diabetes, and preeclampsia were diagnosed more commonly, as was fetal demise due to these maternal complications. Placenta previa and abruptions were more common in women past 35, likely due to vascular disease. As might be expected, the incidence of cesarean section was increased significantly. The final sobering fact was that maternal mortality was increased several times more in older compared to younger pregnant women.

Lehmann and Chism (1987) reported similar findings in 183 women aged 40 or older who were delivered at Charity Hospital in New Orleans. In addition to an increased incidence of pregnancy-induced hypertension and placental abruption, they reported that 6 percent of these women required blood transfusions for hemorrhage and that there was substantively increased deep venous thrombosis and pulmonary embolism. Birthweight less than 2,500 g (17.5 versus 10.5 percent) and more than 4,000 g (7.7 versus 3.3 percent) were almost doubled compared to their general obstetrical population.

Not all investigators paint such a bleak picture. Kirz and colleagues (1985) from Women's Hospital of Long Beach compared pregnancy outcomes in 1,023 women 35 years and older to those in 5,343 women aged 20 to 25. As expected, the incidences of hypertension and diabetes were increased in the older women (about fourfold); however, preterm labor was almost half as common as in the younger women. They, too, confirmed, but could not explain, an almost doubled cesarean delivery rate in the older women. Perhaps expectedly, infants with birthweights more than 4,000 g were encountered more commonly in the older-aged women (16 versus 11 percent). Importantly, this observation held true even if diabetic women were excluded from the analysis.

Fetal and neonatal mortality were noted by Horger and Smythe (1977) to be increased in older women, in part due to preterm births and fetal growth retardation. The stillbirth rate doubled with advancing maternal age from the early 20s to the late 30s and quadrupled by the mid-40s. The neonatal mortality rate had only a mild association with advancing maternal age but chromosomal anomalies increased remarkably with advancing maternal age, especially trisomies 13, 18, and 21 as well as sex chromosome aneuploides. Likewise, Lehmann and Chism (1987) reported a threefold increased perinatal mortality in women 40 or over compared to their general obstetrical population. Conversely, Kirz and co-workers (1985) reported that perinatal mortality rates were similar in women 35 or older compared to those 20 to 25.

The obstetrical and pediatric implications are apparent. These additional risks for the older pregnant woman and her fetus-infant must be anticipated and appropriate interventions planned to lessen these risks.

REFERENCES

Aboul-Khair SA, Crooks J, Turnbull AC, Hytten FE: The physiological changes in thyroid function during pregnancy. Clin Sci 27:195, 1964

Abou-Samra M, Pugeat M, Dechaud H, Nachury L, Tourniaire J: Acute dopaminergic blockage by sulpiride stimulates β-endorphin secretion in pregnant woman. Clin Endocrinol 21:583, 1984

Alvarez H, Caldeyro-Barcia R: Contractility of the human uterus recorded by new methods. Surg Gynecol Obstet 91:1, 1950

Amino N, Tanizawa O, Miyai K, Tanaka F, Hayashi C, Kawashima M, Ichihara K: Changes in serum immunoglobulins IgG, IgA, IgM, and IgE during pregnancy. Obstet Gynecol 52:415, 1978

Andersen JR: Prolactin in amniotic fluid and maternal serum during uncomplicated human pregnancy. Dan Med Bull 29:266, 1982

Anderson GH, Howland T, Domascek P, Streeten DHP: Effect of sodium balance and calcium channel blocking drugs on blood pressure responses. Hypertension 10:239, 1987

Assali NS, Dilts PV, Pentl AA, Kirschbaum TH, Gross SJ: Physiology of the placenta. In Assali NS (ed): Biology of Gestation, Vol I: The Maternal Organism. New York, Academic, 1968

Assali NS, Douglass RA, Baird WW, Nicholson DB, Suyemoto R: Measurement of uterine blood flow and uterine metabolism: IV. Results in normal pregnancy. Am J Obstet Gynecol 66:248, 1953

Assali NS, Rauramo L, Peltonen T: Measurement of uterine blood flow and uterine metabolism: VIII. Uterine and fetal blood flow and oxygen consumption in early human pregnancy. Am J Obstet Gynecol 79:86, 1960

Astedt B: Significance of placenta in depression of fibrinolytic activity during pregnancy. J Obstet Gynaecol Br Commonw 79:205, 1972

Atarashi K, Mulrow PJ, Franco-Saenz R, Snajdar R, Rapp J: Inhibition of aldosterone production by an atrial extract. Science 224:992, 1984

Baboonian C, Griffiths P: Is pregnancy immunosuppressive? Humoral immunity against viruses. Br J Obstet Gynaecol 90:1168, 1983

Bailey RR, Rolleston GL: Kidney length and ureteric dilatation in the puerperium. J Obstet Gynaecol Br Commonw 78:55, 1971

Baldwin GR, Moorthi DS, MacDonnell KF: New lung functions and pregnancy. Am J Obstet Gynecol 127:235, 1977

Baumann G, Puavilai G, Freinkel N, Domont LA, Metzger BE, Levene HB: Hepatic insulin and glucagon receptors in pregnancy: Their role in the enhanced catabolism during fasting. Endocrinology 108:1979, 1981

Bean WB, Cogswell R, Dexter M, Embick JF: Vascular changes of the skin in pregnancy—vascular spiders and palmar erythema. Surg Gynecol Obstet 88:739, 1949

Beaufils M, Uzan S, Donsimoni R, Colau JC: Prevention of pre-eclampsia by early antiplatelet therapy. Lancet 1:840, 1985

Belizan JM, Villar J: The relationship between calcium intake and edema-, proteinuria-, and hypertension-gestosis. Am J Clin Nutr 33:661, 1971

Belizan JM, Villar J, Zalazar A, Rojas L, Chan D, Bryce GF: Preliminary evidence of the effect of calcium supplementation on blood pressure in normal pregnant women. Am J Obstet Gynecol 146:175, 1983

Bellina JH, Dougherty CM, Mickal A: Pyeloureteral dilation and pregnancy. Am J Obstet Gynecol 108:356, 1970

Bender HS, Chickering WR: Minireview: Pregnancy and diabetes: The maternal response. Life Sci 37:1, 1985

Besinger RE, Niebyl JR: Tocolytic agents for the treatment of preterm labor. In Niebyl JR (ed): Drug Use in Pregnancy, 2nd ed. Philadelphia, Lea & Febiger, 1988, Chap 13, p 127

Bieniarz J, Branda LA, Maqueda E, Morozovsky J, Caldeyro-Barcia R: Aortocaval compression by the uterus in late pregnancy: III. Unreliability of the sphymomanometric method in estimating uterine artery pressure. Am J Obstet Gynecol 102:1106, 1968

Blechner JN, Stenger VG, Prystowsky H: Blood flow to the human uterus during maternal metabolic acidosis. Am J Obstet Gynecol 121:789, 1975

Bolton FG, Street MJ, Pace AJ: Changes in erythrocyte volume and shape in pregnancy. Br J Obstet Gynecol 89:1018, 1982

Bonnar J: Hemostatic function and coagulopathy during pregnancy. In Wynn R (ed): Obstetrics and Gynecology Annual. New York, Appleton, 1978, p 195

Borenstein AB: The effect of natriuretic atrial extract on renal hemodynamics and urinary excretion in anesthetized rats. J Physiol 334:133, 1983

Brar HS, Platt LD, DeVore GR, Horenstein J, Medearis AL: Qualitative assessment of maternal uterine and fetal umbilical artery blood flow and resistance in laboring patients by Doppler velocimetry. Am J Obstet Gynecol 158:95, 1988

Broughton-Pipkin F, Meirelles RS: Prostaglandin E$_2$ attenuates the pressor response to angiotensin II in pregnant subjects but not in nonpregnant subjects. Am J Obstet Gynecol 142:168, 1982

Brown MA, Crawford GA, Horgan EA, Gallery EDM: Arginine vasopressin in primigravid human pregnancy: A prospective study. J Repro Med 33:35, 1988

Brown MA, Gallery EDM, Ross MR, Esber RP: Sodium excretion in normal and hypertensive pregnancy: A prospective study. Am J Obstet Gynecol 159:297, 1988

Brown MA, Sinosich MJ, Saunders DM, Gallery EDM: Potassium regulation and progesterone-aldosterone interrelationships in human pregnancy: A prospective study. Am J Obstet Gynecol 155:349, 1986

Brown RD, Strott CA, Liddle GW: Plasma desoxycorticosterone in normal and abnormal human pregnancy. J Clin Endocrinol Metab 35:736, 1972

Browne JCM, Veall N: The maternal placental blood flow in normotensive and hypertensive women. J Obstet Gynaecol Br Emp 60:142, 1953

Browning AJF, Butt WR, Lynch SS, Shakespear RA: Maternal plasma concentrations of β-endorphin and γ-lipotrophin throughout pregnancy. Br J Obstet Gynaecol 90:1147, 1983a

Browning AJF, Butt WR, Lynch SS, Shakespear RA, Crawford JS: Maternal and cord plasma concentrations of β-lipotrophin, β-endorphin, and γ-lipotrophin at delivery: Effect of analgesia. Br J Obstet Gynaecol 90:1152, 1983b

Bryant-Greenwood GD: Relaxin as a new hormone. Endocr Rev 3:62, 1982

Burnett JC: Effects of synthetic ANF on renal function and renin release. Am J Physiol F863, 1984

Burt CC: Forearm and hand blood flow in pregnancy. In Toxaemias of Pregnancy. Ciba Foundation Symposium. Philadelphia, Blakiston, 1950, p 151

Burt RL, Davidson IWF: Insulin half-life and utilization in normal pregnancy. Obstet Gynecol 43:161, 1974

Calloway DH: Nitrogen balance during pregnancy. In Winick M (ed): Nutrition and Fetal Development. New York, Wiley, 1974, Vol 2

Campbell S, Griffin DF, Pearce JM, Diaz-Recasens J, Cohen-Overbeek TE, Willson K, Teague MJ: New Doppler technique for assessing uteroplacental blood flow. Lancet 1:675, 1983

Carsten ME, Regulation of myometrial composition, growth, and activity. In Assali NS (ed): Biology of Gestation, Vol I: The Maternal Organism. New York, Academic, 1968

Casey ML, MacDonald PC: Metabolism of deoxycorticosterone and deoxycorticosterone sulfate in men and women. J Clin Invest 70:312, 1982

Casey ML, Winkel CA, Guerami A, MacDonald PC: Mineralocorticosteroids and pregnancy: Regulation of extraadrenal deoxycorticosterone production by estrogen. J Steroid Biochem 27:1013, 1987

Caton WL, Roby CC, Reid DE, Gibson JG: Plasma volume and extravascular fluid volume during pregnancy and the puerperium. Am J Obstet Gynecol 57:471, 1949

Chard T, Craig PH, Menabawey M, Lee C: Alpha interferon in human pregnancy. Br J Obstet Gynaecol 93:1145, 1986

Chesley LC: Renal function during pregnancy. In Carey HM (ed): Modern Trends in Human Reproductive Physiology. London, Butterworth, 1963

Chesley LC: Renin, angiotensin, and aldosterone in pregnancy. In Chesley LC (ed): Hypertensive Disorders in Pregnancy. New York, Appleton-Century-Crofts, 1978, p 236

Chesley LC: Weight changes and water balance in normal and toxic pregnancy. Am J Obstet Gynecol 48:565, 1944

Chesley LC, Sloan DM: The effect of posture on renal function in late pregnancy. Am J Obstet Gynecol 89:754, 1964

Chesley LC, Talledo OE, Bohler CS, Zuspan FP: Vascular reactivity to angiotensin II and norepinephrine in pregnant and nonpregnant women. Am J Obstet Gynecol 91:837, 1965

Chrétien FC: Ultrastructure and variations of human cervical mucus during pregnancy and the menopause. Acta Obstet Gynecol Scand 57:337, 1978

Christofides ND, Ghatei MA, Bloom SR, Borberg C, Gillmer MDG: Decreased plasma motilin concentrations in pregnancy. Br Med J 285:1453, 1982

Cohen DA, Daughaday WH, Weldon VV: Fetal and maternal virilization associated with pregnancy. Am J Dis Child 136:353, 1982

Cole DEC, Gundberg CM, Stirk LJ, Atkinson SA, Hanley DA, Ayer LM, Baldwin LS: Changing osteocalcin concentrations during pregnancy and lactation: Implications for maternal mineral metabolism. J Clin Endocrinol Metab 65:290, 1987

Combes B, Adams RH: Pathophysiology of the liver in pregnancy. In Assali NS (ed): Pathophysiology of Gestation. New York, Academic, 1971, Vol I

Combes B, Shibata H, Adams R, Mitchell BD, Trammell V: Alterations in sulfobromophthalein sodium-removal mechanisms from blood during normal pregnancy. J Clin Invest 42:1431, 1963

Coopland A, Alkjaersig N, Fletcher AP: Reduction in plasma factor XIII (fibrin stabilization factor) concentration during pregnancy. J Lab Clin Med 73:144, 1969

Cotes PM, Canning CE, Lind T: Changes in serum immunoreactive erythropoietin during the menstrual cycle and normal pregnancy. Br J Obstet Gynecol 90:304, 1983

Crawford RJ, Hudson P, Shine J, Niall HD, Eddy RL, Shows TB: Two human relaxin genes are on chromosome 9. EMBO J 3:2341, 1984

Crisp WE, DeFrancesco A: The hand syndrome of pregnancy. Obstet Gynecol 23:433, 1964

Csapo AI, Pulkkinen MO, Wiest WG: Effects of hysterectomy and progesterone replacement in early pregnant patients. Am J Obstet Gynecol 115:759, 1973

Cunningham FG, Cox K, Gant NF: Further observations on the nature of pressor responsivity to angiotensin II in human pregnancy. Obstet Gynecol 46:581, 1975

Cusson JR, Gutkowska J, Rey E, Michon N, Boucher M, Larochelle P: Plasma concentration of atrial natriuretic factor in normal pregnancy. N Engl J Med 313:1230, 1985

Cutforth R, MacDonald CB: Heart sounds and murmurs in pregnancy. Am Heart J 71:741, 1966

Dahlström H, Ihrman K: A clinical and physiological study of pregnancy in a material from Northern Sweden: IV. Observations on the blood volume during and after pregnancy. Acta Soc Med Upsal 65:295, 1960

Darmady JM, Postle AD: Lipid metabolism in pregnancy. Br J Obstet Gynaecol 89:211, 1982

Davison JM, Hytten FE: Glomerular filtration during and after pregnancy. J Obstet Gynaecol Brit Commonw 81:588, 1974

Davison JM, Hytten FE: The effect of pregnancy on the renal handling of glucose. Br J Obstet Gynaecol 82:374, 1975

Davison JM, Vallotton MB, Lindheimer MD: Plasma osmolality and urinary concentration and dilution during and after pregnancy: Evidence that lateral recumbency inhibits maximal urinary concentrating ability. Br J Obstet Gynaecol 88:472, 1981

Dennis KJ, Bytheway WR: Changes in the body weight after delivery. J Obstet Gynaecol Br Commonw 72:94, 1965

Desoye G, Schweditsch MO, Preiffer KP, Zechner R, Kostner GM: Correlation of hormones with lipid and lipoprotein levels during normal pregnancy and postpartum. J Clin Endocrinol Metab 64:704, 1987

Diczfalusy E, Troen P: Endocrine functions of the human placenta. Vitam Horm 19:229, 1961

Douglas JT, Shah M, Lowe GDO, Betch JF, Forbes CD, Prentice CRM: Plasma fibrinopeptide A and beta-thromboglobulin in pre-eclampsia and pregnancy hypertension. Thromb Haemost 47:54, 1982

Dunlop W: Investigations into influence of posture on renal plasma flow and glomerular filtration rate during late pregnancy. Br J Obstet Gynaecol 83:17, 1976

Dunlop W: Serial changes in renal haemodynamics during normal human pregnancy. Br J Obstet Gynaecol 88:1, 1981

Easterling TR, Schmucker BC, Benedetti TJ: The hemodynamic effects of orthostatic stress during pregnancy. Obstet Gynecol 72:550, 1988

Eddie LW, Bell RJ, Lester A, Geier M, Bennett G, Johnston PD, Niall HD: Radioimmunoassay of relaxin in pregnancy with an analogue of human relaxin. Lancet 1:1344, 1986

Edman CD, Devereux WP, Parker CR, MacDonald PC: Placental clearance of maternal androgens: A protective mechanism against fetal virilization. Gynecol Invest 67 [Abstract], 1979

Edman CD, Toofanian A, MacDonald PC, Gant NF: Placental clearance rate of maternal plasma androstenedione through placental estradiol formation: An indirect method of assessing uteroplacental blood flow. Am J Obstet Gynecol 131:1029, 1981

Efrati P, Presentey B, Margalith M, Rozenszajn L: Leukocytes of normal pregnant women. Obstet Gynecol 23:429, 1964

Enein M, Zina AAA, Kassem M, El-Tabbakh G: Echocardiography of the pericardium in pregnancy. Obstet Gynecol 69:851, 1987

Evans MI, Dougan MB, Moawad AH, Evans WJ, Bryant-Greenwood GD, Greenwood FC: Ripening of the human cervix with porcine ovarian relaxin. Am J Obstet Gynecol 147:410, 1983

Everett RB, Worley RJ, Leveno K, MacDonald PC, Gant NF: The control of vascular reactivity to angiotensin II in human pregnancy. Gynecol Obstet Invest 8:88, 1977

Everett RB, Worley RJ, MacDonald PC, Gant NF: Modification of vascular responsiveness to angiotensin II in pregnant women by intravenously infused 5α-dihydroprogesterone. Am J Obstet Gynecol 131:352, 1978a

Everett RB, Worley RJ, MacDonald PC, Gant NF: Oral administration of theophylline to modify pressor responsiveness to angiotensin II in women with pregnancy-induced hypertension. Am J Obstet Gynecol 132:359, 1978b

Everett RB, Worley RJ, MacDonald PC, Gant NF: Effect of prostaglandin synthetase inhibitors on pressor response to angiotensin II in human pregnancy. J Clin Endocrinol Metab 46:1007, 1978c

Ezimokhai M, Davison JM, Philips PR, Dunlop W: Non-postural serial changes in renal function during the third trimester of normal human pregnancy. Br J Obstet Gynaecol, 88:465, 1981

Faure A, Sutter-Dub MT, Sutter BCJ, Assan R: Ovarian-adrenal interactions in regulation of endocrine pancreatic function in the rat. Diabetologia 24:122, 1983

Fay RA, Hughes AO, Farron NT: Platelets in pregnancy: Hyperdestruction in pregnancy. Obstet Gynecol 61:238, 1983

Fletcher AP, Alkjaersig NK: Thromboembolism and contraceptive medications: Incidence and mechanism. In Salhanick HA, Kipnis DM, Van de Wiele RL (eds): Metabolic Effects of Gonadal Hormones and Contraceptive Steroids. New York, Plenum Press, 1969

Fletcher AP, Alkjaersig NK, Burstein R: The influence of pregnancy upon blood coagulation and plasma fibrinolytic enzyme function. Am J Obstet Gynecol 134:743, 1979

Fletcher JE, Thomas TA, Hill RG: β-Endorphin and parturition. Lancet 1:310, 1980

Fogh-Andersen N, Schultz-Larsen P: Free calcium ion concentration in pregnancy. Acta Obstet Gynecol Scand 60:309, 1981

Freinkel N: Banting lecture 1980: Of pregnancy and progeny. Diabetes 29:1023, 1980

Freinkel N, Dooley SL, Metzger BE: Care of the pregnant woman with insulin-dependent diabetes mellitus. N Engl J Med 313:96, 1985

Fulop M, Brazeau P: Increased ureteral back pressure enhances renal tubular sodium reabsorption. J Clin Invest 49:2315, 1970

Gallery EDM, Brown MA: Control of sodium excretion in human pregnancy. Am J Kidney Dis 9:290, 1987

Gant NF, Chand S, Worley RJ, Andersen GD: Unpublished observations, 1977

Gant NF, Chand S, Worley RJ, Whalley PJ, Crosby UD, MacDonald PC: A clinical test for predicting the development of acute hypertension in pregnancy. Am J Obstet Gynecol 120:1, 1974a

Gant NF, Daley GL, Chand S, Whalley PJ, MacDonald PC: A study of angiotensin II pressor response throughout primigravid pregnancy. J Clin Invest 52:2682, 1973

Gant NF, Daley GL, Chand S, Whalley PJ, MacDonald PC: The nature of pressor responsiveness to angiotensin II in human pregnancy. Obstet Gynecol 43:854, 1974b

Gant NF, Madden JD, Chand S, Worley RJ, Strong JS, MacDonald PC: Metabolic clearance rate of dehydroisoandrosterone sulfate: V. Studies of essential hypertension complicating pregnancy. Obstet Gynecol 47:319, 1976

Gant NF, Madden JD, Siiteri PK, MacDonald PC: A sequential study of the metabolism of dehydroisoandrosterone sulfate in primigravid pregnancy. Excerpta Medica Int Congr Series 273:1026, 1972

Garcia-Bunuel R, Berek JS, Woodruff JD: Luteomas of pregnancy. Obstet Gynecol 45:407, 1975

Gee JBL, Packer BS, Millen JE, Robin ED: Pulmonary mechanics during pregnancy. J Clin Invest 46:945, 1967

Geelhoed GW, Vander AJ: Plasma renin activities during pregnancy and parturition. J Clin Endocrinol 28:412, 1968

Genazzani AR, Facchinetti F, Parrini D: β-Lipotrophin and β-endorphin plasma levels during pregnancy. Clin Endocrinol 141:409, 1981

Goland RS, Wardlaw SL, Stark RI, Frantz AG: Human plasma β-endorphin during pregnancy, labour and delivery. J Clin Endocrinol Metab 52:74, 1981

Gonzalez JG, Elizondo G, Saldivar D, Nanez H., Todd, LE, Villarreal JZ: Pituitary gland growth during normal pregnancy: An in vivo study using magnetic resonance imaging. Am J Med 85:217, 1988

Grace AA, D'Souza V, Menon RK, O'Brien S, Dandona P: Atrial natriuretic peptide concentrations during pregnancy. Lancet 1:1267, 1987

Greiss FC Jr, Wagner WD: Glycosaminoglycans: Their distribution and potential vasoactive action in the nonpregnant and pregnant ovine uterus. Am J Obstet Gynecol 145:1041, 1983

Habicht J, Yarbrough C, Lechtig A, Klein RE: Relationships of birthweight, maternal nutrition and infant mortality. Nutr Rept Intl 7:533, 1973

Hahn PF, Carothers EL, Darby WJ, Martin M, Sheppard CW, Cannon RO, Beam AS, Densen PM, Peterson JC, McClellan GS: Iron metabolism in human pregnancy as studied with the radioactive isotope Fe59. Am J Obstet Gynecol 61:477, 1951

Handwerger S, Quarfordt S, Barrett J, Harman I: Apolipoproteins AI, AII, and CI stimulate placental lactogen release from human placental tissue. J Clin Invest 79:625, 1987

Hankins GDV, Wendel GD, Whalley PJ, Quirk JG Jr: Cardiovascular monitoring in high-risk pregnancy. Perinatol Neonatol 7:29, 1983

Hansen JP: Older maternal age and pregnancy outcome: A review of the literature. Obstet Gynecol Surv 41:726, 1986

Harbert GM, Cornell GW, Littlefield JB, Kayan JB, Thornton WN: Maternal hemodynamics associated with uterine contraction in gravid monkeys. Am J Obstet Gynecol 104:24, 1969

Hellman LM, Rosenthal AH, Kistner RW, Gordon R: Some factors influencing the proliferation of the reserve cells in the human cervix. Am J Obstet Gynecol 67:899, 1954

Hensleigh PA, Woodruff JD: Differential maternal-fetal response to androgenizing luteoma or hyperreactio luteinalis. Obstet Gynecol 33:262, 1978

Herrera E, Lasunción MA, Gomez-Coronado D, Aranda P, López-Luna P, Maier I: Role of lipoprotein lipase activity on lipoprotein metabolism and the fate of circulating triglycerides in pregnancy. Am J Obstet Gynecol 158:1575, 1988

Hershman JM, Starnes WR: Extraction and characterization of a thyrotropic material from the human placenta. J Clin Invest 48:923, 1969

Hirai N, Yanaihara T, Nakayama T, Ishibashi M, Yamaji T: Plasma levels of atrial natriuretic peptide during normal pregnancy and in pregnancy complicated by hypertension. Am J Obstet Gynecol 159:27, 1988

Hodgkinson CP: Physiology of the ovarian veins in pregnancy. Obstet Gynecol 1:26, 1953

Hof RP: The calcium antagonists PY 108-068 and verapamil diminish the effects of angiotensin II: Sites of interaction in the peripheral circulation of anaesthetized cats. Br J Pharmacol 82:51, 1984

Hof RP: Modification of vasopressin- and angiotensin II-induced changes by calcium antagonists in the peripheral circulation of anaesthetized rabbits. Br J Pharmacol 85:75, 1985

Horger EO III, Smythe AR II: Pregnancy in women over forty. Obstet Gynecol 49:257, 1977

Hornnes PJ, Kuhl C: Plasma insulin and glucagon responses to isoglycemic stimulation in normal pregnancy and post partum. Obstet Gynecol 55:425, 1980

Howard BK, Goodson JH, Mengert WF: Supine hypotensive syndrome in late pregnancy. Obstet Gynecol 1:371, 1953

Hubinont CJ, Balasse H, Dufrane SP, Leclercq-Meyer V, Sugar J, Schwers J, Malaisse WJ: Changes in pancreatic B cell function during late pregnancy, early lactation and postlaction. Gynecol Obstet Invest 25:89, 1988

Hudson P, Haley J, John M, Cronk M, Crawford R, Haralambidis J, Gregear G, Shine J, Niall H: Structure of a genomic clone encoding biologically active human relaxin. Nature 301:628, 1983

Huisman A, Aarnoudse JG, Heuvelmans JHA, Goslinga H, Fidler V, Huisjes HJ, Zijlstra WJ: Whole blood viscosity during normal pregnancy. Br J Obstet Gynaecol 94:1143, 1987

Hutchinson DL, Westoner JL, Well DW: The destruction of the maternal and fetal pituitary glands in subhuman primates. Am J Obstet Gynecol 83:857, 1962

Hytten FE, Chamberlain G: Clinical Physiology in Obstetrics. Oxford, Blackwell, 1981

Hytten FE, Leitch I: The Physiology of Human Pregnancy, 2nd ed. Philadelphia, Davis, 1971

Hytten FE, Thomson AM: Maternal physiological adjustments. In Assali NS (ed): Biology of Gestation: The Maternal Organism, Vol I. New York, Academic, 1968

Ihrman K: A clinical and physiological study of pregnancy in material from northern Sweden: VII. The heart volume during and after pregnancy. Acta Soc Med Upsal 65:326, 1960

Illingworth PJ, Jung RG, Howie PW, Tsles TE: Reduction in postprandial energy expenditure during pregnancy. Br Med J 294:1573, 1987

Ingerslev M, Teilum G: Biopsy studies on the liver in pregnancy: II. Liver biopsy on normal pregnant women. Acta Obstet Gynecol Scand 25:352, 1946

Iosif S, Ingemarsson I, Ulmsten U: Urodynamic studies in normal pregnancy and the puerperium. Am J Obstet Gynecol 137:696, 1980

Janbu T, Nesheim B-I: Uterine artery blood velocities during contractions in pregnancy and labour related to intrauterine pressure. Br J Obstet Gynaecol 94:1150, 1987

Jepson JH, Friesen HG: The mechanism of action of human placental lactogen on erythropoiesis. Br J Haematol 15:465, 1968

Kambam JR, Perry SM, Entman S, Smith BE: Effect of magnesium on plasma cholinesterase activity. Am J Obstet Gynecol 159:309, 1988

Kangawa K, Fukuda A, Matsuo H: Structural identification of β- and γ-human atrial natriuretic polypeptides. Nature 313:397, 1985

Kangawa K, Matsu H: Purification and complete amino acid sequence of a human atrial natriuretic polypeptide (α-hANP). Biochem Biophys Res Commun 111:131, 1984

Kasper CK, Hoag MS, Aggelar PM, Stone S: Blood clotting factors in pregnancy: Factor VIII concentrations in normal and AHF-deficient women. Obstet Gynecol 24:242, 1964

Katz R, Karliner JS, Resnik R: Effects of a natural volume overload state (pregnancy) on left ventricular performance in normal human subjects. Circulation 58:434, 1978

Kauppila A, Chatelain P, Kirkinen P, Kivinen S, Ruokonen A: Isolated prolactin deficiency in a woman with puerperal alactogenesis. J Clin Endocrinol Metab 64:309, 1987

Kauppila A, Koskinen M, Puolakka J, Tuimala R, Kuikka J: Decreased intervillous and unchanged myometrial blood flow in supine recumbency. Obstet Gynecol 55:203, 1980

Killam AP, Rosenfeld CR, Battaglia FC, Makowshi EL, Meschia G: Effect of estrogens on the uterine blood flow of oophorectomized ewes. Am J Obstet Gynecol 115:1045, 1973

Killingsworth LM: Plasma protein patterns in health and disease. CRC Crit Rev Clin Lab Sci 11:1, 1979

King JC: Protein metabolism during pregnancy: Symposium on nutrition. Clin Perinatol 2:243, 1975

Kirz DS, Dorchester W, Freeman RK: Advanced maternal age: The mature gravida. Am J Obstet Gynecol 152:7, 1985

Klafen, Palugyay: Arch Gynaekol 131:347, 1927

Kleinert HD, Maack T, Atlas SA, Januszewicz A, Sealy JE, Laragh JH: ANF inhibits angiotensin-, norepinephrine-, and potassium-induced vascular contractility. Hypertension 6:143, 1984

Kletzky OA, Rossman F, Bertolli SI, Platt LD, Mischell DR: Dynamics of human chorionic gonadotropin, prolactin, and growth hormone in serum and amniotic fluid throughout normal human pregnancy. Am J Obstet Gynecol 151:878, 1985

Krause DE, Stembridge VA: Luteomas of pregnancy. Am J Obstet Gynecol 95:192, 1966

Krause PJ, Ingardia CJ, Pontius LT, Malech HL, LoBello TM, Maderazo EG: Host defense during pregnancy: Neutrophil chemotaxis and adherence. Am J Obstet Gynecol 157:274, 1987

Laidlaw JC, Ruse JL, Gornall AG: The influence of estrogen and progesterone on aldosterone excretion. J Clin Endocrinol 22:161, 1962

Landau RL, Lugibihl K: The catabolic and natriuretic effects of progesterone in man. Recent Prog Horm Res 17:249, 1961

Lehmann DK, Chism J: Pregnancy outcome in medically complicated and uncomplicated patients aged 40 years or older. Am J Obstet Gynecol 157:738, 1987

Levy RP, Newman DM, Rejali LS, Barford DAG: The myth of goiter in pregnancy. Am J Obstet Gynecol 137:701, 1980

Lind T: Metabolic changes in pregnancy relevant to diabetes mellitus. Postgrad Med J 55:353, 1979

Lind T, Bell S, Gilmore E, Huisjes HJ, Schally AV: Insulin disappearance rate in pregnant and non-pregnant women, and in non-pregnant women given GHRIH. Eur J Clin Invest 7:47, 1977

Lindheimer MD, Barron WM, Dürr J, Davison JM: Water homeostasis and vasopressin release during rodent and human gestation. Am J Kidney Dis 9:270, 1987a

Lindheimer MD, Richardson DA, Ehrlich EN, Katz AI: Potassium homeostasis in pregnancy. J Repro Med 32:517, 1987b

Lopez-Espinoza I, Dhar H, Humphreys S, Redman CWG: Urinary albumin excretion in pregnancy. Br J Obstet Gynecol 93:176, 1986

Makowski EL, Meschia G, Droegemueller W, Battaglia FC: Distribution of uterine blood flow in the pregnant sheep. Am J Obstet Gynecol 101:409, 1968

Massani ZM, Sanguinetti R, Gallegos R, Raimondi D: Angiotensin blood levels in normal and toxemic pregnancies. Am J Obstet Gynecol 99:313, 1967

Matsuura S, Naden RP, Gant NF, Parker CR, Rosenfeld CR: Effect of hypertonic saline on vascular responses to angiotensin II in pregnancy. Am J Obstet Gynecol 147:231, 1983

McGiff JC, Itskovitz HD: Prostaglandins and the kidney. Circ Res 33:479, 1973

McLennan CE: Antecubital and femoral venous pressure in normal and toxemic pregnancy. Am J Obstet Gynecol 45:568, 1943

McMurray RG, Katz VL, Berry MJ, Cefalo RC: The effect of pregnancy on metabolic responses during rest, immersion, and aerobic exercise in the water. Am J Obstet Gynecol 158:481, 1988

Mendenhall HW: Serum protein concentrations in pregnancy: I. Concentrations in maternal serum. Am J Obstet Gynecol 106:388, 1970

Metcalfe J, McAnulty JH, Ueland K: Cardiovascular physiology. Clin Obstet Gynecol 24:693, 1981

Metcalfe J, Romney SL, Ramsey LH, Reid DE, Burwell CS: Estimation of uterine blood flow in normal human pregnancy at term. J Clin Invest 34:1632, 1955

Migeon CJ, Bertrand J, Wall PE: Physiological disposition of 4-C¹⁴ cortisol during late pregnancy. J Clin Invest 36:1350, 1957

Milne JS, Howie AD, Pack AI: Dyspnoea during normal pregnancy. Brit J Obstet Gynaecol 85:260, 1978

Miyamoto J: Prolactin and thyrotropin responses to thyrotropin-releasing hormone during the peripartal period. Obstet Gynecol 63:639, 1984

Miyamoto S, Shimokawa H, Sumioki H, Touno A, Nakano H: Circadian rhythm of plasma atrial natriuretic peptide, aldosterone, and blood pressure during the third trimester in normal and preeclamptic pregnancies. Am J Obstet Gynecol 158:393, 1988

Möbius W von: Atmung und Schwangerschaft. Munch Med Wochenschr 103:1389, 1961

Muechler EK, Fichter J, Zongrone J: Human chorionic gonadotropin, estriol, and testosterone changes in two pregnancies with hyperreactio luteinalis. Am J Obstet Gynecol 157:1126, 1987

Mueller MN, Kappas A: Estrogen pharmacology: I. The influence of estradiol and estriol on hepatic disposal of sulfobromophthalein (BSP) in man. J Clin Invest 43:1905, 1964

Mulaisho C, Utiger RD: Serum thyroxine-binding globulin: Determination by competitive ligand-binding assay in thyroid disease and pregnancy. Acta Endocrinol 85:314, 1977

Murad SHN, Tabsh KMA, Shilyanski G, Kapur PA, Ma C, Lee C, Conklin KA: Effects of verapamil on uterine blood flow and maternal cardiovascular function in the awake pregnant ewe. Anesth Analg 64:7, 1985

Naden RP, Rosenfeld CR: Effect of angiotensin II on uterine and systemic vasculature in pregnant sheep. J Clin Invest 68:468, 1981

Naden RP, Rosenfeld CR: Systemic and uterine responsiveness to angiotensin II and norepinephrine in estrogen-treated nonpregnant sheep. Am J Obstet Gynecol 153:417, 1985

National Research Council, Food and Nutrition Board: Recommended Dietary Allowances, 8th ed. Washington, DC, National Academy of Sciences, 1974

Newnham JP, Tomlin S, Ratter SJ, Bourne GL, Rees LH: Endogenous opiod peptides in pregnancy. Brit J Obstet Gynaecol 90:535, 1983

Nielsen JH: Effects of growth hormone, prolactin, and placental lactogen on inulin content and release, and deoxyribonucleic acid synthesis in cultured pancreatic islets. Endocrinology 110:600, 1982

Nolten WE, Lindheimer MD, Oparil S, Ehrlich EN: Desoxycorticosterone in pregnancy: I. Sequential studies of the secretory patterns of desoxycorticosterone, aldosterone and cortisol. Am J Obstet Gynecol 132:414, 1978

Nolten WE, Rueckert PA: Elevated free cortisol index in pregnancy: Possible regulatory mechanisms. Am J Obstet Gynecol 139:492, 1981

Noriyoshi K, Matsui K, Ito M, Nakamura T, Yoshimura T, Ushijima H, Maeyama M: Effect of calcium supplementation on the vascular sensitivity to angiotensin II in pregnant women. Am J Obstet Gynecol 153:576, 1985

Oian P, Maltau JM, Noddeland H, Fadnes HO: Oedema-preventing mechanisms in subcutaneous tissue of normal pregnant women. Br J Obstet Gynaecol 92:1113, 1985

Osathanondh R, Tulchinsky D, Chopra IJ: Total and free thyroxine and triiodothyronine in normal and complicated pregnancy. J Clin Endocrinol Metab 42:98, 1976

Ozanne P, Linderkamp O, Miller FC, Meiselman HJ: Erythrocyte aggregation during normal pregnancy. Am J Obstet Gynecol 147:576, 1983

Parisi VM, Salinas JK, Stockmar EJ: Fetal cardiorespiratory responses to maternal administration of nicardipine in the hypertensive ewe. Abstract presented at the Sixth Annual Meeting of the Society of Perinatal Obstetricians, January 1986

Parker CR, Carr BR, Ragland SR, Morrison JC, Herbert WNP, MacDonald PC: Ontogeny of human fetal plasma progesterone, deoxycorticosterone (DOC), and DOC-SO$_4$. Am J Obstet Gynecol 147:955, 1983

Parker CR, Everett RB, Whalley PJ, Quirk JG, Gant NF, MacDonald PC: Hormone production during pregnancy in the primigravid patient: II. Plasma levels of deoxycorticosterone throughout pregnancy of normal women and women who developed pregnancy-induced hypertension. Am J Obstet Gynecol 138:626, 1980

Pasanisi F, Elliott HL, Reid JL: Vascular and aldosterone responses to angiotensin II in normal humans: Effects of nicardipine. J Cardiovasc Pharmacol 7:1171, 1985

Patton PE, Coulam CB, Bergstralh E: The prevalence of autoantibodies in pregnant and nonpregnant women. Am J Obstet Gynecol 157:1345, 1987

Peake SL, Roxburgh HB, Langlois SLP: Ultrasonic assessment of hydronephrosis of pregnancy. Radiology 146:167, 1983

Phelps RL, Metzger BE, Freinkel N: Carbohydrate metabolism in pregnancy: XVII. Diurnal profiles of plasma glucose, insulin, free fatty acids, triglycerides, cholesterol, and individual amino acids in late normal pregnancy. Am J Obstet Gynecol 140:730, 1981

Pipe NGJ, Smith T, Halliday D, Edmonds CJ, Williams C, Coltart TM: Changes in fat, fat free mass and body water in human normal pregnancy. Brit J Obstet Gynaecol 86:929, 1979

Pitkin RM, Reynolds WA, Williams GA, Hargis GK: Calcium metabolism in pregnancy: A longitudinal study. Am J Obstet Gynecol 151:99, 1985

Pitkin RM, Witte DL: Platelet and leukocyte counts in pregnancy. JAMA 242:2696, 1980

Porter DG: Myometrium of the pregnant guinea pig: The probable importance of relaxin. Biol Reprod 7:458, 1972

Porter DG: Relaxin and cervical softening. In Anderson AM, Ellwood DA (eds): The Cervix in Pregnancy and Labour. Edinburgh, Churchill Livingstone, 1980

Potter MG: Observations of the gallbladder and bile during pregnancy at term. JAMA 106:1070, 1936

Pritchard JA: Plasma cholinesterase activity in normal pregnancy and in eclamptogenic toxemias. Am J Obstet Gynecol 70:1083, 1955

Pritchard JA: Changes in the blood volume during pregnancy and delivery. Anesthesiology 26:393, 1965

Pritchard JA, Adams RH: Erythrocyte production and destruction during pregnancy. Am J Obstet Gynecol 79:750, 1960

Pritchard JA, Barnes AC, Bright RH: The effect of the supine position on renal function in the near-term pregnant woman. J Clin Invest 34:777, 1955

Pritchard JA, Hunt CF: A comparison of the hematologic responses following the routine prenatal administration of intramuscular and oral iron. Surg Gynecol Obstet 106:516, 1958

Pritchard JA, Mason RA: Iron stores of normal adults and their replenishment with oral iron therapy. JAMA 190:897, 1964

Pritchard JA, Scott DE: Iron demands during pregnancy. In Iron Deficiency-Pathogenesis: Clinical Aspects and Therapy. London, Academic, 1970, p 173

Rakoczi F, Tallian F, Bagdany S, Gati I: Platelet life-span in normal pregnancy and pre-eclampsia as determined by a non-radioisotope technique. Thromb Res 15:553, 1979

Ratnoff OD, Colopy JE, Pritchard JA: The blood-clotting mechanism during normal parturition. J Lab Clin Med 44:408, 1954

Rechberger T, Uldbjerg N, Oxlund H: Connective tissue changes in the cervix during normal pregnancy and pregnancy complicated by cervical incompetence. Obstet Gynecol 71:563, 1988

Reitz RE, Thomas AD, Woods JR, Weinstein RL: Calcium, magnesium, phosphorus, and parathyroid hormone interrelationships in pregnancy and newborn infants. Obstet Gynecol 50:701, 1977

Rekonen A, Luotola H, Pitkänen M, Kuikka J, Pyörälä M: Measurement of intervillous and myometrial blood flow by an intravenous ^{133}Xe method. Br J Obstet Gynaecol 83:723, 1976

Robinson CJ, Spanos E, James MF, Pike JW, Haussler MR, Makeen AM, Hillyard CJ, MacIntyre I: Role of prolactin in vitamin D metabolism and calcium absorption during lactation in the rat. J Endocrinol 94:443, 1982

Rosenfeld CR: Consideration of the uteroplacental circulation in intrauterine growth. Semin Perinatol 8:42, 1984

Rosenfeld CR, Barton MD, Meschia G: Effects of epinephrine on distribution of blood flow in the pregnant ewe. Am J Obstet Gynecol 124:156, 1976

Rosenfeld CR, Gant NF Jr: The chronically instrumented ewe. A model for studying vascular reactivity to angiotensin II in pregnancy. J Clin Invest 67:486, 1981

Rosenfeld CR, Killam AP, Battaglia FC, Makowski EL, Meschia G: Effect of estradiol-17,β on the magnitude and distribution of uterine blood flow in nonpregnant, oophorectomized ewes. Pediatr Res 7:139, 1973

Rosenfeld CR, Morriss FH Jr, Makowski EL, Meschia G, Battaglia FC: Circulatory changes in the reproductive tissues of ewes during pregnancy. Gynecol Invest 5:252, 1974

Rosenfeld CR, West J: Circulatory response to systemic infusion of norepinephrine in the pregnant ewe. Am J Obstet Gynecol 127:376, 1977

Roti E, Gnudi A, Braverman LE: The placental transport, synthesis and metabolism of hormones and drugs which affect thyroid function. Endocrin Rev 4:131, 1983

Rubi RA, Sala NL: Ureteral function in pregnant women: III. Effect of different positions and of fetal delivery upon ureteral tonus. Am J Obstet Gynecol 101:230, 1968

Russ EM, Raymunt J: Influence of estrogens on total serum copper and caeruloplasmin. Proc Soc Exp Biol Med 92:465, 1956

Russell DH, Durie BGM: Polyamines and biochemical markers of normal and malignant growth. In Progress in Cancer Research and Therapy, Vol 8. New York, Raven Press, 1978

Russell DH, Giles HR, Christian CD, Campbell JL: Polyamines in amniotic fluid, plasma, and urine during normal pregnancy. Am J Obstet Gynecol 132:649, 1978

Russell KP, Rose H, Starr P: Further observations on thyroxine interactions in the newborn at delivery and in the immediate neonatal period. Am J Obstet Gynecol 90:682, 1964

Rutherford AJ, Anderson JV, Elder MG, Bloom SR: Release of atrial natriuretic peptide during pregnancy and immediate puerperium. Lancet 1:928, 1987

Sagnella GA, Markandu ND, Shore AC, MacGregor GA: Effects of changes in dietary sodium intake and saline infusion on immunoreactive atrial natriuretic peptide in human plasma. Lancet 1:1208, 1985

Salvatore CA: Cervical mucus crystallization in pregnancy. Obstet Gynecol 32:226, 1968

Sanborn BM: The role of relaxin in uterine function. In Huszar G (ed): Physiology and Biochemistry of the Uterus in Pregnancy and Labor. Boca Raton, FL, CRC Press, 1986, p 225

Schulman A, Herlinger H: Urinary tract dilatation in pregnancy. Br J Radiol 48:638, 1975

Scott DE, Pritchard JA: Iron deficiency in healthy young college women. JAMA 199:897, 1967

Sherwood OD: Relaxin. In Knobil E, Neil J (eds): The Physiology of Reproduction. New York, Raven Press, 1988, p 585

Shortle BE, Warren MP, Tsin D: Recurrent androgenicity in pregnancy: A case report and literature review. Obstet Gynecol 70:462, 1987

Sjöstedt S: Acid-base balance of arterial blood during pregnancy, at delivery, and in the puerperium. Am J Obstet Gynecol 84:775, 1962

Song CS, Kappas A: The influence of estrogens, progestins and pregnancy on the liver. Vitam Horm 26:147, 1968

Spellacy WN, Buhi WC: Pituitary growth hormone and placental lactogen levels measured in normal term pregnancy and at the early and late postpartum periods. Am J Obstet Gynecol 105:888, 1969

Spellacy WN, Goetz FC: Plasma insulin in normal late pregnancy. New Engl J Med 268:988, 1963

Spencer G: Projections of the population of the United States, by age, sex, and race: 1983–2080. Current Population Reports—Population Estimates and Projections. May 1984, Series P-25, No 952, US Department of Commerce

Spetz S: Peripheral circulation during normal pregnancy. Acta Obstet Gynecol Scand 43:309, 1964

Spitz B, Magness RR, Cox SM, Brown CEL, Rosenfeld CR, Gant NF: Low-dose aspirin: I. Effect on angiotensin II pressor responses and blood prostaglandin concentrations in angiotensin II-sensitive pregnant women. Am J Obstet Gynecol 159:1035, 1988

Steegers EAP, Hein PR, Groeneveld EAM, Jongsma HW, Tan ACITL, Benraad TJ: Atrial natriuretic peptide concentrations during pregnancy. Lancet 1:1267, 1987

Steinetz BG, O'Byrne EM, Kroc RL: The role of relaxin in cervical softening during pregnancy in mammals. In Naftolin F, Stubblefield PG (eds): Dilatation of the Uterine Cervix, Connective Tissue Biology and Clinical Management. New York, Raven Press, 1980

Sternberg WH: Non-functioning ovarian neoplasms. In Grady HG, Smith DE (eds): International Academy of Pathology Monograph, No 3, The Ovary. Baltimore, Williams & Wilkins, 1963

Sturgeon P: Studies of iron requirements in infants: III. Influence of supplemental iron during normal pregnancy on mother and infant: A. The mother. Br J Haematol 5:31, 1959

Sutton FD, Zwillich CW, Creagh E, Pierson DJ, Wiel JV: Progesterone for outpatient treatment of Pickwickian Syndrome. Ann Intern Med 83:476, 1975

Talbert LM, Langdell RD: Normal values of certain factors in the blood clotting mechanism in pregnancy. Am J Obstet Gynecol 90:44, 1964

Taylor DJ, Phillips P, Lind T: Puerperal haematological indices. Br J Obstet Gynaecol 88:601, 1981

Teasdale F: Numerical density of nuclei in the sheep placenta. Anat Rec 185:186, 1976

Terragno NA, Terragno DA, Pacholczyk D, McGiff JC: Prostaglandins and the regulation of uterine blood flow in pregnancy. Nature 249:57, 1974

Tsai CH, deLeeuw NKM: Changes in 2,3-diphosphoglycerate during pregnancy and puerperium in normal women and in β-thalassemia heterozygous women. Am J Obstet Gynecol 142:520, 1982

Tsang RC, Donovan EF, Steichen JJ: Calcium physiology and pathology in the neonate. Pediatr Clin North Am 23:611, 1976

Tsibris JCM, Raynor LO, Buhi WC, Buggie J, Spellacy WN: Insulin receptors in circulating erythrocytes and monocytes from women on oral contraceptives or pregnant women near term. J Clin Endocrinol Metab 51:711, 1980

Tulchinsky D, Hobel CJ: Plasma human chorionic gonadotropin, estrone, estradiol, estriol, progesterone, and 17α-hydroxyprogesterone in human pregnancy: III. Early normal pregnancy. Am J Obstet Gynecol 117:884, 1973

Tygart SG, McRoyan DK, Spinnato JA, McRoyan CJ, Kitay DZ: Longitudinal study of platelet indices during normal pregnancy. Am J Obstet Gynecol 154:883, 1986

Ueland K: Maternal cardiovascular dynamics: VII. Intrapartum blood volume changes. Am J Obstet Gynecol 126:671, 1976

Ueland K, Hansen JM: Maternal cardiovascular dynamics: II. Posture and uterine contractions. Am J Obstet Gynecol 103:1, 1969

Ueland K, Metcalfe J: Circulatory changes in pregnancy. Clin Obstet Gynecol 18:41, 1975

Ulmsten U, Sundström G: Esophageal manometry in pregnant and nonpregnant women. Am J Obstet Gynecol 132:260, 1978

Van Geelen JM, Lemmens WAJG, Eskes TKAB, Martin CB Jr: The urethral pressure profile in pregnancy and after delivery in healthy nulliparous women. Am J Obstet Gynecol 144:636, 1982

Van Wagenen G, Jenkins RH: An experimental examination of factors causing ureteral dilatation of pregnancy. J Urol 42:1010, 1939

Veille JC, Morton MJ, Burry KJ: Maternal cardiovascular adaptations to twin pregnancy. Am J Obstet Gynecol 153:261, 1985

Verkauf BS, Reiter EO, Hernandez L, Burns SA: Virilization of mother and fetus associated with luteoma of pregnancy: A case report with endocrinologic studies. Am J Obstet Gynecol 129:274, 1977

Vierhapper H, Waldhäusl W: Reduced pressor effect of angiotensin II and of noradrenaline in normal man following the oral administration of the calcium-antagonist nifedipine. Eur J Clin Med 12:263, 1982

Vir SC, Love AHG, Thompson W: Serum and hair concentrations of copper during pregnancy. Am J Clin Nutr 34:2382, 1981

Wakitani K, Cole BR, Geller DM, Currie MG, Adams SP, Fok KF, Needleman P: Atriopeptins: Correlation between renal vasodilatation and natriuresis. Am J Physiol 249:F49, 1985

Wallenberg HCS, Dekker GA, Makovitz JW, Rotmans P: Low-dose aspirin prevents pregnancy-induced hypertension and pre-eclampsia in angiotensin-sensitive primigravidae. Lancet 1:1, 1986

Watanabe M, Meeker CI, Gray MJ, Sims EAH, Solomon S: Secretion rate of aldosterone in normal pregnancy. J Clin Invest 42:1619, 1963

Weiner CP, Brandt J: Plasma antithrombin III activity in normal pregnancy. Obstet Gynecol 56:601, 1980

Weisman Y, Harell A, Edelstein S, David M, Spirer Z, Golander A: 1,25-Dihydroxyvitamin D_3 and 24,25-dihydroxyvitamin D in vitro synthesis by human decidua and placenta. Nature 281:317, 1979

Whalley PJ, Roberts AD, Pritchard JA: The effects of posture on renal function during pregnancy in a patient with diabetes insipidus. J Lab Clin Med 58:867, 1961

Wharton LR: Normal pregnancy with living children in women past the age of fifty. Am J Obstet Gynecol 90:672, 1964

Whitehead M, Lane G, Young O, Campbell S, Abeyasekera G, Hillyard CJ, MacIntyre I, Phang KG, Stevenson JC: Interrelations of calcium-regulating hormones during normal pregnancy. Br Med J 283:10, 1981

Widdowson EM: Growth and composition of the fetus and newborn. In Assali NS (ed): Biology of Gestation, Vol II: The Fetus and Neonate. New York, Academic, 1968

Widdowson EM, Spray CM: Chemical development in utero. Arch Dis Child 26:205, 1951

Winkel CA, Parker CR Jr, Milewich L, Simpson ER, Gant NF, MacDonald PC: The conversion of plasma progesterone to desoxycorticosterone (DOC) in men, nonpregnant and pregnant women, and adrenalectomized subjects: Evidence for steroid 21-hydroxylase activity in non-adrenal tissues. J Clin Invest 66:803, 1980

Winters AJ, Colston C, MacDonald PC, Porter JC: Fetal plasma prolactin levels. J Clin Endocrinol Metab 41:626, 1975

Woodfield DG, Cole SK, Allan AGE, Cash JD: Serum fibrin degradation products throughout normal pregnancy. Br Med J 4:665, 1968

Wright HP, Osborn SB, Edmonds DG: Changes in rate of flow of venous blood in the leg during pregnancy, measured with radioactive sodium. Surg Gynecol Obstet 90:481, 1950

Yoshima T, Strott CA, Marshall JR, Lipsett MD: Corpus luteum function early in pregnancy. J Clin Endocrinol Metab 29:225, 1969

Zivný J, Kobilková J, Neuwirt J, Andrasová V: Regulation of erythropoiesis in fetus and mother during normal pregnancy. Obstet Gynecol 60:77, 1982

Part III

SPONTANEOUS LABOR AND DELIVERY

The Normal Pelvis

The mechanisms of labor are essentially processes of accommodation of the fetus to the bony passage through which the fetus must pass. Accordingly, the size and shape of the pelvis are extremely important in obstetrics. In both women and men the pelvis forms the bony ring through which body weight is transmitted to the lower extremities, but in women it assumes a special form that adapts it to childbearing (Fig. 8–1).

The adult pelvis is composed of four bones: the sacrum, the coccyx, and two innominate bones. Each innominate bone is formed by the fusion of the ilium, the ischium, and the pubis. The innominate bones are joined firmly to the sacrum at the sacroiliac synchondroses and to one another at the symphysis pubis. Consideration of the pelvis will be limited to those features of importance in childbearing.

PELVIC ANATOMY: OBSTETRICAL CONSIDERATIONS

The *linea terminalis* demarcates the *false pelvis* from the *true pelvis* (Fig. 8–2). The false pelvis lies above the linea terminalis and the true pelvis below this anatomical boundary. The false pelvis is bounded posteriorly by the lumbar vertebrae and laterally by the iliac fossae, and in front the boundary is formed by the lower portion of the anterior abdominal wall. The false pelvis varies considerably in size among women according to the flare of the iliac bones, but this has no obstetrical significance.

The true pelvis lies beneath the linea terminalis and is the portion important in childbearing. The true pelvis is bounded above by the promontory and alae of the sacrum, the linea terminalis, and the upper margins of the pubic bones, and below by the pelvic outlet. The cavity of the true pelvis can be described as an obliquely truncated, bent cylinder with its greatest height posteriorly, since its anterior wall at the symphysis pubis measures about 5 cm and its posterior wall about 10 cm (Figs. 8–2 to 8–4). With the woman upright, the upper portion of the pelvic canal is directed downward and backward, and its lower course curves and becomes directed downward and forward.

The walls of the true pelvis are partly bony and partly ligamentous. The posterior boundary is the anterior surface of the sacrum, and the lateral limits are formed by the inner surface of the ischial bones and the sacrosciatic notches and liga-

ments. In front the true pelvis is bounded by the pubic bones, the ascending superior rami of the ischial bones, and the obturator foramina, which they partially enclose.

The sidewalls of the true pelvis of the normal adult woman converge somewhat; therefore, if the planes of the ischial bones were extended downward, they would meet near the knee. Extending from the middle of the posterior margin of each ischium are the ischial spines, which are of great obstetrical importance, since the distance between them usually represents the shortest lateral diameter of the pelvic cavity. Moreover, since the ischial spines can be felt readily by vaginal or rectal examination, they serve as valuable landmarks in determining the level to which the presenting part of the fetus has descended into the true pelvis (p. 170).

The sacrum forms the posterior wall of the pelvic cavity. Its upper anterior margin, corresponding to the body of the first sacral vertebra and designated as the promontory, may be felt on vaginal examination and can provide a landmark for clinical pelvimetry (p. 168). Normally the sacrum has a marked vertical and a less pronounced horizontal concavity, which, in abnormal pelves, may undergo important variations. A straight line drawn from the promontory to the tip of the sacrum usually measures 10 cm, whereas the distance along the concavity averages 12 cm.

The appearance of the pubic arch is characteristic. The descending inferior rami of the pubic bones unite at an angle of 90 to 100 degrees to form a rounded arch under which the fetal head may readily pass (Fig. 8–1).

PELVIC INCLINATION

The normal position of the pelvis, in the erect woman, can be reproduced by holding a skeletal specimen with the incisures of the acetabula pointing directly downward. The same result is achieved when the anterior superior spines of the ilium and the pubic tubercles are placed in the same vertical plane (Fig. 8–2).

PELVIC JOINTS

Symphysis Pubis
Anteriorly, the pelvic bones are joined together by the symphysis pubis, which consists of fibrocartilage, and by the superior and inferior pubic ligaments; the latter is frequently designated

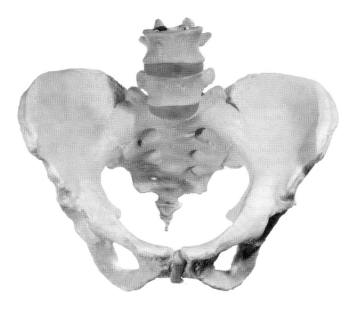

Figure 8–1. Normal female pelvis.

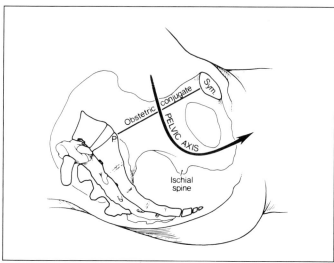

Figure 8–3. The cavity of the true pelvis is comparable to an obliquely truncated, bent cylinder with its greatest height posteriorly. Note the curvature of the pelvic axis.

the *arcuate ligament of the pubis* (Fig. 8–5). The symphysis has a certain degree of mobility, which increases during pregnancy, particularly in multiparas. This fact was demonstrated by Budin (1897), who reported that if a finger was inserted into the vagina of a pregnant woman and she then walked, the ends of the pubic bones could be felt moving up and down with each step.

Sacroiliac Joints
Posteriorly the pelvic bones are joined by the articulations between the sacrum and innominate bones (sacroiliac joints). These joints also have a certain degree of mobility (Fig. 8–6).

Relaxation of the Pelvic Joints
During pregnancy relaxation of these joints is probably the result of hormonal changes. Abramson and co-workers (1934) observed that relaxation of the symphysis pubis commenced in women in the first half of pregnancy and increased during the last 3 months. These investigators observed that regression of relaxation began immediately after parturition and was completed within 3 to 5 months. The symphysis pubis also increases in width during pregnancy (more in multiparas than in primigravidas) and returns to normal soon after delivery. By careful radiographic studies Borell and Fernstrom (1957) demonstrated that the rather marked mobility of the pelvis of women at term was caused by an upward gliding movement of the sacroiliac joint. The displacement, which is greatest in the dorsal lithotomy position, may increase the diameter of the outlet by 1.5 to 2.0 cm.

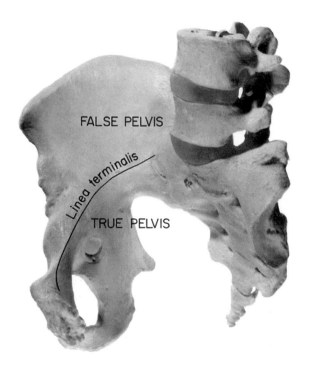

Figure 8–2. Sagittal section of pelvis showing the false and true pelvis.

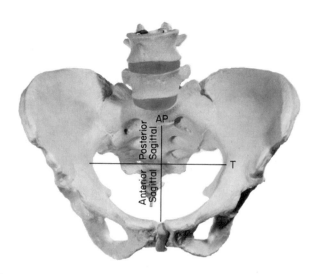

Figure 8–4. Adult female pelvis. Anteroposterior (AP) and transverse (T) diameters of the pelvic inlet are illustrated, as well as the posterior sagittal of the inlet.

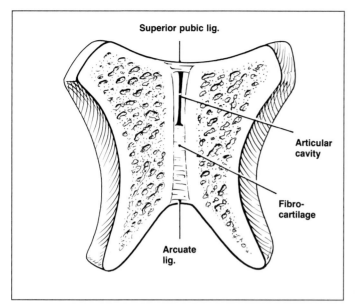

Figure 8–5. Frontal section through symphysis pubis. (*Redrawn from Spalteholz: Hand Atlas of Human Anatomy. Philadelphia, Lippincott, 1933, Vol. 1*)

Because of the elasticity of the pelvic joints in pregnancy, it was formerly thought that positioning the woman in extreme hyperextension increased the obstetrical conjugate. To obtain this objective, the woman was placed on her back with her buttocks extending slightly over the edge of the delivery table and with her legs hanging down by their own weight. This was called the Walcher position. From results of x-ray studies Young (1940) and Brill and Danielius (1941) showed clearly that no appreciable increase in pelvic size results from this position, which is both useless and very uncomfortable.

PLANES AND DIAMETERS OF THE PELVIS

Because of its complex shape, it is difficult to describe the exact location of an object within the pelvis. For convenience, therefore, the pelvis is described as having four imaginary planes: (1) the plane of the pelvic inlet (superior strait), (2) the plane of the pelvic outlet (inferior strait), (3) the plane of the midpelvis (least pelvic dimensions), and (4) the plane of greatest pelvic dimensions.

PELVIC INLET

The pelvic inlet (superior strait) is bounded posteriorly by the promontory and alae of the sacrum, laterally by the linea terminalis, and anteriorly by the horizontal rami of the pubic bones and symphysis pubis (Figs. 8–2 to 8–4, 8–7). The configuration of the inlet of the human female pelvis typically is more nearly round than ovoid. Caldwell and co-workers (1934) identified radiographically a nearly round or *gynecoid* pelvic inlet in approximately 50 percent of the pelves of white women.

Four diameters of the pelvic inlet are usually described: anteroposterior, transverse, and two obliques. The obstetrically important anteroposterior diameter is the shortest distance between the promontory of the sacrum and the symphysis pubis and is designated the *obstetrical conjugate* (Figs. 8–3, 8–4, 8–7). Normally, the obstetrical conjugate measures 10 cm or more, but it may be considerably shortened in abnormal pelves.

The transverse diameter is constructed at right angles to the obstetrical conjugate and represents the greatest distance between the linea terminalis on either side. It usually intersects the obstetrical conjugate at a point about 4 cm in front of the promontory (Fig. 8–4). The segment of the obstetrical conjugate from the intersection of these two lines to the promontory is designated the *posterior sagittal* of the inlet.

Each of the oblique diameters extends from one of the sacroiliac synchondroses to the iliopectineal eminence on the opposite side of the pelvis. They average just under 13 cm and are designated right and left, respectively, according to whether they originate at the right or left sacroiliac synchondrosis.

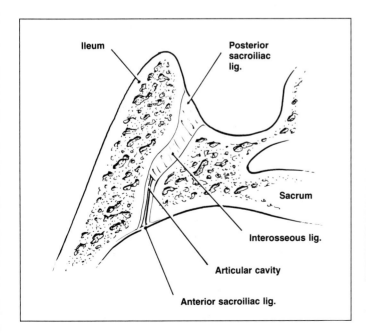

Figure 8–6. Sacroiliac synchondrosis. (*Redrawn from Spalteholz: Hand Atlas of Human Anatomy. Philadelphia, Lippincott, 1933, Vol. 1*)

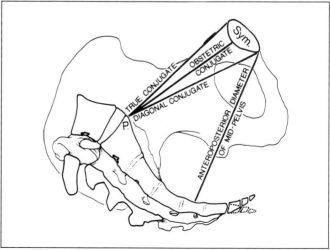

Figure 8–7. Three anteroposterior diameters of the pelvic inlet are illustrated: the true conjugate, the more important obstetrical conjugate, and the clinically measurable diagonal conjugate. The anteroposterior diameter of the midpelvis is also shown (P = sacral promontory; Sym = symphysis pubis).

The anteroposterior diameter of the pelvic inlet that has been identified as the *true conjugate* does not represent the shortest distance between the promontory of the sacrum and symphysis pubis (Fig. 8–7). The shortest distance is the *obstetrical conjugate*, which is the shortest anteroposterior diameter through which the head must pass in descending through the pelvic inlet (Figs. 8–3, 8–4, 8–7).

The obstetrical conjugate cannot be measured directly with the examining fingers; therefore, various instruments have been designed in an effort to obtain such a measurement, but none has proven reliable. For clinical purposes, it is sufficient to estimate the length of the obstetrical conjugate indirectly by measuring the distance from the lower margin of the symphysis to promontory of the sacrum, that is, the *diagonal conjugate* (Fig. 8–7), and subtracting 1.5 to 2 cm from the result, according to the height and inclination of the symphysis pubis (see Pelvic Size and Its Clinical Estimation, p. 168).

MIDPELVIS

The midpelvis at the level of the ischial spines (midplane, or plane of least pelvic dimensions) is of particular importance following engagement of the fetal head in obstructed labor. The interspinous diameter, of 10 cm or somewhat more, is usually the smallest diameter of the pelvis (Fig. 8–8). The anteroposterior diameter, through the level of the ischial spines, normally measures at least 11.5 cm (Fig. 8–7). The posterior component (posterior sagittal diameter) between the sacrum and the intersection with the interspinous diameter is usually at least 4.5 cm.

PELVIC OUTLET

The outlet of the pelvis consists of two approximately triangular areas not in the same plane but having a common base, which is a line drawn between the two ischial tuberosities (Fig. 8–9). The apex of the posterior triangle is at the tip of the sacrum, and the lateral boundaries are the sacrosciatic ligaments and the ischial tuberosities. The anterior triangle is formed by the area under the pubic arch. Three diameters of the pelvic outlet are usually described: the anteroposterior, the transverse, and the posterior sagittal. The anteroposterior diameter (9.5 to 11.5 cm) extends from the lower margin of the symphysis pubis to the tip

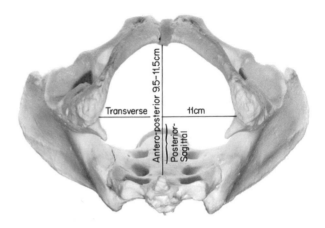

Figure 8–9. Pelvic outlet with diameters marked. Note that the anterior-posterior diameter may be divided into anterior and posterior sagittal diameters.

of the sacrum (Fig. 8–9). The transverse diameter (11 cm) is the distance between the inner edges of the ischial tuberosities. The posterior sagittal diameter extends from the tip of the sacrum to a right-angled intersection with a line between the ischial tuberosities. The normal *posterior sagittal diameter* of the outlet usually exceeds 7.5 cm (Fig. 8–9).

In obstructed labors caused by a narrowing of the midpelvis and/or pelvic outlet, the prognosis for vaginal delivery often depends on the length of the posterior sagittal diameter of the pelvic outlet (Figs. 20–4 and 20–6).

PLANE OF GREATEST PELVIC DIMENSIONS

The *plane of greatest pelvic dimensions* has no obstetrical significance. As the name implies, this plane represents the roomiest portion of the pelvic cavity. It extends from the middle of the posterior surface of the symphysis pubis to the junction of the second and third sacral vertebrae and passes laterally through the ischial bones over the middle of the acetabulum. Its anteroposterior and transverse diameters average about 12.5 cm. Since its oblique diameters terminate in the obturator foramina and the sacrosciatic notches, their length cannot be determined.

PELVIC SHAPES

In the years before the potential hazards of diagnostic x-rays were appreciated, but before antimicrobial drugs and blood transfusions were generally available, the real and immediate risks of cesarean section were formidable. At this time x-ray pelvimetry was used with greater frequency in women with suspected cephalopelvic disproportion or fetal malpresentation. Pelvic radiography was also used as an aid in understanding the general architecture and configuration of the pelvis, as well as its size.

Caldwell and Moloy (1933, 1934) developed a classification of the pelvis that still is used. The classification is based upon the shape of the pelvis, and familiarity with the classification helps the physician to understand the mechanisms of labor in normally and abnormally shaped pelves. This information is useful in helping the physician to manage abnormal labors due to various types of pelvic contractions.

CALDWELL–MOLOY CLASSIFICATION

A line drawn through the greatest transverse diameter of the inlet divides it into anterior and posterior segments. The shapes

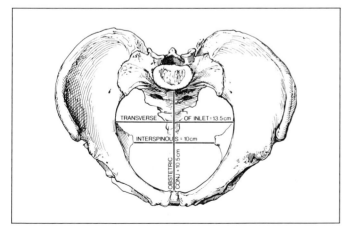

Figure 8–8. Adult female pelvis demonstrating anteroposterior and transverse diameters of the pelvic inlet and transverse (interspinous) diameter of the midpelvis. The obstetrical conjugate normally is greater than 10 cm.

of these segments are important determinants in this method of classification (Fig. 8–10). The character of the posterior segment determines the type of pelvis, and the character of the anterior segment determines the tendency. Many pelves are not pure but mixed types, for example, a gynecoid pelvis with android "tendency," meaning that the posterior pelvis is gynecoid and the anterior pelvis is android in shape.

Gynecoid Pelvis

This type of pelvis has the anatomical characteristics ordinarily associated with the female pelvis. The posterior sagittal diameter of the inlet is only slightly shorter than the anterior sagittal. The sides of the posterior segment are well rounded and wide. Since the transverse diameter of the inlet is either slightly greater than or about the same as the anteroposterior diameter, the inlet is either slightly oval or round. The sidewalls of the pelvis are straight, the spines are not prominent, the pubic arch is wide, and the transverse diameter at the ischial spines is 10 cm or more. The sacrum is inclined neither anteriorly nor posteriorly. The sacrosciatic notch is well rounded and never narrow. Caldwell and co-workers (1939) ascertained the frequency of the four parent pelvic types by study of Todd's collection, and they reported the gynecoid pelvis was found in almost 50 percent of women.

Android Pelvis

The posterior sagittal diameter at the inlet is much shorter than the anterior sagittal, limiting the use of the posterior space by the fetal head. The sides of the posterior segment are not rounded but tend to form, with the corresponding sides of the anterior segment, a wedge at their point of junction. The anterior pelvis is narrow and triangular. The sidewalls are usually convergent, the ischial spines are prominent, and the subpubic arch is narrowed. The bones are characteristically heavy, and the sacrosciatic notch is narrow and high arched. The sacrum is set forward in the pelvis and is usually straight, with little or no curvature, and the posterior sagittal diameter is decreased from inlet to outlet by the forward inclination. Not infrequently there is considerable forward inclination of the sacral tip.

The extreme android pelvis presages a very poor prognosis for vaginal delivery. The frequency of difficult forceps operations and stillbirths increases substantively when there is a small android pelvis. Android-type pelves made up one third of pure-type pelves encountered in white women and one sixth in nonwhite women in the Todd collection.

Anthropoid Pelvis

This type of pelvis is characterized by an anteroposterior diameter of the inlet greater than the transverse, forming more or less an oval anteroposteriorly, with the anterior segment somewhat narrow and pointed. The sacrosciatic notch is large. The sidewalls are often somewhat convergent, and the sacrum usually has six segments and is straight, making the anthropoid pelvis deeper than the other types.

The ischial spines are likely to be prominent. The subpubic arch is frequently somewhat narrow but well shaped. The anthropoid pelvis is said to be more common in nonwhite women, whereas the android form is more frequent in white women. Anthropoid-type pelves make up one fourth of pure-type pelves in white women and nearly one half of those in nonwhite women.

Platypelloid Pelvis

This type of pelvis has a flattened gynecoid shape, with a short anteroposterior and a wide transverse diameter. The latter is set

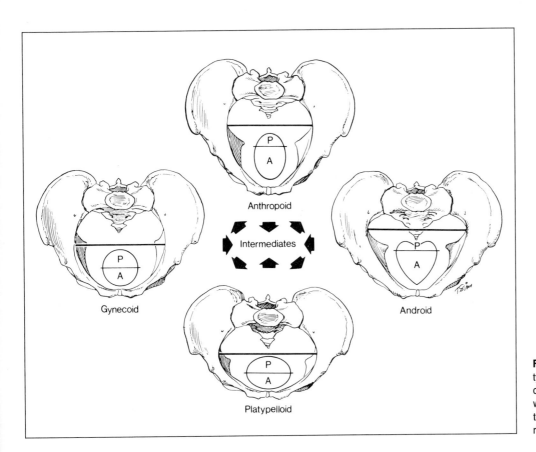

Figure 8–10. The four parent pelvic types of the Caldwell–Moloy classification. A line passing through the widest transverse diameter divides the inlet into posterior (P) and anterior (A) segments.

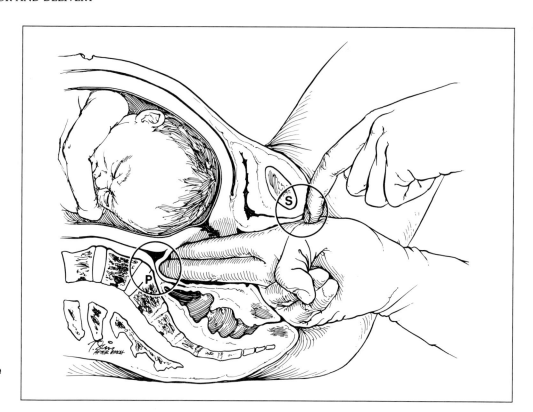

Figure 8–11. Vaginal examination to determine the diagonal conjugate (P = sacral promontory; S = symphysis pubis).

well in front of the sacrum, as in the typical gynecoid form. The angle of the anterior pelvis is very wide, and the anterior puboiliac and posterior iliac portions of the iliopectineal lines are well curved. The sacrum is usually well curved and rotated backward. Thus, the sacrum is short and the pelvis shallow, creating a wide sacrosciatic notch. The platypelloid pelvis is the rarest of the pure varieties and is found in less than 3 percent of women.

Intermediate-type Pelves
Intermediate or mixed types of pelves are much more frequent than pure types.

PELVIC SIZE AND ITS CLINICAL ESTIMATION

PELVIC INLET MEASUREMENTS

Diagonal Conjugate
In many abnormal pelves the anteroposterior diameter of the pelvic inlet (the obstetrical conjugate) is considerably shortened. It is important therefore to determine its length, but this measurement can be obtained only by radiographic techniques. The distance from the sacral promontory to the lower margin of the symphysis pubis (the diagonal conjugate), however, can be measured clinically (Figs. 8–11 to 8–13). **The diagonal conjugate measurement is most important, and every practitioner of obstetrics should be thoroughly familiar with the technique of its measurement and the interpretation of the information gained from its use.**

To obtain this measurement, have the patient placed upon an examining table with her knees drawn up and her feet supported by suitable stirrups. If such an examination cannot be arranged conveniently, she should be brought to the edge of the

bed, where a firm pillow should be placed beneath her buttocks. The examiner introduces two fingers into the vagina, and before measuring the diagonal conjugate, the mobility of the coccyx is evaluated and the anterior surface of the sacrum is palpated. The mobility of the coccyx is tested by palpating it with the fingers in the vagina and attempting to move it to and fro. The anterior surface of the sacrum is then palpated methodically from below upward, and its vertical and lateral curvatures are noted. In normal pelves only the last three sacral vertebrae can be felt without indenting the perineum, whereas in markedly contracted pelves the entire anterior surface of the sacrum usually is readily accessible. Occasionally, the mobility of the coccyx and the anatomical features of the lower sacrum may be defined more easily by rectal examination.

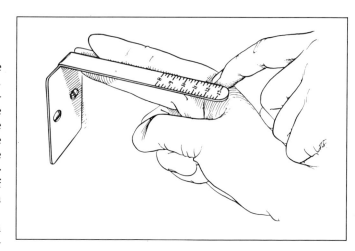

Figure 8–12. Metal scale fastened to wall for measuring the diagonal conjugate diameter as ascertained manually.

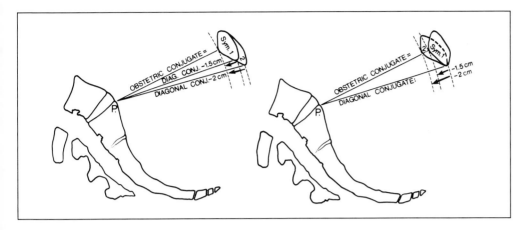

Figure 8–13. Variations in length of diagonal conjugate dependent on height and inclination of the symphysis pubis (P = sacral promontory; Sym = symphysis pubis).

Except in extreme degrees of pelvic contraction, in order to reach the promontory of the sacrum, the elbow must be depressed and, unless the examiner's fingers are unusually long, the perineum forcibly indented by the knuckles of the examiner's third and fourth fingers. The index and the second fingers, held firmly together, are carried up and over the anterior surface of the sacrum, where, by sharply depressing the wrist, the promontory is felt by the tip of the second finger as a projecting bony margin at the base of the sacrum. With the finger closely applied to the most prominent portion of the upper sacrum, the vaginal hand is elevated until it contacts the pubic arch, and the immediately adjacent point on the index finger is marked, as shown in Figure 8–11. The hand is withdrawn, and the distance between the mark and the tip of the second finger is measured. Because measurement using a pelvimeter often introduces an error of 0.5 to 1 cm, it is better to employ a rigid measuring scale attached to the wall, as shown in Figure 8–12. The diagonal conjugate is thus determined and the obstetrical conjugate is computed by deducting 1.5 to 2.0 cm, depending upon the height and inclination of the symphysis pubis, as illustrated in Figure 8–13. If the diagonal conjugate is greater than 11.5 cm, it is justifiable to assume that the pelvic inlet is of adequate size for vaginal delivery of a normal-sized fetus.

Objection to measurement of the diagonal conjugate is sometimes raised on the basis that it is painful to the patient. It probably causes momentary discomfort, but if it is properly performed and deferred until the latter half of pregnancy when the distensibility of the vagina and perineum is greater, the discomfort is minimized.

Transverse contraction of the inlet can be measured only by imaging pelvimetry (p. 170). Such a contraction may exist even in the presence of an adequate anteroposterior diameter.

Engagement

This refers to the descent of the biparietal plane of the fetal head to a level below that of the pelvic inlet (Figs. 8–14, 8–15). When the biparietal, or largest, diameter of the normally flexed fetal head has passed through the inlet, the head is engaged. Although engagement of the fetal head is usually regarded as a phenomenon of labor (and is discussed later in that connection), in nulliparas it commonly occurs during the last few weeks of pregnancy. When it does so, it is confirmatory evidence that the pelvic inlet is adequate for that fetal head.

With engagement, the fetal head serves as an internal pelvimeter to demonstrate that the pelvic inlet is ample for that fetus.

Whether the head is engaged may be ascertained either by rectal or vaginal examination or by abdominal palpation. After gaining experience with vaginal examination, it becomes relatively easy to locate the station of the lowermost part of the fetal head in relation to the level of the ischial spines. If the lowest part of the occiput is at or below the level of the spines, the head is usually, but not always, engaged, since the distance from the plane of the pelvic inlet to the level of the ischial spines is approximately 5 cm in most pelves, and the distance from the biparietal plane of the unmolded fetal head to the vertex is about 3 to 4 cm. Under these circumstances the vertex cannot possibly reach the level of the spines unless the biparietal diameter has passed the inlet or unless there has been considerable elongation of the fetal head because of molding and formation of a caput succedaneum (see Chap. 11, p. 232).

Engagement may be ascertained less satisfactorily by abdominal examination. If, in a term-sized infant, the biparietal plane has descended through the inlet, then that plane so completely fills the inlet that the examining fingers cannot reach the

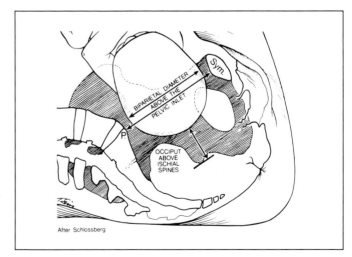

Figure 8–14. When the lowermost portion of the fetal head is above the ischial spines, the biparietal diameter of the head is not likely to have passed through the pelvic inlet and therefore is not engaged (P = sacral promontory; Sym = symphysis pubis).

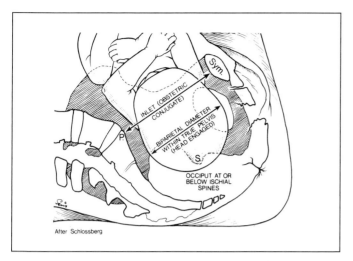

Figure 8–15. When the lowermost portion of the fetal head is at or below the ischial spines, it is usually engaged. Exceptions occur when there is considerable molding or caput formation, or both (P = sacral promontory; Sym = symphysis pubis; S = ischial spine).

lowermost part of the head. Thus, when pushed downward over the lower abdomen, the examining fingers will slide over that portion of the head proximal to the biparietal plane (nape of the neck) and diverge. Conversely, if the head is not engaged, the examining fingers can easily palpate the lower part of the head and will converge (Chap. 9, p. 183).

Fixation of the fetal head is its descent through the pelvic inlet to a depth that prevents its free movement in any direction when pushed by both hands placed over the lower abdomen. Fixation is not necessarily synonymous with engagement. Although a head that is freely movable on abdominal examination cannot be engaged, fixation of the head is sometimes seen when the biparietal plane is still 1 cm or more above the pelvic inlet, especially if the head is molded appreciably.

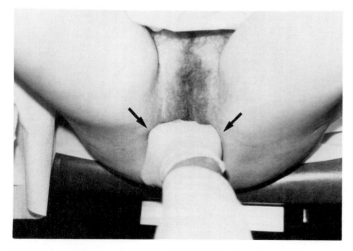

Figure 8–16. Measurement of the biischial diameter. The distance across the top of a closed fist can be measured and this used as a frame of reference to estimate the distance between the ischial tuberosities, indicated by the arrows.

Although engagement is conclusive evidence of an adequate pelvic inlet for the fetus concerned, its absence is by no means always indicative of pelvic contraction. For instance, Bader (1936) reported that labor was entirely normal in 87 percent of the 499 primigravidas with unengaged fetal heads at the onset of labor. Nevertheless, the incidence of contraction of the inlet is higher in this group than in the obstetrical population at large.

PELVIC OUTLET MEASUREMENTS

An important dimension of the pelvic outlet that is accessible for clinical measurement is the diameter between the ischial tuberosities, variously called the *biischial diameter*, the *intertuberous diameter*, and the *transverse diameter of the outlet*. A measurement of over 8 cm is considered normal. The measurement of the transverse diameter of the outlet can be estimated by placing a closed fist against the perineum between the ischial tuberosities, after first measuring the width of the closed fist (Fig. 8–16). Usually the closed fist is wider than 8 cm. The shape of the subpubic arch also can be evaluated at the same time by palpating the pubic rami from the subpubic region toward the ischial tuberosities.

MIDPELVIS ESTIMATION

Clinical estimation of midpelvis capacity by any direct form of measurement is not possible. If the ischial spines are quite prominent, the sidewalls are felt to converge, the concavity of the sacrum is very shallow, and if the biischial diameter of the outlet is less than 8 cm (Chap. 20, p. 381), suspicion is aroused about a contraction in this region, but only by imaging studies can the midpelvis be precisely measured.

IMAGING PELVIMETRY: X-RAY, COMPUTED TOMOGRAPHY, ULTRASOUND, AND MAGNETIC RESONANCE

X-RAY PELVIMETRY

Status of X-ray Pelvimetry
The prognosis for successful vaginal delivery in any given pregnancy cannot be established on the basis of x-ray pelvimetry alone, since the pelvic capacity is but one of several factors that determine the outcome. As enumerated by Mengert (1948), there are at least five factors concerned: (1) size and shape of the bony pelvis, (2) size of the fetal head, (3) force of the uterine contractions, (4) moldability of the fetal head, and (5) presentation and position of the fetus. Only the first of these factors is amenable to reasonably precise radiographic measurement, and it is possible to eliminate only this one factor from the category of the unknown. Today x-ray pelvimetry is no longer considered necessary in the management of a labor with a cephalic fetal presentation in which the mother is suspected of having a contracted pelvis. If vaginal delivery is anticipated for a fetus presenting as a breech (Chap. 19, p. 356), however, x-ray pelvimetry still remains an accepted standard of care in many medical centers (Collea and co-workers, 1980; Gimovsky and associates, 1983; Gordon and colleagues, 1984; Ridley and co-workers, 1982), including Parkland Hospital.

X-ray pelvimetry has the following advantages over manual estimation of pelvic size:

1. It can provide precision to a degree of mensuration un-obtainable clinically. The clinical importance of such precision becomes evident when the shortcomings of the diagonal conjugate measurement are considered. When the diagonal conjugate exceeds 11.5 cm, the anteroposterior dimension of the inlet (the obstetrical conjugate) is very rarely contracted. When the diagonal conjugate is under 11.5, however, it is not always a reliable index of the obstetrical conjugate, since the difference between these two diameters, usually about 1.5 cm, may range from less than 1 to more than 2 cm. For example, two women may have diagonal conjugates of 10.5 cm, but in one the obstetrical conjugate may be 10.2 cm, whereas in the other it may be 8.2 cm. Such information may prove critical during a breech delivery.

2. It can provide exact mensuration of two important diameters not otherwise obtainable, namely, the transverse diameter of the inlet and the interischial spinous diameter (transverse diameter of the midpelvis).

Indications for X-ray Pelvimetry

Because of the expense involved, as well as potential radiation hazards (Table 8–2), radiographic pelvic measurement is not necessary in the great majority of cases (Barton, 1982; Fine, 1980; Hernandez, 1982; Jagani, 1981; Joyce, 1975; Laube, 1981; Lao, 1987; O'Brien and Cefalo, 1982; Parsons and Spellacy, 1985; Poma, 1982; Schussman and Lutz, 1982; Varner, 1980, and all their co-workers). There are, however, certain clinical circumstances in which x-ray pelvimetry is a part of good obstetrical practice. One is the woman with a previous injury or disease likely to affect the bony pelvis. The other is in the case of the fetus presenting breech when vaginal delivery is anticipated.

Before obtaining x-ray or other types of imaging pelvimetry, it is essential to ask two important questions. First, is the information to be obtained likely to affect the subsequent management of labor and delivery? If cesarean section almost certainly is going to be performed regardless of the radiographic information, the use of x-ray pelvimetry is difficult to justify. Second, are other types of imaging techniques available for pelvimetry measurements that can give similar results with lower or no radiation exposure?

Hazards of Diagnostic Radiation

An increasing awareness of the potential hazards of radiation has focused attention on the true value of diagnostic x-rays in obstetrics, as compared with the potential damage to the mother, her fetus, and generations yet unborn. The recognized dangers to the fetus from diagnostic radiation are mutations and increased risk of malignancy later in life. Many, but not all, geneticists and radiobiologists believe, on the basis of animal experimentation, that the only entirely safe dose of irradiation is zero (Brent and Gordon, 1972; Gaulden, 1974). The possibility of childhood malignancy was raised by the report of Stewart and associates in 1956; they identified an increased incidence of leukemia in children of women x-rayed during pregnancy. Since then, there have been several other reports supportive of the thesis that diagnostic radiation absorbed by the fetus increases the risk of subsequent development of leukemia and other malignancies (Bithell and Stewart, 1975; Harvey and associates, 1985; Kneale and Stewart, 1976; MacMahon, 1962; Stewart and co-workers, 1958). A comparison made by Brent (1974) of the apparent risk of leukemia developing in various risk groups is presented in Table 8–1. He showed a relative risk of 1.5 for

TABLE 8–1. RISK OF CHILDHOOD LEUKEMIA AFTER IN UTERO RADIATION EXPOSURE BY PELVIMETRY

Risk Category	Approximate Risk, First 10 Yr	Relative Risk
White children, United States (control)	1:2,800	1
Exposure in utero to x-ray pelvimetry	1:2,000	1.5
Siblings of leukemic children	1:710	4
Identical twin of leukemic child	1:3	1,000

Adapted from Brent RL: J Reprod Med 12:6, 1974.

leukemia developing in children exposed to x-ray pelvimetry. However, Oppenheim and associates (1975) emphasize that increased morbidity and mortality have not been identified uniformly among children exposed prenatally to diagnostic x-rays. If the mother underwent examination because of a medical indication, there was increased morbidity and mortality in the offspring, compared to that found in offspring of healthy women in whom irradiation was for pelvimetry. Finally, the risk of childhood malignancy also may be the consequence of other antenatal factors, such as maternal cigarette smoking (Stjernfeldt and co-workers, 1986), narcotic analgesics (McKinney and associates, 1987), and postnatal factors, such as viral infections (McKinney and associates, 1987).

Certainly not all investigators have reported a risk of leukemia developing in children whose mothers received antepartum x-rays (Table 8–2). **The slight risk from x-ray pelvimetry, however, seems justifiable whenever information critical to the welfare of the fetus or mother is likely to be obtained.**

The concept that x-ray pelvimetry should be limited has been endorsed by the American College of Radiology and the American College of Obstetricians and Gynecologists (1979). The Bureau of Radiological Health of the Food and Drug Administration (U.S. Department of Health and Human Resources, 1980) convened a panel composed of radiologists and obstetricians to examine available information on x-ray pelvim-

TABLE 8–2. CHILDHOOD LEUKEMIA FOLLOWING ANTEPARTUM X-RAYS

Year	Author	Relative Risk	p value
1958	Kaplan	1.37	NS[a]
1958	Stewart	2.00	<0.05
1959	Murray	1.00	NS
1959	Ford	1.66	<0.05
1959	Polhemus and Koch	1.34	<0.05
1960	Court-Brown	0.86	NS
1960	Lewis	0.42	NS
1961	Wells and Steer	0.72	NS
1962	MacMahon	1.52	<0.05
1964	Gunz and Atkinson	1.13	NS
1965	Ager	1.21	NS
1972	Bross and Natarajan	1.40	<0.05
1973	Diamond	2.81	<0.05
1975	Bithell and Stewart	1.41	<0.05
1975	Oppenheim	1.73	NS
1985	Harvey	2.40	0.05

[a]NS = not statistically significant.
Adapted from Klapholz: Evaluation of fetopelvic relationships. In Cohen and Friedman (eds): Management of Labor. Baltimore, University Park Press, 1983, p 33.

etry. A statement concerning the uses of such x-rays was developed and unanimously endorsed by the panel. The statement adopted by the American College of Radiology (1979), written by the panel, is presented below:

> Pelvimetry is not usually necessary or helpful in making the decision to perform a cesarean section. Therefore, pelvimetry should be performed only when the physician caring for the patient feels that pelvimetry will contribute to the decisions concerning diagnosis or treatment. In those few instances, the reason for requesting the pelvimetry should be written on the patient's chart. This statement does not apply to x-ray examinations for purposes other than measurement of the pelvis.

The following statement by the American College of Obstetricians and Gynecologists (1979) was published in the *ACOG Newsletter*:

> X-ray pelvimetry provides limited additional information to physicians involved in the management of labor and delivery. It should not be a prerequisite to clinical decisions concerning obstetrical management. Reasons for requesting x-ray pelvimetry should be individually established.

Other X-ray Examinations

Not only have recommendations been made to limit x-ray pelvimetry exposure, but similar advice has been given to limit diagnostic radiation exposure to the pelvis of any woman at any time in the childbearing years. As emphasized by Brent (1987),

radiation exposure of less than 5 rad, except for carcinogenesis, represents no measurable risk to the embryo.

In 1977, the American College of Obstetricians and Gynecologists, in cooperation with the American College of Radiology, issued a policy statement, *Guidelines for Diagnostic X-ray Examination of Fertile Women.* They agreed that *"Attempts to schedule abdominal x-ray examinations in relation to a woman's menstrual cycle are of little value. The developing ovum is at risk prior to ovulation as well as subsequently. Thus it is erroneous to assume that any time is 'safer' for radiation exposure than another."*

They recommended the following guidelines:

1. The use of x-ray examination should be considered on an individual basis. Concern over harmful effects should not prevent the proper use of radiation exposure when significant diagnostic information can be obtained. Preexamination consultation with a radiologist may be useful in obtaining optimal information from the x-ray exposure.
2. There is no measurable advantage to scheduling diagnostic x-ray examinations at any particular time during a normal menstrual cycle.
3. The degree of risk involved in an x-ray examination if the person is pregnant, or may become pregnant, should be explained to the patient and documented in her record.

COMPUTED TOMOGRAPHY (CT SCANNING)

Status of Computed Tomography

Because of the small but potential risk of childhood malignancy discussed above, digital radiographs obtained with computed

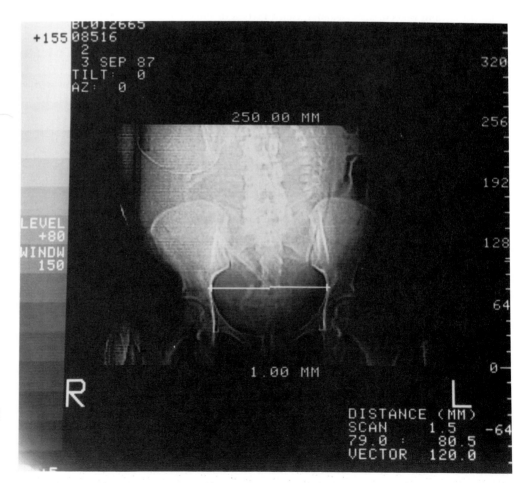

Figure 8–17 A. Anteroposterior view of digital radiograph. Illustrated is the measurement of the transverse diameter of the pelvic inlet using an electronic cursor. The fetal body is clearly outlined.

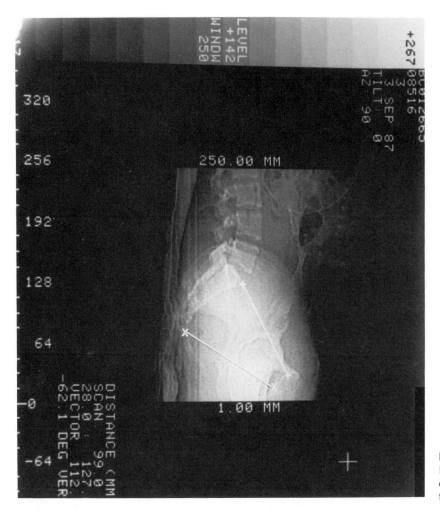

Figure 8–17 B. Lateral view of digital radiograph. Illustrated are measurements of the anteroposterior diameters of the inlet and midpelvis measured using the electronic cursor.

tomographic scanners have been used to measure pelvic diameters in attempts to reduce radiation exposure. The International Commission on Radiological Protection recommended that the radiation dose to the fetus not exceed 1 rad during pregnancy (Reekie and colleagues, 1967). With conventional x-ray pelvimetry the mean gonadal exposure is estimated to be 885 ± 111 millirads (mrad) by the Committee on Radiological Hazards to Patients (Osborn, 1963). Thus, even without additional x-ray views, the average radiation dose approaches the 1 rad value (Varner and associates, 1980).

In 1982 Federle and associates reported that adequate images of the bony pelvis could be obtained utilizing anteroposterior and lateral digital radiographs in a tomogram machine with an average absorbed dose of 22 mrad each and a single computed tomograph at the level of the ischial spines with an average absorbed dose of 380 mrad. This has been confirmed by others (Adam and colleagues, 1985; Claussen and co-workers, 1985; Gimovsky and associates, 1985; Kopelman and co-workers, 1986; Lenke and Shuman, 1986; Surano and co-workers, 1984). Subsequently, Adam and associates (1985) reported that two digital radiographs (anteroposterior and lateral views) usually are sufficient to measure the necessary pelvic diameters, including the interspinous, provided appropriate corrections are made.

Technique for Computed Tomographic Pelvimetry

Views are obtained for anteroposterior and lateral projections, and a single axial tomogram also is obtained at the level of the fovea of the femoral heads, a level accurately selected from the anteroposterior projection. In this projection the fetus presenting as breech also can be evaluated for hyperextension of the head and the type of breech. Electronic calipers are used to measure the transverse diameter of the inlet (anteroposterior view) and the anteroposterior diameters of the inlet and midpelvis from the lateral view (Fig. 8–17A through C). There is little or no distortion or magnification as long as the patient remains at the center of the table. Thus, when the electronic calipers are used, careful positioning of the patient is essential (Federle and co-workers, 1982). Maternal movement is kept at minimum, since maternal or fetal movement may cause artifacts (Brody and associates, 1986). The digital radiograph at the level of the ischial spines can be eliminated in some cases and the interspinous diameter measured when appropriate compensations are made for distortion, as described by Adam and colleagues (1985).

Advantages of Computed Tomographic Pelvimetry

The obvious advantage of this technique is a reduction in radiation exposure with a range of 44 mrad (Adam and associates, 1985) to 425 mrad (Federle and co-workers, 1982). The accuracy

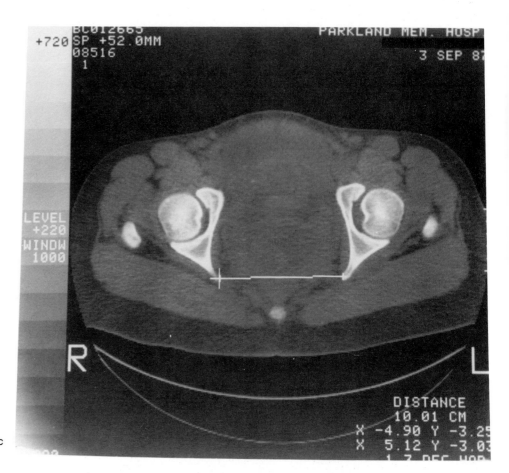

Figure 8–17 C. An axial computed tomographic section through the midpelvis. The level of the fovea of the femoral heads was ascertained from the anteroposterior digital radiograph because it corresponds to the level of the ischial spines. The interspinous diameter is measured using the electronic cursor.

is greater than conventional x-ray pelvimetry and it is easier to perform (Adam and associates, 1985; Gimovsky and co-workers, 1985). The cost is comparable to conventional x-ray pelvimetry.

ULTRASOUND

Despite the significant advances in obstetrics achieved with the use of diagnostic ultrasound, the accurate measurement of maternal pelvic diameters has not been achieved. Unfortunately, all techniques to the present remain complicated, tedious, incomplete, and without immediate clinical utility (Nakano, 1981; Nakano and co-workers, 1977; Vàclavinkovà, 1973, 1976). Morgan and Thurnau (1988) have described a *fetal-pelvic index* calculated from x-ray and ultrasonically derived measurements. Although they report that the use of this index is helpful to predict cephalopelvic disproportion with fetuses weighing more than 4,000 g, their observations are preliminary.

MAGNETIC RESONANCE IMAGING

The advantages of magnetic resonance imaging include lack of ionizing radiation, accurate pelvic measurements, and complete imaging of the fetus, as well as giving the potential for evaluating reasons for soft tissue dystocia (McCarthy, 1986; Stark and co-workers, 1985). Currently this methodology is limited because of expense, time involved for adequate imaging studies, and availability of equipment. At least for now, this new and promising technology is experimental.

OTHER CONSIDERATIONS

Because of their limited clinical applicability, pelvis of the newborn, sexual differences in the adult pelvis, and transformation of the fetal into the adult pelvis are not considered here. These topics have been covered extensively in previous editions of *Williams Obstetrics*. The interested reader is referred to the seventeenth edition, Chapter 11, page 231.

REFERENCES

Abramson D, Roberts SM, Wilson PD: Relaxation of the pelvic joints in pregnancy. Surg Obstet Gynecol 58:595, 1934

Adam PH, Alberge AY, Castellano S, Kassab M, Escude B: Pelvimetry by digital radiography. Clin Radiol 36:327, 1985

Ager EA, Schuman LM, Wallace HM, Rosenfeld AB, Gullen WH: An epidemiological study of childhood leukemia. J Chronic Dis 18:113, 1965

American College of Obstetricians and Gynecologists: Statement of Policy: Guidelines for Diagnostic X-ray Examination of Fertile Women. Chicago, May 1977

American College of Obstetricians and Gynecologists: ACOG Bull 23:10, 1979

American College of Radiology: ACR Bull 35:2, 1979

Bader A: The significance of the unengaged head in primiparous labor. Ber ges Gynak u Geburtsh 31:395 [Abstract], 1936

Barton JJ, Garbaciak JA Jr, Ryan GM: The efficacy of x-ray pelvimetry. Am J Obstet Gynecol 143:304, 1982

Bithell J, Stewart A: Prenatal irradiation and childhood malignancy: A review of British data from the Oxford Survey. Br J Cancer 31:271, 1975

Borell U, Fernstrom I: Movements at the sacroiliac joints and their importance to changes in pelvic dimensions during parturition. Acta Obstet Gynecol Scand 36:42, 1957

Brent RL: Comment on editorial. J Reprod Med 12:6, 1974

Brent RL: Ionizing radiation. Contemp Ob/Gyn 30:20, 1987

Brent RL, Gordon RO: Radiation exposure in pregnancy. Curr Probl Radiol 2:1, 1972

Brill HM, Danielius G: Roentgen pelvimetric analysis of Walcher's position. Am J Obstet Gynecol 42:821, 1941

Brody AS, Saks BJ, Field DR, Skinner SR, Capra RE: Artifacts seen during CT pelvimetry: Implications for digital systems with scanning beams. Radiology 160:269, 1986

Bross IDJ, Natarajan N: Leukemia from low level radiation. N Engl J Med 287:107, 1972

Budin RC: X-radiography of a Naegele pelvis. Obstetrique Par 2:499, 1897

Caldwell WE, Moloy HC: Anatomical variations in the female pelvis and their effect in labor with a suggested classification. Am J Obstet Gynecol 26:479, 1933

Caldwell WE, Moloy HC, D'Esopo DA: Further studies on the pelvic architecture. Am J Obstet Gynecol 28:482, 1934

Caldwell WE, Moloy HC, Swenson PC: The use of the roentgen ray in obstetrics: I. Roentgen pelvimetry and cephalometry; technic of pelviroentgenography. Am J Roentgenol 41:305, 1939

Claussen C, Köhler D, Christ F, Golde G, Lochner B: Pelvimetry by digital radiography and its dosimetry. J Perinat Med 13:287, 1985

Collea JV, Chein C, Quilligan EJ: The randomized management of term frank breech presentation: A study of 208 cases. Am J Obstet Gynecol 137:235, 1980

Court-Brown WM, Doll R, Hill AB: Incidence of leukaemia after exposure to diagnostic x-ray in utero. Br Med J 2:1539, 1960

Diamond EL, Schmerler H, Lilienfeld AM: The relationship of intrauterine radiation to subsequent mortality and development of leukemia in children (a prospective study). Am J Epidemiol 97:283, 1973

Federle MP, Cohen HA, Rosenwein MF, Brant-Zawadzki MN, Cann CE: Pelvimetry by digital radiography: A low-dose examination. Radiology 143:733, 1982

Fine EA, Bracken M, Berkowitz RL: An evaluation of the usefulness of x-ray pelvimetry: Comparison of the Thoms and modified Ball methods with manual pelvimetry. Am J Obstet Gynecol 137:15, 1980

Ford DD, Paterson JCS, Treuting WL: Fetal exposure to diagnostic x-rays and leukemia and other malignant disease in childhood. J Natl Cancer Inst 22:1903, 1959

Gaulden ME: Possible effects of diagnostic x-rays on the human embryo and fetus. J Arkansas Med Soc 70:424, 1974

Gimovsky ML, Wallace RL, Schifrin BS, Paul RH: Randomized management of the nonfrank breech presentation at term. Am J Obstet Gynecol 146:34, 1983

Gimovsky ML, Willard K, Neglio M, Howard T, Zerne S: X-ray pelvimetry in a breech protocol: A comparison of digital radiography and conventional methods. Am J Obstet Gynecol 153:887, 1985

Gordon A, Pinchen C, Walker E, Tudor J: The changing place of radiology in obstetrics. Br J Radiol 57:891, 1984

Gunz FW, Atkinson HR: Medical radiations and leukaemia: A retrospective survey. Br Med J 1:389, 1964

Harvey EB, Boice JD, Honeyman M, Flannery JT: Prenatal x-ray exposure and childhood cancer in twins. N Engl J Med 312:541, 1985

Hernandez E, Rosenshein NB, Goldberg E, King TM: Roentgenographic pelvimetry in single vertex pregnancies. South Med J 75:439, 1982

Jagani N, Schulman H, Chandra P, Gonzalez R, Fleischer A: The predictability of labor outcome from a comparison of birth weight and x-ray pelvimetry. Am J Obstet Gynecol 139:507, 1981

Joyce DN, Giwa-Sagie F, Stevenson GW: Role of pelvimetry in active management of labor. Br Med J 4:505, 1975

Kaplan HS: An evaluation of the somatic and genetic hazards of the medical uses of radiation. Am J Roentgenol Radium Ther Nucl 80:696, 1958

Klapholz H: Evaluation of fetopelvic relationships. In Cohen WR: Friedman EA (eds): Management of Labor. Baltimore, University Park Press, 1983, p 33

Kneale GW, Stewart AM: Mantel-Haenszel analysis of Oxford data: I. Independent effects of several birth factors including fetal irradiation. J Natl Cancer Inst 56:879, 1976

Kopelman JN, Duff P, Karl RT, Schipul AH, Read JA: Computed tomographic pelvimetry in the evaluation of breech presentation. Obstet Gynecol 68:455, 1986

Lao TT, Chin RKH, Leung BFH: Is x-ray pelvimetry useful in a trial of labour after caesarean section? Eur J Obstet Gynecol Reprod Biol 24:277, 1987

Laube DW, Varner MW, Cruikshank DP: A prospective evaluation of x-ray pelvimetry. JAMA 246:2187, 1981

Lenke RR, Shuman WP: Computed tomographic pelvimetry. J Reprod Med 31:958, 1986

Lewis TLT: Leukaemia in childhood after antenatal exposure to x-rays (a survey at Queen Charlotte's Hospital). Br Med J 2:1551, 1960

MacMahon B: Prenatal x-ray exposure and childhood cancer. J Natl Cancer Inst 28:1173, 1962

McCarthy S: Magnetic resonance imaging in obstetrics and gynecology. Magn Reson Imaging 4:59, 1986

McKinney PA, Cartwright RA, Saiu JMT, Mann JR, Stiller CA, Draper GJ, Harley AL, Hopton PA, Birch JM, Waterhouse JAH, Johnston HE: The interregional epidemiological study of childhood cancer (IRESCC): A case control study of aetiological factors in leukaemia and lymphoma. Arch Dis Child 62:279, 1987

Mengert WF: Estimation of pelvic capacity. JAMA 138:169, 1948

Morgan MA, Thurneau GR: Efficacy of the fetal-pelvic index for delivery of neonates weighing 4000 grams or greater: A preliminary report. Am J Obstet Gynecol 158:1133, 1988

Murray R, Heckel P, Hempelmann LH: Leukemia in children exposed to ionizing radiation. N Engl J Med 261:585, 1959

Nakano H: Assessment of dystocia pelvis by ultrasound pelvimetry. Acta Obstet Gynaecol Jpn 7:1077, 1981

Nakano H, Koyanagi T, Nii F, Kumano Y, Kubota S, Sakamoto C, Taki I: Study on the female pelvis by ultrasonic tomography. Acta Obstet Gynaecol Jpn 29:431, 1977

O'Brien WF, Cefalo RC: Evaluation of x-ray pelvimetry and abnormal labor. Clin Obstet Gynecol 25:157, 1982

Oppenheim BE, Briem ML, Meier P: The effects of diagnostic x-ray exposure on the human fetus: An examination of the evidence. Radiology 114:529, 1975

Osborn SB: The implications of the Committee on Radiological Hazards to Patients (Adrian Committee): I. Variations in the radiation dose received by the patient in diagnostic radiology. Br J Radiol 36:230, 1963

Parsons MT, Spellacy WN: Prospective randomized study of x-ray pelvimetry in the primigravida. Obstet Gynecol 66:76, 1985

Polhemus DW, Koch R: Leukemia and medical radiation. Pediatrics 23:453, 1959

Poma PA: X-ray pelvimetry in primiparas: I. Role of physiological maturity. J Natl Med Assoc 74:173, 1982

Poma PA: Value of x-ray pelvimetry in primiparas: II. Influence on management of labor. J Natl Med Assoc 74:267, 1982

Reekie D, Davison M, Davidson JK: The radiation hazard in radiography of the female abdomen and pelvis. Br J Radiol 40:849, 1967

Ridley WJ, Jackson P, Stewart JH, Boyle P: Role of antenatal radiography in the management of breech deliveries. Br J Obstet Gynaecol 89:342, 1982

Schussman LC, Lutz LJ: Hazards and uses in prenatal diagnostic x-radiation. J Fam Pract 3:473, 1982

Stark DD, McCarthy SM, Filly RA, Parer JT, Hricak H, Callen PW: Pelvimetry by magnetic resonance imaging. Am J Radiol 144:947, 1985

Stewart A, Webb J, Giles D, Hewitt D: Malignant disease in childhood and diagnostic irradiation in utero. Lancet 2:447, 1956

Stewart A, Webb J, Hewitt D: A survey of childhood malignancies. Br Med J 1:1495, 1958

Stjernfeldt M, Berglund K, Lindsten J, Ludvigsson J: Maternal smoking during pregnancy and risk of childhood cancer. Lancet 1:1350, 1986

Suramo I, Torniainen P, Jouppila P, Kirkinen P, Lahde S: A low-dose CT-pelvimetry. Br J Radiol 57:35, 1984

US Department of Health and Human Resources: The selection of patients for x-ray examinations: The pelvimetry examination. HHS Pub (FDA) 80:8128, July 1980

Vàclavinkovà V: A method of measuring the interspinous diameter by an ultrasonic technique. Acta Obstet Gynecol Scand 52:161, 1973

Vàclavinkovà V: Ultrasonic pelvimetry: A method for preliminary estimation of the pelvic outlet. Ultrasonics 14:133, 1976

Varner MW, Cruikshank DP, Laube DW: X-ray pelvimetry in clinical obstetrics. Obstet Gynecol 56:296, 1980

Wells J, Steer CM: Relationship of leukemia in children to abdominal radiation of mothers during pregnancy. Am J Obstet Gynecol 81:1059, 1961

Young J: Relaxation of pelvic joints in pregnancy: Pelvic arthropathy of pregnancy. Br J Obstet Gynaecol 47:493, 1940

Attitude, Lie, Presentation, and Position of the Fetus

FETAL ATTITUDE OR POSTURE

In the later months of pregnancy the fetus assumes a characteristic posture sometimes described as *attitude* or *habitus* (Fig. 9–1). As a rule the fetus forms an ovoid mass that corresponds roughly to the shape of the uterine cavity. The fetus becomes folded or bent upon itself in such a manner that the back becomes markedly convex; the head is sharply flexed so that the chin is almost in contact with the chest; the thighs are flexed over the abdomen; the legs are bent at the knees; and the arches of the feet rest upon the anterior surfaces of the legs. Usually the arms are crossed over the thorax or become parallel to the sides, and the umbilical cord lies in the space between them and the lower extremities. This characteristic posture results partly from the mode of growth of the fetus and partly from a process of accommodation to the uterine cavity.

LIE OF THE FETUS

The lie is the relation of the long axis of the fetus to that of the mother and is either *longitudinal* or *transverse.* Occasionally, the fetal and the maternal axes may cross at a 45-degree angle, forming an *oblique* lie, which is unstable and always becomes longitudinal or transverse during the course of labor. Longitudinal lies are present in over 99 percent of labors at term.

PRESENTATION AND PRESENTING PART

The presenting part is that portion of the body of the fetus that is either foremost within the birth canal or in closest proximity to it; that is, the presenting part is that portion of the fetus that is felt through the cervix on vaginal examination. The presenting part determines the presentation. Accordingly, in longitudinal lies, the presenting part is either the fetal head or the breech, creating cephalic and breech presentations, respectively. When the fetus lies with the long axis transversely, the shoulder is the presenting part. Thus, a shoulder presentation is felt through the cervix on vaginal examination.

Cephalic presentations are classified according to the relation of the head to the body of the fetus (Fig. 9–1). Ordinarily the head is flexed sharply so that the chin is in contact with the thorax. In this circumstance the occipital fontanel is the presenting part, although such a presentation is usually referred to as a *vertex* or *occiput presentation.* (The vertex actually lies just in front of the occipital fontanel, and the occiput just behind the fontanel, as illustrated in Fig. 6–8, p. 93.) Much less commonly, the fetal neck may be sharply extended so that the occiput and

back come in contact and the face is foremost in the birth canal (*face presentation*). The fetal head may assume a position between these extremes, partially flexed in some cases, with the anterior (large) fontanel, or bregma, presenting (*sinciput presentation*), or partially extended in other cases, with the brow presenting (*brow presentation*). Perhaps the latter two should not be classified as distinct presentations, since these are usually transient. As labor progresses, sinciput and brow presentations are almost always converted into vertex or face presentations by flexion or extension, respectively.

When the fetus presents as a breech, the thighs may be flexed and the legs extended over the anterior surfaces of the body (*frank breech presentation*) (Fig. 9–2), or the thighs may be flexed on the abdomen and the legs upon the thighs (*complete breech presentation*) (Fig. 9–3), and one or both feet, or one or both knees, are lowermost (*incomplete,* or *footling, breech presentation*) (Fig. 9–4).

POSITION

Position refers to the relation of an arbitrarily chosen portion of the presenting part of the fetus to the right or left side of the maternal birth canal. Accordingly, with each presentation there may be two positions, right or left. The occiput, chin, and sacrum are the determining points in vertex, face, and breech presentations, respectively (Figs. 9–5 to 9–8).

Variety

For still more accurate orientation the relation of a given portion of the presenting part to the anterior, transverse, or posterior portion of the mother's pelvis is considered. Since there are two positions, it follows that there must be six varieties for each presentation (Figs. 9–5 to 9–8).

Nomenclature

Since the presenting part in any presentation may be in either the left or right position, there are left and right occipital, left and right mental, and left and right sacral presentations, abbreviated as LO and RO, LM and RM, and LS and RS, respectively. Since the presenting part in each of the two positions may be directed anteriorly (A), transversely (T), or posteriorly (P), there are six varieties of each of these three presentations (Figs. 9–5 to 9–8).

In shoulder presentations the acromion (or the scapula) is the portion of the fetus arbitrarily chosen to orient it with the maternal pelvis. One example of the terminology sometimes

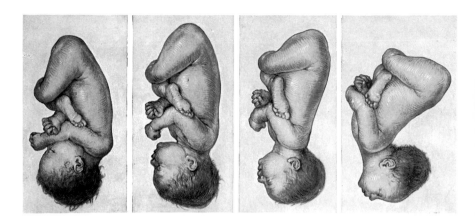

Figure 9–1. Differences in attitude of fetus in vertex, sinciput, brow, and face presentations.

employed for the purpose is illustrated in Figure 9–9. The acromion or back of the fetus may be directed either posteriorly or anteriorly and superiorly or inferiorly (see Chap. 19, p. 361). However, since it is impossible to differentiate exactly the several varieties of shoulder presentation by clinical examination and since such differentiation serves no practical purpose, it is customary to refer to all transverse lies of the fetus simply as shoulder presentations.

Frequency of the Various Presentations and Positions

At or near term the incidence of the various presentations is approximately as follows: vertex, 96 percent; breech, 3.5 percent; face, 0.3 percent; shoulder, 0.4 percent. About two thirds of all vertex presentations are in the left occiput position, and one third in the right.

Although the incidence of breech presentation is only a little over 3 percent at term, it is much greater earlier in pregnancy. White (1956) found the incidence of breech presentation to be 7.2 percent by x-ray examination at the end of the 34th week. A similar frequency was identified sonographically in 1976 by Scheer and Nubar (see Table 19–1). Subsequently, in about one third of nulliparas and two thirds of multiparas, the breech converted to vertex spontaneously before delivery.

Reasons for the Predominance of Cephalic Presentations

Of the several reasons that have been advanced to explain why the fetus at term usually presents by the vertex, the most logical explanation seems to be that this is because the uterus is piriform shaped. Although the fetal head at term is slightly larger than the breech, the entire podalic pole of the fetus, that is, the breech and its flexed extremities, is bulkier than the cephalic pole

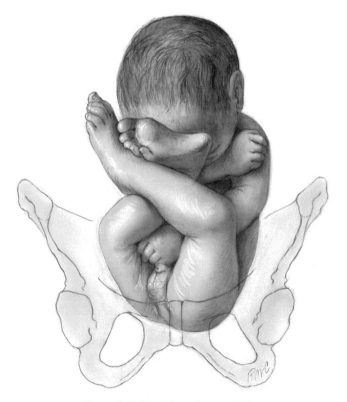

Figure 9–2. Frank breech presentation.

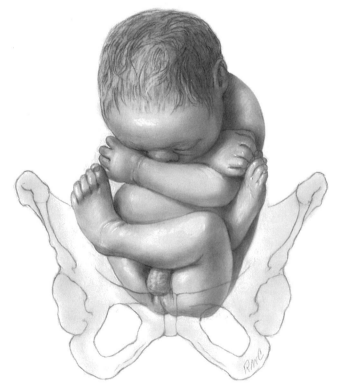

Figure 9–3. Complete breech presentation.

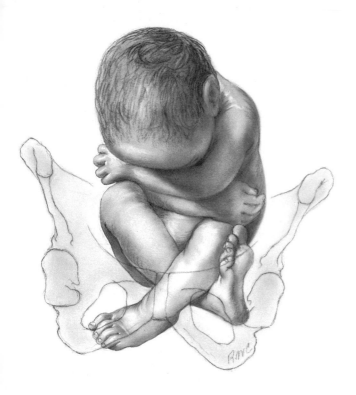

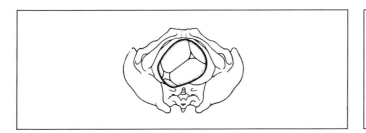

Figure 9–4. Incomplete, or footling, breech presentation.

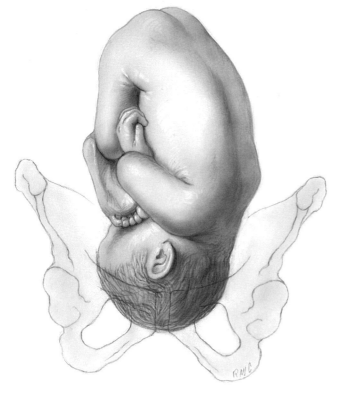

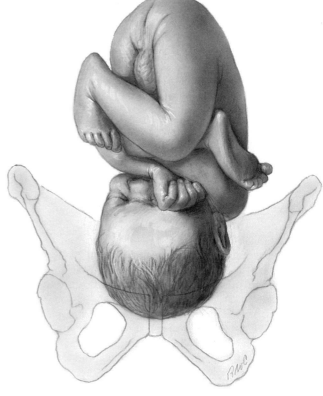

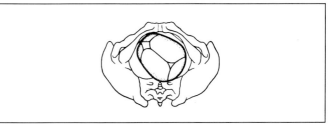

Figure 9–5. Vertex presentation. **A.** Left occipito-anterior. **B.** Left occipito-posterior.

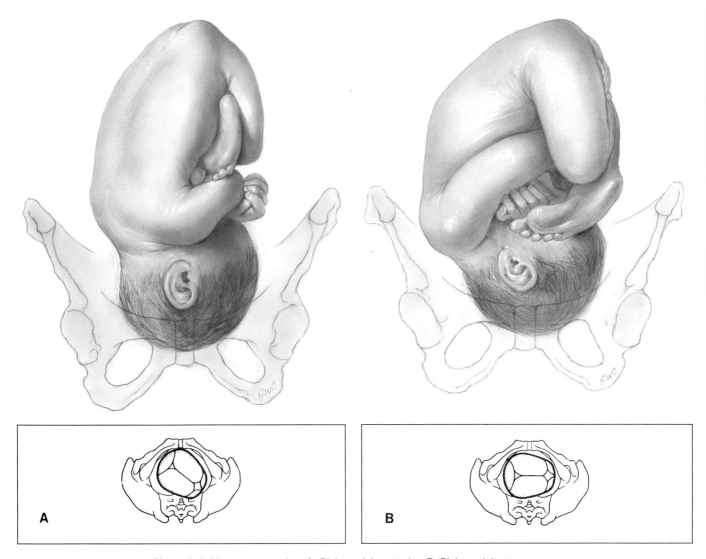

Figure 9–6. Vertex presentation. **A.** Right occipito-anterior. **B.** Right occipito-transverse.

and more movable. The cephalic pole is comprised of the fetal head only, because the upper extremities are removed some distance, are small, and are less protruding than the buttocks and lower extremities combined. Until about the 32nd week, the amnionic cavity is large compared to the fetal mass, and there is no crowding of the fetus by the uterine walls. At approximately this time, however, the ratio of amnionic fluid volume to fetal mass becomes altered by relative diminution of amnionic fluid and by increasing fetal size. As a result, the uterine walls are apposed more closely to the fetal parts, and then the fetal lie is more nearly dependent upon the piriform shape of the uterus. The fetus, if presenting by the breech, often changes polarity in order to make use of the roomier fundus for its bulkier and more movable podalic pole. The high incidence of breech presentation in hydrocephalic fetuses is in accord with this theory, since in this circumstance the cephalic pole of the fetus is definitely larger than the podalic pole. The fetus need not be alive late in pregnancy for polarity to change (Chap. 19, p. 349).

The cause of breech presentation may be some circumstance that prevents normal version from taking place, for example, a septum that protrudes into the uterine cavity. A peculiarity of fetal attitude, particularly extension of the verte-bral column, as occurs in frank breeches, also may prevent the fetus from turning.

DIAGNOSIS OF PRESENTATION AND POSITION OF THE FETUS

There are several diagnostic methods that can be used: abdominal palpation, vaginal examination, combined examination, auscultation, and, in certain doubtful cases, ultrasonography or radiography.

ABDOMINAL PALPATION—LEOPOLD'S MANEUVERS

In order to obtain satisfactory results, the examination should be conducted systematically employing the four maneuvers suggested by Leopold and Sporlin (1894). The mother should be on a firm bed or examining table, with her abdomen bared. During the first three maneuvers, the examiner stands at the side of the bed more convenient to him or her and faces the patient, but the examiner reverses this position and faces her feet for the last maneuver (Fig. 9–10).

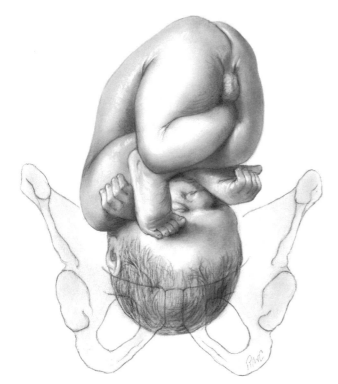

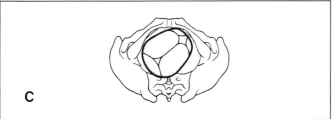

C

Figure 9–6. Vertex presentation. **C.** Right occipito-posterior.

First Maneuver

After outlining the contour of the uterus and ascertaining how nearly the fundus approaches the xiphoid cartilage, the examiner gently palpates the fundus with the tips of the fingers of both hands in order to define which fetal pole is present in the fundus. The fetal breech gives the sensation of a large, nodular body, whereas the head feels hard and round and is more freely movable and ballottable.

Second Maneuver

After the determination of the pole of the fetus that lies in the fundus, the palms of the examiner's hands are placed on either side of the abdomen, and gentle but deep pressure is exerted. On one side, a hard, resistant structure is felt, the back, and on the other, numerous nodulations, the small parts. In pregnant women with thin abdominal walls, the fetal extremities can be differentiated readily, but in obese women only irregular nodulations can be felt. In the presence of obesity or considerable amnionic fluid, the back is felt more easily by making deep pressure with one hand while palpating with the other. By next noting whether the back is directed anteriorly, transversely, or

posteriorly, a more accurate picture of the orientation of the fetus is obtained.

Third Maneuver

Employing the thumb and fingers of one hand, the examiner grasps the lower portion of the maternal abdomen, just above the symphysis pubis. If the presenting part is not engaged, a movable body will be felt, usually the fetal head. The differentiation between head and breech is made as in the first maneuver. If the presenting part is not engaged, the examination is almost complete; with the location of the fetal head, breech, back, and extremities known, all that remains to be defined is the attitude of the head. If by careful palpation it can be shown that the cephalic prominence is on the same side as the small parts, the head must be flexed, and therefore the vertex is the presenting part. When the cephalic prominence of the fetus is on the same side as the back, the head must be extended. However, if the presenting part is deeply engaged, the findings from this maneuver are simply indicative of the fact that the lower pole of the fetus is fixed in the pelvis; the details are then defined by the last (fourth) maneuver.

Fourth Maneuver

The examiner faces the mother's feet and, with the tips of the first three fingers of each hand, makes deep pressure in the direction of the axis of the pelvic inlet. If the head presents, one hand is arrested sooner than the other by a rounded body, the cephalic prominence, while the other hand descends more deeply into the pelvis. In vertex presentations, the prominence is on the same side as the small parts, and in face presentations, on the same side as the back. The ease with which the prominence is felt is indicative of the extent to which descent has occurred. In many instances, when the fetal head has descended into the pelvis, the anterior shoulder of the fetus may be differentiated readily by the third maneuver. In breech presentations, the information obtained from this maneuver is less precise.

Abdominal palpation can be performed throughout the latter months of pregnancy and during the intervals between the contractions of labor. The findings provide information about the presentation and position of the fetus and the extent to which the presenting part has descended into the pelvis. For example, so long as the cephalic prominence is readily palpable, the vertex has not descended to the level of the ischial spines. The degree of cephalopelvic disproportion, moreover, can be gauged by evaluating the extent to which the anterior portion of the fetal head overrides the mother's symphysis pubis. With experience, it is possible to estimate the size of the fetus and even to map out the presentation of the second fetus in a twin gestation.

During labor, palpation also may provide information about the lower uterine segment. When there is obstruction to the passage of the fetus, a pathological retraction ring sometimes may be felt as a transverse or oblique ridge extending across the lower portion of the uterus (see Chap. 18, p. 347). Even in normal cases, the contracting body of the uterus and the passive lower uterine segment may be distinguished by palpation. During a contraction, the upper portion of the uterus is firm or hard, whereas the lower segment feels elastic or almost fluctuant.

VAGINAL EXAMINATION

Before labor, the diagnosis of fetal presentation and position by vaginal examination may be somewhat inconclusive, because

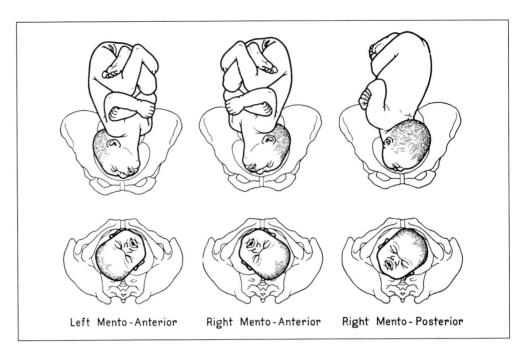

Left Mento-Anterior   Right Mento-Anterior   Right Mento-Posterior

Figure 9–7. Face presentation. Left and right anterior and right posterior positions.

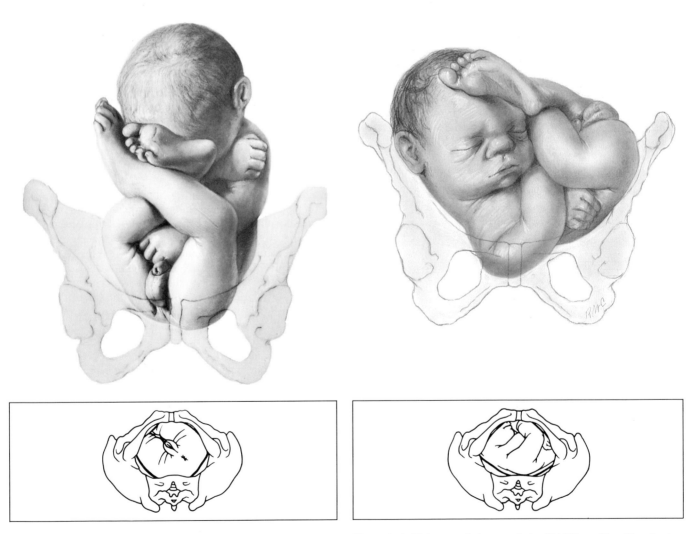

Figure 9–8. Breech presentation. Left sacrum posterior position.

Figure 9–9. Right acromiodorsoposterior (RADP) position. The shoulder of the fetus is to the mother's right, and the back is posterior.

the presenting part must be palpated through the closed cervix and lower uterine segment. During labor, however, after dilatation of the cervix, important information may be obtained. In vertex presentations, the position and variety are recognized by differentiation of the various sutures and fontanels; in face presentations, by the differentiation of the portions of the face; and in breech presentations, by the palpation of the sacrum and ischial tuberosities.

In attempting to determine presentation and position by vaginal examination, it is advisable to pursue a definite routine, comprised of three maneuvers (Figs. 9–11, 9–12):

1. After the woman is prepared appropriately, as described in Chapter 16, two fingers of either gloved hand of the examiner are introduced into the vagina and carried up to the presenting part. The differentiation of vertex, face, and breech then is accomplished readily.

2. If the vertex is presenting, the examiner's fingers are

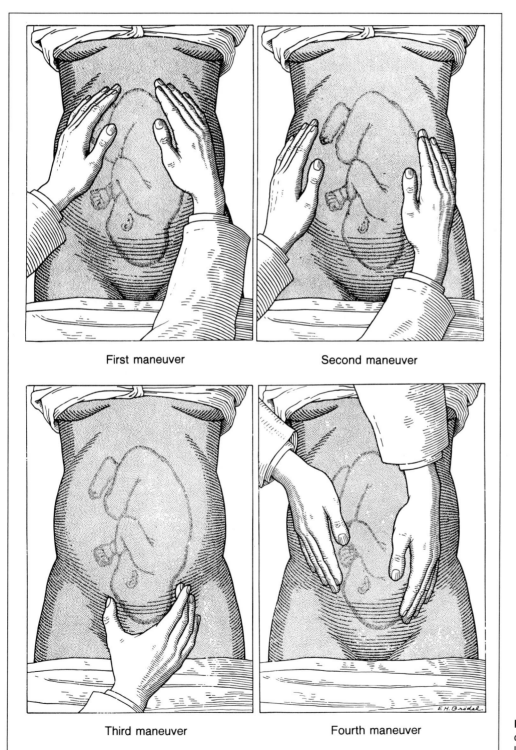

First maneuver

Second maneuver

Third maneuver

Fourth maneuver

Figure 9–10. Palpation in left occiput anterior position (maneuvers of Leopold). See also Figure 9–5A.

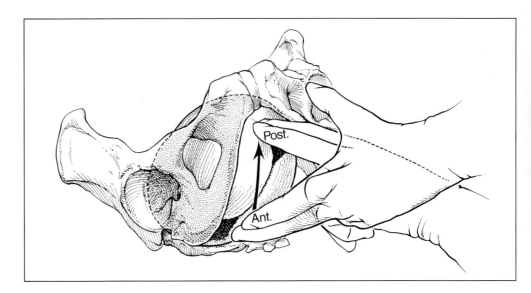

Figure 9–11. Locating the sagittal suture by vaginal examination.

introduced into the posterior aspect of the vagina. The fingers are then swept forward over the fetal head toward the maternal symphysis (Fig. 9–11). During the performance of this movement, the examiner's fingers necessarily cross the sagittal suture. When it is felt, its course is outlined, with small and large fontanels at the opposite ends.

3. The positions of the two fontanels then are ascertained. The examiner's fingers are passed to the anterior extremity of the sagittal suture, and the fontanel encountered there is examined carefully and identified; then by a circular motion, the fingers are passed around the side of the head until the other fontanel is felt and differentiated (Fig. 9–12).

Using these three maneuvers, the various sutures and fontanels are located readily, and the possibility of error is lessened considerably. In face and breech presentations, er-

rors are minimized, since the various parts are distinguished more readily.

AUSCULTATION

Auscultation by itself does not provide very reliable information concerning the presentation and position of the fetus, but the findings of auscultation sometimes reinforce the results obtained by palpation. Ordinarily, the fetal heart sounds are transmitted through the convex portion of the fetus that lies in intimate contact with the uterine wall. Therefore, fetal heart sounds are heard best through the fetal back in vertex and breech presentations and through the fetal thorax in face presentations. The region of the abdomen in which the fetal heart tones are heard most clearly varies according to the presentation and the extent to which the presenting part has descended. In cephalic presentations the point of maximal intensity of fetal heart sounds is usually midway between the maternal umbili-

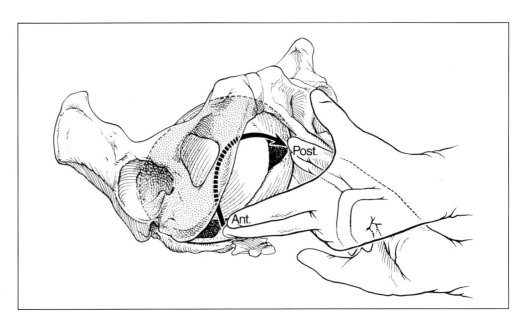

Figure 9–12. Differentiating the fontanels by vaginal examination.

cus and the anterior superior spine of her ilium, whereas in breech presentations it is usually about level with the umbilicus. In occipitoanterior positions the heart sounds usually are heard best a short distance from the midline, in the transverse varieties they are heard more laterally, and in the posterior varieties well back in the mother's flank.

SONOGRAPHY

Improvements in ultrasonographic technique have provided another diagnostic aid of particular value in doubtful cases. In obese women or in women whose abdominal walls are rigid, a sonographic examination may provide information to solve many diagnostic problems and lead to early recognition of a breech or shoulder presentation that might otherwise have escaped detection until late in labor. Employing ultrasonography, the fetal head and body can be located without the potential hazards of radiation (see Chap. 15, p. 283). On some occasions, however, the information obtained radiographically far exceeds the minimal risk from a single diagnostic x-ray exposure.

REFERENCES

Leopold, Sporlin: Conduct of normal births through external examination alone. Arch Gynaekol 45:337, 1894

Scheer K, Nubar J: Variation of fetal presentation with gestational age. Am J Obstet Gynecol 125:269, 1976

White AJ: Spontaneous cephalic version in the later weeks of pregnancy and its significance in the management of breech presentation. Br J Obstet Gynaecol 63:706, 1956

Parturition: Biomolecular and Physiological Processes

OVERVIEW

Parturition: the act of bringing forth or being delivered of young; the act of giving birth; childbirth
Webster's New Twentieth Century Dictionary, 1979.

It can be argued that parturition commences at the time of conception. And there is merit in this argument. Clearly, implantation of the blastocyst in the uterus, rather than in some ectopic site, is essential to parturition. The forceful contractions necessary to propel the fetus through the cervix and birth canal during childbirth are dependent upon prior hypertrophy of the uterine smooth muscle cells. Even the proper orientation of the fetus in the uterine cavity is vital for successful delivery.

It also can be argued, and with equal vigor, that the prevention of parturition is fundamental to the maintenance of pregnancy. Indeed, from the biomolecular and physiological perspective, it is more convenient to consider the parturitional process as encompassing those final events of pregnancy when (1) distinctive morphological and biochemical changes in uterine tissues preparatory for coordinated, forceful contractions begin, (2) labor brings forth the delivery of the fetus, placenta, and fetal membranes, and (3) the morphological and biochemical identity of the uterus is returned to what is characteristic of the nonpregnant state.

PHASES OF PARTURITION

Physiologically and clinically, parturition, as defined, is divisible into three distinctive but overlapping phases. **Phase one of parturition is the time of uterine preparedness for labor. Phase two of parturition is the time of forceful contractions of active labor and delivery. Phase three of parturition is the time of puerperal contraction and involution of the uterus.**

The first phase of parturition is commonly identifiable by distinctive signs of this preparatory process; these include ripening of the cervix, increasing frequency of painless uterine contractions, and uterine irritability. Phase two of parturition begins with *the onset of labor*, i.e., the regular, forceful, painful uterine contractions that bring about cervical dilatation and descent of the fetus, and ends with delivery of the conceptus. The second phase of parturition is divided further into *the three stages of labor* (p. 213). Phase three of parturition begins after delivery of the conceptus, with persistent contraction of the uterus that ensures puerperal hemostasis, and proceeds through complete involution of the uterus, a process that returns this organ to the nonpregnant state (Fig. 10–1).

Parturition, therefore, commences during the final days of gestation, marking the time in pregnancy when the maintenance of pregnancy, *i.e.*, the stronghold on the formation of uterotropins and uterotonins, is relinquished. *Retreat from pregnancy maintenance* and *the initiation of parturition* are synchronous, perhaps synonymous.

Uterotropin is a term used to describe an agent or agents that serve to cause uterine preparedness for labor (Casey and MacDonald, 1988a). In all mammalian species studied, the first phase of parturition involves discrete morphological and biochemical changes in the uterus. Among these alterations are (1) cervical softening and ripening, (2) the development of gap junctions between myometrial cells, (3) an increase in the number of oxytocin receptors in myometrium, and (4) increased contractile responsiveness of the myometrium to uterotonins. These uterine modifications are attributed, arbitrarily, to the action of one or more uterotropins, even though the identity of the agents that effect these modifications is not precisely defined in all cases. In the context of parturition, the term *uterotropin* is not used to describe an agent that causes uterine growth, but neither is it intended to exclude substances that may be important in myometrial cell hypertrophy, *e.g.*, sex steroid hormones.

Uterotonin is a term used to describe substances, for example, prostaglandins and oxytocin, that act to cause myometrial contractions, such as those that are characteristic of active labor, *i.e.*, the second phase of parturition. It is possible, of course, that a particular uterotonin, for example, a prostaglandin, also may be a uterotropin. Some agents known to act as uterotonins are produced within the uterus and are believed to act in a paracrine manner; other uterotonins may be produced in extra-uterine sites and act in an endocrine manner (Casey and Mac-Donald, 1988b,c).

THE ONSET OF PARTURITION: DEFINITION

For purposes of discussion and clarity, we define *the onset of parturition* as that time late in pregnancy when accelerated uterotropin-uterotonin formation begins and the uterine changes that are preparatory to labor commence. According to this definition, accelerated uterotropin-uterotonin formation and *the onset of parturition* are synchronous. There are advantages to the use of this definition: First, according to these criteria, those events that lead to increased uterotropin-uterotonin formation precede parturition. Second, this definition of *the onset of parturition* is synonymous with *retreat from pregnancy maintenance* (Casey and MacDonald, 1988a,c).

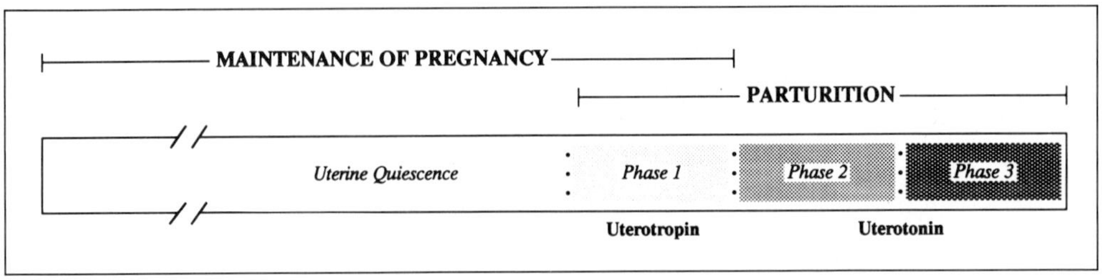

Figure 10–1. The three phases of parturition. Phase 1: uterine preparedness for labor. Phase 2: active labor. Phase 3: uterine contraction and involution.

ORIGIN OF UTEROTROPINS AND UTEROTONINS

There are a number of naturally occurring compounds that will cause uterine contractions. Among the more potent of these uterotonins are prostaglandins, oxytocin, angiotensin II, arginine vasopressin, and bradykinin. Some of these uterotonins are known to be produced in the intrauterine tissues of pregnancy. For example, the uterine decidua and extraembryonic fetal membranes are tissues in which there is a reasonably high enzymatic potential for the formation of PGE_2 and $PGF_{2\alpha}$.

It seems most likely that parturition is initiated in response to uterotropins and uterotonins that are produced within the uterus, *i.e.*, in uterine tissues or else in extraembryonic fetal tissues. A number of bioactive agents, produced in these tissues, accumulate in amnionic fluid during labor. Indeed, it may be that the amnionic fluid constitutes a window through which we can view, with amazing clarity, the procession of the biomolecular events of human parturition (see p. 198). For example, prostaglandins, which are potent uterotonins formed within the uterus during labor, accumulate in the amnionic fluid.

Several of the more likely candidates as uterotropins and uterotonins for parturition, such as the prostaglandins, are extremely potent substances that bring about a variety of profound responses in many tissues. The formation of these compounds within the uterus permits an autocrine or paracrine action (or both), obviating the potential undesirable side-effects that could be effected if the delivery of these agents to myometrium were obliged by way of the systemic circulation. In addition, the half-life of many of these uterotonins in blood is very short. Therefore, the *in situ* formation of uterotonins within the uterus is a metabolically economical manner of ensuring a higher concentration of these agents at the tissue site of action, *viz.*, the myometrium.

Alternatively, selected uterotonins may be produced in extrauterine tissues. An example of such a uterotonin, which could act by an endocrine mechanism and possibly in concert with intrauterine-generated uterotonins, is oxytocin. Indeed, oxytocin may be the principal uterotonin of the third phase of parturition, acting after delivery of the conceptus to cause contraction of the uterus, thereby preventing postpartum hemorrhage.

CONTRACTILITY OF MYOMETRIUM

We do not understand how the transition from *maintenance of pregnancy* (uterine quiescence) to *the onset of labor* (forceful uterine contractions) is accomplished. But more than this, we do not understand how effective uterine quiescence is instituted and maintained for 99 percent of pregnancy in the first place. Contraction is a constitutive property of smooth muscle, and this is certainly true in the case of uterine smooth muscle, *viz.*, the myometrium. In nonpregnant women uterine contractions are

involved in the transport of spermatozoa along the uterine cavity into the fallopian tube. The dysmenorrhea of menstruation is caused, in large measure, by uterine contractions. Intrauterine devices inserted for purposes of contraception commonly provoke such painful uterine contractions as to necessitate their removal. Not infrequently, intense uterine contractions in nonpregnant women cause the delivery of pedunculated submucous leiomyomata through the cervix into the vaginal canal. Indeed, the uterus that is enlarged by leiomyomata has been mistaken on many occasions for the uterus of pregnancy, and the extrusion of a submucous myoma through the cervix has been interpreted as delivery of the fetal head.

UTERINE CHANGES OF PREGNANCY

Stretching, cell replication, inflammation, trauma, and foreign tissue grafts all are known stimulators of prostaglandin formation, and each of these processes is fundamental to pregnancy. During human pregnancy, the uterus increases in size from an organ of about 50 g to one that, at term, weighs more than 1 kg. This comes about by way of a 10-fold increase in myometrial cell size as a consequence of cellular hypertrophy. And during this same time, the volume capacity of the uterus increases by several orders of magnitude. Thus, there is an inherent capacity for the human uterus to contract, and during pregnancy several processes that should provoke such contractions are in place. And even more, the capacity for the formation of selected uterotonins in the intrauterine tissues of human pregnancy is substantial. Nonetheless, pregnancy normally proceeds for about 260 days from the time of implantation.

UTERINE QUIESCENCE OF PREGNANCY

It is no wonder, therefore, that one of the great mysteries of human pregnancy is the almost unbelievable quiescence of the uterus during more than 99 percent of pregnancy. It has been stated that *the uterus is remarkably tolerant of its burden* during this time; today we recognize, perhaps as never before, that this is a phenomenally accurate, even understated, description of the maintenance of pregnancy. Before parturition, pregnancy is a physiological state in which a biomolecular stronghold is placed on the formation of uterotropins and uterotonins in intrauterine tissues to prevent myometrial contraction, *i.e.*, to maintain myometrial quiescence, indeed to prevent parturition (Casey and MacDonald, 1988b).

REGULATION OF PROSTAGLANDIN FORMATION

To gain an appreciation for the effectiveness of the system that operates to maintain pregnancy by restraining uterotonin formation, the amount of $PGF_{2\alpha}$ (administered by intravenous infusion at term) that must reach the uterus to cause the induction of labor has been estimated. The amount computed is very small, namely, 50 pg per g of myometrial tissue per minute, and the amount of $PGF_{2\alpha}$ produced in intrauterine tissues during spontaneous labor is estimated to be only 100 pg per g of myometrial tissue per minute (Casey and MacDonald, 1988b). If this small amount of $PGF_{2\alpha}$ is indeed sufficient to induce labor, it is apparent that there is stringent inhibition of prostaglandin formation in the uterine and extraembryonic fetal tissues during pregnancy before the onset of labor.

From these analyses it also follows that parturition will occur (1) if there is retreat from the *maintenance of pregnancy* or (2) if the systems promoting the maintenance of pregnancy are subverted or overridden by a stimulus, natural or unnatural, for *parturition*, *i.e.*, direct stimulation of uterotropin-uterotonin formation, which seems to be the cause of some forms of preterm labor (p. 208).

CONTEMPORARY ERA OF PARTURITION RESEARCH

The contemporary era of the study of the physiological and biochemical processes involved in the initiation of labor began 25 years ago. At that time reproductive biologists began to define, at the biomolecular level, the processes that are involved in the fetal–maternal communication system of pregnancy. During these 2½ decades, important discoveries have been made and new concepts have been formulated. Most investigators of this era have been seeking to identify the physiological events leading to and involved in spontaneous human parturition at term in the belief that an understanding of these processes would lead to the discovery of the cause of preterm labor and thus its prevention.

Twenty-five years later we optimistically accept the possibility that the cause of preterm labor (at least some forms thereof) may be discovered before we understand fully the cause of labor that commences normally at term; if this pleasant prospect comes to fruition, preterm labor can be used as a model to investigate the mechanisms involved in spontaneous parturition. At that time, we will, in the words of the late Chet Huntley, *"have marched majestically backward from conclusion to fact."*

Today some investigators are optimistic that we can define the biomolecular processes that cause labor in a sizable fraction of human pregnancies that deliver preterm. This optimism is based on the belief that preterm labor is frequently caused by the products of microorganisms, substances that act to induce uterotropin and uterotonin formation in intrauterine tissues (p. 208). If this proposition were proven to be correct, great insights could be gained into the biomolecular processes of parturition, whether occurring prematurely or normally at term.

Notwithstanding this hopeful posture of parturition research, at present our understanding of the biomolecular events involved in the initiation of human labor is incomplete. Nonetheless, several attractive hypotheses have been formulated to explain the nature of the underlying events that lead to the onset of parturition, and there are elements of plausibility for each proposition, yet each also clearly is deficient to some extent. For some time, we have been struggling with three general theorems. Simplistically stated, these can be referred to as (1) the "progesterone withdrawal" hypothesis, (2) the oxytocin theory, and (3) the fetal–maternal communication system postulate (MacDonald and associates, 1978).

There are, of course, many combinations of selected features of each of these three theories in the speculations of most investigators; for example, it is commonly presumed that the mature fetus, in some manner, provides some sort of a signal that initiates the procession of parturitional events. And in all theories proposed, so far as we know, some obligatory role is postulated for systems that include prostaglandin formation, be it a primary or a secondary one.

There is no doubt that the most complete scheme for the physiological sequence of events involved in parturition among mammalian species is that established for parturition in the sheep. Liggins and colleagues (1967, 1973) and other investigators from around the world have developed many of the particulars for the sheep model of parturition in great detail (Challis and Olson, 1988). In fact, the sheep model presently is the "gold standard" of mammalian parturition research. This is true despite the probability that greater progress has been made during the past 25 years in establishing the fundamentals of the endocrinology of human pregnancy than has been made in any other species. The details of the fetal–maternal communication system are defined most clearly in the human, and in many areas we are more knowledgeable about the specific biomolecular processes involved in selected phenomena of parturition in the human than in other animals. Nonetheless, although it has been done in studies of sheep pregnancy and parturition, a plausible horizontal scheme for the sequence of physiological events involved in human parturition has not been developed. In the human a profound conundrum has been faced in defining the cause of labor because there have been no striking endocrinological or metabolic alterations identified that precede the initiation of parturition. In most mammalian species, excepting the primates, fundamental and dramatic endocrinological alterations that precede the onset of parturition are clearly demonstrable.

PROGESTERONE WITHDRAWAL

There is in most mammalian species an unambiguous and usually dramatic decrease in the level of progesterone in maternal blood just before the onset of parturition: *progesterone withdrawal*. This striking endocrine antecedent of parturition occurs in pregnant animals in which progesterone arises from the placenta (*e.g.*, sheep) and in animals in which progesterone arises from the corpus luteum (*e.g.*, goat, rat, rabbit). At the time of progesterone withdrawal, there is in most species a concomitant or parallel surge is estrogen secretion. In these species, therefore, progesterone withdrawal occurs before the commencement of the first phase of parturition.

But in humans and other primates there is no demonstrable withdrawal of progesterone before the onset of parturition, i.e., there is no reduction in the level of progesterone in maternal plasma before labor commences. And in human pregnancy there is no demonstrable increase in estrogen levels in maternal or fetal blood before the onset of labor. Progesterone withdrawal in human pregnancy occurs only after delivery of the conceptus (including the placenta), *i.e.*, after the second phase (but before the third phase) of parturition.

During the past 25 years many investigators have strived to understand the biological meaning of the differences in the endocrine physiology of parturition in primates and other mammalian species. Most students of parturition have reasoned that the fundamental biomolecular events of the parturitional process *per se* are likely to be similar in all mammals irrespective of differences in endocrine physiology that precede or follow the commencement of parturition.

PROGESTERONE WITHDRAWAL AND PROSTAGLANDIN FORMATION

Progesterone withdrawal is known to be followed by increased prostaglandin formation (at least in selected progesterone-dependent tissues); this is true of parturition in species in which this endocrine event precedes the onset of labor; it also is true of progesterone-withdrawal–induced menstruation in women. But regrettably, very little is known of the mechanism(s) by which the withdrawal of progesterone serves to initiate accelerated prostaglandin formation. This is true in both the uterine decidua and endometrium, tissue sites of progesterone action and prostaglandin formation in parturition and menstruation.

It is probable that our ignorance of the biomolecular relationship between these two important discoveries, *viz.*, (1) progesterone withdrawal before the onset of parturition in some species and (2) an obligatory role of prostaglandins in the initiation of parturition in all species, has contributed appreciably to the continuation of our befuddled state as to the cause of human labor. We acknowledge this profound gap in our understanding of the sequence of events in parturition. The relationship between these two important processes of parturition must be defined at the molecular level before the physiological events of parturition in the sheep and human model can be merged or else separated forever.

COMPARISON OF HUMAN AND SHEEP PARTURITION

Two independent observations made 25 years ago have influenced the direction of parturition research. The first of these was the discovery of the mechanism of estrogen formation in human pregnancy. It was known, at that time, that human pregnancy was a hyperestrogenic state of almost unbelievable magnitude (Chap. 5) in which the placenta was virtually the sole source of estrogen. But, it also was known that the human placenta could not synthesize estrogen *de novo*, i.e., from acetate or cholesterol, or even from a C_{21}-steroid precursor such as progesterone. These potential inconsistencies were reconciled by the discovery that the adrenal glands of the human fetus produce prodigious amounts of C_{19}-steroids, which are transported by way of the fetal blood to the placenta, and in trophoblasts these precursors are converted to estrogens. This finding permitted a considerable expansion of the fetal–maternal communication system concept; namely, steroid prehormones of fetal origin serve as substrates for estrogen formation in the human placenta. And the estrogen produced in this manner accounts for the hyperestrogenic state of human pregnancy (Siiteri and MacDonald, 1963).

A short time later, Liggins and associates (1967, 1968) conducted an elegant series of experiments to define the physiological processes involved in the onset of parturition in the sheep. The findings of these studies led them to conclude that the sheep fetus is in control of its own destiny with respect to the timely onset of parturition. In clever and technically demanding investigations they demonstrated, on the one hand, that adrenalectomy or hypophysectomy of the sheep fetus caused a delay in the time of onset of parturition in the ewe. On the other hand, infusion of adrenocorticotropic hormone (ACTH) or cortisol (or else a synthetic glucocorticosteroid) into the sheep fetus brought about the premature onset of labor. Liggins and colleagues concluded, therefore, that brain-pituitary-adrenal function in the fetal sheep serves to provide the signal for the initiation of parturition in that animal model.

Because the role of the human fetal adrenal in supplying precursors for the formation of massive amounts of estrogen by the placenta was understood, and because a relationship between fetal sheep brain-pituitary-adrenal function and the initiation of labor was established, considerable effort has been expended since these discoveries were made in attempts to merge these two sets of findings into one unifying scheme to describe the physiological events that lead to parturition in all mammalian species.

Regrettably, this has not been possible; there are several areas of sharp divergence in the endocrine physiology of human and sheep pregnancy that transpire before the onset of parturition. To this day these differences pose a fundamental impasse that has prevented the development of a unifying scheme that encompasses the antecedent events of parturition in all mammals.

For example, whereas the fetal sheep adrenal is the source of one of the signals (by way of accelerated cortisol secretion) for the commencement of parturition, it is not the source of precursors for estrogen formation in the placenta. Rather, the precursors, *i.e.*, C_{19}-steroids, for estrogen formation in the sheep placenta are produced *de novo* in the trophoblasts.

PHYSIOLOGICAL SEQUENCE OF EVENTS IN SHEEP PARTURITION

The horizontal scheme, *i.e.*, the physiological sequence of events, leading to the initiation of parturition in the sheep model has been defined in appreciable detail (Liggins, 1973; Liggins and associates, 1973). Challis and Olson (1988) have presented an excellent, comprehensive review of the findings of many investigators concerning the details of the physiological sequence of events in sheep parturition.

Late in sheep gestation, at a critical time in fetal organ maturation, there is an increase in the secretion of cortisol by the fetal sheep adrenal cortex in response to fetal pituitary ACTH. Because the levels of immunoreactive ACTH in fetal sheep blood do not increase substantially at this time in gestation, it is believed that the increase in cortisol secretion is caused primarily by an increase in responsiveness of fetal adrenal cells to ACTH. In consequence of the increased responsiveness to ACTH, cortisol secretion by the fetal adrenal increases strikingly. Fetal-produced cortisol acts upon trophoblasts to induce the synthesis of steroid 17α-hydroxylase, the microsomal P-450 monooxygenase enzyme that catalyzes the 17α-hydroxylation of C_{21}-steroids (France and colleagues, 1988). An increase in the activity of this enzyme leads to a redirection of steroid biosynthesis in placenta, and this culminates in decreased progesterone secretion and increased estrogen formation/secretion (Fig. 10–2).

Progesterone withdrawal, together with adequate or increased levels of estrogen, provokes, in some undefined way, increased prostaglandin formation (probably in the sheep equivalent of human decidua), the formation of gap junctions between myometrial cells, sensitization of the uterus to uterotonic agents, cervical ripening, and the commencement of labor, likely in response to the action of $PGF_{2\alpha}$, produced in decidua, on myometrium.

The particulars of fetal-induced progesterone withdrawal

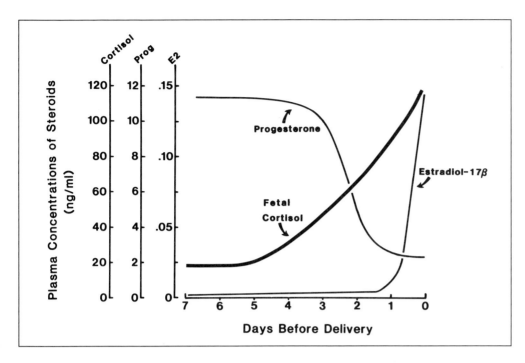

Figure 10–2. Endocrine events in the sheep that herald the onset of parturition. As the levels of fetal plasma cortisol rise, the levels of maternal plasma progesterone decline. Thereafter, there is an increase in estrogen production by the placenta.

and the surge in estrogen formation in the placenta in sheep pregnancy are somewhat more complex than originally believed. In sheep placenta, as in other steroidogenic organs, cholesterol is converted to pregnenolone in a reaction catalyzed by the mitochondrial cholesterol side-chain cleavage enzyme. Before the time of fetal cortisol-induced increase in placental steroid 17α-hydroxylase activity, pregnenolone is converted to progesterone, which is secreted from the trophoblasts. After stimulation of placental 17α-hydroxylase by fetal cortisol, pregnenolone is converted to 17α-hydroxypregnenolone and thence, by the same enzyme, to dehydroisoandrosterone. Steroid 17α-hydroxylation and removal of the C-17,20 side-chain in sheep placenta is accomplished by the same enzyme. In this manner, pregnenolone is diverted from progesterone biosynthesis. Dehydroisoandrosterone, produced from pregnenolone by the action of the enzyme steroid 17α-hydroxylase/17,20-desmolase, is converted to androstenedione (by the action of steroid 3β-hydroxysteroid dehydrogenase) and thence to estrogen in placenta by way of the enzyme reactions catalyzed by aromatase. Progesterone formed from pregnenolone is also acted upon by steroid 17α-hydroxylase to give 17α-hydroxyprogesterone; the formation of 17α-hydroxyprogesterone also contributes to progesterone withdrawal. In this coordinated manner, progesterone secretion is attenuated severely.

Compared with 17α-hydroxypregnenolone, however, 17α-hydroxyprogesterone is a poor substrate for 17,20 desmolase; thus, androstenedione, the immediate precursor of estrogen in sheep placenta, arises primarily from dehydroisoandrosterone and not from 17α-hydroxyprogesterone (France and associates, 1988). Fetal cortisol also acts to cause a modest increase in aromatase activity in the sheep placenta, but aromatase is not the rate-limiting step in estrogen formation; rather, the supply of C_{19}-steroid precursors, *i.e.*, dehydroisoandrosterone (androstenedione), formed de novo in placenta, is rate limiting (France and colleagues, 1987).

Thus, an increase in the synthesis of a single protein (steroid 17α-hydroxylase/17,20 desmolase) in placenta, in response to the action of fetal cortisol, brings about the endocrine events that precede parturition in sheep, *viz.*, progesterone withdrawal and a concomitant increase in placental estrogen secretion.

In sheep, therefore, it seems that the mature fetus provides the initial signal to commence parturition. Another way of viewing these events, however, is to see that the mature sheep fetus induces the sounding of retreat from further maintenance of pregnancy: the fetus provides the signal for initiating progesterone withdrawal, and the decrease in progesterone formation is the result of the redirection of pregnenolone metabolism in fetal trophoblasts. The endocrine antecedents of sheep parturition are presented in diagrammatic form in Figure 10–3.

AREAS OF DIVERGENCE OF HUMAN AND SHEEP PARTURITIONAL PROCESSES

To restate an issue of considerable importance to parturition research, it has always seemed reasonable to presume that we would ultimately learn that the fundamental biomolecular processes involved in parturition are similar among all mammalian species, even though the particulars of the antecedent events (endocrine or otherwise) may differ. But despite this probability and the likelihood of this expectation, crucial differences in key endocrine events that transpire before sheep and human parturition—events that seem to be pivotal in the physiological scheme leading to the onset of labor in each species—have obstructed our realization of this goal.

Among important differences in the endocrinology of human and sheep pregnancy before parturition are the following: (1) in the human there is no appreciable increase in cortisol formation by the fetal adrenal before the onset of labor as there is in the sheep fetus; (2) the infusion of ACTH or cortisol into the fetus does not cause labor in the human as it does in the sheep; (3) dexamethasone treatment in human pregnancy causes a pronounced decrease in estrogen formation (by inhibiting fetal adrenal C_{19}-steroid formation) and no change in the levels of progesterone; in contrast, glucocorticosteroid treatment

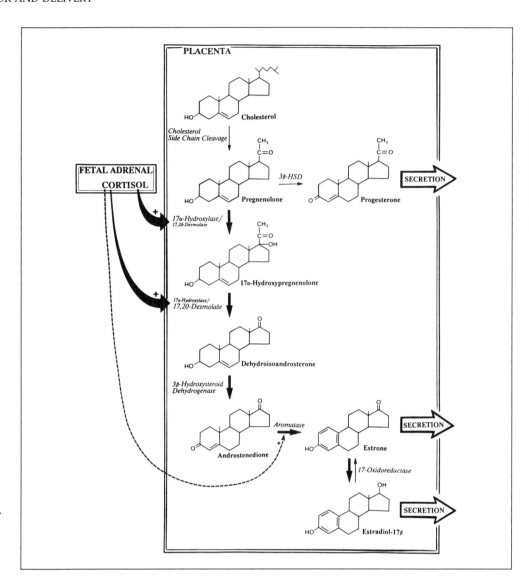

Figure 10–3. Regulation, by the action of fetal cortisol, of placental progesterone and estrogen biosynthesis just prior to the onset of parturition in the sheep.

of the sheep fetus causes an increase in placental estrogen secretion and a decrease in progesterone secretion; (4) in the human there is no decrease in the rate of secretion or the blood levels of progesterone before the onset of labor; in the sheep model there is a precipitous decline in the level of progesterone in plasma of the ewe before the onset of parturition; (5) placental progesterone production in sheep pregnancy is very small compared with that in the human; (6) the sheep fetal adrenal is not the source of placental estrogen precursors as is the case in humans, and estrogen production in sheep pregnancy is small compared with that in the human; (7) steroid 17α-hydroxylase is expressed in sheep (but not in human) placenta; and (8) intrauterine prostaglandin formation during sheep parturition (Liggins, in Discussion: Flower, 1977) is at least 20 times that produced in uterine tissues during human labor (Casey and MacDonald, 1988c).

This last finding may indicate that progesterone-withdrawal–induced parturition eventuates in greater prostaglandin formation than is the case when parturition commences in the absence of progesterone withdrawal. Furthermore, this greater production of prostaglandin may be one reason for the very rapid completion of labor that is characteristic of some mammalian

pregnancies in which parturition commences after progesterone withdrawal, compared with the human, in which progesterone withdrawal does not occur. In equine pregnancy, as a case in the extreme, labor rarely lasts more than 1 hour.

PROGESTERONE AND HUMAN PARTURITION

ORIGIN OF PROGESTERONE IN HUMAN PREGNANCY

Immediately after ovulation in women, the granulosa cells of the follicle (from which the ovum was extruded) are luteinized to form the corpus luteum. This temporary organ within an organ secretes progesterone in prodiguous amounts, but only for a brief time. The life span of the corpus luteum of the nonfertile ovarian cycle of women is about 12 to 14 days, but by 10 days the secretion of progesterone begins to decline abruptly (Chap. 5). With implantation of the blastocyst, however, hCG is produced in the trophoblasts and enters maternal blood by way of the placental arm of the fetal–maternal communication system. Compared with the amount of LH produced by the pituitary, hCG is produced in massive quantities, and this LH surrogate acts to rescue the corpus luteum and to prolong the functional life span of this progesterone-producing organ—a fundamental component of the fetal-induced maternal recognition of pregnancy system in the human (Chap. 2). This important function of the blastocyst (production of hCG) is probably crucial for optimizing conditions for the success of early pregnancy.

Progesterone acts to effect secretory changes in the endometrium, which are believed to be optimal for the implantation of the blastocyst. Progesterone, the "progestation steroid," is important, perhaps essential, to the maintenance of mammalian pregnancy. Nonetheless, the corpus luteum of human pregnancy functions for only a short time, even though the plasma levels of hCG are massive. In fact, corpus luteum function begins to decline by about 6 weeks of gestation (menstrual age), and by 8 weeks there is very little or no progesterone produced by the ovary. Thus, the life span of the corpus luteum during pregnancy is only 4 to 6 weeks, but this is appreciably longer than that of the corpus luteum of the menstrual cycle, which is only 10 to 14 days (Chap. 41).

But as the function of the corpus luteum declines, fetal trophoblasts begin to produce progesterone by way of the efficient uptake and utilization of low-density lipoprotein (LDL)-cholesterol from maternal plasma. Cholesterol, derived from cholesterol esters in the LDL particle, serves as substrate for placental formation of progesterone by way of the synthesis of the steroid intermediate, pregnenolone, which is the immediate precursor of progesterone (Chap. 5).

In the human, progesterone formation by trophoblasts increases rapidly until about 32 to 34 weeks of gestation, at which time a plateau is reached that is maintained for the remainder of pregnancy. Near term, the rate of progesterone formation by the placenta is enormous, about 250 mg per day on average, but in some pregnancies, as much as 600 mg progesterone are produced daily, e.g., in pregnancies with multiple fetuses. For reasons to be described in some detail, we point out now that Little and colleagues (1966) found that the metabolic clearance rate of progesterone from maternal plasma during human pregnancy does not change, being similar to that found in men and non-pregnant women (Billiar and associates, 1974; Lin and co-workers, 1972). Therefore, the blood level of progesterone is directly proportional to its production rate; accordingly, there is no decrease in either the blood level or the production rate of progesterone in human pregnancy before the onset of labor—or during labor for that matter. Stated differently, progesterone withdrawal does not occur in human pregnancy before the onset of parturition; progesterone withdrawal occurs only after delivery of the placenta, i.e., after removal of the tissue site of progesterone formation.

In humans, therefore, progesterone withdrawal occurs between the second and third phases of parturition. Conceptually, this is an interesting point. The third phase of parturition encompasses that time from immediately after delivery of the conceptus until complete involution of the uterus, a process that restores this tissue to the organ of the nonpregnant state. But during this time, i.e., the third phase of parturition, other phenomenally important processes essential to successful parturition, in its broadest sense, are operative. Suckling of the maternal breast by the newborn causes oxytocin secretion or release, and oxytocin may serve as the important uterotonin of the early puerperal period to ensure uterine contractions and the prevention of postpartum hemorrhage. Oxytocin also acts on the myoepithelial cells of the ducts of the breast to cause milk let-down. In an evolutionary sense milk production is essential to successful parturition, the bringing forth of young. An important corollary to this concept is that the best biological endpoint of progesterone withdrawal in all mammalian pregnancies is the initiation of lactogenesis. This is true of those mammals in which progesterone withdrawal occurs before the onset of parturition (e.g., sheep) and in those in which progesterone withdrawal occurs after delivery of the conceptus (e.g., primates, including the human). Thus, progesterone withdrawal occurs before the onset of phase one of parturition in some species, but before the commencement of phase three of parturition in others. But in all species progesterone withdrawal signals the onset of lactogenesis, the limiting step in the final events leading to successful lactation.

PROGESTERONE WITHDRAWAL AND MENSTRUATION

It also is important to remember that there is an important physiological condition in women that is characterized by a precipitous decline in the level of progesterone in blood. This occurs at the end of a nonfertile ovarian cycle; it is clear that progesterone withdrawal at this time is important in the initiation of the cellular and biomolecular processes that cause menstruation. As pointed out in Chapter 3, there is little doubt that fundamentally similar biochemical phenomena are involved in menstruation and parturition; indeed, we suggested in that discussion that **menstruation is the parturition of failed fertility.**

SURGICAL, PATHOLOGICAL, OR PHARMACOLOGICAL WITHDRAWAL OF PROGESTERONE IN HUMAN PREGNANCY

Nonetheless, during normal human pregnancy there is no reduction in progesterone levels in maternal or fetal blood before the onset of spontaneous parturition. But if progesterone withdrawal is artificially effected during human pregnancy, by whatever means, abortion or labor does ensue. Removal of the corpus luteum in early human pregnancy (before 8 weeks gestation) results in abortion. And in other abnormal circumstances, e.g., ectopic pregnancies and fetal demise, a decrease in progesterone formation may precede the onset of uterine contractions and the delivery of a decidual cast (ectopic pregnancy, Chap. 31) or a dead fetus. Progesterone withdrawal, however, is not an immediate accompaniment or result of fetal demise; rather, it may occur many weeks after fetal death (Chap. 5). Pharmacologically induced inhibition of progesterone action or progesterone formation in human pregnancy also causes abortion or increased sensitivity of myometrium to uterotonic agents, or both (Chap. 29). On the other hand, the administration of progesterone to women does not prevent or arrest preterm labor. These issues have been reviewed by Casey and MacDonald (1988a).

OCCULT PROGESTERONE WITHDRAWAL AND HUMAN PARTURITION

Many investigators have searched for some kind of "loophole" to explain this conundrum, viz., the absence of progesterone withdrawal before the onset of human parturition. The evidence in favor of a fundamental role for progesterone withdrawal in the initiation of phase one of parturition in most mammalian species is so clear that many researchers, including ourselves, have asked whether there could be some alternative form of progesterone withdrawal or sequestration or inhibition (or whatever) to explain the initiation of human parturition in the absence of a decrease in the plasma concentration of this steroid. In particular, can there be some sort of hidden or occult* form of progesterone deprivation, even in selected tissues, during human pregnancy that leads to the onset of parturition?

To summarize the findings of the studies of many investigators, there is no substantive evidence for alterations in progesterone metabolism, compartmentalization (sequestration) of progesterone, or for alterations in progesterone-binding protein or receptor numbers to account for some hidden, i.e., occult, form of progesterone withdrawal near the end of human pregnancy. Therefore, we conclude, however reluctantly, that progesterone withdrawal is not a fundamental component of the parturition process of human pregnancy (Casey and MacDonald, 1988a).

LOW PROGESTERONE PRODUCTION AND SUCCESSFUL HUMAN PREGNANCY

Recently an unusual case of human pregnancy relevant to this issue was described. In this woman plasma levels of progesterone after ovulation were quite low. Despite these low levels of progesterone, pregnancy was achieved, and despite low levels of progesterone throughout gestation, this pregnancy progressed to term and ended normally with the spontaneous onset of labor and the delivery of a healthy baby (Parker and associates, 1986). This was the case of a woman with homozygous familial abetalipoproteinemia, i.e., the absence of LDL-cholesterol in plasma. The corpus luteum and the trophoblasts of the human are highly dependent upon plasma LDL for optimal progesterone production; the cholesterol esters contained in the LDL particle serve as a quantitatively important source of cholesterol for the mitochondrial cholesterol side-chain cleavage P-450 enzyme in both tissues (Chap. 5).

PROGESTERONE AND PARTURITION IN PERSPECTIVE

All of these findings taken together have led us to ponder the possibility that the fetus, by way of the fetal–maternal communication system, acts to promote the maintenance of pregnancy by inhibiting the production of uterotropins-uterotonins. Perhaps some of the components of this system of fetal-induced pregnancy maintenance are, more or less, progesterone dependent. Nonetheless, we must surmise that fetal-induced retreat from the maintenance of pregnancy can be sounded with or without progesterone withdrawal as a fundamental component of this mechanism (Casey and MacDonald, 1988b). Accepting that some of the components of this system are progesterone dependent, withdrawal of progesterone is one mechanism by which retreat from pregnancy maintenance could be initiated.

We have acknowledged already that we do not understand how the withdrawal of progesterone causes increased prostaglandin formation during parturition or during menstruation in women and some other primates. But more than this, we also are unable to deduce the mechanism by which progesterone acts to maintain pregnancy in the first place. There is no doubt that our ignorance of the precise mechanism(s) by which pro-

gesterone is operative in the maintenance of pregnancy has retarded our understanding of the physiological process involved in the initiation of parturition in all species.

THE MISSING PIECE OF THE PARTURITION PUZZLE

There is a very important missing piece of the parturition puzzle that should fit between those of progesterone withdrawal and increased uterotropin-uterotonin formation. There must be an intermediate step, one that has not yet been defined. There must be an *intermediate modulator* that acts to cause increased formation of uterotropins-uterotonins, which effect the onset of parturition. And there must be more than one mechanism by which the synthesis of this intermediate modulator can be stimulated. One mechanism is progesterone withdrawal. Another mechanism may be by direct stimulation through the action of an agent that is foreign to the biological system to cause preterm labor. Yet another mechanism must involve fetal-induced retreat from further pregnancy maintenance even with progesterone withdrawal, i.e, spontaneous parturition.

MODULATION OF UTEROTROPIN AND UTEROTONIN FORMATION DURING PARTURITION

It is clear that the same physiological-biochemical-morphological changes that take place in the uterus of some species after progesterone withdrawal also come to pass in the uteruses of pregnant women and other primates just before, or at the time of, the onset of labor. These distinctive morphological and biochemical changes that serve to prepare the uterus for labor during the first phase of parturition occur in all species, irrespective of the specifics of the endocrine antecedents of parturition in that species. And forceful myometrial contractions are characteristic of the labor processes in all mammalian species.

These similarities of the first phase of parturition among species are supportive of the possibility that the intermediate modulator(s) of these events are also the same or similar in all mammalian species, irrespective of the antecedent processes involved. It also seems most reasonable at this time to presume that progesterone withdrawal brings about the generation of an agent or agents that serve to effect increased hydrolysis of glycerophospholipids, the release of free arachidonic acid, and thence the formation of prostaglandins. Knowledge of the identity and regulation of formation of such a putative **intermediate modulator of parturition** could go a long way toward resolving the riddle of parturition initiation among all species (Fig. 10–4).

It also seems reasonable to surmise that preterm labor could be induced by way of the action of agents (for example, a bacterial toxin) that cause an increase in the formation of an intermediate modulator of parturition. A number of tissue stimulants are known that act in a variety of tissues to increase glycerophospholipid hydrolysis and prostaglandin formation. For example, some act by way of stimulating the hydrolysis of phosphatidylinositol, giving rise to free arachidonic acid, diacylglycerols, and inositol phosphates. This metabolic sequence is believed to be an important component of a signal transmission system in many tissues causing activation of protein kinase C, increases in free cytosolic calcium, and the generation of arachidonic acid metabolites. Yet other agents act, at least in part by the activation of phospholipase A_2, causing hydrolysis of phosphatidylcholine and phosphatidylethanolamine with the release of arachidonic acid. Some agent or agents that act to

---

* Occult: to shut off from exposure; to become concealed from view; not revealed, secret, not easily understood; abstruse or mysterious; not manifest or detectable by clinical methods alone. (Webster's Ninth New Collegiate Dictionary.)

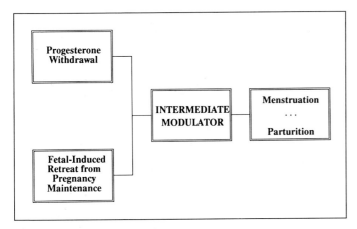

Figure 10–4. Putative intermediate modulator of menstruation and parturition.

stimulate arachidonic acid release must be the intermediate modulator of parturition; possibly this agent is the same in all species, and possibly the same agent is operative in normal spontaneous parturition at term, and in some cases of preterm labor as well.

Later in this chapter (pp. 200–202) we suggest that a candidate for the role of intermediate modulator of parturition is interleukin-1 (IL-1). This potent immunohormone-immunomodulator acts in many tissues to cause increased hydrolysis of glycerophospholipids, release of arachidonic acid, and the formation of prostaglandins and platelet-activating factor. IL-1 acts in an autocrine, paracrine, and endocrine fashion. It is produced in endometrium and in decidua, and the concentration of this cytokine increases strikingly in amnionic fluid during some forms of preterm labor (p. 205).

OXYTOCIN AND HUMAN PARTURITION

OXYTOCIN ACTION AND PARTURITION

Oxytocin means "quick birth." In 1906 uterotonic bioactivity was discovered in extracts of the posterior pituitary. By 1909 the uterotonic property of these extracts was demonstrated after administration to women, and by 1911 these crude preparations were in use in clinical obstetrics. In 1950 Du Vigneaud determined the structure of oxytocin, the uterotonic agent of the posterior pituitary; he was later awarded the Nobel Prize for his pioneering work in the elucidation of peptide structure. Oxytocin is a nonapeptide synthesized in the cell bodies of the supraoptic and paraventricular neurons and transported along the axons to the neural lobe of the posterior pituitary in membrane-bound vesicles for storage and later release. Gainer and colleagues (1988) have presented a learned review of the synthesis and secretion of oxytocin.

A role for oxytocin in the initiation of parturition is supported by a variety of lines of evidence. Oxytocin is known to be a very potent uterotonin, causing (in very low concentrations) uterine contractions in a sensitized uterus. And we have known for more than three quarters of a century that the administration of this potent uterotonic agent will bring about orderly labor in near-term pregnant women in a manner that recapitulates most of the events that are characteristic of the second phase of

spontaneous parturition.

These findings alone were sufficient reasons for conducting in-depth investigations of the role of oxytocin in the initiation of spontaneous parturition. But recent discoveries have provided additional and provocative new evidence supportive of a role of oxytocin in this process. Among the more notable of these findings are that (1) there is a striking increase in the number of oxytocin receptors in myometrial tissue at the end of gestation and (2) oxytocin acts upon endometrial (decidual) tissue to promote the release of prostaglandins. A review of the role of oxytocin in the initiation of labor was presented recently by Soloff (1988).

OXYTOCIN, LUTEOLYSIS, AND PARTURITION

We observed in Chapter 2 that there is an interesting set of analogies between the processes involved in luteolysis at the end of a nonfertile cycle in a number of species (*e.g.*, sheep, cow, and pig) and the initiation of parturition. In these animals the corpus luteum of the nonfertile cycle is *murdered* by the luteolytic action of $PGF_{2\alpha}$ produced in the endometrium. Indeed, one of the components of the fetal-induced maternal recognition of the pregnancy system is the inhibition of endometrial $PGF_{2\alpha}$ formation by a product of the blastocyst (Chap. 2). Today there is evidence that oxytocin, arising in the corpus luteum in some species (*e.g.*, sheep), acts on the endometrium to stimulate $PGF_{2\alpha}$ formation. The $PGF_{2\alpha}$, in turn, acts directly on the corpus luteum to interrupt the function of this progesterone-producing organ, *i.e.*, luteolysis (Flint and Sheldrick, 1985).

In a somewhat similar manner it can be envisioned that oxytocin acts on decidua at the end of pregnancy to induce the formation of uterotropins and uterotonins. If this were true, the action of oxytocin in the initiation of parturition may not be confined singularly to its direct action on myometrium in effecting the uterine contractions of labor.

OXYTOCIN AND THE INITIATION OF PARTURITION

Notwithstanding the importance of all of these exciting new findings with respect to the physiology and biochemistry of oxytocin action, we conclude that all of the evidence, examined critically, is in favor of a primary role of oxytocin during the second stage of labor (after complete dilatation of the cervix, p. 219) and after delivery of the fetus, not before. It is possible that oxytocin also may serve, together with uterotonins produced within the uterus, in a synergistic manner, to ensure fail-safe systems for successful labor.

There are several reasons for rejecting the likelihood of a physiological role for oxytocin in the initiation of spontaneous parturition. As stated, there is little or no evidence that oxytocin is involved in the first phase of parturition, *i.e.*, the preparation of the uterus for labor. The infusion of oxytocin is relatively ineffective in inducing labor in human pregnancies, except those near term; perhaps oxytocin is effective only in those pregnancies in which the first phase of parturition, *i.e.*, the preparation of the uterus for active labor, already is completed. There is no evidence that oxytocin will act to induce gap-junction formation between myometrial cells, and most commonly failures of labor induction with oxytocin in human pregnancy are encountered when there has been no antecedent cervical softening or ripening.

Another important factor that mitigates against the likelihood of a primary role for oxytocin in the initiation of spontaneous parturition is the fact that the levels of oxytocin in maternal blood do not increase before or during labor, at least not until late, *i.e.*, during the second stage of labor.

It has been argued that the increase in oxytocin receptor concentration in myometrium (or decidua or both) late in pregnancy may be so great that oxytocin action is effected with only subtle or even no changes in the levels of circulating oxytocin. Such an increase in oxytocin receptor levels in these tissues immediately before the onset of labor, however, has not been demonstrated; for obvious reasons this would be difficult to accomplish by use of human tissues.

It also has been argued that the metabolic clearance rate (MCR) of oxytocin from plasma is so great that increases in the rate of secretion of oxytocin could occur without detectable increases in the plasma concentration. We find this argument to be the most untenable of all. Oxytocin is a hormone, *i.e.*, oxytocin is transported from its site of synthesis (storage) to tissue sites of action by way of the blood. Unlike prostaglandins and other potential uterotropins and uterotonins, which are produced *in situ* in uterine tissues, oxytocin is not delivered to myometrial cells by autocrine or paracrine mechanisms. Even oxytocin that enters amnionic fluid must first have been secreted into the blood of either the mother or the fetus.

The accuracy of measurements of oxytocin in blood and the rate of clearance of oxytocin from blood are therefore crucial in analyses of the role of this uterotonin in the initiation of parturition (Leake, 1983).

The MCR of oxytocin (MCR-oxy) in the human has been established, and the values obtained by several investigators are similar. The MCR-oxy is about 1,700 to 2,000 L plasma per 24 hours in pregnant women, and this value is not different from that found in men and nonpregnant women (Leake and associates, 1980). This rate of clearance of oxytocin from plasma is somewhat less than that of many steroids, *e.g.*, progesterone, androstenedione, dehydroisoandrosterone, and aldosterone, the blood production rates of which are measured routinely by many investigators.

The secretion rate (SR) of oxytocin in pregnant women before and during labor can be computed as follows: SR-oxy = MCR-oxy · [oxy], where [oxy] is the concentration of oxytocin in plasma. Most investigators find that the plasma concentration of oxytocin in pregnant women is 2 to 10 pg per mL (Leake and colleagues, 1981). Taking a value of 5 pg per mL as representative (and an MCR-oxy as 2,000 L per day), the SR-oxy in pregnant women is 10 μg per day, or about 7 ng per minute. The concentrations of oxytocin in blood do not change during labor, at least until the very end of labor.

The infusion of oxytocin at a rate of 20 ng per min will cause labor in some women (1 μU oxytocin equals 2 pg). This rate of infusion will effect an increase in blood levels of about 3- to 7-fold. In fact, the infusion of oxytocin at constant rates that are less than those required to induce labor causes a predictable increase in the plasma concentrations of oxytocin.

A number of investigators also have been successful in monitoring increases in the levels of oxytocin in blood during breast-suckling–induced increases in oxytocin secretion. The rates of oxytocin secretion during breast feeding are similar to rates of oxytocin infusion that sometimes will induce labor. For all of these reasons, it is difficult to believe that increases in oxytocin secretion of sufficient magnitude to induce labor can go undetected, unless the assay procedure used to quantify oxytocin in blood is woefully inadequate.

OXYTOCIN AND PARTURITION IN PERSPECTIVE

The increase in oxytocin receptors in the uterus before (or during) the onset of labor is an important marker of the preparational events for parturition. Oxytocin may act to maximize the myometrial forces involved in the expulsive phase (second stage) of labor, it may act to ensure uterine contraction and thereby decrease blood loss after delivery, it may act synergistically with other uterotonins produced within the uterus to maintain labor, and it is important in milk let-down during lactation. But there is scant or no evidence that oxytocin is the initiator of human parturition or that oxytocin is the primary uterotonin of human labor.

SUMMARY OF THE STATUS OF KNOWLEDGE OF HUMAN PARTURITION

Presently the greatest body of evidence points against any readily identifiable or even occult form of progesterone withdrawal before the spontaneous onset of human parturition. There is neither a decline in the blood levels or production rate of progesterone before the commencement of parturition nor any substantive evidence for peculiar sequestration, extraglandular production withdrawal, unique metabolism, or failure of progesterone action to herald the onset of labor in the human.

Similarly, the majority of evidence points against an elementary role for oxytocin in the initiation of spontaneous human parturition. There is no doubt that oxytocin is a very potent uterotonin; this naturally occurring stimulant of uterine contractions probably is important in facilitating uterine contractions during the second stage of labor and during the puerperium. But there is little evidence to support a fundamental role of oxytocin in the initiation of parturition. Possibly, endogenous oxytocin serves an adjuvant role during labor in optimizing the parturitional process by acting synergistically with other uterotonins, which are produced in intrauterine tissues, *e.g.*, $PGF_{2\alpha}$. Thereby, a fail-safe system for the maintenance of the active phase of labor is facilitated.

If these deductions are correct, the pieces of the human parturitional puzzle must be assembled in a manner that excludes antecedent progesterone withdrawal or increased oxytocin secretion, if a clear picture of the physiological events of human parturition is to be revealed.

THE CRITICAL UNANSWERED QUESTIONS OF HUMAN PARTURITION

There are (and always have been) three elementary, but as yet still unresolved, questions that are fundamental to an understanding of human parturition; answers to these three inquiries are crucial to a clear definition of the biomolecular processes of spontaneous parturition at term, and possibly to those of preterm labor as well:

1. What are the uterotropin(s) and uterotonin(s) of human parturition?
2. What is (or are) the tissue source(s) of these agents?
3. What is the role of the human fetus in regulating the timing of parturition?

The findings of a large number of studies conducted by many investigators over the past 25 years should be useful in our quest for answers to these three questions. This obtains even though presently we are not able to assemble all of the evidence into a single unifying and complete description of all of the processes involved in the commencement of labor.

PROSTAGLANDINS AND HUMAN PARTURITION

Today there is persuasive evidence that an increase in the rate of prostaglandin formation is intimately involved in some obligatory manner in human parturition. This also is true of prostaglandin formation and labor in all other mammalian species that have been examined. Interestingly, Hertelendy (1983) also demonstrated that prostaglandins are physiologically important in oviposition, *i.e.,* the laying of hard-shelled eggs by birds.

Consider the following. (1) The levels of prostaglandins in amnionic fluid (Fig. 10–5), in maternal blood and urine, and in intrauterine tissues increase strikingly during labor. (2) Prostaglandins (PGE_2 and $PGF_{2\alpha}$), administered at any stage of human pregnancy, will evoke myometrial contractions and abortion or delivery of the fetus. (3) Prostaglandins are effective in promoting labor whether given by mouth, by instillation into the amnionic fluid, by intravenous infusion, or by extraovular injection. (4) Ingestion of inhibitors of prostaglandin synthesis (specifically, inhibitors or arachidonic acid cyclooxygenase activity) by pregnant women leads to prolongation of gestation and lengthens the induction-abortion time interval in women who undergo therapeutic termination of pregnancy induced by instillation of hypertonic saline. (5) Inhibitors of prostaglandin synthesis are also effective in suppressing preterm labor. (6) Prostaglandins are potent uterotonins that also may serve, directly or indirectly, as uterotropins. At the very least, therefore, there is some obligatory biomolecular process involved in parturition that eventuates in the formation of prostaglandin in all species examined. A learned review of the obligatory role for prostaglandin in parturition was presented by Novy and Liggins (1980).

BIOSYNTHESIS OF PROSTAGLANDINS

Van Dorp and colleagues (1964) and Bergstrom and co-workers (1964) demonstrated that arachidonic acid is the obligate precursor for the biosynthesis of prostaglandins of the 2-series. It also seems highly probable that prostaglandins of the 2-series, in particular PGE_2 and $PGF_{2\alpha}$, are important bioactive metabolites of arachidonic acid that are involved in human parturition.

REGULATION OF THE RATE OF PROSTAGLANDIN FORMATION

Most of the arachidonic acid in tissues is esterified in glycerophospholipids. Lands and Samuelson (1968) and Vonkeman and Van Dorp (1968) demonstrated that it is free arachidonic acid, however, that serves as the substrate for prostaglandin formation. Thus, arachidonic acid must be released from these esterified forms before it can be converted into prostaglandins. Heretofore the rate of release of arachidonic acid from glycerophospholipid storage forms was considered the rate-limiting step in prostaglandin formation in several tissues believed to be important in parturition. We now know, however, that in some of the tissues involved directly in parturition, the rate of prostaglandin formation also is regulated by the rate of conversion of arachidonic acid to prostaglandins. Therefore, both processes appear to be important in determining the rate of prostaglandin formation during human parturition (Casey and associates, 1988a). It is evident that knowledge of the mechanism(s) that serves to regulate the rate of synthesis of prostaglandins in intrauterine tissues is fundamental to our understanding of the parturitional processes.

SPECIFICITY OF PROSTAGLANDIN FORMATION IN VARIOUS TISSUES

There is specificity in the biosynthesis of the various prostaglandins among tissues; this is also true in parturition. For example, in some tissues the formation of prostacylin (PGI_2) is dominant (myometrium), whereas in other tissues there may be almost exclusive formation of PGE_2 (amnion and chorion leave) or preferential formation of $PGF_{2\alpha}$ (decidua) (Fig. 10–6). This is an important consideration in defining the tissue site of origin of the prostaglandins that are produced during human labor. This obtains because there is a characteristic pattern and time of appearance of the various prostaglandins (and metabolites thereof) in amnionic fluid and maternal plasma after the onset of parturition.

THE PROSTAGLANDINS PRODUCED DURING HUMAN PARTURITION

As yet there is no convincing evidence for an increase in the rate of formation of prostaglandins in intrauterine tissues before the onset of human parturition. But during labor there is a striking increase in the concentration of both PGE_2 and $PGF_{2\alpha}$ in amnionic fluid (Fig. 10–7). There is also an increase in the concentration of a metabolite of $PGF_{2\alpha}$, namely, 13,14-dihydro-15-keto-$PGF_{2\alpha}$ (PGFM) in amnionic fluid and in maternal blood and urine during labor. On the other hand, there is no firm evidence for an increase in PGE_2 (or metabolites thereof) in maternal blood during labor. Comprehensive reviews of this subject were presented recently (Casey and MacDonald, 1988c; Mitchell, 1988).

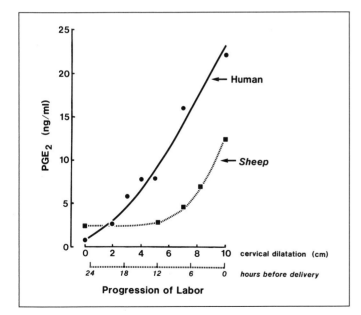

Figure 10–5. Concentration of PGE_2 in amnionic fluid of the human and sheep during labor, as a function of centimeters cervical dilatation or hours before delivery in women and sheep, respectively (*Data from Mitchell: Studies on Prostaglandins in Relation to Parturition in the Sheep. Oxford University, 1976*).

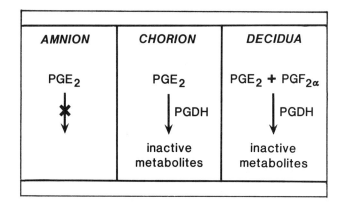

Figure 10–6. Comparison of prostaglandin biosynthesis and metabolism in amnion, chorion laeve, and decidua. The greatest prostaglandin synthase activity is in amnion, in which only PGE_2 is formed; in amnion PGE_2 is not metabolized. In chorion laeve PGE_2 is the principal prostanoid produced, yet in chorion laeve there is considerable NAD^+-dependent PGDH activity. In decidua, PGE_2 and $PGF_{2\alpha}$ are formed; PGDH is active in decidua.

Because $PGF_{2\alpha}$ can be produced in decidua and myometrium, but not in the fetal membranes, **the finding of increased concentrations of $PGF_{2\alpha}$ and PGFM (in amnionic fluid and maternal blood and urine) during human labor is a most important cornerpiece of the human parturition puzzle** (Casey and MacDonald, 1988a,b,c).

THE ROLE OF DECIDUA IN HUMAN PARTURITION

There is appreciable evidence that the prostaglandin that gains access to the myometrium during parturition is principally $PGF_{2\alpha}$ and probably not PGE_2. This conclusion is not based on the relative uterotonic potency of the two prostaglandins but rather upon an analysis of the likelihood of the two prostaglandins actually reaching myometrial cells before metabolism (inactivation). If this deduction is correct, a very important clue is provided as to the tissue source of uterotonin prostaglandin in human parturition; namely, if increased $PGF_{2\alpha}$ formation is a marker of phase two of parturition, the decidua is the likely source of this uterotonin.

Earlier in this book we cited similarities between the cellular and biomolecular processes involved in parturition and in menstruation. In particular we pointed to the fact that both events are characterized by increased formation of $PGF_{2\alpha}$ (Chap. 2 and 3). In the case of menstruation there is no doubt that the $PGF_{2\alpha}$, which is produced in increased amounts, is formed in the endometrium, the tissue precursor of decidua.

Recall that menstruation is induced in response to the withdrawal of progesterone; in this chapter we have also emphasized the importance of progesterone withdrawal in many mammalian species before the onset of parturition. In all mammalian species studied, increased formation of $PGF_{2\alpha}$ is characteristic of the parturitional process. There is also appreciable evidence that in those species in which labor begins after progesterone withdrawal the $PGF_{2\alpha}$ of parturition is formed in decidua (or in the anatomical equivalent thereof).

And whereas progesterone withdrawal does not occur before the onset of human parturition, it still is probable that the $PGF_{2\alpha}$ that is produced during human labor arises in uterine decidua. The decidua, but not the fetal membranes, produces $PGF_{2\alpha}$. Therefore, there are many reasons to surmise that the increased $PGF_{2\alpha}$ formed during labor arises in decidua and that decidual activation is a fundamental feature of the biomolecular processes of parturition. Accordingly, increased $PGF_{2\alpha}$ formation is both a marker of decidual activation and a marker of parturition. Possibly this constitutes a cause-and-effect relationship, *i.e.,* decidual activation brings about parturition.

BIOACTIVE AGENTS IN HUMAN AMNIONIC FLUID DURING LABOR: DECIDUAL ORIGIN

During labor, a number of bioactive agents accumulate in amnionic fluid; the identity of each of these and the particular combination of agents that accumulate are highly suggestive of a decidual source of these potential uterotropins-uterotonins. In fact, these agents in combination appear to constitute a matched biological set.

The accumulation of this set of substances in amnionic fluid during labor is particularly fortuitous. The amnionic fluid compartment constitutes a remarkable repository that may be especially useful for deciphering the biomolecular processes of parturition. This biological fluid not only is contiguous with tissues that are intimately involved in parturition, but also seems to be a medium in which important markers of the labor process are temporarily stored. We choose the term *storage* because the half-life of selected agents in amnionic fluid is much greater than are those of the same compounds in blood. This may be especially true of selected molecules believed to be crucial to the initiation of parturition. For example, the half-life of $PGF_{2\alpha}$ and PGE_2 in blood is only 6 to 8 minutes; but the half-life of PGE_2 and $PGF_{2\alpha}$ in amnionic fluid is 4 to 6 hours. Therefore, during times of rapid intrauterine physiological change, *e.g.,* during parturition, substances accumulate in amnionic fluid. This phenomenon provides us with an opportunity to quantify the initiators of parturition in a relatively accessible and uniquely positioned biological medium.

From the measurement of selected agents in amnionic fluid, information has been provided in support of a working hypothesis to define some of the biomolecular processes of human parturition. This hypothesis is that **decidual activation is synchronous with the initiation of parturition.** A natural extension of this hypothesis is that fetal-induced retreat from pregnancy maintenance brings about decidual activation (Casey and MacDonald, 1988a; 1989).

To develop the fundamentals of this hypothesis further, it also is important to recognize that **the decidua is macrophage-like** in many of its functional properties. It now seems clear, too, that key events known to occur during parturition are nearly exact recapitulations of those that take place in simulated macrophages. We will return to a consideration of the macrophage-like properties of the decidua, and we will develop a decidua-macrophage connection (p. 202), but for now, suffice it to say that during spontaneous labor at term, a set of bioactive agents accumulate in amnionic fluid in high concentrations. The members of this bioactive agent set are **arachidonic acid, prostaglandins, platelet-activating factor (PAF), and selected cytokines.** This same matched set of agents is produced by stimulated macrophages.

Because of one or more particular prostaglandins produced, *e.g.,* $PGF_{2\alpha}$, and because of the particular combination of sub-

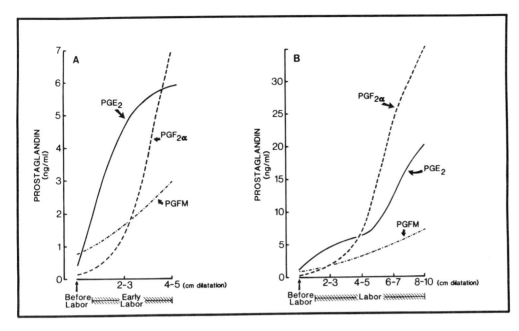

Figure 10–7. Prostaglandins in amnionic fluid during human parturition. **A.** Before and during early labor. **B.** Throughout labor. (*Data from Dray and Frydman: Am J Obstet Gynecol 126:13, 1976; Keirse and Turnbull: J Obstet Gynaecol Br Commonwealth 80:970, 1973; Keirse and associates: J Obstet Gynaecol Br Commonwealth 81:131, 1974; Satoh and co-workers: Am J Obstet Gynecol 133:886, 1979.*)

stances that accumulate in amnionic fluid during labor, it is likely that this bioactive set of agents is produced by an activated, macrophage-like decidua (Casey and MacDonald, 1988a,d).

Arachidonic Acid in Amnionic Fluid During Labor: Decidual Contribution

There is a 5- to 10-fold increase in the concentration of free arachidonic acid in amnionic fluid during labor, and the concentration of this prostaglandin precursor continues to increase as a function of the progress of labor. Moreover, there is a disproportionate increase in the concentration of arachidonic acid in amnionic fluid during labor, compared with that of all other free fatty acids (Keirse and colleagues, 1977; MacDonald and associates, 1974).

Recall that in many tissues the rate of release of arachidonic acid is believed to be the rate-limiting step in prostaglandin formation; increased release of free arachidonic acid is commonly indicative of a type of tissue response that results in increased prostaglandin formation. Therefore, an understanding of the tissue source or sources of free arachidonic acid, which enters amnionic fluid during labor, is very important to an understanding of the regulation of prostaglandin formation and of the tissues that are stimulated during parturition.

Until recently it was believed that the free arachidonic acid, the precursor of prostaglandin that accumulates in amnionic fluid during labor, was released from the fetal membranes. This conclusion was based on the fact that during early labor (less than 5 cm cervical dilatation), the arachidonic acid content of specific glycerophospholipids in both amnion and chorion laeve, which are contiguous with amnionic fluid, is decreased (Okita and co-workers, 1982a). It probably is correct to conclude that, early in labor, the free arachidonic acid that enters amnionic fluid arises, at least in part, by release from glycerophospholipids in the fetal membranes by way of the action of phospholipases in these tissues.

This must be an incomplete explanation for the accumulation of arachidonic acid in amnionic fluid during labor because (1) the arachidonic acid content of the avascular fetal membranes is restored later in labor (Okita, 1981) and (2) the concentration of arachidonic acid in amnionic fluid continues to increase as labor progresses. Thus, there must be another tissue source of arachidonic acid for this compartment during labor.

To evaluate this important issue further, it is important to know that arachidonic acid (an essential fatty acid) that is assimilated into the avascular amnion is derived exclusively from the amnionic fluid. This important discovery came from a study of the content and distribution of arachidonic acid among lipids in the amnions of diamnionic-dichorionic human twin pregnancies. In this study Okita and colleagues (1983a) found that the content and distribution of arachidonic acid in the fused portion of the amnion of these twin pregnancies was the same as that in the nonfused portion of the same amnion and was the same as that in amnions of singleton fetuses. Because the human amnion and chorion laeve are avascular tissues, it follows that the arachidonic acid in the fused portion of amnion must have been assimilated from the amnionic fluid. In this same study the arachidonic acid content of fused chorion laeve was found to be appreciably less (about 50 percent) than that of nonfused chorion laeve and less than that of amnion at all anatomical sites. This is indicative that arachidonic acid in chorion laeve nominally (*i.e.*, in singleton pregnancies) is assimilated from both amnionic fluid and from contiguous maternal decidua or plasma.

Knowing that amnion assimilates arachidonic acid singularly from amnionc fluid, the particulars of arachidonic acid release, metabolism, and accumulation in the fetal membranes–amnionic fluid compartment during labor can be analyzed. In the later stages of labor the arachidonic acid content of the fetal membranes is as great as or greater than that which existed before labor commenced. During labor the free arachidonic acid content of amnionic fluid increases strikingly; therefore, there is a net gain in the arachidonic acid content of the avascular fetal membrane–amnionic fluid compartment before labor is completed.

The net increase in arachidonic acid in this avascular compartment most likely arises by way of the release of arachidonic acid after activation of the macrophage-like decidua. Stimulation of macrophages also causes the release of 50 percent of the arachidonic acid of macrophages. In this regard, therefore, the activation of decidua and the stimulation of macrophages are similar, as reviewed by Casey and MacDonald (1988a; 1989).

Prostaglandins in Amnionic Fluid During Labor: Decidual Contribution

To define the tissue source of prostaglandins produced during parturition, it is helpful to analyze the identity of the particular prostaglandins produced during this time. Such an analysis has been very rewarding because of the specificity of various uterine and extraembryonic fetal tissues for the formation of particular prostaglandins.

To recapitulate, there is a striking increase in the concentration of PGE_2, $PGF_{2\alpha}$, and PGFM in amnionic fluid during labor, and the concentrations of these prostaglandins increase as labor progresses. It is probable that this continuing increase in the concentration of prostaglandins in amnionic fluid as labor continues is in part the result of an accumulation of these compounds in amnionic fluid and is not singularly the consequence of a continually increasing rate of prostaglandin formation as a function of the progress or duration of labor. The level of PGFM in maternal blood also is increased during labor.

It is important to emphasize that there is an accumulation of $PGF_{2\alpha}$ and PGFM in amnionic fluid during labor and of PGFM in maternal blood. Indeed, during the latter part of labor there is a significantly greater amount of $PGF_{2\alpha}$ and PGFM in amnionic fluid, compared with that of PGE_2 (Fig. 10–7). The importance of these observations is that the amnion and chorion laeve do not produce $PGF_{2\alpha}$; rather, they produce PGE_2 almost exclusively. On the other hand, the decidua produces both $PGF_{2\alpha}$ and PGE_2.

These findings are highly suggestive that the $PGF_{2\alpha}$ and PGFM that enter amnionic fluid during labor arise in decidua. Myometrium also produces $PGF_{2\alpha}$ and therefore may contribute to the $PGF_{2\alpha}$ in amnionic fluid. This tissue is unlikely to represent a quantitatively important source of amnionic fluid $PGF_{2\alpha}$, however, because of (1) the ready accessibility of myometrial prostaglandins to blood and (2) the likelihood of reduced myometrial prostaglandin production in response to the action of cortisol, the levels of which are increased in the blood of pregnant women during labor (Casey and colleagues, 1985; Richardson and associates, 1986).

Prostaglandin Metabolism in Decidua

Because of the importance of $PGF_{2\alpha}$ as a marker of decidual activation during parturition, several studies have been conducted to confirm the validity of this proposition. There was a possibility that PGE_2, originating in amnion or chorion laeve or both, may be converted to $PGF_{2\alpha}$, for example, in decidua. The activity of the enzyme that catalyzes the conversion of PGE_2 to $PGF_{2\alpha}$ (PGE_2 9-ketoreductase) is demonstrable in decidual tissue (Niesert and associates, 1986; Schlegel and co-workers, 1984). There are, however, at least four findings that mitigate against this possibility. (1) The specific activity of PGE_2 9-ketoreductase, in decidual tissue and in subcellular fractions of decidual tissue, is very low. (2) The specific activity of this enzyme is appreciably less than that of 15-hydroxyprostaglandin dehydrogenase (PGDH), the enzyme that catalyzes the first step in the inactivation of both PGE_2 and $PGF_{2\alpha}$. (3) PGDH of decidua preferentially catalyzes the metabolism of PGE_2, compared with $PGF_{2\alpha}$. (4) In incubations conducted with intact decidual cells, there is little or no conversion of PGE_2 to $PGF_{2\alpha}$,

reflective of the low activity of PGE_2 9-ketoreductase or limited entry of PGE_2 into decidual cells, or both. These data were reviewed by Casey and MacDonald (1988c).

Therefore, the accumulation of $PGF_{2\alpha}$ and PGFM in amnionic fluid during labor seems to be a marker of decidual prostaglandin formation, and there is no clear-cut evidence of an increase in PGE_2 or metabolites thereof in maternal blood during labor.

PAF in Amnionic Fluid During Labor

Platelet-activating factor (PAF) accumulates in amnionic fluid during labor (Billah and Johnston, 1983; Nishihara and associates, 1984), and PAF biosynthesis in amnion and decidua has been demonstrated (Ban and associates, 1986). The tissue sites of origin of the increased amounts of PAF in amnionic fluid during human labor are not defined. Several suggestions have been made; among these are fetal urine, fetal lung secretions, amnion, and decidua (Angle and associates, 1988; Johnston and colleagues, 1987). It is well established that stimulation of macrophages causes a marked increase in glycerophospholipid hydrolysis, arachidonic acid release, prostaglandin formation (Kunkel and Chensue, 1986), and the production of PAF (Albert and Snyder, 1983). The release of arachidonic acid from 1-alkyl-2-arachidonoyl phosphatidylcholine favors the formation of PAF because the other product of this reaction, viz., 1-alkyl-lysophosphatidylcholine, is the cosubstrate for PAF biosynthesis. The role of PAF in parturition was the subject of a learned review presented by Johnston and associates (1987). Because of the likelihood of increased glycerophospholipid hydrolysis in decidua during labor, it may be that much of the PAF that accumulates in amnionic fluid during labor arises in decidua.

Interleukin-1β in Amnionic Fluid During Labor

During labor, there may be remarkable increase in the concentration of interleukin-1β (IL-1β) in amnionic fluid. Before the onset of labor, there is little or no IL-1β in amnionic fluid at any stage of gestation. But after spontaneous labor at term, IL-1β in concentrations of 100 to 5,000 pg per mL (Cox and associates, 1988a), may be observed. It is likely that this IL-1β arises, at least in part, in macrophage-like decidua.

In tissues that produce IL-1, two forms of this cytokine are synthesized, viz., IL-1α and IL-1β. Originally these two cytokines were distinguished by differences in pI by isoelectric focusing. Now we know that the two IL-1s are the products of two separate genes, the organizational structures of which are quite similar. Nonetheless, there is very little amino acid sequence homology (26 percent) between the two proteins, but in most systems the biological action of IL-1α and IL-1β are indistinguishable and the mature forms of the cytokines (M_r about 17,500) act by way of a common receptor. It is probable that the IL-1β gene evolved more recently; in most tissues IL-1β formation exceeds that of IL-1α by an order of magnitude. So far as we know today, the transcription of the two genes for IL-1 is regulated simultaneously by stimuli that eventuate in increased IL-1 formation. IL-1 is produced principally in macrophages but also in other tissues in response to specific challenges. Dinarello (1986) has presented an excellent review of the origin and actions of IL-1. IL-1 also is known as *endogenous pyrogen* and *lymphocyte-activating factor*, and perhaps in the future we will call it **the intermediate modulator of parturition.** As yet there are no definitive data one way or the other concerning the levels of IL-1α in amnionic fluid.

The accumulation of IL-1β in amnionic fluid during labor is important for several reasons. First, this constitutes another indication that macrophage-like decidua is activated during parturition. It is known that decidua produces IL-1β (Casey and associates, 1988b). Second, the simultaneous accumulation of arachidonic acid, PGF$_{2\alpha}$, PAF, and IL-1β in amnionic fluid during labor is suggestive of a coordinated response of this macrophage-like tissue to a common stimulant (or else release from a state of induced quiescence).

Importantly, IL-1β is known to act to stimulate prostaglandin formation in a number of tissues, including amnion, endometrial stromal cells, and human myometrial cells. **Thus, IL-1β may serve as the intermediate modulator of parturition by acting to stimulate glycerophospholipid hydrolysis, arachidonic acid release, prostaglandin formation, and PAF biosynthesis in uterine and extraembryonic fetal tissues** (Fig. 10–8). Moreover, IL-1β may act in an autocrine fashion on decidua and by a paracrine mechanism in fetal membranes and myometrium (Casey and associates, 1988b; Cox and colleagues, 1988b; Word and co-workers, 1989).

An important consideration in the formation and action of IL-1β is that this cytokine is synthesized as pro-IL-1β (M$_r$ about 31,500), a precursor form in which there is no leader sequence and that, at least at the plasma membrane receptor level, is biologically inactive, or relatively so. Pro-IL-1β thus accumulates in the cytosol, *i.e.*, it is not secreted from the cell. Pro-IL-1β, perhaps at the plasma membrane, after being acted upon by serine proteases (such as plasmin), is converted to lower molecular weight forms, *viz.*, an intermediate (M$_r$ about 23,000) form and thence to the mature (M$_r$ about 17,500) form, the moiety that is found outside the cell of synthesis. The mature (immunohormone-immunomodulator) form of IL-1β acts on responsive cells by way of a specific receptor-mediated process. The regulation of synthesis and processing of IL-1β has been described in detail by Webb and colleagues (1987).

This fascinating (and somewhat puzzling) synthesis and processing of pro-IL-1β gives rise to several interesting possibilities. For example, it is possible, but not proven, that progesterone acts to regulate the synthesis or processing (or both) of IL-1β. Increased levels of IL-1 are found in the blood of women during the luteal phase of the cycle (Cannon and Dinarello, 1985), and it has been shown that macrophages isolated from the peritoneal cavity of women after ovulation produce IL-1, whereas those obtained before ovulation do not (Glover and colleagues, 1987).

It is interesting to ponder the question as to whether progesterone may act to stimulate the synthesis of pro-IL-1β and at the same time act to prevent its processing by stimulating the synthesis of a serine protease inhibitor, *e.g.*, plasminogen activator inhibitor, which is known to be produced in large amounts during human pregnancy. For some time, inexplicable features of progesterone action and prostaglandin formation have been recognized. To wit: progesterone seems to stimulate the potential of some tissues to produce prostaglandin, but at the same time progesterone may serve to prevent the actual formation of prostaglandins (Casey and co-workers, 1980). Perhaps this enigmatic feature of progesterone action and prostaglandin formation is related to progesterone-mediated regulation of IL-1β synthesis and processing.

Other Cytokines in Amnionic Fluid During Labor

In addition to IL-1β, other cytokines are produced by stimulated monocytes/macrophages. To evaluate further the analogies between the responses of activated decidua during parturition and those of stimulated macrophages, cytokines other than IL-1β also should be considered.

The *colony stimulating factors* (CSFs) are glycoproteins that regulate the formation of mature macrophages and granulocytes from immature progenitor cells (Stanley, 1986). Selected CSFs are produced by stimulated macrophages and, in turn, one particular CSF, namely *macrophage CSF* (M-CSF), usually produced in stromal cells of tissues, acts on macrophages and precursors thereof, to promote replication and differentiation of these cells. Uniquely, the receptor for M-CSF, which is the product of the proto-oncogene, *c-fms*, is present in decidual and trophoblastic tissue (Casey ML, personal communication). Heretofore, *c-fms* was believed to be present only in monocytes and macrophages. This represents yet another analogy between macrophages and decidua.

The concentration of M-CSF in mouse uterine tissue during pregnancy is increased strikingly (1,000-fold), compared with that present in the uterus of nonpregnant animals (Bartocci and colleagues, 1986; Rosendaal, 1975). It has been suggested that M-CSF produced in decidua acts on trophoblasts as a growth or differentiating factor (Rettenmier and associates, 1986).

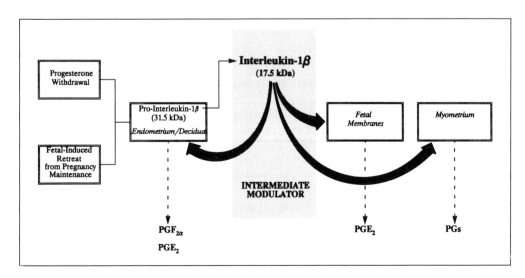

Figure 10–8. IL-1β as the intermediate modulator of parturition. (*Illustration courtesy Dr. L. Casey.*)

Presently it is not possible to deduce the exact role of CSFs in the regulation of decidual function or in the initiation of parturition. There is, however, suspicion that such a role exists, because CSF (type not yet defined) concentrations in amnionic fluid are increased during parturition (Cox SM and Casey ML, personal communication). And it is known that there is a marked increase in the number of neutrophils in the blood of women during labor and in the puerperium, possibly indicating an increase in granulocyte-macrophage (GM)-CSF formation during labor. As yet, it is difficult to place all of these findings concerning CSFs and labor into one coordinated scheme, but the finding of increased concentrations of CSF(s) in amnionic fluid during labor may be another indication of activation of the macrophage-like decidua.

Tumor necrosis factor-α (TNF-α), also known as cachectin, is another cytokine produced by macrophages in response to a variety of challenges, in particular bacterial endotoxin. TNF-α is not found in amnionic fluid of normal pregnancies at any stage of gestation before or after the onset of labor. But TNF-α is found in amnionic fluid of some pregnancies complicated by bacterial endotoxin-induced preterm labor (Casey and associates, 1989; and p. 210).

The Decidua–Macrophage Connection

If the accumulation of arachidonic acid, prostaglandins, PAF, IL-1β, and possibly other cytokines in amnionic fluid during labor is the consequence of the activation of a single tissue, that tissue is most likely decidua, and the simultaneous release of these particular agents is remindful of the coordinated response of stimulated monocytes or macrophages: the decidua–macrophage connection of human parturition.

There is no doubt that the decidua is enriched with bone-marrow–derived macrophages (Bulmer and Johnson, 1984; Nehemiah and colleagues, 1981). But more than this, the decidual cell *per se* is macrophage-like in many functional characteristics. Indeed, the endometrial stromal cell, the progenitor of the decidual cell, is endowed with macrophage-like properties. There are unusual and distinctive properties shared by macrophages and by decidua. Consider the following: the arachidonic acid content of both tissues is especially great; *viz.*, 20 to 25 percent of the fatty acids of both tissues is arachidonic acid. The 1α-hydroxylation of 25-hydroxyvitamin D_3 is demonstrable in both tissues as is the biosynthesis of β-endorphin. Both tissues produce PAF. Both tissues produce the cytokines, IL-1 and TNF-α (Casey and associates, 1988b, 1989). The endometrial stromal cell, the decidua, and the macrophage respond to bacterial endotoxin—lipopolysaccharide (LPS)—by producing prodigious amounts of cytokines and prostaglandins. As stated before, the gene product of *c-fms*, the M-CSF receptor, is present in both macrophages and decidua. Selected macrophage antigens are present in decidua and in endometrial stromal cells, *e.g.*, MAC-1, and the concentration of this protein increases in IL-1–treated endometrial stromal cells. The similarities between selected functional characteristics of macrophages and decidua were reviewed recently (Casey and MacDonald, 1988a,b,c).

Decidual Activation in the Initiation of Parturition

The decidua must be maintained in a state of functional quiescence (at least as regards the initiation of labor) during more than 99 percent of pregnancy; but during parturition, activation of the decidua causes a robust response that includes the formation of a set of bioactive agents, compounds that are likely to be important as uterotropins or uterotonins, or as intermediate modulators of parturition that stimulate the formation of uterotropins and uterotonins.

It is probable that the decidua is always metabolically poised to initiate parturition but is restrained from doing so until fetal retreat from pregnancy maintenance is sounded. Thereby, early parturition, *viz.*, menstruation and abortion, is possible, but it constitutes a fail-safe system that is initiated only when pregnancy maintenance is unsuccessful.

THE AMNION AND HUMAN PARTURITION

As described in Chapter 2, the proximal anatomical parts of the paracrine arm of the fetal–maternal communication system are the amnionic fluid, amnion, chorion laeve, decidua, and myometrium. In the development of the fetal–maternal communication concept of human pregnancy the paracrine arm of this system occupies an important role in pregnancy maintenance and parturition. Scientific explorations of the means by which this system serves to facilitate the maintenance of pregnancy have just begun, but investigators have been evaluating the metabolic function of the fetal membranes in the initiation of parturition for the past 15 years (MacDonald and associates, 1974; for review, Bleasdale and Johnston, 1984).

During the entire human pregnancy the fetus exists in an aqueous environment, *i.e.*, the amnionic fluid, which is bounded by the fetal membranes, *viz.*, the avascular amnion and chorion laeve. At term, the fetal membranes occupy the entire surface area (about 0.6 m^2) of the uterine cavity not occupied by placenta. Direct communication between the fetus and amnion is operative by way of the amnionic fluid, which is enriched in fetal secretions and excretions from kidney, lung, umbilical cord, and skin (Fig.2–1). Anatomically, therefore, the amnion is positioned ideally to receive a fetal signal and to transmit a response to such a signal. The chorion laeve, also a thin membrane of fetal origin, is contiguous with the amnion on one side and with the maternal decidua vera (parietalis) on the other side.

AMNION INVOLVEMENT IN PARTURITION

There is persuasive evidence that the amnion and chorion laeve, as clearly is the case with decidua and myometrium, are stimulated to new levels of metabolic activity during parturition, and insights into the function of the fetal membranes in this process are fundamental to an understanding of the biomolecular events of parturition. There are clinical, anatomical, metabolic, physiological, pathophysiological, and pharmacological sets of data in favor of an active involvement of the fetal membranes in the parturitional process.

PROSTAGLANDIN FORMATION IN AMNION

In attempting to deduce the role of the amnion in parturition, it is important at the outset to recognize that there are curious features of amnion prostaglandin formation. First, **the amnion produces PGE_2 almost exclusively and little or no $PGF_{2\alpha}$**. Second, there is a reasonably large potential capacity for PGE_2 production in amnion. However, third, during all of pregnancy (before the onset of labor), the free arachidonic acid concentration of the extracellular medium of the avascular amnion, *viz.*, the amnionic fluid, is very low. This low extracellular concentration of arachidonic acid delimits the capacity of amnion tissue to produce PGE_2 during pregnancy, at least before labor. After labor commences, the concentration of free arachidonic acid in the amnionic fluid increases and the formation of PGE_2 in amnion is facilitated. We discuss this important issue in greater detail in a later section (p. 204).

ARACHIDONIC ACID CONTENT OF AMNION

Amnion tissue is particularly enriched in arachidonic acid, the obligate precursor of prostaglandins of the 2-series. Approximately 20 percent of the fatty acids of amnion is arachidonic acid, a very high content compared with many other tissues. Arachidonic acid in tissues is almost always esterified in the sn-2 position of glycerolipids; this is true of amnion (Fig. 10–9). Indeed, arachidonic acid is found in the sn-2 position of the majority of the phosphatidylinositol and phosphatidylethanolamine molecules of amnion (Okita and co-workers, 1982a).

LIPASES OF AMNION

The enzymatic release of arachidonic acid commonly involves the hydrolysis of the sn-2 fatty acid of glycerolipids. Prevention of reacylation of free arachidonic acid into phosphatidic acid also may be important in this process. Johnston and colleagues, as reviewed by Bleasdale and Johnston (1984) and Angle and co-workers (1988), found that the lipases of amnion are particularly suited to effect the preferential release of arachidonic acid from glycerophospholipids in this tissue. They demonstrated that there is specificity of the lipases of amnion for arachidonoyl-containing substrates. They also demonstrated that selected lipases (viz., phospholipase A_2 and phospholipase C) of the amnion are calcium-dependent, whereas another enzyme (diacylglycerol kinase), important in the recycling of arachidonic acid back into amnion glycerophospholipid storage forms, is inhibited by calcium (Fig. 10–10). Thus, a coordinated system of enzymatic reactions in amnion is possible for effecting the preferential release of arachidonic acid, which is present in high concentrations in this tissue. These specific mechanisms are regulated by calcium in a manner that favors preserving the free arachidonic acid that is released for PGE_2 formation. Moreover, Johnston and associates found that there is a significant increase in the specific activity of certain of the lipases in amnion late in gestation, compared with the specific activities of these enzymes in these same tissues obtained from early gestation.

ARACHIDONIC ACID METABOLISM IN AMNION DURING LABOR

There is a highly significant, specific decrease in the arachidonic acid content of amnion during early labor. Namely, there is a decrease in the concentration of arachidonic acid in phosphatidylinositol and in (diacyl)phosphatidylethanolamine in amnion that occurs before approximately 5 cm dilatation of the cervix (Okita and colleagues, 1982a). During this same time in labor, the concentration of arachidonic acid and PGE_2 begins to increase in the amnionic fluid. These findings point to the probability of increased amnion production of PGE_2 during early labor.

As labor progresses, however, the arachidonic acid content of amnion is restored. There are several conclusions to be drawn from this finding. For one, this must mean that there is continuous glycerophospholipid turnover in amnion during labor. There is other evidence of increased glycerophospholipid metabolism during this time. There is an increase in the content of palmitic acid in the glycerophospholipids of amnion near the end of labor, diacylglycerols accumulate in the amnion during labor, and the fatty acid content of the diacylglyercols is the same as that of phosphatidylinositol of this tissue, suggestive of increased hydrolysis of phosphatidylinositol (Okita, 1981; Okita and associates, 1982b).

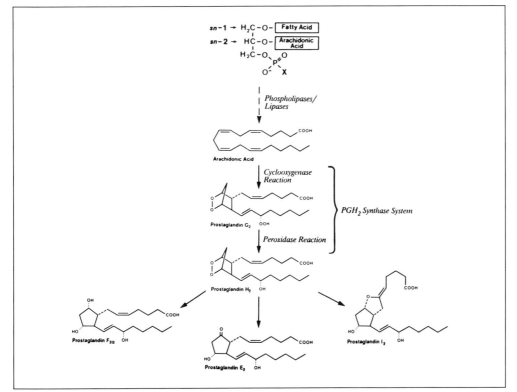

Figure 10–9. Schematic model (general) for the biosynthesis of prostaglandins. Generally, arachidonic acid is released from glycerophospholipids by the action of one or more tissue lipases. The conversion of arachidonic acid to PGH_2 is accomplished by two enzymatic reactions catalyzed by a single protein, namely, PGH_2 synthase. (*Illustration courtesy of Dr. L. Casey.*)

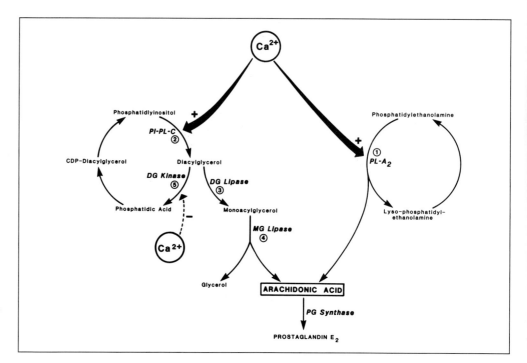

Figure 10–10. Metabolism and enzymatic release of arachidonic acid in human amnion. A Ca^{2+} cycle is proposed, according to Dr. J. M. Johnston, whereby Ca^{2+}, in increased concentrations, favors the release of arachidonate and prevents the recycling of arachidonate back into glycerophospholipids.

PROSTAGLANDIN METABOLISM IN AMNION

There is little or no PGDH activity in amnion (Keirse and Turnbull, 1976; Okazaki and co-workers, 1981); this is the enzyme that catalyzes the first step in the metabolism (inactivation) of prostaglandins. Accordingly the potential for PGE_2 production in amnion is large, and there is limited or no inactivation of PGE_2 in this tissue, as reviewed by Casey and MacDonald (1986).

METABOLIC FATE OF AMNION PGE_2

PGE_2 produced in amnion, which diffuses toward maternal tissues, is likely to be metabolized rapidly by PGDH in chorion laeve or decidua or both. The specific activity of PGDH in chorion laeve is very high (Keirse and Turnbull, 1976; Okazaki and associates, 1981). But the levels of PGE_2 metabolites in maternal plasma do not increase during labor. Perhaps the explanation for this is that (1) most of the PGE_2 and metabolites of PGE_2 produced in amnion and chorion laeve enter amnionic fluid. The small amount of PGE_2 metabolites that reach the maternal circulation are rapidly cleared from maternal plasma. PGE_2 that enters amnionic fluid accumulates in this space because there is no prostaglandin-metabolizing activity in amnionic fluid (Keirse and Turnbull, 1975).

AMNION PROSTAGLANDIN FORMATION DURING LABOR

During the very early phases of labor there is a preferential increase in the concentration of PGE_2 (compared with $PGF_{2\alpha}$) in amnionic fluid, and the increase in the concentration of PGE_2 in amnionic fluid even may precede the onset of clinically detectable labor (Dray and Frydman, 1976). The greater rate of increase of PGE_2 in amnionic fluid during early labor also may be indicative of an amnion (or chorion laeve or both) origin of this PGE_2, because $PGF_{2\alpha}$ and also PGE_2 are produced in decidua (Fig. 10–6). As labor progresses, however, there is a considerably greater increase in the amnionic fluid concentrations of $PGF_{2\alpha}$ and PGFM, which ultimately exceed that of PGE_2 (Reddi and colleagues, 1984; Dray and Frydman, 1976) (Fig. 10–7). Decidua produces $PGF_{2\alpha}$ preferentially (compared with the formation of PGE_2).

REGULATION OF PGE_2 FORMATION IN AMNION

There are two distinct mechanisms by which amnion PGE_2 formation is regulated; these separate regulatory phenomena are important to an understanding of amnion prostaglandin formation before and during labor. The first of these involves alterations in the enzymatic conversion of arachidonic acid to prostaglandin; the second involves the availability of free arachidonic acid (Casey and co-workers, 1987, 1988a).

Stimulation of Amnion PGH_2-Synthase
An agent in human fetal urine has been identified that acts on amnion cells in monolayer culture to cause replication of these cells and an increase in the rate of PGE_2 synthesis. This fetal urinary stimulant acts by way of the epidermal growth factor (EGF) receptors on the amnion. This agent is believed to be EGF or a transforming growth factor-α that is produced in fetal kidney and excreted into amnionic fluid (Casey and co-workers, 1983a; Strickland and associates, 1983).

Agents such as EGF and the fetal kidney-derived growth factor (KDGF) act on amnion to increase PGE_2 formation by inducing an increase in the synthesis of PGH_2-synthase, the enzyme that catalyzes the first reaction in the conversion of arachidonic acid to prostaglandins (Fig. 10–9). These types of stimulants of amnion PGE_2 synthesis do not act to effect the release of arachidonic acid (and do not cause an increase in the specific activities of phospholipase A_2 or phospholipase C). In the absence of free (nonesterified) arachidonic acid in the extracellular environment, these agents do not cause an increase in the formation of PGE_2 (Casey and associates, 1987, 1988a).

The amount of fetal KDGF, *i.e.,* the EGF-like substance in fetal urine, does not increase as a function of gestational age. In particular, there is no increase in the amount of this substance in urine obtained from fetuses delivered after labor, compared with the amount of this substance in urine obtained from fetuses delivered before labor commences. The same is true of urine obtained from fetuses before term. It is likely, therefore, that this agent (KDGF) acts upon amnion (1) to cause an increase in amnion cell replication (to facilitate amnion growth) and (2) to effect a continual high rate of synthesis of PGH_2-synthase. If this should be the case, the release of arachidonic acid or its availability in amnionic fluid during labor would be the rate-limiting factor(s) in the rate of PGE_2 formation in activated amnion during parturition (Casey and associates, 1987, 1988a).

Stimulation of Amnion Arachidonic Acid Release

Therefore, some other, as yet unidentified, agent(s) must act on amnion during labor to cause the release of arachidonic acid, because clearly (1) arachidonic acid is lost from amnion during early labor, and (2) there is increased glycerophospholipid turnover in amnion throughout labor. As suggested previously, these actions on amnion may be brought about by a specific agent, one we referred to as an intermediate modulator of parturition; possibly this agent is IL-1β.

Role of Amnionic Fluid Arachidonic Acid in Amnion Prostaglandin Formation

The formation of PGE_2 in amnion is delimited ultimately by the concentration of free arachidonic acid in the extracellular medium of this tissue, *viz.*, amnionic fluid.

In amnion cells in culture, the capacity for PGE_2 formation is restricted by the availability of free arachidonic acid in the culture medium. Amnion cells, maintained in monolayer culture, produce very little PGE_2, but these cells can be stimulated to produce PGE_2 by a variety of agents, including EGF, KDGF, tumor-promoting phorbol esters, vanadate, and calcium ionophores. The rate of increase in PGE_2 production in treated amnion cells, however, is highly dependent upon arachidonic acid in the medium in which the cells are maintained. Specifically, in the absence of fetal calf serum, which contains arachidonic acid, or in albumin to which arachidonic acid is bound, the rate of PGE_2 formation in amnion cells in response to stimuli is limited (Casey and associates, 1987, 1988a).

These findings are relevant to the in vivo situation of human pregnancy because (1) the concentration of arachidonic acid in amnionic fluid before the onset of labor is very low and (2) the amnion obtains arachidonic acid exclusively from the amnionic fluid. On average, the concentration of arachidonic acid in culture medium that contains fetal calf serum (10 percent) is 3.5 μM. The concentration of arachidonic acid in the amnionic fluid before labor commences is 0.2 μM, and during late labor it is 1 to 4 μM. The apparent Km of amnion cyclooxygenase for arachidonic acid is 1 μM. Thus, prior to labor, when the level of arachidonic acid in amnionic fluid is low, PGE_2 production by amnion is severely restricted. Increased PGE_2 formation in amnion in vivo can be effected only after there is an increase in arachidonic acid concentration in amnionic fluid or with stimulation of release of arachidonic acid from amnion; probably both are required.

In fact, optimal PGE_2 formation in amnion can be achieved only when (1) PGH_2-synthase synthesis is stimulated (EGF-like action), (2) glycerophospholipid turnover is effected, and (3) the concentration of arachidonic acid in the culture medium (or amnionic fluid) is increased (labor: release of arachidonic acid from decidua).

AMNION AND PARTURITION IN PERSPECTIVE

For all of the reasons stated, there is no doubt that the amnion is activated to new levels of metabolic function during human parturition, processes that facilitate maximum PGE_2 production. Nonetheless, there are important reasons to conclude that amnion is not the source of the primary prostaglandin of parturition.

The amnion (and also the chorion laeve) produces PGE_2 almost exclusively, but during labor there is an unequivocal increase in $PGF_{2\alpha}$ or PGFM (or both) in amnionic fluid, maternal blood, and maternal urine (p. 200). Recall that PGE_2 produced in amnion is not converted to $PGF_{2\alpha}$ in decidua. Moreover, during labor it has not been possible to demonstrate a significant increase in the concentration of PGE_2 or metabolites thereof in the maternal compartment, suggesting that amnion PGE_2 may not reach the myometrium. It seems likely, therefore, that the PGE_2 produced in amnion is targeted for action in the fetal membranes or else in the fetus by way of fetal ingestion of PGE_2 in the amnionic fluid.

It is known that manipulation of the fetal membranes by digital examination or by amniotomy causes increased prostaglandin formation. The increase in the prostaglandin formed, however, is that of $PGF_{2\alpha}$ not PGE_2 (Mitchell, 1988). This suggests that manipulation of the membranes gives rise to an increase in decidual $PGF_{2\alpha}$ formation in decidua. These important relationships are discussed in greater detail in a consideration of the role of chorion laeve in parturition (p. 206).

The instillation of PGE_2 or free arachidonic acid (MacDonald and associates, 1974) into the amnionic fluid in the human causes abortion or labor. But it has always been curious that the amount of these agents required to cause labor were extraordinarily large, in fact, orders of magnitude more than is produced during spontaneous labor. And the extraovular instillation of arachidonic acid in the rhesus does not cause labor (Robinson and colleagues, 1979). Perhaps the explanation for these findings is that amnion PGE_2 is not the primary uterotonin of human parturition and PGE_2 formed in the amnion is largely metabolized before reaching the myometrium.

THE INTERMEDIATE MODULATOR OF PARTURITION

It seems relatively clear that an increase in the rate of prostaglandin formation, *viz.*, $PGF_{2\alpha}$ synthesis in decidua and PGE_2 synthesis in decidua and in the fetal membranes, is linked closely to the events of parturition. Therefore, a cogent question is posed; namely, what is the mechanism by which increased prostaglandin formation is induced in decidua and fetal membranes at the time of parturition? The answer to this same question is also central to an understanding of the mechanism by which progesterone withdrawal brings about increased prostaglandin formation: namely, what is the intermediate agent that acts to facilitate prostaglandin formation in response to this endocrine antecedent of parturition (in some species) or menstruation (in primates)?

It may be possible that a single agent acts as **the intermediate modulator of parturition and menstruation**. In particular, there may be a particular agent that acts to cause glycerophospholipid hydrolysis, arachidonic acid release, prostaglandin formation, and PAF production. If this should be true, we suggest that the identity of this agent may be IL-1β, which is produced in decidual tissue and in endometrial stromal cells, the progenitors of decidual cells. IL-1β acts on amnion cells, endometrial stromal cells, and myometrial cells to promote the formation of prostaglandins in each (Figs. 10–4, 10–8). The formation of IL-1β in decidua could promote increased prostaglandin formation in decidua by an autocrine action and could promote increased prostaglandin formation in fetal membranes and myometrium by a paracrine action. These are characteristic of the diversity of IL-1 actions in other tissues.

THE CHORION LAEVE AND HUMAN PARTURITION

Heretofore most investigators have given less attention to the role of the chorion laeve in the events of parturition than they have given to that of the amnion. Perhaps this was because it has been relatively more difficult to work with isolated chorion and chorion laeve cells than with isolated amnion and amnion cells. But as we explore new concepts to explain the biomolecular processes of pregnancy maintenance and parturition, the chorion laeve is clearly a tissue of paramount importance.

The chorion laeve is the fetal tissue of the anatomical core of the paracrine arm of the fetal–maternal communication system, which is believed to be supportive of the maintenance of pregnancy and thence the initiation of labor. The chorion laeve is composed primarily of trophoblasts, i.e., cytotrophoblasts, derived from an extension of the peripheral cells of trophectoderm of the developing blastocyst (Chap. 4). It is therefore a membranous tissue endowed with some of the properties of cytotrophoblast. Moreover, it is the fetal tissue that is in direct cell-to-cell contact with both maternal and fetal tissues. There is unique molecular trafficking between the chorion laeve and the decidua; for example, prolactin produced in decidua is preferentially (perhaps completely) secreted into amnionic fluid and not into the extravascular space of the decidual cells. It is likely that this involves the transfer of prolactin from the decidual cells to the cells of the chorion laeve in this unique transport phenomenon (Chap. 4, p. 56).

ARACHIDONIC ACID METABOLISM IN CHORION LAEVE

There is no doubt that as in the case of decidua and amnion, the chorion laeve is stimulated to new levels of metabolic activity during human parturition. Okita and colleagues (1982a) found that during the course of early labor (before 5-cm cervical dilatation) there is a significant loss of arachidonic acid from two glycerophospholipids of chorion laeve tissue, viz., (diacyl)phosphatidylethanolamine and phosphatidylinositol. As labor progresses the arachidonic acid content of the chorion laeve is restored to levels even greater than those that existed before the onset of labor. There is also fatty acid remodeling of glycerophospholipids of chorion laeve during labor as there is in amnion (Okita, 1981).

The chorion laeve is also avascular; therefore, the arachidonic acid incorporated into chorion laeve must be derived from a tissue source other than fetal blood. From a study of the arachidonic acid composition of chorion laeve tissues of diamnionic-dichorionic twin pregnancies, it was shown that chorion laeve tissue obtains arachidonic acid from both the amnionic fluid (possibly by way of the amnion) and from maternal tissues (blood or decidua). The arachidonic acid composition of

fused chorion laeve in diamnionic-dichorionic twin pregnancies was about one half that found in nonfused chorion laeve tissue and in chorion laeve tissue of singleton pregnancies. On the other hand, the arachidonic acid content of fused and nonfused amnion tissue of diamnionic-dichorionic twin fetal membranes was the same and, in turn, was the same as that found in amnion of singleton pregnancy amnions (Okita and associates, 1983a).

PROSTAGLANDIN PRODUCTION AND METABOLISM IN CHORION LAEVE

As stated before, the chorion laeve, like the amnion, produces almost exclusively PGE_2; in particular, the chorion laeve produces little or no $PGF_{2\alpha}$. But in contrast to the amnion, the chorion laeve is rich in PGDH activity, the initial and rate-limiting enzyme in prostaglandin inactivation (Fig. 10–6.).

CHORION LAEVE AND DECIDUAL $PGF_{2\alpha}$ FORMATION

Fetal chorion laeve is juxtaposed to macrophage-like decidual tissue. Several investigators have found that disruption of this tissue interface causes labor. For example, separation of chorion laeve from decidua by (1) rupture of the membranes, (2) sweeping of the membranes, (3) separation by the instillation of saline, (4) separation by air-filled balloons, or even (5) delivering the fetal membranes together with attached placenta leads to a striking increase in the levels of PGFM in maternal blood and, commonly, labor. These findings were reviewed recently (Casey and MacDonald, 1988b). This strongly suggests that some fundamental interaction between chorion laeve and contiguous decidua serves throughout most of pregnancy to promote decidual quiescence, at least as this pertains to the generation of bioactive products in the decidua.

ROLE OF THE HUMAN FETUS IN THE INITIATION OF PARTURITION

THEORETICAL CONSIDERATIONS

Teleologically it is satisfying, even tantalizing, to believe that the fetus, after key maturational events in vital fetal tissues and organs are initiated or completed, provides a signal to maternal tissues to commence parturition. Because of the attractiveness of this possibility, many investigators, including ourselves, have searched for a fetal trigger that would launch the procession of parturitional events. No such fetal signal has been found in human pregnancy and parturition.

Fetal signals to initiate parturition could be transmitted in one of several ways. In the sheep model the fetus seems to promote retreat from the further maintenance of pregnancy by way of blood-borne fetal cortisol-induced alterations in the biosynthesis of steroidogenic enzymes in the placenta (the endocrine component of the placental arm of the fetal–maternal communication system). The end result is progesterone withdrawal.

Similarly the human fetus may sound retreat from pregnancy maintenance through a fetal blood-borne agent that acts by way of the placental arm of the fetal–maternal communication system. Alternatively a signal could be transmitted from the fetus by way of the fetal lungs or fetal kidneys through secretions or excretions that enter the amnionic fluid (the paracrine arm of the fetal–maternal communication system).

For a variety of reasons it seems unlikely that the initial signal for the commencement of parturition is a uterotropin or uterotonin per se; rather, it is more likely that with maturation of key fetal tissues, there is retreat from support of those systems that serve to effect uterine quiescence throughout most of pregnancy. In this manner the uterotropins and uterotonins are produced in the intrauterine environment in response to the withdrawal of support of pregnancy maintenance (Casey and MacDonald, 1988b).

From this perspective the maintenance of pregnancy involves (above all else) the prevention of formation of bioactive agents that would bring about uterine contractions. If this is true, it is easier to come to grips with the fact that all too commonly there is some intervening factor that can serve to perturbate this system and provoke the premature production of uterotropins and uterotonins, or both, within uterine tissues or extraembryonic fetal membranes, *i.e.*, preterm labor. What we should have been searching for all along, we now believe, is the mechanism by which the fetus promotes withdrawal of the support systems that effect the maintenance of pregnancy.

CLINICAL CORRELATIONS

Speigelberg, in 1882 (cited by Thorburn, 1983), put forward the proposition that the origin of the signal for the initiation of parturition in the human was the fetus. The bovine fetus, the ovine fetus, and the human fetus each appear to participate in the timely onset of labor. Anomalies of the brain of the fetal calf, fetal lamb, and human fetus interfere with the timing of the onset of labor. When there is congenital absence of the pituitary in the bovine fetus, the gestation period is prolonged by several weeks. Adrenal hypoplasia in the bovine fetus also causes prolonged gestation. If, early in pregnancy, the ewe eats the foliage of a plant, *Veratrum californicum,* which grows wild in the northwestern United States, the fetal sheep develops a characteristic cyclopean deformity that is associated with abnormal vascularization of the pituitary from the hypothalamus. In a ewe with such a fetus there is fetal adrenal hypoplasia along with prolonged gestation. Indeed, the pregnancy goes far beyond term, and the sheep fetus continues to persist and ultimately dies *in utero*. These issues have been reviewed by Thorburn (1983) and by Challis and Olson (1988).

In 1898 Rea observed an association between anencephaly in the human fetus and prolonged gestation. In 1933 Malpas extended these observations on an association between anencephaly in the human fetus and prolonged gestation and concluded that this seemed to be attributable to anomalous brain-pituitary-adrenal function. These findings are suggestive that in the human, as in sheep, the fetal adrenal may serve an important role in the timely onset of labor. The adrenal glands of the anencephalic fetus are very small compared with those of normal fetuses. Indeed, the adrenals of the anencephalic fetus at term may weigh only 5 to 10 percent of those of a normal fetus. The smallness of the gland is due largely to failure of development of the fetal zone—the structure that accounts for most of the mass of the human fetal adrenal (Chap. 5).

There is another corollary between the biomolecular events of parturition in the human and those in the sheep model. In the human pregnancy in which there is a fetus with adrenal hypoplasia there also may be prolonged gestation (Anderson and Turnbull, 1973). This condition is reminiscent of that in sheep in which the fetal adrenal has been rendered inactive either by hypophysectomy or adrenalectomy and there is also prolonged gestation.

On the other hand, at this point in the development of analogies between the sheep and human models of parturition initiation there is a divergence of considerable importance. There is no clear-cut increase in cortisol concentration in fetal blood before the onset of parturition in the human—and there is no evidence of a decline in the concentration of progesterone, at least in maternal plasma before or during labor (p. 191).

FETAL CONTRIBUTIONS TO HUMAN PARTURITION: SUMMARY

Today there is only fragmentary evidence that pregnancies with hypoestrogenism (fetal anencephaly, fetal adrenal hypoplasia, and placental sulfatase deficiency) may be associated with prolonged gestation or dysfunctional labor. But with these conditions, prolonged gestation is not universally the case. Normal amounts of estrogen may serve to facilitate the development of optimal parturitional processes, but the regulation of estrogen formation is not the functional key to the timely onset of human parturition. Similarly, other fetal abnormalities that prevent or else attenuate the entry of fetal urine (absence of fetal kidneys) or lung secretions (pulmonary hypoplasia) into amnionic fluid do not cause prolongation of human pregnancy.

SPECULATIONS

Teleologically it seems probable that fetal maturation is central to the fetal-induced retreat from pregnancy maintenance, *i.e.*, the commencement of parturition. It is unlikely, however, that such a momentous process is resident in the molecular maturation of a single fetal organ. There are too many examples of organ abnormalities in the fetuses of human pregnancy that are not associated with aberrations in the timing of parturition for this to be tenable. Yet fetal adrenal maturation in the sheep fetus (and possibly other mammalian fetuses) seems to be a clear means of effecting a signaling system. On the other hand, this system seems a bit indirect, involving as it does an alteration in adrenal cell responsiveness rather than a straightforward increase in pituitary ACTH secretion. We suggest that this adrenal response is but one maturational event that is part of a more generalized developmental milestone of the fetus in response to a specific alteration in fetal metabolism—one as yet not identified, but possibly common to all mammalian fetuses before the retreat from continued pregnancy maintenance, namely, parturition.

PRETERM LABOR

Notwithstanding our ignorance of the precise biomolecular processes involved in birthing, there is no doubt that the timeliness of this momentous happening is among the most important biological determinants in establishing the quality of life of the human species. The parturition process nominally commences about 260 days after implantation of the blastocyst, but all too commonly labor takes place far in advance of the achievement of full fetal maturation; indeed, some 6 to 10 percent of newborns are delivered preterm.

In the United States alone there are at least 250,000 preterm fetuses born each year. It can be argued, and with great persuasion we believe, that an untimely birth is one of the major health hazards of human beings. **There is no doubt that the greatest single cause of neonatal morbidity and mortality is preterm birth.** But more than this, a large number of permanently institutionalized persons are those who are mentally or physically impaired because of an untimely birth. To suffer the agony of lifelong mental and physical impairment is surely one of the greatest tragedies that can beset a person, his or her family, society, and even the economies of the world. An untimely birth may portend grave and horrendous impositions on the most innocent and vulnerable of our society: the newborn. And the sequelae of the complications of an untimely birth can produce lifelong disabilities.

Guaranteeing the optimal quality of life for newborns, who should expect to enjoy 70 to 80 years or more of good health, must be a major goal of scientists, physicians, and economists concerned with the health care needs of all persons. The clinical aspects and the management of preterm labor are discussed in Chapter 38.

INFECTION-ASSOCIATED PRETERM LABOR

There is a large body of epidemiological data suggesting a role for infection in the pathophysiology of preterm labor. Indeed, both intrauterine (chorioamnionitis-deciduitis) and extrauterine (pyelonephritis, pneumonia, appendicitis, peritonitis) infections are associated with an increased incidence of preterm labor. Among most obstetricians there is great suspicion that "silent" infections are also a common accompaniment and cause of preterm labor. In this context silent infection is meant to describe a pregnancy in which infection exists but there is no clinical evidence of this process in the mother-to-be (she is afebrile, for example) and microorganisms cannot be demonstrated in the amnionic fluid (Iams and co-workers, 1987).

Heretofore, most investigators were unwilling to accept infection as the cause of preterm labor unless microorganisms could be demonstrated within the amnionic sac. Before now, this was a reasonable approach to the problem because other indices of infection, establishing an unequivocal relationship between microorganisms and preterm labor, were not available.

BIOMOLECULAR PROCESSES OF INFECTION-INDUCED PRETERM LABOR

Many theories have been advanced to explain the relationship between infection and the premature onset of labor. Among these are the following: inflammation leads to premature rupture of the fetal membranes; bacterial lipases act upon glycerophospholipids in the fetal membranes to effect the release of arachidonic acid, thereby bringing about PGE_2 formation; a general inflammatory response leads to increased uterotonin formation; infection causes premature dilatation of the cervix. Other explanations have also been advanced. None of these proposals, however, is sufficiently specific or testable as to permit the development of a common biomolecular scheme to explain the mechanism(s) by which infection causes the induction of labor prematurely. This is particularly true in the case of "silent" infections in pregnancies in which the fetal membranes are intact.

ANATOMY OF PREGNANCY AND INFECTION

The patency of the reproductive tract of women, while essential for the achievement of pregnancy and delivery of the fetus, may sometimes be problematic in the containment of microbial growth in key intrauterine tissues during pregnancy. The lower pole of the fetal membrane–decidual junction is contiguous with the cervical canal, which is patent to the vagina. To be sure, as pointed out in Chapter 7 (p. 133), there is functional obliteration of the cervical canal by a mucous plug; and there are significant antimicrobial properties associated with cervical mucus.

Nonetheless, this anatomical arrangement provides for a reasonably good opportunity for infection. Microorganisms, from the endocervical canal or vagina, may ascend to colonize tissues at the lower pole of the fetal membranes and contiguous decidua. In fact, it seems reasonable to surmise that the antimicrobial properties of the cervical glands and the macrophage-like decidua (and possibly the fetal membranes and amnionic fluid as well) must be substantial to contain and prevent the spread of infection and penetration of the fetal membranes and the entry of microorganisms into the amnionic fluid. If this should be a correct formulation of the bacteriological homeostasis of intrauterine tissues during pregnancy, it also seems reasonable to assume that the success of these tissues in preventing replication of microorganisms may vary among otherwise normal pregnancies.

SILENT INFECTION AND PRETERM LABOR

And according to this formulation of the problem, "silent" infections, which may involve the outer surface of the amnion or the chorion laeve and decidua, must be common, even though well contained. If bioactive products of microorganisms of such infections should act upon decidua or fetal membranes (or both) to cause accelerated formation of uterotropins and uterotonins, preterm labor would ensue. This sequence of events could come to pass in a pregnancy with intact fetal membranes, in the absence of maternal fever, and in the absence of demonstrable microorganisms in the amnionic fluid.

The rate-limiting factor, with respect to continuation of pregnancy or the initiation of preterm labor, therefore, would be related to the amount and potency of the bioactive microbial product(s) released. Accordingly, the specificity of infection—microorganism(s)—in the pathophysiology of preterm labor could be related to the potency and amount of the toxin produced and not necessarily to the tissue invasiveness or penetrance of the microorganism(s) involved.

Bacterial Toxins and Preterm Labor

Two important considerations have led to a reappraisal of the role of infection as a causative factor in the induction of preterm labor. From these considerations a theorem was developed to describe the biomolecular processes operative in this phenomenon.

1. A set of bioactive agents accumulates in the amnionic fluid during labor. These include free arachidonic acid, prostaglandins, PAF, and IL-1β. This same set of agents is produced by monocytes–macrophages, especially those stimulated by endotoxin (LPS) of gram-negative bacteria.
2. Uterine decidua is macrophage-like, and decidua is a key tissue in the generation of the bioactive agents that accumulate in amnionic fluid during labor.

Hypothesis

These considerations were instrumental in the formulation of a testable hypothesis for an investigation of the biomolecular processes leading to infection-induced preterm labor. In particular, it was deduced that the activation of decidua by one or more products of microorganisms may serve to initiate labor prematurely. Bacterial endotoxin (LPS) acts on macrophages to cause a robust response that includes the outpouring of free arachidonic acid, prostaglandins, PAF, IL-1β, and other cytokines, a response nearly identical to what occurs in intrauterine tissues during spontaneous parturition at term.

The question posed, therefore, was as follows: Does LPS, produced in microorganisms, act upon macrophage-like decidua to cause a response similar to that found in LPS-stimulated macrophages and similar to what occurs when decidua is activated during spontaneous parturition at term? If this were true, bacterial toxins could act to initiate labor prematurely by way of the initiation of the same or a very similar set of events that come about with retreat from pregnancy maintenance, *i.e.*, spontaneous parturition at term. Moreover, this formulation of the basis of infection-induced preterm labor provides an explanation for this occurrence in those circumstances in which microorganisms are replicating outside of the amnionic fluid.

Background
More than 40 years ago it was shown that the administration of LPS to pregnant experimental animals caused abortion or premature delivery of their fetuses. LPS treatment of these pregnant animals was associated with decidual hemorrhage and necrosis (Zahl and Bjerknes, 1943). It also has been demonstrated that many of the sequelae of infection are the result of bacterial toxin-stimulation of monocytes–macrophages. In response to LPS, for example, macrophages release arachidonic acid in large amounts (Kunkel and Chensue, 1986) and a variety of cytokines are produced, including IL-1β and tumor necrosis factor-α (cachectin) (Beutler and Cerami, 1986). The particulars of the macrophage response to LPS have been described in detail (Dinarello, 1986).

Experimental Evidence
To address the possibility that LPS or other bacterial toxins—for example, lipoteichoic acid (LTA), which is produced by group B streptococci—act to cause the generation of uterotropins and uterotonins and thereby preterm labor, two complementary sets of investigations were conducted. First, in vivo studies were performed to evaluate amnionic fluids from pregnancies (fetal membranes intact) complicated by preterm labor for the presence of LPS and cytokines. Second, in vitro studies were conducted to evaluate the possibility that LPS (or LTA) or IL-1β or both, act on uterine and extraembryonic fetal tissues to cause the generation of uterotropins and uterotonins.

At the outset of these studies it was demonstrated that LPS is not a constituent of amnionic fluid of normal pregnancies at any stage of gestation before or after the onset of labor (Cox and co-workers, 1988c). In particular, LPS does not normally accumulate in amnionic fluid during spontaneous labor so long as the fetal membranes are intact. Accordingly, the presence of LPS in amnionic fluid (in pregnancies with intact fetal membranes) is a highly sensitive indicator of infection (Cox and associates, 1988c; Romero and colleagues, 1987).

In these studies, LPS was found in a sizable fraction (about 35 percent) of amnionic fluids obtained from preterm labor pregnancies (that went on to spontaneous delivery) in which the fetal membranes were intact and in which there were no demonstrable microorganisms in the amnionic fluid in the majority (about 85 percent) of cases. And in the majority of such

pregnancies (85 percent), the pregnant women were afebrile (Cox and associates, 1989).

LPS in Amnionic Fluid
At present it is not possible to ascertain how LPS gains access to the amnionic fluid when the fetal membranes are intact. One explanation is that this lipopolysaccharide diffuses through the membranes from its site of origin in microorganisms infecting chorion laeve or decidua (Cox and associates, 1988c); alternatively, microorganisms may have been in the amnionic fluid but the growth of these gram-negative bacteria in this medium was restricted by the antimicrobial actions of the amnionic fluid (Romero and colleagues, 1987). In either case, LPS in amnionic fluid in cases of preterm labor (fetal membranes intact) serves as a sensitive marker of gram-negative infections of intrauterine tissues.

LPS and IL-1β
Confirmation of the important role of LPS in the induction of preterm labor in these pregnancies was obtained by the demonstration that the concentration of IL-1β in these same LPS-positive amnionic fluids of preterm labor pregnancies was elevated strikingly, as were the levels of PGE_2 and $PGF_{2\alpha}$ and PGFM (Cox and co-workers, 1989). Recall that LPS acts on macrophages to cause the outpouring of IL-1β, and IL-1β acts in many tissues to cause arachidonic acid release and prostaglandin formation.

Group B Streptococci and IL-1β
In yet other preterm labor pregnancies with intact fetal membranes viable group B streptococci were identified in the amnionic fluid. In these cases IL-1β levels also were increased, as were the concentrations of prostaglandins (Cox and associates, 1989). Note that in these cases streptococci were present in the amnionic fluid, whereas in most instances when LPS was present in the amnionic fluid, microorganisms could not be demonstrated. Possibly, streptococci penetrate the fetal membranes into the amnionic fluid more readily than do gram-negative organisms; alternatively, amnionic fluid may not interfere with replication of group B streptococci as it does in the case of gram-negative microorganisms. There is evidence in favor of this latter possibility (Hemming and colleagues, 1985).

Notwithstanding the importance of this latter issue, it seems reasonable to surmise that bacterial products, *viz.*, LPS or LTA, arising in microorganisms infecting intrauterine tissues, may act to cause preterm labor by activating decidua and causing a response that is similar to that evoked by bacterial toxins in macrophages, namely, the outpouring of IL-1β.

In turn, IL-1β can serve as the intermediate modulator of preterm labor just as it may serve as the intermediate modulator of spontaneous parturition. IL-1β acts to cause increased prostaglandin formation in decidua, in the fetal membranes, and in myometrium.

Classification of Preterm Labor (Intact Fetal Membranes)
Preterm labor occurring in pregnancies with intact fetal membranes, therefore, is divisible biochemically into two categories: in category 1, IL-1β is present in amnionic fluid in high concentrations; in category 2, IL-1β is not present in amnionic fluid. In the first category of preterm labor pregnancies either LPS or group B streptococci also are identified in the amnionic fluid. In the second category of preterm labor pregnancies neither microorganisms nor bacterial products are identified. In

some of the preterm labor pregnancies of category 1 (LPS and IL-1β present in amnionic fluid), TNF-α also was identified in the same fluids (Cox and associates, 1989). LPS acts on macrophages (Beutler and Cerami, 1986) and on decidua (Casey and associates, 1989) to cause the formation of TNF-α.

IL-1β Formation and Action

In studies conducted *in vitro* it was demonstrated that (1) IL-1β is produced in decidua and in endometrial stromal cells in culture, (2) LPS acts on these tissue to cause the production of IL-1β and prostaglandins, (3) LPS acts on decidua to cause the formation of TNF-α, and (4) IL-1β acts on endometrial stromal cells, decidual tissue, amnion cells, and myometrial smooth muscle cells to cause the formation of prostaglandins.

Conclusions

As yet, too few cases of preterm labor have been studied in the manner described to establish the incidence of bacterial toxin-induced preterm labor. The findings of studies conducted in a single institution only, Parkland Hospital (which serves primarily a socioeconomically depressed population), are suggestive that somewhat more than 50 percent of preterm labor pregnancies (with intact fetal membranes) that go on to spontaneous delivery can be attributed to bacterial toxin-induced decidual activation (Cox and co-workers, 1989).

PREMATURE RUPTURE OF THE MEMBRANES AND PRETERM LABOR

The studies of preterm labor cited were limited to the evaluation of pregnancies with intact membranes. In most institutions, including Parkland Hospital, however, upwards of two thirds of preterm labor pregnancies are those with premature rupture of the membranes as an antecedent or direct accompaniment of preterm labor (Chap. 38).

It has not been possible to study these pregnancies in the same manner as those in which the fetal membranes are intact, however, for two reasons. First, colonization of the fetal membranes may occur after premature rupture and thus cause confusion about the role of infection in the initiation of preterm labor. Second, after rupture of the membranes, the repository, *i.e.*, traplike nature of the amnionic fluid compartment is lost. This makes the evaluation of the presence of cytokines and other putative uterotropins-uterotonins in this space problematic.

RELATIONSHIPS BETWEEN TERM AND PRETERM LABOR

If there should be an intermediate modulator of parturition, *i.e.*, an agent that serves to provoke the formation of uterotropins-uterotonins in uterine and extraembryonic fetal tissues, IL-1β would be likely to be that agent. The levels of IL-1β in amnionic fluid sometimes increase strikingly during spontaneous labor; IL-1β levels in amnionic fluid are also increased with bacterial infections that give rise to the production of LPS or LTA, agents known to act to cause the formation of IL-1β. It is even possible that IL-1β is produced in endometrium after progesterone withdrawal during menstruation and in decidua after progesterone withdrawal that precedes spontaneous parturition in some mammalian species.

But even if IL-1β is not the intermediate modulator of parturition, it seems reasonably certain that some particular agent with very similar properties to those of IL-1β must be involved

in the initiation of parturition irrespective of whether this momentous event occurs spontaneously at term or prematurely in response to extraneous factors, such as bacterial toxins.

PHYSIOLOGY OF UTERINE CONTRACTIONS

The final event in initiating a uterine contraction is an increase in the intracellular concentration of ionic calcium (Ca^{2+}) in myometrial smooth muscle cells in response to the action of a uterotonin. The ATP-energy-dependent translocation of calcium to a stored form in the sarcoplasmic reticulum is associated with uterine relaxation.

THE UTERINE ELEMENTS

The body of the uterus and the cervix, although parts of the same organ, must respond to the uterotropins-uterotonins of parturition in quite different ways. On the one hand, during most of pregnancy, it is essential that the myometrium be dilatable but remain quiescent. On the other hand, the cervix must remain rigid and unyielding. Coincident with the events that are involved in parturition, however, the cervix must soften, yield, and thence dilate. The fundus must be transformed from the relaxed, quiescent organ characteristic of most of pregnancy to one of thunderous contractions of sufficient force and efficiency to drive the fetus through the yielding cervix and on through the birth canal. Failure of a timely interaction between the functions of cervix and fundus portends an unfavorable pregnancy outcome. But despite the apparent reversal of roles between cervix and fundus from before to during labor, there is evidence that both processes are regulated by common agents, the uterotropins-uterotonins of parturition.

Myometrium

The myometrial smooth muscle cells of the fundus are embedded in an extracellular matrix that is comprised principally of collagen fibers. This matrix is believed to facilitate the transmission of forces generated by the contraction of myometrial cells and also may serve to integrate the contractile forces of these cells.

Gap Junctions of Myometrium

Gap junctions are cell-to-cell contacts that are believed to be composed of symmetrical portions of the plasma membranes of two adjacent cells (Fig. 10–11); communication between myometrial cells may be accomplished by way of gap junctions. The proteins within the membranes of the cells in apposition are aligned and thereby create pores between the cytoplasms of the two cells (Garfield, 1983). Thus, a means can be established whereby a pathway is formed between coupled cells to facilitate the passage of current (electrical or ionic coupling) or metabolites (metabolite coupling) between cells. Only recently, however, has it been possible to demonstrate gap junctions in myometrial tissue. From the elegant studies of Garfield (1988) we now know that gap junctions between myometrial cells do develop during labor. In the study of a number of species, including the human, it was found that gap junctions are absent (or very nearly so) throughout pregnancy until term. At term the number of gap junctions per cell increases, and during labor these continue to increase in number and size. The gap junctions begin to disappear within 24 hours of delivery. Gap junc-

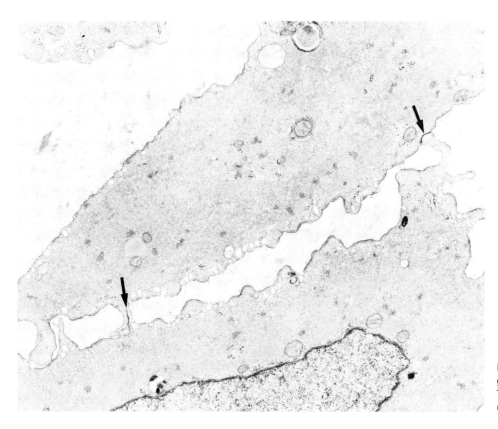

Figure 10–11. Electron photomicrograph of gap junctions in human myometrial cells. Tissue obtained after labor commenced. (*Courtesy of Dr. R. Garfield.*)

tions are present in myometrium during preterm labor, whether the onset of labor is spontaneous or induced.

On the one hand, the factor(s) that prevents the appearance of gap junctions between myometrial cells may be important in the maintenance of uterine quiescence. On the other hand, the rapid appearance of gap junctions at term may facilitate the coordinated contractions of the uterus that are characteristic of labor.

Therefore, the regulation of gap junction formation is a subject of considerable importance. Evidence has been obtained, by in vitro and in vivo studies of experimental animals, that progesterone prevents and estrogen promotes gap junction formation. It is known that protein synthesis is required for the formation of gap junctions. Prostaglandins also are believed to be important in gap junction formation. Inhibition of prostaglandin synthesis inhibits gap junction formation in vitro. Some prostanoids, *e.g.*, PGE_2, $PGF_{2\alpha}$, and thromboxanes and possibly endoperoxides, stimulate gap junction formation whereas others, e.g., prostacyclin (PGI_2), may inhibit gap junction formation. Interestingly (see p. 195), oxytocin does not act to increase gap junction formation (Garfield, 1983).

CELLULAR ORGANIZATION OF MYOMETRIUM

There are unique anatomical features of myometrial muscle (and other smooth muscle) compared with skeletal muscle. Huszar (1983) and Huszar and Roberts (1982) point out that these differences serve to create a peculiar advantage with respect to myometrial contractions and the successful delivery of the fetus. First, the degree of shortening in smooth muscle cells may be one order of magnitude greater than in striated muscle cells with contraction. Second, in smooth muscle cells, forces can be exerted in any direction, whereas the contraction force gener-

ated by skeletal muscle is such as always to be aligned with the axis of the muscle fibers; moreover, smooth muscle is not organized in the same manner as skeletal muscle. In myometrium the thick and thin bundles of filaments are found in long, random bundles throughout the cells. This arrangement facilitates the greater shortening and force-generating capacity of smooth muscle (Huszar, 1983). And there is the advantage that multidirectional force generation in smooth muscle permits versatility in expulsive force directionality that can come to bear irrespective of the lie or presentation of the fetus.

MOLECULAR REGULATION OF SMOOTH MUSCLE CONTRACTIONS

The protein of primary importance in muscle contraction is myosin (M_r about 500,000); the myosin molecule is about 1,600 angstrom units in length and is laid down in thick monofilaments. Functionally, there is a *"head"* and a *"tail"* part of myosin. The globular-shaped head portion is (1) the site of the actin-combining site, where the interaction of myosin and actin occurs and force is thereby generated, (2) the site of ATPase, where ATP is hydrolyzed and chemical energy is converted to physical force, and (3) the site of the low molecular weight (M_r about 20,000) myosin light chains, the phosphorylation of which is the key reaction in contractile regulation, *i.e.*, the actin–myosin interaction in smooth muscle.

In this context it is important to remember that calcium ion (Ca^{2+}) flux either from extracellular or intracellular stores is essential to the generation of muscular contraction. Ca^{2+} is sequestered in intracellular vesicles of the sacroplasmic reticulum. In smooth muscle the interaction of myosin and actin is regulated by enzymatic phosphorylation (or dephosphorylation) of the myosin light chains (Stull and colleagues, 1980).

Specifically the actin–myosin interaction in myometrial cells can take place only after phosphorylation of the myosin light chain. The phosphorylation of the myosin light chain is catalyzed by the enzyme *myosin light chain kinase*; importantly, this enzyme is activated by Ca^{2+} (Fig. 10–12). Agents that effect an increase in intracellular free Ca^{2+} concentration thus promote myometrial smooth muscle contraction. Calcium binds to calmodulin (a calcium-binding regulatory protein, which commonly modulates the action of calcium), which, in turn, binds to and activates myosin light chain kinase.

Circumstances that give rise to decreased intracellular free Ca^{2+} concentration favor relaxation. Dephosphorylation of the myosin light chain by the action of phosphatase also gives rise to muscle relaxation (Fig. 10–12). Actin and nonphosphorylated myosin do not interact. Agents that cause an increase in the intracellular concentration of cyclic adenosine monophosphate (cAMP) promote uterine relaxation. Such agents include

β-adrenergic agonists. It is believed that cAMP acts to cause a decrease in intracellular Ca^{2+}, although the exact mechanism is not defined. Alternatively, it has been proposed that phosphorylation of the enzyme myosin light chain kinase by cAMP-dependent protein kinase causes inactivation of this enzyme, and thereby the phosphorylation of myosin light chains is inhibited (Krall and Korenman, 1977). The decrease in activity of the phosphorylated enzyme is attributable to a decrease in the affinity for calmodulin; the association of calmodulin with myosin light chain kinase is mandatory for activity of this enzyme.

Therefore, it can be envisioned that the regulation of myometrial contractions at the cellular level is attributable to the action of myosin light chain kinase, which is modulated in large measure by calcium. On balance, the dephosphorylation of myosin light chain kinase by way of myosin light chain kinase phosphatase also must be taken into consideration. The relationships between these processes are illustrated diagrammatically in Figure 10–12. The activation of contraction is thus accomplished by way of the interaction of phosphorylated myosin and actin to give phosphorylated actomyosin. The biochemistry and physiology of smooth muscle contractility has been reviewed recently by Stull and associates (1988).

CERVIX

There are three principal structural components in the cervix: smooth muscle, collagen, and connective tissue, *i.e.*, the ground substance. In the ground substance important constituents of cervix, the glycosaminoglycans, *i.e.*, dermatan sulfate and hyaluronic acid, are formed. The smooth muscle content of cervix varies, from upward to downward, from 25 percent to only 6 percent. There is in the human, however, no apparent role for smooth muscle in the cervical "ripening" process; rather, this process seemingly involves changes that occur in collagen and connective tissue; thus, with "ripening," cervical flexibility increases as collagen and protein concentrations decrease.

The glycosaminoglycans also are believed to be important in the processes leading to cervical ripening. Thus, cervical ripening is believed to be associated with two principal events: (1) collagen breakdown or rearrangement of the collagen fibers and (2) an alteration in the relative amounts of the various glycosaminoglycans. Hyaluronic acid is a substance that is associated with the capacity of a tissue to retain water. Near term there is a striking increase in the relative amount of hyaluronic acid in cervix, together with a decrease in cervical dermatan sulfate.

REGULATORY FACTORS IN MYOMETRIAL CONTRACTIONS AND CERVICAL RIPENING

The role of hormones and other factors in the appearance of gap junctions between myometrial cells was discussed on page 210. There appears to be a unique response system whereby gap junctions in myometrial cells, activation of contractions, and cervical ripening can occur in a coordinated manner. Ultimately it seems that prostaglandins occupy a crucial role in these processes. Consider the following: PGE_2 and $PGF_{2\alpha}$ are potent stimuli of myometrial contractions and are believed to act to increase the concentration of intracellular free Ca^{2+}, a process that leads to activation of myosin light chain kinase, phosphorylation of myosin, and thereby, the interaction of phosphorylated myosin and actin (Carsten and Miller, 1983). At the same time PGE_2 and $PGF_{2\alpha}$ act to cause the rapid appearance of myometrial gap junctions, whereas prostacyclin inhibits gap

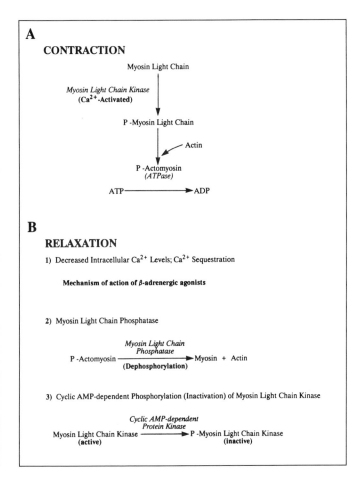

Figure 10–12. Metabolic regulation of smooth muscle contraction (**A**) and relaxation (**B**). Phosphorylation of myosin light chains by way of myosin light chain kinase (a reaction activated by Ca^{2+}) is essential for the association of myosin and actin to give rise to phosphorylated actomyosin, which is an enzyme that catalyzes the conversion of ATP to ADP, a reaction that gives rise to energy that can be converted to force in uterine contractions.

Relaxation is promoted (a) by sequestration of calcium in the sarcoplasmic reticulum, (b) by dephosphorylation of phosphorylated myosin by the action of phosphatase, and (c) by phosphorylation (inactivation) of myosin light chain kinase by a cAMP-dependent protein kinase. (*Illustration courtesy of Dr. L. Casey.*)

junction formation. PGE_2 and $PGF_{2\alpha}$ act to induce the maturational changes of cervical ripening, *i.e.*, activation of collagenase(s) and an alteration in the relative concentration of the glycosaminoglycans. In some species these same events can be recapitulated in response to an alteration in the effective endogenous estrogen-to-progesterone ratio by manipulations that favor estrogen, as reviewed by Huszar (1983). Yet other compounds may serve as active participants in the activation or orchestration of these coordinated events. For example, prostacyclin (PGI_2), which is produced in large amounts by uterine smooth muscle cells, may promote uterine relaxation; relaxin acts to facilitate cervical ripening while maintaining the uterus in a quiescent state, possibly by accelerating prostacyclin formation in myometrium (Casey and associates, personal communication). Much remains to be learned with respect to the biomolecular events of myometrial contractions, but much insight into the very fundamental biochemical aspects of these processes has been acquired in the past 25 years.

THREE STAGES OF LABOR

Customarily, labor (the second phase of parturition) is, and for good clinical reasons, divided into three separate stages.

The *first stage of labor* commences when uterine contractions (myometrial forces) of sufficient *frequency, intensity,* and *duration* to bring about readily demonstrable effacement and dilatation of the cervix are attained. The first stage of labor ends when the cervix is fully dilated, *i.e.*, when the cervix is sufficiently dilated (about 10 cm) to allow passage of the fetal head. The first stage of labor, therefore, is that stage in which *cervical effacement and dilatation* occurs.

The *second stage of labor* begins when dilatation of the cervix is complete and ends with delivery of the infant. The second stage of labor is the stage of *expulsion of the fetus.*

The *third stage of labor* begins with delivery of the infant and ends with the delivery of the placenta and fetal membranes. The third stage of labor is the stage of *separation and expulsion of the placenta.*

In addition to these classic three stages of labor, some obstetricians categorize a period of prelabor and a latent phase of labor (phase 1 of parturition) that precede active labor (stages 1, 2, and 3), which is the second phase of parturition. Hendricks (1970), for example, identified *prelabor* as the period of increased uterine activity that occurs for a few weeks before active labor. During this time the increased uterine activity is believed to facilitate softening of the cervix, some cervical effacement, slight-to-modest cervical dilatation, and expansion of the lower uterine segment, *viz.*, the time of uterine preparedness for labor. Friedman (1955) described a *latent phase of labor* that preceded active labor by several hours (see Chapter 18, p. 341). During the latent phase uterine contractions typically are infrequent, produce some discomfort, and may be irregular; nonetheless, these contractions apparently can generate sufficient force to facilitate slow effacement and dilatation if biochemical changes have occurred that lead to ripening and softening of the cervix.

Some obstetricians also designate a *fourth stage of labor,* which is identified as that period of an hour or so after delivery of the placenta, during which time myometrial contractions and retraction, along with vessel thrombosis, act effectively to control bleeding from the placental implantation site. This is the beginning of the third phase of parturition, which ultimately includes the involution of the uterus, returning this organ to the characteristic tissue of the nonpregnant state.

Prelabor, *i.e.*, the latent phase of labor (phase 1 of parturition), and the fourth stage of labor (phase 3 of parturition) lack the precision of definition and ease of identification that are characteristic of the three stages of active labor (phase 2 of parturition) but are of undoubted importance in successful parturition in women.

CLINICAL COURSE OF LABOR

"LIGHTENING"

A few weeks before the onset of labor, the abdomen of the pregnant woman commonly undergoes a change in shape. The fundal height decreases somewhat; at times this event is described by the mother as "The baby dropped." This phenomenon is the consequence of the development of a well-formed lower uterine segment, the descent of the fetal head to or even through the pelvic inlet, and to some degree to a reduction in the volume of amnionic fluid.

FALSE LABOR

For a variable time before the establishment of true or effective labor, women may experience so-called *false labor.* The uterine contractions of false labor are characterized by irregularity in occurrence and by brevity of duration; most often, the discomfort produced is confined to the lower abdomen and groin. In contrast, the discomfort produced by the uterine contractions that are characteristic of true labor begins first in the fundal region and then radiates over the uterus and through to the lower back.

Uterine irritability that causes discomfort but that does not represent true labor (in that cervical dilatation does not occur) may develop at any time during pregnancy. False labor is observed most commonly late in pregnancy and in parous women. It often stops spontaneously but may proceed rapidly to the effective contractions of true labor. Therefore, the report of relatively infrequent and short-lived, but uncomfortable, uterine contractions cannot be dismissed summarily. All too frequently when this is done, delivery takes place without benefit of the assistance of professional personnel or facilities essential for optimal care of the mother and fetus-infant.

"SHOW"

A rather dependable sign of the impending onset of labor (provided no rectal or vaginal examination has been performed in the preceding 48 hours) is "show" or "bloody show," which consists of the discharge from the vagina of a small amount of blood-tinged mucus, representing the extrusion of the plug of mucus that was filling the cervical canal during pregnancy. "Show" is a late sign, for labor usually ensues during the next several hours to a few days. Normally, only a few drops of blood escape with the mucus plug; more substantial bleeding is suggestive of an abnormal condition.

CHARACTERISTICS OF UTERINE CONTRACTIONS IN LABOR

Unique among physiological muscular contractions, those of labor are painful. Therefore, the common designation in many languages for such a contraction is "pain." The cause of the pain is not known definitely, but several hypotheses have been suggested, as follow: (1) hypoxia of the contracted myometrium (as in angina pectoris), (2) compression of nerve ganglia in the cervix and lower uterus by the tightly interlocking muscle bundles, (3) stretching of the cervix during dilatation, and (4) stretching of the overlying peritoneum. Compression of nerve ganglia in the cervix and lower uterine segment by the contracting myometrium is an especially attractive hypothesis, because paracervical infiltration with a local anesthetic drug typically produces appreciable relief of pain during subsequent uterine contractions (see Chap. 17, p. 335).

Uterine contractions are involuntary and for the most part independent of extrauterine control. Neural blockage from caudal or epidural analgesia, if initiated quite early in labor, is sometimes associated with a reduction in the frequency and intensity of uterine contractions, but not after labor is well established. Moreover, in paraplegic women, there are normal, though painless, contractions as in women after bilateral lumbar sympathectomy. Thus far, attempts to initiate labor in women by electrical stimulation have been only partially successful (Theobald, 1968).

Ivy and co-workers (1931) believed that there are *pacemakers* in the uterus that act to initiate uterine contractions and thereby control the rhythmicity of uterine contractions. As pointed out by Carsten (1968), however, in a comprehensive review of myometrial composition, growth, and activity, the cells that participate in the pacemaker activities, unlike those of the heart, do not differ anatomically from the surrounding myocytes. Pacemaker activity is not confined to a specific site (Wolfs and van Leeuwen, 1979); only a group of highly excitable myometrial cells are required, and uterine activity may commence in a variety of sites. The contractile rhythm of one pacemaker may be such as to reinforce or even to block that of another. Because electric current does not flow easily from one myometrial cell to another, activation of individual myometrial cell membranes almost certainly serves to propagate the impulse throughout the myometrium, possibly by way of myometrial cell gap junctions.

In women, the pacemaker sites in the uterus most often appear to be near the uterotubal junctions.

Mechanical stretching of the cervix enhances uterine activity in several species, including the human. This phenomenon has been referred to as the *Ferguson reflex*. The exact mechanism by which mechanical dilatation of the cervix causes increased myometrial contractility is not clear. Release of oxytocin was suggested as the cause by Ferguson (1941), but this is not proven. Manipulation of the cervix causes a rapid and striking increase in prostaglandin $F_{2\alpha}$ metabolites in blood (Mitchell, 1976).

The interval between contractions diminishes gradually from about 10 minutes at the onset of the first stage of labor to as little as 1 minute or less in the second stage. Periods of relaxation between contractions, however, are essential to the welfare of the fetus, because unremitting contraction of the uterus may interfere with uteroplacental blood flow of sufficient magnitude to produce fetal hypoxia. In the active phase of labor, the duration of each contraction ranges from 30 to 90 seconds, averaging about 1 minute. There is appreciable variability in the intensity of uterine contractions during apparently normal labor, as emphasized by Schulman and Romney (1970). They recorded the amnionic fluid pressures generated by uterine contractions in women during spontaneous labor; the pressures averaged about 40 mm Hg, but varied from 20 to 60 mm Hg.

DIFFERENTIATION OF UTERINE ACTIVITY

With labor, the uterus differentiates into two distinct parts. The actively contracting upper segment becomes thicker as labor advances; the lower portion, comprising the lower segment of the uterus and the cervix, is relatively passive compared with the upper segment, and it develops into a much thinner-walled passage for the fetus. The lower uterine segment is analogous to a greatly expanded and thinned-out isthmus of the uterus of nonpregnant women, the formation of which is not solely a phenomenon of labor. The lower segment develops gradually as pregnancy progresses and then thins remarkably during labor (Figs. 10–13 and 10–14). By abdominal palpation, even be-

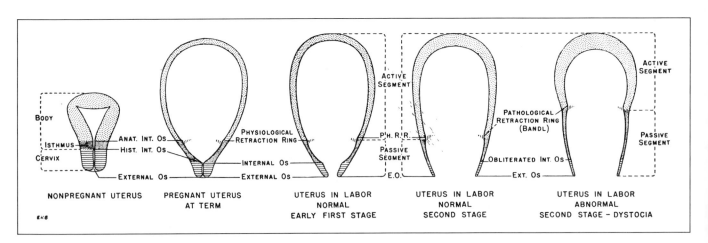

Figure 10–13. Sequence of development of the segments and rings in the uterus in pregnant women at term and in labor. Note comparison between the uterus of a nonpregnant woman, the uterus at term, and the uterus during labor. The passive lower segment of the uterine body is derived from the isthmus; the physiological retraction ring develops at the junction of the upper and lower uterine segments. The pathological retraction ring develops from the physiological ring. Anat. Int. Os = anatomical internal os; Hist. Int. Os = histological internal os; Ph.R.R. = physiological retraction ring; E.O. = external os.

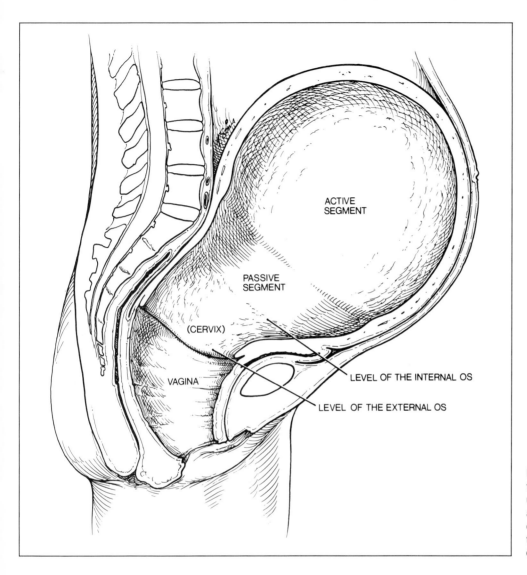

ACTIVE
SEGMENT

PASSIVE
SEGMENT

(CERVIX)

VAGINA

LEVEL OF THE INTERNAL OS

LEVEL OF THE EXTERNAL OS

Figure 10–14. The uterus at the time of vaginal delivery. The active upper segment of the uterus retracts about the fetus as the fetus descends through the birth canal. In the passive lower segment, there is considerably less myometrial tone.

fore rupture of the membranes, the two segments can be differentiated during a contraction. The upper uterine segment is quite firm or hard, whereas the consistency of the lower uterine segment is much less firm. The former represents the actively contracting part of the uterus; the latter is the distended, normally much more passive, portion.

If the entire sac of uterine musculature, including the lower uterine segment and cervix, were to contract simultaneously and with equal intensity, the net expulsive force would be decreased markedly. Therein lies the importance of the division of the uterus into an actively contracting upper segment and a more passive lower segment that differ not only anatomically but also physiologically. The upper segment contracts, retracts, and expels the fetus; in response to the force of the contractions of the upper segment, the ripened lower uterine segment and cervix dilate and thereby form a greatly expanded, thinned-out muscular and fibromuscular tube through which the fetus can pass.

The myometrium of the upper uterine segment does not relax to its original length after contractions; rather, it becomes relatively fixed at a shorter length, the tension, however, remaining the same as before the contraction. The purpose of the ability of the upper portion of the uterus, or active segment, to contract down on its diminishing contents with myometrial ten-

sion remaining constant is to take up slack, *i.e,* to maintain the advantage gained with respect to expulsion of the fetus, and to maintain the uterine musculature in firm contact with the intrauterine contents. As the consequence of retraction, each successive contraction commences where its predecessor left off, so that the upper part of the uterine cavity becomes slightly smaller with each successive contraction. Because of the successive shortening of its muscular fibers with each contraction, the upper uterine segment (active segment, Fig. 10–13) becomes progressively thickened throughout the first and second stages of labor and tremendously thickened immediately after the birth of the baby. The phenomenon of retraction of the upper uterine segment is contingent upon a decrease in the volume of its contents. For its contents to be diminished, particularly early in labor when the entire uterus is virtually a closed sac with only a minute opening at the cervix, there is a requirement that the musculature of the lower segment stretch, permitting increasingly more of the intrauterine contents to occupy the lower segment. Indeed, the upper segment retracts only to the extent that the lower segment distends and the cervix dilates.

The relaxation of the lower uterine segment is by no means complete relaxation, but rather the opposite of retraction. The fibers of the lower segment become stretched with each con-

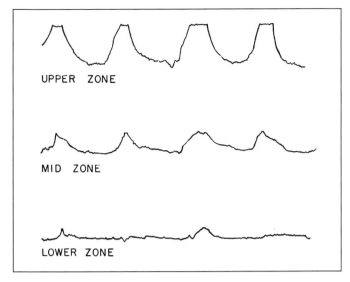

Figure 10–15. Uterine contractions in various parts of the uterus recorded by Reynolds tokodynamometer. The lower zone probably corresponds to the lower uterine segment. The woman studied was a primigravida in active labor; the cervix was 5 cm dilated, and contractions were occurring at about 3-minute intervals. The original tracings have been inked over for clearer reproduction. (*From Reynolds and co-workers: Obstet Gynecol Surv 3:629, 1948.*)

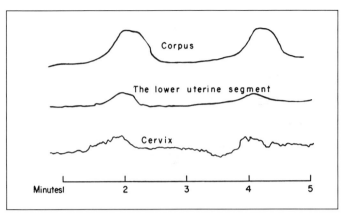

Figure 10–16. Uterine contractions in various parts of the uterus recorded by Karlson by means of intrauterine receptors. The woman studied was in early labor, but from the time this tracing was made, progress of labor was rapid. To permit clearer reproduction, the background of the original record has been eliminated and the tracings have been inked over. (*Modified from Karlson: Acta Obstet Gynecol Scand 28:209, 1949.*)

traction of the upper segment, after which these are not returned to the previous length but rather remain relatively fixed at the longer length; the tension, however, remains essentially the same as before. The musculature still manifests tone, still resists stretch, and still contracts somewhat on stimulation.

The successive lengthening of the muscular fibers in the lower uterine segment, as labor progresses, is accompanied by thinning, normally to only a few millimeters in its thinnest part. As a result of the thinning of the lower uterine segment and the concomitant thickening of the upper, the boundary between the two is marked by a ridge on the inner uterine surface, the *physiological retraction ring*. When the thinning of the lower uterine segment is extreme, as in obstructed labor, the ring is very prominent, forming, in extreme cases, a *pathological retraction ring* (the ring of Bandl), an abnormal condition, the nature of which is illustrated in Figure 10–13, and one that is discussed further in Chapter 18 (p. 347).

From quantitative measurements of the difference in behavior of the upper and lower parts of the uterus during normal labor it was found that there normally is a gradient of diminishing physiological activity from the fundus to the cervix. Several ingenious devices have been used to evaluate uterine forces, including the tokodynamometer, intrauterine receptors, and intramyometrial catheters.

In the tokodynamometer three strain gauges set in heavy brass ring mountings are employed; the three gauges may be placed anywhere on the abdomen. When the uterus contracts, the increased convexity of the local arc of the uterus underlying the ring pushes upward on the gauge and applies a strain to its elements proportional to the local force of the uterine contraction. A record is obtained electrometrically, an example of which is shown in Figure 10–15. It is evident from these tracings that the intensity of each contraction is greater in the fundal zone than in the midzone and greater in the midzone than lower

down. Equally noteworthy is the differential in the duration of the contractions; those in the midzone are much briefer than those above, whereas the contractions in the lower zone are extremely brief and sometimes absent. This subsidence of contractions in the midzone, at a time when the upper zone is still contracting, is indicative that the upper part of the corpus, throughout a substantial portion of each contraction, comes to exert pressure caudally on the more relaxed parts of the uterus. Occasionally, when labor is not progressing, this gradient is absent, and both the intensity and the duration of the contractions may be the same in all three zones.

These findings of Reynolds (1949) were confirmed by Karlson (1949) through the use of an entirely different apparatus. By his technique, the internal pressure in the uterus at any point was measured by means of so-called receptors (metal capsules about 12 mm long with a diameter of 4.5 mm), in the middle of which is a small aperture. On the inner side of this aperture there is a membrane that is sensitive to pressure. Pressure exerted against the window is carried and registered electrometrically; an example of one of Karlson's tracings is shown in Figure 10–16. Here again, there is a gradient of diminishing activity from the fundus to the lower uterine segment. Karlson's other tracings, like those of Reynolds, are indicative that in the absence of this gradient, that is, when the intensity of contraction of the lower segment equals or exceeds that of the fundus, cervical dilatation may cease. Similar results were obtained by Caldeyro-Barcia and associates (1950), who inserted either small intramyometrial balloons or open-ended catheters at various levels and recorded the pressures during contractions.

CHANGE IN UTERINE SHAPE

Each contraction produces an elongation of the uterine ovoid with a concomitant decrease in horizontal diameters. By virtue of this change in shape, there are important effects on the process of labor:

1. The decrease in horizontal diameter produces a straightening of the fetal vertebral column, pressing its upper pole firmly against the fundus of the uterus, whereas the

lower pole is thrust farther downward and into the pelvis. The lengthening of the fetal ovoid thus produced has been estimated as between 5 and 10 cm. The pressure so exerted is known as fetal axis pressure.

2. With lengthening of the uterus, the longitudinal fibers are drawn taut; since the lower segment and cervix are the only parts of the uterus that are flexible, these are pulled upward over the lower pole of the fetus. This effect on the musculature of the lower segment and on the cervix is an important factor in cervical dilatation. The round ligaments also contain smooth muscle, which can contract and pull the uterus forward. These actions, however, are not essential for successful labor and delivery.

OTHER FORCES CONCERNED IN LABOR

INTRA-ABDOMINAL PRESSURE

After the cervix is dilated fully, the force that is principally important in the expulsion of the fetus is that produced by increased intra-abdominal pressure created by contraction of the abdominal muscles simultaneously with forced respiratory efforts with the glottis closed. In obstetrical jargon this usually is referred to as pushing. The nature of the force produced is similar to that involved in defecation, but usually the intensity is much greater. The important role that is served by intra-abdominal pressure in fetal expulsion is most clearly attested to by the labors of women who are paraplegic. Such women suffer no pain, although the uterus may contract vigorously. Cervical dilatation, in large measure the result of uterine contractions acting on a ripened cervix, proceeds normally, but expulsion of the infant is rarely possible except when the woman is instructed to bear down and can do so at the time that the obstetrician identifies uterine contractions. Although increased intra-abdominal pressure is required for the spontaneous completion of labor, it is futile until the cervix is fully dilated. In other words, it is a necessary auxiliary to uterine contractions in the second stage of labor, but pushing accomplishes little in the first stage, except for fatigue of the mother.

Intra-abdominal pressure also may be important in the third stage of labor, especially if the parturient is unattended. After the placenta has separated, its spontaneous expulsion is aided by the mother's bearing down, *i.e.*, by an increase in intra-abdominal pressure.

RESISTANCE

Mechanically, work is the generation of motion against resistance. Labor is work. The forces involved in labor are those of the uterus and the abdomen, which act to expel the fetus, and those that must overcome the resistance offered by the cervix to dilatation and the friction created by the birth canal during passage of the presenting part. In addition, forces of resistance may be exerted by the muscles of the pelvic floor. The work involved in labor, according to Gemzell and colleagues (1957), is only a fraction of the maximal functional capacity of the normal woman.

CHANGES INDUCED IN THE CERVIX

The effective force of the first stage of labor is the uterine contraction, which, in turn, exerts hydrostatic pressure through the membranes against the cervix and lower uterine segment. In the

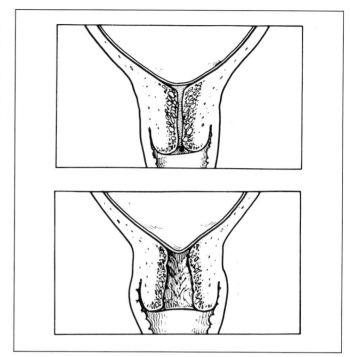

Figure 10–17. Cervix near the end of pregnancy but before labor. Top, primigravida; bottom, multipara.

absence of intact membranes, the presenting part is forced directly against the cervix and lower uterine segment. As the result of the action of these forces, two fundamental changes, *i.e.*, effacement and dilatation, take place in the previously ripened cervix.

THE MECHANISM OF CERVICAL EFFACEMENT

Effacement ("obliteration" or "taking up") of the cervix is the shortening of the cervical canal from a structure approximately 2 cm in length to one in which the canal is replaced by a mere circular orifice with almost paper-thin edges. This process takes place from above downward; it occurs as the muscular fibers in the vicinity of the internal os are pulled upward, or "taken up," into the lower segment, while the condition of the external os remains temporarily unchanged. As illustrated in Figures 10–17 through 10–20, the edges of the internal os are drawn upward several centimeters to become, functionally, part of the lower uterine segment. Effacement may be compared with a funneling process in which the whole length of a narrow cylinder is converted into a very obtuse, flaring funnel with only a small circular orifice for an outlet. As the result of increased myometrial activity during phase 1 of parturition, appreciable effacement of the ripened cervix is sometimes attained before true labor begins. Such effacement usually facilitates expulsion of the mucus plug from the cervical canal as the canal shortens.

THE MECHANISM OF CERVICAL DILATATION

In order for the head of the average fetus at term to pass through the cervix, the canal must dilate to a diameter of about 10 cm. When sufficient dilatation is attained for the fetal head to pass through, the cervix is said to be completely dilated or fully dilated.

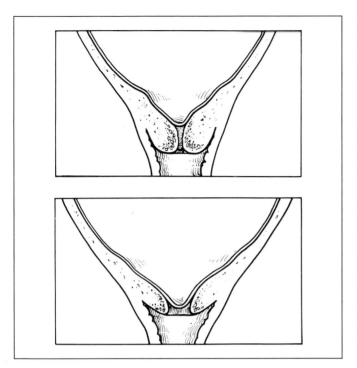

Figure 10–18. Beginning effacement of cervix. Note dilatation of internal os and funnel-shaped cervical canal. Top, primigravida; bottom, multipara.

Compared with the body of the uterus, the lower uterine segment and cervix are regions of lesser resistance. Therefore, during a contraction, these structures are subjected to distension, in the course of which a centrifugal pull is exerted on the cervix (Figs. 10–21 to 10–23). As the uterine contractions act to cause pressure on the membranes, the hydrostatic action of the amnionic sac, in turn, dilates the cervical canal in the manner of a wedge. In the absence of intact membranes, the pressure of the presenting part against the cervix and lower uterine segment is similarly effective. Early rupture of the membranes ("dry birth") does not retard cervical dilatation so long as the presenting part of the fetus is positioned so as to exert pressure against the cervix and lower uterine segment.

The decidua of the lower uterine segment is thin and poorly developed. The slightest movement of the underlying muscle, therefore, might allow the fetal membranes to slip back and forth over the decidua. This loosening of the membranes in the lower segment is a normal feature of early labor and prerequisite to successful cervical dilatation. Membranes that slide readily over the lower segment and partly through the cervix are much more efficacious dilators than are those that are more firmly attached.

There may be no fetal descent during cervical effacement, but as a rule, the station of the presenting part descends somewhat as the cervix dilates. During the second stage descent of the fetal presenting part typically occurs rather slowly but steadily in nulliparas. In multiparas, however, particularly those of high parity, descent may be very rapid.

PATTERN OF CERVICAL DILATATION

Friedman (1978), in his treatise on labor, stated correctly, *"The clinical features of uterine contractions—namely, frequency, intensity, and duration—cannot be relied upon as measures of progression in labor nor as indices of normality. . . . Except for cervical dilatation and fetal descent, none of the clinical features of the parturient patient (woman) appears to be useful in assessing labor progression."* The pattern of cervical dilatation that takes place during the course of normal labor takes on the shape of a sigmoid curve. As

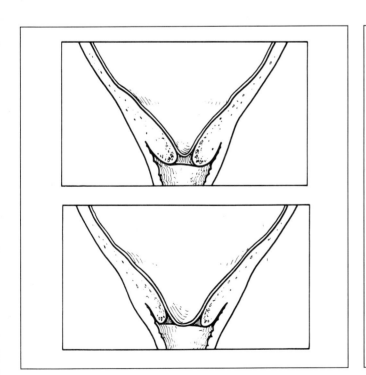

Figure 10–19. Further effacement of cervix. Top, primigravida; bottom, multipara.

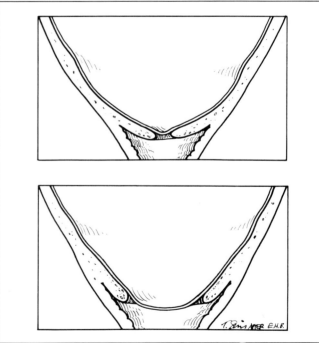

Figure 10–20. Cervical canal obliterated; *i.e.*, the cervix is completely effaced. Top, primigravida; bottom, multipara.

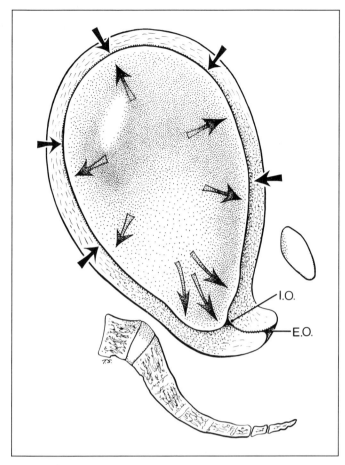

Figure 10–21. Hydrostatic action of membranes in effecting cervical effacement and dilatation. In the absence of intact membranes, the presenting part, applied to the cervix and forming the lower uterine segments, acts similarly. In this and the next two illustrations, note changing relations of the external os (E.O.) and internal os (I.O.).

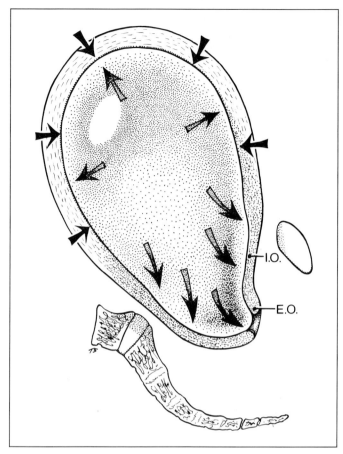

Figure 10–22. Hydrostatic action of membranes at completion of effacement.

depicted in Figure 10–24, two phases of cervical dilatation can be defined: the latent phase and the active phase. The active phase has been subdivided further as the acceleration phase, phase of maximum slope, and the deceleration phase (Friedman, 1978). The duration of the latent phase is more variable and subject to sensitive changes by extraneous factors and by sedation (prolongation of latent phase) and myometrial stimulation (shortening of latent phase). The duration of the latent phase has little bearing on the subsequent course of labor, whereas the characteristics of the accelerated phase usually are predictive of the outcome of a particular labor. Friedman (1978) considers the maximum slope as a "good measure of the overall efficiency of the machine," whereas the nature of the deceleration phase is more reflective of fetopelvic relationships. The completion of cervical dilatation during the active phase of labor is accomplished by cervical retraction about the presenting part of the fetus. After complete cervical dilatation, the second stage of labor commences; thereafter, only progressive descent of the presenting fetal part is available to assess the progress of labor.

PATTERN OF DESCENT

In many nulliparas engagement of the fetal head is accomplished prior to the onset of labor, and further descent does not occur until late in labor. In others in whom engagement of the fetal head initially is not so extensive, further descent occurs

during the first stage of labor. In the descent pattern of normal labor, a typical hyperbolic curve is formed when the station of the fetal head is plotted as a function of the duration of labor. Active descent usually takes place after cervical dilatation has progressed for some time. In nulliparas increased rates of descent are observed ordinarily during the phase of maximum slope of cervical dilatation. At this time, the speed of descent increases to a maximum (Friedman, 1978), and this maximal rate of descent is maintained until the presenting fetal part reaches the perineal floor.

FIRST AND SECOND STAGES OF LABOR

Based upon the findings of a scholarly analysis of the labor patterns of a large number of women, Friedman (1978) also sought to select criteria that would delimit normal labor and thus enable us to identify significant abnormalities of labor. The limits, admittedly arbitrary, appear to be logical and clinically useful.

    The group of women studied were nulliparas and multiparas with no fetopelvic disproportion, no fetal malposition or malpresentation, no multiple pregnancy, and none treated with heavy sedation or conduction analgesia, oxytocin, or operative intervention; all had a normal pelvis and were at term with a vertex presentation and delivered average-sized infants. From

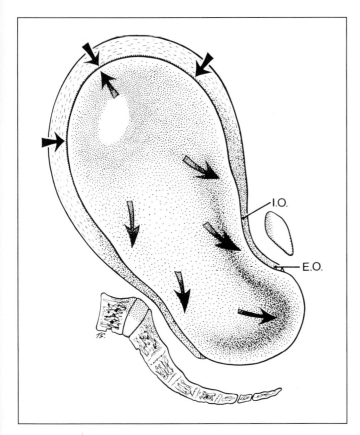

Figure 10–23. Hydrostatic action of membranes at full cervical dilatation.

these studies Friedman developed the concept of three functional divisions of labor—preparatory, dilatational, and pelvic—to describe the physiological objectives of each division (Fig. 10–25). He found that the preparatory division of labor may be sensitive to sedation and conduction analgesia. Although little cervical dilatation occurs during this time, considerable changes take place in the ground substance, *i.e.*, collagen and other connective tissue components, of the cervix (Danforth and colleagues, 1960). The dilatational division of labor, during which time dilatation is occurring at its most rapid rate, is principally unaffected by sedation or conduction analgesia. The pelvic division of labor commences with the deceleration phase of cervical dilatation. The classic mechanisms of labor that involve the cardinal movements of the fetus take place principally during the pelvic division of labor. In actual practice, however, the time of onset of the pelvic division of labor is seldom clearly identifiable separate from the dilatational division of labor. Moreover, the rate of cervical dilatation does not always decelerate as full dilatation is approached; in fact, it may accelerate.

RUPTURE OF MEMBRANES

Spontaneous rupture of the membranes most often occurs sometime during the course of active labor. Typically rupture of the membranes is evident by a sudden gush of a variable quantity of normally clear or slightly turbid, nearly colorless fluid. Less frequently the membranes remain intact until the time of delivery of the infant. If by chance the membranes remain intact until completion of delivery, the fetus is born surrounded by them, and the portion covering the head of the newborn infant is sometimes referred to as the *caul*.

CHANGES IN THE VAGINA AND PELVIC FLOOR

The birth canal is supported and is closed functionally by a number of layers of tissues that together form the pelvic floor.

Figure 10–24. Composite of the average dilatation curve for nulliparous labor based on analysis of the data derived from the patterns traced by a large, nearly consecutive, series of gravidas. The first stage is divided into a relatively flat latent phase and a rapidly progressive active phase. In the active phase, there are three identifiable component parts: an acceleration phase, a linear phase of maximum slope, and a deceleration phase. (*Illustration courtesy of Dr. L. Casey; redrawn from Friedman: Labor: Clinical Evaluation and Management, 2nd ed. New York: Appleton, 1978.*)

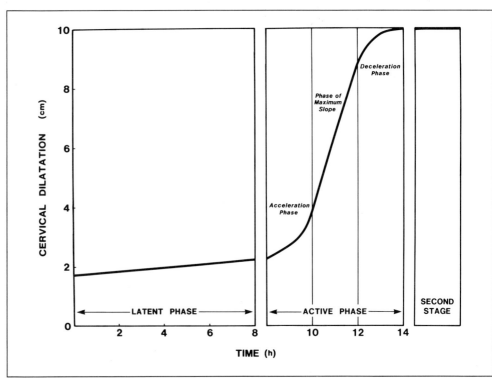

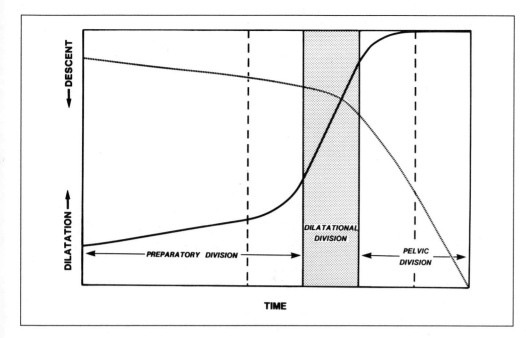

Figure 10–25. Labor course divided functionally on the basis of expected evolution of the dilatation and descent curves into (1) a preparatory division, including latent and acceleration phases, (2) a dilatational division, occupying the phase of maximum slope of dilatation, and (3) a pelvic division, encompassing both deceleration phase and second stage while concurrent with the phase of maximum slope of descent. (*Illustration courtesy Dr. L. Casey; redrawn from Friedman: Labor: Clinical Evaluation and Management, 2nd ed. New York: Appleton, 1978.*)

From within outward these tissues are (1) peritoneum, (2) subperitoneal connective tissue, (3) internal pelvic fascia, (4) levator ani and coccygeus muscles, (5) external pelvic fascia, (6) superficial muscles and fascia, (7) subcutaneous tissue, and (8) skin.

ANATOMY OF THE PELVIC FLOOR

Of these structures the most important are the levator ani and the fascia covering its upper and lower surfaces, which for practical purposes may be considered as the pelvic floor (Fig. 40–6, p. 878). This muscle (or group of muscles) closes the lower end of the pelvic cavity as a diaphragm and thereby a concave upper and a convex lower surface is presented, as illustrated in Figures 10–26 and 10–27. On either side the levator ani consists of a pubic and iliac portion. The former is a band 2 to 2.5 cm in width arising from the horizontal ramus of the pubis, 3 to 4 cm below its upper margin, and 1 to 1.5 cm from the symphysis pubis. Its fibers pass backward to encircle the rectum and possibly give off a few fibers that pass behind the vagina. The greater, or iliac, portion of the muscle arises on either side of the pelvis from the white line (the tendinous arch of the pelvic fascia) and from the ischial spine at a distance of about 5 cm below the margin of the pelvic inlet. The greater part of the muscle passes backward and unites with that from the other side of the rectum; the posterior portions meet in the tendinous raphe in front of the coccyx, with the most posterior fibers attached to the bone itself. The posterior and lateral portions of the pelvic floor, which are not filled out by the levator ani, are occupied by the piriformis and coccygeus muscles on either side (Fig. 40–6, p. 878).

The levator ani varies from 3 to 5 mm in thickness, though its margins encircling the rectum and vagina are somewhat thicker. During pregnancy the levator ani usually undergoes hypertrophy. By vaginal examination the internal margin of the muscle can be felt as a thick band that extends backward from the pubis and encircles the vagina about 2 cm above the hymen. On contraction the levator ani draws both the rectum and vagina forward and upward in the direction of the symphysis pubis and thereby acts to close the vagina, for the more superficial muscles of the perineum are too delicate to serve more than an accessory function.

The internal pelvic fascia, which forms the upper covering of the levator ani, is attached to the margin of the pelvic inlet, where it is joined by the fascia of the iliac fossa and by the transverse fascia of the obturator internus and is attached firmly to the periosteum covering the lateral wall of the pelvis. The white line is indicative of its point of deflection from the periosteum. From there the internal pelvic fascia spreads out over the upper surface of the levator ani and coccygeus muscles.

The inferior fascial covering of the pelvic diaphragm is divided into two parts by a line drawn between the ischial tuberosities. The posterior portion consists of a single layer, which, taking its origin from the sacrosciatic ligament and the ischial tuberosity, passes up over the inner surface of the ischial bones and the obturator internus to the white line, in the formation of which it takes part. From this tendinous structure it is reflected at an acute angle over the inferior surface of the levator ani; the space induced between the latter and the lateral pelvic wall forms the *ischiorectal fossa*. The structure filling out the triangular space between the pubic arch and a line joining the ischial tuberosities is known as the *urogenital diaphragm*, which, exclusive of skin and subcutaneous fat, consists principally of three layers of fascia: (1) the deep perineal fascia, which covers the anterior portion of the inferior surface of the levator ani muscle and is continuous with the fascia just described, (2) the middle perineal fascia, which is separated from the former by a narrow space in which are situated the pubic vessels and nerves, and (3) the superficial perineal fascia, which, together with the layer just described, forms a compartment in which the superficial perineal muscles lie, with the exception of the sphincter ani, the rami of the clitoris, the vestibular bulbs, and the vulvovaginal glands (see Fig. 40–6, p. 878).

The superficial perineal muscles are comprised of the bulbocavernosus, the ischiocavernosus, and the superficial transverse perineal muscles. These muscles are delicately formed and are of no major obstetrical importance except that the su-

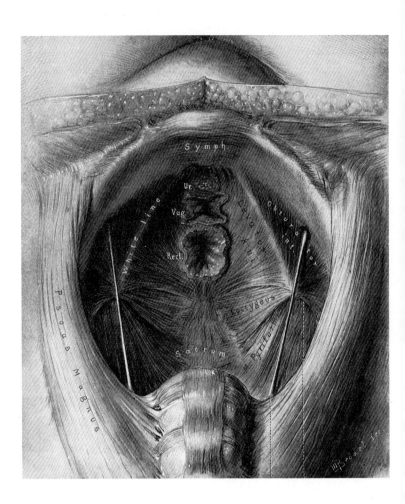

Figure 10–26. The pelvic floor seen from above. Uterus, tubes, ovaries, peritoneum, supporting ligaments, and internal fascial coverings have been removed. Symph = symphysis; Ur = urethra; Vag = vagina; Rect = rectum (*From Kelly: Operative Gynecology. New York: Appleton, 1906.*)

perficial transverse perineal muscles are always torn in the case of perineal lacerations.

In the first stage of labor the membranes and presenting part of the fetus serve a role in dilating the upper portion of the vagina. After the membranes have ruptured, however, the changes in the pelvic floor are caused entirely by pressure that is exerted by the presenting part of the fetus. The most marked change consists of the stretching of the fibers of the levator ani muscles and the thinning of the central portion of the perineum, which becomes transformed from a wedge-shaped mass of tis-

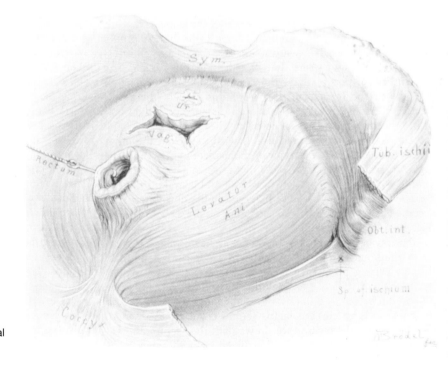

Figure 10–27. The deep muscles of the pelvic floor seen from below. Sym = symphysis; Ur = urethra; Vag = vagina; Sp. of Ischium = ischial spine; Obt. int. = obturator internus muscle; Tub. ischii = ischial tuberosity.

sue 5 cm in thickness to, in the absence of an episiotomy, a thin almost transparent membranous structure that is less than 1 cm in thickness. When the perineum is distended maximally, the anus becomes dilated markedly and presents an opening that varies from 2 to 3 cm in diameter and through which the anterior wall of the rectum bulges.

The extraordinary number and size of the blood vessels that supply the vagina and pelvic floor is such as to cause a great increase in the amount of blood loss when the tissues are torn.

THIRD STAGE OF LABOR

The third stage of labor, which begins immediately after delivery of the fetus, involves the separation and expulsion of the placenta.

THE PHASE OF PLACENTAL SEPARATION

As the baby is born, the uterus spontaneously contracts down on its diminishing contents. Normally, by the time the infant is completely delivered, the uterine cavity is nearly obliterated and the organ consists of an almost solid mass of muscle, the walls of which are several centimeters thick above the lower segment, and the fundus of which lies just below the level of the umbilicus. This sudden diminution in uterine size inevitably is accompanied by a decrease in the area of the placental implantation site (Fig. 10–28). In order for the placenta to accommodate itself to this reduced area, it increases in thickness, but because of limited placental elasticity, it is forced to buckle. The resulting tension causes the weakest layer of the decidua—the spongy layer, or decidua spongiosa—to give way, and cleavage takes place at that site. Therefore, separation of the placenta results primarily from a disproportion created between the unchanged size of the placenta and the reduced size of the underlying implantation site. During cesarean section, this phenomenon may be observed directly when the placenta is implanted posteriorly.

Cleavage of the placenta is facilitated greatly by the nature of the loose structure of the spongy decidua, which may be likened to the row of perforations between postage stamps. As

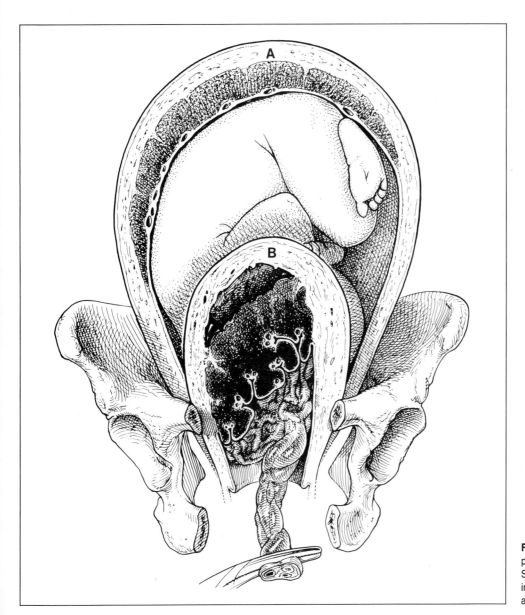

Figure 10–28. Diminution in size of placental site after birth of baby. **A.** Spatial relations before birth of the infant. **B.** Placental spatial relations after birth of the infant.

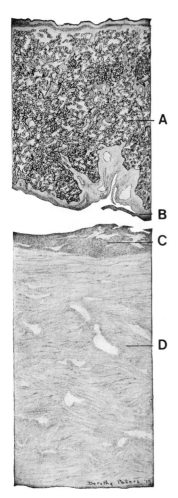

Figure 10–29. Separation of placenta with cleavage of the decidua. **A.** Placenta. **B.** Decidua cast off with placenta. **C.** Decidua retained in utero. **D.** Myometrium.

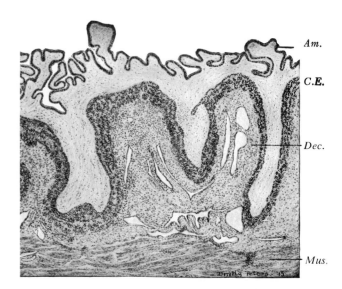

Figure 10–30. Folding of membranes as uterine cavity decreases in size. Am. = amnion; C.E. = epithelium of chorion laeve; Dec. = decidua vera; Mus. = myometrium.

separation proceeds, a hematoma forms between the separating placenta and the remaining decidua. Formation of the hematoma usually is the result, rather than the cause, of the separation, because in some cases bleeding is negligible. The hematoma may, however, accelerate the process of cleavage. Since the separation of the placenta is through the spongy layer of the decidua (see Chap. 4, p. 53), part of the decidua is cast off with the placenta, whereas the rest remains attached to the myometrium (Fig. 10–29). The amount of decidual tissue retained at the placental site varies.

Most investigators have found that placental separation occurs within a very few minutes after delivery. Brandt (1933) and others, based on results obtained in combined clinical and radiographic studies, supported the idea that since the periphery of the placenta is probably the most adherent portion, separation usually begins elsewhere. Occasionally some degree of separation begins even before the third stage of labor commences, probably accounting for certain cases of fetal distress that occur just before expulsion of the infant.

SEPARATION OF AMNIOCHORION

The great decrease in the surface area of the cavity of the uterus simultaneously causes the fetal membranes (amniochorion) and

the parietal decidua to be thrown into innumerable folds that increase the thickness of the layer from less than 1 mm to 3 to 4 mm. The lining of the uterus, as illustrated in Figure 10–30, early in the third stage, indicates that much of the parietal layer of decidua vera is included between the folds of the festooned amnion–chorion laeve.

The membranes usually remain *in situ* until the separation of the placenta is nearly completed. These are then peeled off the uterine wall, partly by the further contraction of the myometrium and partly by traction that is exerted by the separated placenta, which lies in the flabby lower uterine segment or in the upper portion of the vagina. The body of the uterus at that time normally forms an almost solid mass of muscle, the anterior and posterior walls of which, each measuring 4 to 5 cm in thickness, lie in close apposition such that the uterine cavity is almost obliterated.

THE PHASE OF PLACENTAL EXTRUSION

After the placenta has separated from its implantation site, the pressure exerted upon it by the uterine walls causes it to slide downward into the flaccid lower uterine segment or the upper part of the vagina. In some cases the placenta may be expelled from those locations by an increase in abdominal pressure, but women in the recumbent position frequently cannot expel the placenta spontaneously. An artificial means of completing the third stage is therefore generally required. The usual method employed is alternately to compress and elevate the fundus, while exerting minimal traction on the umbilical cord (see Chap. 16, p. 319)

MECHANISMS OF PLACENTAL EXTRUSION

When the central, or usual, type of placental separation occurs, the retroplacental hematoma is believed to push the placenta toward the uterine cavity, first the central portion and then the rest. The placenta, thus inverted and weighted with the hematoma, then descends. Since the surrounding membranes are still attached to the decidua, the placenta can descend only by dragging after it the membranes, which peel off its periphery. Consequently the sac formed by the membranes is inverted, with the glistening fetal surface of the placenta presenting at the vulva. The retroplacental hematoma either follows the placenta or is found within the inverted sac. In this process, known as *the mechanism of Schultze* of placental expulsion, blood from the placental site pours into the inverted sac, not escaping externally until after extrusion of the placenta.

The other method of placental extrusion is known as *the Duncan mechanism*, in which separation of the placenta occurs first at the periphery, with the result that blood collects between the membranes and the uterine wall and escapes from the vagina. In this circumstance the placenta descends to the vagina sideways, and the maternal surface appears first at the vulva.

REFERENCES

Albert DH, Snyder F: Biosynthesis of 1-alkyl-2-acetyl-*sn*-glycero-3-phosphocholine (platelet activating factor) from 1-alkyl-2-acyl-*sn*-glycero-3-phosphocholine by rat alveolar macrophages. Phospholipase A_2 and acetyl transferase activities during phagocytosis and ionophore stimulation. J Biol Chem 258:97, 1983

Anderson ABM, Turnbull AC: Comparative aspects of factors involved in the onset of labor in ovine and human pregnancy. In Klopper A, Gardner J (eds): Endocrine Factors in Labour. London, Cambridge University Press, 1973, p 141

Angle M, Maki N, Johnston JM: Bioactive metabolites of glycerophospholipid metabolism in relation to parturition. In McNellis D, Challis JRG, MacDonald PC, Nathanielsz P, Roberts J (eds): Cellular and Integrative Mechanisms in the Onset of Labor. An NICHD workshop, Ithaca, NY, Perinatology Press, 1988

Ban C, Billah MM, Truong CT, Johnston JM: Metabolism of platelet-activating factor (1-O-alkyl-2-acetyl-*sn*-glycero-3-phosphocholine) in human fetal membranes and decidua vera. Arch Biochem Biophys 246:9, 1986

Bartocci A, Pollard JW, Stanley ER: Regulation of colony-stimulating factor 1 during pregnancy. J Exp Med 164:956, 1986

Bergstrom S, Danielson H, Samuelsson B: The enzymatic formation of prostaglandin E_2 from arachidonic acid: Prostaglandins and related factors. Biochim Biophys Acta 90:207, 1964

Beutler B, Cerami A: Cachectin and tumor necrosis factor as two sides of the same biological coin. Nature 320:584, 1986

Billah MM, Johnston JM: Identification of phospholipid platelet-activating factor (1-O-alkyl-2-acetyl-*sn*-glycero-3-phosphocholine) in human amniotic fluid and urine. Biochem Biophys Res Commun 113:51, 1983

Billiar RB: Jassani M, Little B: The metabolic clearance rate and uterine extraction of progesterone at midgestation. Endocr Res Commun 1:339, 1974

Bleasdale JE, Johnston JM: Prostaglandins and human parturition: Regulation of arachidonic acid mobilization. Rev Perinatol Med 5:151, 1984

Brandt ML: Mechanism and management of the third stage of labor. Am J Obstet Gynecol 25:662, 1933

Bulmer JN, Johnson PM: Macrophage populations in the human placenta and amniochorion. Clin Exp Immunol 57:393, 1984

Caldeyro-Barcia R, Alvarez H, Reynolds SRM: A better understanding of uterine contractility through simultaneous recording with an internal and a seven channel external method. Surg Gynecol Obstet 91:641, 1950

Cannon JG, Dinarello CA: Increased plasma interleukin-1 activity in women after ovulation. Science 227:1247, 1985

Carsten ME: Regulation of myometrial composition, growth, and activity. In Assali NS (ed): Biology of Gestation, Vol I: The Maternal Organism. New York, Academic, 1968

Carsten ME, Miller JD: Regulation of myometrial contractions. In MacDonald PC, Porter JC (eds): Initiation of Parturition: Prevention of Prematurity. Fourth Ross Conference on Obstetric Research, Ross Laboratories. Columbus, OH, 1983, p 166

Casey ML, Cox SM, Beutler B, MacDonald PC: The formation of cytokines in human decidua: The role of decidua in the initiation of both term and preterm labor. Proc Soc Gynecol Invest (Abstract) 35:219, 1988b

Casey ML, Cox SM, Beutler B, Milewich L, MacDonald PC: Cachectin (tumor necrosis factor-α) production in human decidua: Potential role of cytokines in infection-induced preterm labor. J Clin Invest (in press), 1989

Casey ML, Hemsell DL, MacDonald PC, Johnston JM: NAD^+-dependent 15-hydroxyprostaglandin dehydrogenase activity in human endometrium. Prostaglandins 19:115, 1980

Casey ML, Korte K, MacDonald PC: Epidermal growth factor-stimulation of prostaglandin E_2 biosynthesis in amnion cells: Induction of PGH_2 synthase. J Biol Chem 263:7846, 1988a

Casey ML, MacDonald PC: Biomelecular mechanisms in human parturition: Activation of uterine decidua. Proc Symp on Contraception and Mechanisms of Endometrial Bleeding, World Health Organization. Geneva, 1989

Casey ML, MacDonald PC: Biomolecular processes in the initiation of parturition: Decidual activation. Clin Obstet Gynecol 31:533, 1988a

Casey ML, MacDonald PC: Decidual activation: The role of prostaglandins in labor. In McNellis D, Challis JRG, MacDonald PC, Nathanielsz P, Roberts J (eds): Cellular and Integrative Mechanisms in the Onset of Labor. An NICHD workshop. Ithaca, NY, Perinatology Press, 1988c, p 141

Casey ML, MacDonald PC: The initiation of labor in women: Regulation of phospholipid and arachidonic acid metabolism and of prostaglandin production. Semin Perinatol 10:270, 1986

Casey ML, MacDonald PC: The role of a fetal-maternal paracrine system in the maintenance of pregnancy and the initiation of parturition. In Jones CT (ed): Fetal and Neonatal Development. Ithaca, NY, Perinatology Press, (in press) 1988b

Casey ML, MacDonald PC, Mitchell MD: Despite a massive increase in cortisol secretion in women during parturition, there is an equally massive increase in prostaglandin synthesis: A paradox? J Clin Invest 75:1852, 1985

Casey ML, MacDonald PC, Mitchell MD: Stimulation of prostaglandin E_2 production in human amnion cells in culture by a substance(s) in human fetal urine. Biochem Biophys Res Commun 114:1056, 1983a

Casey ML, Mitchell MD, MacDonald PC: Epidermal growth factor-stimulated prostaglandin E_2 production in human amnion cells: Specificity and nonesterified arachidonic acid dependency. Mol Cell Endocrinol 53:169, 1987

Casey ML, Winkel CA, Porter JC, MacDonald PC: Endocrine regulation of parturition. Clin Perinatol 10:709, 1983b

Challis JRG, Olson DM: Parturition. In Knobil E, Neill JD (eds): The Physiology of Reproduction. New York, Raven Press, 1988, p 2177, Vol 2

Cox SM, Casey ML, MacDonald PC: Decidual activation and parturition: Stimulation of prostaglandin production in human uterine decidua by interleukin-1. Proc Endocrine Soc (Abstract) 70:166, 1988b

Cox SM, MacDonald PC, Casey ML: Assay of bacterial endotoxin (lipopolysaccharide) in human amniotic fluid: Potential usefulness in diagnosis and management of preterm labor. Am J Obstet Gynecol 159:99, 1988c

Cox SM, MacDonald PC, Casey ML: Cytokines and prostaglandins in amniotic fluid of preterm labor pregnancies: Decidual origin in response to bacterial toxins [lipopolysaccharide (LPS) and lipoteichoic acid (LTA)]. Proc Soc Gynecol Invest (Abstract) 36, 1989

Cox SM, MacDonald PC, Casey ML: Decidual activation is synchronous with spontaneous parturition and with bacterial endotoxin [lipopolysaccharide (LPS)]-induced preterm labor. Proc Soc Gynecol Invest (Abstract) 35:89, 1988a

Danforth DN, Buckingham JC, Roddick JW: Connective tissue changes incident to cervical effacement. Am J Obstet Gynecol 80:939, 1960

Dinarello CA: Interleukin-1: Amino acid sequences, multiple biological activities, and comparison with tumor necrosis factor (cachectin). Year Immunol 2:69, 1986

Dray F, Frydman R: Primary prostaglandins in amniotic fluid in pregnancy and spontaneous labor. Am J Obstet Gynecol 126:13, 1976

Ferguson JKW: A study of the motility of the intact uterus at term. Surg Gynecol Obstet 73:359, 1941

Flint APF, Sheldrick EL: Ovarian peptides and luteolysis. In Edwards RG, Purdy JM, Steptoe PC (eds): Implantation of the Human Embryo. London, Academic, 1985, p 235

Flower RJ: The role of prostaglandins in parturition, with special reference to the rat. In Knight J, O'Connor M (eds): The Fetus and Birth. Ciba Foundation Symposium 47. Amsterdam, Elsevier, 1977, p 297

France JT, Magness RR, Murry BA, Rosenfeld CR, Mason JI: The regulation of ovine placental steroid 17α-hydroxylase and aromatase by glucocorticoid. Mol Endocrinol 2:193, 1988

France JT, Mason JI, Magness RR, Murry BA, Rosenfeld CR: Ovine placental aromatase: Studies of activity level, kinetic characteristics and effects of aromatase inhibitors. J Steroid Biochem 28:155, 1987

Friedman EA: Graphic appraisal of labor: A study of 500 primigravidas. Bull Sloan Hosp Women 1:42, 1955

Friedman EA: Labor: Clinical Evaluation and Management, 2nd ed. New York, Appleton, 1978

Gainer H, Alstein M, Whitnall MH, Wray S: The biosynthesis and secretion of oxytocin and vasopressin. In Knobil E, Neill J (eds): The Physiology of Reproduction. New York, Raven Press, 1988, p 2265, Vol 2

Garfield RE: Gap junctions: Their development, role, and regulation in the myometrium during parturition. In MacDonald PC, Porter JC (eds): Initiation of Parturition: Prevention of Prematurity. Fourth Ross Conference on Obstetric Research, Ross Laboratories. Columbus, OH, 1983, p 51

Garfield RE: Structural and functional studies of the control of myometrial contractility and labor. In McNellis D, Challis JRG, MacDonald PC, Nathanielsz P, Roberts J (eds): Cellular and Integrative Mechanisms in the Onset of Labor. An NICHD workshop. Ithaca, NY, Perinatology Press, 1988, p 55

Gemzell CA, Robbe H, Stern B, Strom G: Observation on circulatory changes and muscular work in normal labor. Acta Obstet Gynecol Scand 36:75, 1957

Glover DM, Brownstein D, Burchett S, Larsen A, Wilson CB: Expression of HLA class II antigens and secretion of interleukin-1 by monocytes and macrophages from adults and neonates. Immunology 61:195, 1987

Hemming VG, Nagarajan K, Hess LW, Fisher GW, Wilson SR, Thomas LS: Rapid in vitro replication of group B streptococcus in term human amniotic fluid. Gynecol Obstet Invest 19:124, 1985

Hendricks CH: The control of labor. Gynecol Invest (Suppl)1:37, 1970

Hertelendy F: Regulation of oviposition. In MacDonald PC, Porter JC (eds): Initiation of Parturition: Prevention of Prematurity. Fourth Ross Conference on Obstetric Research, Ross Laboratories. Columbus, OH, 1983, p 79

Huszar G: Biology of the myometrium and cervix. In Washaw JB (ed): The Biological Basis of Reproductive and Developmental Medicine. New York, Elsevier, 1983, p 85

Huszar G, Roberts JB: Biochemistry and pharmacology of the myometrium and labor: Regulation at the cellular and molecular levels. Am J Obstet Gynecol 142:225, 1982

Iams JD, Clapp DH, Contox DA, Whitehurst R, Ayers LW, O'Shaughnessy RW: Does extraamniotic infection cause preterm labor: Gas-liquid chromatography studies of amniotic fluid in amnionitis, preterm labor, and normal controls. Obstet Gynecol 70:365, 1987

Ivy AC, Hartman CG, Koff A: The contractions of the monkey uterus at term. Am J Obstet Gynecol 22:388, 1931

Johnston JM, Bleasdale JE, Hoffman DR: Functions of PAF in reproduction and development: Involvement of PAF in fetal lung maturation and parturition. In Snyder F (ed): Platelet-Activating Factor and Related Lipid Mediators. New York, Plenum Press, 1987

Karlson S: On the motility of the uterus during labour and the influence of the motility pattern on the duration of the labour. Acta Obstet Gynecol Scand 28:209, 1949

Keirse MJNC, Flint APF, Turnbull AC: F prostaglandins in amniotic fluid during pregnancy and labour. J Obstet Gynaecol Br Commonw 81:131, 1974

Keirse MJNC, Hicks BR, Mitchell MD, Turnbull AC: Increase in the prostaglandin precursor, arachidonic acid, in amniotic fluid during spontaneous labour. Br J Obstet Gynaecol 84:937, 1977

Keirse MJNC, Mitchell MD, Turnbull AC: Changes in prostaglandin F and 13, 14-dihydro-15-keto-prostaglandin F concentrations in amniotic fluid at the onset of and during labour. Br J Obstet Gynaecol 84:743, 1977

Keirse MJNC, Turnbull AC: E prostaglandins in amniotic fluid during late pregnancy and labour. J Obstet Gynaecol Br Commonw 80:970, 1973

Keirse MJNC, Turnbull AC: Metabolism of prostaglandins within the human pregnant uterus. Br J Obstet Gynaecol 82:887, 1975

Keirse MJNC, Turnbull AC: The fetal membranes as a possible source of amniotic fluid prostaglandins. Br J Obstet Gynaecol 83:146, 1976

Krall JF, Korenman SG: Prevention of preterm labor. In Knight J, O'Connor M (eds): The Fetus and Birth. Amsterdam, Elsevier, 1977, p 319

Kunkel SL, Chensue SW: The role of arachidonic acid metabolites in mononuclear phagocytic cell interaction. Int J Dermatol 25:83, 1986

Lands WEM, Samuelsson B: Phospholipid precursors of prostaglandins. Biochim Biophys Acta 164:426, 1968

Leake RD: Oxytocin. In MacDonald PC, Porter JC (eds): Initiation of Parturition: Prevention of Prematurity. Fourth Ross Conference on Obstetric Research, Ross Laboratories. Columbus, OH, 1983, p 43

Leake RD, Weitzman RE, Fisher DA: Pharmacokinetics of oxytocin in the human subject. Obstet Gynecol 56:701,1980

Leake RD, Weitzman RE, Glatz TH, Fisher DA: Plasma oxytocin concentrations in men, nonpregnant women, and pregnant women before and during labor. J Clin Endocrinol Metab 53:730, 1981

Liggins GC: Premature parturition after infusion of corticotrophin or cortisol into foetal lambs. J Endocrinol 42:323, 1968

Liggins GC: Fetal influences on myometrial contractility. Clin Obstet Gynecol 16:148, 1973

Liggins GC, Fairclough RJ, Grieves SA, Kendall JZ, Knox BS: The mechanism of initiation of parturition in the ewe. Recent Prog Horm Res 29:111, 1973

Liggins GC, Kennedy PC, Holm LW: Failure of initiation of parturition after electrocoagulation of the pituitary of the fetal lamb. Am J Obstet Gynecol 98:1080, 1967

Lin TJ, Billiar RB, Little B: Metabolic clearance of progesterone in the menstrual cycle. J Clin Endocrinol Metab 35:879, 1972

Little B, Tait JF, Tait SA, Erlenmeyer F: The metabolic clearance rate of progesterone in males and ovariectomized females. J Clin Invest 45:901, 1966

MacDonald PC, Porter JC, Schwarz BE, Johnston JM: Initiation of parturition in the human female. Semin Perinatol 2:273, 1978

MacDonald PC, Schultz FM, Duenhoelter JH, Gant NF, Jimenez JM, Pritchard JA, Porter JC, Johnston JM: Initiation of human parturition: I. Mechanism of action of arachidonic acid. Obstet Gynecol 44:629, 1974

Malpas P: Postmaturity and malformation of the fetus. J Obstet Gynaecol Br Emp 40:1046, 1933

Mitchell MD: Sources of eicosanoids within the uterus during pregnancy. In McNellis D, Challis JRG, MacDonald PC, Nathanielsz P, Roberts J (eds): Cellular and Integrative Mechanisms in the Onset of Labor. An NICHD workshop. Ithaca, NY, Perinatology Press, 1988, p 165

Mitchell MD: Studies on prostaglandins in relation to parturition in the sheep. D. Phil. Thesis, Oxford University, 1976

Nehemiah JL, Schnitzer JA, Schulman H, Novikoff AB: Human chorionic trophoblasts, decidual cells and macrophages: A histochemical and electron microscopic study. Am J Obstet Gynecol 140:261, 1981

Niesert S, Christopherson WA, Korte K, Mitchell MD, MacDonald PC, Casey ML: Prostaglandin E_2 9-keto-reductase activity in human decidua vera tissue. Am J Obstet Gynecol 155:1348, 1986

Nishihara J, Ishibashi T, Mai Y, Muramatsu T: Mass spectrometric evidence for the presence of platelet-activating factor (1-O-alkyl-2-sn-glycero-3-phosphocholine) in human amniotic fluid during labor. Lipids 19:907, 1984

Novy MJ, Liggins GC: Role of prostaglandin, prostacyclin, and thromboxanes in the physiologic control of the uterus and in parturition. Semin Perinatol 4:45, 1980

Okazaki T, Casey ML, Okita JR, MacDonald PC, Johnston JM: Initiation of human parturition: XII. Biosynthesis and metabolism of prostaglandins in human fetal membranes and uterine decidua vera. Am J Obstet Gynecol 139:373, 1981

Okita JR: Alternations in arachidonic acid content of specific glycerophospholipids of amnion and chorion laeve during human parturition. Doctoral Dissertation, University of Texas Southwestern Medical School, Dallas, 1981

Okita JR, Johnston JM, MacDonald PC: Source of prostaglandin precursor in human fetal membranes: Arachidonic acid content of amnion and chorion laeve of diamnionic-dichorionic twin placentae. Am J Obstet Gynecol 147:477, 1983a

Okita JR, MacDonald PC, Johnston JM: Initiation of human parturition: XIV. Increase in the diacylglycerol content of amnion during parturition. Am J Obstet Gynecol 142:432, 1982b

Okita JR, MacDonald PC, Johnston JM: Mobilization of arachidonic acid from specific glycerophospholipids of human fetal membranes during early labor. J Biol Chem 247:14029, 1982a

Okita JR, Sagawa N, Casey ML, Snyder JM: A comparison of amnion cells in monolayer culture and amnion tissue. In Vitro 19:117, 1983b

Parker CR Jr, Illingworth DR, Bissonette J, Carr BR: Endocrinology of pregnancy in abetalipoproteinemia: Studies in a patient with homozygous familial hypobetalipoproteinemia. N Engl J Med 314:557, 1986

Rea C: Prolonged gestation, acrania, monstrosity and apparent placenta praevia in one obstetrical case. JAMA 30:1166, 1898

Reddi K, Kambaran SR, Norman RJ, Joubert SM, Philpott RH: Abnormal concentrations of prostaglandins in amniotic fluid during delayed labour in multigravid patients. Br J Obstet Gynaecol 91:781, 1984

Rettenmier CW: Sacca R, Furman WL, Roussel MF, Holt JT, Neinhuis AW, Stanley ER, Sherr CJ: Expression of the human c-fms proto-oncogene product (colony-stimulating factor-1 receptor) on peripheral blood mononuclear cells and choriocarcinoma cell lines. J Clin Invest 77:1740, 1986

Reynolds SRM: Physiology of the Uterus with Clinical Correlations, 2nd ed. New York, Hoeber, 1949

Richardson MR, Mitchell MD, MacDonald PC, Casey ML: Glucocorticosteroid regulation of prostaglandin biosynthesis in human myometrial smooth muscle cells in monolayer culture. J Steroid Biochem 25:521, 1986

Robinson JS, Chapman RL, Challis JR, Mitchell MD: Administration of extra-amniotic arachidonic acid and the suppression of uterine prostaglandin synthesis during pregnancy in the rhesus monkey. J Reprod Fertil 54:369, 1979

Romero R, Kadar N, Hobbins JC, Duff GW: Infection and labor: The detection of endotoxin in amniotic fluid. Am J Obstet Gynecol 157:815, 1987

Rosendaal M: Colony-stimulating factor (CSF) in the uterus of the pregnant mouse. J Cell Sci 19:411, 1975

Satoh K, Yasumizu T, Fukuoka H, Kinoshita K, Kaneko Y, Tsuchiya M, Sakamoto S: Prostaglandin $F_{2\alpha}$ metabolite levels in plasma, amniotic fluid, and urine during pregnancy and labor. Am J Obstet Gynecol 133:886, 1979

Schlegel W, Kruger S, Korte K: Purification of prostaglandin E_2-9-oxoreductase from human decidua vera. FEBS Lett 171:141, 1984

Schulman H, Romney SL: Variability of uterine contractions in normal human parturition. Obstet Gynecol 36:215, 1970

Siiteri PK, MacDonald PC: The utilization of circulating dehydroisoandrosterone sulfate for estrogen synthesis during human pregnancy. Steroids 2:713, 1963

Soloff MS: The role of oxytocin in the initiation of labor, and oxytocin-prostaglandin interactions. In McNellis D, Challis JRG, MacDonald PC, Nathanielsz P, Roberts J (eds): Cellular and Integrative Mechanisms in the Onset of Labor. An NICHD workshop. Ithaca, NY, Perinatology Press, 1988, p 87

Stanley ER: Action of the colony-stimulating factor, CSF-1. In Evered D, Nugent J, O'Connor M (eds): Biochemistry of machrophages. Ciba Foundation Symp 118. New York, Wiley, 1986, p 29

Strickland DM, Saeed SA, Casey ML, Mitchell MD: Stimulation of prostaglandin biosynthesis by urine of the human fetus may serve as a trigger for parturition. Science 220:521, 1983

Stull JT, Blumenthal DK, Cooke R: Regulation of contraction by myosin phosphorylation. A comparison between smooth and skeletal muscles. Biochem Pharmacol 29:2537, 1980

Stull JT, Taylor DA, MacKenzie LW, Casey ML: Biochemistry and physiology of smooth muscle contractility. In McNellis D, Challis JRG, MacDonald PC, Nathanielsz P, Roberts J (eds): Cellular and Integrative Mechanisms in the Onset of Labor. An NICHD workshop. Ithaca, NY, Perinatology Press, 1988, p 17

Theobald GW: Nervous control of uterine activity. Clin Obstet Gynecol 11:15, 1968

Thorburn GD: Past and present concepts on the initiation of parturition. In MacDonald PC, Porter JC (eds): Initiation of Parturition: Prevention of Prematurity. Fourth Ross Conference on Obstetric Research, Ross Laboratories. Columbus, OH, 1983, p 2

van Dorp DA, Beerthuis RK, Nguteren DH, Vonkeman H: The biosynthesis of prostaglandins. Biochim Biophys Acta 90:204, 1964

Vonkeman H, van Dorp DA: The action of prostaglandin synthetase on 2-arachidonoyl-lecithin. Biochim Biophys Acta 164:430, 1968

Webb AC, Rosenwasser LJ, Auron PE: Molecular organization and expression of the prointerleukin-1β gene. In Gillis S (ed): Recombinant Lymphokines and Their Receptors. New York, Marcel Dekker, 1987, p 139

Wolfs GMJA, van Leeuwen M: Electromyographic observations on the human uterus during labour. Acta Obstet Gynecol Scand (Suppl) 90:128, 1979

Word RA, MacDonald PC, Casey ML: Stimulation of prostaglandin (PG) production in human myometrial cells in culture by interleukin-1 (IL-1). Proc Soc Gynecol Invest (Abstract) 36, 1989

Zahl PA, Bjerknes C: Induction of decidua-placental hemorrhage in mice by the endotoxins of certain gram-negative bacteria. Proc Soc Exp Biol Med 54:329, 1943

Mechanism of Normal Labor in Occiput Presentation

The fetus is in the occiput or vertex presentation in approximately 95 percent of all labors. The fetal presentation is most commonly ascertained by abdominal palpation and confirmed sometime before or at the onset of labor by vaginal examination. In the majority of cases the vertex enters the pelvis with the sagittal suture in the transverse pelvic diameter (Caldwell and associates, 1934).

DIAGNOSIS OF OCCIPUT PRESENTATION

OCCIPUT TRANSVERSE POSITIONS

For diagnosis by abdominal examination, the four maneuvers of Leopold are employed (see Fig. 9–10). The fetus enters the pelvis in the left occiput transverse (LOT) position in 40 percent of all labors, compared to 20 percent in the right occiput transverse (ROT) position (Caldwell and associates, 1934). The following findings are obtained for the LOT position by abdominal examination (Figs. 9–5A and 9–10):

- *First maneuver:* Fundus occupied by the breech.
- *Second maneuver:* Resistant plane of the back felt directly to the examiner's right, readily palpated through the mother's left flank (see Fig. 9–10).
- *Third maneuver:* Negative if the head is engaged (biparietal diameter through the pelvic inlet): otherwise, the movable head is detected at or above the pelvic inlet.
- *Fourth maneuver:* Negative if head is engaged: otherwise cephalic prominence on the right.

In the ROT position palpation yields similar information (see Fig. 9–6B), except that the fetal back is in the mother's right flank and the small parts and cephalic prominence are on the left.

On vaginal examination the sagittal suture occupies the transverse diameter of the pelvis more or less midway between the sacrum and the symphysis. In LOT positions the smaller posterior fontanel is to the left in the maternal pelvis and the larger anterior fontanel is directed to the opposite side. In ROT positions the reverse holds true. The fetal heart in right and left positions is usually heard in the right and left flank, respectively, at or slightly below the level of the mother's umbilicus.

OCCIPUT ANTERIOR POSITIONS

In occiput anterior positions (LOA or ROA) the head either enters the pelvis with the occiput rotated 45 degrees anteriorly from the transverse position or subsequently does so. *This degree of anterior rotation produces only slight differences on abdominal examination* (see Figs. 9–5A, 9–6A). The mechanism of labor is usually very similar to that in occiput transverse positions.

OCCIPUT POSTERIOR POSITIONS

The incidence of occiput posterior positions is approximately 20 percent and the right occiput posterior (ROP) is slightly more common than the left (LOP) (Caldwell and associates, 1934). It appears likely from evidence obtained from radiographic studies that posterior positions more often are associated with a narrow forepelvis.

On vaginal or rectal examination in the ROP position the sagittal suture occupies the right oblique diameter, the small fontanel is felt opposite the right sacroiliac synchondrosis, and the large fontanel is directed toward the left iliopectineal eminence (see Fig. 9–6C). In the LOP position the reverse is true (see Fig. 9–5B). In many cases, particularly in the early part of labor, because of imperfect flexion of the head, the large fontanel lies at a lower level than in anterior positions and is more readily felt.

CARDINAL MOVEMENTS OF A LABOR IN OCCIPUT PRESENTATION

Because of the irregular shape of the pelvic canal and the relatively large dimensions of the mature fetal head, it is evident that not all diameters of the head can necessarily pass through all diameters of the pelvis. It follows that a process of adaptation or accommodation of suitable portions of the head to the various segments of the pelvis is required for completion of childbirth. These positional changes in the presenting part constitute the mechanism of labor. *The cardinal movements of labor are (1) engagement, (2) descent, (3) flexion, (4) internal rotation, (5) extension, (6) external rotation, and (7) expulsion.* These movements are illustrated in Figure 11–1.

For purposes of instruction, the various movements are often described as though they occurred separately and independently. In reality the mechanism of labor consists of a combination of movements that are going on at the same time. For example, as part of the process of engagement there is both flexion and descent of the head. It is manifestly impossible for the movements to be completed unless the presenting part descends simultaneously. Concomitantly the uterine contractions

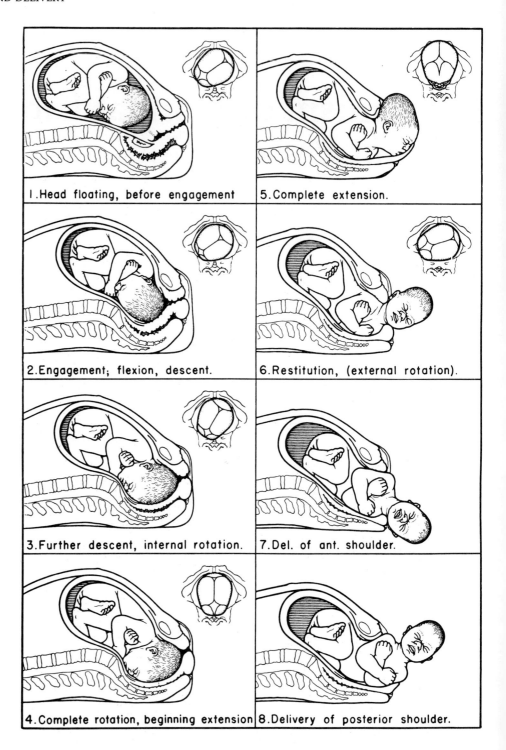

Figure 11–1. Cardinal movements in the mechanism of labor and delivery, left occiput anterior position.

1. Head floating, before engagement
2. Engagement; flexion, descent.
3. Further descent, internal rotation.
4. Complete rotation, beginning extension
5. Complete extension.
6. Restitution, (external rotation).
7. Del. of ant. shoulder.
8. Delivery of posterior shoulder.

effect important modifications in the attitude, or habitus, of the fetus, especially after the head has descended into the pelvis. These changes consist principally of a straightening of the fetus, with loss of its dorsal convexity and closer application of the extremities and small parts to the body. As a result, the fetal ovoid is transformed into a cylinder with normally the smallest possible cross section passing through the birth canal.

ENGAGEMENT

As discussed in Chapter 8, the mechanism by which the biparietal diameter, the greatest transverse diameter of the fetal head in occiput presentations, passes through the pelvic inlet is designated *engagement*. This phenomenon may take place during the last few weeks of pregnancy or may not occur until after the commencement of labor. In many multiparous and some nulliparous women, at the onset of labor the fetal head is freely movable above the pelvic inlet. In this circumstance, the head is sometimes referred to as "floating." A normal-sized head usually does not engage with its sagittal suture directed anteroposteriorly. Instead, the fetal head usually enters the pelvic inlet either in the transverse diameter or in one of the oblique diameters (Caldwell and colleagues, 1934).

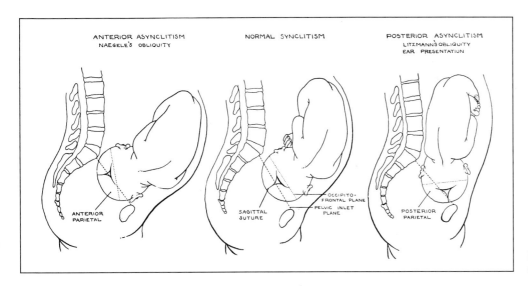

Figure 11–2. Synclitism and asynclitism.

Asynclitism

Although the fetal head tends to accommodate to the transverse axis of the pelvic inlet, the sagittal suture, while remaining parallel to that axis, may not lie exactly midway between the symphysis and sacral promontory. The sagittal suture is frequently deflected either posteriorly toward the promontory or anteriorly toward the symphysis, as shown in Figure 11–2. Such lateral deflection of the head to a more anterior or posterior position in the pelvis is called *asynclitism*. If the sagittal suture approaches the sacral promontory, more of the anterior parietal bone presents itself to the examining fingers and the condition is called *anterior asynclitism*. If, however, the sagittal suture lies close to the symphysis, more of the posterior parietal bone will present and the condition is called *posterior asynclitism*. Moderate degrees of asynclitism are the rule in normal labor, but if severe, they may lead to cephalopelvic disproportion even with an otherwise normal-sized pelvis. Successive changes from posterior to anterior asynclitism facilitate descent by allowing the fetal head to take advantage of the roomiest areas of the pelvic cavity.

DESCENT

The first requisite for birth of the infant is descent. With the nulliparous woman engagement may occur before the onset of labor, and further descent may not necessarily follow until the onset of the second stage of labor. In multiparous women descent usually begins with engagement. Descent is brought about by one or more of four forces: (1) pressure of the amnionic fluid, (2) direct pressure of the fundus upon the breech, (3) contraction of the abdominal muscles, and (4) extension and straightening of the fetal body.

FLEXION

As soon as the descending head meets resistance, whether from cervix, the walls of the pelvis, or the pelvic floor, flexion of the head normally results. In this movement, the chin is brought into more intimate contact with the fetal thorax, and the appreciably shorter suboccipitobregmatic diameter is substituted for the longer occipitofrontal diameter (Figs. 11–3, 11–4).

INTERNAL ROTATION

This movement is a turning of the head in such a manner that the occiput gradually moves from its original position anteriorly toward the symphysis pubis or, less commonly, posteriorly toward the hollow of the sacrum (Figs. 11–5, 11–6). Internal rotation is essential for the completion of labor, except when the fetus is unusually small. Internal rotation, which is always associated with descent of the presenting part, is usually not accomplished until the head has reached the level of the spines and therefore is engaged.

Calkins (1939) studied more than 5,000 patients in labor to ascertain when internal rotation occurs. He concluded that in approximately two thirds of all women, internal rotation is complete by the time the head reaches the pelvic floor; in about one fourth, internal rotation is completed very shortly after the head reaches the pelvic floor; and in about 5 percent, rotation to the anterior does not take place. When rotation fails to occur until the head reaches the pelvic

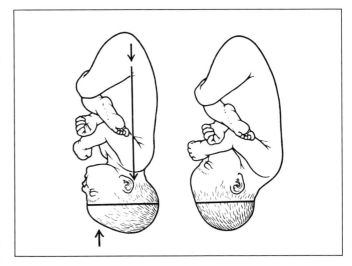

Figure 11–3. Lever action producing flexion of the head; conversion from occipitofrontal to suboccipitobregmatic diameter typically reduces the anteroposterior diameter from nearly 12 cm to 9.5 cm.

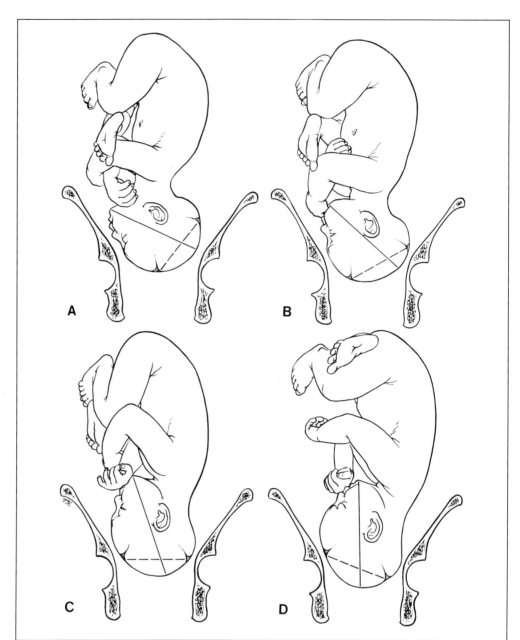

Figure 11–4. Four degrees of head flexion. Indicated by the solid line is the occipitomental diameter, and the broken line connects the center of the anterior fontanel with the posterior fontanel: **A.** Flexion poor. **B.** Flexion moderate. **C.** Flexion advanced. **D.** Flexion complete. Note that with flexion complete, the chin is on the chest and the suboccipito-bregmatic diameter, the shortest anteroposterior diameter of the fetal head, is passing through the pelvic inlet. (*Modified from Rydberg: The Mechanism of Labour. Springfield, IL., Thomas, 1954.*)

floor, it takes place during the next one or two contractions in multiparas, and in nulliparas during the next three to five. Rotation before the head reaches the pelvic floor is definitely more frequent in multiparas than in nulliparas, according to Calkins.

EXTENSION

When, after internal rotation, the sharply flexed head reaches the vulva, it undergoes another movement that is essential to its birth, namely, extension, which brings the base of the occiput into direct contact with the inferior margin of the symphysis pubis. Since the vulvar outlet is directed upward and forward, extension must occur before the head can pass through it. If the sharply flexed head, on reaching the pelvic floor, did not extend but was driven farther downward, it would impinge upon the posterior portion of the perineum and, if the force from behind were sufficiently strong, would eventually be forced through

the tissues of the perineum. When the head presses upon the pelvic gutter, however, two forces come into play. The first, exerted by the uterus, acts more posteriorly, and the second, supplied by the resistant pelvic floor and the symphysis, acts more anteriorly. The resultant force is in the direction of the vulvar opening, thereby causing extension.

With increasing distension of the perineum and vaginal opening, an increasingly large portion of the occiput gradually appears. The head is born by further extension as the occiput, bregma, forehead, nose, mouth, and finally the chin pass successively over the anterior margin of the perineum. Immediately after its birth, the head drops downward so that the chin lies over the maternal anal region.

EXTERNAL ROTATION

The delivered head next undergoes restitution. If the occiput was originally directed toward the left, it rotates toward the left

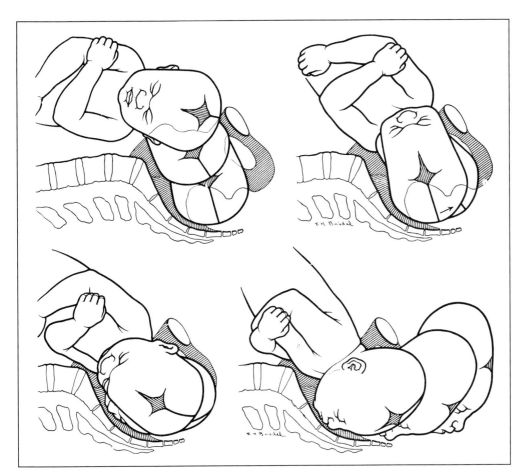

Figure 11–5. Mechanism of labor for the left occiput transverse position, lateral view. Anterior asynclitism at the pelvic brim followed by lateral flexion, resulting in posterior asynclitism after engagement, further descent, rotation, and extension. (*From Steele and Javert: Surg Gynecol Obstet 75:477, 1942.*)

ischial tuberosity; if it was originally directed toward the right, the occiput rotates to the right. The return of the head to the oblique position (restitution) is followed by completion of external rotation to the transverse position, a movement that corresponds to rotation of the fetal body, serving to bring its bisacromial diameter into relation with the anteroposterior diameter of the pelvic outlet. Thus, one shoulder is anterior behind the symphysis and the other is posterior. This movement is apparently brought about by the same pelvic factors that effect internal rotation of the head.

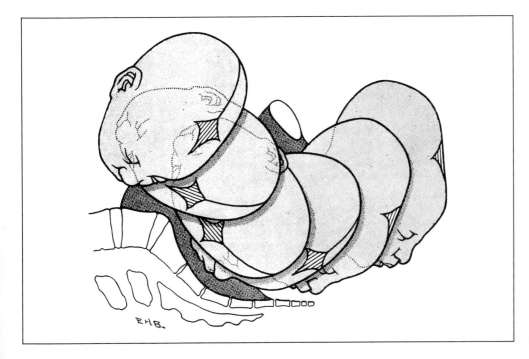

Figure 11–6. Mechanism of labor for left occiput anterior position.

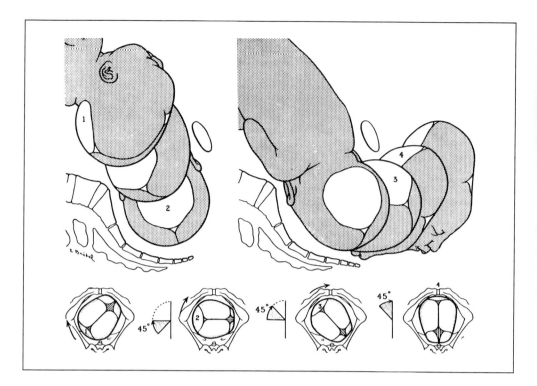

Figure 11–7. Mechanism of labor for right occiput posterior position, anterior rotation.

EXPULSION

Almost immediately after external rotation, the anterior shoulder appears under the symphysis pubis, and the perineum soon becomes distended by the posterior shoulder. After delivery of the shoulders, the rest of the body of the child is quickly extruded.

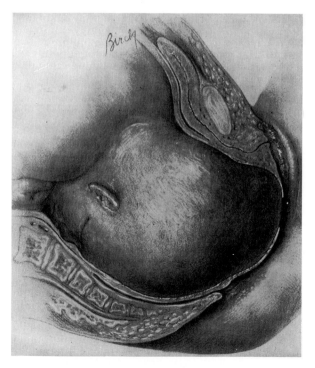

Figure 11–8. Formation of caput succedaneum.

LABOR IN OCCIPUT POSTERIOR POSITIONS

In the great majority of labors in the occiput posterior positions the mechanism of labor is identical to that observed in the transverse and anterior varieties, except that the occiput has to rotate to the symphysis pubis through 135 degrees instead of 90 degrees and 45 degrees, respectively (Fig. 11–7).

With effective contractions, adequate flexion of the head, and a fetus of average size, the great majority of posteriorly positioned occiputs rotate promptly as soon as they reach the pelvic floor, and labor is not appreciably lengthened. In perhaps 5 to 10 percent of cases, however, these favorable circumstances do not occur. For example, with poor contractions or faulty flexion of the head or both, rotation may be incomplete or may not take place at all, especially if the fetus is large. If rotation is incomplete, *transverse arrest* results. If rotation toward the symphysis does not take place, the occiput usually rotates to the direct occiput posterior position, a condition known as *persistent occiput posterior*. Both transverse arrest and persistent occiput posterior represent deviations from the normal mechanisms of labor and are considered further in Chapter 19.

CHANGES IN THE SHAPE OF THE FETAL HEAD

CAPUT SUCCEDANEUM

In vertex presentations the fetal head undergoes important characteristic changes in shape as the result of the pressures to which it is subjected during labor. In prolonged labors before complete dilatation of the cervix, the portion of the fetal scalp immediately over the cervical os becomes edematous, forming a swelling known as the *caput succedaneum* (Fig. 11–8). It usually attains a thickness of only a few millimeters, but in prolonged labors it may be sufficiently extensive to prevent the differentiation of the various sutures and fontanels. More commonly the

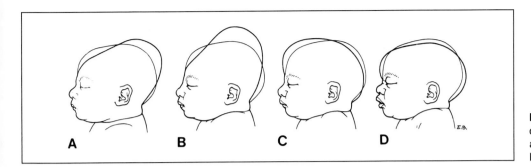

Figure 11–9. Molding of head, cephalic presentations. **A.** Occiput anterior. **B.** Occiput posterior. **C.** Brow. **D.** Face.

caput is formed when the head is in the lower portion of the birth canal and frequently only after the resistance of a rigid vaginal outlet is encountered. Since it occurs over the most dependent portion of the head, in LOT position it is found over the upper and posterior extremity of the right parietal bone, and in ROT positions over the corresponding area of the left parietal bone. It follows that after labor the original position often may be ascertained by noting the location of the caput succedaneum.

MOLDING

Of considerable importance is the degree of molding that the head undergoes. Because the various bones of the skull are not firmly united, movement may occur at the sutures. Ordinarily the margins of the occipital bone, and more rarely those of the frontal bone, are pushed under those of the parietal bones. In many cases one parietal bone may overlap the other, the anterior parietal usually overlapping the posterior. These changes are of greatest importance in contracted pelves, when the degree to which the head is capable of molding may make the difference between successful vaginal delivery and a major obstetrical operation (Fig. 11–9). Molding may account for a diminution in biparietal and suboccipitobregmatic diameters of 0.5 to 1.0 cm, or even more in prolonged labors.

REFERENCES

Caldwell WE, Moloy HC, D'Esopo DA: A roentgenologic study of the mechanism of engagement of the fetal head. Am J Obstet Gynecol 28:824, 1934

Calkins LA: The etiology of occiput presentations. Am J Obstet Gynecol 37:618, 1939

Rydberg: The Mechanism of Labour. Springfield, IL: Thomas, 1954

Steele KB, Javert CT: The mechanism of labor for transverse positions of the vertex. Surg Gynecol Obstet 75:477, 1942

The Newborn Infant

ADAPTATION OF THE NEWBORN TO AIR BREATHING

THE FIRST BREATH OF AIR

As the infant is born and the fetoplacental circulation ceases to function, the infant is subjected to rapid and profound physiological changes (Chap. 6, p. 100). The baby's survival depends upon a prompt and orderly interchange of oxygen and carbon dioxide between his or her new environment and the pulmonary circulation. For efficient interchange, the fluid-filled alveoli of the lungs must fill with air, the air must be exchanged by appropriate respiratory motion, and a vigorous microcirculation must be established in close proximity to the alveoli.

Intrauterine Respiration

Until recently it was widely taught that only at times of hypoxic stress did the fetus breathe in utero. This view was so strongly championed by some eminent fetal physiologists that observations to the contrary most often were promptly rejected as being the consequence of abnormal stimulation, most likely hypoxia, during the course of the experiment. In recent years, however, conclusive evidence of episodic respiratory movements in utero has been obtained during normal human pregnancy. Breathing movements are commonly observed when the fetus is evaluated by ultrasound. Pressure changes during inspiration recorded in monkey fetuses by Martin and co-workers (1974) appear sufficiently intense to induce movement of amnionic fluid into and out of the fetal lungs, as demonstrated in both monkey and human fetuses by Duenhoelter and Pritchard (1976).

INITIATION OF AIR BREATHING

Very soon after birth, the breathing pattern shifts from one of shallow episodic inspirations, which characterizes fetal breathing, to that of regular deeper inhalations. It is now apparent that aeration of the newborn lung is not the inflation of a collapsed structure, but, instead, the rapid replacement of bronchial and alveolar fluid by air.

In the lamb, and presumably in the human infant, residual alveolar fluid after delivery is cleared through the pulmonary circulation and, to a lesser degree, through pulmonary lymphatics (Chernick, 1978). Delay in the removal of fluid from the alveoli probably contributes to the syndrome of *transient tachypnea of the newborn.*

As the fluid is replaced by air, there is considerable reduction in pulmonary vascular compression and, in turn, lowered resistance to blood flow. With the fall in pulmonary arterial blood pressure, the ductus arteriosus normally closes. Closure of the foramen ovale is more variable.

High negative intrathoracic pressures are required to bring about the initial entry of air into fluid-filled alveoli. Normally, from the first breath after birth, progressively more residual air accumulates in the lung, and with each successive breath, lower pulmonary opening pressure is required. In the mature normal infant, by about the fifth breath of air, the pressure-volume changes achieved with each respiration are very similar to those of the normal adult.

Alveolar Surface Tension and Lung Surfactant

The successful filling of the lungs with air and the rapid establishment of a physiological pattern of pressure-volume changes on inspiration and expiration require the presence of surface-active material that will lower surface tension in the alveoli and thereby prevent the collapse of the lung with each expiration (Chap. 6, p. 107). Lack of sufficient surfactant leads to the prompt development of the respiratory distress syndrome (Chap. 33, p. 593).

The Stimuli to Breathe Air

Normally, the newborn infant begins to breathe and cry almost immediately after birth, indicating the establishment of active respiration. All the factors involved in the first breath of air have been difficult to elucidate, undoubtedly because many individually subtle stimuli contribute simultaneously. Some noteworthy explanations follow.

Physical Stimulation

The handling of the infant during delivery and contact with various relatively rough surfaces are believed to provoke respiration through stimuli reaching the respiratory center reflexly from the skin.

Compression of Fetal Thorax at Delivery

The compression of the thorax during the second stage of labor forces some fluid from the respiratory tract. For example, Saunders (1978) found that considerable pressure is often produced by compression of the chest during vaginal delivery and estimated that lung fluid is expelled equivalent to one fourth to one third of ultimate functional residual capacity. While babies born by cesarean section usually cry satisfactorily and sometimes just as quickly as babies born vaginally, they are likely to have more fluid and less gas in their lungs throughout the first 6 hours after birth (Milner and colleagues, 1978). The compression of the thorax incident to vaginal delivery and the expansion that follows delivery may, nevertheless, be an auxiliary factor in the initiation of respiration.

Deprivation of Oxygen and Accumulation of Carbon Dioxide

It was the opinion of Barcroft and associates (1939), based on animal experimentation, that lack of oxygen caused respiration after birth. Observations on both animals and human beings, however, have

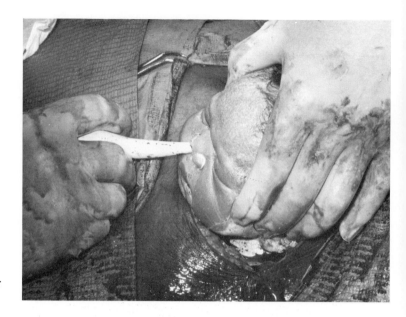

Figure 12–1. Aspirating the nose and mouth immediately after delivery of the head.

shown that profound lack of oxygen produces apnea. If minor degrees of hypoxia produce the first respiration after birth, certain observations become difficult to explain. For example, there is no relation between the concentration of oyxgen in the blood at birth and the onset of respiration except possibly that infants with normal levels of oyxgen breathe more readily than those with extremely low levels, who are often apneic. Blood samples obtained from catheters implanted into fetal vessels of experimental animals for prolonged periods of time without interruption of the pregnancy have revealed that P_{O_2} is low by adult standards. A further decrease in P_{O_2} diminishes or abolishes fetal respiratory motion, whereas elevation of P_{CO_2} increases the frequency and magnitude of fetal breathing movements (Dawes, 1974). The fetus-infant most likely responds to hypoxia and to hypercapnea the same way in utero and after birth.

MANAGEMENT OF DELIVERY

Immediate Care
As the head of the infant is delivered, either vaginally or by cesarean section, the face is immediately wiped and the mouth and nares suctioned (Fig. 12–1). A soft rubber ear syringe or its equivalent inserted with care is quite suitable for the purpose. Before clamping and severing the cord, while the infant is still being held head down, it may be beneficial to aspirate the mouth and pharynx again. Once the cord has been divided, as described in Chapter 16, page 318, the infant is immediately placed supine with the head lowered and turned to the side in a heated unit that has appropriate thermal regulation and is equipped for immediate intensive care (Fig. 12–2). To minimize heat loss, the baby is wiped dry.

Evaluation of the Infant
Before and during delivery, careful considerations must be given to the following determinants of well-being for the infant: (1) health status of the mother, (2) fetal (gestational) age, (3) duration of labor, (4) duration of rupture of the membranes, (5) kinds, amounts, times, and routes of administration of analgesics, (6) kind and duration of anesthesia, and (7) degree of difficulty encountered in effecting delivery. The obstetrician inspects the infant for any visible abnormalities during delivery

and until the cord is severed, and the infant is handed over to a trained associate for further care.

The person immediately in charge of caring for the infant should observe respirations closely and identify the heart rate. The heart rate can be determined by auscultation over the chest or by palpating the base of the umbilical cord. A readily discernible heart beat of 100 or more is acceptable. Persistent bradycardia requires prompt resuscitation. Next, the mouth, nares, and pharynx are carefully suctioned.

Most normal infants take a breath within a few seconds of birth and cry within half a minute. If respirations are infrequent, suction of the mouth and pharynx followed by light slapping of the soles of the feet and rubbing of the back, usually together serve to stimulate breathing. Prolongation of these intervals beyond 1 and 2 minutes, respectively, indicates an abnormality.

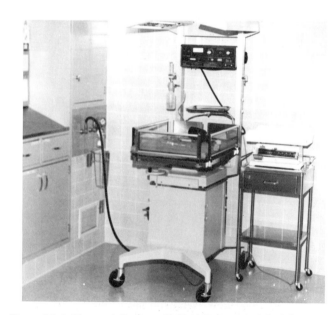

Figure 12–2. Thermostatically controlled infant care unit in delivery room.

Continued lack of breathing indicates either marked central depression or mechanical obstruction and demands active resuscitation. "Tubbing," "jackknifing," and dilatation of sphincters are condemned as wasteful of valuable time and may cause serious injury.

Lack of Effective Respirations

Important causes of failure to establish effective respirations include the following: (1) fetal hypoxemia from any cause, (2) drugs administered to the mother, (3) gross immaturity of the fetus, (4) upper airway obstruction, (5) pneumothorax, (6) other lung abnormalities, either intrinsic (e.g., hypoplasia) or extrinsic (e.g., diaphragmatic hernia), (7) aspiration of amnionic fluid grossly contaminated with meconium, (8) central nervous system injury, and (9) septicemia.

METHODS USED TO EVALUATE THE NEWBORN'S CONDITION

APGAR SCORE

A useful aid in the evaluation of the infant is the Apgar scoring system applied at 1 minute and again at 5 minutes after birth (Table 12–1). In general, the higher the score, up to a maximum of 10, the better is the condition of the infant. The 1-minute Apgar score determines the need for immediate resuscitation. Most infants at birth are in excellent condition, as indicated by Apgar scores of 7 to 10, and require no aid other than perhaps simple nasopharyngeal suction. *Mildly to moderately depressed infants* score 4 to 7 at 1 minute, demonstrating depressed respirations, flaccidity, and pale to blue color. Heart rate and reflex irritability, however, are good. *Severely depressed infants* score 0 to 4, with heart rate slow to inaudible and reflex response depressed or absent. Resuscitation, including artificial ventilation, should be started immediately. Often, babies who need immediate active intervention are obvious. They are flaccid, apneic, and often covered with meconium, and the heart rate is below 100. There is no need for considering further the 1-minute Apgar score. Pharyngeal suction, endotracheal intubation, endotracheal suction, and positive pressure oxygenation should be instituted as soon as possible.

For many years the Apgar score as described above was used to assess the condition of the newborn immediately after birth. The score has been a useful clinical tool to help identify those neonates who might require resuscitation, as well as the effectiveness of any resuscitative measures. Unfortunately, attempts have been made to relate the score to the ultimate long-term outcome of infants. Additionally, for reasons that are not entirely clear, erroneous definitions of asphyxia have been established, based upon the Apgar score alone. Because of these misconceptions, the Committee on Maternal and Fetal Medicine

of the American College of Obstetricians and Gynecologists (1986) and the Committee on Fetus and Newborn of the American Academy of Pediatrics (1986) issued a joint statement on the use and misuse of the Apgar score. Because of the importance of this statement, and with permission from the American College of Obstetricians and Gynecologists, it is now included in its entirety:

Use and Misuse of the Apgar Score

The Apgar score, devised in 1952 by Dr. Virginia Apgar, is a quick method of assessing the state of the newborn (Apgar, 1953; Apgar and co-workers, 1958). The ease of scoring by this method has led to its use in many studies of neonatal outcome. Its misuse, however, as appears in the 9th revision of the International Classification of Disease (ICD-9-CM) Coding, has led to an erroneous definition of asphyxia. Intrapartum asphyxia implies fetal hypercarbia and hypoxemia, which if prolonged will result in metabolic acidemia. Since the intrapartum disruption of uterine or fetal blood flow is rarely, if ever, absolute, asphyxia is an imprecise, general term. Terms such as hypercarbia, hypoxia, metabolic, respiratory, or lactic acidemia are more precise, both for immediate assessment of the newborn and for retrospective assessment of intrapartum management.

Although the Apgar score continues to provide a convenient shorthand for reporting the state of the newborn and the effectiveness of resuscitation, the purpose of this statement is to place the Apgar score in its proper perspective as a tool for assessing asphyxia and predicting future neurological deficit.

Factors That May Affect Apgar Scores

The Apgar score comprises five components: heart rate, respiratory effort, tone, reflex irritability, and color, each of which can be given a score of 0, 1, or 2 [Table 12–1]. Although rarely stated, it is important to recognize that elements of the score such as tone, color, and reflex irritability are partially dependent on the physiologic maturity of the infant. The normal premature infant may thus receive a low score purely because of immaturity, with no evidence of anoxic insult or cerebral depression.

Maternal sedation or analgesia may decrease tone and responsiveness. Neurologic conditions such as muscle disease and cerebral malformations may decrease tone and interfere with respiration. Cardiorespiratory conditions may interfere with heart rate, respiration, and tone. Thus, to equate the presence of a low Apgar score solely with asphyxia or with future neurologic outcome represents a misuse of the score.

Apgar Score and Subsequent Disability

The 1-minute Apgar score may be used to indicate the infant who requires special attention. A low 1-minute score, however, does not correlate with future outcome (Fields and associates, 1983).

The 5-minute Apgar score, particularly the change in the score between 1 and 5 minutes, is a useful index of the effectiveness of resuscitation efforts. However, even a 5-minute score of 0 to 3, although possibly due to hypoxia, is limited in indicating the severity of the problem and correlates poorly with future neurologic

TABLE 12–1. APGAR SCORING SYSTEM

Sign	0	1	2
Heart rate	Absent	Slow (below 100)	Over 100
Respiratory effort	Absent	Slow, irregular	Good, crying
Muscle tone	Flaccid	Some flexion of extremities	Active motion
Reflex irritability	No response	Grimace	Vigorous cry
Color	Blue, pale	Body pink, extremities blue	Completely pink

outcome (Nelson and Ellenberg, 1981). An Apgar score of 0 to 3 at 5 minutes is associated with an increased risk of cerebral palsy, but this risk increases only from 0.3 percent to 1 percent. A 5-minute Apgar score of 7 to 10 is considered normal. Scores of 4, 5, and 6 are intermediate and are not markers of high risk of later neurologic dysfunction. As mentioned, such scores are affected by physiologic immaturity, sedation, the presence of congenital malformations, and other factors.

Because Apgar scores at 1 and 5 minutes correlate poorly with either cause or outcome, these scores alone should not be considered either evidence of or consequent to substantial asphyxia. Therefore, a low 5-minute Apgar score alone does not prove that later cerebral palsy was caused by perinatal asphyxia.

Later Scores

Correlation of the Apgar score with future neurologic outcome increases when the score is 0 to 3 at 10, 15, and 20 minutes (Nelson and Ellenberg, 1981). Although cerebral asphyxia may be brief or transient and may be manifested as a low Apgar score at 5 minutes, substantial cerebral hypoxia leading to cerebral palsy can be presumed only when three criteria are met:

1. Apgar score is 0 to 3 at 10 minutes (in the absence of other cause)
2. Infant remains hypotonic for at least several hours (Sarnat and Sarnat, 1976; Finer and associates, 1983)
3. Infant has seizures (Mellits and colleagues, 1982)

Confirmation of suspected hypoxia (asphyxia) may be obtained by demonstrating metabolic acidemia in umbilical cord blood. The absence of metabolic acidemia in umbilical cord blood makes intrapartum asphyxia unlikely.

Cerebral palsy is the only neurologic deficit clearly linked to perinatal asphyxia. Although mental retardation and epilepsy may accompany cerebral palsy, there is no evidence that these conditions are caused by perinatal asphyxia unless cerebral palsy is also present (U.S. Department of Health and Human Services, 1985). The Apgar score alone cannot establish the occurrence of sufficient hypoxia to cause cerebral palsy. An infant with an Apgar score of 0 to 3 at 5 minutes whose 10-minute score improves to 4 or better has a 99 percent chance of not having cerebral palsy at 7 years of age. It should also be noted that 75 percent of children in whom cerebral palsy has developed had normal Apgar scores at birth (Nelson and Ellenberg, 1981).

In an infant with a low Apgar score, the presence of umbilical cord acidemia in the absence of maternal acidemia, large base deficit, and nucleated erythrocytes in the peripheral blood may provide supporting evidence of asphyxia; liver, renal, and cardiac dysfunction may also provide evidence of asphyxia. To date, however, none of these indications has been convincingly correlated with central nervous system outcome.

Summary

Low Apgar scores at 1 and 5 minutes are excellent indicators for identification of infants needing resuscitation. Although low scores may be evidence of hypoxia, they are influenced by other factors affecting tone, responsiveness, and respiration. Apgar scores alone are not evidence of sufficient hypoxia to result in neurologic damage. In a child who later is found to have cerebral palsy, low 1- or 5-minute Apgar scores provide insufficient evidence that the damage was due to hypoxia. To substantiate that hypoxia led to adverse neurologic outcome, additional perinatal evidence, such as Apgar scores of 0 to 3 at 10 minutes, early perinatal seizures, and prolonged hypotonia, is required. One of these elements alone is insufficient evidence that prolonged or severe asphyxia has occurred. In the absence of such evidence, subsequent neurologic deficits cannot be ascribed to perinatal asphyxia (Brann and Dykes, 1977).

UMBILICAL CORD BLOOD ACID-BASE AND BLOOD GAS MEASUREMENTS

An objective method that might be used to identify hypoxia in the newborn has been sought. It is possible that hypoxia can be confirmed by identifying evidence for metabolic acidemia through umbilical arterial acid-base measurements at birth (Fields and co-workers, 1983; Gilstrap and associates, 1984a, 1984b, 1987; Goldenberg and colleagues, 1984). Normal values for acid-base and blood gas measurements have been reported by Yeomans and associates (1985) and are listed in Table 12–2. These were obtained in neonates who had normal intrapartum fetal heart rate tracings and who were delivered at term from women without complications. Ruth and Raivio (1988) reported similar values. Acidemia has been defined as umbilical arterial pH of less than 7.2 (Gilstrap and associates, 1984a; Seeds, 1978; Wible and colleagues, 1982). Subsequently, however, Yeomans and associates (1988) showed that a pH between 7.10 and 7.19 was associated with a vigorous neonate in 83 percent of cases.

Umbilical cord blood gas and acid-base analysis can be informative and reassuring, but sometimes misleading. For example, an umbilical cord arterial pH above 7.2 is convincing evidence that obstetrical management of labor did not result in fetal asphyxia. The detection of an umbilical cord pH of less than 7.2, however, may be the result of a respiratory, metabolic or mixed acidosis. Most often, these low pHs are not due to metabolic acidemia, and **it is only a metabolic acidosis of severe magnitude and long duration** that results in serious fetal damage. Unfortunately, neither the severity of the acidosis nor any corresponding damage has been well elucidated. Therefore, it is important to ascertain in the acidemic fetus the type of acidosis present and the likely etiology. If such information is not available, an arterial cord blood pH of less than 7.2 can be misleading. Although the precise pH that should be used to identify "significant acidosis" is not known, pH values above 7.2 are generally reassuring with regard to fetal hypoxia. Gilstrap and co-workers (1989) suggest that to diagnose asphyxia requires an arterial pH

TABLE 12–2. UMBILICAL ARTERIAL AND VENOUS pH AND BLOOD GAS DETERMINATIONS AT BIRTH IN 146 NORMAL NEONATES

	Arterial				Venous			
	Mean	SD[a]	Range	SEM[b]	Mean	SD[a]	Range	SEM[b]
pH	7.28	0.05	7.15–7.43	0.004	7.35	0.05	7.24–7.49	0.0004
PCO_2 (mm Hg)	49.2	8.4	31.1–74.3	0.68	38.2	5.6	23.2–49.2	0.46
PO_2 (mm Hg)	18.0	6.2	3.8–33.8	0.50	29.2	5.9	15.4–48.2	0.48
Bicarbonate (mEq per L)	22.3	2.5	13.3–27.5	0.20	20.4	2.1	15.9–24.7	0.17

[a]SD = standard deviation.
[b]SEM = standard error of the mean.
Modified from Yeomans and associates: Am J Obstet Gynecol 151:798, 1985.

TABLE 12–3. UMBILICAL ARTERIAL pH AND BLOOD GAS DETERMINATIONS IN 277 NEWBORNS WITH NORMAL AND ABNORMAL BASELINE FETAL HEART RATE DURING SECOND-STAGE LABOR

| | Second-Stage Labor Baseline Fetal Heart Rate | | | |
Factor[a]	Normal (N = 129)	Tachycardia (N = 32)	Mild Bradycardia (N = 53)	Moderate to Severe Bradycardia (N = 63)
pH	7.29 ± 0.6	7.25 ± .05[b]	7.23 ± .07[b]	7.22 ± .07[b]
PCO_2 (mm Hg)	45 ± 10	46.3 ± 12.1	48.6 ± 10.7	50.7 ± 11.5
PO_2 (mm Hg)	21.2 ± 7.5	20.3 ± 7.0	19.9 ± 7.5	19.9 ± 6.5
HCO_3 (mEq per L)	21.1 ± 3.8	19.8 ± 4.4	19.9 ± 3.8	19.7 ± 3.9
Buffer deficit (mEq per L)	−6.5 ± 8.5	−6.7 ± 3.5	−7.8 ± 3.9	−8.8 ± 4.4[b]
Hgb (g per dL)	15.7 ± 2.5	14.9 ± 3.5	15.5 ± 2.3	15.2 ± 2.8
Arterial pH < 7.20	6%	22%	30%	40%

[a]Data are expressed as mean ± SD.
[b]Statistically significantly different from normals ($P < 0.05$).
Modified from Gilstrap and associates: Obstet Gynecol 70:191, 1987.

less than 7.00, a 1-minute Apgar less than 3, and evidence of organ dysfunction.

Gilstrap and co-workers (1987) correlated the specific type of neonatal acidemia with second-stage labor fetal heart rate abnormalities. *Respiratory acidosis* was defined as umbilical arterial pH less than 7.2, PCO_2 two standard deviations above the mean (65 mm Hg or above), and normal or more commonly elevated umbilical arterial HCO_3 (33.3 mEq per L or higher). *Metabolic acidemia* was defined as arterial pH less than 7.2, normal or low PCO_2 (49.2 mm or less), and HCO_3 within two standard deviations of reported mean values (17.3 mEq per L or lower). *Mixed umbilical arterial acidemia* was defined as all other umbilical arterial PCO_2 and HCO_3 values between those defined for respiratory and metabolic values.

Fetal heart rate tracings were obtained during second-stage labor by scalp electrodes, and fetuses with periodic heart rate abnormalities were excluded. Therefore, they included only fetuses with normal heart rates or those with obvious baseline changes of either bradycardia or tachycardia. They defined mild fetal bradycardia as 90 to 119 beats per minute, moderate bradycardia as 60 to 89 beats per minute, and severe bradycardia as less than 60 beats per minute. Tachycardia was defined as a fetal heart rate greater than 160 beats per minute.

Umbilical arterial acidemia was observed in 40 percent of 63 neonates with moderate and severe bradycardia, in 30 percent of 53 with mild bradycardia, and in 22 percent of 32 with tachy-

cardia, compared to only 6 percent of 129 with a normal heart rate (Table 12–3). Of the 53 acidemic neonates, 55 percent had mixed respiratory-metabolic acidosis, 23 percent had respiratory acidosis, and 21 percent had metabolic acidosis (Table 12–4). Of interest was the finding that 8 of the 12 neonates with metabolic acidosis had had moderate to severe bradycardia during labor. These authors concluded that second-stage labor fetal heart rate abnormalities were predictive for newborns at increased risk for acidemia at birth. However, the severity and duration of metabolic acidemia to produce fetal damage is not known. It is likely that the continued evaluation of umbilical cord blood gas and acid-base measurements will provide data for such assessments that hopefully will correlate with ante- and intrapartum events.

ACTIVE RESUSCITATION

Although resuscitative measures beyond the stimulation provided by suctioning the mouth and nares, patting the feet, and rubbing the back are needed by only a small percentage of infants, more active measures, skillfully performed, are lifesaving for that small group.

Successful active resuscitation requires (1) skilled personnel who are immediately available, (2) a suitably heated, well-lighted, appropriately large work area (Fig. 12–2), (3) equipment to deliver oxygen by intermittent positive pressure through a face mask and to carry out endotracheal intubation with endotracheal suction and positive-pressure oxygenation (Fig. 12–3), and (4) drugs, syringes, needles, and catheters for possible intravenous administration of naloxone (Narcan), sodium bicarbonate, and, rarely, intracardiac injection of epinephrine. The site of every delivery, vaginal or abdominal, must be so equipped for resuscitation, and the equipment should be thoroughly checked before each delivery.

VENTILATION BY MASK

Inadequate respirations that persist much beyond a minute lead to a falling heart rate and decreased muscle tone and call for a quick but careful physical examination, especially of the mouth, nose, pharynx, neck, and chest, and the administration of oxygen. If the mouth and pharynx are free of liquid and foreign material and no physical obstruction to breathing is identified, oxygen may be delivered through a well-fitting mask at a pressure of about 20 cm of water in 1- to 2-second bursts to deliver

TABLE 12–4. CORRELATION OF SECOND-STAGE LABOR BASELINE FETAL HEART RATE AND TYPE OF UMBILICAL ARTERIAL ACIDEMIA

| | Acidemia | | |
	Metabolic	Respiratory	Mixed
Normal (N = 8)	1	3	4
Tachycardia (N = 7)	1	1	5
Mild bradycardia (N = 16)	2	4	10
Moderate to severe bradycardia (N = 25)	8	5	12
Total (N = 56)	12 (21%)	13 (23%)	31 (55%)

From Gilstrap and associates: Obstet Gynecol 70:191, 1987.

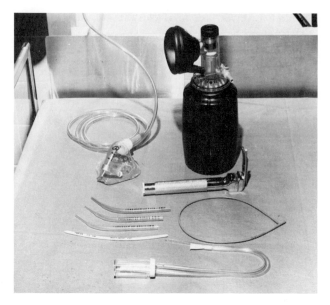

Figure 12–3. Equipment for emergency ventilation of the newborn infant.

oxygen into the bronchi. If this maneuver does not *promptly* stimulate breathing and correct the evidence of hypoxia, tracheal intubation is necessary under direct visualization with an appropriate laryngoscope.

TRACHEAL INTUBATION

The head of the supine infant is kept level. The laryngoscope is introduced into the right side of the mouth and then directed posteriorly toward the oropharynx (Fig. 12–4). The laryngoscope is next gently moved into the space between the base of

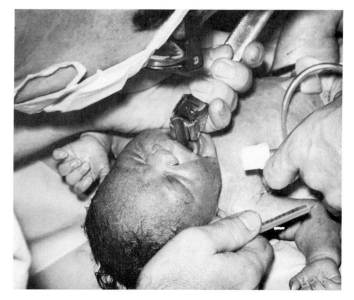

Figure 12–4. Use of laryngoscope to insert tracheal tube under direct vision. Oxygen is being delivered from curved tube held by an assistant.

the tongue and the epiglottis. Gentle elevation of the tip of the laryngoscope will pick up the epiglottis and expose the glottis and the vocal cords. The tracheal tube is introduced through the right side of the mouth and is inserted through the vocal cords until the shoulder of the tube reaches the glottis. Care must be exercised to make sure that the tube is in the trachea and not in the esophagus. The laryngoscope is then removed. Any foreign material encountered in the tracheal tube is immediately removed by suction. Meconium, blood, mucus, and particulate debris in amnionic fluid or in the birth canal may have been inhaled in utero or in the vagina. The resuscitator fills his mouth from an oxygen line and repeatedly puffs oxygen-rich air into the endotracheal tube at 1- to 2-second intervals with force adequate to lift gently the infant's chest wall. Pressures of 25 to 35 cm of water are desired to expand the alveoli yet not cause pneumothorax or pneumomediastinum. Alternatively, intermittent positive-pressure ventilation with oxygen delivered from a bag connected to the tracheal tube is used. If the stomach expands, the tube is almost certainly in the esophagus rather than in the trachea. Once adequate spontaneous respirations have been established, the tube can usually be removed safely.

CAUSES OF PERSISTENT DEPRESSION OF THE NEWBORN

Acidosis

Sodium bicarbonate, 1 mEq per kg, is injected through the umbilical vein of the severely depressed, hypoxic newborn who does not respond promptly to establishment of an airway and positive-pressure oxygen administration. This dose may be repeated if a favorable clinical response is not achieved. It is essential that the infant be ventilated effectively so that carbon dioxide from the bicarbonate can be dissipated. Otherwise, respiratory acidosis will develop, as well as a metabolic acidosis. Further administration of sodium bicarbonate is dependent upon results of measurements of blood gases and pH.

Opioid Drugs

Meperidine (Demerol) and similar drugs given to the mother an hour or less before delivery may cause respiratory depression in the newborn infant. In such cases, naloxone (Narcan) may be given in a dose of 10 μg per kg (Chap. 17, p. 329). If narcotics have not been given within 4 hours, naloxone at 10 times the usual dose (400 μg per kg) provided no benefit in the resuscitation of depressed newborns (Chernick and colleagues, 1988).

Hypovolemia

Some severely depressed newborn infants are hypovolemic. Hypovolemia may occur without fetal hemorrhage having been detected, for example, with sepsis, fetal-to-maternal hemorrhage, trauma to the placenta, cord compression with obstruction of the umbilical vein and pooling of blood in the placenta, and twin-to-twin transfusion. At least partial restoration of intravascular volume and correction of severe anemia are essential for improvement in the volume-depleted infant.

CARDIAC MASSAGE

If fetal heart action was present just before delivery but cannot be demonstrated after birth or if the heart stops after birth, external cardiac massage may be initiated. Immediately, the airway must be cleared, the trachea intubated, and adequate pulmonary ventilation established. External cardiac massage is effected with pressure from two fingers applied to the anterior chest wall in the lower midline at a rate of about 120 per minute. Four compressions of the chest are alternated with each inflation of the lung. A delay of several minutes in cardiac massage most likely will result in an unfortunate outcome, either death or permanent marked impairment of central nervous system function.

Epinephrine may be of value in resuscitating the arrested heart. Epinephrine, 0.1 mL per kg of a 1:10,000 dilution, is injected directly into the heart. A 22- or 24-gauge needle is inserted through the fourth intercostal space just to the left of the sternum, blood is aspirated to assure appropriate position of the needle tip, and the drug is injected as a bolus. Serious trauma from intracardiac injection is always a possibility, but an intravenous injection may never reach the heart.

COMMON ERRORS IN RESUSCITATION OF THE NEWBORN

If resuscitation efforts are not rapidly successful, the apparent failure may be the consequence of an easily correctable technical error. Even the most skilled and experienced operator can experience difficulties, and the possibility of technical errors should always be kept in mind when an infant fails to respond to resuscitation. These common errors include the following:

1. Failure to check resuscitation equipment beforehand
   a. Damaged resuscitation bag
   b. Laryngoscope with dull or flickering light
   c. Unsterile umbilical catheter
2. Use of a cold resuscitation table
3. Unsuccessful intubation
   a. Hyperextension of neck
   b. Inadequate suctioning
   c. Excessive force
4. Inadequate ventilation
   a. Improper head position
   b. Improper application of mask
   c. Placement of tracheal tube into esophagus or right mainstem bronchus
   d. Failure to secure the tracheal tube
5. Failure to detect and determine cause of poor chest movement or persistent bradycardia
6. Failure to detect and treat hypovolemia
7. Failure to perform cardiac massage

ROUTINE NEWBORN CARE

ESTIMATION OF GESTATIONAL AGE

A rapid yet rather precise estimate of gestational age of the newborn infant may be made very soon after delivery by examining (1) sole creases, (2) breast nodules, (3) scalp hair, (4) ear lobe, and (5) in the case of the male, testes and scrotum, as outlined in Table 12–5. A more definitive estimate can be made in a few days with the help of neurological examination (Chap. 38, p. 744). Unfortunately, estimates of gestational age based upon physical and neurological examination of the neonate are frequently unacceptably inaccurate in preterm and growth-retarded infants. (Rosenfeld and associates, 1984; Spinnato and co-workers, 1984). It is unwise to rely on these evaluations alone in such neonates.

CARE OF THE EYES

Because of the possibility of infection of the eyes of the newborn during passage through the vagina of a mother with gonorrhea, Credé, in 1884, introduced the practice of instilling into each eye immediately after birth one drop of a 1 percent solution of silver nitrate, which was later washed out with saline. This procedure led to a marked decrease in the frequency but not the elimination of a *gonococcal ophthalmia* and resulting blindness.

> **Technique for Silver Nitrate Prophylaxis**
>
> As a preliminary precaution, the region about each eye should be irrigated with sterile water applied to the nasal side of the eye and allowed to run off the opposite side. The lower lid should then be drawn down and the 1 percent silver nitrate solution dropped into the lower cul-de-sac. The silver nitrate produces a discernible chemical conjunctivitis in over half the cases, manifested by redness, edema, or discharge, which develops in 24 hours and lasts 2 to 3 days.

Antibiotic Prophylaxis

Penicillin serves as an alternate to silver nitrate in prophylaxis of gonococcal ophthalmia neonatorum. Penicillin ointment in the strength of 100,000 units per g is placed in the eyes of the newborn baby, or penicillin is given parenterally. Some institutions use a single dose of penicillin injected intramuscularly soon after delivery. Penicillin so administered to the neonate also may reduce the frequency of sepsis from group B *Streptococcus* (Siegel and associates, 1982).

Tetracycline ointment containing the antibiotic in a concentration of 1 percent, or erythromycin ointment, 0.5 percent,

---

TABLE 12–5. RAPID ESTIMATION OF GESTATIONAL AGE OF THE NEWBORN

Sites	Gestational age		
	36 Wk or Less	*37 to 38 Wk*	*39 Wk or More*
Sole creases	Anterior transverse crease only	Occasional creases anterior two thirds	Sole covered with creases
Breast nodule diameter	2 mm	4 mm	7 mm
Scalp hair	Fine and fuzzy	Fine and fuzzy	Coarse and silky
Ear lobe	Pliable, no cartilage	Some cartilage	Stiffened by thick cartilage
Testes and scrotum	Testes in lower canal, scrotum small, few rugae	Intermediate	Testes pendulous, scrotum full, extensive rugae

liberally instilled into each eye with the lids held apart, affords effective prophylaxis. Both should serve to prevent, or at least reduce, the incidence of chlamydial conjunctivitis (Dillon, 1986). Laga and colleagues (1988) reported that tetracycline ointment was as effective as silver nitrate solution in preventing gonococcal ophthalmia. Interestingly, while both afforded substantive protection against *Chlamydia trachomatis* infection, approximately 10 percent of exposed infants developed chlamydial conjunctivitis despite prophylaxis.

PERMANENT INFANT IDENTIFICATION

Proper identification of each infant is of prime importance. A foolproof system must be operative at all hours. It should prevent separation of the infant from his or her mother until identification is complete, and it should provide a record easily recognized by the mother, such as an identification band or row of beads that spell the infant's name. It is crucial, furthermore, that a permanent record, such as footprints, be kept on file at the hospital (Fig. 12–5).

The definitive ridges on the palms, fingers, and feet of human beings begin to form several months before birth and remain throughout life. Most hospitals today use footprints rather than fingerprints or palmprints in identifying infants, because the ridges in the feet are more pronounced, and it is easier to obtain prints from them in newborn infants. For the footprint to be satisfactory, close attention must be paid to technique. Too often the ridges are not discrete and, therefore, the print is of no value (Clark and associates, 1981). Footprinting procedures were discontinued at Parkland Hospital in 1985.

SUBSEQUENT CARE

Temperature
The temperature of the infant drops rapidly immediately after birth. If the naked newborn is left exposed in the usual air-conditioned delivery room or nursery, chilling so produced incites shivering and increases oxygen requirements. Conse-

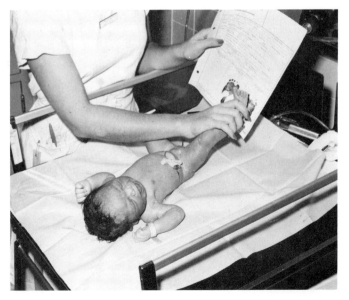

Figure 12–5. Making a permanent record of the newborn infant's footprints.

quently, the infant must be cared for in a warm crib in which temperature control is regulated closely. During the first few days of life, the infant's temperature is unstable, responding to slight stimuli with considerable fluctuations above or below the normal level.

Vitamin K
Routine administration of vitamin K is urged, as described in Chapter 33 (p. 611).

Umbilical Cord
Loss of water from Wharton's jelly leads to mummification of the cord shortly after birth. Within 24 hours it loses its characteristic bluish white, moist appearance and soon becomes dry and black. Gradually the line of demarcation appears just beyond the skin of the abdomen, and in a few days the stump sloughs, leaving a small, granulating wound, which after healing forms the umbilicus. Separation usually takes place within the first 2 weeks, with a range of 3 to 45 days (Novack and colleagues, 1988). The umbilical cord dries more quickly and separates more readily when exposed to the air, and therefore a dressing is not recommended.

Formerly, disregard for asepsis in management of the cord frequently resulted in serious infection transmitted through the umbilical vessels. Even today serious umbilical infections are sometimes encountered, usually, but not always, indicating lack of care. The offending organisms often are *Staphylococcus aureus*, *Escherichia coli*, or group B *Streptococcus*. Since the umbilical stump in such cases may present no outward sign of infection, the diagnosis cannot be made with certainty except by autopsy. Strict aseptic precautions should therefore be observed in the immediate care of the cord. Most apply triple dye or bacitracin ointment (American College of Obstetricians and Gynecologists, 1988). Gladstone and colleagues (1988) found that povidone-iodine applied daily was effective and acceptable.

Neonatal *tetanus* continues to kill infants in developing countries, with neonatal death rates as high as 145 per 1,000 births in Haiti! Hygienic practices applied to the cutting and subsequent management of the umbilical cord serve to eliminate this serious complication. In addition, active immunization of the mother against tetanus with passage of antibody to the fetus can serve to reduce the risk to the infant appreciably.

Care of the Skin
Infants should be promptly patted dry to minimize heat loss caused by evaporation. In most hospitals, not all the vernix caseosa is removed, but the excess, as well as blood and meconium, is gently wiped off. The vernix caseosa is readily absorbed by the baby's skin and disappears entirely within 24 hours. It is unwise to wash a newborn until his or her temperature has stabilized. Handling of the baby is minimized.

Stools and Urine
For the first 2 or 3 days after birth, the contents of the colon are composed of soft, brownish-green *meconium,* which is composed of desquamated epithelial cells from the intestinal tract, mucus, and epidermal cells and lanugo (fetal hair) that have been swallowed with the amnionic fluid. The characteristic color results from bile pigments. During intrauterine life and for a few hours after birth, the intestinal contents are sterile, but bacteria soon gain access. The passage of meconium and urine in the minutes immediately after birth or during the next few hours indicates patency of the gastrointestinal and urinary tracts. Of

all newborn infants, 90 percent pass meconium within the first 24 hours; most of the rest do so within 36 hours. Voiding, although usually occurring shortly after birth, may not occur until the second day of life. Failure of the infant to eliminate meconium or urine after these times suggests a congenital defect, such as imperforate anus or a urethral valve.

After the third or fourth day, as the consequence of ingesting milk, the meconium disappears and is replaced by light yellow homogeneous feces with a characteristic odor. For the first few days the stools are unformed, but soon thereafter they assume the cylindric shape.

Icterus Neonatorum

About one third of all babies, between the second and fifth day of life, develop so-called *physiological jaundice of the newborn.* There is a hyperbilirubinemia at birth of 1.8 to 2.8 mg per dL. It increases during the next few days but with wide individual variation. Between the third and fourth day, the bilirubin in mature infants commonly reaches somewhat more than 5 mg per dL, the concentration at which jaundice usually becomes noticeable. Most of the bilirubin is free, or unconjugated. One cause, but not the sole cause, of the hyperbilirubinemia is immaturity of the hepatic cells, resulting in slight conjugation of bilirubin with glucuronic acid and reduced excretion in bile (Chap. 33, p. 609). Reabsorption of free bilirubin as the consequence of the enzymatic splitting of bilirubin glucuronide by intestinal conjugase activity in the newborn intestine also appears to contribute significantly to the transient hyperbilirubinemia. In preterm infants, jaundice is more common and usually more severe and prolonged than in term infants because of greater hepatic enzymatic immaturity. Infants who are term but small for gestational age, however, metabolize bilirubin in a manner similar to term infants. Increased erythrocyte destruction from any cause contributes to hyperbilirubinemia.

Initial Weight Loss

Because the infant may receive little nutriment for the first 3 or 4 days of life and at the same time produces a considerable amount of urine, feces, and sweat, he or she progressively loses weight until the flow of maternal milk or other feeding has been established. Preterm infants lose relatively more weight and regain their birthweight more slowly than do term infants. Infants that are small for gestational age but otherwise healthy regain their initial weight more quickly when fed than do preterm infants.

If the normal infant is nourished properly, the birthweight is usually regained by the end of the tenth day. Subsequently, the weight typically increases steadily at the rate of about 25 g a day for the first few months, to double the birthweight by 5 months of age and to triple it by the end of the first year.

Feeding

It is advisable, because of the stimulating effect of nursing on mother and baby, to commence regular nursing within the first 12 hours postpartum. Most term infants thrive best when fed at intervals of about 4 hours. Preterm or growth-retarded infants require feedings at shorter intervals. In most instances a 3-hour interval is satisfactory.

The proper length of each feeding depends on several factors, such as the quantity of breast milk, the readiness with which it can be obtained from the breast, and the avidity with which the infant nurses. It is generally advisable to allow the baby to remain at the breast for 10 minutes at first; 4 to 5 minutes are sufficient for some infants, however, and 15 to 20 minutes are required by others. It is satisfactory for the baby to nurse for 5 minutes at each breast for the first 4 days or until the mother has a supply of milk. After the fourth day, the baby nurses up to 10 minutes on each breast. A baby receiving proper nourishment should increase steadily in weight.

Circumcision

There is no absolute medical indication for routine circumcision of the newborn, as emphasized in the report of the Ad Hoc Task Force on Circumcision to the American Academy of Pediatrics (1975). Despite this, Brown and Brown (1987) report that there has been no change in circumcision practice in the United States. They attribute this to cultural rituals rather than to a medical misunderstanding by parents.

The following advantages are commonly claimed for circumcision of the newborn infant: (1) phimosis is prevented, (2) the incidence of balanitis is markedly reduced, (3) penile cancer is virtually eliminated, and (4) it has become traditional to circumcise male infants in the United States. None of these items justifies routine circumcision. Lack of circumcision of the male sex partner does not appear to increase the risk of carcinoma of the cervix, as previously thought.

Circumcision, if it is to be done at all, should not be performed at delivery but rather a day or two later, after the infant has been demonstrated to be healthy. Prematurity, neonatal illness, most congenital anomalies of the penis, and coagulation defects are contraindications to circumcision.

Within the past few years, there has been a flurry of reports critical of routine circumcision. The adverse comments range from psychological trauma to subsequent hypesthesia of the glans. The subjective nature of these allegations makes them difficult to prove. For example, Thompson (1983) cites at least 100 listings from the English-speaking literature referenced in *Index Medicus* from 1975 to 1983, 19 of which were in the journal *Pediatrics*. Perhaps 5 to 10 percent of males will be considered to need circumcision later in life when the cost, emotional trauma, and the risk from anesthesia will be greater. Routine circumcision of the male newborn is not performed at Parkland Hospital.

Anesthesia for Circumcision?

Kirya and Werthmann (1978) raised the question, "Why not anesthesia for neonatal circumcision?" and, in turn, described their experiences with regional nerve block from injected lidocaine. Stang and colleagues (1988) verified that dorsal penile nerve block reduced behavioral distress and modified adrenocortical stress response. Perhaps a more pertinent question is "Why routine neonatal circumcision in the first place?"

Rooming-in

Rooming-in involves keeping the infant in a crib at the mother's bedside rather than in the nursery, thus permitting the mother to take care of the baby. This practice stems in part from a trend to make all phases of childbearing as natural as possible and to foster proper mother-child relationships at an early date. By the end of 24 hours, the mother is generally fully ambulatory, and thereafter, with rooming-in, she can conduct for herself and for the infant practically all routine care. An advantage of this program is the mother's increased ability when she arrives home to assume full care of the baby.

Abnormalities of the Newborn Infant

These are considered throughout the text and especially in Chapters 33 and 38.

REFERENCES

Ad Hoc Task Force on Circumcision: Pediatrics 56:610, 1975

American Academy of Pediatrics: Committee on Fetus and Newborn: Use and abuse of the Apgar Score. Pediatrics 78:1148, 1986

American College of Obstetricians and Gynecologists Committee on Maternal and Fetal Medicine: Use and misuse of the Apgar Score. November 1986

American College of Obstetricians and Gynecologists: Control of Infections in Obstetric and Nursing Areas. Chap 6 In Guidelines for Perinatal Care, 2nd ed., 1988, p 128

Apgar V: A proposal for a new method of evaluation of the newborn infant. Curr Res Anesth Analg 32:260, 1953

Apgar V, Holaday DA, James LS, Weisbrot IM, Berrien C: Evaluation of the newborn infant—second report. JAMA 168:1985, 1958

Barcroft J, Kramer K, Millikan GA: The oxygen in the carotid blood at birth. J Physiol 94:571, 1939

Brann AW Jr, Dykes FD: The effects of intrauterine asphyxia on the full-term neonate. Clin Perinatol 4:149, 1977

Brown MS, Brown CA: Circumcision decision: Prominence of social concerns. Pediatrics 80:215, 1987

Chernick V: Fetal breathing movements and the onset of breathing at birth. Clin Perinatol 5:257, 1978

Chernick V, Manfreda J, DeBooy V, Davi M, Rigatto H, Seshia M: Clinical trial of naloxone in birth asphyxia. J Pediatr 113:519, 1988

Clark DA, Thompson J, Cahill J, Salisbury B: Footprinting the newborn—cost effective? Pediatr Res 15:552, 1981

Credé CSF: Die Verhütung der Augenenzündung der Neugeborenen. Berlin, Hirschwald, 1884

Dawes GS: Breathing before birth in animals or man. N Engl J Med 290:557, 1974

Dillon HC Jr: Prevention of gonococcal ophthalmia neonatorum. N Engl J Med 315:1414, 1986

Duenhoelter JH, Pritchard JA: Fetal respiration: Quantitative measurements of amnionic fluid inspired near term by human and rhesus fetuses. Am J Obstet Gynecol 125:306,1976

Fields LM, Entman SS, Boehm FH: Correlation of the one-minute Apgar score and the pH value of the umbilical arterial blood. South Med J 76:1477, 1983

Finer NN, Robertson CM, Peters KL, Coward JH: Factors affecting outcome in hypoxic-ischemic encephalopathy in term infants. Am J Dis Child 137:21, 1983

Gilstrap LC, Hauth JC, Hankins GDV, Beck AW: Second-stage fetal heart rate abnormalities and type of neonatal acidemia. Obstet Gynecol 70:191,1987

Gilstrap LC, Hauth JC, Toussaint S: Second-stage fetal heart rate abnormalities and neonatal acidosis. Obstet Gynecol 62:209, 1984a

Gilstrap LC, Hauth JC, Schiano S, Connor KD: Neonatal acidosis and method of delivery. Obstet Gynecol 63:681, 1984b

Gilstrap LC, Leveno KJ, Burris J, Williams ML: Birth asphyxia: 1988. Presented at the Society of Perinatal Obstetricians meeting, February, 1989

Goldenberg RL, Huddleston JF, Nelson KG: Apgar scores and umbilical arterial pH in preterm newborn infants. Am J Obstet Gynecol 149:651, 1984

Josten BE, Johnson TRB, Nelson JP: Umbilical cord blood pH and Apgar scores as an index of neonatal health. Am J Obstet Gynecol 157:843, 1987

Kirya C, Werthmann MW Jr: Neonatal circumcision and penile dorsal route nerve block—a painless procedure. J Pediatr 92:998, 1978

Laga M, Plummer FA, Piot P, Datta P, Namaara W, Ndinya-Achola JO, Nzanze II, Maitha G, Ronald AR, Pamba HO, Brunham RC: Prophylaxis of gonococcal and chlamydial ophthalmia neonatorum: A comparison of silver nitrate and tetracycline. N Engl J Med 318:653, 1988

Martin CB Jr, Murata Y, Petrie RH, Parer JT: Respiratory movements in fetal rhesus monkeys. Am J Obstet Gynecol 119:939, 1974

Mellits ED, Holden KR, Freeman JM: Neonatal seizures: II. A multivariate analysis of factors associated with outcome. Pediatrics 70:177, 1982

Milner AD, Saunders RA, Hopkins IE: The effect of delivery by caesarean section on lung mechanics and lung volume in the human neonate. Arch Dis Child 53:545, 1978

Nelson KB, Ellenberg JH: Apgar scores as predictors of chronic neurologic disability. Pediatrics 68:36, 1981

Novack AH, Mueller B, Ochs H: Umbilical cord separation in the normal newborn. Am J Dis Child 142:220, 1988

Rosenfeld C, Gant N, Tyson J: Unpublished observations

Ruth VJ, Raivio KO: Perinatal brain damage: Predictive value of metabolic acidosis and the Apgar score. Br Med J 297:24, 1988

Sarnet HB, Sarnet MS: Neonatal encephalopathy following fetal distress: A clinical and electroencephalographic study. Arch Neurol 33:696, 1976

Saunders RA: Pulmonary/volume relationships during the last phase of delivery and the first postnatal breaths in human subjects. J Pediatr 93:667, 1978

Seeds AE: Maternal-fetal acid-base relationships and fetal scalp-blood analysis. Clin Obstet Gynecol 21:579, 1978

Siegel JD, McCracken GH Jr, Threlkeld N, DePasse BM, Rosenfeld CR: Single-dose penicillin prophylaxis of neonatal group B streptococcal disease. Lancet 2:1426, 1982

Spinnato JA, Sibai BM, Shaver DC, Anderson GD: Inaccuracy of Dubowitz gestational age in low birth weight infants. Obstet Gynecol 63:491, 1984

Stang JH, Gunnar MR, Snellman L, Condon LM, Kestenbaum R: Local anesthesia for neonatal circumcision. Effects on distress and cortisol response. JAMA 259:1507, 1988

Thompson HC: The value of neonatal circumcision. Am J Dis Child 137:939, 1983

US Department of Health and Human Services: The International Classification of Diseases ICD-9-CM, DHHS Publication No (PHS) 80-1260, Washington DC, GPO, 1980

US Department of Health and Human Services; Public Health Service, National Institutes of Health; National Institute of Child Health and Human Development; Freeman JM (ed): Prenatal and Perinatal Factors Associated with Brain Disorders, NIH Publications No 85-1149. Washington DC, GPO, 1985

Wible JL, Petrie RH, Koons A, Perez A: The clinical use of umbilical cord acid-base determinations in perinatal surveillance and management. Clin Perinatol 9:387, 1982

Yeomans ER, Gilstrap LC, Leveno KJ, Burris JS: Meconium in the amniotic fluid and fetal acid-base status. Obstet Gynecol 73:175, 1989

Yeomans ER, Hauth JC, Gilstrap LC III, Strickland DM: Umbilical cord pH, pCO_2 and bicarbonate following uncomplicated term vaginal deliveries. Am J Obstet Gynecol 151:798, 1985

The Puerperium

DEFINITION

Although the puerperium is defined literally as the period of confinement during and just after birth, it has come to include the subsequent weeks during which the reproductive tract returns to a normal nonpregnant state. The plan for follow-up care that has been generally practiced by most obstetricians, at least until recently, has resulted in the first 6 weeks commonly being considered the puerperium. During this time, the reproductive tract returns anatomically to a normal nonpregnant state, which includes those permanent structural changes in the cervix, vagina, and perineum that were acquired as the consequence of labor and delivery. Moreover, by 6 weeks after delivery, or not long thereafter, in most mothers who are not breast feeding, pituitary-ovarian synchrony will have been reestablished appropriate for ovulation.

INVOLUTION OF THE GENITAL AND URINARY TRACTS

INVOLUTION OF THE BODY OF THE UTERUS

Immediately after expulsion of the placenta, the fundus of the contracted body of the uterus is about midway between the umbilicus and symphysis, or slightly higher. The body of the uterus now consists of mostly myometrium covered by serosa and lined by basal decidua. The anterior and posterior walls, in close apposition, each measure 4 to 5 cm in thickness. Because its vessels are compressed by the contracted myometrium, the puerperal uterus on section appears ischemic when compared to the reddish-purple hyperemic pregnant organ. During the next 2 days, the uterus remains approximately the same size and then shrinks, so that within 2 weeks it has descended into the cavity of the true pelvis and can no longer be felt above the symphysis. It normally regains its previous nonpregnant size within about 4 weeks. The rapidity of the process is remarkable. The freshly delivered uterus weighs approximately 1 kg. As the consequence of *involution*, 1 week later it weighs about 500 g, decreasing at the end of the second week to about 300 g, and soon thereafter to 100 g or even less. The total number of muscle cells does not decrease appreciably; instead, the individual cells decrease markedly in size. The mechanism by which the individual muscle cell divests itself of excess cytoplasm, including contractile protein, remains to be elucidated. The involution of the connective tissue framework occurs equally rapidly.

Since the separation of the placenta and membranes involves primarily the spongy layer of the decidua, the basal portion of the decidua remains in the uterus. The decidua that remains has striking variations in thickness, an irregular jagged appearance, and is infiltrated with blood, especially at the placental site.

REGENERATION OF ENDOMETRIUM

Within 2 or 3 days after delivery the decidua remaining in the uterus becomes differentiated into two layers. The superficial layer becomes necrotic, and is sloughed in the lochia. The basal layer adjacent to the myometrium, which contains the fundi of endometrial glands, remains intact and is the source of new endometrium. The endometrium arises from proliferation of the endometrial glandular remnants and the stroma of the interglandular connective tissue.

The process of endometrial regeneration is rapid, except at the placental site. Elsewhere, the free surface becomes covered by epithelium within a week or 10 days, and the entire endometrium is restored during the third week. Sharman (1953), in an extensive study of postpartum uteri, identified fully restored endometrium in all biopsy specimens obtained from the 16th day onward. The endometrium was normal except for occasional hyalinized decidual remnants and leucocytes. The so-called endometritis indentified histologically in the reparative days of the puerperium is but part of the normal process of repair. Similarly, in almost half of postpartum women tubes demonstrate microscopic inflammatory changes of acute salpingitis between 5 and 15 days; however, this is not because of infection (Andrews, 1951).

INVOLUTION OF THE PLACENTAL SITE

According to Williams (1931), complete extrusion of the placental site takes up to 6 weeks. This process is of great clinical importance, for when it is defective, late puerperal hemorrhage may ensue. Immediately after delivery, the placental site is about the size of the palm of the hand, but it rapidly decreases in size. By the end of the second week, it is 3 to 4 cm in diameter. Very soon after termination of labor, the placental site normally consists of many thrombosed vessels (Fig. 13–1) that next undergo typical organization of the thrombus.

If involution of the placental site comprised only these events, each pregnancy would leave a fibrous scar in the endometrium and subjacent myometrium, thus eventually limiting the number of future pregnancies. In his classic investigations, Williams (1931) explained involution of the placental site as follows:

> Involution is not effected by absorption in situ, but rather by a process of exfoliation which is in great part brought about by the undermining of the placental implantation site by the growth of endometrial tissue. This is affected partly by extension and down

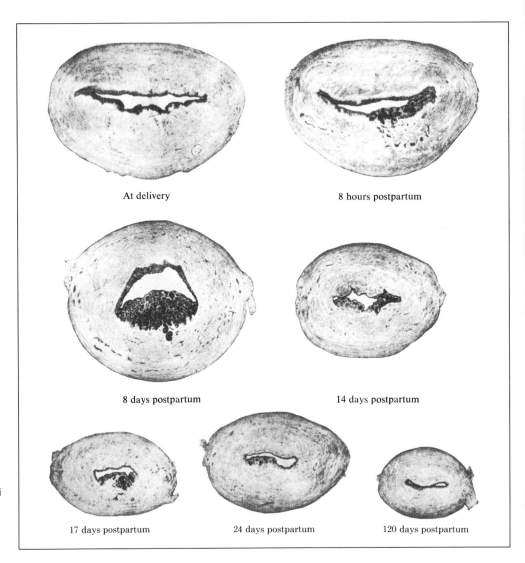

Figure 13–1. Cross-sections of uteri made at the level of the involuting placental site at varying times after delivery. (*From Williams: Am J Obstet Gynecol 22:664, 1931.*)

growth of endometrium from the margins of the placental site and partly by the development of endometrial tissue from the glands and stroma left in the depths of the decidua basalis after the separation of the placenta . . . [;] such a process of exfoliation should be regarded as very conservative, and as a wise provision on the part of nature; otherwise great difficulty might be experienced in getting rid of the obliterated arteries and organized thrombi which, if they remained in situ, would soon convert a considerable part of the uterine mucosa and subadjacent myometrium into a mass of scar tissue with the result that after a few pregnancies it would unlikely be possible for it to go through its usual cycle of changes, and the reproductive career would come to an end.

Anderson and Davis (1968), on the basis of their studies of involution of the placental site, concluded that exfoliation of the placental site is brought about as the consequence of a necrotic slough of infarcted superficial tissues followed by a reparative process not unlike that which takes place on any denuded epithelium-covered structure.

CHANGES IN THE UTERINE VESSELS

A successful pregnancy requires a great increase in uterine blood flow. To provide for this, arteries and veins that transport blood to and from the uterus and those that convey blood within the uterus, especially to the placental site, enlarge remarkably, as do transport vessels to and from the uterus (Chap. 7, p. 130). Within the uterus, growth of new vessels also provides for the marked increase in blood flow. After delivery the caliber of the extrauterine vessels decreases to equal, or at least closely approximate, that of the prepregnant state.

Within the puerperal uterus, for the most part, the blood vessels are obliterated by hyaline changes, and vessels that are smaller develop in their place. The resorption of the hyalinized residue is accomplished by processes similar to those observed in the ovaries subsequent to ovulation and corpus luteum formation. Minor vestiges, however, may persist for years, affording under the microscope a means of differentiating between the uteri of parous and nulliparous women.

CHANGES IN THE CERVIX AND LOWER UTERINE SEGMENT

Immediately after the completion of the third stage of labor, the cervix and lower uterine segment are thin, collapsed, flabby structures. The outer margin of the cervix, which corresponds to the external os, usually is lacerated, especially laterally. The cervical opening contracts slowly. For a few days immediately after labor, it readily admits two fingers, but by the end of the first week, it has become so narrow as to render difficult the introduction of one finger. As the cervical opening narrows, the cervix thickens and a canal is reformed. At the completion of involution, however, the external os does not resume its pregravid appearance completely. It remains somewhat wider, and typically, bilateral depressions at the site of lacerations remain as permanent changes that characterize the parous cervix (Fig. 40–11, p. 880).

After delivery, the markedly thinned-out myometrium of the lower uterine segment contracts and retracts but not as forcefully as the body of the uterus. Over the course of a few weeks the lower segment is converted from a clearly evident structure large enough to contain most of the head of the term fetus to a barely discernible uterine isthmus located between the body of the uterus above and the internal os of the cervix below (Fig. 40–8, p. 879).

VAGINA AND VAGINAL OUTLET

The vagina and vaginal outlet in the first part of the puerperium form a capacious, smooth-walled passage that gradually diminishes in size but rarely returns to the nulliparous dimensions. The rugae reappear by the third week. The hymen is represented by several small tags of tissue, which during cicatrization are converted into the myrtiform caruncles characteristic of parous women.

CHANGES IN THE PERITONEUM AND ABDOMINAL WALL

As the myometrium contracts and retracts after delivery, and for a few days thereafter, the peritoneum covering much of the uterus is formed into folds and wrinkles. The broad and round ligaments are much more lax than in the nonpregnant condition, and they require considerable time to recover from the stretching and loosening to which they have been subjected during pregnancy.

As a result of the rupture of the elastic fibers of the skin and the prolonged distention caused by the enlarged pregnant uterus, the abdominal walls remain soft and flabby for a while. The return to normal of these structures requires several weeks. Recovery is aided by exercise. Except for silvery striae, the abdominal wall usually resumes its prepregnancy appearance, but when the muscles are atonic, it may remain lax. There may be a marked separation, or diastasis, of the rectus muscles. In that condition, the abdominal wall in the vicinity of the midline is formed simply by peritoneum, attenuated fascia, subcutaneous fat, and skin.

CHANGES IN THE URINARY TRACT

Cystoscopic examination soon after delivery shows not only edema and hyperemia of the bladder wall but, frequently, submucous extravasation of blood. In addition, the puerperal bladder has an increased capacity and a relative insensitivity to intravesical fluid pressure. Therefore, overdistention, incomplete emptying, and excessive residual urine must be watched for closely. The paralyzing effect of anesthesia, especially conduction analgesia, and the temporarily disturbed neural function of the bladder are undoubtedly contributory factors. Residual urine and bacteriuria in a traumatized bladder, coupled with the dilated renal pelves and ureters, create optimal conditions for the development of urinary tract infection (Chap. 39, p. 808). The dilated ureters and renal pelves return to the prepregnant state anywhere from 2 to 8 weeks after delivery (Chap. 7, p. 149).

Kerr-Wilson and colleagues (1984) studied the effect of labor on postpartum bladder function using urodynamic techniques. They concluded that, as long as prolonged labors were avoided, and if catheterization was done promptly for bladder distension, there was no evidence for bladder hypotonia. Although they reported that epidural analgesia did not predispose to bladder hypotonia postpartum, Weil and colleagues (1983) found that 35 percent of women who had epidural analgesia had asymptomatic urinary retention. Obviously, careful attention to all postpartum women, with prompt catheterization for those who cannot void, will prevent many urinary problems.

The stretching and dilatation during pregnancy do not cause permanent changes in the renal pelves and ureters unless infection has supervened.

CHANGES IN MAMMARY GLANDS

ANATOMY OF THE BREASTS

The anlagen of the mammary glands are contained in the ectodermal ridges that form on the ventral surface of the embryo and extend from forelimb to hindlimb laterally. The multiple pairs of buds normally all disappear from the embryo except for one pair in the pectoral region that eventually develops into the two mammary glands (Fig. 13–2). At times, however, the buds elsewhere may not completely disappear but, instead, may participate to an amazing degree in the pattern of growth that characterizes the two normal mammary glands (Fig. 28–5).

At midpregnancy each of the two mammary buds in the fetus destined to form the breasts begins to grow and divide, with the formation of 15 to 25 secondary buds that provide the basis for the duct system in the mature breast. Each secondary bud elongates into a cord, bifurcates, and differentiates into two concentric layers of cuboidal cells and a central lumen. The inner layer of cells eventually gives rise to the secretory epithelium, which synthesizes the milk, while the outer layer becomes myoepithelium, which provides the mechanism for milk ejection (Fig. 13–3A,B).

Thelarche, the onset of rapid increase in breast size from estrogen stimulation, begins about the time of puberty when estrogen production rises. The previously infantile mammary glands respond to estrogen with growth and development of the mammary ducts and the deposition of fat. With the onset of ovulation, progesterone is produced, which stimulates development of the alveoli of the mammary glands and sets the stage for future lactation.

Anatomically, each mature mammary gland is composed of 15 to 25 lobes that arose from the secondary mammary buds described above. The lobes are arranged more or less radially and are separated from one another by a varying amount of fat. Each lobe consists of several lobules, which in turn are made up of large numbers of alveoli (Fig. 13–3A,B). Every alveolus is provided with a small duct that joins others to form a single larger duct for each lobe (Fig. 13–3B). These lactiferous ducts make their way to the nipple and open separately upon its surface, where they may be distinguished as minute but distinct orifices. The alveolar secretory epithelium synthesizes the various constituents of the milk (Fig. 13–3C).

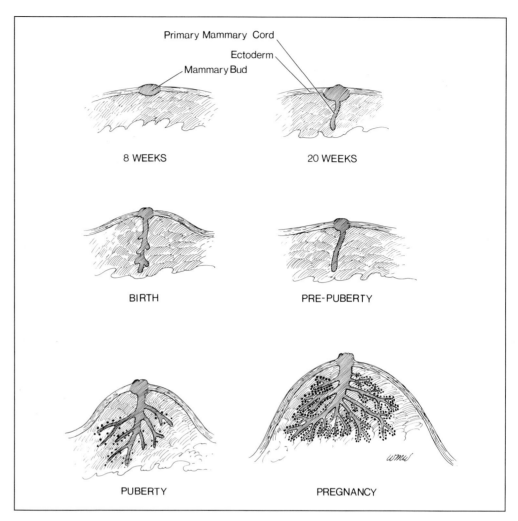

Figure 13–2. Sequential growth of the mammary gland is illustrated from 8 weeks embryonic age through puberty and during pregnancy. (*Courtesy of Dr. John C. Porter.*)

LACTATION

By the second postpartum day a modest amount of colostrum, the liquid secreted by the breasts for the first 5 days after birth of the infant, can be expressed from the nipples.

Colostrum

Compared with the mature milk that is ultimately secreted by the breasts, colostrum contains more protein, much of which is globulin, and more minerals but less sugar and fat. Colostrum nevertheless contains rather large fat globules in so-called colostrum corpuscles, which are thought by some to be epithelial cells that have undergone fatty degeneration and by others to be mononuclear phagocytes containing considerable fat. The secretion of colostrum persists for about 5 days, with gradual conversion to mature milk. Antibodies are readily demonstrable in colostrum. Its content of immunoglobulin A may offer protection to the newborn infant against enteric infection, as described below. Other host resistance factors, as well as immunoglobulins, are present in human colostrum and milk. These include components of complement, macrophages, lymphocytes, lactoferrin, lactoperoxidase, and lysozyme.

Milk

The major components of milk are proteins, lactose, water, and fat. Milk is isotonic with plasma, with lactose accounting for half of the osmotic pressure. The major *proteins* in milk—α-lactalbumin, β-lactoglobulin, and casein—are synthesized in the rough endoplasmic reticulum of the alveolar secretory cell. The essential amino acids are derived from the blood, and nonessential amino acids are derived in part from the blood or synthesized in the mammary gland. Most of the proteins of milk are unique proteins not found elsewhere. Also, prolactin appears to be actively secreted into breast milk (Yuen, 1988).

Major changes that occur 30 to 40 hours postpartum include a sudden increase of lactose concentration. The synthesis of lactose from glucose in the alveolar secretory cells is catalyzed by lactose synthetase. Some lactose spills into the maternal circulation and may be excreted by the kidney and detected in the urine unless specific glucose oxidase is used in testing for glycosuria.

Fatty acids are synthesized in the alveoli from glucose. Fat droplets are secreted by an apocrine-like process (Fig. 13–3A).

All vitamins except vitamin K are present in human milk but in variable amounts (Committee on Nutrition, 1981). The levels of most are increased by maternal dietary supplementation. Since the mother does not provide for the vitamin K requirements of the breast-fed infant, vitamin K administration to the infant soon after delivery is beneficial to prevent hemorrhagic disease of the newborn (Chap. 33, p. 611).

Human milk contains a low concentration of iron. However, iron in human milk is better absorbed than is iron in cow's

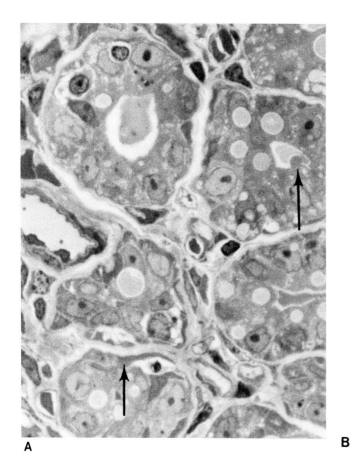

A

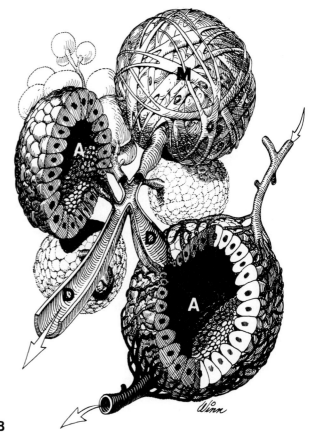

B

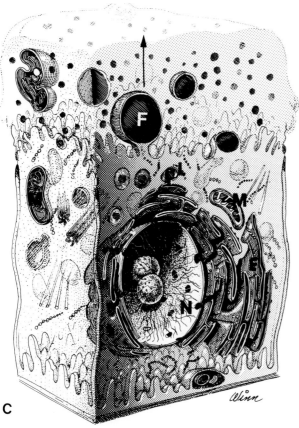

C

Figure 13–3. A. Histology of maternal breast at 32 weeks gestation in preparation for lactation. Secretions are evident in the lumen of each alveolus. Myoepithelial cells are evident around alveoli (*lower left arrow*). Secretions are being delivered by exocytosis into the lumen of one alveolus (*upper right arrow*). **B.** Graphic demonstration of alveolar and ductal system shown in **A.** Note the myoepithelial fibers (M) that surround the outside of the uppermost alveolus. The secretions from the glandular elements are extruded into the lumen of the alveoli (A) and ejected by the myoepithelial cells into the ductal system (D) which empties through the nipple. The arterial blood supply to the alveolus is identified by the upper right arrow and the venous drainage by the arrow beneath. **C.** Individual secretory cell. Two nucleoli are located within the nucleus (N). The endoplasmic reticulum (E) surrounds the nucleus. Mitochondria (M) are evident. Lactose granules (L) and fat droplets (F) migrate to the luminal margin of the cell and are there secreted by exocytosis into an alveolus (*arrow*). (*Courtesy of Dr. John C. Porter.*)

milk. Maternal iron stores do not seem to influence the amount of iron in breast milk. The mammary gland, like the thyroid gland, concentrates iodine, which appears in the milk.

The approximate concentrations of the more important components of human colostrum, human mature milk, and cow's milk are presented in Table 13–1. These concentrations may vary depending on when studied in the puerperium (Karra and colleagues, 1988).

ENDOCRINOLOGY OF LACTATION

The precise humoral and neural mechanisms involved in lactation are obviously complex. Progesterone, estrogen, and placental lactogen, as well as prolactin, cortisol, and insulin, appear to act in concert to stimulate the growth and development of the milk-secreting apparatus of the mammary gland (Porter, 1974). With delivery, there is an abrupt and profound decrease in the levels of progesterone and estrogen, which somehow serves to initiate lactation. It is very likely that lactation is not initiated until the end of pregnancy because the high levels of estrogen and progesterone during pregnancy interfere with the lactogenic actions of prolactin and adrenal steroids.

In otherwise normal circumstances the intensity and the duration of lactation are subsequently controlled in large part by the repetitive stimulus of nursing. Prolactin is essential for lactation; women with extensive pituitary necrosis, as in Sheehan syndrome, do not lactate (Chap. 24, p. 417). Although plasma prolactin falls after delivery to appreciably lower levels than during pregnancy, each act of suckling triggers a rise in prolactin levels (McNeilly and associates, 1983). Presumably a stimulus from the breast curtails the release of prolactin-inhibiting factor from the hypothalamus, which, in turn, induces transiently an increased secretion of prolactin by the pituitary.

The neurohypophysis in pulsatile fashion secretes oxytocin, which stimulates the expression of milk from a lactating breast by causing contraction of myoepithelial cells in the alveoli and small milk ducts. In fact, this mechanism has been utilized to assay oxytocin activity in biological fluids. The ejection, or letting down, of milk is a reflex initiated especially by suckling, which stimulates the neurohypophysis to liberate oxytocin (McNeilly and associates, 1983). It may be provoked just by the cry of the infant or inhibited by fright or stress.

In women who continue lactating but who resume ovulation, there are acute alterations in breast milk composition 5 to 6 days before and 6 to 7 days following ovulation (Hartmann and Prosser, 1984). These changes are abrupt and characterized by increased concentrations of sodium and chloride, along with decreased potassium, lactose, and glucose concentrations. In women who become pregnant but who continue to breast feed, milk composition undergoes progressive alterations suggesting gradual loss of metabolic and secretory breast activity (Hartmann and Prosser, 1984).

IMMUNOLOGICAL CONSEQUENCES OF BREAST FEEDING

Antibodies are present in human colostrum and milk but are poorly absorbed, if at all, from the infant's gut. Indeed, no anti-D antibodies have been detected in the sera of infants fed milk containing a high titer of anti-D antibodies. This circumstance, however, does not mitigate necessarily against the importance of at least some of the antibodies in breast milk. The predominant immunoglobulin in milk is secretory IgA, a macromolecule that is important in antimicrobial processes in the mucous membranes across which it is secreted. In this context, it is envisioned that secretory IgA contained in mother's milk may act locally within the infant's gastrointestinal tract. For example, milk contains secretory IgA antibodies against *Escherichia coli,* and it is known that breast-fed babies are less prone to enteric infections than are bottle-fed babies. It has been suggested that IgA exerts its action by preventing bacterial adherence to epithelial cell surfaces, thus preventing tissue invasion.

In addition to study of the role of antibodies in human milk, much attention is being directed to an elucidation of the role of maternal lymphocytes in breast milk in fetal immunological processes. It has been reported that human milk contains both T and B lymphocytes. Lymphocytes in colostrum undergo blastoid transformation in vitro following exposure to specific antigens. In studies of experimental animals Beer and Billingham (1976) obtained evidence that there is transmission of viable lymphocytes from mother to infant through the breast milk.

The amounts of protective factors in human milk appear to vary appreciably, being much richer in the milk of young women compared to that of older women (Whitehead, 1983).

NURSING

The ideal food for the newborn child is the milk of the mother. Appropriately, the frequency of infant breast feeding in recent years has increased considerably. In one recent survey in the United States carried out by a manufacturer of infant formula, nearly two thirds of women were breast feeding their 1-week-old infants, compared to less than one third 25 years before.

In most instances, even though the supply of milk at first appears insufficient, it becomes adequate if suckling is continued. Nursing also accelerates involution of the uterus, since

TABLE 13–1. APPROXIMATE CONCENTRATIONS (PER dL) OF COMPONENTS OF HUMAN COLOSTRUM, HUMAN MATURE MILK, AND COW'S MILK

	Human Colostrum	Human Mature Milk	Cow's Milk
Water (g)	—	88	88
Lactose (g)	5.3	6.8	5.0
Protein (g)	2.7	1.2	3.3
Casein:lactalbumin ratio	—	1:2	3:1
Fat (g)	2.9	3.8	3.7
Linoleic acid	—	8.3% of fat	1.6% of fat
Potassium (mg)	55	55	58
Sodium (mg)	92	15	138
Chloride (mg)	117	43	103
Calcium (mg)	31	33	125
Magnesium (mg)	4	4	12
Phosphorus (mg)	14	15	100
Iron (mg)	0.09[a]	0.15[a]	0.10[a]
Vitamin A (μg)	89	53	34
Vitamin D (μg)	—	0.03[a]	0.06[a]
Thiamine (μg)	15	16	42
Riboflavin (μg)	30	43	157
Nicotinic acid (μg)	75	172	85
Ascorbic acid (μg)	4.4[b]	4.3[b]	1.6[b]

[a] Poor source.
[b] Just adequate.
From Edwards (ed): Res Reprod, vol 6, 1974.

repeated stimulation of the nipples through release of oxytocin leads to increased contractions of the myometrium.

Drugs Secreted in Milk

Most drugs given to the mother are secreted in the milk. Many factors influence their excretion, including the concentration of drugs in plasma, the degree of protein binding of the drug, plasma and milk pH, degree of ionization, lipid solubility, and molecular weight. Drugs are secreted in milk usually in concentrations no higher than in maternal plasma. Consequently, the amount of drug ingested by the infant typically is small.

The Committee on Drugs of the American Academy of Pediatrics (1983) has provided an extensive list of drugs and other chemicals and their transfer into breast milk and compatibility with breast feeding. Drugs that are contraindicated or those for which temporary cessation of breast feeding is recommended are listed in Table 13–2. Drugs ingested by the mother are also excreted in breast milk, and Chasnoff and colleagues (1987) reported cocaine intoxication in a 2-week-old infant.

CLINICAL ASPECTS OF THE PUERPERIUM

TEMPERATURE

Breast engorgement, which is common on the third or fourth day of the puerperium, was once thought to cause a rise in temperature. This so-called milk fever was regarded as physiological. Although no such entity is clearly recognized today, on occasion perhaps extreme vascular and lymphatic engorgement may result in fever, but it does not last more than 24 hours at the most. **Any rise of temperature in the puerperium implies an infection, most likely somewhere in the genitourinary tract.**

AFTERPAINS

In primiparas the puerperal uterus tends to remain tonically contracted unless blood clots, fragments of placenta, or other foreign bodies are retained in its cavity, causing hypertonic contractions in an effort to expel them. In multiparas especially, the uterus often contracts vigorously at intervals, the contractions giving rise to painful sensations that are known as afterpains and that occasionally are sufficiently severe to require an analgesic. In some mothers, they may last for days. Afterpains are particularly noticeable when the infant suckles, presumably because of the release of oxytocin. Usually, they decrease in intensity and become quite mild by the third day after delivery.

LOCHIA

Beginning early in the puerperium, there is continued sloughing of decidual tissue that results in vaginal discharge of variable quantities, which is termed *lochia*. Microscopically the lochia consists of erythrocytes, shreds of decidua, epithelial cells, and bacteria. Microorganisms are found in lochia pooled in the vagina and are present in most cases even when the discharge has been obtained from the uterine cavity.

For the first few days after delivery, the content of blood in the lochia is sufficient to color it red, or *lochia rubra*. After 3 or 4 days, the lochia becomes progressively paler, or *lochia serosa*. After the 10th day, because of a marked admixture with leucocytes and a reduced fluid content, the lochia assumes a white or yellowish-white color, or *lochia alba*. Foul-smelling lochia suggests, but does not prove, infection.

In some centers it is routine to prescribe an oxytocic agent to promote uterine contractility and presumably diminish bleeding complications and hasten involution. Adams and Flowers (1960) measured the lochia of 120 women during the first 5½ days after delivery. During this period, the lochial weight in nursing and nonnursing women averaged 251 and 277 g, respectively. Similar patients also received 0.2 mg of methylergonovine maleate (Methergine) orally every 4 hours for the first 3 days after delivery. There was no appreciable difference in the amount of lochia between the women who received methylergonovine maleate and those who did not. The morbidity rates during the puerperium were the same, and the height of the fundus was identical in both the treated and untreated groups. The only real observed difference related to the mother's discomfort. Those who received the drug suffered much more from uterine cramping. These investigators concluded that the routine use of such medication was unwarranted. Newton and Bradford (1961) similarly concluded that after the immediate period following delivery, the routine administration of intramuscular oxytocin to normal women was of no value in decreasing blood loss or hastening involution of the uterus.

A reddish color in the lochia may be maintained for a longer period. When it persists for more than 2 weeks, however, it indicates either the retention of small portions of the placenta or imperfect involution of the placental site, or both.

URINE

Diuresis regularly occurs between the second and fifth days, even when intravenous fluids were not vigorously infused during labor and delivery. Normal pregnancy is associated with an appreciable increase in extracellular water. The puerperal diuresis represents a reversal of this process as the fluid-retaining stimuli of pregnancy-induced hyperestrogenism and elevated venous pressure in the lower half of the body are removed and as any residual hypervolemia is dissipated. In preeclampsia,

TABLE 13–2. DRUGS AND CHEMICALS CONTRAINDICATED IN BREAST-FEEDING WOMEN

	Reported Side-Effects
Contraindicated	
Amethopterin	Possible immune suppression; unknown effect on growth or carcinogenesis
Bromocriptine	Suppresses lactation
Cimetidine	May suppress gastric acidity in infant, inhibit drug metabolism, cause central nervous system stimulation
Clemastine	Drowsiness, irritability, poor feeding, high-pitched cry, neck stiffness
Cyclophosphamide	Possible immune suppression; unknown effect on growth or carcinogenesis
Ergotamine	Vomiting, diarrhea, convulsions (doses used in migraine medications)
Gold salts	Rash, renal or hepatic inflammation
Methimazole	Potential for interfering with thyroid function
Phenindione	Hemorrhage
Thiouracils	Decreased thyroid function (does not include propylthiouracil)
Temporary Cessation	
Metronidazole	
Radiopharma-ceuticals	

From the American Academy of Pediatrics: Pediatrics 72:375, 1983.

both retention of fluid antepartum and diuresis postpartum may be greatly increased (Chap. 35, p. 684).

Occasionally, substantial amounts of sugar may be found in the urine during the first weeks of the puerperium. The sugar most likely is lactose, which, fortunately, is not detected by test systems using glucose oxidase.

After a long labor, acetone may be identified in the urine as a consequence of starvation.

BLOOD

Rather marked leucocytosis occurs during and after labor, the leukocyte count sometimes reaching levels as high as 30,000 per μL (Chap. 7, p. 143). The increase is made up predominantly of granulocytes. There is a relative lymphopenia and an absolute eosinopenia.

Normally, during the first few days after delivery, the hemoglobin, hematocrit, and erythrocyte count fluctuate moderately. In general, however, if they fall much below the levels present just before or during early labor, the woman has lost a considerable amount of blood (Chap. 36, p. 695). By 1 week after delivery, the blood volume has returned to near the usual nonpregnant level. Robson and colleagues (1987) showed that cardiac output remains elevated for at least 48 hours postpartum. This most likely is because of increased stroke volume, presumably from increased venous return, since heart rate falls during this time. By 2 weeks these changes have returned to normal for nonpregnancy.

The pregnancy-induced changes in blood coagulation factors persist for variable periods of time after delivery. The elevation of plasma fibrinogen is maintained at least through the first week of the puerperium. As a consequence, the elevated sedimentation rate normally found during much of pregnancy normally remains high during the early puerperium.

LOSS OF WEIGHT

In addition to the loss on the average of about 12 lb as the consequence of evacuation of the contents of the uterus and normal blood loss, there is generally further loss of body weight during the puerperium of about 5 lb. This weight loss is accounted for by fluid lost chiefly through urination, as described above. Chesley and co-workers (1959) demonstrated a decrease in the sodium space of about 2 L, or nearly 5 lb, during the first week after delivery.

CARE OF THE MOTHER DURING THE PUERPERIUM

ATTENTION IMMEDIATELY AFTER LABOR

After delivery of the placenta, the uterus should be firm, with its upper margin just below the umbilicus. As long as it remains in this condition, there is no danger of postpartum hemorrhage from *uterine atony*. To guard against such an occurrence, the uterus should be palpated through the abdominal wall at frequent intervals after the completion of the third stage of labor, that is, delivery of the placenta. If relaxation is detected, the uterus should be massaged through the abdominal wall until it remains contracted. Blood may accumulate within the uterus without external evidence of bleeding. This condition may be detected early by identifying uterine enlargement through frequent palpation of the fundus during the first few hours post-

partum. **Since the likelihood of significant hemorrhage is greatest immediately postpartum, even in normal cases, a trained attendant should remain with the mother for at least 1 hour after completion of the third stage of labor.**

CARE OF THE VULVA

Shortly after completion of the third stage of labor and perineal repair, the draping and soiled linen beneath the mother are removed, provided there is no excessive bleeding or other reason to keep her in the lithotomy position on the delivery table. The external genitalia and buttocks are flushed with soap and water in such a way that all of the liquid drains from the vulva and perineum down over the anus, rather than in the reverse direction. A sterile vulvar pad is then applied over the genitalia and replaced by a clean pad as necessary. After each bowel movement and before any local treatment or examination, the external genitalia should be similarly cleansed.

SUBSEQUENT DISCOMFORT

The discomfort from cesarean section, its causes and its management are considered in Chap. 26, p. 455. During the first few days after vaginal delivery, the mother may be uncomfortable for a variety of reasons, including afterpains, episiotomy and lacerations, breast engorgement, and, at times, postspinal headache. It is prudent to provide codeine, 60 mg, or aspirin, 600 mg, at intervals as frequent as every 3 hours during the first few days after delivery. Uterine contractions are commonly accentuated during nursing, giving rise at times to troublesome afterpains.

The repaired episiotomy or lacerations may be uncomfortable, as discussed in Chapter 16, p. 325. Early application of an icebag to the perineum may minimize the swelling and discomfort. The majority of women also appear to obtain a measure of relief from the periodic application of a local anesthetic spray on the site of episiotomy or laceration. Severe discomfort may mean that a sizable hematoma has formed in the genital tract. Therefore, careful examination is warranted, especially whenever ordinary orally ingested analgesics do not provide appreciable relief. The episiotomy incision is normally firmly healed and nearly asymptomatic by the third week after delivery.

MILD DEPRESSION

It is fairly common for a mother to exhibit some degree of depression a few days after delivery. The transient depression, or "postpartum blues," most likely is the consequence of a number of factors. Prominent in its genesis are (1) the emotional letdown that follows the excitement and fears that most women experience during pregnancy and delivery, (2) the discomforts of the early puerperium that have been described above, (3) fatigue from loss of sleep during labor and postpartum in most hospital settings, (4) anxiety over her capabilities for caring for her infant after leaving the hospital, and (5) fears that she has become less attractive to her husband. In the great majority of cases effective treatment need be nothing more than anticipation, recognition, and reassurance.

As stressed by Robinson and Stewart (1986), this mild disorder is self-limited and usually remits after 2 to 3 days, although it sometimes persists for up to 10 days. Should postpartum blues persist, or worsen, then careful attention is given to searching for symptoms of psychotic depression, which requires prompt consultation (Chap. 28, p. 486). Women particularly susceptible to more severe depression are those with unwanted pregnancies or those with major marital difficulties. Watson and co-workers (1984) reported that 12 percent of women developed clinically relevant depressive disorders by 6 weeks after delivery; however, in 90 percent situational aspects or long-standing problems had important etiological roles.

EARLY AMBULATION

Immediately after World War II, important changes began to take place in the management of the puerperium in the direction of early ambulation. Women are now out of bed well within the first 24 hours after vaginal delivery. The many advantages of early ambulation are confirmed by numerous well-controlled studies. Women state that they feel better and stronger after early ambulation. Bladder complications and constipation are less frequent. Importantly, early ambulation has also reduced materially the frequency of thrombosis and pulmonary embolism during the puerperium. For the first ambulation at least, an attendant should be present to help prevent injury if the woman should become syncopal.

ABDOMINAL WALL RELAXATION

An abdominal binder is unnecessary. Although it was formerly believed to aid involution and help restore the mother's figure, the consensus now is that a binder has no effect on involution. If the abdomen is unusually flabby or pendulous, an ordinary girdle is often more satisfactory than an abdominal binder. Exercises to help restore tone to the abdominal wall may be started at any time after vaginal delivery and as soon as the abdominal soreness diminishes after cesarean section.

DIET

It was formerly customary to restrict the diet of the puerperal woman who has been delivered vaginally, but at present an attractive general diet is recommended. If at the end of 2 hours after vaginal delivery there are no complications likely to necessitate an anesthetic, the patient should be given something to drink if she is thirsty and something to eat if she is hungry. The diet of the lactating mother, compared with that consumed during pregnancy, should be increased somewhat, especially in calories and protein, as recommended by the Food and Nutrition Board of the National Research Council (Table 14–1, p. 263). If the mother does not breast-feed her infant, her dietary requirements are the same as for a normal nonpregnant woman. There is absolutely no rationale for restricting fluids for women who do not desire to nurse.

It is standard practice at Parkland Hospital to continue iron supplementation for at least 1 month after delivery. The hematocrit is also checked at the same time of the first postpartum visit, which is performed routinely during the third week of the puerperium.

BLADDER FUNCTION

The rate of accumulation of urine in the bladder after delivery may be quite variable. In most hospitals, intravenous fluids are nearly always infused during labor and for an hour or so after delivery. Oxytocin, in doses that are antidiuretic, is commonly infused in the intravenous fluid after the third stage of labor. As a consequence of the volume of fluid infused and the sudden withdrawal of the antidiuretic effect of oxytocin, rapid filling of the bladder is common. Moreover, both bladder sensation and the capability of the bladder to empty spontaneously may be appreciably diminished by anesthesia, especially conduction analgesia, and by painful lesions in the genital tract, such as extensive episiotomy, lacerations, or hematomas. It is not surprising, therefore, that urinary retention with overdistention of the bladder is a common complication of the early puerperium. Once overdistention occurs, bladder function becomes further impaired, and ascending infection of the urinary tract is a likely consequence.

Prevention of overdistention demands close observation of the bladder after delivery to ensure that it does not overfill and that with each voiding it empties adequately. The bladder may be palpated as a cystic mass suprapubically, or the enlarged bladder may be evident abdominally only indirectly, the full bladder having elevated the uterine fundus to well above the umbilicus.

If the woman has not voided within 4 hours after delivery, it is likely that she cannot do so. Ambulation to a commode usually should be tried before resorting to catheterization. The woman who has trouble voiding initially is likely to have further trouble. At times, an indwelling catheter is necessary, as described in Chapter 28, p. 483. The likelihood of hematomas of the genital tract must be kept in mind when the woman cannot void following delivery. Whenever the bladder has become overdistended, an indwelling catheter for a day, until the factors causing the retention have for the most part abated, is likely to be beneficial. Harris and colleagues (1977) have shown that 40 percent of such women will develop bacteriuria; thus, a short course of antimicrobial therapy seems reasonable when the catheter is removed.

BOWEL FUNCTION

At times the lack of a bowel movement is no more than the expected consequence of an efficient cleansing enema administered a few hours before delivery and little food being eaten subsequently. With both early ambulation and early feeding of a general diet, constipation has become much less of a problem in the puerperium. Routine prescription of a stool softener is practiced in many clinics.

CARE OF THE BREASTS AND NIPPLES

The nipples require little attention in the puerperium other than cleanliness and attention to fissures. Since dried milk is likely to accumulate and irritate the nipples, cleansing of the areola with water and mild soap is helpful before and after nursing. Occasionally, with irritated nipples, it is necessary to resort to a nipple shield for 24 hours or longer. A nursing brassiere that provides support without constriction is desirable. Suppression of lactation in the woman who does not nurse her infant is considered in Chapter 28, p. 483.

IMMUNIZATIONS

The D negative woman who is not isoimmunized and whose baby is D positive is given 300 μg of anti-D immune globulin shortly after delivery (Chap. 33, p. 603). Women who are not already immune to rubella (Chap. 14, p. 259) are excellent candidates for vaccination before discharge. At Parkland Hospital the mother also receives a tetanus toxoid booster injection at this time, unless it is contraindicated.

TIME OF DISCHARGE

Early ambulation soon after delivery is recommended, as discussed above. If there are no puerperal complications, hospitalization is seldom warranted for more than 3 days for primiparas and 2 days for multiparas. Indeed, because of prohibitive hospitalization costs, many women request discharge after a 1-day stay. This is certainly acceptable as long as physician access is readily available and appropriate neonatal screening is performed for hypothyroidism, phenylketonuria, and other congenital disorders. Following an uncomplicated postoperative cesarean delivery course, these women are usually ready for discharge on the fourth or fifth day.

RETURN OF MENSTRUATION AND OVULATION

If the woman does not nurse her child, the menstrual flow will probably return within 6 to 8 weeks after labor. At times, however, it is difficult clinically to assign a specific date to the first menstrual period after delivery. A minority of women bleed small to moderate amounts intermittently, starting soon after delivery. Menses may not appear so long as the infant is nursed, but great variations are observed, for in lactating women the first period may occur as early as the second or as late as the 18th month after delivery.

Sharman (1966), by means of histological dating of the endometrium, identified ovulation as early as 42 days after delivery, and Perez and associates (1972) did so as early as 36 days. Moreover, a corpus luteum has been observed 6 weeks after delivery at the time of sterilization. The necessity for avoiding delay in instituting contraceptive techniques by the sexually active woman is obvious.

It has long been appreciated that ovulation is much less frequent in women who breast feed compared to those who do not. Nonetheless, pregnancy can occur while lactating. Hefnawi and Badraoui (1977) have provided the following quantitative information for women who nurse. Of 340 lactating Egyptian women who used no contraception after delivery, one fourth had conceived again within the next 12 months. Of those who

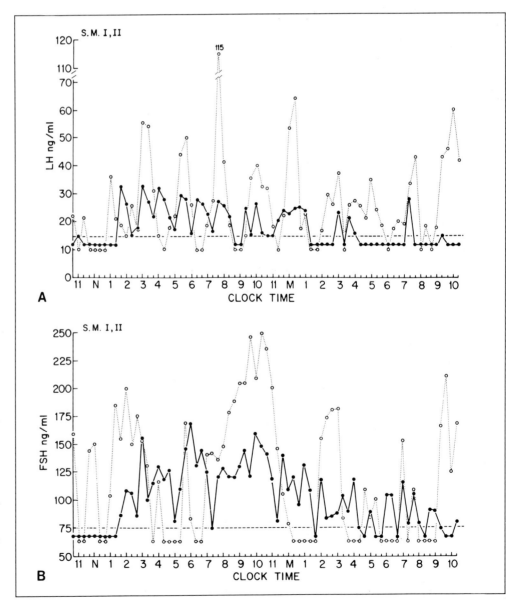

Figure 13–4. A. Comparison of the 24-hour secretory patterns of LH in the lactating woman. The closed circles denote plasma LH levels during the period of amenorrhea. The open circles correspond to the plasma LH concentrations after menses had resumed. **B.** Comparison of the 24-hour secretory patterns of FSH in the lactating woman. The closed circles denote plasma FSH levels during the period of amenorrhea. The open circles correspond to the plasma FSH concentrations after menses had resumed. (*From Madden and co-workers. Am J Obstet Gynecol 132:436, 1978.*)

became pregnant, one fourth had never menstruated since delivery. Onset of menses increased from 8 percent the first month after delivery to 61 percent by 12 months. Among those who menstruated, ovulation, identified by examinations of cervical mucus and endometrial biopsies, rose from 3 percent at 1 month to 59 percent at 12 months.

It is generally thought that amenorrhea during the period of lactation is the consequence of lack of appropriate ovarian stimulation by pituitary gonadotropins. In keeping with this concept, as illustrated by Figure 13–4A and B, the levels of luteinizing hormone (LH) and follicle-stimulating hormone (FSH) in one carefully studied lactating woman were appreciably lower during the time of amenorrhea than they were after the resumption of menstruation (Madden and colleagues, 1978).

Keettel and Bradley (1961), in a much earlier study, noted very low pituitary gonadotropic activity, as anticipated, in the urine of some lactating women with amenorrhea. They also detected by bioassay normal or even elevated amounts of gonadotropins in the urine of others. They concluded that in the latter circumstance the absent or very limited estrogenic affect on the vaginal epithelium, as well as the amenorrhea and anovulation, resulted from the failure of the ovaries to respond to the gonadotropins. The studies of Bonnar and co-workers (1975) have provided an explanation for their observation. In some women in their study who were breast feeding, plasma estrogens did not increase despite a rise in FSH. The lack of response was attributed to an inhibitory effect of the increased prolactin levels on follicular development.

FOLLOW-UP CARE

By the time of discharge from the hospital after a vaginal delivery and a normal in-hospital puerperium, the mother can resume most activities, including bathing, driving, and household functions. Although it has been customary for some obstetricians to recommend that she not resume employment or return to school for several weeks, there is no evidence that to do so earlier causes any physical harm. However, Tulman and Fawcett (1988) reported that only half of women had regained their usual level of energy by 6 weeks postpartum. Women who had been delivered vaginally were twice as likely to have normal energy levels at this time compared to those delivered by cesarean section. Ideally the care and nurturing received by the neonate should be provided by the mother with ample help from the father. For the mother to provide this care, her presence at home with the infant precludes her early return to full-time work or school.

Recommendations as to the time of resumption of sexual intercourse have varied considerably and there is little scientific evidence. Robson and Kumar (1981) longitudinally interviewed 119 nulliparous women throughout pregnancy and for 1 year postpartum to determine aspects of sexuality. They reported that the diminished sexual activity and enjoyment from intercourse seen in latter pregnancy may persist for at least a year after delivery. Only 35 percent of these women resumed intercourse by 6 weeks, and at 3 months, 40 percent of those having intercourse reported pain and discomfort. It is most unlikely that there are increased risks from intercourse as early as 2 weeks after delivery, except perhaps for dyspareunia, which can be minimized by careful repair of the episiotomy (Richardson and associates, 1976).

Delay of examination of the mother until 6 weeks postpartum became routine practice in obstetrics, but from the standpoint of optimal clinical care, the reasons for selecting that time are not altogether clear. Since 1969 at Parkland Hospital puerperal women typically have been given appointments for follow-up examination during the third week following delivery. The third week has proven quite satisfactory both to identify any abnormalities of the later puerperium and to initiate contraceptive practices. Estrogen plus progestin oral contraceptives started at this time have proved effective without increased morbidity. Moreover, the frequencies of uterine perforation, expulsions, and pregnancies when intrauterine devices were inserted during the third week postpartum were no greater than when the devices were inserted 3 months or more postpartum. Family planning technique and follow-up care are discussed further in Chapter 42, (p. 921).

Women who gain weight excessively during pregnancy are more likely to gain extra weight. Greene and colleagues (1988) analyzed data from the Collaborative Perinatal Study, and found that prenatal weight gain in excess of 20 lb was associated with postpartum weight retention.

REFERENCES

Adams H, Flowers CE: Oral oxytocic drugs in the puerperium. Obstet Gynecol 15:280, 1960

American Academy of Pediatrics: Committee on Drugs: The transfer of drugs and other chemicals into human breast milk. Pediatrics 72:375, 1983

Anderson WR, Davis J: Placental site involution. Am J Obstet Gynecol 102:23, 1968

Andrews MC: Epithelial changes in the puerperal fallopian tube. Am J Obstet Gynecol 62:28, 1951

Beer AE, Billingham RE: The Immunobiology of Mammalian Reproduction. Englewood Cliffs, NJ, Prentice-Hall, 1976, p 198

Bonnar J, Franklin M, Nott PN, McNeilly AS: Effect of breastfeeding on pituitary-ovarian function after childbirth. Br Med J 4:82, 1975

Chasnoff IJ, Lewis DE, Squires L: Cocaine intoxication in a breast-fed infant. Pediatrics 80:836, 1987

Chesley LC, Valenti C, Uichano L: Alterations in body fluid compartments and exchangeable sodium in early puerperium. Am J Obstet Gynecol 77:1054, 1959

Committee on Nutrition: Nutrition and lactation. Pediatrics 68:435, 1981

Greene GW, Smiciklas-Wright H, Scholl TO, Karp RJ: Postpartum weight change: How much of the weight gained in pregnancy will be lost after delivery? Obstet Gynecol 71:701, 1988

Harris RE, Thomas VL, Hui GW: Postpartum surveillance for urinary tract infection: Patients at risk of developing pyelonephritis after catheterization. South Med J 70:1273, 1977

Hartmann PE, Prosser CG: Physiological basis of longitudinal changes in human milk yield and composition. Fed Proc 43:2448, 1984

Hefnawi F, Badraoui MHH: The benefits of lactation amenorrhea as a contraceptive. Fertil Steril 28:320, 1977

Karra MV, Kirksey A, Galal O, Bassily NS, Harrison GG, Jerome NW: Zinc, calcium, and magnesium concentrations in milk from American and Egyptian women throughout the first 6 months of lactation. Am J Clin Nutr 47:642, 1988

Keettel WC, Bradbury JT: Endocrine studies of lactation amenorrhea. Am J Obstet Gynecol 82:995, 1961

Kerr-Wilson RJH, Thompson SW, Orr JW, Davis RO, Cloud GA: Effect of labor on the postpartum bladder. Obstet Gynecol 64:115, 1984

Madden JD, Boyar R, MacDonald PC, Porter JC: Analysis of secretory patterns of prolactin and gonadotropins during twenty-four hours in a lactating woman before and after resumption of menses. Am J Obstet Gynecol 132:436, 1978

McNeilly AS, Robinson ICA, Houston MJ, Howie PW: Release of oxytocin and prolactin in response to suckling. Br Med J 286:257, 1983

Newton M, Bradford WM: Postpartal blood loss. Obstet Gynecol 17:229, 1961

Perez A, Vela P, Masnic GS, Potter RG: First ovulation after childbirth: The effect of breastfeeding. Am J Obstet Gynecol 114:1041, 1972

Porter JC: Hormonal regulation of breast development and activity. J Invest Dermatol 63:85, 1974

Richardson AC, Lyon JB, Graham EE, Williams NL: Decreasing postpartum sexual abstinence time. Am J Obstet Gynecol 126:416, 1976

Robinson GE, Stewart DE: Postpartum psychiatric disorders. Can Med Assoc J 134:31, 1986

Robson KM, Kumar R: Maternal sexuality during first pregnancy and after childbirth. Br J Obstet Gynecol 88:882, 1981

Robson SC, Dunlop W, Hunter S: Haemodynamic changes during the early puerperium. Br Med J 294:1065, 1987

Sharman A: Postpartum regeneration of the human endometrium. J Anat 87:1, 1953

Sharman A: Ovulation in the post-partum period. Excerpta Medica International Congress Series, No 133, 1966, p 158

Tulman L, Fawcett J: Return of functional ability after childbirth. Nurs Res 37:77, 1988

Watson JP, Elliott SA, Rugg AJ, Brough DI: Psychiatric disorders in pregnancy and the first postnatal year. Br J Psychol 144:453, 1984

Weil A, Reyes H, Rottenberg RD, Begiun F, Herrmann WL: Effect of lumbar epidural analgesia on lower urinary tract function in the immediate postpartum period. Br J Obstet Gynaecol 90:428, 1983

Whitehead RG: Nutritional aspects of human lactation. Lancet 1:167, 1983

Williams JW: Regeneration of the uterine mucosa after delivery with especial reference to the placental site. Am J Obstet Gynecol 22:664, 1931

Yuen BH: Prolactin in human milk: The influence of nursing and the duration of postpartum lactation. Am J Obstet Gynecol 158:583, 1988

Part IV

MANAGEMENT OF NORMAL PREGNANCY

Prenatal Care

The objective of prenatal care is to assure that every wanted pregnancy culminates in the delivery of a healthy baby without impairing the health of the mother.

SIGNIFICANCE

Before the evolution of modern obstetrics, the pregnant woman usually had but a single antepartum interview with a physician. At that interview often not much more was accomplished than an attempt to anticipate the date of delivery. When next seen by the physician, the woman might be in the throes of an eclamptic convulsion, or suffering severe chills and high fever from pyelonephritis, or struggling to expel a very large but dead fetus. Appropriate antepartum care has proven to be of great value in the prevention of such catastrophes.

Perhaps somewhat paradoxically, it must be emphasized that prenatal care should do no harm, since at times, it has been a two-edged sword. Instead of improving pregnancy outcome, on occasion, the exact opposite was brought about in a variety of ways, including inappropriate dietary advice to achieve rigid weight restriction, the unnecessary prescription of potentially dangerous drugs such as powerful diuretics, and the failure to encourage the immediate reporting of an abnormal event, allowing the pregnant woman to wait to do so at the next scheduled office or clinic visit.

A priori pregnancy should be considered a normal physiological state. Unfortunately, the complexity of the functional and anatomical changes that accompany gestation tends in the minds of some to stigmatize normal pregnancy as a disease process. For example, a hemoglobin concentration of 10.5 g per dL is abnormally low for the woman who is not pregnant, but not for one who is late in the second trimester of pregnancy; a plasma thyroxine level of 16 μg per dL is normal during pregnancy but is very strongly suggestive of hyperthyroidism in the absence of pregnancy unless the women is taking exogenous estrogen. At times pregnancy imposes other changes that when modest in degree are normal, but when more intense are decidedly abnormal. For example, edema of the feet and ankles after ambulation is the normal consequence of regional physical forces imposed by the large pregnant uterus and by gravity. Generalized edema obvious in the face, hands, and abdomen, however, is definitely abnormal. **It is essential for the physician who assumes responsibility for prenatal care to be very familiar with the normal physiological changes, as well as the pathological changes, that may develop during pregnancy.**

Good prenatal care is vital for the accomplishment of the objective stated at the outset, namely, the delivery of a healthy baby from a healthy mother. An attempt has been made in this chapter to delineate many of the ingredients essential to good prenatal care. **Bad prenatal care may be worse than none.** All too often, inappropriate prenatal care provides the expectant mother with an unwarranted sense of security that allows her to ignore signs and symptoms for which, if left to her own instincts, she might have urgently sought advice. Hemminki (1988) has provided a review of the subject.

GENERAL HEALTH CARE

Systematic health care beginning long before pregnancy undoubtedly proves quite beneficial to the physical and emotional well-being of the mother-to-be and, in turn, her child-to-be. Therefore, prenatal care ideally should be a continuation of a regimen of physician-supervised health care already established for the woman. As the consequence of such a program, acquired diseases and developmental abnormalities, for the most part, will have been recognized before pregnancy and appropriate steps taken to eradicate them or, at least, to minimize their deleterious effects. For example, women with diabetes can and should be advised of the probable benefits for the embryo-fetus to be achieved from near normalization of blood glucose levels before conception (Chap. 39, p. 819). In any event, the mother should be evaluated as early in pregnancy as possible and at appropriate intervals thereafter.

TERMINOLOGY

DEFINITIONS

- A *nulligravida* is a woman who is not now and never has been pregnant.
- A *gravida* is a woman who is or has been pregnant, irrespective of the pregnancy outcome. With the establishment of the first pregnancy, she becomes a primigravida and with successive pregnancies a multigravida.

- A *nullipara* is a woman who has never completed a pregnancy beyond an abortion. She may or may not have had a spontaneous or elective abortion(s).
- A *primipara* is a woman who has been delivered once of a fetus or fetuses who reached the stage of viability. Therefore, the completion of any pregnancy beyond the stage of abortion (see Chap. 29, p. 489) bestows parity upon the mother.
- A *multipara* is a woman who has completed two or more pregnancies to the stage of viability. It is the number of pregnancies reaching viability and not the number of fetuses delivered that determines *parity*. Parity is not greater if a single fetus, twins, or quintuplets were delivered, nor lower if the fetus or fetuses were stillborn.

In certain clinics it is customary to summarize the past obstetrical history of a woman by a series of digits connected by dashes as follows: 6–1–2–6. The first digit refers to the number of term infants, the second to the number of preterm infants, the third to the number of abortions, and the fourth to the number of children currently alive. For the example given, 6–1–2–6, the woman has had six term deliveries, one preterm delivery, two abortions, and she has six children currently alive. This series of digits serves to summarize the obstetrical history somewhat better than does the designation *gravida 9, para 7, abortus 2* only when the recipient of the information understands the code.

- A *parturient* is a woman in labor.
- A *puerpera* is a woman who has just given birth.

NORMAL DURATION OF PREGNANCY

The mean duration of pregnancy calculated from the first day of the last normal menstrual period for a large number of healthy women has been identified to be very close to 280 days, or 40 weeks. Three studies are cited: Kortenoever (1950), in an analysis of 7,504 pregnancies, found the average duration to be 282 days. A mean value of 281 days was calculated from the data of the Obstetrical Statistical Cooperative for 77,300 women who underwent spontaneous labor and whose infants weighed at least 2,500 g. Nakano (1972) identified for 5,596 pregnancies in Osaka, Japan, the mean duration to be 279 days from the first day of the last menstrual period, with two standard deviations of ± 17 days. All pregnancies that terminated before 28 weeks gestation were excluded by Nakano, as were breeches and multiple fetuses.

It is customary to estimate the expected date of delivery by adding 7 days to the date of the first day of the last normal menstrual period and counting back 3 months (Naegele's rule). For example, if the woman's last menstrual period began on September 10, the expected date of delivery would be June 17. It is apparent that pregnancy is considered erroneously to have begun about 2 weeks before ovulation if the duration of pregnancy is so calculated from the first day of the last menstrual period. Nonetheless, clinicians persist in using *gestational age* or *menstrual age*, calculated from the first day of the last menstrual period, to identify temporal events in pregnancy; embryologists and other reproductive biologists more often employ *ovulatory age* or *fertilization age*, both of which are typically 2 weeks shorter.

It has become customary to divide pregnancy into three equal parts, or *trimesters*, of slightly more than 13 weeks, or 3 calendar months, each. There are certain major obstetrical problems that cluster in each of these time periods. For example, most spontaneous abortions occur during the first trimester, whereas practically all cases of pregnancy-induced hypertension become clinically evident during the third trimester. However, it is no longer true that no infant will survive if born earlier than the third trimester.

The clinical use of trimesters to describe the duration of a specific pregnancy fosters imprecision and should be abandoned. For example, it is inappropriate in case of uterine hemorrhage to categorize the problem temporally as "third trimester bleeding." Appropriate management for the mother and her fetus will vary remarkably, depending upon whether the bleeding is encountered early or late in the third trimester. **Precise knowledge of the age of the fetus is imperative for ideal obstetrical management!** Therefore, expert attention must be given to this important measurement. The clinically appropriate unit of measure is *Weeks of Gestation Completed*.

GENERAL PROCEDURES

Every word and every act by all who come in contact with the pregnant woman should impress upon her both the importance and the availability of prenatal care for her fetus and herself. All too often, especially in public clinics, the strong impression has been propagated that such care is not really available without great expenditure of physical and emotional effort by her, and, too often, of money beyond her ability to pay. It is tragic when women and their fetuses are denied adequate prenatal care simply because of lack of funds. Over and above the humanitarian aspects, the cost for good prenatal care is modest compared to the expense of caring subsequently for serious, but preventable, complications in the mother, her fetus-infant, or both. For example, at Parkland Hospital not only is the frequency of low-birthweight infants much higher for pregnancies without prenatal care, but also the cost of caring for the newborn whose mother had no prenatal care on average is nearly doubled (Leveno and colleagues, 1985).

It is also unfortunate that, among those who in one way or another come in contact with the pregnant woman who seeks prenatal care, there may be some who display an intolerance for the poor, for the unwed, or for the mother's particular ethnic group. In such circumstances, the best of medical care may go to waste.

INITIAL CARE

Prenatal care should be initiated as soon as there is reasonable likelihood of pregnancy. This may be as early as a few days after a missed menstrual period, especially for the woman who desires an abortion, but it should be no later than the second missed period for anyone.

In order to initiate antepartum care early, a system was developed at Parkland Hospital that has, in general, proved effective. The woman is seen for initial screening any day of the week without an appointment. At this initial visit nurses familiar with obstetrical care identify the following: (1) the probability of pregnancy (including urine testing for human chorionic gonadotropin when indicated), (2) the woman's desire for the pregnancy to continue, (3) any current health problems, (4) any previous major illnesses, including those in previous pregnancies, (5) the outcomes of previous pregnancies, and (6) all medications being taken. The woman is instructed to bring with her at the next visit a few days later all drugs that she has been taking.

Physical evaluation initiated at the initial screening visit by the nurse includes determination of blood pressure, height, and weight.

The following laboratory tests are initiated at the first visit:

- *Blood:* Hemoglobin, hematocrit, red cell indexes, white blood cell count, platelet count, sickle cell screening for black women, glucose and creatinine concentration, serological test for syphilis, identification of blood types and of abnormal antibodies to red cell antigens, and presence of antibody to rubella. The Centers for Disease Control (1988) now recommends routine screening for Hepatitis B antigen.
- *Urine:* Glucose, protein, and quantitative culture of clean catch midstream urine to identify significant bacteriuria.

Physicians are continually available in the clinic and are consulted by the nurse whenever a problem is suspected that might require immediate attention. Any woman who is considering abortion is offered counseling. Moreover, every woman is asked specifically if she wishes to see a physician at this screening visit. Finally, she is given explicit instructions as to how to get help promptly in case a problem develops.

It is difficult to convince the pregnant woman of the importance of prenatal care if, when she seeks it, the physician delays for many weeks her initial care! Even in the absence of identified pregnancy problems, all women are given appointments within 10 days for the completion by a physician of a comprehensive general health evaluation, described below. Previous health records and laboratory data are reviewed at that time.

INITIAL COMPREHENSIVE EVALUATION

GOALS

The major goals are (1) to define the health status of the mother and fetus, (2) to determine the gestational age of the fetus, and (3) to initiate a plan for continuing obstetrical care. Once the health status of the mother and fetus has been defined, the initial plan for subsequent care may range from relatively infrequent routine visits to that of prompt hospitalization because of serious maternal or fetal disease.

History

For the most part, the same essentials go into appropriate history taking from the pregnant woman as elsewhere in medicine. The history should be obtained unhurriedly in a reasonably private setting. This is the best time for the physician and for those who assist in providing care for the expectant mother and her fetus to establish the good rapport so necessary for a successful outcome for the pregnancy. Although it is undesirable for the woman to wait for protracted periods of time before interview, it is worse for her to be hurriedly and indifferently interrogated without having her answers appropriately evaluated. **It is mandatory that all data important to the care of the mother and fetus be clearly recorded so that all members of the health care team who use the record can correctly interpret them.**

The *menstrual history* is extremely important. The woman who spontaneously menstruates regularly every 28 days or so is most likely to ovulate at midcycle. Thus, the gestational age (menstrual age) becomes simply the number of weeks since the onset of the last menstrual period. If her menstrual cycles were

significantly longer than 28 days to 30 days, ovulation more likely occurred well beyond 14 days or, if the intervals were much longer and irregular, chronic anovulation is likely to have preceded some of the episodes of vaginal bleeding identified as menses. In the latter instance, the menstrual data are unreliable for calculating the duration of the gestation. **Without regular, predictable, cyclic, spontaneous menses that suggest ovulatory cycles, accurate dating of pregnancy by physical examination is difficult at best.**

Thus, it is important to ascertain whether or not *steroidal contraceptives* were used before the pregnancy and, if so, when. It is now common, but not necessarily recommended, for women who sustain regularly recurring withdrawal bleeding while using oral contraceptives cyclically to stop their use and to conceive without any further menstrual-like bleeding. Ovulation, however, may not have resumed 2 weeks after the onset of the last withdrawal bleeding but instead at an appreciably later but highly variable date. The difficult problem of predicting the time of ovulation in this circumstance is similar to that in which pregnancy follows delivery or abortion prior to the reestablishment of normal menstrual periods.

The possibility of the presence of an *intrauterine device* should be ascertained, since certain pregnancy complications are increased by its presence in utero (see Chap. 42, p. 930). If present, its fate must also be clearly recorded.

Obstetrical Examination

The cervix is visualized employing a speculum lightly lubricated but only on the outside of each blade. Next, in order to identify cytological abnormalities, a gentle swabbing from the lower half of the cervical canal and then a scraping from the squamocolumnar junction are obtained and spread on slides and fixed immediately in ether-alcohol or by an appropriate aerosol spray. The outer half of the cervical canal is again swabbed slowly to obtain material to culture and identify *Neisseria gonorrhoeae*. The applicator stick is rolled over Trans-Grow or another suitable transport medium while the container is held vertically to prevent loss of the carbon dioxide–enriched air in the culture bottle. The specimens are labeled immediately and accurately.

Bluish-red passive hyperemia of the cervix is characteristic, but not of itself diagnostic, of pregnancy. Dilated, occluded cervical glands bulging beneath the exocervical mucosa, so-called *Nabothian cysts*, may be prominent. If the cervix is dilated appreciably, fetal membranes may be visualized through the cervical canal, implying at least, that expulsion of the products of conception may be imminent.

The character of vaginal secretions is noted. A moderate amount of white mucoid discharge is normal. The presence of foamy yellow liquid in the vagina is strongly suggestive of *Trichomonas*, whereas the presence of a curdlike discharge is consistent with *Candida* infection (p. 273). Material may be swabbed from the vagina for microscopic examination and for culture.

The speculum is removed and the digital pelvic examination is completed by palpation, with special attention given to the consistency, length, and dilatation of the cervix; to the fetal presenting part, especially if late in pregnancy; to the bony architecture of the pelvis; and to any anomalies of the vagina and perineum, including cystocele, rectocele, and relaxed or torn perineum. The vulva and contiguous structures are also carefully inspected. (The pelvic examination is described in more detail in Chapter 16, p. 308.) All cervical, vaginal, and vulvar lesions should be evaluated further by appropriate use of colposcopy, biopsy, culture, or darkfield examination. The perianal region should be visualized and digital rectal examination done to identify hemorrhoids or other lesions.

Between 18 and 32 weeks gestation there is good correlation between the gestational age of the fetus in weeks and the height of the uterine fundus in centimeters when measured as the distance over the abdominal wall from the top of the symphysis pubis to the top of the fundus. During this time period the height in centimeters approximates the gestational age in weeks. Therefore, it is important for the examiner to document carefully the height of the fundus, as described below.

Physical Examination

The general physical examination includes evaluation of the teeth. Repair of carious teeth should be undertaken promptly. Varicose veins should be looked for and, when identified, frequent postural drainage should be urged and elastic support stockings provided to minimize complications.

Further Instructions

After the history and physical examination have been completed, the expectant mother is instructed about diet, relaxation and sleep, bowel habits, exercise, bathing, clothing, recreation, smoking, drug and alcohol ingestion, and follow-up visits, including steps to take if an appointment is missed. Usually it is possible to assure her that she may anticipate an uneventful pregnancy followed by an uncomplicated delivery. **At the same time, she is tactfully instructed about the following danger signals, which must be reported immediately, day or night:**

1. Any vaginal bleeding
2. Swelling of the face or fingers
3. Severe or continuous headache
4. Dimness or blurring of vision
5. Abdominal pain
6. Persistent vomiting
7. Chills or fever
8. Dysuria
9. Escape of fluid from the vagina
10. Marked change in frequency or intensity of fetal movements

Prognosis

All information obtained should be employed to identify accurately the gestational age of the fetus and to anticipate the kinds and the magnitude of morbidity, both maternal and fetal, that may develop subsequently. Often, when morbidity is anticipated, its intensity can be minimized by appropriate care.

High-Risk Pregnancies

Considerable attention has been directed toward identifying complicated or "high-risk" pregnancies, and, indeed, risk-assessment programs have been demonstrated to be effective for identifying most pregnancies at increased risk (Hobel and associates, 1979; Sokol and co-workers, 1977). Creasy and colleagues (1980) have used a risk-scoring system modified after Papiernik and Kaminski (1974) in an attempt to identify women at risk for preterm labor. In this system scores of 1 to 10 are given to a variety of pregnancy factors, including socioeconomic status, reproductive history, daily habits, and current pregnancy complications. Women with scores of 10 or more are considered at high risk for preterm delivery. In practice, one problem inherent in such attempts to identify the high-risk

pregnancy has been a tendency to ignore subsequently the pregnancy that early on had been categorized as low-risk yet proved later to be high-risk. Nonetheless, there are major categories for increased risk that should be identified antepartum and given appropriate consideration in subsequent pregnancy management. These include (1) preexisting medical illness, (2) previous poor pregnancy performance, such as perinatal mortality, preterm delivery, fetal growth retardation, malformations, placental accidents, and maternal hemorrhage, and (3) evidence of maternal undernutrition.

SUBSEQUENT PRENATAL CARE

RETURN VISITS

Traditionally the timing of subsequent prenatal examinations has been scheduled at intervals of 4 weeks until 28 weeks, then every 2 weeks until 36 weeks, and weekly thereafter. Rather often, however, important information can be gained from a more flexible appointment schedule. For example, at midpregnancy, certain clinically discernible events characteristically occur that, when precisely identified, enhance the reliability of the estimate of gestational age of the fetus.

Audible Fetal Heart Sounds

In essentially all pregnancies the fetal heart may be first heard between 16 and 19 weeks of gestation when carefully listened for with a DeLee fetal stethoscope (Fig. 16–2A, B; also see Chap. 2, p. 18). Obviously, the ability of an examiner to hear unamplified fetal heart sounds will depend upon several factors. These include, among others, patient size and the examiner's hearing acuity. Herbert and co-workers (1987) reported that the fetal heart was audible by 20 weeks in 80 percent of women chosen for study because of regular menses. By 21 weeks audible fetal heart sounds were present in 95 percent, and by 22 weeks in all.

Fundal Height

Measurement of the height of the uterine fundus above the symphysis can provide useful information. For example, Jimenez and co-workers (1983) demonstrated that between 20 and 31 weeks of gestation the fundal height in centimeters equaled the gestational age in weeks. Utilizing a tape calibrated in centimeters and applied over the abdominal curvature, they measured the distance from the top of the fundus to the top of the symphysis pubis. The top of the fundus was identified by percussion and by palpation, and the tape was placed there and extended to the top of the symphysis. Quaranta and associates (1981) and Calvert and colleagues (1982) have reported essentially identical observations up to 34 weeks gestation. *The bladder must be emptied before making the measurement.* Worthen and Bustillo (1980), for example, demonstrated that at 17 to 20 weeks gestation the fundal height was 3 cm higher with a full bladder.

GESTATIONAL AGE

For the great majority of pregnancies the most important question to be answered through prenatal examination is, "How old is the fetus?" Fortunately, it is possible to identify the gestational age of the fetus with considerable precision through an appropriately timed, carefully performed clinical examination, coupled with knowledge of the time of onset of the last menstrual period. When the date of onset of the last menstrual period and the fundal height are in repeatedly temporal agreement, the duration of gestation can be firmly established. When gestational age cannot be clearly identified, sonography is likely to be of considerable value (see Chap. 15, p. 283).

Later in pregnancy, previously acquired precise knowledge of gestational age is of considerable importance, since a number of pregnancy complications may develop, for which the optimal treatment will depend on fetal age. For example, with the development of preeclampsia at 38 weeks, very often delivery is the treatment most beneficial to both mother and fetus. However, if the duration of gestation is only 28 weeks when preeclampsia develops, attempts at medical management and delay of delivery may be more beneficial for the quite premature fetus.

PRENATAL SURVEILLANCE

At each return visit steps are taken to identify the well-being of both the expectant mother and her fetus. Certain information, obtained by interrogation and by examination, is especially important in this regard:

Fetal

1. Fetal heart rate(s)
2. Size of fetus(es), actual and rate of change
3. Amount of amnionic fluid
4. Presenting part and station (late in pregnancy)
5. Fetal activity

Maternal

1. Blood pressure, actual and extent of change
2. Weight, actual and amount of change
3. Symptoms, including headache, altered vision, abdominal pain, nausea and vomiting, bleeding, fluid from vagina, and dysuria
4. Distance to uterine fundus from symphysis
5. A carefully performed vaginal examination late in pregnancy often provides valuable information as follows:
   a. Confirmation of the presenting part
   b. Station (depth in the pelvis) of the presenting part (see Chap. 16, p. 308)
   c. Clinical mensuration of the pelvis and an appreciation of its general configuration (see Chap. 8, pp. 168–70).
   d. The consistency, effacement, and dilatation of the cervix. Digital exploration must be conducted with care lest membranes be ruptured or an undiagnosed low-lying placenta be separated, causing severe hemorrhage.

Subsequent Laboratory Tests

If the initial results were quite normal, most of the procedures need not be repeated. Hematocrit determination and the serological test for syphilis, if syphilis prevails in the population cared for, should be repeated at about 28 to 32 weeks gestation. A cervical culture for gonorrhea may be repeated at the time of the pelvic examination near term, especially if gonorrhea is common.

Determination of maternal serum α-fetoprotein concentration at 16 to 18 weeks is recommended by most to screen for open neural tube defects and some chromosomal anomalies. Precise knowledge of gestational age is paramount for accuracy of this screening test (see Chap. 32, p. 584).

For women at risk for gestational diabetes, screening for glucose intolerance is recommended between 24 and 28 weeks

by the American College of Obstetricians and Gynecologists (1986a). Following a 50-g oral glucose challenge, if plasma glucose at 1 hour exceeds 140 mg per dL, then a 3-hour 100-g test is recommended (see Chap. 39, p. 818). Some recommend that all women be given a 1-hour 50-g glucose challenge. For women without risk factors for gestational diabetes we prefer to obtain a random plasma glucose level to rule out overt diabetes.

For pregnant women at high risk for sexually transmitted diseases the American College of Obstetricians and Gynecologists (1985b) recommends that diagnostic testing for *Chlamydia trachomatis* be performed, if possible, at the first prenatal visit and then again in the third trimester (see Chap. 39, p. 853).

Other screening tests may be applied selectively to populations at high risk for the condition sought. For example, serological testing for human immunodeficiency virus should be considered for women who take illicit intravenous drugs or who may be at risk for other reasons (see Chap. 39, p. 857).

Routine urine examination at every clinic visit is rarely warranted. Practically all women who develop preeclampsia develop a significant rise in blood pressure, and many have a sudden gain in weight before overt proteinuria develops. Therefore, in general, after the initial examination proteinuria need only be looked for selectively in those women who develop an increase in blood pressure or marked increase in weight. Fasting and postprandial plasma glucose levels are so much more informative than are tests for glucosuria, especially in the case of the woman with a strong family history of diabetes or of previous large infants or the woman who, during the current pregnancy, has an unusually large fetus. Nonetheless, glucosuria, if detected, should not be ignored.

All pertinent information obtained at each visit must be recorded legibly and be sufficiently descriptive that anyone who uses the pregnancy record at any time can appreciate the significance of the information contained.

NUTRITION DURING PREGNANCY

Throughout most of this century the diets of pregnant women have been the subject of endless discussions that often resulted in considerable contradiction and confusion. Various enthusiasts have urged pregnant women to adhere to a wide variety of diets, ranging from those that emphasized rigid caloric restriction to those that provided unusually large amounts of protein as well as calories. Faulty reasoning led some obstetricians to advise rigid caloric restriction, a recommendation that stemmed primarily from the observation that a prominent feature of preeclampsia and eclampsia was excessive weight gain. It was not generally appreciated that the abnormal weight gain in preeclampsia and eclampsia resulted from edema rather than excessive caloric intake.

Meaningful studies of nutrition in human pregnancy are exceedingly difficult to design. For ethical reasons, dietary deficiency must not be deliberately produced experimentally in pregnant women. In those instances in which severe nutritional deficiencies have been induced as a consequence of social, economic, or political disaster, coincidental events often have created many variables, the effects of which are not amenable to quantification. Some past experiences suggest, however, that in otherwise healthy women a state of near starvation is required to establish clear differences in pregnancy outcome. Such an example is the acute starvation imposed on pregnant women during the occupation of the Netherlands late in World War II.

During the winter of 1944–45 nutritional deprivation of known intensity prevailed in a well-circumscribed area of the Netherlands. As pointed out by Stein and associates (1972), the type and the degree of nutritional deprivation during the famine was identified with a precision unequaled in any large population before or since. At the lowest point, rations reached 450 kcal per day, with generalized undernutrition rather than selective malnutrition. Shortly after the end of the war, Smith (1947) analyzed the outcomes of pregnancies that were in progress during this 6-month period of famine. The median birthweights of infants were decreased about 8 ounces. The birthweights rose again after food became available in a way that indicated that birthweight can be influenced significantly by starvation during the latter half of pregnancy. The perinatal mortality rate, however, was not altered, nor was the incidence of malformations significantly increased.

Smith also identified the frequency of pregnancy toxemia (preeclampsia–eclampsia), defined by three different sets of criteria, to have declined during the "hunger-winter" of 1944–45. Subsequent analyses of this population by Ribeiro and associates (1982) identified an overall decline in maternal blood pressure near delivery during the famine.

Evidence of impaired brain development has been obtained in some animal fetuses whose mothers during pregnancy had been subjected to intense dietary deprivation. These animal studies, in turn, stimulated interest in the subsequent intellectual development of the young adults in the Netherlands whose mothers had been starved during pregnancy. The comprehensive study by Stein and co-workers (1972) was made possible by the fact that practically all males at age 19 undergo compulsory examination for military service. From the extensive analyses, Stein and associates concluded that the severe dietary deprivation during pregnancy caused no detectable effects on the mental performance of the surviving male offspring.

More recently, Nilsen and colleagues (1984) reported no adverse effects of low birthweight on intelligence in Norwegian men who weighed less than 2,500 g at birth from a variety of causes. These young men were evaluated for physical fitness and intelligence at compulsory military induction, and when compared to other 18 year olds, they were indistinguishable except for somewhat smaller size and increased frequency of minor visual defects. The results of intelligence tests were the same for both groups.

Caution must be exercised in extrapolating from one species to another. For example, severe protein deprivation of a few days duration in the pregnant rat, in which gestation is only 21 days and in which total fetal weight represents one fourth of maternal weight, may lead to serious reproductive casualties. In human pregnancy, which lasts 13 times longer and in which fetal weight is only about one twentieth of that of the mother, failure to ingest protein for the same number of days could hardly be expected to produce an insult of the same intensity.

WEIGHT GAIN DURING PREGNANCY

For several years at least, the American College of Obstetricians and Gynecologists (1985a) and others have recommended that pregnant women gain around 10 to 12 kg (22 to 27 lb) during pregnancy. Of the recommended weight, normal physiological events account cumulatively for about 9 kg as fetus, placenta, amnionic fluid, uterine hypertrophy, increase in maternal blood volume, breast enlargement, and dependent maternal edema as the consequence of mechanical factors. The remainder of the 10 to 12 kg appears to be mostly maternal fat. Weight gain of this magnitude has been widely accepted as appropriate until very recently, when uncertainty has surfaced again over what is ideal weight gain for the general obstetrical population. Analyses of data recently provided by the National Center for Health Statistics (1986) that conceivably support even a larger maternal weight gain during pregnancy have been disseminated. Soon

after publication, this extensive report served to stimulate the following recommendation: "*Regardless of how much women weigh before they become pregnant, gaining between 26 to 35 pounds during pregnancy can improve the outcome of pregnancy and reduce their chances for having the pregnancy end in fetal death*" (ACOG Newsletter, 1986). The wisdom of so strong a statement at this time is questioned. Several possible disadvantages as a consequence of the fetus-infant being heavier must be considered. For example, from the standpoint of the fetus, there must be some birthweight above which more birthweight might prove detrimental. The typically heavy fetus-infant of the hyperglycemic mother serves as one worrisome example. Another is the fetus who remains in utero beyond 40 weeks and commonly is larger than if he or she were born sooner. In spite of a higher birthweight, and many times as the direct consequence of the increase in fetal size, both perinatal and maternal morbidity and even mortality are increased. It seems likely that larger fetuses will cause an increased incidence of dystocia with more cesarean deliveries or maternal and fetus-infant birth trauma. Many more problems generated by big babies have been cited recently by Bromovich (1986).

Finally, the lasting effects of obesity acquired through repeated pregnancy in which women accrue twice the weight attributed to physiological changes of pregnancy must be considered.

Therefore, for the woman whose weight is normal before pregnancy, a gain of 20 to 27 pounds appears to be associated with the most favorable outcome of pregnancy (Naeye, 1979). In most pregnant women this result may be achieved by eating, according to appetite, a diet adequate in calories, protein, essential fatty acids, minerals, and vitamins. Seldom, if ever, should maternal weight gain be restricted deliberately below this level. **Indeed, failure of the pregnant woman to gain weight is an ominous sign.**

Eastman and Jackson (1968) carefully evaluated the relation between maternal weight gain and birthweight in term pregnancies and found that, in general, birthweight paralleled maternal weight gain. The full significance of this relationship is best appreciated when the fate of low-birthweight infants is considered. The neonatal mortality rate for chronologically mature white newborns weighing 2,500 g or less was 45.1 per 1,000 live births, in contrast to 6.1 per 1,000 live births for those whose weight exceeded 2,500 g. Undoubtedly, failure of the mother to gain weight was caused in some instances by associated maternal disease rather than just imposed caloric restriction. Nonetheless, in spite of the reported experiences in the Netherlands, alluded to above, observations such as those of Eastman and Jackson, coupled with those from several well-controlled animal studies demonstrating deleterious effects on the offspring when *severe* maternal caloric restriction was imposed, point out that rigid caloric restriction during pregnancy might prove dangerous to the fetus.

A Task Force on Nutrition of the American College of Obstetricians and Gynecologists (1978) has emphasized that the nutritional status of the expectant mother is more likely to be compromised in any of the following circumstances:

1. She is under 16 years of age.
2. She is economically deprived.
3. She is pregnant for the third time within 2 years.
4. Her past reproductive performance has been poor.
5. She consumes a therapeutic diet in the course of management of some preexisting disease.

6. She is a food faddist.
7. She smokes, drinks, or uses hard drugs.
8. She is appreciably underweight at the outset.
9. The hematocrit drops much below 33 or the hemoglobin concentration falls much below 11 g per dL.
10. Her weight gain for any month during the second and third trimesters is less than 2 lb.

RECOMMENDED DIETARY ALLOWANCES

Periodically the Food and Nutritional Board of the National Research Council recommends dietary allowances for women, including those who are pregnant or lactating. Their latest recommendations are summarized in Table 14–1. For certain nutrients, the board made higher recommendations for the nonpregnant teenager compared to older women of reproductive age. Where there is a difference, the recommended value for 15 to 18 years of age is given for each nutrient unless otherwise stated.

CALORIES

A daily caloric increase throughout pregnancy of 300 kcal has been recommended by the Food and Nutrition Board. Calories are necessary for energy production. Whenever caloric intake is inadequate, protein may be metabolized as a source of energy,

rather than being spared for its vital role in growth and development.

The importance of adequate caloric intake was emphasized by a nutrition intervention study in Guatemala that identified infant birthweights to be larger when the at most marginal diets of the mothers were supplemented (Delgado and associates, 1977). In two of four villages a high-protein plus calorie supplement was made available; in the other two villages a drink that provided calories without protein was offered. Birthweights were influenced by the number of calories ingested rather than by the protein content of the supplements. For those pregnancies in which less than 10,000 supplemental kcal were ingested, birthweight averaged 2,986 g and 18.3 percent of the infants weighed less than 2,500 g. For those pregnancies in which more than 20,000 kcal were consumed in the form of supplements, the mean birthweight was 3,120 g, and only 9.4 percent of the infants (half as many) weighed less than 2,500 g at birth.

In a more recent investigation of the impact of caloric supplementation on birthweights of infants of Gambian women a threshold effect was apparent (Prentice and co-workers, 1983, 1988). Food supplementation that provided throughout much of pregnancy somewhat more than 400 kcal per day on average improved birthweights for infants whose mothers were in marked negative energy balance as the consequence of both food shortage and heavy work load. For example, the frequency of low-birthweight infants ($< 2,500$ g) decreased threefold with calorie supplementation of these mothers. However, for women who were in positive energy balance, even though they were consuming only 60 percent of the recommended dietary allowance, supplementation had no demonstrable beneficial effect on birth outcome. These studies serve especially to emphasize the deleterious effect on fetal growth imposed by severe restriction of caloric intake.

TABLE 14–1. RECOMMENDED DAILY DIETARY ALLOWANCES FOR WOMEN 163 CM (64 IN) TALL AND WEIGHING 55 KG (121 LB)

| Nutrient | Nonpregnant | Increase | |
		Pregnant	Lactating
Kilocalories	2,100	300	500
Protein (g)	44[a]	30	20
Vitamin A (RE)[b]	800	200	400
Vitamin D (μg)[c]	7.5	5	5
Vitamin E (mg T.E.)[d]	10	2	3
Ascorbic Acid (mg)	60	20	40
Folacin (mg)[e]	0.4	0.4	0.1
Niacin (mg)[f]	14	2	5
Riboflavin (mg)	1.3	0.3	0.5
Thiamin (mg)	1.1	0.4	0.5
Vitamin B$_6$ (mg)	2.0	0.6	0.5
Vitamin B$_{12}$ (μg)	3.0	1.0	1.0
Calcium (mg)	800	400	400
Phosphorus (mg)	800	400	400
Iodine (μg)	150	25	50
Iron (mg)	18	Supplement[g]	0
Magnesium (mg)	300	150	150
Zinc (mg)	15	5	10

[a] 46 g for under 19 years of age
[b] 1 μg retinol = 1 retinol equivalent (R.E.)
[c] As cholecalciferol; 100 International Units = 2.5 μg of cholecalciferol
[d] T.E. = tocopherol equivalent
[e] Refers to dietary sources ascertained by *Lactobacillus casei* assay; pteroylglutamic acid may be effective in smaller doses
[f] Includes dietary sources of the vitamin plus 1 mg equivalent for each 60 mg of dietary tryptophan
[g] Increased requirement cannot be met by ordinary diets; therefore supplementation recommended (see text)
From Recommended Dietary Allowances, 9th ed., National Academy of Sciences, Washington, D.C., 1979.

Protein

To the basic protein needs of the nonpregnant woman for repair of her tissues are added the demands for growth and repair of the fetus, placenta, uterus and breasts, and increased maternal blood volume. During the last 6 months of pregnancy about 1 kg of protein is deposited, amounting to 5 to 6 g per day on average (Hytten and Leitch, 1971). The Food and Nutrition Board has recommended for young nonpregnant women a protein intake of about 0.9 g per kg per day, but an additional 30 g of protein per day is recommended during pregnancy. This is considerably more than the amount recommended by the World Health Organization.

It is desirable that the majority of the protein be supplied from animal sources, such as meat, milk, eggs, cheese, poultry, and fish, since they furnish amino acids in optimal combinations. Milk and milk products have long been considered nearly ideal sources of nutrients, especially protein and calcium, for pregnant or lactating women. Nonetheless, milk (lactose) intolerance in the form of gastrointestinal disturbances that include bloating, flatulence, and cramps is a problem in some adults. For example, some degree of lactose intolerance was found in 81 percent of black adults, compared with 12 percent of whites, in the studies of Bayless and co-workers (1975). As little as 240 mL of milk caused the unpleasant symptoms.

A "high" protein diet has been urged by some enthusiasts who contend that most problems of pregnancy are amenable to manipulation of maternal diet. The desirability of consuming large amounts of protein must be questioned from the standpoint of economics and, perhaps, of safety. Analyses of several studies by Stein and associates (1978) have failed to demonstrate improvement in birthweight due specifically to a protein-rich supplement. In fact, they were concerned that the reverse might sometimes be the consequence.

Zlatnik and Burmeister (1983) used the maternal urinary urea-to-creatinine ratio to evaluate protein intakes and, in turn, the apparent effects of protein intake on anthropometric indices of the newborn. Little difference in birthweights or other anthropometric indices was identified between the lowest decile of protein intake (0.7 g per kg per day) and the highest decile (1.5 g per kg per day).

Minerals

The intakes recommended by the Food and Nutrition Board for a variety of minerals are presented in Table 14–1 and discussed below. There is good evidence that only one mineral, iron, provides any demonstrated benefit when provided as a supplement to pregnant women. Practically all diets that supply sufficient calories for appropriate weight gain will contain enough of the other minerals to prevent a mineral deficiency if iodized salt is used.

Iron

There are increased iron requirements during pregnancy, the reasons for which are discussed in Chapter 7 (p. 141). Of the approximately 300 mg of iron transferred to the fetus and placenta and the 500 mg incorporated, if available, into the expanding maternal hemoglobin mass, nearly all is utilized during the latter half of pregnancy. During that time, the average iron requirements imposed by the pregnancy itself are about 6 mg a day, and, in addition, there is the need for nearly 1 mg to compensate for maternal excretion, a total of about 7 mg of iron per day (Pritchard and Scott, 1970). Very few women have sufficient iron stores to supply this amount of iron. Moreover, the diet seldom contains enough iron to meet this demand. The recommendation by the Food and Nutrition Board (Table 14–1) of 18 mg of dietary iron per day for nonpregnant women represents the ceiling imposed by caloric requirements. To ingest any more iron from dietary sources would simultaneously provide an undesirable excess of calories. The board has acknowledged that because of small iron stores, the pregnant woman will often be unable to meet the iron requirements imposed by pregnancy, and therefore it has recommended supplementation.

Supplementation with medicinal iron is commonly practiced in the United States and elsewhere, although the merits of this practice continue to be questioned by a minority of investigators, cited below. Scott and co-workers (1970) established that as little as 30 mg of iron supplied in the form of a simple iron salt such as ferrous gluconate, sulfate, or fumarate, taken regularly once each day throughout the latter half of pregnancy, provided sufficient iron to meet the requirements of pregnancy and to protect any preexisting iron stores. Iron, 30 mg daily, as a simple salt, should also provide for the iron requirements of lactation. The pregnant woman may benefit from 60 to 100 mg of iron per day if she is large, has twin fetuses, is late in pregnancy, or takes iron irregularly, or her hemoglobin level is somewhat depressed. The woman who is overtly anemic from iron deficiency responds well to 200 mg of iron per day in divided doses (see Chap. 39, p. 780).

The availability for absorption of iron contained in at least some prenatal vitamin-mineral supplements has been questioned (Seligman and associates, 1983). Undoubtedly, calcium and magnesium compounds included in such mixtures can inhibit iron absorption, as they do when taken as antacids. Inter-

estingly, the reaction of at least one provider of such multi-everything preparations has been to reduce markedly the calcium and magnesium content of their "formulation." Why this approach, rather than adding more iron, is not clear. Presumably, they now consider the previously provided amounts of calcium and magnesium to be superfluous. **A very effective and inexpensive way to avoid impairment of iron absorption by such agents is to prescribe simple iron salts alone!**

Since iron requirements are slight during the first 4 months of pregnancy, it is *not* necessary to provide supplemental iron during this time. Withholding iron supplementation during the first trimester of pregnancy avoids the risk of aggravating nausea and vomiting, which are common at that time. Ingestion of iron at bedtime also appears to minimize the possibility of an adverse gastrointestinal reaction. Moreover, keeping the container of iron tablets in proximity to toothpaste enhances the ability of the expectant mother to remember to ingest the supplement regularly. When she brushes her teeth, she should take an iron tablet! Iron-containing medication must be kept out of the reach of small children lest they ingest a large number of the usually quite attractive tablets or capsules.

Deficiency Versus "Oversufficiency" of Iron

Paintin and co-workers (1966), Taylor and Lind (1976), and a few others at one time or another have insisted that iron supplements stimulate hemoglobin synthesis to an abnormal degree in pregnant women. Moreover, Taylor and Lind questioned whether iron preparations can be given safely to all pregnant women because of a modest increase in mean red cell volume that is likely to follow. A number of studies refute both of these contentions. In brief, evidence has long been available that a higher hemoglobin concentration depends on whether or not the iron is available, irrespective of whether or not the iron is derived from oral supplements, from parenteral injection, or simply from stores (Scott and co-workers, 1970). The similarity of the magnitude of the increases observed in several of the studies performed over the past quarter-century is apparent in Table 14–2 even though the amounts of iron given varied widely. Importantly, the average increase demonstrated almost universally equals the hemoglobin content of 500 mL of donor blood. The presence or absence of this amount at delivery may determine whether or not a mother is transfused. This is especially true for the 20 percent or so of women who are now delivered by cesarean section!

The moderate increase in maternal mean red cell volume that originally concerned Taylor and Lind (1976) has physiological bases: (1) recently synthesized red cells of iron-replete individuals are larger than are older red cells and (2) red cells formed by iron-deficient individuals are smaller yet more rigid than are those of

TABLE 14–2. STUDIES OF THE EFFECTS OF IRON SUPPLEMENTATION DURING PREGNANCY ON HEMOGLOBIN CONCENTRATION, 1958–82

| | Hemoglobin (g per dL) | | |
	Unsupplemented	*Supplemented*	*Difference*
Taylor et al (1982)	11.2	12.7	+1.5
Chanarin et al (1977)	11.2	12.8	+1.6
Taylor and Lind (1976)	11.0	12.3	+1.3
Paintin et al (1966)	10.7	12.0	+1.3
De Leeuw et al (1966)	10.9	12.4	+1.5
Chisholm (1966)	11.2	12.4	+1.2
Pritchard and Hunt (1958)	11.3	12.5	+1.2
Average	11.05	12.40	+1.35

iron-replete subjects (Yip and co-workers, 1983). Their rigidity could impair flow in the microcirculation. It should be pointed out that Taylor and co-workers (1982) have now reversed their previous position and state, *"It is concluded that routine oral iron administration should be recommended during pregnancy, certainly after 28 weeks gestation."*

In some circumstances compromised fetal well-being may be associated with an above-average maternal hemoglobin concentration (Garn and associates, 1981; Koller, 1982). Recently, Murphy and co-workers (1986) reported findings from the Cardiff Births Survey of 54,382 singleton pregnancies and confirmed that women with hemoglobin values greater than 13.2 g per dL at 13 to 18 weeks had excessive perinatal mortality, low birthweight, and preterm delivery. Importantly, pregnancy-induced hypertension was substantively increased in nulliparas with higher hemoglobin levels. Unfortunately, findings such as these have led to the supposition by some that iron ingested prenatally, by stimulating an abnormally high hemoglobin concentration, is actually detrimental and therefore should not be used (Goodlin, 1982). Even vigorous iron administration does not raise the hemoglobin concentration of iron-sufficient women (Taylor and associates, 1982). Almost certainly, reduced blood volume from failure of plasma volume is the important culprit in the genesis of impaired fetal well-being. Failure of the hemoglobin concentration to fall is but one consequence of inadequate expansion. (If hemoglobin concentration per se were an important factor, phlebotomy or even leeches might come into vogue again!)

Calcium

The expectant mother retains about 30 g of calcium during pregnancy, most of which is deposited in the fetus late in pregnancy (Pitkin, 1985). This amount of calcium represents only about 2.5 percent of the total maternal calcium, most of which is in bone, and which can be readily mobilized for fetal growth. Moreover, Heaney and Skillman (1971) demonstrated increased absorption of calcium by the intestine and progressive retention throughout pregnancy. In a few places in the world *osteomalacia* is still recognized in women who are reproducing but only under the very unusual circumstances of almost total avoidance of sunlight coupled with low vitamin D and calcium intake for very long periods. According to Pitkin (1985), bound calcium levels, but not ionized calcium, fall slightly in maternal plasma as the concentration of albumin decreases (Chap. 7, p. 155).

Belizán and colleagues (1988) reviewed the relationship between calcium intake and pregnancy-induced hypertension and found no firm evidence that calcium supplementation was protective. Although widely practiced in the United States, supplementation is unlikely to be of any benefit. One quart of cow's milk provides approximately 1 g of calcium.

Phosphorous

The ubiquitous distribution of phosphorous assures an adequate intake during pregnancy. Plasma levels of inorganic phosphorus do not differ appreciably from nonpregnant levels.

Zinc

Severe zinc deficiency may lead to poor appetite, suboptimal growth, and impaired wound healing. Profound zinc deficiency may cause dwarfism and hypogonadism. It may also lead to a specific skin disorder, *acrodermatitis enteropathica*.

The concentration of zinc in plasma is only about 1 percent of total body zinc. Moreover, zinc in plasma is almost entirely bound to several plasma proteins and to amino acids. Therefore, most often low plasma concentration of zinc is but the consequence of changes in concentration of the various binders in plasma rather than true zinc depletion (Swanson and King, 1983). Even though the concentration is reduced, the total pool of zinc in plasma of normally pregnant women is actually increased as the consequence of the large increase in plasma volume induced by pregnancy. The rationale for increasing the recommended zinc intake during pregnancy (Table 14–1) is not altogether clear. There is no strong evidence at this time that dietary supplementation with zinc in the United States is of any benefit to the expectant mother or fetus. Meadows and co-workers (1981) have reported the concentration of zinc in leucocytes to be lower in mothers of infants small for gestational age, but whether the low zinc concentration is causally related or merely a marker of fetal growth has not been clarified.

Iodine

The use of iodized salt by all pregnant women is recommended to offset the increased need for fetal requirements and probable increased loss through the maternal kidneys. Severe maternal iodine deficiency in expectant mothers predisposes their offspring to endemic cretinism, characterized by multiple severe neurological defects. In parts of New Guinea where this condition was endemic, the intramuscular injection of iodized oil into women very early in pregnancy or before successfully prevented cretinism in the offspring (Pharoah and associates, 1971). The ingestion of iodide in large (pharmacological) amounts during pregnancy may depress thyroid function and induce a sizable goiter in the fetus. The consumption of large amounts of seaweed by food faddists may do the same.

Magnesium

A deficiency in this element as the consequence of pregnancy has not been recognized. Undoubtedly, during prolonged illness with no magnesium intake, the plasma level might become critically low, as it would in the absence of pregnancy. We have observed magnesium deficiency during pregnancy complicated by the consequences of previous intestinal bypass surgery.

Potassium

The concentration of potassium in maternal plasma decreases by about 0.5 mEq per L by midpregnancy (Brown and colleagues, 1986). Since glomerular excretion increases appreciably but potassium excretion remains constant at about 60 mEq per day, its fractional excretion is decreased. Potassium deficiency develops in the same circumstances as when the patient is not pregnant. Prolonged nausea and vomiting may lead to hypokalemia and metabolic alkalosis. A previously rather common cause—the use of diuretics—has nearly disappeared.

Sodium

A deficiency of sodium during pregnancy is most unlikely unless diuretics are prescribed or dietary sodium intake is reduced drastically. In general, salting food to taste will provide an abundance of sodium for the pregnant woman. The concentration of sodium in plasma normally decreases a few milliequivalents during pregnancy. Sodium excretion is unchanged during pregnancy and averages 100 to 110 mEq per day (Brown and colleagues, 1986).

In the not too distant past much was said about the dangers of inciting preeclampsia–eclampsia through sodium ingestion during pregnancy and, by implication at least, of the benefits to be achieved from rigid restriction of sodium intake. Next, sodium restriction by pregnant women was cited as being detrimental, undoubtedly because rigid sodium restriction in pregnant rats caused abnormalities in the dams' adrenals. About this time it was claimed that extra salt in the maternal diet, especially rock salt, prevented preeclampsia–eclampsia (Robinson, 1958). Nonetheless, the ingestion of exorbitant amounts of sodium may prove harmful. However, there is no good evidence that rigorous sodium restriction is beneficial. Indeed, it too may be harmful.

Fluoride

The value of supplemental fluoride during pregnancy has been questioned. Horowitz and Heifetz (1967) investigated the prevalence of caries in temporary and permanent teeth of children with the same postnatal exposure to optimally fluoridated water but different patterns of prenatal exposure. They concluded that there were no meaningful additional benefits from the ingestion of fluoride in water by the expectant mother if the offspring ingested fluoridated water from birth.

Glenn and associates (1982) reported a remarkably lower incidence (99 percent) of caries in children whose mothers ingested 2.2 mg of sodium fluoride daily during pregnancy, compared to those whose mothers used only fluoridated water. They strongly recommended that for structurally superior and caries-free teeth, 2.2 mg of sodium fluoride daily be ingested while fasting, starting during the third month of pregnancy. Obviously, further investigations are needed to confirm the benefits claimed by Glenn and associates and, at the same time, to detect deleterious effects, if any, from the fluoride.

Supplemental fluoride ingested by the lactating woman does not increase the fluoride concentration in her milk, according to Elkstrand (1981).

VITAMINS

Most evidence concerning the importance of vitamins for successful reproduction has been obtained from animal experiments. Typically, severe deficiency has been produced in the animal either by withholding the vitamin completely, beginning long before the time of pregnancy, or by giving a very potent vitamin antagonist. The administration of some vitamins in great excess to pregnant animals has been shown to exert deleterious effects on the fetus and newborn.

The practice of supplying vitamin supplements prenatally is a deeply ingrained habit of many obstetricians, even though scientific evidence to show that the usual vitamin supplements are of benefit to either the mother or her fetus is quite meager. The Committee on Maternal Nutrition of the National Research Council pointed out that in the majority of cases routine pharmaceutical supplementation of vitamin and mineral preparations to pregnant women is of doubtful value, except for iron and possibly folic acid. **Such vitamin and mineral preparations should not be regarded as substitutes for food.**

The increased requirements for vitamins during pregnancy (Table 14–1) can in practically all circumstances be supplied by any general diet that provides adequate numbers of calories and amounts of protein, including protein from animal sources. The possible exception is folic acid during times of unusually large requirements, such as pregnancy complicated by protracted vomiting, hemolytic anemia, or multiple fetuses.

Folic Acid

Whereas the advantages to be gained from supplemental iron during pregnancy are quite straightforward, namely, protection against maternal iron deficiency and anemia, the benefits to be derived from folic acid supplementation are not nearly so distinct. In the 1960s several investigators implicated maternal folate deficiency in a variety or reproductive casualties, including placental abruption, pregnancy-induced hypertension (toxemia of pregnancy), and fetal anomalies. For the most part, these reports have not been confirmed (Emery, 1977; Hall, 1977; Pritchard and co-workers, 1969; Whalley and associates, 1969). To date, no one has been able to reduce unequivocally the frequency of these complications simply by administering folic acid during pregnancy.

The possibility of increased frequency of fetal malformations as the consequence of maternal folate deficiency has long been discussed, especially neural tube defects (Smithells and colleagues, 1980, 1983; White and Moffa, 1984). Some evidence has been presented that ingestion preconceptually as well as prenatally of a polyvitamin preparation that included folic acid reduced the frequency of neural tube defects. Wald and Polani (1984), however, after examining evidence existing prior to 1984, concluded that there is considerable doubt as to whether vitamin supplementation can prevent neural tube defects. The need for a well-controlled study seemed obvious to some but certainly not to everyone. The ethics of such an anterospective study were vigorously debated. Nonetheless, a collaborative study was organized and is under way. The results are awaited.

Molloy and co-workers (1985) carried out an interesting study of folate levels in maternal sera that had been collected early in pregnancy for rubella antibody testing. Folate levels in the frozen sera from pregnancies complicated by neural tube defects were the same as in sera from normal pregnancies.

Evidence is abundant that maternal folate requirements are increased somewhat during pregnancy. In the United States, this increase frequently leads to lowered plasma folate levels, less often to hypersegmentation of neutrophils, infrequently to megaloblastic erythropoiesis, but only rarely to megaloblastic anemia. The amount of folic acid supplement that will prevent these changes varies considerably, depending primarily on the diet consumed by the pregnant woman. Since 1 mg of folic acid orally per day produces a vigorous hematological response in pregnant women with severe megaloblastic anemia, this amount would almost certainly provide very effective prophylaxis (Pritchard and co-workers, 1969). Chanarin and associates (1979) found that as little as 0.1 mg of folic acid per day raises the blood folate levels to the normal nonpregnant range.

Vitamin B_{12}

The level of vitamin B_{12} in maternal plasma decreases variably in otherwise normal pregnancies (Sauberlich, 1978). The decrease, which is thought to result mostly from a reduction in plasma binders rather than depletion, is prevented only in part by supplementation. However, maternal vitamin B_{12} deficiency can develop in special circumstances. Vitamin B_{12} occurs naturally only in foods of animal origin. It is now established that *strict vegetarians* may give birth to infants whose vitamin B_{12} stores are low. Moreover, since breast milk of a vegetarian mother will most likely contain little vitamin B_{12}, the deficiency may become profound in the breast-fed infant (Higginbottom and associates, 1978).

Excessive ingestion of vitamin C can also lead to a functional deficiency of vitamin B_{12}, as described below under the section on vitamin C.

Vitamin B_6

A variety of biochemical changes induced by vitamin B_6 deficiency, including excessive excretion of xanthurenic acid after the ingestion of a tryptophan load, have been summarized by Sauberlich (1978). Several of the changes also accompany otherwise apparently normal pregnancy and have been identified in women who use estrogen-containing oral contraceptives.

Some investigators have related impaired glucose tolerance during pregnancy to altered metabolic pathways induced by low vitamin B_6 levels and, in turn, a lowering of the biological activity of endogenous insulin. However, neither the observations of Perkins (1977) nor those of Gillmer and Mazibuko (1979) provide support for this premise. Gillmer and Mazibuko investigated 13 pregnant women who had abnormal glucose tolerance tests and who excreted elevated amounts of xanthurenic acid after a tryptophan load. Treatment with pyridoxine, 100 mg daily for 2 to 3 weeks, restored the urinary excretion of xanthurenic acid to normal levels for nonpregnant individuals, but improvement in the glucose tolerance test was observed in only 2 of the 13 pregnant women. There was no change in five and deterioration in six subjects.

As the consequence of some of these observations, an appreciable increase in the recommended daily dietary allowance for pyridoxine intake during pregnancy has been urged by some. However, to modify some of the biochemical changes that imply a deficiency of vitamin B_6 during pregnancy requires appreciably more of the vitamin than is now recommended and would be likely to necessitate specific supplementation. For example, Cleary and associates (1975) emphasized that to raise pyridoxal phosphate levels in maternal plasma to those characteristic of normal nonpregnant women required a daily supplement of pyridoxine of more than 2.5 mg. In fact, in some pregnant women daily supplementation with 10 mg did not accomplish this objective. The benefits that might accrue from larger supplements do not appear at this time to warrant so vigorous an undertaking.

> Pyridoxine ingested in large excess can cause dysfunction of the nervous system (Schaumberg and colleagues, 1983). Megadoses of pyridoxine have been implicated in the genesis of a syndrome of progressive sensory ataxia and profound distal limb impairment of position and vibration sense. It is now apparent that a number of vitamins when consumed in large doses can prove toxic. It is unlikely that either the pregnant woman or her fetus is immune to such risks.

The recommendation of the National Research Council calls for 2.0 mg of pyridoxine daily for nonpregnant women and 2.6 mg per day when pregnant or lactating.

Vitamin C

The recommended dietary allowance for vitamin C during pregnancy is 80 mg per day, or about one third more than when nonpregnant (Table 14–1). A reasonable diet should readily provide this amount. The maternal plasma level declines during pregnancy while the cord level is higher, a phenomenon that is observed with most water-soluble vitamins.

The ingestion of 1 g or more of vitamin C for the prophylaxis of the common cold has become commonplace, even though there is no good evidence that vitamin C when so used is of any benefit. There is evidence that it may prove harmful during pregnancy. Scurvy has been identified in normally fed infants whose mothers had ingested large doses of vitamin C during pregnancy (Cochrane, 1965). Large doses of vitamin C can also interfere with vitamin B_{12} absorption and metabolism. This problem may not be overcome by supplementation with vitamin B_{12} (Herbert and Jacob, 1974).

PRAGMATIC NUTRITIONAL SURVEILLANCE

While the science of nutrition continues in its perpetual struggle to identify the ideal amounts of protein, calories, vitamins, and minerals for the pregnant woman and her fetus, those directly responsible for their care may best discharge their duties as follows:

1. In general, advise the expectant mother to eat what she wants in amounts she desires and salted to taste.
2. Make sure that there is ample food to eat, especially in the case of the socioeconomically deprived woman.
3. Make sure by serially weighing every expectant mother that she is gaining weight, with a goal of at least 20 lb.
4. At each prenatal visit, explore the food intake by dietary recall to uncover the ingestion of any bizarre diet. In this way the occasional nutritionally absurd diet will be discovered—for example, the ingestion of a peck of grapes per day or a pound of Argo Gloss Starch.
5. Give tablets of simple iron salts that provide 30 to 60 mg of iron daily.
6. Recheck the hematocrit or hemoglobin concentration at 28 to 32 weeks, so as to detect any significant decrease.

GENERAL HYGIENE

EXERCISE

In general, it is not necessary for the pregnant woman to limit exercise, provided she does not become excessively fatigued or risk injury to herself or her fetus. The current enthusiasm for jogging has also attracted a number of pregnant women to the endeavor. In fact, several women, even late in pregnancy, have run safely in marathons. Hall and Kaufman (1987) reported that pregnant women who exercised regularly had a lower cesarean section rate and length of hospitalization.

Hauth and co-workers (1982) studied fetal heart rate reactivity throughout the third trimester of pregnancy in seven women who jogged at least 1.5 miles three times a week before and during pregnancy. Upon completion of a run the women immediately climbed three flights of stairs to undergo evaluation. Fetal heart reactivity was evident in spite of the vigorous, very recent maternal exercise, and appreciable fetal tachycardia so induced, persisted for up to one half hour. Carpenter and colleagues (1988) observed that submaximal exercise was not followed by fetal bradycardia; however, it was common after maximal exercise.

With some pregnancy complications, the mother and her fetus may benefit from a very sedentary existence; for example, women with pregnancy-induced hypertension appear to do so (see Chap. 35, p. 676), as do women pregnant with two or more fetuses (see Chap. 34, p. 643) and women suspected of having a growth-retarded fetus (see Chap. 38, p. 771).

The American College of Obstetricians and Gynecologists (1986b) recommends that women who are accustomed to aerobic exercise before pregnancy should continue this during pregnancy. It cautions against starting new aerobic exercise programs or intensifying training efforts. For example, in women who previously were sedentary, aerobic activity more strenuous than walking is not recommended.

EMPLOYMENT

It is estimated that nearly one half of all women of childbearing age in the United States are now in the labor force, and even larger proportions of socioeconomically less fortunate women are working. According to the report of Naeye and Peters (1982), working during pregnancy can be deleterious to pregnancy outcome. They identified birthweights of infants whose mothers worked during the third trimester to be 150 to 400 g less than those of newborns whose mothers did not work, even though the length of gestation was the same for both groups. Reduction in birthweight was greatest for mothers who were underweight before pregnancy and whose weight gain during pregnancy was low, for mothers who were hypertensive, and for mothers whose work required standing. The data analyzed by them were collected between 1959 and 1966 and therefore these results were possibly influenced by the widespread practice of dietary restrictions and use of drugs then in vogue to try to control weight gain and dependent edema.

Manshande and colleagues (1987) reported a sevenfold increased low-birthweight incidence in women from Zaire who worked hard in the fields. However, Berkowitz and associates (1983) and Murphy and co-workers (1984) did not find physical activity to be detrimental to pregnancy; in fact, they suggested that the opposite is more likely true. It is apparent that the problems associated with attempts to compare pregnancy performance in women who do and do not work during pregnancy are numerous. Benefits for working pregnant women are likely to minimize possible adverse effects that might otherwise accrue from working (Saurel and Kaminski, 1983).

Common sense dictates that any occupation that subjects the pregnant woman to severe physical strain should be avoided. Ideally, no work or play should be continued to the extent that undue fatigue develops. Adequate periods of rest should be provided during the working day. Women with previous complications of pregnancy that are likely to be repetitive (for example, low-birthweight infants) probably should minimize physical work.

Travel

The restriction of travel to short trips had been a rule for obstetrical patients until World War II, when many women found it necessary to follow their husbands regardless of distance or mode of travel. The data compiled during that era are consistent with the conclusion that travel by the woman without complications has no harmful effect on pregnancy. Travel in properly pressurized aircraft offers no unusual risk. At least every 2 hours, the pregnant woman should walk about. Perhaps the greatest risk with travel, especially international travel, is the development of a pregnancy complication remote from facilities adequate for treatment of the complication.

Bathing

There is no objection to bathing during pregnancy or the puerperium. During the last trimester, the heavy uterus usually upsets the balance of the pregnant woman and increases the likelihood of her slipping and falling in the bathtub. For that reason, tub baths at the end of pregnancy may be inadvisable.

Clothing

The clothing worn during pregnancy should be practical and nonconstricting. Intricate, expensive supporting girdles are no longer used routinely. The increasing mass of the breasts may make them pendulous and painful. In such instances, well-fitting supporting brassieres are indicated. Constricting garters should be avoided during pregnancy because of the interference with venous return and the aggravation of varicosities. Backache and pressure associated with lordotic posture and a pendulous abdomen may be relieved by a properly fitted maternity girdle. There is no real reason for insisting that the pregnant woman wear only low-heeled shoes, unless she develops backache from the increased lordosis that results from shoes with high heels or if she is unable to maintain good balance.

Bowel Habits

During pregnancy, bowel habits tend to become more irregular, presumably because of generalized relaxation of smooth muscle and compression of the lower bowel by the enlarging uterus early in pregnancy or by the presenting part of the fetus late in pregnancy. In addition to the discomfort caused by the passage of hard fecal material, bleeding and painful fissures in the edematous and hyperemic rectal mucosa may develop. There is also greater frequency of *hemorrhoids* and, much less commonly, of prolapse of the rectal mucosa.

Women whose bowel habits are reasonably normal in the nonpregnant state may prevent constipation during pregnancy by close attention to bowel habits, sufficient quantities of fluid, and reasonable amounts of daily exercise, supplemented when necessary by a mild laxative, such as prune juice, milk of magnesia, bulk-producing substances, or stool-softening agents. The use of nonabsorbable oil preparations has been discouraged because of their possible interference with the absorption of lipid-soluble vitamins. The use of harsh laxatives and enemas is not recommended.

COITUS

Whenever abortion or preterm labor threatens, coitus should be avoided. Otherwise it has been generally accepted that in healthy pregnant women sexual intercourse usually does no harm before the last 4 weeks or so of pregnancy. It has long been the custom of many obstetricians to recommend abstinence from intercourse during the last 4 weeks of pregnancy, a recommendation undoubtedly not followed in many instances.

> The risks versus possible benefits from intercourse late in pregnancy have not been clearly delineated. Pugh and Fernandez (1953), for example, did not find that intercourse caused preterm labor, rupture of the membranes, bleeding, or infection. They concluded that it is not necessary to abstain from coitus during the final weeks of gestation.
>
> Goodlin and associates (1972) were more concerned about possible injurious effects from intercourse late in pregnancy. They identified transient fetal bradycardia with increased uterine tension during maternal orgasms induced by vulval and vaginal manipulation at 39 weeks gestation. The painful uterine contractions ceased within 15 minutes after the last orgasm. Whether such changes commonly accompany orgasm and whether they are harmful to the fetus are not definitely known. They also reported the incidence of orgasm after 32 weeks to have been significantly higher for women who subsequently delivered prematurely. Grudzinkas and co-workers (1979) found no association between gestational age at delivery and the frequency of coitus during the last 4 weeks of pregnancy. However, women who were sexually active in the last 4 weeks showed a higher incidence of fetal distress.
>
> Naeye (1979) using data from the Collaborative Perinatal Project, investigated the impact of coitus during the month before delivery, and reported that amnionic fluid infections and perinatal mortality

were significantly increased if mothers reported intercourse once or more weekly. On the other hand, Mills and associates (1981) identified no increase in premature rupture of the membranes, low birthweight, or perinatal death among selected women who had sexual intercourse throughout pregnancy. Their study was biased, however, by the exclusion from potential risk of a large number of cases in which intercourse had been interdicted late in pregnancy because of a history of premature birth, spontaneous abortion, bleeding, uterine scar, hypertension, twins, or stillbirth.

On occasion, the couple's sexual drive in the face of admonishment against intercourse late in pregnancy has led to unusual sexual practices with disastrous consequences. Aronson and Nelson (1967) for instance, describe fatal cases of air embolism late in pregnancy as a result of air blown into the vagina during cunnilingus. Other near-fatal cases have been described (Bernhardt and associates, 1988).

Douches

If douching in pregnancy is desirable because of excessive cervical and vaginal secretions, the following precautions should be observed:

1. Hand bulb syringes must absolutely be forbidden, since several deaths in pregnancy from air embolism have followed their use (Forbes, 1944).
2. The douche bag should be placed not more than 2 feet above the level of the hips to prevent high fluid pressure.
3. The nozzle should not be inserted more than 3 inches through the vulva.

Care of Breasts and Abdomen

Special care of the breasts during pregnancy is often advised to increase the ability to nurse by toughening the nipples and thereby reduce the incidence of cracking and by effecting enlargement and eversion of the nipples. From the available data it is concluded that ointments, massage, and traction on the nipples do not always improve these functions, but such practices are usually harmless. Massages and ointments do not alter significantly the incidence of striae on the breasts or abdomen. In general, the extent of striation is proportional to the size of the uterus and the weight gain of the woman.

Care of the Teeth

Examination of the teeth should be included in the prenatal general physical examination. Pregnancy rarely is a contraindication to needed dental treatment. The concept that dental caries are aggravated by pregnancy is unfounded.

Immunization

There has been some concern over the safety of various immunization techniques during pregnancy. The recommendations of the American College of Obstetricians and Gynecologists (1982) with appropriate updating for specific immunizations during pregnancy are summarized in Table 14–3.

SMOKING

Mothers who smoke during pregnancy frequently bear smaller infants than do nonsmokers. There is also evidence that smoking mothers have a significantly greater number of unsuccessful pregnancies because of an increase in perinatal deaths. Goldstein (1977) estimated that about 4,600 infants die in the United States every year because their mothers smoke. Many of the data to support these statements were presented in the publication, *Smoking and Health, Report to the Surgeon General of the Public Health Service* (1979).

To explain these adverse effects from smoking, various investigators have implicated the following: (1) carbon monoxide and its functional inactivation of fetal and maternal hemoglobin, (2) vasoconstrictor action of nicotine causing reduced perfusion of the placenta, (3) reduced appetite and, in turn, reduced calorie intake by women who smoke, (4) decreased plasma volume in mothers who smoke, and (5) an unexplained peculiarity in certain women that persists even when they do not smoke.

Astrup and associates (1972), Socol and co-workers (1982), and Bureau and colleagues (1982) implicated carbon monoxide in the genesis of low birthweight on the basis of their studies on women, monkeys, and rabbits. D'Souza and co-workers (1978) identified the hemoglobin level in cord blood to average 17.8 g per dL if the mother smoked during pregnancy, compared to 16.3 g per dL if she did not smoke; a plausible explanation to account for these differences in hemoglobin concentrations is bone marrow stimulation from chronic fetal hypoxia. Low birthweight has been described, however, for infants whose mothers did not smoke, but rather had chewed tobacco (Krushna, 1978). Lehtovirta and Forss (1978) reported intervillous blood flow to be acutely reduced during smoking and for 15 minutes afterwards. Monheit and associates (1983) did not alter significantly either uterine or umbilical hemodynamics by infusing nicotine acutely into pregnant sheep in doses that produced blood levels of the alkaloid substantially greater than those reported in humans while smoking. Moreover, Jouppila and

---

TABLE 14–3. SUMMARY OF RECOMMENDATIONS FOR IMMUNIZATION DURING PREGNANCY

Live Virus Vaccines	Inactivated Bacterial Vaccines	Hyperimmune Globulins
Measles—contraindicated	Cholera—to meet international travel requirements	Hepatitis B—postexposure prophylaxis: give along with hepatitis B vaccine initially, then vaccine alone at 1 and 6 months
Mumps—contraindicated	Meningococcus—same as nonpregnant	Rabies—postexposure prophylaxis
Poliomyelitis—not routine; increased risk exposure	Plague—selective vaccination of exposed persons	Tetanus—postexposure prophylaxis
Rubella—contraindicated	Typhoid—travel to endemic areas	Varicella—same as nonpregnant
Yellow fever—travel to high-risk areas only		
Inactivated Virus Vaccines	**Toxoids**	**Pooled Immune Serum Globulins**
Influenza—serious underlying diseases	Tetanus-Diphtheria—same as nonpregnant	Hepatitis A—postexposure prophylaxis
Rabies—same as nonpregnant		Measles—postexposure prophylaxis

Modified from the American College of Obstetricians and Gynecologists, Technical Bulletin No. 64, May 1982.

co-workers (1983) found no significant change in human fetal blood flow in the thoracic aorta or umbilical vein during and immediately following the mother smoking a cigarette.

Rush (1974) and Davies and co-workers (1976) have contended that lower birthweight of infants whose mothers smoke is primarily the consequence of lower pregnancy weight gain by smoking mothers. However, Haworth and co-workers (1980) identified birthweights to be lower for infants whose mothers smoked than for those whose mothers did not, even though maternal weight gain and dietary intake were the same for both groups.

Boomer and Christensen (1982) identified evidence for increased high maternal hematocrits and low-birthweight infants in pregnancies of women who smoked. They considered these events to reflect most likely the decrease in plasma volume among pregnant women who smoked described by Pirani and MacGillivray (1978). Brown and colleagues (1988) described that extensive placental calcification at 37 weeks was doubled (36 versus 14 percent) in smokers. Yerushalmy (1972) implicated the smoker and not the smoke in the genesis of low birthweight. He reported lower birthweights for infants whose mothers had not yet smoked when the infants were born but who began to smoke subsequently. Most other investigators have not confirmed Yerushalmy's findings. Interestingly, the incidence of preeclampsia has been reported to be somewhat lower in women who smoke (Duffus and MacGillivray, 1968; Underwood and co-workers, 1967).

Hardy and Mellits (1973) could not identify any harmful long-term effects in children of smoking mothers even though they weighed on the average 250 g less and were shorter at birth. Butler and Goldstein (1973), however, based on a sample of several thousand children 7 to 11 years of age, found slight retardation for reading, mathematics, and general ability in children whose mothers smoked during pregnancy.

In view of the obvious dangers to people who smoke, cigarettes should be avoided completely by women, irrespective of any deleterious effects on pregnancy.

ALCOHOL

Excessive ingestion of alcohol by the expectant mother is likely to produce abnormalities in the fetus. Chronic alcoholism can lead to fetal maldevelopment, commonly referred to as the *fetal alcohol syndrome,* the features of which are discussed in detail in Chapter 32 (p. 567). Women with chronic and severe drinking problems must be discouraged from becoming pregnant until these problems are brought under control. Serious consideration should be given to early pregnancy termination in alcoholic women.

Differences of opinion persist in regard to the possible adverse effects on the fetus from social drinking. (Sulaiman and colleagues, 1988). Evidence has been presented, however, that a linear relationship between alcohol consumption and fetal damage exists (Chap. 32, p. 567). From the evidence available the best advice to the woman pregnant or about to become pregnant would seem to be "Don't consume alcohol." Hopefully, the adverse effects of alcohol on pregnancy do not linger after the woman stops drinking.

CAFFEINE

In 1980 the Food and Drug Administration advised pregnant women to limit caffeine intake. The Fourth International Caffeine Workshop concluded shortly thereafter that there was no evidence that caffeine increased teratogenic or reproductive risk (Dews and colleagues, 1984). In small laboratory animals caffeine is not a teratogen, but it does potentiate mu-

tagenic effects of radiation and some chemicals if given in massive doses. Infused intravenously into sheep, it decreases uterine blood flow by 5 to 10 percent (Conover and colleagues, 1983).

Most studies of human pregnancy report no association between caffeine consumption and birth defects or low birthweight (Kurppa and co-workers, 1983; Leviton, 1988; Linn and colleagues, 1982).

"HARD" DRUGS

Chronic use by the expectant mother of "hard" drugs, including opium derivatives, barbiturates, and amphetamines, in large doses, is harmful to the fetus. Intrauterine distress, low birthweight, and serious compromise as the consequence of drug withdrawal soon after birth have been well documented. Often the mother who uses hard drugs does not seek prenatal care, and even if she does, she may not admit to the use of such substances. Detection of scars from venipunctures may be the first clue. As emphasized elsewhere (see Chap. 32, p. 567), the management of pregnancy and delivery and successful care of the newborn infant may be extremely difficult (Edelin and associates, 1988). Early abortion should be considered for the addicted pregnant woman who wants to try to "kick the habit."

The effects of maternal marijuana smoking on the human embryo and fetus are not known. Maternal administration of Δ^9-tetrahydrocannabol in large amounts is teratogenic in some animals at least.

MEDICATIONS

With rare exception, any drug that exerts a systemic effect in the mother will cross the placenta to reach the embryo and fetus. Some drugs commonly ingested during pregnancy, and their possible adverse fetal effects, are considered in detail in Chapter 32 (p. 562).

All physicians should develop the habit early of ascertaining the likelihood of pregnancy before prescribing drugs for any woman, since a number of medications in common use can be injurious to the embryo and the fetus. Package inserts provided by pharmaceutical companies and approved by the Food and Drug Administration should be consulted before drugs are prescribed for pregnant women. **If a drug is administered during pregnancy, the advantages to be gained must clearly outweigh any risks inherent in its use.**

COMMON COMPLAINTS

NAUSEA AND VOMITING

Nausea and vomiting are common complaints during the first half of pregnancy. Typically nausea and vomiting commence between the first and second missed menstrual period and continue until about the time of the fourth missed period. Nausea and vomiting are usually worse in the morning but may continue throughout the day.

The genesis of pregnancy-induced nausea and vomiting is not clear. Possibly the hormonal changes of pregnancy are responsible. Chorionic gonadotropin, for instance, has been implicated on the basis that its levels are rather high at the same time that nausea and vomiting are most common. Moreover, in women with hydatidiform mole, in which levels of chorionic gonadotropin typically are very much higher than in normal pregnancy, nausea and vomiting are often prominent clinical features. However, Soules and co-workers (1980) found no relationship between the serum levels of chorionic gonadotropin and the incidence and severity of nausea and vomiting in pregnant women, including those with a hydatidiform mole. Depue and colleagues (1987) also found no association with serum chorionic gonadotropin levels; however, they reported significantly increased plasma estradiol and sex hormone binding globulin-binding capacity. They hypothesized that vomiting in early pregnancy is stimulated by rapid rises in plasma estradiol concentrations.

Emotional factors undoubtedly can contribute to the severity of the nausea and vomiting of pregnancy. Very infrequently vomiting may be so severe that dehydration, electrolyte and acid-base disturbances, and starvation become serious problems.

Seldom is the treatment of nausea and vomiting of pregnancy so successful that the affected expectant mother is afforded complete relief. However, the unpleasantness and discomfort usually can be minimized. Eating small feedings at more frequent intervals but stopping short of satiation is of value. Since the smell of certain foods often precipitates or aggravates the symptoms, such foods should be avoided as much as possible.

For several years at Parkland Hospital a combination of doxylamine succinate plus pyridoxine (Bendectin) was given for pregnancy-induced nausea and vomiting. The preparation is no longer available, however, as the consequence of legal pressures (Chap. 32, p. 564). We prescribe currently either promethazine, perchloperazine, or trimethylperazine suppositories for severe nausea and vomiting.

> There has been considerable lay publicity that suggested, at least, that the use of Benedectin causes fetal malformations, and lawsuits have been initiated based on this assumption. However, data have been published from at least nine series of pregnant women who used Benedectin early in pregnancy and in none was there a significant increase in the frequency of malformations among infants exposed in utero (see Chap. 32, p. 564).

A great variety of other agents has been recommended for treatment. Fairweather (1968), for example, in his comprehensive review of nausea and vomiting in pregnancy, tabulated such bizarre and diverse treatments as hibernotherapy, intravenously administered honey, husband's blood, and the husband's sex hormone (testosterone). These are mentioned only to illustrate the extent to which humankind has gone to try to cope with the aggravation from nausea and vomiting induced somehow by early pregnancy.

Fortunately, effective psychological support can be offered in the form of reassurance to the pregnant woman that these symptoms nearly always will disappear by the fourth month and, moreover, that pregnancies in which nausea and vomiting occur are more likely to have a favorable outcome than are those without nausea and vomiting (Yerushalmy and Milkovich, 1965).

The syndrome of nausea and vomiting of great intensity and requiring hospitalization for successful management is referred to as *hyperemesis gravidarum*. Prompt correction of fluid and electrolyte imbalances usually relieves the symptoms (Chap. 39, p. 829). Today therapeutic abortion is rarely required.

BACKACHE

Backache occurs to some extent in some pregnant women. Minor degrees follow excessive strain or fatigue and excessive bending, lifting, or walking. Mild backache usually requires little more than elimination of the strain and occasionally a lightweight maternity girdle.

Severe backaches should not be attributed simply to pregnancy until a thorough orthopedic examination has been conducted. Muscular spasm and tenderness, which are often classified clinically as acute strain or fibrositis, respond well to analgesics, heat, and rest.

In some women motion of the symphysis pubis and lumbosacral joints, and general relaxation of pelvic ligaments may be demonstrated. In severe cases the pregnant woman may be unable to walk or even remain comfortable without support furnished by a heavy girdle and prolonged periods of rest. Occasionally, anatomical defects are found, either congenital or traumatic, that may precipitate the complaints. Pain caused by herniation of an intervertebral disc occurs during pregnancy with about the same frequency as at other times.

VARICOSITIES

Varicosities, generally resulting from congenital predisposition, are exaggerated by prolonged standing, pregnancy, and advancing age. Usually varicosities become more prominent as pregnancy advances, as weight increases, and as the length of time spent upright is prolonged. As discussed in Chapter 7 (p. 147), femoral venous pressure becomes appreciably increased as pregnancy advances.

The symptoms produced by varicosities vary from cosmetic blemishes on the lower extremities and mild discomfort at the end of the day to severe discomfort that requires prolonged rest with the feet elevated.

The treatment of varicosities of the lower extremities is generally limited to periodic rest with elevation of the legs, or elastic stockings, or both. Surgical correction of the condition during pregnancy generally is not advised, although the symptoms rarely may be so severe that injection, ligation, or even stripping of the veins is necessary in order to allow the pregnant woman to remain ambulatory. In general, these operations should be postponed until after delivery. Varicosities of the vulva may be aided by application of a foam rubber pad suspended across the vulva by a belt of the type used with a perineal pad. Rarely, large varicosities may rupture, resulting in profuse hemorrhage.

A severe case of massive varicosities that involved both legs and the vulva of a woman of high parity is demonstrated in Figure 14–1. Treatment during pregnancy consisted of elastic stockings, frequent elevation of the legs throughout the day to provide drainage, and avoidance of injury to the affected parts. (A leg varix had ruptured with severe hemorrhage, necessitating transfusion shortly before this pregnancy.) Delivery was accomplished spontaneously without laceration. Aggressive ambulation with elastic support stockings was initiated soon after delivery and after tubal sterilization. Surgical intervention with extensive vein stripping was performed late in the puerperium.

Occasionally, *superficial thrombophlebitis* complicates preexisting varicose veins. Treatment is discussed in Chapter 28, (p. 477).

HEMORRHOIDS

Varicosities of hemorrhoidal veins occasionally first appear during pregnancy. More often, pregnancy causes an exacerbation or recurrence of previous symptoms. The development or aggravation of hemorrhoids during pregnancy is related undoubt-

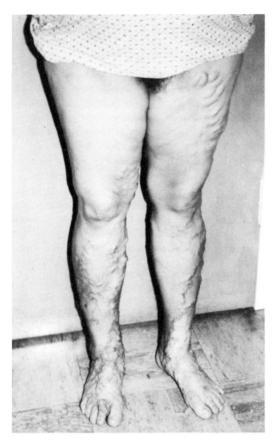

Figure 14–1. Massive varices during pregnancy in a multiparous woman. Well-fitting support hose provided considerable relief until surgical correction was performed late in the puerperium.

edly to increased pressure in the hemorrhoidal veins caused by obstruction of venous return by the large pregnant uterus, and to the tendency toward constipation during pregnancy. Usually pain and swelling are relieved by topically applied anesthetics, warm soaks, and agents that soften the stool. Thrombosis of a hemorrhoidal vein can cause considerable pain, but the clot can usually be evacuated by incising the wall of the involved vein with a scalpel under topical anesthesia.

Bleeding from hemorrhoidal veins occasionally may result in loss of sufficient blood to cause iron-deficiency anemia. The loss of only 15 mL of blood results in the loss of 6 to 7 mg of iron, an amount equal to the daily requirements for iron during the latter half of pregnancy. If bleeding is persistent, hemorrhoidectomy may be required. In general, however, hemorrhoidectomy is not desirable during pregnancy, since most often hemorrhoids become asymptomatic soon after delivery.

HEARTBURN

Heartburn, one of the most common complaints of pregnant women, usually is caused by reflux of gastric or duodenal contents into the lower esophagus (Feeney, 1982). The increased frequency of regurgitation during pregnancy most likely results from the upward displacement and compression of the stomach by the uterus combined with decreased gastrointestinal motility. In some pregnant women, the cardia actually herniates through the diaphragm.

In most pregnant women symptoms are mild and relieved by a regimen of more frequent but smaller meals and avoidance of bending over or lying flat. Antacid preparations may provide considerable relief. Aluminum hydroxide, magnesium trisilcate, or magnesium hydroxide, alone or in combination (for example, Amphojel, Gelusil, Maalox, and milk of magnesia), should be used in preference to sodium bicarbonate. The pregnant woman who tends to retain sodium can become edematous as the result of ingestion of excessive amounts of sodium bicarbonate. Antacids that contain magnesium and aluminum hydroxides impair absorption of iron somewhat but otherwise appear to be quite innocuous.

PICA

Occasionally during pregnancy bizarre cravings for strange foods develop and at times for materials hardly considered edible, such as laundry starch, clay, and even dirt. For example, at Parkland Hospital, interrogation of recently delivered mothers in a single day disclosed that the following items were craved and consumed by them during the current pregnancy: Argo Gloss Starch, flour, baking powder, baking soda, clay, baked dirt, powdered bricks, and frost scraped from the refrigerator (pagophagia).

The ingestion of starch (amylophagia) or clay (geophagia) or related items is practiced more often by socioeconomically less privileged pregnant women. It is unlikely that the craving for these materials is the consequence of hunger but is rather in large part a social custom.

The desire for dry lump starch, clay, chopped ice, or even refrigerator frost has been considered by some to be triggered by severe iron deficiency. Although women with severe iron deficiency sometimes crave these items, and although the craving is usually ameliorated after correction of the iron deficiency, not all pregnant women with pica are necessarily iron-deficient.

Minnich and associates (1968) found that the ingestion of clay, especially Turkish clay and to a lesser extent clays from Georgia and Mississippi, impaired absorption of iron. In Dallas, however, we were unable to demonstrate that either of two Texas clays studied or Argo Gloss Starch reduced absorption of iron significantly (Talkington and associates, 1970).

The consumption of starch in sufficient quantities to provide a significant portion of the calories ingested or to cause ptyalism is not healthful nor is the ingestion of clay to the extent that the intestine is sufficiently filled to cause obstruction of labor or fecal impaction. Nonetheless, it is quite unlikely that either laundry starch or clay free of parasites is distinctly harmful to the pregnancy if consumed in moderation and if the diet is nutritionally adequate.

PTYALISM

Women during pregnancy are occasionally distressed by profuse salivation. The cause of the ptyalism sometimes appears to be stimulation of the salivary glands by the ingestion of starch. This cause should be looked for and eradicated if found.

FATIGUE

Early in pregnancy, most women complain of fatigue and desire for excessive periods of sleep. The condition usually remits spontaneously by the fourth month of pregnancy and has no special significance.

HEADACHE

Headache early in pregnancy is a frequent complaint. A few cases may result from sinusitis or ocular strain caused by refractive errors. In the vast majority, however, no cause can be demonstrated. Treatment is largely symptomatic. By the middle of pregnancy, most of these headaches decrease in severity or disappear. The pathological significance of headaches as the consequence of pregnancy-induced hypertension that develops later in pregnancy is considered in Chapter 35, p. 672).

LEUCORRHEA

Pregnant women commonly develop increased vaginal discharge, which in many instances has no pathological cause. Increased formation of mucus by cervical glands in response to hyperestrogenemia is undoubtedly a contributing factor. If the secretion is troublesome, the woman may be advised to douche with water mildly acidified with vinegar. The precautions for douching listed on page 269 should be stressed.

Occasionally, troublesome leucorrhea is the result of an infection caused by *Trichomonas vaginalis* or *Candida albicans*.

Trichomonas vaginalis

This organism can be identified in as many as 20 percent of women during prenatal examination; however, the infection is symptomatic in a much smaller percentage of pregnant women. Trichomonal vaginitis is characterized by foamy leucorrhea with pruritis and irritation. Trichomonads are readily demonstrated in fresh vaginal secretions as flagellated, pear-shaped, motile organisms that are somewhat larger than leucocytes.

It has been suggested that *Trichomonas vaginalis* is a cause of preterm labor. However, Mason and Brown (1980) found no difference in birthweights of infants from mothers with or without vaginal infestation with the organism.

Metronidazole (Flagyl) has proved effective in eradicating *Trichomonas vaginalis*. The drug may be administered orally or vaginally. When ingested by the mother, metronidazole crosses the placenta and enters the fetal circulation. The possibility of teratogenicity had been raised if metronidazole were ingested during the first trimester; however, earlier described chromosomal abnormalities following metronidazole therapy for Crohn's disease are now thought by the investigators to have been the consequence of sulphasalazine and not metronidazole. In a more recent report they found no increase in frequency of chromosomal aberrations after 4 months of therapy (Mitelman and associates, 1980). Finally, Rosa and colleagues (1987) found no increased frequency of birth defects in 1,020 women given metronidazole during the first trimester.

Candida albicans

Candida (Monilia) can be cultured from the vagina in about 25 percent of women approaching term. Asymptomatic vaginal candidiasis probably requires no treatment. However, it may sometimes cause an extremely profuse irritating discharge. Miconazole nitrate, 2 percent, in a vaginal cream, has been claimed to be highly effective for the treatment of candidiasis during pregnancy (McNellis and co-workers, 1977). Candidiasis is likely to recur, thereby requiring repeated treatment during pregnancy, but usually it subsides at the end of gestation.

Serious fetal infections with *Candida* occur but are rare when compared to the high prevalence of *Candida* in the maternal vagina. Penetration of the fetal membranes, even without gross rupture and invasion of the umbilical cord, can lead to an intense inflammatory response in the fetus, with a high mortality rate. The presence of a foreign body such as an intrauterine device in the maternal reproductive tract appears to enhance the risk of fetal infection (Whyte and associates, 1982).

REFERENCES

American College of Obstetricians and Gynecologists: Immunization During Pregnancy. Technical Bulletin, No 64, May 1982

American College of Obstetricians and Gynecologists: Standards for Obstetric-Gynecologic Services. Washington, DC, American College of Obstetricians and Gynecologists, 1985a

American College of Obstetricians and Gynecologists: Gonorrhea and Chlamydial Infections. Technical Bulletin, No 89, November 1985b

American College of Obstetricians and Gynecologists: ACOG Newsletter 30:9, 1986

American College of Obstetricians and Gynecologists: Management of Diabetes Mellitus in Pregnancy. Technical Bulletin, No 92, March 1986a

American College of Obstetricians and Gynecologists: Women and Exercise. Technical Bulletin, No 87, September 1986b

Aronson ME, Nelson PK: Fatal air embolism in pregnancy resulting from an unusual sex act. Obstet Gynecol 30:127, 1967

Astrup P, Olsen HM, Trolle D, Kjeldsen K: Effect of moderate carbon-monoxide-exposure on fetal development. Lancet 2:1220, 1972

Bayless TM, Rothfeld B, Massa C, Wise L, Paige D, Bedine M: Lactose and milk intolerance: Clinical implications. N Engl J Med 292:1156, 1975

Berkowitz GS, Kelsey JL, Holford TR, Berkowitz RL: Physical activity and the risk of spontaneous preterm delivery. J Reprod Med 28:581, 1983

Bernhardt TL, Goldmann RW, Thombs PA, Kindwall EP: Hyperbaric oxygen treatment of cerebral air embolism from orogenital sex during pregnancy. Crit Care Med 16:729, 1988

Boomer AL, Christensen BL: Antepartum hematocrit, maternal smoking and birth weight. J Reprod Med 27:387, 1982

Bromovich P: Big babies. Brit Med J 293:1387, 1986

Brown HL, Miller JM, Khawli O, Gabert HA: Premature placental calcification in maternal cigarette smokers. Obstet Gynecol 71:914, 1988

Brown MA, Sinosich MJ, Saunders DM, Gallery ED: Potassium regulation and progesterone-aldosterone interrelationships in human pregnancy: A prospective study. Am J Obstet Gynecol 155:349, 1986

Bureau MA, Monette J, Shapcott D, Paré C, Mathieu J-L, Lippé J, Blovin D, Berthiaume Y, Begin R: Carboxyhemoglobin concentration in fetal cord blood and in blood of mothers who smoked during labor. Pediatrics 69:371, 1982.

Butler NR, Goldstein H: Smoking in pregnancy and subsequent child development. Br Med J 3:573, 1973

Calvert JP, Crean EE, Newcombe RG, Pearson JF: Antenatal screening of measurement of symphysis-fundus height. Br Med J 285:846, 1982

Carpenter MW, Sady SP, Hoegsberg B, Sady MA, Haydon B, Cullinane EM, Coustan DR, Thompson PD: Fetal heart rate response to maternal exertion. JAMA 259:2006, 1988

Center for Disease Control: Influenza vaccine: Preliminary statement. Ann Intern Med 89:373, 1978

Center for Disease Control: Prevention of perinatal transmission of hepatitis B virus: Prenatal screening of all pregnant women for hepatitis B surface antigen. 37:341, 1988

Chanarin I, McFayden IR, Kyle R: The physiological macrocytosis of pregnancy. Brit J Obstet Gynaecol 84:504, 1977

Chisholm M: A controlled clinical trial of prophylactic folic acid and iron in pregnancy. J Obstet Gynaecol Brit Commonw 73:191, 1966

Cleary RE, Lumeng L, Li Y-K: Maternal and fetal plasma levels of pyridoxal phosphate at term: Adequacy of vitamin B_6 supplementation during pregnancy. Am J Obstet Gynecol 121:25, 1975

Cochrane WA: Overnutrition in prenatal and neonatal life: A problem? Can Med Assoc J 93:893, 1965

Conover WB, Key TC, Resnik R: Maternal cardiovascular response to caffeine infusion in the pregnant ewe. Am J Obstet Gynecol 145:534, 1983

Creasy RK, Gummer BA, Liggins GC: System for predicting spontaneous preterm birth. Obstet Gynecol 55:692, 1980

Davies DP, Gray OP, Ellwood PC, Abernathy M: Cigarette smoking in pregnancy: Associations with maternal weight gain and fetal growth. Lancet 1:385, 1976

De Leeuw NK, Lowenstein L, Hsieh YS: Iron deficiency and hydremia in normal pregnancy. Medicine 45:201, 1966

Delgado H, Lechug A, Yarbrough C, Martorell R, Klein RE, Irwin M: Maternal nutrition—Its effects on infant growth and development and birthspacing. In Moghissi KS, Evans TN (eds): Nutritional Impacts on Women. Hagerstown, MD, Harper & Row, 1977, p 133

Depue RH, Bernstein L, Ross RK, Judd HL, Henderson BE: Hyperemesis gravidarum in relation to estradiol levels, pregnancy outcome, and other maternal factors: A seroepidemiologic study. Am J Obstet Gynecol 156:1137, 1987

Dews P, Grice HC, Neims A, Wilson J, Wurtman R: Report of Fourth International Caffeine Workshop, Athens, 1982. Food Chem Toxicol 22:163, 1984

D'Souza SW, Black PM, Williams N, Jennison RF: Effect of smoking during pregnancy upon the haematological values of cord blood. Br J Obstet Gynaecol 85:495, 1978

Duffus G, MacGillivray I: The incidence of preeclamptic toxemia in smokers and non-smokers. Lancet 1:994, 1968

Eastman NJ, Jackson E: Weight relationships in pregnancy: I. The bearing of maternal weight gain and pre-pregnancy weight on birth weight in full term pregnancies. Obstet Gynecol Surv 23:1003, 1968

Edelin KC, Gurganious L, Golar K, Oellerich D, Kyei-Aboagye K, Hamid MA: Methadone maintenance in pregnancy: Consequences to care and outcome. Obstet Gynecol 71:399, 1988

Ekstrand J: No evidence of transfer of fluoride from plasma to breast milk. Br Med J 283:761, 1981

Emery AEH: Folates and fetal central-nervous-system malformations. Lancet 1:703, 1977

Fairweather DV: Nausea and vomiting in pregnancy. Am J Obstet Gynecol 102:135, 1968

Feeney JG: Heartburn in pregnancy (editorial). Br Med J 284:1138, 1982

Food and Nutrition Board Position Paper on the Relationship of Nutrition to Brain Development and Behavior. Washington, DC, National Academy of Sciences, 1973

Forbes G: Air embolism as complication of vaginal douching in pregnancy. Br Med J 2:529, 1944

Gant NF, Scott DE, Pritchard JA: Unpublished observations

Garn SM, Keating MT, Falkner F: Hematological status and pregnancy outcomes. Am J Clin Nutr 34:115, 1981

Gillmer MDG, Mazibuko D: Pyridoxine treatment of chemical diabetes in pregnancy. Am J Obstet Gynecol 133:499, 1979

Glenn FB, Glenn WD III, Duncan RC: Fluoride tablet supplementation during pregnancy for caries immunity: A study of the offspring produced. Am J Obstet Gynecol 143:560, 1982

Goldstein H: Smoking in pregnancy: Some notes on the statistical controversy. Br J Prevent Soc Med 31:13, 1977

Goodlin RC: Why treat "physiologic" anemias of pregnancy? J Reprod Med 27:639, 1982

Goodlin RC, Keller DW, Raffin M: Orgasm during late pregnancy: Possible deleterious effects. Obstet Gynecol 38:916, 1971

Goodlin RC, Schmidt W, Creevy DC: Uterine tension and fetal heart rate during maternal orgasm. Obstet Gynecol 39:125, 1972

Grudzinkas JG, Watson C, Chard T: Does sexual intercourse cause fetal distress? Lancet 2:692, 1979

Hall DC, Kaufmann DA: Effects of aerobic and strength conditioning on pregnancy outcomes. Am J Obstet Gynecol 157:1199, 1987

Hall MH: Folates and the fetus. Lancet 1:648, 1977

Hardy JB, Mellits ED: Does maternal smoking during pregnancy have a long-term effect on the child? Lancet 2:1332, 1973

Hauth JC, Gilstrap LC III, Widmer K: Fetal heart rate reactivity before and after maternal jogging during the third trimester. Am J Obstet Gynecol 142:545, 1982

Haworth JC, Ellestad-Sayed JJ, King J, Dilling LA: Fetal growth retardation in cigarette-smoking mothers is not due to decreased maternal food intake. Am J Obstet Gynecol 137:719, 1980

Heaney RP, Skillman TG: Calcium metabolism in normal human pregnancy. J Clin Endocrinol 33:661, 1971

Hemminki E: Content of prenatal care in the United States. A historic perspective. Med Care 26:199, 1988

Herbert V, Jacob E: Destruction of vitamin B_{12} by ascorbic acid. JAMA 230:241, 1974

Herbert WNP, Bruninghaus HM, Barefoot AB, Bright TG: Clinical aspects of fetal heart auscultation. Obstet Gynecol 69:574, 1987

Higginbottom MC, Sweetman L, Nyhan WL: A syndrome of methylmalonic aciduria, homocystinuria, megaloblastic anemia and neurologic abnormalities in a vitamin B_{12}-deficient breast-fed infant of a strict vegetarian. N Engl J Med 299:317, 1978

Hobel CJ, Youkeles L, Forsythe A: Prenatal and intrapartum high-risk screening: II. Risk factors reassessed. Am J Obstet Gynecol 135:1051, 1979

Horowitz HS, Heifetz SB: Effects of prenatal exposure to fluoridation on dental caries. Public Health Rep 82:297, 1967

Hytten FE, Leitch I: The Physiology of Human Pregnancy, 2nd ed. Oxford, Blackwell, 1971

Jimenez JM, Tyson JE, Reisch JS: Clinical measures of gestational age in normal pregnancies. Obstet Gynecol 61:438, 1983

Jouppila P, Kirkinen P, Eik-Nes S: Acute effect of maternal smoking on the human fetal blood flow. Br J Obstet Gynaecol 90:7, 1983

Koller O: The clinical significance of hemodilution during pregnancy. Obstet Gynecol Surv 37:649, 1982

Kortenoever ME: Pathology of pregnancy: Pregnancy of long duration and postmature infant. Obstet Gynecol Surv 5:812, 1950

Krushna K: Tobacco chewing in pregnancy. Br J Obstet Gynaecol 85:726, 1978

Kurppa K, Holmberg PC, Kuosma E, Saxen L: Coffee consumption during pregnancy and selected congenital malformations: A nationwide case-control study. Am J Public Health 73:1397, 1983

Lehtovirta P, Forss M: The acute effect of smoking on intervillous blood flow of the placenta. Br J Obstet Gynaecol 85:729, 1978

Leveno KJ, Cunningham FG, Roark ML, Nelson SD, Williams ML: Prenatal care and the low birth weight infant. Obstet Gynecol 66:599, 1985

Leviton A: Caffeine consumption and the risk of reproductive hazards. J Reprod Med 33:175, 1988

Linn S, Schoenbaum SC, Monson RR, Rosner B, Stubblefield PG, Ryan KJ: No association between coffee consumption and adverse outcomes of pregnancy. N Engl J Med 306:141, 1982

Manshande JP, Eeckels R, Manshande-Desmet V, Vlietinck R: Rest versus heavy work during the last weeks of pregnancy: Influence on fetal growth. Br J Obstet Gynaecol 94:1059, 1987

Mason PR, Brown I McL: Trichomonas in pregnancy. Lancet 2:1025, 1980

McNellis D, McLeod M, Lawson J, Pasquale SA: Treatment of vulvovaginal candidiasis in pregnancy. Obstet Gynecol 50:674, 1977

Meadows NJ, Ruse W, Smith MF, Day J, Keeling PW, Scopes JW, Thompson RP, Bloxam DL: Zinc and small babies. Lancet 2:1135, 1981

Mills JL, Harlap S, Harley EE: Should coitus late in pregnancy be discouraged? Lancet 2:136, 1981

Minnich V, Okcuoglu A, Tarcon Y, Arcasoy A, Cin S, Yorukoglu O, Renda F, Demirag B: Pica in Turkey: II. Effect of clay upon iron absorption. Am J Clin Nutr 21:78, 1968

Mitelman F, Strombeck B, Ursing B: No cytogenic effect of metronidazole. Lancet 1:1249, 1980

Molloy AM, Kirke P, Hillary I, Weir DG, Scott JM: Maternal serum folate and vitamin B_{12} concentration in pregnancies associated with neural tube defects. Arch Dis Child 50:660, 1985

Monheit AG: Maternal and fetal cardiovascular effects of nicotine infusion in pregnant sheep. Am J Obstet Gynecol 145:290, 1983

Murphy JF, Newcomb RG, O'Riodan J, Coles EC, Pearson JF: Relation of haemoglobin levels in first and second trimesters of outcome of pregnancy. Lancet 1:993, 1986

Murphy JF, Dauncey M: Employment in pregnancy. Lancet 1:1163, 1984

Naeye RL: Coitus and associated amniotic-fluid infections. N Engl J Med 301:1198, 1979

Naeye R: Weight gain and the outcome of pregnancy. Am J Obstet Gynecol 135:3, 1979

Naeye RL, Peters EC: Working during pregnancy: Effects on the fetus. Pediatrics 69:724, 1982

Nakano R: Post-term pregnancy. Acta Obstet Gynecol Scand 51:217, 1972

National Center for Health Statistics: Maternal weight gain and the outcome of pregnancy—United States, 1980. In: Advance Data from Vital and Health Statistics, DHHS Publication No (PHS) 86-1922, Washington, DC, Government Printing Office, 1986

Nielsen ST, Finne PH, Bergs JO, Stamnes O: Males with low birthweight examined at 18 years of age. Acta Paediatr Scand 73:168, 1984

Paintin DB, Thomson AM, Hytten FE: Iron and the haemoglobin level in pregnancy. J Obstet Gynaecol Br Commonw 73:181, 1966

Papiernik E, Kaminski M: Multifactorial study of the risk of prematurity at 32 weeks of gestation: A study for the frequency of 30 predictive characteristics. J Perinat Med 2:30, 1974

Perkins RP: Failure of pyridoxine to improve glucose tolerance in gestational diabetes mellitus. Obstet Gynecol 50:370, 1977

Pharoah POD, Buttfield IH, Hetzel BS: Neurological damage to the fetus resulting from severe iodine deficiency during pregnancy. Lancet 1:308, 1971

Pirani BBK, MacGillivray I: Smoking during pregnancy: Its effects on maternal metabolism and fetoplacental function. Br J Obstet Gynaecol 52:257, 1978

Pitkin RM: Calcium metabolism in pregnancy and the perinatal period: A review. Am J Obstet Gynecol 151:99, 1985

Prentice AM, Cole TJ, Foord FA, Lamb WH, Whitehead RG: Increased birthweight after prenatal dietary supplementation of rural women. Am J Clin Nutr 46:912, 1987

Prentice AM, Whitehead RG, Watkinson, M, Lamb WH, Cole TJ: Prenatal dietary supplementation of African women and birth-weight. Lancet 1:489, 1983

Pritchard JA, Hunt CF: A comparison of the hematologic responses following the routine prenatal administration of intramuscular and oral iron. Surg Gynecol Obstet 106:516, 1958

Pritchard JA, Scott DE: Iron demands during pregnancy. In Hallberg L, Harwerth H-G, Vannotti A (eds): Iron Deficiency: Pathogenesis, Clinical Aspects, Therapy. New York, Academic, 1970

Pritchard JA, Scott DE, Whalley PJ: Folic acid requirements in pregnancy induced megaloblastic anemia. JAMA 208:1163, 1969

Pritchard JA, Whalley PJ: High risk pregnancy and reproductive outcome. In Gluck L (ed): Modern Perinatal Medicine. Chicago, Year Book, 1974

Pugh WE, Fernandez FL: Coitus late in pregnancy. Obstet Gynecol 2:636, 1953

Quaranta P, Currell R, Redman CWG, Robinson JS: Prediction of small-for-date infants by measurements of symphysial-fundal height. Br J Obstet Gynaecol 88:115, 1981

Recommended Dietary Allowances, 9th ed. Food and Nutrition Board, Washington, DC, National Research Council, National Academy of Sciences, 1979

Ribeiro MD, Stein Z, Susser M, Cohen P, Neugut R: Prenatal starvation and maternal blood pressure. Am J Clin Nutr 35:535, 1982

Robinson M: Salt in pregnancy. Lancet 1:178, 1958

Rosa FW, Baum C, Shaw M: Pregnancy outcomes after first trimester vaginitis drug therapy. Obstet Gynecol 69:751, 1987

Rush D: Lower weight gain among smokers explains most of the effect of smoking on birthweight. Pediatr Res 8:450, 1974

Sauberlich HE: Vitamin indices. In Laboratory Indices of Nutritional Status in Pregnancy. Washington DC, National Research Council Committee on Nutrition of the Mother and Preschool Child, National Academy of Sciences, 1978, p 109

Saurel MJ, Kaminski M: Pregnant women at work. Lancet 1:475, 1983

Schaumberg H, Kaplan J, Windebank A, Vick N, Rasmus S, Pleasure D, Brown MJ: Sensory neuropathy from pyridoxine abuse. N Engl J Med 309:445, 1983

Scott DE, Pritchard JA, Saltin A-S, Humphreyes SM: Iron deficiency during pregnancy. In Hallberg L, Harwerth H-G, Vannotti A (eds): Iron Deficiency: Pathogenesis, Clinical Aspects, Therapy. New York, Academic, 1970

Seligman PA, Caskey JH, Frazier JL, Zucker RM, Podell ER, Allen RH: Measurements of iron absorption from prenatal multivitamin-mineral supplements. Obstet Gynecol 61:356, 1983

Smith CA: Effects of maternal undernutrition upon the newborn infant in Holland (1944–1945). Am J Obstet Gynecol 30:229, 1947

Smithells RW, Sellar MJ, Harris R, Fielding DW, Schorah CJ, Nevin NC, Sheppard S, Read AP, Walker S, Wild J: Further experience of vitamin supplementation for prevention of neural tube defect recurrences. Lancet 1:1027, 1983

Smithells RW, Sheppard S, Schorah CJ, Seller MJ, Nevin NC, Harris R, Read AP: Possible prevention of neural-tube defects by periconceptual vitamin supplementation. Lancet 1:339, 1980

Socol ML, Manning FA, Murata Y, Druzin ML: Maternal smoking causes fetal hypoxia: Experimental evidence. Am J Obstet Gynecol 142:214, 1982

Sokol RJ, Rosen MG, Stojkov J, Chik J: Clinical application of high-risk scoring on an obstetric service. Am J Obstet Gynecol 128:652, 1977

Soules MR, Hughes CL Jr, Garcia JA, Livengood CH, Prystowski MR, Alexander E III: Nausea and vomiting of pregnancy: Role of human chorionic gonadotropin and 17-hydroxyprogesterone. Obstet Gynecol 55:696, 1980

Stein Z, Susser M, Rush D: Prenatal nutrition and birth weight: Experiments and quasi-experiments in the past decade. J Reprod Med 21:287, 1978

Stein Z, Susser M, Saenger G, Marolla F: Nutrition and mental performance. Science 178:708, 1972

Sulaiman ND, Florey C, Taylor DJ, Ogston SA: Alcohol consumption in Dundee primigravidas and its effects on outcome of pregnancy. Br Med J 296:1500, 1988

Swanson CA, King JC: Reduced serum zinc concentration during pregnancy. Obstet Gynecol 62:313, 1983

Talkington KM, Gant NF, Scott DE, Pritchard JA: Effect of ingestion of starch and some clays on iron absorption. Am J Obstet Gynecol 108:262, 1970

Task Force Report: American College Obstet Gynecol Assessment of Maternal Nutrition. Chicago, American College of Obstetricians and Gynecologists, 1978

Taylor DJ, Lind T: Haemotological changes during normal pregnancy: Iron induced macrocytosis. Br J Obstet Gynaecol 83:760, 1976

Taylor DJ, Mallen C, McDougall N, Lind T: Effect of iron supplementation on serum ferritin levels during and after pregnancy. Br J Obstet Gynaecol 89:1011, 1982

Underwood PB, Hester LL, Lafitte T Jr, Gregg KV: The relationship of smoking empirically related to pregnancy outcome. Obstet Gynecol 29:1, 1967

Whalley PJ, Scott DE, Pritchard JA: Maternal folate deficiency and pregnancy wastage: I. Placental abruption. Am J Obstet Gynecol 105:670, 1969

White JA, Moffa AM: Periconceptional supplementation of folic acid and the incidence of open neural tube defects in golden hamster embryos. Presented before the Society for Gynecological Investigation, San Francisco, March 21–24, 1984

Whyte RK, Hussain Z, deSa D: Antenatal infections with *Candida* species. Arch Dis Child 57:528, 1982

Worthen N, Bustillo M: Effect of urinary bladder fullness on fundal height measurements. Am J Obstet Gynecol 138:759, 1980

Yerushalmy J: Infants with low birth weight born before their mothers started to smoke cigarettes. Am J Obstet Gynecol 112:277, 1972

Yerushalmy J, Milkovich L: Evaluation of the teratogenic effect of meclizine in man. Am J Obstet Gynecol 93:553, 1965

Yip R, Mohandas N, Clark MR, Jain S, Shohet SB, Dallman PR: Red cell membrane stiffness in iron deficiency. Blood 62:99, 1983

Zlatnik RJ, Burmeister LF: Dietary protein in pregnancy: Effect on anthropometric indices of the newborn. Am J Obstet Gynecol 146:199, 1983

Techniques to Evaluate Fetal Health

Until relatively recently, the intrauterine sanctuary of the fetus was held to be inviolate. The mother was the patient to be cared for; the fetus was but another, albeit transient, maternal organ. The philosophy prevailed that "good maternal care" would automatically provide what was best for the products of conception. Ideally, labor would not occur until the fetus weighed more than 2,500 g (once the widely accepted definition of fetal maturity), except in instances of gross developmental abnormality when, it was hoped, the embryo or nonviable fetus might be expelled spontaneously. If, however, spontaneous abortion did not ensue, society decreed the only alternative to be that the parents, or at times some governmental agency, must try to care for the subsequently liveborn but malformed offspring.

During the past two decades, remarkably detailed knowledge of the human fetus and his or her immediate environment has accumulated (see Chap. 6). As did maternal health earlier in this century, fetal health, or fetal medicine, has come to be appreciated not merely as an exciting arena for research but as a clinical discipline with great potential for favorably influencing the quality of human offspring. Indeed, the fetus is no longer regarded as a maternal appendage ultimately to be shed at the whim of biological forces beyond control. Instead, the fetus has achieved the status of the second patient, a patient who usually faces much greater risks of serious morbidity and mortality than does the mother.

It is now possible not only to identify but to quantify with some precision physical abnormalities and functional derangements that afflict the fetus. Moreover, in some instances treatment can be implemented—surgical as well as medical—while the fetus continues to mature in utero.

The many advances in diagnosis and treatment that now clearly establish the fetus as a patient have also contributed remarkably to legal considerations involving the fetus. Fetal legal rights are emerging; for example, in some courts, the fetus has been allowed to file suit. Moreover, law-enforcement officials and the judiciary are now more inclined to think of the fetus as a person deserving protection against criminal acts performed against him or her. Interestingly, not too long ago in Dallas a fetus killed in a motor vehicle accident a few minutes before birth at term was not a victim of manslaughter in the eyes of the law-enforcement officials; in fact, the fetus could not even qualify as a traffic fatality.

DIAGNOSTIC MODALITIES

A variety of techniques that may be of value to assess fetal health are considered in this chapter. In the past, attempts were made to predict fetal health by measuring a number of fetally derived hormones and enzymes in maternal plasma, urine, or both. In general, however, these have proved to be unsatisfactory, and subsequently other noninvasive technological developments have been used. Ultrasound techniques, including use of Doppler technology, have assumed a prime role in fetal health evaluation. These technologies include fetal, placental, and amnionic fluid imaging as well as assessment of fetal heart rate and its reaction to a variety of stimuli. X-ray and magnetic resonance imaging have been used, but much less often. Invasive techniques used to evaluate the fetus began with amniocentesis to study amnionic fluid. This was followed by fetoscopy and amnioscopy, which proved cumbersome. Both have now been superseded by techniques for ultrasonic fetal visualization and direct sampling of fetal blood. Thus, modern technology allows for biophysical assessment of the fetus, giving further credence to the specialty of fetal medicine.

The use of newer biochemical, biophysical, and electronic procedures should be regarded, *as their value is proved,* as worthy additions to existing clinical procedures already available to help identify the fetus at risk. It is emphasized at the outset that these procedures may impose some risk of morbidity and mortality to the fetus and the mother, or impose significant expense, or both. Therefore, their use should provide benefits that clearly outweigh both the potential risks and the costs. Certainly the physician who orders them must be prepared to acknowledge the results and to use them objectively.

There is no doubt that pregnancy outcomes have improved during the time that most, if not all, the techniques described in this chapter have been available to try to identify the presence or absence of fetal well-being. In 1969, for the first time, the perinatal death rate dropped below 30 per 1,000. It has continued to fall and in 1985 was estimated to be 14.7 per 1,000 births. Although tempting, it is inappropriate to ascribe the dramatic decrease solely to the availability of more techniques to evaluate fetal health. A multiplicity of important factors have undoubtedly contributed to this accomplishment:

1. Less unplanned and unwanted pregnancies as the consequence of federally funded family planning programs and the legalization of elective abortion.
2. Pregnant women taking better advantage of antepartum care.
3. The prevention or selective abortion of some pregnancies in which the fetus or neonate would have been at increased risk of dying.
4. More liberal use of hospitalization in an attempt to prolong gestation safely.
5. Greater attention paid to the fetus, including the use of a variety of techniques to monitor the fetal condition.

6. Increased use of cesarean delivery to minimize fetal trauma and asphyxia.
7. Availability of excellent neonatal care.
8. As was emphasized by Schifrin (1979), Factor X, or *tender loving care* for mother and fetus-neonate.

AMNIOCENTESIS

The ability to enter the amnionic sac without appreciable risk to the mother or fetus has influenced obstetrical care remarkably. The aspiration of a sample of amnionic fluid provides for a variety of diagnostic tests that are indicative of fetal well-being or lack thereof. A very comprehensive listing of abnormalities of the fetus that are amenable to detection with the aid of appropriate analysis of amnionic fluid has been provided by Roberts and co-workers (1983).

TECHNIQUES

Beginning early in the second trimester, after the exocoelomic space between amnion and chorion has been obliterated, the chorion laeve has fused with the uterine decidua, and the uterus is enlarged sufficiently to be easily palpated above the symphysis, amnionic fluid may be aspirated transabdominally. After locally anesthetizing the abdominal wall, a 20- or 22-gauge needle 3 to 6 inches long, depending upon the thickness of the abdominal wall, the size of the uterus, and the site of puncture, is carefully inserted into the amnionic sac. When cells from amnionic fluid are desired for culture, up to 30 mL of amnionic fluid is withdrawn at 15 to 18 weeks gestation (Chap. 32, p. 582).

Risks

The three major risks from amniocentesis are readily deduced: (1) trauma to the fetus, to the placenta, or, less often, to the umbilical cord or to maternal structures; (2) infection; and (3) abortion or preterm labor. Surgical asepsis is mandatory to avoid infection not only in the mother and fetus but also in the aspirated amnionic fluid, especially when it is to be used for cell culture or microbiological studies.

As well as causing hemorrhage into the placenta and into the amnionic sac (Fig. 15–1), perforation of the placenta may lead to significant transfer of fetal blood to the mother, which may incite or enhance maternal isoimmunization and, in turn, hemolytic disease in the fetus. Therefore, sonographic localization of the placenta before amniocentesis is recommended to reduce the likelihood of perforating the placenta during insertion of the needle, but, unfortunately, it does not always preclude fetal to maternal bleeding. Consequently, anti-D globulin is commonly administered to nonsensitized Rh(D) negative women at the time of amniocentesis (see Chap. 33, p. 604).

Suprapubic amniocentesis decreases the risk of placental perforation (Fig. 15–2). The experiences of Leach and co-workers (1978) further attest to the suprapubic site being the most favorable one for amniocentesis performed late in pregnancy. Whether such a low puncture site enhances the risk of a leak of amnionic fluid is not clear. It has been our experience that if late in pregnancy the fetus can be easily palpated immediately beneath the proposed site of transabdominal puncture, the placenta is implanted elsewhere. If, however, fetal parts cannot be easily palpated immediately beneath the proposed site of puncture, ultrasonic localization of the placenta is indicated.

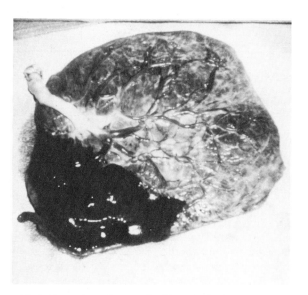

Figure 15–1. Hemorrhage from perforation of a fetal vessel in the placenta at the time of amniocentesis.

Trauma to the umbilical cord is more likely if the cord is around the neck of the fetus and entry into the amnionic space is attempted adjacent to the fetal head and shoulder. Injury to the fetus is more common when the volume of amnionic fluid is small compared to the size of the fetus, or when the amnionic fluid is thick and does not flow freely through the needle. These later conditions are more likely to be encountered late in pregnancy and especially in the postterm pregnancy. Whenever the possibility exists of the placenta implanted beneath the proposed site of puncture, or when amnionic fluid volume appears to be restricted, amniocentesis should be performed with the aid of direct ultrasonic guidance. Repeated taps after failure to obtain amnionic fluid increase the risk of trauma to the fetus.

After amniocentesis, the fetus who is sufficiently mature to have reasonable potential for survival if delivered should be carefully evaluated for evidence of deterioration by close monitoring of the fetal heart rate, especially if the tap was thought possibly to be traumatic. Immediately after delivery all infants should be carefully examined for any evidence of needle puncture.

Several attempts have been made to identify the overall risk of amniocentesis performed near midpregnancy for the purpose of detecting hereditary disease or congenital defects in the fetus. In one study (National Institute of Child Health and Human Development, 1976), no significant differences were found in fetal loss rate, birthweights, birth defects, neonatal complications, or growth and development at 1 year of age. The overall fetal loss was 3.5 percent for the amniocentesis group and 3.2 percent for the control group. The overall accuracy of prenatal diagnosis was 99.4 percent. Similar results were obtained in a Canadian study (Simpson and colleagues, 1976). However, in a British study (Working Party on Amniocentesis, 1978), a significantly higher fetal loss rate—2.6 percent—was identified in the amniocentesis group, compared to an unusually low value of 1.1 percent in the control group. Of concern, there was an apparent increase in certain abnormalities in the newborn infants, especially respiratory problems at birth and orthopedic postural deformities. These abnormalities suggest that amniocentesis, at times, resulted in loss of amnionic fluid volume

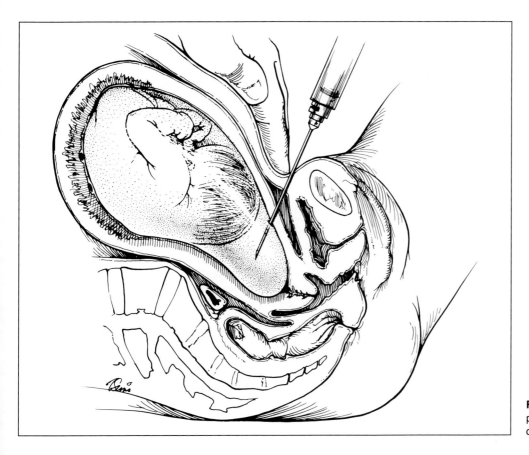

Figure 15–2. Amniocentesis late in pregnancy, performed suprapubically.

sufficient to restrict pulmonary excursion and to create abnormal fetal postures. In all studies, complications were greater when a large needle (18-gauge or larger) was used and when more than two taps were needed to obtain fluid.

Poreco and co-workers (1983), at a center in San Diego, analyzed the outcomes for more than 2,300 pregnancies in which midtrimester amniocentesis was performed, and they estimated the procedure-related loss to have been 0.6 to 0.9 percent. Gillberg and associates (1982) evaluated 62 children at 5 to 7 years of age whose mothers had undergone amniocentesis at midpregnancy and for this small group identified no increase in neurodevelopmental disorders, orthopedic problems, or respiratory abnormalities.

Bloody Tap

Blood contaminating the amnionic fluid may complicate appreciably the techniques for study and the interpretation of the results. Erythrocytes may inhibit the replication in culture of fetal cells from amnionic fluid. Moreover, blood may change the apparent level of various constituents of amnionic fluid under study, especially α-fetoprotein from fetal blood. Gibbons and co-workers (1974) studied the effects of adding up to 4 percent maternal blood to fresh amnionic fluid, which was then promptly centrifuged. The addition to amnionic fluid of blood concentrations of 1 percent or more produced a lowering of the lecithin-to-sphingomyeline (L/S) ratio, a direction of change that would lead to the prediction of a less mature fetus for reasons considered below. Buhi and Spellacy (1975) identified maternal serum to have an L/S ratio of 1:3 to 1:5, and they found that its addition to amnionic fluid influenced the ratio accordingly; meconium also lowered the L/S ratio somewhat. In general, if

the "hematocrit" of the spun amnionic fluid exceeds 3 percent, the sample should be considered unsatisfactory for measurement of L/S ratio. **Minute amounts of fetal, but not maternal, blood can lead to falsely high levels of α-fetoprotein in amnionic fluid.** Therefore, if the amnionic fluid appears bloody, it should not be used for such analysis if the red cells are of fetal origin.

AMNIONIC FLUID SURFACTANT (FETAL LUNG MATURITY)

Amniocentesis was initially employed primarily to estimate the concentration of bilirubin or bilirubin-like pigment in amnionic fluid and thereby to identify hemolytic disease in the fetus (see Chap. 33, p. 605). Currently, it probably is used most often to determine the relative concentration of surfactant-active phospholipids to identify the fetus who has or has not developed lung maturity.

So-called type II pneumonocytes of fetal lung alveoli produce surface-active phospholipids that are essential for the maintenance of effective respiration immediately after birth (see Chap. 6, p. 107). Without appropriate surfactant activity, the lung literally collapses with each expiration because of the high surface tension at air-fluid interfaces, and the syndrome of idiopathic respiratory distress develops (see Chap. 33, p. 593).

The specific lecithin dipalmitoyl phosphatidylcholine plus phosphatidylinositol and especially phosphatidylglycerol are critically important in the formation and stabilization of the surface-active layer that prevents alveolar collapse and the development of respiratory distress. These compounds are contained in lamellar bodies that are released from the type II cell into the alveolar space from which appreciable amounts are transported to the surrounding amnionic fluid. An important consequence of the containment of most of the surfactant in the lamellar bodies is that after too vigorous centrifugation the precipitate is likely to contain most of the lecithin, with most of the sphingomyelin remaining in the supernatant and thus giving a falsely low lecithin-to-sphingomyelin ratio.

Several tests used to estimate pulmonary surfactant, and thus to predict respiratory distress, have been reviewed in detail by Weiner and Weinstein (1987).

Lecithin-to-Sphingomyelin (L/S) Ratio

Measurement of the L/S ratio demands a well-monitored laboratory, since slight variations in technique can appreciably affect the accuracy of the results. Especially critical steps are centrifugation at appropriate speed, acetone precipitation, and densitometric measurement of the charred lecithin and sphingomyelin. If the analysis is not to be performed promptly, the specimen should be refrigerated.

Before 34 weeks gestation, lecithin and sphingomyelin are present in amnionic fluid in similar concentrations. At about 34 weeks, the concentration of lecithin relative to sphingomyelin begins to rise (Fig. 15–3).

It was shown by Gluck and co-workers (1971), and soon confirmed by others, that for pregnancies of unknown duration but otherwise uncomplicated, the risk of respiratory distress in the newborn is very slight whenever the concentration of lecithin in amnionic fluid is at least twice that of sphingomyelin, whereas there is increased risk of respiratory distress when the L/S ratio is below 2. Harvey and colleagues (1975) combined the data from 25 reports in which L/S ratios were measured by similar techniques on amnionic fluid collected within 72 hours of delivery. With an L/S ratio greater than 2, the risk of respiratory distress was found to be slight unless the mother had diabetes (see Chap. 39, p. 821). If the L/S ratio was 1.5 to 2.0, respiratory distress was identified in 40 percent, and if below 1.5, in 73 percent. Although 73 percent of infants developed respiratory distress when the L/S ratio was below 1.5, it proved fatal in but 14 percent.

The experiences at Parkland Hospital have been that respiratory distress did not develop in some instances in which the L/S ratio was as low as 0.6. Moreover, infants for whom the L/S ratio in amnionic fluid was as low as 0.3 have survived after

suffering respiratory distress (Herbert and colleagues, 1979). When the L/S ratio was greater than 0.5, deaths from respiratory distress were actually quite low. Obviously, there are times when the risk to the fetus from a hostile intrauterine environment will be greater than the risk of death from respiratory distress, even though the L/S ratio is less than 2.

Unfortunately, with some pregnancy complications, for example, class A and B maternal diabetes (Quirk and Bleasdale, 1986), erythroblastosis fetalis, fetal-neonatal sepsis, or most any event that causes the infant to be metabolically seriously compromised at birth, an L/S ratio of 2 does not necessarily preclude the development of respiratory distress.

Phosphatidylglycerol

Surfactant action insufficient to prevent respiratory distress, even though the L/S ratio is 2, is thought to be due in part to lack of phosphatidylglycerol and its enhancement of surface-active properties. The identification of phosphatidylglycerol in amnionic fluid provides considerable assurance, but not necessarily an absolute guarantee, that respiratory distress will not develop (Whittle and co-workers, 1982).

Phosphatidylglycerol has not been detected in blood, meconium, or vaginal secretions; consequently, these contaminants do not confuse the interpretation. Importantly, the absence of phosphatidylglycerol is not necessarily a strong indicator that respiratory distress is likely to develop after delivery; its absence serves to indicate only that the infant *may* develop respiratory distress.

A rapid (15-minute) immunological agglutination test (Amniostat-FLM) to identify phosphatidylglycerol in amnionic fluid samples is available commercially. Its accuracy for identifying phosphatidylglycerol, and, in turn, the improbability of the neonate developing respiratory distress syndrome, has been found satisfactory by Garite and associates (1983) and Saad and colleagues (1987).

Foam Stability (Shake) Test

To reduce the time and effort inherent in precise measurement of the L/S ratio, the foam stability test, or so-called shake test, was introduced by Clements and associates (1972). The test depends upon the ability of surfactant in amnionic fluid, when mixed appropriately with ethanol, to generate stable foam at the air-liquid interface. The technique takes no more than 30 minutes to complete.

> Into one chemically clean 13 × 100-mm glass tube with a Teflon-lined plastic screw cap are added 1.0 mL of recently collected amnionic fluid and 1 mL of 95 percent ethanol (prepared by diluting 19.0 parts absolute alcohol with 1 part of distilled water); 0.5 mL of amnionic fluid, 0.5 mL of 0.9 percent saline, and 1 mL of the 95 percent ethanol are added to another tube. Each tube is vigorously shaken for 15 seconds and placed upright in a rack for 15 minutes. The persistence of an intact ring of bubbles at the air-liquid interface after 15 minutes is considered a positive test.

If the ring of foam persists for 15 minutes, the risk of respiratory distress is very low. For example, Schlueter and co-workers (1979) identified only one instance of respiratory distress developing out of 205 pregnancies in which the test was positive for amnionic fluid diluted with an equal volume of saline. There are, however, two problems with the test: (1) slight contamination of amnionic fluid, reagents, or glassware, or errors in measurement, may alter the test results markedly; and (2) a false negative test is rather common—that is, failure of

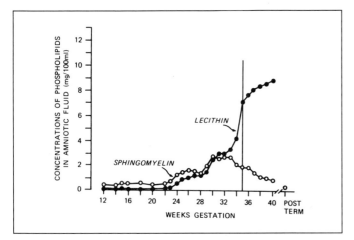

Figure 15–3. Changes in mean concentrations of lecithin and sphingomyelin in amnionic fluid during gestation in normal pregnancy. (*From Gluck and Kulovich: Am J Obstet Gynecol 115:541, 1973.*)

the ring of foam to persist intact for 15 minutes in the tube containing diluted amnionic fluid is not necessarily predictive of respiratory distress. This is explicable, at least in our experiences, since an L/S ratio of 4 to 6 or higher is necessary for a positive shake test, whereas respiratory distress is uncommon if the ratio is at least 2.

Lumadex–FSI Test
This test represents a commercially available kit that uses the principle of foam stability to identify surfactant activity in amnionic fluid. It also has been found to be reliable (Sher and Statland, 1983; Herbert and associates, 1984).

Fluorescent Polarization (Microviscometry)
Another approach to the identification of surfactant activity in amnionic fluid has been evaluated by Barkai and associates (1982, 1988) for normal and abnormal pregnancies. The microviscosity of lipid aggregates in the amnionic fluid may be assayed by mixing the fluid with a specific fluorescent dye that incorporates into the hydrocarbon region of the lipids in surfactant. The intensity of the fluorescence induced by polarized light is then measured. The technique is rapid and appears simple to perform but the instrument is expensive.

Amnionic Fluid Absorbance at 650 nm
The degree of absorbance of light of 650 nm wavelength has been reported to correlate well with the L/S ratio in amnionic fluid (Sbarra and co-workers, 1977). Tsai and associates (1983) reported the test to have been most informative at low absorbance and high absorbance; between these extremes, however, false positive and false negative values proved troublesome. Moreover, Khouzami and associates (1983) reported that differences in centrifugation altered appreciably light absorbance by the amnionic fluid.

Other Amnionic Fluid Indicators of Fetal Maturity

Evaluation of many other constituents or properties of amnionic fluid has been suggested to try to identify fetal maturity. Those that have been cited often are the concentration of creatinine, the osmolality, and the presence of appropriate amounts of cells that are lipid-stainable. Although these constituents or properties change as the fetus matures, the rate and the degree of change are often so slight or so variable that their measurements do not provide an acceptable level of precision for identification of fetal maturity. Moreover, results that imply functional maturity of one organ system should not be interpreted to imply functional maturity of another. For example, remarkable variation was demonstrated for quintuplets born at Parkland Hospital 222 days after the onset of the last menstrual period. Within the limits of measurement the creatinine concentration and the osmolality were identical in amnionic fluid from each sac, 2 mg per dL and 265 mOsm per L, respectively. These values implied fetal maturity as pointed out below. At the same time the L/S ratio in the amnionic fluid from each sac ranged from less than 2 to greater than 5. Respiratory distress was associated with the low but not the high L/S ratios.

Amnionic Fluid Bilirubin
Hemolysis yields bilirubin, most of which remains unconjugated by the fetus. How unconjugated bilirubin reaches the amnionic fluid from the fetus is uncertain, as there is essentially none in the fetal urine and the fetal skin appears to be impermeable to free bilirubin during the latter half of pregnancy. The respiratory tract and the amnion over the placenta and umbilical cord are possible but unproven pathways. The concentration of bilirubin in amnionic fluid normally falls progressively during the latter half of pregnancy, usually to become essentially zero as the fetus reaches maturity. Typically, the bilirubin levels and the rate of decrease during the last several weeks of pregnancy are so slight and problems inherent in analysis are sufficiently great to preclude its use as a sensitive test of fetal maturity. In case of fetal hemolytic disease, however, the concentration of bilirubin for any given fetal age usually reflects the intensity of the hemolysis (see Fig. 33–7, p. 607).

It is not always appreciated that bilirubin in the amnionic fluid need not be of fetal origin. An elevated maternal plasma concentration of free bilirubin, as, for example, with sickle cell anemia, is reflected in an elevation in the amnionic fluid.

Amnionic fluid supernatant is best analyzed for bilirubin using a continuous-recording spectrophotometer. There is a characteristic absorption peak at 450 nm, the correct height of which, when measured as an increase in optical density above baseline, is proportional to the bilirubin concentration (Fig. 33–6, p. 606). In current symbolism, the value is usually expressed as Δ OD 450. Measurement of bilirubin by ordinary chemical methods is not satisfactory because of the low concentration in amnionic fluid.

Amnionic Fluid Creatinine
During the latter half of pregnancy, the concentration of creatinine in amnionic fluid slowly rises until near term, when the increase is more rapid. The rise is the consequence of increased excretion of creatinine by the maturing fetal kidneys. A level of 2 mg per dL in amnionic fluid not treated to remove nonspecific chromogens most often indicates fetal maturity. There are two problems inherent in the test: (1) pulmonary function may prove to be mature even though the creatinine concentration is less than 2 mg per dL; (2) an increase in maternal plasma creatinine will cause an increase in the amnionic fluid creatinine although the fetus is not mature.

Amnionic Fluid Osmolality
Early in pregnancy, the osmolality of amnionic fluid and fetal serum are the same. From 20 weeks onward, however, the osmolality of amnionic fluid decreases at the rate of approximately 1 mOsm per L per week, presumably as the consequence of dilution by nonprotein nitrogen-rich, but hypotonic, fetal urine. The rate of decrease in osmolality, however, is too gradual and too variable to allow a precise prediction of fetal maturity.

Lipid-Staining of Cells in Amnionic Fluid
Staining of amnionic fluid aspirate with Nile blue sulfate discloses two categories of cells or cell particles. Blue-stained bodies represent shed fetal epithelial cells, while the orange-stained bodies originate from sebaceous glands. In the later stages of gestation, an increase in orange bodies appears to reflect maturity of the sebaceous glands. Two major problems arise from the use of the Nile blue sulfate technique to identify fetal maturity: (1) the orange-colored bodies tend to clump, which makes quantification difficult; (2) lower percentages of orange-colored bodies do not necessarily indicate prematurity.

AMNIOCENTESIS TO IDENTIFY INHERITED DISORDERS

Amniocentesis allows retrieval of fetal somatic cells and fluid that can be used to identify the cytogenetic constitution of the fetus or to assess a variety of abnormal biochemical processes. These are discussed in detail in Chapter 33.

AMNIOSCOPY

Saling (1973) has reported extensively on the visualization of amnionic fluid through the membranes when the cervix is sufficiently dilated. Amnioscopy to identify meconium staining of amnionic fluid may be of value in late pregnancy complicated by (1) maternal hypertension, (2) apparently prolonged pregnancy, (3) suspected fetal growth retardation, (4) previous unexplained stillbirth, and (5) lack of orderly cervical dilatation or descent of the presenting part during the first stage of labor. The following problems are associated with amnioscopy: (1) the cervix must be accessible for visualization—that is, neither too far posterior nor too far anterior; (2) the cervix must be dilated enough to visualize the membranes and the fluid behind them; (3) the membranes may be ruptured inadvertently during the examination; and (4) the intravaginal and intracervical manipulations may lead to infection of the products of conception and the upper genital tract. Amnioscopy to try to visualize amnionic fluid for meconium staining has not become very popular in the United States.

Use of an amnioscope to obtain fetal blood is illustrated in Figure 15–13.

FETAL BLOOD SAMPLING

FETAL SCALP BLOOD SAMPLING

Fetal scalp blood sampling is dependent upon ruptured membranes and therefore is used for intrapartum fetal surveillance. The technique, indications, and limitations are discussed on page 300.

FETOSCOPICALLY DIRECTED BLOOD SAMPLING

Direct fetal blood sampling using a fetoscope was introduced by Valenti in 1973 and Hobbins and Mahoney in 1974. Others since have documented the efficacy of the technique (Cao and colleagues, 1982; Rodeck and co-workers, 1978, 1980, 1984), but have noted commonly that fetal blood samples are diluted with amnionic fluid. Rodeck and Campbell (1979) and MacKenzie and Maclean (1980) subsequently sampled fetal blood directly by aspirating fetal blood from the umbilical vein at its placental insertion. Use of the fetoscope requires advanced technical expertise and is associated with a fetal loss of approximately 5 percent.

PERCUTANEOUS UMBILICAL BLOOD SAMPLING (CORDOCENTESIS)

In 1982, Bang and associates reported umbilical vein blood sampling and direct transfusion of a severely anemic D-isoimmunized fetus. They also obtained umbilical blood at 23 weeks from another fetus with a known chromosomal anomaly. Subsequently, the Paris group further developed the technique and expanded indications for its use (Daffos and associates, 1983a and b; Forestier and colleagues, 1988).

Technique for Umbilical Cord Blood Sampling
Daffos and colleagues (1983a) use a 20-gauge spinal needle, 10 to 13 cm in length, filled with a 3.8 percent sodium citrate solution with an attached 2 mL disposable syringe containing 0.1 mL of the same anticoagulant. The anterior abdominal wall is prepared and a local anesthetic is injected into the skin and anterior abdominal wall. With a real-time transducer held stationery, the needle is inserted through the abdominal and uterine walls, and the progress of the needle tip is followed into the umbilical vein.

Hobbins and associates (1985) use a 25-gauge spinal needle with a stylet. They stress the importance of identifying the site of insertion of the umbilical cord into the placenta. Rotating the ultrasound transducer 90 degrees to the long axis of the umbilical cord allows a cross-sectional view approximately 1 to 2 cm from its placental insertion. The operator then may follow the needle tip directly into the umbilical vein.

Daffos and associates (1985) described three approaches to the umbilical cord (Fig. 15–4): (A) with the placenta anterior, the needle is introduced transplacentally, without entering the amnionic cavity, to puncture the umbilical cord at its base; (B) with a posterior placenta, the needle passes through the placenta to penetrate the umbilical cord 1 to 2 cm from its insertion; (C) when the placenta is fundal and lateral, the needle passes transplacentally through the amnionic fluid before puncturing the umbilical cord 1 to 2 cm from its insertion.

After blood is obtained, a second syringe without anticoagulant is attached to the needle and blood is aspirated and transferred to appropriate tubes. Surprisingly, after needle withdrawal, the duration of bleeding from the umbilical cord usually is very short and can be monitored ultrasonically. Daffos and co-workers (1985) recommend continuous fetal heart rate monitoring for a few minutes after the procedure and a repeat ultrasound examination one hour later to ensure that there was no further bleeding or hematoma formation. In cases of oligohydramnios, the cord can be punctured at any site since it is less likely to move away as the needle is introduced. Confirmation that fetal blood has been obtained is made using a Coulter Channelyzer to detect the larger fetal red blood cells.

Using a 20-gauge needle, Daffos and associates (1985) reported a 1.1 percent fetal death rate and a 0.8 percent abortion rate with the first 606 umbilical cord samplings. They were successful on the first attempt in 588 cases (97 percent), and a second attempt was successful in the remaining 18 cases.

Normal Fetal Blood Values
One of the many advantages of this technique is the ability to establish normal fetal blood values throughout gestation. Shown in Figure 15–5 are normal fetal hemoglobin values from 16 through 26 weeks gestation. These range from about 11 g per dL at 16 weeks gestation to 15 g per dL at 35 weeks.

Soothill and colleagues (1986b) reported that fetal blood gas and acid-base values change with gestational age. Thus it is necessary to know gestational age as well as local (altitude and laboratory) ranges. It is likely that other fetal blood values will vary with gestational age. For example, despite a fall in oxygen tension with advancing age, fetal oxygen content remains constant because of increasing hemoglobin concentration. Furthermore, fetal values may be altered if the mother has been sedated (Soothill, 1986b). Finally, fetal blood carbon dioxide tension and plasma lactate concentrations increase with gestational age, but at present, normal preterm values have not been established (Soothill and associates, 1987a and b).

Indications for Fetal Blood Sampling
The earliest attempts at umbilical blood sampling arose from a need to evaluate the hemoglobin concentration of the D-isoimmunized fetus and to have intravenous access for fetal transfusion (Bang, 1982). Today, one accepted management of fetal hemolytic disease includes umbilical blood sampling and direct intraumbilical vein transfusion, either with or without additional red blood cells injected into the fetal peritoneal cavity (see Chap. 33, p. 606).

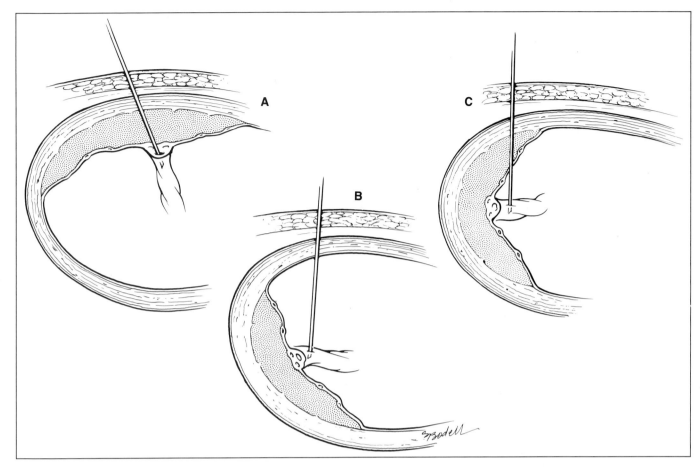

Figure 15–4. Umbilical cord blood sampling. Access to the umbilical artery or vein varies, depending upon both the placental location and the position of cord insertion into the placenta. **A.** With an anterior placenta, the needle may traverse the placenta. **B.** With a posterior implantation, the needle usually passes through the amnionic fluid before penetrating an umbilical vessel. **C.** With a lateral or fundal placenta, the needle may pass through the placenta and amnionic cavity to enter the umbilical vessel. (Redrawn after Queenan and King: Contemp Ob/Gyn 30:51, 1987.)

Percutaneous umbilical blood sampling has revolutionized the fields of human fetal physiology, diagnosis, and therapy. The indications for fetal blood sampling are increasing rapidly, and any list will be outdated by the time of its publication. While genetic indications are expanding most rapidly, the diagnosis and treatment of fetal hypoxia and isoimmunization also are being done. These and other current indications are presented in Table 15–1.

SONOGRAPHY

The impact of the use of ultrasonography on the practice of obstetrics has been profound! Given but one choice from the many biochemical and biophysical techniques that have been developed in more recent years to try to improve pregnancy outcome, sonography would seem the best. Methods for evaluating the health of the fetus that apply pulse–echo ultrasound are now widely employed for the very good reasons summarized below and illustrated frequently throughout this text. Sonographic techniques that are now available, when carefully performed and accurately interpreted, can supply vital information about the status of the fetus, with no known risks from ultrasound.

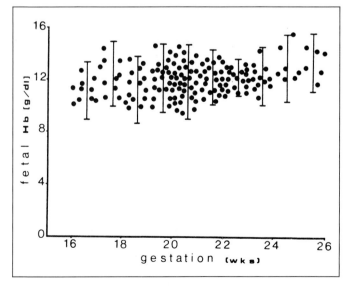

Figure 15–5. Reference range (mean + 2SD) and distribution of individual values for fetal hemoglobin concentration from 153 pregnancies not complicated by fetal hemolysis. (*From Nicolaides and colleagues: Am J Obstet Gynecol 155:90, 1986b, with permission.*)

TABLE 15–1. SOME INDICATIONS FOR FETAL BLOOD SAMPLING

Indication	Reference
Diagnosis and management of isoimmunization	
Rh disease (C and D factors)	Berkowitz, 1986a and 1986b; de Crespigny, 1985; Frigoletto, 1986; Grannum, 1986;Ludomirski, 1987; Nicolaides, 1986b; Seeds and Bowes, 1986
Kell sensitization	Berkowitz, 1986a; Copel, 1986; Hobbins, 1985
Diagnosis of fetal infection	
Toxoplasmosis	Daffos, 1988a; Desmonts, 1985; Forestier, 1984b
Other viral infections	Daffos, 1985
Diagnosis of fetal blood factor abnormalities	
Hemophilia A	Daffos 1985; Hobbins, 1985
Hemophilia B	Daffos, 1985
Factor V deficiency	Daffos, 1985
Thrombocytopenia	Daffos, 1985; Hobbins, 1985
Treatment of fetal blood abnormalities	
Thrombocytopenia	Daffos, 1984c; Daffos, 1988b
Rapid karyotyping for fetal chromosomal number	Daffos, 1984a, 1985; Nicolaides, 1986a; Ludomirski, 1987
Diagnosis of fetal genetic diseases	Daffos, 1985; Daffos, 1984a
Adrenoleukodystrophy	
β-thalassemia	
Duchenne muscular dystrophy	
Familial hypercholesterolemia	
Immunodeficiency	
Pyropoikolocytosis	
Sickle cell disease	
Triose phosphate isomerase deficiency	
Diagnosis of fetal hypoxia (distress)	
Fetal growth retardation	Soothill, 1986a; Pearce and Chamberlain, 1987
Assessment of fetal well-being	Soothill, 1986a; Nicolaides, 1986c; Nicolaides, 1987b
Treatment of fetal hypoxia	Nicolaides 1987a
Monitor fetal drug therapy	Forestier, 1984a
Assess fetal organ function	
Kidney	Suggested by Ludomirski, 1987

Intermittent high-frequency sound waves are generated by applying an alternating current to a transducer made of a piezoelectric material. The transducer is "connected" to the abdominal wall by placing a coupling agent—usually water-soluable gel—on the skin to diminish the loss of ultrasound waves at the interface between the transducer and the skin. In static systems the transducer so applied emits a pulse of sound waves that passes through soft tissue until an interface between the structures of different tissue densities is reached. When this occurs, some of the energy, proportional to the difference in densities at the interface, is reflected, or echoed, back to the transducer. This, in turn, stimulates the transducer while in the listening state to generate a small electrical voltage that is then amplified and displayed on a screen.

With real-time ultrasonography, the transducers employed generate multiple pulse–echo systems that are activated in sequence and thereby detect movement, including breathing, cardiac actions, and vessel pulsations.

CLINICAL APPLICATION

Sonography has proved valuable for monitoring the products of conception in a variety of ways that include the following:

1. Very early identification of intrauterine pregnancy.

2. Demonstration of the size and the rate of growth of the amnionic sac and the embryo, and, at times, resorption or expulsion of the embryo.

3. Identification of multiple fetuses, including conjoined twins.

4. Measurements of the fetal head, abdominal circumference, femur, and other anatomical landmarks to help identify the duration of gestation for the normal fetus or, when measured sequentially, to help identify the growth-retarded fetus.

5. Comparison of fetal head and chest or abdominal circumference to identify hydrocephaly, microcephaly, or anencephaly.

6. Detection of fetal anomalies such as abnormal distention of the fetal bladder, ascites, polycystic kidneys, renal agenesis, ovarian cysts, intestinal obstruction, diphragmatic hernia, meningomyelocele, intracranial, cardiac, or limb defects.

7. Demonstration of hydramnios or oligohydramnios by comparing the size of the fetus to the amnionic space surrounding the fetus.

8. Identification of the location, size, and "maturity" of the placenta.

9. Demonstration of placental abnormalities such as hy-

datidiform mole, molar degeneration, and anomalies such as chorioangioma.

10. Identification of uterine tumors or anomalous development.
11. Detection of a foreign body such as an intrauterine device, blood clot, or retained placental fragment.

FETAL SURVEILLANCE USING REAL-TIME SONOGRAPHY

It is established that the fetus breathes throughout most of pregnancy (see Chap. 6, p. 116). The movements can be witnessed with real-time sonography. Using real-time sonography fetal heart beat has been demonstrated as early as 7 weeks gestation, trunk movement as early as 8 weeks, and limb movement as early as 9 weeks (Shawker and associates, 1980). Filling and intermittent emptying of the fetal urinary bladder are especially obvious with real-time sonography. Sonographic confirmation of fetal movement, fetal tone, fetal breathing, and the presence of normal amounts of amnionic fluid provides evidence of fetal well-being (see Biophysical Profile, page 293). Real-time sonography especially has allowed surgical amelioration in utero of some defects identified sonographically—for example, hydrocephaly.

The already widespread use of sonography in obstetrics and its potential for identification of fetal abnormalities and for providing reassurance of fetal well-being have stimulated several questions that are difficult to answer: Should sonography be used in all pregnancies and, if so, when should it be initiated, how often should it be repeated, and how vigorous an examination for possible fetal abnormalities should be carried out? Who should actually perform the examination? Who should directly supervise the examination? Who should interpret the results of the examination? What should be the responsibilities of the practicing obstetrician? In what circumstances should sonography be performed under the supervision of and interpreted by the certified obstetrical specialist who is highly trained in sonography? When should these tasks be the responsibility of a radiologist who has been certified in sonography?

Some of these questions have been addressed and partially answered. The American College of Obstetricians and Gynecologists (1988) recommended that ultrasound examinations be performed by "a trained professional," and the targeted examinations, which are done for suspected defective fetuses, should be performed by an operator with "expertise in more sophisticated scanning."

The issue of universal ultrasound screening is again only partially answered. Thacker (1985), for example, reviewed four published prospective and randomized studies on the effectiveness of universal ultrasound screening in early pregnancy and concluded that the published results failed to support the usefulness of such a screening procedure for all pregnant women. However, Waldenström and colleagues (1988), using a single scan at approximately 15 weeks gestation, found that the incidence of labor inductions for all reasons was 5.9 percent in the screened versus 9.1 percent in the control patients.

In the United States, sonography is not used routinely. The National Institutes of Health Consensus Conference on ultrasound imaging in pregnancy concluded that ultrasonic studies during pregnancy appeared to be safe, but that they should be performed only when specifically indicated (Shearer, 1984).

DOPPLER ULTRASOUND

Doppler ultrasound detects the movement of red blood cells in vessels, and this principle is used to assess directly or indirectly a variety of altered measurements of blood flow within maternal and fetal vessels. For example, using the Doppler effect, the velocity of blood in a vessel can be measured. Copel and associates (1988) recently reviewed this subject, and portions are included in this brief review.

DOPPLER EFFECT

The Doppler effect is based upon the concept that pitch or sound frequency changes as an object moves past a listener, or if the object is stationary as the listener moves. An example of this concept is the changing sound of a train whistle moving past a stationary listener. With sensitive equipment, the frequency of the sound changes can be measured, and sound at a fixed frequency can be directed toward a moving object, such as moving red blood cells. This is the outgoing (or original) sound frequency (f_o). When the sound is returned from the moving object to the source, the frequency is different or deviated from the original (fd). This alteration in sound frequency is referred to as the *Doppler shift* and is dependent upon a number of factors (Fig. 15–6).

In the equation shown in Figure 15–6, f_o is the original frequency of the ultrasound beam (in obstetrical imaging this is usually 3 to 5 MHz), v is the velocity of blood in the vessel studied, θ is the incident angle between the ultrasound beam and the vessel, and c is the speed of sound (in tissue = 1,540 m per sec). The cosine remains close to 1 as long as the angle of insonation is kept low; but at higher angles, especially more

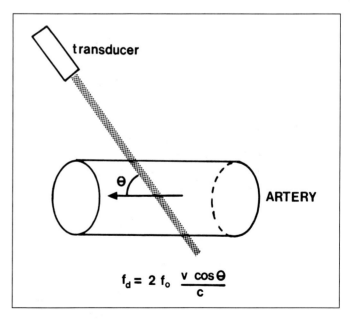

Figure 15–6. Dopper equation. Ultrasound emanating from transducer with initial frequency (f_o) strikes blood moving at velocity (v). Reflected frequency (fd) is dependent on the cosine of angle θ between beam of sound and vessel and the speed of sound through tissue (c). (*From Copel and associates: Williams Supplement No 16, Appleton & Lange, January/February 1988.*)

than 60 degrees, this factor has a significant impact on the calculation.

The Doppler principle has been used for some years in obstetrical practice. At physiological blood velocities and medical ultrasound frequencies, Doppler shifts from 100 to 10,000 Hz are audible to the human ear. This led to the development of external electronic fetal monitors and pocket Doppler stethoscopes used to auscultate the fetal heart. The type of Doppler ultrasound used in these applications is *continuous wave* (CW), so named because two transducers are used—one to transmit and the other to receive the reflected signals—both operating continuously.

Continuous Doppler Wave

Continuous Doppler wave machines are used commonly to auscultate fetal heart sounds. Also, many of the currently available Doppler waveform spectrum analyzers use continuous-wave techniques for identification of characteristic fetal and maternal waveform shapes.

Pulsed Doppler Wave

Pulsed Doppler wave machines consist of a combination of conventional imaging ultrasound and Doppler. For example, imaging ultrasound machines usually operate with a *duty cycle* that has "time on" versus "time off" of about 1/1,000. That is, the machine transmits the signal 0.1 percent of the time, and for the remaining 99.9 percent of the time it receives returning echoes. Doppler can be integrated into such a system in either of two ways, and both involve *pulsed Doppler*, consisting of rapidly alternating the imaging and Doppler modes along with superimposition of a selected Doppler sample volume onto the two-dimensional image seen on the screen of the machine. The location of this sample volume is controlled by a *range-gate* that varies the timing of when the returning signals are sought. Listening for longer or shorter periods of time allows variation in the size of the sample volumes as well.

DETERMINATION OF VOLUME FLOW

Actual volume-flow measurements within a specific vessel can be made. They may be calculated using the formula:

$$\text{Volume flow} = \frac{\text{velocity} \times \text{cross-sectional area of the vessel}}{\text{fetal weight}}$$

$$= \text{mL per min per kg}$$

Velocity can be calculated from the formula in Figure 15–6 and expressed as:

$$\text{Velocity} = \frac{fd \times c}{2f_o \times \cos\theta}$$

(cross-sectional area of a vessel $= \pi \times \text{radius}^2$).

Unfortunately, multiple small errors can significantly alter the calculation of volume flow. These include the shape of the column of blood, measurement of the incident angle, determination of cross-sectional area, and the varying diameters of some vessels.

DETERMINATION OF INDEXED FLOW FROM WAVEFORM ANALYSIS

Doppler arterial waveforms in nonpregnant humans are characterized by high systolic velocity and little or no diastolic velocity. Exceptions are the carotid and cerebral vessels, which have continuous diastolic blood flow seen on waveform analysis. During pregnancy, maternal and fetal vessels perfusing the placenta assume waveforms indicative of continuous diastolic flow.

Doppler waveforms of vessels have been described in a variety of ways, but all are based upon the relationship between systole and diastole. The most common measurements are some variation of the systolic/diastolic ratio. Ratios have been used to reduce the same potential error factors in the numerator and denominator. These measurements are intended to relate peak flow at systole to that at end-diastole, and the ratio is calculated from the height of the systolic and diastolic peaks. The use of a ratio obviates most problems of measuring the angle of insonation (Schulman and associates, 1986). Thus, indirectly determined indices are not measurements of actual flow; however, they provide useful information about flow.

Systolic/Diastolic Ratio

The systolic/diastolic ratio is the simplest index to calculate and also is known as the *S/D ratio*, the *A/B ratio*, or the *Stuart index*. It is calculated by dividing the maximal systolic Doppler shift by the end-diastolic shift; and it is most often determined from measurements of the maternal uterine or the fetal umbilical artery, using either pulsed or continuous-wave Doppler (Fig. 15–7). In both vessels, the index gradually decreases as gestation progresses. Since larger fetal vessels have low or absent diastolic flow, the S/D ratio is not useful for assessing fetal aortic blood flow.

Pourcelot or Resistance Index

The Pourcelot index is calculated from the difference in systolic and diastolic shifts divided by the systolic value ($[S-D]/S$. It also may be expressed as $1-[D/S]$). The index is best used in studies of umbilical and uterine arteries, since low diastolic values limit or prevent its use in the fetal aorta or other vessels without significant continuous diastolic flows.

Pulsatility Index

The pulsatility index is the most difficult one to use, and a uniform method for calculating it has not been established. It usually is figured as ($[S-D]/\text{mean}$), which requires digitized waveform analysis for calculating the mean of the frequencies represented. Because of the mean value in the denominator, this index can be used for low- or no-diastolic flow vessels such as the fetal descending aorta.

TECHNIQUES FOR SPECIFIC VESSELS

Uterine and Arcurate Arteries

Placental circulation is characterized by high volume flow, with an extensive diastolic component. Uterine blood flow increases from 50 mL per min shortly after conception, to 500 to 750 mL per min by term. The Doppler waveform shape is unique, characterized by high diastolic velocities similar to those in systole and highly turbulent flow, with many different velocities apparent (Fig. 15–7). With this degree of diastolic flow, indices **de-**

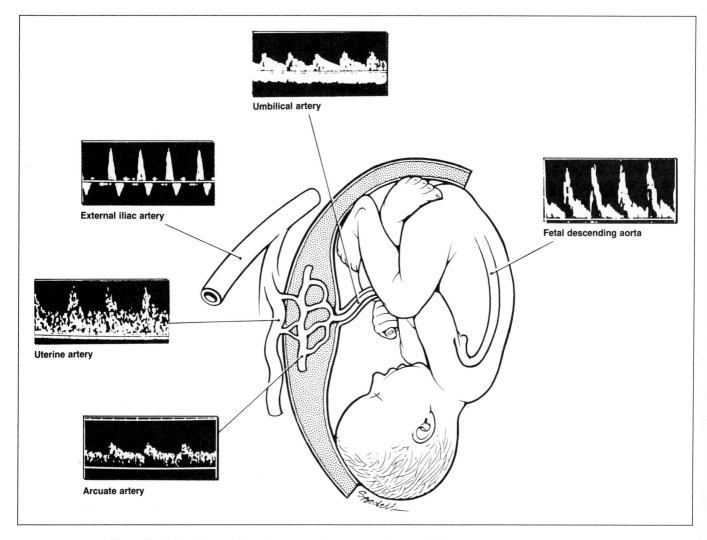

Figure 15–7. Doppler waveforms from normal pregnancy. Shown clockwise are normal waveforms from the maternal arcuate, uterine, and external iliac arteries, and from the fetal umbilical artery and descending aorta. Reversed end-diastolic flow velocity is apparent in the external iliac artery, whereas continuous diastolic flow characterizes the uterine and arcuate vessels. Finally, note the greatly diminished end-diastolic flow in the fetal descending aorta. (*Modified from Copel and associates: Williams Supplement No 16, Appleton & Lange, January/February 1988.*)

crease as term approaches—that is, diastolic velocity increases with advancing gestation. A failure of this pattern to appear or the presence of a notch in the waveform at end-systole has been reported with fetal growth retardation (Schulman and associates, 1986).

Either continuous-wave or pulsed Doppler systems can be used to evaluate the uterine artery using the indices described above. Regardless of the one used for either uterine or arcuate vessels, the most distal signals should be sampled. The internal iliac arteries are easily identified because they do not have diastolic flow (Fig. 15–7). For other vessels, any absence of late-diastolic flow, or reversal of flow, is considered abnormal. As mentioned, the various indices applied to umbilical artery analysis **decrease** during the latter phases of normal pregnancy (Al-Ghazali, 1988; Fitzgerald, 1984; Griffin, 1983; Schulman, 1984; Thompson, 1988; and their co-workers).

Umbilical Vein

The intraabdominal portion of the umbilical vein is relatively straight, and the flow tends to be constant rather than pulsating. Therefore, the umbilical vein is a reasonable vessel for measuring volume flow rather than indexed flow. An intensity-weighted mean Doppler shift must be used since flow is parabolic. Umbilical vein blood-flow measurements in several studies ranged from 110 to 125 mL per kg per minute (Table 15–2).

Fetal Descending Aorta

The fetal descending aorta receives the majority of right-ventricular output via the ductus arteriosus, while the majority of left-ventricular output supplies the fetal head and upper arms (Goodwin, 1976). Flow in the descending aorta is highly pulsatile, with little diastolic flow. The straight course of the aorta also makes it amenable to volume flow studies. Indexed flow mea-

TABLE 15–2. VOLUME FLOW MEASUREMENTS OF UMBILICAL VENOUS BLOOD FLOW

Investigator	No. of Studies	Flow (mL/kg/min)
Eik-Nes (1980)	20	110 ± 6 (SEM)
Eik-Nes (1982)	27	115 ± 7 (SEM)
Griffin (1983)	45	122 ± 42 (2 SD)
Van Lierde (1984)	20	117 ± 16 (1 SD)
Erskine (1985)	68[a]	125 ± 7.5 (SEM)

SEM = Standard error of the mean; SD = Standard deviation.
[a]Longitudinal study of 15 women.
Modified from Copel and associates: Williams Supplement No 16, Appleton & Lange, January/February 1988.

surement is limited to the pulsatility index because of the lack of diastolic flow. Measurements of fetal descending aorta blood flow range from 185 to 246 mL per kg per minute (Table 15–3).

Carotid Artery and Cerebral Blood Flow

Attempts have been made to measure fetal cerebral blood flow in order to explain why fetal head growth is spared in some forms of fetal growth retardation. If there is preferential blood flow to the brain, there should be maintenance, or even augmentation, of cerebral blood flow. Currently, the carotid arteries are the only cerebral vessels that can be identified reliably, but they are too narrow to measure accurately. Thus, preliminary findings are interpreted with caution since it is not always possible to be sure that comparable vessels are studied.

CLINICAL APPLICATIONS OF DOPPLER ULTRASOUND

Applications of this technology are discussed in relation to its use in the diagnosis and management of a variety of pregnancy complications and their management is presented throughout this book.

FETAL CARDIAC FUNCTION

The measurement of fetal cardiac function has immediate clinical importance as well as research implications.

TABLE 15–3 VOLUME FLOW MEASUREMENTS OF FETAL DESCENDING AORTA BLOOD FLOW

Investigator	No. of Studies	Flow (mL/kg/min)
Eik-Nes (1982)	33	185 ± 8 (SEM)
Marsál (1984)	64	238 ± 40 (SD)
Van Lierde (1984)	20	216 ± 24 (SD)
Griffin (1985)	75	246 ± 60 (SD)
Erskine (1985)	71[a]	206 ± 72 (SD)
Eldridge (1985)	77[b]	184 ± 35 (SD)
Lauren (1987)	21	238 ± 46 (SD)

SEM = Standard error of the mean; SD = Standard deviation.
[a]Longitudinal study of 15 women.
[b]Longitudinal study of 16 women.
Modified from Copel and associates: Williams Supplement No 16, Appleton & Lange, January/February 1988.

Cardiac Output

Doppler techniques that measure fetal cardiac output are extremely difficult to apply because of fetal movement and technical factors discussed above. However, with combined use of two-dimensional ultrasound and Doppler echocardiography, initial results appear promising. Reed and colleagues (1986a and b) reported that mean right-ventricular output was 307 mL per kg per minute and left-ventricular output was 232 mL per kg per minute (right to left ventricular output ratio 55:45). Kenny and co-workers (1986) measured combined ventricular outputs, and they calculated this to be approximately 450 mL per kg per minute at term. DeSmedt and associates (1987) reported a slightly higher value for combined ventricular output.

Ductus Arteriosus

Functional applications of fetal Doppler echocardiography have been reported by Huhta and colleagues (1987). They assessed ductus arteriosus constriction in both lamb and human fetuses. Reversible ductal constriction was observed in three fetuses whose mothers received indomethacin for treatment of preterm labor. Such changes were not observed in 25 normal pregnancies.

Fetal Arrhythmias

Using a variety of techniques, several groups have reported convincing evidence that fetal cardiac arrhythmias can be diagnosed and appropriately treated (Kleinman, 1985, 1986; Reed, 1987; Steinfeld, 1986; Strasburger, 1986; and their colleagues). In most instances these diagnostic techniques consist of two-dimensional real-time ultrasound examinations to identify cardiac anatomy and accurate placement of M-mode echocardiographic beams. M-mode echocardiography appears to be especially useful in diagnosing fetal cardiac arrhythmias and in assessing ventricular wall function. Functional outputs by atria and ventricles as well as timing of these events can be measured using pulsed-Doppler methods. Reed and associates (1987) presented evidence of improved (ventricular) cardiac output after conversion of supraventricular tachycardias to normal sinus rhythms. They also were able to confirm that the Frank-Starling mechanism (increased diastolic volume results in increased stroke volume) is operative even in the fetus!

Other Fetal Cardiac Applications

Silverman and associates (1985) used combined cardiac ultrasound examinations, cross-sectional M-mode echocardiography, and pulsed Doppler to diagnose arterioventricular valvar incompetence in fetuses with nonimmune hydrops. These workers also were able to diagnose some congenital structural cardiac anomalies that caused hydrops.

FETAL WELL-BEING

The use of Doppler measurements of blood flow is considered in the discussion of specific clinical conditions. These include fetal growth retardation (Chap. 38, p. 769), postterm pregnancy (Chap. 38, p. 762), and pregnancy-induced hypertension (Chap. 35, p. 671).

A recurring theme in the practical applications of Doppler ultrasound is the search to distinguish normal from abnormal pregnancies. Soothill and colleagues (1986a) correlated the severity of hypoxia in growth-retarded fetuses using mean descending aorta blood velocity. Hypoxic fetuses had lower aortic velocities. The relationships between mean aortic velocity and fetal pH, P_{CO_2}, and lactic acidemia were insufficient to permit good correlations based alone on Doppler-derived information. There was, however, a good relationship observed between mean aortic velocity and the degree of hypoxia. Following maternal oxygen therapy, there was a return of aortic velocities toward normal and an improvement in fetal blood gases (Nicolaides and associates, 1987a). Conversely, a randomized trial, in which the results of umbilical artery Doppler studies were either given or withheld from managing clinicians, failed to demonstrate any difference in Apgar scores, nursery stay, or duration of ventilatory support (Trudinger and colleagues, 1987). Newnham and associates (1989) reported similar results. What remains to be accomplished is to evaluate the efficacy of Doppler studies in the assessment of those specific fetal conditions in which blood-flow abnormalities might be expected to result in fetal compromise.

RADIOGRAPHY, AMNIOGRAPHY, AND FETOGRAPHY

A variety of diagnostic radiological techniques have been applied in attempts to evaluate the status of the fetus. It is of interest to note the reduction in the use of diagnostic x-ray that has taken place since the advent of sonography. Whitehouse and associates, for example, reported for their department in 1958 that more than half of the x-ray requests for obstetrical conditions were for determination of fetal age or for placental localization. With the advent of sonography, both determinations are now performed sonographically, with much greater precision and probably greater safety.

X-RAY

An x-ray of the abdomen and pelvis after 16 weeks gestation most often will identify fetal skeletal parts. Usually during the latter half of pregnancy the presenting fetal part is easily identified, the number of fetuses can be quantified, and gross skeletal abnormalities such as anencephaly and marked hydrocephaly are obvious. During the second half of pregnancy characteristic x-ray changes in the fetus are usually evident some time after death (see Chap. 2, p. 21).

Neither the age nor the size of the fetus can be identified with precision by use of simple radiography. Studies that have shown the best correlation between fetal age and the time of appearance of *lower limb ossification centers* typically have evaluated the limb radiologically after birth. Identification of ossification centers radiologically while in utero is often difficult if not impossible.

AMNIOGRAPHY

Radiopaque agents may be injected into the amnionic sac to identify certain characteristics of the amnionic fluid, fetus, and placenta. Amniography, using water-soluble, iodinated radiocontrast material, such as Urografin or Hypaque to opacify the amnionic fluid, may be employed to demonstrate abnormal amounts of amnionic fluid, the abnormally located placenta, the soft-tissue silhouette of the fetus, and, after a few hours of swallowing, the fetal gastrointestinal tract.

Hydatidiform moles very often produce a diagnostic honeycombed x-ray pattern when water-soluble, iodinated contrast material is injected into the uterine cavity. However, sonography provides a simpler and usually more accurate technique for identification of a hydatidiform mole (Fig. 31–17, p. 547).

FETOGRAPHY

Fetography involves the use of a heavily iodinated, lipid-soluble agent such as Ethiodol. When injected into the amnionic sac, the iodinated lipid adheres to the vernix on the skin of the almost-mature fetus and thereby may outline the fetus much more vividly than do water-soluble radiopaque agents.

Sonography carefully performed usually provides most of the information that may be afforded by amniography or fetography without using diagnostic x-rays, invading the amnionic sac, or injecting potentially harmful chemical agents.

MAGNETIC RESONANCE IMAGING

Equipment essential for organ and body imaging using magnetic resonance is available in many medical centers. This technology has been used for imaging of structural and anatomical fetal defects (Lowe, 1985; Powell, 1988; Smith, 1983; Symonds, 1984; and co-workers). **We have found it particularly useful for definition of maternal anatomy with suspected intraabdominal or retroperitoneal disease.** Finally, fetal *function* can be assessed since magnetic resonance detects some enzyme defects.

Use of magnetic resonance imaging during pregnancy appears to be safe, however the conclusion of the National Institutes of Health Consensus Development Conference (Marx, 1987) was that *"pregnant women, especially early in pregnancy, not undergo the procedure unless they have a clear medical need that cannot be resolved by other means."*

HORMONE AND ENZYME ASSAYS

Pregnancy-induced changes in a variety of hormones and enzymes have been extensively investigated with the hope of discovering practical tests to ascertain fetal age and fetal well-being.

Placental Lactogen and Estriol

Human placental lactogen (hPL) in maternal plasma and, especially, estriol in maternal plasma or urine have been claimed to provide important predictive information concerning fetal well-being or lack thereof. The use and abuse of measurements of these hormones are considered in Chapter 5, along with their production, distribution, metabolic functions, and clearance.

At present there appears to be no clinical use for these assays in the management of complicated pregnancies. They are mentioned only for historical purposes, since their usefulness as tests of fetal well-being has been superceded by more sensitive and specific tests using electronic fetal heart rate monitoring, sonography, or combinations of these two biophysical techniques.

Chorionic Gonadotropin

This hormone, normally produced by trophoblast and of clinical value for identifying early pregnancy, is considered in Chapters 2 and 5 (pp. 15, 67, respectively). Its measurement to identify persistent trophoblastic neoplasia is discussed in Chapter 31 (p. 549).

Other Hormonal Tests

Measurements of *progesterone levels* in maternal plasma have uncovered no constant pattern of change in pregnancies complicated by hypertension, diabetes, Rh isoimmunization, fetal growth retardation, or impending fetal death.

Measurement of the increase in *urinary estriol* excretion following intravenous injection of dehydroisoandrosterone has been evaluated as a test of placental function but has not been established to have clinical value.

The metabolic clearance rate of *dehydroisoandrosterone sulfate* for young women destined to develop pregnancy-induced hypertension is somewhat greater early in pregnancy and then significantly lower than in normal pregnant women (Gant and associates, 1971). Measurement of the metabolic clearance rate of dehydroisoandrosterone sulfate has not been demonstrated to have practical clinical utility.

Enzymes of Fetal Origin in Maternal Serum

The activities of a number of enzymes change appreciably in maternal serum during pregnancy. Measurements of heat-stable and total alkaline phosphatase, oxytocinase, and diamine oxidase have been urged by some to monitor fetal well-being, or to identify fetal maturity, or to do both. Such measurements, in general, have provided little information of value clinically.

FETAL MOVEMENT AND WELL-BEING

Normally, throughout the second half of pregnancy expectant mothers are cognizant of frequent movement by the fetus. Ehrström (1979) identified fetal movements in normal pregnancies to increase from a median value of 86 per 12 hours in the 24th week to a maximum of 132 in the 32nd week. Activity then decreased to a median 12-hour value of 107 movements during the 40th week. Conners and associates (1988) reported similar results and emphasized that there was considerable individual variation among normal pregnancies.

REDUCED FETAL MOVEMENTS

The fetus who late in pregnancy is felt by the mother to move consistently is most often healthy. Conversely, a sudden decrease in fetal movements is an ominous sign of loss of fetal well-being. The absolute number of movements per day appears to be less important in prognosis than is the degree of change in the frequency of fetal movements. In the case of cessation of fetal movements, fetal heart sounds have been

observed commonly to disappear within the next 24 hours. Sadovsky and Polishuk (1977) found loss of fetal movements to be more reliable than urinary estriol for predicting impending fetal death. Moreover, such assessment allows the mother to participate actively in the monitoring of fetal well-being.

ANTEPARTUM BIOPHYSICAL ASSESSMENT OF FETAL WELL-BEING

Two techniques have emerged in which changes in the fetal heart rate are used to evaluate fetal well-being. One is commonly referred to as the *contraction stress test* and the other as the *nonstress test*, or fetal heart acceleration test. A third antepartum test of fetal well-being that has gained widespread acceptance is the *biophysical profile*. The profile consists of a nonstress test plus three to five other assessments of fetal well-being, which include amnionic fluid volume, fetal respiratory motions, fetal tone, fetal movement, and placental grading. Four of the last five parameters can only be obtained with real-time ultrasound equipment as well as expertise on the part of the operator. These tests were reviewed by Leveno and Cunningham (1988).

CONTRACTION STRESS TEST

Hammacher (1966) appears to have been the first to suggest that the fetal heart rate response to uterine contractions be used antepartum as a test of fetal well-being. Subsequently, in this country, Ray and co-workers (1972), and many others since, have recommended the use of the contraction stress test, or oxytocin challenge test, for this purpose.

Technique

The contraction stress test usually takes 1 to 2 hours when performed as follows: With the mother lying on her back, but with her head and shoulders raised somewhat and turned toward her side, the fetal heart rate is recorded from an externally placed detector. Most often an ultrasound transducer (Fig. 15–8) is used because both phonocardiography and fetal electrocardiography when attempted through maternal tissue usually

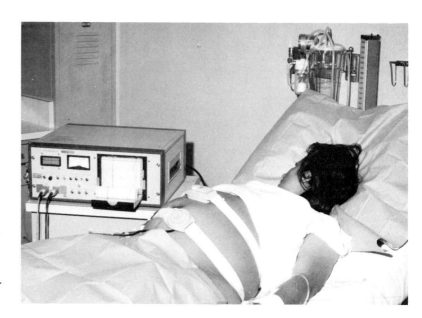

Figure 15–8. External tococardiography. The upper detector strapped to the abdomen senses uterine contractions from the change in the curvature of the abdomen. The lower one detects fetal heart rate action using the Doppler principle and ultrasound. During the monitoring, the mother should not be restricted to the supine position.

prove unsatisfactory. Uterine activity is identified with an external tocographic transducer. As the uterus contracts and moves forward, a sensor pin attached to a strain gauge is pushed in by the change in shape of the abdominal wall. The change in electric current so generated is amplified and recorded. Although actual intrauterine pressure is not recorded, the onset, the time of maximum intensity, and the cessation of the contraction can be identified with reasonable precision. In order to detect any reduction in placental perfusion as the consequence of aortocaval compression by the pregnant uterus while the mother is recumbent and thereby avoid a false positive test, the maternal blood pressure is recorded initially and at least every 10 minutes thereafter during the procedure.

Baseline uterine activity and fetal heart rate are recorded for 15 to 20 minutes. If, by chance, spontaneous uterine contractions that last 40 to 60 seconds and recur approximately three times in 10 minutes are detected, the response of the fetal heart rate to the contractions is evaluated as described below. In the absence of demonstrable spontaneous uterine activity usually oxytocin is administered intravenously. The initial rate of infusion of 0.5 mU per minute through a constant-speed infusion pump is doubled every 15 to 20 minutes until uterine contractions lasting 40 to 60 seconds with a frequency of three per 10 minutes are established.

Nipple Stimulation Test

To avoid the difficulties associated with the intravenous infusion of oxytocin, yet stimulate the uterus to contract somewhat, the breast stimulation, or more correctly, *the nipple stimulation test*, has been employed (Huddleston and associates, 1984; Lenke and Nemes, 1984). The basis for the test presumably was that tactile stimulation of the nipple would stimulate the release of exogenous oxytocin from the neurohypophysis, although Ross and co-workers (1984) were unable to detect a surge of oxytocin into the plasma of women whose uterus contracted in association with nipple stimulation.

Indications and Contraindications

The following conditions may contraindicate the use of oxytocin—and perhaps nipple stimulation—to perform a contraction stress test: (1) threatened preterm labor, (2) placenta previa, (3) hydramnios, (4) multiple fetuses, (5) rupture of the membranes, (6) previous preterm labor, and (7) previous classical cesarean section. Otherwise, the proponents of the contraction stress test recommend that it be implemented during the third trimester whenever the fetus is suspected of being in jeopardy. If the test is negative, it has usually been repeated weekly thereafter as long as it remained negative.

Interpretation

Freeman (1975) categorized the results of the contraction stress test as follows:

- *Positive:* There is consistent and persistent late deceleration of the fetal heart rate—that is, slowing of the heart rate develops sometime after the onset of the uterine contraction, the nadir for the heart rate is reached after the peak of uterine contraction, and recovery occurs after the contraction is completed (p. 292 and Fig. 15–9).
- *Negative:* At least three contractions in 10 minutes, each lasting at least 40 seconds, are identified without late deceleration of the fetal heart rate.

- *Suspicious:* There are inconsistent late decelerations that do not persist with subsequent contractions.
- *Hyperstimulation:* If uterine contractions are more frequent than every 2 minutes, or last longer than 90 seconds, or persistent uterine hypertonus is suspected, late deceleration does not necessarily indicate uteroplacental disease.
- *Unsatisfactory:* The frequency of contractions is less than three per 10 minutes or the tracing is poor.

False Negative Tests

It is now apparent that a negative contraction stress test *usually, but not always,* is compatible with uteroplacental function sufficient to maintain the fetus alive in utero for at least another week. For example, in one study Evertson and associates (1978) identified the fetal death rate from all causes to be 7 out of 680, or 1 percent, within the next 7 days after a negative contraction stress test. In another study, Gal and co-workers (1979) reported three antepartum fetal deaths among 584 pregnancies within 1 week of a negative oxytocin challenge test. We have documented fetal death within 48 hours of the completion of the third 8-hour infusion of oxytocin administered to try to effect labor. The 24 hours of infusion were electronically monitored continuously. Careful review of all tracings failed to provide any evidence compatible with a positive test (Chap. 38, Fig. 38–9).

False Positive Tests

The high false positive rate with the contraction stress test is troublesome. To avoid prematurely interrupting pregnancy when the test is positive, most advocates of the test recommend the application of other tests, including assessment of fetal heart rate accelerations in response to fetal movement (see Nonstress Test, following). Most often, the fetus is not in serious jeopardy if the fetal heart rate accelerates with fetal movement and the contraction stress test is usually repeated within 24 hours (Grundy and associates, 1984). Others recommend a biophysical profile (see below) or at least an ultrasonic evaluation of amnionic fluid volume before deciding that the contraction stress test is falsely positive. The presence of a positive contraction stress test along with a nonreactive fetal heart rate pattern is associated with serious fetal malformations often enough that real-time ultrasound screening for fetal anomalies is recommended by some (Freeman and co-workers, 1982a; Manning and associates, 1985).

NONSTRESS TEST

Fetal movement typically is accompanied by transient acceleration of the fetal heart rate. This phenomenon, observed and reported by Hammacher and associates (1968), Kubli and co-workers (1969), and by many others, serves as the basis for the "nonstress test" or fetal heart acceleration test.

Technique

An ultrasonic transducer to detect fetal heart beat is placed as described for the oxytocin test. Each time fetal movement is felt by the mother she presses a button to record the instant of movement on the same moving paper strip that the heart rate is recorded.

Interpretation

The test is generally considered normal when two or more fetal movements are accompanied by acceleration of the fetal heart rate of 15 beats per minute for at least 15 seconds duration

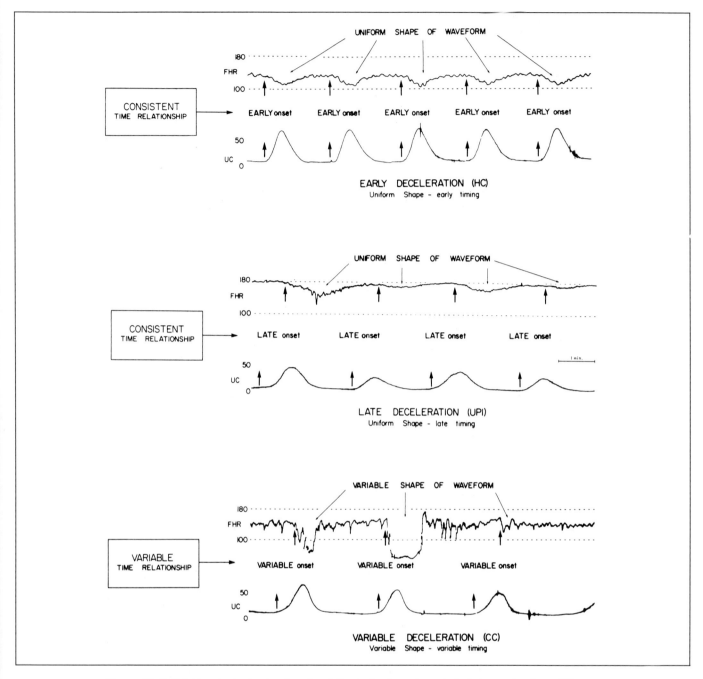

Figure 15–9. Fetal heart rate decelerations in relation to the time of onset of uterine contractions. HC = head compression; UPI = uteroplacental insufficiency; CC = cord compression. (*From Hon: An Atlas of Fetal Heart Rate Patterns. New Haven, CT, Harty, 1968.*)

within a 20-minute period (Fig. 15–10). A nonreactive tracing is one without acceptable fetal heart rate accelerations over a 40-minute period. These are the most widely accepted criteria for a normal test, but at least 15 and possibly more variations of this definition have been reported. Absent fetal motion is considered unsatisfactory for testing, but if prolonged, it is ominous if not occurring during a period of fetal sleep. Smith and associates (1986) described the *fetal acoustic stimulation test,* in which they used an artificial larynx placed against the maternal abdomen to "awaken the fetus" and reduced the number of falsely nonreactive tests.

A heart rate tracing with a spontaneous variable deceleration of at least 15 beats per minute for 15 seconds or longer, usually associated with oligohydramnios, is suggestive of umbilical cord jeopardy and should be followed by an assessment of amnionic fluid volume or delivery (Phelan and associates, 1981). A prolonged (greater than 1 minute) and severe (below 90 beats per minute or 40 beats below baseline) deceleration regardless of type, was reported by Druzin and co-workers (1981) to be associated with a high incidence of intrapartum fetal distress. They recommended delivery when such a deceleration was detected. This pattern of deceleration apparently

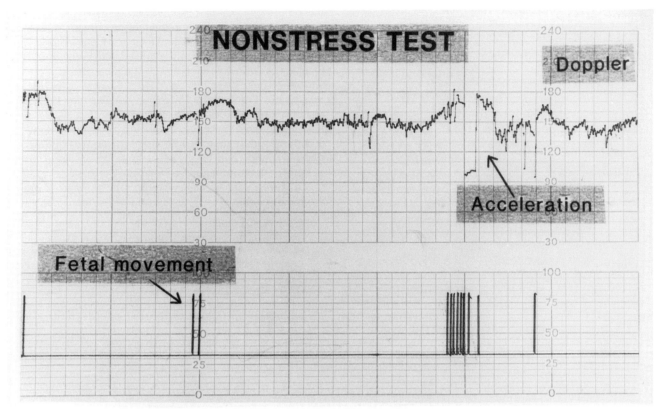

Figure 15–10. Reactive nonstress test. Notice increase of fetal heart rate to more than 15 beats per minute for longer than 15 seconds following fetal movements, indicated by the vertical marks on the lower part of the recording. (*Photo courtesy of Dr. K. Leveno.*)

may be seen with either a contraction stress test or with a nonstress test.

The fetus who does not accelerate his or her heart rate over a longer period is likely to be quite sick. Leveno and colleagues (1983) reported 27 pregnancies from the High Risk Unit at Parkland Hospital in which heart rate acceleration was absent or less than 10 beats per minute over 80-minutes. All were associated with features of uteroplacental insufficiency that included fetal growth retardation (74 percent), oligohydramnios (81 percent), fetal acidosis (41 percent), meconium-stained amnionic fluid (30 percent), and placental infarctions (93 percent). In this series, four fetuses were stillborn, and despite delivery by cesarean section before labor, seven of the other 16 neonates died.

Several investigators have reported that acceleration of the fetal heart rate during and immediately after fetal movement is as good a prognosticator of fetal well-being as a negative contraction stress test. Observations reported to date imply that acceleration of the fetal heart with fetal movement most often, *but certainly not always,* indicates that the fetus will survive in utero for at least one more week.

Biophysical Profile

Manning and associates (1980) were the first to report the use of a biophysical profile to assess fetal well-being. The test they originally described consists of a nonstress test with an additional four observations made with the use of real-time ultrasound. The five components of their biophysical profile are:

1. A reactive nonstress test.
2. Fetal breathing movements consisting of one or more episodes within 30 minutes and lasting 30 seconds or more.
3. Fetal movement consisting of three or more discrete body or limb movements within 30 minutes.
4. Fetal tone defined as one or more episodes of limb extension with return to flexion within 30 minutes.
5. Adequate amnionic fluid volume defined as one or more 1 cm or larger pockets of fluid two perpendicular planes.

For each of the five components, a normal observation is given a score of 2 and an abnormal observation is given a score of 0. As shown in Table 15–4, **in the absence of oligohydramnios,** a score of 8 or 10 is normal, a score of 6 is equivocal, and a score of 4 or less is abnormal (Manning and associates, 1985, 1987a). Baskett (1988) emphasized that falsely abnormal tests are more common in preterm fetus.

Oligohydramnios

The importance of oligohydramnios detected by the biophysical profile is evident. Although the identification of diminished amnionic fluid alone is not, at present, considered as a single test of fetal well-being, it may assume such a role in the future. In 1981, Manning and co-workers suggested that quantitative estimation of amnionic fluid volume could be used to identify fetal growth retardation, and Crowley and associates (1984) later recommend its use to identify postterm pregnancies. Because of its association with postterm pregnancy and fetal growth retardation, oligohydramnios is discussed in detail in Chapter 38.

TABLE 15–4. BIOPHYSICAL PROFILE SCORING: MANAGEMENT PROTOCOL

Score	Interpretation	Recommended Management
10	Normal nonasphyxiated fetus	No fetal indication for intervention; repeat test weekly except in diabetic and postterm pregnancy, in which it is done twice weekly
8/10 normal fluid	Normal nonasphyxiated fetus	No fetal indication for intervention; repeat testing as above
8/10 decreased fluid	Chronic fetal asphyxia suspected	Deliver
6	Possible fetal asphyxia	Deliver if amnionic fluid volume abnormal; if normal fluid at > 36 wk with favorable cervix—delivery; if < 36 wk or L/S ratio < 2 or cervix unfavorable then repeat test in 24 hr; if repeat test ≤ 6— deliver; if repeat test > 6 observe and repeat tests as above
4	Probably fetal asphyxia	Repeat testing same day; if score ≤ 6 then deliver
0–2	Almost certain fetal asphyxia	Deliver

From Manning and co-workers: Am J Obstet Gynecol 157:880, 1987a, with permission.

"Modified" Biophysical Profile

Manning and associates (1987b) have modified their original biophysical profile by selective use of the nonstress test. Specifically, they now assess the fetus ultrasonically, and if all four parameters are normal, they do not perform the nonstress test. A normal test score is then 8 of 8. They observed no instances of a nonreactive nonstress test when all four of the sonographically derived measurements were normal, but recommended nonstress testing if any were abnormal, and especially if amnionic fluid volume was decreased. They reported that if respirations were abnormal, 35 percent of nonstress tests were nonreactive, whereas if amnionic fluid was decreased, then 87 percent of tests were nonreactive.

The advantage cited by these workers for performing sonography first is that there are fewer false-positive tests. In fact, they reported that approximately 97 percent of the tests were normal. Additionally, more than 90 percent of these could be performed in 10 minutes or less. They also maintained that there was no loss of accuracy in testing by omitting the nonstress test under these conditions, since fetal movements, breathing, tone, and heart rate variability are central nervous system regulated and as such are acute biophysical variables. That is, if one is abnormal, others also are likely to be abnormal. By contrast, decreased amnionic fluid volume probably reflects a chronic condition associated with fetal stress and shunting of

blood flow away from the kidney, with decreased urine volume and in turn a decreased amnionic fluid volume.

Since 1985, the false-negative rate of about 1 per 1,000 for a structurally normal nonisoimmunized fetus has not been altered by the selective omission of the nonstress test (Manning and associates, 1985, 1987b). However, since five of the eight fetal deaths they reported occurred within 7 days of a normal test in which the nonstress test was not performed, the authors now recommend twice-weekly testing in women with diabetes and postterm pregnancy and "more frequent testing" for pregnancies complicated by growth retardation or proteinuric hypertension (Manning and co-workers, 1987a).

Manning and associates interpret the biophysical profile as outlined in Table 15–4. They add the following clarification:

> A biophysical profile scoring of 8 was achieved in two ways: Either four or five variables were normal, or more recently, if the first four variables monitored by dynamic ultrasound methods (movement, tone, breathing, and qualitative amnionic fluid volume) were normal. When the test score was normal, Manning and associates (1985) advocated conservative therapy. Exceptions to this are the postterm pregnancy with a fetus with a normal score but with a favorable cervix, growth-retarded fetuses with proven pulmonary maturity and a favorable cervix, insulin-dependent diabetic women at 37 weeks or greater and proven pulmonary maturity, the class A diabetic at term with a favorable cervix, women with a previous abdominal delivery of a recurrent etiology and proven fetal pulmonary maturity, and patients with unstable hypertension or other medical disorders that pose a serious threat to maternal health (Manning and associates, 1987a).

Divon and colleagues (1988) identified late decelerations in 56 fetuses during biophysical profile testing in 1,322 high-risk women. The profile score was 8 or above in 44 of the 56 patients, 6 in eight patients, and 4 or less in the remaining four patients. Cesarean sections were performed in all women whose fetuses had a score of 4 or less and in five of the eight women whose fetuses had scores of 6. Even in the patients with biophysical profile scores of 8, the cesarean section rate was 25 percent (11 of 44). The authors concluded that the identification of spontaneous late decelerations during biophysical profile testing was associated with significant fetal morbidity regardless of the score.

Other Biophysical Profile Tests

Other variations of the original biophysical profile have been reported. For example, Shime and co-workers (1984) omit fetal tone from their biophysical profile and Vintzileos and associates (1983) add a sixth factor for placental grading. Both groups use a grading score for each variable of 2, 1, or 0, and Shime adds a complex scoring system to the nonstress test. The advantages of these scoring systems over the original biophysical profile reported by Manning and associates remain to be confirmed. Eden and colleagues (1988) begin with the nonstress test, and if reactive, they assess only amnionic fluid volume that they consider normal if a 2 cm pocket is identified.

OTHER ANTEPARTUM FETAL HEART RATE TESTS

Read and Miller (1977) reported that sound of 105 to 120 decibels intensity delivered for 5 seconds through a microphone closely applied to the lower abdomen of the mother evoked acceleration of the fetal heart rate in instances where the oxytocin challenge test was negative. However, no response to the sound was frequently associated with a suspicious or positive oxytocin challenge test. Serafini and associates (1984) and Smith and co-workers (1986) reported similar results from acoustic stimulation studies. Smith and colleagues (1988) have concluded that a reactive test evoked by acoustic stimulation is as reliable as a reactive nonstress test. Harrigan and Marino (1978) claimed that acceleration of the fetal heart rate in response to insertion of the needle during transabdominal amniocentesis is a favorable sign of fetal well-being, with the reverse usually being true for decelerations that accompany amniocentesis.

VALUE OF ANTEPARTUM TESTS USING FETAL HEART RATE AND OTHER BIOPHYSICAL PARAMETERS

These tests are now widely applied at least in the United States. However, arguments persist as to the relative merits of the contraction stress test, the nonstress test, and the biophysical profile to identify the fetus whose well-being might be deteriorating in utero. The nonstress test appears to be favored by many because it is easier to perform; however, there is no unanimity of opinion as to which is the best test to evaluate fetal well-being. Each test evaluates different endpoints.

The contraction stress test apparently is a more sensitive, or certainly an earlier, indicator of fetal jeopardy. For example, Murata and co-workers (1982) reported that in hypoxic monkeys late decelerations preceded the loss of fetal heart rate reactivity. Clinically this appears to be true, since Freeman and associates (1982b), in a large prospective but nonrandomized trial comparing the contraction stress and nonstress tests, reported that there were eightfold fewer stillbirths when the contraction stress test was the primary fetal surveillance method. Finally, once a nonreactive nonstress test is present, serious fetal compromise already may have occurred (Leveno and associates, 1983). There are no randomized trials in which the efficacy of one method versus the other has been compared (Thacker and Berkelman, 1986).

False-Positive Tests

Thacker and Berkelman (1986), in an extensive and scholarly review, emphasized that the false-positive rates for all three tests were excessively high for fetal mortality and morbidity, with generally poor sensitivities and specificities for the stress tests. Only four randomized controlled trials have been used to evaluate the nonstress test, but insufficient numbers of patients have been studied. No randomized controlled trials as yet have been reported for the contraction stress test or the biophysical profile.

False-Negative Tests

The likelihood of a fetus dying within 1 week of a normal or reassuring test has been low, and generally it is less than 1 per 1,000. Manning and associates (1987a) reported the false-negative rate of 0.7 per 1,000 for the biophysical profile, and Freeman and co-workers (1982a) reported a fetal death rate of zero for the contraction stress test and 1.4 per 1,000 for the nonstress test. Unfortunately, such universally good results are not always obtained (Thacker and Berkelman, 1986).

Frequency of Testing

No firm guidelines can be made with respect to a fixed testing interval. Certainly in the face of clinical deterioration of the mother, more frequent testing than every 7 days seems reasonable. Additionally, testing more frequently than every 7 days now is recommended by some for women with suspected post-

term pregnancies, connective tissue diseases, chronic hypertension, suspected fetal growth retardation, and in women who previously have sustained a fetal loss due to a recurring medical or obstetrical complication.

It is not always fully appreciated that considerable obstetrical art in other forms has been applied by the proponents of these tests to achieve the excellent fetal outcomes that they most often have reported to try to validate the importance of the test in pregnancy management. Therefore, it is not surprising that a few groups have reported that failure to use one or the other test imposed no detectable penalty upon the fetus or neonate even though the pregnancy was high risk (Brown and co-workers, 1982; Lumley and associates, 1983). Interestingly, in one institution subsequent to a controlled study in which no benefits from antenatal fetal heart monitoring were identified, there was a 16-fold increase in antenatal monitoring (Lumley and associates, 1983). Importantly, earlier recommendations that included performance of fetal heart rate testing at weekly intervals in pregnancies considered to be high risk may no longer be valid, as mentioned above.

In summary, the following statements seem appropriate: (1) A week can prove to be a dangerously long time in the life of a fetus! (2) Anything that focuses attention on the fetus is likely to improve care. (3) No test of fetal well-being, including cardiotocographic and biophysical profile tests, provides complete reassurance no matter how meticulously performed and interpreted. (4) Finally, the false positive rates of all these tests are excessively high and the specificity and sensitivity extremely variable among medical centers.

ANTEPARTUM BIOPHYSICAL ASSESSMENT OF FETAL WELL-BEING AT PARKLAND HOSPITAL

There is no specific biophysical test or testing interval applied in a routine manner in the antepartum clinics at Parkland Hospital. Initial fetal assessments are clinical. If the pregnant woman or her fetus are judged to be at risk, the patient is referred to a complications clinic or directly to the labor suite. In either case, the woman is evaluated by an experienced team of obstetricians and a plan of management is outlined, which usually consists either of delivery or admission to an antepartum unit in the hospital.

If the pregnant woman with a fetus judged to be at risk is at or near term, oxytocin induction of labor most often is initiated. Prior to induction, an ultrasonic examination of the fetus frequently is performed.

When the woman is admitted to another hospital unit, she may be assigned to a routine antepartum unit or the High Risk Pregnancy Unit. If admitted to the High Risk Unit, fetal movement counts are begun and an ultrasonic evaluation of the fetus usually is done. Subsequent management is based upon repeated clinical assessments of both the fetus and the mother as well as a selective and specific use of antepartum fetal heart rate monitoring.

Antepartum fetal heart rate testing at Parkland Hospital is based upon the following rationale: (1) the presence of fetal heart rate accelerations following fetal movement do *not* reliably predict fetal health and (2) the *absence of fetal heart accelerations* for 80 to 90 minutes or the presence of significant decelerations is associated with a high incidence of fetal jeopardy, especially if this pattern has evolved from a previously normal picture (Leveno and associates, 1983). Therefore, antepartum electronic fetal heart rate monitoring at Parkland Hospital is *not* done to predict continuing fetal health; conversely, it is done to identify when there is possible fetal jeopardy. **This distinction is extremely important. Specifically, it is our contention that fetal heart rate accelerations do not predict fetal well-being for a definable time period, and this renders outpatient monitoring impractical since the fetus may deteriorate rapidly in women not evaluated clinically on a daily basis.**

On the High Risk Pregnancy Unit at Parkland Hospital, fetal heart rate monitoring is done every 7 days in selected high-risk women. Daily fetal heart rate monitoring is done for pregnancies with (1) oligohydramnios, (2) prematurely ruptured membranes, and (3) maternally perceived decreased fetal activity (Leveno and Cunningham, 1988).

The method consists of placing the women in a semi-Fowler position and recording blood pressure at the beginning of the session. A 20-minute fetal heart rate recording is performed with the woman noting spontaneous fetal movements by pressing an event marker. The interpretation of the fetal heart rate recording is as outlined.

1. A heart rate acceleration of more than 10 beats per minute is considered normal. Neither the number of accelerations nor their duration is considered.
2. The heart rate tracing must be of good technical quality. Tracings with Doppler "drop out" *or* electronic "jitter" are unacceptable.
3. If the recording quality is either technically unsatisfactory in the first 20 minutes *or* accelerations are not seen, the recording is continued after 20 minutes, for a total of 40 minutes.
4. If, after 40 minutes, the tracing is still technically unsatisfactory, the test should be repeated later the same day.
5. If, after the first 40 minutes, accelerations are not seen in a good-quality record, a *physician* should personally repeat the tracing by sitting at the bedside and recording the fetal heart rate for an *additional* 40 minutes.
6. The lack of fetal heart rate accelerations for 80 to 90 minutes in a good-quality record is considered an ominous finding.
7. Significant decelerations of any type require clinical reevaluation.
8. A sinusoidal fetal heart rate pattern should be considered as indicative of fetal anemia often associated with hydrops owing to a number of various etiologies.
9. A transient late deceleration may be the result of supine hypotension; therefore, the blood pressure should be checked and the position changed if there is hypotension.

Delivery should be considered if there are significant spontaneous decelerations or if there are no fetal heart rate accelerations observed for 90 minutes. This antepartum fetal heart rate assessment does not replace obstetrical judgment. Accelerations of the fetal heart do not predict fetal well-being for 7 days and indicate only that the fetal heart is capable of accelerating at the time of the recording. The presence of fetal heart rate accelerations does not preclude the possibility that the fetus is in a precarious intrauterine environment. **Therefore, the assessment of antepartum fetal heart rate is used to identify fetuses in jeopardy and not to predict continuing fetal health.**

The above technique for assessing fetal well-being has been used at Parkland Hospital for more than a decade in more than 1,000 selected high-risk pregnancies. In 115 insulin-dependent diabetic women in which the protocol outlined above was used as part of the management, Leveno and Whalley (1982) observed that an abnormal test result occurred in only one patient. Unfortunately, two fetal deaths occurred 1 and 4 days after normal fetal heart rate accelerations were observed, again emphasizing that the procedure is used when possible to identify fetal jeopardy and not to predict continuing fetal health.

INTRAPARTUM SURVEILLANCE OF THE FETUS

A goal to be constantly pursued during labor is the preservation of fetal well-being by early detection and relief of fetal distress. To monitor means simply to watch or check on a person or thing. In the minds of many people in obstetrics, however, the word "monitor" has come to mean specifically surveillance of the fetal heart and uterine activity by some sort of an electronic detecting and recording device. It is sometimes forgotten that clinical monitoring has produced meritorious results when conscientiously applied during labor and delivery by appropriately trained individuals (Haverkamp and colleagues, 1976, 1979; Leveno and colleagues, 1986).

ELECTRONIC MONITORING OF FETAL HEART RATE AND UTERINE CONTRACTIONS

With each uterine contraction, there is a temporary variable reduction in the flow of oxygenated maternal blood through the placental intracotyledonary spaces. Hon (1974) aptly pointed out that labor is a stress test for the fetus who may be handicapped by (1) intrinsic fetal disease, (2) placental disease, (3) cord compression, (4) maternal disease, (5) drugs administered for analgesia and anesthesia, or (6) maternal hypotension from the supine position, conduction analgesia, or both. To detect fetal distress during labor, he and others urged that continuous beat-to-beat recording of the fetal heart rate be made concomitant with the pressure changes generated by the uterine contractions. To this end, Hon and others perfected sophisticated electronic detection and recording equipment that is widely used for monitoring the fetal heart and uterine contractions (Fig. 15–8).

INTERNAL MONITORING OF FETAL HEART RATE

The fetal heart rate may be identified beat to beat by attaching a unipolar electrode directly to the fetus and another electrode to the mother and, after appropriate filtration and amplification, recording each contraction of the fetal heart on a time-calibrated moving-strip recorder.

The spiral electrode in common use, developed by Hon and associates (1972), is shown in Figure 15–11. Electrical contact with the fetus is established by twisting the driving tube, which propels the spiral electrode through the skin. To be able to attach the electrode to the fetus, the cervix must be dilated at least 1 cm, and, of course, the membranes above the cervix must be ruptured. It is important that the electrode be attached to the fetus at a relatively benign site, avoiding such critical areas as the fontanels and suture lines of the head, as well as the face and genitalia. Thus it is imperative that not only the presenting part be identified but that the site of attachment be known precisely.

The electrocardiographic signal picked up by the electrode inserted through the fetal skin is amplified sufficiently that typically the fetal R wave can be identified by a threshold detector

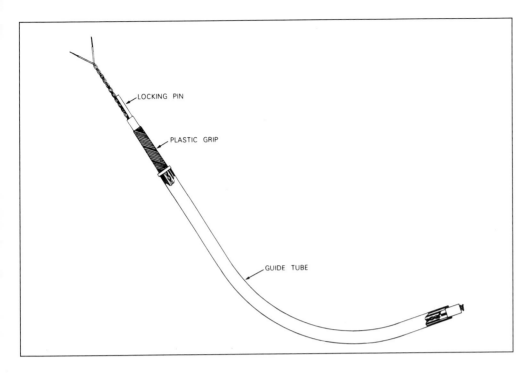

LOCKING PIN

PLASTIC GRIP

GUIDE TUBE

Figure 15–11. Spiral electrode with guide tube. (*From Hon co-workers: Obstet Gynecol 40:362, 1972.*)

that excludes all artifacts of lesser intensity. Good electrode placement that provides a high-amplitude fetal electrocardiographic signal yields the best "signal-to-noise" ratio. In practice, each detected R wave (and any electronic noise of equal intensity) is recorded on a calibrated moving paper strip.

INTRAUTERINE PRESSURE MEASUREMENTS

Measurements of intrauterine pressure—that is, the pressure of amnionic fluid, between and during contractions—are made by directly coupling the fluid to some sort of recording device. In clinical practice, a fluid-filled plastic catheter is positioned in

utero so that the distal tip is located in amnionic fluid above the presenting fetal part (Fig. 15–12A, B). First, a plastic catheter guide that contains the distal portion of the catheter is inserted just through the cervical internal os and the fluid-filled catheter is then gently pushed beyond the guide into the uterine cavity. To minimize risk to the placenta from the catheter tip, when the site of placental implantation is known, the tip of the catheter inserter should be positioned so that the catheter is likely to be inserted away from the placental site. The opposite end of the catheter, filled with saline, is connected to a strain-gauge pressure sensor adjusted to the same level as the catheter tip in the uterus. The amplified electrical signal produced in the strain-

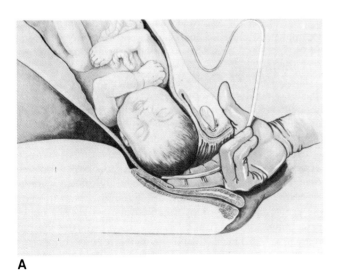

A

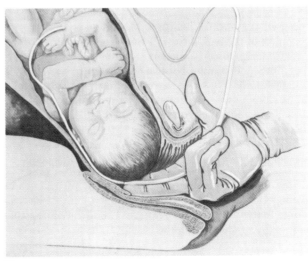

B

Figure 15–12. A. A sagittal view demonstrating placement of the catheter guide and catheter just within the cervix. **B.** A sagittal view showing the catheter inserted beyond the guide and within the amnionic sac. (*From Chan, Paul, Toews: Obstet Gynecol 41:7, 1973.*)

gauge by variations in pressure within the fluid system is recorded on a calibrated moving paper strip, usually simultaneously with the recording of the fetal heart rate. Free communication between amnionic fluid and fluid in the catheter is essential for meaningful pressure measurements. If the catheter tip becomes obstructed, it usually can be relieved by injecting a small volume of sterile saline from a syringe through the catheter. To avoid damage to the transducer, it must be isolated from the system during this maneuver.

EXTERNAL (INDIRECT) ELECTRONIC MONITORING

The necessity for rupture of the membranes and invasion of the uterus may be avoided by use of external detectors to discover fetal heart action and identify uterine activity (Fig. 15–8). External monitoring does not provide the precision of measurement of fetal heart rate afforded by internal monitoring or any quantification of uterine pressure.

The fetal heart rate may be detected in a number of ways through the maternal abdominal wall overlying the uterus. The easiest technique to use during the antepartum and early intrapartum periods employs the *ultrasound Doppler principle.* Ultrasonic waves undergo a shift in frequency as they are reflected from moving fetal heart valves and from fetal blood cells ejected in pulsatile fashion by cardiac systole. The unit for detecting fetal heart action consists of a transducer that emits ultrasound, typically with a frequency of 2 megahertz, and a sensor to detect a shift in frequency of the reflected sound. The detector is placed on the abdomen at a site where fetal heart action is best detected. A coupling gel must be applied to the maternal skin, since air conducts ultrasound poorly. The device is held in position by an abdominal belt (Fig. 15–8).

Phonocardiography using a sensitive microphone may be tried to detect the sound generated by fetal heart action. Unfortunately, in clinical practice, extraneous sounds often create technical difficulties that limit the utility of this technique. The fetal *electrocardiogram* may, at times, be detected through electrodes attached to the maternal abdomen. The signal strength is typically quite weak and therefore is difficult to separate from extraneous electrical interference, including the maternal electrocardiogram.

Remote Display from Electronic Monitors

Observation of the fetal heart rate and uterine contraction patterns of laboring women by means of centrally located electronic display units is becoming popular. Although this enables one individual to observe these recorded functions at a distance from the laboring women, other aspects of intrapartum surveillance that are equally important may be neglected as a consequence.

TERMINOLOGY TO DESCRIBE FETAL HEART RATE

Since the fetal heart rate is rarely fixed but, instead, shows frequent periodic variations, standardized terminology has been proposed to try to describe more precisely both baseline activity and periodic variations from the baseline (Freeman and Garite, 1981):

Baseline fetal heart rate refers to the modal rate that prevails apart from any periodic accelerations or decelerations associated with uterine contractions. A baseline rate between 120 and 160 beats per minute is considered *normal,* a rate of 100 to 120 *mild bradycardia,* and a rate of less than 100 *marked bradycardia.*

Tachycardia is considered *mild* if the baseline rate is between 161 and 180 beats per minute and *marked* if 180 or more.

Periodic fetal heart rate refers to deviations from baseline that are related to uterine contractions. *Acceleration* refers to an increase in fetal heart rate above baseline and *deceleration* to a decrease below the baseline rate. Three major patterns of deceleration are described: (1) *Uniform patterns of deceleration* reflect the shape of the simultaneously recorded uterine contractions. With the uniform pattern of *early deceleration,* the onset, nadir, and recovery of the fetal heart rate to baseline coincide with the onset, peak, and end of the uterine contraction. Early decelerations are usually attributed to compression of the fetal head, although the stimulus to early deceleration may be more ominous. With the other uniform pattern, that of *late deceleration,* the onset of slowing occurs as the contraction intensity peaks, the nadir in heart rate is reached well after the peak, and recovery is not achieved until after the uterine contraction has terminated (Fig. 15–9). Late decelerations are likely to be the consequence of uteroplacental insufficiency. (2) *Variable patterns of deceleration, or nonuniform decelerations,* are characterized by a decrease in heart rate beginning at no fixed time in relation to the uterine contractions and by waveforms that differ in shape from those of the uterine contractions and from each other, and may be nonrepetitive (Fig. 15–9). Variable decelerations are most often the consequence of cord compression. (3) *Combined (mixed) patterns of deceleration,* as the term implies, exhibit the characteristics of both of the patterns described above.

The *pattern of early deceleration* characterized by slowing of the heart rate at the onset of the contraction (Fig. 15–9), is likely to be the consequence of a transient increase in intracranial pressure from head compression, which stimulates the vagus nerve, thereby slowing the heart. Early decelerations may, however, have a more ominous origin. Mendez-Bauer and coworkers (1978), for example, demonstrated early deceleration to be, at times, the consequence of compression of the umbilical cord. Prompt sterile vaginal examination to identify the status of the cervix and the presenting part, and to rule out prolapsed cord, is indicated. Treatment includes ascertaining that the mother is reclining comfortably on her side and checking the monitor, especially if external, to ensure that it is functioning properly. Early decelerations from head compression may be eliminated by the administration of atropine to the mother; however, this is not recommended. Early decelerations that are severe and prolonged or persistent, and certainly if accompanied by gross meconium staining of the amnionic fluid, must not be ignored.

The *pattern of late deceleration* (Fig. 15–9) is likely to be the consequence of hypoxia and associated metabolic derangement and acidosis from uteroplacental insufficiency. A fetus acidotic from any other causes, examples of which include prolonged and repetitive cord occlusion or fetal sepsis from chorioamnionitis, also may show this pattern. After termination of the uterine contractions, the heart rate may return to or rise transiently above normal baseline in the less severely affected fetus, or remain low in the severely affected fetus. The fetus stressed to an intermediate degree may demonstrate tachycardia between contractions. Delivery can be safely delayed only if the uteroplacental insufficiency is promptly corrected, as, for example, the relief of uterine overactivity by immediately stopping oxytocin stimulation or by correcting maternal hypotension and thereby improving uteroplacental perfusion. Otherwise, most often prompt delivery is indicated.

The *pattern of variable deceleration (nonuniform deceleration)* is likely to be the consequence of compression of the umbilical cord. Vaginal examination should be undertaken promptly to search for cord prolapse and determine the degree of cervical dilatation and the station and position of the presenting part. The position of the mother should then be changed so that she is lying on her side or turned to the opposite side. If decelerations persist or worsen, either immediate measurement of fetal scalp blood pH (p. 282) or prompt delivery is indicated. Since this heart rate pattern signifies umbilical cord compression, it usually recurs. In such women, there is anticipation of an increased likelihood of abdominal delivery. Therefore, should serious umbilical cord compression recur and persist, there should be no delay in performing an emergency cesarean section.

It is becoming apparent that various deceleration patterns do not always reflect the causes ascribed to them. Although the classification presented has served as a guide to the interpretation of various patterns of fetal heart rate responses during labor, its rigid application, unfortunately, has led, at times, to erroneous diagnosis and treatment.

Beat-to-Beat Variability

Later in pregnancy there is normally a beat-to-beat variation in the fetal heart rate; that is, the time interval between the same locus, for example, the R wave, in consecutive electrical systoles is not fixed. The variation was attributed by Hon (1974) to the continuous interaction of sympathetic and parasympathetic nerve action on the heart. However, Dalton and associates (1983) demonstrated that in the sheep fetus, at least, sympathetic blockade has little effect on fetal heart rate variability and, although parasympathetic blockade reduces variability, it does not abolish it.

Absence of beat-to-beat variability in some circumstances late in pregnancy may be indicative of fetal compromise. In fact, Boehm (1977) maintained that fetal heart rate variability has become the most important aspect of the overall clinical evaluation of the fetus in utero. Gilstrap and associates (1987) subsequently reported that fetal acidosis, defined as a pH of less than 7.2, was unlikely as long as fetal heart rate beat-to-beat variability was present. It should be emphasized, however, that an otherwise normal preterm fetus or the fetus who is "asleep" may not demonstrate beat-to-beat variability. Moreover, medications in doses commonly used during labor and in preparation for delivery may ablate beat-to-beat variability. These include meperidine, morphine, alphaprodine, barbiturates, conduction analgesia, general anesthesia, diazepam, phenothiazines, atropine, scopolamine, and perhaps magnesium sulfate in large doses (Babaknia and Niebyl, 1978; Boehm, 1977; Cohen and Schifrin, 1977). Unfortunately, recordings made with externally applied detecting devices are unreliable for identifying the presence or absence of beat-to-beat variation.

Sinusoidal Fetal Heart Rate Pattern

A sinusoidal fetal heart rate pattern, especially when marked, can prove to be an ominous sign of fetal deterioration. For example, Katz and co-workers (1983) observed that with sinusoidal oscillations of more than 25 beats per minute, death of the fetus or newborn infant was very common (six out of nine died); but when the sinusoidal oscillations were less than 25 per minute, the outcome was very much better (82 out of 83 survived). A marked sinusoidal pattern of fetal heart rate has been identified frequently in fetuses who were severely anemic. Lowe and co-workers (1984) observed the development of sinusoidal fetal heart rate patterns in two fetuses following intraperitoneal

transfusions. In one, the pattern disappeared as the blood was absorbed from the peritoneal cavity. The second fetus did not absorb the intraperitoneal blood, and the persistent sinusoidal fetal heart rate led to cesarean section with an ultimately successful outcome.

Several drugs have been reported to produce a sinusoidal fetal heart rate pattern. Gray and associates (1978) observed the development of a sinusoidal fetal heart rate pattern in nearly one half of pregnancies in which the mothers received alphoprodine (Nisentil) for relief of labor discomfort. In this particular circumstance fetal outcome did not appear to be adversely affected by the presence of a sinusoidal heart rate pattern. Epstein and associates (1982) described a sinusoidal fetal heart rate pattern following maternal administration of meperidine, with reversal of the pattern when naloxone was administered. Butophanol (Stadol) also has been reported to induce sinusoidal heart rate patterns in the fetus (Angel and associates, 1984; Hatjis and Meis, 1986).

Persistent Fetal Tachycardia or Bradycardia

Tachycardia without deceleration may be the consequence of febrile illness, a response to hypoxia, or rarely a reaction to fetal thyrotoxicosis. Gilstrap and associates (1987) identified umbilical arterial blood acidemia (pH < 7.2) in 7 of 32 neonates (22 percent) with tachycardia during second-stage labor. They defined tachycardia as 160 beats per minute or greater. Pure metabolic acidemia or respiratory acidemia were noted in two neonates and the remaining five had mixed metabolic-respiratory acidemia. None of these acidemic neonates needed resuscitation.

Mild bradycardia without deceleration or acceleration is not necessarily evidence for fetal distress. Young and associates (1979) found no evidence of acidosis during labor and delivery in several fetuses who demonstrated persistent bradycardia in the range of 100 to 120 beats per minute, and the neonatal outcomes were good. Interestingly, an occiput posterior or transverse position was identified in each instance. They ascribed the mild bradycardia to a vagal response induced by persistent head compression in the occiput posterior position. Umbilical arterial blood acidemia (pH < 7.2) was identified by Gilstrap and co-workers (1987) in 16 of 53 neonates (30 percent), with mild bradycardia defined by 90 to 119 beats per minute and detected during second-stage labor. Two each of the acidemic neonates had pure metabolic or respiratory acidemia and the remaining 12 had mixed metabolic-respiratory acidemia. None of these acidemic neonates required resuscitation.

These workers also noted umbilical arterial blood acidemia in 25 of 63 neonates (40 percent), with moderate to severe bradycardia defined as less than 90 beats per minute. Eight neonates had metabolic acidemia and four had respiratory acidosis. The remaining 13 neonates had mixed metabolic-respiratory acidosis. Only one of the neonates with pure metabolic acidosis required resuscitation. More severe bradycardia may be the consequence of congenital heart lesions or severe hypoxia. An association has been identified between heart block in the fetus and newborn infant and maternal collagen vascular diseases, especially lupus erythematosus (Chap. 39, p. 838). Viral infections of the fetus also may cause congenital heart block (Lewis and co-workers, 1980). We also have observed that fetal bradycardia accompanies marked maternal hypothermia; the heart rate rose from 90 to 136 when the mother became euthermic. Fetal bradycardia also has been associated with sudden lowering of the blood pressure from excessive administration of antihypertensive drugs to severely hypertensive women.

An important cause of presumed fetal bradycardia is fetal death, with the *maternal* heart rate being recorded by the monitor but erroneously considered to be the fetal heart rate (Odendaal, 1976). An illustration of this phenomenon is seen in Figure 36–9 (p. 708). Maternal tachycardia, as occurs with sepsis or with concealed hemorrhage from abruptio placentae, may, at times, spuriously provide a recording of what appears to be a normal fetal heart rate even though the fetus is dead. **Especially before performing any heroic treatment on the basis of electronic monitoring data, it is always wise to listen carefully to the fetal heart with an appropriate stethoscope while simultaneously checking the maternal pulse rate. Another approach is to look for fetal heart motion with real-time ultrasound.**

Fetal Cardiac Arrhythmias

Intermittently recurring cardiac arrythmias of ectopic origin may cause concern. The experience of Sugarman and associates (1978), as well as the earlier reports of others, however, indicate that the arrhythmias are likely to be innocuous. The generally favorable neonatal outcome is not improved by pregnancy intervention or attempts at pharmacologic treatment in utero unless evidence of fetal heart failure (hydrops) is present.

Normal Fetal Heart Rate Pattern

The absence of an ominous fetal heart rate pattern is generally, but not absolutely, predictive of a good fetal outcome. Hayashi and Fox (1975) and others documented cardiac arrest and death of a fetus without detecting a preceding ominous fetal heart rate pattern.

FETAL SCALP BLOOD SAMPLING

Measurements of the pH of appropriately collected capillary blood may help to identify the fetus in serious distress. A suitably illuminated endoscope is inserted through the sufficiently dilated cervix and ruptured membranes so as to press firmly against fetal skin, usually the scalp (Fig. 15–13). The skin is wiped clean with a cotton swab; it may be sprayed with ethyl chloride to induce hyperemia, and coated with a silicone gel to cause the blood to accumulate as discrete globules. An incision

is made through the skin to a calibrated depth with a special blade on an appropriately long handle. As a drop of blood forms on the surface, it is immediately collected into a heparinized glass capillary tube and the pH of the blood is promptly measured. The pH of fetal capillary blood usually is lower than arterial blood and approaches that of venous blood.

Saling (1964) initially proposed a pH of 7.20 as the critical value for identification of serious fetal distress, while Mann (1978) and some others recommended immediate delivery whenever scalp blood pH was 7.25 or less. Zalar and Quilligan (1979) recommended the following protocol to try to confirm fetal distress through use of fetal scalp sampling: If the pH is greater than 7.25, labor is observed. If the pH is between 7.20 and 7.25, the pH measurement is repeated within 30 minutes. If the pH is less than 7.20, another scalp blood sample is immediately collected and the mother is taken to an operating room and prepared for surgery. Cesarean section is promptly performed if the low pH is confirmed. Otherwise, labor is allowed to continue and scalp blood samples are repeated periodically. The obstetrician must be careful not to allow the time for repetition of laboratory tests to lead to dangerous clinical procrastination.

Adhering too closely to a critical pH value may in actual practice prove disadvantageous, since it will tend to allay suspicion of early hypoxic acidosis. A fall in pH is a relatively late effect of hypoxia, and when samples of fetal blood are obtained intermittently, detection of hypoxia of rapid onset may be unduly delayed. It must also be kept in mind that the pH of fetal capillary blood need not accurately reflect the degree of hypoxia in the fetus, since the pH will be influenced appreciably by that of the mother. The severely hypoxic fetus becomes overtly acidotic, which is reflected by a low blood pH except when the mother is alkalotic—for example, from hyperventilation. Conversely, the fetus may have a low blood pH without being remarkably hypoxic if the mother is acidotic. Rooth and associates (1973) emphasized the impact of maternal pH on fetal scalp blood pH. They suggested that clinically important fetal acidosis be identified by demonstrating the value for the fetus to be at least 0.20 pH units less than that of the mother.

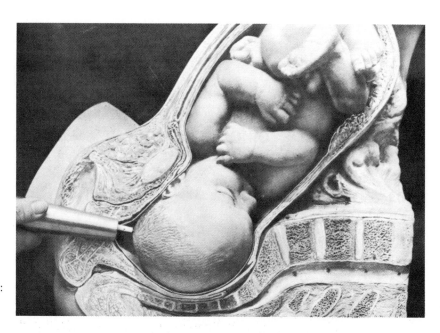

Figure 15–13. The technique of fetal scalp sampling utilizing an amnioscope. Note end of endoscope displaced from fetal vertex approximately 2 cm to show disposable blade against the fetal scalp before incision. (*From Hamilton and McKeown. In Wynn RM (ed): Obstetrics and Gynecology Annual: 1973. New York, Appleton, 1974.*)

Clark and Paul (1985) maintain that while fetal scalp sampling remains a valuable clinical tool in select cases, the technique should be deemphasized in general clinical practice. They believe that *"the properly trained clinician may pursue an approach for the detection of fetal distress that does not include scalp blood sampling without either compromising his ability to detect fetal distress or significantly increasing the cesarean section rate."* Fetal heart rate acceleration in response to vibroacoustic stimulation has been recommended as a substitute for scalp sampling by some (Edersheim and colleagues, 1987), but not by all (Richards and associates, 1988). Fetal scalp blood sampling was never used widely at Parkland Hospital and has not been available for several years.

COMPLICATIONS FROM INTERNAL ELECTRONIC AND PHYSIOCHEMICAL MONITORING

There are potential dangers inherent in monitoring the fetal heart rate by direct application of an electrode to the fetus, measuring uterine pressure by inserting an indwelling catheter into the uterine cavity, or incising the fetal scalp to measure blood pH. A strong orientation toward universal use of internal monitoring techniques is likely to predispose to *early amniotomy* and its potential dangers, including cord prolapse, infection, and possibly more stress to the fetus when not cushioned by amnionic fluid during labor. In this regard the studies performed in late gestation in monkeys by Gabbe and associates (1976) and similar studies in sheep serve to reemphasize the protective cushion against cord compression provided by amnionic fluid. Acute reduction in amnionic fluid volume led to variable decelerations. Restoration of the amnionic fluid volume eliminated the abnormal pattern.

Another potential morbidity is *trauma.* Injury to the fetal scalp induced by the electrode is rarely a major problem, although application at some other site, for example, the eye in case of a face presentation, can prove serious. A fetal vessel in the placenta may be ruptured inadvertently by the placement of the catheter. Trudinger and Pryse-Davies (1978) observed four such accidents, two of which led to death of the fetus or newborn infant from exsanguination. Moreover, they identified one instance of severe cord compression from entanglement with the intrauterine catheter. Others have had similar experiences. Penetration of the placenta causing hemorrhage and perforations of the uterus during insertion of the catheter has led to serious morbidity, as well as spurious recordings that resulted in inappropriate management of labor and delivery.

Both the fetus and the mother may be at increased risk of *infection* as the consequence of internal electronic monitoring. Scalp wounds from the electrode may become infected by organisms of the vaginal flora (Okada and associates, 1977). Infection of the newborn infant with *Herpes hominis* type 2 virus has been identified following the use of scalp electrodes; systemic viral disease, as well as chronic scalp infection, resulted. Infants born after internal electronic monitoring appear more likely to have been colonized by maternal group B streptococcus.

An increase in maternal infections following the use of internal electronic monitoring is not a common finding. Perhaps a decrease in the frequency and therefore the number of vaginal examinations for the woman who is being monitored offsets the risk imposed by rupture of the membranes and the placement and persistence of the catheter and wires in utero.

Although external monitoring techniques obviate the necessity of ruptured membranes and invasion of the uterus, as well as direct trauma to the fetus, their use, unless meticulously guarded against, commonly results in the mother lying in the supine position most of the time so as to protect the placement of the external detectors. The supine position, by causing aortocaval compression, is likely to be deleterious to the fetus if the fetus is already in jeopardy for other reasons, fetal or maternal.

Three troublesome complications resulting from fetal scalp blood sampling are infection, blade breakage, and bleeding. If vaginal bleeding is encountered at any time following scalp blood sampling, fetal bleeding must be ruled out. Marked deficiencies of vitamin K-dependent coagulation factors have been implicated in the genesis of such hemorrhage in some infants (Hull, 1972), and hemophilia has been subsequently diagnosed in a few others. The negative pressure from use of a vacuum extractor to effect delivery after scalp blood sampling may incite troublesome hemorrhage.

ASSESSMENT OF RESULTS FROM ELECTRONIC MONITORING

In the United States, Hon, Quilligan, Paul, and Freeman are prominent among the names of obstetricians who have long championed continuous electronic recording of the fetal heart during labor. They observed somewhat lower perinatal mortality rates at Los Angeles County Hospital for labors in which the fetal heart rate was continuously recorded, despite the fact that the group so monitored was selected because of pregnancy complications recognized to predispose to a poorer outcome for the fetus (Paul and colleagues, 1977). Beard (1974) in Great Britain considered electronic monitoring limited only to so-called high-risk pregnancies to be unsound, and urged that electronic monitoring be used for all labors. In his experience, in terms of the number of fetuses who became acidotic during labor, there was little difference between the identified high-risk pregnancies and those considered normal. He emphasized that only by so monitoring all labors would intrapartum asphyxial damage be eliminated.

Although many groups have stated, or at least implied, that fetal mortality rates were reduced significantly as the consequence of continuous electronic monitoring, some studies have demonstrated similarly good outcomes for pregnancies using systematic clinical monitoring. For example, in one series of studies in Denver, trained nursing personnel clinically monitored the mother and fetus in a standardized fashion throughout labor until the actual delivery of the infant (Haverkamp and co-workers, 1976, 1979). The fetal heart was routinely checked every 15 minutes during the first stage, every 5 minutes during the second stage, and more often if an abnormality was suspected. Uterine contractions were frequently evaluated by palpation and the mother was observed continuously. In the group so monitored clinically, the Apgar scores were as high as in the group routinely subjected to continuous electronic monitoring, while the cesarean section group was appreciably lower.

In Oxford, England, the results of two systems of obstetrical care for apparently low-risk pregnancies have been compared with the conclusion drawn that care of one mother by one midwife during labor and delivery without electronic fetal monitoring produced results as good as or better than were achieved with electronic monitoring and a consultant team of obstetricians directly responsible for intrapartum management (Klein and co-workers, 1983). They were favorably impressed by the simplicity, yet safety, of delivery of low-risk parturients that could be achieved with such labor management.

Leveno and associates (1986) studied the effects of using intrapartum electronic fetal monitoring in all pregnancies (universal) versus such monitoring only in pregnancies in which the fetus was judged to be at high risk (selective). Perinatal outcomes that include intrapartum stillbirths, low Apgar scores, a need for newborn resuscitation, admission to the neonatal intensive-care unit, and neonatal seizures were not significantly different between the two groups. The incidence of cesarean section for fetal distress was slightly but significantly increased in these low-risk women universally monitored. A discussion on fetal monitoring also is presented in Chapter 16 (p. 310).

It cannot be overemphasized that the techniques for continuous recording of fetal heart rates and uterine pressures do not by themselves provide continuous surveillance of the fetus. Appropriately trained personnel must be immediately available to activate the electronic techniques, to inspect and analyze almost continuously the data that are being recorded, and to act promptly on the findings.

For many, but not all, obstetrical services the increasing use of electronic fetal monitoring has been accompanied by an appreciable increase in cesarean section rate (Antenatal Diagnosis, 1979; Prentice and Lind, 1987). Whether the two phenomena are directly related is not clear in many instances. However, in the case of the two studies by Haverkamp and co-workers cited above, cesarean section with electronic monitoring of labor, when compared to clinical monitoring carried out as described, was either two times or three times as high, depending upon whether or not scalp sampling to measure fetal blood pH was performed in conjunction with electronic monitoring.

CLINICAL MONITORING

The status of the fetus can often be satisfactorily monitored clinically by appropriately trained individuals who closely adhere to the guidelines that follow and that are emphasized in Chapter 16 (p. 312). In summary, the fetal heart rate is carefully determined at close intervals during and immediately after a uterine contraction until the infant is actually delivered; the frequency and intensity of uterine contractions are carefully estimated; and the rates of cervical dilatation and descent of the presenting part are determined periodically.

Normally, the fetal heart rate between contractions will average about 140 and will range from no less than 120 to no more than 160 beats per minute. Typically, the fetal heart rate drops somewhat with the onset of a uterine contraction but recovers promptly as the contraction ends. The fetal heart rate may be determined using a specialized stethoscope or an instrument that uses the Doppler principle with ultrasound to detect fetal heart action.

INTRAPARTUM SURVEILLANCE OF THE FETUS AT PARKLAND HOSPITAL

In about 60 percent of labors, the fetus is monitored clinically as described above and in Chapter 16. Continuous electronic monitoring currently is reserved for the following circumstances:

1. Variations in the fetal heart rate detected by auscultation *and for which immediate delivery is not considered necessary.*

2. Meconium in amnionic fluid.
3. Induction or augmentation of labor with oxytocin.
4. Previous cesarean delivery.
5. Increased likelihood of uteroplacental insufficiency or compromised fetus:
   a. Hypertension.
   b. Bleeding.
   c. Preterm and postterm pregnancies.
   d. Small fetus, probably growth-retarded.
   e. Abnormal presentations.
   f. Previous unexplained stillbirth.
   g. Sickle cell hemoglobinopathies.
   h. Hemolytic disease of the fetus.
   i. Diabetes.

Although the application of continuous electronic monitoring cannot by itself be credited for any remarkable reduction in intrapartum or neonatal mortality at Parkland Hospital, it has provided an elegant means of demonstrating to physicians in training, medical students, nurses, physicians' assistants, and others the normal and abnormal forces of labor and the cardiac responses of the fetus during this important event.

REFERENCES

Al-Ghazali W, Chapman MG, Allan LD: Doppler assessment of the cardiac and uteroplacental circulations in normal and complicated pregnancies. Br J Obstet Gynaecol 95:575, 1988

American College of Obstetricians and Gynecologists: Antepartum Fetal Surveillance. Technical Bulletin, No 107, August 1987

American College of Obstetricians and Gynecologists: Ultrasound in Pregnancy. Technical Bulletin No 116, May 1988

Angel JL, Knuppel RA, Lake M: Sinusoidal fetal heart rate pattern associated with intravenous butophanol administration: A case report. Am J Obstet Gynecol 149:465, 1984

Antenatal Diagnosis. Report of a Consensus Development Conference Sponsored by the National Institute of Child Health and Human Development, NIH Publication Number 79—1973. Washington, DC, US Government Printing Office, 1979

Babaknia A, Niebyl JR: The effect of magnesium sulfate on fetal heart rate baseline variability. Obstet Gynecol 51 (Suppl):2, 1978

Bang J, Bock JE, Trolle D: Ultrasound-guided fetal intravenous transfusion for severe rhesus haemolytic disease. Br Med J 284:373, 1982

Barkai G, Mashiach S, Lanzer D, Kayam Z, Brish M, Goldman B: Determination of fetal lung maturity from amniotic fluid microviscosity in high-risk pregnancy. Obstet Gynecol 59:615, 1982

Barkai G, Reichman B, Modan M, Goldman B, Serr DM, Mashiach S: The influence of abnormal pregnancies on fluorescence polarization of amniotic fluid lipids. Obstet Gynecol 72:39, 1988

Baskett TF: Gestational age and fetal biophysical assessment. Am J Obstet Gynecol 158:332, 1988

Beard RW: The detection of fetal asphyxia in labor. Pediatrics 53:157, 1974

Berkowitz RL, Chitkara U, Goldberg JD, Wilkins I, Chervenak FA, Lynch L: Intrauterine intravascular transfusions for severe red blood cell isoimmunization: Ultrasound-guided percutaneous approach. Am J Obstet Gynecol 155:574, 1986a

Berkowitz RL, Chitkara U, Goldberg JD, Wilkins I, Chervenak FA: Intravascular transfusion in utero: The percutaneous approach. Am J Obstet Gynecol 154:622, 1986b

Boehm FH: FHR variability: Key to fetal well-being. Contemp Ob/Gyn 9:57, 1977

Brown VA, Sawers RS, Parsons RJ, Duncan SLB, Cooke ID: The value of antenatal cardiotocography in the management of high-risk pregnancy: A randomized controlled trial. Br J Obstet Gynaecol 89:716, 1982

Buhi WC, Spellacy WN: Effect of blood or meconium on the determination of the amniotic fluid lecithin/sphinomyelin ratio. Am J Obstet Gynecol 121:321, 1975

Cao A, Furbetta M, Angius A, Ximenes A, Rosatelli C, Turveri T, Scalas MT, Falchi AM, Angioni G, Caminiti F: Hematological and obstetrical aspects of antenatal diagnosis of β thalassemia—experience with 200 cases. J Med Genet 19:81, 1982

Clark SL, Paul RH: Intrapartum fetal surveillance: The role of fetal scalp sampling. Am J Obstet Gynecol 153:717, 1985

Clements JA, Platzker ACG, Tierney DF, Hobel CL, Creasy RK, Margolis AJ, Thibeault DW, Tooley WH, Oh W: Assessment of the risk of respiratory distress syndrome by a rapid test for surfactant in amniotic fluid. N Engl J Med 286:1077, 1972

Cohen WR, Schifrin BS: Diagnosis and treatment of fetal distress. In Bolognese RJ, Schwarz RH (eds): Perinatal Medicine. Baltimore, Williams & Wilkins, 1977, p 131

Connors G, Natale R, Nasello-Paterson C: Maternally perceived fetal activity from twenty-four weeks' gestation to term in normal and at risk pregnancies. Am J Obstet Gynecol 158:294, 1988

Copel JA, Grannum PA, Hobbins JC, Cunningham FG: Doppler ultrasound in obstetrics. Williams Supplement No 16. Appleton & Lange, January/February 1988

Copel JA, Scioscia A, Grannum PA, Romero R, Reece EA, Hobbins JC: Percutaneous umbilical blood sampling in the management of Kell isoimmunization. Obstet Gynecol 67:299, 1986

Crowley P, O'Herlihy C, Bowlan P: The value of ultrasound measurements of amniotic fluid volume in the management of prolonged pregnancies. Br J Obstet Gynaecol 91:444, 1984

Daffos F, Capella-Pavlovsky M, Forestier F: A new procedure for fetal blood sampling in utero: Preliminary results of 53 cases. Am J Obstet Gynecol 146:985, 1983a

Daffos F, Capella-Pavlovsky M, Forestier F: Fetal blood sampling in the umbilical cord using a needle guided by ultrasound: Report of 66 cases. Prenat Diagn 3:271, 1983b

Daffos F, Capella-Pavlovsky M, Forestier F: Fetal blood sampling during pregnancy with the use of a needle guided by ultrasound: A study of 606 consecutive cases. Am J Obstet Gynecol 153:655, 1985

Daffos F, Forestier F, Capella-Pavlovsky M: Fetal blood sampling during the third trimester of pregnancy. Br J Obstet Gynaecol 91:118, 1984a

Daffos F, Forestier F, Capella-Pavlovsky M, Thulliez P, Aufrant C, Valenti D, Cox WL: Prenatal management of 746 pregnancies at risk for congenital toxoplasmosis. N Engl J Med 318:271, 1988a

Daffos F, Forestier F, Kaplan C, Cox W: Prenatal diagnosis and management of bleeding disorders with fetal blood sampling. Am J Obstet Gynecol 158:939, 1988b

Daffos F, Forestier F, Grangeot-Keros L, Capella-Pavlovsky M, Lebon P, Chartier M: Prenatal diagnosis of congenital toxoplasmosis. Lancet 2:1, 1984b

Daffos F, Forestier F, Muller JY, Reznikoff-Etievant M, Habibi B, Capella-Pavlovsky M, Maigret P, Kaplan C: Prenatal treatment of alloimmune thrombocytopenia. Lancet 2:632, 1984c

Dalton KJ, Dawes GS, Patrick JE: The autonomic nervous system and fetal heart rate variability. Am J Obstet Gynecol 146:456, 1983

de Crespigny L, Robinson HP, Quinn M, Doyle L, Ross A, Cauchi M: Ultrasound-guided fetal blood transfusion for severe rhesus isoimmunization. Obstet Gynecol 66:529, 1985

deSmedt MCH, Visser GHA, Meijboom EJ: Fetal cardiac output estimated by Doppler echocardiography during mid- and late gestation. Am J Cardiol 60:338, 1987

Desmonts G, Daffos F, Forestier F, Cappela-Pavlovsky M, Thulliez P, Chartier M: Prenatal diagnosis of congenital toxoplasmosis. Lancet 1:500, 1985

Divon MY, Guidetti DA, Cantu U, Sklar AJ, Lev-Gur M, Merkatz IR: Fetal biophysical profile scoring: The significance of fetal heart rate late decelerations. Abstract No 199. Presented at the 35th Annual Meeting of the Society of Gynecologic Investigation, March 17–20, 1988

Druzin ML, Gratacos J, Keegan KA, Paul RH: Antepartum fetal heart rate testing: VII. The significance of fetal bradycardia. Am J Obstet Gynecol 139:194, 1981

Eden RD, Seifert LS, Kodack LD, Trofatter KF, Killam AP, Gall SA: A modified biophysical profile for antenatal fetal surveillance. Obstet Gynecol 71:365, 1988

Edersheim TG, Hutson JM, Druzin ML, Kogut EA: Fetal heart rate response to vibratory acoustic stimulation predicts fetal pH in labor. Am J Obstet Gynecol 157:1557, 1987

Ehrström C: Fetal movement monitoring in normal and high-risk pregnancy. Acta Obstet Gynecol (Suppl) 80:1, 1979

Eik-Ness SH, Brubakk AO, Ulstein MK: Measurement of human fetal blood flow. Br Med J 1:283, 1980

Eik-Ness SH, Marsal K, Brubakk AO, Kristofferson K, Ulstein M: Ultrasonic measurement of human fetal blood flow. J Biomed Eng 4:28, 1982

Eldridge MW, Berman W, Greene ER: Serial echo-Doppler measurements of human fetal abdominal aortic blood flow. J Ultrasound Med 4:453, 1985

Epstein H, Waxman A, Gleicher N, Lauersen NH: Meperidine-induced sinusoidal fetal heart rate pattern and its reversal with naloxone. Obstet Gynecol (Suppl) 59:22, 1982

Erskine RLA, Ritchie JWK: Quantitative measurement of fetal blood flow using Doppler ultrasound. Br J Obstet Gynecol 92:600, 1985

Evertson LR, Gauthier RJ, Collea JV: Fetal demise following negative contraction stress tests. Obstet Gynecol 51:671, 1978

Fitzgerald DE, Stuart B, Drumm JE, Duignan NM: The assessment of the feto-placental circulation with continuous wave Doppler ultrasound. Ultrasound Med Biol 10:371, 1984

Forestier F, Cox WL, Daffos F, Rainaut M: The assessment of fetal blood samples. Am J Obstet Gynecol 158:1184, 1988

Forestier F, Daffos F, Capella-Pavlovsky M: Low molecular weight heparin (PK 10169) does not cross the placenta during the second trimester of pregnancy: Study by direct fetal blood sampling under ultrasound. Thromb Res 34:557, 1984a

Forestier F, Daffos F, Capella-Pavlovsky M: Hematological values of 163 fetuses between 18 and 30 weeks of gestation: Their application to prenatal diagnosis of infectious diseases. Blood 64:44A, 1984b

Freeman RK: The use of the oxytocin challenge test for antepartum clinical evaluation of utero-placental respiratory function. Am J Obstet Gynecol 121:481, 1975

Freeman RK, Anderson G, Dorchester W: A prospective multi-institutional study of antepartum fetal heart rate monitoring: I. Risk of perinatal mortality and morbidity according to antepartum fetal heart rate test results. Am J Obstet Gynecol 143:771, 1982a

Freeman RK, Anderson G, Dorchester W: A prospective multi-institutional study of antepartum fetal heart rate monitoring: II. Contraction stress test versus nonstress test for primary surveillance. Am J Obstet Gynecol 143:778, 1982b

Freeman RK, Garite TJ: Fetal Heart Rate Monitoring. Baltimore, Williams & Wilkins, 1981, p 63

Frigoletto FD, Greene MF, Benacerraf BR, Barss VA, Saltzman DH: Ultrasonographic fetal surveillance in the management of the isoimmunized pregnancy. N Engl J Med 315:430, 1986

Gabbe SG, Ettinger BB, Freeman RK, Martin CB: Umbilical cord compression associated with amniotomy: Laboratory observations. Am J Obstet Gynecol 126:353, 1976

Gal D, Neuhoff S, Lilling MI, Tancer ML: False negative oxytocin challenge test: Report of three cases. Am J Obstet Gynecol 133:111, 1979

Gant NF, Hutchinson HT, Siiteri PK, MacDonald PC: Study of the metabolic clearance rate of dehydroisoandrosterone sulfate in pregnancy. Am J Obstet Gynecol 111:555, 1971

Garite TJ, Yabusaki KK, Moberg LJ, Symons JL, White T, Itano M, Freeman RK: A new rapid slide agglutination test for amniotic fluid phosphatidylglycerol. Am J Obstet Gynecol 147:681, 1983

Gibbons JM Jr, Huntley TE, Corral AG: Effect of maternal blood contamination on amniotic fluid analysis. Obstet Gynecol 44:657, 1974

Gillberg C, Rasmussen P, Wahlström J: Long-term follow-up of children born after amniocentesis. Clin Genetics 21:69, 1982

Gilstrap LC III, Hauth JC, Hankins GDV, Beck AW: Second-stage fetal heart rate abnormalities and type of neonatal acidemia. Obstet Gynecol 70:191, 1987

Gluck L, Kulovich MV: Lecithin/sphingomyelin ratios in amniotic fluid in normal and abnormal pregnancy. Am J Obstet Gynecol 115:539, 1973

Gluck L, Kulovich MV, Borer RC Jr, Brenner PH, Anderson GG, Spellacy WN: Diagnosis of the respiratory distress syndrome by amniocentesis. Am J Obstet Gynecol 109:440, 1971

Goodwin J: The fetal circulation. In Goodwin JW, Gooden JO, Chance GW (eds): Perinatal Medicine. Baltimore, Williams & Wilkins, 1976, p 143

Grannum PA, Copel JA, Plaxe SC, Scioscia AL, Hobbins JL: In utero exchange transfusion by direct intravascular injection in severe erythroblastosis fetalis. N Engl J Med 314:1431, 1986

Gray JH, Cudmore DW, Luther ER, Martin TR, Gardner AJ: Sinusoidal fetal heart rate pattern associated with alphaprodine administration. Obstet Gynecol 52:678, 1978

Griffin D, Cohen-Overbeek T, Campbell S: Fetal and utero-placental blood flow. Clin Obstet Gynecol 10:565, 1983

Griffin DR, Teague MJ, Tallet P, Willson K, Bilardo C, Massini L, Campbell S: A combination ultrasonic linear array scanner and pulsed Doppler velocimeter for the estimation of blood flow in the foetus and adult abdomen: II. Clinical evaluation. Ultrasound Med Biol 11:37, 1985

Grundy H, Freeman RK, Lederman S, Dorchester W: Nonreactive contraction stress test: Clinical significance. Obstet Gynecol 64:337, 1984

Hammacher K: Früherkennung intrauteriner gefahrenzustände durch electrophonokardiographie und fokographie. In Elert R, Hüter KA (eds): Prophylaxe Frühkindlicher Hirnshäden. Stuttgart, Georg Thieme, 1966, p 120

Hammacher K, Hüter KA, Bokelmann J, Werners PH: Foetal heart frequency and perinatal condition of the foetus and newborn. Gynaecologia 166:349, 1968

Harrigan JT, Marino JF: Fetal heart rate reaction to amniocentesis as an indicator of fetal well-being. Am J Obstet Gynecol 132:49, 1978

Harvey D, Parkinson CE, Campbell S: Risk of respiratory-distress syndrome. Lancet 1:42, 1975

Hatjis CG, Meis PJ: Sinusoidal fetal heart rate pattern associated with butophanol administration. Obstet Gynecol 67:377, 1986

Haverkamp AD, Orleans M, Langendoerfer S, McFee JG, Murphy J, Thompson HE: A controlled trial of the differential effects of intrapartum fetal monitoring. Am J Obstet Gynecol 143:399, 1979

Haverkamp AD, Thompson HE, McFee JG, Cetrulo C: The evaluation of continuous fetal heart rate monitoring in high-risk pregnancy. Am J Obstet Gynecol 125:310, 1976

Hayashi RH, Fox ME: Unforeseen sudden intrapartum fetal death in a monitored labor. Am J Obstet Gynecol 122:786, 1975

Herbert WNP, Chapman JE, Cefalo RC: Reliability of the foam stability index test in assessing fetal lung maturation. Presented at the annual meeting of the Society for Perinatal Obstetricians, San Antonio, TX, February 2–4, 1984

Herbert WNP, Tyson JE, Jimenez JM: Absence of hyaline membrane disease at low lecithin to sphingomyelin ratios. Pediatr Res 13:497, 1979

Hobbins JC, Grannum PA, Romero R, Reece EA, Mahoney MJ: Percutaneous umbilical blood sampling. Am J Obstet Gynecol 152:1, 1985

Hobbins JC, Mahoney MJ: In utero diagnosis of hemoglobinopathies. N Engl J Med 209:1065, 1974

Hon EH: Fetal heart rate monitoring. In Gluck L (ed): Modern Perinatal Medicine. Chicago, Year Book, 1974

Hon EH, Paul RH, Hon RW: Electronic evaluation of fetal heart rate. XI. Description of spiral electrode. Obstet Gynecol 40:362, 1972

Huddleston JF, Sutliff JG, Robinson D: Contraction stress test by intermittent nipple stimulation. Obstet Gynecol 63:669, 1984

Huhta JC, Moise KJ, Fisher DJ, Sharif DS, Wasserstrum N, Martin C: Detection and quantitation of constriction of the fetal ductus arteriosus by Doppler echocardiography. Circulation 75:406, 1987

Hull MGR: Perinatal coagulopathies complicating fetal blood sampling. Br Med J 3:319, 1972

Katz M, Meizner I, Shani N, Insler V: Clinical significance of sinusoidal fetal heart rate pattern. Br J Obstet Gynaecol 90:832, 1983

Kenny JF, Plappert T, Doubilet P, Saltzman DH, Cartier M, Zollars L, Leatherman GF, St John Sutton MG: Changes in intracardiac blood flow velocities and right and left ventricular stroke volumes with gestational age in the human fetus: A prospective Doppler echocardiographic study. Circulation 74:1208, 1986

Khouzami VA, Beck JC, Sullivant H, Johnson JWC: Amniotic fluid absorbance at 650 nm: Its relationship to lecithin/sphingomyelin ratio and neonatal pulmonary sufficiency. Am J Obstet Gynecol 147:552, 1983

Klein M, Lloyd I, Redman C, Bull M, Turnbull AC: A comparison of low-risk pregnant women booked for delivery in two systems of care: Shared-care (consultant) and integrated general practice unit: II. Labour and delivery management and neonatal outcome. Br J Obstet Gynaecol 90:123, 1983

Kleinman CS, Copel JA, Weinstein EM, Santalli TV Jr: In utero diagnosis and treatment of fetal supraventricular tachycardia. Semin Perinatol 9:113, 1985

Kleinman CS, Weinstein EM, Copel JA: Pulsed Doppler analysis of human fetal blood flow. Clin Diagn Ultrasound 17:173, 1986

Kubli FW, Kaeser O, Hinselmann M: Diagnostic management of chronic placental insufficiency. In Pecile A, Finzi C (eds): The Foeto-Placental Unit. Amsterdam, Excerpta Medica, 1969, p 323

Laurin J, Lingman G, Marsal K, Persson P: Fetal blood flow in pregnancies complicated by intrauterine growth retardation. Obstet Gynecol 69:895, 1987

Leach G, Chang A, Morrison J: A controlled trial of puncture sites for amniocentesis. Br J Obstet Gynaecol 85:328, 1978

Lenke RR, Nemes JM: Use of nipple stimulation to obtain contraction stress test. Obstet Gynecol 63:345, 1984

Leveno KJ, Cunningham FG: Forecasting fetal health. Williams Supplement No 19. Appleton & Lange, August/September 1988

Leveno KJ, Cunningham FG, Nelson S, Roark M, Williams ML, Guzick D, Dowling S, Rosenfeld CR, Buckley A: A prospective comparison of selective and universal electronic fetal monitoring in 34,995 pregnancies. N Engl J Med 315:615, 1986

Leveno KJ, Whalley PJ: Dilemmas in the management of pregnancy complicated by diabetes. Med Clin North Am 66:1325, 1982

Leveno KJ, Williams MJ, DePalma RT, Whalley PJ: Perinatal outcome in absence of antepartum fetal heart rate acceleration. Obstet Gynecol 61:347, 1983

Lewis PE, Cefalo RC, Zaritsky AL: Fetal heart block due to cytomegalo-virus. Am J Obstet Gynecol 136:967, 1980

Lowe TW, Leveno KJ, Quirk JG Jr, Santos-Ramos R, Williams ML: Sinusoidal fetal heart rate pattern after intrauterine transfusion. Obstet Gynecol 64:21S, 1984

Lowe TW, Weinreb J, Santos-Ramos R, Cunningham FG: Magnetic resonance imaging in human pregnancy. Obstet Gynecol 66:629, 1985

Ludomirski A, Nemiroff R, Johnson A, Ashmead GG, Weiner S, Bolognese RJ: Percutaneous umbilical blood sampling: A new technique for prenatal diagnosis. J Reprod Med 32:276, 1987

Lumley J, Lester A, Anderson I, Renou P, Wood C: A randomized trial of weekly cardiotocography in high-risk obstetric patients. Br J Obstet Gynaecol 90:1018, 1983

MacKenzie IZ, Maclean DA: Pure fetal blood from the umbilical cord obtained at fetoscopy: Experience with 125 consecutive cases. Am J Obstet Gynecol 138:1214, 1980

Mann L: Intrapartum fetal monitoring: Scalp blood pH is a useful tool. Contemp Ob/Gyn 11:25, 1978

Manning FA, Hill LM, Platt LD: Quantitative amniotic fluid volume determined by ultrasound: Antepartum detection of intrauterine growth retardation. Am J Obstet Gynecol 139:254, 1981

Manning FA, Morrison I, Harman CR, Lange IR, Menticoglou S: Fetal assessment based on fetal biophysical profile scoring: Experience in 19,221 referred high-risk pregnancies: II. An analysis of false-negative fetal deaths. Am J Obstet Gynecol 157:880, 1987a

Manning FA, Morrison I, Lange IR, Harman CR, Chamberlain PFC: Fetal biophysical profile scoring: Selective use of the nonstress test. Am J Obstet Gynecol 156:709, 1987b

Manning FA, Morrison I, Lange IR, Harman CR, Chamberlain PFC: Fetal assessment based on fetal biophysical profile scoring: Experience in 12,620 referred high-risk pregnancies: I. Perinatal mortality by frequency and etiology. Am J Obstet Gynecol 151:343, 1985

Manning FA, Platt LD, Sipos L: Antepartum fetal evaluation: Development of a fetal biophysical profile. Am J Obstet Gynecol 136:787, 1980

Marsál K, Lindblad A, Lingman G, Eik-Nes SH: Bloodflow in the fetal descending aorta: Intrinsic factors affecting fetal blood flow, i.e., fetal breathing movements and cardiac arrhythmia. Ultrasound Med Biol 10:339, 1984

Marx JL: Imaging technique passes muster. Science 238: 888, 1987

Mendez-Bauer C, Ruiz Canesco A, Andujar Ruiz M, Menendez A, Arroya J, Gardi RD, Sastry V, Zamarriego Crespo J: Early decelerations of the fetal heart rate from occlusion of the umbilical cord. J Perinat Med 6:69, 1978

Murata Y, Martin CB Jr, Ikenoue T, Hashimoto T, Taira S, Sagawa T, Sakata H: Fetal heart rate accelerations during the course of intrauterine death in chronically catheterized rhesus monkeys. Am J Obstet Gynecol 144:218, 1982

National Institute of Child Health and Human Development, National Registry for Amniocentesis Study Group: Midtrimester amniocentesis for prenatal diagnosis: Safety and accuracy. JAMA 236:1471, 1976

Newnham J, Patterson L, James I, Diepeveen D, Reid S: Doppler flow velocity waveform analysis: A prospective double-blind evaluation of its efficacy as a screening test in pregnancy. Presented at the Society for Gynecologic Investigation, San Diego, California, March 1989

Nicolaides KH, Campbell S, Bradley RJ, Bilardo CM, Soothill PW, Gibb D: Maternal oxygen therapy for intrauterine growth retardation. Lancet 1:942, 1987a

Nicolaides KH, Rodeck CH, Gosden CM: Rapid karyotyping in non-lethal malformations. Lancet 1:283, 1986a

Nicolaides KH, Rodeck CH, Mibashan RS, Kemp JR: Have Liley charts outlived their usefulness? Am J Obstet Gynecol 155:90, 1986b

Nicolaides KH, Rodeck CH, Soothill PW, Campbell S: Ultrasound-guided sampling of umbilical cord and placental blood to assess fetal wellbeing. Lancet 1:1065, 1986c

Odendaal HJ: False interpretation of fetal heart rate monitoring in cases of intrauterine death. S Afr Med J 50:1963, 1976

Okada DM, Chow AW, Bruce VT: Neonatal scalp abscess and fetal monitoring: Factors associated with infection. Am J Obstet Gynecol 129:185, 1977

Paul RH, Huey JE Jr, Yaeger CF: Clinical fetal monitoring. Postgrad Med 61:160, 1977

Pearce JM, Chamberlain GVP: Ultrasonically guided percutaneous umbilical blood sampling in the management of intrauterine growth retardation. Br J Obstet Gynaecol 94:318, 1987

Person P-H, Kullander S: Long-term experience of general ultrasound screening in pregnancy. Am J Obstet Gynecol 146:942, 1983

Phelan JP, Lewis PE Jr, Paul RH: Fetal heart rate decelerations during a nonstress test. Obstet Gynecol 57:228, 1981

Poreco R, Young PE, Resnik R, Cousins L, Jones OW, Richards T, Kernahan C, Matson M: Reproductive outcome following amniocentesis for genetic indications. Am J Obstet Gynecol 143:653, 1983

Powell MC, Worthington BS, Buckley JM, Symonds EM: Magnetic resonance imaging (MRI) in obstetrics. II. Fetal anatomy. Br J Obstet Gynaecol 95:38, 1988

Prentice A, Lind T: Fetal heart rate monitoring during labour—too frequent intervention, too little benefit? Lancet 2:1375, 1987

Quirk JG, Bleasdale JE: Fetal lung maturation in the pregnancy complicated by diabetes mellitus. In DiRenzo GC, Hawkins PR (eds): Perinatal Medicine: Updates and Controversies. New York, Cortina International, 1986, p 117

Ray M, Freeman R, Pine S, Hesselgesser R: Clinical experience with the oxytocin challenge test. Am J Obstet Gynecol 114:1, 1972

Read JA, Miller FC: Fetal heart rate acceleration in response to acoustic stimulation as a measure of fetal well-being. Am J Obstet Gynecol 129:512, 1977

Reed KL, Meijboom EJ, Sahn DJ, Scagnelli SA, Valdes-Cruz LM, Shenker L: Cardiac Doppler flow velocities in human fetuses. Circulation 73:41, 1986a

Reed KL, Sahn DJ, Marx GR, Anderson CF, Shenker L: Cardiac Doppler flow during fetal arrhythmias: Physiological consequences. Obstet Gynecol 70:1, 1987

Reed KL, Sahn DJ, Scagnelli S, Anderson CF, Shenker L: Doppler echocardiographic studies of diastolic function in the human fetal heart: Changes during gestation. J Am Coll Cardiol 8:391, 1986b

Richards DS, Cefalo RC, Thorpe JM, Salley M, Rose D: Determinants of fetal heart rate response to vibroacoustic stimulation in labor. Obstet Gynecol 71:535, 1988

Roberts NS, Dunn LK, Weiner S, Godmilow L, Miller R: Midtrimester amniocentesis: Indications, techniques, risks and potential for prenatal diagnosis. J Reprod Med 28:167, 1983

Rodeck CH: Fetoscopy guided by real-time ultrasound for pure fetal blood samples fetal skin samples and examination of the fetus in utero. Br J Obstet Gynaecol 87:449, 1980

Rodeck CH, Campbell S: Sampling pure fetal blood by fetoscopy in second trimester of pregnancy. Br Med J 2:728, 1978

Rodeck CH, Campbell S: Umbilical cord insertion as a source of pure fetal blood for prenatal diagnosis. Lancet 1:1244, 1979

Rodeck CH, Nicolaides KH, Warsof SL, Fysh WJ, Gamsu HR, Kemp JR: The management of severe rhesus isioimmunization by fetoscopic intravascular transfusions. Am J Obstet Gynecol 150:769, 1984

Rooth G, McBride R, Ivy BJ: Fetal and maternal pH measurements. Acta Obstet Gynecol Scand 52:47, 1973

Ross MG, Leake RD, Ervin G, Sicon J, Fisher DA: Breast stimulation contraction test. Presented at the annual meeting of the Society of Perinatal Obstetricians, San Antonio, February 2–4, 1984

Saad SA, Fadel HE, Fahmy K, Nelson GH, Moustafa M, Davis HC: The reliability and clinical use of a rapid phosphatidylglycerol assay in normal and diabetic pregnancies. Am J Obstet Gynecol 157:1516, 1988

Sadovsky E, Polishuk WZ: Fetal movements in utero: Nature, assessment, prognostic value, time of delivery. Obstet Gynecol 50:49, 1977

Saling EZ: Die Blutgasverhältnisse und der saure Basen-Haushalt der Feten bei ungerstörtem geburtsablauf. Z Geburtsh Gynaekol 161:262, 1964

Saling EZ, Dudenhausen JW: The present situation of clinical monitoring of the fetus during labor. J Perinat Med 1:75, 1973

Sbarra AJ, Michlewitz H, Selvaraj RJ, Mitchell GW, Cetrulo CL, Kelley EC, Kennedy JL, Herschell MJ, Paul BB, Louis F: Relation between optical density at 650 nm and L/S ratio. Obstet Gynecol 50:723, 1977

Schifrin BS: The non-stress test. Presented at the Seventy-eighth Ross Conference on Pediatric Research (Obstetrical Decisions and Neonatal Outcome), San Diego, CA, May 30, 1979

Schlueter MA, Phibbs RH, Creasy RK, Clements JA, Tooley WH: Antenatal prediction of graduated risk of hyaline membrane disease by amniotic fluid foam test for surfactant. Am J Obstet Gynecol 134:761, 1979

Schulman H, Fleischer A, Farmakides G, Bracero L, Rochelson B, Grunfeld L: Development of uterine artery compliance in pregnancy as detected by Doppler ultrasound. Am J Obstet Gynecol 155:1031, 1986

Schulman H, Fleischer A, Stern W, Farmakides G, Jagani N, Blattner P: Umbilical velocity wave ratios in human pregnancy. Am J Obstet Gynecol 148:985, 1984

Seeds JW, Bowes WA Jr: Ultrasound-guided fetal intravascular transfusion in severe rhesus immunization. Am J Obstet Gynecol 154:1105, 1986

Serafini P, Lindsay MBJ, Nagey DA, Pupkin MJ, Tseng P, Crenshaw C Jr: Antepartum fetal heart rate response to sound stimulation: The acoustic stimulation test. Am J Obstet Gynecol 148:41, 1984

Shawker TH, Schuette WH, Whitehouse W, Rifka SM: Early fetal movement: A real-time ultrasound study. Obstet Gynecol 55:194, 1980

Shearer MH: Revelations: A summary and analysis of the NIH Consensus Development Conference on ultrasound imaging in pregnancy. Birth 11:23, 1984

Sher G, Statland BE: Assessment of fetal pulmonary maturity by the Lumadex foam stability index test. Obstet Gynecol 61:444, 1983

Shime J, Gare DJ, Andrews J, Bertrand M, Salgado J, Whillans G: Prolonged pregnancy: Surveillance of the fetus and the neonate and the course of labor and delivery. Am J Obstet Gynecol 148:547, 1984

Silverman NH, Kleinman CS, Rudolph AM, Copel JA, Weinstein EM, Enderlein MA, Golbus M: Fetal atrioventricular valve insufficiency associated with nonimmune hydrops: A two-dimensional echocardiographic and pulsed Doppler ultrasound study. Circulation 72:825, 1985

Simpson H, Dallaire L, Miller J, Simonovitch L, Hamerton J: Prenatal diagnosis of genetic disease in Canada: Report of a collaborative study. Can Med Assoc J 115:739, 1976

Smith CV, Phelan JP, Broussard P, Paul RH: Fetal acoustic stimulation testing: II. Predictive value of a reactive test. J Reprod Med 33:217, 1988

Smith CV, Phelan JP, Platt LD, Broussard P, Paul RH: Fetal acoustic stimulation testing: II. A randomized clinical comparison with the nonstress test. Am J Obstet Gynecol 155:131, 1986

Smith FW, Adam AH, Phillips WDP: NMR imaging in pregnancy. Lancet 1:61, 1983

Soothill PW, Nicolaides KH, Bilardo CM, Campbell S: Relation of fetal hypoxia in growth retardation to mean blood velocity in the fetal aorta. Lancet 2:1118, 1986a

Soothill PW, Nicolaides KH, Campbell S: Prenatal asphyxia, hyperlacticaemia, hypoglycaemia, and erythroblastosis in growth retarded fetuses. Br Med J 294:1051, 1987a

Soothill PW, Nicolaides KH, Rodeck CH, Campbell S: The effect of gestational age on blood gas and acid-base values in human pregnancy. Fetal Ther 1:166, 1986b

Soothill PW, Nicolaides KH, Rodeck CH, Clewell WH, Lindridge J: Relationship of fetal hemoglobin and oxygen content to lactate concentration in Rh isoimmunized pregnancies. Obstet Gynecol 69:268, 1987b

Steinfeld L, Rappaport HL, Rossbach HC, Martinez E: Diagnosis of fetal arrhythmias using echocardiographic and Doppler techniques. J Am Coll Cardiol 9:1425, 1986

Strasburger JF, Huhta JC, Carpenter RJ, Garson A Jr, McNamara DG: Doppler echocardiography in the diagnosis and management of persistent fetal arrhythmias. J Am Coll Cardiol 7:1386, 1986

Sugarman RG, Rawlinson KF, Schifrin BS: Fetal arrhythmias. Obstet Gynecol 52:301, 1978

Symonds EM, Johnson IR, Kean DM, Worthington BS, Pipkin FB, Hawkes RC, Gyngell M: Imaging the pregnant human uterus with nuclear magnetic resonance. Am J Obstet Gynecol 148:1136, 1984

Thacker SB, Berkelman RL: Assessing the diagnostic accuracy and efficacy of selected antepartum fetal surveillance techniques. Obstet Gynecol Surv 41:121, 1986

Thompson RS, Trudinger BJ, Cook CM, Giles WB: Umbilical artery velocity waveforms: Normal reference values for A/B ratio and Pourcelot ratio. Br J Obstet Gynaecol 95:589, 1988

Trudinger BJ, Cook CM, Giles WB, Thompson RS: Umbilical artery flow velocity waveforms in high-risk pregnancy: Randomised control trial. Lancet 1:188, 1987

Trudinger BJ, Pryse-Davies J: Fetal hazards of the intrauterine pressure catheter: Five case reports. Br J Obstet Gynaecol 85:567, 1978

Tsai MY, Josephson MW, Knox GE: Absorbance of amniotic fluid at 650 nm as a fetal lung maturity test: A comparison with the lecithin/sphingomyelin ratio and tests for desaturated phosphatidylcholine and phosphatidylglycerol. Am J Obstet Gynecol 146:963, 1983

Valenti C: Antenatal detection of hemoglobinopathies: A preliminary report. Am J Obstet Gynecol 115:851, 1973

Van Lierde M, Oberweis D, Thomas K: Ultrasonic measurement of aortic and umbilical blood flow in the human fetus. Obstet Gynecol 63:801, 1984

Vintzileos AM, Campbell WA, Ingardia CJ, Nochimson DJ: The fetal biophysical profile and its predictive value. Obstet Gynecol 62:271, 1983

Waldenström U, Axelsson O, Nilsson S, Eklund G, Fall O, Lindeberg S, Sjödin Y: Effects of routine one-stage ultrasound screening in pregnancy: A randomised controlled trial. Lancet 2:586, 1988

Weiner SA, Weinstein L: Fetal pulmonary maturity and antenatal diagnosis of respiratory distress syndrome. Obstet Gynecol Surv 42:75, 1987

Whitehouse WM, Simmons CS, Evans TN: Reduction of radiation hazard in obstetric roentgenography. Am J Roentgenol 80:690, 1958

Whittle MJ, Wilson AI, Whitfield CR, Paton RD, Logan RW: Amniotic fluid phosphatidylglycerol and the lecithin/sphingomyelin ratio in the assessment of fetal lung maturity. Br J Obstet Gynaecol 89:727, 1982

Working Party on Amniocentesis: An assessment of the hazards of amniocentesis: Report to the MRC Br J Obstet Gynaecol (Suppl) 85:2, 1978

Young BK, Katz M, Klein SA, Silverman F: Fetal blood and tissue pH with moderate bradycardia. Am J Obstet Gynecol 135:45, 1979

Zalar RW, Quillivan EJ: The influence of scalp sampling on the cesarean section rate for fetal distress. Am J Obstet Gynecol 135:239, 1979

Conduct of Normal Labor and Delivery

PSYCHOLOGICAL CONSIDERATIONS

The pregnant woman very often approaches labor with two major fears: "Will my baby be all right?" and "Will labor and delivery be very painful?" Her concerns should also be uppermost in the minds of everyone who participates in caring for the mother and her fetus. All things possible should be done to make the answer to the first question, "Yes" and to the second, "No."

Is labor easy because a woman is calm, or is she calm because her labor is easy? Is a woman pained and frightened because her labor is difficult, or is her labor difficult and painful because she is frightened? After scrutinizing many cases, the late British obstetrician Read concluded: *"Fear is in some way the chief pain-producing agent in otherwise normal labor."* Quite likely, fear may exert a deleterious effect on the quality of uterine contractions and on cervical dilatation.

It is not an easy task to dispel the age-old fear of pain during labor and delivery, but from the first prenatal visit a conscious effort should be made on the part of all persons involved in the care of the mother and her unborn child to make the point that labor and delivery are normal physiological processes. Everyone who is involved in caring for the mother and her fetus must demonstrate professional competence but also instill the feeling that he or she is the mother's friend and friend of her unborn baby, sincerely desirous of sparing her all possible pain within the limit of safety for her and her child. Physicians, nurses, and students should note especially that the morale of a woman in labor may sometimes be destroyed by careless remarks or actions. Casual comments outside the labor room are often overheard by her and misinterpreted. Laughter is frequently interpreted as directed toward her.

PHYSIOLOGICAL CHILDBIRTH

To eliminate the harmful influence of fear in labor, there has developed a school of thought that emphasizes the advantages of "natural childbirth" or "physiological childbirth." Natural or physiological childbirth entails antepartum education that emphasizes elimination of fear, exercises to promote relaxation, muscle control, and breathing; and adroit management throughout labor with a professional attendant skilled in reassurance of the mother constantly in attendance.

Cook (1982), in his monograph on natural childbirth, emphasized that the natural order results in very high maternal, fetal, and neonatal death rates and uncounted forms of morbidity. He stressed that it was medical intervention in this *natural*

process that resulted in the dramatic drop in mortality. He supported many of the natural childbirth movement's goals of education, husbands in the delivery room, breast feeding, and limitation of unnecessary sedation and analgesia, but he also discussed frankly the risks to both mother and fetus of placing the parents' desire for a *meaningful experience* before the needs of the fetus-infant. He concluded that as long as the *outcome* of childbirth is not subjugated to the *experience,* these reforms likely will be incorporated into patient care.

Most proponents of physiological childbirth have never claimed that labor can be made devoid of pain or that delivery should be conducted without anesthetic aids. With natural childbirth, most women experience some pain, and analgesics and anesthetics are not withheld when they are indicated. Physiological, or psychoprophylactic, childbirth also is considered in Chapter 17, p. 328.

ADMITTANCE PROCEDURES

The woman should be urged to report early in labor rather than to procrastinate until delivery is imminent for fear that she might be experiencing false labor. Early admittance to the labor and delivery unit is especially important if, during antepartum care, the gravida, her fetus, or both have been identified as being at risk.

IDENTIFICATION OF LABOR

Although the differential diagnosis between false and true labor is difficult at times, it usually can be made on the basis of the following features:

Contractions of True Labor

- Occur at regular intervals
- Intervals gradually shorten
- Intensity gradually increases
- Discomfort in back and abdomen
- Cervix dilates
- Not stopped by sedation

Contractions of False Labor

- Occur at irregular intervals
- Intervals remain long
- Intensity remains unchanged

- Discomfort chiefly in lower abdomen
- Cervix does not dilate
- Usually relieved by sedation

The general condition of the mother and her fetus must be quickly but accurately ascertained by means of history and physical examination. Inquiry is made as to the frequency and intensity of the uterine contractions and when they first become uncomfortable. The degree of discomfort that the mother displays is noted. The heart rate, presentation, and size of the fetus are evaluated abdominally. **The fetal heart rate should be checked especially at the end of a contraction and immediately thereafter to identify pathological slowing of the fetal heart rate** (Chap. 15, p. 296). Inquiries are made about the status of the fetal membranes and if there has been any vaginal bleeding. The questions of whether fluid has leaked from the vagina and, if so, how much and when the leakage first commenced are also addressed.

ADMITTANCE VAGINAL EXAMINATION

Most often, *unless there has been bleeding in excess of bloody show*, a vaginal examination under aseptic conditions is performed as described below. Careful attention to the following items is essential in order to obtain the greatest amount of information and to minimize bacterial contamination from multiple examinations:

1. *Amnionic fluid.* If there is a question of rupture of the membranes, the vulva and vaginal introitus are cleansed, a sterile speculum is carefully inserted, and fluid is sought in the posterior vaginal fornix. Any fluid is observed for vernix or meconium and, if the source of the fluid remains in doubt, it is collected on a swab for further study as described below.
2. *Cervix.* Softness, degree of effacement (length), extent of dilatation, and location of the cervix with respect to the presenting part and vagina are ascertained as described below. The presence of membranes with or without amnionic fluid below the presenting part often can be felt by careful palpation and the membranes visualized if they are intact and the cervix is dilated somewhat.
3. *Presenting part.* The nature of the presenting part should be positively determined and, ideally, its position as well, as described in Chapter 9 (p. 184).
4. *Station.* The degree of descent of the presenting part into the birth canal is identified as described below and, if the fetal head is high in the pelvis (above the level of the ischial spines), the effect of firm fundal pressure on descent of the fetal head is tested.
5. *Pelvic architecture.* The diagonal conjugate, ischial spines, pelvic sidewalls, and sacrum are reevaluated for adequacy (see Chapter 8, p. 168).
6. *Vagina and perineum.* The distensibility of the vagina and the firmness of the perineum are assessed.

Cervical Effacement

The degree of effacement of the cervix usually is expressed in terms of the length of the cervical canal compared to that of an uneffaced cervix (see Chapter 10, p. 217). When the length of the cervix is reduced by one half, it is 50 percent effaced; when the cervix becomes as thin as the adjacent lower uterine segment, it is completely, or 100 percent, effaced.

Cervical Dilatation

The amount of cervical dilatation is ascertained by estimating the average diameter of the cervical opening. The examining finger is swept from the margin of the cervix on one side to the opposite side, and the diameter traversed is expressed in centimeters. The cervix is said to be dilated fully when the diameter of the opening measures 10 cm, for the presenting part of a term-size infant usually can pass through a cervix so widely dilated (see Chapter 10, p. 218).

Position of the Cervix

The relationship of the cervical os to the fetal head is categorized as posterior, midposition, or anterior. A posterior position is suggestive of preterm labor.

Station

When conducting a vaginal examination, it is valuable to identify the level of the presenting fetal part in the birth canal. The ischial spines are about halfway between the pelvic inlet and the pelvic outlet. When the lowermost portion of the presenting fetal part is at the level of the ischial spines, it is designated as being at zero (0) station. The long axis of the birth canal above the ischial spines is arbitrarily divided into thirds. If the presenting part is at the level of the pelvic inlet, it is at −3 station; if it has descended one third the distance from the pelvic inlet to the ischial spines, it is at −2 station; if it has reached a level two thirds the distance from the inlet to the spines, it is at −1 station. The long axis of the birth canal between the level of the ischial spines and the outlet of the pelvis is similarly divided into thirds. If the level of the presenting part in the birth canal is one third or two thirds of the distance between the ischial spines and the pelvic outlet, it is at +1 station or +2 station, respectively. When the presenting fetal part reaches the perineum, its station is +3. If the vertex is at 0 station or below, most often engagement of the head has occurred; that is, the biparietal plane of the head has passed through the pelvic inlet. **If the head is unusually molded, or if there is an extensive formation of caput, or both, engagement might not have taken place even though the vertex is at 0 station or even lower.** Progressive cervical dilatation with no change in the station of the presenting part, in a woman of low parity, implies fetopelvic disproportion.

> An alternative method for designating the station of the fetal head has been used by some obstetricians (Friedman, 1978). Five levels, rather than three levels, are identified above and below the ischial spines. Each of the five levels differs from the adjacent level by approximately 1 cm. A change in station of 1 cm implies precision of mensuration that is not achievable in clinical practice. It is important that the two systems not be confused in the course of management of labor.

Detection of Ruptured Membranes

The pregnant woman should be instructed during the antepartum period to be aware of leakage of fluid from the vagina and to report such an occurrence promptly. Rupture of the membranes is significant for three reasons: First, if the presenting part is not fixed in the pelvis, the possibility of prolapse of the cord and cord compression is greatly increased. Second, labor is likely to occur soon if the pregnancy is at or near term. Third, if the fetus remains in utero upward of 24 hours or more after the rupture of the membranes, there is likelihood of serious intrauterine infection.

A firm diagnosis of rupture of the membranes is not always easy to make unless amnionic fluid is seen or felt escaping from the cervical os by the examiner. Although several diagnostic tests for the detection of ruptured membranes have been recommended, none is completely reliable. Perhaps the most widely employed procedures involve testing the acidity or alkalinity of the vaginal fluid. The basis for these tests is the fact that normally the pH of the vaginal secretion ranges between 4.5 and 5.5, whereas that of the amnionic fluid is usually 7.0 to 7.5.

Nitrazine Test

The use of the indicator nitrazine for the diagnosis of ruptured membranes was first suggested by Baptisi (1938) and is a simple and fairly reliable method. Test papers are impregnated with the dye, and the color of the reaction is interpreted by comparison with a standard color chart. The pH of the vaginal secretion is estimated by inserting a sterile cotton-tipped applicator deeply into the vagina and then touching it to a strip of the nitrazine paper and comparing the color of the paper with the chart. Color changes are interpreted as follows:

Probably Intact Membranes

- Yellow   pH 5.0
- Olive-yellow   pH 5.5
- Olive-green   pH 6.0

Ruptured Membranes

- Blue-green   pH 6.5
- Blue-gray   pH 7.0
- Deep-blue   pH 7.5

Baptisi (1938) pointed out that a false reading is likely to be encountered in women with intact membranes who have an unusually large amount of bloody show, since blood, like amnionic fluid, is not acidic. A more extended study of the nitrazine test by a slightly different technique was made by Abe (1940), who found the nitrazine test to be correct in 98.9 percent of women with known rupture of membranes and in 96.2 percent of women with intact membranes. In clinical practice, however, these tests will not yield such accurate results because they are used in questionable cases in which the amount of fluid is small and therefore more susceptible to a change in pH by admixed blood and vaginal secretions.

OTHER ADMITTANCE PROCEDURES

Vital Signs and Review of Pregnancy Record

The maternal blood pressure, temperature, pulse, and respiratory rate are checked for any abnormality, and these are recorded. The Pregnancy Record is promptly reviewed to identify complications. Any problems identified previously during the antepartum period, as well as any that were anticipated, should be prominently displayed in the Pregnancy Record, along with the plan of management.

Preparation of Vulva and Perineum

The woman is placed on a bedpan with her legs widely separated. While washing the region, the attendant holds a sponge to the woman's introitus to prevent wash water from running into the vagina. Scrubbing is directed from above downward and away from the introitus. Attention should be paid to careful cleansing of the vulvar folds during this procedure. As the scrub sponge passes over the anal region, it is discarded immediately. In many hospitals the hair on the lower half of the vulva and the perineum is removed either by shaving or by clipping.

Vaginal Versus Rectal Examinations

Ideally, after the vulvar and perineal regions have been prepared properly, and the examiner has donned sterile gloves, the thumb and forefinger of one hand separate the labia widely to expose the vaginal opening and prevent the examining fingers from coming in contact with the inner surfaces of the labia. The index and second fingers of the other hand are then introduced into the vagina (Fig. 16–1A–C). During vaginal examination, a precise routine of evaluation as described in the section on Admittance Vaginal Examination should be followed. It is important not to withdraw the fingers from the vagina until the examination is completed.

Rectal examinations were once considered to be much safer than vaginal because they were less likely to carry bacteria from the introitus into the cervix and then the uterus. A vaginal examination, *properly performed with appropriate preparation and care,* is probably not much more likely than a rectal examination to carry pathogenic bacteria through the dilating cervix into the uterus. In spite of past reports that vaginal examinations during labor do not contribute to morbidity, clinical experience in certain circumstances strongly supports the opposite view, especially in cases of early rupture of the membranes followed by repeated vaginal examinations casually performed by multiple examiners.

Enema

Early in labor, a cleansing enema is generally given to minimize subsequent contamination by feces, which otherwise may be a problem, especially during delivery. A ready-to-use enema solution of sodium phosphates in a disposable container (Fleet enema) has proved satisfactory at Parkland Hospital. Enemas are not used to stimulate labor.

Laboratory

When the woman is admitted in labor, most often the hematocrit, or hemoglobin concentration, should be rechecked. The hematocrit can be measured easily and quickly. Blood may be collected in a plain tube from which a heparinized capillary tube is filled immediately. By employing a small microhematocrit centrifuge in the labor-delivery unit, the value can be obtained in 3 minutes. A labeled tube of blood is allowed to clot and is kept on hand for blood group and screen, if needed, or otherwise used for routine serology. A voided urine specimen, as free as possible of debris, is examined for protein and glucose.

MANAGEMENT OF THE FIRST STAGE OF LABOR

As soon as possible after admittance, the remainder of the general physical examination is completed. The physician can reach a conclusion about the normalcy of the pregnancy only when all the examinations have been completed. The physician must then draw upon the information obtained from these results, as well as all information previously compiled during the antepartum period. A rational plan for monitoring labor can then be established based on the needs of the fetus and the mother. If no abnormality is identified or suspected, the mother should be

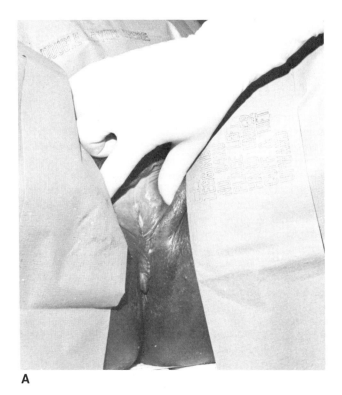

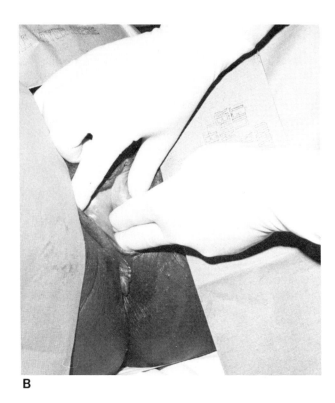

Figure 16–1. A. Vaginal examination. The labia are separated with a sterile gloved hand. B. Vaginal examination. The first and second fingers of the other sterile gloved hand are carefully inserted through the introitus.

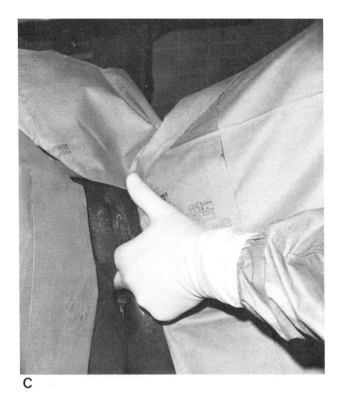

Figure 16–1. C. During vaginal examination, the fourth and fifth fingers should not contact the anus.

assured that all is well. Although the average duration of the first stage of labor in nulliparous women is about 8 hours and in parous women about 5 hours, there is marked individual variation. Most often, therefore, any precise statement as to the duration of her labor is unwise. Obstetricians and others who venture to make precise statements will find that their predictions are likely to be faulty and the mother and family are made more anxious needlessly.

MONITORING FETAL WELL-BEING DURING LABOR

The word *monitor* currently is equated in the minds of some only with continuous electronic recording of the fetal heart rate and intrauterine pressures. The desirability, let alone the necessity, of electronic monitoring for *all* labors has certainly not been established, as will be discussed subsequently.

It is mandatory, however, that for a good pregnancy outcome, a well-defined program be established that provides careful surveillance of the well-being of both the mother and the fetus. All observations must be appropriately recorded. The frequency, intensity, and duration of uterine contractions, and the response of the fetal heart rate to the contractions, are of considerable concern. These features can be promptly evaluated in logical sequence.

Fetal Heart Rate

The heart rate of the fetus may be identified with a suitable stethoscope or any of a variety of Doppler ultrasonic devices (Fig. 16–2A, B). Changes in the fetal heart rate that are most likely to be ominous almost always are detectable immediately after a uterine contraction. Therefore, it is imperative that the

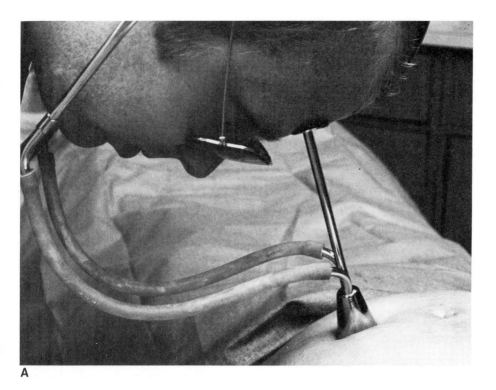

A

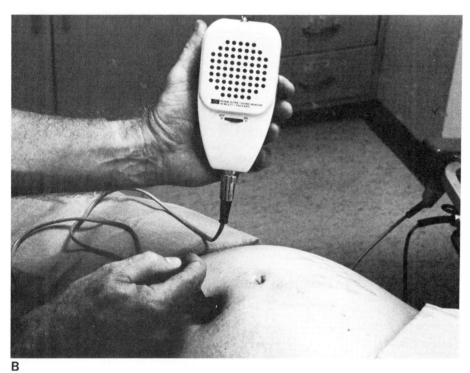

B

Figure 16–2. A. Monitoring the fetal heart rate with a DeLee–Hillis fetoscope. The bell of the stethoscope is firmly applied to the uterine wall to improve the transmission of sound. **B.** Monitoring the fetal heart rate by use of ultrasound and the Doppler effect. The transducer may be held in an appropriate place on the abdomen by a comfortable rubber strap, yet allow the mother to be free to move about.

fetal heart be monitored by auscultation immediately after a contraction. To avoid confusing maternal and fetal heart actions, the maternal pulse should be counted as the fetal heart rate is counted. Otherwise, maternal tachycardia may be misinterpreted as a normal fetal heart rate.

Fetal distress, i.e., loss of fetal well-being, is suspected if the fetal heart rate immediately after a contraction is repeatedly below 120 per minute. Fetal distress very likely exists if the rate is heard to be less than 100 per minute, even though there is recovery to a rate in the 120 to 160 range before the next contraction. When decelerations of this magnitude are found after a contraction, the fetus may be in jeopardy and further labor, if allowed, is often best monitored electronically, as described in Chapter 15.

The appropriate frequency of fetal heart rate auscultation is not known. In the 17th edition of this book, auscultation every 15 minutes was recommended; however, this is impractical with less than one-to-one nursing. In a subsequent study at Parkland

Hospital, Leveno and associates (1986) showed in low-risk pregnancies that auscultation at least every 30 minutes resulted in perinatal outcomes similar to those obtained with continuous electronic fetal monitoring. As emphasized by the American College of Obstetricians and Gynecologists (1988), there is no evidence that listening at intervals longer than every 15 minutes is deleterious. Thus, during the first stage of labor, in the absence of any abnormalities, the fetal heart is best checked immediately after a contraction at least every 30 minutes. For women with pregnancies at high risk, most recommend continuous electronic monitoring; however, intermittent auscultation every 15 minutes during the first stage is an acceptable alternative.

> The findings of the study by Benson and associates (1968) have been quoted widely as evidence that auscultation of the fetal heart during labor is unreliable for detecting fetal distress save in an extreme degree. Their study by design ignored the determination of the fetal heart rate for at least the first 30 seconds after a contraction, a critical period for identifying ominous decelerations (see Chap. 15, p. 298). Moreover, the protocol for evaluating the fetal heart every 15 minutes during the first stage of labor and every 5 minutes during the second stage frequently was not followed.

Uterine Contractions

The examiner with the palm of the hand lightly on the uterus determines the time of onset of the contraction. The intensity of the contraction is gauged from the degree of firmness the uterus achieves. At the acme of effective contractions, the finger or thumb cannot readily indent the uterus. Next, the time that the contraction disappears is noted. This sequence is repeated in order to evaluate the frequency, duration, and intensity of uterine contractions. It is inappropriate simply to describe ongoing uterine contractions, or labor, as "good." "Good" uterine contractions can be identified only retrospectively—that is, if the contractions produced orderly effacement and dilatation of the cervix with descent of the presenting part followed by uncomplicated delivery of an uncompromised infant.

Attendance in Labor

Ideally, the person who performs these measurements is able to remain with the mother throughout labor to provide psychological support as well as to discern promptly any fetal or maternal abnormalities. Haverkamp and co-workers (1976, 1979) demonstrated that an equally satisfactory outcome for the fetus can be achieved without continuous electronic monitoring of the fetal heart rate, continuous intrauterine pressure recording, and fetal scalp blood pH measurement *if the mother and fetus are closely attended by appropriately trained labor room personnel.*

The concept that universal electronic fetal monitoring will not improve pregnancy outcome was confirmed by Leveno and co-workers (1986) in a prospective comparison of selective versus universal electronic fetal monitoring in 34,995 pregnancies delivered at Parkland Hospital. Pregnancy outcomes in which universal electronic fetal monitoring was used (13,956 of 17,586 women, or 79 percent) were compared to those in which selective electronic monitoring was used when the fetus was judged to be at high risk (6,420 of 17,409 women, or 37 percent). Major risk factors included oxytocin stimulation of labor, dysfunctional labor, abnormalities of the fetal heart rate, or meconium-stained amnionic fluid. In alternate months, either 7 ("selective monitoring") or 19 ("universal monitoring") fetal monitors were made available in the delivery unit. Perinatal outcomes as reflected by

intrapartum fetal deaths, low Apgar scores, assisted ventilation of the neonates, admissions to the neonatal intensive care unit, and incidence of neonatal seizures were not significantly different between the two groups (Table 16–1). There was, however, a small but significantly increased incidence of cesarean sections for fetal distress in the low-risk women who were universally monitored compared to those selectively monitored (Table 16–2). These authors stressed that many women judged to be at low risk at the onset of labor subsequently were assigned to a high-risk category and thus were electronically monitored. They concluded that clinical monitoring is mandatory for all laboring women, and that this type of "screening" procedure for fetuses considered to be at low risk was as efficacious as universal electronic fetal monitoring.

Given a choice, most women probably would prefer the reassurance of the nearly continuous presence of the obstetrician or of a compassionate well-trained obstetrical associate to that of a metal cabinet and its wires and tubes that invade her and her fetus. However, because of the ease of operation, the constant threat of legal action, and simply because the trend to continuous electronic fetal monitoring has become almost an accepted reality, it seems highly unlikely that there will be less continuous electronic fetal monitoring. It is important to note, however, that the monitor itself is not a mystical talisman. Electronic monitors are merely extensions of doctors' and nurses' eyes and hands. All information obtained from these mechanical devices are of no value unless processed through the human brain in a timely and appropriate fashion. **Simply stated, the physician or nurse must be present to interpret the information gathered from electronic monitors.** There is no reason, in most instances, why the machine and health care providers cannot be combined to provide a safe and a compassionate environment for the laboring woman.

MATERNAL MONITORING AND MANAGEMENT DURING LABOR

Maternal Position During Labor

The normal mother and fetus need not be confined to bed early in labor prior to use of analgesia. A comfortable chair may be beneficial psychologically and perhaps physiologically. In bed, the mother should be allowed to assume the position she finds most comfortable, which will be lateral recumbency most of the time. She must not be restricted to lying supine.

TABLE 16–1. COMPARISON OF TYPES OF OUTCOME THAT SUGGESTED FETAL ASPHYXIA IN SELECTIVE-MONITORING MONTHS AND UNIVERSAL-MONITORING MONTHS

Outcome[a]	Selective Monitoring	Universal Monitoring
Fetuses alive upon admission to labor and delivery	17,410	17,641
Fetal deaths in labor and delivery (≥ 500 g)	25 (1.4/1,000)	30 (1.7/1,000)
Assisted ventilation of neonate	1,259 (7.2%)	1,315 (7.5%)
5-minute Apgar score ≤ 5	293 (1.7%)	296 (1.7%)
Neonates admitted to intensive care nursery	(428 (2.5%))	460 (2.6%)
Neonates with seizures	45 (2.6/1,000)	53 (3.0/1,000)

[a] Any differences in outcome between groups are not significant.
Modified from Leveno and co-workers: N Engl J Med 315:615, 1986.

TABLE 16–2. MATERNAL AND NEONATAL OUTCOMES WITH SELECTIVE VERSUS UNIVERSAL MONITORING IN 14,618 LOW-RISK PREGNANCIES[a]

Outcome	Selective Monitoring (N = 7,330) No. (%)	Universal Monitoring (N = 7,288) No. (%)	p Value[b]
Abnormal fetal heart rate	196 (2.7)	551 (7.6)	< 0.01
Cesarean section for fetal distress	28 (0.4)	64 (0.9)	< 0.01
Intrapartum fetal deaths	None	None	NS
Neonatal deaths	5 (0.1)	4 (0.1)	NS
Assisted ventilation of newborn	102 (1.4)	119 (1.6)	NS
5-minute Apgar score ≤ 5	14 (0.2)	18 (0.2)	NS
Admission to intensive care nursery	17 (0.2)	25 (0.3)	NS
Neonates with seizures	3 (0.04)	1 (0.01)	NS

[a] Low-risk defined as single fetus in cephalic presentation; spontaneous, uncomplicated labor; and birthweight more than 2,500 g.
[b] NS = not significant.
Modified from Leveno and co-workers: N Engl J Med 315:615, 1986.

Subsequent Vaginal Examinations

During the first stage of labor, the need for subsequent vaginal examinations to identify the status of the cervix and the station and position of the presenting part will vary considerably. When the membranes rupture, the examination should be repeated immediately if the fetal head was not definitely engaged at the previous vaginal examination. In any event, the fetal heart rate should be checked immediately and during the next uterine contraction to help detect cord compression.

Analgesia

Most often, analgesia is initiated on the basis of the woman's discomfort, a uterine contraction pattern of established labor, and cervical dilatation of at least 2 cm. The kinds of analgesia, the amounts, and the frequency of administration should be based on the need to allay pain on the one hand and the likelihood of delivering a depressed infant on the other (see Chap. 17, p. 328).

The timing, the method of administration, and the size of initial and subsequent doses of systemically acting analgesic agents are based to a considerable degree on the anticipated interval of time until delivery. A repeat vaginal examination is often appropriate, therefore, before administering more analgesia. With the onset of symptoms characteristic of the second stage of labor, that is, an urge to bear down or "push," the status of the cervix and the presenting part should be reevaluated.

Maternal Vital Signs

The mother's temperature, blood pressure, and pulse are evaluated every 1 to 2 hours. The blood pressure is taken between contractions. The blood pressure normally rises during a contraction (Kjeldsen, 1979). If membranes have been ruptured for many hours before the onset of labor, or if there is a borderline elevation, the temperature should be checked hourly during labor. Moreover, with prolonged rupture of the membranes, the pregnancy should be considered to be at high risk.

Amniotomy

If the membranes are intact, there is great temptation even during normal labor to perform amniotomy. The presumed ben-

efits are more rapid labor, earlier detection of instances of meconium staining of amnionic fluid, and the opportunity to apply an electrode to the fetus and insert a pressure catheter into the uterine cavity. Rosen and Peisner (1987) reported that *spontaneous* rupture of the membranes during labor was followed by a shorter duration of labor when compared to *artificial* rupture or no rupture. When membranes were artifically ruptured, there was a slightly shorter labor than recorded with intact membranes. Amniotomy may shorten the length of labor slightly but there is no evidence that shorter labor is necessarily beneficial to the fetus or to the mother. Indeed, the reverse may be true (Caldeyro-Barcia and associates, 1974). If amniotomy is performed, aseptic technique should be attempted and the fetal head must not be dislodged from the pelvis to hasten the escape of amnionic fluid; to do so invites prolapse of the umbilical cord.

Oral Intake

In essentially all circumstances, food and oral fluids should be withheld during active labor and delivery. Gastric emptying time is remarkably prolonged once labor is established and analgesics are administered. As a consequence, ingested food and most medications remain in the stomach and are not absorbed, but they can be vomited and aspirated (see Chap. 17, p. 331).

Intravenous Fluids

Although it has become customary in many hospitals to establish an intravenous infusion system routinely early in labor, there is seldom any real need for such in the normally pregnant woman at least until analgesia is administered. An intravenous infusion system is advantageous during the immediate puerperium in order to administer oxytocin prophylactically and at times therapeutically when uterine atony persists. Moreover, with longer labors the administration of glucose, some salt, and water to the otherwise fasting woman at the rate of 60 to 120 mL per hour is efficacious to combat dehydration and acidosis.

Urinary Bladder Function

Bladder distension must be avoided, since it can lead both to obstructed labor and to subsequent bladder hypotonia and infection. In the course of each abdominal examination, the suprapubic region should be palpated in order to detect a filling bladder. If the bladder is readily palpated above the symphysis, the woman should be encouraged to void. At times she can ambulate with assistance to a toilet and successfully void, even though she could not void on a bedpan. If the bladder is distended and she cannot void, catheterization is indicated. It is likely, however, to be less traumatic to catheterize again during labor, if needed, than to leave an indwelling catheter in place.

ACTIVE MANAGEMENT OF LABOR

As the cesarean delivery rate began to increase during the 1970s, O'Driscoll and colleagues (1984) proposed that their active labor management scheme described as early as 1970 would decrease this trend. Active management, at least as defined by the Irish investigators, includes artificial amniotomy upon detection of painful uterine contractions accompanied by passage of blood-stained mucus or complete cervical effacement regardless of dilatation. Afterwards, frequent cervical examinations are made and oxytocin is given if cervical dilatation does not progress at least 1 cm per hour. Oxytocin administration is more aggressive than described in Chapter 18, and 6 mU per minute are infused initially. If necessary, this is increased by 6 mU per minute every 15 minutes, not to exceed 40 mU per minute. While this plan was associated with a very low cesarean delivery rate in nulliparas—about 5 percent—there was a sevenfold increased incidence of intrapartum fetal death and a twofold increased incidence of infants with seizures when compared to contemporaneous obstetrical data from Parkland Hospital (Leveno and colleagues, 1985). Thorp and associates (1988) reported no adverse perinatal effects of high-dose oxytocin given to 612 nulliparas.

While Turner (1988) and Akoury (1988) and their co-workers were able to decrease the primary cesarean section rate with such management, Cohen and associates (1987) reported no differences in two populations randomly assigned to routine versus active management. If the primary section rate is 30 percent, then we agree with Boylan and Frankowski (1986) that active intervention may be successful in lowering it.

MANAGEMENT OF SECOND STAGE

IDENTIFICATION

With full dilatation of the cervix, which signifies the onset of the second stage of labor, the woman typically begins to bear down and with descent of the presenting part she develops the urge to defecate. Uterine contractions and the accompanying expulsive forces may last 1½ minutes and recur at times after a myometrial resting phase of no more than a minute.

DURATION

The median duration of the second stage (from complete dilatation of the cervix to delivery) is 50 minutes in nulliparas and 20 minutes in multiparas, but it can be highly variable. In a woman of higher parity with a stretched vagina and perineum, two or three expulsive efforts after the cervix is fully dilated may suffice to complete the delivery of the infant. Conversely, in a woman with a contracted pelvis or a large fetus, or with impaired expulsive efforts from conduction analgesia or intense sedation, the second stage may become abnormally long.

Fetal Heart Rate

For the low-risk fetus, the heart rate should be auscultated at least every 15 minutes, whereas in those at high risk, 5-minute intervals are recommended (American College of Obstetricians and Gynecologists, 1988). Slowing of the fetal heart rate induced by head compression is common during a contraction and the accompanying maternal expulsive efforts. If recovery of the fetal heart rate is prompt after the contraction and expulsive efforts cease, labor is allowed to continue. Not all instances of slowing of the fetal heart during the second stage of labor are the consequence of head compression, however. The vigorous force generated within the uterus by its contraction and by the woman's expulsive efforts may reduce placental perfusion appreciably. Descent of the fetus through the birth canal and the consequent reduction in uterine volume may trigger some degree of premature separation of the placenta, with further compromise of fetal well-being. Descent of the fetus is more likely to tighten a loop or loops of umbilical cord around the fetus, especially the neck, sufficiently to obstruct umbilical blood flow. Prolonged, uninterrupted expulsive efforts by the mother can be dangerous to the fetus in this circumstance. Maternal tachycardia, which is common during the second stage, must not be mistaken for a normal fetal heart rate.

Maternal Expulsive Efforts

In most cases, bearing down is reflex and spontaneous in the second stage of labor, but occasionally the woman does not employ her expulsive forces to good advantage and coaching is desirable. Her legs should be half-flexed so that she can push with them against the mattress. Instructions should be to take a deep breath as soon as the next uterine contraction begins and, with her breath held, to exert downward pressure exactly as though she were straining at stool. She should not be encouraged to "push" beyond the time of completion of each uterine contraction. Instead, she and her fetus should be allowed to rest and recover from the combined effects of the uterine contraction, breath holding, and considerable physical effort.

Usually, bearing down efforts are rewarded by increasing bulging of the perineum—that is, by further descent of the fetal head. The mother should be informed of such progress, for encouragement at this stage is very important. During this period of active bearing down, the fetal heart rate auscultated immediately after the contraction is likely to be slow but should recover to normal range before the next expulsive effort.

As the head descends through the pelvis, small particles of feces are frequently expelled by the mother. As they appear at the anus, they should be sponged downward, away from the vagina, with large pledgets soaked in diluted soap solution. As the head descends still farther, the perineum begins to bulge and the overlying skin becomes tense and glistening. Now the scalp of the fetus may be visible through the vulvar opening (Fig. 16–3). At this time, or before in instances where little perineal resistance to expulsion is anticipated, the woman and her fetus are prepared for delivery.

Preparation for Delivery

Actual delivery of the fetus can be accomplished with the mother in a variety of positions. The most widely used and often the most satisfactory one is the dorsal lithotomy position on a delivery table with leg supports. In placing the legs in leg-holders, care should be taken not to separate the legs too widely or place one leg higher than the other. The popliteal

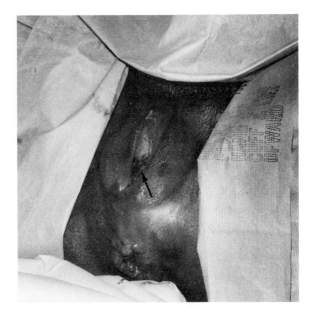

Figure 16–3. Scalp (arrow) appearing at vulva during a contraction.

region should rest comfortably in the proximal portion and the heel in the distal portion of the leg-holder. Too often the leg is forced to conform to the existing setting. Cramps in the leg may develop in the second stage of labor in part because of pressure by the fetal head on nerves in the pelvis. Such cramps may be relieved by changing the position of the leg or by brief massage, but leg cramps should never be ignored.

No one should be permitted in the delivery room without a scrub suit, a mask covering both nose and mouth, and a cap that completely covers the hair. Preparation for actual delivery entails thorough vulvar and perineal scrubbing and covering with sterile drapes in such a way that only the immediate area about the vulva is exposed (Fig. 16–4A, B).

Scrubbing and Gloving

Since sterile rubber gloves are punctured easily or tear occasionally, the necessity for meticulously cleaning the hands before putting on gloves is apparent. Even with these precautions, the possibility of disseminating bacteria within the genital tract is not eliminated entirely, since the organisms may be carried up from the vaginal outlet by the gloved finger.

In the past, the major reason for care in scrubbing, gowning, and gloving was to protect the laboring woman from the introduction of infectious agents. Although this reason remains valid, concern today also must be extended to the health-care providers, because of the threat of exposure to the lethal *human immunodeficiency virus*. Recommendations for protection of those who care for women during labor and delivery are summarized in Chapter 39, (p. 858).

SPONTANEOUS DELIVERY

DELIVERY OF THE HEAD

With each contraction, the perineum bulges increasingly and the vulvovaginal opening becomes more and more dilated by the fetal head (Fig. 16–5), gradually forming an ovoid and finally an almost circular opening. With the cessation of each contraction, the opening becomes smaller as the head recedes. As the head becomes increasingly visible, the vaginal outlet and vulva are stretched further until they ultimately encircle the

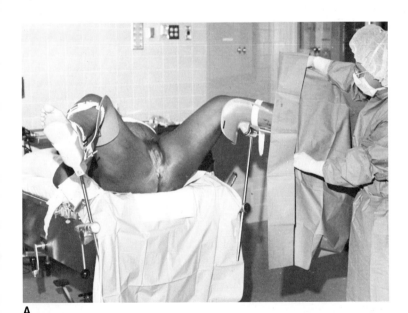

A

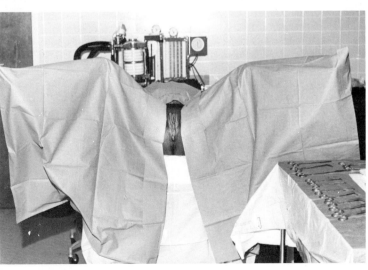

B

Figure 16–4. A. The vulva, perineum, and adjacent regions have been thoroughly scrubbed. Sterile disposable drapes are being applied. **B.** The field is sterile-draped in preparation for delivery.

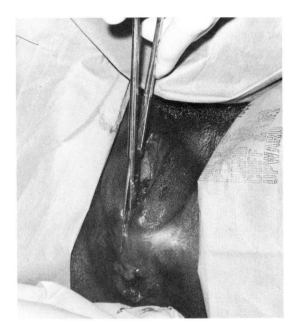

Figure 16–5. Vulva partially distended by fetal head. Midline episiotomy being made.

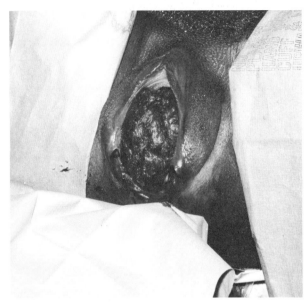

Figure 16–6. Birth of head. The occiput is being kept close to the symphysis by moderate pressure to the fetal chin at the tip of the maternal coccyx.

largest diameter of the baby's head (Fig. 16–6). This encirclement of the largest diameter of the fetal head by the vulvar ring is known as *crowning*.

Unless an episiotomy has been made, as described on page 323, the perineum by now is extremely thin and, in the case of the nulliparous woman especially, is almost at the point of rupture with each contraction. At the same time the anus becomes greatly stretched and protuberant, and the anterior wall

of the rectum may be easily seen through it. Failure to perform an episiotomy by this time invites perineal lacerations and some degree of permanent relaxation of the pelvic floor with its possible sequelae of cystocele, rectocele, and uterine prolapse.

Ritgen Maneuver

By the time the head distends the vulva and perineum during a contraction sufficiently to open the vaginal introitus to a diam-

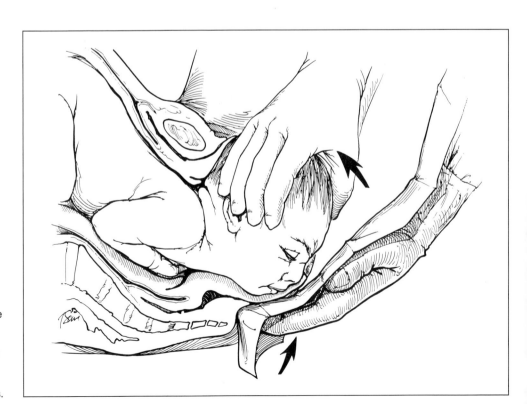

Figure 16–7. Near completion of the delivery of the fetal head by the modified Ritgen maneuver. Moderate upward pressure is applied to the fetal chin by the posterior hand covered with a sterile towel while the suboccipital region of the fetal head is held against the symphysis.

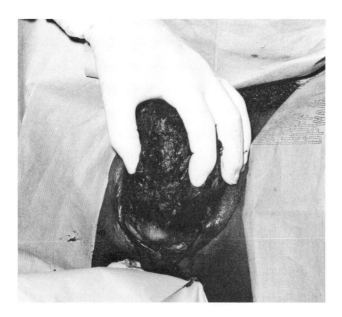

Figure 16–8. Pressure is applied through the towel covering the hand to the underside of the chin of the infant as soon as the occiput is beyond the symphysis. This extends the head. At the same time, the fingers of the other hand simultaneously elevate the scalp to help extend the head.

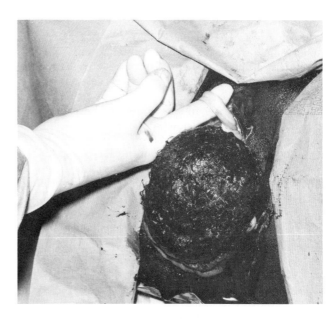

Figure 16–10. Cord identified around the neck. It readily slipped over the head.

eter of 5 cm or so, it is desirable to drape a towel over one gloved hand to protect it from the anus and then exert forward pressure on the chin of the fetus through the perineum just in front of the coccyx, while the other hand exerts pressure superiorly against the occiput (Fig. 16–7). Although this maneuver is simpler than that originally described by Ritgen (1855), it is customarily designated the Ritgen maneuver, or the modified Ritgen maneuver. It allows the physician to control the delivery of the head. It also favors extension, so that the head is delivered with its smallest diameters passing through the introitus and over the perineum (Fig. 16–8). The head is delivered slowly with the base

of the occiput rotating around the lower margin of the symphysis pubis as a fulcrum, while the bregma (anterior fontanel), brow, and face pass successively over the perineum (Fig. 16–9).

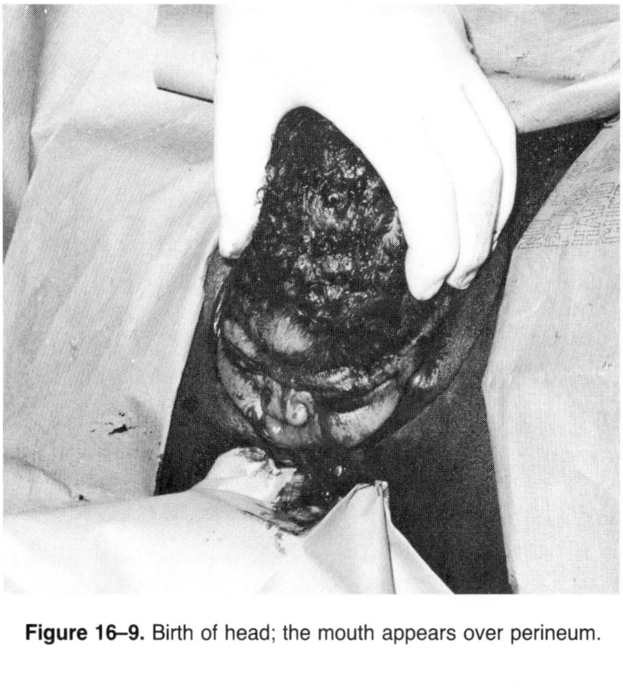

Clearing the Nasopharynx

To minimize the likelihood of aspiration of amnionic fluid debris and blood that might occur once the thorax is delivered and the infant can inspire, the face is quickly wiped and the nares and mouth are aspirated as demonstrated in Figure 12–1 (p. 236).

Nuchal Cord

Next the finger should be passed to the neck of the fetus to ascertain whether it is encircled by one or more coils of the umbilical cord (Fig. 16–10). Coils occur in about 25 percent of cases and ordinarily do no harm. If a coil is felt, it should be drawn down between the fingers and, if loose enough, slipped over the infant's head. If it is applied too tightly to the neck to be slipped over the head, it should be cut between two clamps and the infant delivered promptly.

DELIVERY OF SHOULDERS

After its birth, the head falls posteriorly, bringing the face almost into contact with the anus. As described in Chapter 11, the occiput promptly turns toward one of the maternal thighs so that the head assumes a transverse position. The successive movements of restitution and external rotation indicate that the bisacromial diameter (transverse diameter of the thorax) has rotated into the anterioposterior diameter of the pelvis.

In most cases, the shoulders appear at the vulva just after external rotation and are born spontaneously. Occasionally, a delay occurs and immediate extraction may appear advisable. In that event, the sides of the head are grasped with the two hands and *gentle* downward traction applied until the anterior shoulder appears under the pubic arch. Then, by an upward movement, the posterior shoulder is delivered and the anterior

Figure 16–9. Birth of head; the mouth appears over perineum.

shoulder usually drops down from beneath the symphysis. An equally effective method entails completion of delivery of the anterior shoulder before that of the posterior (Fig. 16–11).

The rest of the body almost always follows the shoulders without difficulty, but in case of prolonged delay its birth may be hastened by *moderate* traction on the head and moderate pressure on the uterine fundus. Hooking the fingers in the axillae should be avoided, however, since this may injure the nerves of the upper extremity, producing a transient or possibly even a permanent paralysis. Traction, furthermore, should be exerted only in the direction of the long axis of the infant, for if applied obliquely it causes bending of the neck and excessive stretching of the brachial plexus.

Immediately after extrusion of the infant, there is usually a gush of amnionic fluid, often tinged with blood but not grossly bloody.

CLAMPING THE CORD

The umbilical cord is cut between two clamps such as pean clamps placed 4 or 5 cm from the fetal abdomen, and later an umbilical cord clamp is applied 2 or 3 cm from the fetal abdomen. A plastic clamp that is safe, efficient, easy to sterilize, and fairly inexpensive is shown in Figure 16–12.

Timing of Cord Clamping

If after delivery the infant is placed at the level of the vaginal introitus or below and the fetoplacental circulation is not immediately occluded by clamping the cord, as much as 100 mL of blood may be shifted from the placenta to the infant.

Yao and Lind (1969, 1974) measured the residual volume of placental blood in response to positioning the infant at precisely measured distances above or below the introitus for varying periods of time before clamping the cord. They observed that placing the infant within 10 cm above or below the introitus for 3 minutes before clamping the cord resulted in the shift of about 80 mL of blood from the placenta to the infant. Lowering the newborn to 40 cm below the introitus for only 30 seconds before clamping effected the same degree of transfer. If the infant was held at 50 or 60 cm above the introitus, however, transfer of blood to the infant was negligible even after 3 minutes.

One benefit to be derived from placental transfusion is the fact that the hemoglobin in 80 mL of placental blood that shifts to the fetus eventually provides about 50 mg of iron to the infant's stores and no doubt reduces the frequency of iron-deficiency anemia later in infancy. In the presence of accelerated destruction of erythrocytes, as occurs with maternal alloimmunization, the bilirubin formed from the added erythrocytes con-

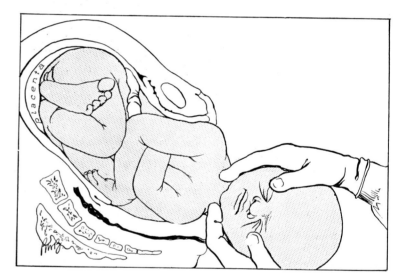

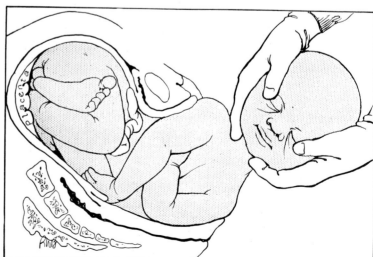

Figure 16–11. *Gentle* downward traction to bring about descent of anterior shoulder (top). Delivery of anterior shoulder completed; *gentle* upward traction to deliver the posterior shoulder (bottom).

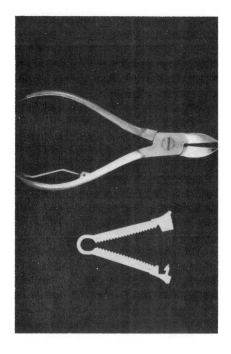

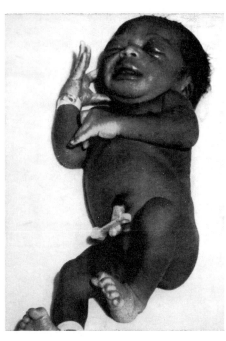

Figure 16–12. Plastic cord clamp. These clamps lock in place and cannot slip. They are removed on the second or third day simply by cutting the plastic at the loop, or they can be allowed to drop off with the cord.

tributes further to the danger of hyperbilirubinemia (see Chap. 33, p. 603). Although theoretically the risk of circulatory overloading from gross hypervolemia is formidable, especially in preterm infants, the addition of placental blood to the infant's circulation does not ordinarily cause difficulty. Exceptions include the growth-retarded fetus (Chap. 38, p. 773) or one of a diabetic mother (Perrine and associates, 1986) in whom polycythemia may be a serious complication.

Our policy is to clamp the cord after first thoroughly clearing the infant's airway, all of which usually takes about 30 seconds. The infant is not elevated above the introitus at vaginal delivery nor much above the maternal abdominal wall at cesarean section. The cord is then clamped.

MANAGEMENT OF THE THIRD STAGE

Immediately after delivery of the infant, the height of the uterine fundus and its consistency are ascertained. As long as the uterus remains firm and there is no unusual bleeding, watchful waiting until the placenta is separated is the usual practice. No massage is practiced; the hand is simply rested on the fundus frequently, to make certain that the organ does not become atonic and filled with blood behind a separated placenta.

SIGNS OF PLACENTAL SEPARATION

Since attempts to express the placenta prior to its separation are futile and possibly dangerous, it is most important that the following signs of placental separation be recognized:

1. The uterus becomes globular and, as a rule, firmer. This sign is the earliest to appear.
2. There is often a sudden gush of blood.
3. The uterus rises in the abdomen because the placenta, having separated, passes down into the lower uterine segment and vagina, where its bulk pushes the uterus upward.

4. The umbilical cord protrudes farther out of the vagina, indicating that the placenta has descended.

These signs sometimes appear within about a minute after delivery of the infant and usually within 5 minutes. When the placenta has separated, the physician first ascertains that the uterus is firmly contracted. The mother, if she is not anesthetized, may be asked to bear down, and the intraabdominal pressure so produced may be adequate to expel the placenta. If these efforts fail, or if spontaneous expulsion is not possible because of anesthesia, the physician, again having made certain that the uterus is contracted firmly, exerts pressure with the hand on the fundus to propel the detached placenta into the vagina, as depicted and described in Figure 16–13.

DELIVERY OF THE PLACENTA

Placental expression should never be forced before placental separation lest the uterus be turned inside out. *Inversion of the uterus* is one of the grave accidents associated with delivery (see Chap. 24, p. 422). As pressure is applied to the body of the uterus (Fig. 16–13), the umbilical cord is kept slightly taut. The uterus is lifted cephalad with the abdominal hand. This maneuver is repeated until the placenta reaches the introitus.

Traction on the cord, however, must not be used to pull the placenta out of the uterus. As the placenta passes through the introitus, pressure on the uterus is stopped. The placenta is then gently lifted away from the introitus (Fig. 16–14). Care is taken to prevent the membranes from being torn off and left behind. If the membranes start to tear, they are grasped with a clamp and removed by gentle traction (Fig. 16–15). The placenta should be examined carefully to ascertain whether it has been delivered in its entirety from the uterine cavity.

Manual Removal of Placenta

If at any time there is brisk bleeding and the placenta cannot be delivered by these techniques, manual removal of the placenta is indicated, with safeguards described in Chapter 24 (p. 417).

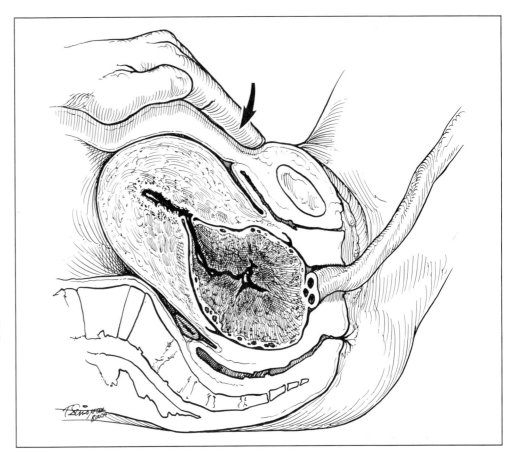

Figure 16–13. Expression of placenta. Note that the hand is *not* trying to push the fundus of the uterus through the birth canal! As the placenta leaves the uterus and enters the vagina, the uterus is elevated by the hand on the abdomen (arrow) while the cord is held in position. The mother can aid in the delivery of the placenta by bearing down. As the placenta reaches the perineum the cord is lifted, which, in turn, lifts the placenta out of the vagina. Adherent membranes are eased away from thin attachments so as to prevent their being torn off and retained in the birth canal.

Occasionally, the placenta will not separate promptly. A question to which there is no definite answer concerns the length of time that should elapse in the absence of bleeding before the placenta is manually removed. Manual removal of the placenta is rightfully practiced much sooner and more often than in the past. In fact, some obstetricians practice routine manual removal of any placenta that has not separated spontaneously by the time they have completed delivery of the infant and care of the cord. The majority, however, do not resort so promptly to manual removal of the placenta, although the procedure must be performed whenever bleeding is excessive.

Routine manual removal of the placenta has proved to be a safe procedure only in the following circumstances: (1) if few vaginal

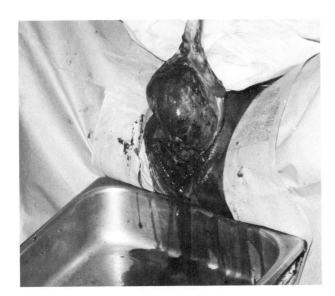

Figure 16–14. The placenta is removed from the vagina by lifting the cord.

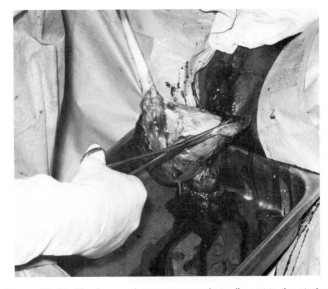

Figure 16–15. Membranes that were somewhat adherent to the uterine lining are separated by gentle traction with a ring forceps.

examinations were performed during labor and if they likely were accompanied by a minimum of bacterial contamination; (2) if the vulva, perineum, and adjacent regions were carefully prepared and draped prior to delivery; (3) if delivery was accomplished without contaminating the genital tract; and (4) if regional or general anesthesia is satisfactory. In other circumstances, since the risks of immediate manual removal of the placenta outweigh the advantages, the procedure should be restricted to instances in which hemorrhage threatens.

"FOURTH STAGE" OF LABOR

The placenta, membranes, and umbilical cord should be examined for completeness and for anomalies, as described in Chapter 31.

The hour immediately following delivery of the placenta is a critical period and has been designated by some obstetricians as the "fourth stage of labor." Even though oxytocics are administered, as described below, postpartum hemorrhage as the result of uterine relaxation is most likely to occur at this time. As emphasized in Chapter 13 (p. 252), it is mandatory that the uterus be evaluated very frequently throughout this period by a competent attendant, who places a hand frequently on the fundus and massages it at the slightest sign of relaxation. At the same time, the vaginal and perineal region is also inspected frequently to allow prompt identification of any excessive bleeding.

OXYTOCIC AGENTS

After the uterus has been emptied and the placenta has been delivered, the primary mechanism by which hemostasis is achieved at the placental site is vasoconstriction produced by a well-contracted myometrium (see Chap. 36, p. 696). Oxytocin (Pitocin, Syntocinon), ergonovine maleate (Ergotrate), and methylergonovine maleate (Methergine) are employed in various ways in the conduct of the third stage of labor, principally to stimulate myometrial contractions and thereby reduce the blood loss.

OXYTOCIN

The synthetic form of the octapeptide oxytocin is commercially available in the United States as Syntocinon and Pitocin; 1 mg of oxytocin is equal to about 500 USP units. Each milliliter of injectable oxytocin contains 10 USP units of oxytocin, which is not effective by mouth. The half-life of intravenously infused oxytocin is very short, perhaps 3 minutes.

Before delivery, the spontaneously laboring uterus is very likely to be exquisitely sensitive to oxytocin. Even with an intravenous dose of a few milliunits per minute, the pregnant uterus may contract so violently as to kill the fetus, rupture itself, or both (see Chap. 18, p. 345). After delivery of the fetus, these dangers no longer exist. Nonetheless, at this time there are other potentially grave dangers from inappropriate use of oxytocin.

Cardiovascular Effects

Deleterious effects may on occasion follow the intravenous injection of a bolus of oxytocin. Hendricks and Brenner (1970), for example, demonstrated with the rapid intravenous injection of 5 units (0.5 mL) of oxytocin that the uterus contracted tetanically for several minutes but maternal blood pressure decreased simultaneously. In one dramatic instance of hypotension from uterine bleeding following delivery of twins, they noted that the injection of 5 units of oxytocin intravenously was followed promptly by a further decrease in blood pressure from 70/42 to 44/26 mm Hg (Fig. 16–16). After rapid administration of 500 mL of saline, the blood pressure increased and the mother again became responsive.

Secher and co-workers (1978) consistently found in healthy women after an intravenous bolus of 10 units of oxytocin a transient but marked fall in arterial blood pressure that was followed rapidly by an abrupt increase in cardiac output. They too concluded that these hemodynamic changes could be dangerous to women whose circulation was already compromised by hypovolemia or who had cardiac disease that limits cardiac output or is complicated by right-to-left shunts. Oxytocin should not, therefore, be given intravenously as a large bolus, but rather as a much more dilute solution by continuous intravenous infusion as described on page 322, or be injected intramuscularly in a dose of 10 units.

Antidiuresis

Another important adverse effect of oxytocin is antidiuresis, caused primarily by reabsorption of free water. Abdul-Karim and Assali (1961) demonstrated clearly that in both pregnant and nonpregnant women oxytocin has considerable antidiuretic activity. In women who are undergoing diuresis in response to the administration of water, the continuous intravenous infusion of 20 mU of oxytocin per minute usually produces a demonstrable decrease in urine flow. When the rate of infusion is

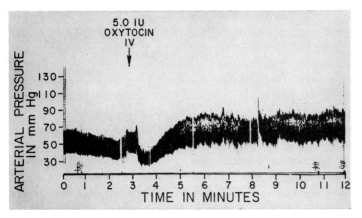

Figure 16–16. Adverse effect of the intravenous bolus of 5 units of oxytocin in a case of postpartum hemorrhage 18 minutes postdelivery. The hypotension worsened to a level of 44/26 mm Hg until saline was infused rapidly. (*From Hendricks and Brenner: Am J Obstet Gynecol 108:751, 1970.*)

raised to 40 mU per minute, urinary flow is strikingly reduced. With doses of this magnitude, it is possible to produce water intoxication if the oxytocin is administered in a large volume of electrolyte-free aqueous dextrose solution (Liggins, 1962; Whalley and Pritchard, 1963; Eggers and Fliegner, 1979).

The hyponatremic, hypoosmotic state is not limited to just the mother. Schwartz and Jones (1978), for example, described convulsions in both the mother and her newborn infant following the administration of 6.5 liters of 5 percent dextrose solution and 36 units of oxytocin predelivery. The concentration of sodium in cord plasma was 114 mEq per L.

In general, if oxytocin is to be administered at a relatively high rate of infusion for a considerable period of time, increasing the concentration of the hormone is preferable to increasing the rate of flow of the more dilute solution. The antidiuretic effect of intravenously administered oxytocin disappears within a few minutes after the infusion is stopped. Oxytocin injected intramuscularly in doses of 5 to 10 units (0.5 to 1 mL) every 15 to 30 minutes also causes antidiuresis, but the possibility of water intoxication is not nearly so great, since large volumes of electrolyte-free aqueous solution are not required as a vehicle (Whalley and Pritchard, 1963).

ERGONOVINE AND METHYLERGONOVINE

Ergonovine is an alkaloid obtained either from ergot, a fungus that grows on rye and some other grains, or synthesized in part from lysergic acid. Methylergonovine is a very similar alkaloid made from lysergic acid. The alkaloids are dispensed as the maleate (Ergotrate and Methergine, respectively) either in solution for parenteral use or in tablets for oral use.

Effects

There is no convincing evidence of any appreciable difference in the actions of ergonovine and methylergonovine; therefore, they will be considered together. Whether given intravenously, intramuscularly, or orally, ergonovine and methylergonovine are powerful stimulants of myometrial contraction, exerting an effect that may persist for hours. The sensitivity of the pregnant uterus to ergonovine and methylergonovine is very great. In pregnant women, an intravenous dose of as little as 0.1 mg, or an oral dose of only 0.25 mg, results in the tetanic contraction that occurs almost immediately after intravenous injection of the drug and within a few minutes after intramuscular or oral administration. Moreover, the response is sustained with little tendency toward relaxation. The tetanic effect of ergonovine and methylergonovine is effective for the prevention and control of postpartum hemorrhage but is very dangerous for the fetus and the mother prior to delivery.

The parenteral administration of these alkaloids, especially by the intravenous route, sometimes initiates transient but severe hypertension. Such a reaction is most likely to occur when conduction analgesia is used for delivery and in women who are prone to develop hypertension. Browning (1974) vividly described four instances of serious side effects postdelivery attributable to 0.5 mg of ergonovine administered intramuscularly. Two women promptly became severely hypertensive, the third became hypertensive and convulsed, and the fourth suffered a cardiac arrest. Because of the frequency of hypertension among our obstetrical population, these alkaloids are not used routinely at Parkland Hospital.

Oxytocics During and After Delivery

Oxytocin, ergonovine, and methylergonovine are all employed widely in the conduct of the normal third stage of labor, but the timing of their administration differs in various institutions. Oxytocin, and especially ergonovine, given before delivery of the placenta will decrease blood loss somewhat. Of considerable concern, the use of oxytocin, and especially ergonovine or methylergonovine, before delivery of the placenta may entrap an undiagnosed and therefore undelivered second twin. This may prove injurious, if not fatal, to the entrapped fetus. In most cases following uncomplicated vaginal delivery, the third stage of labor can be conducted with reasonably small blood loss without using alkaloids of ergot.

If an intravenous infusion is in place, standard practice at Parkland Hospital has been to add 20 units (2 mL) of oxytocin per liter, which is administered after delivery of the placenta at a rate of 10 mL per minute for a few minutes until the uterus remains firmly contracted and the bleeding is controlled. Then the infusion rate is reduced to 1 to 2 mL per minute until the mother is ready for transfer from the recovery suite to the postpartum unit, when the infusion is usually discontinued.

LACERATIONS OF THE BIRTH CANAL

Lacerations of the vagina and perineum are classified as first, second, or third degree. Such lacerations most often are preventable with an appropriate episiotomy and avoidance of midforceps delivery.

First-degree lacerations involve the fourchet, the perineal skin, and vaginal mucous membrane but not the underlying fascia and muscle.

Second-degree lacerations (Fig. 16–17) involve, in addition to

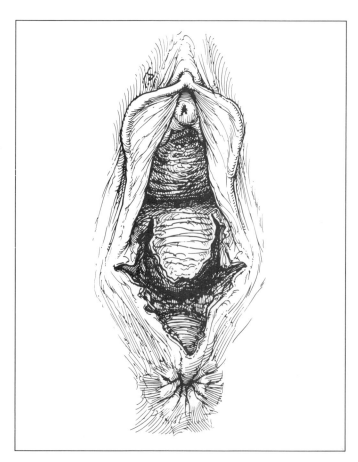

Figure 16–17. Deep second-degree laceration of perineum and vagina.

skin and mucous membrane, the fascia and muscles of the perineal body but not the rectal sphincter. These tears usually extend upward on one or both sides of the vagina, forming an irregular triangular injury.

Third-degree lacerations extend through the skin, mucous membrane, and perineal body, and involve the anal sphincter. Not infrequently, these third-degree lacerations may also extend a distance up the anterior wall of the rectum.

A so-called *fourth-degree laceration* is distinguished by some. This designation is applied to third-degree tears that extend through the rectal mucosa to expose the lumen of the rectum. The term *fourth-degree laceration* will not be used in the ensuing discussion. Instead, when third-degree lacerations with rectal wall extensions are mentioned, they will be so designated. Tears in the region of the urethra are also likely to occur unless an adequate episiotomy is performed, and they may bleed profusely.

Since the repair of perineal tears is virtually the same as that of episiotomy incisions, albeit often less satisfactory because of irregular lines of tissue cleavage, the technique of repairing lacerations is discussed in the following section.

EPISIOTOMY AND REPAIR

Episiotomy, in a strict sense, is incision of the pudenda. Perineotomy is incision of the perineum. In common parlance, however, episiotomy is often used synonymously with perineotomy, a practice that will be followed here. The incision may be made in the midline (median or midline episiotomy), or it may begin in the midline but be directed laterally and downward away from the rectum (mediolateral episiotomy).

PURPOSES OF EPISIOTOMY

Except for cutting the umbilical cord, episiotomy is the most common operation in obstetrics. The reasons for its popularity among obstetricians are clear. It substitutes a straight, neat surgical incision for the ragged laceration that otherwise frequently results. It is easier to repair and heals better than a tear. With mediolateral episiotomy, the likelihood of lacerations into the rectum is reduced.

More recently, the advantages provided by episiotomy have been questioned by some individuals (Thacker and Banta, 1983). One commonly cited but unproven benefit of routine episiotomy is that it prevents pelvic relaxation—that is, cystocele, rectocele, and urinary incontinence. Obviously, if the perineal incision is made at the time of maximal distension, then this benefit might be limited. Gass and colleagues (1986), as well as Thorp and co-workers (1987), recommended that routine episiotomy be reevaluated since it possibly was associated with an increased incidence of anal sphincter and rectal tears. Reynolds and Yudkin (1987) studied nearly 25,000 deliveries at the John Radcliffe Hospital in Oxford, and reported that the episiotomy rate in nulliparas decreased from 73 percent in 1980 to 45 percent in 1984. During this same time, the incidence of second-degree tears increased from 7 to 20 per 1,000, but the incidence of third-degree lacerations was unchanged at about 5 per 1,000.

The important questions for the obstetrician concerning episiotomy are:

1. How long before delivery should it be performed?
2. Should a median or mediolateral incision be made?

3. Should the incision be sutured before or after expulsion of the placenta?
4. What are the best suture materials and technique to employ?

Timing of Episiotomy

If episiotomy is performed unnecessarily early, bleeding from the gaping wound may be considerable during the interim between the incision and the birth of the baby. If episiotomy is performed too late, the muscles of the perineal floor already will have undergone excessive stretching, and one of the objectives of the operation is defeated. It is common practice to perform episiotomy when the head is visible during a contraction to a diameter of 3 to 4 cm (Fig. 16–5).

In this connection, the question arises whether episiotomy should be performed before or after the application of forceps. Application and articulation of forceps with widely separated shanks, as with Simpson forceps, may cause tearing of the introitus (see Chap. 25, p. 426). The application of those with narrow overlapping shanks, such as Tucker McLane forceps, before episiotomy is not likely to be so traumatic. Although it is slightly more awkward to perform episiotomy with the forceps in place, blood loss from the episiotomy is somewhat less with this technique, since immediate traction on the forceps can be exerted, and the resultant tamponade of the perineal floor by the fetal head is effected earlier than could otherwise be achieved.

Midline Versus Mediolateral Episiotomy

The advantages and disadvantages of the two types of episiotomies may be enumerated as follows:

Median Episiotomy

1. Easy to repair
2. Faulty healing rare
3. Less painful in puerperium
4. Dyspareunia rarely follows
5. Anatomical end results almost always excellent
6. Blood loss less
7. Extension through the anal sphincter and into rectum is rather common

Mediolateral Episiotomy

1. More difficult to repair
2. Faulty healing more common
3. Pain in one third of cases for a few days
4. Dyspareunia occasionally follows
5. Anatomical end results more or less faulty in some 10 percent of cases (depending on operator)
6. Blood loss greater
7. Extension through sphincter is uncommon

With proper selection of cases, it is possible to secure the advantages of median episiotomy and at the same time reduce to a minimum its one disadvantage, the greater risk of third-degree extension. The size of the perineal body is related to the likelihood of third-degree laceration, since the accident is naturally more likely if the perineal body is short. The possibility of extension of a median episiotomy into the rectal sphincter is also much greater when the fetus is large, when the occiput is posterior, in midforceps deliveries, and in breech deliveries. It is good practice, in general, to use mediolateral episiotomy in the

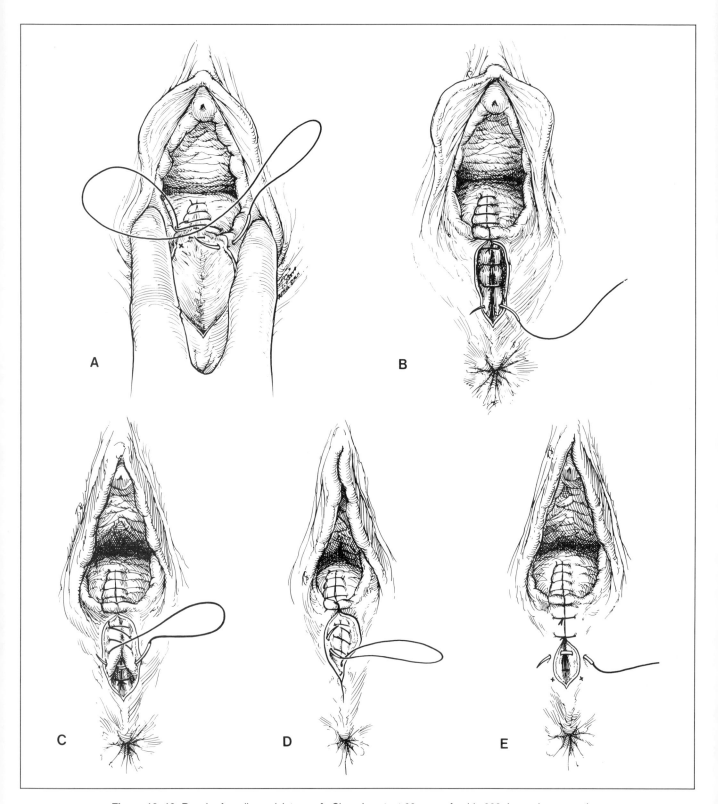

Figure 16–18. Repair of median episiotomy. **A.** Chromic catgut 00, or preferably 000, is used as a continuous suture to close the vaginal mucosa and submucosa. **B.** After closing the vaginal incision and reapproximating the cut margins of the hymenal ring, the suture is tied and cut. Next three or four interrupted sutures of 00 or 000 catgut are placed in the fascia and muscle of the incised perineum. **C.** A continuous suture is now carried downward to unite the superficial fascia. **D.** Completion of repair. The continuous suture is carried upward as a subcuticular stitch. (An alternative method of closure of skin and subcutaneous fascia is illustrated in E.) **E.** Completion of repair of median episiotomy. A few interrupted sutures of 000 chromic catgut are placed through the skin and subcutaneous fascia and loosely tied. This closure avoids burying two layers of catgut in the more superficial layers of the perineum.

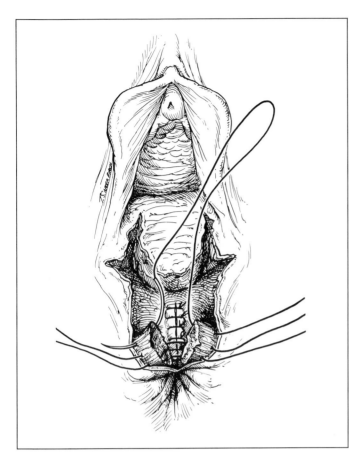

Figure 16–19. Repair of complete perineal tear. The rectal mucosa has been repaired with interrupted, fine chromic catgut sutures. The torn ends of the sphincter ani are next approximated with two or three interrupted chromic catgut sutures. The wound is then repaired, as in a second-degree laceration or an episiotomy.

circumstances mentioned but to employ the median incision otherwise. Even with this selection of cases, however, the total number of third-degree lacerations sustained with this policy is probably greater than with routine mediolateral episiotomy. In any case, sharply pointed scissors should not be used lest they inadvertently penetrate the rectum.

Benyon (1974) described her experiences with a policy of mandatory midline episiotomy. Of 1,166 nulliparas who underwent a midline episiotomy, there was extension through the sphincter with involvement of *the rectum in 8 percent*. The technique of repair was similar to that described below. She emphasized that the episiotomies and repairs were performed primarily by house officers in training. Following repair, there was no special emphasis on bowel action. Suppositories, rectal tubes, and enemas were not allowed and rectal examinations were avoided. All were followed after primary repair and in only one woman was a rectovaginal fistula subsequently identified. Therefore, a third-degree laceration as the consequence of a median episiotomy need not be a major catastrophe. Despite its one drawback, the median episiotomy is a satisfactory procedure for most deliveries.

Timing of the Repair of Episiotomy

The most common practice is to defer repair of the episiotomy until after the placenta has been delivered. This policy permits the obstetrician to give undivided attention to the signs of placental separation and to deliver the organ just as soon as it has separated. Early delivery of the placenta is believed to decrease the loss of blood from the implantation site, since it prevents the development of extensive retroplacental bleeding. A further advantage of this practice is that the episiotomy repair is not interrupted or disrupted by the obvious necessity of delivering the placenta, especially if manual removal must be performed.

Technique

There are many ways to close the episiotomy incision, but *hemostasis and anatomical restoration without excessive suturing are essential* for success with any method. A technique that is commonly employed in episiotomy repair is shown in Figure 16–18A–E. The suture material ordinarily used is 000 chromic catgut.

Third-Degree Laceration

The technique of repairing a third-degree laceration with extension into the wall of the rectum is shown in Figure 16–19. Various techniques have been recommended, but in all instances it is essential to approximate the torn edges of the rectal sphincter with sutures approximately 0.5 cm apart. This muscular layer then is covered with a layer of fascia. Finally, the cut ends of the anal sphincter are isolated, approximated, and sutured together with two or three interrupted stitches. The remainder of the repair is the same as for an episiotomy. If the rectal mucosa was involved, stool softeners should be prescribed for a week. Enemas, of course, should be avoided. The value of prophylactic antibiotics has not been established.

Pain After Episiotomy

For the relief of episiotomy pain, a heat lamp has been a standard remedy, but during the summer months especially it may produce more discomfort than relief. An ice collar applied early tends to reduce swelling and allay discomfort. Aerosol sprays containing a local anesthetic are helpful at times. Analgesics such as codeine give considerable relief. **Since pain may be a signal of a large vulvar, paravaginal, or ischiorectal hematoma or perineal cellulitis, it is essential to examine these sites carefully if pain is severe or persistent.** Management of these complications is discussed in Chapter 28.

REFERENCES

Abdul-Karim R, Assali NS: Renal function in human pregnancy: V. Effects of oxytocin on renal hemodynamics and water and electrolyte excretion. J Lab Clin Med 57:522, 1961

Abe T: The detection of the rupture of fetal membranes with the nitrazine indicator. Am J Obstet Gynecol 39:400, 1940

Akoury HA, Brodie G, Caddick R, McLaughin VD, Pugh PA: Active management of labor and delivery in nulliparous women. Am J Obstet Gynecol 158:255, 1988

American College of Obstetricians and Gynecologists: Guidelines for Perinatal Care. Washington, 1988, p 67

Baptisti A: Chemical test for the determination of ruptured membranes. Am J Obstet Gynecol 35:688, 1938

Benson RC, Shubeck F, Deutschberger J, Weiss W, Berendes H: Fetal heart rate as a predictor of fetal distress. A report from the Collaborative Project. Obstet Gynecol 32:259, 1968

Benyon CL: Midline episiotomy as a midline procedure. J Obstet Gynaecol Br Commonw 81:126, 1974

Boylan PC, Frankowski R: Dystocia, parity, and the cesarean problem. Am J Obstet Gynecol 155:455, 1986

Browning DJ: Serious side effects of ergometrine and its use in routine obstetric practice. Med J Austral 1:957, 1974

Caldeyro-Barcia R, Schwarcz R, Belizan JM, Martell M, Nieto F, Sabatino H, Tenzer SM: Adverse perinatal effects of early amniotomy during labor. In Gluck L (ed): Modern Perinatal Medicine. Chicago, Year Book, 1974

Cohen CR, O'Brien WF, Lewis L, Knuppel RA: A prospective randomized study of the aggressive management of early labor. Am J Obstet Gynecol 157:1174, 1987

Cook WA: Natural Childbirth: Fact and Fallacy. Chicago, Nelson-Hall, 1982

Eggers TR, Fliegner JR: Water intoxication and syntocinon intoxication. Aust NZ J Obstet Gynaecol 19:59, 1979

Freidman EA: Labor, Clinical Evaluation and Management, 2nd ed. New York, Appleton, 1978

Gass MS, Dunn C, Styes SJ: Effect of episiotomy on the frequency of vaginal outlet lacerations. J Reprod Med 31:240, 1986

Haverkamp AD, Orleans M, Langendoerfer S, McFee J, Murphy J, Thompson HE: A controlled trial of the differential effects of intrapartum fetal monitoring. Am J Obstet Gynecol 134:399, 1979

Haverkamp AD, Thompson HE, McFee JG, Cetrulo C: The evaluation of continuous fetal heart rate monitoring in high risk pregnancy. Am J Obstet Gynecol 125:310, 1976

Hendricks CH, Brenner WE: Cardiovascular effects of oxytocic drugs used postpartum. Am J Obstet Gynecol 108:751, 1970

Kjeldsen J: Hemodynamic investigations during labour and delivery. Acta Obstet Gynecol Scand (Suppl) 89:1, 1979

Leveno KJ, Cunningham FG, Nelson S, Roark M, Williams ML, Guzick D, Dowling S, Rosenfeld CR, Buckley A: A prospective comparison of selective and universal electronic fetal monitoring in 34,995 pregnancies. N Engl J Med 315:615, 1986

Leveno KJ, Cunningham FG, Pritchard JA: Cesarean section: An answer to the House of Horne. Am J Obstet Gynecol 153:838, 1985

Liggins GC: Treatment of missed abortion by high dosage syntocinon intravenous infusion. J Obstet Gynaecol Br Commonw 69:277, 1962

O'Driscoll K, Foley M, MacDonald D: Active management of labor as an alternative to cesarean section for dystocia. Obstet Gynecol 63:485, 1984

Perrinne SP, Greene MF, Lee PDK, Cohen RA, Faller DV: Insulin stimulates cord erythroid progenitor growth: Evidence for an aetiological role in neonatal polycythaemia. Br J Haematol 64:503, 1986

Reynolds JL, Yudkin PL: Changes in the management of labour: II. Perineal management. Can Med Assoc J 136:1045, 1987

Ritgen G: (Concering his method for protection of the perineum. Monatschrift für Geburtskunde 6:21, 1855.) See English translation, Wynn RM: Am J Obstet Gynecol 93:421, 1965

Rosen MG, Peisner DB: Effect of amniotic membrane rupture on length of labor. Obstet Gynecol 70:604, 1987

Schwartz RH, Jones RWA: Transplacental hyponatremia due to oxytocin. Br Med J 1:152, 1978

Secher NJ, Arnso P, Wallin L: Haemodynamic effects of oxytocin (Syntocinon) and methylergometrine (Methergin) on the systemic and pulmonary circulations of pregnant anaesthetized women. Acta Obstet Gynecol Scand 57:97, 1978

Thacker SB, Banta HD: Benefits and risks of episiotomy: An interpretive review of the English language literature, 1860–1980. Obstet Gynecol Surv 38:232, 1983

Thorp JA, Boylan PC, Parisi VM, Heslin EP: Effects of high-dose oxytocin augmentation on umbilical cord blood gas values in primigravid women. Am J Obstet Gynecol 159:670, 1988

Thorp JM Jr, Bowes WA Jr, Brame RG, Cefalo R: Selected use of midline episiotomy: Effect of perineal trauma. Obstet Gynecol 70:260, 1987

Turner MJ, Brassil M, Gordon H: Active management of labor associated with a decrease in the cesarean section rate in nulliparas. Obstet Gynecol 71:150, 1988

Whalley PJ, Pritchard JA: Oxytocin and water intoxication. JAMA 186:601, 1963

Yao AC, Lind J: Effect of gravity on placental transfusion. Lancet 2:505, 1969

Yao AC, Lind J: Placental transfusion. Am J Dis Child 127:128, 1974

Analgesia and Anesthesia

The nulliparous woman during labor may encounter the most pain that she has ever experienced, but fortunately, it often proves to be the most rewarding. Pain relief in labor presents unique problems. These may be best appreciated by comparing several important differences between obstetrical and surgical analgesia and anesthesia:

1. *Fetus-Infant.* In surgical procedures, there is but one patient to consider, whereas during labor there are two patients: mother and fetus. The respiratory center of the fetus is highly vulnerable to sedative and anesthetic drugs. Thus, when these agents are given to the laboring woman, they rapidly traverse the placenta and may cause respiratory depression in the newborn infant.
2. *Indications.* Analgesia is essential to the safe, satisfactory, and humane performance of surgical procedures, and it also is essential for many abnormal deliveries. While analgesia is not absolutely necessary for all spontaneous vaginal deliveries, it may relieve unnecessary suffering.
3. *Duration.* In most surgical cases, analgesia is required for only a few hours. Obstetrical analgesia may be required for 12 hours or even longer.
4. *Effects on Labor.* Analgesic agents should exert little or no deleterious effect on uterine contractions and voluntary expulsive efforts. If they do, labor may be prolonged and postpartum hemorrhage may be an added risk.
5. *Timing.* Surgical patients most often can be prepared for anesthesia by withholding food and fluids for several hours. Labor begins without warning, and obstetrical anesthesia may be required within a few hours of a full meal. Moreover, gastric emptying is delayed during pregnancy and prolonged even more during labor, especially after analgesics are given. Vomiting with aspiration of gastric contents is a constant threat and often a major cause of serious maternal morbidity and mortality.

Because of these inherent difficulties, as yet no completely safe and satisfactory method of pain relief has been developed for obstetrics. Therefore, the advantages of pain relief in labor must offset its disadvantages. In fact, analgesia and anesthesia, when employed by skilled personnel, actually may be beneficial rather than detrimental to both fetus and mother. For example, adequate pain relief often forestalls inappropriate operative interventions. The relief of pain itself, however desirable, does not justify the use of inappropriate procedures administered by poorly trained individuals using inadequate equipment.

Pain relief during labor and delivery is a benefit-versus-risk issue. Specifically, complications related to analgesia administration are associated with 1 to 8 percent of maternal deaths (Endler and colleagues, 1988; Gabel, 1987; Kaunitz and associates, 1985; Lehmann and co-workers, 1987). With the introduction of obstetrical anesthesia as a special priority, however, the maternal mortality rate from anesthetic-related accidents in Massachusetts decreased more than sevenfold over 30 years (Sachs and associates, 1987). Unfortunately, there has been almost no increase in availability of obstetrical anesthesia services in the past 25 years (Gibbs and colleagues, 1986).

GENERAL PRINCIPLES

OBSTETRICAL ANESTHESIA SERVICES

The American College of Obstetricians and Gynecologists and the American Society of Anesthesiologists (ACOG Newsletter, 1988) issued a joint statement concerning anesthesia care for obstetrics. They recommend that a qualified person be readily available to administer an appropriate anesthetic and to maintain support of vital functions in an obstetrical emergency. In larger facilities with high-risk patients, 24 hour in-house anesthesia is recommended. Another important recommendation was that hospitals providing obstetrical care should be capable of performing a cesarean section within 30 minutes from the time the decision is made. Improved interpersonal relationships between obstetricians and anesthesiologists were stressed.

The Joint Commission on Accreditation of Hospitals urged that skilled personnel and appropriate equipment be available immediately to provide obstetrical anesthesia: *"Obstetric anesthesia must be considered as emergency anesthesia demanding a competence of personnel and equipment similar to or greater than that required for elective procedures."* The benefits to society to be derived from modifying existing priorities were stated succinctly by Jacoby (1974): *"Young women with babies are far more important to society than old people with irreversible disease. If we cannot do justice to both, then we should concentrate on the obstetrical patients."*

PRINCIPLES OF PAIN RELIEF

The three essentials of obstetrical pain relief are simplicity, safety, and preservation of fetal homeostasis. With respect to the latter, the most important is the transfer of oxygen, which is dependent on the concentration of inhaled oxygen, uterine blood flow, the oxygen gradient across the placenta, and umbilical blood flow. Impaired fetal oxygenation most often is the consequence of either compression of the umbilical cord or prolonged or repeated decreases in placental perfusion. Prominent causes of reduced placental perfusion include hypertonic uterine contractions, severe pregnancy-induced hypertension, hemorrhage, premature separation of the placenta, and hypotension from spinal or epidural analgesia.

The woman who is given any form of analgesia should be closely supervised. Without close supervision, she may fall out of bed or vomit and aspirate gastric contents. Similarly, assiduous attention to blood pressure and anesthetic levels should follow administration of all spinal and epidural analgesia.

The obstetrician should master an effective method of parenteral analgesia such as provided by meperidine (Demerol) plus promethazine (Phenergan), and become expert in local, pudendal, and low spinal (saddle block) analgesia. Continuous lumbar epidural analgesia also may be administered by the obstetrician when he or she has been properly trained and in appropriately selected circumstances. General anesthesia such as that produced by the combination of thiopental (Pentothal), nitrous oxide, succinylcholine, and a halogenated agent should be immediately available for laparotomy, but also should be administered only by those with special training.

NONPHARMACOLOGICAL METHODS OF PAIN CONTROL

As mentioned in Chapter 16 (p. 307), the proper psychological management of the pregnant woman throughout pregnancy and labor is a valuable basic tranquilizer. **Fear potentiates pain.** A woman who is free from fear, and who has confidence in the obstetrical staff who cares for her, usually has a relatively comfortable first stage of labor. In such instances, the laboring woman usually requires only modest amounts of analgesia.

Great benefits can be obtained by women and their spouses—or "significant others"—who attend childbirth preparation classes. Pregnant women who are taught what to expect regarding pain with labor generally have less fear regarding childbirth. Conversely, women who attempt natural childbirth, but who eventually request intrapartum analgesia, should never be allowed to feel as if they have failed.

Read (1944) emphasized that the intensity of pain during labor is related in large measure to emotional tension. He urged that women be well informed about the physiology of parturition and the various hospital procedures to which they will be subjected during labor and delivery. Lamaze (1970) subsequently described his psychoprophylactic method, which emphasized childbirth as a natural physiological process. Both taught that pain can be minimized by appropriate training in breathing and correct psychological support. Read and Lamaze have had a considerable impact on the reduction of potent analgesic, sedative, and amnestic drugs used during labor as well as the reduction that has occurred in the use of general anesthesia for delivery. The presence of a supportive spouse or other family member, of conscientious labor attendants, and of a considerate obstetrician who instills confidence contributes greatly to accomplishing this goal.

Although psychoprophylaxis will not be universally successful, it should be available for those who desire it and are willing to make the effort. At the same time, women who attempt psychoprophylaxis but find the discomforts of labor too great should not be denied the relief provided by appropriate analgesics. It is not unusual for Lamaze-prepared women in the United States to be given a narcotic during labor and conduction analgesia for delivery (Hughey and colleagues, 1978). As stated above, it is paramount that these women not be allowed to consider themselves "failures."

Acupuncture

Although the contemporary American woman is likely to be subjected to a multitude of needle punctures during labor and delivery, there are few reports concerned with formal application of acupuncture. Bonica (1974) commented that in one small group of obstetrical patients, relief of pain was good in about one third, partial in one third, and poor in one third. Of 21 laboring women studied by Wallis and co-workers (1974), 19 regarded acupuncture as unsuccessful in providing sufficient analgesia for labor and delivery.

ANALGESIA AND SEDATION DURING LABOR

With cervical dilatation and uterine contractions that cause discomfort, medication for pain relief with a narcotic such as meperidine, plus one of the tranquilizer drugs such as promethazine, usually is indicated. The mother should rest quietly between contractions with a successful program of analgesia and sedation. In this circumstance, discomfort usually is felt at the acme of an effective uterine contraction, but the pain is not unbearable. Finally, she should not recall labor as a horrifying experience. Appropriate drug selection and administration should accomplish these objectives for the great majority of women in labor, without risk to them or their infants.

MEPERIDINE AND PROMETHAZINE

Meperidine, 50 to 100 mg, with promethazine, 25 mg, may be administered intramuscularly at intervals of 3 to 4 hours. In general, a small dose given more frequently is preferable to a large one administered less often. Then, if delivery follows during the next hour or so after the injection, the neonate is less likely to be depressed by the medication. The size of the mother must be taken into account in determining the size of the dose.

A more rapid effect is achieved by giving these drugs intravenously, but in general, not more than 50 mg of meperidine or more than 25 mg of promethazine should be given at one time by this route. Whereas analgesia is maximal about 45 minutes after an intramuscular injection, it develops in about 5 minutes following intravenous administration. The depressant effect in the fetus follows closely behind the peak analgesic effect in the mother.

Effect of Meperidine on Labor

There is no convincing evidence that meperidine prolongs labor. In fact, Riffel and co-workers (1973) evaluated the effects of meperidine alone and meperidine plus promethazine on labor; they observed not a decrease but a slight increase in uterine activity following injection of these drugs. DeVoe and co-workers (1969) previously reported similar observations.

OTHER DRUGS

Other narcotic analgesics such as alphaprodine (Nisentil) and butorphanol (Stadol) have been used to provide pain relief during labor. A great variety of sedative and tranquilizer agents have been administered with such narcotics or, at times, alone. It is important to recognize that all narcotics and tranquilizers rapidly cross the placenta and may produce significant neonatal respiratory depression.

The synthetic narcotic butorphanol, given in 1 to 2 mg doses, compares favorably with 40 to 60 mg of meperidine (Quilligan and colleagues, 1980). Neonatal respiratory depression is reported to be less than with meperidine, but care must be taken that the two drugs are not given contiguously since butorphanol antagonizes the narcotic effects of meperidine. Furthermore, Angel and colleagues (1984), and Hatjis and Meis (1986), described a sinusoidal fetal heart rate pattern following butorphanol administration.

Morphine is no longer used during labor. It was used in the past along with scopolamine to produce so-called *twilight sleep.* The combination produced excellent analgesia and amnesia, but the mother occasionally became quite excited and delirious, and she hallucinated. Moreover, at birth the infant often was apneic.

NARCOTIC ANTAGONISTS

Meperidine or other narcotics used during labor may impair respiratory function in the newborn. **Prompt ventilation is mandatory.** Naloxone hydrochloride (Narcan) is a narcotic antagonist capable of reversing respiratory depression induced by opioid narcotics by displacing the narcotic from specific receptors in the central nervous system. Unfortunately, it concomitantly inhibits the analgesia and euphoria produced by the narcotic. In fact, withdrawal symptoms may be precipitated in recipients who are physically dependent on narcotics. The suggested dose for the newborn infant is 10 μg per kg injected into the umbilical vein, which usually acts within 2 minutes with an effective duration of at least 30 minutes. Since the depressant action of meperidine may persist beyond this time, the injection of naloxone may have to be repeated.

In the absence of narcotics, naloxone exhibits little, if any, adverse activity and thereby differs from levallorphan (Lorphan) and nalorphine (Nalline). These latter two compounds may, in fact, enhance respiratory depression not caused by narcotic drugs. Thus, naloxone is the drug of choice for treating narcotic depression in the newborn. Although narcotic antagonists may help relieve respiratory depression from opioid drugs in the newborn, it is best to avoid, whenever possible, the administration of narcotics to the mother in doses that cause serious respiratory depression in the newborn.

GENERAL ANESTHESIA

Without exception, all anesthetic agents that depress the maternal central nervous system cross the placenta and depress the fetal central nervous system. Another constant hazard with any general anesthetic is aspiration of gastric contents and particulate matter that will obstruct airways. Fasting before the time of anesthesia is not always an effective safeguard, since fasting gastric juice, even though free of particulate matter, is likely to be strongly acidic and thus can produce fatal aspiration pneumonitis. At the same time, tracheal intubation is valuable to ensure a satisfactory airway and minimize the risk of aspiration. Failed attempted tracheal intubation is uncommon but has emerged as a major cause of anesthesia-related maternal deaths (Endler and colleagues, 1988).

With inhalation, the concentration of the anesthetic agent increases in the lungs of the pregnant woman somewhat more rapidly because the functional residual capacity and residual volume of the lungs are reduced (see Chap. 7, p. 147). For the same reason, residual oxygen in the lung after expiration is appreciably less, a factor of importance when there is delay in intubation and oxygenation after injection of a muscle relaxant. **Trained personnel and specialized equipment are mandatory for the safe use of general anesthesia.**

INHALATION ANESTHESIA

GAS ANESTHETICS

Nitrous oxide (N_2O) is the only anesthetic gas in current use for obstetrical analgesia and anesthesia in the United States. It may be used to provide pain relief during labor as well as at delivery. This agent produces analgesia and altered consciousness, but by itself does not provide true anesthesia. Nitrous oxide does not prolong labor or interfere with uterine contractions. Satisfactory analgesia often is obtained with a concentration of 50 percent nitrous oxide and 50 percent oxygen, but its satisfactory use requires that personnel be in close attendance. During the second stage of labor, when a uterine contraction begins, a well-fitting clear mask is placed on the woman's face and she is encouraged to take three deep breaths and then to bear down.

Nitrous oxide is commonly used as part of a balanced general anesthesia that is popular for cesarean section and some forceps deliveries. It is given along with oxygen in a 50:50 mixture, and a short-acting barbiturate (usually thiopental) is given intravenously along with a muscle relaxant (usually succinylcholine) just prior to tracheal intubation. With this technique, high concentrations of potent inhalational anesthetics are avoided.

Cyclopropane

At one time, cyclopropane was popular in obstetrical practice. There are several disadvantages inherent in the use of cyclopropane for abdominal or vaginal delivery. The gas is highly explosive and always must be given in a closed system. It is not likely to relax the myometrium sufficiently to allow intrauterine manipulation of the fetus. Finally, unless the time of anesthesia is kept very short, resuscitation of the infant is required.

VOLATILE ANESTHETICS

Halothane (Fluothane), enflurane (Ethrane), and isoflurane (Forane) are used to supplement nitrous oxide during maintenance of general anesthesia. These halogenated hydrocarbons cross the placenta readily and are capable of producing narcosis in the fetus.

Halothane is a potent, nonexplosive agent of limited use for obstetrical anesthesia. It produces remarkable uterine relaxation and should be restricted to those very uncommon situations in which uterine relaxation is a requisite rather than a hazard. It is one of the anesthetic agents of choice for the now very uncommon procedures of internal podalic version of the second twin, breech decomposition, and replacement of the acutely inverted uterus. As soon as the maneuver has been completed, halothane administration should be stopped and immediate efforts made to promote myometrial contraction and retraction to minimize hemorrhage from the placental implantation site. Because of its cardiodepressant and hypotensive effects, halothane may intensify the adverse effects of maternal hypovolemia. Halothane rarely has been associated with *hepatitis* and *massive hepatic necrosis*. This may be due to a hypersensitivity reaction.

Enflurane and *isoflurane* are used by some because of possible halothane hepatotoxicity. In doses that provide analgesia, they are likely to cause unconsciousness. Also, like halothane, they cause myometrial depression and increased hemorrhage. In fact, we now use isoflurane preferentially to induce uterine relaxation for version and extraction of the second twin. Enflurane should not be given to anyone suspected of impaired renal function.

Methoxyflurane is pleasant to take and may be self-administered in low concentration to provide analgesia during the first and second stages of labor and during delivery. Overdose may be a major complication when methoxyflurane is self-administered for analgesia. Unless the woman is kept under very close surveillance, she may, at times, cover the inhaler and her head with a pillow or sheet and thereby increase appreciably the concentration inhaled. Methoxyflurane, especially in higher concentrations, may depress myometrial contractility and thereby increase blood loss from the placental implantation site. There is also convincing evidence of dose-related methoxyflurane nephrotoxicity. Thus, the total dose administered must be carefully controlled. This agent is rarely used today.

Nitrous oxide and oxygen given for balanced general anesthesia have been associated with some degree of maternal awareness when these women were interviewed postpartum (Hodgkinson and colleagues, 1978; Warren and associates, 1983). For this reason, as well as to be able to increase the inspired concentration of oxygen, many anesthesiologists recommend the addition of one of the halogenated agents in concentrations of less than 1 percent (Warren and colleagues, 1983). Gilstrap and associates (1987), however, reported that such practices in women undergoing cesarean delivery were associated with substantively increased blood loss, presumably from intraoperative uterine atony. Those given halothane, enflurane, or isoflurane were twice as likely (35 versus 17 percent) to experience a hematocrit fall postpartum of 8 volumes percent or more. Importantly, 18 percent of 114 women given one of the halogenated agents required blood transfusions, compared to only 1 of 179 given nitrous oxide-oxygen or conduction analgesia.

Ether

Since, in the hands of inexperienced personnel, the margin of safety was usually greater with diethyl ether than with any other general anesthetic, it enjoyed considerable popularity in former years. Ether is unpleasant to the mother, it depresses the fetus-infant, it causes uterine relaxation and enhances postpartum hemorrhage, and it is explosive. For all these reasons, it is seldom used in the United States.

Trichloroethylene

This compound is no longer available in this country. When a closed-circuit system with soda lime was used to provide anesthesia, trichloroethylene formed toxic products. Moreover, deaths were recorded when trichloroethylene was self-administered for analgesia during labor.

ANESTHETIC GAS EXPOSURE AND PREGNANCY OUTCOME

Sufficient data have been accumulated to create concern over the welfare of the embryo and fetus of pregnant women who work in operating rooms where they are exposed chronically to anesthetic gases. In some reports but not all, the spontaneous abortion rate of female workers exposed was about twice that for unexposed personnel and the minor malformation rate in children of exposed male workers was slightly greater (Knill-Jones and colleagues, 1975). In England and Wales, a comparison has been made between pregnancy outcomes of women doctors exposed to anesthetic gases during pregnancy and those working but not so exposed (Pharah and colleagues, 1977). Conception while the woman was actively engaged in practicing anesthesiology resulted in slightly smaller babies (3,347 versus 3,388 g), an increased frequency of cardiovascular malformations (1.4 versus 0.4 percent), and of stillbirths (1.7 versus 0.8 percent). Spontaneous abortions were the same in both groups (13.8 percent). However, Ericson and Källen (1979) found no differences in pregnancies of operating-room workers in Sweden. From Denmark, Husum and co-workers (1983) detected no effects from long-term exposure to trace concentrations of waste anesthetic gases. Sister chomatid exchanges and structural chromosomal aberrations in lymphocytes were no more common in operating-room personnel than in unexposed control subjects.

INTRAVENOUS DRUGS DURING ANESTHESIA

Thiopental

Intravenous thiopental (Pentothal) is widely used in conjunction with other agents for general anesthesia in obstetrics. The drug offers the advantages of ease and extreme rapidity of induction, ample oxygenation, ready controllability, minimal postpartum bleeding, and prompt recovery with minimal risk of vomiting. The first and last of these advantages make it very popular with patients. Thiopental and similar compounds are poor analgesic agents, and the administration of sufficient drug given alone to maintain analgesia in the mother may cause appreciable newborn depression. Thus, thiopental is not used as the sole anesthetic agent, but is given in a dose that induces sleep along with a muscle relaxant, usually succinylcholine, and nitrous oxide plus oxygen inhaled through a tracheal tube.

General anesthesia should not be induced until all steps preparatory to actual delivery have been completed, so as to minimize transfer of the anesthetic agent to the fetus and, in turn, avoid respiratory depression in the newborn. General anesthesia, however, need not cause appreciable neonatal depression. Zagorzycki and Brinkman (1982) compared the status of infants immediately after cesarean delivery whose mothers received either epidural analgesia or general anesthesia, the technique for which consisted of preoxygenation, thiopental (4 mg per kg), muscle relaxant, nitrous oxide (50 percent), and halothane (0.5 percent). No difference was found in Apgar scores at 1 and 5 minutes. No appreciable differences in mean scores or in the frequency of scores below 7 were evident.

When the time from induction of anesthesia to delivery is prolonged appreciably, there is an increased likelihood of neonatal depression. Often the delay is the consequence of obstetrical difficulties necessitating manipulation of the uterus and the fetus, leading to fetal depression.

Ketamine

This drug is seldom used in obstetrics. The intravenous injection of 1 mg per kg of ketamine will produce appreciable analgesia. It usually causes a rise in blood pressure, which is not desirable in the already hypertensive woman. Unpleasant delirium and hallucinations commonly are induced by this agent. Ketamine may cause newborn respiratory depression and hypertonus sufficient to impair efforts at ventilation.

ASPIRATION DURING GENERAL ANESTHESIA

Pneumonitis from inhalation of gastric contents has been the most common cause of anesthetic death in obstetrics. A survey in Great Britain reported by Crawford (1972) identified inhalation of gastric contents to be associated with at least half of all maternal deaths. The aspirated material from the stomach may contain undigested food and thereby cause airway obstruction that, unless promptly relieved, may prove rapidly fatal. Gastric juice is likely to be free of particulate matter during fasting, but it is extremely acidic and capable of inducing a lethal chemical pneumonitis. The aspiration of strongly acidic gastric juice is probably more common and perhaps even more dangerous than is the aspiration of gastric contents that contain particulate matter which is buffered somewhat by food.

PROPHYLAXIS

Important to effective prophylaxis are (1) fasting for at least 6 and preferably 12 hours before anesthesia, (2) use of agents to reduce gastric acidity during the induction and maintenance of general anesthesia, (3) skillful tracheal intubation accompanied by pressure on the cricoid cartilage to occlude the esophagus, and (4) at completion of the operation, extubation with the mother awake and lying on her side with head lowered.

Fasting
Steps should be taken to lessen the likelihood of danger from aspiration of both particulate matter as well as acidic gastric secretions. These measures should be included also for women for whom conduction analgesia is planned. For elective obstetrical procedures, fasting for 12 hours usually rids the stomach of undigested food but not necessarily of acidic liquid. Sutherland and colleagues (1986) studied women undergoing early pregnancy termination or minor gynecological surgery, and they showed that despite overnight fasting, the mean stomach juice volume was 20 mL with a pH of 1.6. In women at term undergoing elective cesarean section, Lewis and Crawford (1987) showed that women given a light meal of only tea and toast had twice the volume of gastric contents as fasted controls at 4 hours, and particulate matter was identified in 20 percent. Gastric emptying in labor is even more retarded, and women in early labor should be advised to fast before coming to the hospital, and certainly thereafter. **Despite these precautions, it should be assumed that any woman in labor has both gastric particulate matter as well as acidic contents.** If general anesthesia is used soon after eating, then it is our practice to insert a nasogastric tube during surgery, and with irrigation, the likelihood of vomiting and aspiration during extubation is lessened.

Antacids
The practice of administering antacids shortly before induction of anesthesia probably has done more to decrease mortality from obstetrical anesthesia than any other single practice. It is essential that the antacid disperse promptly throughout all of the gastric contents to neutralize the hydrogen ion effectively; but it is equally important that the antacid, if aspirated, not incite comparably serious pulmonary problems.

Gibbs and colleagues (1984) reported that 30 mL of 0.3 M sodium citrate with citric acid (Bicitra), given about 45 minutes before surgery, neutralized gastric contents (mean volume 70 mL) in nearly 90 percent of women undergoing cesarean section. For several years now at Parkland Hospital, we have routinely administered 30 mL of Bicitra within a few minutes of the anticipated time of anesthesia induction, either general or by major regional block. If more than 30 minutes have passed since the first dose was given and anesthesia induction, then a second dose is given.

Magnesium hydroxide, or milk of magnesia, also effectively neutralizes gastric acid (Wheatley and colleagues, 1979). In theory, 1 mL will neutralize nearly 3 mEq of acid, or about 25 mL of gastric juice with a pH of 1.0, and its favorable effects last long enough for cesarean section to be completed. Gibbs and associates (1979) demonstrated in dogs that pulmonary instillation of a suspension of milk of magnesia and aluminum hydroxide can induce pneumonitis; however, we have observed no long-term effects on the respiratory tract in those instances in which women aspirated the compound.

Cimetidine, given sometime before general anesthesia for delivery, also has been recommended (Hodgkinson and colleagues, 1983); but at least 60 minutes are required after parenteral administration to decrease gastric acidity to relatively safe levels. Therefore, in emergency situations, either an antacid or antacid plus cimetidine should be used (Moir, 1983).

Intubation
Various positions have been tried to minimize aspiration before and during tracheal intubation and cuff inflation, but the disadvantages from positions other than supine outweigh any advantage. Cricoid pressure from the time of induction of anesthesia until intubation should be performed by a trained associate. In special instances, intubation may be performed with the mother awake. In these cases, local anesthesia usually is applied, yet it may obtund the laryngeal reflex sufficiently to allow aspiration.

Extubation
At the completion of the surgical procedure, the tracheal tube may be safely removed only if the woman is conscious and has been placed in the lateral recumbent position with her head lowered.

PATHOLOGY

Aspiration pneumonitis associated with obstetrical anesthesia was described by Mendelson in 1946. Teabeaut (1952) demonstrated experimentally that if the pH of aspirated fluid was below 2.5, severe chemical pneumonitis developed. Of interest, in one study the pH of gastric juice of nearly half of women tested intrapartum without treatment was below 2.5 (Taylor and Pryse-Davies, 1966). The right mainstem bronchus usually offers the simplest pathway for aspirated material to reach the lung parenchyma, and therefore the right lower lobe is most often involved. In severe cases, there is bilateral widespread involvement.

The woman who aspirates may develop evidence of respiratory distress immediately or as long as several hours after aspiration, depending in part upon the material aspirated, the severity of the process, and the acuity of the attendants. Aspiration of a large amount of solid material causes obvious signs of airway obstruction. Smaller particles without acidic liquid may lead to patchy atelectasis and later to bronchopneumonia.

When highly acidic liquid is inspired, tachypnea, bronchospasm, rhonchi, rales, atelectasis, cyanosis, tachycardia, and hypotension are likely to develop. At the sites of injury, protein-rich fluid containing numerous erythrocytes exudes from capillaries into the lung interstitium and alveoli to cause decreased pulmonary compliance, shunting of blood, and severe hypoxemia (see Chap. 39, p. 807). Radiographic changes may not appear immediately and they may be quite variable. Therefore, a chest x-ray alone should not be used to exclude aspiration of a significant amount of strongly acidic gastric contents.

TREATMENT

In recent years, the methods recommended for treatment of aspiration have changed appreciably, indicating that previous therapy was not very successful. Suspicion of aspiration of gastric contents demands very close monitoring of the patient for evidence of any pulmonary damage.

Suction and Bronchoscopy

As much as possible of the inhaled fluid should be immediately wiped out of the mouth and removed from the pharynx and trachea by suction. We do not practice saline lavage, which, rather than being beneficial, probably further disseminates the acid throughout the lung. If large particulate matter is inspired, prompt bronchoscopy may be indicated to relieve airway obstruction. Otherwise, bronchoscopy not only is unnecessary but may contribute to morbidity and mortality.

Corticosteroids

There has been considerable enthusiasm for administering corticosteroids in pharmacological doses in an attempt to maintain cell integrity in the presence of strong acid. There is no clinical evidence that such therapy is unequivocally beneficial (Bynum and Pierce, 1976). Furthermore, experimental evidence is not consistent with the conclusion that appreciable benefits accrue from the use of corticosteroids. Nonetheless, the clinical impression of some has been that the immediate intravenous administration of 500 mg of methylprednisolone sodium succinate (Solu-Medrol), with repeated doses of 250 mg every 8 hours for 24 hours, is beneficial.

Oxygen and Ventilation

Oxygen delivered through a tracheal tube in increased concentration by intermittent positive pressure often is required to raise and maintain the arterial P_{O_2} at 60 mm Hg. Frequent suctioning is necessary to remove secretions including edema fluid. Mechanical ventilation that produces positive end-expiratory pressure may prove lifesaving by preventing the complete collapse of the now surfactant-poor lung on expiration and, partially at least, the outpouring of protein-rich fluid from pulmonary capillaries into the interstitium and alveoli.

Antimicrobials

Although the likelihood of bacterial contamination and infection from aspiration is appreciable, the use of antimicrobials prophylactically is controversial (Bynum and Pierce, 1976). Barlett and associates (1974) identified anaerobic bacteria in 50 of 54 cases of pneumonia caused by aspiration. They concluded that anaerobes play a key role in most cases of infection after aspiration, and they suggested the use of clindamycin or chloramphenicol for those anaerobes not sensitive to penicillin. We do not give antimicrobials unless there is clinical evidence of infection.

An extensive review of the aspiration syndrome has been provided by Cohen (1982).

REGIONAL ANALGESIA

A variety of nerve blocks have been developed over the years to provide pain relief for the woman in labor and at delivery. Since they are designed to be implemented without loss of consciousness (anesthesia), they are correctly referred to as regional analgesics.

SENSORY INNERVATION OF GENITAL TRACT

UTERINE INNERVATION

Pain in the first stage of labor is generated largely from the uterus. Visceral sensory fibers from the uterus, cervix, and upper vagina traverse through *Frankenhäuser's ganglion,* which lies just lateral to the cervix, into the pelvic plexus, and then to the middle and superior hypogastric plexuses. From there, the fibers travel in the lumbar and lower thoracic sympathetic chains to enter the spinal cord through the white rami communicantes associated with the 10th, 11th, and 12th thoracic and 1st lumbar nerves. Early in the first stage of labor, the pain of uterine contractions is transmitted through predominantly the 11th and 12th thoracic nerves.

The motor pathways to the uterus leave the spinal cord at the level of the 7th and 8th thoracic vertebrae. Theoretically, any method of sensory block that does not also block the motor pathways to the uterus can be used for analgesia during labor.

LOWER GENITAL TRACT INNERVATION

Although painful contractions of the uterus continue during the second stage of labor, much of the pain of vaginal delivery arises in the lower genital tract. Painful stimuli from the lower genital tract are transmitted primarily through the *pudendal nerve,* the peripheral branches of which provide sensory innervation to the perineum, anus, and the more medial and inferior parts of the vulva and clitoris. The pudendal nerve passes across the posterior surface of the sacrospinous ligament just as the ligament attaches to the ischial spine (Fig. 17–1). The sensory nerve fibers of the pudendal nerve are derived from the ventral branches of the 2nd, 3rd, and 4th sacral nerves.

ANESTHETIC AGENTS

A variety of compounds are currently used in obstetrics to induce local or regional analgesia. Some of the more commonly used local anesthetics, along with their usual concentration,

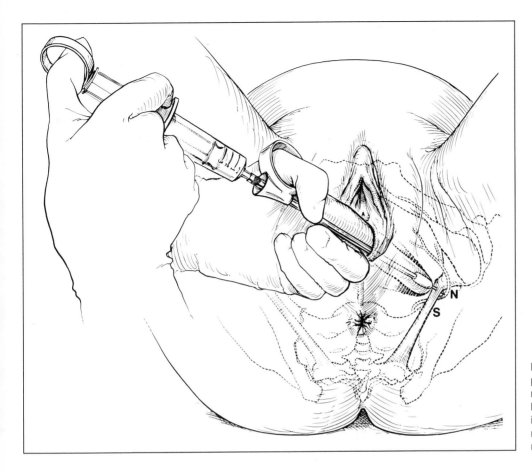

Figure 17–1. Local infiltration of the pudendal nerve. Transvaginal technique showing the needle extended beyond the needle guard and passing through the sacrospinous ligament (S) to reach the pudendal nerve (N).

doses, and duration of actions are shown in Table 17–1. **The physician is cautioned to study carefully the package insert for each product before use.** Some preparations suitable for epidural analgesia are not suitable for subarachnoid injection because the preservative may cause inflammation. Some preparations contain a dilute solution of epinephrine to prolong the action of the anesthetic or to produce symptoms when a test

dose is inadvertently given intravenously. We find that there is sufficient flexibility in the choice of plain solutions, and thus we avoid the potential hazard of severe hypertension from epinephrine. The dose of each agent varies widely, and is dependent upon the indicated nerve block and physical status of the woman. When the dose is increased, onset, duration, and quality of analgesia are enhanced, but only incremental dosage of

TABLE 17–1. SOME LOCAL ANESTHETIC AGENTS USED IN OBSTETRICS

| Anesthetic Agent | Plain Solutions | | | | |
	Usual Concentration (%)	Usual Volume (mL)	Usual Dose (mg)	Average Duration (min)	Clinical Use
Amino-esters					
2-Chloroprocaine	1–2	20–30	400–600	15–30	Infiltration Pudendal block
	2–3	15–25	300–750	30–60	Epidural for cesarean section
	2	8–10	160–200	30–60	Epidural for labor analgesia
Tetracaine	0.2	—	4	75–150	Low spinal block with 6% glucose
	0.5	—	7–10	75–150	Spinal for cesarean section with 5% glucose
Amino-amides					
Lidocaine	1	20–30	200–300	30–60	Infiltration Pudendal block
	1.5	8–10	120–150	60–90	Epidural for labor analgesia
	1.5–2	15–30	300–450	60–90	Epidural for cesarean section
	5	1–2	50–75	45–60	Spinal for cesarean section with 7.5% glucose
Bupivacaine	0.5	10–20	50–100	90–150	Epidural for cesarean section
	0.25	8–10	20–25	60–90	Epidural for labor analgesia

small-volume boluses allows safety through careful monitoring for early warning signs of toxicity.

While appropriate use of these anesthetics almost always proves to be safe for mother and fetus-infant, the potential exists for toxic reactions that may prove life threatening to both. **Administration of these agents must be followed by appropriate monitoring for adverse reactions, and equipment and personnel to manage these reactions must be immediately available.**

Most often, serious toxicity follows injection of an anesthetic into a vessel, but it may be induced by administration of excessive amounts, usually because of a miscalculated dose. Since many of these agents are manufactured in more than one concentration and ampule size to be used for specific local or regional blocks, a thorough knowledge of the ones selected for use is essential for safety. Two manifestations of systemic toxicity from local anesthetics are those of the central nervous and cardiovascular systems. Because both are life threatening and may follow any route of administration, they are considered now.

CENTRAL NERVOUS SYSTEM TOXICITY

Symptoms include lightheadedness, dizziness, tinnitus, bizarre behavior, slurred speech, metallic taste, numbness of the tongue and mouth, muscle fasciculation and excitation, loss of consciousness, and generalized convulsions. Quickly and simultaneously the convulsions should be controlled, an airway established, and oxygen delivered. Succinylcholine abolishes the peripheral manifestations of the convulsions and allows tracheal intubation. Thiopental or diazepam acts centrally to inhibit convulsions. In the few instances in which it has been tried at Parkland Hospital, magnesium sulfate administered according to the regimen for eclampsia (Chap. 35, p. 679) also has controlled effectively the convulsions. Fetal distress, manifested by either late heart rate decelerations or persistent bradycardia, may develop as the consequences of maternal hypoxia and lactic acidosis induced by convulsions. With arrest of the convulsions, administration of oxygen, and application of other supportive measures, the fetus is likely to recover more quickly in utero than if immediately delivered by cesarean section. Moreover, maternal well-being usually is better served by waiting until the intensity of the hypoxia and the metabolic acidosis have diminished. Personnel and facilities for instituting cardiopulmonary resuscitation should be available immediately for both the mother and the infant.

CARDIOVASCULAR TOXICITY

Cardiovascular manifestations from local anesthetic toxicity do not always follow central nervous system involvement. Generally, they develop later than those from cerebral toxicity, since they are induced by higher blood levels of drug. They also are characterized by stimulation and depression. First there is hypertension and tachycardia, soon followed by hypotension and cardiac arrhythmias. The hypotension and arrhythmias contribute appreciably to impaired uteroplacental perfusion and fetal distress. Hypotension is initially managed by turning the woman onto her side to avoid aortocaval compression. A balanced salt solution is infused rapidly along with intravenously administered ephedrine. **The temptation to perform emergency cesarean section for fetal distress must be resisted, since this may prove fatal for the mother if done before she is resuscitated.**

As with convulsions, the fetus is likely to recover more quickly in utero once maternal cardiac output is reestablished.

Inadvertent intravenous injection of local anesthetic is likely to cause these adverse effects. Another mechanism is repeated injections of the drug at multiple sites, resulting in an increase in total dose. Such an example is the administration of an ineffective epidural, followed by pudendal block that was not satisfactory for repairing an episiotomy or lacerations, followed by local infiltration. The physician must be aware of the upper limit of safety for the local anesthetics used.

LOCAL INFILTRATION

This technique is of no value for analgesia during labor, but has been employed for delivery. Local infiltration is of especial value in the following circumstances: (1) before episiotomy and delivery, (2) after delivery into the site of lacerations to be repaired, and (3) around the episiotomy wound if adequate analgesia is lacking. From the standpoint of safety, local infiltration analgesia is preeminent. Unfortunately, from the standpoint of effectiveness, too often the incision or repair is begun before enough local anesthetic agent has been given or time allowed to establish analgesia.

PUDENDAL BLOCK

A tubular director that allows 1.0 to 1.5 cm of a 15 cm-long 22-gauge needle to protrude beyond its tip is used to guide the needle into position over the pudendal nerve (Fig. 17–1). The end of the director is placed against the vaginal mucosa just beneath the tip of the ischial spine. The needle is pushed beyond the tip of the director into the mucosa and a mucosal wheal is made with 1 mL of 1 percent lidocaine solution or an equivalent dose of another local anesthetic with similar high-tissue penetration and rapid action. **Aspiration is attempted before this and all subsequent injections to guard against intravascular infusion.** The needle is then advanced until it touches the sacrospinous ligament, which is infiltrated with 3 mL of lidocaine. The needle is advanced farther through the ligament, and as it pierces the loose areolar tissue behind the ligament, the resistance of the plunger decreases. Another 3 mL of the anesthetic solution is injected into this region. Next, the needle is withdrawn into the guide, the tip of the guide is moved to just above the ischial spine, and the needle is inserted through the mucosa. After again aspirating to avoid intravascular injection, the rest of 10 mL of solution is deposited. Most obstetricians elect to perform pudendal block bilaterally so that discomfort of perineal distension with delivery is minimal.

Within 3 to 4 minutes of the time of injection, the successful pudendal block will allow pinching of the lower vagina and posterior vulva bilaterally without pain. It is often of benefit before pudendal block to infiltrate the fourchet, perineum, and adjacent vagina directly at the site where the episiotomy is to be made with 5 to 10 mL of 1 percent lidocaine solution. Then, if delivery occurs before pudendal block becomes effective, an episiotomy can be made without pain. By the time of the repair, the pudendal block usually has become effective.

Pudendal block usually works well and is an extremely safe and relatively simple method of providing analgesia for spontaneous delivery. In 1986, at Parkland Hospital, nearly 25 percent of 12,000 women delivered vaginally were managed effectively with bilateral pudendal block and local analgesia. Some of these women had been given epidural analgesia during labor. Pudendal block, however, is not likely to provide adequate analgesia for forceps delivery or when delivery requires manipulation. Moreover, analgesia limited to pudendal block usually is inadequate for women in whom complete visualization of the cervix and upper vagina or manual exploration of the uterine cavity are indicated. Under these circumstances, the addition of an intravenously administered narcotic analgesic such as 50 mg of meperidine may provide appreciable, although not total, relief from the pain of examination. **With such an approach, caution must be exercised not to give narcotics and sedatives in doses or combinations that might so obtund the woman that she would suffer airway obstruction or aspiration.**

COMPLICATIONS

Intravascular injection of a local anesthetic agent may cause serious systemic toxicity characterized by stimulation of the cerebral cortex leading to convulsions as described above. A troublesome hematoma, the consequence of perforation of a blood vessel, is most likely to occur when there is defective coagulation such as that induced by heparin or by severe placental abruption. Rarely, a severe infection may originate at the injection site. The infection may spread to the region posterior to the hip joint, into the gluteal musculature or into the retropsoal space (Svancarek and associates, 1977). Death or severe permanent impairment in some survivors have been recorded (Wenger and Gitchell, 1973).

PARACERVICAL BLOCK

This technique serves to relieve the pain of uterine contractions, but since the pudendal nerves are not blocked, additional analgesia is required for delivery. Usually lidocaine or chloroprocaine, 5 to 10 mL of a 1 percent solution, is injected at 3 and 9 o'clock. Since the anesthesia is relatively short acting, paracervical block may have to be repeated during labor.

COMPLICATIONS

While good to excellent pain relief is usually achieved from paracervical block during the first stage of labor, *fetal bradycardia* is a worrisome complication that has been reported in 10 to 70 percent of such blocks. Bradycardia usually develops within 10 minutes and may last up to 30 minutes. Several investigators stress that bradycardia is not a sign of fetal asphyxia, since it is usually transient and the newborns are in most instances vigorous at birth. There are reports, however, in which fetal scalp blood pH and Apgar scores were found at times to be low and a few fetuses have died. The effect may be the consequence of transplacental transfer of the anesthetic agent or its metabolites and, in turn, a depressant effect on the heart. However, Greiss (1976) and Fishburne (1979) and their associates, based on studies in pregnant ewes, believe that fetal bradycardia results from decreased placental perfusion as the consequence of drug-induced uterine artery vasoconstriction and myometrial hypertonus. For these reasons, paracervical block should not be used in situations of potential fetal compromise (Carlsson and colleagues, 1987).

SPINAL (SUBARACHNOID) BLOCK

Introduction of a local anesthetic into the subarachnoid space to effect spinal block has long been used for uncomplicated cesarean section and for vaginal delivery of normal women of low parity. Because of the smaller subarachnoid space during pregnancy, the same amount of anesthetic agent in the same volume of solution produces much higher blockade in parturients than in nonpregnant women. The smaller space is the consequence most likely of engorgement of the internal vertebral venous plexus, which in turn is the consequence of compression by the uterus of the inferior vena cava and adjacent large veins.

VAGINAL DELIVERY

Low spinal block is a popular form of analgesia for delivery. The level of analgesia extends to the 10th thoracic dermatome, which corresponds to the level of the umbilicus. Blockade to this level provides excellent relief from the pain of uterine contractions. The term *saddle block* has been incorrectly applied to this level of analgesia, since the area of skin anesthetized is appreciably greater than that which would be in contact with a saddle.

Nearly all local anesthetic agents have been used for spinal analgesia, but for many years one that has proved quite satisfactory for vaginal delivery is tetracaine (Pontocaine) in a dose of 4 mg already dissolved in 2 mL of a 6 percent solution of dextrose in water (Table 17–1). With 4 mg of tetracaine, satisfactory anesthetic in the lower vagina and the perineum persists for about an hour. Lidocaine given in a hyperbaric solution also produces excellent spinal analgesia and has the advantage of a shorter duration. Neither is administered for vaginal delivery until the cervix is fully dilated and all other criteria for safe forceps delivery have been fulfilled (see Chap. 25, p. 427). Spinal analgesia is not recommended before this time because of the frequency of disruption of orderly labor by the anesthetic and, as the consequence, an often unnecessarily complicated delivery traumatic to the infant and the mother. Preanalgesic intravenous hydration with a liter of crystalloid solution will prevent hypotension in many cases.

CESAREAN SECTION

For cesarean section, a higher level of spinal sensory blockade is essential to at least the level of the 8th thoracic dermatome, which is just below the xiphoid process of the sternum. **Since a larger area is to be anesthetized, a somewhat larger dose of anesthetic agent is necessary, and this increases the frequency and the intensity of toxic reactions.** Depending upon the mother's size, 8 to 10 mg of tetracaine or 50 to 75 mg of lidocaine are administered. The addition of 0.2 mg of morphine improves pain control during delivery and postoperatively (Abouleish and colleagues, 1988). Undue delay between intrathecal injection of anesthetic agent and delivery of the infant should be avoided if a safe dose of the anesthetic drug is to be used, yet have spinal analgesia of sufficient intensity and duration to allow completion of abdominal delivery without serious discomfort. Therefore, catheterization of the bladder and shaving of the operative field should be done before the anesthetic is administered. Preanalgesic intravenous volume expansion usually prevents dangerous hypotension.

COMPLICATIONS WITH SPINAL ANALGESIA

A number of complications may follow induction of spinal analgesia, and it is imperative that close clinical monitoring of vital signs be performed. This includes assessment of the level of analgesia, which should stabilize by 10 to 20 minutes.

Hypotension

Maternal hypotension may develop very soon after injection of the analgesic agent. This is the consequence of vasodilatation from sympathetic blockade compounded by obstructed venous return caused by uterine compression of the vena cava and adjacent large veins. Importantly, in the supine position, even in the absence of maternal hypotension, at least as measured in the brachial artery, placental blood flow may be reduced significantly. Important to prophylaxis and to treatment of spinal hypotension are (1) uterine elevation and displacement to the left of the abdomen, (2) acute hydration with a balanced salt solution, and (3) at the first sign of a decrease in blood pressure after hydration, the intravenous injection of 10 to 15 mg of ephedrine.

Total Spinal Blockade

Complete spinal blockade with respiratory paralysis may complicate spinal analgesia. Most often, total spinal blockade is the consequence of administration of a dose of analgesic agent far in excess of that tolerated by pregnant women. Hypotension and apnea promptly develop and must be immediately treated to prevent cardiac arrest. In the undelivered woman, the uterus is displaced laterally to minimize aortovenal compression. Effective ventilation is established, through a tracheal tube when possible, to protect against aspiration. When the woman is hypotensive, intravenous fluids are given and ephedrine may be helpful to increase cardiac output. Elevation of the legs will increase venous return and help reverse hypotension. Preparations should be made for cardiac resuscitation in the event of cardiac arrest.

Anxiety and Discomfort

It is imperative that everyone in the operating room remember that the woman under regional analgesia is awake. Great care must be exercised over what is said and how the many activities associated with care of the mother and fetus are performed, lest the mother interpret remarks or actions as an indication that she or her fetus may be in jeopardy or that there is inappropriate concern for her welfare. The woman usually is aware of surgical manipulation, identifying each maneuver as a feeling of pressure. She is painfully aware of any manipulation above the level of the spinal sensory blockade.

At times, the degree of pain relief from spinal analgesia is inadequate. In this circumstance, a significant measure of relief can be provided before delivery by administering 50 to 70 percent nitrous oxide with oxygen. Immediately after clamping the cord, a variety of techniques can be employed to provide effective analgesia. Morphine, meperidine, or fentanyl given intravenously at this time often provide excellent analgesia and euphoria as the operation is completed.

Spinal (Postpuncture) Headaches

Leakage of cerebrospinal fluid from the site of puncture of the meninges is thought to be the major factor in the genesis of spinal headache. Presumably, when the woman sits or stands, the diminished volume of cerebrospinal fluid allows traction on pain-sensitive central nervous system structures. The likelihood of this unpleasant complication can be reduced by using a small-gauge spinal needle and avoiding multiple punctures of the meninges. Placing the woman absolutely flat on her back for

several hours has been recommended to prevent postspinal headache, but there is no good evidence that this procedure is very effective. Vigorous hydration has been claimed to be of value, but also without compelling evidence to support its use. Application of a *blood patch* is effective; a few mL of the woman's blood without anticoagulant is injected epidurally at the side of the dural puncture. Saline similarly injected in larger volumes also has been claimed to provide relief. Abdominal support with a girdle or abdominal binder does seem to afford relief and is worth trying. Typically, the headache is remarkably improved by the third day and absent by the fifth.

Bladder Dysfunction

With spinal analgesia, bladder sensation is likely to be obtunded and bladder emptying impaired for the first few hours after delivery. As a consequence, bladder distension is a frequent complication of the puerperium, especially if appreciable volumes of intravenous fluid have been or are being administered. Combinations of (1) infusion of a liter or more of fluid, (2) neural blockade from epidural or spinal analgesia, (3) antidiuretic effect of oxytocin infused for a time after delivery and then stopped, (4) discomfort from a sizable episiotomy, (5) failure to observe the woman very closely for bladder distension, and (6) failure to relieve bladder distension promptly by catheterization are very likely to lead to quite troublesome bladder dysfunction and urinary tract infection.

Oxytocics and Hypertension

Paradoxically, hypertension from ergonovine (Ergotrate) or methylergonovine (Methergine) injected following delivery is most common in women who have received a spinal or epidural block.

Arachnoiditis and Meningitis

No longer are the ampules of local anesthetic stored in alcohol, formalin, or other highly toxic preservatives or solutes. Needles and catheters are now rarely subjected to cleaning by chemical treatment so that they can be reused. Instead, disposable equipment is used, and these current practices, coupled with strict aseptic technique, have made meningitis and arachnoiditis rarities.

Continuous Spinal Analgesia

Use of continuous spinal analgesia, in which an indwelling catheter is inserted into the subarachnoid space, allows the anesthetic agent to be administered in fractional doses. This technic minimizes the likelihood of many of the serious adverse effects that may promptly follow a larger dose of anesthetic by single injection, especially total spinal block. Also, for longer procedures, the drug can be replenished as needed. A hole through the meninges large enough initially for a needle containing the indwelling catheter and the perpetuation of the hole by the continued presence of the catheter are very likely to predispose to troublesome postspinal headache.

CONTRAINDICATIONS TO SPINAL ANALGESIA

The common serious complication from spinal block is hypotension. The supine position late in pregnancy commonly predisposes to a reduction in return of blood from veins below the level of the large pregnant uterus and, in turn, a reduction in cardiac output (see Chap. 7, p. 144). Moreover, sympathetic blockade from spinal analgesia usually is extensive, and it leads to further pooling of blood in dilated blood vessels below the blockade. Obstetrical complications that in themselves predispose to maternal hypovolemia and hypotension are contraindications to the use of spinal block. A severe decrease in blood pressure can be predicted when subarachnoid analgesia is used in the presence of hemorrhage or severe pregnancy-induced or aggravated hypertension. **The woman with preeclampsia is exquisitely sensitive to the hypotensive effects caused by subarachnoid block.** Even those who recommend epidural analgesia for women with severe preeclampsia believe that spinal block is contraindicated in these cases (Malinow and Ostheimer, 1987).

The cardiovascular effects of spinal block in the presence of acute blood loss but in the absence of the hemodynamic effects of pregnancy have been investigated by Kennedy and co-workers (1968). In 15 nonpregnant volunteers, spinal analgesia to the 5th thoracic sensory level was induced twice, the second time after a phlebotomy of 10 mL per kg. In the case of subarachnoid block without hemorrhage, the mean arterial blood pressure fell 10 percent while cardiac output rose slightly. In the case of hemorrhage without subarachnoid block, the mean blood pressure fell to the same degree and again the cardiac output rose slightly. However, when there was subarachnoid block after the modest hemorrhage, the mean arterial pressure fell nearly 30 percent and cardiac output fell 15 percent. Undoubtedly, the presence of a large pregnant uterus serves in the supine position to magnify appreciably these deleterious changes from spinal analgesia after overt hemorrhage.

Disorders of coagulation and defective hemostasis preclude the use of spinal analgesia. Subarachnoid puncture is contraindicated when the skin or underlying tissue at the site of needle entry is infected. Neurological disorders are usually considered to be a contraindication, if for no other reason than exacerbation of the neurological disease might be attributed to injection of the anesthetic agent.

EPIDURAL (PERIDURAL) ANALGESIA

Relief from the pain of uterine contractions and delivery, vaginal or abdominal, can be accomplished by injecting a suitable local anesthetic agent into the epidural or peridural space. The epidural space, in effect, is a potential area that contains areolar tissue, fat, lymphatics, and the internal venous plexus, which becomes engorged during pregnancy so that it reduces appreciably the volume of the space. It is limited peripherally by the ligamentum flavum and centrally by the dura matter, and it extends from the base of the skull to almost the end of the sacrum. The portal of entry into the epidural space for obstetrical analgesia is through either a lumbar intervertebral space (*lumbar epidural analgesia*) or through the sacral hiatus and sacral canal (*caudal epidural analgesia*). Although one injection may be used, much more often these are repeated through an indwelling plastic catheter, or they are given by continuous infusion using a volumetric pump.

CONTINUOUS LUMBAR EPIDURAL BLOCK

Complete analgesia for the pain of labor and vaginal delivery necessitates a block from the 10th thoracic to 5th sacral dermatomes. For abdominal delivery, the block is essential beginning at the 8th thoracic level and extending to the 1st sacral dermatome. The spread of the epidurally injected anesthetic agent will depend upon the location of the catheter tip as well as the dose, concentration, and volume of anesthetic agent used

(Table 17–1), and whether the woman is placed in the head-down, horizontal, or head-up position. It is important that the meninges not be perforated, otherwise the anesthetic enters the subarachnoid space, and in the much larger dose used to achieve epidural analgesia, it rapidly will produce total spinal blockade.

Before any injection of the local anesthetic agent, a *test dose* is given and the woman observed for features of toxicity from intravascular injection and signs of spinal blockade from subarachnoid injection. If there is no evidence for these, then a full dose is given carefully and analgesia is maintained by intermittent boluses of similar volume, or small volumes of the drug are delivered continuously by infusion pump. The addition of small doses of a short-acting narcotic, either fentanyl or sufentanil, was shown to improve analgesic efficacy for labor or cesarean delivery (Chestnut and colleagues, 1988; Phillips, 1988; Preston and associates, 1988).

When vaginal delivery is anticipated in 10 to 15 minutes, a rapidly acting agent is given through the epidural catheter to effect perineal analgesia.

Caudal Analgesia

At the lower end of the sacrum, on its posterior surface, there is a foramen resulting from the nonclosure of the laminae of the last sacral vertebra. It is screened by a thin layer of fibrous tissue. This foramen, called the sacral hiatus, leads to the caudal canal or space, which is actually the lowest extent of the epidural, or peridural space. Through the caudal space, a rich network of sacral nerve passes downward after having emerged from the dural sac several centimeters cephalad. The dural sac separates the caudal canal from the spinal cord and its surrounding fluid.

A suitable anesthetic solution that fills the caudal canal may abolish the sensation of pain carried via the sacral nerves and anesthetize the pelvis, producing analgesia suitable for vaginal delivery. Higher levels with continuous caudal technique provide analgesia both in the first and second stages and for delivery. Caudal analgesia is infrequently used today.

COMPLICATIONS

Both lumbar and caudal epidural analgesia for labor and delivery may provide most pleasant relief from the pain of labor. There are certain problems inherent in their use and, as with spinal blockade, it is imperative that close monitoring, including the level of analgesia, be performed by trained personnel.

Inadvertent Spinal Blockade

Puncture of the dura, along with inadvertent subarachnoid injection, is always a potential complication, so personnel and facilities must be immediately available to manage the complications of high spinal block. Postspinal headache is a less serious but troublesome complication of inadvertent entry.

Ineffective Analgesia

The extent to which pain relief during labor can be obtained with lumbar epidural analgesia varies. In the best of circumstances, according to Crawford (1979), about 85 percent of parturient women are free of pain, 12 percent experience partial relief, and 3 percent have no relief. Nonetheless, establishment of effective pain relief with maximum safety takes time. Consequently, in cases of rapid labor, the potential for pain relief is not realized. Epidural analgesia for women of higher parity in active labor is likely to prove not worth the risk and expense.

If the epidural analgesia is allowed to dissipate before another injection of anesthetic drug, subsequent pain relief may be delayed, incomplete, or both.

At times, perineal analgesia for delivery is difficult to obtain, especially with the lumbar epidural technique. When this condition is encountered, Akamatsu and Bonica (1974) recommended use of a second catheter to achieve low caudal block. Insertion of a second catheter, of course, increases many of the risks being described. For this problem, others have suggested addition of a low spinal or pudendal block, or systemic analgesia.

Hypotension

By blocking sympathetic tracts, epidurally injected analgesic agents may cause hypotension. In the nonhypertensive and normally hypervolemic pregnant women, hypotension induced by epidural analgesia usually can be prevented by rapid infusion of a balanced salt solution or treated successfully as described for spinal analgesia. Despite these precautions, hypotension is the most common side effect. Brizgys and colleagues (1987) studied 583 consecutive women given epidural analgesia for cesarean section and reported that hypotension followed in 32 percent, even after volume expansion with 1 L of lactated Ringer's solution. In another group of women, similarly prehydrated but also given 25 mg of intramuscular ephedrine prophylactically, the incidence was 25 percent (Fig. 17–2). Although there were no differences in umbilical arterial and venous P_{O_2} and P_{CO_2}, neonates born to women with hypotension had a lower mean pH.

It is important that with each injection of analgesic the blood pressure be measured every 2 minutes for the next 20 minutes. Brizgys and colleagues (1987) showed that rapid correction of hypotension with crystalloid infusion, left uterine displacement, and intravenous ephedrine resulted in delivery of healthy infants.

Central Nervous Stimulation

Convulsions are an uncommon but serious complication, the immediate management of which has been described above.

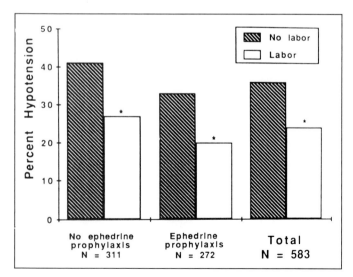

Figure 17–2. The incidence of hypotension following epidural analgesia given for cesarean section. Asterisk indicates significant difference between women with and without labor. (*From Brizgys and colleagues: Anesthesiology 67:782, 1987.*)

TABLE 17–2. EFFECT OF EPIDURAL ANALGESIA ON THE METHOD OF VAGINAL DELIVERY IN 1,377 WOMEN DELIVERED DURING JULY 1984 AT JEFFERSON DAVIS HOSPITAL, HOUSTON, TEXAS

Method of Delivery	Epidural Analgesia Percent (N = 296)	Other Analgesia Percent (N = 822)
Spontaneous	72	96
Outlet Forceps	23[a]	3
Midforceps	5[a]	1

[a] $P < 0.005$ compared to other analgesia group.
Adapted from Cox and colleagues: Texas Med 83:45, 1987.

Effect on Labor

Epidural block induced prior to well-established labor may be followed by desultory labor. The precise role played by epidural analgesia in this phenomenon is not clear, since this sequence of events also is seen in its absence. Lowensohn and co-workers (1974) reported significant depression of uterine activity for about 30 minutes following the epidural injection of lidocaine. Akamatsu and Bonica (1974) suggested that epinephrine injected with the anesthetic agent may impair labor. During the second stage of labor, epidural analgesia that provides effective pain relief is likely to reduce appreciably maternal expulsive efforts. As a consequence, an epidural block may lead to delay or, less frequently, to failure of descent of the presenting part and spontaneous rotation to the occiput anterior position. Therefore, as reported by Chestnut (1987), Cox (1987), and Kaminski (1987) and their colleagues, with epidural analgesia there is likely to be an increased incidence of midforceps deliveries and forceps rotations (Table 17–2; also Chap. 25, p. 425).

SAFETY

The relative safety of epidural analgesia is attested to by the extraordinary experiences reported by Crawford (1985) from the Birmingham Maternity Hospital in England. From 1968 through 1985, nearly 26,000 women were given epidural analgesia for labor, and there were no maternal deaths. He outlined the significant complications encountered, and he divided these into the categories shown in Table 17–3. As expected, the nine potentially life-threatening complications followed either inadvertent intravenous or intrathecal injections of lidocaine, bupivacaine, or both.

CONTRAINDICATIONS

As with spinal analgesia, the contraindications include actual or anticipated serious maternal hemorrhage, overt hypertension, infection at or near the sites for puncture, and suspicion of neurological disease. Rolbin and colleagues (1988) advise against epidural analgesia if the platelet count is below 100,000 per μL.

Disagreements persist over the use of epidural analgesia in the presence of hypertension (Malinow and Ostheimer, 1987). Some obstetrical anesthesiologists urge regional analgesia for women with overt hypertension (Gutsche and Cheek, 1987; Moir, 1986). Marx (1974) contends that by use of regional blockade maternal circulatory and cerebrospinal fluid pressure responses to painful uterine contractions are reduced and the

TABLE 17–3. COMPLICATIONS WITH LUMBAR EPIDURAL ANALGESIA GIVEN DURING LABOR TO 26,490 WOMEN AT BIRMINGHAM MATERNITY HOSPITAL, ENGLAND

Complication Category	Example	Outcome
Potentially life-threatening (1:3,000)	Intravenous injection (3)	Loss of consciousness
	Intrathecal injection (6)	1 cardiac arrest (recovered)
Serious, not life-threatening (1:13,000)	Epidural space fibrosis (1)	Laminectomy (improved)
	Epidural abscess (1)	Laminectomy (recovered)
Moderately serious	Prolonged hypotension (2)	Recovered
During labor (1:2,000)	Severe hypertension, headache (1)	Recovered
	Failed analgesia, paresis (1)	Recovered
After delivery (1:2,000)	Backache, leg pain (1)	Recovered
	Numbness and weakness (2)	Recovered

Data from Crawford: Anaesthesia 40:1219, 1985.

hazard of hypertensive crisis is minimized. The intrigue for the use of regional analgesia in hypertensive states complicating pregnancy undoubtedly stems from the fact that the mother is hypertensive and the blood pressure very often is lowered by regional analgesia. This attitude prevails even though the mechanism by which the blood pressure is lowered is probably no more physiological than phlebotomy. Shnider and Levinson (1979) emphasized *"Sudden falls in blood pressure can rapidly produce fetal distress and demise as the uteroplacental circulation becomes further compromised."* For these reasons, in over 300 consecutive cases of antepartum or intrapartum eclampsia at Parkland Hospital, spinal and epidural blockade have been deliberately avoided. Instead, local or pudendal block plus nitrous oxide–oxygen analgesia are used for vaginal deliveries and general analgesia with thiopental, succinylcholine, and nitrous oxide–oxygen is used for the occasional difficult vaginal delivery and for cesarean sections. Perinatal and maternal mortality rates have been very low in these pregnancies complicated by eclampsia (Pritchard and co-workers, 1984).

In many medical centers, a more liberal view of epidural analgesia is taken. This undoubtedly stems from the availability of continuous anesthesia coverage by physicians with expertise in obstetrical analgesia and anesthesia. As discussed in Chapter 35, (p. 686), if epidural analgesia is to be used for women with severe preeclampsia–eclampsia, specially trained anesthesiologists and obstetricians should be responsible for the woman and her fetus (American College of Obstetricians and Gynecologists, 1988; Moore and colleagues, 1985).

EPIDURAL OPIATE ANALGESIA

Injection of opiates into the epidural space to relieve pain was described in 1979 by Wang and colleagues. This method of relieving pain from labor is becoming popular, especially since complications with this technique are less worrisome than those seen with epidural injections of local anesthetics. The mechanism of action of opiates given epidurally is from their interaction with specific receptors in the dorsal horn and dorsal roots. The few systemic symptoms encountered are from low levels of the drug following vascular absorption.

Fentanyl is commonly employed for this purpose, and has been the most widely studied. Following doses of 100 μg given through an epidural catheter, analgesia is apparent within 5 to 10 minutes, it is maximal by 20 minutes, and lasts for 60 to 90 minutes (Cousins and Mather, 1984). A most attractive feature of this method is that there are minimal cardiovascular effects, since there is no sympathetic blockade. There is also no motor paresis, but the drug does not provide adequate analgesia for second-stage labor pain, episiotomy, or delivery.

Adverse effects of epidural fentanyl are principally from its systemic absorption. If given intravascularly during the epidural injection, then respiratory depression may be encountered immediately. Most other side effects are encountered 1 to 3 hours later, and are thought to be due to the effects of fentanyl on the central nervous system as it is carried cephalad within the cerebrospinal fluid. These effects include nausea and vomiting, pruritus, urinary retention, and late-onset respiratory depression. Naloxone, given in doses of 40 to 80 μg intravenously, usually will abolish these symptoms without affecting the analgesic action.

When given intravenously, fentanyl quickly crosses the placenta, and drug levels are 20 to 40 percent of those in the mother (Craft and colleagues, 1983). Unless given very close to delivery or in excessive doses, fentanyl administered epidurally to the mother is unlikely to cause newborn respiratory depression. If it does, then naloxone is given.

More recently, a combination of epidural fentanyl with bupivacaine has been advocated (Gibson, 1986). The advantages cited are that smaller bupivacaine doses are needed, and thus worrisome side effects, including hypotension, are less commonly encountered. At least three randomized studies have shown improved efficacy of fentanyl or sufentanil added to epidurally administered bupivacaine given for labor or cesarean section (Chestnut and colleagues, 1988; Phillips, 1988; Preston and associates, 1988).

REFERENCES

Abouleish E, Rawal N, Fallow K, Hernandez D: Combined intrathecal morphine and bupivacaine for cesarean section: Anesth Analg 67:370, 1988

Akamatsu TJ, Bonica JJ: Spinal and extradural analgesia-anesthesia for parturition. Clin Obstet Gynecol 17:183, 1974

American College of Obstetricians and Gynecologists: ACOG and ASA recommend obstetric anesthesia goals. Newsletter, September 1988, p 9

American College of Obstetricians and Gynecologists: Obstetric anesthesia and analgesia. Technical Bulletin, No 112, January 1988

Angel JL, Knuppel RA, Lake M: Sinusoidal fetal heart rate pattern associated with intravenous butorphanol administration: A case report. Am J Obstet Gynecol 149:465, 1984

Bartlett JG, Gorbach SL, Finegold SM: The bacteriology of aspiration pneumonia. Am J Med 56:202, 1974

Bonica JJ: Acupuncture anesthesia in the People's Republic of China: Implications for American Medicine. JAMA 229:1317, 1974

Brizgys RV, Dailey PA, Shnider SM, Kotelko DM, Levinson G: The incidence and neonatal effects of maternal hypotension during epidural anesthesia for cesarean section. Anesthesiology 67:782, 1987

Bynum LJ, Pierce AK: Pulmonary aspiration of gastric contents. Am Rev Respir Dis 114:1129, 1976

Carlsson B-M, Johansson M, Westin B: Fetal heart rate pattern before and after paracervical anesthesia. A prospective study. Acta Obstet Gynecol Scand 66:391, 1987

Chestnut DH, Owen CL, Bates JN, Ostman LG, Choi WW, Geiger MW: Continuous infusion epidural analgesia during labor: A randomized, double-blind comparison of 0.625% bupivacaine/0.0002% fentanyl versus 0.125% bupivacaine. Anesthesiology 68:754, 1988

Chestnut DH, Vandewalker GF, Owen CI, Bates JN, Choi WW: The influence of continuous epidural bupivacaine analgesia on the second stage of labor and method of delivery in nulliparous women. Anesthesiology 66:774, 1987

Cohen SE: The aspiration syndrome. Clin Obstet Gynecol 9:235, 1982

Cousins MJ, Mather LE: Intrathecal and epidural administration of opioids. Anesthesiology 61:276, 1984

Cox SM, Bost JE, Faro S, Carpenter RJ: Epidural anesthesia during labor and the incidence of forceps delivery. Tex Med 83:45, 1987

Craft JB, Coaldrake LA, Bolan JC, Mondino M, Mazel P, Gilman RM, Shokes LK, Woolf WA: Placental passage and uterine effects of fentanyl. Anesth Analg 62:894, 1983

Crawford JS: Maternal mortality associated with anesthesia. Lancet 2:918, 1972

Crawford JS: Continuous lumbar epidural analgesia for labour and delivery. Br Med J 1:72, 1979

Crawford JS: Some maternal complications of epidural analgesia for labour. Anesthesia 40:1219, 1985

DeVoe SJ, DeVoe K Jr, Rigsby WC, McDaniels BA: Effects of meperidine on uterine contractility. Am J Obstet Gynecol 105:1004, 1969

Endler GC, Mariona FG, Sokol RJ, Stevenson LB: Anesthesia-related maternal mortality in Michigan, 1972 to 1984. Am J Obstet Gynecol 159:187, 1988

Ericson A, Källen B: Survey of infants born in 1973 or 1975 to Swedish women working in operating rooms during their pregnancies. Anesth Analg 58:302, 1979

Fishburne JI Jr, Greiss FC Jr, Hopkinson R, Rhyne AL: Response of the gravid uterine vasculature to arterial levels of local anesthetic agents. Am J Obstet Gynecol 133:753, 1979

Gabel HD: Maternal mortality in South Carolina from 1970 to 1984: An analysis. Obstet Gynecol 69:307, 1987

Gibbs CP, Banner TC: Effectiveness of Bicitra® as a preoperative antacid. Anesthesiology 61:97, 1984

Gibbs CP, Krischer J, Peckham BM, Sharp H, Kirschbaum TH: Obstetric anesthesia: A national survey. Anesthesiology 65:298, 1986

Gibbs CP, Schwartz DJ, Wynne JW, Hood CI, Kuck EJ: Antacid pulmonary aspiration in the dog. Anesthesiology 51:380, 1979

Gibson WP: Epidural fentanyl for labor pain. Contemp Ob/Gyn 28:111, 1986

Gilstrap LC, Hauth JC, Hankins DG, Patterson AR: Effect of type of anesthesia on blood loss at cesarean section. Obstet Gynecol 69:328, 1987

Greiss FC Jr, Still JG, Anderson SG: Effects of local anesthetic agents on the uterine vasculatures and myometrium. Am J Obstet Gynecol 124:889, 1976

Gutsche BB, Cheek TG: Anesthetic considerations in preeclampsia-eclampsia. In Shnider SM, Levinson G (eds): Anesthesia for Obstetrics, 2nd ed. Baltimore, Williams & Wilkins, 1987, p 225

Hatjis CG, Meis PJ: Sinusoidal fetal heart rate pattern associated with butorphanol administration. Obstet Gynecol 67:377, 1986

Hodgkinson R, Bhatt M, Kim SS, Grewal G, Marx GF: Neonatal neurobehavioral tests following cesarean section under general and spinal anesthesia. Am J Obstet Gynecol 132:670, 1978

Hodgkinson R, Glassenberg R, Joyce TH, Coombs DW, Ostheimer GW, Gibbs CP: Comparison of cimetidine (Tagamet) with antacid for safety and effectiveness in reducing gastric acidity before elective cesarean section. Anesthesiology 59:86, 1983

Hughey MJ, McElin TW, Young T: Maternal and fetal outcome of Lamaze prepared patients. Obstet Gynecol 51:643, 1978

Husum B, Wulf HC, Norgaard T: Sister chromatid exchanges and structural chromosome aberrations in lymphocytes in operating room personnel. Acta Anaesthesiol Scand 27:262, 1983

Jacoby J: Anesthesia for normal vaginal delivery. Anesth Rev 1:11, 1974

Kaminski HM, Stafl A, Aiman J: The effect of epidural analgesia on the frequency of instrumental obstetric delivery. Obstet Gynecol 69:770, 1987

Kaunitz AM, Hughes JM, Grives DA, Smith JC, Rochat RW, Kaffrissen ME: Causes of maternal mortality in the United States. Obstet Gynecol 65:605, 1985

Kennedy WF Jr, Bonica JJ, Akamatsu TJ, Ward RJ, Martin WE, Grinstein A: Cardiovascular and respiratory effects of subarachnoid block in the presence of acute blood loss. Anesthesiology 29:29, 1968

Knill-Jones RP, Newman BJ, Spence AA: Anaesthetic practice and pregnancy. Lancet 2:807, 1975

Lamaze F: Painless Childbirth: Psychoprophylactic Method. Chicago, Henry Regnery, 1970

Lehmann DK, Mabie WC, Miller JM Jr, Pernoll ML: The epidemiology and pathology of maternal mortality: Charity Hospital of Louisiana in New Orleans, 1965–1984. Obstet Gynecol 69:833, 1987

Lewis M, Crawford JS: Can one risk fasting the obstetric patient for less than 4 hours? Br J Anaesth 59:312, 1987

Liddicoat R: The effects of maternal antenatal decompression treatment on infant mental development. S Afr Med J 42:203, 1968

Lowensohn RI, Paul RH, Fales S, Yeh S-Y, Hon EH: Intrapartum epidural anesthesia: An evaluation of effects on uterine activity. Obstet Gynecol 44:388, 1974

Malinow AM, Ostheimer GW: Anesthesia for the high-risk parturient. Obstet Gynecol 69:951, 1987

Marx GF: Obstetric anesthesia in the presence of medical complications. Clin Obstet Gynecol 17:165, 1974

Mendelson CL: The aspiration of stomach contents into the lungs during obstetric anesthesia. Am J Obstet Gynecol 52:191, 1946

Moir DD: Cimetidine, antacids, and pulmonary aspiration. J Anesthesiol 59:81, 1983

Moir DD: Local anaesthetic techniques in obstetrics. Br J Anaesth 58:747, 1986

Moore TR, Key TC, Reisner LS, Resnick R: Evaluation of the use of continuous lumbar epidural anesthesia for hypertensive pregnant women in labor. Am J Obstet Gynecol 152:104, 1985

Pharah POD, Alberman E, Doyle P: Outcome of pregnancy among women in anesthetic practice. Lancet 1:34, 1977

Phillips G: Continuous infusion epidural analgesia in labor: The effect of adding sufentanil to 0.125% bupivacaine. Anesth Analg 67:462, 1988

Preston PG, Rosen MA, Hughes SC, Glosten B, Ross BK, Daniels D, Shnider SM, Dailey PA: Epidural anesthesia with fentanyl and lidocaine for cesarean section: Maternal effects and neonatal outcome. Anesthesiology 68:938, 1988

Pritchard JA, Cunningham FG, Pritchard SA: The Parkland Memorial Hospital protocol for treatment of eclampsia: Evaluation of 245 cases. Am J Obstet Gynecol 148:951, 1984

Quilligan EJ, Keegan KA, Donahue MJ: Double-blind comparison of intravenously injected butorphanol and meperidine in parturients. Int J Gynaecol Obstet 18:363, 1980

Read GD: Childbirth Without Fear. New York, Harper, 1944, p 192

Riffel HD, Nochimson DJ, Paul RH, Hon EHG: Effects of meperidine and promethazine during labor. Obstet Gynecol 42:738, 1973

Rolbin SH, Abbott D, Musclow E, Papsin F, Lie LM, Freedman J: Epidural anesthesia in pregnant patients with low platelet counts. Obstet Gynecol 71:918, 1988

Sachs BP, Brown DA, Driscoll SG, Schulman E, Acker D, Ransil BJ, Jewett JF: Maternal mortality in Massachusetts: Trends and prevention. N Engl J Med 316:667, 1987

Schultz JH, Luthe W: Autogenic Training. New York, Grune & Stratton, 1959

Shnider SM, Levinson G: Anesthesia for Obstetrics. Baltimore, Williams & Wilkins, 1979

Sutherland AD, Stock JG, Davies JM: Effects of preoperative fasting on morbidity and gastric contents in patients undergoing day-stay surgery. Br J Anaesth 58:876, 1986

Svancarek W, Chirino O, Schaefer G Jr, Blythe JG: Retropsoas and subgluteal abscesses following paracervical and pudendal anesthesia. JAMA 237:892, 1977

Taylor G, Pryse-Davies J: The prophylactic use of antacids in the prevention of the acid pulmonary aspiration syndrome. Lancet 1:288, 1966

Teabeaut JR II: Aspiration of gastric contents: An experimental study. Am J Pathol 28:51, 1952

Wallis L, Shnider SM, Palahniuk RJ, Spivey HT: An evaluation of acupuncture analgesia in obstetrics. Anesthesiology 41:596, 1974

Wang JK, Nauss LE, Thomas JE: Pain relieved by intrathecally applied morphine in man. Anesthesiology 50:149, 1979

Warren TM, Datta S, Ostheimer GW, Naulty JS, Weiss JB, Morrison JA: Comparison of the maternal and neonatal effects of halothane, enflurane, and isoflurane for cesarean delivery. Anesth Analg 62:516, 1983

Wenger DR, Gitchell RG: Severe infections following pudendal block anesthesia: Need for orthopaedic awareness. J Bone Joint Surg [AM] 55:202, 1973

Wheatley RG, Kallus FT, Reynolds RC, Giesecke AH: Milk of magnesia is an effective pre-induction antacid in obstetrical anesthesia. Anesthesiology 50:514, 1979

Zagorzycki MT, Brinkman CR III: The effect of general and epidural anesthesia upon neonatal Apgar scores in repeat cesarean section. Surg Gynecol Obstet 155:641, 1982

Part V

ABNORMALITIES OF LABOR AND DELIVERY

Dystocia Due to Abnormalities of the Expulsive Forces and Precipitate Labor

Dystocia (literally, difficult labor) is characterized by abnormally slow progress of labor. It is the consequence of four distinct abnormalities that may exist singly or in combination:

1. Abnormalities of the expulsive forces, either uterine forces insufficiently strong or appropriately coordinated to efface and dilate the cervix (uterine dysfunction) or inadequate voluntary muscle effort during the second stage of labor (Chap. 18).
2. Abnormalities of presentation, position, or development of the fetus (see Chap. 19).
3. Abnormalities of the maternal bony pelvis—that is, pelvic contraction (see Chap. 20).
4. Abnormalities of the birth canal other than those of the bony pelvis that form an obstacle to fetal descent (see Chap. 21).

Pelvic contraction is often accompanied by uterine dysfunction, and the two together constitute the most common cause of dystocia. Similarly, faulty presentation or unusual fetal size or shape may be accompanied by uterine dysfunction. *As a generalization, uterine dysfunction is common whenever there is disproportion between the presenting part of the fetus and the birth canal.*

UTERINE DYSFUNCTION

As described in Chapter 10 (p. 213), the *first stage of labor* has commonly, but somewhat artificially, been divided into two distinct phases: the *latent phase* and the *active phase*. Typically, the latent phase (*prodromal labor*) will be of several hours duration, during which time the cervix undergoes softening and effacement but only slight dilatation. This phase of cervical change is characterized by uterine contractions of mild intensity, short duration, and variable frequency. The phase of more rapid cervical dilatation, or the active phase, follows. During the active phase, or what has long been called simply labor, the cervix dilates more rapidly at 1 to 2 cm per hour

and there is descent of the presenting part through the birth canal (Fig. 18–1).

The active phase of labor has been subdivided further into three additional divisions or phases: the acceleration phase, the phase of maximum slope, and the deceleration phase. It must be emphasized that the acceleration and deceleration phases may never be identified during rapid labor. In fact, to anticipate a deceleration phase in labor can result in the delivery of many babies under less than optimal circumstances! Friedman (1980) emphasized this when he stated that the deceleration phase *"is an artifact in the sense that nothing is actually slowing down, but rather, the cervix is now being retracted cephalad around the fetal presenting part, and therefore is no longer being actively dilated by the forces of uterine contraction."*

The descent of the presenting part normally begins well before the cervix reaches full dilatation and proceeds until the presenting part reaches the perineum. It should be noted that this pattern is highly variable. The fetal presenting part in nulliparous women may be at the +1 or even +2 station before the onset of labor, whereas in parous women, descent of the presenting part may not begin until the cervix is nearly fully dilated.

The sigmoid curve for cervical dilatation and the slope of fetal descent, at best, should be considered as *idealized visual aids* to help understand the temporal relationships of cervical dilatation and the descent of the presenting part (Fig. 18–1).

Failure of the cervix to dilate or of the presenting part to descend is cause for concern. Prolongation of either the *first or second stage of labor* may result in increased perinatal and maternal morbidity. Any delay in cervical dilatation during the first stage or prolongation of the second stage of labor should alert the obstetrician to possible danger.

Uterine dysfunction in any phase of cervical dilatation is characterized by lack of progress, for one of the prime characteristics of normal labor is its progression. Friedman (1978) defined prolongation of the latent phase as 20 hours in nulliparas and 14 hours in multiparas, and a protracted active phase as cervical dilatation of less than 1.2 cm per hour in nulliparas and 1.5 cm in multiparas (Fig. 18–1; Table 18–1). The diagnosis of

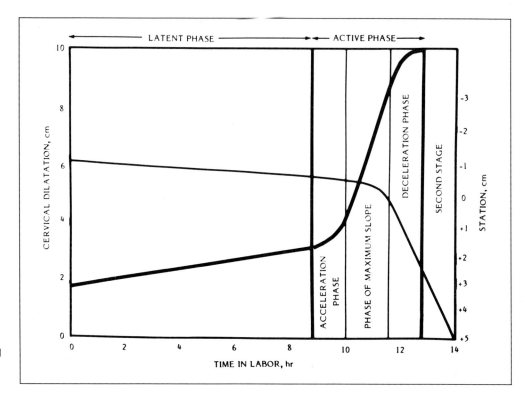

Figure 18–1. Composite of cervical dilatation and fetal descent curves illustrating their interrelationship and their component phases. (*Courtesy of Cohen and Friedman, 1983.*)

uterine dysfunction in the latent phase is difficult and sometimes can be made only in retrospect. One of the most common errors is to treat women for uterine dysfunction who are not yet in active labor.

There have been three significant advances in the treatment of uterine dysfunction: (1) the realization that undue prolongation of labor may contribute to perinatal morbidity and mortality; (2) the use of very dilute intravenous infusion of oxytocin in the treatment of certain types of uterine dysfunction; and (3) the more frequent use of cesarean section to effect delivery rather than difficult midforceps delivery when oxytocin fails or its use is inappropriate (Table 18–2).

TYPES OF DYSFUNCTION

Reynolds and co-workers (1948) emphasized that the uterine contractions of labor are normally characterized by a gradient of myometrial activity, being greatest and lasting longest at the fundus (fundal dominance) and diminishing toward the cervix (see Chap. 10, p. 214). Caldeyro-Barcia and his colleagues in Montevideo (1950) advanced the work of Reynolds by inserting small balloons into the myometrium at various levels. With the balloons attached to strain-gauge transducers, they demonstrated that there was, in addition to a gradient of activity, a time differential in the onset of the contractions in the fundus,

TABLE 18–1. ABNORMAL LABOR PATTERNS, DIAGNOSTIC CRITERIA, AND METHODS OF TREATMENT

Labor Pattern	Diagnostic Criterion		Preferred Treatment	Exceptional Treatment
	Nulliparas	*Multiparas*		
Prolongation Disorder				
(Prolonged latent phase)	> 20 hr	> 14 hr	Therapeutic rest	Oxytocin or cesarean sections for urgent problems
Protraction Disorders				
1. Protracted active phase dilatation	< 1.2 cm/hr	< 1.5 cm/h		
2. Protracted descent	< 1.0 cm/hr	< 2 cm/hr	Expectant and support	Cesarean section for CPD[a]
Arrest Disorders				
1. Prolonged deceleration phase	> 3 hr	> 1 hr	Without CPD: oxytocin	Rest if exhausted
2. Secondary arrest of dilatation	> 2 hr	> 2 hr		
3. Arrest of descent	> 1 hr	> 1 hr	With CPD: cesarean section	Cesarean section
4. Failure of descent	No descent in deceleration phase or second stage of labor			

[a]CPD: Cephalopelvic disproportion.
Modified from Cohen and Friedman, 1983.

TABLE 18–2. NEONATAL APGAR SCORES BY LABOR PATTERN IN NULLIPARAS AND PERINATAL MORTALITY BY DELIVERY METHOD

Labor Pattern	Percent of Apgar Scores Less than 5		Perinatal Mortality per 1,000 by Delivery Method		
	At 1 min	At 5 min	Spontaneous	Low Forceps	Midforceps
Normal	12.7	3.2	1.5	2.8	10.8[a]
Prolongation disorder	12.9	4.6	0.0	0.0	10.8[a]
Protraction disorders	23.7[a]	3.1	0.0	12.0[a]	28.5[a]
Arrest disorders	25.2[a]	8.0[a]	16.1[a]	24.4[a]	38.3[a]

[a]Statistically significant, p < 0.01.
Modified from Cohen and Friedman, 1983.

midzone, and lower segments of the uterus. Larks (1960) described the exciting stimulus as starting in one cornu and then several milliseconds later in the other, the excitation waves then joining and sweeping over the fundus and down the uterus.

The group in Montevideo (Caldeyro-Barcia, 1950) made another significant contribution to the understanding of uterine dysfunction. By inserting a polyethylene catheter through the abdominal wall into the amnionic fluid, they ascertained that the lower limit of pressure of contractions required to dilate the cervix is 15 mm Hg, a figure in keeping with the findings of Hendricks and coworkers (1959), who reported that a normal spontaneous uterine contraction often exerts a pressure of about 60 mm Hg. From these observations, it is possible to define two types of uterine dysfunction. In one, *hypotonic uterine dysfunction*, there is no basal hypertonus and uterine contractions have a normal gradient pattern (synchronous), but the slight rise in pressure during a contraction is insufficient to dilate the cervix at a satisfactory rate. This type of uterine dysfunction usually occurs during the active phase of labor, after the cervix has dilated to more than 4 cm. In the other, *hypertonic uterine dysfunction*, or *incoordinate uterine dysfunction*, either basal tone is elevated appreciably or the pressure gradient is distorted, perhaps by contraction of the midsegment of the uterus with more force than the fundus or by complete asynchronism of the impulses originating in each cornu, or a combination of these two. This type of dysfunction is typically encountered in the latent phase of labor.

In hypotonic uterine dysfunction, contractions become less frequent and the uterus is easily identable even at the acme of a contraction. Contractions of the hypertonic or incoordinate variety are typically much more painful yet ineffective. As discussed below, hypotonic dysfunction often responds favorably to treatment with oxytocin. The opposite is most often true of the hypertonic variety, in which the abnormal pattern of uterine contractions is more likely to become accentuated and the tone of the uterine muscle increased. Exceptions have been documented, however, in which a uterus with basal hypertonus and frequent, incoordinate contractions did convert to orderly physiological contractions, apparently in response to intravenous oxytocin (Caldeyro-Barcia, 1957). In general, the likelihood of such a response is low and the risk of enhancing the hypertonus is considerable (Cohen and Friedman, 1983).

ETIOLOGY

Pelvic contraction and fetal malposition are common causes of uterine dysfunction. That moderate degrees of pelvic contraction and fetal malposition may cause hypotonic uterine dysfunction is of great clinical importance. Overdistention of the uterus, as with twins and with hydramnios, may contribute to the condition. *In many—perhaps one half—of instances, however, the cause of uterine dysfunction is unknown* (Seitchik and co-workers, 1987). The main fault seldom lies within a cervix that is too rigid to dilate. In elderly nulliparas, and in women with cervical fibrosis from some cause, however, excessive rigidity of the cervix may be a factor in the production of dystocia.

COMPLICATIONS

Undue procrastination too often leads to an unfortunate outcome, whereas intervention too early results in needless cesarean deliveries. Fetal and neonatal deaths are accompaniments of intrauterine infection, which commonly develops in prolonged dysfunctional labor. Although it may be wise for the mother's protection to treat these intrauterine infections with antibiotics, such therapy may be of less value in protecting the fetus. Maternal exhaustion may occur if labor is greatly prolonged; however, supportive therapy with adequate intravenous fluids should be initiated and delivery effected before these complications appear. Difficult labors and deliveries are more likely to leave psychological scars on the mothers, as emphasized by Jeffcoate (1961), as well as Steer (1950). Both found that difficult labor exerted a definite deleterious effect upon future childbearing. These investigators showed that, although more than two thirds of their patients had additional children after spontaneous delivery, only one third did so after midforceps operations.

TREATMENT OF HYPOTONIC UTERINE DYSFUNCTION

Two questions must be answered before a plan for treatment can be formulated: (1) Has the woman actually been in active labor? If there has been rhythmic uterine activity of sufficient intensity to produce some discomfort and the cervix has been observed to undergo distinct changes in effacement *and* in dilatation to 4 cm at least, it is correct to conclude that there has been real, albeit abnormal, labor. (2) Is there cephalopelvic disproportion? Uterine dysfunction is often a protection against some degree of pelvic contraction or abnormalities of fetal size or presentation. Fortunately, the uterus does not typically persist in spontaneous activity that would lead to rupture. Instead, the usual forces of labor are replaced by hypotonic uterine dysfunction.

Most often, once the diagnosis of active labor followed by hypotonic uterine dysfunction has been made and the head is well fixed in the pelvis, the membranes, if intact, should be ruptured and ideally an intrauterine pressure catheter and fetal scalp electrode placed. Close observation may be employed for

30 to 60 minutes to see if the amniotomy will improve the quality of contractions. Next, a decision must be made whether to stimulate labor with oxytocin or to effect cesarean delivery. The presence of meconium in the amnionic fluid may be an ominous sign, and this observation makes close monitoring of fetal heart rate and the uterine contraction pattern even more critical.

The choice of whether to augment labor with *hypotonic uterine dysfunction* has been for many years an empirical decision based largely upon clinical judgment as to fetal size, presentation, and position as well as clinical assessment of pelvic size. In practice, x-ray pelvimetry provides little help (Joyce and associates, 1975; Barton and co-workers, 1982; Anderson, 1983), and in some cases may result in an increased and unnecessary cesarean section rate (Bottoms and associates, 1987).

Oxytocin Stimulation

It should be ascertained that the birth canal is most likely adequate for the size of the fetal head and that the fetal head is well flexed so as to utilize its smallest diameters to negotiate the birth canal (biparietal and suboccipitobregmatic diameters). A contracted pelvis is most *unlikely* when all of the following criteria are met:

1. The diagonal conjugate is normal.
2. The pelvic sidewalls are nearly parallel.
3. The ischial spines are not prominent.
4. The sacrum is not flat.
5. The subpubic angle is not narrow.
6. The occiput is known to be the presenting part.
7. The fetal head is engaged or descends through the pelvic inlet with fundal pressure.

If these criteria are not met, the alternatives are cesarean delivery or possibly oxytocin stimulation. If oxytocin is used, it is mandatory that the fetal heart rate and the contraction pattern frequency, intensity, duration, and timing in relation to the fetal heart rate be observed closely. If fetal heart action is monitored discontinuously, it is imperative that it be checked *immediately following* contractions rather than waiting a minute or more afterward (see Chap. 15, p. 302).

Technique for Intravenous Oxytocin

Ten units of oxytocin are thoroughly mixed with 1 L of aqueous solution, usually 5 percent glucose in water or, preferably, a balanced salt solution. More dilute solutions can be prepared by doubling the amount of diluent or halving the amount of oxytocin. Although more dilute solutions have been found effective by numerous authors, the mixture (10 U per L) is easy to prepare, safe, effective, and likely to cause the least confusion in preparation and administration. Since the oxytocin solution contains 10 mU per mL, its rate of flow is easily calculated. Use of a constant infusion pump enhances the precision of the dosage delivered, especially in the lower range, and is recommended. A needle, *with the flow shut off*, is inserted into an arm vein, or preferably into an already well-functioning intravenous infusion line, and the flow started to deliver no more than 1 mU per minute (Seitchik and Castillo, 1982).

For *augmentation* of labor in true hypotonic dysfunction, 1 mU of oxytocin should not initiate tetanic uterine contractions, although one should be prepared to stop the flow in the event that the uterus is overly sensitive to the drug. The flow can be increased gradually at not greater than 30-minute intervals to yield no more than 10 mU per minute, according to Seitchik and

Castillo (1982). It is rarely necessary to exceed this rate in the treatment of uterine dysfunction. For the *induction* of labor, if a flow rate of 30 to 40 mU per minute fails to initiate satisfactory uterine contractions, greater rates are not likely to do so.

The Parkland Hospital protocol for oxytocin administration, for either induction or augmentation of labor, calls for oxytocin to be infused initially at 1 mU per minute. If contractions do not ensue, then this is increased by 1 mU per minute every 20 minutes until 8 mU per minute is reached. If contractions have not then become apparent, the delivery rate is increased by 2 mU increments every 20 minutes until 20 mU per minute are being given. These higher doses are seldom needed for successful augmentation, but may be necessary for induction of labor. If there is still no uterine activity at these higher concentrations, then the need for induction is reassessed and the dosage may be increased in 20-minute increments until 40 mU per minute are reached. At Parkland Hospital, approximately 20 percent of labors are induced or stimulated using oxytocin, and from 1983 to 1987, more than 11,000 women have been given oxytocin according to this protocol (K. Leveno, unpublished observations). Hyperstimulation resulting in fetal heart rate abnormalities has been very uncommon. The American College of Obstetricians and Gynecologists (1987) recommends increasing the dose at 30- to 60-minute intervals by 1 to 2 mU per minute.

Experience from the San Antonio investigators is that the biological plasma half-time is sufficiently prolonged that continuous infusion is followed by rising plasma oxytocin concentrations for 40 minutes (Seitchik and colleagues, 1984). Foster and co-workers (1988) examined the effects of oxytocin augmentation in 174 nulliparas, 92 in whom oxytocin dosage was escalated at 15-minute intervals and 82 in whom it was increased at 30-minute intervals. The number of cesarean sections (17 percent) and induction-delivery intervals (about 7 hours) were similar for both groups, however the infusion was stopped more often (18 versus 7 percent) for hyperstimulation in those women in whom oxytocin infusion was increased at 15-minute intervals. Thorp and associates (1988) used high-dose oxytocin for active management of labor (see Chap. 16) and reported no adverse fetal sequelae when oxytocin was begun at 4 mU per minute and increased by 4 mU every 15 minutes.

The mother should never be left alone while the oxytocin infusion is running. Uterine contractions must be evaluated continually and oxytocin shut off immediately if contractions exceed 1 minute in duration or if the fetal heart rate decelerates significantly. When either occurs, immediate discontinuation of the oxytocin nearly always corrects the disturbances, preventing harm to mother and fetus. The oxytocin concentration in plasma rapidly falls, since the mean half-life oxytocin is approximately 5 minutes.

It always must be kept in mind that oxytocin has potent antidiuretic action. Whenever 20 mU per minute or more of oxytocin is infused, free water clearance by the kidney decreases markedly. If aqueous fluids, especially dextrose in water, are infused in appreciable amounts along with the oxytocin, there exists the possibility of water intoxication that may lead to convulsions, coma, and even death (see Chap. 16, p. 321).

At Parkland Hospital, the following precautions are exercised with the use of oxytocin to treat hypotonic dysfunction:

1. The woman must be in true labor, not false or prodromal labor. The evidence of labor is progressive effacement and dilatation of the cervix. Although progress has

ceased, labor must have progressed 3 to 4 cm dilatation. One of the most common mistakes in obstetrics is to try to stimulate labor in women who have not been in active labor.

2. There must be no other discernible evidence of mechanical obstruction to safe delivery.

3. Use of oxytocin is generally avoided in cases of abnormal presentations of the fetus and of marked uterine overdistention such as gross hydramnios, a large singleton fetus, or multiple fetuses.

4. Women of high parity (more than 5), in general, are not given oxytocin because their uteri rupture more readily than those of women of lower parity (Chap. 23, p. 409). Oxytocin usually is withheld from women with a previous uterine scar (see Chap. 26. p. 446).

5. The condition of the fetus must be good, as evidenced by normal heart rate and lack of heavy contamination of the amnionic fluid with meconium. A dead fetus is, of course, no contraindication to oxytocin unless there is overt fetopelvic disproportion or a transverse lie.

6. The obstetrician must note the time of the first contraction after administration of the drug and be prepared to discontinue its use if a tetanic contraction occurs. It is imperative that hyperstimulation of the uterus be avoided. The frequency, intensity, and duration of contractions, and uterine tone between contractions, must not exceed those of normal spontaneous labor.

7. Continuous electronic monitoring of the fetal heart and uterine activity is conducted. Internal scalp electrode and pressure monitoring devices are used as soon as it is prudent to insert them.

Oxytocin is a powerful drug, and it has killed or maimed mothers through rupture of the uterus and even more babies through hypoxia from markedly hypertonic uterine contractions. The intravenous administration of oxytocin, however, has brought about a distinct advance in both its efficacy and safety. Failure to treat uterine dysfuntion exposes the mother to increased hazards from maternal exhaustion, intrapartum infection, and traumatic operative delivery. At the same time, failure to treat uterine dysfunction may expose the fetus to an appreciably higher risk of death, whereas the risk from intravenous oxytocin should be negligible when used appropriately. (Niswander and colleagues, 1966; Friedman and co-workers, 1979). Serious accidents, nevertheless, may accompany its use unless the precautions mentioned here are rigidly observed. The ruptured uterus illustrated in Figure 18–2 should serve as a warning to the physician of the need for these precautions. In this case, oxytocin was administered to a multiparous woman who was 38 years of age. Inasmuch as no other abnormalities were present, it must be assumed that the aging uterine muscle had been previously stretched repeatedly in other labors and could not stand the stress produced by the oxytocin.

One characteristic of intravenous oxytocin is that when successful, it acts promptly, leading to noticeable progress with little delay. For any given rate of infusion the plasma level reaches a plateau after about 30 to 40 minutes as the rate of infusion and rate of destruction by oxytocinase achieve equilibrium. Therefore, the drug need not be used for an indefinite period of time to stimulate labor. It should be employed for no more than a few hours (O'Driscoll and co-workers, 1984; Seitchik and Castillo, 1982); if, by then, the cervix has not changed appreciably and if predictably easy

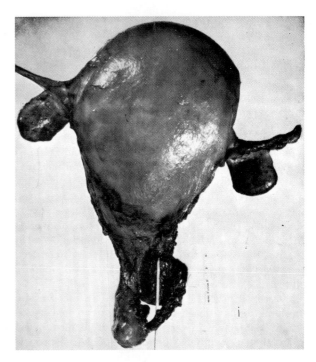

Figure 18–2. Rupture of the lower uterine segment resulting from stimulation by dilute intravenous oxytocin in a 38-year-old multipara.

vaginal delivery is not imminent, cesarean delivery should be performed. On the other hand, oxytocin should not be used to force cervical dilatation at a rate that exceeds normal (Cohen and Friedman, 1983). Ready resort to cesarean section in cases where oxytocin fails or in which there are contraindications to its use has served to diminish perinatal mortality and morbidity appreciably.

In years past, oxytocin was available in tablets that contained up to 200 units of the drug, and these were placed next to the buccal mucosa. Absorption was erratic and overstimulation was common. Oxytocin is available in nasal spray, but it is not intended for labor induction. **Oxytocin administration by any route other than in a dilute intravenous solution as described above is not recommended.**

Prostaglandins

Prostaglandins $F_{2\alpha}$ and E_2 are potent uterotonic agents that are capable of inducing and augmenting labor. The possibility of uterine hypertonus following oral or intravenous administration is worrisome, but it has not been a major problem in studies of labor induction using prostaglandin E_2 given orally (Cunningham and co-workers, 1976; Hauth and associates, 1977; Lange and co-workers, 1983).

Considerable efficacy has been claimed for vaginal prostaglandin E_2 suppositories, pessaries, and gels as well as intracervical gels when they are used to "ripen" unfavorable crevices or to induce labor (Bernstein, 1987; Buchanan, 1984; Ekman-Ordeberg, 1985; Macer, 1984; MacKenzie, 1984; Mainprize, 1987; Prins, 1983; and their many co-workers). Although vaginal prostaglandin E_2 has been reported not to alter fetal circulation (Lindblad and associates, 1985), rupture of the uterus has been reported (Claman and associates, 1984). Because of such risks, it seems wise that attempts at cervical ripening should include continuous electronic uterine activity and fetal heart rate monitoring.

At present, none of these agents has been approved by the Food and Drug Administration for such uses in the United States.

TREATMENT OF HYPERTONIC UTERINE DYSFUNCTION

Such dysfunction is characterized by uterine pain that appears to be out of proportion to the intensity of contractions and certainly out of proportion to their effectiveness in effacing and dilating the cervix. This type of uterine dysfunction characteristically occurs prior to the cervix reaching a dilatation of 4 cm or more. Because of the relative infrequency of this variety of dysfunctional labor, it has attracted little attention as a clinical entity, and thus its role in perinatal morbidity may be overlooked. **Placental abruption must always be considered as a possible cause of uterine hypertonus.**

Oxytocin is rarely, if ever, indicated in the presence of uterine hypertonus with a living fetus. Cesarean delivery should be employed if fetal distress is suspected. If the membranes are intact and there is no other evidence of fetopelvic disproportion, administration of morphine or meperidine will relieve pain and rest the mother as well as arrest the abnormal uterine activity. When she awakes, it is hoped, more effective labor will be evident. As mentioned earlier, it is important that such management does not lead to undue procrastination and unappreciated fetal distress, including the defecation of copious amounts of meconium into the amnionic fluid, and, in turn, serious meconium aspiration by the fetus (see Chap. 33, p.595 Tocolytic agents, such as ritodrine, have been used, presumably with some success, especially in other countries.

ATTEMPTS AT PRECISE CLASSIFICATION AND MANAGEMENT OF LABOR DISORDERS

In an attempt at precision, Friedman (1978) divided labor disorders into three divisions: prolonged latent phase disorders, protraction disorders, and arrest disorders. The prolonged latent phase is a single entity; the protraction disorders are two in number and consist of two further divisions, a protracted active dilatation phase and protracted descent. The arrest of labor disorders are four in number and consist of prolonged deceleration phase, secondary arrest of dilatation, arrest of descent, and failure of descent. These labor disorders and the diagnostic criteria to establish their diagnoses and treatments are listed in Table 18–1.

The diagnosis of a prolonged latent phase is based upon the passage of excessive time with failure of the cervix to dilate past 3 to 4 cm. Unfortunately, this diagnosis is most often made in retrospect. Also, this disorder of labor is almost impossible to distinguish from false labor. The causes of this form of labor disorder are discussed elsewhere (p. 343), but in summary the most frequent causes are related to the early use of excessive narcotic and/or sedative analgesics and the use of regional epidural analgesia (Friedman and Sachtleben, 1961). Thus, treatment usually consists of allowing these drugs to be metabolized and cleared from the maternal circulation if sufficient time is available—that is, the membranes have not been ruptured for an excessive period of time and the fetal and maternal patients are both in no specific danger. If this is not effective, 85 percent of such patients will respond to an oxytocin infusion.

As simple as these diagnoses and managements may seem, the problem remains that a prolonged latent phase may be due to (1) *injudicious use of analgesics*, (2) *false labor*, (3) *hypertonic uterine dysfunction*, or (4) *"unknown" reasons*. Thus, if analgesic causes are not present and if delivery is not mandated for fetal and/or maternal reasons, Friedman (1978) recommends heavily sedating the patient with narcotics. When the patient awakens in 6 to 7 hours she usually will be in progressive labor if the disorder was due to *hypertonic uterine dysfunction* or will not be in labor if she had been in false labor. In those 2 to 3 percent of patients who revert to the same pattern as before the sedation, a diagnosis of *hypertonic uterine dysfunction* is most likely.

The two protraction disorders are closely related and should be considered together. The diagnosis is established when the cervix fails to dilate at the rates listed in Table 18–1 or when the presenting part fails to descend at the rates listed in the same table but progress continues. The major cause(s) of these disorders is unknown but approximately one third of cases are due to varying degrees of cephalopelvic disproportion.

Treatment of the protraction disorders is not clearly established except in cases where cephalopelvic disproportion can be documented; then, delivery by cesarean section is indicated. In other circumstances, Friedman (1978) recommends supportive measures such as hydration and psychological support but maintains that even with oxytocin stimulation the rate of dilatation of the cervix and the rate of descent of the presenting part cannot be accelerated.

This view of passive support is opposed by O'Driscoll and colleagues (1983, 1984), who actively intervene if cervical dilatation is not achieved at a specific rate. They discourage the use of intravenous oxytocin in multiparous but not in nulliparous patients, and the use of midforceps in patients who have experienced either prolongation or arrest patterns of dysfunctional labor. Cohen and Friedman (1983) also discourage the use of midforceps in such labors (Table 18–2).

The arrest disorders are considered to be present (Table 18–2) when there is no cervical dilatation for 2 hours, when the deceleration phase is prolonged, or when there is failure of the presenting part to descend for greater than 1 hour or longer. Friedman (1978) maintains that approximately one half of these patients have "insurmountable obstruction" and recommends the judicious use of intravenous oxytocin but cautions that such efforts, while effective in dilating the cervix and ultimately resulting in vaginal delivery, may subject the fetus to substantial risks of hypoxic injury as well as birth trauma. O'Driscoll and associates (1983, 1984) strongly disagree with this approach. They aggressively stimulate such labors in nulliparous patients but not in multiparas. Others, including us, take a less aggressive approach.

At Parkland Hospital, our approach has been to assess the quality of uterine contractions with an internal pressure catheter. An adequate contraction pattern is considered to be at least three contractions per 10 minutes lasting at least 45 seconds with an amplitude of 50 mm Hg or more. An arrest pattern in the face of such contractions is unlikely to respond to an oxytocin augmentation and cesarean section is performed instead. If, however, the contraction pattern is inadequate, oxytocin augmentation is performed as previously discussed under treatment of hypotonic dysfunction and techniques of intravenous oxytocin (see p. 344). A similar approach with excellent results was reported by Bottoms and co-workers (1987), who recommend amniotomy and oxytocin augmentation in such cases. They reported that 50 percent of arrest disorders resolve with amniotomy or ambulation or both, even without oxytocin; and that 71 percent of those in which oxytocin was used delivered spontaneously or with low forceps.

INADEQUATE VOLUNTARY EXPULSIVE FORCE

With achievement of full cervical dilatation the great majority of women cannot resist the urge to "bear down" or "push" each time the uterus contracts. Typically, the laboring woman inhales deeply, closes her glottis, and contracts her abdominal musculature repetitively with vigor to generate appreciably increased intra-abdominal pressure throughout the time that the uterus is contracting. The combined force created by the contractions of the uterus and the abdominal musculature propels the fetus down the vagina and, in the case of spontaneous delivery, through the vaginal outlet.

CAUSES OF INADEQUATE EXPULSIVE FORCES

At times, the magnitude of the force created by the contraction of the abdominal musculature is sufficiently compromised to prevent spontaneous vaginal delivery. Conduction analgesia—lumbar epidural, caudal, or intrathecal—is likely to reduce the reflex urge for the woman to "push," and, at the same time, may impair her ability to contract the abdominal muscles sufficiently to increase intra-abdominal pressure. General anesthesia, with loss of consciousness, certainly imposes these adverse effects, as does *heavy* sedation.

In some instances, the inherent urge to "push" that develops in most women as the cervix becomes fully dilated is overridden by the intensification of pain that is created by bearing down. Rarely, insufficient expulsive efforts may be the consequence of long-standing paralysis of the abdominal musculature, as may occur after poliomyelitis or transection of the spinal cord.

MANAGEMENT

Careful selection of the kind of analgesia and the timing of its administration are very important if compromise of voluntary expulsive efforts is to be avoided. With rare exception, intrathecal analgesia or general anesthesia should not be administered until all conditions for a safe, outlet forceps delivery have been met—that is, the fetal head is engaged, the sagittal suture is in the anteroposterior position, and the occiput distends the perineum and protrudes somewhat through the vaginal introitus with a contraction. With continuous epidural analgesia, it may be necessary to allow the paralytic effects to wear off so that the mother in response to coaching can generate intra-abdominal pressure sufficient to move the fetal head into position appropriate for outlet forceps delivery. The alternatives—a possibly difficult midforceps vaginal delivery or cesarean delivery—are unsatisfactory choices in the absence of any evidence of fetal distress.

For the woman who cannot bear down appropriately with each contraction because of great discomfort, analgesia is likely to be of considerable benefit. Perhaps the safest for both fetus and mother is nitrous oxide, mixed with an equal volume of oxygen and provided during the time of each uterine contraction. At the same time, appropriate encouragement and instruction are most likely to be of benefit.

LOCALIZED ABNORMALITIES OF UTERINE ACTION

PATHOLOGICAL RETRACTION AND CONSTRICTION RINGS

Very rarely, localized rings or constrictions of the uterus develop in association with prolonged rupture of the membranes and protracted labors. The most common type is the so-called *pathological retraction ring of Bandl,* an exaggeration of the normal retraction ring described in Chapter 10 (p. 214), and is often, but not always, the result of obstructed labor, with marked stretching and thinning of the lower uterine segment. In such a situation, the ring may be clearly evident as an abdominal indentation and signifies impending rupture of the lower uterine segment (Fig. 19–13). Localized constrictions of the uterus are rarely seen today, since prolonged obstructed labor is no longer compatible with acceptable obstetrical practice. They may, however, still occur occasionally as hourglass constrictions of the uterus following the birth of the first of twins. In such a situation, they can sometimes be relaxed and delivery effected with appropriate general anesthesia, but on occasion prompt cesarean section offers a better prognosis for the second twin (see Chap. 34, p. 646).

Missed Labor

In rare instances, uterine contractions commence at or near term and, after continuing for a variable time, disappear without leading to the birth of the child. The fetus then dies and may be retained in utero for months or years undergoing mummification. This condition is known as missed labor. If uterine contractions disappear without leading to the birth of the child, and especially if the infant dies and is retained, abdominal pregnancy is a much more likely diagnosis than is missed labor. Management of prolonged retention of a fetus dead in utero is discussed in Chapter 36 (p. 716) and of extrauterine (abdominal) pregnancy in Chapter 30 (p. 526).

PRECIPITATE LABOR AND DELIVERY

Precipitate—that is, extremely rapid—labor and delivery may result from an abnormally low resistance of the soft parts of the birth canal, from abnormally strong uterine and abdominal contractions, or, *very rarely,* from the absence of painful sensations and thus a lack of awareness of vigorous labor.

MATERNAL EFFECTS

Precipitate labor and delivery are seldom accompanied by serious maternal complications if the cervix is appreciably effaced and easily dilated, the vagina has been previously stretched, and the perineum is relaxed. However, vigorous uterine contractions combined with a long, firm cervix and a vagina, vulva, or perineum that resists stretch may lead to rupture of the uterus or extensive lacerations of the cervix, vagina, vulva, or perineum. It is in these later circumstances that the rare condition *amnionic fluid embolism* is most likely to occur (see Chap. 36, p. 719). **The uterus that contracts with unusual vigor before delivery is likely to be hypotonic after delivery with hemorrhage from the placental implantation site as the consequence** (see Chap. 24, p. 415).

EFFECTS ON FETUS AND NEONATE

Perinatal mortality and morbidity from precipitate labor may be increased considerably for several reasons. First, the tumultuous uterine contractions, often with negligible intervals of relaxation, prevent appropriate uterine blood flow and oxygenation of the fetal blood. Second, the resistance of the birth canal to expulsion of the head may cause intracranial trauma, although this must be rare. Moreover, Acker and colleagues (1988) reported that Erb-Duchenne palsy was associated with such labors in a third of cases. Third, during an unattended birth, the infant may fall to the floor and be injured or may need resuscitation that is not immediately available.

TREATMENT

Unusually forceful spontaneous uterine contractions are not likely to be modified to a significant degree by the administration of analgesia. Importantly, if tried, the dose should be such that the infant at birth is not further depressed by the maternally administered analgesia. The use of general anesthesia with agents that impair uterine contractibility, such as halothane and isoflurane, is often excessively heroic. Certainly, any oxytocic agents being administered should be stopped immediately. Tocolytic agents, such as ritodrine and parenteral magnesium sulfate may prove effective. It is indefensible to lock the mother's legs or hold the baby's head back directly to try to delay delivery. Such maneuvers may damage the infant's brain.

REFERENCES

Acker DB, Gregory KD, Sachs BP, Friedman EA: Risk factors for Erb-Duchenne palsy. Obstet Gynecol 71:389, 1988

American College of Obstetricians and Gynecologists: Induction and augmentation of labor. Technical Bulletin, No 110, November 1987

Anderson N: X-ray pelvimetry: Helpful or harmful? J Fam Pract 17:405, 1983

Barton JJ, Garbaciak JA Jr, Ryan GM: The efficacy of x-ray pelvimetry. Am J Obstet Gynecol 143:304, 1982

Bernstein P, Leyland N, Gurland P, Gare D: Cervical ripening and labor induction with prostaglandin E$_2$ gel: A placebo-controlled study. Am J Obstet Gynecol 156:336, 1987

Bottoms SF, Hirsch VJ, Sokol RJ: Medical management of arrest disorders of labor: A current overview. Am J Obstet Gynecol 156:939, 1987

Buchanan D, Macer J, Yonekura ML: Cervical ripening with prostaglandin E$_2$ vaginal suppositories. Obstet Gynecol 63:659, 1984

Caldeyro-Barcia R: Oxytocin and pregnant human uterus. Proceedings of the 4th Pan-American Congress on Endocrinology. Buenos Aires, 1957

Caldeyro-Barcia R, Alvarez H, Reynolds SRM: A better understanding of uterine contractility through simultaneous recording with an internal and a seven channel external method. Surg Obstet Gynecol 91:641, 1950

Claman P, Carpenter RJ, Reiter A: Uterine rupture with the use of vaginal prostaglandin E$_2$ for induction of labor. Am J Obstet Gynecol 150:889, 1984

Cohen W, Friedman EA (eds): Management of Labor. Baltimore, University Park Press, 1983

Cunningham FG, Cox K, Hauth JC, Strong JD, Whalley PJ: Oral prostaglandin E$_2$ for labor induction in high-risk pregnancy. Am J Obstet Gynecol 125:881, 1976

Ekman-Ordeberg G, Uldbjerg N, Ulmsten U: Comparison of intravenous oxytocin and vaginal prostaglandin E$_2$ gel in women with unripe cervixes and premature rupture of the membranes. Obstet Gynecol 66:307, 1985

Foster TCS, Jacobson JD, Valenzuela GJ: Oxytocin augmentation of labor: A comparison of 15- and 30-minute dose increment intervals. Obstet Gynecol 71:147, 1988

Friedman EA: Cervical function in human pregnancy and labor. In Naftolin F, Stubblefield PG (eds): Dilatation of the Uterine Cervix: Connective Tissue Biology and Clinical Management. New York, Raven, 1980

Friedman EA: Labor: Clinical Evaluation and Management, 2nd ed. New York, Appleton, 1978

Friedman EA, Sachtleben MR: Dysfunctional labor: I. Prolonged latent phase in the nullipara. Obstet Gynecol 17:135, 1961

Friedman EA, Sachtleben MR, Wallace AK: Infant outcome following labor induction. Am J Obstet Gynecol 133:718, 1979

Hauth JC, Cunningham FG, Whalley PJ: Early labor initiation with oral PGE$_2$ after premature rupture of the membranes at term. Obstet Gynecol 49:523, 1977

Hendricks CH, Quilligan EJ, Tyler AB, Tucker GJ: Pressure relationships between intervillous space and amniotic fluid in human term pregnancy. Am J Obstet Gynecol 77:1028, 1959

Jeffcoate TNA: Prolonged labor. Lancet 2:61, 1961

Joyce DN, Giwa-Asagie F, Stevenson GW: Role of pelvimetry in active management of labor. Br Med J 4:505, 1975

Lange AP, Westergaard JG, Secher NJ, Pedersen GT: Labor induction with prostaglandins. Acta Obstet Gynecol Scand (Suppl) 113:177, 1983

Larks SD: Electrohysterography. Springfield, IL, Thomas, 1960

Lindblad A, Ekman G, Marsál K, Ulmsten U: Fetal circulation 60 to 80 minutes after vaginal prostaglandin E$_2$ in pregnant women at term. Arch Gynecol 237:31, 1985

Macer J, Buchanan D, Yonekura ML: Induction of labor with prostaglandin E$_2$ vaginal suppositories. Obstet Gynecol 63:664, 1984

MacKenzie IZ, Bradley S, Embrey MP: Vaginal prostaglandins and labour induction for patients previously delivered by cesarean section. Br J Obstet Gynaecol 91:7, 1984

Mainprize T, Nimrod C, Dodd G, Persaud D: Clinical utility of multiple-dose administration of prostaglandin E$_2$ gel. Am J Obstet Gynecol 156:341, 1987

Niswander KR, Turoff BB, Romans J: Developmental status of children delivered through elective induction of labor. Obstet Gynecol 27:15, 1966

O'Driscoll K, Foley M: Correlation of decrease in perinatal mortality and increase in cesarean section rates. Obstet Gynecol 61:1, 1983

O'Driscoll K, Foley M, MacDonald D: Active management of labor as an alternative to high cesarean section rate for dystocia. Obstet Gynecol 63:485, 1984

Prins RP, Bolton RN, Mark C III, Neilson DR, Watson P: Cervical ripening with intravaginal prostaglandin E$_2$ gel. Obstet Gynecol 61:459, 1983

Reynolds SRM, Heard OO, Bruns P, Hellman LM: A multichannel strain-gauge tokodynamometer: An instrument for studying patterns of uterine contractions in pregnant women. Bull Johns Hopkins Hosp 82:446, 1948

Seitchik J, Amico J, Robinson AG, Castillo M: Oxytocin augmentation of dysfunctional labor: IV. Oxytocin pharmacokinetics. Am J Obstet Gynecol 150:225, 1984

Seitchik J, Castillo M: Oxytocin augmentation of dysfunctional labor: I. Clinical data. Am J Obstet Gynecol 144:899, 1982

Seitchik J, Holden AEC, Castillo M: Spontaneous rupture of the membranes, function dystocia, oxytocin treatment, and the route of delivery. Am J Obstet Gynecol 156:125, 1987

Shepherd J, Pearce JMF, Sims CD: Induction of labour using prostaglandin E$_2$ pessaries. Br Med J 2:108, 1979

Steer CM: Effect of type of delivery on future childbearing. Am J Obstet Gynecol 60:395, 1950

Thorp JA, Boylan PC, Parisi VM, Heslin EP: Effects of high-dose oxytocin augmentation on umbilical cord blood gas values in primigravid women. Am J Obstet Gynecol 159:670, 1988

19

Dystocia Due to Abnormalities in Presentation, Position, or Development of the Fetus

BREECH PRESENTATION

INCIDENCE

Breech presentation is common remote from term, as demonstrated in Table 19–1. Most often, however, some time before the onset of labor the fetus turns spontaneously to a vertex presentation so that breech presentation persists in only about 3 to 4 percent of singleton deliveries. For example, 3 percent of 49,156 singleton infants delivered from 1983 through 1986 at Parkland Hospital presented as breech (Table 19–2).

ETIOLOGY

As term approaches, the uterine cavity, for reasons that are not entirely clear, most often accommodates the fetus in a longitudinal lie with the vertex presenting. Breeches are much more common at the end of the second trimester of pregnancy than at or near term. (Table 19–1). Factors other than gestational age that appear to predispose to breech presentation include uterine relaxation associated with great parity, multiple fetuses, hydramnios, oligohydramnios, hydrocephalus, anencephalus, previous breech delivery, uterine anomalies, and tumors in the pelvis.

Implantation of the placenta in either cornual-fundal region of the uterus has been suspected of predisposing to breech presentation. Fianu and Vaclavinkova (1978) provided sonographic evidence of a very much higher prevalence of implantation of the placenta in the cornual-fundal region for breech presentations (73 percent) than for vertex presentations (5 percent). The frequency of breech presentation also is increased with placenta previa, but only a small minority of cases of breech presentation are associated with placenta previa. No strong positive correlation has been shown between breech presentation and a contracted pelvis in most recent reports.

A live fetus is *not* required for a fetus to change presentations spontaneously. For example, a woman was admitted to Parkland Hospital at term with a fetus known to be dead, confirmed by the lack of fetal heart sounds with Doppler examination and also by the lack of heart action seen with real-time sonography. The presentation was cephalic at the time of the first oxytocin induction, which proved unsuccessful. Three days later, at the time of the second attempt at induction of labor, the fetus was in a breech presentation. Three days later, at the time

of a third and successful induction of labor, the fetus was again in a vertex presentation!

SIGNIFICANCE

In the persistent breech presentation, an *increased* frequency of the following complications can be anticipated: (1) perinatal morbidity and mortality from difficult delivery; (2) low birthweight from prematurity, growth retardation, or both; (3) prolapsed cord; (4) placenta previa; (5) fetal anomalies and developmental abnormalities that appear after the newborn period; (6) uterine anomalies and tumors; (7) multiple fetuses; and (8) operative intervention, especially cesarean section.

DIAGNOSIS

The varying relations between the lower extremities and buttocks of the fetus in breech presentations form the categories of frank breech, complete breech, and incomplete breech presentations (Figs. 9–2 to 9–4, pp. 178–79). With a *frank breech* presentation, the lower extremities are flexed at the hips and extended at the knees and thus the feet lie in close proximity to the head. A *complete breech* presentation differs from a frank breech presentation in that one or both knees are flexed rather than both extended. With *incomplete breech* presentation, one or both hips are not flexed and one or both feet or knees lie below the breech, that is, a foot or knee is lowermost in the birth canal. The frank breech appears most commonly when the diagnosis is established radiologically near term.

Abdominal Examination

Typically, with the first maneuver of Leopold the hard, round, readily ballottable fetal head is found to occupy the fundus of the uterus (Fig. 19–1). The second maneuver indicates the back to be on one side of the abdomen and the small parts on the other. On the third maneuver, if engagement has not occurred—that is, the interotrochanteric diameter of the fetal pelvis has not passed through the pelvic inlet—the breech is movable above the pelvic inlet. After engagement, the fourth maneuver shows the firm breech to be beneath the symphysis. The heart sounds of the fetus are usually heard loudest slightly above the umbilicus, whereas with engagement of the fetal head the heart sounds are loudest below the umbilicus.

349

TABLE 19–1. FETAL PRESENTATION AT VARIOUS GESTATIONAL AGES DETERMINED SONOGRAPHICALLY

Gestation (Wk Inclusive)	Total (No.)	Cephalic (%)	Breech (%)	Other (%)
21–24	264	54.6	33.3	12.1
25–28	367	61.9	27.8	10.4
29–32	443	78.1	14.0	7.9
33–36	638	88.7	8.8	2.5
37–40	463	91.5	6.7	1.7

From Scheer and Nubar: Am J Obstet Gynecol 125:269, 1976.

Vaginal Examination

The diagnosis of a frank breech presentation is confirmed vaginally by palpating its characteristic components. Both ischial tuberosities, the sacrum, and the anus are usually palpable, and after further descent, the external genitalia may be distinguished.

Especially when labor is prolonged, the buttocks may become markedly swollen, rendering differentiation of face and breech very difficult; the anus may be mistaken for the mouth, and the ischial tuberosities for the malar eminences. Careful examination, however, should prevent that error, for the finger encounters muscular resistance with the anus, whereas the firmer, less yielding jaws are felt through the mouth. Furthermore, the finger, upon removal from the anus, is sometimes stained with meconium. The mouth and malar eminences form a triangular shape, while the ischial tuberosities and anus are in a straight line. The most accurate information, however, is based on the location of the sacrum and its spinous processes, which establishes the diagnosis of position and variety.

In complete breech presentations, the feet may be felt alongside the buttocks, and in footling presentations, one or both feet are inferior to the buttocks (Fig. 19–2). In footling presentations, the foot can readily be identified as right or left on the basis of the relation to the great toe. When the breech has descended farther into the pelvic cavity, the genitalia may be felt; if not markedly edematous, they may permit identification of fetal sex.

X-Ray, Computed Tomography, and Ultrasonic Examinations

Sonography ideally should be used to confirm a clinically suspected breech presentation and to identify, if possible, any fetal anomalies. Unfortunately, sonography usually cannot be used to identify the relationship of the lower extremities to the fetal

TABLE 19–2. FETAL PRESENTATION IN 49,156 SINGLETON PREGNANCIES AT PARKLAND HOSPITAL, 1983–86

Presentation	Number	Percent	Incidence
Cephalic	47,497	96.6	—
Breech	1,468	3.0	—
Transverse	117	0.24	1 : 420
Face	41	0.08	1 : 1,200
Compound	22	0.05	1 : 2,235
Brow	11	0.02	1 : 4,470

Data courtesy of Dr. K. Leveno.

pelvis. This information often is essential in planning the route of delivery (see Chap. 22, p. 394).

If delivery by cesarean section is planned without exception, there are few justifications for x-rays. If, however, the woman is in labor and vaginal delivery is considered, the type of breech presentation is of considerable importance (see Chap. 22, p. 394). In this instance, radiation exposure may be reduced considerably by using computed tomographic pelvimetry (Kopelman and associates, 1986). These imaging techniques can be used to provide information about the type of breech presentation, presence or absence of a flexed fetal head, and accurate measurements of the pelvis (see Chap. 8, p. 172).

LABOR

There are fundamental differences between labor and delivery in cephalic and breech presentations as described in Chapter 22. With a cephalic presentation, once the head is delivered, typically the rest of the body follows without difficulty. With a breech, however, successively larger and very much less compressible parts of the fetus are born.

Spontaneous complete expulsion of the fetus who presents as a breech, as described below, is seldom successfully accomplished. As the rule, either cesarean delivery (see Chap. 26) or vaginal delivery that requires skilled participation by the obstetrician is essential for a favorable outcome (see Chap. 22).

PROGNOSIS

With breech presentation, compared to cephalic presentation, both the mother and the fetus are at greater risk but to nowhere near the same degree. Schutte and colleagues (1985) reported that even after correction for gestational age, congenital defects, and birthweight, in an analysis of 57,819 pregnancies in the Netherlands, perinatal mortality was higher in breech than in vertex infants. They concluded that *"it is possible that breech presentation is not coincidental but is a consequence of poor fetal quality, in which case medical intervention is unlikely to reduce the perinatal mortality associated with breech presentation to the level associated with vertex presentation."*

The possibility that the breech presentation might be a factor identifying an already abnormal fetus has been suggested before by Hytten (1982) and by Suzuki and Yamamuro (1985). This concept was strengthened even more by the report of Nelson and Ellenberg (1986), who observed that a third of the children with cerebral palsy who were in the breech presentation at birth had major noncerebral malformations.

Maternal

Because of the greater frequency of operative delivery, including cesarean section, there is a higher maternal morbidity and slightly higher mortality for pregnancies complicated by persistent breech presentation (Collea, 1980). This risk likely is increased even more if an emergency cesarean section is performed instead of an elective cesarean section (Bingham and Lilford, 1987). Labor usually is not prolonged; Hall and Kohl (1956), in a large series of cases, reported the median duration of labor to be 9.2 hours for nulliparas and 6.1 hours for multiparas.

Fetus-Infant

The prognosis for the fetus in a breech presentation is considerably worse than when in a vertex presentation. The major contributors to this perinatal loss are preterm delivery, congenital anomalies, and birth trauma. Brenner and associates (1974) provided a careful analysis of the characteristics and perils to the fetus from breech presentation. They determined the overall

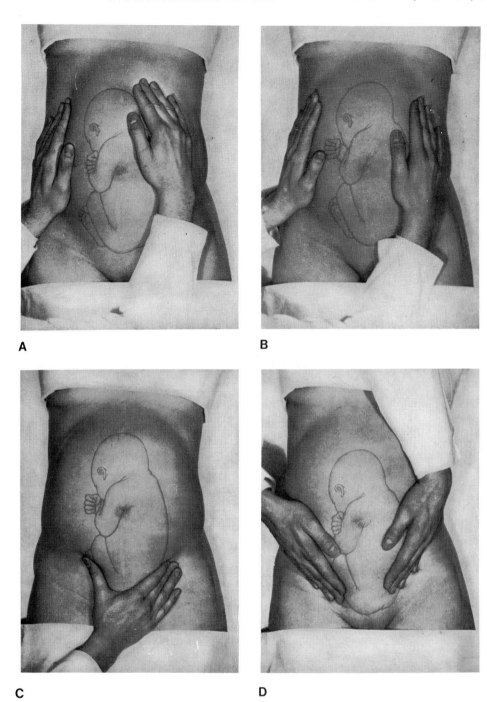

Figure 19–1. Palpation in left sacroanterior position. **A.** First maneuver. **B.** Second maneuver. **C.** Third maneuver. **D.** Fourth maneuver.

mortality rate for 1,016 breech deliveries to be 25.4 percent compared to 2.6 percent for nonbreech deliveries at the University Hospitals of Cleveland. At every stage of gestation, they identified antepartum, intrapartum, and neonatal deaths to be significantly greater among breeches and the average Apgar scores to be lower for those who survived. During the latter half of pregnancy, the birthweight at any gestational age was somewhat less for breech infants than for nonbreech infants. Congenital abnormalities were identified in 6.3 percent of breech deliveries compared to 2.4 percent in nonbreech deliveries.

Tank and associates (1971) examined the character of serious traumatic vaginal delivery. At autopsy, the organs most frequently found to be injured were, in order of frequency, the brain, spinal cord, liver, adrenal glands, and spleen. It is of interest that, in retrospective analysis of cases of "idiopathic" adrenal calcification, breech delivery was very common. Other sites of injuries from vaginal delivery included the brachial plexus; the pharynx, in the form of tears or pseudodiverticula from the obstetrician's finger in the mouth as part of the Mauriceau maneuver (see Chap. 22, Fig. 22–8, p. 399); and the bladder, which might be ruptured if distended. Traction might injure the sternomastoid muscle and, if not appropriately treated, lead to torticollis (see Chap. 33, p. 623).

Similar results were reported from the Los Angeles Women's Hospital by Gimovsky and Paul (1982). They observed an overall mortality rate for all breech presentations of 8.5 percent

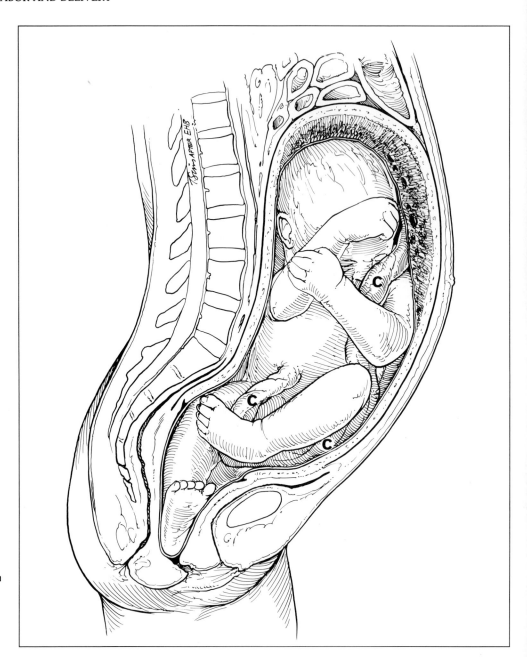

Figure 19–2. Double-footling breech presentation in labor with membranes intact. Note possibility of umbilical cord accident at any instant, especially after rupture of membranes (C = umbilical cord).

compared to a 2.2 percent rate for cephalic presentations. These results were obtained despite a cesarean delivery rate of 74 percent for all breech presentations. Thus, even with liberal use of cesarean section and after exclusion of very preterm fetuses or fetuses with severe congenital anomalies, there still remained a relative twofold risk for the infant delivered as a breech compared to the overall population.

Green and associates (1982) reported distressing results obtained for breeches managed during 1963–72 at the Royal Victoria Hospital in Montreal compared to the 1978–79 time period. In the decade 1963–72, the cesarean section rate was 22 percent compared to 94 percent for 1978–79. In spite of the significant increase in cesarean section rates, rates of fetal asphyxia remained the same, despite a *trend* toward decreased fetal trauma and death. The authors concluded that cesarean section alone could not guarantee a good infant outcome because the *"maneuvers of extracting a breech by cesarean section are similar to*

that associated with the delivery of a breech via the vaginal route." A similar warning that cesarean section alone cannot assure a better outcome was presented by Calvert (1980), who urged a more liberal use of large uterine incisions for breeches.

Because of the confusing nature of compounding variables in trying to ascertain the safest method of breech delivery for both maternal and fetal patients, several studies have been conducted to contrast outcomes obtained for term versus preterm infants and within such groups to contrast outcomes obtained for different types of breech presentations.

TERM FETUS

Rovinsky and associates (1973), at Mount Sinai Hospital in New York City, looked especially at the risks associated with breech presentation for singleton fetuses who weighed 2,500 g or more and were considered to be at or near term. The overall perinatal mortality rate for more than 2,000 such infants was 3.2 percent compared to 0.84 percent for infants with a cephalic presentation at or near term. Major congenital anomalies were identified in 2.1 percent of those presenting as breech versus 0.8 percent in those that were vertex. In one third of the perinatal deaths, breech presentation or delivery, or both were thought to be etiological factors. Mortality and morbidity rates from trauma were understandably lowest in infants who weighed 2,500 to 3,000 g and highest among those who weighed 4,000 g or more. Morbidity from trauma was progressively higher as the amount of obstetrical manipulation required to effect vaginal delivery increased. As might be expected, mortality and morbidity rates from trauma were higher when less experienced obstetricians delivered the breech.

In the Mount Sinai experiences, the incidence of overt prolapse of the cord among frank breeches at term was three times greater (1.7 percent) than for term vertex presentations; for complete and footling breeches, however, cord prolapse was 20 times greater (10.9 percent). Moreover, the incidence of fetal distress of undetermined cause in term breeches was 6.4 percent, or eight times greater than for term vertex presentations. No perinatal deaths were attributable to either breech presentation or delivery among the 425 (19.8 percent) that were delivered by cesarean section.

According to Rovinsky and associates, in retrospect it is likely that the deaths of 17 infants at term who succumbed as the consequence of labor and vaginal delivery, or about 1 percent of all term breech deliveries, would have been prevented by cesarean section. It is also pertinent that Brenner and co-workers (1974) identified in their study the perinatal mortality rate for fetuses of 32 weeks or greater gestational age and alive at the onset of labor to be 3.4 percent for those who were delivered vaginally and 0 percent for those who were delivered by cesarean section.

Collea and colleagues (1980) reported the results of a *prospective study* designed to identify the optimal method of delivery of the fetus who presented as a frank breech at term. Of those women who were randomly selected as candidates for vaginal delivery, 46 percent were promptly excluded from further consideration because of possible fetopelvic disproportion based on x-ray pelvimetry. Of the 60 infants who eventually delivered vaginally, all survived although two sustained injury to the brachial plexus. In this study there were no perinatal deaths, but 73 (49.3 percent) of the 148 women who delivered by cesarean section had significant morbidity compared to only 4 (6.7 percent) of the 60 women who delivered vaginally. Similar results have been reported by Watson and Benson (1984) and by Flanagan and associates (1987).

Gimovsky and associates (1983) published the preliminary results of a prospective study designed to identify the optimal method of delivery of the fetus who presented as a *nonfrank* breech at term. One hundred five women with nonfrank breech presentations in labor were entered into the study. Seventy (67 percent) were placed in the group to receive a trial of labor and 35 (33 percent) underwent elective cesarean section. Of those placed in the labor group, 31 (44 percent) delivered vaginally and 39 (56 percent) required cesarean section. The largest single reason for a cesarean section being performed in the trial of labor group was inadequate pelvic dimensions observed by x-ray pelvimetry (23 of the 39, or 59 percent). Neonatal morbidity assessed by Apgar scores, cord blood pH, birth injury, and hospital stay was essentially the same for infants delivered vaginally or by cesarean section, except for the one infant who died

following a vaginal delivery. This infant death was attributed to inadequate resuscitation. Maternal morbidity in terms of fever, blood transfusions, wound infections and length of hospital stay was significantly greater among women delivered by cesarean section. While this report is an interesting preliminary evaluation of vaginal delivery of nonfrank breeches, the 1 death out of 31 patients allowed to deliver vaginally is in essence "one too many." This rate, if maintained, would be equivalent to a fetal death rate of 32 per 1,000. The long-term results in this continuing study may, of course, be much more favorable after additional patients are studied.

In the retrospective study by Fortney and colleagues (1986), in which outcome variables were analyzed for 10,749 breech deliveries from 86 hospitals throughout the world, the inescapable conclusion was that vaginal delivery of footling breeches, at term, was associated with a prohibitive perinatal mortality. They also reported that perinatal mortality increased significantly in vaginally delivered breeches weighing more than 3,500 g, regardless of the type of breech.

PRETERM FETUS

Vaginal delivery as a breech may be much more hazardous to the preterm infant than previously thought. Ingemarsson and associates (1978) compared neonatal mortality and the frequency of subsequent developmental abnormalities in 42 preterm breech infants delivered by cesarean section versus 48 preterm infants who were delivered vaginally. For those delivered vaginally, 6 (14.6 percent) succumbed and developmental abnormalities were detected at 12 months of age in 10 (24 percent) of the survivors, compared to 2 deaths (4.8 percent) and 1 with developmental abnormalities (2.5 percent) among those who were delivered by cesarean section.

Kauppila and associates (1981) reported from Finland that from 1967 to 1976, infant mortality was significantly higher in breech than in cephalic deliveries and that perinatal mortality and neonatal mortality were 1.8-fold and 2.9-fold greater, respectively. The causes of death were primarily intracranial hemorrhage, fetal asphyxia, and prolapsed cord. However, during the last 5 years of the study, even with an increasing cesarean section rate, this policy did not improve the prognosis for 1,500 to 2,499 g infants. For infants less than 1,500 g, there was a higher incidence of cerebral hemorrhage when delivered vaginally, especially if the infant was a footling breech. They concluded that vaginal delivery of infants 1,500 g and larger was justified *if proper fetal monitoring and prompt operative capabilities were present for signs of fetal distress.* With added complications such as hypertension, diabetes, fetal growth retardation, and footling breech presentations, primary cesarean section should be undertaken. For infants less than 1,500 g, primary cesarean section was recommended. Crowley and Hawkins (1980) reviewed 11 papers published between 1975 and 1979 and reported that with weights between 1,000 and 1,500 g (28 to 31 weeks gestation) cesarean section seemed to confer an advantage in survival.

In a review of the method of delivery for very low-birthweight infants, Westgren and Paul (1985b) summarized mortality rates in vaginally versus cesarean-delivered breech infants weighing less than 1,500 g. Their summary included the results of their own study (Westgren and colleagues, 1985a) plus those previously reported in 13 earlier publications. The mortality rate for 5,026 vaginally delivered infants was 45 percent; it was 18 percent for 4,298 infants delivered by cesarean section. Furthermore, in each report, morbidity was greater in the vaginally delivered infants. Finally, Doyle and associates (1985) reported that very-low-birthweight infants (500 to 1,499 g) delivered by cesarean section not only were more likely to survive but also had significantly fewer handicaps at 2 years of age.

Morales and Koerten (1986) reported that intracranial hemorrhage and mortality were reduced significantly in abdominally delivered breech infants weighing less than 1,500 g, when compared to those delivered vaginally. Bodmer and associates (1986) reported that head entrapment in vaginally delivered infants weighing less than 1,000 g was a significant cause of neonatal mortality. Unfortunately, they also concluded that despite cesarean section, newborn depression and mortality were not always prevented. Luterkort and Marsàl (1987) reported that vaginally delivered breech and cephalic infants had a lower umbilical cord pH compared to infants delivered by cesarean section. They concluded, however, that vaginal delivery of selected term breeches was not associated with an increased risk of fetal asphyxia.

The rather universal acceptance of primary cesarean section for infants less than 2,000 g has been questioned by two groups of investigators. Cox and associates (1982) compared 1973–74 and 1979–80 morbidity and mortality figures for breech infants under 2,500 g delivered at Coventry Maternity Hospital. In 1979–80 a neonatal intensive care unit was operating for the first time and the cesarean section rate had increased from 20 to 42 percent. The stillbirth rate had declined from 24.7 percent to 11.1 percent and the neonatal mortality rate (corrected for lethal congenital abnormalities) had decreased from 23.9 percent to 8.7 percent. Infant survival had increased from 66 to 82 percent. However, the long-term survival rates for *normal* babies in the two periods were 63.1 and 64.1 percent, respectively. The 1973–74 period had 1/21.5 handicapped survivors compared to 1/4.6 in 1979–80. The authors concluded that the perinatal mortality rate had decreased but the increased survival rate was accounted for by the survival of handicapped infants. They further speculated that the increased overall survival rate might have been the result of the neonatal intensive care unit rather than the consequence of the increased cesarean section rate. Effer and associates (1983) reported that perinatal mortality decreased by 20 percent from 1976 to 1980 in very-low-birthweight infants. During the same time the increased cesarean section rate (12 to 49 percent) was thought to be responsible for the improved outcome. The changes were most marked in the less than 1,000 g weight group. Survival and cesarean section rates for vertex infants of similar birthweights and gestational ages were analyzed for the same years. **A similar or greater reduction in mortality rate (85 to 45 percent) was noted in the very-low-birthweight vertex infants, while the cesarean section rate only increased from 14.2 percent to 22.2 percent.** The authors concluded that no clear interpretation of this study was possible but that any hypothesis must include the possibility that the increased cesarean section rate might be incidental and in no way related to the observed improved outcome and that *"as yet unidentified perinatal care practices, other than cesarean section, may be more likely to affect outcome in this high-risk group."*

At Parkland Hospital, when delivery is indicated or when there is active labor, our practice is to perform a cesarean section for any live fetus presenting breech who weighs less than 2,000 g and more than 700 g (26 weeks gestation). We agree with Thiery (1987) and conclude that, despite the arguments advanced that no prospective study has been performed for breech fetuses in this weight range delivered vaginally versus by cesarean section, the evidence presented above is sufficient to support this practice.

PROPHYLAXIS

Whenever a breech presentation is recognized during the third trimester, an attempt may be made to substitute a vertex presentation by *external version* (Chap. 22). External version is more readily accomplished in multiparous women with lax abdominal walls than in nulliparous women. Because of possible trauma, anesthesia should never be used.

External version, if properly and gently performed, carries little danger, according to Ranney (1973), who reported his experiences with gentle attempts at external cephalic version in 860 instances of either breech presentation or, less often, transverse lie. The initial attempt was successful 781 times. Although many of the 781 fetuses reverted to an abnormal presentation, repeat attempts at conversion were usually successful. The failure rate during the third trimester increased as pregnancy advanced, with a marked rise after the 36th week. During the study, the overall frequency of breech delivery was only 0.6 percent, or about one sixth the expected frequency. No trauma to the fetus was identified. There was no increase in the frequencies of placental abruption or of hemolytic disease in the newborn infants, although these have been reported by others. Ranney believes that successful version relatively early in the third trimester, as well as lowering the risk associated with vaginal delivery, may reduce the likelihood of preterm delivery, which is more common with breech presentation.

Based on their experiences with 491 pregnancies in which the fetus presented other than cephalic, Ylikorkala and Hartikainen-Sorri (1977) also concluded that a breech presentation any time during the third trimester warrants attempts at external version. These Finnish workers always used ultrasound to confirm the presentation of the fetus and location of the placenta. In some instances they administered tocolytic or analgesic drugs but never anesthesia. They were able to convert the presentation of the fetus to that of vertex in three fourths of their attempts with no serious morbidity identified. The incidence of breech presentation decreased to 2.9 percent from the previous value of 4.5 percent. Interestingly, the mean duration of pregnancy was no greater after successful external version than in those pregnancies in which attempts were unsuccessful. Similar results, using sonography, continuous fetal heart rate monitoring, and tocolytic agents are presented in Table 19–3.

Enthusiasm for external cephalic version is not shared by all. The complications cited in Table 19–3 are not inconsequential. Moreover, Chapman and associates (1978) described spinal cord transection in utero after an unsuccessful attempt at external cephalic version. Marcus and associates (1975) identified significant fetomaternal hemorrhage in 6 of 100 pregnancies and Gjóde (1980) reported fetomaternal bleeds in 14 of 50 women during the first attempt at external version. Gjóde recommends that immunoprophylaxis with anti-D globulin be given *prior* to attempting external version in pregnant women who are Rh$_0$ (D) negative (see Chap. 33, p. 603). Stine and co-workers (1985) reported a maternal death due to amnionic fluid embolus and one unexplained fetal death. Kasule and associates (1985) reported three perinatal deaths, two due to abruption and one to prematurely ruptured membranes and vaginal delivery. In this study, however, attempted versions were begun after 30 weeks gestation.

TABLE 19–3. RESULTS OF EXTERNAL CEPHALIC VERSION FOR BREECH PRESENTATIONS PERFORMED LATE IN PREGNANCY

Study	Tocolysis	Attempts	Successes (%)	Successful Version Vertex at Delivery	Control Patients Vertex at Delivery	Complications
Brocks (1984)	Yes	130	53 (41)	53 (100)	8/56 (14)	None
Dyson (1986)	Yes	158	122 (77)	122 (100)	5/40 (12)	Fetal bradycardia during version— 7 patients
Morrison (1986)	Yes	304	207 (68)	201 (97)	Not Done	None
Stine (1985)	Yes	148	108 (73)	95/102 (93)[a]	4/23 (17)	Fetomaternal bleed in 4% 1 fetal death unexplained 1 maternal mortality due to amnionic fluid embolus
Totals		740	490 (67)	471/483 (97)	17/119 (14)	

[a] 6 patients lost to follow-up.

PROBLEMS WITH VAGINAL DELIVERY

Major problems do arise from vaginal delivery of a fetus in a breech presentation. Delivery of the breech draws the umbilicus and attached cord into the pelvis, which compresses the cord. Therefore, once the breech has passed beyond the vaginal introitus, the abdomen, thorax, arms, and head must be delivered promptly. This involves the delivery of successively less readily compressible parts. With a term fetus, some degree of molding of the fetal head may be essential for the head to negotiate the birth canal successfully. In this unfortunate circumstance, the alternatives with vaginal delivery are both unsatisfactory; delivery may be delayed many minutes while the aftercoming head accommodates to the maternal pelvis, but hypoxia and acidosis become severe; or delivery is forced, causing trauma from compression, traction, or both, to the brain, spinal cord, skeleton, and abdominal viscera.

With a preterm fetus, the disparity between the size of the head and the buttocks is even greater than with a larger fetus. At times, the buttocks and lower extremities of the preterm fetus will pass through the cervix and be delivered, and yet the cervix will not be adequately dilated for the head to escape without trauma to the infant (Bodmer and associates, 1986). In this circumstance, Dührssen incisions of the cervix may be tried (see Chap. 25, p. 438). Even so, trauma to the fetus and mother may be appreciable, and hypoxia in the fetus may prove harmful. The frequency of prolapsed cord is increased when the fetus is small or the breech is not a frank breech.

RECOMMENDATIONS FOR DELIVERY

A diligent search for any other complication, actual or anticipated, that might further justify delivery by cesarean section has become a feature of many obstetricians' philosophy for managing delivery in breech presentations. To try to minimize infant mortality and morbidity, cesarean section is now commonly used in the following circumstances to deliver all but the extremely immature fetus whose potential for survival is negligible.

1. Breech presentation and a large fetus.
2. Breech presentation and any degree of contraction or unfavorable shape of the pelvis.
3. Breech presentation and a hyperextended head.
4. Breech presentation not in labor, with maternal or fetal indications for delivery such as pregnancy-induced hypertension or rupture of the membranes for 12 hours or more.
5. Breech presentation and uterine dysfunction.
6. Footling breech presentation.
7. Breech presentation, an apparently healthy but preterm fetus of 26 weeks or more gestation, with the mother in either active labor or in need of delivery.
8. Breech presentation and severe fetal growth retardation.
9. Breech presentation and previous perinatal death or children suffering from birth trauma.
10. Breech presentation and a request by the mother for sterilization.

Large Fetus

The experiences of Rovinsky and associates (1973) and Fortney and colleagues (1986) have been that morbidity and mortality rates for the fetus at term increase with birthweight. Therefore, the fetus estimated to weigh 3,500 g (8 pounds) or more often will benefit from delivery by cesarean section even though the mother's pelvis appears adequate. This allows for underestimation of fetal weight, a relatively common phenomenon when the fetus is large. With the head free in the uterine fundus, sonographic measurements of the biparietal diameter to estimate fetal size, unfortunately, are more likely to be erroneous than with a vertex presentation, as is pointed out in Chapter 20 (p. 377). Nonetheless, the obstetrician could feel much more secure about the estimate of fetal size if there were good agreement about the clinical and sonographic estimates.

Unfavorable Pelvis

In contrast to labor with a cephalic presentation, there is no time for molding of the aftercoming head. Therefore, a moderately contracted pelvis that had not previously caused problems in delivery of an average-size fetus who presented as a vertex might prove dangerous if the fetus were presenting as a breech. Rovinsky and colleagues (1973) urge not only accurate measurements of the pelvic dimensions but also precise evaluation of the pelvic architecture rather than reliance on pelvic indexes. Gynecoid (round) and anthropoid (elliptical) pelves are favorable configurations, but platypelloid (anteroposteriorly flat) and android (heart-shaped) pelves are not (see Chap. 8, p. 167). The platypelloid pelvis typically is narrowed anteroposteriorly, which is unfavorable for the aftercoming head. The android pelvis has a narrow forepelvis, which renders the inlet less favorable than the pelvic diameters would suggest.

Hyperextension of Fetal Head

In perhaps 5 percent or fewer cases of breech presentation at or near term, the fetal head may be in extreme hyperextension (Fig. 19–3). Most often, the cause of hyperextension is not apparent, but vaginal delivery may result in injury to the cervical spinal cord. In general, evidence for marked hyperextension of the fetal head after labor has begun is considered an indication of cesarean delivery (Svenningsen and associates, 1985).

No Labor or Uterine Dysfunction

Induction of labor in women with a breech presentation is defended by some and condemned by others. Brenner and colleagues (1974) noted no significant differences in mortality rates and Apgar scores between cases with induced labor and those

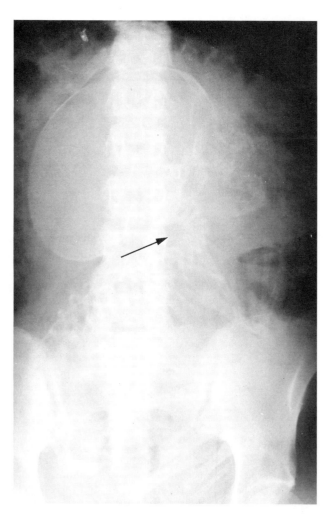

Figure 19–3. Radiological demonstration of a complete breech presentation with a markedly hyperextended cervical spine (*arrow*) and head. Delivery by cesarean section resulted in a normal newborn infant.

with spontaneous labor. In instances in which oxytocin was used to augment labor, however, infant mortality rates were higher and Apgar scores were lower. Gimovsky and Paul (1982) observed that augmentation of labor was followed by vaginal delivery in two of nine women, both multiparous, but one of the two deliveries resulted in entrapment of the aftercoming head. The general policy at Parkland Hospital is to resort to cesarean delivery, rather than oxytocin to induce or augment labor, unless the fetus is previable or has a severe anomaly.

Footling Breech Presentations

The possibility of compression of a prolapsed cord or a cord entangled around the extremities as the breech fills the pelvis, if not before, is a threat to the fetus (Fig. 19–2).

Preterm Delivery

If the fetus is preterm, the aftercoming head may be trapped by a cervix that is sufficiently effaced and dilated to allow passage of the thorax but not the less compressible head. The consequences of vaginal delivery in this circumstance all too often have been both hypoxia and physical trauma, both of which are especially deleterious to the preterm infant. Delivery of the apparently healthy, although preterm, fetus by cesarean section reduces the risks of hypoxia, birth trauma, and their sequelae.

Previous Pregnancy Wastage

The compelling desire to minimize any likelihood of trauma to the fetus may lead to the decision to perform cesarean section.

Desire for Sterilization

For the woman with a breech presentation who desires sterilization, the risk of cesarean section to accomplish delivery and sterilization is no greater, and probably less, than the summation of risks from vaginal breech delivery followed by anesthesia and celiotomy for sterilization.

VAGINAL DELIVERY

Vaginal delivery should be relatively safe for a frank breech presentation if (1) the pelvis is in no way contracted when examined by imaging pelvimetry [a previous cephalic delivery by itself is not proof that the pelvis may not be "contracted" for a breech delivery (Bistoletti, 1981)]; (2) the fetus is judged not to be unusually large (less than 8 pounds) when examined independently by two or more trained examiners or when estimated ultrasonically; (3) spontaneous labor is demonstrated to effect orderly effacement and dilatation of the cervix and descent of the breech through the birth canal; and (4) individuals skilled in breech delivery, in providing appropriate anesthesia, and in infant resuscitation are in immediate attendance. Even when every attempt is made to fulfill these criteria, the outcome for the infant is not always as good as when cesarean section is performed (Collea and co-workers, 1980; Gimovsky and Paul, 1982; Schutte and colleagues, 1985).

The physician who might naively champion any childbirth outside of a hospital setting either is not aware of the hazards of breech delivery in such a setting or is totally insensitive to the welfare of the fetus and the mother. The techniques and precautions for vaginal delivery are detailed in Chapter 22.

CESAREAN SECTION

There is little question that perinatal mortality and morbidity from trauma and hypoxia can be reduced by liberal use of cesarean section. Even for fetuses at term (2,500 g or more), Rovinsky and associates (1973) concluded from their analyses that cesarean section improved the outcome for the fetus. During the 17-year period studied by them, the use of cesarean section for breech delivery increased dramatically.

This same trend in most training institutions toward delivery by cesarean section of the majority of fetuses that present as a breech means that one important criterion for safe vaginal delivery is becoming more and more difficult to fulfill: most resident training programs within the near future will not provide sufficient opportunity for acquisition of skills essential for successful vaginal breech delivery.

Our policy at Parkland Hospital has been liberal use of cesarean section for delivery of the fetus presenting as breech. Even recently, the cesarean delivery rate for breech presentation has increased remarkably. For example, for singleton breech fetuses, the rate was 76 percent in 1983, 78 percent in 1984, 76 percent in 1985, 82 percent in 1986, and 83 percent in 1987.

SUMMARY

The fetus in the breech position is likely to benefit from cesarean section carried out early in labor but at the expense of an appreciable increase in maternal morbidity and a slight increase in maternal mortality. It is anticipated that the prevailing enthusiasm for offspring of the highest quality but of limited number will continue to result in frequent use of cesarean section for breech delivery.

FACE PRESENTATION

In a face presentation, the head is hyperextended so that the occiput is in contact with the fetal back and the chin (mentum) is the presenting part.

INCIDENCE

Cruikshank and White (1973) reported an incidence of 1 in 600, or 0.17 percent; the Obstetrical Statistical Cooperative identified a similar frequency of 0.2 percent. Of nearly 50,000 singleton infants delivered at Parkland Hospital from 1983 through 1986, 41—or 1 in 1,200—presented as a face (Table 19–2).

DIAGNOSIS

Although abdominal findings may be suggestive, the clinical diagnosis of face presentation must rest on vaginal examination. On vaginal palpation, the distinctive features of the face are the mouth and nose, the malar bones, and particularly the orbital ridges. It is possible to mistake a breech presentation for a face, since the anus may be mistaken for the mouth and the ischial tuberosities for the malar prominences. The fetal anus is always on a line with the ischial tuberosities, however, whereas the fetal mouth and malar prominences form the corners of a triangle. The radiographic demonstration of the hyperextended head with the facial bones at or below the pelvic inlet is quite characteristic (Fig. 19–4).

ETIOLOGY

The causes of face presentations are numerous, generally stemming from any factor that favors extension or prevents flexion of the head. Extended positions of the head, therefore, occur more frequently when the pelvis is contracted or the fetus is very

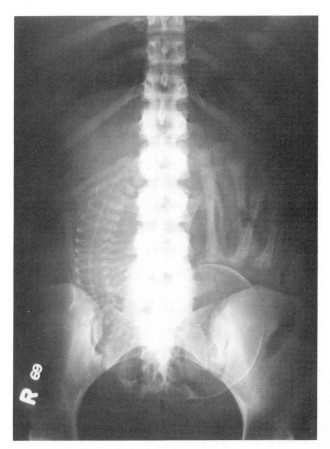

Figure 19–4. Radiograph showing face presentation. Note marked hyperextension of head and spine of fetus.

large. In a series of 141 face presentations studied by Hellman and co-workers (1950), the incidence of inlet contraction was 39 percent. This high incidence of pelvic contraction, as well as large infants, must be kept in mind when considering the successful management of face presentation.

In multiparous women, the pendulous abdomen is another factor that predisposes to face presentation. It permits the back of the fetus to sag forward or laterally, often in the same direction in which the occiput points, thus promoting extension of the cervical and thoracic spine.

In exceptional instances, marked enlargement of the neck or coils of cord about the neck may cause extension. Anencephalic fetuses naturally present by the face because of faulty development of the cranium.

Mechanism

Face presentations are rarely observed above the pelvic inlet. The brow generally presents and is converted to a face presentation after further extension of the head during descent through the pelvis.

The mechanism of labor in these cases consists of the cardinal movements of descent, internal rotation, and flexion, and the accessory movements of extension and external rotation. Descent is brought about by the same factors as in vertex presentations. Extension results from the relation of the fetal body to the deflected head, which is converted into a two-armed lever, the longer arm of which extends from the occipital condyles to the occiput. When resistance is then encountered,

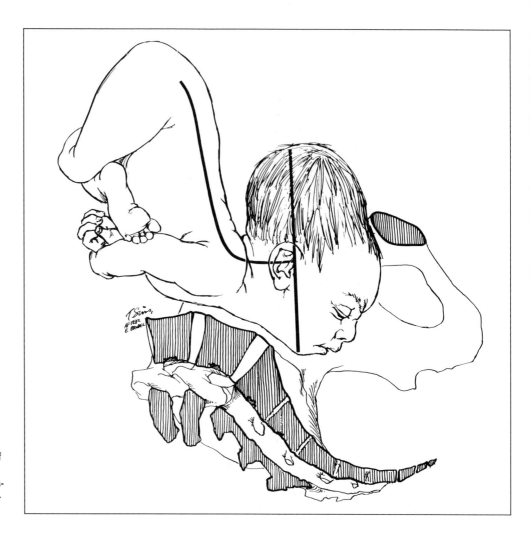

Figure 19–5. Face presentation. The occiput is on the longer end of the head lever. The chin is directly posterior. Vaginal delivery is impossible unless the chin rotates anteriorly.

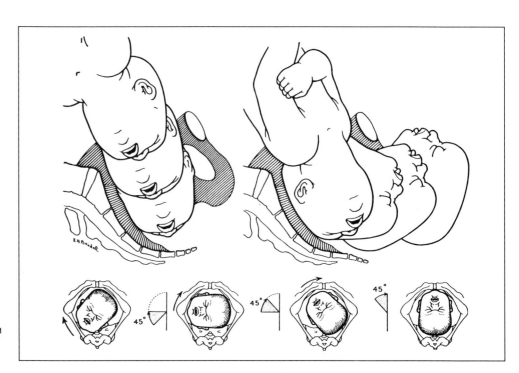

Figure 19–6. Mechanism of labor for right mentoposterior position with subsequent rotation of mentum anterior and delivery.

the occiput must be pushed toward the back of the fetus while the chin descends (Fig. 19–5).

The object of internal rotation of the face is to bring the chin under the symphysis pubis. Unless the head is unusually small, natural delivery cannot otherwise be accomplished. Only in this way can the neck subtend the posterior surface of the symphysis pubis. If the chin rotates directly posteriorly, the relatively short neck cannot span the anterior surface of the sacrum, which measures about 12 cm in length (Fig. 19–5). Hence, the birth of the head is manifestly impossible unless the shoulders enter the pelvis at the same time, an event that is out of the question except when the fetus is extremely small or macerated. Internal rotation in a face presentation results from the same factors as in vertex presentations.

After anterior rotation and descent, the chin and mouth appear at the vulva, the undersurface of the chin presses against the symphysis, and the head is delivered by flexion (Fig. 19–6). The nose, eyes, brow (bregma), and occiput then appear in succession over the anterior margin of the perineum. After the birth of the head, the occiput sags backward toward the anus. In a few moments, the chin rotates externally to the side toward which it was originally directed, and the shoulders are born as in vertex presentations.

Edema may sometimes distort the face sufficiently to obliterate the features and lead to erroneous diagnosis of breech presentation (Fig. 19–7). At the same time, the skull undergoes considerable molding, manifested by increase in length of the occipitomental diameter of the head (Fig. 19–5).

TREATMENT

In the absence of a contracted pelvis and with effective spontaneous labor and no evidence of fetal distress, successful vaginal delivery will usually follow. If labor is allowed, careful monitoring of the fetal heart is probably better done with external devices so as to avoid damage to the face and eyes. As pointed out above, face presentations among term-size fetuses occur more commonly when there is some degree of contraction of the pelvic inlet. Therefore, cesarean section often proves to be the best method for their delivery.

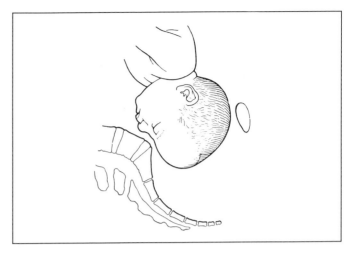

Figure 19–8. Brow posterior presentation.

Other methods of management of face presentations are rarely, if ever, indicated in modern obstetrics. Outmoded are attempts to convert manually a face to a vertex presentation, manual or forceps rotation of a persistently posterior chin to a mentum anterior position, and internal podalic version and extraction. All are likely to be unduly traumatic to both fetus and mother.

BROW PRESENTATION

Brow presentation is rare, and we have encountered it in only 11 cases in nearly 50,000 singleton fetuses delivered over a 4-year period (Table 19–2). With a brow presentation, that portion of the fetal head between the orbital ridge and the anterior fontanel presents at the pelvic inlet. The fetal head thus occupies a position midway between full flexion (occiput) and full extension (mentum or face). Except when the fetal head is small or the pelvis is unusually large, engagement of the fetal head and subsequent delivery cannot take place as long as the brow presentation persists.

ETIOLOGY

The causes of persistent brow presentation are essentially the same as those of face presentation. The brow presentation is commonly unstable and converts to a face or an occiput presentation. Cruikshank and White (1973), for example, observed either flexion to an occiput presentation or extension to a face presentation to take place in two thirds of cases in which the presentation was initially that of the brow.

DIAGNOSIS

The presentation may be recognized by abdominal palpation when both the occiput and chin can be easily palpated, but vaginal examination is usually necessary. The frontal sutures, large anterior fontanel, orbital ridges, eyes, and root of the nose can be felt on vaginal examination. Neither mouth nor chin is within reach however (Figs. 19–8, 19–9).

MECHANISM

The mechanism of labor varies greatly with the size of the fetus. With a very small fetus and a large pelvis, labor is generally

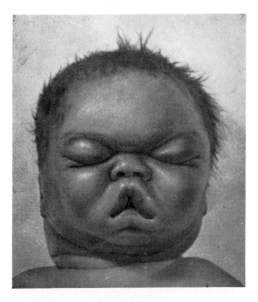

Figure 19–7. Edema in face presentation.

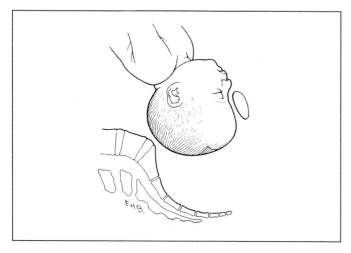

Figure 19–9. Brow anterior presentation.

easy. With larger fetuses, however, it is usually very difficult, since engagement is impossible until after marked molding that shortens the occipitomental diameter or, more commonly, either flexion to an occiput presentation or extension to a face presentation.

The considerable molding essential for delivery of the fetus where the brow presentation persists characteristically deforms the head. The caput succedaneum is over the forehead and may be so extensive that identification of the brow by palpation is impossible. In these instances, the forehead is prominent and squared, and the occipitomental diameter is diminished.

PROGNOSIS

In the transient varieties of brow presentation, the prognosis depends upon the ultimate presentation. When the brow presentation persists, the prognosis is poor for vaginal delivery of an uncompromised infant unless the fetus is small or the birth canal is huge.

TREATMENT

The principles underlying the treatment of brow presentations are much the same as those for a face presentation. If, by chance, spontaneous labor is progressing without any evidence of distress in the closely monitored fetus and without unduly vigorous uterine contractions, no interference is necessary. If labor becomes either unduly vigorous or, more likely, ineffective, or if fetal distress is suspected, prompt cesarean section is indicated.

TRANSVERSE LIE

In this condition, the long axis of the fetus is approximately perpendicular to that of the mother. When the long axis forms an acute angle, an *oblique lie* results. An oblique lie is usually only transitory, however, for either a longitudinal or transverse lie commonly results when labor supervenes. For this reason, the oblique lie is termed *unstable lie* in Great Britain.

In transverse lies, the shoulder is usually over the pelvic inlet, with the head lying in one iliac fossa and the breech in the other. This condition is referred to as a *shoulder* or an *acromion*

presentation. The side of the mother toward which the acromion is directed determines the designation of the lie as right or left acromial. Moreover, since in either position the back may be directed anteriorly or posteriorly, superiorly or inferiorly, it is customary to distinguish varieties as dorsoanterior and dorsoposterior.

INCIDENCE

Transverse lie occurred once in 322 singleton deliveries (0.3 percent) at both the Mayo Clinic and the University of Iowa Hospitals (Johnson, 1964; Cruikshank and White, 1973). At Parkland Hospital, we encountered a transverse lie in 117 of nearly 50,000 singleton fetuses delivered over a 4-year period, for an incidence of 1 in 420 (Table 19–2).

ETIOLOGY

The common causes of transverse lie are (1) unusual relaxation of the abdominal wall resulting from great multiparity, (2) preterm fetus, (3) placenta previa, (4) abnormal uterus, and (5) contracted pelvis. The incidence of transverse lie increases with parity, occurring approximately 10 times more frequently in patients of parity of four or more than in nulliparous women. Relaxation of the abdominal wall with a pendulous abdomen allows the uterus to fall forward, deflecting the long axis of the fetus away from the axis of the birth canal into an oblique or transverse position. Placenta previa and pelvic contraction act similarly. A transverse or oblique lie occasionally develops in labor from an initial longitudinal position, the head or breech migrating to one of the iliac fossae.

DIAGNOSIS

The diagnosis of a transverse lie is usually readily made, often by inspection alone. The abdomen is unusually wide from side to side, whereas the fundus of the uterus extends scarcely above the umbilicus.

On palpation, with the first Leopold maneuver no fetal pole is detected in the fundus. On the second maneuver, a ballottable head is found in one iliac fossa and the breech in the other. The third and fourth maneuvers are negative unless labor is well advanced and the shoulder has become impacted in the pelvis (Figs. 19–10, 19–11). At the same time, the position of the back is readily identified. When the back is anterior, a hard resistance plane extends across the front of the abdomen; when it is posterior, irregular nodulations representing the small parts are felt in the same location (Figs. 19–10, 19–11).

On vaginal examination, in the early stages of labor, the side of the thorax, if it can be reached, may be recognized by the "gridiron" feel of the ribs above the pelvic inlet. When dilatation is further advanced, the scapula and the clavicle are distinguished on opposite sides of the thorax. The position of the axilla indicates the side of the mother toward which the shoulder is directed. Later in labor, the shoulder becomes tightly wedged in the pelvic canal, and a hand and arm frequently prolapse into the vagina and through the vulva (Figs. 19–12, 19–13).

COURSE OF LABOR

The spontaneous birth of a fully developed infant is manifestly impossible in a persistent transverse lie, since expulsion cannot be effected unless both the head and trunk of the fetus enter the pelvis at the same time. At term, therefore, both the fetus and

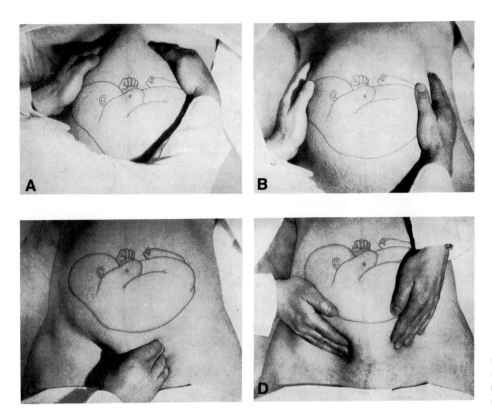

Figure 19–10. Palpation in transverse lie, right acromiodorsoanterior position. **A.** First maneuver. **B.** Second maneuver. **C.** Third maneuver. **D.** Fourth maneuver.

the mother will die unless appropriate measures are instituted.

After the rupture of the membranes, if the mother is left to herself, the fetal shoulder is forced into the pelvis, and the corresponding arm frequently prolapses (Fig. 19–13). After some descent, the shoulder is arrested by the margins of the pelvic inlet, with the head in one iliac fossa and the breech in the other. As labor continues, the shoulder is firmly impacted in the upper part of the pelvis. The uterus then contracts vigorously in an unsuccessful attempt to overcome the obstacle. After a time, a retraction ring rises increasingly higher and becomes more marked. The situation is referred to as neglected transverse lie. If not vigorously and properly treated, the uterus eventually ruptures, and the mother and fetus die.

If the fetus is quite small and the pelvis is large, spontaneous delivery may occur despite persistence of the abnormal lie. In such cases, the fetus is compressed with the head forced against the abdomen. A portion of the thoracic wall below the shoulder thus becomes the most dependent part, appearing at the vulva. The head and thorax then pass through the pelvic cavity at the same time, and the fetus, which is doubled upon itself (*conduplicato corpore*), is expelled. Such a mechanism obviously is possible only in the case of very small infants and occasionally when the second preterm fetus in a twin pregnancy is born.

PROGNOSIS

Labor with shoulder presentation increases the maternal risk and adds tremendously to the fetal hazard. Most maternal deaths from this complication occur in neglected cases from spontaneous rupture of the uterus or traumatic rupture consequent upon late and ill-advised version and extraction. Even with the best of care, however, the chance of maternal death will be increased slightly for four reasons: (1) the frequent as-

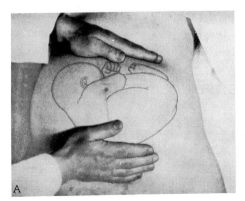
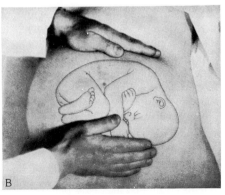

Figure 19–11. Transverse lie, palpation of back in dorsoanterior (**A**) and in dorsoposterior (**B**) positions.

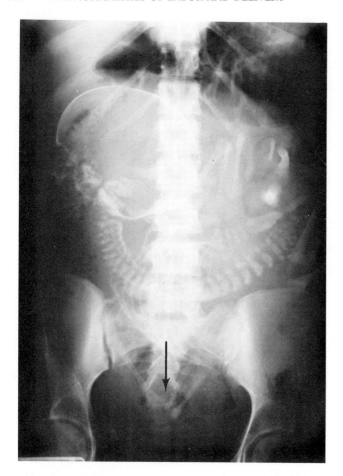

Figure 19–12. Radiograph of a transverse lie, which illustrates an elbow (arrow) at the level of the cervix.

sociation of transverse lie with placenta previa, (2) the increased likelihood of cord accidents, (3) the almost inevitable necessity of major operative interferences, and (4) the likelihood of sepsis after rupture of the membranes and extrusion of the arm through the vagina.

MANAGEMENT

In general, the onset of active labor in a woman with a transverse lie is an indication for cesarean section. Once labor is well established, attempts at conversion to a longitudinal lie by abdominal manipulation are not likely to be successful. Before labor or early in labor, with the membranes intact, attempts at external version are worthy of a trial in the absence of other obstetrical complications that point toward cesarean section. Phelan and co-workers (1986) recommend such an attempt only after 39 weeks gestation because of the high (83 percent) spontaneous conversion to a longitudinal lie. If during early labor the fetal head can be maneuvered by abdominal manipulation into the pelvis, it should be held there during the next several contractions to try to fix the head in the pelvis. The fetal heart rate must be closely checked during this time. If these measures fail in the woman in labor, cesarean section should be performed promptly.

Because neither the feet nor the vertex of the fetus occupies the lower uterine segment, a low transverse incision into the uterus may lead to difficulty in extraction of a fetus entrapped in the body of the uterus above the level of incision. Therefore, a vertical incision generally is favored. The treatment of neglected transverse lie entails support in the form of antimicrobials, fluid therapy, and transfusion, if needed. Delivery may be accomplished abdominally by cesarean section or cesarean section-hysterectomy, as indicated (see Chap. 26, pp. 441, 453).

COMPOUND PRESENTATION

In a compound presentation, an extremity prolapses alongside the presenting part with both presenting in the pelvis simultaneously (Fig. 19–14).

INCIDENCE

Goplerud and Eastman (1953) identified a hand or arm prolapsed alongside the head once in every 700 deliveries. Much less common was prolapse of one or both lower extremities alongside a vertex presentation or a hand alongside a breech presentation. We have identified compound presentations in only 22 of nearly 50,000 singleton fetuses delivered from 1983 through 1986, an incidence of 1 in 2,235 (Table 19–2).

ETIOLOGY

As expected, the causes of compound presentations are conditions that prevent complete occlusion of the pelvic inlet by the fetal head. In Goplerud and Eastman's series, the incidence of preterm delivery was twice the expected rate. Often, however, no cause is demonstrable.

PROGNOSIS

Although the reported perinatal loss is increased, a major portion of the wastage is contributed by preterm delivery, prolapsed cord, and traumatic obstetrical procedures.

MANAGEMENT

In most cases, the prolapsed part should be left alone, since most often it will not interfere with labor. In Goplerud and Eastman's series of 50 cases not associated with prolapse of the cord, 24, or almost one half, had no treatment. Normal delivery ensued in all, with the loss of one infant. If the arm is prolapsed alongside the head, the condition should be observed closely to ascertain whether the arm rises out of the way with descent of the presenting part. If it fails to do so and if it appears to prevent descent of the head, the prolapsed arm should be gently pushed upward and the head simultaneously downward by fundal pressure.

With a compound presentation, electronic fetal heart rate monitoring and intrauterine pressure monitoring are preferable. If there is fetal distress or uterine dysfunction, then cesarean section is done.

PERSISTENT OCCIPUT POSTERIOR POSITIONS

Most often, occiput posterior positions undergo spontaneous anterior rotation followed by uncomplicated delivery. In 10 percent or fewer cases, spontaneous rotation does not occur. Although the precise reasons for failure of spontaneous rotation are not known, transverse narrowing of the midpelvis undoubtedly plays a role.

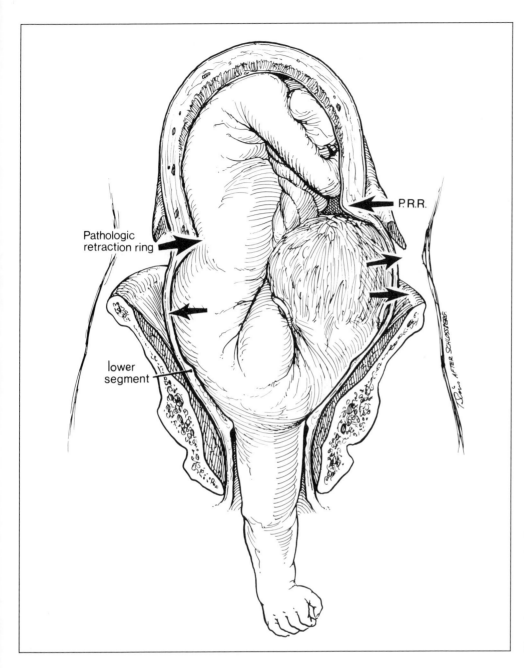

Figure 19–13. Neglected shoulder presentation. A thick muscular band to form a pathological retraction ring has developed just above the very thin lower uterine segment. The force generated during a uterine contraction is directed centripetally at and above the level of the pathological retraction ring. This serves to stretch further and possibly to rupture the very thin lower segment below the retraction ring. P.R.R. = pathological retraction ring.

The conduct of labor and delivery with the occiput posterior need not differ remarkably from that with the occiput anterior. The status of the fetus is probably best monitored, however, by continuous electronic techniques. Progress of labor may be ascertained by checking the rate and extent of cervical dilatation and the descent of the fetal head through the birth canal. In most instances, delivery can usually be accomplished without great difficulty once the head reaches the perineum.

The possibilities for vaginal delivery are (1) await spontaneous delivery, (2) forceps delivery with the occiput directly posterior, (3) forceps rotation of the occiput to the anterior position and delivery, or (4) manual rotation to the anterior position followed by spontaneous or forceps delivery.

SPONTANEOUS DELIVERY

If the pelvic outlet is roomy and the vaginal outlet and perineum are somewhat relaxed from previous vaginal deliveries, rapid spontaneous delivery will often take place. If the vaginal outlet is resistant to stretch and the perineum is firm, the deceleration portion of the labor curve or the second stage of labor, or both, may be prolonged appreciably before spontaneous delivery will occur (see Chap. 18, p. 342). During each expulsive effort, with the occiput posterior, the head is driven against the perineum to a much greater degree than when the occiput is anterior. Therefore, forceps delivery often is indicated. A generous episiotomy is usually needed for either spontaneous or forceps delivery.

FORCEPS DELIVERY AS AN OCCIPUT POSTERIOR

The need for more traction compared to forceps deliveries from the occiput anterior position can be minimized by making a larger episiotomy. In most instances, a mediolateral incision should be made to avoid lacerations into the anus and rectum. The use of forceps and a large episiotomy warrant more com-

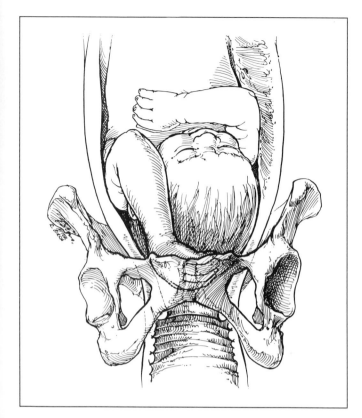

Figure 19–14. Compound presentation. The left hand is lying in front of the vertex. With further labor, the hand and arm may retract from the birth canal and the head descend normally.

plete analgesia than may be achieved with pudendal block and local perineal infiltration. The forceps are applied bilaterally along the occipitomental diameter, as described in Chapter 25 (p. 434).

It is important to identify the infrequent case in which the protrusion of fetal scalp through the introitus is the consequence of marked elongation of the fetal head from molding combined with the formation of a large caput. In this circumstance, the head may not even be engaged—that is, the biparietal diameter has not yet passed through the pelvic inlet. Labor characteristically has been long in such a case and, in turn, descent of the head has been slow. Careful palpation above the symphysis discloses the fetal head to be present above the pelvic inlet. Prompt cesarean section is the appropriate method of delivery. It may be necessary at the time of operation to have an associate insert a sterile gloved hand into the vagina to dislodge the head upward.

FORCEPS ROTATION

If the head is engaged, the cervix fully dilated, and the pelvis is adequate, forceps rotation may be attempted if the operator is sufficiently skilled. These circumstances are most likely to prevail when expulsive efforts of the mother during the second stage are ineffective, as, for example, with continuous regional analgesia. Rotation by the so-called Scanzoni maneuver or with Kielland forceps is described in Chapter 25 (p. 434).

MANUAL ROTATION

The requirements for forceps rotation must be met. When the hand is introduced to locate the posterior ear and thus confirm

the posterior position, the occiput often rotates toward the anterior position. The head may be grasped with the fingers over the posterior ear and the thumb over the anterior ear and an attempt made to rotate the occiput to the anterior position (see Chap. 25, p. 433).

OUTCOME

Phillips and Freeman (1974) reviewed the extensive experiences with occiput posterior positions at Grady Memorial Hospital, Atlanta, Georgia. Basic management of the persistent occiput posterior position was similar to that for the occiput anterior position, namely, delivery without manual or forceps rotation. Compared to the occiput anterior position, labor was prolonged on the average 1 hour in parous women and 2 hours in nulliparous women. The perinatal mortality rate of 2.2 percent did not differ significantly from the 1.8 percent for the occiput anterior group. No significant rise in Apgar scores of less than 7 was found. Extension of the episiotomy, however, was increased appreciably. Phillips and Freeman (1974) comment that midline episiotomies are not acceptable for occiput posterior deliveries and, instead, adequate mediolateral incisions should be made.

At Parkland Hospital, either manual rotation to the anterior position followed by forceps delivery, or forceps delivery from the occiput posterior position, is used to effect delivery. When neither can be done with relative ease, cesarean section usually is performed.

PERSISTENT OCCIPUT TRANSVERSE POSITION

In the absence of an abnormality of the pelvic architecture, the occiput transverse position is most likely a transitory one as the occiput rotates to the anterior position. If hypotonic uterine dysfunction, either spontaneous or the consequence of conduction analgesia, does not develop, spontaneous rotation is usually soon completed, thus allowing the choice of spontaneous delivery or delivery with outlet forceps.

DELIVERY

If rotation ceases because of lack of uterine action and in the absence of pelvic contraction, vaginal delivery usually can be readily accomplished in a number of ways: The occiput may be manually rotated anteriorly or posteriorly and forceps delivery carried out from either the anterior or posterior position. Another approach recommended by some is to apply forceps of the Kielland type to the head in the occiput transverse position (see Chap. 25, p. 435), rotate the occiput to the anterior position, and then deliver the head with either the same forceps or with standard outlet forceps. If the failure of spontaneous rotation of the head is caused by hypotonic uterine dysfunction *without cephalopelvic disproportion*, dilute oxytocin may be infused while the fetal heart rate and the uterine contractions are closely monitored.

The genesis of the occiput transverse position is not always so simple, nor is the treatment so benign. With the platypelloid (anteroposteriorly flat configuration) pelvis and the android (heart-shaped) pelvis, there may not be adequate room for rotation of the occiput to either the anterior or the posterior position. With the android pelvis, the head may not even be engaged, yet the scalp may be visible through the vaginal introitus as the consequence of considerable molding and caput formation. This situation is fraught with danger to both the fetus and mother. If forceps are tried for delivery, it is imperative that undue force not be applied but, instead, delivery be accomplished by cesarean section.

FETAL MACROSOMIA

Birthweights rarely exceed 11 pounds (5,000 g), although in 1979 the birth of an infant who weighed 16 pounds (7,300 g) was widely reported in the United States. Postpartum, delayed glucose metabolism was detected in the mother. She had previously given birth to several infants who weighed 9 and 10 pounds. Certainly one of the largest infants on record weighed 23.75 pounds (10,800 g), as reported by Beach in 1879 (Barnes, 1957).

Several factors, alone or in combination, may be operative in the genesis of macrosomia. These include (1) large size of the parents, especially the mother; (2) multiparity; (3) diabetes in the mother; (4) maternal obesity; (5) prolonged gestation; and (6) previous delivery of an infant weighing more than 4,000 g (Houchang and co-workers, 1980).

With large fetuses, dystocia may arise because the head becomes not only larger but harder and less moldable with increasing weight. Moreover, after the head has passed through the pelvic canal, dystocia may be caused by the arrest of even larger shoulders at either the pelvic brim or outlet (Fig. 19–15).

INCIDENCE

It is common practice to designate all newborn infants weighing 4,000 g or more as macrosomic. The incidence of these infants in more than 104,000 deliveries in the Obstetrical Statistical Cooperative was 5.3 percent, and the incidence of infants weighing 4,500 g or more was 0.4 percent. Interestingly, among the often socioeconomically deprived, predominantly young population with a relatively low prevalence of diabetes cared for at Parkland Hospital, the frequency of birth weights of 4,000 g or more among 22,000 deliveries was 5.8 percent. Moreover, this number appears to be increasing.

DIAGNOSIS

Inasmuch as the clinical estimation of the size of the fetus may be inaccurate, the diagnosis of macrosomia is often not made until after fruitless attempts at delivery. Nevertheless, competent clinical examination should enable experienced examiners to arrive at a fairly accurate estimate. Sonographic evaluation of the dimensions of the head, thorax, and abdomen often enhances appreciably the confidence of the estimate (Wladimiroff and colleagues, 1978).

Serious dystocia may arise when an excessively large head attempts to pass through a normal pelvis, just as when the head of an average-size fetus is arrested by a definitely contracted pelvic inlet. At times, the head is delivered without great difficulty but the large shoulder girdle becomes entrapped. Dystocia from a large shoulder girdle is discussed subsequently.

PROGNOSIS

Since macrosomic infants are more often born to multiparous mothers and to women with diabetes, both the maternal and fetal risks are increased. In a report on 766 infants who weighed over 4,500 g, Sack (1969) cited a perinatal loss of 7 percent. More distressing, 16 percent of the infants were severely depressed at birth, 11 percent had severe neurological complications, and 4.5 percent of those who survived the perinatal period were dead before the age of 7 years.

SHOULDER DYSTOCIA

Shoulder dystocia is a serious complication of delivery. The problem is that the head is delivered, causing the cord to be drawn into the pelvis and compressed before it is realized there is an arrest to the delivery of the shoulders.

INCIDENCE, ETIOLOGY, AND CONTRIBUTING FACTORS

In 1960, Swartz reported that the incidence of shoulder dystocia was 0.15 percent for all fetus-infants weighing more than 2,500

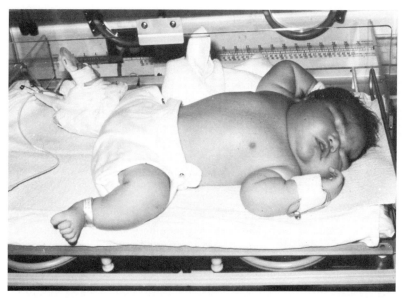

Figure 19–15. This infant weighed 6,065 g and was delivered by cesarean section. The mother had gestational diabetes.

g and 1.7 percent for those who weighed more than 4,000 g. Unfortunately, the etiology of shoulder dystocia is fetal macrosomia and not simply an increase in fetal weight to above an arbitrarily defined weight of 4,000 g. Thus, fetal macrosomia is an *increase in body size in relation to head size*, the result often but not always being a larger shoulder girdle than fetal head. The ponderal index (Chap. 38, p. 766) of such infants most often is increased, making a predictable diagnosis of fetal macrosomia extremely difficult and a *reliable prediction of shoulder dystocia impossible*. Any maternal or fetal factor that contributes to an increased incidence of fetal macrosomia also naturally increases the incidence of shoulder dystocia.

For convenience, factors that contribute to shoulder dystocia can be separated into antepartum and intrapartum considerations. It is important, however, to realize that in clinical practice each of these factors may influence the incidence of shoulder dystocia as an independent variable or in a multivariate manner. Unfortunately, clinical practice is rarely limited to a single variable, and thus single or isolated factors cannot be considered in making clinical decisions concerning the possibility of shoulder dystocia.

ANTEPARTUM CONTRIBUTING FACTORS

Maternal Obesity
Maternal obesity alone is difficult to separate from gestational diabetes or overt diabetes, however Johnson and colleagues (1987) reported that in pregnant women weighing more than 250 pounds the incidence of shoulder dystocia was 5.1 percent compared to 0.6 percent for control women who weighed less than 200 pounds. Spellacy and co-workers (1985) reported that for women weighing more than 90 kg, birthweight distribution was 8.2 percent for 2,500 to 3,499 g infants; 33 percent for 4,500 to 4,999 g infants; and 50 percent for infants who weighed more than 5,000 g. Shoulder dystocia was identified in 0.3 percent of the 2,500 to 3,499 g infants; 7.3 percent of the 4,500 to 4,999 g infants; and 14.6 percent of the larger infants. Parks and Ziel (1978) reported that maternal pre- or early pregnancy weight above 90 kg was associated with 5.5 percent of infants weighing more than 4,500 g, compared to 1.9 percent in control women. They reported that excessive weight gain during pregnancy was not associated with an increased incidence of 4,500 g or heavier neonates. Shoulder dystocia was identified in 13.6 percent of infants who weighed more than 4,500 g, compared to 1.7 percent of control patients.

Diabetes Mellitus
The association of macrosomia with mild diabetes mellitus is well established and was a significantly important contributing factor to shoulder dystocia reported in the studies discussed above. Similar results have been reported by Berne and associates (1985) in Sweden, Klebe and co-workers (1986) in Denmark, and Cousins and colleagues (1985) in the United States. The incidences of shoulder dystocia in these studies were 2.5, 5, and 16.7 percent, respectively, versus 1.7 percent for controls.

Postterm Pregnancy
The fact that many fetuses continue to grow after 42 weeks (Chap. 38, p. 759) now is well recognized. The association of an increased incidence of shoulder dystocia in postterm pregnancy has been reported by Golditch (1978), Spellacy (1985), Acker (1985), Johnson (1987), Eden (1987), and all their co-workers.

INTRAPARTUM CONTRIBUTING FACTORS

At least three intrapartum factors have been reported to be associated with an increased incidence of shoulder dystocia: (1) prolonged second stage of labor, (2) oxytocin induction or augmentation of labor, and (3) the use of midforceps or a vacuum extraction during delivery.

Prolonged Second Stage of Labor
Benedetti and Gabbe (1978) reported that with a prolonged second stage of labor and a midpelvic delivery (vacuum extraction or midforceps delivery), the incidence of shoulder dystocia was 4.6 percent compared to 0.16 percent in the absence of a prolonged second stage of labor. Acker and co-workers (1985) reported an increased incidence of shoulder dystocia in 4,000 g and larger infants if there was a prolongation or arrest of labor (see Chap. 18, p. 346). Acker and colleagues (1986) also reported an increased incidence of shoulder dystocia in normal weight infants (2,500 to 3,000 g) born to women in whom labor was complicated by an arrest disorder.

Oxytocin Induction
Since shoulder dystocia is the consequence of macrosomia, it is not surprising that oxytocin may be associated with an increased incidence. Large infants often are associated with dysfunctional labors, and oxytocin frequently is indicated in many forms of dysfunctional labor (see Chap. 18). Also, the treatment for postterm pregnancy is delivery, and this is accomplished by labor induction. Finally, a postterm gestation often is associated with increased macrosomia and shoulder dystocia.

Midforceps and Vacuum Extraction
For many of the same reasons discussed under oxytocin induction or augmentation, there is a significant increase in the incidence of shoulder dystocia with midforceps or vacuum extractions. As described earlier, Benedetti and Gabbe (1978) reported such an association, and subsequently other investigators have done so as well (Levine and co-workers, 1984; McFarland and associates, 1986).

PREDICTION AND PREVENTION OF SHOULDER DYSTOCIA

It seems reasonable that identification of the ante- and intrapartum factors associated with an increased incidence of shoulder dystocia might enable the clinician accurately to predict its occurrence. If so, cesarean section then could be done to prevent both maternal and infant morbidity associated with a complicated vaginal delivery. In fact, Elliott and associates (1982) observed that a transthoracic diameter for an infant of a diabetic mother of 1.4 cm greater than the biparietal diameter served as a predictor of significant fetomaternal disproportion and as such correlated with the possibility of shoulder dystocia. This work was the extension of their previous work with Houchang and associates (1980, 1982), who obtained these measurements in newborns over 4,000 g. As a result of this study, they reported that a chest-minus-head diameter difference of 1.6 cm or more or a shoulder-minus-head diameter of 4.8 cm or more indicated a high likelihood of shoulder dystocia. They recommended that if such measurements were obtained in fetuses likely to develop shoulder dystocia, one of two choices of management should be planned. The first choice should be cesarean section. If vaginal delivery was considered as the second plan,

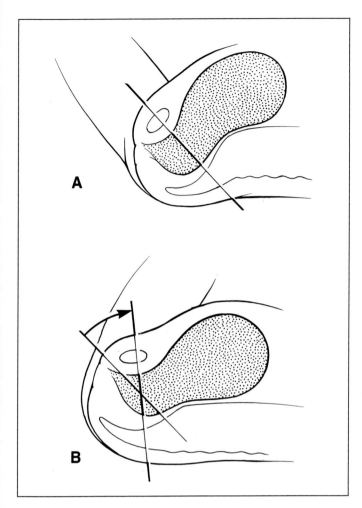

Figure 19–16. The McRoberts maneuver. The maneuver consists of (**A**) removing the woman's legs from the stirrups and (**B**) sharply flexing them upon her abdomen.

the following conditions should be met: (1) a physician experienced in the management of shoulder dystocia should attend the delivery; (2) appropriate anesthesia support personnel should be present for the delivery; and (3) pediatric support personnel should be present in order to minimize the sequelae of a potentially traumatic delivery.

Kitzmiller and associates (1987) used computed tomography to measure fetal shoulder width in 22 diabetic women within 2 days of birth. Their preliminary observations were that a width of 14 cm correlated with a birthweight of more than 4,200 g, with a positive predictive value of 78 percent and a negative predictive value of 100 percent.

Gross and colleagues (1987b) looked at the problem of predictability in a critical manner. Specifically, they studied 394 women delivered of infants whose birthweights were greater than 4,000 g, and used three-way discriminant analysis to determine if a model could be developed to predict women in each of three groups: (1) no shoulder dystocia; (2) shoulder dystocia without trauma; and (3) shoulder dystocia with trauma. Three factors contributed significantly: birthweight, prolonged deceleration phase of labor, and length of the second stage. While 94 percent of cases *without* shoulder dystocia could be predicted, only 16 percent of the shoulder dystocias associated with trauma could be predicted using their mathematical model. They concluded that *"the occurrence of shoulder dystocia cannot be predicted from clinical characteristics or labor abnormalities. . . ."* Acker and associates (1988) arrived at a similar conclusion.

FETAL CONSEQUENCES

Shoulder dystocia, if not appropriately managed, may be associated with significant fetal morbidity and mortality. Benedetti and Gabbe (1978) reported that of 19 neonates with shoulder dystocia, 5 had a fractured humerus or clavicle, 3 had Erb's palsy, and 1 had an abnormal neurological examination. Similar results have been reported by Levine (1984), Coustan (1984), Spellacy (1985), McFarland (1986), and their co-workers. Prompt

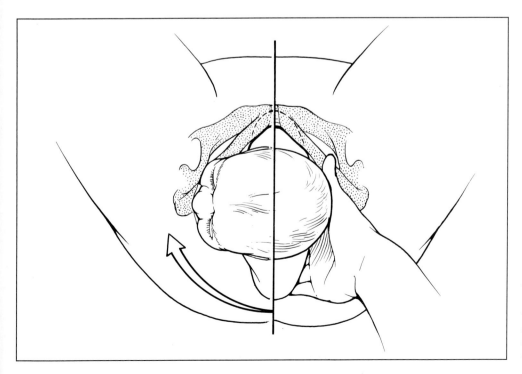

Figure 19–17. Woods' maneuver. The operator's hand is placed behind the posterior shoulder of the fetus. The shoulder then is progressively rotated 180 degrees in a corkscrew manner so that the impacted anterior shoulder is released.

physiotherapy may improve brachial nerve damage in some but not all cases of Erb's palsy (see Chap. 33, p. 62). While fractures and brachial nerve damage are serious consequences, severe asphyxia and death also may result. McCall (1962) described 105 cases of shoulder dystocia, and there were 8 perinatal deaths with at least 2 directly related to shoulder dystocia. In the surviving infants were 7 cases of brachial plexus injury and 21 cases of asphyxia. Of 46 survivors who could be traced, 2 were mentally retarded, 5 were slow learners, and 2 had speech defects.

Maternal Consequences

Postpartum hemorrhage, usually from uterine atony but also from vaginal and cervical lacerations, remains the major mater-

nal risk (Benedetti and Gabbe, 1978; Parks and Zicl, 1978). Puerperal infection remains a problem, but significant infection largely can be prevented with the use of perioperative broad-spectrum antimicrobials (see Chap. 27).

MANAGEMENT

Because shoulder dystocia cannot be predicted, there always will be the unexpected case, despite a carefully obtained history that may identify the likelihood of a shoulder dystocia developing and despite the possibility of sonographic evidence used to identify candidates in whom this complication is likely to occur. Therefore, the practitioner of obstetrics *must* be well versed in the management principles of this occasionally devastating complication.

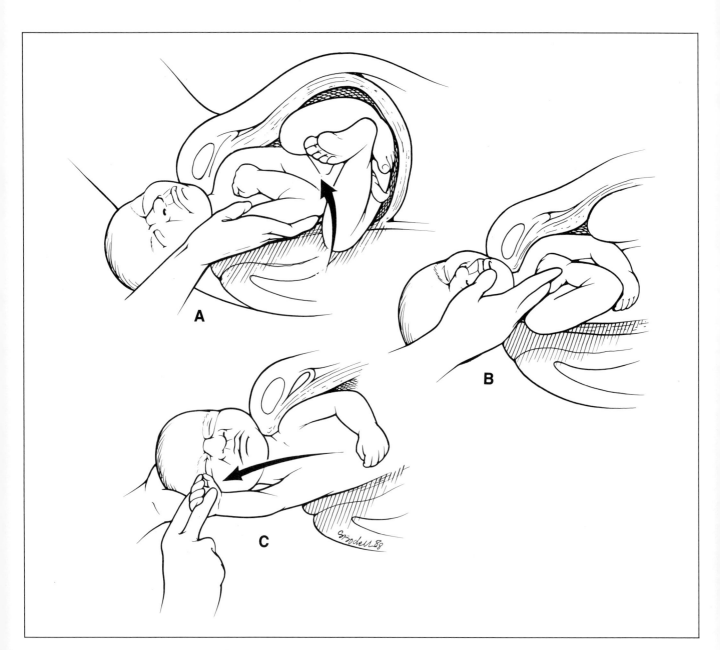

Figure 19–18. Shoulder dystocia with impacted anterior shoulder of the fetus. **A.** The operator's hand is introduced into the vagina along the fetal posterior humerus, which is splinted as the arm is swept across the chest, keeping the arm flexed at the elbow. **B.** The fetal hand is grasped and the arm extended along the side of the face. **C.** The posterior arm is delivered from the vagina.

Reduction in the interval of time from delivery of the head to delivery of the body is of great importance to survival, but overly vigorous traction on the head or neck, or excessive rotation of the body, may cause serious damage to the infant.

A large mediolateral episiotomy and adequate anesthesia are necessary and should be accomplished expeditiously. The next step is to clear the infant's mouth and nose. Having completed the above steps, a variety of methods or techniques have been described to free the anterior shoulder from its impacted position beneath the maternal symphysis pubis. The most popular techniques include:

1. Suprapubic pressure. Resnik (1980), as well as others, recommended moderate suprapubic pressure by an assistant while downward traction is applied to the fetal head.
2. The McRoberts maneuver was described by Gonik and associates (1983). It is named for William A. McRoberts, Jr., who

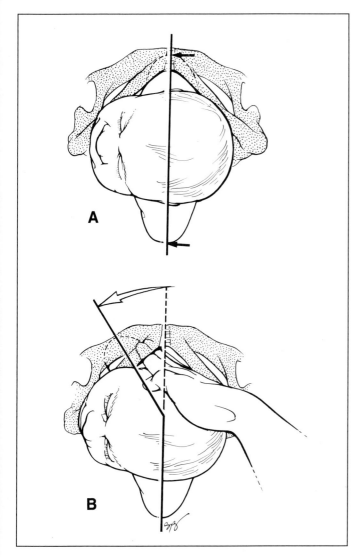

Figure 19–19. Rubin's (second) maneuver. **A.** The shoulder-to-shoulder diameter is shown as the distance between the two small arrows. **B.** The most easily accessible fetal shoulder (the anterior is shown here) is pushed toward the anterior chest wall of the fetus. Most often, this results in abduction of both shoulders, reducing the shoulder-to-shoulder diameter and freeing the impacted anterior shoulder.

popularized its use at the University of Texas Health Science Center at Houston/Hermann Hospital. The maneuver consists of removing the woman's legs from the stirrups and sharply flexing them upon her own abdomen (Fig. 19–16). This supposedly results in a straightening of the sacrum relative to the lumbar vertebrae with accompanying rotation of the symphysis pubis toward the patient's head and a decrease in the angle of pelvic inclination (see Chap. 8). This maneuver does not increase the dimensions of the pelvis, but the cephalic rotation of the pelvis frees the impacted anterior shoulder. Pollack and associates (1985) reported the successful use of this maneuver in 24 of 25 cases of shoulder dystocia.

3. Woods (1943) reported that, by progressively rotating the posterior shoulder 180 degrees in a corkscrew fashion, the impacted anterior shoulder could be released. This is frequently referred to as the Woods corkscrew maneuver (Fig. 19–17).
4. Delivery of the posterior shoulder consists of carefully sweeping the posterior arm of the fetus across the chest, followed by delivery of the arm. The shoulder girdle then is rotated into one of the oblique diameters of the pelvis with subsequent delivery of the anterior shoulder (Fig. 19–18).
5. Rubin (1964) recommended two maneuvers. First, the fetal shoulders are rocked from side to side by applying force to the mother's abdomen. If this is not successful, the most easily accessible fetal shoulder is pushed toward the anterior surface of the fetus's chest. This most often results in abduction of both fetal shoulders. This in turn produces a smaller shoulder-to-shoulder diameter and displacement of the anterior shoulder from behind the symphysis pubis (Fig. 19–19).
6. Chavis (1979) described the use of a shoulder horn instrument consisting of a concave blade with a long handle, which is slipped between the symphysis and the impacted anterior shoulder. The instrument is then used like a shoehorn as a lever with the symphysis pubis as a fulcrum.
7. Hibbard (1982) recommended that pressure be applied to the infant's jaw and neck in the direction of the mother's rectum, with strong fundal pressure applied by an assistant as the anterior shoulder is freed. **This is a potentially dangerous procedure.** It must be remembered that strong fundal pressure applied at the wrong time may result in even further impaction of the anterior shoulder. Furthermore, Gross and associates (1987a) reported that fundal pressure in the absence of other maneuvers **"resulted in a 77 percent complication rate and was strongly associated with (fetal) orthopedic and neurologic damage."**
8. Sandberg (1988) reported the Zavanelli maneuver for cephalic replacement into the pelvis and then cesarean section. The first part of the maneuver consists of returning the head to the OA or OP position if the head has rotated from either position. The second step is to flex the head and slowly push it back into the vagina, following which a cesarean delivery is performed. O'Leary and Gunn (1985), while commenting on Sandberg's report, urged that the maneuver simply be called cephalic replacement. They reported success with the technique in four cases of shoulder dystocia. In three cases, they administered 0.25 mg of terbutaline subcutaneously to the mother to produce uterine relaxation.
9. Deliberate fracture of the clavicle by pressing the anterior clavicle against the ramus of the pubis can be done to free the shoulder impaction. The fracture will heal rapidly and is not nearly as serious as a brachial nerve injury, asphyxia, or death.
10. Cleidotomy consists of cutting the clavicle with scissors or other sharp instruments and is usually used on a dead fetus (Schramm, 1983). Symphysiotomy also has been successfully applied and the technique was described by Hartfield (1986).

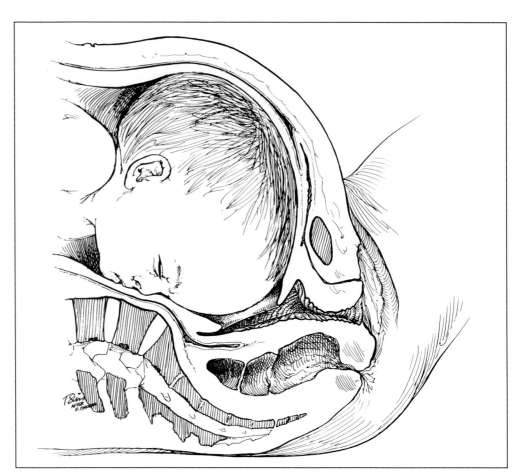

Figure 19–20. Severe dystocia from hydrocephalus, cephalic presentation. Note the disparity between the small size of the face and the rest of the cranium.

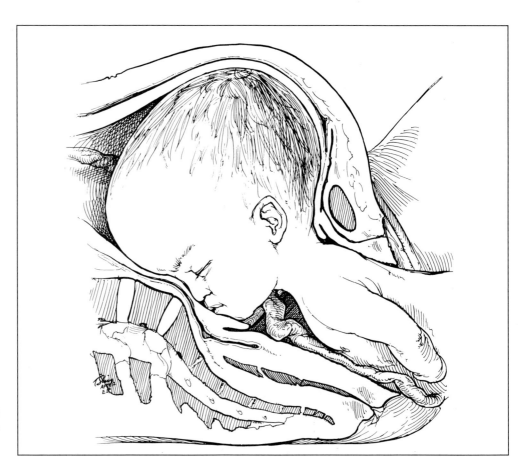

Figure 19–21. Severe dystocia from hydrocephalus, breech presentation. Note the distension of the lower uterine segment.

At Parkland Hospital, our first maneuver to free the impacted shoulder is simple abdominal pressure applied over the symphysis. If this is not successful, the McRoberts maneuver is added. If still unsuccessful, the posterior fetal arm and shoulder are delivered or the shoulder girdle is rotated into the oblique position. In the exceptional case when none of the above is possible, it seems reasonable to attempt the cephalic replacement technique, or as a last effort, to deliberately fracture the clavicle.

HYDROCEPHALUS AS A CAUSE OF DYSTOCIA

Internal hydrocephalus, or excessive accumulation of cerebrospinal fluid in the ventricles of the brain with consequent enlargement of the cranium, occurs in about one in 2,000 fetuses and accounts for about 12 percent of all severe malformations found at birth. Associated defects are common, with spina bifida occurring in about one third of cases. Not infrequently, the circumference of the head exceeds 50 cm, and sometimes reaches 80 cm. The volume of fluid is usually between 500 and 1,500 mL, but as much as 5 L may accumulate. Breech presentation is found in about one third of these cases. Whatever the presentation, gross cephalopelvic disproportion is the rule, with serious dystocia the usual consequence (Figs. 19–20, 19–21).

DIAGNOSIS

Since the treatment of this complication of labor is usually straightforward, early diagnosis is the key to success. In this condition particularly, an empty bladder facilitates both abdominal and vaginal examination. In cephalic presentations, a broad, firm mass above the symphysis is evident from abdominal examination. The thickness of the abdominal wall usually prevents detection of the thin, elastic, hydrocephalic cranium. The high head forces the body of the infant upward, with the result that the fetal heart is often loudest above the umbilicus, a circumstance leading to the suspicion of a breech presentation. Vaginally, the broader dome of the head feels tense, but more careful palpation may disclose very large fontanels, wide suture lines, and an indentable, thin cranium characteristic of hydrocephalus. Radiography or sonography provides confirmation by the demonstration of a large, globular head (Figs. 19–22, 19–23).

Hydrocephalus is somewhat more difficult to diagnose radiographically with a breech presentation, since the radio-

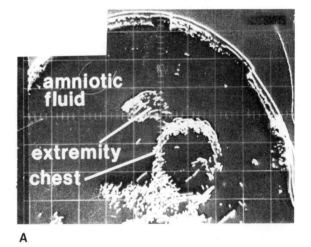

A

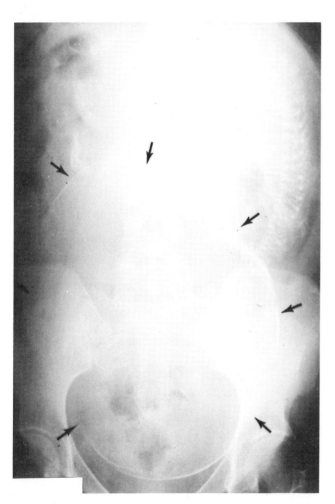

Figure 19–22. Radiograph demonstrating severe hydrocephalus, further outlined by arrows; 2,300 mL of cerebrospinal fluid were aspirated transvaginally (Figs. 19–24, 19–25).

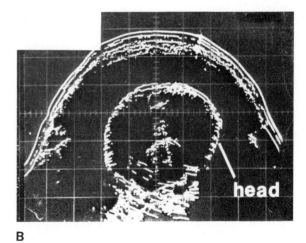

B

Figure 19–23. Sonograms of a fetus with hydrocephalus and associated hydramnios. Visible in **A** are the thorax, an extremity, and an excessive amount of amnionic fluid. In **B,** the head is remarkably enlarged compared to the thorax. (*Courtesy of Dr. R. Santos.*)

graphic outline of a normal fetal head often appears enlarged to a degree suggestive of hydrocephalus. This results from the fetal head lying more anterior than with a cephalic presentation and the divergence of x-rays inherent in diagnostic radiography. Therefore, in breech presentations hydrocephalus may not have been considered until it is found that the head cannot be extracted. The mistake may be avoided by paying particular attention to the following criteria: (1) the face of the hydrocephalic infant is small in relation to the large head; (2) the hydrocephalic cranium tends to be globular, whereas the normal head is ovoid; and (3) the shadow of the hydrocephalic cranium is often very thin or scarcely visible.

The difficulties inherent in radiological diagnosis are obviated by the use of sonography to compare the diameter of the lateral ventricles to the biparietal diameter of the head, and to evaluate the thickness of the cerebral cortex, as well as to compare the size of the head to that of the thorax and abdomen (Clark and associates, 1985). Sonography also can be used to identify the extremely rare cases in which the enlargement of the fetal head is due to a congenital brain tumor (Wakai and co-workers, 1984). The marked difference between the size of the hydrocephalic head and the thorax is apparent in the sonograms in Figures 19–23A and B.

PROGNOSIS

Rupture of the uterus is a danger and may occur before complete dilatation of the cervix. Hydrocephalus predisposes to rupture not only because of the obvious disproportion but also because the great transverse diameter of the cranium overdistends the lower uterine segment. When fetal hydrocephalus is overlooked, the maternal mortality rate is lamentably high.

TREATMENT

Most often, the size of the hydrocephalic head must be reduced if the head is to pass through the birth canal. With a cephalic presentation, as soon as the cervix is dilated 3 cm or so, the huge ventricles may be tapped transvaginally with a needle. An 8-inch-long, 17-gauge needle usually used for intrauterine transfusion has proved quite satisfactory for promptly removing appreciable volumes of cerebrospinal fluid. In the case illustrated in Figures 19–22, 19–24, and 19–25, 2,300 mL of cerebrospinal fluid were removed. With cesarean section, it is also desirable at times to remove cerebrospinal fluid just before incising the uterus in order to circumvent dangerous extensions of a low transverse or vertical incision and to avoid deliberately creating a very long vertical incision to the uterus.

With a breech presentation, labor can be allowed to progress and the breech and trunk are delivered. With the head over the inlet and the face toward the mother's back, the needle is inserted transvaginally just below the anterior vaginal wall and into the aftercoming head through the widened suture line. To protect the birth canal from the needle as it is passed toward the head, the more distal part of the needle, including the point, may be covered with a segment of sterile plastic tubing about 6 inches long cut from an intravenous infusion set.

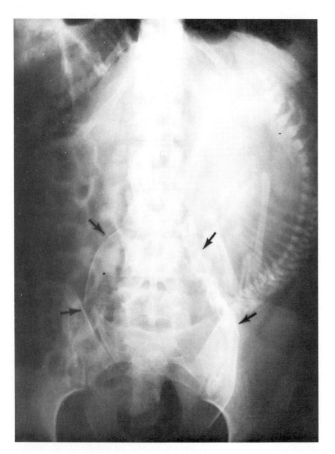

Figure 19–24. Radiograph from same case as in Figure 19–22 after 2,300 mL of cerebrospinal fluid had been removed.

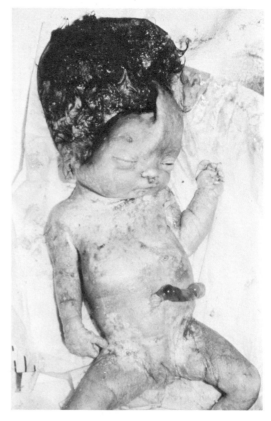

Figure 19–25. Hydrocephalic infant delivered spontaneously after removal of 2,300 mL of cerebrospinal fluid.

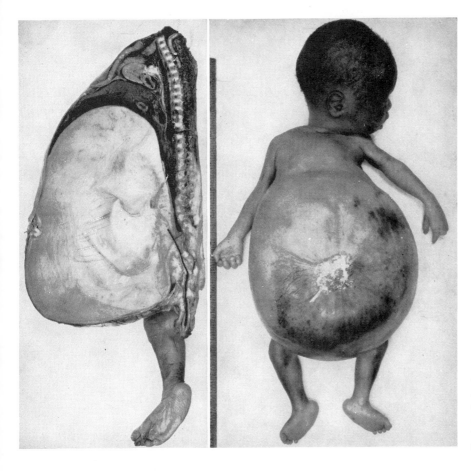

Figure 19–26. Fetus at 28 weeks with immensely distended bladder. Delivery was made possible by expression of fluid from bladder through perforation at umbilicus. Median sagittal section shows interior of bladder and compression of organs of abdominal and thoracic cavities. A black thread has been laid in the urethra. (*From Savage: Am J Obstet Gynecol 29:276, 1935.*)

Alternatively, fluid may be withdrawn through a needle inserted transabdominally into the fetal head. After the bladder is emptied and the skin is cleansed, the needle is inserted in the midline somewhat below the maternal umbilicus and inferior to the top of the fetal skull. The transabdominal approach to remove cerebrospinal fluid also can be used in the event of a cephalic presentation before trying to stimulate labor with oxytocin. The transabdominal approach also has been applied successfully in the breech fetus using ultrasound to guide the needle (Osathanondh, 1980).

The antepartum identification of fetal hydrocephaly has resulted in the successful "shunt" of the ventricles in such an

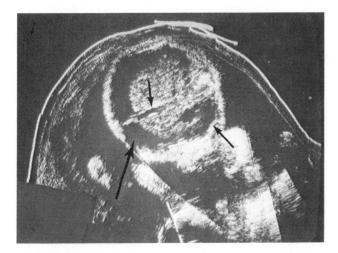

Figure 19–27. Ascites demonstrated sonographically in a transverse scan of the fetal abdomen. The larger lower arrow points to the peritoneal cavity with ascites; the smaller upper arrow overlies the liver and points to the ductus venosus; the smaller arrow to the right is directed toward the stomach. (*Courtesy of Dr. R. Santos.*)

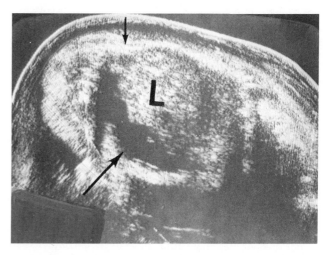

Figure 19–28. A longitudinal scan of the fetal body shown in Figure 19–27. The larger lower arrow is directed toward the peritoneal cavity distended with fluid; the upper smaller arrow points to the spinal column; L = liver. (*Courtesy of Dr. R. Santos.*)

affected fetus. However, not all attempts have been successful, not only because of mechanical problems, but also because many of these fetuses can be expected to have *multiple* abnormalities, many of which are lethal (see Chap. 32, p. 576). *This technique is highly experimental at present and should be attempted only in centers capable of screening likely candidates, performing the procedure, and providing adequate neonatal and surgical support for the baby.*

LARGE FETAL ABDOMEN AS A CAUSE OF DYSTOCIA

Enlargement of the fetal abdomen sufficient to cause grave dystocia is usually the result of a *greatly distended bladder* (Fig. 19–26), *ascites, or enlargement of the kidneys or liver.* Occasionally, the abdomen of a fetus affected with *edema* may attain such proportions that spontaneous delivery is impossible. Enlargement of the fetal abdomen may escape detection until fruitless attempts at delivery have demonstrated an obstruction. An enlarged abdomen and intra-abdominal accumulation of fluid can be diagnosed in utero by careful sonographic examination (Figs. 19–27, 19–28).

TREATMENT

If the abdominal enlargement is not discovered until the fetal head has been delivered, decompression of the fetal abdomen often becomes a necessity. The maternal bladder is emptied and the suprapubic area is cleansed. A large-gauge long needle, as described for hydrocephalus, is inserted through the midline of the maternal abdomen into the fetal abdomen. Fluid in the fetal bladder or peritoneal cavity promptly escapes. The decompression may be aided by use of continuous suction. As the fetal abdomen approaches normal dimensions, the delivery is readily completed. At times, as with severe hydrops fetalis, ascites will be accompanied by such severe edema of the abdominal wall and so great an enlargement of the liver that removal of the peritoneal fluid provides insufficient decompression for easy delivery. Such cases, fortunately, are becoming extremely rare.

If the diagnosis of gross enlargement of the fetal abdomen is made before delivery, the decision must be made whether or not to perform a cesarean section (Clark and associates, 1985). In general, the prognosis is very poor for the fetus with abdominal enlargement so marked as to cause dystocia, irrespective of route of delivery.

CONJOINED TWINS

The embryological bases of incomplete twinning is considered in Chapter 34. For practical purposes, three groups of conjoined twins may be distinguished: (1) incomplete double formations at the upper or lower half of the body (diprosopus dipagus); (2) twins that are united at the upper or lower end of the body (craniopagus, ischiopagus, or pygopagus); and (3) conjoined twins united at the trunk (thoracopagus and dicephalus).

Although twins may be diagnosed antenatally, conjoining is not always identified until difficulty is encountered in attempting delivery. Since such pregnancies seldom go to term, conjoined twins may not exceed greatly the size of a normal fetus. Also, the connection between the halves is sometimes sufficiently flexible to allow vaginal delivery. Harper and co-

workers (1980) reported a 300-year review of the obstetrical, morphopathological, neonatal, and surgical problems associated with xiphopagus conjoined twins.

REFERENCES

Acker DB, Gregory KD, Sachs BP, Friedman EA: Risk factors for Erb-Duchenne palsy. Obstet Gynecol 71:389, 1988

Acker DB, Sachs BP, Friedman EA: Risk factors for shoulder dystocia in the average-weight infant. Obstet Gynecol 67:614, 1986

Acker DB, Sachs BP, Friedman EA: Risk factors for shoulder dystocia. Obstet Gynecol 66:762, 1985

Barnes AC: An obstetric record from The Medical Record. Obstet Gynecol 9:237, 1957

Benedetti TJ, Gabbe SG: Shoulder dystocia. A complication of fetal macrosomia and prolonged second stage of labor with mid-pelvic delivery. Obstet Gynecol 52:526, 1978

Berne C, Wibell L, Lindmark G: Ten-year experience of insulin treatment in gestational diabetes. Acta Paediatr Scand 320:85, 1985

Bingham P, Lilford RJ: Management of the selected term breech presentation: Assessment of the risks of selected vaginal delivery versus cesarean section for all cases. Obstet Gynecol 69:965, 1987

Bistoletti P, Nisell H, Palme C, Lagercrantz H: Term breech delivery: Early and late complications. Acta Obstet Gynecol Scand 60:165, 1981

Bodmer B, Benjamin A, McLean FH, Usher RH: Has use of cesarean section reduced the risks of delivery in the preterm breech presentation? Am J Obstet Gynecol 154:144, 1986

Brenner WE, Bruce RD, Hendricks CH: The characteristics and perils of breech presentation. Am J Obstet Gynecol 118:700, 1974

Brocks V, Philipsen T, Secher NJ: A randomized trial of external cephalic version with tocolysis in late pregnancy. Br J Obstet Gynaecol 91:653, 1984

Calvert JP: Intrinsic hazard of breech presentation. Br Med J 281:1319, 1980

Chapman GP, Weller RO. Normand ICS, Gibbens D: Spinal cord transection in utero. Br Med J 2:398, 1978

Chavis WM: A new instrument for the management of shoulder dystocia. Int J Gynaecol Obstet 16:331, 1979

Clark S, DeVore GR, Platt LD: The role of ultrasound in the aggressive management of obstructed labor secondary to fetal malformations. Am J Obstet Gynecol 152:1042, 1985

Collea JV, Chein C, Quilligan EJ: The randomized management of term frank breech presentation: A study of 208 cases. Am J Obstet Gynecol 137:235, 1980

Cousins L, Dattel B, Hollingsworth D, Hulbert D, Zettner A: Screening for carbohydrate intolerance in pregnancy: A comparison of two tests and reassessment of a common approach. Am J Obstet Gynecol 153:381, 1985

Coustan DR, Imarah J: Prophylactic insulin treatment of gestational diabetes reduces the incidence of macrosomia, operative delivery, and birth trauma. Am J Obstet Gynecol 150:836, 1984

Cox C, Kendall AC, Hommers M: Changed prognosis of breech-presenting low birthweight infants. Br J Obstet Gynaecol 89:881, 1982

Crowley, P, Hawkins DF: Premature breench delivery: The Cesarean section debate. J Obstet Gynaecol 1:2, 1980

Cruikshank DP, White CA: Obstetric malpresentations: Twenty years' experience. Am J Obstet Gynecol 116:1097, 1973

Doyle LW, Rickards AL, Ford GW, Pepperell RJ, Kitchen W: Outcome for the very low birth-weight (500–1,499 g) singleton breech: Benefit of Cesarean section. Aust N Z J Obstet Gynaecol 25:259, 1985

Dyson DC, Ferguson JE II, Hensleigh P: Antepartum external cephalic version under tocolysis. Obstet Gynecol 67:63, 1986

Eden RD, Seifert LS, Winegar A, Spellacy WN: Perinatal characteristics of uncomplicated postdate pregnancies. Obstet Gynecol 69:296, 1987

Effer SB, Saigal S, Rand C, Hunter DJS, Stoskopf B, Harper AC, Nimrod C, Milner R: Effect of delivery method on outcomes in the very low-birth weight breech infant: Is the improved survival related to cesarean section or other perinatal care maneuvers? Am J Obstet Gynecol 145:123, 1983

Elliott JP, Garite TJ, Freeman RK, McQuown DS, Patel JM: Ultrasonic prediction of fetal macrosomia in diabetic patients. Obstet Gynecol 60:159, 1982

Fianu S, Vaclavinkova V: The site of placental attachment as a factor in the aetiology of breech presentation. Acta Obstet Gynecol Scand 57:371, 1978

Flanagan TA, Mulchahey KM, Korenbrot CC, Green JR, Laros RK Jr: Management of term breech presentation. Am J Obstet Gynecol 156:1492, 1987

Fortney JA, Higgins JE, Kennedy KI, Laufe LE, Wilkens L: Delivery type and neonatal mortality among 10,749 breeches. AJPH 76:790, 1986

Gimovsky ML, Paul RH: Singleton breech presentation in labor. Am J Obstet Gynecol 143:733, 1982

Gimovsky ML, Wallace RL, Schifrin BS, Paul RH: Randomized management of the nonfrank breech presentation at term: A preliminary report. Am J Obstet Gynecol 146:34, 1983

Gjøde P, Rasmussen K, Jørgensen J: Fetomaternal bleeding during attempts at external version. Br J Obstet Gynaecol 87:571, 1980

Golditch IM, Kirkman K: The large fetus: Management and outcome. Obstet Gynecol 52:26, 1978

Gonik B, Stringer CA, Held B: An alternate maneuver for management of shoulder dystocia. Am J Obstet Gynecol 145:882, 1983

Goplerud J, Eastman NJ: Compound presentation: Survey of 65 cases. Obstet Gynecol 1:59, 1953

Green JE, McLean F, Smith LP, Usher R: Has an increased cesarean section rate for term breech delivery reduced the incidence of birth asphyxia, trauma, and death? Am J Obstet Gynecol 142:643, 1982

Gross SJ, Shime J, Farine D: Shoulder dystocia: Predictors and outcome: A five-year review. Am J Obstet Gynecol 156:334, 1987a

Gross TL, Sokol RJ, Williams T, Thompson K: Shoulder dystocia: A fetal-physician risk. Am J Obstet Gynecol 156:1408, 1987b

Hall JE, Kohl SG: Breech presentation: A study of 1456 cases. Am J Obstet Gynecol 72:977, 1956

Harper RG, Kenigsberg K, Sia CG, Horn D, Stern D, Bongiovi V: Xiphopagus conjoined twins: A 300-year review of the obstetric, morphopathologic, neonatal, and surgical parameters. Am J Obstet Gynecol 137:617, 1980

Hartfield VJ: Symphysiotomy for shoulder dystocia. Am J Obstet Gynecol 155:228, 1986

Hellman LM, Epperson JWW, Connally F: Face and brow presentation: The experience of the Johns Hopkins Hospital, 1896 to 1948. Am J Obstet Gynecol 59:831, 1950

Hibbard LT: Coping with shoulder dystocia. Contempt Ob/Gyn 20:229, 1982

Houchang D, Dorchester W, Thorosian A, Freeman RK: Macrosomia—maternal, fetal, and neonatal implications. Obstet Gynecol 55:420, 1980

Houchang D, Komatsu G, Dorchester W, Freeman RK, Bosu SK: Large-for-gestational age neonates: Anthropometric reasons for shoulder dystocia. Obstet Gynecol 60:417, 1982

Hytten FE: Breech presentation: Is it a bad omen? Br J Obstet Gynaecol 89:879, 1982

Johnson CE: Transverse presentation of the fetus. JAMA 187:642, 1964

Johnson SR, Kolberg BH, Varner MW: Maternal obesity and pregnancy. Surg Gynecol Obstet 164:431, 1987

Kasule J, Chimbira THK, Brown I McL: Controlled trial of external cephalic version. Br J Obstet Gynaecol 92:14, 1985

Kauppila O, Grönroos M, Avs P. Aittoniemi P. Kuoppala M: Management of low birth weight breech delivery: Should cesarean section be routine? Obstet Gynecol 57:289, 1981

Kitzmiller JL, Mall JC, Gin GD, Hendricks SK, Newman RB, Scheerer L: Measurement of fetal shoulder width with computed tomography in diabetic women. Obstet Gynecol 70:941, 1987

Klebe JG, Espersen T, Allen J: Diabetes mellitus and pregnancy. A seven-year material of pregnant diabetics, where control during pregnancy was based on a centralized ambulant regime. Acta Obstet Gynecol Scand 66:235, 1987

Kopelman JN, Duff P, Karl RT, Schipul AH, Read JA: Computed tomographic pelvimetry in the evaluation of breech presentation. Obstet Gynecol 68:455, 1986

Lazer S, Biale Y, Mazer M, Lewenthal H, Insler V: Complications associated with the macrosomic fetus. J Reprod Med 31:501, 1986

Levine MG, Holroyde J, Woods JR, Siddiqi TA, Scott MacH, Miodovnik M: Birth trauma: Incidence and predisposing factors. Obstet Gynecol 63:792, 1984

Luterkort M, Marsàl K: Umbilical cord acid-base state and Apgar score in term breech neonates. Acta Obstet Gynecol Scand 66:57, 1987

Marcus RG, Crewe-Brown H, Krawitz S, Katz J: Feto-maternal haemorrhage following successful and unsuccessful attempts at external cephalic version. Br J Obstet Gynaecol 82:578, 1975

McCall JO: Shoulder dystocia: A study of after effects. Am J Obstet Gynecol 83:1486, 1962

McFarland LV, Raskin M, Daling JR, Benedetti TJ: Erb/Duchenne's palsy: A consequence of fetal macrosomia and method of delivery. Obstet Gynecol 68:784, 1986

Morales WJ, Koerten J: Obstetric management and intraventricular hemorrhage in very-low-birthweight infants. Obstet Gynecol 68:35, 1986

Morrison JC, Myatt RE, Martin JN Jr, Meeks GR, Martin RW, Bucovaz ET, Wiser WL: External cephalic version of the breech presentation under tocolysis. Am J Obstet Gynecol 154:900, 1986

Nelson KB, Ellenberg JH: Antecedents of cerebral palsy: Multivariate analysis of risk. N Engl J Med 315:81, 1986

O'Leary JA, Gunn D: Cephalic replacement for shoulder dystocia. Am J Obstet Gynecol 153:592, 1985

Osathanondh R, Birnholz JC, Altman AM, Driscoll SG: Ultrasonically guided transabdominal encephalocentesis. J Reprod Med 25:125, 1980

Parks DG, Ziel HK: Macrosomia: A proposed indication for primary cesarean section. Obstet Gynecol 52:407, 1978

Phelan JP, Boucher M, Mueller E, McCart D, Horenstein J, Clark SL: The non-laboring transverse lie: A management dilemma. J Reprod Med 31:184, 1986

Phillips RD, Freeman M: The management of the persistent occiput posterior position: A review of 552 consecutive cases. Obstet Gynecol 43:171, 1974

Pollack NB, O'Leary JA: McRoberts maneuver for shoulder dystocia: A survey. Thesis, University Hospital of Jacksonville, Jacksonville, FL, 1985, p 6

Ranney B: The gentle art of external cephalic version. Am J Obstet Gynecol 116:239, 1973

Resnik R: Management of shoulder girdle dystocia. Clin Obstet Gynecol 23:559, 1980

Rovinsky JJ, Miller JA, Kaplan S: Management of breech presentation at term. Am J Obstet Gynecol 115:497, 1973

Rubin A: Management of shoulder dystocia. JAMA 189:835, 1964

Sack RA: The large infant: A study of maternal, obstetric and newborn characteristics; including a long-term pediatric follow-up. Am J Obstet Gynecol 104:195, 1969

Sandberg EC: The Zavanelli maneuver extended: Progression of a revolutionary concept. Am J Obstet Gynecol 158:1347, 1988

Schramm M: Impacted shoulders—A personal experience. Aust N Z J Obstet Gynaec 23:28, 1983

Schutte MF, van Hemel OJS, van de Berg C, van de Pol A: Perinatal mortality in breech presentations as compared to vertex presentations in singleton pregnancies: An analysis based upon 57,819 computer-registered pregnancies in the Netherlands. Eur J Obstet Gynecol Reprod Biol 19:391, 1985

Spellacy WN, Miller MS, Winegar A, Peterson PQ: Macrosomia—Maternal characteristics and infant complications. Obstet Gynecol 66:158, 1985

Stine LE, Phelan JP, Wallace R, Eglinton GS, Van Dorsten JP, Schifrin BS: Update on external cephalic version performed at term. Obstet Gynecol 65:642, 1985

Susuki S, Yamamuro T: Fetal movement and fetal presentation. Early Hum Dev 11:255, 1985

Svenningsen NW, Westgren M, Ingemarsson I: Modern strategy for the term breech delivery—A study with a 4-year follow-up of the infants. J Perinat Med 13:117, 1985

Swartz DP: Shoulder girdle dystocia in vertex delivery; clinical study and review. Obstet Gynecol 15:194, 1960

Tank ES, Davis R, Holt JF, Morley GW: Mechanism of trauma during breech delivery. Obstet Gynecol 38:761, 1971

Thiery M: Management of breech delivery. Eur J Obstet Gynecol Reprod Biol 24:93, 1987

Wakai S, Arai T, Nagai M: Congenital brain tumors. Surg Neurol 21:597, 1984

Watson WJ, Benson WL: Vaginal delivery for the selected frank breech infant at term. Obstet Gynecol 64:638, 1984

Westgren LMR, Songster G, Paul RH: Preterm breech delivery: Another retrospective study. Obstet Gynecol 66:481, 1985a

Westgren M, Paul RH: Delivery of the low birth weight infant by cesarean section. Clin Obstet Gynecol 28:752, 1985b

Wladimiroff JW, Bloemsma CA, Wallenburg HCS: Ultrasonic diagnosis of the large-for-dates infant. Obstet Gynecol 52:285, 1978

Woods CE: A principle of physics is applicable to shoulder delivery. Am J Obstet Gynecol 45:796, 1943

Ylikorkala O, Hartikainen-Sorri A: Value of external version in fetal malpresentation in combination with use of ultrasound. Acta Obstet Gynecol Scand 56:63, 1977

Dystocia Due to Pelvic Contraction

Any contraction of the pelvic diameters that diminishes the capacity of the pelvis can create dystocia during labor. Pelvic contractions may be classified as follows:

1. Contraction of the pelvic inlet
2. Contraction of the midpelvis
3. Contraction of the pelvic outlet
4. Generally contracted pelvis (combinations of the above)

CONTRACTED PELVIC INLET

DEFINITION

The pelvic inlet is usually considered to be contracted if its shortest *anteroposterior diameter is less than 10.0 cm or if the greatest transverse diameter is less than 12.0 cm.* The anteroposterior diameter of the pelvic inlet is commonly approximated by measuring manually the diagonal conjugate, which is about 1.5 cm greater. Therefore, inlet contraction usually is defined as a *diagonal conjugate of less than 11.5 cm.* (The errors inherent in the use of this measurement are discussed in Chapter 8, p. 169.)

Using clinical and, at times, imaging pelvimetry (Chapter 8, p. 170), it is important to identify the shortest anteroposterior diameter through which the fetal head must pass. Occasionally, the body of the first sacral vertebra is displaced forward so that the shortest distance may actually be between this false, or abnormal, sacral promontory and the symphysis pubis.

The biparietal diameter of the fetal head at term has been identified by sonography before delivery to *average* from 9.5 to as much as 9.8 cm in different clinic populations; therefore, it might prove difficult or even impossible for some fetuses to pass through an inlet with an anteroposterior diameter of less than 10 cm. Mengert (1948) and Kaltreider (1952), employing x-ray pelvimetry, demonstrated that the incidence of difficult deliveries is increased to a similar degree when either the anteroposterior diameter is decreased below 10 cm or the transverse diameter of the inlet is decreased below 12 cm. When both diameters are contracted, the incidence of obstetrical difficulty is much greater than when only one diameter is contracted. The configuration of the pelvic inlet also is an important determinant of the adequacy of any pelvis, independent of actual measurements of the anteroposterior and transverse diameters and of calculated "areas" (see Fig. 8–10, and Caldwell–Moloy Classification, p. 167).

A small woman is likely to have a small pelvis, but at the same time, she is more likely to have a small infant. Thoms (1937), in a study of 362 primigravid women, found the average weight of the offspring to be significantly lower (278 g) in women with small pelves than in those with medium or large pelves. In veterinary obstetrics, it frequently has been observed that in most species maternal size rather than paternal size is the important determinant of fetal size.

SIZE OF FETAL HEAD

Clinical, radiological, and ultrasonic techniques have been used with varying degrees of success to identify the size of the fetal head relative to that of the pelvic inlet.

Clinical Estimation

Impression of the fetal head into the pelvis, as described by Müller (1880), may provide useful information. In an occiput presentation, the obstetrician grasps the brow and the suboccipital region through the abdominal wall with his or her fingers and makes firm pressure downward in the axis of the pelvic inlet. Pressure on the fundus by an assistant at the same time is usually helpful. The effect of the forces on the descent of the head can be evaluated by palpation with a sterile gloved hand in the vagina. If no disproportion exists, the head readily enters the pelvis and vaginal delivery can be predicted. Inability to push the head into the pelvis, however, does not necessarily indicate that vaginal delivery is impossible. A clear demonstration of a flexed fetal head that overrides the symphysis pubis is presumptive evidence of disproportion.

Radiologic Estimation

In general, measurements of the diameters of the fetal head by radiographic techniques have been disappointing.

Sonographic Measurements

Measurement of the fetal biparietal diameter and head circumference by ultrasonic means allows precise measurement. The freely floating fetal head, as in breech presentations, may, unfortunately, move sufficiently during sonographic examination to invalidate the measurement. Additionally, the head of the fetus in the breech presentation may be elongated in the occipitofrontal diameter (dolichocephaly) (Kasby and Poll, 1982).

This dolichocephalic, or co-called breech head (Fig. 20–1), also may be observed in multifetal gestations and in cases of oligohydramnios (Berkowitz and Hobbins, 1982). Such an observation may lead the sonographer to underestimate fetal weight and gestational age. When a dolichocephalic head is observed, a head circumference measurement will result in a more accurate estimation of fetal size.

PRESENTATION AND POSITION OF THE FETUS

A contracted pelvic inlet plays an important part in the production of abnormal presentations. In normal nulliparous women,

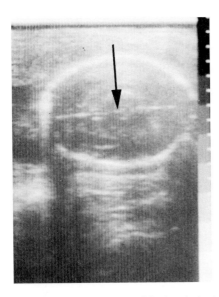

Figure 20–1. Ultrasonic transverse scan of the head of a fetus presenting as breech. The arrow is perpendicular to the linear midline structures of the head. The biparietal diameter is significantly smaller than the occipitofrontal diameter. This dolichocephalic or so-called breech head may also develop from crowding in multifetal gestations and from oligohydramnios. (*Courtesy of Dr. R. Santos.*)

the presenting part commonly descends into the pelvic cavity before the onset of labor at term. When the pelvic inlet is considerably contracted, however, descent usually does not occur until after the onset of labor, if it occurs at all. Vertex presentations still predominate, but since the head floats freely over the pelvic inlet or rests more laterally in one of the iliac fossae, very slight influences may cause the fetus to assume other presentations. **For example, face and shoulder presentations occur three times more frequently in women with contracted pelves, and prolapse of the cord and of the extremities occurs four to six times more frequently.**

COURSE OF LABOR

When the pelvic deformity is sufficiently pronounced to prevent the head from readily entering the inlet, the course of labor is prolonged and, often, effective spontaneous labor is never achieved, resulting in serious maternal and fetal effects.

MATERNAL EFFECTS

While maternal and fetal effects resulting from inlet contraction are arbitrarily divided in the subsequent discussion, it must be remembered that bony dystocia may result in serious consequences to either or both patients.

Abnormalities in Cervical Dilatation

Normally, dilatation of the cervix is facilitated by the hydrostatic action of the unruptured membranes or, after their rupture, by the direct application of the presenting part against the cervix. In contracted pelves, however, when the head is arrested in the pelvic inlet the entire force exerted by the uterus acts directly upon the portion of membranes that overlie the dilating cervix. Consequently, early spontaneous rupture of the membranes is more likely to result.

After rupture of the membranes, the absence of pressure by the fetal head against the cervix and lower uterine segment

predisposes to less effective uterine contractions. Hence, further dilatation of the cervix may proceed very slowly or not at all. Cibils and Hendricks (1965) reported that the mechanical adaptation of the passenger to the bony passage plays an important part in determining the efficiency of uterine contractions. The better the adaptation, the more efficient are the contractions. Since adaptation is poor in the presence of a contracted pelvis, prolongation of labor often results. **With degrees of pelvic contractions incompatible with vaginal delivery, the cervix seldom dilates satisfactorily. Thus, the behavior of the cervix has a prognostic value in regard to the outcome of labor in women with inlet contraction.**

Danger of Uterine Rupture

Abnormal thinning of the lower uterine segment creates a serious danger during a prolonged labor. When the disproportion between the head and the pelvis is so pronounced that engagement and descent do not occur, the lower uterine segment becomes increasingly stretched, and the danger of its rupture becomes imminent. In such cases, a *pathological retraction ring* may develop and can be felt as a transverse or oblique ridge extending across the uterus somewhere between the symphysis and the umbilicus. Whenever this condition is noted, prompt delivery is urgently indicated. Unless cesarean section is employed to terminate labor, there is the great danger of rupture of the uterus, as well as serious compromise of fetal well-being.

Production of Fistulas

When the presenting part is firmly wedged into the pelvic inlet but does not advance for a considerable time, portions of the birth canal lying between it and the pelvic wall may be subjected to excessive pressure. As the circulation is impaired, the resulting necrosis may become manifest several days after delivery by the appearance of vesicovaginal, vesicocervical, or rectovaginal fistulas. Formerly, when operative delivery was deferred as long as possible, such complications were frequent, but today they are rarely seen. Most often, pressure necrosis follows a very prolonged second stage of labor.

Intrapartum Infection

Infection is another serious danger to which the mother and the fetus are exposed in labors complicated by prolonged rupture of the membranes. The danger of infection is increased by repeated vaginal examinations and other intravaginal and intrauterine manipulations. If the amnionic fluid becomes infected, fever may or may not develop during labor.

FETAL EFFECTS

Prolonged labor in itself is deleterious to the fetus. In women with labors of more than 20 hours or in women with a second stage of labor of more than 3 hours, Hellman and Prystowsky (1952) found, in general, a significant increase in perinatal mortality rates. If the pelvis is contracted and there is associated early rupture of membranes and intrauterine infection, the risk to the infant, as well as the mother, is compounded. Intrapartum infection is not only a serious complication for the mother but also an important cause of fetal and neonatal death, as bacteria in amnionic fluid can make their way through the amnion and invade the walls of the chorionic vessels, thus giving rise to fetal bacteremia. Pneumonia, caused by aspiration of infected amnionic fluid by the fetus, is another serious consequence.

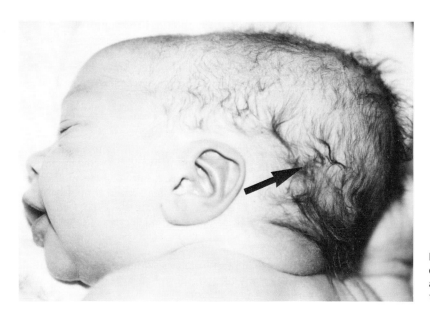

Figure 20–2. Considerable molding of the head and caput formation in a very recently delivered infant. The arrow is directed toward the appreciable scalp edema that overlies the occiput, i.e., caput succedaneum.

Caput Succedaneum Formation

A large *caput succedaneum* frequently develops on the most dependent part of the head during labor if the pelvis is contracted. The caput succedaneum (Fig. 20–2) may assume considerable proportions and lead to serious diagnostic errors. **The caput may reach almost to the pelvic floor while the head is still not engaged, that is, the biparietal diameter has not passed through the pelvic inlet. An inexperienced physician may make premature and unwise attempts at forceps delivery.** Typically, the large caput disappears within a few days after birth.

Molding of the Fetal Head

Under the pressure of strong uterine contractions, the bones of the skull overlap one another at the major sutures, a process referred to as *molding* (Figs. 20–2, 33–12). As a rule, the median margin of the parietal bone that is in contact with the sacral promontory is overlapped by that of its fellow; the same result occurs with the frontal bones. The occipital bone, however, is pushed under the parietal bones. These changes are frequently accomplished without obvious detriment to the child, although when the distortion is marked it may lead to tentorial tears and, when blood vessels are torn, to fatal intracranial hemorrhage (Fig. 33–14). Such *molding* of the fetal head may produce a diminution of 0.5 cm or so in the biparietal diameter without cerebral injury, but when greater degrees of molding occur, the likelihood of intracranial injury increases.

Coincident with the molding of the head, the parietal bone, which was in contact with the promontory, may show signs of having been subjected to marked pressure, sometimes becoming very much flattened. Accommodation more readily occurs when the bones of the head are imperfectly ossified. This important process may provide one explanation for the differences in the course of labor in two apparently similar cases in which the pelvis and the head present identical measurements. In one case, the head is softer and more readily molded, and spontaneous delivery results. In the other, the more ossified head retains its original shape and operative interference is required for its delivery.

Characteristic pressure marks may form upon the scalp, covering the portion of the head that passes over the promontory of the sacrum. From their location, it is frequently possible to ascertain the movements that the head has undergone in passing through the pelvic inlet. Much more rarely, similar marks appear on the portion of the head that has been in contact with the symphysis pubis. Such marks usually disappear a few days after birth, although in exceptional instances severe pressure may lead to necrosis of the scalp.

Fractures of the skull are occasionally encountered, usually following forcible attempts at delivery, though sometimes they may occur with spontaneous delivery. The fractures are of two varieties, either a shallow groove or a spoon-shaped depression just posterior to the coronal suture (Fig. 20–3). The former is relatively common, but since it involves only the external plate of the bone, it is not very dangerous. The latter, however, if not surgically corrected, may lead to death of the neonate, because it extends through the entire thickness of the skull and gives rise upon its inner surface to projections that exert injurious pressure upon the brain and may cause hemorrhage. Accordingly, as soon as feasible after delivery, it is advisable to elevate or remove the depressed portion of the skull.

Prolapse of the Cord

A serious fetal complication is prolapse of the cord, which is facilitated by imperfect adaptation between the presenting part and the pelvic inlet. Unless prompt delivery is accomplished, fetal death may result. Katz and associates (1988) have reported, however, that rapid filling of the urinary bladder with 500 to 700 mL of normal saline to elevate the presenting fetal part and intravenous ritodrine to produce uterine relaxation prior to cesarean seciton resulted in improved neonatal outcome.

PROGNOSIS

The prognosis for successful vaginal delivery of a term-sized fetus in cases of severe inlet contraction with an anteroposterior diameter of less than 9 cm is nearly hopeless. For the borderline group in which the anteroposterior diameter is slightly below 10 cm, the prognosis for vaginal delivery is influenced significantly by a number of variables, including the following:

1. The presentation is of extreme importance. All presentations but the occiput are unfavorable.
2. The size of the fetus is of obvious importance. Despite many advances in sonography, estimates of fetal size at term, especially the head, often are imprecise.
3. Not only the diameters of the pelvic inlet but also its configuration plays an important role. With an android configuration (Fig. 8–10), for any given anteroposterior diameter of the inlet, there is less available space, especially in the forepelvis.
4. The frequency and intensity of spontaneous uterine contractions are informative. Uterine dysfunction, typically infrequent contractions of low intensity, is common with significant disproportion. The uterus does not often self-destruct.
5. The behavior of the cervix in labor has great prognostic significance. In general, orderly spontaneous progression to full dilatation indicates that vaginal delivery most likely will be successful.
6. Extreme asynclitism and appreciable molding of the head without engagement are unfavorable prognostic signs.
7. Knowledge of the outcome of previous labor and delivery at term is helpful as well as previous infant weights.
8. Finally, the prognosis for successful vaginal delivery is altered by coincidental conditions that impaire uteroplacental perfusion, for example, preeclampsia. In such circumstances, uterine contractions sufficient to dilate the cervix and propel the fetus through the birth canal are much more likely to compromise further an already decreased placental perfusion to such a degree that the fetus is distressed.

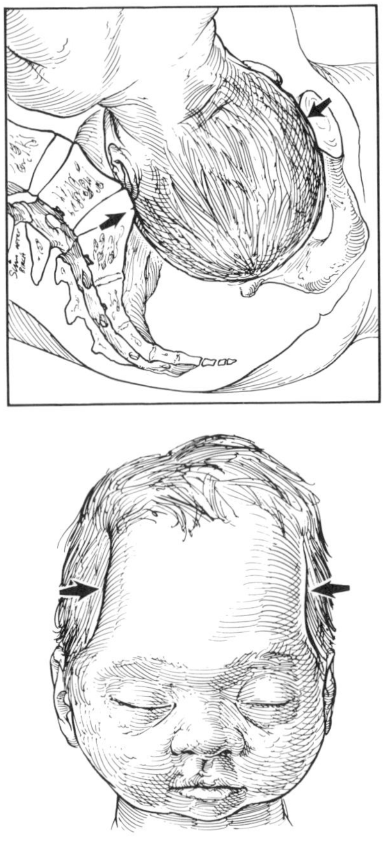

TREATMENT

The management of inlet contraction is determined principally by the prognosis for safe vaginal delivery. If, on the basis of the criteria reviewed, a delivery that is safe for both mother and child cannot be anticipated, cesarean section should be done. Today it is so rare to employ craniotomy that even dead fetuses are often delivered by cesarean section in cases of contraction of the pelvis. Only in a minority of instances can a prognosis be reached before the onset of labor. A carefully managed trial of labor is desirable in most instances. Women with inlet contraction are particularly likely to have both weak uterine contractions during the first stage of labor and a need for vigorous voluntary expulsive efforts during the second stage. Therefore, in general, the use of conduction analgesia should be avoided. The course of labor should be monitored closely and the prognosis established as soon as reasonably possible. Although signs of impending uterine rupture should always be looked for if the contractions are strong, the danger of this accident occurring is remote in primigravid women. With greater parity, however, the likelihood of rupture of the uterus increases. Finally, the administration of oxytocin in the presence of any form of pelvic contraction, unless the fetal head has unequivocally passed the point of obstruction, can be catastrophic for both the fetus and the mother.

CONTRACTED MIDPELVIS

DEFINITION

The obstetrical plane of the midpelvis extends from the inferior margin of the symphysis pubis, through the ischial spines, and touches the sacrum near the junction of the fourth and fifth vertebrae. A transverse line theoretically connecting the ischial spines divides the midpelvis into anterior and posterior portions. The former is bounded anteriorly by the lower border of the symphysis pubis and laterally by the ischiopubic rami. The posterior portion is bounded dorsally by the sacrum and laterally by the sacrospinous ligament, forming the lower limits of the sacrosciatic notch. Average midpelvis measurements are as follows: transverse (interspinous), 10.5 cm; anteroposterior (from the lower border of the symphysis pubis to the junction of the fourth and fifth sacral vertebrae), 11.5 cm; and posterior sagittal (from the midpoint of the interspinous line to the same point on the sacrum), 5 cm. Although the definition of midpelvic contractions has not been established with the same precision possible for inlet contractions, the midpelvis likely is contracted when the sum of the interischial spinous and posterior sagittal diameters of the midpelvis (normally, 10.5 plus 5 cm, or 15.5 cm) falls to 13.5 or below. This concept has been emphasized by Chen and Huary (1982) in evaluating possible midpelvic contraction. There is reason to suspect that midpelvic contraction exists whenever the interischial spinous diameter is less than 10 cm. When it is smaller than 9 cm, the midpelvis is contracted. The preceding definitions of midpelvic contraction do not, of course, imply that dystocia will necessarily occur in

Figure 20–3. Depression of the skull (*arrows*) caused by labor with contracted pelvic inlet.

such a pelvis, but simply that it may develop, depending also upon the size and shape of the forepelvis, and the size of the fetal head, as well as the degree of midpelvic contraction.

IDENTIFICATION

Although there is no precise manual method of measuring midpelvic contraction, a suggestion of midpelvic contraction can sometimes be obtained by ascertaining on vaginal examination that the spines are prominent, that the pelvic side walls converge, or that the sacrosciatic notch is narrow. Eller and Mengert (1947), moreover, pointed out that the relationship between the intertuberous and interspinous diameters of the ischium is sufficiently constant that narrowing of the interspinous diameter can be anticipated when the intertuberous diameter is narrow. A normal intertuberous diameter, however, does not always exclude a narrow interspinous diameter (Chap. 8, p. 170).

PROGNOSIS

Midpelvic contraction probably is more common than inlet contraction and frequently is a cause of transverse arrest of the fetal head and of potentially difficult midforceps operations.

TREATMENT

In the management of labor complicated by midpelvic contraction, the main injunction is to allow the natural forces of labor to push the biparietal diameter beyond the potential interspinous obstruction. Forceps operations may be very difficult when applied to a head, the greatest diameter of which has not yet passed a contracted midpelvis. This difficulty may be explained on two grounds: (1) pulling on the head with forceps destroys flexion, whereas pressure from above increases it and (2) although the forceps blades occupy a space of only a few millimeters, this diminishes further the available space. Only when the head has been allowed to descend to such an extent that the perineum is bulging and the vertex is actually visible is it reasonably certain that the head has passed the obstruction. It is then usually safe to apply forceps. Strong suprafundal pressure should not be used to try to force the head past the obstruction.

The use of forceps to affect delivery in midpelvic contraction, usually undiagnosed, has been responsible for much of the stigma attached to the midforceps operation. Midforceps delivery, therefore, is contraindicated in any case of midpelvic contraction in which the biparietal diameter of the fetal head has not passed beyond the level of contraction. Otherwise, the perinatal mortality and morbidity rates associated with the operation are prohibitive.

The vacuum extractor (see Chapter 25, p. 437) has been reported to be of advantage in some cases of midpelvic contraction *after the cervix has become fully dilated.* Traction need not cause deflection of the fetal head and the vacuum extractor does not occupy space, as do forceps. **As with forceps, the vacuum extractor should not be applied unless the biparietal diameter has passed the pelvic obstruction.** Oxytocin, of course, has no place in the treatment of dystocia caused by midpelvic contraction.

CONTRACTED PELVIC OUTLET

DEFINITION AND INCIDENCE

Contraction of the pelvic outlet is usually defined as diminution of the interischial tuberous diameter to 8 cm or less. The pelvic outlet may be likened roughly to two triangles (Figs. 20–4 through 20–7). The interischial tuberous diameter constitutes the base of both. The sides of the anterior triangle are the pubic rami, and its apex the inferior posterior surface of the symphysis pubis. The posterior triangle has no bony sides but is limited at its apex by the tip of the last sacral vertebra (not the tip of the coccyx). Floberg and associates (1987) reported that outlet contractions were found in 0.9 percent of 1,429 unselected term primigravidas cared for in their hospital in Stockholm.

PROGNOSIS

It is apparent in Figure 20–4 that diminution in the intertuberous diameter with consequent narrowing of the anterior triangle must inevitably force the fetal head posteriorly. Whether delivery can take place, therefore, depends partly on the size of the posterior triangle or, more specifically, the interischial tuberous diameter and the posterior sagittal diameter of the outlet, as demonstrated in Figures 20–4 through 20–7. A contracted outlet may cause dystocia not so much by itself as through the often associated midpelvic contraction. *Outlet contraction without concomitant midplane contraction is rare.*

Even when the disproportion between the size of the fetal head and the pelvic outlet is not sufficiently great to give rise to severe dystocia, it may play an important part in the production of perineal tears. With increasing narrowing of the pubic arch, the occiput cannot emerge directly beneath the symphysis pubis but is forced increasingly farther down upon the ischiopubic rami. In extreme cases, the head must rotate around a line

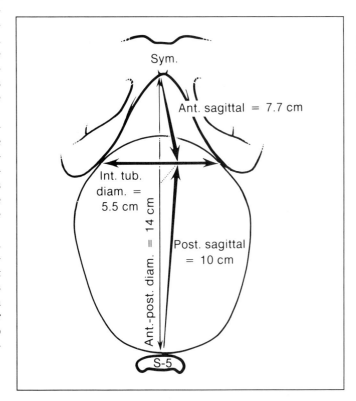

Figure 20–4. Diagram of pelvic outlet of case shown in Figure 20–5. Even though the intertuberous diameter is quite narrow (5.5 cm), vaginal delivery is possible because of the long (10 cm) posterior sagittal diameter. (Int. tub. diam. = intertuberous diameter; Sym. = symphysis pubis; S-5 = fifth sacral vertebra.)

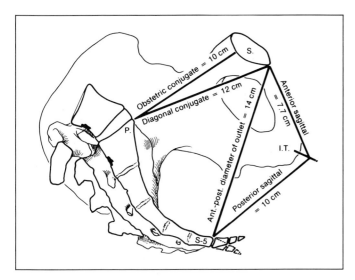

Figure 20–5. Diagram of the lateral view of the same pelvis depicted in Figure 20–4. The long (10 cm) posterior sagittal diameter may allow the fetal head to negotiate the narrow (5.5 cm) intertuberous diameter (IT = ischial tuberosity; S = symphysis pubis; P = sacral promontory).

joining the ischial tuberosities. The perineum, consequently, must become increasingly distended and thus exposed to great danger of disruption. An extensive mediolateral episiotomy is usually indicated.

GENERALLY CONTRACTED PELVIS

PROGNOSIS

Since the contraction involves all portions of the pelvic canal, labor is not rapidly completed after the fetal head has passed the pelvic inlet. The prolongation of labor is caused not only by the resistance offered by the pelvis but also in many instances by the faulty spontaneous uterine contractions that frequently accompany diminution in the size of the pelvis and a fetus of average or larger size.

PELVIC FRACTURES AND PREGNANCY

Speer and Peltier (1972) reviewed their experiences and those of others with pelvic fractures and pregnancy. As expected, trauma from automobile collisions was the most common cause of fracture. With bilateral fractures of the pubic rami, compromise of the capacity of the birth canal by callus formation or malunion was very common. The experiences at Parkland Memorial Hospital are that a history of previous fracture of the pelvis warrants careful review of previous x-rays and possibly computed tomographic pelvimetry later in pregnancy, unless cesarean section is to be performed for another reason (Chap. 8, p. 172).

RARE PELVIC CONTRACTIONS

Due to the relative safety of cesarean section, rare pelvic contractions do not result in the same maternal and fetal consequences as in earlier times. Therefore, the descriptions and

illustrations of these many and varied pelvic contractions have been omitted from this edition (see *Williams Obstetrics*, Editions 10 through 17). It is important to note, however, that potentially lethal problems other than pelvic abnormalities may be encountered in dwarfs, and in women with poliomyelitis, kyphoscoliosis, and those who are small and dysmorphic. These dangers include, but *are not limited* to pulmonary and cardiovascular abnormalities. For this reason, a brief description of the kyphotic pelvis is presented as a prototype of problems associated with many of the rare forms of pelvic contraction.

Kyphotic Pelvis

Kyphosis, or humpback, when involving the lower portion of the vertebral column, is usually associated with a characteristically funnel-shaped distortion. The effect exerted upon the pelvis by kyphosis differs according to its location. When the gibbus, or hump, is situated in the thoracic region, there is usually a compensatory pronounced lordosis beneath it, so that the pelvis itself is little changed. When situated at the junction of the thoracic and lumbar portions of the vertical column, however, its effect upon the pelvis becomes manifest. It is further accentuated when the kyphosis is lower down and is most marked when it is at the lumbrosacral junction. If the vertebral defect is in the lumbosacral region, the upper arm of the gibbus may overlie the inlet.

Diagnosis

The diagnosis is usually obvious, for the external deformity is readily visible and should at once suggest the possibility of a funnel pelvis. On palpation of the pubic arch, transverse narrowing of the pelvic outlet is observed, whereas by internal examination the lengthening of the obstetrical conjugate is found. In lumbosacral

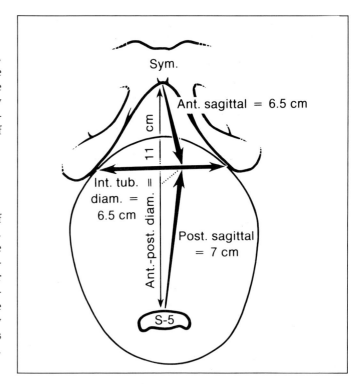

Figure 20–6. Diagram of pelvic outlet in which the intertuberous diameter is narrow (6.5 cm) *and* the posterior sagittal diameter is quite short (7 cm), precluding vaginal delivery of most term-size fetuses (Int. tub. diam. = intertuberous diameter; Sym. = symphysis pubis; S-5 = fifth sacral vertebra).

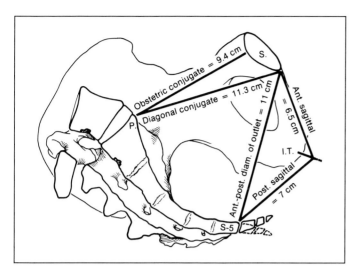

Figure 20–7. Diagram of lateral view of the pelvis from the same case depicted in Figure 20–6. Note the short (7 cm) posterior sagittal diameter (IT = ischial tuberosity; S = symphysis pubis; S-5 = fifth sacral vertebra; P = sacral promontory)

kyphosis, there is no longer a promontory, and the bodies of the lower lumbar vertebrae overhang the superior strait. In this type of deformity, therefore, particular attention should be devoted to the length of the "pseudoconjugate," the distance from the upper margin of the symphysis pubis to the nearest portion of the vertebral column. Occasionally, the condition may be mistaken for spondylolisthesis.

Effect upon Labor

The mechanical conditions favor abnormal positions of the fetus. Generally when the distance between the ischial tuberosities is less than 8 cm, labor becomes difficult or impossible, according to the degree of transverse contraction of the outlet. In such cases, the dystocia is more pronounced than in typical funnel pelves presenting identical measurements, because the anterior displacement of the tip of the sacrum is inevitably associated with shortening of the posterior sagittal diameter.

Effect upon the Heart

In 50 fatal cases of kyphoscoliosis associated with pregnancy that were collected by Jensen (1938), at least 31 were caused by heart failure, far more than resulted from pelvic dystocia. Because of the collapse of the vertebral column, the volume of the thoracic cage in thoracic kyphoscoliosis is diminished, with consequent pressure exerted on the lungs and heart. As a result, the vital capacity is

decreased to one half the normal value, as shown by the studies of Chapman and co-workers (1939). This reduction applies to both the absolute and relative vital capacities. In five patients with thoracic kyphoscoliosis studied by them, the vital capacity was from 35 to 53 percent of the total pulmonary volume, whereas in the normal women studied, the fraction was 57 to 69 percent of the total. The ratio of residual air to vital capacity was 1.3 in kyphoscoliotic patients and 0.6 in the normal subjects. In other words, in these deformed women, the usual mechanism of respiration is altered by the greater limitation of costal movement. The ribs move only ineffectively, and breathing is accomplished largely by movements of the diaphragm. Partial collapse and infection are natural results of these poorly aerated lungs.

Prognosis and Treatment

The kyphoscoliotic patient is severely handicapped in childbearing. If the condition is entirely thoracic, cardiac complications are a threat; if the condition is entirely lumbar, midpelvic contraction is common, and if the condition is lower down, contraction may be extreme. When the gibbus is thoracolumbar, both heart and pelvis may be sources of difficulty.

The prognosis here, as in all other types of contracted pelves, depends not only upon the dimensions of the pelvis but upon the progress of labor. If labor is prolonged with dimensions below the critical levels, delivery is best accomplished by cesarean section.

REFERENCES

Berkowitz RL, Hobbins JC: How head shape affects BPD. Contemp Ob/Gyn 19:35, 1982

Chapman EM, Dill DB, Graybiel A: Decrease in functional capacity of lungs and heart resulting from deformities of the chest: Pulmonocardiac failure. Medicine 18:167, 1939

Chen H-Y, Huang S-C: Evaluation of midpelvic contraction. Int Surg 67:516, 1982

Cibils LA, Hendricks CH: Normal labor in vertex presentation. Am J Obstet Gynecol 91:385, 1965

Eller WC, Mengert WF: Recognition of mid-pelvic contraction. Am J Obstet Gynecol 53:252, 1947

Floberg J, Belfrage P, Ohlsén H: Influence of pelvic outlet capacity on labor: A prospective pelvimetry study of 1429 unselected primiparas. Acta Obstet Gynecol Scand 66:121, 1987

Hellman LM, Prystowsky H: Duration of the second stage of labor. Am J Obstet Gynecol 63:1223, 1952

Jensen J: The Heart in Pregnancy. St Louis, Mosby, 1938, pp 333–341

Kaltreider DF: Criteria of midplane contraction. Am J Obstet Gynecol 63:392, 1952

Kasby CB, Poll V: The breech head and its ultrasound significance. Br J Obstet Gynaecol 89:106, 1982

Katz Z, Shoham (Schwartz) Z, Lancet M, Blickstein I, Mogilner BM, Zalel Y: Management of labor with umbilical cord prolapse: A 5-year study. Obstet Gynecol 72:278, 1988

Mengert WF: Estimation of pelvic capacity. JAMA 138:169, 1948

Müller: On the frequency and etiology of general pelvic contraction. Arch Gynaek 16:155, 1880

Speer DP, Peltier LF: Pelvic fractures and pregnancy. J Trauma 12:474, 1972

Thoms H: The obstetrical significance of pelvic variations: A study of 450 primiparous women. Br Med J 2:210, 1937

Dystocia Due to Soft Tissue Abnormalities of the Reproductive Tract

VULVAR ABNORMALITIES

Complete *atresia of the vulva* or the lower portion of the vagina is usually congenital and, unless corrected by operative measures, precludes conception. More frequently, vulvar atresia is incomplete, resulting from adhesions or scars following injury or infection. The defect may present a considerable obstacle to delivery, but the resistance is usually overcome eventually by the continued pressure exerted by the fetal head, commonly at the cost of deep perineal tears.

Whenever the vulvovaginal outlet is small, rigid, and inelastic, dystocia and extensive lacerations are likely unless prevented by adequate episiotomy. The vulva may become extremely edematous, but dystocia rarely results from edema alone. Thrombi and hematomas about the vulva, although more common during the puerperium, occasionally form late in pregnancy before or during labor and may give rise to difficulty (see Chapter 28, p. 482). Inflammatory lesions or tumors near the vulva may have a similar effect. For example, extensive perineal inflammation and scarring from hidradenitis suppurativa, lymphogranuloma venereum, or Crohn's disease may create difficulty with both vaginal delivery as well as episiotomy or laceration repair. Rarely, *condylomata acuminata* may be so extensive as to make vaginal delivery undesirable (see Chapter 39, p. 858). Such deliveries usually can be accomplished without extensive lacerations or hemorrhage, but predelivery eradication of the lesions is possible using local applications of 85 percent trichloroacetic acid and laser vaporization (Schwartz and associates, 1988). *Bartholin cysts* rarely are large enough to contribute to dystocia.

VAGINAL ABNORMALITIES

Complete *vaginal atresia* is nearly always congenital and, unless corrected operatively, forms an effective bar to pregnancy. Incomplete atresia is either a manifestation of faulty development or results from postnatal accidents.

Occasionally, the vagina is divided by a *longitudinal septum*, which may be complete, extending from the vulva to the cervix, or more often incomplete, limited to either the upper or lower portion of the canal. Since such conditions are frequently associated with other abnormalities in development of the genital tract, their detection should always prompt careful examination

to ascertain whether there is a coexistent uterine and/or renal deformity (see Chapter 37, p. 729). A complete longitudinal septum usually does not cause dystocia, since the half of the vagina through which the fetus descends gradually dilates satisfactorily. An incomplete septum, however, occasionally interferes with descent of the head or breech, over which the septum may become stretched as a band of varying thickness. Such structures are usually torn through spontaneously but occasionally are sufficiently resistant that either they must be divided or cesarean section must be performed.

Occasionally, the vagina may be obstructed by an *annular stricture* or band of congenital origin. These are unlikely to interfere seriously with delivery, however, since they usually soften as pregnancy advances and yield before the oncoming head, requiring incision in only extreme cases.

Sometimes the upper portion of the vagina is separated from the rest of the canal by a *transverse septum* with a small opening. Some of these are associated with in utero exposure to diethylstilbestrol (see Chap. 37, p. 736). Such a stricture is occasionally mistaken for the upper limit of the vaginal vault and, at the time of labor, the opening in the septum is erroneously considered to be an undilated external os. On careful examination, however, the obstetrician can pass a finger through the opening and feel the cervix or on rectal examination can palpate the cervix through the anterior rectal wall above the level of the vaginal septum. After the external os has become completely dilated, the head impinges upon the septum and causes it to bulge downward. If the septum does not yield, slight pressure upon its opening will usually lead to further dilatation, but cruciate incisions may be required occasionally to permit delivery.

Atresia can result from scarring, the consequence of injury or inflammation. Following an infection in which much of the lining of the vagina sloughs, the vaginal lumen during healing may be almost entirely obliterated. Atresia may result from the corrosive action of abortifacients inserted into the vagina. Injuries that lead to extensive scarring, for example, the trauma that may ensue during rape of a child by an adult male, may also cause vaginal atresia.

The effects of atresia vary greatly. In most cases, because of the softening of the tissues incident to pregnancy, the obstruction is gradually overcome by the pressure exerted by the presenting part; less often, manual or hydrostatic dilatation or incisions may become necessary. If, however, the structure is so resistant that spontaneous dilatation appears improbable, cesarean section should be performed at the onset of labor.

A *Gartner duct cyst* may protrude into the vagina and even through the introitus and possibly be confused with a cystocele. A *cystocele* may be managed successfully by emptying the bladder, using a catheter and upward manual pressure on the prolapsed anterior vaginal wall. A Gartner duct cyst may or may not slip above the presenting part. If not, the cyst may be aspirated aseptically.

Among the rare causes of serious dystocia are *neoplasms*, such as *fibroma, carcinoma,* or *sarcoma,* arising from the vaginal walls or adjacent structures.

Tetanic contraction of the levator ani, rarely, may seriously interfere with descent of the head. In that condition, analogous to vaginismus in nonpregnant women, a thick, ringlike structure completely encircles and markedly constricts the vagina about midway between the cervix and the vulva. Ordinarily, the obstruction yields when regional analgesia is administered by epidural or subarachnoid block.

CERVICAL ABNORMALITIES

ATRESIA AND STENOSIS

Complete atresia of the cervix is incompatible with conception. In pregnancy, therefore, complete *cervical atresia* could only occur after conception.

Cicatrical *stenosis of the cervix* may follow extensive cauterization or difficult labor associated with infection and considerable destruction of tissue. For example, of the ten cases of severe cervical dystocia following treatment of the cervix reported by Gibbs and Moore (1968), previous conization was responsible in six. Cryotherapy and laser therapy are less likely to produce stenosis. Rarely, cervical stenosis is caused by extensive infiltration by carcinoma or syphilitic ulceration and induration. Occasionally, it has resulted from corrosives, such as potassium permanganate tablets, used in an attempt to produce abortion. Amputation of the cervix, with suturing to effect hemostasis and promote reepithelialization, may lead to stenosis, although cervical incompetence is much more likely.

Ordinarily, because of the softening of the tissues during pregnancy, the stenosis gradually yields during labor. In rare instances, however, the stenosis may be so pronounced that dilatation appears improbable, and cesarean section should be employed to effect delivery.

In cases of *conglutination* of the cervical os, the cervical canal at the time of labor undergoes complete obliteration through effacement while the cervical os remains extremely small. Thus the presenting part is separated from the vagina by only a thin layer of cervical tissue. Ordinarily, complete dilatation promptly follows pressure with the fingertip, although in rare instances manual dilatation or cruciate incisions may be required.

CARCINOMA OF THE CERVIX

Dystocia may be a consequence of extensive infiltration of the cervix by carcinoma since dilatation is likely to be inadequate even when uterine contractions remain forceful. With less involvement, the cervix will usually dilate. The effects of carcinoma of the cervix upon pregnancy and vice versa, as well as appropriate treatment, are discussed in Chapter 37, p. 728.

UTERINE DISPLACEMENTS

ANTEFLEXION

Marked anteflexion of the enlarging pregnant uterus is usually associated with diastasis recti and a pendulous abdomen (see Chapter 37, p. 737). When the abnormal position of the uterus prevents the proper transmission of the force of uterine contractions to the cervix, cervical dilatation, as well as engagement of the presenting part, is impeded. Marked improvement may follow maintenance of the uterus in an approximately normal position by means of a properly fitting abdominal binder.

RETROFLEXION

As stated in Chapter 37 (p. 737), persistent retroflexion of the pregnant uterus usually is incompatible with advanced pregnancy. If spontaneous or artificial reposition does not occur, the woman either aborts or develops symptoms caused by incarceration of the uterus before the end of the fourth month. In very exceptional instances, however, pregnancy may proceed, in which event the adherent fundus remains applied to the floor of the pelvis, with the anterior wall stretching to accommodate the products of conception. In this condition, known as *sacculation*, the head of the fetus may occupy the displaced fundus, with the cervix drawn up so high that the external os lies above the upper margin of the symphysis pubis (Jackson and associates, 1988). Consequently, during labor the contractions tend to force the infant through the most dependent portion of the uterus, with the cervix dilating only partially. Spontaneous delivery is impossible and rupture of the uterus may occur. For these reasons, cesarean section affords the best method of delivery and at the same time facilitates repositioning of the uterus.

Previous Operative Correction
Fortunately, operative correction of the retroverted uterus has fallen into disrepute. The one indication may be to bring the

TABLE 21–1. ULTRASONICALLY MEASURED CHANGES IN MYOMAS DURING PREGNANCY

	Small Myomas[a] (N = 111)			Large Myomas[b] (N = 51)		
Trimester	**No Change** No. (%)	**Increase** No. (%)	**Decrease** No. (%)	**No Change** No. (%)	**Increase** No. (%)	**Decrease** No. (%)
First	7 (58)	5 (42)	0	1 (20)	4 (80)	0
Second	42 (55)	23 (30)	11 (15)	11 (38)	4 (14)	14 (48)
Third	14 (61)	1 (4)	8 (35)	5 (29)	2 (12)	10 (59)

[a] Small myomas 2.0–5.9 cm.
[b] Large myomas 6.0–11.9 cm.
Modified from Lev-Toaff and co-workers: Radiology 164:375, 1987.

TABLE 21–2. COMPLICATIONS RELATED TO MYOMAS AND THEIR LOCATION

	Method of Delivery[a]			Pregnancy Complication		
		Cesarean Section				
Source	Vaginal	Elective	Indicated	Abortion	Fetal Growth Retardation	Preterm Labor
Winer-Muram and associates (1984)	68/79 (86)	—	11/79 (14)	10/89 (11)	3/79 (4)	5/79 (6)
Uterine corpus	47/68 (66)	10/68 (15)	11/68 (16)	6/68 (9)	Not stated	
Lev-Toaff and co-workers (1987)						
Lower uterine segment	21/45 (47)	9/45 (20)	15/45 (33)	None	Not stated	

[a] Percentages are in parentheses.

retroflexed uterus into the anterior position as part of an operation for extensive pelvic endometriosis. Uterine suspension accomplished by shortening the round ligaments does not adversely affect subsequent labor. If, as part of the operation, the bladder is advanced on the anterior wall of the uterus, urinary frequency, as well as bladder discomfort, may be troublesome during pregnancy. When this situation exists, cesarean section must be carried out very carefully because of the abnormally distorted anatomy.

Pregnancy is contraindicated following the Watkins interposition operation, an operation once performed by some to try to correct a cystocele. Pregnancy after fixation of the fundus of the uterus to the anterior abdominal wall to try to correct either uterine prolapse or uterine retroversion may be complicated by considerable discomfort as the pregnant uterus enlarges. Hopefully, both the Watkins interposition operation and fixation of the uterus to the abdominal wall have been eliminated from contemporary gynecological surgery.

UTERINE MYOMAS

A myoma may be located immediately beneath the endometrial or decidual surface of the uterine cavity (*submucous myoma*), immediately beneath the uterine serosa (*subserous myoma*), or be confined to the myometrium (*intramural myoma*). An intramural myoma, as it grows, may develop a significant subserous or submucous component, or both. Submucous and subserous myomas may, at times, be attached to the uterus by only a stalk (*pedunculated myoma*).

As in the nonpregnant state, pedunculated subserous myomas may undergo torsion with necrosis to the extent that the myoma is detached from the uterus. At times, a subserous myoma may become parasitic, and much or all of its blood is supplied through a highly vascularized omentum.

Myomas during pregnancy or the puerperium occasionally undergo "red," or "carneous," degeneration that, in actuality, is *hemorrhagic infarction*. The symptoms and signs of red degeneration are focal pain, with tenderness on palpation and sometimes low-grade fever. Moderate leukocytosis is common. On occasion, the parietal peritoneum overlying the infarcted myoma becomes inflamed and a peritoneal "rub" develops. Red degeneration is difficult to differentiate at times from appendicitis, placental abruption, ureteral stone, or pyelonephritis, but the sonographic findings to be discussed below likely will prove to be helpful in establishing the correct diagnosis. Treatment consists of analgesia such as codeine. Most often, the signs and symptoms abate within a few days.

Myomas may become infected during the course of puerperal metritis or septic abortion, and are especially likely to do so if the myoma is located immediately adjacent to the placental implantation site or if an instrument such as a sound or curette perforates the myoma. If the myoma is infarcted, the risk of infection is increased and the likelihood of cure of the infection, except by hysterectomy, is reduced.

EFFECTS OF PREGNANCY ON MYOMAS

Until recently, it was widely believed that myomas almost always increased in size during pregnancy, likely as a consequence of estrogen stimulation. In fact, based upon ultrasonic monitoring of the size and position of myomas, Lev-Toaff and co-workers (1987) observed that only about one half changed significantly in size during pregnancy. Specifically, during the first trimester, myomas of all sizes either remained unchanged or increased in size. During the second trimester, smaller myomas (2 to 6 cm) usually remained unchanged or *increased* in size, whereas larger myomas become smaller. Regardless of *initial* myoma size, during the third trimester, myomas usually remained unchanged or decreased in size (Table 21–1). The importance of these observations is that an accurate prediction of myoma growth in pregnancy cannot be made.

EFFECTS OF MYOMA LOCATION AND NUMBER ON PREGNANCY

The likelihood of cesarean section is increased especially if a myoma is located in the lower uterine segment (Table 21–2; Figs. 21–1 and 21–2). Also, the risk of malposition and preterm labor is increased when there are multiple myomas, and the risk of retained placenta is increased when there is a lower uterine segment tumor (Lev-Toaff and co-workers, 1987).

TABLE 21–3. PREGNANCY COMPLICATIONS AND RELATIONSHIP OF MYOMA TO PLACENTA

Complications	No Contact[a]	Contact
Minor complications		
Bleeding or pain	5/54 (9)	8/35 (23)
Major complications		
Abortion	1/54 (2)	9/35 (26)
Preterm labor	0	5/35 (14)
Postpartum hemorrhage	0	4/35 (11)
Total complications	6/54 (11)	26/35 (74)

[a] Percentages are in parentheses.
Modified from Winer-Muram and associates: Can Assoc Radiol 35:168, 1984.

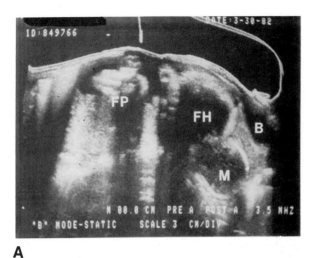 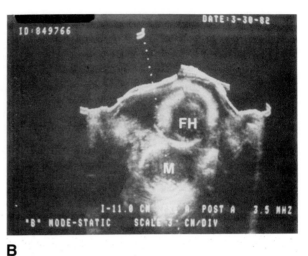

A   **B**

Figure 21–1. A. Longitudinal sonographic view of fetus and large myoma filling the pelvis. Note similarity of appearance of the fetal head (FH) to the myoma (M). The maternal bladder (B) and fetal parts (FP) are easily seen. **B.** The same case as shown in Figure 21–1A. Transverse sonographic view of the pelvis. (*Sonograms courtesy of Dr. R. Santos.*)

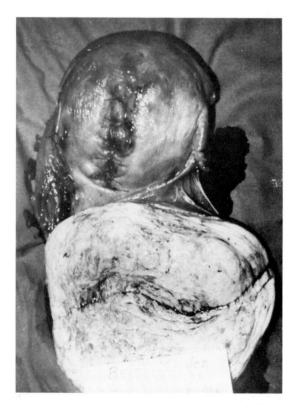

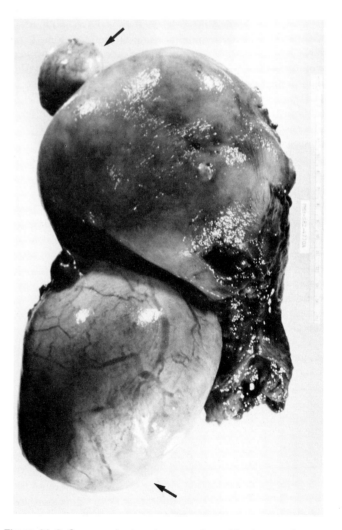

Figure 21–2. Same case as shown in Figures 21–1A and 21–1B. Cesarean hysterectomy specimen. The upper mass is the body of the uterus that was just emptied by cesarean section. The lower mass is a huge myoma arising low in the uterus and now incised. The infant weighed 3,250 g and the uterus with myoma weighed 2,900 g. Red degeneration was not found. Delivery 2 years before had also been by cesarean section.

Figure 21–3. Cesarean hysterectomy specimen. The large pedunculated myoma (*lower arrow*) filled the birth canal almost completely and prevented vaginal delivery of near-term large twins. A small myoma (*upper arrow*) protrudes from the fundus. A vertical incision was made in the lower uterine segment for the delivery.

Interestingly, the incidence of abortion, fetal growth retardation, and preterm labor do not appear to be increased appreciably unless the placenta is implanted over or adjacent to a myoma (Table 21–2, 21–3). In cases of placental contact with uterine myomas, however, the incidence of uterine bleeding, abortion, preterm labor, and postpartum hemorrhage are increased, compared to cases in which the placenta is not in contact with a myoma.

Lev-Toaff and associates (1987) described six echotextures of myomas in pregnancy and presented examples. She and her colleagues reported that these patterns could change as pregnancy advanced, but the development of a heterogeneous pattern or anechoic/cystic spaces on follow-up studies was associated in 7 of 10 patients with severe abdominal pain compared to 12 instances of abdominal pain in 103 women without these changes. Thus, these ultrasonic changes appear to confirm the presence of infarction or degeneration of myomas.

The conclusions derived from these reports appear clearly defined: (1) the growth of myomas cannot be predicted; (2) the implantation of the placenta over or in contact with a myoma increases the likelihood of abortion, preterm labor, and postpartum hemorrhage; (3) multiple myomas are associated with an increased incidence of fetal malposition and preterm labor; (4) degeneration of myomas apparently is associated with a characteristic sonographic pattern; and (5) the incidence of cesarean section is increased. It seems reasonable to perform serial ultrasonic examinations during pregnancy in women with uterine myomas.

Cervical Myoma

Myomas in the cervix or in the lower uterine segment may obstruct labor and may be confused with the fetal head. Sonograms from such a case and a picture of the uterus are shown in Figures 21–1A, B and 21–2. Myomas that lie within or contiguous to the birth canal earlier in pregnancy may be carried upward as the uterus enlarges, with relief of obstruction to vaginal delivery. Even though relief was not provided in the cases demonstrated in Figures 21–1 through 21–3, a decision regarding the method of delivery usually should not be made before the onset of labor.

Myomectomy

This procedure should be limited to those tumors with discrete pedicles that can be easily clamped and ligated. Otherwise, myomas should not be dissected from the uterus, during pregnancy or delivery, for bleeding may be profuse and at times the uterus may have to be sacrificed. Typically, the myomas will undergo remarkable involution after delivery. In myomas resected during pregnancy or the puerperium there are often bizarre changes in the nuclei of the smooth muscle cells, changes that may be confused with sarcoma.

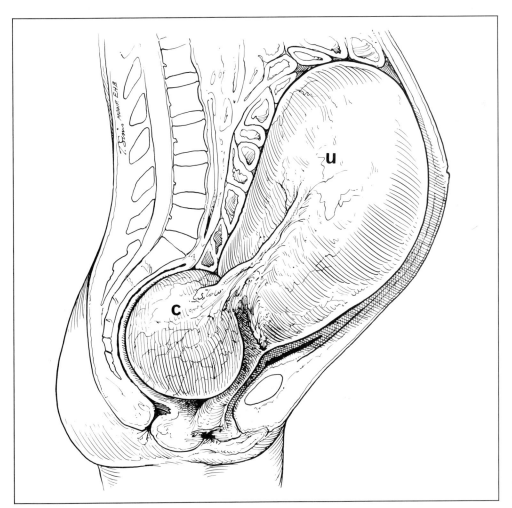

Figure 21–4. Ovarian cyst filling most of true pelvis and causing dystocia. C = ovarian cyst; U = pregnant uterus.

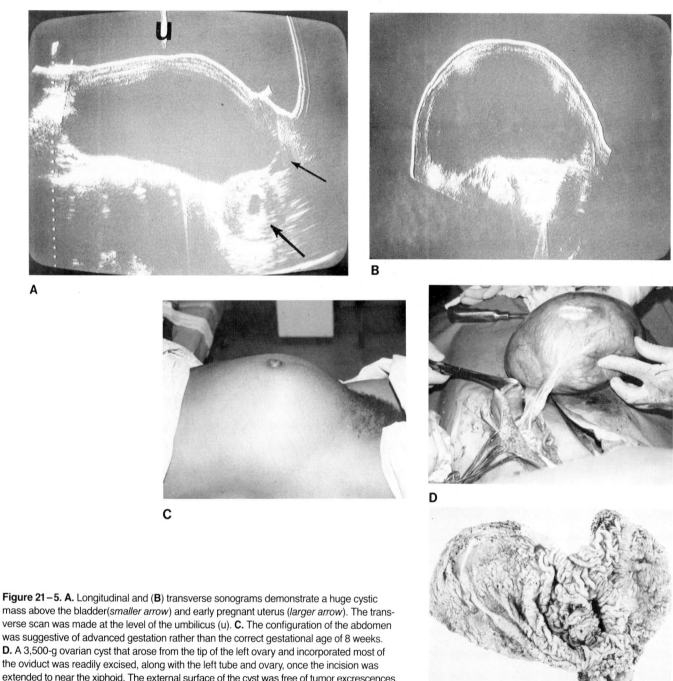

Figure 21–5. A. Longitudinal and (**B**) transverse sonograms demonstrate a huge cystic mass above the bladder(*smaller arrow*) and early pregnant uterus (*larger arrow*). The transverse scan was made at the level of the umbilicus (u). **C.** The configuration of the abdomen was suggestive of advanced gestation rather than the correct gestational age of 8 weeks. **D.** A 3,500-g ovarian cyst that arose from the tip of the left ovary and incorporated most of the oviduct was readily excised, along with the left tube and ovary, once the incision was extended to near the xiphoid. The external surface of the cyst was free of tumor excrescences. **E.** The cyst was unilocular as evident in the sonograms. (*Courtesy of Dr. R. Santos.*)

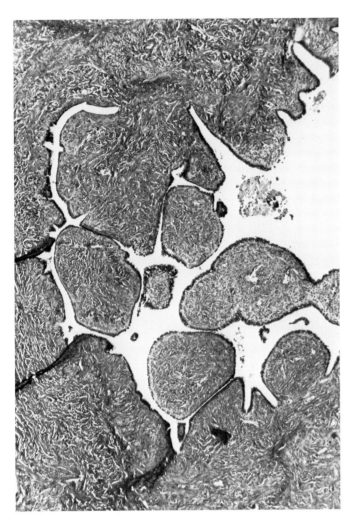

Figure 21–5. F. The histologic diagnosis was serous cystadenofibroma.

When myomectomy results in a defect through or immediately adjacent to the endometrium, subsequent pregnancies should be delivered by cesarean section, preferably before active labor has begun.

OVARIAN TUMORS

BENIGN OVARIAN TUMORS

Ovarian tumors may be serious complications of pregnancy, may undergo torsion, and may pose insuperable obstacles to vaginal delivery. Moreover, even after spontaneous labor and delivery, they may give rise to disturbances during the puerperium.

Although all varieties of ovarian tumors may complicate pregnancy and labor, the most common are cystic (Fig. 21–4). Beischer and associates (1971) noted that of 164 ovarian tumors diagnosed during pregnancy, one fourth were cystic teratomas, and one fourth were mucinous cystadenomas. Four of the 164 (2.4 percent) were malignant. Hopkins and Duchon (1986) reported an incidence of adnexal masses of 1 in 556 pregnancies. Benign cystic teratomas and corpus luteum cysts each accounted for about a third of these. Interestingly, two women had corpus luteum cysts persisting into the third trimester and one very large mass ruptured postpartum. The most frequent and next

most serious complication of ovarian cysts during pregnancy is torsion. The incidence of the accident was 12 percent in Booth's series (1963). Torsion is most common in the first trimester. The cyst may rupture and extrude its contents into the peritoneal cavity as the consequence of torsion, or during spontaneous labor, or during surgical removal. This event is not likely to be as devastating with serous cystomas as with dermoid cysts. Rupture of the latter may be followed by serious, even fatal, granulomatous peritonitis. When the tumor blocks the pelvis, it may lead to rupture of the uterus or the tumor may be forced into the vagina, the rectum, or the intervening rectovaginal septum.

An ovarian tumor complicating pregnancy is often entirely unsuspected. Careful examination of all pregnant women would eliminate a large proportion, but not all, of these errors. If an ovarian tumor does not occupy the pelvis, diagnosis through physical examination is especially difficult, since the abdominal enlargement may be attributed to a pregnancy more advanced than indicated by menstrual data, to multiple fetuses, or to hydramnios, and the true condition may not be recognized until after labor. Usually sonography can provide accurate differentiation between uterine enlargement and an extrauterine cystic mass. A dramatic instance is presented in Figure 21–5.

Early in pregnancy an ovary may be somewhat enlarged, creating suspicion of neoplasm. Ovaries less than 6 cm in diameter are usually increased in size as the consequence of corpus luteum formation. In fact, Thornton and Wells (1987) reported that with the advent of high-resolution sonography a conservative approach to management of ovarian cysts might be adopted based upon their sonographic characteristics. They recommend resection of all cysts suspected of rupture, torsion, or obstruction of labor, and those over 10 cm in diameter because of the increased risk of cancer in these large cysts. Cysts 5 cm or less could be left alone. Cysts between 5 and 10 cm in diameter also could be managed expectantly if they had a simple cystic ultrasonic appearance. If, however, the 5- to 10-cm cysts contained septae or nodules, or if there were solid components, then the cysts should be resected. In contrast, Hess and colleagues (1988) recommend elective resection of any ovarian mass that is 6 cm or larger in diameter which persists after 16 weeks gestation. They reported a markedly better fetal-neonatal outcome in such patients compared to those in which an emergency procedure was required for resection of a ruptured, twisted, or infarcted cyst.

In view of the increased incidence of abortion during early pregnancy, the safest time to perform laparotomy is during the fourth month of gestation (Hess and associates, 1988; Struyk and Treffers, 1984), provided the operation can be postponed until that time. When the diagnosis is not made until late in pregnancy, it is usually advisable, except in the case of known or suspected malignant tumors, to delay laparotomy until fetal viability has been achieved. If the ovarian cyst is not impacted, it is preferable usually to permit spontaneous labor and remove the tumor later in the puerperium. If the tumor is impacted in the pelvis, cesarean section should be performed, followed by resection of the tumor.

CARCINOMA OF THE OVARY

Malignant ovarian neoplasms are rare in pregnancy. Only 41 cases were found in a literature survey by Valenti (1960), who, along with Amico (1957), believed that the natural course of the disease is influenced by pregnancy. This incidence may increase, however, with the recognition of borderline malignant

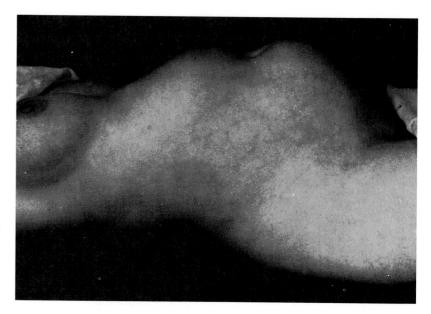

Figure 21–6. Dystocia caused by distension of the bladder. This woman was sent to the hospital after 3 days of ineffectual labor at home. The cervix was thought to have been completely dilated for 24 hours. After catheterization of the greatly distended bladder, which yielded over 1,000 mL of urine, the baby's head descended at once and delivery was accomplished easily.

tumors (Thornton and Wells, 1987). The acknowledgment of this category of ovarian malignancy now appears to be well established, and the risk of bilateral ovarian disease is 30 percent for serous borderline tumors (Julian and Woodruff, 1982) and 3 percent for mucinous borderline tumors (Hart and Norris, 1973).

If cancer is discovered at the time of laparotomy, the treatment should be the same as in the nonpregnant patient. In some circumstances, it is justifiable to remove the tumor and allow the pregnancy to continue when a few more weeks would assure viability of the delivered infant. Even then, delivery should usually be by cesarean section, with decision regarding further surgery and chemotherapy based on the results of clinical and histological examination.

PELVIC MASSES OF OTHER ORIGINS

Labor may be obstructed by pelvic masses of various origins sufficiently large to render delivery difficult or even impossible. A *distended bladder*, with or without a cystocele, may obstruct delivery, as demonstrated in Figure 21–6. However, a less severely distended bladder apparently often does not delay the normal progress of labor (Kerr-Wilson and co-workers, 1983; Read and colleagues, 1980). A large *cystocele* or *rectocele*, though occasionally offering slight resistance to labor, can generally be replaced during delivery. Tumors of the bladder may impede passage of the fetus, though rarely seriously enough to require operative delivery. *Pelvic ectopic kidney* is a rare complication of pregnancy. However, a *transplanted kidney* is usually placed in the pelvis. Although vaginal delivery is usually possible, such a kidney may block the birth canal and sustain injury during passage of the fetus. Most women with an ectopic kidney will deliver vaginally without hazard, but if the kidney is entirely intrapelvic, as is often the case with transplanted kidneys, abdominal delivery is safer.

In rare instances, an enlarged spleen may prolapse into the pelvic cavity and obstruct labor. Echinococcal cysts have been found in the pelvis. An old extrauterine gestation may obstruct the pelvic canal, interfering with the delivery of a subsequent intrauterine fetus. An *enterocele* rarely gives rise to dystocia. The herniated intestine can usually be replaced and the obstacle temporarily overcome, but when reduction is impossible, cesarean section is safer than forcing the fetus over a large irreducible hernia. Tumors or inflammation arising from the lower part of the rectum or pelvic connective tissue also may give rise to dystocia.

REFERENCES

Amico JC: Pregnancy complicated by primary carcinoma in the ovary. Am J Obstet Gynecol 74:920, 1957

Beischer NA, Buttery BW, Fortune DW, Macafee CAJ: Growth and malignancy of ovarian tumors in pregnancy. Aust N Z J Obstet Gynecol 11:208, 1971

Booth RT: Ovarian tumors in pregnancy. Obstet Gynecol 21:189, 1963

Gibbs CE, Moore, SF: The scarred cervix in pregnancy and labor. Gen Pract 37:85, 1968

Hart WR, Norris HJ: Borderline and malignant mucinous tumors of the ovary: Histologic criteria and clinical behavior. Cancer 31:1031, 1973

Hess LW, Peaceman A, O'Brien WF, Winkel CA, Cruikshank DW, Morrison JC: Adnexal mass occurring with intrauterine pregnancy: Report of fifty-four patients requiring laparotomy for definitve management. Am J Obstet Gynecol 158:1029, 1988

Hopkins MP, Duchon MA: Adnexal surgery in pregnancy. J Reprod Med 31:1035, 1986

Jackson D, Elliott JP, Pearson M: Asymptomatic uterine retroversion at 36 weeks' gestation. Obstet Gynecol 71:466, 1988

Julian CG, Woodruff JD: The biological behavior of low-grade papillary serous carcinoma of the ovary. Obstet Gynecol 40:860, 1972

Kerr-Wilson RHJ, Parham GP, Orr JW Jr: The effect of a full bladder on labor. Obstet Gynecol 62:319, 1983

Lev-Toaff AS, Coleman BG, Arger PH, Mintz MC, Arenson RL, Toaff ME: Leiomyomas in pregnancy: Sonography study. Radiology 164:375, 1987

Read JA, Miller FC, Yeh S-Y, Platt LD: Urinary bladder distension: Effect on labor and uterine activity. Obstet Gynecol 56:565, 1980

Schwartz DB, Greenberg MD, Daoud Y, Reid R: Genital condylomas in pregnancy: Use of trichloroacetic acid and laser therapy. Am J Obstet Gynecol 158:1407, 1988

Struyk AP, Treffers PE: Ovarian tumors in pregnancy. Acta Obstet Gynecol Scand 63:421:1984

Thornton JG, Wells M: Ovarian cysts in pregnancy: Does ultrasound make traditional management inappropriate? Obstet Gynecol 69:717, 1987

Valenti C: On carcinoma of the ovary in pregnancy. Minerva Ginecol 9:4, 1960

Winer-Muram HT, Muram D, Gillieson MS: Uterine myomas in pregnancy. J Assoc Can Radiol 35:168, 1984

Techniques for Breech Delivery

The indications for vaginal versus cesarean delivery for breech presentations have been considered in Chapter 19 (p. 355). Labor and techniques for vaginal delivery of the breech presentation are considered below.

MECHANISM OF LABOR

Unless there is disproportion between the size of the fetus and the pelvis, engagement and descent of the breech in response to labor usually takes place with the bitrochanteric diameter of the breech in one of the oblique diameters of the pelvis. The anterior hip usually descends more rapidly than the posterior hip, and when the resistance of the pelvic floor is met, internal rotation usually follows, bringing the anterior hip toward the pubic arch and allowing the fetal bitrochanteric diameter to occupy the anteroposterior diameter of the pelvic outlet. Rotation usually takes place through an arc of 45 degrees. If, however, the posterior extremity is prolapsed, it always rotates to the symphysis pubis, ordinarily through an arc of 135 degrees, but occasionally in the opposite direction past the sacrum and the opposite half of the pelvis through an arc of 225 degrees.

After rotation, descent continues until the perineum is distended by the advancing breech, while the anterior hip appears at the vulva and is stemmed against the pubic arch. By lateral flexion of the body, the posterior hip is then forced over the anterior margin of the perineum, which retracts over the buttocks, thus allowing the infant to straighten out when the anterior hip is born. The legs and feet follow the breech and may be born spontaneously, although the aid of the obstetrician is usually required.

After the birth of the breech, there is slight external rotation, with the back turning anteriorly as the shoulders are brought into relation with one of the oblique diameters of the pelvis. The shoulders then descend rapidly and undergo internal rotation, with the bisacromial diameter occupying the anteroposterior diameter of the inferior strait. Immediately following the shoulders, the head, which is normally sharply flexed upon the thorax, enters the pelvis in one of the oblique diameters and then rotates in such a manner as to bring the posterior portion of the neck under the symphysis pubis. The head is then born in flexion, with the chin, mouth, nose, forehead, bregma (brow), and occiput appearing in succession over the perineum. Usually the breech engages in the transverse diameter of the pelvis, with the sacrum directed anteriorly or posteriorly. The mechanism of labor in the transverse position differs only in that internal rotation occurs through an arc of 90 degrees.

Infrequently, rotation occurs in such a manner that the back of the infant is directed toward the vertebral column instead of toward the abdomen of the mother. Such rotation should be prevented if possible. Although the head may be delivered by allowing the chin and face to pass beneath the symphysis, the slightest traction on the body may cause extension of the head. Extension, if uncorrected, increases the diameters of the head, which must pass through the pelvis.

VAGINAL DELIVERY OF BREECH

There are three general methods of breech delivery through the vagina:

- **Spontaneous breech delivery:** The infant is expelled entirely spontaneously without any traction or manipulation other than support of the infant. This form of delivery of mature infants is rare.
- **Partial breech extraction:** The infant is delivered spontaneously as far as the umbilicus, but the remainder of the body is extracted.
- **Total breech extraction:** The entire body of the infant is extracted by the obstetrician.

Since the technique of breech extraction differs in complete and incomplete breeches on the one hand, and frank breeches on the other, it is necessary to consider these conditions separately. (The varieties of breech presentation are illustrated in Figs. 9–2 through 9–4, pp. 178–79.)

MANAGEMENT OF LABOR

A woman admitted in labor with a breech presentation deserves the immediate attention of nursing and medical personnel since both mother and fetus are at considerably increased risk compared to a woman with a cephalic presentation (Chap. 19, p. 350). A rapid assessment should be made to establish the stage of labor, the status of the fetal membranes, and the condition of the fetus. An intravenous infusion is established, the hematocrit determined, and a group and screen done to detect antibodies since these women have a high likelihood of undergoing operative delivery. Continuous electronic monitoring of fetal heart rate and uterine contractions is commenced. An immediate recruitment of the necessary nursing and medical personnel to accomplish a vaginal or abdominal delivery also should be done.

Stage of Labor

Assessment of cervical dilatation and effacement and the station of the fetal part presenting are essential in planning the route of delivery. If labor is too far advanced, insufficient time may be available to obtain imaging pelvimetry, and this alone may force the decision for abdominal rather than vaginal delivery. Regardless, the time available to accomplish all necessary nursing and medical procedures is the first priority to be established in the laboring woman with a breech presentation.

Fetal Condition

The presence or absence of gross fetal abnormalities such as hydrocephaly or anencephaly can be ascertained rapidly with the use of sonography or x-ray examination. Such efforts will help to ensure that a cesarean section is not done under emergency conditions, thereby increasing maternal risks, for an anomalous infant. If a vaginal delivery is planned, the fetal head should be well flexed. Sometimes this is difficult to ascertain from sonography. Most often, however, computed tomographic pelvimetry will be adequate to document flexion of the fetal head (Chap. 8, p. 172), but if not, a plain film of the abdomen will suffice.

Intravenous Infusion and Laboratory Values

An intravenous infusion through an indwelling catheter should be started as soon as the woman arrives in the labor suite. Possible emergency induction of anesthesia or hemorrhage from lacerations or uterine atony from halogenated anesthetics are but two of many reasons for an immediate intravenous access route which can be used to administer medications or fluids, including blood.

Electronic Fetal Monitoring

We prefer continuous electronic monitoring of fetal heart rate and uterine contractions which is started immediately. When membranes are ruptured, the risk of umbilical cord prolapse is increased appreciably (Chap. 19, p. 353). Therefore, a vaginal examination should follow rupture of the membranes to check for umbilical cord prolapse. Special attention should be directed to the fetal heart rate for the first 5 to 10 minutes following rupture to ensure there has not been an occult cord prolapse. After rupture, internal electronic monitoring of fetal heart rate and uterine contractions is preferable because of the more reliable information provided by these techniques.

Recruitment of Nursing and Medical Personnel

Increased help is required for managing labor and delivery of a breech. The requirements for a delivery team are listed below. For labor, one-on-one nursing should be maintained due to the risk of umbilical cord prolapse or occlusion, and the physician also must be readily available should there be an emergency.

Route of Delivery

The obstetrician should decide the route of delivery as soon as possible after admission. The choice of abdominal or vaginal delivery is based upon the type of breech, flexion of the fetal head, fetal size, and the size of the maternal pelvis. The indications and contraindications for vaginal delivery of a breech are discussed in detail in Chapter 19, p. 355.

TIMING OF DELIVERY

In general, preparations for breech extraction should be initiated by the time that the buttocks or the feet appear at the vulva. It is essential that the delivery team include (1) an obstetrician skilled in the art of breech extraction, (2) an associate who is also scrubbed and gowned to assist with the delivery, (3) an anesthesiologist who can quickly induce appropriate general anesthesia when needed, (4) an individual trained to resuscitate the infant effectively, including tracheal intubation, and (5) someone to provide general assistance.

Delivery is easier and, in turn, perinatal morbidity and mortality are lower when the breech of the fetus is allowed to deliver spontaneously to the umbilicus. If fetal distress develops before this time, however, a decision must be made whether to perform a total breech extraction or, more likely, a cesarean section. It must be remembered that, for a favorable outcome with any breech delivery, at the very minimum the birth canal must be sufficiently large to allow passage of the fetus without trauma and the cervix must be effaced and fully dilated. If these conditions are lacking, cesarean section nearly always is the more appropriate method of delivery.

EXTRACTION OF COMPLETE OR INCOMPLETE BREECH

During total breech extraction of a complete or incomplete breech presentation, the obstetrician's hand is introduced through the vagina and both feet of the fetus grasped; the ankles are held with the second finger lying between them. The feet are brought with gentle traction through the vulva. If difficulty is experienced in grasping both feet, first one foot should be drawn down the vagina to, but not through, the introitus and then the other foot is so manipulated (Fig. 22–1).

Now both feet are grasped and pulled through the vulva simultaneously. Unless there is considerable relaxation of the perineum, an *episiotomy* is made. The episiotomy is an important adjunct to any type of breech delivery. A mediolateral episiotomy is usually preferred with a term-sized infant because it furnishes greater room and is less likely to extend into the rectum.

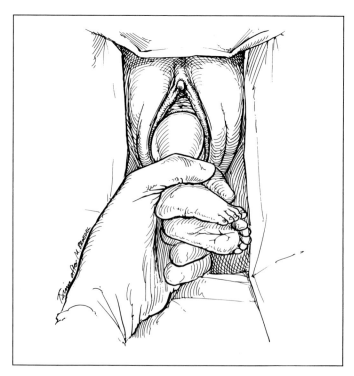

Figure 22–1. Breech extraction. Traction on the feet and ankles.

As the legs begin to emerge through the vulva, they should be wrapped in a sterile towel to obtain a firmer grasp, for the vernix caseosa renders them slippery and difficult to hold. Many obstetricians prefer the towel to be moistened. The sterile water or normal saline used should be warm but not so hot as to burn the infant. Downward gentle traction is then continued.

As the legs emerge, successively higher portions are grasped, first the calves and later the thighs (Fig. 22–2). When the breech appears at the vulva, *gentle traction* is applied until the hips are delivered. As the buttocks emerge, the back of the infant usually rotates to the anterior. The thumbs of the operator are then placed over the sacrum and the fingers over the hips, and *gentle downward traction* is continued until the costal margins, and then the scapulas become visible (Figs. 22–3 and 22–4). As traction is exerted and the scapulas become visible, the back of the infant tends to turn spontaneously toward the side of the mother to which it was originally directed (Fig. 22–4). If turning is not spontaneous, slight rotation should be added to the traction, with the object of bringing the bisacromial diameter of the fetus into the anteroposterior diameter of the pelvic outlet.

A cardinal rule in successful breech extraction is to employ steady, gentle, downward traction until the lower halves of the scapulas are delivered outside the vulva, making no attempt at delivery of the shoulders and arms until one axilla becomes visible. Frequently, failure to follow this rule will make an otherwise easy procedure difficult. The appearance of one axilla indicates that the time has arrived for delivery of the shoulders. Provided the arms are maintained in flexion, it makes little difference which shoulder is delivered first. Occasionally, while plans are made to deliver one shoulder, the other is born spontaneously.

There are two methods of delivery of the shoulders: (1) With the scapulas visible, the trunk is rotated in such a way that the anterior shoulder and arm appear at the vulva and can easily be released and delivered first. In Figure 22–4, the operator is shown rotating the trunk of the fetus counterclockwise to deliver the right shoulder and arm. The body of the fetus is then rotated in the reverse direction to deliver the other shoulder and arm. (2) If trunk rotation was unsuccessful, the posterior shoulder must be delivered first. The feet are grasped in one hand and drawn upward over the groin of the mother toward which the ventral surface of the fetus is directed; in this manner, leverage is exerted upon the posterior shoulder, which slides out over the perineal margin, usually followed by the arm and hand (Fig. 22–5). Then, by depressing the body of the fetus, the anterior shoulder emerges beneath the pubic arch, and the arm and hand usually follow spontaneously (Fig. 22–6). Thereafter, the back tends to rotate spontaneously in the direction of the

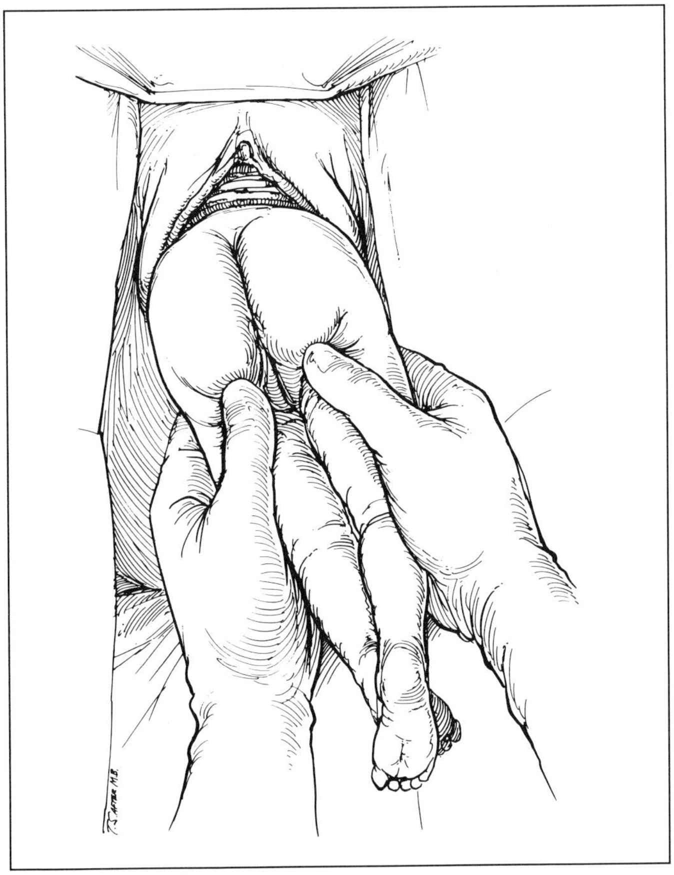

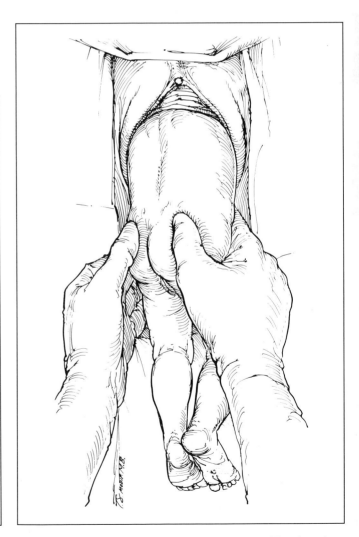

Figure 22–2. Breech extraction. Traction on the thighs. A warm, moist towel is most often applied over the fetal parts to reduce slippage from vernix as traction is applied and to keep the exposed parts warm.

Figure 22–3. Breech extraction. Extraction of the body. The obstetrician's hands are applied over, but not above, the infant's pelvis. Rotation is not attempted until the scapulas are clearly visible.

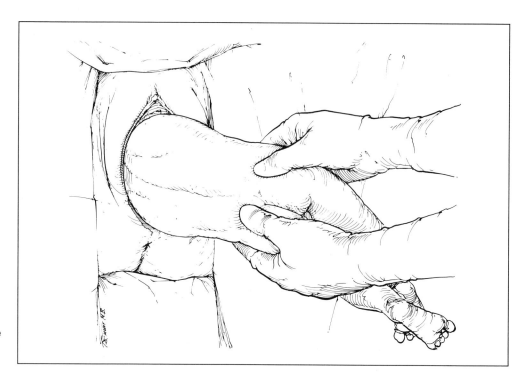

Figure 22–4. Breech extraction. The scapulas are visible and the body is rotating.

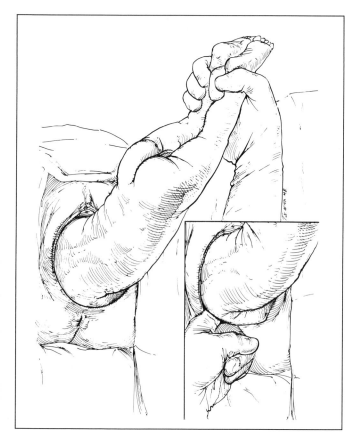

Figure 22–5. Breech extraction. Upward traction to effect delivery of the posterior shoulder, followed by freeing the posterior arm (*insert*).

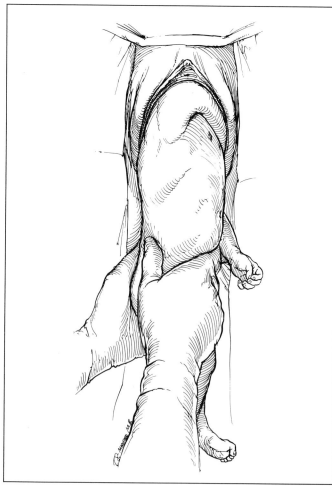

Figure 22–6. Breech extraction. Delivery of the anterior shoulder by downward traction. The anterior arm may then be freed the same way as the posterior arm in Figure 22–5.

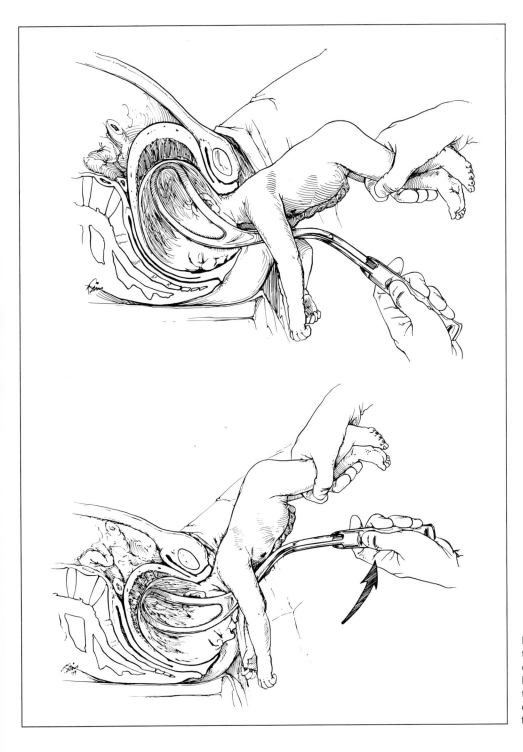

Figure 22–7. A. Forceps applied to the aftercoming head. The head has entered the pelvis and forceps have been applied (see Figs. 22–11 through 22–16). **B.** Forceps delivery of aftercoming head. Note the direction of movement (*arrow*).

mother's symphysis. If upward rotation fails to occur, it is effected by manual rotation of the body. Delivery of the head may then be accomplished.

Unfortunately, however, the process is not always so simple, and it is sometimes necessary first to free and deliver the arms. These maneuvers are much less frequently required today, presumably because of adherence to the principle of continuing traction without attention to the shoulders until an axilla becomes visible. Attempts to free the arms immediately after the costal margins emerge should be avoided.

Since there is more space available in the posterior and lateral segments of the normal pelvis than elsewhere, the posterior arm should be freed first. Since the corresponding axilla is already visible, upward traction upon the feet is continued, and two fingers of the obstetrician's other hand are passed along the humerus until the elbow is reached (Fig. 22–5). The fingers are now used to splint the arm, which is swept downward and delivered through the vulva. To deliver the anterior arm, depression of the fetal body of the infant is sometimes all that is required to allow the anterior arm to slip out spontaneously. In

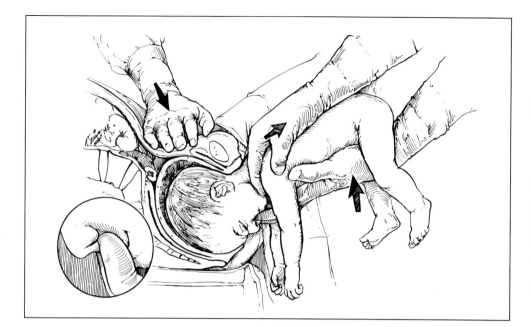

Figure 22–8. Delivery of aftercoming head using the Mauriceau maneuver. Note that as the fetal head is being delivered, flexion of the head is maintained by suprapubic pressure provided by an assistant and simultaneously by pressure on the maxilla (*insert*) by the operator as traction is applied.

other instances, the anterior arm can be swept down over the thorax using two fingers as a splint. Occasionally, however, the body must be seized with the operator's thumbs over the scapulas and rotated to bring the undelivered shoulder near the closest sacrosciatic notch. The legs are then carried upward to bring the ventral surface of the infant to the opposite groin of the mother; subsequently, the arm can be delivered as described previously.

If the arms have become extended over the head, their delivery, although more difficult, can usually be accomplished by the maneuvers just described. In so doing, particular care must be taken to carry the operator's fingers up to the elbow and to use the fingers as a splint, for if the operator's fingers are merely hooked over the fetal arm, the humerus or clavicle is exposed to great danger of fracture. Infrequently, one or both fetal arms is found around the back of the neck (*nuchal arm*), and delivery is still more difficult. If the nuchal arm cannot be freed in the manner described, extraction may be facilitated by rotating the fetus through half a circle in such a direction that the friction exerted by the birth canal will serve to draw the elbow toward the face. Should rotation of the fetus fail to free the nuchal arm, it may be necessary to push the fetus upward in an attempt to release them. If the rotation is still unsuccessful, the nuchal arm is often forcibly extracted by hooking a finger over it. In that event, fracture of the humerus or clavicle is very common. Fortunately, good union almost always follows appropriate treatment.

After the shoulders are born, the head usually occupies an oblique diameter of the pelvis with the chin directed posteriorly. The fetal head may then be extracted either with forceps, as described below and illustrated in Figures 22–7A, B and 22–11 through 22–16, which is the method preferred by many obstetricians and is described subsequently, or by the so-called *Mauriceau maneuver* (Fig. 22–8) (Mauriceau, 1721).

Employing the Mauriceau maneuver to help flex the head, the operator's index and middle finger of one hand are applied over the maxilla, while the fetal body rests upon the palm of the hand and forearm, which is straddled by the fetal legs. Two

fingers of the operator's other hand are then hooked over the fetal neck, and grasping the shoulders, downward traction is applied until the suboccipital region appears under the symphysis. Gentle *suprapubic pressure* simultaneously applied by an assistant helps keep the head flexed. The body of the fetus is then elevated toward the mother's abdomen, and the mouth, nose, brow, and eventually the occiput emerge successively over the perineum. *Gentle traction* should be exerted by the fingers over the shoulders. At the same time, appropriate suprapubic pressure applied by an assistant, as shown in Figure 22–8, is helpful in delivery of the head.

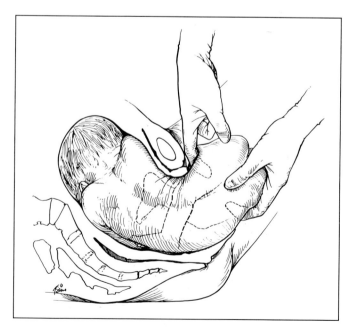

Figure 22–9. Extraction of a frank breech using fingers in groins.

In many cases, the *Pinard maneuver* aids materially in bringing down the feet. In that procedure, two fingers are carried up along one extremity to the knee to push it away from the midline. Spontaneous flexion usually follows, and the foot of the fetus is felt to impinge upon the back of the hand. The fetal foot may then be readily grasped and brought down (Fig. 22–10). As soon as the buttocks are born, first one leg and then the other are drawn out and extraction is accomplished as described under the section on Extraction of Complete or Incomplete Breech (p. 394).

FORCEPS TO AFTERCOMING HEAD

Piper forceps (Figs. 22–7A, B, 22–11 through 22–16) should be applied when the Mauriceau maneuver cannot be easily accomplished, or they may be applied electively instead of the Mauriceau procedure. The blades of the forceps should not be applied to the aftercoming head until it has been brought into the pelvis by gentle traction, combined with suprapubic pressure, and is engaged (Fig. 22–7). As shown in Figure 22–16, suspension of the body of the fetus in a towel keeps the arms out of the way and prevents excessive abduction of the trunk.

ENTRAPMENT OF THE AFTERCOMING HEAD

Occasionally, especially with small preterm fetuses, the incompletely dilated cervix will not allow delivery of the aftercoming head. Prompt action is necessary if a living infant is to be delivered. With gentle traction on the fetal body, the cervix, at times, may be manually slipped over the occiput. If this maneuver is not readily successful, Dührssen incisions can be made in the cervix. Iffy and colleagues (1986) described "abdominal rescue" for a 2,050-g first twin whose fully deflexed head prevented its vaginal delivery after the arms had been delivered. Emergency classical cesarean section resulted in an Apgar 3/7 infant who remained neurologically normal despite a small subarachnoid hemorrhage detected by computed tomographic scans. This is one of the few indications for Dührssen incisions in modern obstetrics (see Chap. 25, p. 438).

Bracht Maneuver

In an effort to stimulate the forces of nature, Bracht (1936) employed a maneuver whereby the breech was allowed to deliver spontaneously to the umbilicus. The baby's body was then held, not pressed, against the mother's symphysis. The force applied in

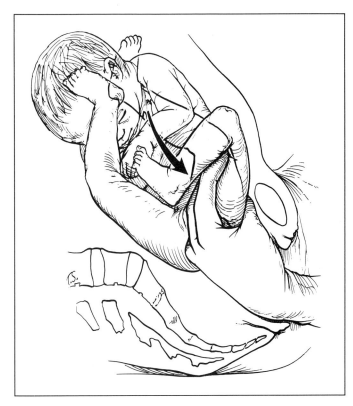

Figure 22–10. Pinard maneuver sometimes used in case of a frank breech presentation to deliver a foot into the vagina.

EXTRACTION OF FRANK BREECH

At times, extraction of a frank breech may be accomplished by *moderate* traction exerted by a finger in each groin and facilitated by a generous episiotomy (Fig. 22–9). If moderate traction does not effect delivery of the breech, and cesarean section is not used, vaginal delivery can only be accomplished by *breech decomposition.* This procedure involves intrauterine manipulation to convert the frank breech into a footling breech. The procedure is more readily accomplished if the membranes were ruptured recently but becomes extremely difficult if considerable time has elapsed after the escape of the amnionic fluid and the uterus has become tightly contracted over the fetus.

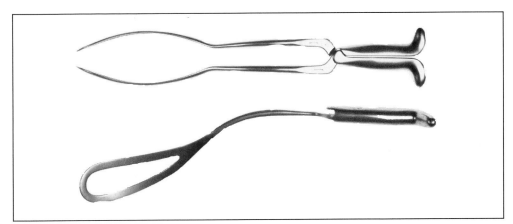

Figure 22–11. Piper forceps.

this procedure should be equivalent to that of gravity. The mere maintenance of this position, added to the effects of uterine contractions and moderate suprapubic pressure by an assistant, often suffices to complete delivery spontaneously. The *Bracht maneuver* has been popular in Europe but has not gained wide acceptance in the United States. The procedure was thoroughly reviewed by Plentl and Stone (1953).

ANESTHESIA FOR BREECH DELIVERY

It is wise to allow the breech to deliver spontaneously to the umbilicus. Analgesia for episiotomy and intravaginal manipulations that are needed for breech extraction can usually be accomplished with pudendal block and local infiltration of the perineum (see Chap. 17, p. 332). The inhalation of nitrous oxide plus oxygen provides further relief from pain. If for any reason general anesthesia is desired, it can be quickly induced with thiopental plus a muscle relaxant and maintained with nitrous oxide.

Continuous epidural analgesia (see Chap. 17, p. 337) has been advocated by some as ideal for women in labor with a breech presentation. According to Crawford and Weaver (1982) such a block provides some protection for the fetal head during the second stage of labor as well as during delivery by abolishing the bearing-down reflex and by inducing pelvic muscle relaxation. Confino and colleagues (1985) reviewed the outcomes of 371 normally formed singleton breech fetuses delivered vaginally. About 25 percent of these women had been given continuous epidural analgesia but it was quite worrisome that oxytocin augmentation was necessary to effect delivery in half of them. Although the first stage of labor was not longer than in a control group not given epidural analgesia, the second stage was significantly prolonged in women whose fetuses weighed more than 2,500 g. In fact, it was doubled if the fetus weighed more than 3,500 g. There was one neonatal death from trauma that followed full breech extraction for a prolapsed cord under epidural analgesia. For the above reasons, we are reluctant to recommend continuous epidural analgesia for these women.

Anesthesia for decomposition and extraction must provide sufficient relaxation to allow intrauterine manipulations. Although successful decomposition has been accomplished using epidural, caudal, or spinal analgesia, increased uterine tone may render the operation difficult. Under such conditions, halothane or one of the other halogenated anesthetic agents may be used to relax the uterus, as well as provide analgesia. The safeguards cited for the use of these agents in Chapter 17 (p. 329) must be followed.

PROGNOSIS

With complicated breech deliveries, there are increased maternal risks. Manual manipulations within the birth canal increase the risk of maternal infection. Intrauterine maneuvers, especially with a thinned-out lower uterine segment, or delivery of the aftercoming head through an incompletely dilated cervix, may cause rupture of the uterus, lacerations of the cervix, or both. Such manipulations may also lead to extensions of the episiotomy and deep perineal tears. Anesthesia sufficient to induce appreciable uterine relaxation may cause uterine atony and, in turn, postpartum hemorrhage from the placental implantation site. Even so, the prognosis, in general, for *the mother* whose fetus is delivered by breech extraction is probably somewhat better than with cesarean section.

For *the fetus*, the outlook is less favorable and it becomes more serious the higher the presenting part is situated at the beginning of the breech extraction. In addition to the increased risk of tentorial tears and intracerebral hemorrhage, which are inherent in breech delivery, the perinatal mortality rate is increased by the greater probability of other trauma during extraction. With incomplete breech presentations, moreover, prolapse of the umbilical cord is much more common than in vertex presentations and this complication further worsens the prognosis for the infant.

Fracture of the humerus and clavicle cannot always be avoided when freeing the arms, and fracture of the femur may be sustained during difficult frank breech extractions. Hemato-

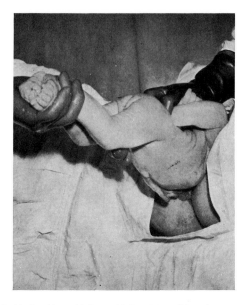

Figure 22–12. Position of infant with head in pelvis prior to application of Piper forceps.

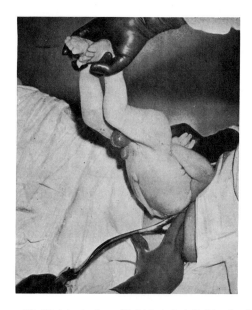

Figure 22–13. Introduction of left blade to left side of pelvis.

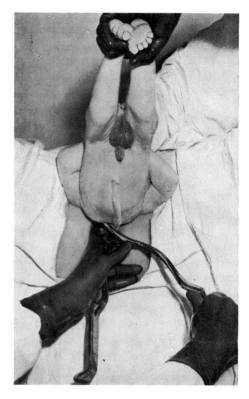

Figure 22–14. Introduction of right blade, completing application.

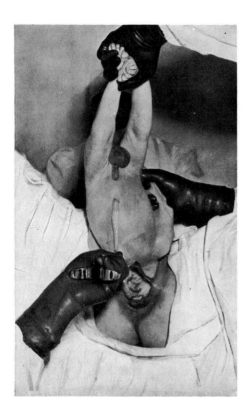

Figure 22–15. Forceps locked and traction applied; chin, mouth, and nose emerging over perineum.

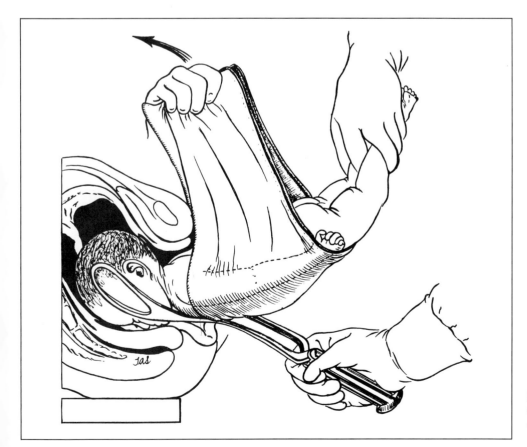

Figure 22–16. Management of fetal arms in breech extraction. (*From Savage: Obstet Gynecol 3:55, 1954.*)

mas of the sternocleidomastoid muscles occasionally develop after the operation, though they usually disappear spontaneously. More serious problems, however, may follow separation of the epiphyses of the scapula, humerus, or femur. Exceptionally, paralysis of the arm follows pressure upon the brachial plexus by the fingers in exerting traction, but more frequently it is caused by overstretching the neck while freeing the arms. When the fetus is forcibly extracted through a contracted pelvis, spoon-shaped depressions or actual fractures of the skull, generally fatal, may result. Occasionally, even the fetal neck may be broken when great force is employed. Perinatal morbidity and mortality are considered in greater detail in Chapter 19 (p. 350).

VERSION

Version, or turning, is an operation in which the presentation of the fetus is altered artificially, either substituting one pole of a longitudinal presentation for the other, or converting an oblique or transverse lie into a longitudinal presentation.

According to whether the head or breech is made the presenting part, the operation is designated cephalic or podalic version, respectively. It is also named according to the method by which it is accomplished. Thus, in *external version*, the manipulations are performed exclusively through the abdominal wall; in *internal version*, the entire hand is introduced into the uterine cavity.

EXTERNAL CEPHALIC VERSION

The object of this procedure is to convert a less favorable presentation to that of a vertex.

Indications

If a breech or shoulder presentation (transverse lie) is diagnosed in the last weeks of pregnancy, its conversion into a vertex may be attempted by external maneuvers, provided there is no marked disproportion between the size of the fetus and the pelvis. Cephalic version is thought by some, but not all, obste-

tricians to be a frequently successful technique with little morbidity (see Chap. 19, p. 354) and therefore should be attempted in order to avoid the increased perinatal mortality that attends breech delivery. If the fetus lies transversely, a change of presentation is the only alternative to cesarean section except for the extremely small and usually previable fetus.

According to Fortunato and colleagues (1988), external cephalic version is more likely to be successful if: (1) The presenting part has not descended into the pelvis. (2) There is a normal amount of amnionic fluid. (3) The fetal back is not positioned posteriorly. (4) The patient is not obese. The fetal heart action must be continuously monitored, usually with a Doppler sound instrument, so that the obstetrician can continuously hear the fetal heart rate during the procedure. Sonography, when immediately available, often proves helpful. Anesthesia should never be used, lest undue force be applied.

In the early stages of labor, before the membranes have ruptured, the same indications apply. They may then be extended to oblique presentations as well, although these unstable lies usually convert spontaneously to longitudinal lies as labor progresses. External cephalic version can rarely be effected, however, after the cervix has become fully dilated or the membranes have ruptured.

Technique

Cephalic version is performed solely by *external manipulations* (Fig. 22–17). In the technique recommended, the presentation and position of the fetus are carefully ascertained and documented by sonography. Each hand then grasps one of the fetal poles. The pole that is to be converted into the presenting part is then gently stroked toward the pelvic inlet while the other is moved in the opposite direction. This procedure should always be performed with continuous fetal heart rate monitoring and in a labor and delivery unit where a rapid cesarean can be performed should fetal distress develop. After version has been completed, the fetus will tend to return to its original position unless the presenting part is fixed in the pelvis. During labor, however, the head may be pressed into the pelvic inlet and held here firmly until it becomes fixed under the influence of uterine

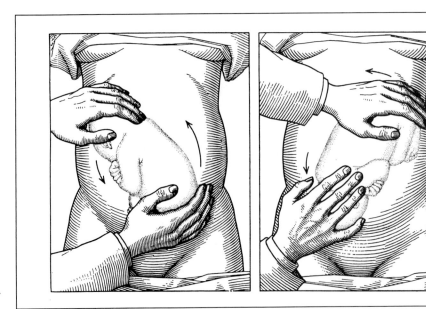

Figure 22–17. External cephalic version.

contractions. Most authors recommend that external version be conducted after uterine relaxation is established with tocolytic agents and especially after failed attempts without tocolytics (Hofmyer, 1983; Van Dorsten and co-workers, 1981, 1982; Ylikorkalo and Hartikainen-Sorri, 1977). Robertson and associates (1987) reported, however, that ritodrine tocolysis did not improve their success.

INTERNAL PODALIC VERSION

This maneuver consists of turning the fetus by the obstetrician inserting a hand into the uterine cavity, seizing one or both feet, and drawing them through the cervix while pushing transabdominally the upper portion of the fetal body in the opposite direction. The operation is followed by breech extraction.

Indications

There are very few, if any, indications for internal podalic version other than for delivery of the second twin. The technique for delivering the second twin is described in Chapter 34, p. 646. Very occasionally, this procedure may be justified when the cervix is fully dilated, the membranes are intact, and the fetus in a transverse lie is small or dead, and usually both. The possibility of serious trauma to the fetus and mother during internal podalic version from a cephalic presentation is apparent from Figures 34–19 and 34–20 (p. 648).

REFERENCES

Bracht E: (Manual aid in breech presentation.) Z. Geburthshilfe Gynaekol 112:271, 1936

Confino E, Ismajovich B, Rudick V, David MP: Extradural analgesia in the management of singleton breech delivery. Br J Anaesth 57:892, 1985

Crawford JS, Weaver, JB: Anaesthetic management of twin and breech deliveries. Clin Obstet Gynecol 9:291, 1982

Fortunato SJ, Mercer LJ, Guzick DS: External cephalic version with tocolysis: Factors associated with success. Obstet Gynecol 72:59, 1988

Hofmyer GJ: Effect of external cephalic version in late pregnancy on breech presentation and cesarean section rate: A controlled trial. Br J Obstet Gynaecol 90:392, 1983

Iffy L, Apuzzio JJ, Cohen-Addad N, Zwolska-Demczuk B, Francis-Lane M, Olenczak J: Abdominal rescue after entrapment of the aftercoming head. Am J Obstet Gynecol 154:623, 1986

Mauriceau F: (The method of delivering the woman when the infant presents one or two feet first.) Traite des Maladies des Femmes Grosses, 6me ed. 1721, pp 280–285

Pinard A: On version by external maneuvers. Paris, Traite de Palper abdominal, 1889

Plentl AA, Stone RE: Bracht maneuver. Obstet Gynecol Surv 8:313, 1953

Robertson AW, Kopelman JN, Read JA, Duff P, Magelssen DJ, Dashow EE: External cephalic version at term: Is a tocolytic necessary? Obstet Gynecol 70:896, 1987

VanDorsten JP: Safe and effective external cephalic version with tocolysis. Contemp Ob/Gyn 19:44, 1982

VanDorsten JP, Schifrin BS, Wallace RL: Randomized control trial of external cephalic version with tocolysis in late pregnancy. Am J Obstet Gynecol 141:417, 1981

Ylikorkalo O, Hartikainen-Sorri A: Value of external version in fetal malpresentation in combination with use of ultrasound. Acta Obstet Gynecol Scand 56:63, 1977

Injuries to the Birth Canal

INJURIES TO THE PELVIC FLOOR AND VAGINA

PERINEAL LACERATIONS

All except the most superficial perineal lacerations are accompanied by varying degrees of injury to the lower portion of the vagina. Such tears may reach sufficient depth to involve the rectal sphincter and may extend to varying depths through the walls of the vagina. Bilateral lacerations into the vagina are usually unequal in length and separated by a tongue-shaped portion of vaginal mucosa (see Figs. 16–17 through 16–19). Their repair should form part of every operation for the restoration of a lacerated perineum. Suturing of just the external integument without approximation of underlying perineal and vaginal fascia and muscle will lead to relaxation of the vaginal outlet and may contribute to rectocele and cystocele formation, as well as uterine prolapse.

VAGINAL LACERATIONS

Isolated lacerations involving the middle or upper third of the vagina but unassociated with lacerations of the perineum or cervix are less commonly observed. Vaginal lacerations in this location are usually longitudinal, resulting from injuries sustained during a forceps operation, although occasionally they accompany spontaneous delivery. Such lacerations frequently extend deep into the underlying tissues and may give rise to copious hemorrhage, which, however, is usually readily controlled by appropriate suturing. They may be overlooked unless thorough inspection of the upper vagina is performed or at least careful attention is paid to bleeding from the genital tract in the presence of a firmly contracted uterus. **Bleeding while the uterus is firmly contracted is strong evidence of genital tract laceration, retained placental fragments, or both.**

Lacerations of the anterior vaginal wall in close proximity to the urethra are relatively common. If superficial and not bleeding, repair is not indicated; otherwise, in order to achieve hemostasis, closure is required. If such lacerations are extensive, difficulty in voiding can be anticipated and an indwelling catheter placed.

INJURIES TO LEVATOR ANI

Injuries to the levator ani as a result of overdistention of the birth canal may result in separation of muscle fibers or in the diminution in their tonicity sufficient to interfere with the function of the pelvic diaphragm. In such cases, the woman may develop pelvic relaxation. If these injuries involve the pubococcygeus muscle, urinary incontinence may supervene.

The likelihood of such injuries is minimized by appropriate episiotomy.

INJURIES TO THE CERVIX

ETIOLOGY

Traumatic lesions of the upper third of the vagina are uncommon by themselves but are often associated with extensions of deep cervical tears. In rare instances, however, the cervix may be entirely or partially avulsed from the vagina, with colporrhexis in the anterior, posterior, or lateral fornices. Such lesions usually follow difficult forceps deliveries performed through an incompletely dilated cervix with the forceps blades applied over the cervix. The cervical tears may extend to involve the lower uterine segment and uterine artery and its major branches, and even through the peritoneum. Fortunately, such extensive traumatic lesions are rare in modern obstetrical practice. They may be totally unsuspected, but much more often they become manifest by excessive external hemorrhage or by the formation of a retroperitoneal hematoma which begins within the leaves of the broad ligaments. These extensive tears of the vaginal vault should be carefully explored. If there is the slightest question of perforation of the peritoneum, or of retroperitoneal or intraperitoneal hemorrhage, laparotomy should be performed. In the presence of damage of this severity, intrauterine exploration for possible rupture is, of course, also mandatory. Formerly, treatment of these lacerations by packing was recommended, *often with poor outcome;* however, surgical repair is much more satisfactory. Effective anesthesia, vigorous blood replacement, and capable assistance are mandatory for a satisfactory outcome.

Cervical lacerations up to 2 cm must be regarded as inevitable in childbirth. Such tears, however, heal rapidly and are rarely the source of any difficulty. In healing, they cause a significant change in the shape of the external os from round before cervical effacement and dilatation to appreciably elongated laterally after delivery and recovery from effacement and dilatation.

Occasionally, during labor the edematous anterior lip of the cervix may be caught and compressed between the head and the symphysis pubis. If ischemia is severe, the cervical lip may undergo necrosis and separation. In still rarer instances, the entire vaginal portion may be avulsed from the rest of the cervix. Such *annular* or *circular detachment of the cervix* probably occurs only in neglected labors or in pregnant women receiving excessive doses of oxytocin.

In all traumatic lesions involving the cervix, there is usually no appreciable bleeding until after birth of the infant, when hemorrhage may then be profuse. Slight cervical tears heal spontaneously. Extensive lacerations have a similar tendency, but perfect union rarely results. As the consequence of such tears, eversion of the cervix with exposure of the delicate mucus-producing endocervical glands is frequently the cause of persistent leucorrhea. If the leucorrhea persists after the puerperium, treatment with cryotherapy is usually beneficial. If a Papanicolaou smear has not been obtained during pregnancy, it should be obtained and the results reviewed before treatment is initiated.

DIAGNOSIS

A deep cervical tear should always be suspected in cases of profuse hemorrhage during and after the third stage of labor, particularly if the uterus is firmly contracted. For a definitive diagnosis to be made, however, a thorough examination is necessary. Because of the flabbiness of the cervix immediately after delivery, digital examination alone is often unsatisfactory. The extent of the injury can be fully appreciated only after adequate exposure and visual inspection of the cervix. The best exposure is gained by the use of right-angle vaginal retractors by an assistant while the operator grasps the patulous cervix with a ring forceps as shown in Figure 23–1, and described below.

In view of the frequency with which deep tears follow major operative procedures, the cervix should be inspected routinely at the conclusion of the third stage after all difficult deliveries, even if there is no bleeding. Annular detachment of the vaginal portion of the cervix should be suspected whenever an irregular mass of tissue with a circular central opening is cast off before or after birth of the infant.

TREATMENT

Deep cervical tears should be repaired immediately. Treatment varies with the extent of the lesion. When the laceration is limited to the cervix, or even when it extends somewhat into the vaginal fornix, satisfactory results are obtained by suturing the cervix after bringing it into view at the vulva. Visualization is best accomplished when an *assistant* makes firm downward pressure on the uterus while the operator exerts traction on the

lips of the cervix with fenestrated ovum or sponge forceps. The vaginal walls are held apart with retractors manipulated with the aid of the assistant (Fig. 23–1). Since the hemorrhage usually comes from the upper angle of the wound, it is advisable to apply the first suture at the angle and suture outward. If there are associated vaginal lacerations, these are repaired after the cervical tears. Tamponade with gauze packs will retard hemorrhage from these lesions while cervical lacerations are repaired. Interrupted chromic catgut sutures should be employed, since they do not have to be removed. The physician must remember that overzealous suturing to try to restore the normal appearance of the cervix may lead to stenosis during involution of the uterus.

RUPTURE OF THE UTERUS

FREQUENCY

It is apparent from the tabulations provided by Schrinsky and Benson (1978) that the incidence of rupture of the uterus varies appreciably among institutions, ranging from 1 in 100 deliveries to 1 in 11,000. Although the frequency of uterine rupture from all causes has probably not decreased remarkably during the past several decades, the etiology of rupture has changed appreciably and the outcome has improved significantly.

Recently, Eden and associates (1986) reviewed the experience with uterine rupture over a 53-year period at Duke University. Surprisingly, the incidence of uterine rupture did not decrease appreciably, and from 1931 to 1950 it was 1 in 1,281 deliveries compared to 1 in 2,251 from 1973 to 1983.

ETIOLOGY

Uterine rupture may develop as a result of preexisting injury or anomaly, or it may complicate labor in a previously unscarred uterus. An extensive classification of the etiology of uterine rupture is presented in Table 23–1.

Currently, the most common cause of uterine rupture is separation of a previous cesarean section scar, and this is probably increasing with the developing trend of allowing a trial of

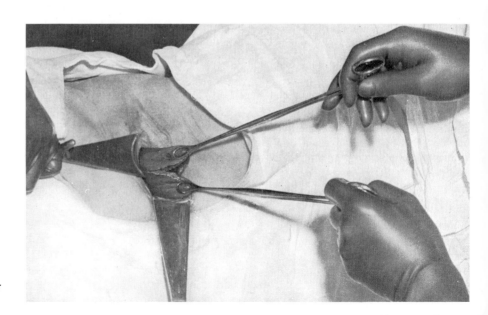

Figure 23–1. Cervical laceration exposed for repair.

TABLE 23–1. CLASSIFICATION OF CAUSES OF UTERINE RUPTURE

Uterine Injury or Anomaly Sustained Before Current Pregnancy	Uterine Injury or Abnormality During Current Pregnancy
1. Surgery involving the myometrium 　　Cesarean section or hysterotomy 　　Previously repaired uterine rupture 　　Myomectomy incision through or to the endometrium 　　Deep cornual resection of interstitial oviduct 　　Metroplasty 2. Coincidental uterine trauma 　　Abortion with instrumentation—curette, sounds 　　Sharp or blunt trauma—accidents, bullets, knives 　　Silent rupture in previous pregnancy 3. Congenital anomaly 　　Pregnancy in undeveloped uterine horn	1. Before delivery 　　Persistent, intense, spontaneous contractions 　　Labor stimulation—oxytocin or prostaglandins 　　Intra-amnionic instillation—saline, prostaglandins 　　Perforation by internal uterine pressure catheter 　　External trauma—sharp or blunt 　　External version 　　Uterine overdistension—hydramnios, multiple pregnancy 2. During delivery 　　Internal version 　　Difficult forceps delivery 　　Breech extraction 　　Fetal anomaly distending lower segment 　　Vigorous uterine pressure during delivery 　　Difficult manual removal of placenta 3. Acquired 　　Placenta increta or percreta 　　Gestational trophoblastic neoplasia 　　Adenomyosis 　　Sacculation of entrapped retroverted uterus

labor following prior transverse cesarean section(s). Shiono and colleagues (1987) from the National Institute of Child Health and Human Development reported that in 1979 a trial of labor was allowed in 2.1 percent of women with prior cesarean delivery, and by 1984 the rate had increased to 8 percent. Flamm (1988) and Phelan (1987) and their colleagues each reported more than 1,500 such women and the incidence of overt uterine rupture was 0.2 to 0.5 percent.

Other common predisposing factors to uterine rupture are previous traumatizing operations or manipulations such as curettage or perforation (Fedorkow and colleagues, 1987). Excessive or inappropriate uterine stimulation with oxytocin, a previously common cause, seems to be decreasing. Generally, the previously untraumatized, spontaneously laboring uterus will not persist in contracting so vigorously as to destroy itself.

From 1963 to 1983, there were 24 cases of uterine rupture at Duke University (Eden and colleagues, 1986). Only 21 percent had rupture of a previous cesarean scar, and the remainder were about equally distributed among the following causes: midforceps delivery, breech version and extraction, precipitous delivery, inappropriate oxytocin administration, and prolonged labor.

DEFINITIONS

It is customary to distinguish between *complete* and *incomplete* rupture of the uterus, depending on whether the laceration communicates directly with the peritoneal cavity or is separated from it by the visceral peritoneum over the uterus or that of the broad ligament. An incomplete rupture may, of course, become complete at any instant.

It is important to differentiate between *rupture of a cesarean section scar* and *dehiscence of a cesarean section scar*. Rupture refers, at the minimum, to separation of the old uterine incision throughout most of its length, with rupture of the fetal membranes so that the uterine cavity and the peritoneal cavity communicate. In these circumstances, all or part of the fetus is usually extruded into the peritoneal cavity. In addition, there is

usually bleeding, often massive, from the edges of the scar or from an extension of the rent into previously uninvolved uterus. By contrast, with dehiscence of a cesarean section scar, the fetal membranes are not ruptured and the fetus is not extruded into the peritoneal cavity. Typically, with dehiscence the separation does not involve all of the previous uterine scar, the peritoneum overlying the defect is intact, and bleeding is absent or minimal. Dehiscence occurs gradually, whereas ruptures are very likely to be symptomatic and, at times, fatal. With labor or intrauterine manipulations, a dehiscence may become a rupture.

COMPARISON OF CLASSICAL AND LOWER-SEGMENT CESAREAN SECTION SCARS

The behavior of a classical scar, that is, a uterine incision through the body of the pregnant uterus rather than the lower uterine segment, in any subsequent pregnancy differs from that of a scar confined to the lower uterine segment. First, the probability of rupture of a classical scar is several times greater than that of a lower segment scar. Second, if a classical scar does rupture, the accident takes place before labor in about one third of the cases. Rupture not infrequently takes place several weeks before term. In fact, Lazarus (1978) described disruption of a previous classical cesarean section scar at 12 weeks' gestation with marked hemorrhage and hypovolemia. Therefore, delivery by subsequent cesarean section cannot prevent such ruptures. Lower-segment scars *that are confined to the noncontractile portion of the uterus* rarely, if ever, rupture before labor.

The statistics available are insufficient to permit a precise calculation of the maternal mortality rate that attends rupture of a cesarean section scar. However, rupture following a trial of labor in a woman with a prior transverse incision has not been associated with maternal deaths, and typically, perinatal loss is very low (Flamm and colleagues, 1988; Phelan and associates, 1987). In 24 cases of uterine rupture from 1963 to 1983, Eden and associates (1986) reported one maternal death and a 46 percent perinatal loss.

Dehiscence of a lower-segment cesarean section scar is much more frequent than actual rupture, especially if the previous uterine incision was transverse. It is remarkable that these separated scars, covered only by the peritoneum, in many instances appear to cause no difficulty in labor or subsequently.

RUPTURE OF A CESAREAN SECTION SCAR

The current trend in obstetrical practice is to encourage a trial of labor in anticipation of vaginal delivery in women who have previously been delivered by one transverse cesarean section (American College of Obstetricians and Gynecologists, 1988). Even more recently, women with two, and even three prior operations have been allowed to labor, either spontaneously or with oxytocin stimulation. The main drawback to this plan is that separation of the previous scar complicates about 1 in 200 trials of labor. From 1984 through 1987, nearly 1,200 women at Parkland Hospital have been allowed a trial of labor following one prior transverse cesarean section and we have encountered only one complete uterine rupture (K. Leveno, unpublished observations). This complication is discussed in detail in Chapter 26 (p. 445).

EXPERIENCES AT PARKLAND HOSPITAL

The experience at this institution has been that antepartum and during early labor, separation of the low transverse uterine incision is almost always limited to dehiscence without an appreciable increase in maternal or perinatal morbidity. Separation of a vertical scar, however, is more likely to result in severe hemorrhage, with an increased perinatal morbidity and mortality.

In another sample of 354 cases, in the great majority of which the previous uterine incision was of the low transverse variety, 211, or 60 percent, were considered to be in labor at the time of repeat cesarean section. There were two instances of uterine dehiscence and one of rupture of the scar. One dehiscence involved a previous low transverse uterine incision. The dehiscence was extended to effect delivery of the healthy infant and then the uterus was closed without much difficulty, using two layers of continuous chromic catgut. In the second case, the dehiscence of the lower vertical incision was not repaired. Instead, cesarean hysterectomy was performed to comply with the woman's request for sterilization. In one case of uterine rupture, a defect believed to be uterine was felt suprapubically during a uterine contraction. With her last two cesarean sections, a vertical uterine incision was made that apparently included some of the upper segment. At laparotomy, the separated vertical scar was covered by a hematoma of about 400 mL that was entrapped beneath the serosa and overlying adherent omentum. Blood had also infiltrated throughout the left broad ligament to the lateral wall of the pelvis. An infant who weighed 2,950 g, with an Apgar score of 8 at 5 minutes, was delivered through the ruptured scar. Hysterectomy was performed with some difficulty because of dense adhesions (Fig. 23–2).

Another woman, in whom the cervix was fully dilated and the occiput at +2 station when she was admitted to the Labor-Delivery Unit, was promptly delivered using forceps, although she had previously undergone cesarean section. Immediate exploration of the uterus was conducted, as should be done in every case of previous cesarean section. Extensive separation of the vertical cesarean section scar with appreciable hemorrhage was identified and the uterus was removed (Fig. 23–3). Both mother and infant survived.

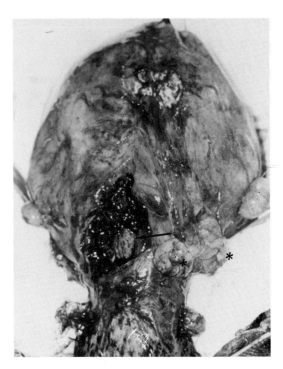

Figure 23–2. Ruptured vertical cesarean section scar (*arrow*) identified at time of repeat cesarean section early in labor; *asterisks* indicate some of the sites of densely adherent omentum.

HEALING OF THE CESAREAN SECTION SCAR

Little information on this subject has been garnered from studies of cesarean section scars. Williams (1921) believed that the uterus heals by regeneration of the muscular fibers and not by scar tissue formation. He based his conclusion on the findings of histological examination of the site of the incision and on two principal observations: First, upon inspection of the unopened uterus at the time of repeated cesarean sections one usually finds no trace of the former incision or, at most, an almost invisible linear scar. Second, when the uterus is removed, often no scar is visible after fixation, or only a shallow vertical furrow in the external and internal surfaces of the anterior uterine wall is seen, with no trace of scar tissue between them. Schwarz and co-workers (1938), however, concluded that healing occurs mainly by the proliferation of fibroblasts. They studied the site of the incision in the human uterus some days after cesarean section, as well as in the uteri of guinea pigs, rabbits, and dogs, and they observed that as the scar shrinks, the proliferation of connective tissue becomes less obvious. Their conclusions appear to be justified by their histological studies, particularly in cases of adequate approximation of the myometrial edges. If the cut surfaces are closely apposed, the proliferation of connective tissue is minimal, and the normal relation of smooth muscle to connective tissue is gradually reestablished, accounting for the occasional absence of even a trace of a former incision. Even when the healing is so poor that marked thinning has resulted, the remaining tissue is often entirely muscular (Fig. 23–4). The fundamental weakness appears to stem from failure to approximate the inner margins of the incision or from formation of a hematoma or abscess in the immediate vicinity. The impact of uterine infection following a previous cesarean section and rupture during subsequent pregnancy appears to be negligible.

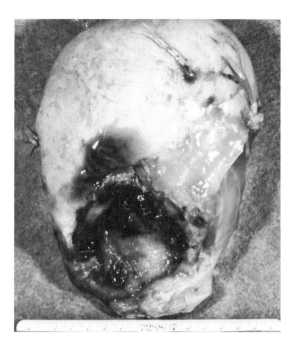

Figure 23–3. Rupture of uterus identified immediately after vaginal delivery; the previous delivery was by cesarean section with a vertical uterine incision.

RUPTURE OF THE UNSCARRED UTERUS

TRAUMATIC RUPTURE

Although the uterus is surprisingly resistant to blunt trauma, pregnant women sustaining blunt trauma to the abdomen should be watched carefully for signs of a ruptured uterus. The experiences at Parkland Hospital, however, have been that rupture of the spleen or traumatic placental abruption, although rare, is more common. Wounds that penetrate the abdomen are much more likely to involve the large pregnant uterus.

Unfortunately, oxytocin stimulation of labor has been a rather common cause of traumatic rupture, especially in women of high parity (Awais and Lebherz, 1970). In the past, traumatic rupture during delivery was most often produced by internal podalic version and extraction. Other causes of traumatic rupture include difficult forceps delivery, breech extraction (Figs. 23–5 and 23–6), and unusual fetal enlargement, such as hydrocephalus. Ruptured uterus caused by strong fundal pressure to try to accomplish vaginal delivery is particularly reprehensible.

SPONTANEOUS RUPTURE OF UTERUS

This catastrophe is more likely to occur in women of high parity. Fuchs and colleagues (1985) reviewed pregnancy outcomes of 5,787 women para 7 or greater and found that uterine rupture was 20 times more likely than in women of lower parity. For this reason, oxytocin should rarely be given to undelivered women of high parity. Similarly, in women of high parity, a trial of labor in the presence of cephalopelvic disproportion, or abnormal presentation such as a brow, may prove dangerous not only to the fetus but also to the mother. Rarely, placenta accreta may result in uterine rupture (see Chapter 31), and Kyodo and colleagues (1988) reported complete separation with expulsion of a live fetus complicating a molar pregnancy.

PATHOLOGICAL ANATOMY

The role in uterine rupture of excessive stretching of the lower uterine segment with the development of a pathological retraction ring is stressed in Chapter 18, p. 347. Rupture of the previously intact uterus at the time of labor most often involves the thinned-out lower uterine segment. The rent, when it is in the immediate vicinity of the cervix, frequently extends transversely or obliquely. Usually, the tear is longitudinal when it occurs in the portion of the uterus adjacent to the broad ligament (Fig. 23–6). Although developing primarily in the lower uterine segment, it is not unusual for the laceration to extend farther upward into the body of the uterus or downward through the cervix into the vagina. At times, the bladder may

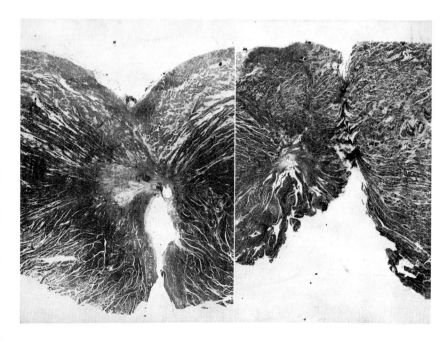

Figure 23–4. Photomicrographs of two poorly healed cesarean section scars.

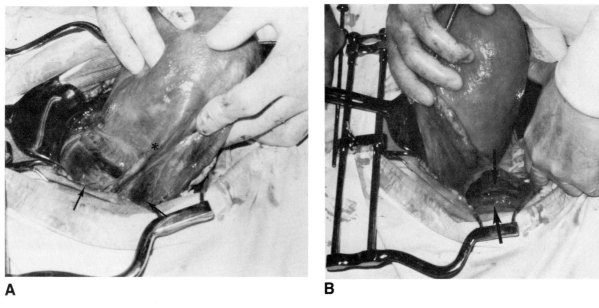

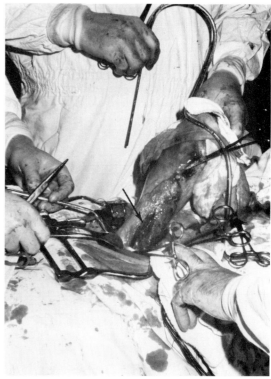

Figure 23–5. A. Rupture of uterus with breech delivery; extensive bleeding beneath uterine serosa and bladder, and in left broad ligament (*arrow*). Asterisk identifies left round ligament. **B.** The broad ligament has been opened and the ureter (*upper arrow*) identified medial to the iliac vessels (*lower arrow*). **C.** Extent of rupture (*arrow*) of lateral wall of uterus is now apparent.

also be lacerated. After complete rupture, the uterine contents escape into the peritoneal cavity, unless the presenting part is firmly engaged, when only a portion of the fetus may be extruded from the uterus.

Incomplete ruptures, that is, those in which the peritoneum is intact, frequently extend into the broad ligament. In such circumstances, the hemorrhage tends to be less rapid than in complete ruptures, the blood accumulating between the leaves of the broad ligament, with the formation of a large retroperitoneal hematoma that may involve sufficient blood loss

to cause death. More frequently, fatal exsanguination supervenes after rupture of the hematoma relieves the tamponading effect of the intact broad ligament. With incomplete rupture, the products of conception may remain within the uterus or assume a position between the leaves of the broad ligament.

Apparent spontaneous rupture of the uterus at times follows manipulations that may very well have caused unappreciated injury to the uterus. Three cases of rupture at Parkland Hospital fall in this category. In one, the previous pregnancy had terminated in an induced septic abortion. During the next

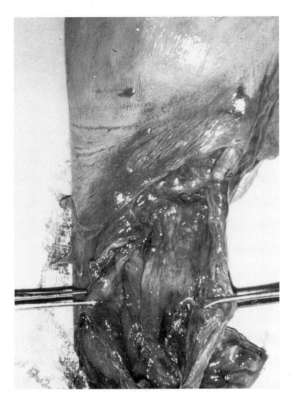

Figure 23–6. Close-up view of resected uterus to show site of rupture observed in Figure 23–5.

pregnancy, at laparotomy following rupture of the uterus, omentum was adherent to the fundus at the site of uterine rupture, strongly suggesting that previous perforation of the uterus had occurred. In the second case, vigorous curettage had followed delivery of a hydatidiform mole and histologically myometrial fragments were identified in the curettings. In this woman's next pregnancy, the uterus ruptured early in labor, the left uterine artery was severed, and rapid exsanguination followed. In the third case, an intrauterine device had been removed by use of a laparoscope with considerable difficulty from the uterine fundus. In the next pregnancy a rent developed in the fundus early in labor, with expulsion of the fetus and placenta, causing fetal death. Taylor and Cummings (1979) described spontaneous rupture of the uterus of a primigravid woman before the onset of labor. The uterine fundus had been traumatized previously by a trocar inserted for laparoscopy.

Instances of uterine rupture have been observed in which hemorrhage was slight. The rupture did not involve large arteries and the emptied uterus contracted well after expulsion of the fetus and placenta into the peritoneal cavity. Less commonly, one or both uterine arteries have been totally avulsed, but spasm develops that prevents exsanguinating hemorrhage. In very rare cases, the fetus may be extruded into the peritoneal cavity while the placenta remains functional within the uterus and the gestation continues as a *uteroabdominal pregnancy* (Badwy, 1962).

CLINICAL COURSE

Prior to circulatory collapse from hemorrhage, the symptoms and physical findings may appear bizarre unless the possibility of rupture of the uterus is kept in mind. As an example, a woman was transferred to Parkland Hospital near term with the diagnosis of pulmonary embolism. She stated that she had been treated for such following a previous pregnancy. She complained of pain on inspiration and shortness of breath, as well as abdominal pain thought to be labor. The symptoms directed to the chest were not the consequence of an embolus, however, but rather of hemoperitoneum from a ruptured uterus, with blood irritating the diaphragm and causing the pain referred to the chest (see Chapter 30, p. 517).

If the accident occurs during labor, the woman, usually after a period of premonitory signs, at the acme of a uterine contraction suddenly complains of a sharp, shooting pain in the abdomen and may cry out that "something ripped" or "something tore" inside her. Immediately after these symptoms and signs have appeared, there is cessation of uterine contractions, and the woman, until that point in intense agony, suddenly experiences much relief. At the same time, there may be external hemorrhage, although it is often slight.

Not all women experience these classical findings of uterine rupture. In some, the appearance is identical to that of placental abruption. In others, rupture is unaccompanied by appreciable pain and tenderness. Also, since most women in labor are given something for discomfort, either narcotics or lumbar epidural analgesia, pain and tenderness may not be readily apparent and the condition becomes evident either because of signs of fetal distress or maternal hypovolemia from concealed hemorrhage, or both.

In some cases in which the fetal presenting part had entered the pelvis with labor, there is *loss of station* detected by pelvic examination. If the fetus is partly or totally extrauterine, abdominal palpation or vaginal examination is helpful in identifying the presenting part, which has moved away from the pelvic inlet. A firm, rounded body, the contracted uterus, may, at times, be felt alongside the fetus. Often fetal parts are more easily palpated than usual. On vaginal examination, it is sometimes possible to palpate a tear in the uterine wall through which the fingers can be passed into the peritoneal cavity, where the viscera may be felt. **Failure to detect the tear by no means proves its absence.** In suspected cases, it is imperative that thorough examination be performed by an experienced examiner before the suspicion is abandoned. At times, either abdominal paracentesis in the flank or culdocentesis is indicated to identify hemoperitoneum. After delivery, culdocentesis can be performed through the posterior fornix into the cul-de-sac. The posterior lip of the cervix is grasped and a long 15-gauge needle is inserted beneath it through the fornix while the cervix is lifted anteriorly.

PROGNOSIS

The chances for fetal survival are dismal; the mortality rates found in various studies range between 50 and 75 percent. However, if the fetus is alive at the time of the accident, the only chance of continued survival is afforded by immediate delivery, most often by laparotomy. Otherwise, hypoxia from both the separation of the placenta and maternal hypovolemia is inevitable. If untreated, most of the women die from hemorrhage or less often later from infection, although spontaneous recovery has been noted in exceptional cases. Prompt diagnosis, immediate operation, the availability of large amounts of blood, and antibiotic therapy have improved greatly the prognosis for women with rupture of the pregnant uterus.

IMMEDIATE TREATMENT

The life of the woman will depend most often on the speed and efficiency with which hypovolemia can be corrected and hemorrhage controlled. Whenever rupture of the uterus is diagnosed, it is mandatory that the following functions be carried out, immediately and simultaneously: (1) Two effective, large-bore intravenous infusion catheters are established, and crystalloid solution, either lactated Ringer's or saline, is infused vigorously; (2) type-specific whole blood is obtained in large quantities, beginning with at least 10 U if possible, and its rapid infusion begun as soon as possible; (3) a surgical team, including anesthesia personnel, is assembled with the operating room set up with instruments necessary to perform cesarean hysterectomy; (4) pediatric personnel skilled in neonatal resuscitation should be present.

It is emphasized that hypovolemic shock may not be quickly reversible until arterial bleeding has been surgically controlled; therefore, delay in starting surgery for these reasons is not acceptable. Instead, blood must be infused vigorously and the laparotomy begun. In desperate cases, compression applied to the aorta may help to reduce the bleeding. Oxytocin administered intravenously may incite contraction of the myometrium and, in turn, vessel constriction, thereby reducing the bleeding.

Clamping the ovarian vessels immediately adjacent to the uterus will help to conserve blood. Techniques for monitoring the adequacy of the circulation, blood and blood-fraction replacement therapy, and the recognition and treatment of coagulation defects are considered in detail in Chapter 36.

HYSTERECTOMY VERSUS REPAIR

Hysterectomy is usually required, but in highly selected cases suture of the wound may be performed.

As part of the overall problem of rupture of the uterus, Mokgokong and Marivate (1976), based on a review of 335 cases treated in Durban, South Africa, considered the merits of hysterectomy compared to suture of the laceration. Maternal mortality was 7 percent and fetal mortality was 80 percent. Three fourths of the cases involved women with previously unscarred uteri. Common specific causes of rupture of the previously unscarred uterus were cephalopelvic disproportion, fetal malpresentation, obstetrical instrumentation, oxytocin stimulation, and internal podalic version. The uterine tears were usually longitudinal and lateral, often involving the uterine artery or its major branches. They concluded that total hysterectomy, especially with longitudinal tears, is the surgical procedure of choice, although transverse lower segment lacerations may be dealt

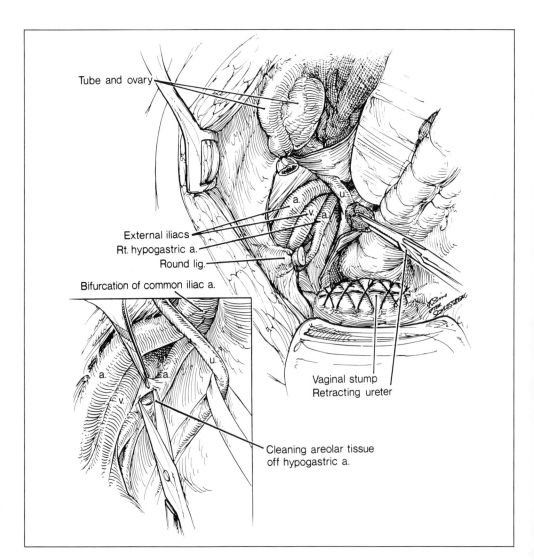

Figure 23–7. Ligation of the right hypogastric artery. The areolar sheath covering the artery is being opened (*lower left*) (a. = artery; lig. = ligament; rt. = right; u. = ureter; v. = vein).

with adequately by repair of the rent. The frequency of subsequent successful pregnancies following repair of the rent was not provided.

Sheth (1968) reported the findings in a series of 66 cases in which repair of a uterine rupture was elected rather than hysterectomy. In 25 instances, the repair was accompanied by tubal sterilization. Thirteen of the 41 mothers who did not have tubal sterilization had a total of 21 subsequent pregnancies, but uterine rupture recurred in 4 instances.

In the presence of a large hematoma in the broad ligament, identification and ligation of the uterine vessels can be extremely difficult. In general, efforts to control hemorrhage by clamping indiscriminately at the site of rupture involving the lower segment should be avoided. To do otherwise often leads to clamping and ligation of the ureter, bladder, or both. With uterine ruptures involving the lower uterine segment, bleeding vessels must be visualized free of surrounding tissue before clamping, or the ureter and bladder must be demonstrated to be remote from the tissue that is clamped. In some cases, the transected uterine artery has retracted laterally and is displaced to the pelvic sidewall by the hematoma that resulted. Placement of clamps to control bleeding carries little risk when rupture involves the body of the uterus remote from the ureters and bladder. The broad ligament may be entered and the ascending uterine artery and veins safely clamped. Usually, the ovarian vessels should be promptly clamped adjacent to the uterus.

Ligation of the hypogastric arteries at times reduces the hemorrhage appreciably. This operation is more easily performed if the midline abdominal incision is extended upward above the umbilicus. With adequate exposure, ligation is accomplished by opening the peritoneum over the common iliac artery and dissecting down to the bifurcation of the external iliac and hypogastric arteries. The areolar sheath covering the hypogastric artery is incised longitudinally and a right-angle clamp is carefully passed just beneath the artery. Care must be taken not to perforate contiguous large veins, especially the hypogastric vein. Suture, usually nonabsorbable, is then inserted into the open clamp, the jaws are locked, the suture is carried around the vessel, and the vessel is securely ligated (Figs. 23–7 and 23–8). Pulsations in the external iliac artery, if present before tying the ligature, should be present afterward as well. If not, pulsations must be identified after arterial hypotension has been successfully treated in order to assure that the blood flow through the external iliac vessel has not been compromised by the ligature. An important mechanism of action with hypogastric ligation, apparently, is reduction of pulse pressure in those arteries distal to the ligation. It is of interest that bilateral ligation of the hypogastric arteries per se does not appear to interfere seriously with subsequent reproduction. Mengert and associates (1969) documented successful pregnancies in five women after bilateral hypogastric artery ligation. In three, the ovarian arteries were also ligated.

In some women, pelvic vessel bleeding may continue even after hypogastric artery ligation. In some cases, angiographically directed arterial embolization with Gelfoam or a similar substance has been described to successfully arrest hemorrhage (Greenwood and colleagues, 1987).

GENITAL TRACT FISTULAS FROM PARTURITION

In obstructed labor, the tissues of various parts of the genital tract may be compressed between the fetal head and the bony pelvis. If the pressure is brief, it is without significance, but if it is prolonged, necrosis results, followed in a few days by sloughing and perforation (Chap. 20, p. 378).

In most such cases, the perforation occurs between the vagina and the bladder, giving rise to a vesicovaginal fistula. Less frequently, the anterior lip of the cervix is compressed against the symphysis pubis, and an abnormal communication is eventually established between the cervical canal and the bladder, a vesicocervical fistula. If the woman has no infection, the fistula may heal spontaneously. More often it persists, requiring subsequent repair.

Rarely, the posterior wall of the uterus may be subjected to so much pressure against the promontory of the sacrum that necrosis results, and a fistula communicating with the cul-de-sac develops.

REFERENCES

American College of Obstetricians and Gynecologists: Committee on Obstetrics: Maternal and Fetal Medicine: Guidelines for vaginal delivery after a previous cesarean birth. Number 64, October, 1988

Awais GM, Lebherz TB: Ruptured uterus, a complication of oxytocin induction and high parity. Obstet Gynecol 36:465, 1970

Badwy AH: Abdominal pregnancy in a previously ruptured uterus. Lancet 1:510, 1962

Eden RD, Parker RT, Gall SA: Rupture of the pregnant uterus: A 53-year review. Obstet Gynecol 68:671, 1986

Fedorkow DM, Nimrod CA, Taylor PJ: Ruptured uterus in pregnancy: A Canadian hospital's experience. Can Med Assoc J 137:27, 1987

Flamm BL, Lim OW, Jones C, Fallon D, Newman LA, Mantis JK: Vaginal birth after cesarean section: Results of a multicenter study. Am J Obstet Gynecol 158:1079, 1988

Fuchs K, Peretz B-A, Marcovici R, Paldi E, Timor-Tritsh I: The "grand multipara"—Is it a problem? A review of 5785 cases. Int J Gynaecol Obstet 23:321, 1985

Greenwood LH, Glickman MG, Schwartz PE, Morese SS, Denny DF: Obstetric and nonmalignant gynecologic bleeding: Treatment with angiographic embolization. Radiology 164:155, 1987

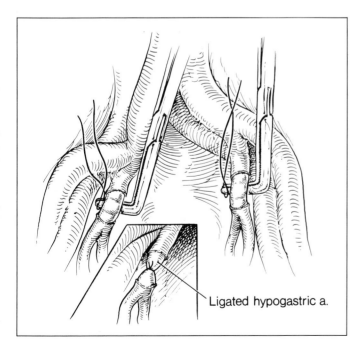

Figure 23–8. Ligation of both hypogastric arteries. After the covering sheath has been opened and the artery has been carefully freed from the immediately adjacent veins, a ligature is carried beneath the artery with a right angle clamp and firmly tied (a. = artery).

Ligated hypogastric a.

Kyodo Y, Inatomi K, Abe T, Kudo K: A case report of destructive mole after uterine rupture. Am J Obstet Gynecol 158:1182, 1988

Lazarus EJ: Early rupture of the gravid uterus. Am J Obstet Gynecol 132:224, 1978

Mengert WJ, Burchell RC, Blumstein RW, Daskal JL: Pregnancy after bilateral ligation of the internal iliac and ovarian arteries. Obstet Gynecol 34:664, 1969

Mokgokong ER, Marivate M: Treatment of the ruptured uterus. Afr Med J 50:1621, 1976

Phelan JP, Clark SL, Diaz F, Paul RH: Vaginal birth after cesarean. Am J Obstet Gynecol 157:1510, 1987

Schrinsky DC, Benson RC: Rupture of the pregnant uterus: A review. Obstet Gynecol Surv 33:217, 1978

Schwarz O, Paddock R, Bortnick AR: The cesarean scar: An experimental study. Am J Obstet Gynecol 36:962, 1938

Sheth SS: Results of treatment of rupture of the uterus by suturing. J Obstet Gynaecol Br Commonw 75:55, 1968

Shiono PH, Fielden JG, McNellis D, Rhoads GG, Pearse WH: Recent trends in cesarean birth and trial of labor rates in the United States. JAMA 257:494, 1987

Taylor PJ, Cummings DC: Spontaneous rupture of a primigravid uterus. J Reprod Med 22:169, 1979

Williams JW: A critical analysis of 21 years' experience with cesarean section. Bull Johns Hopkins Hosp 32:173, 1921

Abnormalities of the Third Stage of Labor

POSTPARTUM HEMORRHAGE

DEFINITION

Postpartum hemorrhage has most often been defined as loss of blood in excess of 500 mL during the first 24 hours after birth of the infant. Through quantitative measurements of puerperal blood loss, however, the incongruity of this definition has been clearly demonstrated, as blood loss resulting from vaginal delivery is *frequently* somewhat more than 500 mL. Newton (1966), for example, measured the amount of hemoglobin shed by 105 women from the time of vaginal delivery through the next 24 hours and ascertained that the average blood loss was at least 546 mL. If appropriate allowance was made for the maternal blood discarded with the placenta, as well as that not measured because of incomplete recovery of shed hemoglobin, the blood loss during the first 24 hours averaged about 650 mL. Moreover, Pritchard and associates (1962) and DeLeeuw and co-workers (1968) demonstrated that erythrocytes equivalent to approximately 600 mL of blood are lost from the maternal circulation during vaginal delivery and the next several hours. Therefore, blood loss somewhat in excess of 500 mL by accurate measurement is not necessarily an abnormal event for vaginal delivery. Pritchard and associates noted that about 5 percent of women delivering vaginally lost more than 1,000 mL of blood, according to their measurements. These same workers observed that estimated blood loss commonly is only about one half the actual loss. Moreover, based on an estimated blood loss greater than 500 mL, postpartum hemorrhage has been found in about 5 percent of deliveries. An estimated blood loss in excess of 500 mL in many institutions, therefore, may call attention to mothers who are bleeding excessively and warn the physician that dangerous hemorrhage is imminent. Hemorrhage after the first 24 hours is designated as *late postpartum hemorrhage* and is discussed in the section Hemorrhages During the Puerperium in Chapter 28 (p. 482).

SIGNIFICANCE

Postpartum hemorrhage is the most common cause of serious blood loss in obstetrics. As a direct factor in maternal mortality, it is the cause of about one fourth of the deaths from obstetrical hemorrhage from postpartum hemorrhage, placenta previa, placental abruption, ectopic pregnancy, hemorrhage from abortion, and rupture of the uterus (Kaunitz and colleagues, 1985).

IMMEDIATE CAUSES

The many factors of importance, singly or in combination, in the genesis of early postpartum hemorrhage are listed in Table 24–1. The two most common causes of immediate hemorrhage are hypotonic myometrium (*uterine atony*) and lacerations of the vagina and cervix. Retention of part or all of the placenta, a less common cause, may produce either immediate or delayed hemorrhage, or both. It is uncommon for an episiotomy alone to cause severe postpartum hemorrhage, although blood so lost averages about 200 mL and, at times, is much more (Odell and Seski, 1947).

PREDISPOSING FACTORS

In the majority of cases, postpartum hemorrhage can be predicted well in advance of delivery. Examples in which trauma is likely to lead to postpartum hemorrhage include delivery of a large infant, midforceps delivery, forceps rotation, delivery through an incompletely dilated cervix, Dührssen incisions of the cervix, any intrauterine manipulation, and perhaps vaginal delivery after cesarean section or other uterine incisions. Uterine atony causing hemorrhage can be anticipated whenever an anesthetic agent is used that will relax the uterus. Halothane and other halogenated compounds are prominent examples (Gilstrap and colleagues, 1987). The overdistended uterus is very likely to be hypotonic after delivery. Thus the woman with a large fetus, multiple fetuses, or hydramnios is prone to hemorrhage from uterine atony. Blood loss with delivery of twins, for example, averages nearly 1,000 mL, or nearly twice that associated with delivery of a singleton, and may be much greater (Pritchard, 1965). The woman whose labor is characterized by uterine activity that is either remarkably vigorous or barely effective is also likely to bleed excessively from uterine atony after delivery. Similarly, labor either initiated or augmented with oxytocin is more likely to be followed by postdelivery uterine atony and hemorrhage. The woman of high parity is at increased risk of hemorrhage from uterine atony. Fuchs and colleagues (1985) described the outcomes of 5,785 women of para 7 or greater. They reported that the 2.7 incidence of postpartum hemorrhage in these women was increased fourfold compared to their general obstetrical population. However, Eidelman and colleagues (1988) found no such associations when they compared 889 women of para 6 or more to their general population. The risk is even greater if she previously had suffered a postpartum hemorrhage. Commonly, mismanagement of the third stage of labor involves an attempt to hasten delivery of the placenta short of manual removal. **Constant kneading and**

TABLE 24–1. PREDISPOSING FACTORS AND CAUSES OF IMMEDIATE POSTPARTUM HEMORRHAGE

Trauma to the Genital Tract
  Large episiotomy, including extensions
  Lacerations of perineum, vagina, or cervix
  Ruptured uterus

Bleeding from Placental Implantation Site
  Hypotonic myometrium—uterine atony
    Some general anesthetics—halogenated hydrocarbons
    Poorly perfused myometrium—hypotension
      Hemorrhage
      Conduction analgesia
    Overdistended uterus—large fetus, twins, hydramnios
    Following prolonged labor
    Following very rapid labor
    Following oxytocin-induced or augmented labor
    High parity
    Uterine atony in previous pregnancy
    Chorioamnionitis
  Retained placental tissue
    Avulsed cotyledon, succenturiate lobe
    Abnormally adherent—accreta, increta, percreta

Coagulation Defects
  Intensify all of the above

squeezing of the uterus that is already contracted are likely to impede the physiological mechanism of placental detachment, with incomplete placental separation and increased blood loss as the consequence.

CLINICAL CHARACTERISTICS

Postpartum hemorrhage before delivery of the placenta is called third-stage hemorrhage. Contrary to general opinion, whether bleeding occurs before or after delivery of the placenta or at both times, there may be no sudden massive hemorrhage but rather a steady bleeding that at any given instant appears to be moderate but persists until serious hypovolemia develops. Especially with hemorrhage after delivery of the placenta, the constant seepage may, over a period of a few hours, lead to enormous loss of blood. The effects of hemorrhage depend to a considerable degree upon the nonpregnant blood volume, the magnitude of pregnancy-induced hypervolemia, and the degree of anemia at the time of delivery. A treacherous feature of postpartum hemorrhage is the failure of the pulse and blood pressure to undergo more than moderate alterations until large amounts of blood have been lost, as emphasized in Chapter 36 (p. 697). The normotensive woman may actually become somewhat hypertensive in response to hemorrhage, at least initially. Moreover, the already hypertensive woman may be interpreted to be normotensive although remarkably hypovolemic. Tragically, the hypovolemia may not be recognized until very late.

As emphasized in Chapter 35 (p. 662), the woman with severe preeclampsia usually has lost the hypervolemia characteristic of normal pregnancy, and thus, she is frequently very sensitive or even intolerant of what may be considered normal blood loss. **Therefore, when excessive hemorrhage is even suspected in the woman with severe pregnancy-induced hypertension, efforts should be made immediately to identify those** clinical and laboratory findings that would prompt vigorous crystalloid and blood replacement (Chap. 36, p. 697).

In instances in which the fundus has not been adequately monitored after delivery, the blood may not escape vaginally but may collect instead within the uterus. The uterine cavity may thus become distended by 1,000 mL or more of blood while an inattentive attendant fails to identify the large uterus or, having done so, erroneously massages a roll of abdominal fat. The care of the postpartum uterus, therefore, must not be left to an inexperienced person.

DIAGNOSIS

Except possibly when an intrauterine and intravaginal accumulation of blood is not recognized, or in some instances of uterine rupture with intraperitoneal bleeding, the diagnosis of postpartum hemorrhage should be obvious. The differentiation between bleeding from uterine atony and from lacerations is tentatively made on the condition of the uterus. If bleeding persists despite a firm, well-contracted uterus, the cause of the hemorrhage most probably is lacerations. Bright red blood also suggests lacerations. **To ascertain the role of lacerations as a cause of bleeding, careful inspection of the vagina, cervix, and uterus is essential.** Sometimes bleeding may be caused by both atony and trauma, especially after major operative delivery. In general, inspection of the cervix and vagina should be performed after every delivery to prevent hemorrhage from cervical or vaginal lacerations. Anesthesia should be adequate to prevent discomfort to the mother during such an examination and there should be no contamination of the lower genital tract from the adjacent perineum. Examination of the uterine cavity, the cervix, and all of the vagina is essential after breech extraction, after internal podalic version, and upon completion of a vaginal delivery in a woman who previously underwent cesarean section. The same is true when unusual bleeding is identified during the second stage of labor.

PROGNOSIS

Women with postpartum hemorrhage should not die, even though hysterectomy may be required in some instances. To obtain this objective, however, requires assiduous attention to all women immediately postpartum, an effective blood bank, and alert action by an experienced obstetrical team. Although death from postpartum hemorrhage is rare in current obstetrical practice in modern hospitals, it is common under less favorable conditions.

There are other hazards associated with postpartum hemorrhage. A particularly serious complication is renal failure from prolonged hypotension in which renal perfusion is not reestablished promptly. Conversely, there are complications that follow appropriate treatment with blood transfusions. These include immediate reactions caused by donor-recipient incompatibilities and, rarely, pulmonary edema from alveolar-capillary injury. Late complications include clinically apparent transfusion-related hepatitis, most often non-A, non-B, which develops in as many as 1 percent of women transfused. Probably another 5 percent of women transfused will develop anicteric non-A, non-B hepatitis, and its long-term sequelae are as yet unclear (Chap. 39, p. 831). The incidence of human immunodeficiency virus infection has been estimated as low as 1 in 250,000 (Bove, 1987) to as high as 1 in 40,000 (Ward and colleagues, 1988) from screened donors.

SHEEHAN SYNDROME

Severe intrapartum or early postpartum hemorrhage is on rare occasions followed by Sheehan syndrome, which, in the classic case, is characterized by failure in lactation, amenorrhea, atrophy of the breasts, loss of pubic hair and axillary hair, superinvolution of the uterus, hypothyroidism, and adrenal cortical insufficiency. The exact pathogenesis of Sheehan syndrome is not well understood since such endocrine abnormalities in most women who hemorrhage severely are not evident. In some but not all instances of Sheehan syndrome, varying degrees of necrosis of the anterior pituitary gland with impaired secretion of one or more of its trophic hormones account for the endocrine abnormalities. The anterior pituitary of some women who develop hypopituitarism after puerperal hemorrhage does respond to various releasing hormones, however, which implies, at least, impaired hypothalamic function rather than pituitary necrosis. Moreover, confirmatory histological evidence of hypothalamic involvement has been provided by Whitehead (1963), who, in some cases, identified specific atrophic changes in the hypothalamic nuclei. Lactation after delivery usually, but not always, excludes extensive pituitary necrosis. In some women, failure to lactate may not be followed until many years later by other symptoms of pituitary insufficiency.

The incidence of Sheehan syndrome was originally estimated to be 1 per 10,000 deliveries (Sheehan and Murdoch, 1938), and it appears to be equally rare today in the continental United States, although 100 cases were identified in two decades in one hospital in Puerto Rico (Haddock and colleagues, 1972). Perhaps the application of the many tests of hypothalamic and pituitary function now available will identify milder forms of the syndrome to be much more prevalent (Grimes and Brooks, 1980). A schema of sequential stimulation tests for Sheehan syndrome has been provided by DiZerega and coworkers (1978).

Diabetes Insipidus

Severe hemorrhage at and immediately after delivery has been implicated in the development of diabetes insipidus without apparent anterior pituitary deficiency. The lesion is rare; in fact, Collins and associates (1979) claim to have reported the first case.

MANAGEMENT OF THIRD-STAGE BLEEDING

Some bleeding is inevitable during the third stage of every labor as the result of transient partial separation of the placenta. As the placenta separates, the blood from the implantation site may escape into the vagina immediately ("Duncan mechanism") or it may be concealed behind the placenta and membranes ("Schultze mechanism") until the placenta is delivered.

In the presence of any external hemorrhage during the third stage, the uterus should be massaged if it is not firmly contracted. If the signs of placental separation have appeared (see Chap. 16, p. 319), expression of the placenta should be attempted by manual pressure on the fundus of the uterus. Descent of the placenta is indicated by the cord becoming slack. If bleeding continues, manual removal of the placenta is mandatory.

TECHNIQUE OF MANUAL REMOVAL

When this operation is necessary, adequate analgesia or anesthesia is mandatory. Aseptic surgical technique should be employed and a sterile glove that covers the forearm to the elbow is recommended. After grasping the fundus of the uterus through the abdominal wall with one hand, the other hand with the long glove is introduced into the vagina and passed into the uterus, along the umbilical cord. As soon as the placenta is reached, its margin is located and the ulnar border of the hand insinuated between it and the uterine wall (Fig. 24–1). Then with the back of the hand in contact with the uterus, the placenta is peeled off its uterine attachment by a motion similar to that employed in separating the leaves of a book. After its complete separation, the placenta should be grasped with the entire hand, which is then gradually withdrawn. Membranes are removed at the same time by carefully teasing them from the decidua, using ring forceps to grasp them as necessary. Some prefer to wipe out the uterine cavity with a sponge. If this is done, it is imperative that a sponge not be left in the uterus or vagina.

MANAGEMENT AFTER DELIVERY OF PLACENTA

Irrespective of the method of delivery of the placenta, the fundus should always be palpated afterwards to make certain that the uterus is well contracted. If it is not firm, vigorous fundal massage is indicated. In some institutions 0.2 mg of ergonovine (Ergotrate) or methylergonovine (Methergine) is routinely administered either intravenously or intramuscularly. More commonly, because hypertension occasionally develops following administration of these compounds, they are given only if there is excessive bleeding not controlled by an intravenous infusion of oxytocin and uterine massage. Most often 20 U of oxytocin in 1,000 mL of lactated Ringer's or normal saline solution proves effective when administered intravenously at approximately 10 mL per minute (200 mU of oxytocin per minute) simultaneously

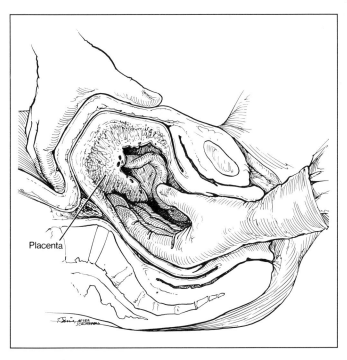

Placenta

Figure 24–1. Manual removal of placenta. The fingers are alternately abducted, adducted, and advanced until the placenta is completely detached.

with effective uterine massage. Oxytocin should never be given as an undiluted bolus dose as serious hypotension may follow (see Chap. 16, p. 321). If oxytocin given by rapid infusion does not prove effective, then methylergonovine (Methergine), 0.2 mg administered intramuscularly or intravenously, may stimulate the uterus to contract and retract sufficiently to control hemorrhage from the placental implantation site. Any superior therapeutic effects of ergot derivatives over oxytocin are speculative, and if intravenously administered they may cause dangerous hypertension, especially in the woman with preeclampsia. More recently, the 15-methyl derivative of prostaglandin $F_{2\alpha}$ (Prostin/15M) has been approved by the Food and Drug Administration for use in treatment of postpartum hemorrhage from uterine atony, and preliminary experiences seem favorable (Buttino and Garite, 1986; Hayashi and colleagues, 1984). The initial recommended dose is 250 μg (0.25 mg) given intramuscularly and this is repeated if necessary at 15- to 90-minute intervals. A high incidence of chorioamnionitis or an abnormally adherent placenta has been reported in women in whom the drug was ineffective. In our experiences, continued bleeding after administration of prostaglandin often is from an unrecognized genital tract laceration, including in some cases, uterine rupture. Prostin/15M was associated with a hypertensive response in less than 5 percent of women in clinical trials, and in most cases it was difficult to attribute to Prostin/15M. At Parkland Hospital we have encountered serious hypertension in a few women so treated. Hankins and colleagues (1988) observed that the intramuscular derivative was associated with arterial oxygen desaturation that developed within 15 minutes and that the decrease averaged 10 percent.

If bleeding persists despite these procedures, no time should be lost in haphazard efforts to control hemorrhage, but the following management should be initiated immediately:

1. Employ bimanual uterine compression (Fig. 24–2). (This procedure will control most hemorrhage.)
2. Obtain help!

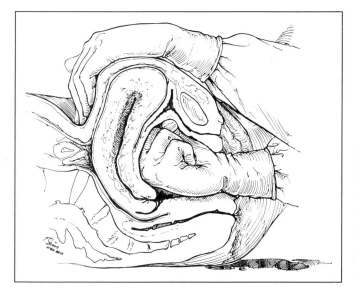

Figure 24–2. Bimanual compression of the uterus and massage with the abdominal hand usually will effectively control hemorrhage from uterine atony.

3. Begin transfusion of blood. The blood group of every obstetrical patient should be known, if possible, before labor, and an indirect Coombs' test done to detect erythrocyte antibodies. If the latter is negative, then cross-matching of blood is not necessary (Chap. 36, p. 698), but in an extreme emergency, type-specific whole blood may be given.
4. Explore the uterine cavity manually for retained placental fragments or lacerations.
5. Thoroughly inspect the cervix and vagina after adequate exposure.
6. Add a second intravenous route using a large bore intravenous catheter so that oxytocin can continue to be given at the same time as blood is being received.
7. Adequacy of cardiac output and arterial filling can be evaluated by monitoring urine output. Put a Foley catheter in the patient's bladder (see Obstetrical Hemorrhage, Chapter 36, p. 697).

The technique of bimanual compression (Fig. 24–2) consists simply of massage of the posterior aspect of the uterus with the abdominal hand and massage through the vagina of the anterior uterine aspect with the other fist, the knuckles of which contact the uterine wall. Packing the uterus was an alternative procedure that formerly enjoyed greater popularity. **The recently pregnant uterus cannot be satisfactorily packed immediately after delivery because it dilates under the packing, with further concealed hemorrhage that may be fatal.**

Blood transfusion should be initiated immediately in any case of postpartum hemorrhage in which abdominal massage of the uterus and oxytocic agents fail to control the bleeding. With transfusion and simultaneous manual compression of the uterus and oxytocin infused intravenously, additional measures are rarely required. If the operator's hand tires, an associate can relieve.

HEMORRHAGE FROM RETAINED PLACENTAL FRAGMENTS

Immediate postpartum hemorrhage is seldom caused by retained small placental fragments, but a remaining piece of placenta is a common cause of bleeding late in the puerperium. Inspection of the placenta after delivery must be routine. If a portion of placenta is missing, the uterus should be explored and the placental fragment removed, particularly in the face of continuing postpartum bleeding. Retention of a succenturiate lobe (see Figs. 4–15 and 4–16) is an occasional cause of postpartum hemorrhage. The late bleeding that may result from a placental polyp is discussed in Chapter 28, (p. 483).

HEMORRHAGE FROM LACERATIONS

If rupture of the uterus is identified, laparotomy, and, most often hysterectomy, is mandatory for a favorable outcome (see Chap. 23, p. 412). Lacerations of the cervix and the vaginal vault sometimes cause profuse bleeding. **Anytime that bleeding persists in the presence of a firmly contracted intact uterus, hemorrhage from lacerations of the cervix, vagina, or uterus should be suspected.** In any case of protracted hemorrhage, moreover, even though the obstetrician is certain that uterine atony is the cause, inspection of the cervix and vagina is a necessary precaution to avoid overlooking a serious laceration. Uterine tears may cause persistent bleeding that distends the uterine cavity to cause in addition uterine atony. Proper exposure of the cervix and upper vagina to repair such lacerations usually requires an associate. Two retractors are inserted into the vagina, the walls of which are separated widely. Ring forceps are then placed on the anterior and posterior lips of the cervix, which is carefully inspected, especially laterally (see Chap. 23, Fig. 23–1). Lacerations that are bleeding should be promptly repaired. Either interrupted single sutures or figure-of-eight sutures are employed, with the highest one placed slightly above the apex of the tear, because bleeding from cervical lacerations usually arises from a vessel at this point.

HYSTERECTOMY

If rupture of the uterus is identified, hysterectomy is life-saving (see Chap. 23, p. 412). With an apparently intact uterus, and when other measures to combat postpartum hemorrhage fail, the question of hysterectomy arises. If performed without initiating blood replacement in a woman who is profoundly hypovolemic, hysterectomy may hasten death. On the other hand, hysterectomy should not be delayed unduly. Vigorous transfusion therapy should be initiated and surgery promptly begun. This approach will prevent deaths in cases in which all other measures to arrest hemorrhage fail. A technique is described in Chapter 26, p. 453.

PLACENTA ACCRETA, INCRETA, AND PERCRETA

In most instances, the placenta separates spontaneously from its implantation site during the first few minutes after delivery of the infant. The precise reason for delay in detachment beyond this time is not always obvious, but quite often it seems to be due to inadequate uterine contraction and retraction. Very infrequently, the placenta is unusually adherent to the implantation site, with scanty or absent decidua, so that the physiological line of cleavage through the spongy layer of decidua is lacking. As a consequence, one or more cotyledon of the placenta are firmly bound to the defective decidua basalis or even to the myometrium. When the placenta is densely anchored in this fashion, the condition is called placenta accreta.

DEFINITIONS

The term *placenta accreta* is used to describe any implantation of the placenta in which there is abnormally firm adherence to the uterine wall. As the consequence of partial or total absence of the decidua basalis and imperfect development of the fibrinoid layer (*Nitabuch layer*), the placental villi are attached to the myometrium (*placenta accreta*) (see Fig. 24–3), actually invade the myometrium (*placenta increta*), or even penetrate through the myometrium (*placenta percreta*) (Fig. 24–4). The abnormal adherence may involve all of the cotyledons (total placenta accreta), a few to several cotyledons (partial placenta accreta), or a single cotyledon (focal placenta accreta).

SIGNIFICANCE

An abnormally adherent placenta, although an uncommon condition, assumes considerable significance clinically because of morbidity and, at times, mortality from severe hemorrhage, uterine perforation, and infection. The true frequencies of placenta accreta, increta, and percreta are unknown. Breen and associates (1977), for example, reviewed reports of this condition published since 1891. The incidence varied from 1 in 540 deliveries to 1 in 70,000 deliveries, with an average incidence of approximately 1 in 7,000. Read and co-workers (1980) reported an incidence of 1 per 2,562 deliveries and concluded that the clinical picture today "is one of higher reported incidence, lower parity, greater incidence of associated placenta previa. . . ." and decreasing maternal and perinatal mortality.

ETIOLOGICAL FACTORS

Abnormal adherence of the placenta is found most often in circumstances where decidual formation was likely to have been

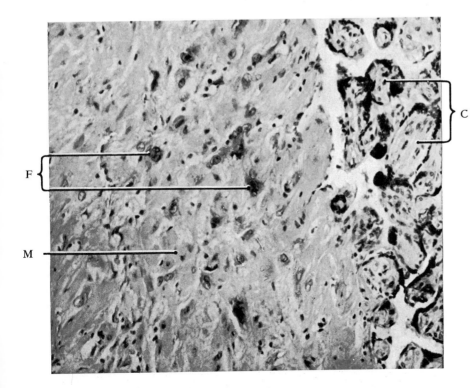

Figure 24–3. Photomicrograph of uterine wall in a case of placenta accreta. Notice the absence of decidua with chorionic villi in contact with the myometrium (C = chorionic villi; F = trophoblastic giant cells; M = myometrium).

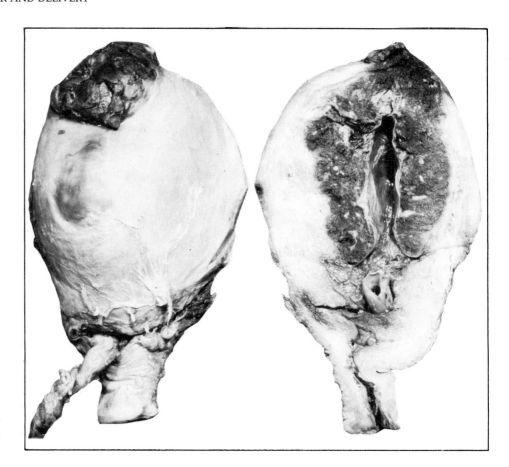

Figure 24–4. Placenta percreta. On the left, the placenta is fungating through the fundus above the old classical cesarean section scar. In the opened specimen on the right, the variable penetration of the fundus by the placenta is evident. (*From Morrison: Obstetrics and Gynecology Annual. New York, Appleton-Century-Crofts, 1978, p 113.*)

defective, for example, implantations in the lower uterine segment, or over a previous cesarean section scar or other previous incisions into the uterine cavity, or after uterine curettage. Fox (1972), in his review of 622 reported cases of placenta accreta collected between 1945 and 1969, noted the following characteristics: (1) placenta previa was identified in one third of affected pregnancies; (2) one fourth of the women had been delivered previously by cesarean section; (3) nearly one fourth of the women had previously undergone curettage; and (4) one fourth of them were gravida 6 or more. A similar result was observed by Read and co-workers for patients studied in the 1970s. However, the overall incidence and parity had decreased, likely due to limiting family size.

CLINICAL COURSE

Antepartum hemorrhage is common, but in the great majority of cases the antepartum bleeding is the consequence of a coexisting placenta previa. Invasion of the myometrium by placental villi at the site of a previous cesarean section scar may lead to rupture of the uterus during labor or even before (Berchuck and Sokol, 1983). Archer and Furlong (1987) described a woman who presented with an acute abdomen from massive hemoperitoneum caused by placenta percreta at 21 weeks' gestation. In women whose pregnancies go to term, however, labor is most likely to be normal in the absence of an associated placenta previa or an involved uterine scar.

The problems associated with delivery of the placenta and subsequent developments will vary appreciably, depending upon the site of implantation, the depth of penetration into the myometrium, and the number of cotyledons involved. It is very likely that the focal placenta accreta with implantation in the

upper segment of the uterus develops much more often than is recognized. The involved cotyledon is either pulled off the myometrium with perhaps somewhat excessive bleeding from that part of the implantation site, or the cotyledon is torn from the placenta and adheres to the implantation site with increased bleeding, immediately or later. This is probably the mechanism of formation of many so-called placental polyps (see Chap. 28, p. 483 and Fig. 28–2).

With more extensive involvement, however, hemorrhage becomes profuse as delivery of the placenta is attempted. Successful treatment depends upon immediate blood replacement therapy, as described under Obstetrical Hemorrhage in Chapter 36, (p. 698), and nearly always prompt hysterectomy.

With total involvement of the placenta (total placenta accreta), there may be very little or no bleeding from the uterus, at least until manual removal of the placenta is attempted. At times, traction on the umbilical cord will invert the uterus as described below. Moreover, usual attempts at manual removal of the placenta will not succeed, since a cleavage plane between the maternal surface of the placenta and the uterine wall cannot be developed. The safest treatment in this circumstance is prompt hysterectomy. Such a case is illustrated in Figures 24–5A through C.

The possibility exists that placenta increta might be diagnosed antepartum. Tabsh and co-workers (1982), as well as Cox and associates (1988), described a case of placenta previa in which they were also able to identify placenta increta ultrasonically from *the lack of the usual subplacental sonolucent space*. These investigators hypothesize that the presence of this normal subplacental sonolucent area represents the decidua basalis and the underlying myometrial tissue. The absence of this sono-

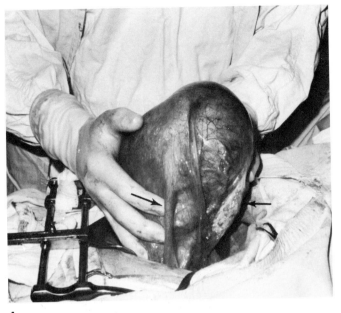

A

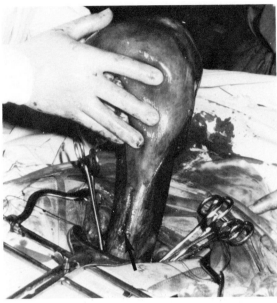

B

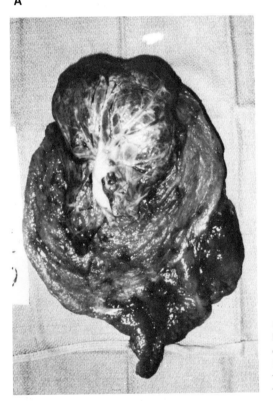

C

Figure 24–5. A. Hysterectomy for placenta accreta. The uterine fundus contains the adherent placenta. Arrows point to round ligament (*left*) and ovary (*right*) separated by the oviduct. **B.** The infundibulopelvic ligaments, broad ligaments, and cardinal ligaments have been resected. The incision in the lower segment (*arrow*) is used to palpate the margin of the cervix to identify where to enter the vagina. **C.** The uterus has been opened anteriorly to show the adherent placenta (placenta accreta).

lucent area is consistent with the presence of a placenta increta. Pasto and associates (1983) confirmed that the *absence* of a subplacental sonolucent or "hypoechoic retroplacental zone" is consistent with the presence of placenta increta.

Placenta percreta is more likely to be life threatening than is placenta accreta or placenta increta, and can cause intra-abdominal antepartum hemorrhage (Cario and colleagues, 1983) or intrapar-

tum hemorrhage, as exemplified by a case reported by Collins and associates (1978). During repeat cesarean section, severe hemorrhage began as the uterine serosa adjacent to the bladder was incised. The placenta had perforated the lower segment of the uterus and actually grown into the bladder. Removal of the placenta resulted in a 7-cm hole in the bladder. The massive hemorrhage was treated with 11 liters of blood. The infant was anemic from blood loss consequent to incision of the placenta to effect

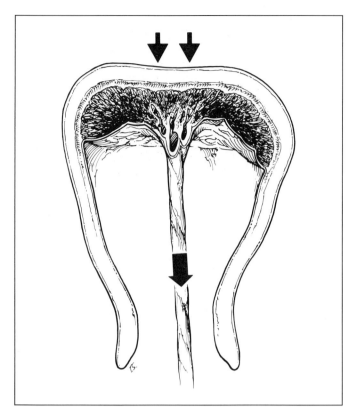

Figure 24–6. Most likely site of placental implantation in cases of uterine inversion. With traction on the cord and the placenta still attached, the likelihood of inversion is obvious.

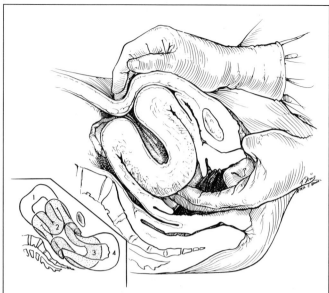

Figure 24–7. Incomplete inversion of the uterus. The diagnosis is made by abdominal palpation of the craterlike depression and vaginal palpation of the fundal wall in the lower segment and cervix. Shown in the *insert* are progressive degrees of inversion.

delivery. The mother promptly developed diabetes insipidus without evidence of anterior pituitary dysfunction.

In the 622 published cases reviewed by Fox (1972), the most common form of "conservative" management was manual removal of as much placenta as possible and then packing of the uterus. **One fourth of the women died,** that is, four times as many as when treatment consisted of immediate hysterectomy. He noted that "conservative" treatment of placenta accreta in at least four instances was followed by an apparently normal pregnancy.

INVERSION OF THE UTERUS

ETIOLOGY

Complete inversion of the uterus after delivery of the infant is almost always the consequence of strong traction on an umbilical cord that is attached to a placenta implanted in the fundus of the uterus (Fig. 24–6). Contributing to uterine inversion are a tough cord that does not readily break away from the placenta, combined with fundal pressure and a relaxed uterus, including the lower segment and cervix. Placenta accreta may be implicated although uterine inversion can occur without the placenta being so firmly adherent. At times, the inversion may be incomplete (Fig. 24–7).

The exact frequency of this complication is not known. Kitchin and co-workers (1975) reported an incidence of 1 in 2,284 deliveries. Platt and Druzin (1981) reported 28 cases in 60,052 deliveries, for an incidence of 1 in 2,148 deliveries. These same investigators suggested that parenteral magnesium sulfate, which was administered to patients with pregnancy-induced hypertension, might have played a role in the etiology of this complication. Pritchard (1982) suggested that the inexperience of personnel performing the deliveries appeared to be a more important factor!

CLINICAL COURSE

Inversion of the uterus following the third stage of labor is most often associated with immediate life-threatening hemorrhage, and without prompt treatment, it may be fatal (Fig. 24–8). It has been stated that shock tends to be disproportionate to blood loss (Greenhill and Friedman, 1974). Careful evaluation of the effects from transfusion of large volumes of blood in such cases does not support this concept, but, instead, makes it very apparent that blood loss in such circumstances was often massive but greatly underestimated. It is not unusual for even the woman who has received several units of blood because of hypotension to become anemic subsequently when isovolemic. Such outcomes are difficult to reconcile with the concept of shock out of proportion to blood loss (Platt and Druzin, 1981; Watson and associates, 1980).

TREATMENT

Delay in treatments increases the mortality rate appreciably. It is imperative that a number of steps be taken immediately and simultaneously:

1. Assistance, including an anesthesiologist, is summoned immediately.
2. The freshly inverted uterus with placenta already separated from it may often be replaced simply by immedi-

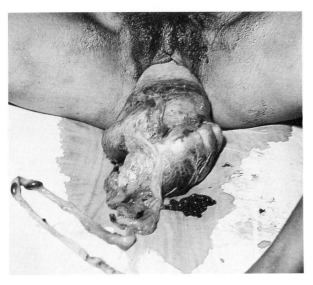

Figure 24–8. A fatal case of inverted uterus following delivery at home. The placenta was firmly adherent to its implantation site in the fundus (placenta accreta.)

4. If attached, the placenta is not removed until the infusion systems are operational, fluids are being given, and anesthesia, preferably halothane, has been administered. More recently, tocolytic drugs have been successfully used for this purpose. Terbutaline, ritodrine, and magnesium sulfate have all been used for uterine relaxation and repositioning (Catanzarite and associates, 1986; Kovacs and DeVore, 1984; Thiery and Delbeke, 1985). To remove the placenta before this time increases the hemorrhage. In the meantime, the inverted uterus, if prolapsed beyond the vagina, is replaced within the vagina.

5. After removing the placenta, the palm of the hand is placed on the center of the fundus with the fingers extended to identify the margins of the cervix. Pressure is then applied with the hand so as to push the fundus upward through the cervix.

6. Oxytocin is *not* given until after the uterus is restored to its normal configuration.

As soon as the uterus is restored to its normal configuration, the anesthetic agent used to provide relaxation is stopped and simultaneously oxytocin is started to contract the uterus while the operator maintains the fundus in normal relationship. Initially, bimanual compression, as illustrated in Figure 24–2, will aid in the control of further hemorrhage until uterine tone is recovered. After the uterus is well contracted, the operator continues to monitor the uterus transvaginally for any evidence of subsequent inversion, although this occurrence is quite unlikely.

ately pushing on the fundus with the palm of the hand and fingers in the direction of the long axis of the vagina.

3. Preferably two intravenous infusion systems are made operational, and lactated Ringer's solution and especially whole blood are given to refill the intravascular compartment and support cardiac output.

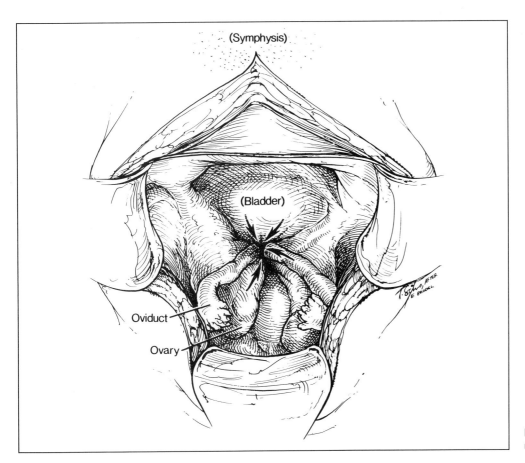

Figure 24–9. Completely inverted uterus viewed from above.

SURGICAL INTERVENTION

Most often, the inverted uterus can be restored to its normal position by the techniques described above. For example, Kitchin and associates (1975) identified 11 "spontaneous" puerperal inversions among 25,000 deliveries, and in each instance the uterus was promptly replaced vaginally without significant morbidity other than hemorrhage from the uterus while in the inverted state. If the uterus cannot be reinverted by vaginal manipulation because of a dense constriction ring, as illustrated in Figure 24–9, laparotomy is imperative. The fundus may then be simultaneously pushed upward from below and pulled from above. A traction suture well placed in the inverted fundus may be of aid. If the constriction ring still prohibits reposition, it is carefully incised posteriorly to expose the fundus. A graphic outline of this surgical technique has been reported (vanVugt and associates, 1981). After replacement of the fundus, the anesthetic agent used to relax the myometrium is stopped, oxytocin infusion is begun, and the uterine incision is repaired. Following restoration of the uterus, the adjacent viscera are carefully examined for trauma.

REFERENCES

Archer GE, Furlong LA: Acute abdomen caused by placenta percreta in the second trimester. Am J Obstet Gynecol 157:146, 1987

Berchuck A, Sokol RJ: Previous cesarean section, placenta increta, and uterine rupture in second-trimester abortion. Am J Obstet Gynecol 145:766, 1983

Bove JR: Transfusion-associated hepatitis and AIDS—What is the risk? N Engl J Med 317:242, 1987

Breen JL, Neubecker R, Gregori CA, Franklin JE Jr: Placenta accreta, increta, and percreta: A survey of 40 cases. Obstet Gynecol 49:43, 1977

Buttino L, Garite TJ: The use of 15 methyl F$_{2\alpha}$ prostaglandin (prostin 15M) for the control of postpartum hemorrhage. Am J Perinatol 3:241, 1986

Cario GM, Adler AD, Morris N: Placenta percreta presenting as intra-abdominal antepartum hemorrhage: Case report. Br J Obstet Gynaecol 90:491, 1983

Catanzarite VA, Moffitt KD, Baker ML, Awadalla SG, Argubright KF, Perkins RP: New approaches to the management of acute puerperal uterine invasion. Obstet Gynecol 68:7S, 1986

Collins ML, O'Brien P, Tabrah N: Placenta previa percreta with bladder invasion. JAMA 240:1749, 1978

Cox SM, Carpenter RJ, Cotton DB: Placenta percreta: Ultrasound diagnosis and conservative surgical management. Obstet Gynecol 72:452, 1988

DeLeeuw NKM, Lowenstein L, Tucker EC, Dayal S: Correlation of red cell loss at delivery with changes in red cell mass. Am J Obstet Gynecol 84:1271, 1968

DiZerega G, Kletzky OA, Mishell DR Jr: Diagnosis of Sheehan's syndrome using a sequential stimulation test. Am J Obstet Gynecol 132:348, 1978

Eidelman AI, Kamar R, Schimmel MS, Bar-On E: The grandmultipara: Is she still a risk? Am J Obstet Gynecol 158:389, 1988

Fox H: Placenta accreta, 1945–1969. Obstet Gynecol Surv 27:475, 1972

Fuchs K, Peretz B-A, Marcovici R, Paldi E, Timor-Tritsh I: The "grand multipara"—Is it a problem? A review of 5785 cases. Int J Gynaecol Obstet 23:321, 1985

Gilstrap LC, Hauth JC, Hankins GDV, Patterson AR: Effect of type of anesthesia on blood loss at cesarean section. Obstet Gynecol 69:328, 1987

Greenhill JP, Friedman EA: Biological Principles and Modern Practice of Obstetrics. Philadelphia, Saunders, 1974, p 687

Grimes HG, Brooks MH: Pregnancy in Sheehan's syndrome. Report of a case and review. Obstet Gynecol Surv 35:481, 1980

Haddock L, Vega LA, Aguilo F, Rodriguez O: Adrenocortical, thyroidal and human growth hormone reserve in Sheehan's syndrome. Johns Hopkins Med J 131:80, 1972

Hankins GDV, Berry GK, Scott RT Jr, Hood D: Maternal arterial desaturation with 15-methyl prostaglandin F$_2$ alpha for uterine atony. Obstet Gynecol 65:605, 1985

Hayashi RH, Castillo MS, Noah ML: Management of severe postpartum hemorrhage with a prostaglandin F$_{2\alpha}$ analogue. Obstet Gynecol 63:806, 1984

Kaunitz AM, Hughs JM, Grimes DA, Smith JC, Rochat RW, Kafrissen ME: Causes of maternal mortality in the United States. Obstet Gynecol 65:605, 1985

Kitchin JD III, Thiagarajah S, May HV Jr, Thornton WN Jr: Puerperal inversion of the uterus. Am J Obstet Gynecol 123:51, 1975

Kovacs BW, DeVore GR: Management of acute and subacute puerperal uterine inversion with terbutaline sulfate. Am J Obstet Gynecol 150:784, 1984

Magil M: PGF$_{2\alpha}$ for postpartum hemorrhage—How well does it work? Contemp Ob/Gyn 23:111, 1984

Newton M: Postpartum hemorrhage. Am J Obstet Gynecol 94:711, 1966

Odell LD, Seski A: Episiotomy blood loss. Am J Obstet Gynecol 54:51, 1947

Pasto ME, Kurtz AB, Rifkin MD, Cole-Beuglet C, Wapner RJ, Goldberg BB: Ultrasonographic findings in placenta increta. J Ultrasound Med 2:155, 1983

Platt LD, Druzin ML: Acute puerperal inversion of the uterus. Am J Obstet Gynecol 141:187, 1981

Pritchard JA: Changes in the blood volume during pregnancy and delivery. Anesthesiology 26:393, 1965

Pritchard JA: Magnesium sulfate and uterine inversion. Am J Obstet Gynecol 143:725, 1982

Pritchard JA, Baldwin RM, Dickey JC, Wiggins KM: Blood volume changes in pregnancy and the puerperium: II. Red blood cell loss and changes in apparent blood volume during and following vaginal delivery, cesarean section, and cesarean section plus total hysterectomy. Am J Obstet Gynecol 84:1271, 1962

Read JA, Cotton DB, Miller FC: Placenta accreta: Changing clinical aspects and outcome. Obstet Gynecol 56:31, 1980

Sheehan HL, Murdoch R: Postpartum necrosis of the anterior pituitary: Pathological and clinical aspects. Br J Obstet Gynaecol 45:456, 1938

Tabsh KMA, Brinkman CR III, King W: Ultrasound diagnosis of placenta increta. J Clin Ultrasound 10:288, 1982

Thiery M, Delbeke L: Acute puerperal uterine inversion: Two-step management with a β-mimetic and a prostaglandin. Am J Obstet Gynecol 153:891, 1985

van Vugt PJH, Baudoin P, Blom VM, van Duersen TBM: Inversio uteri puerperalis. Acta Obstet Gynecol Scand 60:353, 1981

Ward JW, Holmberg SD, Allen JR, Cohn DL, Critchley SE, Kleinman SH, Lenes BP, Ravenholt O, Davis JR, Quinn MG, Jaffee HW: Transmission of human immunodeficiency virus (HIV) by blood transfusions screened as negative for HIV antibody. N England J Med 318:473, 1988

Watson P, Besch N, Bowes WA Jr: Management of acute and subacute puerperal inversion of the uterus. Obstet Gynecol 55:12, 1980

Whitehead R: The hypothalamus in post-partum hypopituitarism. J Pathol Bact 86:55, 1963

OPERATIVE OBSTETRICS

Forceps Delivery and Related Techniques

Obstetrical forceps are designed for extraction of the fetus. The intriguing history of the early development and use of these instruments is presented at the end of this chapter.

GENERAL DESIGN

Forceps vary considerably in size and shape but consist basically of two crossing *branches* that are introduced separately into the vagina. Each branch is maneuvered into appropriate relationship with the fetal head and then articulated. Basically, each branch has four components. These are the *blade*, the *shank*, the *lock*, and the *handle*. Each blade has two curves, the *cephalic* and the *pelvic*. The cephalic curve conforms to the shape of the fetal head and the pelvic curve with that of the birth canal. The blades are oval to elliptical in outline and some varieties are fenestrated rather than solid to permit a more firm hold on the fetal head.

The cephalic curve (Fig. 25–1) should be large enough to grasp the fetal head firmly without compression, but not so large that the instrument slips. The pelvic curve (Fig. 25–1) corresponds more or less to the axis of the birth canal but varies considerably among different instruments. The blades are connected to the handles by the shanks, which give the requisite length to the instrument.

The kind of articulation, or *forceps lock*, varies among different instruments. The common method of articulation consists of a socket located on the shank at the junction with the handle and into which fits a socket similarly located on the opposite shank (Figs. 25–1 and 25–2). This form of articulation is commonly referred to as the *English lock*. A *sliding lock* is used in some forceps, for example, Kielland forceps (Fig. 25–3) and Barton forceps, in which a single U-shaped receptacle mounted midway on the left shank accepts the shank of the right branch. The sliding lock allows the shanks to move forward and backward independently. The components of a quite different type of lock, the *French lock*, are a threaded eye bolt screwed partway into a threaded hole in the left shank and a notch in the right shank that articulates with the eye bolt. After each branch has been applied to the fetal head, the notch is moved over the stem of the eye bolt and the eye bolt is tightened to lock the branches firmly together.

DEFINITIONS AND CLASSIFICATION

Forceps used to aid in the delivery of a fetus presenting by the vertex are classified as follows, according to the level and position of the head in the birth canal at the time the blades are applied:

Low forceps (outlet forceps) operations are those in which the instrument is applied after the fetal head has reached the perineal floor, the sagittal suture is in the anteroposterior diameter of the outlet, and the scalp is visible at the vaginal introitus.

Midforceps operations are those in which forceps are applied before the criteria for low forceps are met but after engagement of the fetal head has taken place. Clinical evidence of engagement is usually afforded by the descent of the lowermost part of the skull to or below the level of the ischial spines, since the distance between the level of the ischial spines and the pelvic inlet is ordinarily greater than the distance from the biparietal diameter to the leading part of the fetal head (see Chap. 8, p. 169). Especially after vigorous labor, elongation of the fetal head from the combination of a marked degree of molding and caput formation will create the erroneous impression that the head is engaged even though the biparietal diameter has not passed through the pelvic inlet (see Chap. 20, p. 379).

Because the definition of midforceps may include many stations of the fetal head, the Maternal Fetal Medicine Committee of the American College of Obstetricians and Gynecologists (1988) recently reclassified forceps applications as follows:

1. **Outlet forceps.** The fetal skull has reached the perineal floor, the scalp is visible between contractions, the sagittal suture is in the anterior-posterior diameter or in the right or left occiput anterior or posterior position, but not more than 45 degrees from the midline.
2. **Low forceps.** The leading edge of the skull is station +2 (in centimeters) or more. Rotations are divided into 45 degrees or less and more than 45 degrees.
3. **Midforceps.** The head is engaged but the leading edge of the skull is above +2 station (in centimeters).

The danger of trauma to the fetus and the mother from low forceps delivery by this definition will vary remarkably depend-

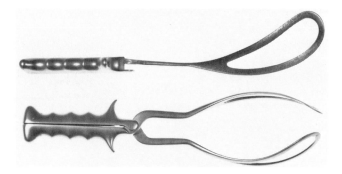

Figure 25–1. Simpson forceps. Note the ample pelvic curve in the single blade above and cephalic curve evident in the articulated blades below. The fenestrated blade and the wide shank in front of the English-style lock characterize the Simpson forceps.

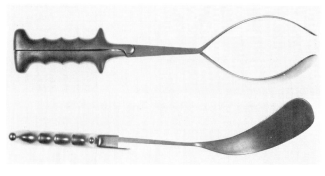

Figure 25–2. Tucker–McLane forceps. The blade is solid and the shank is narrow.

ing upon the circumstances preceding delivery. **It is emphasized that station here is measured in centimeters (0 to +5), rather than by dividing the lower pelvis into thirds (see Chap. 16, p. 308).** At times, the fetal head, as the consequence of appropriate uterine contractions and voluntary expulsive efforts of the mother, will descend to lie firmly against the perineum with the sagittal suture anteroposterior; subsequent to anesthesia for delivery, however, the fetal head will recede somewhat from the perineum and the sagittal suture will revert to an oblique position. Forceps delivery with episiotomy in this circumstance is very likely to be a benign procedure. On the other hand, if the fetal head has *never* reached the perineum and the sagittal suture has never achieved the anteroposterior position, low forceps delivery, by this definition, may prove traumatic to fetus, mother, or both.

High forceps operations are those in which forceps are applied before engagement. High forceps delivery has no place in obstetrics.

INCIDENCE

During much of the first half of this century, polarization of opinions over the use of forceps in obstetrics resulted in two very distinct schools of thought. One school vigorously maintained that forceps delivery should be accomplished as soon as the fetal head was engaged and the cervix fully dilated (or, at times, dilatable). The other contended with equal vigor that spontaneous delivery should be awaited. It was shown subsequently by objective analysis that there was increased perinatal mortality and morbidity and maternal morbidity from midforceps delivery; however, more recent studies to be cited do not confirm these associations. Moreover, there may be less perinatal and maternal morbidity with truly outlet forceps delivery and an adequate episiotomy compared to delayed spontaneous delivery without episiotomy.

In general, the incidence of forceps operations in any given institution will depend upon the attitude of the staff, the kinds of analgesia and anesthesia used for labor and delivery, and the parity of the obstetrical population. For example, at Parkland Hospital, the incidence of forceps delivery is about 5 percent for all women delivered vaginally, and 95 percent of these operations are outlet forceps. This incidence is undoubtedly influenced by the size of our busy obstetrical service in which junior housestaff and nurse midwives perform most of the uncomplicated deliveries and in which only about 2 percent of women are given lumbar epidural analgesia for labor.

FUNCTIONS AND CHOICE OF THE FORCEPS

The forceps may be used as a tractor or a rotator, or both. Its most important function is traction, although, particularly in transverse and posterior positions of the occiput, forceps may be employed successfully for rotation. Any properly shaped instrument will give satisfactory results, provided it is used intelligently. For general purposes, either Simpson or Tucker–McLane forceps are quite useful. In general, Simpson forceps are used to deliver the fetus with a molded head such as is common in nulliparous women. The Tucker–McLane instrument is used for the fetus with a rounded head, which is more characteristically seen in multiparous patients. In some circumstances, more specialized forceps may be preferable, for example, in some cases of *deep transverse arrest*. (When the progress of labor ceases with the fetal head in the transverse position, well down in the pelvis with the occiput below the spines, the situation is referred to as deep transverse arrest.) If there is no cephalopelvic disproportion, transverse arrest may be overcome with oxytocin stimulation, with resulting descent of the head to the perineum and spontaneous anterior rotation. **If, however, there are indications for prompt delivery, as in instances of fetal distress, but safe vaginal delivery without delay cannot be anticipated, then cesarean section should be used.**

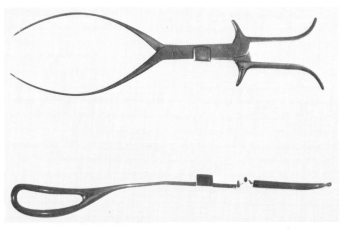

Figure 25–3. Kielland forceps. The characteristic features are the sliding lock, a minimal pelvic curvature, and light weight.

FORCES EXERTED BY THE FORCEPS

Obstetricians have long been interested in the forces exerted by the forceps blades on the fetal skull and maternal tissues. If excessive, these forces can be damaging to both the woman and her fetus. From experiments conducted on women in labor more than a century ago, Joulin (1867) estimated that a pull in excess of 60 kg might damage the fetal skull. These crude studies and subsequent ones have furnished only a gross approximation, for the force produced by the forceps on the fetal skull is a complex function of both pull and compression by the forceps and of friction produced by the maternal tissues.

INDICATIONS FOR THE USE OF FORCEPS

The termination of labor by forceps, provided it can be accomplished without trauma, is indicated in any condition threatening the mother or fetus that is likely to be relieved by delivery. Such maternal indications include heart disease, acute pulmonary edema, intrapartum infection, or exhaustion. Fetal indications include prolapse of the umbilical cord, premature separation of the placenta, and abnormalities in fetal heart rate indicative of fetal jeopardy.

ELECTIVE AND OUTLET FORCEPS

The vast majority of forceps operations performed in this country today are elective forceps. Within the past decade, lumbar epidural analgesia for labor and delivery has become very popular in the United States. Epidural injection of anesthetic agents usually also induces motor blockade sufficient to inhibit maternal expulsive efforts. In order to effect delivery, outlet forceps then are indicated (see Chap. 17, p. 338).

The fact that the methods employed to relieve pain frequently necessitate forceps delivery is not an indictment of the procedures, provided the obstetrician adheres strictly to the definition of outlet forceps. The fetal head must be on the perineal floor with the sagittal suture no more than 45 degrees. In these circumstances, forceps delivery preceded by episiotomy is a simple and safe operation. By allowing the woman in labor ample time, the criteria for outlet forceps can usually be met despite the effects of analgesia. *However, if the head does not descend and rotate, any forceps operation performed is not an outlet forceps procedure.* If anterior rotation is the only criterion not met for outlet forceps, then delivery usually can be accomplished safely; however, in general, the head is higher before rotation occurs. In this latter circumstance, the operation is at least low forceps by the Maternal Fetal Medicine Committee definition (p. 425). To maximize safety for mother and fetus, therefore, forceps should not be used *electively* until the criteria for outlet forceps are fulfilled.

"PROPHYLACTIC" FORCEPS DELIVERY

In a minority of nulliparous women, marked resistance of the perineum and the vaginal introitus may sometimes present a serious obstacle to the passage of the fetus, even when the expulsive forces are normal. In such cases, an episiotomy and outlet forceps delivery are beneficial to mother and fetus. Since it was held widely at the time that prolonged pressure of the fetal head against a rigid perineum might result in fetal brain damage, DeLee (1920) recommended the "prophylactic forceps" operation. In this scheme, interference is elective with knowledge that it is not absolutely necessary and that spontaneous delivery may be forthcoming within 15 minutes. There is no evidence that such "prophylatic forceps" are beneficial in the otherwise normal labor and delivery.

Prophylactic Low Forceps for Small Fetuses

Bishop and associates (1965), after analyzing data from the Collaborative Perinatal Project, suggested that prophylactic outlet forceps delivery improved neonatal outcome in low-birthweight infants. There appeared to be improved mental and motor performance at 8 months and improved neurological function at 1 year of age in low-birthweight infants delivered by low forceps rather than spontaneously. Dewhurst (1976) and Hobel and associates (1980) recommended this approach in the management of preterm and small fetuses, apparently based upon the report of Bishop.

Subsequently, the practice of prophylactic forceps for the delivery of small fetuses has been questioned. Haesslein and Goodlin (1979) reported that the incidence of intraventricular hemorrhage in vertex infants 800 to 1,350 g was two times as high in neonates delivered electively by low forceps as in infants delivered spontaneously. O'Driscoll and associates (1981) reported that in preterm infants only those delivered by outlet forceps suffered traumatic intracranial hemorrhage at birth. It is fair to point out that these studies were retrospective and undoubtedly had inherent biases. For example, the effects of labor itself in the genesis of intraventricular hemorrhage must be considered (see Chap. 38, p. 755). Fairweather (1981) reported no significant differences in outcomes in neonates who weighed 500 to 1,500 g delivered spontaneously or by low forceps. Schwartz and colleagues (1983) reported similar findings. More recently, Anderson and associates (1988) presented preliminary findings consistent with the view that forceps delivery was protective against progression of periventricular hemorrhage in vaginally delivered neonates who weighed less than 1,750 g.

At present, there appears to be no obvious advantage to outlet forceps delivery of a small fetus and the real possibility of harm exists with their use. In such cases, the obstetrician should perform an appropriately large episiotomy in an attempt to increase the size of the vaginal outlet and perineum, thus hopefully ensuring the least trauma to the infant. If the perineum and vaginal introitus are already relaxed, an incision is not necessary.

PREREQUISITES FOR APPLICATION OF FORCEPS

There are at least six prerequisites for the successful application of forceps.

1. **The head must be engaged and preferably deeply engaged.** Application of the blades before engagement, that is, high forceps, is an extremely difficult operation, often entailing brutal trauma to the maternal tissues and death of a large proportion of the babies. Many years ago, when cesarean section was also a highly dangerous operation, high forceps might have had a place in operative obstetrics. Delivery by high forceps should never be done today, however, and is mentioned here only to be condemned. Even after engagement occurs, the higher the station of the fetal head, the more difficult and traumatic the forceps delivery becomes. Moreover, whenever the blades are applied before the head has reached the perineal floor, it is common to find the head decidedly higher than was

believed to be the case from the findings of vaginal examination. This occurs because of extensive caput succedaneum formation and molding. These difficulties of midforceps operation may be encountered even in the presence of a valid maternal indication for forceps delivery. For instance, it is generally agreed that women with heart disease should be spared, as much as safely possible, the effort of bearing down during the second stage of labor. Such efforts, however, may prove much less harmful than a difficult midforceps delivery. Therefore, forceps should not be used until the station of the head is low enough to ensure a nontraumatic operative procedure. The same generalization applies to forceps for fetal distress when the head is not close to the perineal floor. Granted that the fetal heart rate in such a case may suggest that the infant is in jeopardy, it may still be judicious to allow more time for the head to descend rather than superimpose the trauma of a difficult midforceps operation on an already distressed infant. If delivery is mandatory, cesarean section is preferable to a difficult and damaging forceps operation.

2. **The fetus must present either by the vertex or by the face with the chin anterior.** The use of forceps is not applicable, of course, to transverse lies (shoulder presentation), nor is it intended for the breech.

3. **The position of the head must be precisely known so that the forceps can be appropriately applied to the fetal head.** So-called pelvic application can be dangerous.

4. **The cervix must be completely dilated before the application of forceps.** Even a small rim of cervix may offer great resistance when traction is applied, causing extensive cervical lacerations that may reach the lower uterine segment. If prompt delivery becomes imperative before complete dilatation of the cervix, cesarean section is preferable.

5. **Before forceps application, the membranes must be ruptured to permit a firm grasp of the head by the blades of the forceps.**

6. **There should be no disproportion between the size of the head and that of the pelvic inlet, the midpelvis or the outlet.**

TECHNIQUES OF OUTLET FORCEPS OPERATIONS

PREPARATIONS FOR OPERATION

In the absence of previously instituted adequate continuous conduction analgesia, a decision as to the type of analgesia or anesthesia is made based on factors considered especially in Chapter 17. In many cases, pudendal block will not provide sufficient analgesia for forceps delivery. If spinal analgesia is to be used, the anesthetic agent is introduced before placing the woman in the lithotomy position for delivery. If general anesthesia is to be used, the woman is placed in the lithotomy position, the perineum is cleansed and draped, and the obstetrician is ready to perform the forceps delivery before administering the anesthetic.

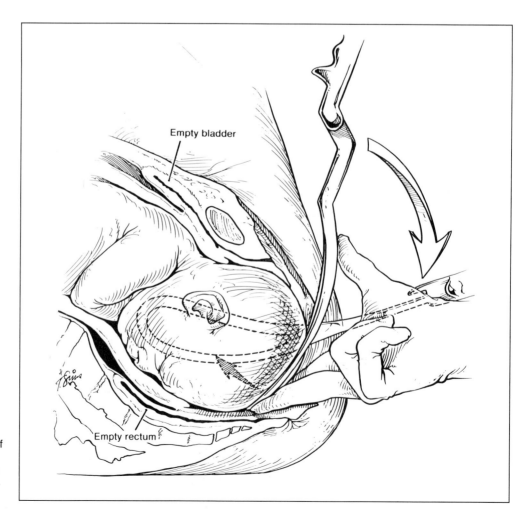

Figure 25–4. The fetus is presenting as vertex with the occiput anterior and crowning. The application of the left blade of the Simpson forceps is shown. Next, the right blade is applied and the blades are articulated.

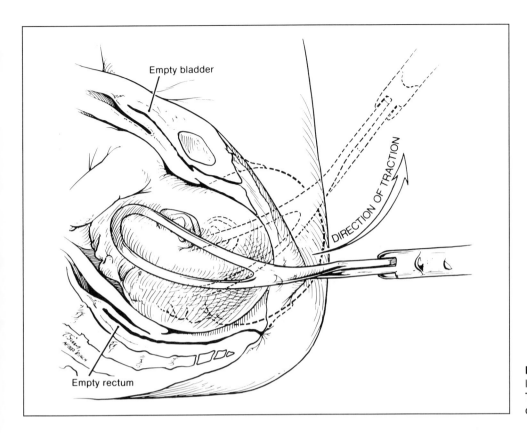

Figure 25–5. Occiput anterior. Delivery by outlet forceps (Simpson). The direction of gentle traction for delivery of the head is indicated.

The woman's buttocks should be brought to the edge of the delivery table, and her legs held in position by appropriate stirrups. She is scrubbed and draped as described in Chapter 16 (p. 309). The bladder should be emptied by catheterization if a midforceps delivery is planned.

APPLICATION OF FORCEPS

Forceps are constructed so that their cephalic curve is closely adapted to the sides of the fetal head (Fig. 25–4). The biparietal diameter of the fetal head corresponds to the greatest distance between the appropriately applied blades. Consequently, the head of the fetus is perfectly grasped only when the long axis of the blades corresponds to the occipitomental diameter, with the tips of the blades lying over the cheeks, while the concave margins of the blades are directed toward either the sagittal suture (occiput anterior position) or the face (occiput posterior position). Consideration must be given to the degree of molding. Thus applied, the forceps should not slip, and traction may be applied most advantageously as illustrated in Figure 25–5. When forceps are applied obliquely, however, with one blade over the brow and the other over the opposite mastoid region, the grasp is less secure, and the fetal head is exposed to injurious pressure (Fig. 25–6). With most forceps, if one blade is applied over the brow and the other over the occiput, the instrument cannot be locked (Fig. 25–7), or, if locked, the blades slip off when traction is applied (Fig. 25–8), causing appreciable trauma. For these reasons, the forceps must be applied directly to the sides of the head along the *occipitomental diameter*, in what is termed the biparietal or bimalar application.

IDENTIFICATION OF POSITION

Precise knowledge of the exact position of the fetal head is essential to a proper cephalic application. With the head low down in the pelvis, diagnosis of position is made by examina-

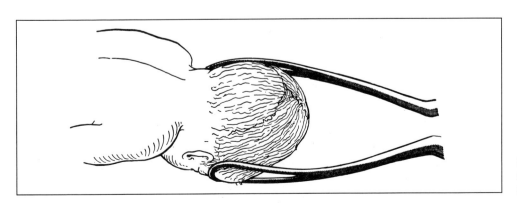

Figure 25–6. Incorrect application of forceps over brow and mastoid region.

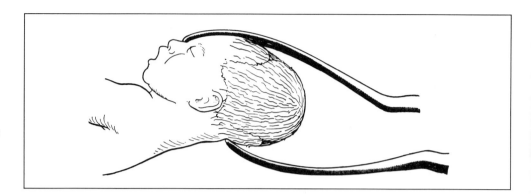

Figure 25–7. Incorrect application of forceps, one blade over the occiput and the other over the brow. Note that the forceps cannot be locked.

tion of the sagittal suture and the fontanels, but when it is at a higher station, an absolute diagnosis can be made by locating the posterior ear.

The term *pelvic application* is employed when the left blade is applied to the left and right blade to the right side of the woman's pelvis, irrespective of the position of the fetal head. It follows that the head is grasped satisfactorily only when the sagittal suture happens to be directly anteroposterior. Pelvic application is likely to be injurious to the fetus and should not be practiced.

OUTLET FORCEPS DELIVERY

Delivery by outlet forceps is illustrated in Figures 25–9 through 25–16. With the head at the low station required in the definition of outlet forceps, the obstacle to delivery is usually insufficient expulsive forces, appreciable resistance of the perineum, or both. In such circumstances, the sagittal suture occupies the anteroposterior diameter of the pelvic outlet, with the small (posterior) fontanel directed toward either the symphysis pubis or the concavity of the sacrum. In either event, the forceps, if applied to the sides of the pelvis, grasps the head ideally. The left blade is introduced by the left hand into the left side of the pelvis and then the right blade is introduced by the right hand into the right side of the pelvis, as follows: Two fingers of the right hand are introduced inside the left, posterior portion of the vulva and into the vagina beside the fetal head. The handle of the left branch is then grasped between the thumb and two fingers of the left hand, as in holding a pen, and the tip of the blade is gently passed into the vagina between the fetal head and the palmar surface of the fingers of the right hand, which

serve as a guide. The handle and branch are held at first almost vertically, but as the blade adapts itself to the fetal head, they are depressed, eventually to a horizontal position. The guiding fingers are then withdrawn, and the handle is left unsupported or held by an assistant. Similarly, two fingers of the left hand are then introduced into the right, posterior portion of the vagina to serve as a guide for the right blade, which is held in the right hand and introduced into the vagina. These guiding fingers are then withdrawn and the horizontally positioned branches are articulated, usually without difficulty. Otherwise, first one and then the other blade should be gently maneuvered until the handles are repositioned to effect easy articulation.

Appropriateness of Application

The application is now checked before any traction is applied. For the occiput anterior position, appropriately applied blades are equidistant from the sagittal suture. In the occiput posterior position the blades are equidistant from the midline of the face and brow. If cervical tissue has been grasped, the forceps should be loosened and, if possible, the incompletely retracted cervix pushed up over the head. Otherwise, labor is allowed to continue or cesarean section is performed.

Traction with Forceps

When it is certain that the blades are placed satisfactorily and the cervix is not entrapped, gentle, intermittent, horizontal traction is exerted until the perineum begins to bulge. Traction with forceps is always applied gently and never with excessive force. As the vulva is distended by the occiput, the handles are gradually elevated, eventually pointing almost directly upward as the parietal bones emerge. With the fetal head in the occiput

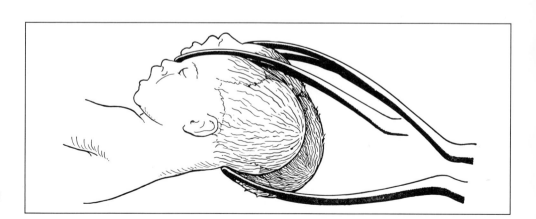

Figure 25–8. Forceps applied **incorrectly** as in Figure 25–7. Note extension of head and tendency of blades to slip off with traction.

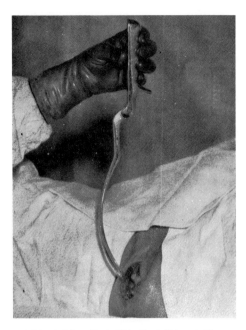

Figure 25–9. The left handle held in the left hand. Simpson forceps.

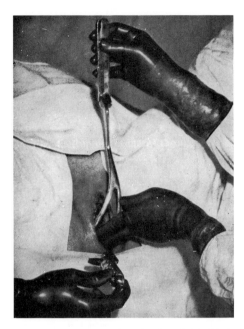

Figure 25–11. Left blade in place; introduction of right blade by right hand.

anterior position, this maneuver takes advantage of the smallest diameters of the fetal head and brings the suboccipital region beneath the symphysis. As the handles are raised, the head is extended. Episiotomy is rarely performed immediately prior to application of the blades but most often when forceps traction on the head begins to distend the perineum. During upward traction, the four fingers should grasp the upper surface of the handles and shanks, while the thumb exerts the necessary force upon their lower surface, as shown in Figure 25–15.

During the birth of the head, spontaneous delivery should be simulated as closely as possible, employing minimal force.

Traction should therefore be intermittent, and the head should be allowed to recede in intervals, as in spontaneous labor. Except when urgently indicated, as in severe fetal distress, delivery should be sufficiently slow, deliberate, and gentle to prevent undue compression of the fetal head. With this in mind, it is preferable to apply traction with each uterine contraction.

After the vulva has been well distended by the head and the brow can be felt through the perineum, the delivery may be completed in several ways. Some obstetricians keep the forceps in place, in the belief that greatest control of the advance of the head is thus maintained. The thickness of the blades may at

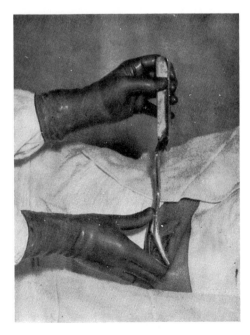

Figure 25–10. Introduction of left blade into left side of pelvis.

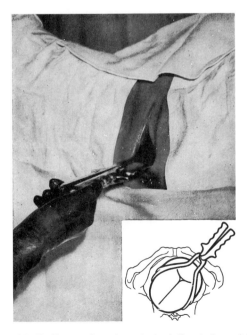

Figure 25–12. Forceps have been locked. (Inset shows LOA.)

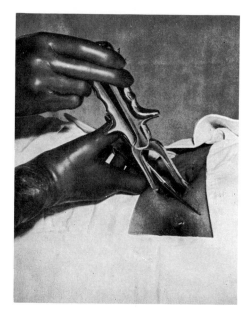

Figure 25–13. Median or mediolateral episiotomy may be performed at this point. Left mediolateral episiotomy shown here.

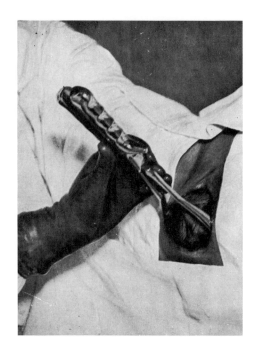

Figure 25–15. Upward traction.

times add to the distension of the vulva, however, thus increasing the likelihood of laceration or necessitating a large episiotomy. In such cases, the forceps are removed and delivery is completed by the modified Ritgen maneuver (Fig. 25–16), slowly extending the head by using upward pressure upon the chin through the posterior portion of the perineum, while covering the anus with a towel to minimize contamination from the bowel. If the forceps are removed prematurely, the modified Ritgen maneuver may prove to be a tedious and inelegant procedure.

LOW AND MIDFORCEPS OPERATIONS

When the head lies above the perineum, the sagittal suture usually occupies an oblique or transverse diameter of the pelvis. In such cases, the forceps should always be applied to the sides of the head. The application is best accomplished by introducing two or more fingers into the vagina to a sufficient depth to feel the posterior fetal ear, over which, whether right or left, the first blade should be applied.

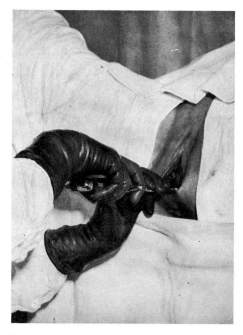

Figure 25–14. Horizontal traction; operator seated.

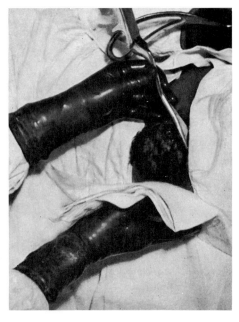

Figure 25–16. Disarticulation of branches of forceps. Beginning modified Ritgen maneuver.

LEFT OCCIPUT ANTERIOR POSITION

In left occiput anterior positions, the right hand, introduced into the left posterior segment of the vagina, should identify the posteriorly located left ear and at the same time serve as a guide for introduction of the left branch of the forceps, which is held in the left hand and applied over the left ear. The guiding hand is then withdrawn, and the handle is held by an assistant or left unsupported, the blade usually retaining its position without difficulty. Two fingers of the left hand are then introduced into the right posterior portion of the pelvis, but no attempt is yet made to reach the anteriorly located right ear, which lies near the right iliopectineal eminence. The right branch of the forceps, held in the right hand, is then introduced along the left hand as a guide. It must then be applied over the anterior ear of the fetus by gently sweeping the blade anteriorly until it lies directly opposite the blade that was introduced first. Of the two branches, when articulated, one occupies the posterior and the other the anterior extremity of the left oblique diameter.

RIGHT OCCIPUT ANTERIOR POSITION

In right positions, the blades are introduced similarly but in opposite directions, for in those cases the right ear of the fetus is the posterior ear, over which the first blade must be placed accordingly. After the blades have been applied to the sides of the head, the left handle and shank lie above the right. Consequently, the forceps does not immediately articulate. Locking of the branches is easily effected, however, by rotating the left around the right to bring the lock into proper position.

OCCIPUT TRANSVERSE POSITIONS

If the occiput is in a transverse position, the forceps are introduced similarly, with the first blade applied over the posterior ear, and the second rotated anteriorly to a position opposite the first. In this case, one blade lies in front of the sacrum and the other behind the symphysis. The conventional Simpson or Tucker–McLane forceps (Figs. 25–1 and 25–2) or the specialized Kielland (Fig. 25–3) or Barton forceps may be used.

ROTATION FROM ANTERIOR AND TRANSVERSE POSITIONS

When the occiput is obliquely anterior, it gradually rotates spontaneously to the symphysis pubis as traction is exerted.

When it is directed transversely, however, in order to bring it anteriorly a rotary motion of the forceps is required. The direction of rotation, of course, varies with the position of the occiput. Rotation counterclockwise from the left side toward the midline is required when the occiput is directed toward the left, and in the reverse direction when it is directed toward the right side of the pelvis. Infrequently, particularly when the Barton forceps are used in transverse positions in anteroposteriorly flattened (platypelloid) pelves, rotation should not be attempted until the fetal head has reached or approached the pelvic floor. Premature attempts at anterior rotation under such conditions may result in injury to the fetus and maternal soft parts. Regardless of the original position of the head, delivery is eventually effected by exerting traction downward until the occiput appears at the vulva; the rest of the operation is completed as described.

In exerting traction before the head appears at the vulva, one or both hands may be employed. To avoid excessive force, the operator should sit with his arms flexed and elbows held closely against the thorax, since the obstetrician's body weight must not be applied.

OCCIPUT POSTERIOR POSITIONS

OBLIQUELY POSTERIOR POSITIONS

Prompt delivery may at times become necessary when the small (occipital) fontanel is directed toward one of the sacroiliac synchondroses, namely, in right occiput posterior and left occiput posterior positions. When delivery is required in either instance, the head is often imperfectly flexed. In some cases, when the hand is introduced into the vagina to locate the posterior ear, the occiput rotates spontaneously toward the anterior, indicating that manual rotation of the fetal head might be easily accomplished.

MANUAL ROTATION FROM POSTERIOR POSITIONS

The requirements for forceps must be met. A hand with the palm upward is inserted into the vagina and the fingers are brought in contact with that side of the fetal head that is to be pushed toward the anterior position while the thumb is placed over the opposite side of the head (Fig. 25–17A, B). With the

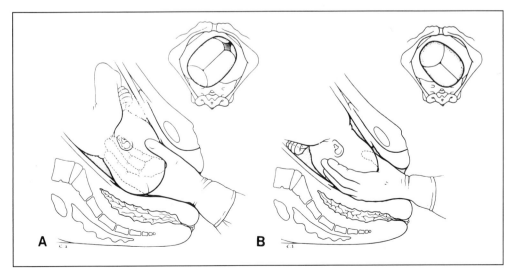

Figure 25–17. A. Manual rotation, left hand in position grasping the head. **B.** Manual rotation accomplished to ROA. Note that with rotation to the ROA position the fetal head may become more flexed. (*Both A and B from Douglas and Stromme: Operative Obstetrics, 3rd ed. New York, Appleton-Century-Crofts, 1976.*)

occiput in a right posterior position, the left hand is used to rotate the occiput anteriorly in a clockwise direction; the right hand is used for the left occiput posterior position. At the beginning of the rotation, it may be helpful to dislodge the head *slightly* upward in the birth canal but the head must not be disengaged. After the occiput has reached the anterior position, labor may be allowed to continue or, more commonly, forceps used to effect delivery. First one blade is applied to that side of the head which is held by the fingers to help maintain the occiput in the anterior position. The other blade is immediately applied and delivery accomplished as described for occiput anterior forceps delivery.

FORCEPS DELIVERY AS OCCIPUT POSTERIOR

If manual rotation cannot be accomplished easily, application of the blades to the head in the posterior position and delivery from the occiput posterior position is the safest procedure (Fig. 25–18). In many of these cases, the cause of the persistent occiput posterior position and of the difficulty in accomplishing rotation is an anthropoid pelvis, the architecture of which predisposes to posterior delivery and opposes rotation. When the occiput is directly posterior, horizontal traction should be applied until the root of the nose is under the symphysis. The handles should then be slowly elevated until the occiput gradually emerges over the anterior margin of the perineum. Then, by imparting a downward motion to the instrument, the nose, face, and chin successively emerge from the vulva. The extraction is more difficult than when the occiput is anterior, and because of greater distension of the vulva, a larger episiotomy is

needed in order to prevent perineal lacerations which are common without such an episiotomy (Fig. 25–18).

FORCEPS ROTATIONS FROM POSTERIOR POSITIONS

Tucker–McLane, Simpson, or Kielland forceps may be used to try to rotate the fetal head. The occiput may be rotated 45 degrees to the posterior position or 135 degrees to the anterior (Fig. 25–19). If rotation is performed with Tucker–McLane or Simpson forceps, the head must be flexed, but this is not necessary with Kielland instruments since they have a more straightened pelvic curve. Forceps rotations should be performed under the guidance of those who are experienced in these operations. In rotating the occiput anteriorly with forceps, the pelvic curvature, originally directed upward, at the completion of rotation is inverted and directed posteriorly. Attempted delivery with the instrument in that position is likely to cause serious injury to maternal soft parts. To avoid such trauma, it is essential to remove and reapply the instrument as described in the following text.

SPECIAL FORCEPS MANEUVERS

SCANZONI–SMELLIE MANEUVER

The double application of forceps, which was first described by Smellie (1752) and about a century later by Scanzoni (1853), has produced satisfactory results in some hands, but it is rarely necessary and is generally employed in only a small percentage

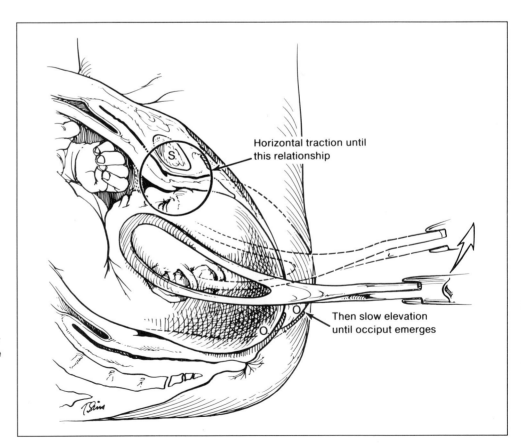

Figure 25–18. Occiput directly posterior. Low forceps (Simpson) delivery as an occiput posterior (O = occiput; S = symphysis). The *arrow* illustrates the point at which time the head should be flexed after the bregma passes under the symphysis. It is evident that to prevent serious perineal lacerations an extensive episiotomy is most often required.

Horizontal traction until this relationship

Then slow elevation until occiput emerges

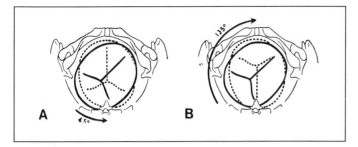

Figure 25–19. Rotation of obliquely posterior occiput to sacrum (**A**) and symphysis pubis (**B**).

of all obliquely posterior occipital positions. Because the right posterior variety is much more frequent, the steps of the operation in that case are detailed.

In the first application, the blades of the forceps are applied to the sides of the head with the pelvic curve toward the face of the fetus, whereas in the second application the pelvic curve is directed toward the occiput. For the first application, the right hand is passed into the vagina posteriorly and the rear ear is located. The left blade is applied over the ear and held in position by an assistant, while the operator's left hand is passed into the right side of the vagina to control the introduction of the right blade, which is then rotated anteriorly until it lies over the left ear and opposite the first blade. The forceps is then locked and the handles elevated to flex the fetal head. Rotation may be facilitated by dislodging the fetal head very slightly upward. *The head must not be disengaged from the pelvis.* To compensate for the pelvic curvature in Tucker–McLane forceps, or others with a pelvic curvature, the handles of the forceps are gently rotated clockwise through an arc that extends well lateral to the circumference of the birth canal (Fig. 25–19). This serves to rotate the fetal head about the occipitomental diameter. With an appropriate initial forceps application, it is often possible to rotate the head completely to the occiput anterior position without undue force.

Once the occiput is rotated anteriorly, it is necessary to remove and reapply the forceps as described for an occiput anterior delivery. The forceps are unlocked and the branch now on the left side of the pelvis (right branch) is removed by gently pulling the handle simultaneously downward and inward. During this maneuver, the other branch is held in position anteriorly by an assistant to help stabilize the occiput in an anterior position. The right branch is now inserted immediately after the remaining branch has been removed. During this time, the occiput will typically rotate back to a right occiput anterior position. After reapplication, some difficulty may arise in proper articulation, since the handle of the left branch lying above the right cannot be locked, but this can be readily overcome by rotating the handle of the left branch around the right to bring the lock into proper position. In left occiput posterior position, the blades are applied similarly but in the reverse order.

ROTATION WITH KIELLAND FORCEPS

Before attempts are made to perform any forceps operations, but especially with midforceps rotations, the station of the fetal head must be accurately ascertained to be at, or preferably below, the level of the ischial spines. Too often in these cases there has been extreme molding of the fetal head, and the caput

succedaneum has descended to below the ischial spines, giving the erroneous impression that the head is engaged when actually the occiput is above the spines. **Forceps application under these circumstances is classified as high and are never to be attempted under any circumstances.**

Kielland (1916) described a forceps with narrow, somewhat bayonet-shaped blades that he claimed could readily be applied to the sides of the head in the occiput transverse position and surpassed all other models as a rotator (Fig. 25–3). He held that his forceps was particularly useful when the station of the fetal head was high and when the sagittal suture was directed transversely. The Kielland forceps has almost no pelvic curve, but does have a sliding lock and is very light. On each handle is a small knob that indicates the direction of rotation.

There are two methods of applying the anterior blade of Kielland forceps. In the first, *which may prove dangerous,* the anterior blade is introduced first with its cephalic curve directed upward and, after it has entered sufficiently far into the uterine cavity, it is turned through 180 degrees to adapt the cephalic curvature to the head. Kielland advised a safer "wandering" or "gliding" method of application for the anterior blade when the uterus is tightly contracted about the head and the lower uterine segment is stretched and thin. In such cases, when the pelvis is slightly contracted, it is dangerous to introduce the anterior blade with its cephalic curvature directed upward to be followed by rotation of the blade. In the wandering or gliding method, the anterior blade is introduced at the side of the pelvis over the brow or face to an anterior position, with the handle of the blade held close to the opposite maternal buttock throughout the maneuver. The second blade is introduced posteriorly and the branches are locked. Since most cases amenable to Kielland forceps rotation are those in which there is deep transverse arrest (the fetal head is deep in the pelvis with the occiput well below the level of the ischial spines), rotation usually is accomplished by unwedging the fetal head from the pelvis by a small amount of upward pressure. From this slightly higher station, the rotation is accomplished. **The head should not be pushed high enough to allow disengagement since the cord may prolapse.**

Rubin and Coopland (1970) summarized the experiences with Kielland's forceps rotation at Winnipeg General Hospital. Of the 1,000 consecutive cases surveyed, almost exactly one half were occiput posterior and the remainder were occiput transverse. Rotation was accomplished successfully in 970. The same forceps were nearly always used for delivery, followed by reapplication when necessary. There were eight perinatal deaths, including four with serious anomalies. Injuries to the infant were considered mostly minor. There were 27 injuries that were not minor, however, including seven fractured skulls.

INJURY FROM MIDFORCEPS OPERATIONS

With any midforceps application, and especially those in which rotations are done, serious trauma may result to both fetus and mother unless considerable care is exercised. In a scholarly and extensive (108 references) review of midforceps delivery, Richardson and co-workers (1983) proposed three prerequisites for the uses of midforceps: (1) midforceps must rationally be needed as an alternate method of delivery to cesarean section; (2) midforceps must be proven to be associated with a lower maternal morbidity rate than cesarean section; and (3) midforceps should improve fetal outcome or, at the least, not result in fetal harm.

With respect to the first requirement, there appears to be little doubt that there is a need for such a method in cases of fetal distress, maternal exhaustion, prolapsed umbilical cord, and cases of secondary labor arrest due to conduction analgesia.

The issue of maternal morbidity following the use of midforceps procedures compared to cesarean section is not clearcut. The use of midforceps is not a benign procedure (O'Driscoll and associates, 1981) for either mother or infant; however, neither is cesarean section (see Chapter 26). Cesarean sections are associated with significantly increased maternal morbidity and mortality when compared to vaginal deliveries. Likewise, midforceps deliveries are associated with a higher incidence of maternal morbidity, usually assessed by lacerations and increased blood loss, when compared to women delivered by low or outlet forceps (Dierker and associates, 1985; Gilstrap and colleagues, 1984). However, it must be concluded that midforceps procedures carry less morbidity for the mother than does cesarean section. The same cannot be said for the fetus.

Damage to the fetus with a midforceps application can result in trauma and death immediately or long-term morbidity in the form of cerebral palsy and lowered intelligence. The immediate consequences of midforceps rotations have recently been reviewed by several groups whose reports included control series. Hughey and colleagues (1978) compared 458 midforceps operations to 17 cesarean section deliveries. The women delivered by cesarean section were selected when the cervix was completely dilated and the occiput failed to rotate to the anterior position from transverse or posterior position. Using a "perinatal morbidity index," an unfavorable result of 30 percent was reported for the fetuses delivered by midforceps versus a zero percent morbidity with cesarean section. Bowes and Bowes (1980) compared the fetal outcome in midforceps deliveries to fetal outcome in patients delivered by cesarean section or by vacuum extraction. Morbid events were identified in 14 of 71 midforceps deliveries (20 percent) compared to two morbid events in the 37 cesarean sections (5.4 percent) and three instances of fetal trauma occurring in 15 vacuum extractions (20 percent). Chiswick and James (1979) have looked carefully at neonatal morbidity and mortality following vaginal delivery with Kielland forceps or cesarean section after attempts at vaginal delivery with these forceps. Birth trauma was evident in 15 percent of infants delivered with forceps. Neonatal mortality, most often from tentorial tears, was 3.5 percent. Factors significantly associated with the use of Kielland forceps were nulliparity, short maternal stature, induction of labor, late engagement of the fetal head, slow dilatation of the cervix, and epidural analgesia during labor (James and Chiswick, 1979).

Gilstrap and colleagues (1984) retrospectively compared immediate maternal and neonatal outcomes of 234 women delivered by midforceps with those of women delivered either spontaneously, by outlet forceps, or by cesarean section. Importantly, forceps were not applied unless the fetal head was *below* zero station, or had descended to lower than +1 station (of 3 stations) in the case of transverse arrest. Almost 60 percent of women delivered by midforceps had epidural analgesia. They assessed neonatal acid-base status by measuring cord blood pH, and found no difference in the incidence of neonatal acidosis between the groups when indications for delivery were matched. Likewise, they found no excessive trauma to fetuses delivered by midforceps.

Dierker and associates (1985) provided a retrospective review of 176 midforceps deliveries at Cleveland Metropolitan General Hospital, and compared these to all other deliveries during the study period, 1976 through 1982. Epidural analgesia was associated with slightly more than half of the cases with midforceps. Although cephalohematomas were identified more commonly in neonates delivered by midforceps (7 percent), they found no increased incidence of low Apgar scores, seizures, shoulder dystocia, or brachial or facial nerve palsy when these infants were compared to the general obstetrical population.

Long-term morbidity for the newborn delivered by midforceps in terms of cerebral palsy appears to be increased (Eastman and co-workers, 1962; Fuldner, 1957), but this has not been universally observed (Steer and Boney, 1962). For example, the issue of intelligence following midforceps delivery is unsettled and is likely to remain so because of the multitude of variables affecting intelligence such as gender, mother's education, race, and socioeconomic status. Broman and co-workers (1975), controlling for socioeconomic status, race, and gender but *not* fetal weight, reported that infants delivered by midforceps had slightly higher IQ scores at 4 years of age than children delivered spontaneously. There were no significant differences among the IQ scores by type of delivery. Nilsen (1984) evaluated 18-year-old men drafted into the Norwegian Army and reported that those delivered by Kielland forceps had higher IQ scores than those who were delivered either spontaneously or by vacuum extraction or cesarean section.

The results published by Friedman and associates (1977, 1984) are in contrast to those reported by Broman and colleagues, and these have been the most controversial because data from the Collaborative Perinatal Project was used by both groups of investigators. In their second report, Friedman and co-workers (1984) described intelligence assessments at least up to 7 years of age, and concluded that those children who had been delivered by midforceps had lower mean IQ scores compared to children who were delivered by outlet forceps.

Dierker and colleagues (1986) assessed the long-term outcome of children delivered by midforceps as described in the study cited above and compared them to children who had been delivered by cesarean section performed for dystocia. These children were assessed at a minimum of 2 years of age, and the authors found no increased morbidity associated with delivery by midforceps.

CONCLUSIONS REGARDING MORBIDITY FROM MIDFORCEPS

There can be no doubt that midforceps delivery performed inappropriately, or by an unsupervised inexperienced operator, can result in considerable maternal as well as fetal trauma. Studies in which these morbid events were reported to be substantively increased were done earlier and at times when cesarean section rates were still around 5 percent. Moreover, many of these earlier studies undoubtedly included forceps applications that would, in all likelihood, never be attempted today. By contrast, in two of the more recent studies, the authors appropriately emphasize that all (Gilstrap, 1984) or the majority (Dierker, 1986) of midforceps deliveries were done with the fetal vertex at +1 or lower station. ("Station" in these studies divided the pelvis into three measurements from spines to outlet.) It is unlikely that midforceps deliveries included in the Collaborative Perinatal Project during the 1960s were this conservative. Finally, the impact of the popular use of epidural analgesia on the incidence of midforceps deliveries cannot be discounted. The majority of such cases result from inadequate maternal expulsive forces against a relaxed pelvic sling, and thus they are not usually associated with true dystocia. Although it is prudent in these cases to allow a longer second stage of labor, in some women delivery is indicated. Midforceps rotations in such circumstances are likely to be safer than in women with prolonged labors and midpelvic arrest unassociated with conduction analgesia.

It seems fair to conclude that midforceps operations can be performed with safety for the mother and fetus if the basic guidelines set forth in this chapter are carefully observed. The operator must be experienced, and in general, forceps rotations or deliveries from zero station, even though the fetal head is likely engaged, should be avoided. If the fetal head is at a lower station in the pelvis, then forceps may be used safely for those indications previously elucidated. In this scheme, *difficult* midforceps deliveries are avoided, along with their adverse outcomes.

TRIAL FORCEPS AND FAILED FORCEPS

In *trial forceps*, the operator attempts low or midforceps delivery with the full knowledge that a certain degree of disproportion at the midpelvis may make the procedure incompatible with safety for the fetus. With an operating room both equipped and staffed for immediate cesarean section, and after a good forceps application has been achieved, firm downward pulls on the instrument are made. If no descent occurs, the procedure is abandoned and cesarean section is performed (Douglass and Kaltreider, 1953).

The term *failed forceps* is usually applied to a case in which a forceps delivery was anticipated and a vigorous but unsuccessful attempt was made to deliver with forceps. The three fundamental factors responsible for such a failure are disproportion, incomplete cervical dilatation, and malposition of the fetal head. Most but not all such cases stem from inexperience and ignorance of obstetrical fundamentals. In most areas of the United States, these cases are becoming less frequent.

While the term *failed forceps* frequently carries a negative connotation, it may also be used to describe abandonment of carefully planned *trial forceps*. Boyd and colleagues (1986) described 53 cases of failed forceps among 6,524 nulliparas, and by their definition, failed forceps included those cases in which there was difficulty with forceps application, and thus did not include any traction efforts. Over 75 percent of these nulliparous women had been given epidural analgesia for labor, and the incidence of midforceps was almost 20 percent, of which 4 percent were classified as failed forceps. They documented more adverse outcomes whenever any operative delivery was performed, but found no differences in outcomes of infants delivered successfully by midforceps when compared to those delivered by cesarean section following failed forceps or failure to progress in the second stage of labor. Lowe (1987) reported similar results and stressed the awareness that forceps application should not be considered a commitment to vaginal delivery.

Rather than using the term failed forceps, it seems preferable to instead place a detailed narrative report in the hospital record—which is better if typewritten—describing the indications for attempting midforceps and the events that followed.

FORCEPS IN FACE PRESENTATIONS

In face presentations with the chin directed toward the symphysis, the application of forceps is occasionally used to effect vaginal delivery. The blades are applied to the sides of the head along the occipitomental diameter, with the pelvic curve directed toward the neck. Downward traction is exerted until the chin appears under the symphysis. Then, by an upward movement, the face is slowly extracted, the nose, eyes, brow, and occiput appearing in succession over the anterior margin of the perineum (Fig. 25–20). Forceps should not be applied to the *mentum posterior presentation*, since delivery cannot be effected.

VACUUM EXTRACTOR

There have been numerous attempts in the past to attach a traction device by suction to the fetal scalp. The theoretic advantages of the vacuum extractor over forceps include the fact that insertion of space-occupying steel blades within the vagina and positioning the blades precisely over the fetal head, as is required for safe forceps delivery, can be avoided, the fetal head can be rotated without impinging upon maternal soft tissues, and there is great reduction in intracranial pressure during traction. All previously described instruments were unsuccessful until Malmström (1954) applied a new principle, namely, traction on a metal cap so designed that the suction creates an artificial caput, or *chignon*, within the cup that holds firmly and allows adequate traction. This cup is now replaced by sialistic material; however, as emphasized by Duchon and associates (1988), high-pressure vacuum generates large amounts of force regardless of the cup used.

In spite of some early enthusiasm in the United States, the vacuum extractor is not used extensively now, partly because of reports of fetal damage, such as lacerations and abrasions of the scalp, cephalohematomas, intracranial hemorrhage, and death

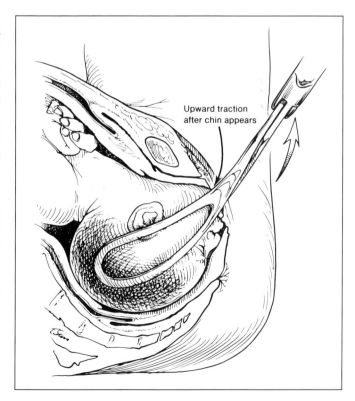

Upward traction after chin appears

Figure 25–20. Face presentation, mentum (chin) anterior. Delivery with low forceps (Simpson).

of infants. In contrast to the American hesitancy, there has been an enthusiastic reception in other parts of the world, although the enthusiasm has waned in at least some foreign institutions (Punnonen and associates, 1986).

There have been a few reports from the United States in which the vacuum extractor was used. In one recent study, the authors concluded that vacuum extraction had replaced midforceps deliveries at their institution (Broekhuizen and colleagues, 1987). In this report, as well as in the studies reported by Baerthlein (1986), Berkus (1985), and Vacca (1983) and their colleagues, it was concluded that vacuum extraction was safer than forceps for the mother, and at least as safe as forceps for the fetusinfant. These conclusions were reached despite the fact that two of these studies reported one fetal-neonatal death from cerebral hemorrhage associated with vacuum extraction. If the operator is inexperienced, Herabutya and colleagues (1988) reported that there were fewer complications with vacuum extraction compared to Kielland forceps for deep transverse arrest.

The tendency to attempt vacuum deliveries at stations higher than usually attempted with forceps is worrisome. Broekhuizen and colleagues (1987) reported that 3.5 percent of vacuum deliveries were performed with the vertex above zero station and another 20 percent were at zero station. If the vacuum instrument is to be used, the same indications for its use should be carefully applied as for any forceps delivery.

GLOSSARY

Craniotomy

The term *craniotomy*, as used in obstetrics, means an operation to collapse the fetal head for the purpose of facilitating its delivery. Widespread prenatal care, more astute management of pelvic contraction, antibiotics, and improvements in cesarean section have rendered craniotomy an exceedingly rare operation in modern obstetrics. As indicated in Chapter 19 (p. 371), cases of hydrocephalus are managed better by needle puncture and drainage.

Dührssen (Cervical) Incisions

When immediate delivery is desirable before the cervix is fully dilated, multiple radial incisions may be made in the cervix and repaired immediately after delivery. These incisions are usually called Dührssen incisions, after the German obstetrician who described them in 1890 (Dührssen, 1890). While the complications may be formidable, the technique of the operation is simple: Three incisions, corresponding approximately to the hours of 2, 6, and 10 on the face of a clock, are made with scissors. Delivery is then effected by forceps or breech extraction, depending on the presentation. The operation should never be done unless the cervix is fully effaced and more than 7 cm dilated, lest profuse or even fatal hemorrhage result. The procedure is, of course, contraindicated in placenta previa.

Most obstetricians now consider the operation obsolete. It is included here only because of the rare posibility of its use in fetal distress when the head of a fetus presenting as breech is trapped by the cervix deep in the pelvis and the cervix is almost fully dilated.

Although the incisions themselves are simple to perform, the procedure involves major potential hazards, and cesarean section is most often preferable. For instance, in cases of uterine dysfunction in which the cervix is not yet fully dilated, the head is usually well above the pelvic floor, and a difficult midforceps operation, with its attendant trauma to mother and fetus, is often required. In such circumstances, severe maternal hemorrhage is common. Moreover, poor anatomical results, such as deep scars and adhesions between the cervix and the vaginal mucosa, are likely to be a result.

Manual Dilatation of the Cervix

In practice, there is no such procedure as "manual dilatation of the cervix." What actually occurs when it is attempted is manual laceration of the cervix. The operation has no place in obstetrics.

Symphysiotomy and Pubiotomy

Symphysiotomy is the division of the pubic symphysis with a wire saw or knife to effect an increase in the capacity of a contracted pelvis sufficient to permit the passage of a living child. In pubiotomy, the pubis is severed a few centimeters lateral to the symphysis: Because of interference with subsequent locomotion, bladder injuries, and hemorrhage, and because of the greater safety of cesarean section, these two operations have been abandoned in the United States. Symphysiotomy is still performed in parts of Africa and elsewhere, especially when it may be impossible to follow a patient in a subsequent pregnancy. Since, in these circumstances, a woman delivered by cesarean section for a mildly contracted pelvis might well die with a ruptured uterus in her next pregnancy, symphysiotomy may be indicated in such a case in an attempt to produce sufficient enlargement of the pelvis to allow vaginal delivery. Hartfield (1973) described a technique for subcutaneous symphysiotomy and summarized his experiences.

History of Forceps

Crude forceps are an ancient invention, several varieties having been described by Albucasis, who died in 1112. Since their inner surfaces were provided with teeth to penetrate the head, however, it appears that they were intended for use only on dead fetuses.

The true obstetrical forceps was devised in the latter part of the 16th century or the beginning of the 17th century by a member of the Chamberlen family. The invention was not made public at the time, but was preserved as a family secret through four generations, not becoming generally known until the early part of the 18th century. Previously, version had been the only method that permitted the operative delivery of an unmutilated child. When that operation was impossible, imperative delivery was accomplished with hooks and crochets, which usually led to the destruction of the child. Thus, before the invention of forceps, the use of instruments was synonymous with the death of the child, and frequently of the mother as well.

William Chamberlen, the founder of the family, was a French physician who fled from France as a Huguenot refugee and landed at Southhampton in 1569. He died in 1596, leaving a large family. Two of his sons, both of whom were named Peter, and designated the elder and younger, respectively, studied medicine and settled in London. They soon became successful practitioners, devoting a large part of their attention to midwifery, in which they became very proficient. They attempted to control the instruction of midwives and, to justify their pretensions, claimed that they could successfully deliver patients when all others failed.

The young Peter died in 1626 and the elder in 1631. The elder left no male children, but the younger was survived by several sons, one of whom, born in 1601, was likewise named Peter. To distinguish him from his father and uncle, he is usually spoken of as Dr. Peter, since the other two did not possess that title. He was well educated, having studied at Cambridge, Heidelberg, and Padua, and on his return to London was elected a Fellow of the Royal College of Physicians. He was most successful in the practice of his profession and counted among his patients many members of the royal family and nobility. Like his father and uncle, he attempted to monopolize control of the midwives, but his pretensions were set aside by the authorities. These attempts gave rise to much discussion, and many pamphlets were written about the mortality of women in labor attended by men. He answered them in a pamphlet entitled "A Voice in Ramah, or the Cry of Women and Children as Echoed Forth in the Compassions of Peter Chamberlen." He was a man of considerable ability, combining some of the virtues of a

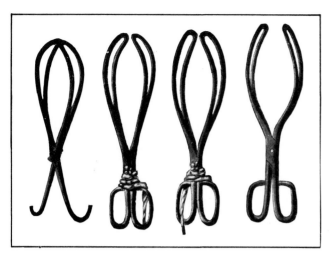

Figure 25–21. Chamberlen forceps.

religious enthusiast with many of the devious qualities of a quack. He died at Woodham Mortimer Hall, Moldon, Essex, in 1683, the place remaining in the possession of his family until well into the succeeding century. He was formerly considered the inventor of the forceps, a fact now known to be incorrect.

Dr. Peter Chamberlen left a very large family, and three of his sons, Hugh, Paul, and John, became physicians who devoted special attention to the practice of midwifery. Of them, (Hugh 1630–?) was the most important and influential. Like his father, he was a man of considerable ability who took a practical interest in politics. Since some of his views were out of favor, he was forced to leave England for Paris, where in 1673 he attempted to sell the family's secret to Mauriceau for 10,000 lires, claiming that with forceps he could deliver in a very few minutes the most difficult case. Mauriceau placed at his disposal a rachitic dwarf whom he had been unable to deliver, and Chamberlen, after several futile hours of strenuous effort, was obliged to acknowledge his inability to do so. Notwithstanding his failure, he maintained friendly relations with Mauriceau, whose book he translated into English. In his preface he refers to the forceps in the following words: "My father, brothers, and myself (though none else in Europe as I know) have by God's blessing and our own industry attained to and long practiced a way to deliver women in this case without prejudice to them or their infants."

Some years later he went to Holland and sold his secret to Roger Roonhuysen. Shortly afterward the Medical-Pharmaceutical College of Amsterdam was given the sole privilege of licensing physicians to practice in Holland, to each of whom, under the pledge of secrecy, was sold Chamberlen's invention for a large sum. The practice continued for a number of years until Vischer and Van de Poll purchased and made public the secret, whereupon it was discovered that the device consisted of only one blade of the forceps. Whether that was all Chamberlen sold to Roonhuysen, or whether the Medical-Pharmaceutical College had swindled the purchasers, is not known.

Hugh Chamberlen left a considerable family, and one of his sons, Hugh (1664–1728), practiced medicine. He was a highly educated, respected, and philanthropic physician, who numbered among his patients members of the best families in England. He was an intimate friend of the Duke of Buckingham, who had a statue erected in Chamberlen's honor in Westminster Abbey. During the later years of his life he allowed the family secret to leak out, and the instrument soon came into general use.

For more than 100 years Dr. Peter Chamberlen was considered the inventor of the forceps, but in 1813 Mrs. Kemball, the mother of Mrs. Codd, who was the occupant of Woodham Mortimer Hall at the time, found in the garret a trunk containing numerous letters and instruments, among them four pairs of forceps together with several levers and fillets. As the drawings indicate (Fig. 25–21) the forceps were in different stages of development, one pair hardly applicable to the living woman, although the others were useful instruments. Aveling (1882), who carefully investigated the matter, believes that the three pairs of available forceps were used, respectively, by the three Peters, and that in all probability the first was devised by the elder Peter, son of the original William. The forceps came into general use in England during the lifetime of Hugh Chamberlen, the younger. The instrument was employed by Drinkwater, who died in 1728, and was well known to Chapman and Giffard.

In 1723, Palfyn, a physician of Ghent, exhibited before the Paris Academy of Medicine a forceps he designated *mains de fer*. It was crudely shaped and impossible to articulate. In the discussion following its presentation, De la Motte stated that it would be impossible to apply it to the living woman, and added that if by chance anyone should happen to invent an instrument that could be so used, and kept it secret for his own profit, he deserved to be exposed upon a barren rock and have his vitals plucked out by vultures. He had little knowledge at the time he spoke such an instrument had been in the possession of the Chamberlen family for nearly 100 years.

The Chamberlen forceps, a short, straight instrument with only a cephalic curve, is perpetuated in the short forceps of today. It was used, with but little modification, until the middle of the 18th century, when Levret, in 1747, and Smellie, in 1751, independently added the pelvic curve and increased the length of the instrument. Levret's forceps was longer, with a more decided pelvic curve than that of Smellie. From these two instruments, the long forceps of the present day are descended.

As soon as forceps became public property, they were subjected to various modifications. As early as 1798, Mulder's atlas included illustrations of nearly 100 varieties. The modifications attempted in improving the instrument are pictured in Witkowski's *Obstetrical Arsenal*, illustrating several hundred forceps but representing only a small fraction of those devised. The monograph of Das contains excellent historical sketches of the development of the instrument. It is remarkable, however, that little advance was made over the instruments of Levret and Smellie until Tarnier, in 1877, clearly enunciated the principle of axis traction. These forceps were designed to cope with very high stations of the fetal head and contracted pelves. Such problems today, however, are generally solved by other means. Episiotomy, furthermore, has eliminated many of the difficulties stemming from the pelvic curve, and severe traction at the fenestra, as in the axis-traction forceps, is therefore unnecessary and probably undesirable (Rhodes, 1958).

Except for two specialized forceps, those of Barton and Kielland, very little that is both new and useful in modern obstetrics has been added to the development of the instrument in over 200 years.

REFERENCES

American College of Obstetricians and Gynecologists: Committee on Obstetrics: Maternal and Fetal Medicine: Obstetric Forceps. No 59, February 1988

Anderson GD, Bada HS, Sibai BM, Korone SB: Obstetrical factors related to progression of periventricular hemorrhage in the preterm newborn. Abstract No 401. Presented at the 35th Annual Meeting of the Society for Gynecologic Investigation, Baltimore, March 1988

Aveling JH: The Chamberlens and the Midwifery Forceps. London, Churchill, 1882

Baerthlein WC, Moodley S, Stinson SK: Comparison of maternal and neonatal morbidity in midforceps delivery and midpelvis vacuum extraction. Obstet Gynecol 67:594, 1986

Barton LG, Caldwell WE, Studdiford WE: A new obstetrical forceps. Am J Obstet Gynecol 15:16, 1928

Berkus MD, Ramamurthy RS, O'Connor PS, Brown K, Hayashi RH: Cohort study of silastic obstetric vacuum cup deliveires: I. Safety of the instrument. Obstet Gynecol 66:503, 1985

Bishop E, Israel L, Briscoe C: Obstetric influences on the premature infants' first year of development: A report from the Collaborative Study of Cerebral Palsy. Obstet Gynecol 26:628, 1965

Bowes WA, Bowes C: Current role of midforceps operations. Clin Obstet Gynecol 23:549, 1980

Boyd ME, Usher RH, McLean FH, Norman BE: Failed forceps. Obstet Gynecol 68:779, 1986

Broekhuizen FF, Washington JM, Johnson F, Hamilton PR: Vacuum extraction versus forceps delivery: Indications and complications, 1979 to 1984. Obstet Gynecol 69:338, 1987

Broman SH, Nichols PL, Kennedy WA: Preschool IQ: Prenatal and Early Developmental Correlates. Hillside, NJ, Lawrence Erlbaum, 1975

Chiswick ML, James DK: Kielland's forceps: Association with neonatal morbidity and mortality. Br Med J 1:7, 1979

DeLee JB: The prophylactic forceps operation. Am J Obstet Gynecol 1:34, 1920

Dewhurst C (ed): Integrated Obstetrics and Gynecology for Postgraduates, 2nd ed. Oxford, Blackwell, 1976, p 440

Dierker LJ, Rosen MG, Thompson K, Debanne S, Linn P: The midforceps: Maternal and neonatal outcomes. Am J Obstet Gynecol 152:176, 1985

Dierker LJ, Rosen MG, Thompson K, Lynn P: Midforceps deliveries: Long-term outcome of infants. Am J Obstet Gynecol 154:764, 1986

Douglas RG, Stromme WB: Operative Obstetrics, 3rd ed. New York, Appleton, 1976

Douglass LH, Kaltreider DF: Trial forceps. Am J Obstet Gynecol 65:889, 1953

Duchon MA, DeMund MA, Brown RH: Laboratory comparison of modern vacuum extractors. Obstet Gynecol 72:155, 1988

Dührssen A: On the value of deep cervical incisions and episiotomy in obstetrics. Arch Gynaekol 37:27, 1890

Eastman NJ, Kohl SG, Maisel JE, Kaveler F: The obstetrical background of 753 cases of cerebral palsy. Obstet Gynecol Surv 17:459, 1962

Fairweather D: Obstetric management and follow-up of the very low-birth-weight infant. J Reprod Med 26:387, 1981

Friedman EA, Sachtleben MR, Bresky PA: Dysfunctional labor: XII. Long-term effects on the fetus. 127:779, 1977

Friedman EA, Sachtleben-Murray MR, Dahrouge D, Neff RK: Long-term effects of labor and delivery on offspring: A matched-pair analysis. Am J Obstet Gynecol 150:941, 1984

Fuldner RV: Labor complication and cerebral palsy. Am J Obstet Gynecol 74:159, 1957

Gilstrap LC, Hauth JC, Schiano S, Connor KD: Neonatal acidosis and method of delivery. Obstet Gynecol 63:681, 1984

Haesslein H, Goodlin R: Survey of the tiny newborn. Am J Obstet Gynecol 134:192, 1979

Hartfield VJ: Subcutaneous symphysiotomy—Time for a reappraisal? Aust NZ J Obstet Gynaecol 13:147, 1973

Herabutya Y, O-Preasertsawat P, Boonrangsimant P: Kielland's forceps or ventouse—a comparison. Br J Obstet Gynaecol 95:483, 1988

Hobel C, Oakes G: Special considerations on the management of preterm labor. Clin Obstet Gynecol 23:147, 1980

Hughey MJ, McElin JW, Lussky R: Forceps operation in perspective: I. Midforceps rotation operations. J Reprod Med 20:253, 1978

James DK, Chiswick ML: Kielland's forceps: Role of antenatal factors in prediction of use. Br Med J 1:10, 1979

Joulin M: Study on the use of force in obstetrics. Arch Gen Med, 6th Series 9:149, 1867

Kielland C: On the application of forceps to the unrotated head, with description of a new model of forceps. Monatsschrift fur Geburtschilfe und Gynealkologie 43:48, 1916

Lowe B: Fear of failure: A place for the trial of instrumental delivery. Br J Obstet Gynaecol 94:60, 1987

Malmström T: The vacuum extractor, an obstetrical instrument. Acta Obstet Gynecol Scand (Suppl) 4:33, 1954

Nilsen ST: Boys born by forceps and vacuum extraction examined at 18 years of age. Acta Obstet Gynecol Scand 63:549, 1984

O'Driscoll K, Meagher D, MacDonald D, Geoghegan F: Traumatic intracranial haemorrhage in firstborn infants and delivery with obstetric forceps. Br J Obstet Gynaecol 88:577, 1981

Punnonen R, Aro P, Kuukankorpi A, Pystynen P: Fetal and maternal effects of forceps and vacuum extraction. Br J Obstet Gynaecol 93:1132, 1986

Richardson DA, Evans MI, Cibils LA: Midforceps delivery: A critical review. Am J Obstet Gynecol 145:621, 1983

Rubin L, Coopland AT: Kielland's forceps. Can Med Assoc J 103:505, 1970

Scanzoni FW: Lehrbuch der Geburtshülfe, 3rd ed. Vienna, Seidel, 1853, pp 838–840

Schwartz DB, Miodovnik M, Lavin JP Jr: Neonatal outcome among low birth weight infants delivered spontaneously or by low forceps. Obstet Gynecol 62:283, 1983

Smellie W: A Treatise on the Theory and Practice of Midwifery. London, Wilson & Durham, 1752

Steer CM, Boney W: Obstetric factors in cerebral palsy. Am J Obstet Gynecol 83:526, 1962

Vacca A, Grant A, Wyatt G, Chalmers T: Portsmouth operative delivery trial: A comparison vacuum extraction and forceps delivery. Br J Obstet Gynaecol 90:1107, 1983

Cesarean Section and Cesarean Hysterectomy

CESAREAN SECTION

DEFINITION

Cesarean section, or cesarean delivery, is defined as delivery of the fetus through incisions in the abdominal wall (laparotomy) and the uterine wall (hysterotomy). This definition does not include removal of the fetus from the abdominal cavity in case of rupture of the uterus or abdominal pregnancy.

INDICATIONS

The indications for cesarean section are discussed in detail throughout the text wherever the fetal or maternal complications that might necessitate cesarean section are presented. The early history of cesarean section is considered at the end of this chapter. In general, cesarean section is used whenever it is believed that further delay in delivery would seriously compromise the fetus, the mother, or both, yet vaginal delivery is unlikely to be accomplished safely.

FREQUENCY

The rate for delivery by cesarean section has increased at an accelerated pace for the past 20 years in the United States and other developed countries (Notzan and co-workers, 1987). In the United States, the rate increased from 4.5 percent in 1965 to 23 percent in 1985 and this was documented in all parts of the country and for women of all ages. The reasons for this marked increase are not completely understood but some explanations include:

1. There has been *reduced parity* and almost half of pregnant women are nulliparas. Therefore, an increased number of cesarean sections might be expected for those conditions that are more common in nulliparous women, especially dystocia and pregnancy-induced hypertension.
2. *Older-aged women are having children.* In 1980, approximately 20 percent of births in the United States were in women 30 years or older, but in 1985, this was 25 percent (Taffel and co-workers, 1987). The frequency of cesarean section increases with advancing age for American and Canadian women (Martel and associates, 1987; Taffel and co-workers, 1987).
3. *Electronic fetal monitoring* likely increases the chances of detecting fetal distress and probably results in an increased number of cesarean sections.

4. *Breeches* are delivered more frequently by cesarean section. For example, in 1985, 79 percent of all breeches were delivered by cesarean section (Taffel and associates, 1987).
5. There are *fewer forceps deliveries* today. Between 1972 and 1980, forceps deliveries declined from 37 percent to 18 percent, corresponding to an increased cesarean section rate from 7 percent to 17 percent (Placek and colleagues, 1983).
6. *Repeat cesarean sections* have contributed significantly to the total increase in cesarean deliveries.
7. There is increasing concern for *malpractice suits.* In 1985, 73 percent of fellows of the American College of Obstetricians and Gynecologists reported that at least one malpractice claim had been filed against them! According to Haynes de Regt and colleagues (1986), private nulliparous patients are much more likely to undergo cesarean delivery than clinic patients if dystocia, malpresentation, or fetal distress is diagnosed.

In 1980, Bottoms and colleagues concluded that the major indications for cesarean section that needed to be reassessed were dystocia and repeat operations. Between 1980 and 1985, more than three fourths of the 16.5 to 22.7 percent increase in the cesarean section rate was the consequence of repeat sections and dystocia (Table 26–1). The contribution of each indication to the total section rate is a function of two variables: (1) the **change in incidence** of the indication and (2) the **change in the cesarean section rate** for the indication. As shown in Table 26–2, in 1980, 51 percent of all deliveries had one or more complications, but by 1985 this had increased to 64 percent. Dystocia was diagnosed in 7.2 percent and 10.2 percent of women in 1980 and 1985, respectively, a 42 percent increase in the incidence of this complication.

In Table 26–3 it can be seen that cesarean delivery was performed in 67 percent of women diagnosed with dystocia in 1980 and 65 percent in 1985. However, since this diagnosis was made more often (Table 26–2), the actual rate increased from 4.8 in 1980 to 6.6 in 1985 (Table 26–1), which is an increase of 29 percent.

There was a decrease of 3 percent in the number of repeat cesarean sections from 1980 to 1985 (Table 26–3); however, the percentage of all women delivered by repeat cesarean section increased from 5.1 percent to 8.4 percent (Table 26–2). This resulted in an actual increase in the rate of repeat cesarean sections from 4.9 percent in 1980 to 7.9 in 1985, an increase of 48 percent (Table 26–1).

TABLE 26-1. COMPARISON OF 1980 AND 1985 CESAREAN SECTION RATES AND INCREASES IN RATES FOR SELECTED INDICATIONS IN THE UNITED STATES

	1980		1985		Increase 1980–1985	
Indication	Rate[a]	%	Rate	%	Rate	%
Repeat section	4.9	30	7.9	35	3.0	48
Dystocia	4.8	30	6.6	29	1.8	29
Fetal distress	0.8	5	1.8	8	1.0	16
Breech	2.0	12	2.3	10	0.3	5
All other	4.0	24	4.1	18	0.1	2
Totals	16.5	100	22.7	100	6.2	100

[a] Cesarean sections per 100 deliveries for stated indication.
Modified from Taffel and associates: Am J Public Health 77:955, 1987.

Therefore, as predicted by Bottoms and associates (1980), the increase in cesarean sections in the United States is not likely to decline unless repeat cesarean sections and those done for dystocia are reduced. As described subsequently, the safety and efficacy of vaginal delivery after cesarean section has been established. It is interesting that the percentage of cesarean sections for all complications except breech has decreased (Table 26–3). If this trend continues it is likely that an overall reduction in cesarean section rates will be achieved (Anderson and Lomas, 1984; Shiono and co-workers, 1987; Taffel and associates, 1987).

Regardless of the indications cited for cesarean section, the increased frequency has been accompanied by an absolute decrease in perinatal mortality. While it is true that the increase in cesarean section rate may have resulted in a lowering of perinatal mortality, many other factors as well may have contributed, for example, better prenatal care, electronic fetal heart rate monitoring, and advances in neonatal care.

In support of the concept that the increased rate of cesarean section was *not* responsible for the observed decrease in perinatal mortality was the report by O'Driscoll and Foley (1983). These authors studied the correlation of decreases in perinatal mortality and the increase in cesarean section rates from 1965 to 1980 in the United States and at the National Maternity Hospital in Dublin, Ireland. (Fig. 26–1). They reported that while cesarean section rates were increasing in the United States from less than 5 percent in 1965 to more than 15 percent in 1980, in Dublin among more than 108,000 infants born during the same period of time, the cesarean section rate remained virtually unchanged at 4.2, 4.2, 4.1, and 4.8 percent in 1965, 1970, 1975, and 1980, respectively. Despite the unchanged rate in cesarean sections in Dublin, perinatal mortality fell from 42.1 to 36.5, 24.0, and 16.8

per 1,000 infants born during the same years. These authors concluded that these results were compatible with the view that the increased rate of cesarean sections reported in the United States had not contributed significantly to the simultaneously observed reduction in perinatal mortality.

The lower cesarean section rate in Dublin was attributed to lower frequencies of cesarean section for dystocia, repeat cesarean section, and breech delivery (Table 26–4). O'Driscoll and associates (1969, 1973, 1984) attributed their apparent success to a more aggressive management of dystocias with oxytocin in nulliparous patients whose uteri they considered to be *"almost immune to rupture except by manipulation,"* to allowing patients with previous low transverse cesarean sections a trial of labor which proved successful in 60 percent, and to a liberal trial of labor in breech presentations (Chap. 22).

Although the results reported from Dublin appear impressive, the results pertain to perinatal mortality but not morbidity. To address this, Leveno and associates (1985) compared perinatal outcomes at Parkland Hospital to those at the National Maternity Hospital. The primary cesarean section rate was 4.4 percent in Dublin and it was 10.1 percent in Dallas. However, the more liberal use of cesarean section, especially for dystocia or for fetal jeopardy, was associated with a **sevenfold decreased incidence of intrapartum fetal death and a twofold decreased incidence of neonatal seizures.** Because perinatal morbidity is much more difficult to assess, such results are still to be reported from Europe, Australia, and the United States.

It seems unlikely that such low cesarean section rates as those reported from Dublin will be seen in the United States. One reason for this is the prevailing enthusiasm for small families, which likely will result in many women, whose first infants were delivered by cesarean section, electing to have a

TABLE 26-2. PERCENTAGE COMPLICATIONS FOR ALL DELIVERIES IN THE UNITED STATES 1980 AND 1985

Complication	1980	1985	Percent Change 1980 and 1985
Repeat section	5.1	8.4	+65
Dystocia	7.2	10.2	+42
Fetal distress	1.2	3.9	+225
Breech	3.1	2.9	−6
All others (normals)	34.6	38.5	+11
All deliveries (vaginal and section) with one or more complications[a]	51	64	+25

[a] Totals do not equal 100 percent because of overlap in some categories.
Modified from Taffel and associates, Am J Public Health 77:955, 1987.

TABLE 26-3. PERCENTAGE OF DELIVERIES BY CESAREAN SECTION FOR VARIOUS INDICATIONS IN UNITED STATES, 1980 AND 1985

Complication	1980	1985	Percent Change 1980–85
Previous section	97	93	−3
Dystocia	67	65	−2
Fetal distress	63	46	−27
Breech	66	79	+20
All other	11.4	11.7	−6

Modified from Taffel and associates, Am J Public Health 77:955, 1987.

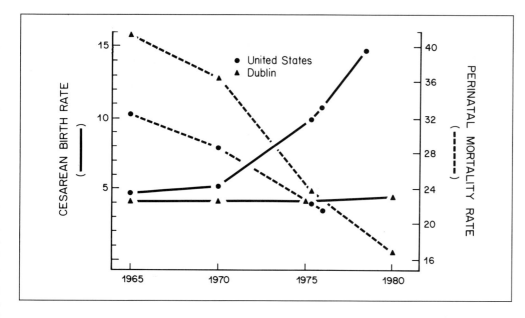

Figure 26–1. Cesarean birth rates per 100 deliveries are represented by *solid lines* and perinatal mortality rates per 1,000 deliveries by *broken lines* for the United States (*circles*), according to Bottoms and co-workers (1980) and for the National Maternity Hospital, Dublin (*triangles*). (*Modified from O'Driscoll and Foley, 1983.*)

repeat cesarean section with tubal sterilization. Another reason is the reluctance to allow vaginal delivery of breech presentations. Even if the liberal standards applied to frank breech presentations and recommended by Collea and associates (1980) were applied, we could expect only a 15 to 30 percent decrease in the cesarean section rate for all breeches (see Chap. 19, p. 353). However, vaginal delivery subsequent to cesarean section is safe and efficacious, and will likely become more popular. Therefore, a reduction or certainly a cessation in the rate of increase in cesarean sections probably will follow.

The final answers with respect to the frequency, indications, results in terms of safety to the mother and fetus, and the legal, ethical, and economic consequences of cesarean section are unlikely to become apparent for several years. To the credit of the obstetrical community these questions continue to be addressed (National Institutes of Health, 1980). There are now several reports by clinical investigators of attempts to reduce the incidence of cesarean section without increasing perinatal mortality and morbidity. These efforts appear to have been successful in university or teaching hospitals and are sometimes referred to as *active management of labor*, which is described in Chapter 16 (p. 313). It is unproved if the application of so-called

active management can be transferred to community hospitals with comparable safety where large numbers of house officers, nurses, and ancillary services are not always readily available as in most teaching hospitals.

MATERNAL MORTALITY

The most remarkable report of the safety of cesarean delivery is that from the Boston Hospital for Women (Frigoletto and associates, 1980). These authors reported a zero maternal mortality rate in 10,231 cases. Certainly, maternal and perinatal mortality and morbidity are typically higher with cesarean delivery than with vaginal delivery, in part because of the complication that led to the cesarean section and in part because of increased risks inherent in the abdominal route of delivery.

Maternal mortality from cesarean section is less than 1 per 1,000. Petitti (1983) reviewed nearly 400,000 cesarean sections performed in the United States from 1965 through 1978 and reported that maternal death followed 1 in 1,635 operations. She rightfully emphasizes that only about half of these are directly attributable to the cesarean section itself. For example, Sachs and co-workers (1988) attributed as a direct cause only 7 of 27 deaths following more than 121,000 cesarean sections performed in Massachusetts from 1976 through 1984. While this mortality rate was 22 per 100,000 for all cesarean sections, it was only 5.8 per 100,000 for deaths directly due to cesarean delivery. However, even this relatively low operative mortality rate must be considered as excessive when one understands that the majority of these deaths occur in young, healthy women undergoing a "normal physiological process."

The major threats to women undergoing cesarean section have been anesthesia, severe sepsis, and thromboembolic episodes. Each of these areas has been or will be considered in great detail. However, it is worth emphasizing that aspiration pneumonia, which had previously been the leading cause of cesarean section deaths at Parkland Hospital, has been avoided completely since the routine practice of ingesting 30 mL of milk of magnesia, or more recently a solution of sodium citrate and citric acid (see Chap. 17, p. 331). Despite such efforts to decrease mortality, it is unlikely that deaths from either cesar-

TABLE 26-4. FREQUENCY OF CESAREAN DELIVERIES ACCORDING TO DIAGNOSTIC INDICATION[a]

Indication	United States[b] (1978)	Dublin[c] (1980)
Dystocia	4.7	0.7
Repeat cesarean	4.7	1.1
Breech	1.8	0.6
Fetal distress	0.8	0.5
Others	3.2	1.9
Total	15.2	4.3

[a] Expressed as percent of all births.
[b] Figures for the United States were calculated from the National Institutes of Health Consensus Statement based on data from New York City.
[c] Figures for Dublin refer to the National Maternity Hospital.
From O'Driscoll and Foley, 1983.

ean or vaginal delivery can be reduced more in severely compromised women who elect, rightly or not, to pursue pregnancies despite their already tenuous medical status. Therefore, one must consider whether the death was related to a complication of the delivery per se or due at least in part to an underlying factor, such as heart disease. It is reasonable to assume that if the frequency of cesarean deliveries can be reduced without compromising the fetus, significant reductions not only in cesarean section mortality rates but in overall maternal mortality rates as well may be achieved. Thus, a major challenge in obstetrics is to answer correctly the question *"Can a significant reduction in cesarean section rate be achieved without increasing perinatal mortality* and *morbidity?"*

MATERNAL MORBIDITY

Even when morbidity and mortality associated with the problem that led to cesarean section are excluded, maternal morbidity is more frequent and likely to be more severe following cesarean section than following vaginal delivery (Rubin and co-workers, 1981). The common causes of morbidity from cesarean delivery remain infection, hemorrhage, and injury to the urinary tract. (Baskett and McMillen, 1981; Danforth, 1985).

PERINATAL MORTALITY

The frequency of stillbirth and neonatal mortality will depend, of course, on the underlying reason for the cesarean section and the gestational age of the fetus. Although the decreasing perinatal mortality rate observed since the mid-1960s in many instances has been associated with and even been attributed to the marked increase in cesarean section rates in the United States, O'Driscoll and Foley (1983), as mentioned earlier, have questioned this assumption. Specifically, they reported similar and equally dramatic decreases in perinatal mortality rates in patients delivered at the National Maternity Hospital in Dublin without an increase in cesarean section rates (Fig. 26–1).

PERINATAL MORBIDITY

Birth trauma in general is much less likely with cesarean section than with vaginal delivery; however, cesarean section is not a guarantee against fetal injury. For example, the head of a preterm breech can be entrapped in a small transverse uterine incision that was judged incorrectly to be large enough for delivery. Such an error in judgment may result in injury to the fetal spinal cord or brain and may result in either extension of the uterine incision into the uterine vessels or lower uterine segment or both. Finally, the fetus can be wounded during the incision into the uterus.

It is important to emphasize that fetal morbidity has been decreased dramatically with the use of cesarean section in instances of certain breech presentations (Chap. 19, p. 350), transverse lie of the fetus, and placenta previa. Also of importance is the fact that the opportunities for obstetricians-in-training to develop and *maintain* the skills necessary to accomplish successfully a potentially difficult breech delivery or to do an internal podalic version for a second twin have diminished greatly and for sound reasons (Chap. 34, p. 647).

Although respiratory distress has been claimed to be higher for repeat cesarean section than for vaginal delivery, it is unlikely that there is a significant difference when gestational ages of the fetuses are identical and fetal hypoxia and acidosis are avoided. The methods employed to avoid anesthetic causes of fetal hypoxia and acidosis are discussed in Chapter 17.

TIMING OF REPEAT CESAREAN SECTION

There are advantages to a predetermined time for carrying out repeat cesarean sections. For example, the family can better arrange for assistance in caring for other children while the mother is hospitalized and for the care of the mother and infant after leaving the hospital. Importantly, a competent team can be assembled more easily to provide optimal care, including anesthesia, infant resuscitation if needed, and subsequent care of the newborn. Conversely, with emergency repeat cesarean section, an operating room may not be immediately available, or the mother may have very recently eaten, which increases the anesthetic risk. Of considerable importance when dealing with a gravida with a previous cesarean section is whether a vertical uterine incision was made that might rupture with the onset of labor, resulting in the death of the fetus and serious morbidity or even death of the mother. The likelihood of these disastrous consequences from rupture of a transverse scar in the lower uterine segment is very low.

Iatrogenic Preterm Delivery

Elective termination of pregnancy with the delivery of a preterm infant has been a major problem at some institutions. This unfortunate circumstance has led to the strong recommendation by some that amniocentesis with appropriate studies on the amnionic fluid be performed before any elective delivery (Flaksman and co-workers, 1978; Gluck, 1977). This approach is not without complications, however, for at times, trauma to the placenta or fetus is caused by attempts to obtain amnionic fluid, which may be of scant volume in pregnancies at or near term. Moreover, after an unsuccessful attempt at amniocentesis, the fetus has been known to succumb in utero awaiting a subsequent and hopefully successful attempt at aspiration of amnionic fluid. Sonography at the time of amniocentesis diminishes the risk somewhat but adds further to the cost.

The guidelines for timing repeat cesarean section at Parkland Hospital do not include mandatory amniocentesis to measure the amnionic fluid lecithin/sphingomyelin (L/S) ratio. Instead, the following information is used to identify fetal maturity: (1) the date of onset of the last normal spontaneous menstrual period if accurately known, (2) ultrasonic estimates of fetal age performed in the first trimester or soon thereafter, (3) serial measurements of uterine fundal height begun before midpregnancy, (4) the time when fetal heart sounds were first heard with an unamplified fetoscope, and (5) the estimated fetal size. Delivery is carried out after 38 completed weeks of gestation, based on the last normal menstrual period, without measuring the L/S ratio if the fetal heart was heard at a time when the fundal height was 18 to 20 cm, if the gestational age at the same time calculated from the normal last menstrual period was 18 to 20 weeks, or if fetal heart tones have been heard for 20 weeks with a fetoscope, and if the fetus is estimated by each of two experienced examiners to weigh as much as did the previous term infant, or more than 3,000 g when the previous infant was preterm or growth retarded. Delivery is postponed if there is discordance that implies a lower gestational age and there are no compelling reasons, maternal or fetal, to effect delivery before the onset of labor, such as a previous vertical incision in the uterus or strong suspicion of retarded fetal growth.

With this approach, about 60 percent of repeat cesarean

sections have been performed at Parkland Hospital at a scheduled time, and respiratory distress has not been a problem in those pregnancies terminated by scheduled repeat cesarean section before the onset of labor.

For women with uncertain or unverified menstrual periods, and in whom early gestational dating by ultrasound was not performed, timing of delivery must be determined either by assuring pulmonary maturity with determination of the L/S ratio or by awaiting spontaneous labor.

CONTRAINDICATIONS

In modern obstetrical practice, there are virtually no contraindications to cesarean section. Cesarean section is seldom indicated, however, if the fetus is dead or too premature to survive. Exceptions to this generalization include pelvic contraction of such a degree that vaginal delivery by any means is impossible, most cases of placenta previa, and most cases of neglected transverse lie. Conversely, whenever the maternal coagulation mechanism is seriously impaired, delivery that minimizes incisions—vaginal delivery—is preferable in most instances (Chap. 36).

VAGINAL DELIVERY SUBSEQUENT TO CESAREAN SECTION

There is no doubt that vaginal delivery most often will prove to be safe following a previous cesarean section. Numerous reports have been published in the past few years that confirm the earlier reports by Riva and Teich (1961), Douglas and co-workers (1963), and McGarry (1969) that attest to the safety and efficacy of vaginal delivery in women who previously had cesarean sections. Flamm (1985), in an excellent review, summarized results from 21 reports including his own. He reported that of 6,258 women who underwent a trial of labor, 5,356 were delivered vaginally (86 percent) and without a maternal mortality. There were five fetal losses and one uterine dehiscence of a previous vertical incision. With an incidence of one maternal mortality per 1,000 cesarean sections, this approach likely saved five mothers and apparently did not increase perinatal mortality.

Even with these successful outcomes, several areas of management remain controversial:

1. How many cesarean sections can be done before it is unsafe to allow a trial of labor?
2. What is the incidence of uterine rupture or scar dehiscence?
3. Following vaginal delivery, should uterine exploration be performed routinely? If so, what should be done if a uterine defect is discovered?
4. If the patient had a cesarean section for a recurrent problem such as cephalopelvic disproportion, should a trial of labor be allowed?
5. Can epidural analgesia be used safely for a trial of labor?
6. Can oxytocin be used safely to induce or augment labor?
7. Should women with multifetal gestation be allowed a trial of labor?
8. What standards should be established for obstetrical services before a trial of labor is justified?

Number and Type of Cesarean Sections

Vaginal delivery subsequent to a cesarean section can be safely carried out for women who have had one previous low trans-

verse uterine incision without an extension. Series have been published in which trials of labor were allowed in women with more than one cesarean section. In most of these reports, the outcomes have been good and the complications minimal (Farmakides, 1987; Flamm, 1988; Mootabar, 1984; Paul, 1985; Phelan, 1988; Porreco and Meir, 1983; Pruett, 1988; and all their colleagues). In order to draw valid conclusions, more patients will have to be studied. If a trial of labor is planned for a woman with more than one previous cesarean section, the responsibility for assuring adequate medical and nursing personnel and technical support (see below) remains with the physician. At Parkland Hospital we continue to limit a trial of labor to those women with a single previous low-transverse cesarean section documented by operative report not to have had an extension of the uterine incision.

Uterine Scar Separation

The issue that most often has prevented physicians from allowing women to undergo a vaginal delivery following a cesarean section has been the fear of uterine rupture or dehiscence. O'Sullivan and co-workers in 1981 reviewed over 8,000 deliveries reported in the literature and added several hundred patients of their own. They reported that frank rupture of the uterus or uterine dehiscence, at least, occurred in 1.8 percent of women undergoing cesarean section compared to only 0.5 percent for women undergoing vaginal delivery. O'Sullivan and colleagues concluded that vaginal delivery not only was as safe as an elective repeat cesarean section but was in fact the preferred method of management in carefully selected patients. Their conclusions have been confirmed (Flamm, 1985; Placek and Taffel, 1988).

Uterine Exploration

After vaginal delivery in a woman with a previous cesarean section, the uterine cavity should be explored. While some do not advocate routine exploration, it seems wise for at least two reasons. First, with a communication between the vagina and peritoneal cavity, infection could be life threatening. Second, if a defect is present but undetected, rational consideration about a subsequent vaginal delivery cannot be made.

The issues to be assessed at the time of uterine exploration are whether there is a defect and, if so, is it connected with the peritoneal cavity? If it is contiguous with the peritoneal cavity or if there is excessive bleeding, laparotomy is performed promptly and the defect repaired or hysterectomy performed. If there is a defect discovered in the uterine wall which does not open into the peritoneum and it is small and not bleeding, repair may be unnecessary. Under these circumstances, the woman is observed closely with frequent vital signs and serial hematocrit determinations. Most such patients do well without uterine repair. What then about a subsequent pregnancy in such a woman with a known uterine defect? There is very little valid information, although Paul and associates (1985) continue to study this problem at Los Angeles County Hospital. Because of these uncertainties, at Parkland Hospital, if a uterine defect is discovered, an immediate laparotomy and repair is usually performed.

Recurrent Indications for Cesarean Section

This issue was controversial until Seitchik and Ramakrishna (1982) reported that women previously delivered by cesarean section for "dystocia" could subsequently be delivered vaginally. This is now established (Ollendorff and associates, 1988).

Flamm (1985) reviewed 13 studies and classified their indications for cesarean section as recurrent (cephalopelvic disproportion or failure to progress) or other nonrecurring causes. Success, defined as vaginal delivery, was 61 percent in 1,064 women with recurring causes and 78 percent of 1,808 with nonrecurring causes. Flamm and associates confirmed these initial results (1988). Some reports published between 1984 and 1986 are presented in Table 26–5. The overall prognosis for vaginal delivery was 72 percent, and success could be anticipated in 63 percent of women who had cesarean sections for dystocia compared to 79 percent of those without recurring indications. Duff and colleagues (1988) confirmed these findings and reported that 68 percent of women with a prior cesarean section for dystocia delivered vaginally compared to 81 percent who had previously undergone abdominal delivery for other indications. Not surprisingly, in most of these studies, the authors reported even better success rates for women who had been delivered vaginally before their cesarean section.

Epidural Analgesia

Most often, epidural analgesia is not withheld in women undergoing a trial of labor. Whereas Ruddick and co-workers (1984) reported a woman in whom uterine rupture was accompanied by pain despite epidural analgesia, Uppington (1983) reported another woman who felt no pain with rupture. In both, oxytocin was given and fetal distress rapidly developed following uterine rupture so that neither case was missed. The risk of epidural analgesia inhibiting maternal cardiovascular responses to hemorrhage from sympathetic blockade has not been adequately studied; however, the possibility is worrisome.

Between 1980 and 1984, Flamm (1985) reported that 38 percent of 1,692 women were given epidural analgesia for a trial of labor. There were no maternal or fetal deaths, but the two cases of uterine rupture cited above were recorded. Both fetuses survived because of early recognition of fetal distress in both and continuous abdominal pain in one of the two women. Finally, the incidence of midforceps deliveries is increased in women who are given epidural analgesia (Chap. 17, p. 338), and the need for oxytocin augmentation following an epidural block is increased appreciably. Because of these uncertainties, we are reluctant to use epidural analgesia in these women allowed a trial of labor.

If epidural analgesia is used, internal electronic monitoring of fetal heart rate and intrauterine pressure is recommended along with **continuous bedside attendance by an obstetrical nurse or the physician.**

Oxytocin Use

The issue of the safety of oxytocin induction or augmentation of labor is not clearly resolved. Flamm (1985) reported 69 percent successful vaginal deliveries of 581 trials of labor in which oxytocin was used for women with previous cesarean sections. There were no maternal or perinatal deaths, but there were two uterine ruptures. One uterine rupture per 300 labors seems excessive, and if oxytocin is used, strict criteria should be followed including internal electronic monitoring of fetal heart rate and intrauterine pressures and a limitation of the total dose of oxytocin (Clark, 1984; Paul, 1985; Vengadasalam, 1986; and their co-workers).

Multifetal Gestation

Any condition that results in overdistension of the uterus poses a risk of rupturing a uterine scar. Thus, labor should not be allowed in these women. The same is true for abnormalities in fetal lie and position with the *possible exception* of a frank breech presentation.

Guidelines for a Trial of Labor

The question is not whether a woman can deliver vaginally following a previous cesarean section but rather the criteria that should be applied and rigidly adhered to in order to allow her to labor and attempt a vaginal delivery. Specific guidelines have been revised by the American College of Obstetricians and Gynecologists (1988). The Committee again stressed the availability of personnel to appropriately deal with emergencies that may arise. **Unlike prior recommendations, it is now felt that women with one prior transverse cesarean section should be counseled to undergo a trial of labor.** Those with two prior cesarean sections are not discouraged from a trial of labor provided there is no other contraindication. The Committee further concluded that oxytocin induction or augmentation and epidural analgesia are not contraindicated. Unanswered issues include prior low vertical incisions (prior classical incisions contraindicate a trial of labor), twins, breeches, and the singleton fetus with an estimated weight of more than 4,000 g.

If a woman is to undergo a trial of labor following a cesarean section, appropriate technical support must be available in the hospital. There should be an adequate blood bank staffed 24 hours a day with compatible blood available promptly. Electronic fetal heart rate and intrauterine pressure monitoring should be available. There should be adequate facilities and personnel to begin an emergency cesarean section within 30 minutes from the time the decision is made.

TABLE 26-5. OUTCOME FOR A TRIAL OF LABOR RELATED TO THE INDICATION FOR A PREVIOUS CESAREAN SECTION

Study	Overall Success for Trial of Labor[a]	Indication for Primary Cesarean Section			
		Dystocia[b]	Breech	Fetal Distress	Other Nonrecurring
Clark (1984)	240/308 (78)	39/61 (64)	81/94 (86)	31/38 (61)	69/92 (75)
Jarrell (1985)	142/216 (66)	42/78 (54)	54/72 (75)		
Mootabar (1984)	161/296 (54)	77/163 (47)			75/123 (61)
Paul (1985)	614/751 (82)	245/319 (77)	103/135 (91)	56/67 (84)	
Vengadasalam (1986)	176/271 (65)	38/82 (46)	33/42 (79)	68/91 (75)	37/56 (52)
Totals	1,333/1,842 (72)	441/703 (63)	291/343 (85)	155/196 (79)	181/271 (67)
			Total nonrecurring = 627/810 (79)		

[a] Numbers in parentheses are percentages.
[b] Includes cephalopelvic disproportion and failure to progress.

The obstetrician in his or her zeal to abandon the old adage *"Once a cesarean section, always a cesarean section,"* should avoid substituting the even more inappropriate motto *"Once a cesarean delivery, never again a cesarean delivery!"*

TECHNIQUE OF CESAREAN SECTION

TYPE OF UTERINE INCISION

The so-called classical cesarean incision, a vertical incision into the body of the uterus above the lower uterine segment and reaching the uterine fundus, is seldom used. Most always the incision is made in the lower uterine segment transversely (Kerr technique; Kerr, 1926) or, less often, vertically (Krönig technique; Krönig, 1912). The lower segment transverse incision has the advantage of requiring only modest dissection of the bladder from the underlying myometrium. If the incision extends laterally, the laceration may involve large branches of the uterine artery and vein. The low vertical incision may be extended upward so that in those circumstances where much more room is needed, the incision can be carried into the body of the uterus; otherwise, it is a less desirable incision. More extensive dissection of the bladder is necessary to keep the vertical incision within the lower uterine segment. Moreover, if the vertical incision extends downward, it may tear through the cervix into the vagina and possibly involve the bladder. If, on the other hand, it is extended upward into the body of the uterus, closure, including satisfactory reperitonealization, is more difficult. Importantly, it has been the experience of most obstetricians that during the next pregnancy the vertical incision is much more likely to rupture, especially during labor, than is the lower segment transverse incision (Chap. 23, p. 408).

Lower Segment Transverse Incision

For a cephalic presentation, most often a transverse incision through the lower uterine segment is the operation of choice. Generally, the transverse incision (1) results in less blood loss, (2) is easier to repair, (3) is located at a site least likely to rupture with extrusion of the fetus into the abdominal cavity during a subsequent pregnancy, and (4) does not promote adherence of bowel or omentum to the incisional line.

Preparation for Incision

Hair is shaved from the abdominal wall from the level of the mons pubis to somewhat above the umbilicus and laterally to about the level of the iliac crests. The bladder is emptied through an indwelling catheter and continuously drained during and after the procedure. The operative field is thoroughly scrubbed with a suitable detergent, and then all of the abdomen is covered with sterile drapings.

If general anesthesia is to be employed, all of the above steps are carried out and the operating team is fully prepared to operate before induction of anesthesia. If continuous conduction analgesia is to be used, it is necessary before scrubbing and draping the abdomen to insert the catheter into the epidural or caudal space. If single-dose intrathecal (spinal) analgesia is to be used, it is injected just before scrubbing and draping the abdomen.

CHOICE OF ABDOMINAL INCISIONS

An infraumbilical midline vertical incision is quickest to make. The abdominal wall is opened in layers from just above the upper margin of the symphysis to near the umbilicus. The incision should be of sufficient length to allow the infant to be delivered without difficulty, but no longer. Therefore, its length should vary with the estimated size of the fetus. Sharp dissection is performed to the level of the anterior rectus sheath, which is freed of subcutaneous fat to expose a strip of fascia in the midline about 2 cm wide. Some surgeons prefer to incise the rectus sheath with the scalpel throughout the length of the fascial incision. Others prefer to make a small opening and then incise the visualized fascial layer with scissors. There seems to be less bleeding with the latter approach, as well as reduced risk of inadvertently incising underlying structures, especially bowel. The rectus and the pyramidalis muscles are separated in the midline by sharp and blunt dissection to expose transversalis fascia and peritoneum.

The transversalis fascia and properitoneal fat are carefully dissected, beginning near the upper pole of the incision, to reach the underlying peritoneum. The peritoneum near the upper end of the incision is elevated with two hemostats placed about 2 cm apart. The tented fold of peritoneum between the clamps is visualized and palpated to rule out the inclusion of omentum, bowel, or bladder, and only then is the peritoneum carefully opened. In women who have had previous intra-abdominal surgery, including cesarean section, omentum or even bowel may be adherent to the undersurface of the peritoneum. The peritoneum is incised superiorly to the upper pole of the incision and downward to just above the peritoneal reflection over the bladder.

Troublesome bleeding sites anywhere in the abdominal incision are clamped as encountered but are not ligated until later, unless the hemostats are in the way. Bleeding vessels should not be ignored, however, for it is essential that there be no active bleeding when the wound is closed.

With the Pfannenstiel type of incision, the skin and subcutaneous tissue are incised using a lower transverse, slightly curvilinear incision. The incision is made at the level of the pubic hairline and is extended somewhat beyond the lateral borders of the rectus muscles. After the subcutaneous tissue has been separated from the underlying fascia for 1 cm or so on each side, the fascia is incised transversely the full length of the incision. The superior and inferior edges of the fascia are grasped with suitable clamps. First, the inferior margin is elevated by the assistant as the operator separates the fascial sheath from the underlying rectus muscles by blunt dissection with the scalpel handle. Then the superior fascial margin is elevated and the rectus sheath freed from the rectus muscles. Blood vessels coursing between the muscles and fascia are clamped, severed, and ligated. It is imperative that meticulous hemostasis be achieved. The separation is carried to near the umbilicus sufficient to permit an adequate midline longitudinal incision of the peritoneum. The rectus muscles are separated from each other and from the underlying transversalis fascia and peritoneum. The peritoneum is opened as discussed above under the description of the vertical midline incision. Closure in layers is carried out the same as with a vertical incision, except that many operators, in trying to prevent hematoma formation, place beneath the fascia small Penrose drains that exit from each angle of the fascial closure.

The cosmetic advantage of the transverse skin incision is apparent. Moreover, the incision is said to be stronger, with less likelihood of dehiscence or hernia formation. There are, nonetheless, disadvantages in the use of the transverse incision. Exposure of the pregnant uterus and appendages is not as good as with a vertical incision. Whenever more room is needed, the

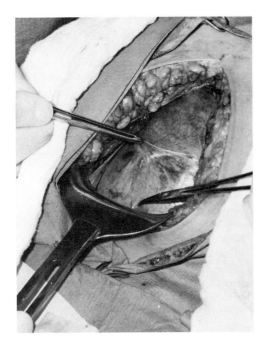

Figure 26–2. The loose vesicouterine serosa is grasped in the forceps. The hemostat tip points to the upper margin of the bladder. The retractor is firm against the symphysis.

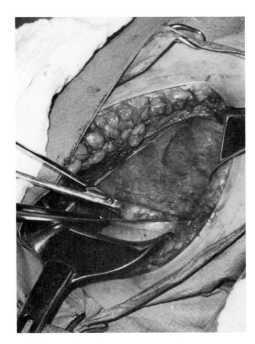

Figure 26–3. The loose serosa above the upper margin of the bladder is being elevated and incised laterally.

vertical incision can be rapidly extended around and above the umbilicus, whereas the Pfannenstiel incision cannot. If the woman is obese, the operative field is even more restricted. Therefore, Pfannenstiel's incision tends to be used for thin women by operators who have achieved technical expertise, while the vertical incision is used almost to the exclusion of the transverse incision whenever rapid delivery is indicated, the woman is obese, or the operator is developing his or her skills. It is not appropriate to compare the vertical incision under these more adverse conditions to the transverse incision carried out under much more favorable circumstances. Finally, at the time of repeat cesarean section, reentry through Pfannenstiel's incision is likely to be more time consuming, which, at times, can be detrimental to the fetus.

UTERINE INCISION

The uterus is quickly but carefully palpated to identify the size and the presenting part of the fetus and to determine the direction and degree of rotation of the uterus. Commonly, the uterus is found to be dextrorotated so that the left round ligament is more anterior and closer to the midline than the right. It may be levorotated, however. Some operators prefer to lay a moistened laparotomy pack in each lateral peritoneal gutter to absorb amnionic fluid and blood that escape from the opened uterus. This technique is especially valuable in order to help localize the spread of infected amnionic fluid.

The typically rather loose reflection of peritoneum (serosa) above the upper margin of the bladder and overlying the anterior lower uterine segment is grasped in the midline with forceps (Fig. 26–2) and incised with a scalpel or scissors. Scissors, inserted between the serosa and myometrium of the lower uterine segment, are pushed laterally from the midline, while partially opening the blades intermittently, to separate a 2-cm-wide strip of serosa, which is then incised. As the lateral margin on each side is approached, the scissors are aimed somewhat more cephalad (Fig. 26–3). The lower flap of peritoneum is elevated and the bladder is gently separated by blunt dissection from the underlying myometrium (Fig. 26–4). In general, the separation of bladder should not exceed 5 cm in depth and usually less. It is possible, especially with an effaced, dilated cervix, to dissect downward so deeply as inadvertently to expose and then enter the underlying vagina rather than the lower uterine segment (Goodlin and co-workers, 1982). The developed bladder flap is held downward beneath the symphysis with a bladder retractor, such as that used with a Balfour self-retaining retractor.

The uterus is opened through the lower uterine segment about 2 cm above the detached bladder. The uterine incision can be made by a variety of techniques. Each is initiated by incising with a scalpel the exposed lower uterine segment transversely

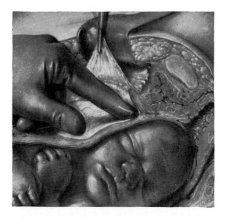

Figure 26–4. Low-segment cesarean section. Cross-section showing dissection of bladder off uterus to expose lower uterine segment.

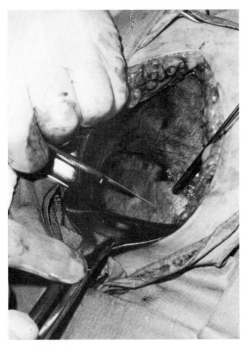

Figure 26–5. The myometrium is being carefully incised to avoid cutting the fetal head.

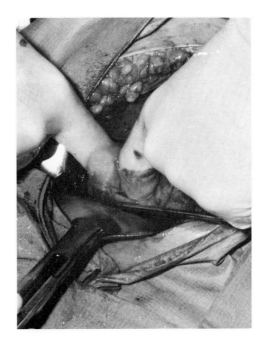

Figure 26–7. The index fingers inserted through the incised lower uterine segment exert moderate pressure laterally to extend the opening in the uterus.

for 2 cm or so half-way between the lateral margins. This must be done carefully so as to cut completely through the uterine wall but not deeply enough to wound the underlying fetus (Figs. 26–5 and 26–6). Suctioning of the operative field by an assistant is especially important. Once the uterus is opened, the incision can be extended by cutting laterally and then slightly upward with bandage scissors, or when the lower uterine segment is thin, the entry incision can be extended by simply spreading the incision, using lateral pressure applied with each index finger (Fig. 26–7), or a combination of these techniques can be used (Fig. 26–8). Exposure is aided by placement of a Richardson retractor into the wound and retracting the abdom-

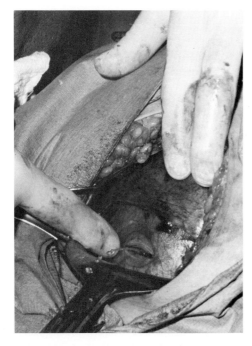

Figure 26–6. The uterine cavity has been entered. Amnionic fluid is escaping through the incision.

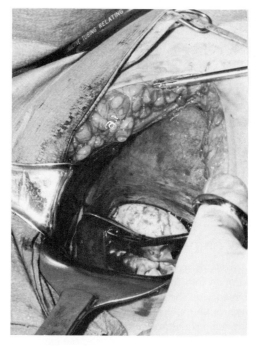

Figure 26–8. Bandage scissors are used to complete the transverse incision when resistance to spreading is encountered.

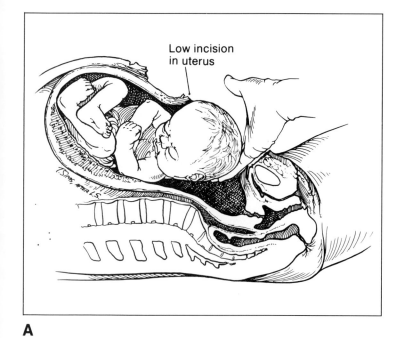

A

B

Figure 26–9. A. Immediately after incising uterus and fetal membranes, the operator's fingers are insinuated between the symphysis pubis and the fetal head until the posterior surface is reached. The head is carefully lifted anteriorly and, as necessary, superiorly to bring it from beneath the symphysis forward through the uterine and abdominal incisions.
B. As the fetal head is lifted through the incision, pressure is usually applied to the uterine fundus through the abdominal wall to help expel the fetus.

inal wall laterally as the incision is extended toward that side. *It is very important to make the uterine incision large enough to allow delivery of the head and trunk of the fetus without either tearing into or having to cut into the uterine arteries and veins that course through the lateral margins of the uterus.* If it appears that the uterine incision is going to be too small, some extra room may be obtained by curving the incision upward bilaterally so as to avoid the lateral uterine vessels. The membranes are incised if this was not done previously. If the placenta is encountered in the line of incision, it must either be detached or incised. Especially when the placenta is incised, fetal hemorrhage may be severe; therefore, the cord should be clamped as soon as possible in such cases.

DELIVERY OF THE INFANT

The retractors are removed, and if the vertex is presenting, a hand is slipped into the uterine cavity between the symphysis and fetal head, and the head is gently elevated with the fingers and palm through the incision (Fig. 26–9 A, B) aided by modest transabdominal fundal pressure. To minimize aspiration by the fetus of amnionic fluid and its contents, the exposed nares and mouth are aspirated with a bulb syringe before the thorax is delivered. The shoulders are then delivered using gentle trac-

tion plus fundal pressure. The rest of the body readily follows.

After a long labor with cephalopelvic disproportion, the fetal head may be rather tightly wedged in the birth canal. Upward pressure exerted through the vagina by the sterile-gloved hand of an associate will readily dislodge the head and allow its delivery above the symphysis.

As soon as the shoulders are delivered (Fig. 26–10), an intravenous infusion containing about 20 U of oxytocin per liter is allowed to flow at a brisk rate of 10 mL per minute until the uterus contracts satisfactorily, and then the rate is reduced to 2 to 4 mL per minute. The cord is promptly clamped with the infant held at the level of the abdominal wall, and the infant is given to the member of the team who will conduct resuscitative efforts as they are needed. A sample of cord blood is obtained from the placental end of the cord.

If the fetus is not presenting as a vertex, or if there are multiple fetuses, and usually with delivery of a very immature fetus from a woman who has had no labor, a vertical incision through the lower segment may, at times, prove to be advantageous. The fetal legs must be carefully distinguished from the arms to avoid premature extraction of an arm and a difficult delivery of the rest of the fetus.

The uterine incision is observed for any vigorously bleeding

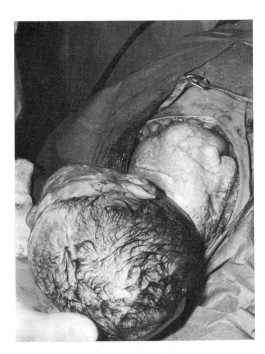

Figure 26–10. Just as the shoulders are delivered, intravenous oxytocin infusion is started.

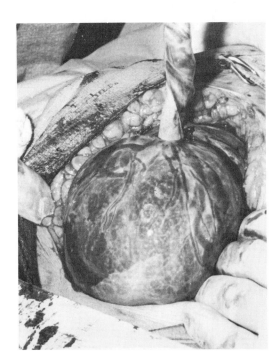

Figure 26–11. Placenta bulging through uterine incision as uterus contracts.

sites. These are promptly clamped, depending upon size and location, with Pennington forceps, short-handled ring forceps, or similar instruments. The placenta is promptly removed manually, unless it is separating spontaneously (Fig. 26–11). Fundal massage, begun as soon as the fetus is delivered, reduces bleeding and hastens delivery of the placenta.

REPAIR OF UTERUS

After delivery of the placenta, the uterus may be lifted through the incision onto the draped abdominal wall and the fundus covered with a moistened laparotomy pack. Uterine exteriorization often has advantages that outweigh any disadvantages. The relaxing uterus can be recognized quickly and massage applied. The incision and bleeding points are more easily visualized and repaired, especially if there have been extensions laterally. Adnexal exposure is superior and thus tubal sterilization easier. The principal disadvantage is from discomfort and vomiting caused by traction in the woman given spinal or epidural analgesia. Hershey and Quilligan (1978) reported that febrile morbidity was not increased if exteriorization for closure was routinely performed.

Immediately after delivery and inspection of the placenta, the uterine cavity is inspected and is wiped out with a gauze pack to remove shreds of membranes, vernix, clots, or other debris. If the cervical canal is not known to be patent, it should be probed with a long clamp to assure patency. The contaminated clamp is discarded from the field.

The upper and lower cut edges and each angle of the uterine incision are carefully examined for bleeding vessels. The lower margin of an incision made through a thinned-out lower uterine segment may be so thin as to be ignored inadvertently. At the same time, the posterior wall of the lower uterine segment may occasionally buckle anteriorly in such a way as to suggest that it is the lower margin of the incision. Incorporation of the posterior wall into the closure must be avoided.

The uterine incision may be closed with either one or two layers of continuous chromic suture. Individually clamped large vessels are best ligated with a suture ligature. Concern has been expressed by some that sutures through the decidua may lead to endometriosis in the scar and a weak scar. In actuality, this is a rare complication. The initial stitch is placed just beyond one angle of the uterine incision. A running-lock suture is then carried out, with each stitch penetrating the full thickness of the myometrium. It is important to select carefully the site of each stitch and, once the needle penetrates the myometrium, not to withdraw it. This minimizes the perforation of unligated vessels and subsequent bleeding from such sites. The running-lock suture is continued just beyond the opposite angle of the incision.

Especially when the lower segment is thin, satisfactory approximation of the cut edges usually can be obtained with one layer of suture. When but one layer of suture is to be used, both hemostasis and closure may be better effected by tying the first running-lock suture at about the middle of the incision, placing a new suture beyond the opposite angle of the uterine incision in the same way as the first, and closing the remainder of the incision with a running-lock stitch. If approximation is not satisfactory after a single-layer continuous closure or if bleeding sites persist, either another layer of suture may be placed so as to achieve approximation and hemostasis, or sites of unsatisfactory approximation or lack of hemostasis can be treated with individual figure-of-eight or mattress sutures.

After the operator is certain that there is no further bleeding after closure of the uterine incision, the cut edges of the serosa overlying the uterus and bladder are approximated with a continuous 00 chromic catgut suture (Figs. 26–12 and 26–13). The lower edge of peritoneum should not be carried above the bladder, especially if the procedure is repeated during subsequent cesarean sections. To do so may lead to bladder discomfort and undue urinary frequency during later pregnancies, as well as

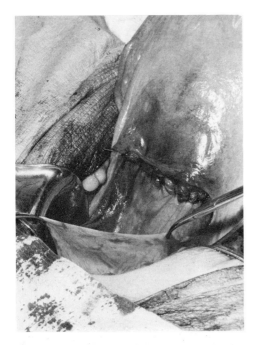

Figure 26–12. The myometrial incision has been closed. The lower edge of the cut serosa is identified in the clamps.

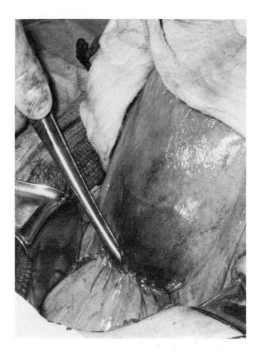

Figure 26–13. The cut margins of the serosa have been approximated to reperitonealize the uterus.

difficult dissection of an unusually adherent overlapped peritoneum with subsequent cesarean section or hysterectomy.

TUBAL STERILIZATION

If tubal sterilization is to be performed, it is done now. The failure rate after the following technique is low (Husbands and associates, 1970):

1. Visualize the fallopian tube in its entirety, being certain to identify the fimbriated ends.
2. Grasp the midportion in a Babcock clamp at a site where the mesosalpinx is seen to be free of veins.
3. Perforate the mesosalpinx immediately beneath the fallopian tube with a fine hemostat and then open the jaws to separate the mesosalpinx from the tube for at least 2 cm.
4. Ligate the separated segment proximally and distally with individual pieces of 0 chromic suture so as to isolate a segment of at least 2 cm.
5. Excise the isolated segment, identify it, and submit it for histological examination.
6. Observe sites of resection for bleeding and, if found, clamp and ligate with fine suture. This technique is described in Chapter 42, p. 936.

ABDOMINAL CLOSURE

Laparotomy packs, if used, are removed, and the gutters and cul-de-sac are emptied of blood and amnionic fluid by gentle suction. If general anesthesia is used, the interior of the abdominal cavity is systematically palpated, as a rule, to evaluate the abdominal contents. With conduction analgesia, however, this may produce considerable discomfort. The uterus is reexamined and compressed to express any blood within it.

As soon as the sponge and instrument counts are found to be correct, the abdominal wall is closed. As each layer is closed, bleeding sites are located, clamped, and ligated. Continuous 00 chromic catgut suture is used to close the peritoneum, including the overlying transversalis fascia (Fig. 26–14). The rectus muscles are allowed to fall into place, and the overlying rectus

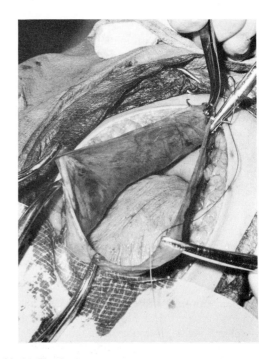

Figure 26–14. The firmly contracted uterus is visible through the uterine incision. The cut margins of the parietal peritoneum are elevated, and closure has been intitiated.

fascia is closed with interrupted 0 nonabsorbable sutures that are placed well lateral to the cut fascial edges and no more than 1 cm apart. The subcutaneous tissue usually need not be closed separately if it is 2 cm or less in thickness, and the skin is closed with vertical mattress sutures of 000 or 0000 silk or equivalent suture or skin clips. If there is more adipose tissue than this or if clips or subcuticular closure is to be used, a few interrupted 000 plain catgut sutures are used to obliterate dead space and reduce tension on the skin edges.

The abdominal wall in most circumstances need only be covered with a light dressing consisting of three 4 × 4 sponges unfolded once and fastened with three pieces of 1-inch tape.

CLASSICAL CESAREAN SECTION

On occasion, it may be necessary to use a classical cesarean section to effect delivery, for example: (1) if the lower uterine segment cannot be exposed or entered safely because the bladder is densely adherent from previous surgery, or if a myoma occupies the lower uterine segment, or if there is invasive carcinoma of the cervix, (2) when there is a transverse lie of a large fetus, especially if the membranes are ruptured and the shoulder is impacted in the birth canal, (3) in some cases of placenta previa with anterior implantation of the placenta, especially if sterilization is to be performed (Chap. 36, p. 715), (4) in some cases of low-birthweight fetuses in which the lower uterine segment is not thinned out.

Incisions

The abdominal incision usually needs to extend somewhat higher than for a lower segment cesarean section. (Originally the classical incision extended to very near the top of the uterine fundus; therefore, in order to expose the uterus, the abdominal incision typically was made just below, lateral to, and above the umbilicus.) The vertical incision into the uterus is initiated with a scalpel beginning above the level of the attached bladder. It is essential to incise through the uterine wall but not lacerate the fetus. Brisk bleeding during entry may make visualization difficult. Once sufficient room is made with the scalpel, the incision is extended cephalad with bandage scissors until it is sufficiently long to permit delivery of the fetus. Numerous large vessels that bleed profusely are commonly encountered within the myometrium. As soon as the fetus has been removed, these vessels may best be clamped and eventually ligated with sutures of chromic catgut. As soon as the fetus has been delivered, oxytocin is administered and the placenta delivered, as described above under Lower Segment Transverse Incision.

Repair of Uterus

The uterus may be lifted through the incision and placed on the abdominal wall. The uterine incision is closed in such a manner that the cut edges are evenly and completely coapted and hemorrhage is controlled. One method employs a layer of continuous 0 or 1 chromic catgut to approximate the inner halves of the incision. The outer half of the uterine incision is then closed with similar chromic catgut suture, using either a continuous stitch or figure-of-eight sutures. Each stitch should be placed sufficiently deep into the myometrium that it will not pull out. No unnecessary needle tracts should be made lest myometrial vessels be perforated with hemorrhage or hematoma formation. To achieve good approximation and to prevent the suture from tearing through the myometrium, it is essential that an assistant compress the myometrium on each side of the wound medially

as each suture is placed and tied. The edges of the uterine serosa, if not already so, are approximated with continuous 00 chromic catgut. The operation is completed as described above under Lower Segment Transverse Incision.

EXTRAPERITONEAL CESAREAN SECTION

Early in this century, Frank (1907) and Latzko (1909) recommended extraperitoneal cesarean section rather than cesarean hysterectomy as a method of managing pregnancies with infected uterine contents. The goal of the operation was to open the uterus extraperitoneally by dissecting through the space of Retzius and then along one side and beneath the bladder to reach the lower uterine segment. The writings of Waters (1940) and Norton (1946) helped to popularize the operation in this country at midcentury. Enthusiasm for the procedure was transient, however, probably in large part because of the availability of a variety of effective antibacterial agents. The increased frequency in recent years of cesarean section, accompanied by either an actual increase in frequency and intensity of troublesome infections or at least a reawareness of the problem, has rekindled interest in the use of extraperitoneal cesarean section. Perkins (1977), for example, demonstrated some enthusiasm for the procedure but, at the same time, carefully explained the limitations of the procedure as well as the benefits that might be derived from its use. He favors the technique described by Douglas and Stromme (1965), who modified the techniques of Latzko and Norton.

POSTMORTEM CESAREAN SECTION

Both Weber (1970) and Arthur (1978) stressed that a satisfactory outcome for the fetus is dependent upon (1) anticipation of death of the mother, (2) fetal age of more than 28 weeks, (3) personnel and appropriate equipment immediately available, (4) continued postmortem ventilation and cardiac massage for the mother, (5) prompt delivery, and (6) effective resuscitation of the infant. While a few infants have survived with no apparent physical or intellectual compromise, others have not been so fortunate. In more recent years, the capability of life-support systems to maintain some level of vegetative function for long periods of time and the reluctance of physicians to pronounce a patient dead have decreased further the likelihood of delivering an infant that will survive and thrive following a postmortem cesarean section. However Field and co-workers (1988) reported the successful delivery by cesarean section of an infant whose mother, though brain dead, was maintained for 10 weeks on life-support systems in order for fetal maturation to occur.

CESAREAN HYSTERECTOMY

INDICATIONS

The indications for cesarean hysterectomy have been discussed in connection with the various conditions that sometimes require the operation. In summary, intrauterine infection, a grossly defective scar, a markedly hypotonic uterus that does not respond to oxytocics, prostaglandins, and massage, inadvertent laceration of major uterine vessels, significant myomas, severe dysplasia or carcinoma in situ of the cervix, and placenta accreta or increta often may best be treated by immediate hysterectomy if cesarean section is being performed. The major deterrents to use of cesarean hysterectomy are increased blood loss and the frequency of damage to the urinary tract in the form of trauma to the ureters and more commonly to the bladder (Plauche and colleagues, 1981).

TECHNIQUE

After delivery of the infant by either classical or lower segment cesarean section, supracervical or preferably total hysterectomy, usually with retention of adnexa, can be carried out according to standard operative techniques. *Although all vessels to the gravid uterus are appreciably larger than those of the nonpregnant organ,* hysterectomy is usually facilitated by the ease of development of tissue planes. Blood loss commonly is appreciable; however, with cesarean hysterectomy performed primarily for sterilization, blood loss averages about 1,500 mL, or about 500 mL more than with cesarean section (Pritchard, 1965).

As the infant's shoulders are delivered, oxytocin is infused intravenously until the uterus is removed. The major bleeding vessels are clamped and ligated quickly. The placenta is removed, and optionally to try to prevent excessive bleeding, a dry laparotomy pack is placed in the cavity over the implantation site before closing the uterine incision with either a continuous suture or a few interrupted sutures. If the incision is not bleeding appreciably, some choose not to close it.

The uterus is elevated out of the abdominal cavity, and the round ligaments close to the uterus are divided between Heaney or Kocher clamps and doubly ligated. Either size 0 or 1 sutures may be used. The incision in the vesicouterine serosa, made to mobilize the bladder for cesarean section, is extended laterally and upward through the anterior leaf of the broad ligament to reach the incised round ligaments. Any actively bleeding vessels must be clamped and tied to minimize blood loss. The posterior leaf of the broad ligament adjacent to the uterus is perforated just beneath the fallopian tubes, utero-ovarian ligaments, and ovarian vessels, and these are then doubly clamped close to the uterus and severed; the lateral pedicle is doubly suture ligated. The pedicles adjacent to the uterus may be ligated and the clamps removed from the operative field. The posterior leaf of the broad ligament is next divided inferiorly toward the cardinal ligaments. Again, any bleeding vessels are discretely clamped and ligated. Next, the bladder and attached peritoneal flap are dissected from the lower uterine segment and retracted out of the operative field. Usually this can be accomplished easily with gentle blunt dissection, using gauze over the fingers. If the bladder flap is unusually adherent, as it may be after previous cesarean sections, careful sharp dissection with scissors may be necessary.

Special care is necessary from this point on to avoid injury to the ureters, which pass beneath the uterine arteries. The ascending uterine artery and veins on either side are identified and near their origin are doubly clamped immediately adjacent to the uterus and divided. The vascular pedicle is doubly suture ligated.

Supracervical Hysterectomy

To perform a subtotal hysterectomy, it is necessary only to amputate the body of the uterus at this level. The cervical stump may be closed with interrupted catgut sutures. If there is persistent oozing of blood or the likelihood of infection, the cervix may be dilated and a drain inserted into the vagina. Reperitonealization is performed as for total hysterectomy.

Total Hysterectomy

To perform a total hysterectomy, it is necessary to mobilize the bladder much more extensively in the midline and laterally.

This will help carry the ureters caudad as the bladder is retracted beneath the symphysis and will also prevent cutting or suturing of the bladder during excision of the cervix and closure of the vagina. The bladder is dissected free for about 2 cm below the lowest margin of the cervix to expose the uppermost part of the vagina. If the cervix is no more than slightly effaced, the cervicovaginal junction can be identified by palpation between the fingers of one hand in the cul-de-sac and the fingers of the other hand anteriorly. If the cervix is appreciably effaced and dilated, this maneuver usually cannot be performed satisfactorily. In this circumstance, the uterine cavity may be entered anteriorly in the mid-line either through the lower pole of the incision made for delivery of the fetus or through a stab wound made at the level of the ligated uterine vessels. A finger is directed inferiorly through the incision to identify the free margin of the dilated, effaced cervix and the anterior vaginal fornix. The contaminated glove is removed by the circulating nurse and the hand regloved. Another useful method to identify the cervical margins is to place four metal skin clips at 12, 3, 6, and 9 o'clock on the cervical edges prior to the laparotomy. Obviously the likelihood of cesarean hysterectomy already would have been considered.

The cardinal ligaments, the uterosacral ligaments, and the many large vessels the ligaments contain are systematically doubly clamped with Heaney-type curved clamps, Ochsner-type straight clamps, or similar instruments. The clamps are placed as close to the cervix as possible without including the cervix. It is imperative that not too large a volume of tissue be included in each clamp. The tissue between the pair of clamps is incised, and the lateral pedicle, which invariably is vascular, is suture ligated appropriately. These steps are repeated until the level of the lateral vaginal fornix is reached. In this way, the descending branches of the uterine vessels are clamped, cut, and ligated as the cervix is dissected from the cardinal ligaments posteriorly.

Immediately below the level of the cervix, a curved clamp is swung in across the lateral vaginal fornix, and the tissue is incised medially to the clamp. The excised lateral vaginal fornix commonly is simultaneously doubly ligated and sutured to the stump of the cardinal ligament. The entire cervix is then excised from the vagina, while an assistant systematically grasps the full thickness of the cut margins of the vagina with straight Ochsner or similar clamps.

The cervix is inspected to insure that it has been completely excised, and the vagina is repaired. Some operators prefer to close the vagina using figure-of-eight chromic catgut sutures. Perhaps the majority prefer to achieve hemostasis by using a running-lock stitch of chromic catgut suture placed through the mucosa and adjacent endopelvic fascia around the circumference of the vagina. The open vagina may promote drainage of the fluids that would otherwise accumulate and contribute to hematoma and abscess formation.

The peritoneal gutters and the cul-de-sac are emptied of blood and other debris. All sites of incision from the upper pedicle (fallopian tube and ovarian ligament) to the vaginal vault and bladder flap are carefully examined for bleeding. Any bleeding sites that are identified are clamped carefully and ligated appropriately. Care is necessary lest the ureter be compromised by such a hemostatic ligature.

The pelvis is reperitonealized. One method employs a continuous chromic suture starting with the tip of the ligated pedicle of fallopian tube and ovarian ligament, which is inverted retroperitoneally. Sutures are then placed continuously so as to approximate the leaves of the broad ligament, to bury the stump of the round ligament, to approximate the cut edge of the vesicouterine peritoneum over the vaginal vault posteriorly to the cut edge of peritoneum above the cul-de-sac, to approximate the leaves of the broad ligament on the opposite side, and to bury the stump of the round ligament and finally the pedicle of fallopian tube and ovarian ligament.

The abdominal wall normally is closed in layers, as previously described under Lower Segment Transverse Incision. In case of sepsis, the abdominal wound may be closed with permanent nonreactive sutures through the peritoneum and fascia in a single layer, while the subcutaneous tissue and skin are not closed until later.

Appendectomy and Oophorectomy

The benefits compared to the risks from incidental appendectomy at the time of cesarean section or hysterectomy continue to be argued. Lacking are results of a study that demonstrate clearly the puerperal morbidity and mortality rates are not increased by appendectomy.

During cesarean hysterectomy, a decision as to the fate of the ovaries has to be made. Should the clamp be placed across the ovarian ligament and fallopian tube medial to the ovary or across the infundibulopelvic ligament just lateral to the ovary and tube? For women who are approaching menopause, the decision is not difficult, but few women who undergo cesarean hysterectomy are approaching the menopause. In general, preservation of the ovaries is favored by most obstetricians unless the ovaries are diseased.

PERIPARTUM MANAGEMENT

PREOPERATIVE CARE

The woman scheduled for repeat cesarean section typically is admitted the day before surgery and evaluated by the obstetrician who will perform surgery and the anesthesiologist who will provide anesthesia. The hematocrit is rechecked, and if the indirect Coombs' test is positive, then 1,000 mL of compatible whole blood or its equivalent in blood fractions is reserved. A sedative, such as secobarbital 100 mg may be given at bedtime the night before the operation. In general, no other sedatives, narcotics, or tranquilizers are administered until after the infant is born. Oral intake is stopped at least 8 hours before surgery. An antacid, such as Bicitra 30 mL, given shortly before the induction of a general anesthesia, minimizes the risk of lung destruction from gastric acid should aspiration occur (Chap. 17, p. 331). The authors strongly recommend this be done routinely, even when regional conduction analgesia will be used; at times it is necessary to switch to, or at least supplement, the regional analgesia with inhalation anesthesia.

INTRAVENOUS FLUIDS

The requirements for intravenous fluids, including blood during and after cesarean section, can vary considerably. The woman of average size with a hematocrit of 33 or more and a normally expanded blood volume and extracellular fluid volume most often tolerates an actual blood loss of up to 1,500 mL without difficulty. The concept that prevailed in some institutions not too long ago that blood loss should be matched milliliter for milliliter by blood transfusion is not tenable, but neither is disregard for excessive bleeding. Careful attention must be paid to blood loss so as to avoid both underestimation and overestimation. Unappreciated bleeding through the vagina during the procedure or bleeding concealed in the uterus after its closure or both commonly lead to underestimation. Blood loss averages about 1 L but is quite variable (Pritchard, 1965; Wilcox and co-workers, 1959).

Intravenously administered fluids consist of lactated Ringer's solution or similar solution and 5 percent dextrose in water. Typically, 1 to 2 L that contain electrolyte are infused during and immediately after the operation. As the shoulders of the infant are delivered, oxytocin, 20 units per L, is added to the infusion, which is then infused for a few minutes at a brisk rate (10 mL per min) until the uterus is well contracted. Throughout the procedure, and subsequently while in the recovery area, the blood pressure and urine flow are monitored closely to ascertain that perfusion of vital organs is satisfactory.

RECOVERY SUITE

It is very important that the uterus remain firmly contracted. In the recovery suite, the amount of bleeding from the vagina must be closely monitored, and the uterine fundus must be identified by palpation frequently to assure that the uterus is remaining firmly contracted. Unfortunately, as the patient awakens from general anesthesia or the conduction analgesia fades, palpation of the abdomen is likely to produce considerable discomfort. This can be made much more tolerable by giving an effective analgesic intramuscularly, such as meperidine (Demerol) 75 mg or morphine 10 mg. A thick dressing with an abundance of adhesive tape over the abdomen interferes with fundal palpation and massage and later causes discomfort as the tape and perhaps skin are removed. Deep breathing and coughing are encouraged.

Once the mother is fully awake, bleeding is minimal, the blood pressure is satisfactory, and urine flow is at least 30 mL per hour, she may be returned to her room.

SUBSEQUENT CARE

Her subsequent care must include the following.

Analgesia

For the woman of average size, meperidine 75 mg is given intramuscularly as often as every 3 hours as needed for discomfort, or morphine 10 mg is similarly administered. If she is small, 50 mg, or if large, 100 mg of meperidine is more appropriate. An antiemetic, for example, promethazine 25 mg, is usually given along with the narcotic.

Vital Signs

The patient is now evaluated at least hourly for 4 hours at the minimum, and blood pressure, pulse, urine flow, amount of bleeding, and status of the uterine fundus are checked at these times. Abnormalities are reported immediately. Thereafter, for the first 24 hours, these are checked at intervals of 4 hours, along with the temperature.

Fluid Therapy and Diet

Unless there has been pathological constriction of the extracellular fluid compartment (diuretics, sodium restriction, vomiting, high fever, prolonged labor without adequate fluid intake), the puerperium is characterized by the excretion of fluid that was retained during pregnancy and became superfluous once delivery was accomplished. Moreover, with the typical cesarean section or uncomplicated cesarean hysterectomy, significant sequestration of extracellular fluid in bowel wall and bowel lumen does not occur, unless it was necessary to pack the bowel away from the operative field or peritonitis develops. Thus, the woman who undergoes cesarean section is rarely a candidate for the development of fluid sequestration in the so-called third space. Quite the contrary, she normally begins surgery with a physiological third space that she acquired during normal pregnancy, namely, the physiological edema of pregnancy that she mobilizes and excretes after delivery. Therefore, large volumes of intravenous fluids during and subsequent to surgery are not needed to replace sequestered extracellular fluid. As a generalization, 3 L of fluid, including lactated Ringer's solution, should prove adequate during surgery and the first 24 hours thereafter. If urine output falls below 30 mL per hour, however, the patient should be reevaluated promptly. The cause of the oliguria may range from unrecognized blood loss to an antidiuretic effect from infused oxytocin (Chap. 16, p. 321). In the absence of extensive intra-abdominal manipulation or sepsis, the woman nearly always should be able to tolerate oral fluids the day after surgery. If not, an intravenous infusion can be continued or restarted. By the second day after surgery, the great majority of women tolerate a general diet.

Bladder and Bowels
The catheter most often can be removed from the bladder by 12 hours after the operation or, more conveniently, the morning after the operation. Subsequent ability to empty the bladder before overdistention develops must be monitored as with a vaginal delivery. Bowel sounds usually are not heard the first day after surgery, they are faint the second day, and they are active the third day. Gas pains from incoordinate bowel action may be troublesome the second and third postoperative days. Frequently, a rectal suppository followed by defecation or, if that fails, an enema provides appreciable relief.

Ambulation
In most instances, by the first day after surgery the patient, with assistance, should get out of bed briefly at least twice. Ambulation can be timed so that a recently administered analgesic will minimize the discomfort. By the second day she may walk to the bathroom with assistance. With early ambulation, venous thrombosis and pulmonary embolism are uncommon.

Wound Care
The incision is inspected each day. Thus, a relatively light dressing without an abundance of tape is advantageous. Normally the skin sutures (or skin clips) are removed on the fourth day after surgery. By the third postpartum day, bathing by shower is not harmful to the incision.

Laboratory
The hematocrit is routinely measured the morning after surgery. It is checked sooner when there was unusual blood loss or when there is oliguria or other evidence to suggest hypovolemia. If the hematocrit is significantly decreased from the preoperative level, it is repeated, and a search is instituted to identify the cause of the decrease. If the lower hematocrit is stable, the mother can ambulate without any difficulty, and if there is little likelihood of further blood loss, hematological repair in response to iron therapy is preferred to transfusion.

Breast Care
Breast feeding can be initiated by the day after surgery. If the mother elects not to breast feed, a breast binder that supports the breasts without marked compression will usually minimize discomfort. Bromocriptine for suppression of lactation has proved to be effective for this purpose. The major disadvantage of bromocriptine remains its high cost. The patient is more comfortable using this drug than using a breast binder, and the suppression of lactation removes one possible source of postpartum fever (Chap. 28, p. 483).

DISCHARGE FROM THE HOSPITAL

Unless there are complications during the puerperium, the mother may be safely discharged from the hospital on the fourth or fifth postpartum day. The mother's activities during the following week should be restricted to self-care and care of her baby with assistance. It is advantageous to perform the initial postpartum evaluation during the third week after delivery rather than at the more traditional time of 6 weeks, for the reasons presented in Chapters 13 and 42.

PROPHYLACTIC ANTIMICROBIALS

Febrile morbidity is rather frequent after cesarean section and and appears to be more common among indigent than affluent women. Since the development of antimicrobial agents, numerous attempts have been made to document the value, if any, of prophylactically administered antibiotics. During the early antibiotic era, various claims for and against such a practice were made. Subsequently, many reports have appeared in which febrile morbidity was shown to be reduced appreciably when antibiotics were administered prophylactically. The issue of prophylactic antibiotics following cesarean section has been addressed by numerous investigators (Gall, 1979; Gibbs and colleagues, 1973; Green and associates, 1978; Kreutner and colleagues, 1979; Wong and associates, 1978).

At Parkland Hospital a group of women at high risk for serious pelvic infection following cesarean delivery has been identified (Cunningham and associates, 1978). It was shown that 85 percent of women in labor with membranes ruptured for longer than 6 hours who then underwent cesarean delivery developed serious infection. The incidence was much less (29 percent) in women who underwent cesarean section after laboring with membranes intact. Moreover, these investigators noted that associated complications such as wound abscesses and pelvic phlegmons were encountered in less than 1 percent of women with intact membranes, compared to 30 percent of women whose membranes ruptured more than 6 hours before cesarean section. In addition, bacteremia was four times more common in those women whose membranes ruptured longer than 6 hours before surgery and who subsequently demonstrated infection.

Subsequently DePalma and colleagues (1980, 1982) evaluated therapeutic intervention in this high-risk group of nulliparous women who underwent cesarean delivery because of cephalopelvic disproportion. Since the frequency of pelvic infection was 85 percent without therapy, they considered intervention with antimicrobials to be treatment rather than prophylaxis. They observed that the administration of penicillin plus gentamicin or of cefamandole alone as soon as the cord was clamped, followed by two more doses of the same medications given at intervals of 6 hours, resulted in a dramatic reduction in morbidity from infection. Postoperative metritis, for example, was decreased from 85 to 20 percent. Importantly, associated complications, such as pelvic phlegmons, incisional abscesses, and pelvic thrombophlebitis, also decreased dramatically (Fig. 26–15).

Duff (1987) recently reviewed 25 randomized clinical trials in which it was demonstrated that one or three doses of an antimicrobial given at the time of cesarean section were found to decrease infection morbidity appreciably. For women in labor or with ruptured membranes, he recommends a single 2-g dose of ampicillin or a first-generation cephalosporin after delivery of the infant. A second dose in 3 to 4 hours is given if surgery is prolonged more than 90 minutes. Currently, our practice at Parkland Hospital is to administer a single-dose of a broad-spectrum antimicrobial such as a cephalosporin or an extended-spectrum penicillin. These regimens have been proven equally effective and they should be chosen by virtue of patient allergies, local availability, cost, and physician comfort with their individual use.

In the very high-risk women shown in Figure 26–15, almost 25 percent developed metritis despite the three-dose perioperative antimicrobial regimen. For women at lower risk, the clinical infection rate is correspondingly less. It is our experience, in most cases at least, that these women with failed prophylaxis tend to have milder infections which usually do not manifest until the third or fourth postoperative day. Treatment is discussed in Chapter 27 (p. 463).

It is emphasized that the woman with clinically diagnosed chorioamnionitis should be given continuous antimicrobial therapy postoperatively until she is afebrile.

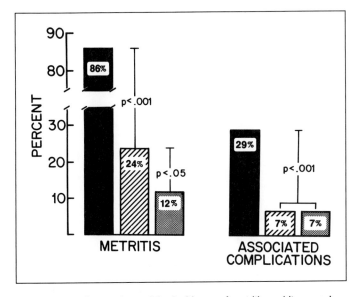

Figure 26–15. Comparison of the incidence of metritis and its associated complications (pelvic phlegmons, incisional abscesses, and pelvic thrombophlebitis) according to treatment management in 642 high-risk women undergoing cesarean section. The *solid bars* represent infections in women not given antimicrobials unless signs and symptoms of infection developed (N = 128). The *hatched bar* represents the outcomes following three-dose perioperative antimicrobials (N = 305). The *speckled bars* represent outcomes obtained by administering antimicrobials from the time of cesarean section until 4 days postpartum (N = 209). (*From DePalma and associates: Obstet Gynecol 60:53, 1982.*)

HISTORICAL

The origin of the term *cesarean section* is obscure. Three principal explanations have been suggested.

1. According to legend, Julius Caesar was born in this manner, with the result that the procedure became known as the "Caesarean operation." Several circumstances weaken this explanation, however. First, the mother of Julius Caesar lived for many years after his birth. Even as late as the 17th century, the operation was almost invariably fatal, according to the most dependable writers of that period. It is thus improbable that Caesar's mother could have survived the procedure in 100 B.C. Second, the operation, whether performed on the living or dead, is not mentioned by any medical writer before the Middle Ages. Historical details of the origin of the family name Caesar are found in Pickrell's monograph (1935).

2. It has been widely believed that the name of the operation is derived from a Roman law, supposedly created by Numa Pompilius (eighth century B.C.), ordering that the procedure be performed upon women dying in the last few weeks of pregnancy in the hope of saving the child. This explanation then holds that this *lex regia*, as it was called at first, became the *lex caesarea* under the emperors, and the operation itself became known as the *caesarean* operation. The German term *Kaiserschnitt* reflects this derivation.

3. The word *caesarean*, as applied to the operation, was derived sometime in the Middle Ages from the Latin verb *caedere*, "to cut." An obvious cognate is the word *caesura*, a cutting, or pause, in a line of verse. This explanation of the term *caesarean* seems most logical, but exactly when it was first applied to the operation is uncertain. Since "section" is derived from the Latin verb *seco*, which also means "cut," the term *caesarean section* seems tautological.

It is customary in the United States to replace the *æ* in the first syllable of *caesarean* with the letter *e*; in Great Britain and Australia, however, the "ae" is still retained.

From the time of Virgil's Aeneas to Shakespeare's Macduff, poets have repeatedly referred to persons "untimely ripped" from their mother's womb. Ancient historians, such as Pliny, moreover, say that Scipio Africanus (the conqueror of Hannibal), Martius, and Julius Caesar were all born thus. In regard to Julius Caesar, Pliny adds that it was from this circumstance that the surname(?) rose by which the Roman emperors were known. Birth in this extraordinary manner, as described in ancient mythology and legend, was believed to confer supernatural powers and elevate the heroes so born above ordinary mortals.

In evaluating these references to abdominal delivery in antiquity, it is pertinent that no such operation is even mentioned by Hippocrates, Galen, Celsus, Paulus, Soranus, or any other medical writer of the period. If cesarean section were actually employed at that time, it is particularly surprising that Soranus, whose extensive work written in the second century A.D. covers all aspects of obstetrics, does not refer to cesarean section. In Genesis (11:21) it is written: "And the Lord God caused a deep sleep to fall upon Adam, and he slept: and he took one of his ribs, and closed up the flesh instead thereof." Are we to conclude from this statement that general anesthesia and thoracic surgery were known in pre-Mosaic times? It would probably be just as logical to draw comparable conclusions about the beginnings of cesarean section from the myths and fantasies that have come down to us.

Several references to abdominal delivery appear in the Talmud, compiled between the second and sixth centuries A.D., but whether they had any background in terms of clinical usage is conjectural. There can be no doubt, however, that cesarean section on the dead was first practiced soon after the Christian Church gained dominance, as a measure directed at baptism of the child. Faith in the validity of some of these early reports is rudely shaken, however, when they glibly state that a living, robust child was obtained 8 to 24 *hours* after the death of the mother.

Some of the early reports of cesarean section on the living excite similar skepticism. The case often cited as representing the first cesarean section performed on a living woman is that attributed to a German gelder named Jacob Nufer, who is said to have carried out the operation on his wife in the year 1500. Not only did his wife survive (a miracle in itself) but she lived to give birth to two subsequent children after normal labors, in a period when suturing of the uterine wound during cesarean section was unknown. The case was not reported until almost a hundred years later (1591) by an author who based his description on hearsay handed down through three generations.

Cesarean section on the living was first recommended, and the current name of the operation used, in the celebrated work of François Rousset entitled "Traité Nouveau de l'Hystérotomotokie ou l'Enfantement Césarien," published in 1581. Rousset had never performed or witnessed the operation; his information was based chiefly on letters from friends. He reported 14 successful cesarean sections, a fact in itself difficult to accept. When it is further stated that 6 of the 14 operations were performed on the same woman, the credulity of the most gullible is exhausted.

The apocryphyal nature of most early reports on cesarean section has been stressed because many of them have been accepted without question. Authoritative statements by dependable obstetricians about early use of the operation, however, did not appear in the literature until the mid-17th century, as for instance in the classic work of the great French obstetrician, François Mauriceau, first published in 1668. These statements show without doubt that the operation was employed on the living in rare and desperate cases during the latter half of the 16th century and that it was usually fatal. Details of the history of cesarean section are to be found in Fasbender's classic text (1906).

The appalling maternal mortality rate of cesarean section continued until the beginning of the 20th century. In Great Britain and Ireland, the maternal death rate from the operation had mounted in 1865 to 85 percent. In Paris, during the 90 years ending in 1876, not a single successful cesarean section had been performed. Harris (1879) noted that as late as 1879 cesarean section was actually more successful when performed by the patient herself or when the abdomen was ripped open by the horn of a bull. He collected from the literature 9 such cases with 5 recoveries, and contrasted them with 12 cesarean sections performed in New York City during the same period, with only 1 recovery.

The turning point in the evolution of cesarean section came in 1882, when Max Sänger, then a 28-year-old assistant of Credé in the University Clinic at Leipzig, introduced suturing of the uterine wall. The long neglect of so simple an expedient as uterine suture was not the result of oversight but stemmed from a deeply rooted belief that sutures in the uterus were superfluous as well as harmful by virtue of serving as the site for severe infection. In meeting these objections Sänger, who had himself used sutures in only one case, documented their value, not from the sophisticated medical centers of Europe but from frontier America. There, in outposts from Ohio to Louisiana, 17 cesarean sections had been reported in which silver wire sutures had been used, with the survival of eight mothers, an extraordinary record in those days. In a table included in his monograph, Sänger gives full credit to these frontier surgeons for providing the supporting data for his hypothesis. The problem of hemorrhage was the first and most serious problem to be solved. Details are found in Eastman's review (1932).

Although the introduction of uterine sutures reduced the mortality rate of the operation from hemorrhage, generalized peritonitis remained the dominant cause of death; hence, various types of operations were devised to meet this scourge. The earliest was the Porro procedure (1876), in use before Sänger's time, that combined subtotal cesarean hysterectomy with marsupialization of the cervical stump. The first extraperitoneal operation was described by Frank in 1907 and, with various modifications, as introduced by Latzko (1909), and by Waters (1940), was employed until recent years.

In 1912, Krönig contended that the main advantage of the extraperitoneal technique consisted not so much in avoiding the peritoneal cavity as in opening the uterus through its thin lower segment and then covering the incision with peritoneum. To accomplish this end, he cut through the vesical reflection of the peritoneum from one round ligament to the other and separated it and the bladder from the lower uterine segment and cervix. The lower portion of the uterus was then opened through a vertical median incision, and the child was extracted by forceps. The uterine incision was then closed and buried under the vesical peritoneum. With minor modifications, this low-segment technique was introduced into the United States by Beck (1919) and popularized by DeLee (1922) and others. A particularly important modification was recommended by Kerr in 1926, who preferred a transverse rather than a longitudinal uterine incision. The Kerr technique is the most commonly employed type of cesarean section today.

A monograph on the history of cesarean section by Trolle (1982) is recommended.

REFERENCES

American College of Obstetricians and Gynecologists Committee on Maternal and Fetal Medicine: Guidelines for vaginal delivery after a previous cesarean birth October 1988

American College of Obstetricians and Gynecologists: Professional liability insurance and its effect: Report of a survey of ACOG's membership. (Prepared by Needham, Porter, and Novelli), Washington, DC, American College of Obstetricians and Gynecologists, November 1985

Anderson GM, Lomas J: Determinants of the increasing cesarean birth rate: Ontario data 1979 to 1982. N Engl J Med 311:887, 1984

Arthur RK: Postmortem cesarean section. Am J Obstet Gynecol 132:175, 1978

Baskett TF, McMillen RM: Cesarean section: Trends and morbidity. Can Med Assoc J 125:723, 1981

Beck AC: Observations on a series of cases of cesarean section done at the Long Island College Hospital during the past six years. Am J Obstet Gynecol 79:197, 1919

Bottoms SF, Rosen MG, Sokol RJ: The increase in the cesarean birth. N Engl J Med 302:559, 1980

Clark SL, Eglinton GS, Beall M, Phelan JP: Effect of indication for previous cesarean section on subsequent delivery outcome in patients undergoing a trial of labor. J Reprod Med 29:22, 1984

Collea JV, Chein C, Quilligan EJ: The randomized management of term frank breech presentation: A study of 208 cases. Am J Obstet Gynecol 137:235, 1980

Cunningham FG, Hauth JC, Strong JD, Kappus SS: Infectious morbidity following cesarean section: Comparison of two treatment regimens. Obstet Gynecol 52:656, 1978

Danforth DN: Cesarean section. JAMA 253:811, 1985

DeLee JB, Cornell EL: Low cervical cesarean section (laparotrachelotomy). JAMA 79:109, 1922

DePalma RT, Cunningham FG, Leveno KJ, Roark ML: Continuing investigation of women at high risk for infection following cesarean delivery: The three-dose perioperative antimicrobial therapy. Obstet Gynecol 60:53, 1982

DePalma RT, Leveno KJ, Cunningham FG, Pope T, Kappus SS, Roark ML, Nobles BJ: Identification and management of women at high risk for pelvic infection following cesarean section. Obstet Gynecol 55:185S, 1980

Douglas RG, Birnbaum SJ, MacDonald FA: Pregnancy and labor following cesarean section. Am J. Obstet Gynecol 86:961, 1963

Douglas RG, Stromme WB: Operative Obstetrics, 2nd ed. New York, Appleton, 1965, pp. 449–452

Duff P: Prophylactic antibiotics for cesarean delivery: A simple cost-effective strategy for prevention of postoperative morbidity. Am J Obstet Gynecol 157:794, 1987

Duff P, Southmayd K, Read JA: Outcome of trial of labor in patients with a single previously low transverse cesarean for dystocia. Obstet Gynecol 71:380, 1988

Eastman NJ: The role of Frontier America in the development of cesarean section. Am J Obstet Gynecol 24:919, 1932

Farmakides G, Duvivier R, Schulman H, Schneider E, Biordi J: Vaginal birth after two or more previous cesarean sections. Am J Obstet Gynecol 154:565, 1987

Fasbender H: Geschichte der Geburlshufe. Jena, 1906, pp 979–1010

Field DR, Gates EA, Creasy R, Jonsen A, Laros R: Maternal brain death during pregnancy: Medical and ethical issues. JAMA 260:816, 1988

Flaksman RS, Vollman JH, Benfield DG: Iatrogenic prematurity due to elective termination of the uncomplicated pregnancy: A major perinatal health care problem. Am J Obstet Gynecol 132:885, 1978

Flamm BL: Vaginal birth after cesarean section: Controversies old and new. Clin Obstet Gynecol 28:735, 1985

Flamm BL, Lim OW, Jones C, Fallon D, Newman LA, Mantis JK: Vaginal birth after cesarean section: Results of a multicenter study. Am J Obstet Gynecol 158:1079, 1988

Frank F: Suprasymphysial delivery and its relation to other operations in the presence of contracted pelvis. Arch Gynaekol 81:46, 1907

Frigoletto FD Jr, Ryan KJ, Phillippe M: Maternal mortality rate associated with cesarean section: An appraisal. Am J Obstet Gynecol 136:969, 1980

Gall SA: The efficacy of prophylactic antibiotics in cesarean section. Am J Obstet Gynecol 134:506, 1979

Gibbs RS, Hunt JE, Schwarz RJ: A follow-up study on prophylactic antibiotics in cesarean section. Am J Obstet Gynecol 117:419, 1973

Gluck L: Iatrogenic RDS and amniocentesis. Hosp Pract 12:11, 1977

Goodlin RC, Scott JC Jr, Woods RE, Anderson JC: Laparoelytrotomy or abdominal delivery without uterine incision. Am J Obstet Gynecol 144:990, 1982

Green SL, Sarubbi FA, Bishop EH: Prophylactic antibiotics in high-risk cesarean section. Obstet Gynecol 51:569, 1978

Harris RP: Lessons from a study of the cesarean operation in the City and State of New York. Am J Obstet 12:82, 1879

Haynes de Regt RH, Minkoff HL, Feldman J, Schwarz RH: Relation of private or clinic care to the cesarean birth rate. N Engl J Med 315:619, 1986

Hershey DW, Quilligan EJ: Extraabdominal uterine exteriorization at cesarean section. Obstet Gynecol 52:189, 1978

Husbands ME Jr, Pritchard JA, Pritchard SA: Failure of tubal sterilization accompanying cesarean section. Am J Obstet Gynecol 107:966, 1970

Jarrell MA, Ashmead GG, Mann LI: Vaginal delivery after cesarean section: A five-year study. Obstet Gynecol 65:628, 1985

Kerr JMM: The technic of cesarean section with special reference to the lower uterine segment incision. Am J Obstet Gynecol 12:729, 1926

Kreutner AK, Del Bene VE, Delamar D, Bodden JL, Loadholt CB: Perioperative cephalosoporin prophylaxis in cesarean section: Effect on endometritis in the high-risk patient. Am J Obstet Gynecol 134:925, 1979

Krönig B: Transperitonealer Cervikaler Kaiserschnitt. In Doderlein A, Krönig B (eds): Operative Gynakologie, 1912, p 879

Latzko W: Ueber den extraperitonealen Kaiserschnitt, Zentralbl Gynaekol 33:275, 1909

Leveno KJ, Cunningham FG, Pritchard JA: Cesarean section: An answer to the House of Horne. Am J Obstet Gynecol 153:838, 1985

Martel M, Wacholder S, Lippman A, Brohan J, Hamilton E: Maternal age and primary cesarean section rates: A multivariate analysis. Am J Obstet Gynecol 156:305, 1987

McGarry JA: The management of patients previously delivered by caesarean section. J Obstet Gynaecol Br Commonw 76:137, 1969

Mootabar H, Dwyer JF, Surur F, Dillon TF: Vaginal delivery following previous cesarean section in 1983. Int J Gynaecol Obstet 22:155, 1984

National Institutes of Health: Consensus Development Conference Summary, Vol 3, No 6, 1980

Norton JF: A paravesical extraperitoneal cesarean section technique. Am J Obstet Gynecol 51:519, 1946

Notzon FC, Placek PJ, Taffel SM: Comparisons of national cesarean-section rates. N Engl J Med 316:386, 1987

O'Driscoll K, Foley M: Correlation of decrease in perinatal mortality and increase in cesarean section rates. Obstet Gynecol 61:1, 1983

O'Driscoll K, Foley M: MacDonald D: Active management of labor as an alternative to cesarean section for dystocia. Obstet Gynecol 63:485, 1984

O'Driscoll K, Jackson RJA, Gallagher JT: Prevention of prolonged labor. Br Med J 2:477, 1969

O'Driscoll K, Stronge JM, Minogue M: Active management of labour. Br Med J 3:135, 1973

Ollendorff DA, Goldberg JM, Minogue JP, Socol ML: Vaginal birth after cesarean section for arrest of labor: Is success determined by maximum cervical dilatation during the prior labor? Am J Obstet Gynecol 159:636, 1988

O'Sullivan MJ, Fumia F, Holsinger K, McLeod AGW: Vaginal delivery after cesarean section. Clin Perinatol 8:131, 1981

Paul RH, Phelan JP, Yeh S-Y: Trial of labor in the patient with a prior cesarean birth. Am J Obstet Gynecol 151:297, 1985

Perkins RP: Extraperitoneal section: A viable alternative. Contemp Ob/Gyn 9:55, 1977

Petitti DB: Maternal mortality and morbidity in cesarean section. Clin Obstet Gynecol 28:763, 1985

Phelan JP, Clark SL, Diab F, Paul RH: Vaginal birth after cesarean. Am J Obstet Gynecol 157:1510, 1987

Pickrell K: An inquiry into the history of cesarean section. Bull Soc Med Hist (Chicago) 4:414, 1935

Placek PJ, Taffel SM: Vaginal birth after cesarean (VBAC) in the 1980s. Am J Public Health 78:512, 1988

Placek PJ, Taffel SM, Keppel KG: Maternal and infant characteristics associated with cesarean section delivery. Department of Health and Human Services, Publication No (PHS) 84-1232, Hyattsville, MD: National Center for Health Statistics, December 1983

Plauché WC, Gruich FG, Bourgeois MO: Hysterectomy at the time of cesarean section: Analysis of 108 cases. Obstet Gynecol 58:459, 1981

Pliny the Elder: Natural History. Cambridge, MA. Harvard University Press, 1942, Book VII, Chap IX. Translated by H Rackham

Porreco RP, Meier RP: Trial of labor in patients with two or more previous cesarean sections. J Reprod Med 28:770, 1983

Porro E: Della Amputazione Utero-ovarica, Milan, 1876

Pritchard JA: Changes in the blood volume during pregnancy and delivery. Anesthesiology 26:393, 1965

Pruett KM, Kirshon B, Cotton DB, Poindexter AN III: Is vaginal birth after two or more cesarean sections safe? Obstet Gynecol 72:163, 1988

Riva HL, Teich JC: Vaginal delivery after cesarean section. Am J Obstet Gynecol 81:501, 1961

Rousset F: Traité Nouveau de l'Hystérotomotokie ou l'Enfantement Césaerien. Paris, Denys deVal, 1581

Rubin GL, Peterson HB, Rochat RW, McCarthy BJ, Terry JS: Maternal death after cesarean section in Georgia. Am J Obstet Gynecol 139:681, 1981

Ruddick V, Niv D, Hetman-Peri M, Geller E, Avni A, Golan A: Epidural analgesia for planned vaginal delivery following previous cesarean section. Obstet Gynecol 64:621, 1984

Sachs BP, Yeh J, Acker D, Driscoll S, Brown DAJ, Jewett JF: Cesarean section-related maternal mortality in Massachusetts, 1954–1985. Obstet Gynecol 71:385, 1988

Sänger M: Der Kaiserschnitt bei Uterusfibromen. Leipzig, 1882

Seitchik J, Ramakrishna RV: Cesarean delivery in nulliparous women for failed oxytocin-augmented labor: Route of delivery in subsequent pregnancy. Am J Obstet Gynecol 143:393, 1982

Shiono PH, McNellis D, Rhoads GG: Reasons for the rising cesarean delivery rates: 1978–1984. Obstet Gynecol 69:696, 1987

Taffel SM, Placek PJ, Liss T: Trends in the United States cesarean section rate for the 1980–1985 rise. Am J Public Health 77:955, 1985

Trolle D: The History of Cesarean Section. Copenhagen, University Library, CA Reitzel Booksellers, 1982

Uppington J: Epidural analgesia and previous cesarean section. Anaesthesia 38:336, 1983

Vengadasalam D: Vaginal delivery following cesarean section. Singapore Med J 37:396, 1986

Waters EG: Supravesical extraperitoneal cesarean section: Presentation of a new technique. Am J Obstet Gynecol 39:423, 1940

Weber CE: Postmortem cesarean section: Review of the literature and case reports. Am J Obstet Gynecol 110:158, 1970

Wilcox CF, Hunt AB, Owen CA: The measurement of blood lost during cesarean section. Am J Obstet Gynecol 77:772, 1959

Wong R, Gee CL, Ledger WJ: Prophylactic use of cefazolin in monitoring obstetric patients undergoing cesarean section. Obstet Gynecol 51:407, 1978

Part VII

ABNORMALITIES OF THE PUERPERIUM

27

Puerperal Infection

DEFINITION

Puerperal infection is bacterial infection of the genital tract after delivery. Previously used but less satisfactory synonyms are puerperal fever, puerperal sepsis, and childbed fever. Infection, along with preeclampsia and obstetrical hemorrhage, for many decades of this century formed the lethal triad of causes of maternal deaths (Chap. 1, p. 2). Fortunately, more recently, maternal death from infection has become less common (Rochat and colleagues, 1988; Sachs and associates, 1988).

PUERPERAL MORBIDITY

Since most temperature elevations in the puerperium are caused by pelvic infection, the incidence of fever after childbirth is a reliable index of the incidence of these infections. For this reason, it has been customary to group all puerperal fevers under the general term "puerperal morbidity" and to estimate the frequency of puerperal infection on this basis. Several definitions have been based on the degree of pyrexia reached. The Joint Committee on Maternal Welfare was convened in 1919 (Mussey and colleagues, 1935), and several years later modified European standards and defined puerperal morbidity as a *"Temperature 38.0°C (100.4°F) or higher, the temperature to occur on any two of the first 10 days postpartum, exclusive of the first 24 hours, and to be taken by mouth by a standard technique at least four times daily."* This remains the most commonly employed standard in the United States, and while it suggests that all puerperal fevers are the consequence of pelvic infection, temperature elevations may be the result of other causes, such as pyelonephritis, respiratory infection, or breast engorgement.

HISTORY

The earliest reference to puerperal infection is found in the 5th century B.C. works of Hippocrates, and in his discussion of women, *De Muliebrum Morbis,* he described the condition and attributed it to retention of bowel contents. By 200 A.D., Celsus and Galen had written in support of the theories of Hippocrates, and they recommended purgation. It was not until the late 1500s that putrefaction of the lochia, or uterine inflammation, were suspected as the cause of childbed fever, and both were linked to a difficult labor. William Harvey (1651) aptly described the placental implantation site as a "vast internal ulcer" which may lead to gangrene. In 1659, Willis

wrote on the subject of *febris puerperarum,* although the English term *puerperal fever* was probably first employed by Strother in 1716.

The theory of *milk metastasis* of Puzos (1686) followed next and predominated for a hundred years, but in the 1700s uterine inflammation was again thought to cause febrile morbidity. John Leake (1772) first suggested that contagious nature of puerperal infection, and Alexander Hamilton positively stated this position in 1781. Alexander Gordon of Aberdeen, in a treatise on epidemic puerperal fever in 1795, discussed the infectious and contagious nature of the disease, antedating the papers of Holmes (1855) and Semmelweis (1861) by a half-century. Charles White (1773) of Manchester postulated that puerperal fever was dependent on lochial stagnation, and advised complete isolation of infected women.

It was not until the mid-1800s that such views were becoming acceptable. In 1843, Oliver Wendell Holmes presented *The Contagiousness of Puerperal Fever* before the Boston Society for Medical Improvement, in which he clearly showed that at least the epidemic forms of the infection could always be traced to the lack of proper precautions on the part of the physician or nurse. Four years later, Semmelweis, then an assistant at the Vienna Lying-In Hospital, began a careful inquiry into the causes of the frightful mortality rate following delivery in that institution, as compared with the relatively small number of women who died as a result of infection following home delivery. He concluded that the morbid process was essentially a wound infection caused by the introduction of septic material by the examining finger. He issued stringent orders that physicians, students, and midwives disinfect their hands with chlorine water, the forerunner of Dakin's solution, before examining parturient women. Despite immediate and surprising results in which the mortality rate fell from over 10 percent to 1 percent, both his work and that of Holmes were ridiculed by many of the most prominent physicians of the time. His discovery remained unappreciated until Lister's teachings in 1867 regarding antisepsis, and the development of bacteriology by Pasteur.

The history of puerperal infection is discussed in detail in the monographs of Eisenmann (1837), Burtenshaw (1904), and Peckham (1935). Willson (1988) provided a review of cesarean section infections.

PREDISPOSING CAUSES

In general, the likelihood of serious postpartum pelvic infection is related to the length of membrane rupture before delivery, the number of cervical examinations, intrauterine manipulation for delivery of the fetus and placenta, and the size and number

461

of incisions and lacerations. It is generally accepted that puerperal infection is much more common in women from populations of lower socioeconomic status compared to middle- or upper-class patients. The precise reasons for these differences is unclear but needs to be diligently investigated.

Several other factors during pregnancy or delivery have been implicated in the genesis of puerperal infection and are discussed below.

ANTEPARTUM FACTORS

Anemia, poor nutrition, and sexual intercourse have long been considered to predispose to puerperal sepsis, although the evidence is mostly indirect. Despite no strong direct evidence to implicate these in the genesis of puerperal infection, anemia and poor nutrition should be prevented or appropriately corrected, and sexual intercourse should probably be avoided near term, and especially if there is membrane rupture.

Anemia

The evidence that anemia increases the likelihood of infection is not decisive (Cook and Lynch, 1986). The results obtained from both animal and in vitro experiments are consistent with the view that iron-deficiency anemia does not predispose to infection, and some believe it may actually prevent infection. For example, transferrin appears to have significant antibacterial action, and transferrin is increased in iron-deficiency anemia. Moreover, growth of a variety of pathogenic bacteria in vitro is inhibited by lack of iron. Finally, there is no impairment of wound healing in animals previously made iron deficient.

Nutrition

The role of nutrition in the genesis of infection is also unclear, although cell-mediated immunity has been reported impaired in malnourished laboratory animals. In vitro lymphocyte responses to antigens are depressed in iron-deficiency anemia as well as kwashiorkor (Joynson and associates, 1972). Kulapongs and co-workers (1974), however, found no such defect in studies of children with severe iron-deficiency anemia.

Sexual Intercourse

An increased incidence of puerperal infection resulting from sexual intercourse has not been clearly demonstrated. If, however, the membranes were ruptured at the time of coitus or were to rupture very soon thereafter, the infection rate most likely would be increased. Moreover, preterm delivery has been reported to be more frequent in women who had intercourse late in gestation, and the etiology may possibly be the consequence of infection (Naeye, 1979).

Prematurely Ruptured Membranes and Preterm Labor

Silent chorioamnionic infection has emerged as a possible explanation for many previously unexplained cases of preterm labor (Minkoff, 1983). For example, Leigh and Garite (1986) reported that 12 percent of women with preterm labor and intact membranes had occult amnionic fluid infection. Others have reported even higher rates. Prematurely ruptured membranes also appear to be associated with covert membrane infection, at least in some cases. Certainly, these conditions seem to be associated with increased puerperal infections.

INTRAPARTUM FACTORS

At least three significant intrapartum factors are implicated in the genesis of puerperal infection. They are iatrogenic introduction of pathogenic bacteria into the upper genital tract, trauma that devitalizes tissue, and hemorrhage. There is no doubt that the first two are of considerable importance.

Bacterial Contamination

The normally sterile upper genital tract is colonized in at least two ways. First, bacteria already present on the pudenda and in the vagina and cervix may be carried into the uterine cavity during the course of examination, insertion of fetal monitoring devices, or operative manipulation. Since no vaginal or cervical manipulation can be carried out with absolute asepsis, every cervicovaginal examination must be carefully considered in terms of benefits to be achieved versus the risks of bacterial contamination. Second, the gloves or instruments may be contaminated by virulent organisms as the result of droplet infection. Because the nasopharynx is the most common course of extraneous bacteria brought to the birth canal, obstetrical personnel in the delivery room usually wear masks that cover the nose and mouth.

Trauma

Lacerations provide portals of entry for pathogenic bacteria and devitalized tissue serves as an excellent culture medium. The most graphic example is that of delivery by cesarean section, which increases substantively the puerperal infection rate. For example, at Parkland Hospital, nearly half of all women undergoing cesarean section, but who are not given perioperative antimicrobials, developed pelvic infections postpartum (Cunningham and colleagues, 1978). Similar results from the University of Washington Hospital were reported by Wager and co-workers (1980). As discussed in Chapter 26 (p. 456), prophylactic antimicrobials given perioperatively drastically reduce the frequency of post-cesarean infections.

Blood Loss

It is not so clear whether hemorrhage per se is of great significance in the pathogenesis of infection. The trauma that led to hemorrhage and the manipulations associated with its control, along with repair of traumatized tissue, certainly predispose to infection. Hematomas that often form in these circumstances early and frequently become infected and enhance the likelihood of troublesome sepsis.

PATHOLOGY

After completion of the third stage of labor, the site of placental attachment is raw and elevated, dark red, and about 4 cm in diameter. Its surface is made nodular by the numerous veins that are normally occluded by thrombi. This site provides an excellent culture medium for bacteria and it is the most likely portal of entry for pathogenic organisms. Also at this time the entire decidua is peculiarly susceptible to bacterial invasion since it is less than 2 mm in thickness, is infiltrated with blood, and now has numerous small openings. Because the cervix rarely escapes some degree of laceration in labor, it offers easy access for bacterial invasion as do vulvar, vaginal, and perineal incisions or lacerations. Finally, the uterine incision for cesarean delivery is a most important portal of entry.

Thus, many puerperal infections are actually wound infections. The inflammatory process may manifest as cellulitis localized in these wounds or it may extend through the lymphatics to other pelvic tissues.

BACTERIOLOGY

Organisms that invade the placental implantation site, incisions, and lacerations that are the consequence of labor and delivery are typically those that normally colonize the cervix, vagina, and perineum. Most of these bacteria are of relatively low virulence, and seldom initiate infection in healthy tissues. Although more virulent bacteria may be introduced from exogenous sources, in modern obstetrics an epidemic of serious puerperal sepsis rarely develops, as virulent bacteria are not usually carried from person to person during labor, delivery, or early in the puerperium. However, an epidemic from group A β-hemolytic streptococcus has been well documented in the past 20 years (Jewett and associates, 1968).

COMMON PATHOGENS

In the great majority of instances of puerperal infection, the bacteria responsible for the infection are those that normally reside in the bowel and also commonly colonize the perineum, vagina, and cervix. Bacteria commonly responsible for female genital tract infections are shown in Table 27–1. Usually multiple species of bacteria are isolated, and although typically considered to be of relatively low virulence, these bacteria may become pathogenic as a result of hematomas and devitalized tissue. Whatever the mechanism, their pathogenicity now is enhanced sufficiently to cause uterine infection with extensive pelvic cellulitis, abscesses, peritonitis, and suppurative thrombophlebitis.

Although the cervix and lower genital tract routinely harbor such bacteria, the uterine cavity is usually sterile before rupture of the amnionic sac. As the consequence of labor and delivery and associated manipulations, the amnionic fluid and perhaps the uterus commonly become contaminated with anaerobic and aerobic bacteria. For example, Gilstrap and Cunningham (1979), from cultures of amnionic fluid obtained at cesarean section performed in women in labor with membranes ruptured more than 6 hours, identified the following bacteria: anaerobic and aerobic organisms in 63 percent, anaerobes alone in 30 percent, and aerobes alone in 7 percent. Predominant anaerobic organisms were gram-positive cocci (*Peptostreptococcus* and *Peptococcus* species), 45 percent; *Bacteroides* species, 9 percent; and *Clostrid-*

TABLE 27–1. BACTERIA COMMONLY RESPONSIBLE FOR FEMALE GENITAL INFECTIONS

Aerobes
  Group A, B, and D streptococci
  Enterococcus
  Gram-negative bacteria—*Escherichia coli*, *Klebsiella*, and *Proteus* species
  Staphylococcus aureus

Anaerobes
  Peptococcus species
  Peptostreptococcus species
  Bacteroides bivius, *B. fragilis*, *B. disiens*
  Clostridium species
  Fusobacterium species

Other
  Mycoplasma hominis
  Chlamydia trachomatis

From the American College of Obstetricians and Gynecologists: Antimicrobial Therapy for Obstetric Patients. Technical Bulletin No 117, June 1988.

---

ium species, 3 percent. Gram-positive aerobic cocci were also common (*Streptococcus faecalis*, 14 percent, and group B *Streptococcus*, 8 percent). *Escherichia coli*, a gram-negative rod, comprised 9 percent of isolates. An average of 2.5 organisms was identified from each specimen. These observations serve to emphasize the polymicrobial nature of genital tract infections associated with delivery, and especially cesarean section. Gibbs (1987) has reemphasized the importance of these organisms, and reported an increasing prevalence of *Bacteroides bivius* as a cause of female pelvic infection. Walmer and colleagues (1988) more recently provided evidence for the role of enterococci in the pathogenesis of these infections.

Chlamydia trachomatis has been implicated as a cause of late-onset, indolent metritis that may develop in a third of women who had antepartum chlamydial cervical infection (Ismail and co-workers, 1985; Wager and colleagues, 1980). However, chlamydiae have not been isolated from women at the time these infections developed, and their role in its pathogenesis is not verified. The role of genital mycoplasma is even less clear, but some have implicated these organisms in the etiology of puerperal metritis (Blanco and colleagues, 1983; Lamey and associates, 1982; Platt and co-workers, 1980). *Gardnerella vaginalis*, a common constituent of normal vaginal flora, was shown by Gibbs and colleagues (1987) to lack a pathogenic role in puerperal infections.

BACTERIAL CULTURES

Precise identification of the bacteria responsible specifically for any puerperal infection may be quite difficult. Even though satisfactory techniques have been described in which double-lumen catheters are used to obtain specimens from the uterine cavity, the results are difficult to interpret since potentially pathogenic bacteria commonly are found in cultures from the uterine cavity taken during the puerperium in women without clinical disease. Gibbs and associates (1975), like Hite and co-workers (1947) three decades before, cultured one or more pathogens from swabbings of the uterine cavity in 70 percent or more of clinically healthy puerperal women. For these reasons, we do not obtain genital tract cultures routinely in these women before beginning treatment for puerperal infection.

Appropriately performed anaerobic and aerobic blood cultures obtained before antimicrobials are given may be useful to identify some of these pathogens. Blood cultures were positive in 13 percent of women treated at Parkland Hospital for pelvic infections that followed cesarean section (Cunningham and colleagues, 1979), and 24 percent of those from Los Angeles County Hospital (diZerega and co-workers, 1979).

PRINCIPLES OF ANTIMICROBIAL TREATMENT

Although few, if any, antimicrobial regimens are effective against all of these putative pathogens, treatment is directed against at least most of the polymicrobial and mixed flora that typically cause puerperal infections (Table 27–1). Fortunately, selection of an agent(s) effective against those most common usually proves suitable. Since, as described above, material for culture frequently is impractical to obtain, antimicrobial therapy is empirical.

β-Lactam antimicrobials have spectra that include activity against many anaerobic pathogens and they have been used successfully for decades to treat these infections. Many of the popular and effective multiagent regimens include a drug from this group, although some are effective when used alone. Examples include some cephalosporins (cefoxitin, cefoperazone, cefotetan, cefotaxime, and others) and extended-spectrum penicillins (piperacillin and mezlocillin). β-Lactam antimicrobials are inherently safe, and except for allergic reactions, they are free of major toxicity. Another advantage is the cost-effectiveness of administering only one drug. The β-lactamase inhibitors, clavulinic acid and sulbactam, have been combined with ampicillin, amoxicillin, and ticarcillin to extend their spectra, and these will likely prove effective.

In 1979, diZerega and colleagues compared the effectiveness of clindamycin plus gentamicin or penicillin G plus gentamicin given for treatment of pelvic infections following cesarean section. Women given the clindamycin-gentamicin regimen had a favorable response 95 percent of the time, and this regimen is now considered to be the standard by which others are measured. Unfortunately, clindamycin, like most other regimens effective against anaerobic flora, may induce *pseudomembranous colitis* by overgrowth of resistant enterotoxin-producing *Clostridium difficile*. If severe, such colitis may be life-threatening and treatment with vancomycin is given along with supportive measures. Recently, Walmer and colleagues (1988) have provided evidence that enterococcal infections may be associated with clinical failure of the clindamycin-gentamicin regimen. While 93 percent of women from whom enterococci were not isolated responded to this regimen, only 82 percent with enterococcal infections responded. The incidence of wound infection was much higher in those women with (16 percent) compared to those without (3 percent) enterococci.

Although many recommend that serum gentamicin levels periodically be monitored, we have not found it necessary to measure peak and trough serum concentrations in most women. However, its potential nephrotoxicity and ototoxicity are worrisome in the event of diminished glomerular filtration. For these reasons, frequently we give a combination of clindamycin with a second-generation cephalosporin, for example, cefoxitin. Others have recommended a combination of clindamycin and aztreonam, a monobactam compound with limited activity against gram-negative aerobic pathogens (American College of Obstetricians and Gynecologists, 1988).

Metronidazole has superior in vitro activity against most anaerobes and it is recommended by some to be given intravenously in combination with either gentamicin or tobramycin, especially if an abscess is suspected.

Chloramphenicol remains a potent antimicrobial in vitro against most anaerobes that cause pelvic infections. Given intravenously along with one of the β-lactam antimicrobials, it provides excellent coverage for severe pelvic sepsis. It can be given safely with impaired renal function, but unfortunately deaths due to irreversible bone marrow suppression follow in about 1 in 20,000 courses of therapy. As with any of these regimens, its benefits must be weighed against these adverse effects.

Duff (1986) and Ledger (1988) have provided reviews of antimicrobial use in women with puerperal infections.

INFECTIONS OF THE PERINEUM, VAGINA, AND CERVIX

Surprisingly, infections of perineal wounds, including episiotomy incisions and repaired lacerations, are relatively uncommon considering the degree of bacterial contamination that accompanies delivery. Sweet and Ledger (1973) reported only 21 infected episiotomies (0.35 percent) among nearly 6,000 women delivered vaginally at the University of Michigan and Wayne County Hospitals. Similarly, during a 6-month survey of nearly 5,000 vaginal deliveries at Parkland Hospital, in only 22 women (0.4 percent) was perineal cellulitis identified (M. Roark and G. Cunningham, unpublished observations).

PATHOGENESIS AND CLINICAL COURSE

Localized infection of the episiotomy wound is the most common puerperal infection of the external genitalia. The apposing wound edges become red, brawny, and swollen. The sutures often then tear through the edematous tissues, allowing the necrotic wound edges to gape, with the result that serous, serosanguineous, or frankly purulent material exudes. In this manner, complete breakdown of the site frequently follows. Local pain and dysuria, with or without urinary retention, are common symptoms. In extreme cases, the entire vulva may become edematous, ulcerated, and covered with exudate. Provided drainage is good, these superficial infections are fortunately seldom severe; however, if purulent materal is confined within a closed space by suture, infection may be accompanied by chills and impressive fever.

Vaginal lacerations are common, especially after traumatic operative delivery, and these may become infected directly or by extension from the perineum. The mucosa becomes edematous and hyperemic and may then become necrotic and slough. Parametrial extension may result in lymphangitis.

Cervical infection is probably more common than appreciated since lacerations are common and the cervix normally harbors potentially pathogenic organisms. Moreover, since deep cervical lacerations often extend directly into the tissue at the base of the broad ligament, infections may readily cause lymphangitis, parametritis, and bacteremia.

TREATMENT

Infected perineal wounds, like other infected surgical wounds, should be treated by establishing drainage. Sutures are removed and the infected wound opened. Failure to do this may lead not only to extension of the infections into the paracervical and paravaginal connective tissue, but to a worse ultimate anatomical result. One of the broad-spectrum antimicrobial regimens discussed above and listed in Table 27–1 should be given. Relief of pain is afforded by effective analgesics and an indwelling bladder catheter is placed if there is urinary retention. Hauth and colleagues (1986) described early repair of episiotomy separations, stressing that infection must be managed beforehand.

Necrotizing Fasciitis

A rare but frequently fatal complication of perineal and vaginal wound infections is deep soft tissue infection involving muscle and fascia. Such infections may extend from any infection adjacent to myofascial edges, and this includes surgical incisions or other wounds. They are seen also with vulvar infections in diabetic and immunocompromised women, but they develop rarely in otherwise healthy women. While Golde and Ledger (1977) reported only one case of necrotizing fasciitis of an episiotomy incision complicating nearly 110,000 deliveries at Los Angeles County Hospital from 1967 through 1976, Shy and Eschenbach (1979) reported that these infections were responsible for 20 percent of 15 maternal deaths in King County, Washington over the same period.

Bacteria causing these serious perineal infections are similar to those causing other pelvic infections, but anaerobes predominate. Gram-positive anaerobic cocci or *Clostridium perfringens* are usually isolated along with aerobic cocci or *E. coli*, but group B streptococcus has been reported (Sutton and colleagues, 1985).

Necrotizing fasciitis of the episiotomy site may involve any of the several superficial or deep perineal fascial layers, and thus it may extend to the thighs, buttocks, and abdominal wall (Shy and Eschenbach, 1979). Although some infections may develop within a day of delivery, they more commonly do not cause symptoms until 3 to 5 days. Clinical symptoms vary, and frequently it is difficult to differentiate superficial perineal infections from deep fascial ones. A high index of suspicion, with surgical exploration if the diagnosis is uncertain, may be lifesaving. Stamenkovic and Lew (1984) recommend biopsy of the fascial edges with frozen section microscopical examination when the diagnosis is uncertain. Certainly, if myofasciitis progresses, the woman becomes very ill from septicemia, there is profound hemoconcentration from capillary leakage with circulatory failure, and death soon follows. Cases of marked vulvar edema that have developed postpartum as described by Finkler and colleagues (1987) probably represent variants of this infection.

Aggressive surgical treatment is indicated and includes wide debridement of all infected tissue. As shown in Figure 27–1, this may include extensive vulvar debridement with unroofing and excision of abdominal, thigh, or buttock fascia.

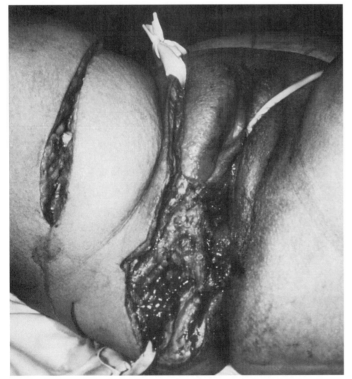

Figure 27–1. Necrotizing fasciitis complicating episiotomy infection. Three days postpartum this woman had severe perineal pain and edema of the episiotomy site. Prompt extensive debridement was carried out. Bacteria cultured from the infected episiotomy included *Escherichia coli*, *Streptococcus viridans*, group D streptococcus, *Corynebacterium* species, *Bacteroides fragilis*, and *Clostridium* species. Blood cultures were positive for *Bacteroides fragilis*.

Split-thickness skin grafts are later used to repair the defects. **Mortality is virtually universal without surgical treatment, and it approaches 50 percent even if aggressive excision is performed.**

Similar infections may develop in abdominal surgical incisions following cesarean section. Prompt diagnosis and aggressive surgical debridement are likewise mandatory for survival.

METRITIS WITH PELVIC CELLULITIS

Postpartum uterine infection has been called by various terms, which include *endometritis*, *endomyometritis*, and *endoparametritis*. Since the infection actually involves the decidua, myometrium, and parametrial tissues, we prefer the term *metritis with pelvic cellulitis*. Uterine infections are relatively uncommon following uncomplicated vaginal delivery, but they continue to be a major problem in women delivered by cesarean section. Sweet and Ledger (1973) reported that the incidence of postpartum uterine infections after vaginal delivery was 2.6 percent, and that this was not different between indigent and more socioeconomically advantaged women. In a 6-month survey during 1984 of nearly 5,000 women delivered vaginally at Parkland Hospital, only 1.3 percent were given treatment for metritis. A similar incidence was recorded in another survey in 1987 (M. Roark and G. Cunningham, unpublished observations). However, when women at high risk, defined by prolonged membrane rupture and labor, multiple cervical examinations, and internal fetal monitoring, were analyzed separately, the incidence of metritis after vaginal delivery increased to nearly 6 percent.

Cesarean section places the woman at extraordinary risk for developing uterine infection. The incidence of metritis following surgical delivery varies with socioeconomic factors, and over the years has been substantively altered by the common use of perioperative antimicrobials (Chap. 26, p. 456). Prior to common use of antimicrobial prophylaxis, Sweet and Ledger (1973) reported an overall incidence of 13 percent amongst affluent women undergoing cesarean section at the University of Michigan Hospital; however, it was 27 percent in indigent women delivered at Wayne County Hospital. We found an overall incidence of about 50 percent in women delivered by cesarean section at Parkland Hospital (Cunningham and associates, 1978). When risk factors for infection were analyzed, duration of labor and membrane rupture, multiple cervical examinations, and internal fetal monitoring were found to be important determinants of infection morbidity. Women with all of these factors delivered for cephalopelvic disproportion, who were not given perioperative prophylaxis, had an incidence of serious pelvic infection that was nearly 90 percent (DePalma and colleagues, 1982; Gilstrap and Cunningham, 1979).

PATHOGENESIS

Puerperal uterine infection involves primarily the endometrium, or more exactly the decidua, and adjacent myometrium. During the first few hours to a few days after delivery, bacteria successfully invade the decidua that remains, usually at the placental site. The term *metritis* is more descriptive than endometritis, because the inflammatory response is almost certain to include the underlying myometrium. The appearance of the infected decidua varies widely. In some cases, the necrotic mucosa sloughs, the debris is abundant, and the discharge is foul, profuse, bloody, and sometimes frothy. In others, the discharge is scant. Uterine involution may be retarded. Microscopic sections may show a superficial layer of necrotic material containing bacteria and a thick zone of leucocytic infiltration.

The pathogenesis of uterine infection following cesarean section is that of an infected surgical incision, and bacteria that colonized the cervix and vagina gain access to amnionic fluid during labor, following which they invade devitalized uterine tissue postpartum (Gilstrap and Cunningham, 1979). Invariably with uterine infections that follow cesarean sections, and probably in most of those after vaginal delivery, parametrial cellulitis develops. As shown in Figure 27–2, infection of the pelvic retroperitoneal fibroareolar connective tissue may develop in three main ways:

1. It may be caused by the lymphatic transmission of organisms from an infected cervical laceration, uterine incision for cesarean section, or a uterine laceration. Although lacerations of the perineum or vagina may cause localized cellulitis, the process is usually limited to the paravaginal tissue, rarely extending deeply into the pelvis.
2. It may be caused by direct extension of cervical lacerations into the connective tissue at the base of the broad ligaments. This tissue may be exposed to direct invasion by pathogenic vaginal organisms. A similar outcome may be seen in cases of criminal abortion when a sharp instrument has created a false passage into the paracervical connective tissue.
3. Pelvic cellulitis may be secondary to pelvic thrombophlebitis, which almost always is accompanied by some degree of cellulitis. If the thrombus becomes purulent, the venous wall may undergo necrosis and large numbers of organisms gain access to the surrounding connective tissue.

CLINICAL COURSE

Although not usually classified as mild or severe, the clinical picture of metritis varies with the extent of the disease, and whenever fever persists postpartum, uterine infection should be suspected. The degree of temperature elevation is probably proportional to the extent of the infection, and when confined to the endometrium (decidua), the cases are mild and there is minimal fever. More commonly, the temperature is at least 39°C, if not higher. Chills may accompany fever and suggest bacteremia, which may be documented in nearly 20 percent of women with uterine infection following cesarean delivery (di-Zerega and colleagues, 1979; Gilstrap and Cunningham, 1979). The pulse rate typically follows the temperature curve.

The woman usually complains of abdominal pain, and afterpains may be bothersome. There is tenderness on one or both sides of the abdomen and parametrial tenderness is elicited upon bimanual examination. Even in the early stages, an offensive odor may develop, long regarded as an important sign of uterine infection. However, in many women, foul-smelling lochia without other evidence for infection is found. Conversely, some infections, and notably those due to group A β-hemolytic streptococci, are frequently associated with scanty, odorless lochia. Leucocytosis may range from 15,000 to 30,000 cells per μL, but in view of the physiological leukocytosis of the early puerperium, these findings are difficult to interpret.

If the process is localized to the uterus, the temperature may return to normal even without antimicrobial treatment. Indeed, localized metritis may be misdiagnosed as a urinary infection or incorrectly attributed to severe breast engorgement or pulmonary atelectasis. Without treatment, parametritis follows an indolent course and ultimately may undergo suppuration; however, with appropriate antimicrobial therapy resolution usually is prompt.

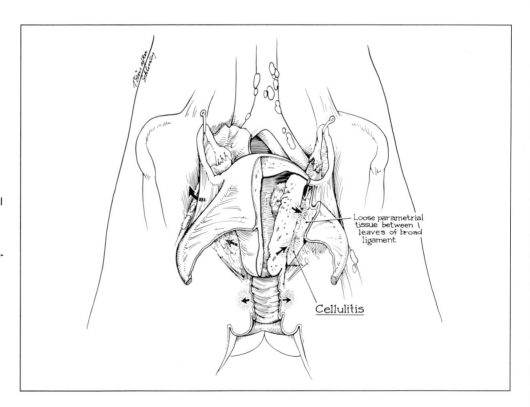

Figure 27–2. Pelvic cellulitis (parametritis) from extension of puerperal infection. Bacteria may enter the parametrial tissue between the leaves of the broad ligament by direct extension or by lymphatic transmission from cervical lacerations or foci of trauma within the uterus, including the site of placental implantation or cesarean section incision. Bacterial spread also may develop across the wall of an infected vein. Lacerations of the perineum or vagina usually cause only localized cellulitis, but may extend to pelvic lymphatics.

TREATMENT OF METRITIS

Treatment for metritis is given with a broad-spectrum antimicrobial(s). For mild cases following vaginal delivery, an oral agent may suffice. However, for moderately to severely infected women, and this includes those delivered by cesarean section, intravenous therapy is indicated. Improvement will follow in 48 to 72 hours in nearly 90 percent of women treated with one of the regimens discussed on page 463. Persistence of fever after this interval mandates a careful search for causes of refractory pelvic infection, although nonpelvic sources occasionally are found. Complications of metritis that cause persistent fever despite appropriate antimicrobial therapy include parametrial phlegmons, surgical incision and pelvic abscesses, and septic pelvic thrombophlebitis.

Peritonitis

Rarely, uterine infection extends by way of the lymphatics to reach the abdominal cavity to cause peritonitis (Fig. 27–3). This complication is rarely seen today with prompt therapy, but may be encountered with infections following cesarean section when there is uterine incisional necrosis and dehiscence. Rarely, late in the course of pelvic cellulitis, a parametrial abscess may rupture and produce catastrophic generalized peritonitis.

Generalized peritonitis is a grave complication, and typically, fibrinopurulent exudate binds loops of bowel to one another, and locules of pus may form between the loops. The cul-de-sac and subdiaphragmatic space may then be sites for abscess formation.

Clinically, puerperal peritonitis resembles surgical peritonitis except that abdominal rigidity is usually less prominent. Pain may be severe. Marked bowel distension is a consequence of paralytic ileus. It is important to identify the cause of the generalized peritonitis. If the infection began in the uterus and extended into the peritoneum, the treatment is usually medical. Conversely, peritonitis as the consequence of a lesion of the bowel or its appendages should be treated surgically. Antimicrobial therapy should include those agents most likely effective against *Peptostreptococcus*, *Peptococcus*, *Bacteroides*, *Clostridia*, and aerobic coliforms. Intravenous fluid and electrolyte replacement are extremely important since with generalized peritonitis large amounts of fluid are sequestered in the lumen and the wall of the gastrointestinal tract and, at times, in the peritoneal cavity. Vomiting, diarrhea, and fever also contribute appreciably to fluid and electrolyte loss. The volumes of fluid and the amounts of electrolytes necessary to replace what is sequestered in the abdomen, aspirated from the gut, and lost through diaphoresis are usually quite large but must not be so massive as to produce circulatory overload. Since paralytic ileus is usually a prominent feature, the gastrointestinal tract should be decompressed by continuous nasogastric suction. Oral feeding is withheld throughout the course of treatment until bowel function returns and flatus is expelled. Drugs to stimulate peristalsis are of no value.

Purulent exudate between loops of bowel, or between bowel and other organs, may cause intestinal kinking, following which symptoms of mechanical bowel obstruction will supervene. Frequently, surgical decompression is necessary. Surgery is not indicated early in the course of the disease, although abscesses may form at various sites and need to be drained, and mechanical intestinal obstruction may need to be relieved.

Adnexal Infections

Most often with puerperal infections the fallopian tubes are involved only with perisalpingitis without subsequent tubal occlusion and sterility. Primary gonococcal salpingitis during the

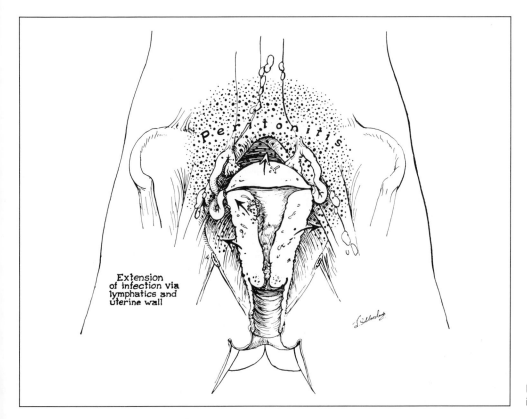

Figure 27–3. Extension of puerperal infection to cause peritonitis.

puerperium is rare. An *ovarian abscess* may develop as a complication of puerperal infection, presumably from bacterial invasion through a rent in the ovarian capsule (Wetchler and Dunn, 1985). We have encountered only two in the past 15 years at Parkland Hospital. The abscess is usually unilateral and women typically present one to several weeks after delivery. In many cases, rupture causes peritonitis, which prompts surgical exploration. Unless peritonitis is apparent, initially intravenous antimicrobial agents are given, but surgical drainage usually becomes necessary.

Toxic Shock Syndrome

This is an acute febrile illness with severe multisystem derangement and a case-fatality rate of 10 to 15 percent. The illness usually is characterized by fever, headache, mental confusion, diffuse macular erythematous rash, subcutaneous edema, nausea, vomiting, watery diarrhea, and marked hemoconcentration. Renal failure followed by hepatic failure, disseminated intravascular coagulation, and circulatory collapse may follow in rapid sequence. During recovery, the rash-covered areas undergo desquamation. *Staphylococcus aureus* has been recovered from almost all of afflicted persons, and a staphylococcal exotoxin, termed *toxic shock syndrome toxin-1*, and formerly called both *enterotoxin F* and *pyrogenic exotoxin C*, causes the syndrome by provoking profound endothelial injury. Recently, McGregor and colleagues (1988) described almost identical findings in women with infection complicated by *Clostridium sordelli* colonization.

The syndrome develops most commonly in young women, and usually is associated with menstruating women who use tampons; however, the syndrome has been reported in a variety of other clinical situations (Reingold and co-workers, 1982). Nearly 10 percent of pregnant women have vaginal colonization with *S. aureus,* and thus it is not surprising that the disease has been reported in postpartum women (Guernot and co-workers, 1982; Lauter and Tom, 1982). It also has been described in a mother-and-newborn pair (Green and LaPeter, 1982). An excellent review of the problem was provided by Wager (1983).

Principal therapy for the toxic shock syndrome is supportive while allowing reversal of capillary endothelial injury. In severe cases, this requires massive fluid replacement, mechanical ventilation with positive end-expiratory pressure, and renal dialysis. Antimicrobial therapy with specific antistaphylococcal drugs is given; however, their role in the resolution is uncertain.

PARAMETRIAL PHLEGMON

CLINICAL COURSE AND PATHOGENESIS

In some women, and almost exclusively in those in whom metritis follows cesarean delivery, parametrial cellulitis is intensive and forms an area of induration termed a *phlegmon,* within the leaves of the broad ligament (Fig. 27–4). Although such areas of cellulitis more often are unilateral, they need not be so.

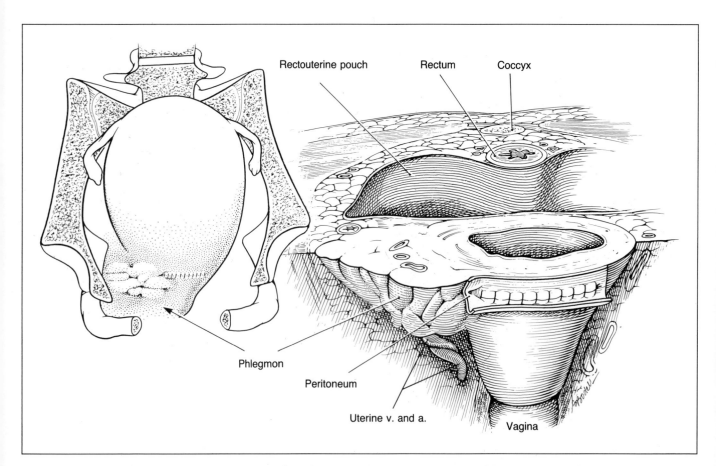

Figure 27–4. Parametrial phlegmon. Cellulitis in the right parametrium begins adjacent to the cesarean section incision and extends to the pelvic sidewall. On pelvic examination, a phlegmon is palpable as a firm, three-dimensional mass.

Cellulitis may remain limited to the base of the broad ligament, but if the inflammatory reaction is more intense, cellulitis extends along natural lines of cleavage. The most common form of extension is directly laterally, along the base of the broad ligament, with a tendency to extend to the lateral pelvic wall. The uterus is pushed toward the opposite side and is fixed. Occasionally, high intraligamentous exudates spread from the region of the uterine cornua to the iliac foss. Retrocervical cellulitis involves the rectovaginal septum with the development of a firm mass posterior to the cervix. With cesarean section incisions, involvement of the connective tissue anterior to the cervix results in cellulitis of the space of Retzius with extension upward, beneath the anterior abdominal wall, as high as the umbilicus. Rarely, the process may extend out through the sciatic foramen into the thigh.

Although a palpable phlegmon probably develops more frequently when appropriate antimicrobial therapy has been delayed, it remains the most common cause of persistent fever despite prompt and adequate treatment of pelvic infections that complicate cesarean section (DePalma and colleagues, 1982).

Fortunately rare, intensive cellulitis of the uterine incision may cause necrosis and separation with extrusion of purulent material into the peritoneal cavity (see p. 467). Frequently, the first symptoms of peritonitis are those of *adynamic ileus*, which usually is absent or mild following uncomplicated cesarean section. **Puerperal metritis with pelvic cellulitis is typically a retroperitoneal infection, and evidence for peritonitis should alert the physician of the possibility of uterine incisional necrosis with dehiscence, or less commonly a bowel injury or other lesion.**

TREATMENT

In the majority of women who develop a parametrial phlegmon, clinical response follows continued treatment with one of the intravenous antimicrobial regimens previously discussed. As long as the initial regimen has been appropriately chosen, and if there is no evidence for clinical deterioration, especially peritonitis, then the same regimen may be continued, or an alternate regimen chosen. Women with a phlegmon usually remain febrile for 5 to 7 days, and in some cases, even longer. Absorption of the induration follows, but it may take several weeks to dissipate completely.

Surgery is reserved for women in whom uterine incisional necrosis is suspected. Hysterectomy and surgical debridement usually are difficult, and often there is appreciable blood loss. Frequently, the cervix and lower uterine segment are involved

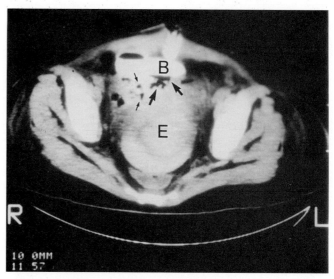

Figure 27–5. Pelvic computed tomograph showing uterine necrosis with gas (*arrows*) in the infected cesarean section incision. B = bladder; E = endometrial cavity.

with an intensive inflammatory process that extends to the pelvic sidewall to encompass one or both ureters, and supracervical hysterectomy should be considered. The adnexae are seldom involved, and depending on their appearance, one or both ovaries may be conserved.

Imaging Studies

Evaluation of pelvic infections using sonography has been less than satisfactory since ultrasound generally is poor for soft tissue imaging. Frequently, these areas of cellulitis have ultrasonic characteristics suggesting an abscess, but as discussed above, surgical drainage of a phlegmon is inadvisable. Recently, Brown and colleagues (1988) reported the use of computed tomography to assess refractory pelvic infections. Sometimes, as shown in Figure 27–5, uterine incisional dehiscence is detected. However, it is important that x-ray findings be interpreted along with clinical findings since apparent uterine separations seen radiographically may resolve spontaneously. These are presumed to represent infection without dehiscence, or perhaps even normal healing.

Pelvic Abscess

Rarely, despite prompt and appropriate antimicrobial treatment given for metritis, a parametrial phlegmon will suppurate, form-

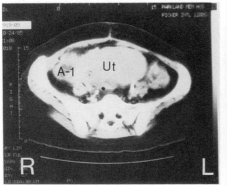
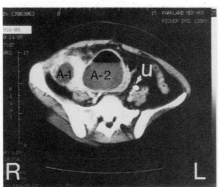

Figure 27–6. Pelvic computed tomograph showing two large pelvic abscesses. **A.** One abscess cavity (*A-1*) is within the right broad ligament adjacent to the puerperal uterus (*Ut*). **B.** The large abscess in the center (*A-2*) is bounded caudad by the uterine fundus and the smaller cavity (*A-1*) on the patient's right. The left ureter (*U*) is shown by the arrow.

A   **B**

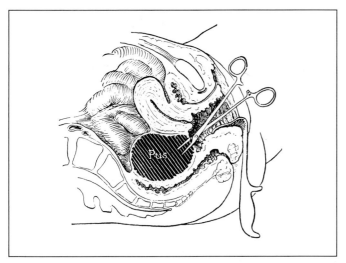

Figure 27–7. Drainage of rectovaginal septal abscess by culpotomy.

posteriorly through the retroperitoneal space to the rectovaginal septum, where surgical drainage is easily effected (Fig. 27–7).

SEPTIC PELVIC THROMBOPHLEBITIS

PATHOGENESIS

Puerperal infection may extend along venous routes with resultant thrombophlebitis (Figs. 27–2 and 27–8). Halban and Kohler (1919) performed autopsies in 163 women who died from puerperal infection before the antimicrobial era, and reported that 82, or slightly more than half, had pelvic thrombophlebitis. In 36 women, it was the only mode of extension identified, whereas in 46 there was coexisting lymphangitis. A similar, but slightly lower, figure (35 percent) was cited by Collins and colleagues (1951) for the period 1937–1946, which encompassed early use of chemotherapy.

Bacterial infection of the placental site causes thrombosed myometrial veins which in turn support anaerobic bacteria proliferation. The ovarian veins may then become involved since they drain the upper uterus, which most often includes veins draining the placental site (Fig. 27–9). The process is usually unilateral and probably more frequent on the right side (Munsick and Gillanders, 1981), from where it may extend into the vena cava. Septic phlebitis of the left ovarian vein may extend to the renal vein, and Bahnson and colleagues (1985) recently documented such a case using computed tomography.

As described by Collins and co-workers (1951), other pelvic

ing a fluctuant broad ligament mass that may point above Poupart's ligament. In these circumstances the woman may not have worsening of symptoms, but fever persists. Should the abscess rupture into the peritoneal cavity, life-threatening peritonitis may develop (p. 467). More likely, these will dissect anteriorly and may be amenable to needle drainage directed by computed tomography (Fig. 27–6). Occasionally they dissect

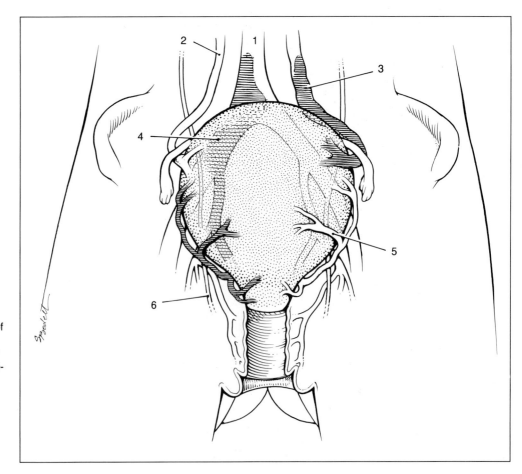

Figure 27–8. Routes of extension of septic pelvic thrombophlebitis. Any or all pelvic vessels and the inferior vena cava may be involved: (1) inferior vena cava, (2) right ovarian vein, (3) clot in left ovarian vein, (4) clot in right common iliac vein, which extends from the uterine and hypogastric veins and into the inferior vena cava, (5) left uterine vein, and (6) right ureter.

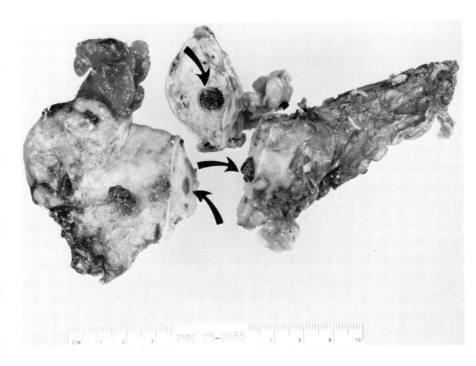

Figure 27–9. Ovarian vein thrombophlebitis. Resected thrombosed right ovarian vein plus right oviduct.

veins may be involved. Brown and colleagues (1986) reported 11 consecutive cases of septic thrombophlebitis diagnosed using computed tomography and magnetic resonance imaging over a 15-month period at Parkland Hospital. In five of these women, the iliofemoral vessels were involved, usually along with the vena cava. In six, an ovarian vein was thrombosed, but in only one woman was the ovarian vein involved along with iliofemoral vessels. Conversely, vena caval thrombosis was documented to accompany ovarian or iliofemoral thrombophlebitis.

CLINICAL FINDINGS

The usual clinical presentation of the woman with septic thrombophlebitis has been described by Schulman (1969) and Gibbs (1976). These women usually experience most aspects of clinical improvement of their pelvic infection following antimicrobial treatment; however, they continue to have hectic fever spikes. They usually do not appear clinically ill, and frequently are asymptomatic unless chills accompany fever. This clinical picture was aptly termed "enigmatic fever" by Dunn and Van-Voorhis (1967).

Munsick and Gillanders (1981) identified the following clinical features from review of cases of ovarian vein thrombophlebitis: The cardinal symptom was pain that developed typically on the second or third postpartum day with or without fever. Pain was present in the lower abdomen, the flank, or both. In some cases, but not all, a tender mass was palpable just beyond

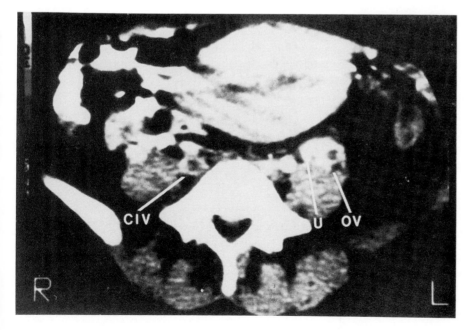

Figure 27–10. Septic pelvic thrombophlebitis. Pelvic computed tomograph on day 13 from a woman with persistent fever since day 6 following vaginal delivery and manual removal of placenta. The left ureter (*U*) is filled with contrast, and there is the characteristic appearance of a thrombus in the right common iliac vein (*CIV*) and a thrombus with surrounding inflammation in the left ovarian vein (*OV*). (*From Brown and colleagues: Obstet Gynecol 68:789, 1986.*)

the uterine cornu. Usually thrombophlebitis involved the right ovarian vein, but in a few instances it involved both ovarian veins overlaid by inflamed peritoneum.

DIAGNOSIS AND TREATMENT

Variable degrees of pelvic thrombophlebitis probably accompany most cases of metritis and parametrial cellulitis, and thus, initial treatment is directed at both, and it is usually successful. For women with persistent fever, with or without a palpable parametrial mass, computed tomography or magnetic resonance may disclose pelvic phlebitis (Figs. 27–10 and 27–11). Before these methods were available to confirm clinical suspicions of venous involvement, the *heparin challenge test* was advocated. Supposedly, after intravenous heparin was given, there was lysis of fever, and this was taken as diagnostic of pelvic phlebitis and heparin treatment continued (Cohen and colleagues, 1983; Duff and Gibbs, 1983; Josey and Staggers, 1974; Munsick and Gillanders, 1981). However, Brown and colleagues (1986) recently questioned this, since they showed that despite withholding heparin from 6 of 11 women with proven pelvic thrombophlebitis, continued antimicrobial therapy resulted in clinical resolution. Conversely, in the five women

given heparin along with antimicrobial drugs, the prolonged febrile course was not appreciably abbreviated, and in fact, three of these women had fever for more than 10 days after heparin was given.

In response to treatment, thrombosis of the involved veins usually limits the infection, and the clot undergoes organization. Rarely, the thrombus may suppurate, while the surrounding venous wall becomes edematous and necrotic. Pulmonary embolization, at least large enough to cause sudden death, is rare. In advanced cases, which are quite rare today, small septic emboli may reach the terminal branches of the pulmonary circulation, resulting in pleural effusions, pulmonary infarctions, and abscesses. In these cases, consideration should be given to a vena caval filter or surgical ligation (Maull and colleagues, 1978).

BACTEREMIA AND SEPTICEMIC SHOCK

Infections that most commonly cause bacteremia and septic shock in obstetrical patients are septic abortion (Chap. 29, p. 507), antepartum pyelonephritis (Chap. 39, p. 809), and puerperal sepsis. As discussed above, the latter is more common with infections following cesarean section, and although 15 to 20 percent of these women have bacteremia, their general good health probably explains the low incidence of septic shock (Blanco and colleagues, 1981).

ETIOLOGY

Most pelvic infections are polymicrobial and thus, septic shock may be due to a large variety of pathogens. Most commonly, bacteria that cause shock are from members of the endotoxin-producing *Enterobacteriaceae* family, especially *E. coli*. Pathogens that less often cause shock are aerobic and anaerobic streptococci and *Bacteroides* and *Clostridium* species.

PATHOGENESIS

Endotoxin is a lipopolysaccharide that is released upon lysis of the bacterial cell wall. There are probably other bacterial substances that result in mediator release with activation of complement, kinins, or the coagulation system (Chap. 36, p. 699). Release of vasoactive mediators produces selective vasodilation with maldistribution of blood flow. Leucocyte and platelet aggregation cause capillary plugging. Vascular endothelial injury causes profound capillary leakage and interstitial fluid accumulation. The end results of this cascade of pathophysiological events, shown in Figure 27–12, cause the septic shock syndrome. Clinical shock, as described by Parker and Parrillo (1983), results primarily from decreased systemic vascular resistance which is not compensated fully by increased cardiac output. Hypoperfusion results in lactic acidosis, decreased oxygen extraction, and end-organ dysfunction (Table 27–2). This is sometimes referred to as *multiple organ failure syndrome* (Carrico and colleagues, 1986).

HEMODYNAMIC CHANGES IN SEPTIC SHOCK

A greater understanding of the septic shock syndrome has been made possible by equipment that allows direct measurement of hemodynamic functions, and the pathophysiology has been elucidated by the elegant clinical studies of Parker and Parrillo and their colleagues (1983) at the National Institutes of Health. According to their observations, if initially circulating volume is

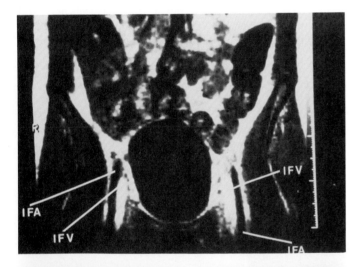
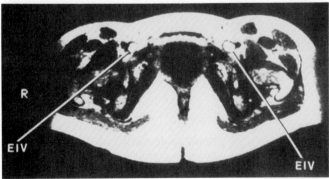

Figure 27–11. A. Coronal magnetic resonance imaging section showing thrombi in both iliofemoral venous systems (*IFV*). By comparison, flowing blood in the iliofemoral arteries (*IFA*) appears dark (repetition time = 1.0 sec; echo time = 28 msec). **B.** Transverse magnetic resonance imaging section of Figure 27–11A showing bilateral external iliac venous (*EIV*) thrombi (repetition time = 1.5 sec; echo time = 56 msec.) (*From Brown and colleagues: Obstet Gynecol 68:789, 1986.*)

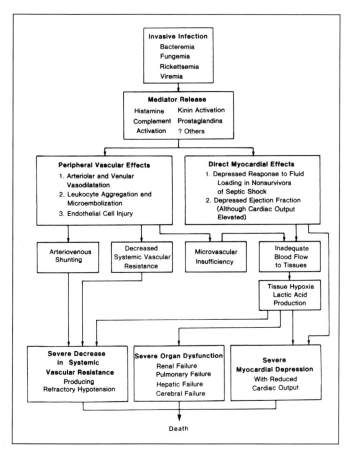

Figure 27–12. Pathogenesis of septic shock in humans (*From Parker and Parrillo: JAMA 250:3325, 1983.*)

restored, then septic shock can be characterized as a high cardiac output, low vascular resistance condition. Concomitantly, pulmonary hypertension develops. Paradoxically, patients with severe sepsis are likely to have myocardial depression despite high cardiac output (Ognibene and co-workers, 1988).

Most generally healthy women with sepsis complicating obstetrical infections respond well to fluid resuscitation, given along with intensive antimicrobial therapy, and if indicated, removal of infected tissue. If hypotension is not corrected following vigorous fluid infusion, then the prognosis is poor. Lack of response may be due to severe and unresponsive vascular insufficiency, or it may be due to myocardial depression. Lee and colleagues (1988) described two maternal deaths in 10 women with low cardiac output unresponsive to fluid resuscitation. Another poor prognostic sign is when reversal of hypotension follows intravenous fluid administration, but end-organ dysfunction continues with renal, pulmonary, and cerebral failure.

DIAGNOSIS

Whenever serious bacterial infection is suspected, blood pressure and urine flow should be monitored closely. Septic shock, as well as hemorrhagic shock, should be considered whenever there is evidence of hypotension or oliguria. In the absence of other evidence of active hemorrhage, if hypotension and oliguria are not improved by the rapid administration of at least a liter of lactated Ringer's solution, it is likely that the shock is caused by infectious agents.

TREATMENT

When shock from sepsis is suspected, prompt and aggressive treatment includes the following: (1) careful monitoring of vital signs to include urinary output and other measures of organ perfusion, (2) vigorous intravenous fluid infusion to restore circulating volume, (3) administration of empirical antimicrobial drugs selected to provide a spectrum that includes all suspected pathogens, and if indicated, (4) surgical intervention after the woman's condition has been stabilized.

As discussed above, these women have enormous fluid requirements because of peripheral vasodilation and capillary endothelial damage with fluid extravasation. Central to their management is administration intravenously of crystalloid fluids, such as lactated Ringer's solution. Rapid infusion with as many as 4 to 6 L may be required to restore renal perfusion in severely affected women. Because of the vascular leak, these women are usually hemoconcentrated, and if the hematocrit is 30 or less, then whole blood is given along with crystalloid to maintain the hematocrit at about 30 or perhaps slightly higher.

If aggressive volume replacement is not promptly followed by urinary output of at least 30 mL and preferably 50 mL per hour, as well as other indicators of improved perfusion, then a flow-directed pulmonary artery catheter is inserted. By using hemodynamic monitoring, the effects of fluid therapy on cardiac function are assessed directly. In women who are seriously ill, the pulmonary capillary endothelium is likely damaged, with leakage into the alveoli causing pulmonary edema, also referred to as the *adult respiratory distress syndrome* (Chap. 39, p. 807). This must be differentiated from heart failure from overly vigorous fluid therapy.

Broad-spectrum antimicrobials are administered in large doses after appropriate cultures are taken. These include blood cultures, along with specimens of exudates that are not contaminated by normal flora. For women with infected abortions or those with deep fascial infections, a Gram-stained smear may be helpful in identifying *Clostridium perfringens.*

SURGICAL TREATMENT

In seriously ill women, continuing sepsis may prove fatal. Thus, debridement of necrotic tissue or drainage of purulent material

TABLE 27–2. MULTIORGAN EFFECTS WITH SEPSIS AND SHOCK

Organ System	Clinical and Laboratory Findings
Central nervous	Confusion
Hypothalamus	Hypothermia, hyperthermia
Cardiovascular	Vasodilatation and hypotension, increased cardiac output (early), myocardial depression (decreased ejection fraction), hypotension, tachyarrhythmias
Pulmonary	Arteriovenous shunting with hypoxemia and tachypnea, alveolar-capillary leakage with pulmonary edema
Gastrointestinal	Vomiting, diarrhea
Liver	Toxic hepatitis, jaundice
Kidney	Oliguria, renal failure
Hematological	Thrombocytopenia, leucopenia, leucocytosis, consumptive coagulopathy

Modified from The American College of Obstetricians and Gynecologists: Septic Shock. Technical Bulletin No. 75, March 1984.

is crucial to survival for these women. Therefore, a meticulous search is made for such foci.

For women with infected abortions, the products of conception must be removed promptly by curettage. According to Pritchard and Whalley (1971), as well as others, hysterectomy is seldom indicated unless the uterus has been lacerated or is obviously intensely infected (Fig. 27–13). Since bacterial shock can become clinically apparent several hours after evacuation of infected products from the uterus, careful monitoring must be continued.

For women with pyelonephritis, continuing sepsis usually is from urinary obstruction caused by calculi or a perinephric abscess or phlegmon, and flank exploration may be indicated (Chap. 39, p. 811). In some cases, end-stage pyonephrosis is found as a source of continuing sepsis and nephrectomy is performed.

Puerperal infections that cause sepsis which may be amenable to surgical treatment are those in which there is appreciable infection of devitalized tissue. Examples include deep myofascial infections of the episiotomy site or abdominal surgical incision (see Necrotizing Fasciitis, p. 464). In women with persistent infections following cesarean section, the uterine incision may undergo necrosis and deshicence with subsequent peritonitis. Another source may be from a ruptured parametrial or intraabdominal abscess. **Any woman with a puerperal infection who is suspected of developing peritonitis should be carefully evaluated for uterine incisional necrosis and separation or for bowel perforation.**

ADJUNCTIVE THERAPY

Pressor Agents

Vasoactive drugs are not given unless aggressive fluid treatment fails to correct hypotension and perfusion abnormalities. If central filling pressure measurements indicate that fluid replacement is adequate, then vasoactive drugs are given. One commonly used is dopamine hydrochloride, which when given in doses of 2 to 10 μg per kg per minute stimulates cardiac β-receptors to increase cardiac output. Doses of 10 to 20 μg per kg per minute cause α-receptor stimulation and increase blood pressure. At doses of more than 20 μg per kg per minute, α-receptor stimulation predominates, but seldom is dopamine needed at these higher doses.

Oxygenation and Ventilation

Oxygen is administered by mask in an attempt to improve ongoing tissue hypoxia. As the septic shock syndrome progresses, and intravascular volume is restored, there may be substantive pulmonary capillary endothelial damage with leakage into alveoli. The resultant pulmonary edema, termed *adult respiratory distress syndrome*, causes hypoxemia, which worsens tissue hypoxia and acidosis. When this is severe, and adequate oxygenation cannot be maintained by increased oxygen delivered by a nonrebreathing mask, then tracheal intubation and mechanical ventilation that delivers positive end-expiratory pressure may prove to be lifesaving.

Adrenocortical Steroids

If control of the infection by antimicrobials and the infusion of blood and aqueous fluids do not result in prompt improvement, corticosteroids are recommended by some. Recently, however, the results of two large clinical studies have shown that methylprednisolone given in large doses within a few hours of sepsis did not improve early or late morbidity or mortality (Bone and colleagues, 1987; Veterans Administration Study Group, 1987).

Heparin

Coagulation defects are common in severe cases of septic shock. The genesis of these abnormalties is extremely complex and difficult to dissect in clinical studies. The concept that intravascular coagulation occludes the microcirculation and consumes coagulation factors and causes hemorrhage has led some to recommend that heparin be used in these circumstances. To date, no clinical trial has been reported to show that the benefits from heparin outweigh the risks. Moreover, animal studies of gram-negative sepsis point out that inhibition of intravascular coagulation by heparin does not necessarily lower mortality (Corrigan and co-workers, 1974). Control of disseminated intravascular coagulation is dependent upon control of the inciting disease, which includes antimicrobial therapy and debridement.

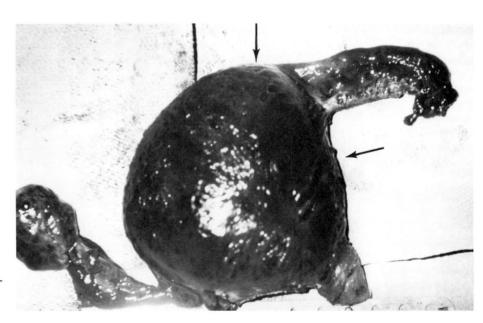

Figure 27–13. The numerous rents in the serosa of the uterus (*arrows*) were the consequence of gas formation plus intensive necrosis from *Clostridium perfringens*.

DIFFERENTIAL DIAGNOSIS OF FEVER

Most fevers after childbirth are caused by genital tract infection, especially if the preceding labor was attended by extensive vaginal or uterine manipulation, prolonged membrane rupture, or intrauterine electronic monitoring. Regardless, every postpartum woman whose temperature rises to 38°C (100.4°F) should be evaluated to rule out extrapelvic causes of fever and to establish the diagnosis of puerperal infection. Filker and Monif (1979) reported that 6.5 percent of 1,000 consecutive women had fever of this magnitude postpartum. Only 21 percent of febrile women delivered vaginally were found to have infection in contrast to 72 percent of those delivered by cesarean section. Common extragenital causes of puerperal fever include *respiratory complications, pyelonephritis, intense breast engorgement, bacterial mastitis, thrombophlebitis,* and in cases of laparotomy, *wound abscess.*

Respiratory complications are most often seen within the first 24 hours following delivery, and almost invariably are in women delivered by cesarean section or given general anesthesia for vaginal delivery. Complications include atelectasis, aspiration pneumonia, or occasionally, bacterial pneumonia. Atelectasis is best prevented with the use of routine coughing and deep breathing on a fixed schedule, usually every 4 hours for at least 24 hours following the administration of general anesthesia, and especially when laparotomy was performed. It is conjectural whether atelectasis, per se, causes fever. Because of severe sequelae, the possibility of aspiration must be suspected, and these women most often will develop a high spiking fever, varying degrees of respiratory wheezing, and in most instances, obvious signs of hypoxemia.

Pyelonephritis may be difficult to diagnose postpartum. In the typical case, bacteriuria, pyuria, costovertebral angle tenderness, and spiking temperature clearly indicate pyelonephritis; however, the clinical picture varies. For example, in the puerperal woman the first sign of renal infection may be a temperature elevation but costovertebral angle tenderness may not develop until later. The clinical diagnosis is confirmed by demonstrating bacteriuria microscopically and by urine culture obtained by catheterization. Empirical therapy is begun immediately without waiting for culture results.

Breast engorgement may occasionally result in a brief temperature elevation which rarely exceeds 38.5°C (101°F) in the first few postpartum days (Chap. 28, p. 483). The fever characteristically lasts no longer than 24 hours. In contrast, the elevated temperature of bacterial mastitis is usually sustained and associated with mammary signs and symptoms that become overt within 24 hours.

Abdominal incisional abscesses usually cause fever beginning on the fourth postoperative day or so. In most cases, these are preceded by uterine infections and they cause persistent fever despite adequate antimicrobial therapy. Organisms causing these infections are usually the same as those isolated from amnionic fluid at the time of cesarean section (Emmons and colleagues, 1988; Gilstrap and Cunningham, 1979), but hospital-acquired pathogens must be suspected. Antimicrobial therapy is given and surgical drainage performed, with careful inspection to ensure that the fascia is intact, and if not, secondary closure is performed. *Necrotizing fasciitis* is an uncommon but frequently fatal complication of these incisional infections, and extensive myofascial debridement may be lifesaving (p. 464).

Superficial or deep venous thrombophlebitis of the legs may cause temperature elevations in the puerperal woman. The diagnosis is made by the observation of a painful, swollen leg, usually accompanied by calf tenderness, or occasionally femoral triangle area tenderness. Treatment is given with intravenous heparin therapy (Chap. 28, p. 477).

REFERENCES

American College of Obstetricians and Gynecologists: Septic shock. Tech Bull No 75, March 1984

American College of Obstetricians and Gynecologists: Antimicrobial therapy for obstetric patients. Tech Bull No 117, June 1988

Bahnson RR, Wendel EF, Vogelzang RL: Renal vein thrombosis following puerperal ovarian vein thrombophlebitis. Am J Obstet Gynecol 152:290, 1985

Blanco JD, Gibbs RS, Castaneda YS: Bacteremia in obstetrics: Clinical course. Obstet Gynecol 58:621, 1981

Blanco JD, Gibbs RS, Malherbe H, Strickland-Cholmley M, St Clair PJ, Castaneda YS: A controlled study of genital mycoplasmas in amniotic fluid from patients with intra-amniotic infection. J Infect Dis 147:650, 1983

Bone RC, Fisher CJ Jr., Clemmer TP, Slotman GJ, Metz CA, Balk RA: A controlled clinical trial of high-dose methylprednisolone in the treatment of severe sepsis and septic shock. N Engl J Med 317:653, 1987

Brown CEL, Lowe TW, Cunningham FG, Weinreb JC: Puerperal pelvic thrombophlebitis: Impact on diagnosis and treatment using x-ray computed tomography and magnetic resonance imaging. Obstet Gynecol 68:789, 1986

Brown CEL, Harrell R, Setiawan H, Cunningham FG: Use of pelvic x-ray computed tomography (CT) to evaluate pelvic infection: Infectious Disease Society in Obstetrics and Gynecology. [Abstract 13] Aspen, Colorado, August 1988

Brown TK, Munsick RA: Puerperal ovarian vein thrombophlebitis: A syndrome. Am J Obstet Gynecol 109:263, 1971

Burtenshaw JH: The fever of the puerperium. NY and Philadelphia Med J, June/July 1904

Carrico CJ, Meakins JL, Marshall JC, Fry D, Maier RV: Multiple-organ-failure syndrome. Arch Surg 121:196, 1986

Cohen MB, Pernoll ML, Gevirtz CM, Kernstein MD: Septic pelvic thrombophlebitis: An update. Obstet Gynecol 62:83, 1983

Collins CG, McCallum EA, Nelson EW, Weinstein BB, Collins JH: Suppurative pelvic thrombophlebitis: I. Incidence, pathology, etiology; II. Symptomatology and diagnosis; III. Surgical techniques: A study of 70 patients treated by ligation of the inferior vena cava and ovarian veins. Surgery 30:298, 1951

Cook JD, Lynch SR: The liabilities of iron deficiency. Blood 68:803, 1986

Corrigan JJ Jr: Disseminated intravascular coagulation. South Med J 67:474, 1974

Cunningham FG, Hauth JC, Strong JD, Kappus SS: Infectious morbidity following cesarean: Comparison of two treatment regimens. Obstet Gynecol 52:656, 1978

DePalma RT, Cunningham FG, Leveno KJ, Roark ML: Continuing investigation of women at high risk for infection following cesarean delivery. Obstet Gynecol 60:53, 1982

diZerega G, Yonekura L, Roy S, Nakamura RM, Ledger WJ: A comparison of clindamycin-gentamicin and penicillin-gentamicin in the treatment of postcesarean section endomyometritis. Am J Obstet Gynecol 134:238, 1979

Duff P: Pathophysiology and management of postcesarean endomyometritis. Obstet Gynecol 67:269, 1986

Duff P, Gibbs RS: Pelvic vein thrombophlebitis: Diagnostic dilemma and therapeutic challenge. Obstet Gynecol Surv 38:365, 1983

Dunn LJ, Van Voorhis LW: Enigmatic fever and pelvic thrombophlebitis. N Engl J Med 276:265, 1967

Eisenmann GE: Die Wundfieber und die Kindbettfieber. Erlangen, 1837

Emmons SL, Krohn M, Jackson M, Eschenbach DA: Development of wound infections among women undergoing cesarean section. Obstet Gyencol 72:559, 1988

Filker R, Monif GRG: The significance of temperature during the first 24 hours postpartum. Obstet Gynecol 53:359, 1979

Finkler NJ, Safon LE, Ryan KJ: Bilateral postpartum vulvar edema associated with maternal death. Am J Obstet Gynecol 156:1188, 1987

Gibbs RS: Microbiology of the female genital tract. Am J Obstet Gynecol 156:491, 1987

Gibbs RS: Treatment of refractory postpartum fever. Clin Obstet Gynecol 19:83, 1976

Gibbs RS, O'Dell TN, MacGregor RR, Schwarz RH, Morton H: Puerperal endometritis: A prospective microbiologic study. Am J Obstet Gynecol 121:919, 1975

Gibbs RS, Weiner MH, Walmer K, St Clair PJ: Microbiologic and serologic studies of *Gardnerella vaginalis* in intra-amniotic infection. Obstet Gynecol 70:187, 1987

Gilstrap LC III, Cunningham FG: The bacterial pathogenesis of infection following cesarean section. Obstet Gynecol 53:545, 1979

Gordon A: A Treatise on Epidemic Puerperal Fever of Aberdeen. London, CG & J Robinson, 1795

Green SL, LaPeter KS: Evidence for postpartum toxic-shock syndrome in a mother-infant pair. Am J Med 72:169, 1982

Guerinot GT, Gitomer SD, Sanko SR: Postpartum patient with toxic shock syndrome. Obstet Gynecol 59:43S, 1982

Halban J, Köhler R: Die pathologische Anatomie des Puerperalprozesses. Vienna and Leipzig, 1919

Hamilton A: A Treatise on Midwifery. London, 1781

Hauth JC, Gilstrap LC III, Ward SC, Hankins GDV: Early repair of an external sphincter ani muscle and rectal mucosal dehiscence. Obstet Gyencol 67:806, 1986

Hippocrates: Liber Prior de Muliebrum Morbis

Hite KE, Hesseltine HC, Goldstein L: A study of the bacterial flora of the normal and pathologic vagina and uterus. Am J Obstet Gynecol 53:233, 1947

Holmes OW: Puerperal Fever as a Private Pestilence. Boston, Ticknor & Fields, 1855

Ismail MA, Chandler AE, Beem ME: Chlamydial colonization of the cervix in pregnant adolescents. J Reprod Med 30:549, 1985

Jewett JF, Reid DE, Safon LE, Easterday CL: Childbed fever: A continuing entity. JAMA 206:344, 1968

Josey WE, Staggers SR Jr: Heparin therapy in septic pelvic thrombophlebitis: A study of 46 cases. Am J Obstet Gynecol 120:228, 1974

Joynson DHM, Jacobs A, Walter DM, Dolby AE: Defect of cell-mediated immunity in patients with iron-deficiency anaemia. Lancet 2:1058, 1972

Kulapongs P, Suskind R, Vithayasai V, Olsen RE: Cell-mediated immunity and phagocytosis and killing function in children with severe iron-deficiency anaemia. Lancet 2:689, 1974

Lamey JR, Eschenbach DA, Mitchell SH, Blumhagen JM, Foy HM, Kenny GE: Isolation of mycoplasmas and bacteria from the blood of postpartum women. Am J Obstet Gynecol 143:104, 1982

Lauter CB, Tom WW: Spiking fever and rash in a postpartum patient. Hosp Pract, 17:163, 1982

Leake J: Practical Observations on the Child-bed Fever; Also on the Nature and Treatment of Uterine Haemorrhages, Convulsions, and Such Other Acute Disease, As Are Most Fatal to Women During the State of Pregnancy. London, J Walter, 1772

Ledger WJ: A historical review of pelvic infections. Am J Obstet Gynecol 158:687, 1988

Lee W, Clark SL, Cotton DB, Gonik B, Phelan J, Faro S, Giebel R: Septic shock during pregnancy. Am J Obstet Gynecol 159:401, 1988

Leigh J, Garite TJ: Amniocentesis and the management of premature labor. Obstet Gynecol 67:500, 1986

Lister J: On the antiseptic principle in the practice of surgery. Br Med J 2:246, 1867

McGregor JA, Soper D, Lovell G: A toxic shock-like syndrome caused by clostridia sordelli affecting postpartum women: Infectious Disease Society in Obstetrics and Gynecology. [Abstract 30] Aspen, Colorado, August 1988

Maull KI, Van Nagell JR, Greenfield LJ: Surgical complications of ovarian vein thrombosis. Am J Surg 44:727, 1978

Minkoff H: Prematurity: Infection as an etiologic factor. Obstet Gynecol 62:137, 1983

Munsick RA, Gillanders LA: A review of the syndrome of puerperal ovarian vein thrombophlebitis. Obstet Gynecol Surv 36:57, 1981

Mussey RD, DeNormandie RL, Adair FL: The American Committee on Maternal Welfare, Inc: Its organization, purposes and activities. Am J Obstet Gynecol 28:754, 1935

Naeye RL: Coitus and associated amniotic fluid infections. N Engl J Med 301:1198, 1979

Ognibene FP, Parker MM, Natanson C, Shelhamer JH, Parrillo JE: Depressed left ventricular performance. Response to volume infusion in patients with sepsis and septic shock. Chest 93:903, 1988

Parker MM, Parrillo JE: Septic shock: Hemodynamics and pathogenesis. JAMA 250:3324, 1983

Peckham CH: A brief history of puerperal infection. Bull Hist Med 3:187, 1935

Platt R, Lin J-SL, Warren JW, Rosner B, Edelin K, McCormack WM: Infection with Mycoplasma hominis in postpartum fever. Lancet 2:1217, 1980

Pritchard JA, Whalley PJ: Abortion complicated by Clostridium perfringens infection. Am J Obstet Gynecol 111:484, 1971

Puzos N: Première mémoire sur les depots laiteux, in Traités des accouchements, 1686, p 341

Reingold AL, Shands KN, Dan BB, Broome CV: Toxic-shock syndrome not associated with menstruation: A review of 54 cases. Lancet 2:1, 1982

Rochat RW, Koonin LM, Atrash HK, Jewett JF, and the Maternal Mortality Collaborative: Maternal mortality in the United States: Report from the Maternal Mortality Collaborative. Obstet Gynecol 72:91, 1988

Sachs BP, Brown DA, Driscoll SG, Schulman E, Acker D, Ransil BJ, Jewett JF: Hermorrhage, infection, toxemia, and cardiac disease, 1954–85: Causes for their declining role in maternal mortality. Am J Public Health 78:671, 1988

Schulman H: Use of anticoagulants in suspected pelvic infection. Clin Obstet Gynecol 12:240, 1969

Semmelweis IP: Die Aetiologie, der Begriff u. die Prophylaxis des Kindbettfiebers. Pest, Vienna and Leipzig, 1861

Shy KK, Eschenbach DA: Fatal perineal cellulitis from an episiotomy site. Obstet Gynecol 52:293, 1979

Stamenkovic I, Lew PD: Early recognition of potentially fatal necrotizing fasciitis: The use of frozen-section biopsy. N Engl J Med 310:1689, 1984

Strother E: Critical Essay on Fevers. London, 1716

Sutton GP, Smirz LR, Clark DH, Bennett JE: Group B streptococcal necrotizing fasciitis arising from an episiotomy. Obstet Gynecol 66:733, 1985

Veterans Administration Systemic Sepsis Cooperative Study Group: Effect of high-dose glucocorticoid therapy on mortality in patients with clinical signs of systemic sepsis. N Engl J Med 317:659, 1987

Wager GP: Toxic shock syndrome: A review. Am J Obstet Gynecol 146:93, 1983

Wager GP, Martin DH, Koutsky L, Eschenbach DA, Daling JR, Chiang WT, Alexander ER, Holmes KK: Puerperal infectious morbidity: Relationship to route of delivery and to antepartum Chlamydia trachomatis infection. Am J Obstet Gynecol 138:1028, 1980

Walmer D, Walmer KR, Gibbs RS: Enterococci in post-cesarean endometritis. Obstet Gynecol 71:159, 1988

Wetchler SJ, Dunn LJ: Ovarian abscess. Report of a case and a review of the literature. Obstet Gynecol Surv 40:476, 1985

White C: Treatise on the management of pregnancy and lying-in women and the means of curing but more especially of preventing the principal disorders to which they are liable. London, EC Dilly, 1773

Willis T: Diatribae duae medico-philosophical . . . de febribus . . . London, T Raycroft, 1659

Willson JR: The conquest of cesarean section related infections: A progress report. Obstet Gyencol 72:519, 1988

Other Disorders of the Puerperium

THROMBOEMBOLIC DISEASE

According to the Consensus Conference sponsored by the National Institutes of Health (1986), the likelihood of venous thromboembolism in normal pregnancy and the puerperium is increased by a factor of 5 when compared to nonpregnant women of similar age. Certainly, venous thrombosis and pulmonary embolism remain a major cause of maternal death in the United States. Kaunitz and colleagues (1985) found that thrombotic pulmonary embolism directly caused 13 percent of 2,067 non-abortion-related maternal deaths in the United States from 1974 through 1978. Similarly, Sachs and associates (1987) reported pulmonary embolism to be now the second most common cause of maternal mortality in Massachusetts. Thromboembolic diseases are considered here because traditionally they were considered unique to the puerperium; however, this is no longer true.

In more recent years, there has been a decrease in the frequency of deep venous thrombosis and thromboembolism during the puerperium but perhaps an increase antepartum. Henderson and co-workers (1972), for example, described 20 cases that developed antepartum among 29,770 pregnancies, but during the same period, only 16 were identified postpartum.

Undoubtedly, the frequency of venous thromboembolic disease during the puerperium decreased remarkably when early ambulation became widely practiced. Until as late as the 1950s, it was common practice after delivery to prohibit ambulation for up to 1 week or more. **Stasis is probably the strongest single predisposing event to deep vein thrombosis, and, therefore, should be kept to a minimum.** Antecedent events that might possibly predispose to deep vein thrombosis during the antepartum period include the use of oral contraceptives before conception and the great prevalence of women working during pregnancy at jobs in which they sit for long periods of time.

Venous thrombosis traditionally has been classified as *thrombophlebitis* if an inflammatory response was apparent, or *phlebothrombosis* if such evidence was lacking. The inflammatory response presumably would anchor the clot more firmly and prevent embolism. Unfortunately, contiguous with and proximal to an adherent clot there may form appreciable thrombus that is not adherent and therefore can easily detach and embolize. Thrombosis with a significant potential for generating pulmonary emboli may take place in the deep veins of the leg, thigh, and pelvis. A thrombosis that involves only the superficial veins of the leg or thigh is very unlikely to generate a pulmonary embolus.

SUPERFICIAL VENOUS THROMBOSIS

Antepartum or postpartum thrombosis limited strictly to the superficial veins of the saphenous system is treated with analgesia, elastic support, and rest. If it does not soon clear, or if deep venous involvement is suspected, heparin is given intravenously, as described below, until the process clears.

DEEP VENOUS THROMBOSIS IN THE LEG

In a carefully conducted prospective investigation in which thrombosis was confirmed by venography, Bergqvist and colleagues (1983) from Sweden reported that the incidence of antepartum deep venous thrombosis was 7 per 1,000. The experience, however, of most American and other European workers is that the incidence is much lower, and is probably about 1 to 2 per 1,000 (Weiner, 1985). Barss and colleagues (1985) confirmed by venography 11 cases at Brigham and Women's Hospital from 1981 to 1984, during which time 27,000 women were delivered. Our experiences at Parkland Hospital are similar, and we have observed that the incidence of deep venous thrombosis, both antepartum and postpartum, has decreased. This decrease likely is due in part to improved techniques to confirm as well as exclude thrombosis diagnosed clinically.

The signs and symptoms with deep venous thrombosis involving the lower extremity vary greatly, depending in large measure upon the degree of occlusion and the intensity of the inflammatory response.

Classic puerperal thrombophlebitis involving the lower extremity, sometimes called *phlegmasia alba dolens* or *"milk leg,"* is abrupt in onset, with severe pain and edema of the leg and thigh. The venous thrombosis typically involves much of the deep venous system from the foot to the iliofemoral region. Reflex arterial spasm sometimes causes a pale, cool extremity with diminished pulsations. Seldom is the reaction to deep venous thrombosis this intense, however. There may be appreciable volume of clot yet little reaction in the form of pain, heat, or swelling. Conversely, calf pain, either spontaneous or in response to squeezing, or to stretching the Achilles tendon (Homans' sign), may be caused by a strained muscle or a contusion. The latter may be common during the early puerperium as the consequence of inappropriate contact between the calf and the delivery table leg holders.

Venography or *phlebography* remains the standard for confirmation of the clinical diagnosis of deep venous thrombosis. In most studies it has been shown that by using this technique at least half of clinically suspected cases do not have a thrombosis, thereby obviating the need for anticoagulation and its hazards. Venography is not without complications, and indeed the method itself may induce thrombosis. Therefore, there has been renewed interest in noninvasive methods to confirm the clinical diagnosis, but unfortunately, none has been proven as effective as venography in pregnant women. In nonpregnant patients, *impedance plethysmography* apparently has promise, both as a screening method as well as for diagnosis. In a study from Amsterdam (Huisman and colleagues, 1986), 471 consecutive patients in whom deep venous thrombosis was clinically suspected were screened with serial impedance plethysmography, and if positive, they underwent venography. All patients in whom plethysmography was normal did well without treatment. By contrast, in those with abnormal plethysmographic findings, thrombi were confirmed in 92 percent using venography. Thus it may be reasonable to use impedance plethysmography for screening in pregnant women in whom thrombosis is suspected, but if the examination is abnormal, then venography is recommended.

In some clinics, Doppler flow measurements and impedance plethysmography are used for screening. Since the diagnosis of deep venous thrombosis effectively commits a pregnant woman to some scheme of anticoagulation for the duration of pregnancy, as well as an indeterminate time postpartum, venography is used to substantiate the diagnosis at Parkland Hospital.

Treatment of deep venous thrombosis consists of heparin given intravenously as described below, bed rest, and analgesia. Most often, the pain is soon relieved by these measures. Seldom is thrombectomy or sympathetic nerve blockade warranted. After the signs and symptoms have completely abated, graded ambulation should be started, with the legs well wrapped in elastic bandages, or, better, well-fitting elastic stockings, and the heparin continued. Recovery to this stage usually takes about 7 to 10 days.

For women who are *postpartum* and suffering their first attack, who have no obvious chronic vascular disease, and who are observed to be completely asymptomatic while fully ambulatory, anticoagulant therapy may be discontinued. Most often signs and symptoms of deep venous thrombosis do not recur. If, however, symptoms and signs do recur, therapy is promptly restarted but is not stopped when relief is obtained. Instead, prolonged anticoagulant therapy is continued on an outpatient basis. After discharge from the hospital, long-term treatment is maintained either with self-administered, subcutaneously injected heparin, or with warfarin.

During the past several years, considerable controversy has arisen concerning the most effective agent to use in long-term therapy to prevent recurrent thrombophlebitis and thromboembolization. Hull and co-workers (1982a) reported that heparin was as effective as oral warfarin when heparin was administered subcutaneously every 12 hours with the dose adjusted to prolong the partial thromboplastin time to 1½ times the control value when measured 6 hours after injection. Furthermore, the heparin therapy was associated with a lower risk of bleeding. Subsequently, Hull and colleagues (1982b) reported that by decreasing the dosage of warfarin so that the prothrombin time was not decreased below specified levels, bleeding complications from warfarin could be reduced to the level achieved with heparin and that the effectiveness of the two agents were comparable.

In the absence of pregnancy it seems reasonable to consider warfarin the drug of choice for long-term treatment or prophylaxis when appropriate consideration is given to the cost of heparin, the problem of administration, the possibility of heparin-induced thrombocytopenia (Chong and associates, 1982; Galle and co-workers, 1978) and the possibility of osteope-

nia with fractures (DeSwiet and colleagues, 1983; Wise and Hall, 1980).

Thrombosis, Antepartum

Thrombosis antepartum involving the deep venous system is especially difficult to manage satisfactorily. As discussed above, when deep venous thrombosis is suspected, it is reasonable to use Doppler or impedance plethysmography to help establish or exclude the diagnosis. If these findings are positive or equivocal, then we agree with Weiner (1985) that ascending venography is recommended. Otherwise, the woman will either have to undergo prolonged anticoagulation with its attendant risks, or run the risk of pulmonary embolism.

Therapy with intravenous heparin usually soon controls active disease, but thrombosis, perhaps with embolization, may recur antepartum, intrapartum, or postpartum unless anticoagulation is continued throughout these periods.

Anticoagulation, Antepartum

Administration of heparin on an outpatient basis can be difficult. All things considered, the best treatment regimen for prophylaxis against recurrence of deep venous thrombosis is self-administered heparin injected subcutaneously in doses of 5,000 U two or three times a day (National Institutes of Health, 1986). With so-called low-dose heparin treatment that provides 10,000 to 15,000 U of heparin subcutaneously per day, there is some increase in the risk of recurrent thrombosis and possibly embolism compared to that with larger doses, but a much lower risk of hemorrhage. The regimen described above by Hull and co-workers (1982a) utilizing subcutaneous adjusted dose heparin every 12 hours also appears to be effective and safe. Aspirin and other drugs that impair platelet function increase the risk of hemorrhage, even with "low-dose" heparin, and therefore should be avoided.

Warfarin and related compounds that inhibit the synthesis of vitamin K–dependent coagulation factors cross the placenta and thereby also impair the coagulation mechanism of the fetus. Moreover, there is evidence that warfarin may be teratogenic if used early in pregnancy (Chapter 32, p. 565). The administration of warfarin during the first 8 weeks of gestation may result in congenital malformations, which include nasal hypoplasia, ophthalmological abnormalities, and retarded development (Shaul and Hall, 1977). Whether the malformations are the consequence of microhemorrhages in embryonic cartilage or a more complex teratogenic action is not known. It also must be remembered that a variety of drugs acts to enhance or inhibit the action of warfarin.

Because of the mechanical forces that develop during labor, the fetus is at increased risk of hemorrhage, especially intracranial hemorrhage, at this time. Therefore, if warfarin has been used as an anticoagulant during the antepartum period, the drug should be stopped weeks before the anticipated time of delivery and anticoagulation with heparin initiated.

PELVIC VENOUS THROMBOSIS

During the puerperium, a thrombus may form transiently in any of the dilated pelvic veins, and possibly does so relatively often. Without associated thrombophlebitis, these thrombi likely do not incite clinical signs or symptoms unless the thrombosis is extensive or pulmonary embolism follows. Unfortunately, these vessels appear to be the source of many of the massive and fatal pulmonary emboli that develop without warning in the puerperium, although some undoubtedly arise from the deep venous system of the legs.

Symptomatic puerperal pelvic thrombosis most commonly is associated with uterine infection, and this is discussed in Chapter 27 (p. 470). The diagnosis of pelvic thrombophlebitis has improved remarkably with the use of computed tomography. As described by Brown and colleagues (1986), pelvic vein thrombosis may occur alone or in combination with the ovarian, iliofemoral, or inferior caval venous systems. Most often this is associated with a septic course, and resolves in most cases with intensive antimicrobial therapy.

ANTICOAGULATION AND ABORTION

The treatment of deep venous thrombosis with heparin does not preclude termination of pregnancy by careful curettage (see Chapter 29, p. 502). After all of the products of conception are removed without trauma to the reproductive tract, heparin can be restarted in therapeutic doses at the termination of the procedure without undue risk. If abdominal hysterotomy is to be performed, those precautions presented below for cesarean section are applicable. Experiences are lacking in which hypertonic saline or a prostaglandin has been used as an abortifacient in the presence of effective anticoagulation. The same is true for laparoscopic tubal sterilization. In both circumstances, it is anticipated that serious bleeding might be induced.

ANTICOAGULATION AND DELIVERY

Labor and delivery may induce severe hemorrhage in the fetus if the mother has very recently been treated with warfarin. The effects of warfarin may be reversed by the slow intravenous administration of vitamin K_1 in a dose of 10 mg. The activities of the vitamin K–dependent clotting factors usually increase to safe levels within 8 hours in the mother, but less rapidly in the fetus. Maternal transfusion of plasma or a plasma fraction rich in factors II, VII, IX, and X (prothrombin complex) will correct the deficiency immediately in the mother but, unfortunately, not in the fetus. Hepatitis may be transmitted with this plasma fraction.

Heparin does not cross the placenta. The effects of heparin on blood loss at delivery will depend upon a number of variables, including the following: (1) the dose, route, and time of administration; (2) the magnitude of incisions and lacerations; (3) the intensity of myometrial contraction and retraction once the products of conception have been delivered; and (4) the presence of other coagulation defects. The experiences at Parkland Hospital have been that measured blood loss is not greatly increased with vaginal delivery if the midline episiotomy is modest in depth, there are no lacerations of the genital tract, and the uterus promptly becomes firmly contracted and remains so after delivery of the placenta. Such ideal circumstances do not always prevail during and after vaginal delivery, however. Mueller and Lebherz (1969), for example, described 10 women with antepartum thrombophlebitis treated with heparin. Three who continued to receive heparin during labor and delivery bled remarkably and developed severe postpartum hemorrhage with large hematomas. Blood replacement of 1,500, 2,500, and 4,500 mL was essential, as was repeated drainage of the hematomas. Therefore, in general, heparin therapy should be stopped during the time of labor and delivery. If the uterus is well contracted and there has been negligible trauma to the lower genital tract, it can soon be restarted. Otherwise, a delay of 2 or 3 days may be prudent. Protamine sulfate administered

intravenously most often will promptly and effectively reverse the effect of heparin but, of course, will be of no benefit for hematomas already formed. Protamine sulfate, if used, should not be given in excess of the amount needed to neutralize the heparin. Excess protamine has an anticoagulant effect.

Serious bleeding is likely when heparin in usual therapeutic doses is administered to a woman who has undergone cesarean section within the previous 72 hours. After that, the risk of bleeding decreases with time so that by 1 week in the otherwise uncomplicated case there is slight risk. Again, preexisting defects in the hemostatic mechanism, such as thrombocytopenia, or impaired platelet function as induced by aspirin, enhance the likelihood of hemorrhage with heparin.

The woman who has very recently suffered a pulmonary embolism and who must be delivered by cesarean section presents a serious problem since reversal of anticoagulation may be followed by another embolus, and surgery while she is fully anticoagulated frequently results in life-threatening hemorrhage or troublesome hematomas. In this situation, consideration at the time of cesarean section should be given for ligation of the vena cava below the renal veins as well as the left ovarian vein near its insertion into the renal vein. Alternatively, before surgery, a vena caval filter device may be placed using either the jugular or femoral approach as discussed subsequently. With either treatment, strong consideration should be given to tubal sterilization.

PULMONARY EMBOLISM

In many cases, but certainly not all, clinical evidence for deep venous thrombosis of the legs precedes pulmonary embolization. In others, especially those that arise from deep pelvic veins, the woman is usually asymptomatic until symptoms of embolization develop. The reported incidence of pulmonary embolism associated with pregnancy has varied widely, and has been reported to be from 1 in 2,700 deliveries (Stamm, 1960) to less than 1 in 7,000 deliveries (Mengert, 1945). Our recent experiences are more consonant with Mengert's earlier observations from Parkland Hospital and indicate that pulmonary embolism is quite uncommon.

Chest discomfort, shortness of breath, air hunger, tachypnea, or obvious apprehension are signs and symptoms that should alert the physician to a strong likelihood of pulmonary embolism during the puerperium. Bell and associates (1977) carefully analyzed the clinical findings in a large number of individuals with angiographically identified pulmonary embolism. The most common abnormality was a respiratory rate of greater than 16 per minute. They emphasized that its frequency was so striking that a lower respiratory rate should rule against the diagnosis. Physical examination of the chest may or may not yield findings such as an accentuated pulmonic valve second sound, rales, or friction rub. Right axis deviation may or may not be evident in the electrocardiogram.

Even with massive pulmonary embolism, signs, symptoms, and laboratory data to support the diagnosis of pulmonary embolism may be deceivingly unspecific, as borne out in a cooperative study sponsored by the National Heart and Lung Institute (Wenger and colleagues, 1972). Ninety patients were identified by pulmonary angiography to have massive embolism. Although at least two lobar arteries were obstructed, the classic triad indicative of pulmonary embolism—hemoptysis, pleuritic chest pain, and dyspnea—was noted in only 20 percent of the subjects. Furthermore, there is no definitive laboratory blood test that is diagnostic (Hirsch, 1981).

Great controversy still exists with respect to the safest, least invasive technique that can most accurately diagnose a pulmonary embolus. Some investigators believe that ventilation-perfusion/scintiphotography is adequate in the majority of young patients without evidence of underlying cardiopulmonary disease (Ruckley, 1982; Sassahara and co-workers, 1983; Viamonte and associates, 1980). However, these techniques utilize radioactive agents administered intravenously and they may not provide a definite diagnosis. Hull and associates (1983) reported that ventilation scanning increased the probability of pulmonary embolus in patients with *large perfusion defects and ventilation mismatches* but a ventilation-perfusion match was *not* helpful in ruling out pulmonary embolism. Pulmonary angiography was necessary in most patients with perfusion abnormalities because the diagnosis of pulmonary embolism could not be made or excluded with sufficient accuracy in such patients.

At Parkland Hospital, we vigorously pursue verification of the clinical diagnosis of pulmonary embolism. Initial evaluation includes a chest radiograph, and if this is not suggestive of another diagnosis, then a ventilation-perfusion lung scan is performed. If the scan is completely normal, this is taken as evidence against an embolism and the workup is considered complete. Conversely, an unequivocally positive result, in concert with a chest radiograph showing no explicable abnormalities, is considered diagnostic of embolization and therapy is begun. For cases in which the diagnosis is still doubtful after these measures, then pulmonary angiography is performed, and *filling defects* or *vessel cutoff* are considered diagnostic for embolization.

The possibility of pulmonary embolism must always be kept in mind, especially during the puerperium. If the woman develops an embolus during her hospital stay, the diagnosis is more likely to be made and appropriate therapy started. Embolism may occur weeks after delivery, however, with no intervening symptoms. Under these circumstances, it is easy to ascribe the symptoms to some other cause, especially anxiety. A woman readmitted to Parkland Hospital provides an example:

A somewhat elderly, multiparous woman was admitted near term with total placental abruption and massive bleeding. Treatment included cesarean section and 15 U of whole blood. Eight days later, after a benign postpartum course, she was discharged. Three weeks after delivery she was awakened during the night by chest pain. In the morning she went to a physician who considered her to be "apprehensive and hyperventilating secondary to grief reaction." Rebreathing into a paper bag and diazepam were prescribed but gave no relief. The same day she came to Parkland Hospital, where supporting evidence of pulmonary embolism was readily uncovered, including tachypnea, splinting of the left side of the chest on inspiration, abnormal chest x-ray, pulmonary perfusion defects demonstrated by lung scan in regions free of infiltrate, and, while breathing room air, an arterial blood P_{O_2} of 62 mm Hg and pH of 7.52. Treatment with heparin intravenously every 4 hours was promptly started. At no time was there clinical evidence of thrombosis in the lower extremities and phlebograms were negative. Presumably the emboli came from the pelvis. She promptly recovered.

HEPARIN DOSAGE

In general, for deep venous thrombosis or pulmonary embolism, whether antepartum or postpartum, therapy with heparin in appropriate doses is effective. Considerable controversy exists as to which regimen is best, and several are widely used, effective, and considered acceptable (Mohr and colleagues, 1988; Weiner, 1985). Heparin is commonly administered by continuous intravenous infusion, and most recommend starting with a dose of 1,000 U per hour. Intermittent intravenous injections of 5,000 U every 4 hours or 7,500 U every 6 hours are preferred by others. Finally, heparin may be given subcutaneously in doses of 10,000 U every 8 hours or 20,000 Units every 12 hours. The common theme of these regimens is that the total daily heparin dose is between 25,000 and 40,000 U.

Barss and colleagues (1985) reported the use of a subcutaneous pump to deliver heparin continuously to six women for a mean of 20 weeks before delivery. The heparin dose was adjusted to maintain the partial thromboplastin time 1 to 1.5 times baseline, and the mean daily dose was nearly 40,000 U. Significant bleeding complications developed in four women and three were given blood transfusions. They correctly concluded that further studies of optimum dose and duration were needed.

The most serious complication with any of these regimens is hemorrhage, which is more likely if there has been recent surgery or lacerations, such as with delivery. Troublesome bleeding is also more likely if the heparin dosage is excessive. Conversely, thrombus extension or embolization are more likely if heparin dosage is inadequate. Unfortunately, management schemes to identify by laboratory testing whether heparin dosage is sufficient to inhibit further thrombosis, yet not cause serious hemorrhage, have been discouraging (Moser, 1987).

Whole blood clotting times have long been used and more recently measurement of the plasma partial thromboplastin time has been popularized. The two tests often correlate poorly. An important test that will aid in detecting hemorrhage, but tends to be forgotten, is the frequent measurement of the hematocrit. Careful clinical evaluation will usually provide the best information concerning adequacy of dosage. Clinical improvement without hemorrhage is the desired goal.

It is important to remember that heparin is being administered whenever blood is to be drawn or medications are ordered to be given parenterally. Serious hemorrhage may occur, especially when arterial blood is drawn for blood gas analyses.

Therapy with heparin as described may be discontinued in the postpartum woman after 10 days to 2 weeks if the disease process has clearly abated and there is no evidence of underlying chronic venous abnormalities that would predispose to venous thrombosis and no evidence of underlying cardiopulmonary dysfunction. If anticoagulation is to be protracted and a switch to warfarin therapy is the plan, it is recommended by some that treatment with heparin and warfarin should overlap for 6 days after the prothrombin time has reached the therapeutic level (Walsh, 1983; Wessler and Gitel, 1979). However, Gallus and colleagues (1986) evaluated this prospectively and reported no adverse sequelae when heparin was discontinued after the prothrombin time was considered therapeutically prolonged.

If the woman is undelivered, there is appreciable risk of recurrence of the venous thrombosis sometime during the subsequent antepartum, intrapartum, and postpartum periods unless an anticoagulant—preferably heparin—is continued. Therefore, anticoagulation should be continued, unless ligation or clipping of the inferior vena cava and left ovarian vein has been carried out, as discussed below.

There are insufficient data to conclude which regimen is best to provide the safest maximal effect against recurrent antepartum pulmonary embolism. This was recently considered in detail at the National Institutes of Health Consensus Conference (1986), and it was concluded that the woman with either deep venous thrombosis or pulmonary embolism in a *prior* pregnancy should be given prophylactic subcutaneous heparin in doses of 5,000 U, either two or three times daily throughout pregnancy. This also has been our practice at Parkland Hospital for many years for women recovering from antepartum pulmonary embolism, and the recurrence of documented embolization has been rare.

VENA CAVAL INTERRUPTION

In the very infrequent circumstances where heparin therapy fails to prevent recurrent pulmonary embolism from the pelvis or legs, or when embolism develops from these sites despite heparin given for their treatment, then vena caval interruption is indicated. In the past, vena caval ligation or plication was performed; however, this procedure, which requires extensive surgical dissection in an area that is highly vascular during pregnancy, is probably best replaced by use of a *vena caval filter*. Hux and colleagues (1986) recently described the use of the Greenfield filter in five pregnant women and another who was 3 days postpartum. A radiograph shown in Figure 28–1 demonstrates the correct placement of the filter above the renal veins. Their indications for filter placement, which is inserted through either the jugular or femoral vein, were either bleeding, thrombocytopenia, or recurrent embolization in these women, who had been anticoagulated with heparin. A complication of this method is perforation of the vena cava during insertion (Greenfield and Alexander, 1985).

Vena caval ligation is employed today more often when there is concurrent obstetrical surgery, for example, cesarean section. Ligation is performed below the level of the renal veins, but above the entry of the right ovarian vein; therefore, the left ovarian vein must be ligated below its entry into the left renal vein. Serrated Teflon clips applied to the vena cava are also effective (Couch and associates, 1975). In spite of previous reports suggesting that obstruction of the vena cava causes placental abruption, there are several reports of successful ligation performed antepartum, with favorable outcomes for the mother and usually the fetus (Stone and colleagues, 1968). Caval and ovarian vein ligation for treatment of septic emboli from the pelvis is considered in Chapter 27 (p. 470).

DISEASES AND ABNORMALITIES OF THE UTERUS

SUBINVOLUTION

Subinvolution is an arrest or retardation of involution, the process by which the puerperal uterus is normally restored to its original proportions. Subinvolution is accompanied by prolongation of the period of lochial discharge and sometimes by profuse hemorrhage. It may be followed by prolonged leucorrhea and irregular or excessive uterine bleeding. The diagnosis is established by bimanual examination. The uterus is larger and softer than normal for the particular period of the puerperium. Among the recognized causes of subinvolution are retention of placental fragments and pelvic infection. Since most cases of subinvolution result from local causes, they are usually amenable to early diagnosis and treatment. Ergonovine (Ergotrate) or methyl ergonovine (Methergine), 0.2 mg every 3 to 4 hours for 24 to 48 hours, has been recommended by some, but its efficacy is questionable. On the other hand, metritis usually promptly responds to oral antimicrobial therapy. Since Wager and colleagues (1980) reported that almost a third of cases of late postpartum uterine infection are caused by *Chlamydia trachomatis*, then tetracycline therapy may be appropriate.

POSTPARTUM CERVICAL EROSIONS

Cervical erosions, or eversions, are a complication of the late postpartum period. Shallow cauterization or cryotherapy can be

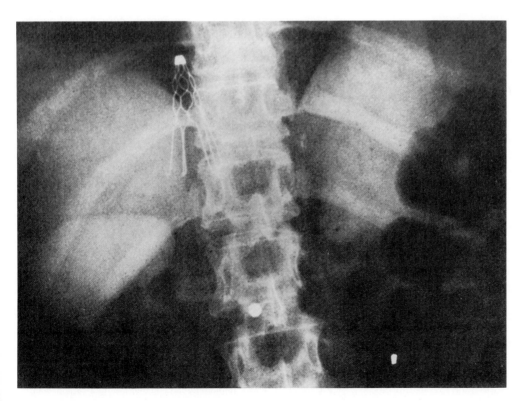

Figure 28–1. X-ray showing placement of Greenfield filter. (*From Hux and colleagues: Am J Obstet Gynecol 155:734, 1986.*)

used to remove persistent exuberant granulations or the delicate exposed endocervical columnar epithelium, without causing stenosis of the endocervix.

RELAXATION OF THE VAGINAL OUTLET AND PROLAPSE OF THE UTERUS

Extensive lacerations of the perineum during delivery, if not properly repaired, are commonly followed by relaxation of the vaginal outlet. Even when external lacerations are not visible, overstretching or submucosal tears may lead to marked relaxation. The changes in the pelvic supports during parturition predispose, moreover, to prolapse of the uterus and to urinary stress incontinence. These conditions may escape detection unless an examination is made at the end of the puerperium and unless the patients are subjected to long-term follow-up.

In general, operative correction should be postponed until the desired number of children has been achieved, unless, of course, serious disability, notably urinary stress incontinence, results in symptoms sufficient for the patient to demand intervention.

HEMORRHAGES DURING THE PUERPERIUM

PUERPERAL HEMATOMAS

Blood may escape into the connective tissue beneath the skin covering the external genitalia or beneath the vaginal mucosa to form vulvar and vaginal hematomas. The condition usually follows injury to a blood vessel without laceration of the superficial tissues, and may occur with spontaneous, as well as operative, delivery. Occasionally, the hemorrhage is delayed, perhaps as a result of sloughing of a vessel that had become necrotic from prolonged pressure.

Less frequently, the torn vessel lies above the pelvic fascia. In that event, the hematoma develops above it. In its early stages, the hematoma forms a rounded swelling that projects into the upper portion of the vaginal canal and may almost occlude its lumen. If the bleeding continues, it dissects retroperitoneally and thus may form a tumor palpable above the Poupart ligament, or it may dissect upward, eventually reaching the lower margin of the diaphragm.

VULVAR HEMATOMAS

Vulvar hematomas, particularly those that develop rapidly, may cause excruciating pain, which is often the first symptom that is noticed (Fig. 28–2). Hematomas of moderate size may be absorbed spontaneously. The tissues overlying the hematoma may give way as a result of necrosis caused by pressure, and profuse hemorrhage may follow. In other cases, the contents of the hematoma may be discharged in the form of large clots.

In the subperitoneal variety, the extravasation of blood beneath the peritoneum may be massive and occasionally fatal. Death may also follow secondary intraperitoneal rupture. Occasionally, rupture into the vagina leads to infection of the hematoma and potentially fatal sepsis.

A vulvar hematoma is readily diagnosed by severe perineal pain and the sudden appearance of a tense, fluctuant, and sensitive tumor of varying size covered by discolored skin. When the mass develops adjacent to the vagina, it may temporarily escape detection, but symptoms of pressure, if not pain, and inability to void should soon lead to a vaginal examination

and the discovery of a round, fluctuant tumor encroaching on the lumen. When the hematoma extends upward between the folds of the broad ligament, it may escape detection unless a portion of the tumor can be felt on abdominal palpation or unless evidence of anemia or infection appears.

The prognosis is usually favorable, though bleeding into very large hematomas has led to death.

Treatment

Smaller vulvar hematomas identified after leaving the delivery room may be treated expectantly. If, however, the pain is severe, or if they continue to enlarge, as they often do, the best treatment is prompt incision and evacuation of the blood with ligation of the bleeding points. The cavity can then be obliterated with mattress sutures. **With hematomas of the genital tract, blood loss is nearly always considerably more than the clinical estimate.** Hypovolemia and severe anemia should be prevented by adequate blood replacement. Broad-spectrum antibiotics are of value.

The subperitoneal and supravaginal varieties are more difficult to treat. They can be evacuated by incision of the perineum, but unless there is complete hemostasis, which is difficult to achieve by this route, laparotomy is advisable.

LATE POSTPARTUM HEMORRHAGE

Occasionally, serious uterine hemorrhage develops in the latter part of the first week, or later in the puerperium. Hemorrhage most often is the result of abnormal involution of the placental site, but it may be caused also by retention of a portion of the placenta. Usually, the retained piece of placenta undergoes necrosis with deposition of fibrin, and may eventually form a so-called *placental polyp* (Fig. 28–3). As the eschar of the polyp detaches from the myometrium, hemorrhage may be brisk.

The observations of Lee and associates (1981) provide an estimate of the incidence of late postpartum hemorrhage. Of 3,822 women delivered during 1 year at Henry Ford Hospital, 27 women, or 0.7 percent, had significant uterine bleeding after the first 24 postpartum hours. In 20 of these women the uterus was judged to be empty by sonographic evaluation, and importantly, only 1 woman had definite retained placental tissue.

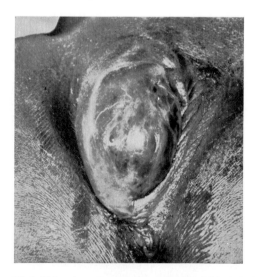

Figure 28–2. Vulvar hematoma bulging into the right vaginal wall.

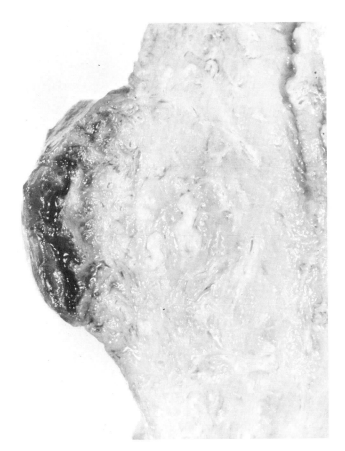

Figure 28–3. Placental polyp. Hysterectomy was performed because of prolonged bleeding, which resulted in severe anemia, in a woman who wanted no more pregnancies.

It generally has been accepted that with late postpartum hemorrhage from the uterus, prompt curettage is necessary. The experiences at Parkland Hospital, however, have been that curettage subsequent to late puerperal hemorrhage most often did not remove identifiable placental tissue. Hemorrhage was initiated by the separation of the retained products of conception that, in turn, were flushed out by the brisk hemorrhage. Lee and co-workers (1981) support this observation and present evidence that the use of sonography can exclude retained placental fragments as the cause of delayed postpartum hemorrhage in the majority of cases. Curettage, rather than reducing hemorrhage, is more likely to traumatize the implantation site and incite more bleeding, at times to such a degree that hysterectomy must be performed. Especially where there is good reason to preserve the uterus for future childbearing, initial treatment may best be directed to control of the bleeding, using intravenous oxytocin, ergonovine, methylergonovine, or prostaglandins (Andrinopoulos and Mendenhall, 1983; Goldstein and co-workers, 1983). If the bleeding subsides, the woman is simply observed, and if the bleeding stops, she is discharged. In general, curettage is carried out only if appreciable bleeding persists or recurs after such management. It is imperative that the physician inform the patient that if a curettage is performed under these conditions, the possibility of a hysterectomy is real. Furthermore, the physician must provide arrangements for adequate blood, appropriate anesthesia, and surgical assistance.

DISEASE OF THE URINARY TRACT

The puerperal bladder is not so sensitive to intravesical fluid tension as in the nonpregnant state. Moreover, it has become commonplace in modern obstetrics to establish an intravenous infusion system during labor in women. After delivery, the infusion system is then used to administer oxytocin during the first hour or so after delivery, if not longer. The oxytocin induces potent antidiuresis until the time the oxytocin is stopped, after which there is a prompt diuresis. The bladder then fills rapidly and may overdistend to a remarkable degree. General anesthesia, and especially conduction analgesia with the temporarily disturbed neural control of the bladder, are important contributory factors. The woman in this circumstance may, in time, void small volumes of urine ("overflow incontinence"), misleading attendants into believing she is voiding normally. Inspection of the abdomen will disclose the uterine fundus to be much higher than it should be, with an overlying cystic mass, the distended bladder.

As stated above, trauma to the genital tract, especially with large hematoma formation, may cause urinary retention. Therefore, pelvic examination should be performed whenever urinary retention is identified.

The combination of residual urine and bacteriuria introduced by catheterization into a traumatized bladder presents the optimal conditions for the development of infection of the urinary tract. The initial symptoms include dysuria, frequency, and urgency. Signs and symptoms of infection will subsequently vary, depending upon whether the infection is localized to the bladder or ascends to involve the upper urinary tract. After urine has been obtained for culture, treatment should consist of appropriate antibiotic or chemotherapeutic agents, as discussed in Chapter 39 (p. 809).

In cases of overdistention of the bladder, it is usually best to leave an indwelling catheter in place for at least 24 hours so as to empty the bladder completely and prevent prompt recurrence, as well as to allow recovery of normal bladder tone and sensation. When the catheter is removed, it is necessary subsequently to demonstrate ability to void appropriately. If the woman cannot void after 4 hours, she should be catheterized and the volume of urine measured. If there is more than 200 mL of urine, it is apparent that the bladder is not functioning appropriately. The catheter should be left in place and the bladder drained for another day. If less than 200 mL of urine is obtained, the catheter can be removed and the bladder rechecked subsequently as described.

In general, the first time the woman voids spontaneously after removal of an indwelling catheter inserted because of previous inability to void and gross overdistention, she should be immediately catheterized for residual urine. If the volume exceeds 200 mL, constant drainage should be reinstituted and those steps in management just outlined should be resumed. Harris (1979) has shown that almost 40 percent of women catheterized for postpartum urinary retention will develop bacteriuria that persists for at least 2 days following catheter removal. Antimicrobial therapy usually prevents this from happening (Garibaldi and associates, 1974; Harris, 1979) and it is our practice to give one-dose therapy at catheter removal.

DISORDERS OF THE BREASTS

ENGORGEMENT OF THE BREASTS

For the first 24 to 48 hours after the development of the lacteal secretion, it is not unusual for the breasts to become distended, firm, and nodular. This condition, commonly known as engorged breasts, or "caked breasts," often causes considerable pain and may be accompanied by a transient elevation of temperature. The disorder represents an exaggeration of the normal venous and lymphatic engorgement of the breasts, which is a regular precursor of lactation. It is not the result of overdistension of the lacteal system with milk.

Puerperal fever from breast engorgement is common. Such fevers are particularly worrisome if infection cannot be excluded in women who have recently undergone cesarean delivery. Roser (1966) observed that 18 percent of otherwise normal women had postpartum fever from breast engorgement. The duration of fever was from 4 to 16 hours and their temperatures ranged from 38 to 39°C. Similarly, Almeida and Kitay (1986) reported that 13 percent of postpartum women had fever from this cause, and it ranged from 37.8 to 39°C. In both studies, the incidence and severity of breast engorgement, and fever associated with it, were lower if treatment was given for lactation suppression. It is emphasized that other causes of fever, especially those due to infection, must be excluded.

Treatment consists of supporting the breasts with a binder or brassiere, applying an ice bag, and, if necessary, orally administering 60 mg of codeine sulfate or another analgesic. Pumping of the breast or manual expression of milk may be necessary at first (Fig. 28–4), but in a few days the condition is usually alleviated and the infant is able to nurse normally.

SUPPRESSION OF LACTATION

When, for a variety of reasons, the infant is not to be breast-fed, suppression of lactation becomes important. Listed in Table 28–1 are a variety of methods that have been used to suppress lactation, as well as their effectiveness and side effects. Perhaps the simplest method consists in support with a comfortable binder, application of cold packs, and mild analgesics for pain. Usually, all signs and symptoms will disappear in a few days if the breasts are not stimulated by pumping. Hormones, particularly estrogens, either alone or combined with testosterone, were formerly widely used for this purpose (Harrison, 1979). A single intramuscular injection of 4 mL of long-acting steroid esters in the form of estradiol valerate and testosterone

TABLE 28–1. EFFICACY OF SOME COMMONLY USED METHODS TO SUPPRESS LACTATION

Method	Symptoms Despite Treatment (%)			Possible Risks and Side Effects
	Minor	*Severe*	*Rebound*	
Breast support, binding, analgesia	84–100	16–28	0	None
Diethylstilbestrol	17–34	4–13	38–40	Thromboembolism
Quinestrol or chlorotrianisene	7	0–9	4–7	Thromboembolism
Deladumone OB	7	2–26	26	Thromboembolism, hirsutism
Bromocriptine	2–26	0–9	0–24	Hypotension, nausea, headache, dizziness, strokes, early ovulation

Modified from Blakemore: Lactation suppression is a matter of choice. Contemp Ob/Gyn 28:39, 1986

enanthate (Deladumone), administered at the time of delivery, is claimed to be effective.

Several estrogens that have been used to try to suppress lactation have been shown to predispose to venous thrombosis and thromboembolism (Niebyl and colleagues, 1979; Tindall, 1968; Turnbull, 1968). Moreover, their effect of lactation may be one of delay rather than effective suppression. Niebyl and co-workers (1979) challenged their use on the bases of increased risk of thromboembolism and questionable benefit. These agents have not been used at Parkland Hospital, even though the majority of mothers still do not breast-feed their infants.

Bromocriptine, a dopamine agonist, stimulates the production of prolactin inhibitory factor, which, in turn, causes a fall in plasma prolactin and the suppression of lactation. When 2.5 mg of bromocriptine is given twice daily for 14 days, severe breast engorgement is prevented in 75 to 98 percent of women, but 25 percent have rebound engorgement when therapy is completed (Blakemore, 1986). An association has been reported with bro-

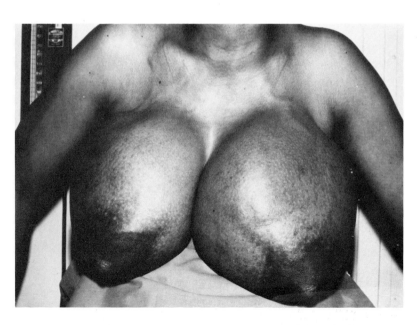

Figure 28–4. Pathological breast engorgement 3 days after delivery. Pumping of the breasts, uplift support, and analgesia provided relief. (*Courtesy of Dr. J. Duenhoelter.*)

mocriptine therapy and hypertension, seizures, and stroke. Considering the widespread use of the drug for lactation suppression, these complications are fortunately uncommon.

An alternative regimen is to prescribe bromocriptine only after severe mammary engorgement develops. This method has not been evaluated objectively in clinical trials, but from our experiences at Parkland Hospital, it is very effective. Defoort and colleagues (1987) presented preliminary evidence for the efficacy of a 50-mg intramuscular dose of bromocriptine for lactation suppression. Melis and co-workers (1988) described the efficacy of a single dose of the long-acting ergot derivative, cabergoline.

MASTITIS

Parenchymatous inflammation of the mammary glands is a rare complication antepartum but is occasionally observed during the puerperium and lactation.

The symptoms of suppurative mastitis seldom appear before the end of the first week of the puerperium and, as a rule, not until the third or fourth week. Marked engorgement usually precedes the inflammation, the first sign of which is chills or actual rigor, soon followed by a rise in temperature and an increase in pulse rate. The breast becomes hard and reddened, and the patient complains of pain. In some cases, the constitutional symptoms attending a mammary abscess are severe. Local manifestations may be so slight as to escape observation, however; such cases are usually mistaken for puerperal infection. In still another group of women, the infection pursues a subacute or almost chronic course. The breast is somewhat harder than usual and more or less painful, but constitutional symptoms are either lacking or very slight. In such circumstances, the first indication of the true diagnosis is often afforded by the detection of fluctuation.

Thomsen and co-workers (1983, 1984) reported that if breast milk has a leucocyte count of more than 10^6 per mL in conjunction with more than 10^3 bacteria per mL identified by culture, infection was likely. Interestingly, in a third of asymptomatic women breast milk was colonized by more than 10^3 bacteria per mL.

Etiology

By far the most common offending organism is *Staphylococcus aureus*. The immediate source of the staphylococci that cause this mastitis is nearly always the nursing infant's nose and throat. At the time of nursing, the organism enters the breast through the nipple at the site of a fissure or abrasion, which may be quite small. Whether the bacteria commonly cause mastitis simply by entering the lactiferous ducts of the breast with completely intact integument is not clear. In cases of true mastitis, the offending organism can nearly always be cultured from breast milk. A case of toxic shock syndrome has been reported in a woman with a puerperal breast abscess (Dixey and associates, 1982). *Staphylococcus aureus* was cultured from the abscess.

Suppurative mastitis among nursing mothers has at times reached epidemic levels. Such outbreaks most often coincide with the appearance of a new strain of antibiotic-resistant *Staphylococcus* or the reappearance of one previously identified. Typically, the infant becomes infected as he comes in contact with the nursery personnel who carry the organism. The attendants' hands are the major source of contamination of the newborn. Especially in a crowded, understaffed nursery, it is a simple matter for the personnel inadvertently to transfer staphylococci from one colonized newborn infant to another. The colonization of staphylococci in the infant may be totally asymptomatic or may locally involve the umbilicus or the skin, but occasionally the organisms may cause a life-threatening systemic infection.

Prevention

Safeguards to prevent colonization of the newborn with virulent strains of staphylococci necessitate exclusion from the care of the infant and mother by all personnel with a known or suspected staphylococcal lesion. Also, as a matter of daily routine, close inspection should be made of every infant, with prompt isolation of any who appear to be developing an infection of the cord or of the skin. Frequent use of soap or detergent for hand-scrubbing by personnel is essential. At the first sign of an outbreak, all personnel should be checked with appropriate cultures and phage-typing of swabbings of the posterior nares to identify carriers of more virulent strains of staphylococci.

Treatment

Antimicrobials have markedly improved the prognosis of acute puerperal mastitis. Provided that appropriate antibiotic therapy is started before suppuration begins, the infection can usually be aborted within 48 hours. Before initiating any antibiotic therapy, milk should be expressed from the affected breast onto a swab and promptly cultured. By so doing, the offending organism can be identified and its bacterial sensitivity ascertained. At the same time, the results of such cultures also provide information that is mandatory for a successful program of surveillance of nosocomial infections. The initial choice of antibiotic will undoubtedly be influenced to a considerable degree by the current experiences with staphylococcal infections at the institution in which the woman is receiving care. If, at the time, most staphylococcal infections are caused by organisms sensitive to penicillin, treatment with penicillin G is likely to be curative. Erythromycin is given to women who are penicillin-sensitive. If the infection is caused by resistant, penicillinase-producing staphylococci, or if resistant organisms are suspected while awaiting the results of culture, a penicillinase-resistant compound should be used. It is important that treatment not be discontinued too soon. Even though clinical response may be prompt and striking, treatment should be continued for at least 10 days.

Nursing should be discontinued when a diagnosis of suppurative mastitis is made, for it may be quite painful and the milk is infected; moreover, the infant often harbors the organisms and can therefore cause reinfection. Since the infant is almost always colonized by the offending organism, the infant should be observed very closely for signs of infection. Once established, resistant staphylococcal infections tend to spread and recur among the family for protracted periods of time.

In the case of frank abscesses, drainage, in addition to antibiotic therapy, is essential. The incision should be made radially, extending from near the areolar margin toward the periphery of the gland, to avoid injury to the lactiferous ducts. In early cases, a single incision over the most dependent portion of the area of fluctuation is usually sufficient, but multiple abscesses require several incisions. The operation should be performed under general anesthesia, and a finger should be inserted to break up the walls of the locules. The resulting cavity is loosely packed with gauze, which should be replaced at the end of 24 hours by a smaller pack. If the pus has been thoroughly evacuated, the cavity of the abscess is obliterated and a complete cure is sometimes effected with great rapidity.

GALACTOCELE

Very exceptionally, as the result of the clogging of a duct by inspissated secretion, milk may accumulate in one or more lobes of the breast. The amount is ordinarily limited, but an excess may form a fluctuant mass that may give rise to pressure symptoms. They may resolve spontaneously or require aspiration.

SUPERNUMERARY BREASTS

One in every few hundred women has one or more accessory breasts (*polymastia*). The supernumerary breasts may be so small as to be mistaken for pigmented moles, or, when without a nipple, for a lipoma. They rarely attain considerable size. They are likely to be situated in pairs on either side of the midline of the thoracic or abdominal walls, usually below the main breasts; they are also found in the axillae, and more rarely on other portions of the body such as the shoulder, flank, groin, or thigh. The number of supernumerary breasts varies greatly. When arranged symmetrically, two or four are most common, although ten have been described.

Polymastia has no obstetrical significance, although occasionally the enlargement of supernumerary breasts in the axillae may result in considerable discomfort. Frequently, a tongue of mammary tissue extends out into the axilla from the outer margin of a normal breast, whereas an isolated fragment is sometimes found in the same location. Such structures undergo hypertrophy during pregnancy (Fig. 28–5). When lactation has been established, they may become swollen and painful. Ordinarily, they soon undergo regression and give no further trouble.

ABNORMALITIES OF THE NIPPLES

The typical nipple is cylindrical, projecting well beyond the general surface of the breast; its exterior is slightly nodular but not fissured. Variations, however, are not uncommon, some sufficiently pronounced to interfere seriously with suckling.

In some women, the lactiferous ducts open directly into a depression at the center of the areola. In marked cases of depressed nipple, nursing is out of the question. When the depression is not very deep, the breast may occasionally be made available by use of a breast pump.

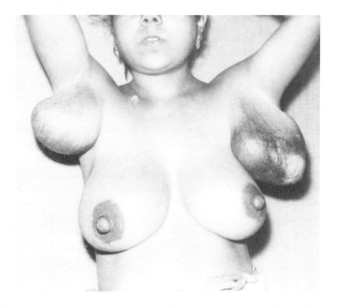

Figure 28–5. Pregnancy with huge bilateral hypertrophic axillary tail of the breasts. (*Courtesy of Dr. P. Bhattacharaya.*)

More frequently, the nipple, although not depressed, is so greatly inverted that it cannot be used for nursing. In such a case, daily attempts should be made during the last few months of pregnancy to draw the nipple out, using traction with the fingers. Since the maneuver is rarely successful, however, if the nipples cannot be made available by temporary use of an electric pump, suckling must be discontinued.

Nipples that are normal in shape and size may become fissured and therefore particularly susceptible to injury from the child's mouth during suckling. In such cases, the fissures almost invariably render nursing painful, sometimes with a deleterious influence upon the secretory function. Moreover, such lesions provide a convenient portal of entry for pyogenic bacteria. For these reasons, every effort should be made to heal such fissures, particularly by protecting them from further injury with a nipple shield and topical medication. If such measures are of no avail, the child should not be permitted to nurse on the affected side. Instead, the breast should be emptied regularly with a suitable pump until the lesions are completely healed.

ABNORMALITIES OF SECRETION

There are marked individual variations in the amount of milk secreted, many of which are dependent not upon the general health and appearance of the woman but upon the development of the glandular portions of the breasts. A woman with large breasts may produce only a small quantity of milk, whereas another with small, flat breasts may produce an abundant supply. Very rarely, there is complete lack of mammary secretion (*agalactia*). As a rule, it is possible to express a small amount from the nipple on the third or fourth day of the puerperium. Occasionally, the mammary secretion is excessive (*polygalactia*).

Formerly, persistent lactation or galactorrhea (together with anemorrhea and signs of estrogen deficiency) was referred to as the Chiari-Frommel syndrome. It was believed that this disorder was a pregnancy-induced derangement in the hypothalamic-pituitary control of prolactin and gonadotropin secretion. A similar set of symptoms commencing independent of pregnancy was described by Ahumada and co-workers (1932) and by Argonz and Del Castillo (1953). With the development of sensitive and accurate radioimmunoassays for prolactin and with the development of polytomography for evaluating the contents of the sella turcica, it has been demonstrated that microadenomas of the pituitary are the most common cause of galactorrhea, amenorrhea, and estrogen deficiency. Thus, the development of this triad should alert the physician to the likelihood of the existence of a microadenoma of the pituitary irrespective of whether the signs and symptoms begin in the puerperal period or remote from pregnancy.

POSTPARTUM PSYCHOSIS

As discussed in Chapter 13 (p. 252), mild and transient depression, called *postpartum blues*, is common within the first week or so after delivery. Frequently, this does not develop until the woman returns home, but in any case it is mild and self-limited. Depression thereafter, especially if severe, is not a normal accompaniment of childbearing and it requires investigation.

There is no evidence that pregnancy per se causes depressive illness, or any other psychotic disorder, although its circumstances might certainly precipitate an underlying disease. For example, Watson and colleagues (1984) observed that 9 of 15 women with affective disorders identified within 6 weeks of delivery had prior psychiatric disturbances. Women with previous postpartum psychosis are reported to have a 50 percent recurrence risk in subsequent pregnancies (Vandenbergh, 1980). Other risk factors include admission by the woman that her pregnancy was not wanted, or that she feels unloved by her mate.

Signs and symptoms of postpartum depression are no different than those of other depressive disorders. Particularly worrisome are suicidal thoughts, paranoid delusions, and threats of violence to the woman's children (Vandenbergh, 1980).

Treatment of suspected serious mental illness is given in consultation with a psychiatrist familiar with these syndromes. Often, hospitalization is warranted, especially if severe depression is accompanied by suicidal ruminations.

OBSTETRICAL PARALYSIS

Pressure on branches of the sacral plexus during labor is demonstrated by complaints of intense neuralgia or cramplike pains extending down one or both legs as soon as the head begins to descend the pelvis. As a rule, the compression is rarely severe enough to give rise to grave lesions. In some instances, however, the pain continues after delivery and is accompanied by paralysis of the muscles supplied by the external popliteal nerve (the flexors of the ankles and the extensors of the toes). Occasionally, the gluteal muscles are affected to a lesser extent. In modern obstetrics, paralysis of this kind is rare. Footdrop results from improper positioning of patients in stirrups or leg holders.

Separation of the symphysis pubis or one of the sacroiliac synchondroses during labor may be followed by pain and marked interference with locomotion.

REFERENCES

Adrinopoulos GC, Mendenhall HW: Prostaglandin F$_{2a}$ in the management of delayed postpartum hemorrhage. Am J Obstet Gynecol 146:217, 1983

Ahumada JC, Del Castillo EB: Amenorrhea and galactorrhea. Bol Soc Obstet Ginec 11:64, 1932

Almeida OD, Kitay DZ: Lactation suppression and puerperal fever. Am J Obstet Gynecol 154:940, 1986

Argonz J, Del Castillo EB: A syndrome characterized by esogenic insufficiency, galoctorrhea and decreased gonadotropin. J Clin Endocrinol 13:79, 1953

Barss VA, Schwartz PA, Green MF, Phillippe M, Saltzman D, Frigoletto FD: Use of the subcutaneous heparin pump during pregnancy. J Reprod Med 30:899, 1985

Bhattacharaya P: Pregnancy with huge bilateral hypertrophic axillary tail of the breast: Case report. Br J Obstet Gynaecol 90:874, 1983

Bell WR, Simon TL, DeMets DL: The clinical features of submassive and massive pulmonary emboli. Am J Med 62:355, 1977

Bergqvist A, Bergqvist D, Hallbook T: Deep vein thrombosis during pregnancy. A prospective study. Acta Obstet Gynecol Scand 62:443, 1983

Blakemore K: Lactation suppression is a matter of choice. Contemp Ob/Gyn 28:39, 1986

Brown CEL, Lowe TW, Cunningham FG, Weinreb JC: Puerperal pelvic thrombophlebitis: Impact on diagnosis and treatment using x-ray computed tomography and magnetic resonance imaging. Obstet Gynecol 68:789, 1986

Chong BH, Pitney WR, Castaldi PA: Heparin-induced thrombocytopenia: Association of thrombotic complications with heparin-dependent IgG antibody that induces thromboxane synthesis and platelet aggregation. Lancet 2:1246, 1982

Couch NP, Baldwin SS, Crane C: Mortality and morbidity rates after inferior vena caval clipping. Surgery 77:106, 1975

Defoort P, Thiery M, Baele G, Clement D, Dhont M: Bromocriptine in an injectable retard form for puerperal lactation suppression: Comparison with estrandron prolongatum. Obstet Gynecol 70:866, 1987

DeSwiet M, Ward PD, Fiddler J. Horsman A, Katz D, Letsky E, Peacock M, Wise PH: Prolonged heparin therapy in pregnancy causes bone demineralization. Br J Obstet Gynaecol 90:1129, 1983

Dixey JJ, Swanson DC, Williams TD, Rusin MH, Crook SJ, Midgley J, deSaxe MJ: Toxic-shock syndrome: Four cases in a London hospital. Br Med J 285:342, 1982

Galle PC, Muss HB, McGrath KM, Stuart JJ, Homesley HD: Thrombocytopenia in two patients treated with low-dose heparin. Obstet Gynecol 52:9S, 1978

Gallus A, Jackaman J, Tillett J, Mills W, Wycherley A: Safety and efficacy of warfarin started early after submassive venous thrombosis or pulmonary embolism. Lancet 2:1293, 1986

Garibaldi RA, Burke JP, Dickman ML, Smith CB: Bacteriuria during indwelling uretheral catheterization. N Engl J Med 291:215, 1974

Goldstein AI, Kent DR, David A: Prostaglandin E$_2$ vaginal suppositories in the treatment of intractable late-onset postpartum hemorrhage: A case report. J Reprod Med 28:425, 1983

Greenfield LJ, Alexander EL: Current status of surgical therapy for deep vein thrombosis. Am J Surg 150:64, 1985

Harris RE: Postpartum urinary retention: Role of antimicrobial therapy. Am J Obstet Gynecol 133:174, 1979

Harrison RG: Suppression of lactation. Semin Perinatol 3:287, 1979

Henderson SR, Lund CJ, Creasman WT: Antepartum pulmonary embolism. Am J Obstet Gynecol 112:476, 1972

Hirsh J: Blood tests for the diagnosis of venous and arterial thrombosis. Blood 57:1, 1981

Huisman MV, Büller HR, Ten Cate JW, Vreeken J: Serial impedance plethysmography for suspected deep venous thrombosis in outpatients: The Amsterdam general practitioner study. N Engl J Med 314:823, 1986

Hull R, Delmore T, Carter C, Hirsch J, Genton E, Gent M, Turpie G, Laughlin D: Adjusted subcutaneous heparin versus warfarin sodium in the long-term treatment of venous thrombosis. N Engl J Med 306:189, 1982a

Hull R, Hirsh J, Jay R, Carter C, England C, Gent M, Turpie AGG, Loughlin D, Dodd P, Thomas M, Taskob G, Ockelford P: Different intensities of oral anticoagulant therapy in the treatment of proximal-vein thrombosis. N Engl J Med 307:1676, 1982b

Hull RD, Hirsh J, Carter CJ, May RM, Dodd PE, Ockelford PA, Coates G, Gill GJ, Turpie G, Doyle DJ, Büller HR, Raskob GE: Pulmonary angiography, ventilation lung scanning, and venography for clinically suspected pulmonary embolism with abnormal perfusion lung scan. Ann Intern Med 98:891, 1983

Hux CH, Wapner RJ, Chayen B, Rattan P, Jarrell B, Greenfield L: Use of the Greenfield filter for thromboembolic disease in pregnancy. Am J Obstet Gynecol 155:734, 1986

Lee CY, Madrazo B, Drukker BH: Ultrasonic evaluation of the postpartum uterus in the management of postpartum bleeding. Obstet Gynecol 58:227, 1981

Kaunitz AM, Hughes JM, Grimes DA, Smith JC, Rochat RW, Kafrissen ME: Causes of maternal mortality in the United States. Obstet Gynecol 65:605, 1985

Melis GB, Mais V, Paoletti AM, Beneventi F, Gambacciani M, Fioretti P: Prevention of puerperal lactation by a single oral administration of the new prolactin-inhibiting drug, cabergoline. Obstet Gynecol 71:311, 1988

Mengert WF: Venous ligation in obstetrics. Am J Obstet Gynecol 50:467, 1945

Mohr DN, Rhu JH, Litin SC, Rosenow EC III: Recent advances in the management of venous thromboembolism. Mayo Clin Proc 63:281, 1988

Moser KM: Pulmonary thromboembolism. Braunwald E, Isselbacher JK, Petersdorf RG, Wilson JD, Martin JB, Fauci AS (eds): In Harrison's Principles of Internal Medicine. McGraw-Hill, New York, 1987, Chap 211, p 1105

Mueller MJ, Lebherz TB: Antepartum thrombophlebitis. Obstet Gynecol 34:867, 1969

Munsick RA, Gillanders LA: A review of the syndrome of puerperal ovarian vein thrombophlebitis with some original observations on ovarian venous blood-flow postpartum. Obstet Gynecol Surv 36:57, 1981

National Institutes of Health Consensus Development Conference: Prevention of venous thrombosis and pulmonary embolism. JAMA 256:744, 1986

Niebyl JR, Bell WR, Schaaf ME, Blake DA, Dubin NH, King TM: The effect of chlorotrianisene on postpartum lactation suppression on blood coagulation factors. Am J Obstet Gynecol 143:518, 1979

Roser DM: Breast engorgement and postpartum fever. Obstet Gynecol 27:73, 1966

Ruckley CV: Management of pulmonary embolism. Br Med J 285:831, 1982

Sachs BP, Brown DAJ, Driscoll SG, Schulman E, Acker D, Ransil BJ, Jewett JF: Maternal mortality in Massachusetts: Trends and prevention. N Engl J Med 316:667, 1987

Sassahara AA, Sharma VRK, Barsamian EM, Schoolman M, Cella G: Pulmonary thromboembolism: Diagnosis and treatment. JAMA 249:2945, 1983

Scurr J, Stannard P, Wright J: Extensive thrombo-embolic disease in pregnancy treated with a Kimray Greenfield vena cava filter. Br J Obstet Gynaecol 88:778, 1981

Shaul WL, Hall JG: Multiple congenital anomalies associated with oral anticoagulants. Am J Obstet Gynecol 127:191, 1977

Stamm H: Obstetrical and gynecological mortality due to embolism in Central Europe and Scandinavia. Geburtshilfe Frauenheilkd 20:675, 1960

Stone SR, Whalley PJ, Pritchard JA: Inferior vena cava and ovarian vein ligation during late pregnancy. Obstet Gynecol 32:267, 1968

Thomsen AC, Espersen T, Maigaard S: Course and treatment of milk stasis, noninfectious inflammation of the breast, and infectious mastitis in nursing women. Am J Obstet Gynecol 149:492, 1984

Thomsen AC, Hansen KB, Møller BR: Leukocyte counts and microbiologic cultivation in the diagnosis of puerperal mastitis. Am J Obstet Gynecol 146:938, 1983

Tindall VR: Factors influencing puerperal thromboembolism. J Obstet Gynaecol Br Commonw 75:1324, 1968

Turnbull AC: Puerperal thromboembolism and the suppression of lactation. J Obstet Gynaecol Br Commonw 75:1321, 1968

Vandenbergh RL: Postpartum depression. Clin Obstet Gynecol 23:1105, 1980

Viamonte M Jr, Koolpe H, Janowitz W, Hildner F: Pulmonary thromboembolism—Update. JAMA 243:2229, 1980

Wager GP, Martin DH, Koutsky L, Eschenbach DA, Daling JR, Chiang WT, Alexander ER, Holmes KK: Puerperal infectious morbidity: Relationship to route of delivery and to antepartum *Chlamydia trachomatis* infection. Am J Obstet Gynecol 138:1028, 1980

Walsh PN: Oral anticoagulant therapy. Hosp Pract 18:101, 1983

Watson JP, Elliott SA, Rugg AJ, Brough DI: Psychiatric disorders in pregnancy and the first postnatal year. Br J Psychol 144:453, 1984

Weiner CP: Diagnosis and management of thromboembolic disease during pregnancy. Clin Obstet Gynecol 28:107, 1985

Wenger NK, Stein PD, Willis PW III: Massive acute pulmonary embolism: The deceivingly nonspecific manifestations. JAMA 220:843, 1972

Wessler S, Gitel SN: Heparin: New concepts relevant to clinical use. 53:525, 1979

Wise PH, Hall AJ: Heparin-induced osteopenia in pregnancy. Br Med J 281:110, 1980

Abortion

DEFINITION

Abortion is the termination of pregnancy by any means before the fetus is sufficiently developed to survive. When abortion occurs spontaneously, the term *miscarriage* has been applied by laypersons.

In the United States this definition is confined to the termination of pregnancy before 20 weeks gestation based upon the date of the first day of the last normal menses. Another commonly used definition is the delivery of a fetus-neonate that weighs less than 500 g. In some European countries, this definition is less than 1,000 g.

SPONTANEOUS ABORTION

INCIDENCE

The incidence of spontaneous abortion has commonly been quoted as 10 percent of all pregnancies (Tietze, 1953; United Nations, 1954). This figure was derived from data that had at least two areas of instability, namely, failure to include early and therefore unrecognized abortions and the inclusion of illegally induced abortions that were claimed to be spontaneous.

The incidence of spontaneous abortion is difficult to determine precisely. First, agreement has to be reached as to when pregnancy actually begins. Does penetration of the ovum by a sperm constitute a pregnancy? Does cellular division of the fertilized ovum to form a blastocyst signal the onset of a pregnancy? Or does pregnancy begin with the invasion of the endometrium by the blastocyst? Second, the precision of the techniques that are used to identify a pregnancy are of obvious importance. With the use of a test that can detect minute amounts of human chorionic gonadotropin (hCG), the frequency of abortion will be higher than if the diagnosis is dependent upon histological confirmation of shed trophoblast.

Miller (1980), Edmonds (1982), Whittaker (1983), and their co-workers designed studies to overcome some of these problems. They measured serial values for chorionic gonadotropin in plasma or urine in normally ovulating women beginning 21 to 25 days after the first day of the last normal menses. A diagnosis was made of clinical and chemical pregnancy as defined in Table 29–1. Although there was considerable variation in the percentage of clinically diagnosed pregnancies in the series by Whittaker and co-workers (92 percent) compared to the other two series (43 and 67 percent), this difference likely was due to a less sensitive assay for β-hCG. Regardless, there were several important findings: (1) There is a remarkably successful conception rate, ranging from 24 to 60 percent with an average of 35 percent per cycle. (2) Of all conceptions, only 66 percent are recognized clinically and 13 percent of these eventually abort, a figure very close to that of 10 to 15 percent that has been accepted widely in the past. (3) The true abortion rate is between 20 and 62 percent with an average of 43 percent. This figure is similar to the 40 percent estimated by Hertig and associates (1959), who used morphological techniques. This subject is discussed in detail also in Chapter 41 (p. 895).

Since as many as 30 percent of abortions go unrecognized, this means that a majority occur very early. Indeed, Simpson and associates (1987) reported that in women with a sonographically confirmed live fetus at 8 weeks gestation, subsequent fetal loss was only 3.2 percent. Similar observations have been reported by Stabile and associates (1987) and by Mackenzie and co-workers (1988). Therefore, unrecognized losses occur early and clinically recognized losses likely contain a number of abortions in which the fetus died earlier than 8 weeks but the products were not expelled until later.

The above information has clinical importance when the physician is attempting to identify the cause(s) of recurrent abortion or when considering chorionic villus sampling (Chap. 32, p. 586). As discussed subsequently, genetic abnormalities of the conceptus are major causes of early pregnancy wastage, which appears to be a *natural means of biological selectivity*.

PATHOLOGY

Hemorrhage into the decidua basalis and necrotic changes in the tissues adjacent to the bleeding usually accompany abortion. The ovum becomes detached in part or whole and, presumably acting as a foreign body in the uterus, stimulates uterine contractions that result in expulsion. When the sac is opened, fluid is commonly found surrounding a small macerated fetus, or, alternatively, there may be no visible fetus in the sac, the so-called *blighted ovum*. Visualized through the dissect-

TABLE 29–1. SUBSEQUENT ABORTION RATES FOLLOWING LABORATORY AND CLINICAL DIAGNOSIS OF PREGNANCY

Investigator	Number of Cycles Studied	Pregnancies Diagnosed[a]		Pregnancies Diagnosed Clinically (%)	Pregnancies Aborted (%)	
		Laboratory[b]	Clinical		Clinically	Total[c]
Miller (1980)	623	152 (24)	102 (16)	102/152 (67)	14/102 (14)	64/152 (42)
Edmonds (1982)	198	118 (60)	51 (26)	51/118 (43)	6/51 (12)	73/118 (62)
Whittaker (1983)	226	92 (41)	85 (38)	85/92 (92)	11/85 (13)	18/92 (20)
Totals	1,047	362 (35)	238 (23)	238/362 (66)	31/238 (13)	155/362 (43)

[a] Number (percentage): Number is value of pregnancies diagnosed either by β-hCG titer or by clinical means, and percentage is number divided by number of cycles studied.
[b] Radioimmunoassays for β-subunit of human chorionic gonadotropin (β-hCG). A diagnosis of pregnancy was made by sampling plasma 21 and 25 days after previous menses by Miller and Whittaker and in urine 21 days after last menses by Edmonds. Pregnancy was diagnosed by a single β-hCG value of 5 μg per L or two values of 2 μg per L, Miller; 56 IU per L, Edmonds; and 16 mU per mL, Whittaker.
[c] Numerator is number of pregnancies diagnosed only by laboratory techniques minus the number of clinical pregnancies diagnosed plus the number of clinically identified abortions.

ing microscope, the placental villi often appear thick and distended with fluid, the ends of the villous branches resembling little sausage-shaped sacs. Such fluid-filled villi are undergoing molar degeneration with the imbibition of tissue fluid (Chap. 31, p. 541).

Blood or carneous mole is an ovum that is surrounded by a capsule of clotted blood. The capsule is of varying thickness, with degenerated chorionic villi scattered through it. The small, fluid-containing cavity within appears compressed and distorted by the thick walls of old blood clot. This type of specimen is associated with an abortion that occurs rather slowly, so that blood is allowed to collect between the decidua and chorion and to coagulate and form layers.

Tuberous mole and *tuberous subchorial hematoma of the decidua* are names applied to the same lesion. The characteristic feature is a grossly nodular amnion resulting from its elevation by localized hematomas of varying size between the amnion and the chorionic membranes.

In abortions after the fetus has attained considerable size, several outcomes are possible. The retained fetus may undergo *maceration*. In such circumstances, the bones of the skull collapse, the abdomen becomes distended with a blood-stained fluid, and the entire fetus takes on a dull reddish color. At the same time, the skin softens and peels off in utero or at the slightest touch, leaving behind the corium. The internal organs degenerate and undergo necrosis, becoming friable and losing their capacity for taking up the usual histological stains. The amnionic fluid may be absorbed when the fetus becomes compressed upon itself and desiccated to form a *fetus compressus*. Occasionally, the fetus eventually becomes so dry and compressed that it resembles parchment, the so-called *fetus papyraceus* (see Fig. 34–12, p. 638). This latter outcome is relatively frequent in twin pregnancy, if one fetus has died at an early period and the other has gone on to full development.

RESUMPTION OF OVULATION

Ovulation may occur as early as 2 weeks after an abortion. Lähteenmäki and Luukkainen (1978) detected a surge of luteinizing hormone (LH) 16 to 22 days after abortion in 15 of 18 women studied. Moreover, the plasma progesterone level, which had plummeted after the abortion, increased soon after the LH surge. These hormonal events are in excellent temporal agreement with the histological changes observed in endometrial biopsies and the rise in basal body temperature after abor-

tion, as described previously by Boyd and Holmstrom (1972). Therefore, it is important that effective contraception be initiated soon after abortion. The use of various contraceptive techniques following abortion is discussed in Chapter 42.

ETIOLOGIES OF SPONTANEOUS ABORTION

More than 80 percent of abortions occur in the first 12 weeks of pregnancy and the rate decreases rapidly thereafter (Harlap and associates, 1980). Chromosomal anomalies cause at least half of these early abortions and steadily and rapidly decrease thereafter (Fig. 29–1). The risk of spontaneous abortion appears to increase with parity as well as with maternal and paternal age (Warburton and Fraser, 1964; Wilson and associates, 1986). The frequency of clinically recognized abortion increases from 12 percent in women less than 20 years of age to 26 percent in those over age 40. The effect of advancing maternal age is illustrated in Figure 29–2. For the same paternal ages, the increase is from 12 to 20 percent. Finally, the incidence of abortion is in-

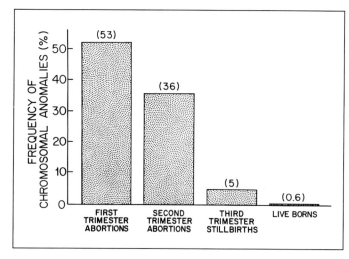

Figure 29–1. Frequency of chromosomal anomalies in abortuses and stillbirths for each trimester compared to the frequency of chromosomal anomalies in liveborn infants. The percentage for each group is shown in parentheses. (*Data adapted from Warburton (p. 261) and Fantel (p. 71) and their co-workers. In Porter IH, Hook EB, eds: Human Embryonic and Fetal Death. New York, Academic, 1980.*)

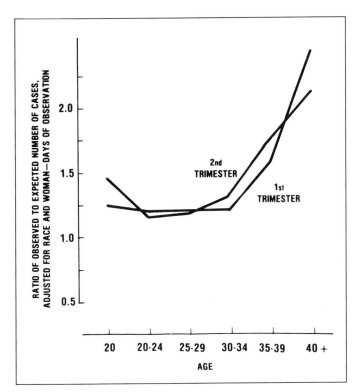

Figure 29-2. First and second trimester spontaneous abortions by maternal age. (*From Harlap and colleagues. In Porter IH, Hook EB (eds): Human Embryonic and Fetal Death. New York, Academic, 1980, p. 145.*)

creased if a woman conceives within three months of a livebirth (Harlap and associates, 1980).

The exact mechanisms responsible for abortion are not always apparent but in the very early months of pregnancy, spontaneous expulsion of the ovum is nearly always preceded by death of the embryo or fetus. For this reason, etiological considerations of early abortion involve ascertaining whenever possible the cause of fetal death. In the subsequent months, the fetus frequently does not die in utero before expulsion and other explanations for its expulsion must be invoked. Fetal death may be caused by abnormalities in the ovum-zygote or by systemic disease of the mother, and, rarely perhaps, of the father.

ABNORMAL DEVELOPMENT OF THE ZYGOTE

The most common morphological finding in early spontaneous abortions is an abnormality of development of the zygote, embryo, the early fetus, or at times, the placenta. In an analysis of 1,000 spontaneous abortions, Hertig and Sheldon (1943) observed pathological ("blighted") ova in which the embryo was degenerated or absent in 49 percent (Fig. 29-3).

Poland and co-workers (1981) morphologically identified disorganization of growth in 40 percent of abortuses (both embryos and fetuses) that were expelled spontaneously before 20 weeks of pregnancy. Among embryos (less than 30 mm crown-rump length), the frequency of abnormal morphological development was 70 percent. Of the embryos on which tissue culture and chromosomal analyses were performed, 60 percent were demonstrated to have a chromosomal abnormality. For fetuses

(30 to 180 mm crown-rump length) the frequency was 25 percent.

Abnormal fetal development, especially in the first trimester, may be classified into that with an abnormal number of chromosomes (aneuploidy) or development with a normal chromosomal component (euploidy).

Aneuploid Abortion

It is now appreciated that chromosomal abnormalities are common among embryos and early fetuses that are aborted spontaneously and account for much or most of early pregnancy wastage. From several studies it is apparent that 50 to 60 percent of early spontaneous abortions are associated with a chromosomal anomaly of the conceptus (Table 29-2).

Autosomal trisomy is a most frequently identified chromosomal anomaly associated with first-trimester abortions (Table 29-2). It can be the result of an isolated nondisjunction, a maternal or paternal **balanced translocation,** or a balanced chromosomal inversion (Chap. 32, p. 570). Translocations may be identifed in either parent and appropriate prenatal diagnostic procedures initiated in subsequent pregnancies to identify abnormal fetuses that may be aborted to prevent delivery of an abnormal infant. **Balanced chromosomal inversions** also may be identifed in couples with recurrent abortions.

Trisomies for all autosomes except chromosome number 1 have been identified in tissue from abortuses, but autosomes 13, 16, 18, 21, and 22 are most common. All of these latter trisomies have been reported in livebirths, but many others have been reported in stillborns. Advancing maternal age is associated with an increased incidence of these defects, especially D and G group trisomies, and chorionic villus sampling or amniocentesis is indicated for prenatal diagnosis in women past 35 years of age (Chap. 32, p. 581).

Monsomy X (45,X) is the next most common chromosomal abnormality and is compatible with liveborn (Turner syndrome) females who often thrive. It is not clear why some fetuses abort, but in those that do, there appear to be increased renal abnormalities.

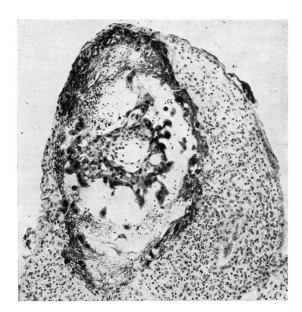

Figure 29-3. Abnormal ovum. A cross-section of a defective ovum showing an empty chorionic sac embedded within a polypoid mass of endometrium. (*From Hertig and Rock: Am J Obstet Gynecol 47:149, 1944.*)

TABLE 29–2. CHROMOSOMAL FINDINGS IN HUMAN ABORTUSES

Chromosomal Studies	Percent	
	Kajii and associates (1980)	Simpson (1986)
Normal (euploid)		
46XY and 46XY	46	54
Abnormal (aneuploid)		
Autosomal trisomy	31	22
Monosomy X(45,X)	10	9
Triploidy	7	8
Tetraploidy	2	3
Structural anomaly	3	2
Double trisomy	2	0.7
Triple trisomy	0.4	NL
Others-XXY, monosomy 21	0.8	NL
Autosomal monosomy G	NL	0.1
Mosaic trisomy	NL	1.3
Sex chromosome polysomy	NL	0.2
Abnormality not specified	NL	0.9

NL = not listed.

From Kajii and associates: Human Genet 55:87, 1980, and Simpson: CREOG Basic Science Monographs in Obstetrics and Gynecology. Washington, D.C., American College of Obstetricians and Gynecologists, 1986.

For reasons that also are not apparent, Turner syndrome is associated with a younger maternal age.

Triploidy is often associated with hydropic placental degeneration. Incomplete hydatidiform moles may have fetal development which is triploid or trisomic for chromosome number 16 (see Chap. 31, p. 542). The incomplete or partial hydatidiform mole is not usually malignant. The fetuses associated with these frequently abort early and the few who are carried longer are all grossly malformed. Triploidy may be caused by (1) dispermy, which likely is the most common mechanism in the human, (2) failure in sperm meiosis resulting in a diploid sperm, or (3) failure in egg meiosis in which either the first or second polar body is retained. Interestingly, advanced maternal and paternal age do not appear to be associated with this abnormality.

Tetraploid abortuses are rarely liveborn and most often are aborted very early in gestation, so little morphological information is available.

Chromosomal structural abnormalities are unusual causes of abortion and have been identified only since the development of banding techniques. Some of these infants are liveborn with balanced translocations and can be normal. This is analogous in many respects to what is observed in 45,X fetuses.

Autosomal monosomy is extremely rare and is incompatible with human life.

Sex chromosomal polysomy (47,XXX or 47,XXY) is unusual in abortus material but is commonly seen in livebirths. The 47,XXY variety is termed Kleinefelter syndrome and the 47,XXX variety is termed the "super female." Both have well-described phenotypic and mental profiles.

Euploid Abortion

Chromosomally normal abortuses usually are lost later in gestation. Kajii and co-workers (1980) reported that three-fourths of aneuploid abortions occurred at or before 8 weeks, while euploid abortions peaked at about 13 weeks. Stein and associates (1980) presented evidence that the incidence of euploid abortions increases dramatically after maternal age 35 years. The reasons for this are unknown. In fact, the reason(s) for euploid abortions generally are unknown but there appear to be at least two possibilities: (1) a genetic abnormality such as an isolated mutation or polygenic factors and (2) a variety of maternal factors which will be discussed subsequently.

A *genetic mechanism* has been proposed by Simpson (1980). He observed that only approximately 0.5 percent of liveborn infants have chromosomal abnormalities while at least 2 percent of livebirths have diseases associated with a single-gene mutation or a polygenic mechanism of inheritance. He reasoned that these more common defects could produce abortions by altering various fetal functions or by altering differentiation.

MATERNAL FACTORS

Maternal diseases usually are associated with euploid abortion. These losses peak at 13 weeks, and because of the later time, an etiology that is amenable to correction may be established in some cases. Thus, an etiology of midtrimester abortion should be sought. A variety of diseases, mental conditions, and developmental abnormalities have been implicated in euploidic abortion, although the evidence is not convincing in all instances. Nevertheless, a brief discussion of many of these conditions is presented, and emphasis is placed upon therapy in conditions where it has been shown efficacious.

Infections

Some chronic infections have been either implicated or strongly suspected of causing abortion. In particular, *Brucella abortus*, well known as a cause of chronic abortion in cattle, has been implicated. Many investigators studied this organism and concluded that it has no significance in human abortion.

Listeria monocytogenes (Rappaport and colleagues, 1960) and *Toxoplasma* (Ruffolo and associates, 1962) can cause abortion, although they appear to be less important in the United States than in other parts of the world. Presented in Figure 29–4 is a sonogram of a gestational sac lacking an embryo in a woman who had symptomatic *Listeriosis* proven by blood culture. She aborted spontaneously 5 days later.

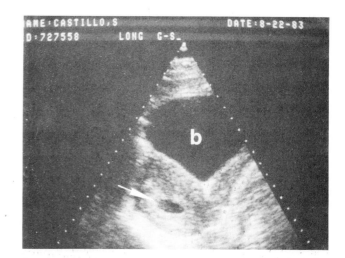

Figure 29–4. Longitudinal sector scan 7 weeks after the last menstrual period showing a gestational sac (*arrow*) devoid of any evidence of an embryo (b = bladder). *Listeria monocytogenes* was cultured from the blood of the febrile patient. She aborted spontaneously 5 days later. (*Courtesy of Dr. R. Santos.*)

The isolation of *Mycoplasma hominis* and *Ureaplasma urealyticum* from the genital tract of some women who have aborted has led to the hypothesis that mycoplasma infections involving the genital tract may be abortifacient. Serological evidence supportive of a role for the organisms in the genesis of abortion has been provided by Quinn and co-workers (1983b). They also reported improvement in pregnancy outcome following treatment with erythromycin (1983a). Their success rate, however, of 83 percent to 85 percent is similar to what has been achieved repeatedly with widely varied treatment regimens.

Of the two organisms, *Ureaplasma urealyticum* appears to be the major offender. Stray-Pedersen and associates (1978) demonstrated an increased incidence of positive uterine cultures for this organism in repeat aborters compared to control subjects (28 versus 7 percent). There were no differences in the organisms cultured from the cervix in the repeat aborters compared to control subjects. Treatment of these women and their sexual partners with doxycyline improved subsequent pregnancy outcomes, but a controlled study was not conducted.

Syphilis rarely if ever causes abortion. *Chlamydia trachomatis,* a common sexually transmitted disease, apparently also does not cause abortion (Quinn and associates, 1987). The evidence that *genital herpes* might cause abortion is weak, but Nahmias and co-workers (1971) reported that if genital herpes occurred in the first 20 weeks of pregnancy, the abortion rate was increased.

Specific therapies for these sexually transmitted diseases are discussed in Chapter 39.

Chronic Debilitating Diseases

In early pregnancy, chronic wasting diseases such as tuberculosis or carcinomatosis seldom have caused abortion; instead, the patient often dies undelivered. In later pregnancy, preterm labor may be induced by severe systemic maternal illness. Hypertension is seldom associated with abortion before 20 weeks' gestation, but rather may lead to fetal death and preterm delivery. Maternal diabetes has been found by some, but not others, to predispose to spontaneous abortion.

Endocrine Effects

An increased incidence of abortion has been attributed to hyperthyroidism, diabetes mellitus, and progesterone deficiency. *Hypothyroidism* does not appear to be associated with an increased incidence (Montoro and associates, 1981). *Diabetes mellitus* does not cause abortion if there is good glucose control (Crane and Wahl, 1981). Inadequate glucose control, however, may increase the incidence of abortion (Sutherland and Pritchard, 1986). *Progesterone deficiency* due to insufficient secretion of the corpus luteum or the placenta has been associated with an increased incidence of abortion. Since progesterone maintains the decidua, its deficiency would theoretically interfere with nutrition of the conceptus and thus contribute to its death.

It has been suggested that abnormal levels of one or more hormones might help to forecast abortion or even serve as therapeutic guides. Unfortunately, reduced levels of these hormones usually are the consequence rather than the cause of irreversible damage to the fetoplacental unit (Salem and co-workers, 1984). There are now well-documented cases of luteal phase defects (Horta and co-workers, 1977), but they appear to be uncommon. The issue of how to make the diagnosis either by serum progesterone measurements or endometrial biopsy as well as the best therapy with either clomiphene citrate or progesterone has been recently reviewed by Lee (1987). Check and

co-workers (1987a, b) reported that administration of progesterone alone is effective as long as there is ultrasonic evidence of normal follicular maturation and normal estrogen production. As yet, there is no convincing evidence in well-controlled, randomized studies that progesterone therapy is efficacious. Rock (1985), Ressequie (1985), Check (1986), and their co-workers presented evidence that *progesterone* therapy is not associated with increased fetal malformations.

Nutrition

At this time, it appears most likely that only very severe general malnutrition predisposes to increased likelihood of abortion. There is no conclusive evidence, however, that dietary deficiency of any one nutrient or moderate deficiency of all nutrients is an important cause of abortion. The nausea and vomiting that develop rather commonly during early pregnancy, and any inanition so induced, rarely are followed by spontaneous abortion. In fact, the reverse is more likely to be true (see Chapter 14, p. 271).

Most micronutrients have been reported at one time or another to have been of value in reducing the risk of spontaneous abortion. However, the evidence presented in support of such claims has been weak to nonexistent.

Recreational Drugs and Environmental Toxins

A variety of different agents have been reported to be associated with an increased incidence of abortion. As might be expected, as adequate information is gained, not all of these reports have been confirmed.

Tobacco has been identified to be associated with increased euploidic abortion (Harlap and Shiono, 1980). This increased risk was reported to be twofold compared to controls, and was independent of maternal age and alcohol ingestion (Kline and associates, 1980). *Alcohol* has been implicated in increasing spontaneous euploidic abortion even when consumed "in moderation" (Harlap and Shiano, 1980; Kline and co-workers, 1980). Increased euploidic abortion is strong evidence that both tobacco and alcohol are embryotoxins.

Radiation in sufficient doses is a recognized abortifacient. The human dose is not precisely known but a minimum lethal dose is believed to be about 5 rads. At the time of implantation, it is likely that a much lower dose of radiation could induce abortion.

Contraceptives have in the past been associated with an increased incidence of abortion; however, there now appears to be no such association. This is true for oral contraceptives and spermicidal agents used in contraceptive creams and jellies. Intrauterine devices, however, are associated with an increased incidence of septic abortion after contraceptive failure (Chap. 42, p. 931).

Environmental toxins such as anesthetic gases have been suspected to increase the incidence of spontaneous abortions (see Chap. 17, p. 330), but Axelsson and associates (1982) report that abortion rates in such women are *not* increased. In most instances, there is little valid information to indict any specific agent; however, there is good evidence that arsenic, lead, formaldehyde, benzene, and ethylene oxide may cause increased abortion (Barlow and Sullivan, 1982).

Immunological Factors

There are two major mechanisms of immunological abnormalities associated with abortion: autoimmune and alloimmune mechanisms.

Autoimmune mechanisms are those by which a cellular or humoral response is directed against a specific site within the host. Connective tissue disorders such as lupus erythematosus have been reported to be associated with increased abortion and fetal death (Chap. 39, p. 838). The antiphospholipid antibodies, including the lupus anticoagulant and other anticardiolipin antibodies, are other examples. Both of these antiphospholipid antibodies are directed against platelets and vascular endothelium which results in vascular destruction, thrombosis, abortion, and placental destruction (see Chap. 39, p. 839).

Allogenecity is used to describe genetic dissimilarities between animals of the same species. The human fetus is an allogenic transplant that is tolerated by the mother for reasons that are incompletely understood; however, several immunological mechanisms are reported to prevent fetal rejection. These mechanisms include, but likely are not limited to, histocompatibility factors, circulating blocking factors, local suppressor factors, and maternal or antipaternal antileucocytotoxic antibodies (Scott and associates, 1987). Therefore, some possible causes of recurrent abortion may be related to an abnormal maternal immune response which is turned against antigens on placental or fetal tissues. There is strong evidence that maternal-fetal *histoincompatibility* is essential to successful human pregnancy and that if mother and fetus are "too compatible" then reproduction failure develops. In some cases of recurrent abortion, there is an increased sharing of maternal and paternal human lymphocyte antigens (HLA). The strongest association is between the HLA-DR locus (Thomas and associates, 1985) and the HLA-DQ locus (Coulam and co-workers, 1987).

Thomas and associates (1985) suggested that the defect resulting in abortion might not be the consequence of a *too-similar immunological response*, but rather a genetic result from the sharing of alleles between husband and wife of recessive lethal genes linked to the HLA locus. Coulam and associates (1987) believe that the failure of Caudle and associates (1983) and Oksenberg and co-workers (1984) to document the HLA-DR and HLA-DQ similarities between couples is likely due to a small sample size and the fact that these investigators did not classify recurrent aborters into primary and secondary cases. The association between sharing the two HLA loci DQ and DR is greatest in couples with recurrent abortions who have no living children.

Maternal circulating blocking antibodies to paternal antigens appear to be essential to the maintenance of normal pregnancy. A failure of the mother to synethesize such blocking antibodies that protect the fetus from her own antibodies directed against paternal antigens shared by the fetus might result in abortion. These blocking antibodies apparently are of immunoglobulin G (IgG) origin and may act in several ways (Fig. 29–5): (1) by being directed against maternal lymphocytes to prevent them from reacting with receptors in fetal tissue, (2) by reacting with antigen-specific receptors on the fetal allograft and thereby blocking recognition of the foreign antigens by maternal lymphocytes, or (3) anti-idiotypic blocking antibodies could bind to antigen receptors and block maternal lymphocytes from attacking the target fetal cells (Scott and colleagues, 1987).

These blocking factors can be detected using a mixed lymphocyte reaction. Scott and associates (1987) reported that such blocking factors were usually found in pregnant and nulliparous women. They were not usually found in women with recurrent abortions and were not identified in nulligravidas. The question remains whether these blocking antibodies are responsible for, rather than the result of, pregnancy. Even so,

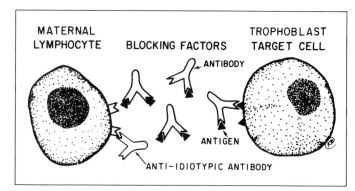

Figure 29–5. The potential role of blocking factors in preventing lymphocyte–target cell recognition. Blocking factors in pregnancy may be complexes of antibody and small-molecular-weight antigen. These complexes may interact with the antigen receptor on the maternal lymphocyte surface or with antigen on the surface of the trophoblast. Blocking factors also may be anti-idiotypic antibodies that react with receptors on the maternal lymphocytes. (*From Scott and colleagues: Obstet Gynecol 70:645, 1987.*)

therapies have been devised to stimulate the development of such blocking antibodies in attempts to prevent recurrent abortions.

Local suppressor factors likely are essential to normal pregnancy and their absence may be involved in the mechanism of recurrent abortion. Suppressor T cells are lymphocytes that produce soluble factors that suppress immune responses. These are present in decidua of normal pregnancies but absent in some abortions (Daya and associates, 1985), however, there is currently no clinical method of evaluating suppressor cells in the decidua of women with recurrent abortion.

Maternal antipaternal antileucocytotoxic antibodies increase in early pregnancy and then decrease near term (Taylor and Hancock, 1975). Scott and associates (1987) noted that it may be the failure of the mother to develop these antibodies that results in recurrent abortion. They emphasize, however, that it is unclear whether the absence of these maternal cytotoxic antibodies to paternal human lymphocyte antigens is a significant marker for women with recurrent abortion.

Therapeutic approaches for correction of the abnormal immune responses discussed above are directed at inducing normal maternal immune responses to paternal antigens or paternal HLA antigens inherited by the fetus. Two methods have been tried. In the first, immunizations are made against paternal leucocytes, and in the second, third-party donor leucocytes or blood transfusions are used. This last procedure has all the current disadvantages of any blood transfusion so other antigenic sources are used including trophoblastic membrane antigens (McIntyre and Faulk, 1986), frozen donor lymphocytes (Denegri and associates, 1986), and even sperm antigens (Johnson and co-workers, 1986).

Successes claimed for these methods have been questioned because of the lack of proper control subjects. However, Mowbray and co-workers (1985, 1987) used the paternal lymphocyte immunization regimen only in women without cytotoxic antibodies and those without other known causes for recurrent abortion. They reported a significant improvement in livebirths in treated versus untreated women. According to Scott and co-workers (1987), over 200 immunized women have been delivered of live infants without a marked increase in fetal abnormalities or pregnancy complications. In their excellent review they stressed that it is still unclear which women are most likely to benefit from immunotherapy, what source of antigen should be chosen for immunization, and how it should be administered. They emphasized that long-term consequences of such therapy are unknown and that such studies should be conducted in research centers equipped to answer these questions.

Aging Gametes

The age of both sperm and egg may influence the spontaneous abortion rate. Guerrero and Rojas (1975) noted an increased incidence of abortion relative to successful pregnancies when insemination occurred four days before or three days after the time of shift in basal body temperature. They concluded, therefore, that aging of the gametes within the female genital tract before fertilization increased the chance of abortion. Animal experiments also are consistent with this observation.

Laparotomy

The trauma of laparotomy may occasionally provoke abortion. In general, the nearer the site of surgery is to the pelvic organs, the more likely is abortion to occur. Ovarian cysts and pedunculated myomas may, however, be removed during pregnancy most often without interfering with the gestation. Peritonitis increases the likelihood of abortion. The administration of progesterone or other progestational agents for the first week or 10 days after operation have been prescribed to diminish the probability of abortion, although the efficacy of these agents remains questionable.

Physical and Emotional Trauma

Both physicians and laypersons are inclined to seek a simple explanation for commonplace medical phenomena. They may relate the abortion to a recent fall or blow or perhaps a fright. Multiple examples of trauma that failed to interrupt the pregnancy are forgotten. Only the particular event apparently related temporally to the abortion is remembered. Most spontaneous abortions, however, occur some time after death of the embryo or fetus. If abortion were caused typically by trauma, it would likely not be a recent accident but an event that had occurred some weeks before the abortion, as a rule.

In a review of personality factors associated with recurrent abortion, Tupper and Weil (1962) found that there were two types: the basically immature woman and the independent, frustrated woman. Results suggest that supportive therapy is as effective—or as ineffective—as anything else in preventing subsequent pregnancy loss.

Uterine Defects

Abnormalities of the uterus can be separated into those that are acquired and those that are developmental and the consequence of spontaneous abnormalities (müllerian anomalies) or induced abnormalities from diethylstilbestrol (DES) exposure.

Acquired uterine defects associated with abortion are *leiomyomas* and *intrauterine adhesions*. Even large and multiple uterine leiomyomas are not usually associated with abortion, and their location apparently is more important than size (Chap. 21, p. 387). Submucous, but not intramural or subserous, myomas are more likely to cause abortion. Even so, leiomyomas should be regarded as a causative factor only if the remainder of the clinical investigation is negative and a hysterogram shows a filling defect in the endometrial cavity. Myomectomies to remove such tumors often result in a scarred uterus which may rupture during a subsequent pregnancy either before or during labor. The only certain method to assess the possibility that a leiomyoma might be associated with abortion is to allow pregnancy.

Intrauterine adhesions (synechiae or Asherman syndrome) most frequently are the result of curettage for an infected or missed abortion or for postpartum complications (Schenker and Margalioth, 1982). The condition is due to the destruction of large areas of endometrium. This, in turn, results in amenorrhea and recurrent abortions believed to be due to insufficient endometrium to support implantation of the conceptus. The recommended treatment is lysis of the adhesions via hysteroscope and placement of an intrauterine contraceptive device to prevent recurrence of synechiae. Continous high-dose estrogen therapy also is recommended for 60 to 90 days. March and Israel (1981) reported a decrease in abortions from more than 80 to less than 15 percent with such therapy.

Developmental uterine defects are the consequence of abnormal müllerian duct formation or fusion. Müllerian abnormalities may be spontaneous or induced by in utero exposure to *diethylstilbestrol* (DES). Müllerian abnormalities and their management are discussed in detail in Chapter 37. Women with a unicornate uterus and women with either a septate or bicornate uterus have the highest abortion rates (Buttram and Gibbons, 1979). The obvious therapy is to resect the septum or unify the uterus; however, even after such corrective surgery and especially in a woman with a unicornate uterus, cervical cerclage appears to be of benefit (Chap. 37, p. 736).

As summarized in Table 29–3, in utero exposure to DES is associated with structural and functional abnormalities of the

TABLE 29–3. UNFAVORABLE PREGNANCY OUTCOMES IN WOMEN EXPOSED TO DIETHYLSTILBESTROL (DES) IN UTERO COMPARED TO CONTROL SUBJECTS

Author	Spontaneous Abortion[a]			Ectopic Pregnancy[a]			Preterm Labor[a]		
	DES	Control	Relative Risk	DES	Control	Relative Risk	DES	Control	Relative Risk
Barnes (1980)	57/220 (26)	36/224 (17)	1.6	8/220 (4)	3/224 (1.3)	2.8	17/220 (8)	10/224 (5)	1.7
Cousins (1980)	5/43 (12)	8/56 (14)	0.8	2/43 (5)	0/56 (—)	4.7	8/20 (40)	0/28 (—)	40
Herbst (1981)	24/114 (21)	14/128 (11)	1.9	8/114 (7)	0/128 (—)	7.0	23/114 (20)	8/128 (6)	3.2
Mangan (1982)	30/154 (18)	26/308 (8)	2.2	8/164 (5)	1/308 (0.3)	16.3	12/164 (7)	7/308 (2)	3.2
Totals	116/541 (21)	84/216 (12)	1.8	26/541 (5)	4/716 (0.6)	8.0	60/518 (12)	25/688 (4)	3.2

[a] Numbers in parentheses are percentages.

reproductive tract and significantly increases abortions and poor pregnancy performance. Kaufman and associates (1984) reported that abortion rates were increased in such women even when they did not have an abnormally shaped uterus. The reason for this is not known, but may be the consequence of an overall reduction in uterine size (Haney and colleagues, 1979).

Ludmir and associates (1987) reported that prophylactic cervical cerclage resulted in prolonging pregnancy in women with diethylstilbestrol-induced uterine defects. They also reported that there were perinatal deaths in women without cerclages, but not in those with cerclages. The differences were not significant. If prophylactic cerclage is not performed for all women, then it likely should be done in those with a strong history of painless cervical dilation and rupture of the membranes and rapid expulsion of the fetus. Even one such episode in a DES-exposed patient should be sufficient evidence to establish a presumptive diagnosis of cervical incompetence.

PATERNAL FACTORS

Even less is known about the role of the paternal factors in the genesis of spontaneous abortion. Certainly, chromosome translocations in sperm can lead to a zygote with too little or too much chromosomal material, resulting in abortion.

CATEGORIES AND TREATMENT OF SPONTANEOUS ABORTION

It is convenient to consider the clinical aspects of spontaneous abortion under five subgroups: threatened, inevitable, incomplete, missed, and recurrent abortion.

THREATENED ABORTION

A threatened abortion is presumed when any bloody vaginal discharge or vaginal bleeding appears during the first half of pregnancy. A threatened abortion may or may not be accompanied by mild cramping pain resembling that of a menstrual period or by low backache. This definition of threatened abortion makes it an extremely commonplace occurrence, since one out of four or five pregnant women has vaginal spotting or heavier bleeding during the early months of gestation. Of those women who bleed in early pregnancy, approximately one half abort. The bleeding of threatened abortion is frequently slight, but it may persist for days or weeks. Unfortunately, an increased risk of suboptimal pregnancy outcome in the form of preterm delivery, low birthweight, and perinatal death persists (Batzofin and associates, 1984; Funderburk and colleagues, 1980). However, the risk of birth of a malformed infant does not appear to be increased significantly.

Some bleeding about the time of expected menses may be physiological, analogous to the *placental sign* described by Hartman (1929) in the rhesus monkey. In these animals, there is always at least microscopic bleeding. The blood apparently makes its way from ruptured blood vessels and eroded uterine epithelium into the uterine cavity. Bleeding begins most commonly 17 days after conception, or about 4½ weeks after the last menses. In many of Hartman's animals, this bleeding could be observed grossly for several days. In the woman, furthermore, lesions of the cervix are likely to bleed in early pregnancy, especially postcoitum. Polyps presenting at the external cervical os as well as decidual reaction in the cervix tend to bleed in early

gestation. Lower abdominal pain and persistent low backache do not accompany bleeding from these causes.

Since most physicians consider any bleeding in early pregnancy to be indicative of threatened abortion, any treatment of so-called threatened abortion has considerable likelihood of apparent success. Most women who are in fact actually threatening to abort probably progress into the next stage of the process no matter what is done. If, however, the bleeding is attributable to one of the unrelated causes mentioned above, it is likely to disappear, regardless of treatment.

The woman should be instructed to notify her physician immediately whenever vaginal bleeding occurs during pregnancy. If the bleeding is slight, and no cause is ascertained through careful inspection of the vagina and cervix, she should be so informed. If an intrauterine device is still present and the "string" is visible, the device should be removed for the reasons cited above and in Chapter 42 (p. 932).

Usually, but not always, bleeding begins first, and cramping abdominal pain follows a few hours to several days later. The pain of abortion may be anterior and clearly rhythmic, simulating mild labor; it may be a persistent low backache, associated with a feeling of pelvic pressure; or it may be a dull, midline, suprasymphyseal discomfort, accompanied by a tenderness over the uterus. Whichever form the pain takes, the prognosis for continuation of the pregnancy in the presence of bleeding and pain is poor. However, in some women with pain who threaten to abort, the bleeding ceases, the pain resolves, and a normal pregnancy results. It may therefore be reasonable not to intervene to complete the abortion if the woman desires to continue the pregnancy. Little immediate harm should occur, but it is important to remember that the higher perinatal mortality rates are observed in women whose pregnancies were complicated early by threatened abortion.

Each woman should be examined thoroughly, for there is always the possibility that the cervix is already dilated and that abortion is inevitable, or that there is a serious complication such as extrauterine pregnancy or torsion of an unsuspected ovarian cyst. The patient may be kept at home in bed with analgesia given to help relieve the pain, but, in general, if the symptoms are more severe, she should be hospitalized. If the bleeding persists, she must be reexamined and the hemoglobin concentration or hematocrit should be rechecked. If blood loss is sufficient to cause anemia, evacuation of the products of conception is generally indicated. If bleeding is so great as to cause hypovolemia, termination of the pregnancy is mandatory.

Women with threatened abortion have been treated by some physicians with progesterone intramuscularly or with a wide variety of synthetic progestational agents orally or intramuscularly. Some of the progestins, particularly those structurally related to testosterone, may result in virilization of the female fetus. Of even greater importance is the lack of evidence of effectiveness of progestational agents in preventing most abortions. "Success" from their use often results in no more than a missed abortion.

Occasionally, as previously mentioned, in threatened abortion, slight hemorrhage may persist for weeks. It then becomes essential to decide whether there is any possibility of continuation of the pregnancy. If quantitative measurements of chorionic gonadotropin over several days do not demonstrate an increase in concentration, the outlook is *almost* hopeless. Importantly, the presence of chorionic gonadotropin in blood or urine does not indicate whether the fetus is alive or dead. If the uterus, when accurately measured over a period of time, does not increase in size, or becomes smaller, it is safe to conclude that the fetus is dead. An increase in uterine size indicates that the fetus is still alive or that a hydatidiform mole is present (see Chap. 31, p. 545).

The demonstration by sonography of a distinct, well-formed gestational ring with central echoes from the embryo implies that the products of conception are reasonably healthy. A gestational sac with no central echoes from an embryo or fetus implies, but does not prove, death of the conceptus (Fig. 29–4). When abortion is inevitable, the mean diameter of gestational sac is frequently smaller than appropriate for the gestational age. Moreover, at 6 weeks' gestation and thereafter fetal heart action should be discernible using real-time ultrasound. Most often, a single examination is insufficient, however, to determine the likelihood of abortion. Serial sonographic observations to document lack of fetal growth are useful. After death of the conceptus, the uterus should be emptied. Some women may elect abortion before it is absolutely certain that the fetus is dead, rather than face further uncertainty and procrastination.

If bleeding and pain persist unabated for 6 hours, it is probably best to face the inevitability of abortion and either perform a dilation and curettage during the first 14 weeks of pregnancy, or, if much more advanced, encourage its completion by stimulating uterine contractions with oxytocin or a prostaglandin until the bulk of the products of conception are expelled. All tissue passed should be carefully studied to determine whether the abortion is complete as well as to ascertain whether the abortion is euploidic or aneuploidic (p. 491). Unless all of the fetus and placenta can be positively identified, curettage most often is indicated.

INEVITABLE ABORTION

Inevitability of abortion is signaled by gross rupture of the membranes in the presence of cervical dilatation. Under these conditions, abortion is almost certain. Rarely, a gush of fluid from the uterus occurs during the first half of pregnancy without serious consequence. The fluid may have previously collected between the amnion and chorion to escape with rupture of the chorion while the initial defect in the amnion has completely healed. Most often, however, either uterine contractions begin promptly, resulting in expulsion of the products of conception, or infection develops.

With obvious gross rupture of the membranes during the first half of pregnancy, the possibility of salvaging the pregnancy is very unlikely. If in early pregnancy the sudden discharge of fluid, suggesting rupture of the membranes, occurs before any pain or bleeding, the woman may be put to bed and observed for further leakage of fluid, bleeding, cramping, or fever. If after 48 hours there has been no further escape of amnionic fluid, no bleeding or pain, and no fever, she may get up and, except for any form of vaginal penetration, continue her usual activities. If, however, the gush of fluid is accompanied or followed by bleeding and pain, or if fever ensues, abortion should be considered inevitable and the uterus emptied.

INCOMPLETE ABORTION

The fetus and placenta are likely to be expelled together in abortions occurring before the 10th week, but separately thereafter. When the placenta, in whole or in part, is retained in the uterus, bleeding ensues sooner or later, to produce the main sign of incomplete abortion. With abortions of pregnancies that are more advanced, bleeding is often profuse and may occasionally be massive to the point of producing profound hypovolemia. If the placenta is partly attached and partly separated, the splintlike action of the attached portion of the placenta interferes with myometrial contraction in the immediate vicinity. The vessels in the denuded segment of the placental site, deprived of the constriction provided by the contraction and retraction of the myometrium, bleed profusely.

In instances of incomplete abortion, it is often unnecessary to dilate the cervix before curettage. In many cases, the retained placental tissue simply lies loose in the cervical canal and can be lifted from an exposed external os with ovum or ring forceps. The suction curettage technique, as described below, is effective for evacuating the uterus, especially if the procedure is to be performed with only local cervical analgesia and moderate systemic analgesia such as meperidine. A woman with a more advanced pregnancy or who is actively bleeding should be hospitalized and the retained tissue removed without delay. Hemorrhage from incomplete abortion is occasionally severe but rarely fatal. Treatment of such hemorrhage is described in Chapter 36 (p. 697). Fever is not a contraindication to curettage once appropriate antibiotic treatment has been started (see Septic Abortion, p. 507).

MISSED ABORTION

The term *missed abortion* refers to the prolonged retention of a fetus who died during the first half of pregnancy. A missed abortion has been defined as the retention of dead products of conception in utero for 4 to 8 weeks or more. The rationale for this time period for the diagnosis of a missed abortion is not clear, but it certainly serves no useful clinical purpose. In the typical instance, early pregnancy appears to be normal, with amenorrhea, nausea and vomiting, breast changes, and growth of the uterus. Upon death of the ovum there may or may not be vaginal bleeding or other symptoms denoting a threatened abortion. For a time, the uterus then seems to remain stationary in size but usually the mammary changes regress. The patient is likely to lose a few pounds in weight. Thereafter, from careful palpation and measurement of the uterus, it becomes apparent that it has not only ceased to enlarge but it is becoming smaller, as a result of absorption of amnionic fluid and maceration of the fetus. Many patients have no symptoms during this period except persistent amenorrhea. If the missed abortion terminates spontaneously, and most do, the process of expulsion is quite the same as in any abortion. The product, if retained several weeks after fetal death, is a shriveled sac containing a greatly macerated embryo (Fig. 29–6).

Occasionally, after prolonged retention of the dead products of conception, serious coagulation defects develop, especially when the gestation had reached the second trimester before the fetus died. The woman may note troublesome bleeding from the nose or gums and especially from sites of slight trauma. The pathogenesis and treatment of the coagulation defects and any attendant hemorrhage in instances of prolonged retention of a dead fetus are considered in Chapter 36 (p. 716).

The reason why some abortions do not terminate after death of the fetus, while others do, is not clear. The use of more potent progestational compounds to treat threatened abortion, however, may contribute to a missed abortion. For example, Piver and colleagues (1967) treated 57 women for threatened abortion with Depo-Provera (injectable medroxyprogesterone acetate), following which more than one third of the women

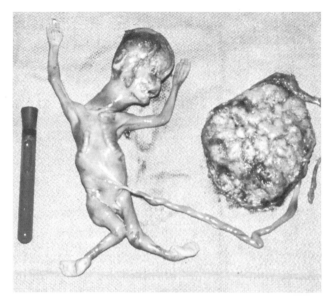

Figure 29–6. Immature fetus retained dead in utero with placenta for many weeks. Characteristics thick, opaque amnionic fluid is contained in the stoppered tube.

retained a dead fetus for more than 8 weeks. Moreover, Smith and co-workers (1978) observed that 73 percent of women who were given hormonal treatment because they threatened to abort did abort, but on the average 20 days later, whereas 67 percent of those who received no hormonal support aborted on the average 5 days later. They concluded that the progestational agents did not improve the outcome in threatened abortion. Instead, the hormones only prolonged the problem by delaying the inevitable.

RECURRENT SPONTANEOUS ABORTION

Recurrent spontaneous abortion has been defined by various criteria of number and sequence, but probably the most generally accepted definition today refers to *three or more consecutive spontaneous abortions.*

Repeated spontaneous abortions are likely to be chance phenomena in the majority of cases. Support for this view is provided by the observation that in the past the employment of any of a great variety of unrelated but presumed therapeutic modalities was followed by a successful pregnancy outcome 70 percent to 90 percent of the time.

It is important to differentiate spontaneous abortions that result from problems within the zygote from those much less common abortions that are due to maternal factors. In early abortions there is likely to be a nonrecurring aneuploidic abnormality of the conceptus that is responsible for the abortion. In late abortions fetal development is more likely to have been euploidic with a maternal abnormality causing the abortion.

Several investigators now recommend karyotyping the parents after they have experienced two or three spontaneous abortions. When karyotyping is performed, chromosomal banding techniques should be applied.

Prognosis
With the exception of the antiphospholipid antibodies and an incompetent cervix, the apparent cure rate after as many as

three spontaneous abortions will range between 70 and 85 percent no matter what treatment is used. In other words, the loss rate will be higher, but not a great deal higher, than that anticipated for pregnancies in general. In fact, Warburton and Fraser (1964) reported that the likelihood of recurrent abortion was 25 to 30 percent regardless of the number of previous abortions. Poland and associates (1977) noted that if a woman previously had delivered a liveborn infant, the risks for each recurrent abortion were approximately 30 percent, but if the woman had no liveborn infants and had experienced at least one fetal loss (spontaneous abortion, fetal or neonatal death), the risk of abortion was 46 percent. Following a successful delivery, the likelihood of an abnormal child is not increased; however, the risk for preterm and small for gestational age infants is increased significantly in such women (Reginald and co-workers, 1987).

Treatment
Specific treatments for recurrent abortions are discussed above under Etiologies of Spontaneous Abortion.

INCOMPETENT CERVIX

DEFINITION AND DIAGNOSIS

The term *incompetent cervix* is applied to a rather discrete obstetrical entity. It is characterized by painless dilatation of the cervix in the second trimester or early in the third trimester of pregnancy, with prolapse of membranes through the cervix and ballooning of the membranes into the vagina, followed by rupture of the membranes and subsequent expulsion of a fetus that is so immature that it is likely to succumb. Unless effectively treated, this same sequence of events tends to repeat itself in each pregnancy. Thus the presumptive diagnosis can usually be made if a woman has experienced spontaneous rupture of membranes and appreciable cervical dilatation without the usual discomfort of labor.

Attempts at a more precise diagnosis of cervical incompetence have not been successful. Numerous methods have been described in the nonpregnant woman to make the diagnosis, usually by documenting a more widely dilated internal cervical os than is normal. The methods have included hysterography, pull-through techniques of inflated Foley catheter balloons, and acceptance without resistance at the internal os of specifically sized cervical dilators (Ansari and Reynolds, 1987). During pregnancy, unsuccessful attempts have been made to predict premature dilation of the cervix using sonographic techniques (Witter, 1984). The diagnosis, however, remains difficult and is a clinical one based upon a history of a carefully observed and recorded sequence of events which includes painless cervical dilatation and spontaneous rupture of the membranes.

ETIOLOGY

Although the cause of cervical incompetence is obscure, previous trauma to the cervix, especially in the course of dilatation and curettage, conization, cauterization, or amputation, appears to be a factor in many cases. In other instances, abnormal cervical development, including that following exposure to stilbestrol in utero (p. 495), plays a role.

The cervical dilatation characteristic of this condition seldom becomes prominent before the 16th week, since before that time the products of conception are not sufficiently large to efface and dilate the cervix except when there are painful uterine contractions. Abortion from incompetence of the cervix is an entirely different and distinct entity from spontaneous abortion in the first trimester, since it results from different factors, presents a different clinical picture, and requires different management. Whereas spontaneous abortion in the first trimester is an extremely common complication of pregnancy, incompetence of the cervix is relatively rare.

TREATMENT

The treatment of the apparently incompetent cervix is surgical. The surgical treatment consists of reinforcing the weak cervix by some kind of pursestring suture. It is best performed after the first trimester but before cervical dilatation of 4 cm is reached, if possible. Bleeding, uterine contractions, or ruptured membranes are contraindications to surgery.

Preoperative Evaluation

Cerclage should be delayed until after 14 weeks gestation so that early abortions due to other factors will be completed. There is no general agreement as to how late in pregnancy the procedure should be performed. Certainly, the more advanced the pregnancy, the more likely surgical intervention will stimulate preterm labor or membrane rupture. For these reasons, some prefer bed rest rather than cerclage after midpregnancy. We seldom perform cerclage after 20 weeks, and certainly the procedure should not be performed after 26 weeks, but instead bed rest is recommended.

Sonography to exclude major fetal anomalies and to confirm a living fetus is mandatory. Cervical cytology should be negative. Obvious cervical infection should be treated, and cultures for gonorrhea, chlamydia, and group B streptococci are recommended by some, and with a positive culture, both sexual partners are treated as described in Chapter 39 (p. 850). For at least a week before and after surgery, there should be no sexual intercourse.

If there is a question as to whether cerclage should be performed, the woman is placed at decreased physical activity. Proscription of sexual intercourse is essential, and frequent cervical examinations should be conducted, preferably weekly, in order to assess cervical effacement and dilation. Unfortunately, rapid effacement and dilation of the cervix can occur even with such precautions (Witter, 1984). Finally, cerclage does not always prevent preterm delivery and, in fact, preterm labor may follow a cerclage or as the result of infection or ruptured membranes induced by the procedure.

Cerclage Procedures

Two main types of operation are in current use during pregnancy. One is a very simple procedure as recommended by McDonald (1963) and illustrated in Figure 29–7. The other is the more complicated Shirodkar operation (1955). There is less trauma and blood loss with the McDonald procedure during placement of the suture than with the Shirodkar procedure.

Success rates approaching 85 percent to 90 percent are achieved with both the McDonald and the Shirodkar techniques (Kuhn and Pepperell, 1977). Thus, there appears to be little reason for performing the more complicated Shirodkar procedure. The success rate has been higher when cervical dilatation was slight and prolapse of the membranes was minimal to absent. This is due, in part at least, to the fact that some cases so treated were not truly cases of cervical incompetence.

Charles and Edward (1981) identified complications, especially infection, to be much less frequent when cerclage was performed by 18 weeks' gestation. When cerclage was done much after 20 weeks there was a high incidence of premature rupture of the membranes, chorioamnionitis, and intrauterine infection. No evidence has been presented that the use of antibiotics around the time of the procedure reduces the risk of infection. Any suggestion of infection (fever, uterine tenderness, fetal or maternal tachycardia) should be investigated. They recommend amniocentesis to substantiate a diagnosis of chorioamnionitis before antibiotic therapy. With clinical infection, the suture should be cut and the uterus emptied.

There is no good evidence that prophylactic antibiotics to try to prevent infection, or either progestational agents or betamimetic drugs to try to prevent uterine contractions, are of any adjunctive value (Thomason and co-workers, 1982). In the event that the operation fails and signs of imminent abortion or delivery develop, it is urgent that the suture be released at once, since failure to do so promptly may result in grave sequelae. Rupture of the uterus or the cervix may be the consequence of vigorous uterine contractions with the ligature in place. If the membranes rupture in the absence of labor, the likelihood of serious infection in the fetus or the mother is increased appreciably if the suture is left in situ and delivery is delayed (Kuhn and Pepperell, 1977).

Following the Shirodkar operation the suture can be left in place if it remains covered by mucosa, and cesarean section can be performed near term (a plan designed to prevent the necessity of repeating the cerclage procedure in subsequent pregnancies). Otherwise, the Shriodkar suture is released and vaginal delivery is permitted.

> Treatment of an incompetent cervix by transabdominal cerclage placed at the level of the uterine isthmus has been recommended in some instances (Herron and Parer, 1988; Olsen and Tobiassen, 1982). The procedure requires laparotomy for placement of the suture and another laparotomy for its removal or for delivery of the pregnancy products or both. We have had little experience with this operation. Obviously, the potential for trauma and other complications initially and subsequently is much greater with this procedure than with the McDonald procedure.

INDUCED ABORTION

THERAPEUTIC ABORTION

DEFINITION

Therapeutic abortion is the *termination of pregnancy before the time of fetal viability for the purpose of safeguarding the health of the mother.*

LEGAL ASPECTS

Until the United States Supreme Court decision of 1973, only therapeutic abortions could be legally performed in most states. The most common legal definition of therapeutic abortion until then was termination of pregnancy before the period of fetal viability for the purpose of saving the *life* of the mother. Not too

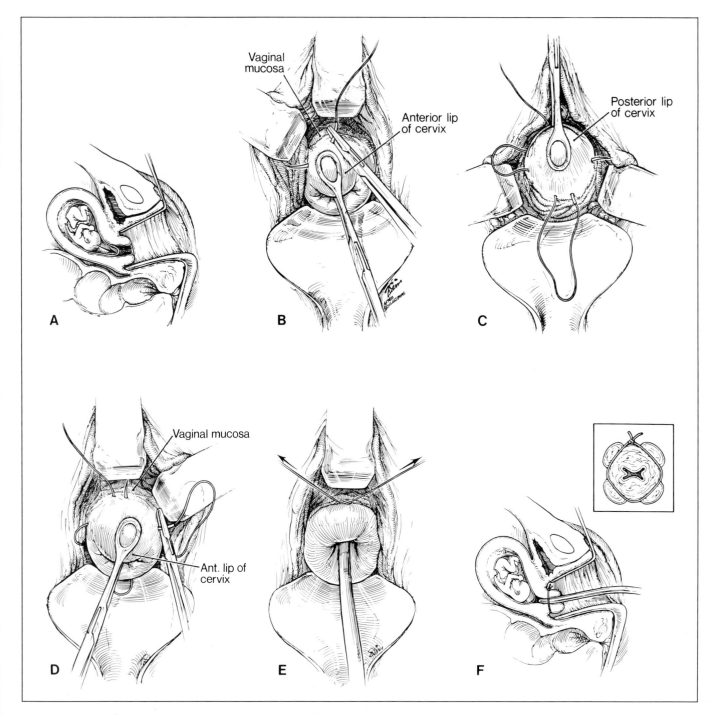

Figure 29–7. Incompetent cervix treated with McDonald cerclage procedure. **A.** Somewhat dilated cervical canal and beginning prolapse of membranes (*arrow*). **B.** Start of the cerclage procedure with a suture of number 2 monofilament proline being placed superiorly in the body of the cervix very near the level of the internal os. **C.** Continuation of the placement of the suture in the body of the cervix so as to encircle the os. **D.** Completion of encirclement. **E.** The suture is tightened around the cervical canal sufficiently to reduce the diameter of the canal to 5 to 10 millimeters and is then securely tied. In the illustration the *small* dilator has been placed just through the level of ligation to maintain patency of the canal when the suture is tied. A second suture similarly placed but somewhat higher may be of value especially if the first is not in close proximity to the internal os. **F.** The effect of the suture placement on the cervical canal is apparent.

long before the Supreme Court decision, a few states extended the law to read "to prevent serious or permanent bodily injury to the mother" or "to preserve the life or health of the woman." A few states allowed abortion if the pregnancy otherwise was likely to result in the birth of an infant with grave malformation.

Contrary to popular belief, the stringent abortion laws that were in effect until 1973 were of fairly recent origin. Abortion before quickening (the term applied to the first definite perception of fetal movement, which most often occurs between 16 and 20 weeks of gestation) was either lawful or widely tolerated in both the United States and Great Britain until 1803. In that year, as part of a general restructuring of British criminal law, a basic criminal abortion statute was enacted that made abortion before quickening illegal. The Roman Catholic Church's traditional condemnation of abortion did not receive the ultimate sanction of universal law (excommunication) until 1869 (Pilpel and Norwich, 1969).

The British law of 1803 became the model for similar laws in the United States, but it was not until 1821 that Connecticut enacted the nation's first abortion law. Subsequently, throughout the nation abortion became illegal except to save the life of the mother. Since therapeutic abortion *to save the life of the woman* is rarely necessary or definable, it follows that the great majority of such operations previously performed in this country went beyond the letter of the law.

INDICATIONS

Some of the indications for therapeutic abortion are discussed with the diseases that commonly led to the operation. A well-documented indication is persistent heart disease in the wake of previous cardiac decompensation. Another commonly accepted indication is advanced hypertensive vascular disease. Still another is invasive carcinoma of the cervix. Although it is impossible to predict what the future acceptable indications for therapeutic abortion will be, the therapeutic abortion policy formerly established by the American College of Obstetricians and Gynecologists seems most rational.

According to this policy, therapeutic abortion may be performed for the following medical indications:

1. When continuation of the pregnancy may threaten the life of the woman or seriously impair her health. In determining whether or not there is such a risk to health, account may be taken of the woman's total environment, actual or reasonably foreseeable.
2. When pregnancy has resulted from rape or incest. In this case the same medical criteria should be employed in the evaluation of the patient.
3. When continuation of the pregnancy is likely to result in the birth of a child with severe physical deformities or mental retardation.

ELECTIVE (VOLUNTARY) ABORTION

DEFINITION

Elective or voluntary abortion is the interruption of pregnancy before viability at the request of the women but not for reasons of impaired maternal health or fetal disease. The great majority of abortions now being done belong in this category. At present, there is approximately one elective abortion for every three live births in this country.

LEGALITY

The legality of elective abortion was established by the United States Supreme Court in its decision in the case of *Roe v. Wade*. The pregnant woman, Ms. Roe, attempted to obtain an abortion in Texas in 1969, where the performance of any abortion was illegal by state law except when done to save the life of the mother. Ms. Roe's pregnancy was the consequence of a gang rape. In spite of millions of abortions that have been performed subsequently as the consequence of the Supreme Court ruling, Ms. Roe's pregnancy was not aborted. In fact, at the time of the Supreme Court decision the child was 4 years old!

United States Supreme Court Decision

The Supreme Court decision voided the abortion statute of the State of Texas, but, as a consequence, nearly all state laws relative to abortion were affected. Moreover, the court's decision went on explicitly to define the extent to which the states might regulate abortion:

(a) For the stage prior to approximately the end of the first trimester, the abortion decision and its effectuation must be left to the medical judgment of the pregnant woman's attending physician.

(b) For the stage subsequent to approximately the end of the first trimester, the State, in promoting its interest in the health of the mother, may, if it chooses, regulate the abortion procedures in ways that are reasonably related to maternal health.

(c) For the stage subsequent to viability the State, in promoting its interest in the potential of human life, may, if it chooses, regulate, and even proscribe, abortion, except where necessary, in appropriate medical judgment, for the preservation of the life or health of the mother.

Fetal Viability

The term *viable* is widely used to identify a reasonable potential for subsequent survival if the fetus were to be removed from the uterus. Termination of pregnancy before 38 weeks' gestation but after the fetus has achieved some potential for survival is referred to as preterm delivery. The gestational age at which the fetus upon delivery ceases to be an abortus and becomes an infant is most difficult to define. In many states, a birth certificate is prepared for any pregnancy at 20 weeks' gestational age or more, or for any fetus that weighs 500 g or more.

The United States Supreme Court in its ruling on the legality of abortion used the term *viability* but did not define it. Moreover, the Court stated:

We need not resolve the difficult question of when life begins. When those trained in the respective disciplines of medicine, philosophy, and theology are unable to arrive at any consensus, the judiciary, at this point in the development of man's knowledge, is not in a position to speculate as to the answer.

The smallest surviving infant has been considered by some to be the one reported to Munro (1939). The infant was alleged to weigh about 400 g. The precision of measurement of the infant's weight on the village grocer's scales and the duration of gestation, which was said to be "2 months premature," are suspect. In recent times infants have been reported, at least by newspapers and television, to have survived although their birthweight was somewhat less than 500 g (see Chap. 38, p. 745).

Controversy Since the U.S. Supreme Court Decision

Numerous attempts have been made by the passage of several local and state laws to obstruct the woman's constitutional right to reach and carry out decisions with her physician concerning abortion. Virtually all such local and state laws have been overturned by federal district courts, and the United States Supreme Court has reaffirmed the earlier decision reached in *Roe v. Wade.*

The opponents and proponents of elective abortion are influenced by a wide range of issues—ethical, moral, legal, and even the issue of national security. For example, Mumford (1982), after citing several internationally prominent political and military figures, concluded as follows: (1) world population growth is a threat to the security of all nations, (2) abortion is essential to effective control of population growth, (3) abortion is a national security issue, and (4) as availability of legal abortion in the United States grows, so does the availability of abortion in the developing world.

Fortunately, there are effective contraceptive techniques for avoiding the birth of an unwanted child that are much more acceptable to most than is abortion. Hopefully, the opponents of abortion will support programs for providing effective contraception and thereby avoid abortion. Unfortunately, strong opponents of abortion, all too frequently, also oppose the dissemination and application of effective contraceptive techniques.

COUNSELING BEFORE ELECTIVE ABORTION

There are, in fact, only three choices available to the woman considering an abortion. The choices, simply stated, are continued pregnancy with its risks and responsibilities, continued pregnancy with its risks and with adoption arranged, or the choice of abortion with its risks. In some instances, the pregnant woman may well want to avoid abortion and allow the pregnancy to continue if social and economic problems can be resolved. Especially in these circumstances, knowledgeable and compassionate counselors are invaluable.

TECHNIQUES FOR ABORTION

The various techniques for performing abortion currently in use are outlined and discussed below.

Techniques for Accomplishing Abortion

  I. *Surgical*
    A. Cervical dilatation followed by evacuation of uterine contents
      1. Curettage
      2. Vacuum aspiration (suction curettage)
      3. Dilatation and evacuation
    B. Laparotomy
      1. Hysterotomy
      2. Hysterectomy
  II. *Medical*
    A. Oxytocin intravenously
    B. Intra-amnionic hyperosmotic fluids
      1. 20 percent saline
      2. 30 percent urea
    C. Prostaglandins E_2, $F_{2\alpha}$, and prostaglandin analogues
      1. Intra-amnionic injection
      2. Extraovular injection
      3. Vaginal insertion
      4. Parenteral injection
      5. Oral ingestion
    D. Various combinations of the above
    E. Antiprogesterone RU 486

SURGICAL TECHNIQUES FOR ABORTION

The products of conception may be removed surgically through an appropriately dilated cervix or transabdominally by either hysterotomy or hysterectomy. These techniques were recently reviewed by the American College of Obstetricians and Gynecologists (1987).

TRANSCERVICAL EVACUATION

Surgical abortion through the cervix is performed by first dilating the cervix and then evacuating the products of conception by mechanically scraping out the contents (curettage) or by the technique of vacuum aspiration (suction curettage), or both. The likelihood of complications, including uterine perforation, cervical laceration, hemorrhage, incomplete removal of the fetus and placenta, and infection increases after the first trimester, and especially after about 16 weeks. For this reason, dilatation and curettage or vacuum aspiration is best performed before the duration of pregnancy has exceeded that limit.

In the absence of maternal systemic disease, pregnancies are usually terminated by dilatation and evacuation without hospitalization. When an abortion is not performed in a hospital setting, it is imperative that the capabilities for effective cardiopulmonary resuscitation be immediately available and that hospitalization can be promptly facilitated whenever needed.

Laminaria Tents

Mechanical dilatation of the "undilated and uneffaced" cervix at the time of abortion is a potentially traumatic procedure. The risk of trauma can be minimized by inserting into the cervical canal an agent that will slowly swell and thus slowly dilate the cervix. Laminaria tents, illustrated in Figure 29–8, are used commonly to help dilate the cervix for abortion. They are made from the stems of *Laminaria digitata* or *Laminaria japonica*, a brown seaweed obtained from northern ocean waters. The stems are cut, peeled, shaped, dried, sterilized, and packaged according to size (small, 3 to 5 mm in diameter; medium, 6 to 8 mm; and large, 8 to 10 mm). The strongly hygroscopic laminaria are thought to act by drawing water from proteoglycan complexes, causing them to dissociate and thereby allowing the cervix to soften and dilate.

> A synthetic hygroscopic dilator made of hydrogel polymer has become available. It is claimed to dilate the cervix more rapidly than those made of traditional seaweed (Blumenthal, 1988; Chvapil and co-workers, 1982). Also, Lamicel, a polyvinyl alcohol polymer sponge impregnated with anhydrous magnesium sulfate ($Mg\ SO_4$) has been used recently as a synthetic laminaria tent and reported to be efficacious by Nicolaides and co-workers (1983). The magnesium levels in plasma described by them before and during its use are probably too low to be compatible with life, but presumably they are in error since no complications were noted in the subjects.

The cleansed cervix is grasped anteriorly with a tenaculum. The cervical canal is carefully sounded, without rupturing the membranes, to identify the length of the canal so as to gain some impression of its diameter and the resistance of the internal os. A laminaria of appropriate size is then inserted so that the tip passes just beyond the internal os using a uterine packing forceps or a radium capsule forceps (see Fig. 29–8). Later, usually after 6 hours, the laminaria will have swollen and thereby dilated the cervix sufficiently to allow easier mechanical dilatation and curettage. The laminaria may cause cramping but

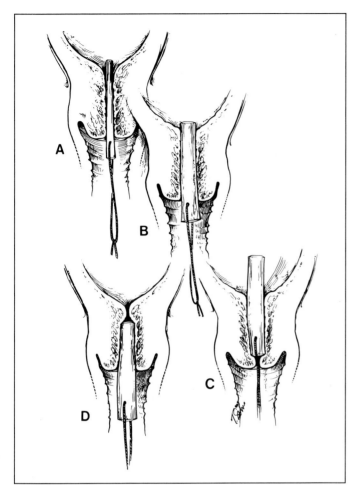

Figure 29–8. Insertion of laminaria prior to dilatation and curettage. **A.** Laminaria immediately after being appropriately placed with its upper end just through the internal os. **B.** The swollen laminaria and dilated, softened cervix about 18 hours later. **C.** Laminaria inserted too far through the internal os; the laminaria may rupture the membranes. **D.** Laminaria not inserted far enough to dilate the internal os.

the pain can be managed easily with 60 mg of codeine orally every 3 to 4 hours. Aspirin likely should not be administered with the codeine for two reasons: (1) aspirin is an antipyretic and might obscure the early signs of uterine infection and (2) aspirin is a prostaglandin synthase inhibitor that might prevent the local production of prostaglandins which are likely to result in cervical effacement and uterine contractions.

Rather than using a laminaria to effect softening of the cervix and thereby minimize trauma to the cervix from mechanical dilatation, prostaglandin pessaries (suppositories) have been inserted into the vagina against the cervix 3 hours or so before attempting dilatation. Chen and associates (1983) reported good results from so applying 1 mg of the prostin 16, 16-dimethyl-trans-Δ_2 prostaglandin E_1 methyl ester. Several newer prostaglandin products have been used to induce labor or to efface the cervix prior to induction of labor. Many of these same products also have been used to prepare the cervix prior to mechanical dilatation for induction of abortion. The products and their routes of administration are discussed in Chapter 18 (p. 345).

Subsequent Dilatation and Evacuation

At the time of abortion the laminaria is removed by grasping the attached thread, and the vulva, vagina, and cervix are cleansed.

The size and position of the uterus are carefully reevaluated through bimanual pelvic–abdominal examination. The anterior lip of the cervix is grasped with a multitoothed tenaculum and a local anesthetic is injected into the body or the cervix. Commonly, 5 mL of 1 or 2 percent solution of lidocaine is injected bilaterally. Alternatively, a paracervical block may be used (see Chap. 17, p. 335). The usual precautions for use of local anesthetics must be observed since deaths have resulted from their use in abortion.

The uterus is *carefully* sounded to identify the status of the internal os and to confirm the size of the uterus and the attitude of the fundus. The cervix is further dilated with Hegar or Pratt dilators until a vacuum aspirator suction curet of appropriate diameter can be inserted. As shown in Figure 29–9, the fourth and fifth fingers of the hand introducing the dilator should rest on the woman's perineum and buttocks as the dilator is pushed through the internal os. This provides a further safeguard against uterine perforation.

Suction curettage is then used to aspirate most, if not all, of the pregnancy products. The vacuum aspirator is moved over the surface systematically in order to cover eventually all the uterine cavity. Once this has been done and no more tissue is aspirated, the procedure is terminated. Gentle curettage with a sharp curet is then utilized if it is thought that any placenta or fetal fragments remain in the uterus. A sharp curet is more efficacious and its dangers need not be greater than those of the dull instrument. Perforations of the uterus rarely occur on the downstroke of the curet, but they may occur when any instrument is introduced into the uterus. A curet, however, is a dangerous instrument if injudicious force is applied to it. As shown in Figure 29–10, the necessary manipulations should be carried out with the thumb and forefingers only.

It is reemphasized that morbidity, immediate and remote, will be kept to a minimum if (1) the cervix is adequately dilated (without trauma to the cervix) before attempting to remove the products of conception, (2) the removal of the products of conception is accomplished without perforating the uterus, and (3) all of the products of conception (but not the decidua basalis) are removed.

Uterine Perforation

Accidental perforation of the uterus may occur during sounding of the uterus, dilatation, or curettage. The reported incidence of uterine perforation associated with elective abortion varies. Two important determinants of this complication are the skill of the physician and the position of the uterus, with a much greater likelihood of perforation if the physician is inexperienced and the uterus is retroverted.

Generally, the accident of uterine perforation is easy to recognize, as the instrument passes without hindrance obviously further than it could have if uterine perforation had not occurred. Observation may be sufficient therapy if the rent in the uterus is small, as when produced by a uterine sound or narrow dilator. Such small defects often heal readily without complication.

Considerable intra-abdominal damage can be caused by instruments passed through a uterine defect into the peritoneal cavity. This is especially true for suction and sharp curets. In this circumstance, laparotomy to examine the abdominal contents, especially the bowel, is the safest course of action. We have cared for a woman transferred to us after much of her right ureter had been removed at the time of attempted abortion using suction curettage! Similar cases have been observed by

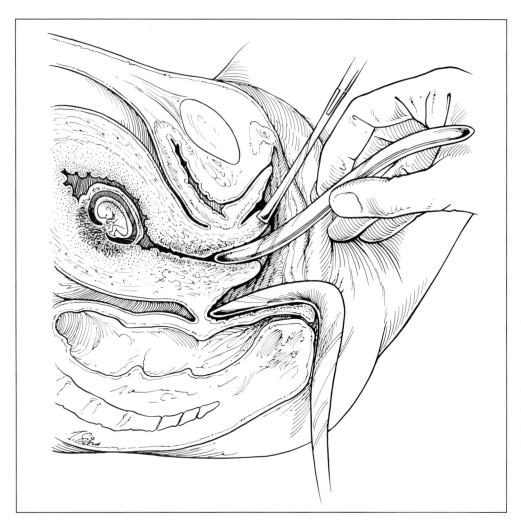

Figure 29–9. Dilatation of cervix with Hegar dilator. Note that the fourth and fifth fingers rest against the perineum and buttocks, lateral to the vagina. This maneuver is a most important safety measure because if the cervix relaxes abruptly, these fingers prevent a sudden and un-controlled thrust of the dilator, a common cause of perforation of the uterus.

others (Keegan and Forkowitz, 1982). Nonetheless, vacuum aspiration is generally preferable to mechanical curettage for abortion since it is quicker, has a lower perforation rate, induces somewhat less blood loss at operation, and there are fewer infections afterward. Especially in more advanced abortions, additional mechanical curettage as a second procedure may be necessary.

Some women may subsequently demonstrate cervical incompetence or uterine synechiae. The possibility of these complications should be explained to those contemplating abortion. In general, the risk of these complications is very slight, however. Unfortunately, more advanced abortion performed by curettage may induce sudden, severe consumptive coagulopathy, which can prove fatal. This complication is considered further in Chapter 36 (p. 699).

Menstrual Aspiration

Aspiration of the endometrial cavity using a flexible 5- or 6-mm Karman cannula and syringe within 1 to 3 weeks after failure to menstruate has been variously referred to as menstrual extraction, menstrual induction, instant period, atraumatic abortion, and miniabortion. Problems include the woman not being pregnant, the implanted zygote being missed by the curet, the failure to recognize an ectopic pregnancy, and rarely, uterine perforation.

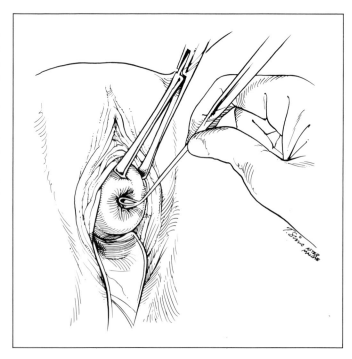

Figure 29–10. Introduction of the sharp curet. Note that the instrument is held merely with the thumb and forefinger; in the upward movement of the curet, only the strength of these two fingers should be used.

A positive pregnancy test will serve to eliminate a needless procedure on a nonpregnant woman whose period has been delayed for other reasons. Munsick (1982) recommends the following technique for identifying placenta in the aspirate: The syringe contents are placed in a clear plastic container and examined with back lighting. Tap water is added and the blood-stained liquid is decanted until tissue becomes visible. The tissue is then removed and immersed in clear water. Placenta is macroscopically soft, fluffy, feathery, and villous. If there is doubt as to whether the tissue is placenta or decidua, microscopic examination of a small piece under a cover glass with high light contrast will allow differentiation. Placental villi are obvious.

Anti-D Immunoglobulin

Treatment of D-negative women after abortion with anti-D immunoglobulin is recommended, since about 5 percent of D-negative women sustaining abortion otherwise become immunized (Chap. 33, p. 603).

HYSTEROTOMY AND HYSTERECTOMY

In a few circumstances, abdominal hysterotomy or hysterectomy for abortion is preferable to either dilatation and curettage or medical induction. If significant uterine disease is present, hysterectomy may provide ideal treatment. If sterilization is to be performed, either hysterotomy with interruption of tubal continuity or hysterectomy may on occasion be more advisable than curettage or medical induction followed by partial resection of the oviducts (see Chap. 42, p. 940). At times, hysterotomy or hysterectomy becomes necessary because of failure of medical induction during the second trimester.

The techniques employed for hysterotomy are similar to those for cesarean section (see Chap. 26, p. 453), except that the abdominal and uterine incisions are appreciably smaller. If further reproduction is anticipated, the smallest uterine incision that will allow removal of the fetus and placenta should be made away from the fundus, and the uterine wound carefully repaired.

Following abortion by abdominal hysterotomy, the potential for rupture during subsequent pregnancies is appreciable, especially during labor. Therefore, most obstetricians believe that in those women with previous hysterotomies, cesarean section is indicated for subsequent obstetric deliveries. After hysterotomy, Clow and Crompton (1973) identified 14 thin scars out of 31 evaluated in the subsequent pregnancy. Although Higginbottom (1973) believed that hysterotomy for abortion compared favorably with other methods of pregnancy termination, of the 242 patients reviewed by him, 12 required blood transfusion, 3 developed deep venous thrombosis, 1 had a pulmonary embolism, 1 had a repeat laparotomy for intestinal obstruction, and 2 subsequently required curettage for retained products of conception. **Nottage and Liston (1975), based on a review of 700 hysterotomies, rightfully concluded that the operation is now outdated as a routine method for terminating pregnancy.**

MEDICAL INDUCTION OF ABORTION

Very few effective, yet safe, abortifacient drugs have been discovered, although throughout history many naturally occurring substances have been tried by women desperate not to be pregnant. Serious systemic illness or even death, but not abortion, often was the result.

OXYTOCIN

Successful induction of second-trimester abortion is possible with high doses of oxytocin administered in small volumes of intravenous fluids. One regimen that we have found effective is to add ten 1-mL ampoules of oxytocin (10 IU per mL) to 1,000 mL of lactated Ringers' solution. This solution contains 100 mU of oxytocin per mL. An intravenous infusion is started at 0.5 mL per minute (50 mU per minute). The rate of infusion is increased at 20- to 30-minute intervals up to a maximum rate of 2 mL per minute (200 mU per minute). If effective contractions are not established at this infusion rate, then the concentration of oxytocin is increased in the infused solution. It is safest to discard all but 500 mL of the remaining solution which contains a concentration of oxytocin of 100 mU per mL. To this 500 mL is added an additional five ampoules of oxytocin and the resulting solution now will contain 200 mU per mL and the rate of infusion is reduced to 1 mL per minute (200 mU per minute). A resumption of a progressive rate increase is commenced up to a rate of 2 mL per minute (400 mU per minute) and left at this rate for an additional 4 to 5 hours or until the fetus is expelled.

After each increase in infusion rate, careful attention must be directed to the frequency and intensity of the uterine contractions since each increase in infusion rate *markedly* increases the amount of oxytocin infused. If the induction is unsuccessful, serial inductions on a daily basis for 2 to 3 days almost always are successful. The chance of a successful induction with high-dose oxytocin is enhanced greatly by the use of laminaria tents (p. 502) inserted the night before induction.

Once the cervix has undergone any degree of effacement and dilatation, either spontaneously or as the consequence of some other agent such as a prostaglandin, intravenously administered oxytocin is much more likely to prove effective for evacuating the products of conception.

There are complications from the use of oxytocin. If appreciable volumes of electrolyte-free solution are administered along with oxytocin, water intoxication may develop (see Chap. 16, p. 322). Rupture of the uterus from oxytocin infused during the first half of pregnancy has been documented in women of high parity (Peyser and Toaff, 1972) but is very unlikely. Rupture of the cervix or isthmus is well documented in instances in which oxytocin was given after intra-amnionic prostaglandin $F_{2\alpha}$. A large bolus of oxytocin intravenously may produce troublesome hypotension (see Chap. 16, p. 321).

INTRA-AMNIONIC HYPEROSMOTIC SOLUTIONS

In order to effect abortion during the second trimester, 20 to 25 percent saline, or 30 to 40 percent urea, has been injected into the amnionic sac to stimulate uterine contractions and cervical dilatation. These techniques are used less often than before. In 1983, only 2 percent of abortions were induced by intra-amnionic instillation techniques (Centers for Disease Control, 1986). Use of hypertonic dextrose has been abandoned because of its relative ineffectiveness as well as the occasional occurrence of serious infection, including *Clostridium perfringens* sepsis.

Mechanism of Action

The mechanism of action of the hyperosmotic agents when placed in the amnionic sac is not clear. Most often, but not always, the fetus is killed, but this does not explain their action, nor does myometrial stretch from an increased intrauterine volume appear to be an important factor. The hypertonic solutions damage the fetal membranes, likely resulting in the liberation of phospholipases. These lipases cleave arachidonic acid from its storage sites in the fetal membranes. The liberated arachidonic acid then is free to be converted into prostaglandins which cause uterine contractions and cervical dilatation (Chap. 10, p. 203).

Hypertonic Saline

Intra-amnionically injected hypertonic saline was used as an abortifacient by the Japanese after World War II but later abandoned because of maternal morbidity and mortality. In spite of documented serious complications, hypertonic saline became popular in the United States for midtrimester abortion once the pregnancy had advanced beyond the 15th week and the amnionic sac could be entered by transabdominal amniocentesis. Serious complications, including death, have been documented. The specific complications are (1) hyperosmolar crisis following the entry of the hypertonic saline into the maternal circulation, (2) cardiac failure, (3) septic shock, (4) peritonitis, (5) hemorrhage, (6) disseminated intravascular coagulation, and (7) water intoxication. Moreover, myometrial necrosis has followed injection of hypertonic saline that apparently remained in contract with the myometrium; cervical and isthmic fistulas and lacerations have been described; and gross rupture of the body of the uterus has been described (Horwitz, 1974). Use of laminaria tents to prevent such cervical trauma has been recommended, but fistula formation has been documented following the use of such tents (Lischke and Gordon, 1974). Serious disruption of the coagulation mechanism characterized by the changes of disseminated intravascular coagulation have been reported repeatedly with use of hypertonic saline for abortion (see Chap. 36, p. 723).

According to the American College of Obstetricians and Gynecologists (1987), intra-amnionic instillation as a method of midtrimester abortion has been largely replaced by dilatation and evacuation. Benefits cited included speed, cost, and less pain and emotional trauma.

Hyperosmotic Urea

Urea, 30 to 40 percent, dissolved in 5 percent dextrose solution, has been injected into the amnionic sac, followed by intravenous oxytocin, about 400 mU per minute. Urea plus oxytocin is as efficacious as an abortifacient as hypertonic saline, but less likely to be toxic. Urea plus prostaglandin $F_{2\alpha}$ injected into the amnionic sac is similarly effective.

PROSTAGLANDINS

Because of shortcomings of other medical methods of inducing abortion, prostaglandins are now widely used to terminate pregnancies, especially in the second trimester.

Mechanism of Action

Compounds commonly used are prostaglandins E_2, prostaglandin $F_{2\alpha}$, and certain analogues, especially 15-methylprostaglandin $F_{2\alpha}$ methyl ester. The probable mode of action of the prostaglandins on the uterus and cervix is considered in some detail in Chapter 10, p. 210).

Technique

Prostaglandins can act effectively on the cervix and uterus when (1) placed in the vagina in the form of a suppository immediately adjacent to the cervix, (2) administered as a gel through a catheter into the cervical canal and lowermost uterus extraovularly, or (3) injected into the amnionic sac by amniocentesis (Embrey, 1981). These three approaches reduce appreciably, but do not eliminate, the unpleasant systemic effects, especially gastrointestinal, that accompany oral or parenteral administration of prostaglandins. At the same time these three routes of administration cause cervical softening, uterine contractions, cervical dilatation, and expulsion of the products of conception in the great majority of cases, although repeated doses of the prostaglandin may be required.

Prostaglandin vaginal suppositories applied to the cervix are also used by some in lower dose during the first and even early in the second trimesters to ripen, that is, soften and dilate somewhat, the cervix before terminating the pregnancy by curettage (MacKenzie and Fry, 1981; Niloff and Stubblefield, 1982) (Chap. 18, p. 345). A troublesome feature with prostaglandin-induced abortions is the expulsion of a fetus with signs of life. The legal implications associated with expulsion of a living abortus may be profound. Although the purpose of abortion is to destroy the fetus before viability— statutes continue to be enacted to protect the abortus.

ANTIPROGESTERONE RU 486

A recently developed oral antiprogesterone RU 486 has been used in clinical experiments to effect abortions in early human gestation, either alone (Grimes and associates, 1988) or in combination with oral prostaglandins (Cameron and Baird, 1988). The clinical efficacy of this compound remains to be proven.

CONSEQUENCES OF ELECTIVE ABORTION

MATERNAL MORTALITY

It is apparent that serious morbidity and even mortality have followed some elective abortions. Nonetheless, legally induced abortion is a relatively safe surgical procedure, especially when performed during the first 2 months of pregnancy. The risk of death from abortion performed during the first 2 months is about 0.6 per 100,000 procedures (Centers for Disease Control, 1986). The relative risk of dying as the consequence of abortion is approximately doubled for each 2 weeks of delay after 8 weeks of gestation. Atrash and colleagues (1988) reported that the proportion of abortion-related deaths caused by general anesthesia has increased from 8 percent in 1975 to 29 percent in 1985. This likely reflects an absolute decrease in deaths from nonanesthetic complications. LeBolt and co-workers (1982) estimated that, during the 1970s at least, the overall risk of death from legal abortion was no more than one seventh the risk from childbirth.

IMPACT ON FUTURE PREGNANCIES

Hogue (1986), in a scholarly review of the impact of elective abortion upon subsequent pregnancy outcome, summarized data from more than 200 publications in 11 languages citing more than 150 studies from 21 countries. Hogue emphasized that the method of inducing abortion must be considered and that women chosen as control subjects should be primigravid since a parous woman has a reduced risk of complications in subsequent pregnancies. The following conclusions were derived from the data:

1. *Fertility* is not altered by an elective abortion. The only possible exception is the small risk of developing pelvic infection following termination.
2. *Vacuum aspiration* for a first pregnancy results in no increased incidence of midtrimester spontaneous abortions, preterm deliveries, or low-birthweight infants in subsequent pregnancies when compared to primigravid controls. However, *dilatation and curettage* in primigravidas results in an increased risk for subsequent ectopic pregnancy, midtrimester spontaneous abortion, and low-birthweight infants.
3. *Subsequent ectopic* pregnancies are not increased if the first termination is done by vacuum aspiration. Possible exceptions are in women with pre-existing *Chlamydia trachomatis* infection or those who develop postabortion infection.
4. *Multiple elective abortions* may increase various risks in subsequent pregnancies but there is insufficient information available to accurately address this. There is a trend toward a higher incidence of preterm delivery and delivery of low-birthweight infants.
5. *Placenta previa* has been reported to be increased following elective abortion (Barrett and associates, 1981), but Hogue discounted the study because of a failure to control for maternal age.
6. *Induced midtrimester abortions* apparently carry little risk to subsequent pregnancies if injection techniques are used. The risk of subsequently delivering a low-birthweight infant is increased following saline- versus prostaglandin-induced midtrimester terminations, but the difference is not significant (Meirik and Nygren, 1984). Similarly, the risk of subsequent low-birthweight infants is increased following *dilatation and evacuation* however, this difference also is not significant. Unfortunately, there are not enough procedure-specific data available to form valid conclusions regarding the risks to future pregnancies following any midtrimester abortion.

Hogue's (1986) review supplies overwhelming proof that forceful dilatation of the cervix by any procedure, whether in a first- or second-trimester abortion, predisposes a subsequent pregnancy to increased risks. If an elective abortion is to be performed, this risk factor should be kept in mind.

SEPTIC ABORTION

Serious complications of abortion have been most often, but certainly not always, associated with criminal abortion. Severe hemorrhage, sepsis, bacterial shock, and acute renal failure all have developed in association with legal abortion but at a very much lower frequency.

Sepsis from abortion is most often caused by pathogenic organisms of the bowel and vaginal flora. Infection most commonly is confined to the uterus in the form of metritis, but parametritis, peritonitis (localized and general), and septicemia are by no means rare. Of 300 cases of febrile abortions at Parkland Hospital shortly before the United States Supreme Court decision legalizing abortion, a positive blood culture was found

in one fourth. The organisms that were identified are listed in Table 29–4.

Treatment of the infection included prompt evacuation of the products of conception. Although mild infections can be treated successfully with broad-spectrum antibiotics in the usual dosage, any serious infection should be attacked with great vigor from the very start.

For septic abortion complicated by persistent, apparently resistant infection, or with evidence of overwhelming sepsis, high-dose broad-spectrum antimicrobials are given intravenously (see Chap. 27, p. 463). An example is clindamycin given along with gentamicin; however, several other regimes are equally effective.

SEPTIC SHOCK

Endotoxemia and exotoxemia are likely to cause severe and even fatal shock. Septic shock, which fortunately now is rare, was previously seen most often in women of reproductive age in connection with induced abortion, although it can occur as a result of infection in the genital or urinary tracts at any time during pregnancy or the puerperium. This complication is discussed in detail in Chapter 27 (p. 472).

ACUTE RENAL FAILURE

Persistent renal failure in abortion usually stems from multiple effects of infection and of hypovolemia. Less commonly, it has been induced by toxic compounds employed to produce abortion, such as soap, pHisohex, or Lysol. Whereas very severe forms of bacterial shock are frequently associated with the intense renal damage, the milder forms rarely lead to overt renal failure. Early recognition of this very serious complication is most important. The word "serious" is used advisedly in connection with acute renal failure in abortion, for the maternal mortality before the extensive use of dialysis exceeded 75 percent (Knapp and Hellman, 1959).

Renal failure is likely to be most intense when the cause of the sepsis includes *Clostridium perfringens* with the production of a very potent hemolytic exotoxin. In our experience, whenever intense hemoglobinemia complicated clostridial infection, renal failure was the rule. At the outset, plans should be made to initiate effective dialysis early, before metabolic deterioration becomes severe.

TABLE 29–4. BACTERIA PRESENT IN 76 CASES OF SEPTIC ABORTION WITH POSITIVE BLOOD CULTURES

Organisms Cultured	Frequency (%)
Anaerobic	63
Peptostreptococcus (anaerobic streptococcus)	41
Bacteroides	9
Clostridium perfringens	4
Aerobic	37
Escherichia coli	14
Pseudomonas	9
β-hemolytic streptococcus	4
Enterococcus	3
Combination	7

From Smith, Southern, and Lehmann: Obstet Gynecol 35:704, 1970.

REFERENCES

American College of Obstetricians and Gynecologists: Methods of midtrimester abortion. Tech Bull No 109, October 1987

Ansari AH, Reynolds RA: Cervical incompetence: A review. J Reprod Med 32:161, 1987

Atrash HK, Cheek TG, Hogue CJR: Legal abortion mortality and general anesthesia. Am J Obstet Gynecol 158:420, 1988

Axelsson G, Rylander R: Exposure to anesthetic gases and spontaneous abortion: Response bias in a postal questionnaire study. Int J Epidemiol 11:250, 1982

Barlow S, Sullivan FM: Reproductive hazards of industrial chemicals: An evaluation of animal and human data. New York, Academic, 1982

Barnes AB, Colton T, Gunderson J, Noller KL, Tilley BC, Strama T, Townsend DE, Hatab P, O'Brien PC: Fertility and outcome of pregnancy in women exposed in utero to diethylstilbestrol. N Engl J Med 302:609, 1980

Barrett JM, Boehm FH, Killam AP: Induced abortion: A risk factor for placenta previa. Am J Obstet Gynecol 141:769, 1981

Batzofin JH, Fielding WL, Friedman EA: Effect of vaginal bleeding in early pregnancy on outcome. Obstet Gynecol 63:515, 1984

Blumenthal PD: Prospective comparison of dilapan and laminaria for pretreatment of the cervix in second-trimester induction abortion. Obstet Gynecol 72:243, 1988

Buttram VC, Gibbons WE: Müllerian anomalies: A proposed classification (an analysis of 144 cases). Fertil Steril 32:40, 1979

Boyd EF Jr, Holmstrom EG: Ovulation following therapeutic abortion. Am J Obstet Gynecol 113:469, 1972

Cameron IT, Baird DT: Early pregnancy termination: a comparison between vacuum aspiration and medical abortion using prostaglandin (16,16 dimethyl-trans-Δ_2-PGE$_1$ methyl ester) or the antiprogestogen RU 486. Br J Obstet Gynaecol 95:271, 1988

Caudle MR, Rote NS, Scott JR, DeWitt C, Barney MF: Histocompatibility in couples with recurrent spontaneous abortion and normal fertility. Fertil Steril 39:793, 1983

Centers for Disease Control: Abortion surveillance: Preliminary analysis—United States, 1982–1983. MMWR 35:7SS, 1986

Charles D, Edward WR: Infectious complications of cervical cerclage. Am J Obstet Gynecol 141:1065, 1981

Check JH, Adelson HG: The efficacy of progesterone in achieving successful pregnancy: II. In women with pure luteal phase defects. Int J Fertil 32:139, 1987a

Check JH, Chase JS, Wu C-H, Adelson HG, Teichman M, Rankin A: The efficacy of progesterone in achieving successful pregnancy: I. Prophylactic use during luteal phase in anovulatory women. Int J Fertil 32:135, 1987b

Check JH, Rankin A, Teichman M: The risk of fetal anomalies as a result of progesterone therapy during pregnancy. Fertil Steril 45:575, 1986

Chen JK, Edler MG: Preoperative cervical dilatation by vaginal pessaries containing prostaglandin E$_1$ analogue. Obstet Gynecol 62:339, 1983

Chvapil M, Droegemueller W, Meyer T. Mascalka R, Stoy V, Suciu T: New synthetic laminaria. Obstet Gynecol 60:729, 1982

Clow WM, Crompton AC: The wounded uterus: Pregnancy after hysterotomy. Br Med J 1:321, 1973

Coulam CB, Moore SB, O'Fallon WM: Association between major histocompatibility antigen and reproductive performance. Am J Reprod Immunol Microbiol 14:54, 1987

Cousins L, Karp W, Lacey C, Lucas WE: Reproductive outcome of women exposed to diethylstilbestrol in utero. Obstet Gynecol 56:70, 1980

Crane JP, Wahl N: The role of maternal diabetes in repetitive spontaneous abortion. Fertil Steril 36:477, 1981

Daya S, Clark DA, Devlin C, Jarrell J: Preliminary characterization of two types of suppressor cells in the human uterus. Fertil Steril 55:778, 1985

Denegri JF, Altin M, McConnachi P, Peterson J, Benny WB, Zouves CG, Wilson D: Immunotheraphy of primary immunological aborters: Rationale for the use of pooled cyropreserved purified normal peripheral blood mononuclear cells. Am J Reprod Immunol Microbiol 12:65, 1986

Edmonds DK, Lindsay KS, Miller JF, Williamson E, Wood PJ: Early embryonic mortality in women. Fertil Steril 38:447, 1982

Embrey MP: Prostaglandins in human reproduction. Br Med J 283:1563, 1981

Fantel AG, Shepard TH, Vadheim-Roth C, Stephens TD, Coleman C: Embryonic and fetal phenotypes: Prevalence and other associated factors in a large study of spontaneous abortion. In Porter IH, Hook EM (eds): Human Embryonic and Fetal Death. New York, Academic, 1980, p. 71

Funderburk SJ, Guthrie D, Meldrum D: Outcome of pregnancies complicated by early vaginal bleeding. Br J Obstet Gynecol 87:100, 1980

Grimes DA, Mishell DR Jr, Shoupe D, Lacarra M: Early abortion with a single dose of the antiprogestin RU-486. Am J Obstet Gynecol 158:1307, 1988

Guerrero R, Rojas OI: Spontaneous abortion and aging of human ova and spermatozoa. N Engl J Med 293:573, 1975

Haney AF, Hammond CB, Soules MR, Creasman WT: Diethylstilbestrol-induced upper genital tract abnormalities. Fertil Steril 31:142, 1979

Harlap S, Shiono PH: Alcohol, smoking, and incidence of spontaneous abortions in the first and second trimester. Lancet 2:173, 1980

Harlap S, Shiono PH, Ramcharan S: A life table of spontaneous abortions and the effects of age, parity and other variables. In Porter IH, Hook EB (eds): Human Embryonic and Fetal Death. New York, Academic, 1980, p 145

Hartman CG: Uterine bleeding as an early sign of pregnancy in the monkey (Macaca rhesus), together with the observation on fertile period of menstrual cycle. Bull Johns Hopkins Hosp 44:155, 1929

Herbst AL, Hubby MM, Azizi F, Makii MM: Reproductive and gynecologic surgical experience in diethylstilbestrol-exposed daughters. Am J Obstet Gynecol 141:1019, 1981

Herron MA, Parer JT: Transabdominal cerclage for fetal wastage due to cervical incompetence. Obstet Gynecol 71:865, 1988

Hertig AT, Rock J, Adams EC, Menkin M: Thirty-four fertilized human ova, good, bad, and indifferent, recovered from 210 women of known fertility: A study of biologic wastage in early human pregnancy. Pediatrics 23:202, 1959

Hertig AT, Sheldon WH: Minimal criteria required to prove prima facie case of traumatic abortion or miscarriage: An analysis of 1,000 spontaneous abortions. Ann Surg 117:596, 1943

Higginbottom J: Termination of pregnancy by abdominal hysterotomy. Lancet 1:937, 1973

Hogue CJR: Impact of abortion on subsequent fecundity. Clin Obstet Gynaecol 13:95, 1986

Horta JLH, Fernandez JG, DeSota LB: Direct evidence of luteal insufficiency in women with habitual abortion. Obstet Gynecol 49:705, 1977

Horwitz DA: Uterine rupture following attempted saline abortion with oxytocin in a grand multiparous patient. Obstet Gynecol 43:921, 1974

Johnson PM, Chia KV, Risk JM: Immunological question marks in recurrent spontaneous abortion. In Clark DA, Croy BA (eds): Reproductive Immunology. New York, Elsevier, 1986, p 239

Kajii T, Ferrier A, Niikawa N, Takahara H, Ohama K, Avirachan S: Anatomic and chromosomal anomalies in 639 spontaneous abortions. Hum Genet 55:87, 1980

Kaufman RH, Noller K, Adam E, Irwin J, Gray M, Jefferies JA, Hilton J: Upper genital tract abnormalities and pregnancy outcome in diethylstilbestrol-exposed progeny. Am J Obstet Gynecol 148:973, 1984

Keegan GT, Forkowitz MJ: A case report: Ureterouterine fistula as a complication of elective abortion. J Urol 128:137, 1982

Kline J, Stein ZA, Shrout P, Susser M: Drinking during pregnancy and spontaneous abortion. Lancet 2:176, 1980

Kline J, Stein Z, Susser M, Warburton D: Environmental influences on early reproductive loss in a current New York study. In Porter IH, Hook EB (eds): Human Embryonic and Fetal Death. New York, Academic, 1980, p 225b

Knapp RC, Hellman LM: Acute renal failure in pregnancy. Am J Obstet Gynecol 78:570, 1959

Kuhn RPJ, Pepperell RJ: Cervical ligation: A review of 242 pregnancies. Aust N Z J Obstet Gynaecol 17:79, 1977

Lähteenmäki P, Luukkainen T: Return of ovarian function after abortion. Clin Endocr 8:123, 1978

LeBolt SA, Grimes DA, Cates W Jr. Mortality from abortion: Are the populations comparable? JAMA 248:188, 1982

Lee CS: Luteal phase defects. Obstet Gynecol Surv 42:267, 1987

Lischke JH, Gordon HR: Cervicovaginal fistula complicating induced midtrimester abortion despite laminaria tent insertion. Am J Obstet Gynecol 120:852, 1974

Ludmir J, Landon MB, Gabbe SG, Samuels P, Mennuti MT: Management of the diethylstilbestrol-exposed pregnant patient: A prospective study. Am J Obstet Gynecol 157:665, 1987

MacKenzie IZ, Fry A: Prostaglandin E$_2$ pessaries to facilitate first trimester aspiration termination. Br J Obstet Gynaecol 88:1033, 1981

Mackenzie WE, Holmes DS, Newton JR: Spontaneous abortion rate in ultrasonographically viable pregnancies. Obstet Gynecol 71:81, 1988

Mangan CE, Borow L, Burtnett-Rubin MM, Egan V, Giuntoli RL, Mikuta JJ: Pregnancy outcome in 98 women exposed to diethylstilbestrol in utero, their mothers, and unexposed siblings. Obstet Gynecol 59:315, 1982

March CM, Israel R: Gestational outcome following hysteroscopic lysis of adhesions. Fertil Steril 36:455, 1981

McDonald IA: Incompetent cervix as a cause of recurrent abortion. J Obstet Gynaecol Br Commonw 70:105, 1963

McIntyre JA, Faulk WP: Trophoblast antigens in normal and abnormal human pregnancy. Clin Obstet Gynecol 29:976, 1986

Meirik O, Nygren K-G: Outcome of first delivery after 2nd trimester two-step induced abortion: Controlled historical cohort study. Acta Obstet Gynecol Scand 63:45, 1984

Miller JF, Williamson E, Glue J, Gordon YB, Grudzinskas JG, Sykes A: Fetal loss after implantation: A prospective study. Lancet 2:554, 1980

Montoro M, Collea JV, Frasier D, Mestman J: Successful outcome of pregnancy in women with hypothyroidism. Ann Intern Med 94:31, 1981

Mowbray JF, Gibbings C, Liddell H, Reginald PW, Underwood JL, Beard RW: Controlled trial of treatment of recurrent spontaneous abortion with paternal cells. Lancet 1:941, 1985

Mowbray JF, Underwood JL, Michel M, Forbes PB, Beard RW: Immunization with paternal lymphocytes in women with recurrent miscarriage. Lancet 1:680, 1987

Mumford SD: Abortion: A national security issue. Am J Obstet Gynecol 142:951, 1982

Munro JS: Premature infant weighing less than one pound at birth who survived and developed normally. Can Med Assoc J 40:69, 1939

Munsick RA: Clinical test for placenta in 300 consecutive menstrual aspirations. Obstet Gynecol 60:738, 1982

Nahmias AJ, Josey WE, Naib ZM, Freeman MG, Fernandez RJ, Wheeler JH: Perinatal risk associated with maternal genital herpes simplex virus infection. Am J Obstet Gynecol 11:825, 1971

Nicolaides KH, Welch CC, Koullapis EN, Filshie GM: Cervical dilatation by Lamicel—Studies on the mechanism of action. Br J Obstet Gynaecol 90:1060, 1983

Niloff JM, Stubblefield PG: Low-dose vaginal 15 methyl prostaglandin $F_{2\alpha}$ for cervical dilatation prior to vacuum curettage abortion. Am J Obstet Gynecol 142:596, 1982

Nottage BJ, Liston WA: A review of 700 hysterectomies. Br J Obstet Gynaecol 82:310, 1975

Oksenberg JR, Persitz E, Amar A, Brautbar C: Maternal-paternal histocompatibility: Lack of association with habitual abortions. Fertil Steril 42:389, 1984

Olsen S, Tobiassen T: Transabdominal isthmic cerclage for the treatment of incompetent cervix. Acta Obstet Gynecol 61:473, 1982

Peyser MR, Toaff R: Rupture of uterus in the first trimester caused by high-concentration oxytocin drip. Obstet Gynecol 40:371, 1972

Pilpel HF, Norwich KP: When should abortion be legal? New York, Public Affairs Committee Inc, No 429, 1969

Piver MS, Bolognese RJ, Feldman JD: Long-acting progesterone as a cause of missed abortion. Am J Obstet Gynecol 97:579, 1967

Poland BJ, Miller JR, Harris M, Livingston J: Spontaneous abortion: A study of 1961 women and their abortuses. Acta Obstet Gynecol Scand (Suppl) 102:1, 1981

Poland BJ, Miller JR, Jones DC, Trimble BK: Reproductive counseling in patients who have had a spontaneous abortion. Am J Obstet Gynecol 127:685, 1977

Quinn PA, Petric M, Barking M, Butany J, Derzko C, Gysler M, Lie KI, Shewchuck AB, Shuber J, Ryan E, Chipman ML: Prevalence of antibody to *Chlamydia trachomatis* in spontaneous abortion and infertility. Am J Obstet Gynecol 156:291, 1987

Quinn PA, Shewchuk AB, Shuber J, Lie KI, Ryan E, Chipman ML, Nocilla DM: Efficacy of antibiotic therapy in preventing spontaneous pregnancy loss among couples colonized with genital mycoplasmas. Am J Obstet Gynecol 145:239, 1983a

Quinn PA, Shewchuck AB, Shuber J, Lie KI, Ryan E, Sheu M, Chipman ML: Serologic evidence of *Ureaplasma urealyticum* infection in women with spontaneous pregnancy loss. Am J Obstet Gynecol 145:245, 1983b

Rappaport F, Rubinovitz M, Toaff R, Krocheck N: Genital listerosis as a cause of repeated abortion. Lancet 1:1273, 1960

Reginald PW, Beard RW, Chapple J, Forbes PB, Liddell HS, Mowbray JF, Underwood JL: Outcome of pregnancies progressing beyond 28 weeks gestation in women with a history of recurrent miscarriage. Br J Obstet Gynaecol 94:643, 1987

Ressequie L, Hick JF, Bruen JA, Noller KL, O'Fallon WM, Kurland LT: Congenital malformations among offspring exposed in utero to progestins, Olmsted County, Minnesota, 1936–1974. Fertil Steril 43:514, 1985

Rock JA, Wentz AC, Cole KA, Kimball AW Jr, Zacur HA, Early SA, Jones GS: Fetal malformations following progesterone therapy during pregnancy: A preliminary report. Fertil Steril 44:17, 1985

Ruffolo EH, Wilson RB, Weed LA: *Listeria monocytogenes* as a cause of pregnancy wastage. Obstet Gynecol 19:533, 1962

Salem HT, Ghaneimah SA, Shaaban MM, Chard T: Prognostic value of biochemical tests in the assessment of fetal outcome in threatened abortion. Br J Obstet Gynecol 91:382, 1984

Schenker JG, Margalioth EJ: Intrauterine adhesions: An updated appraisal. Fertil Steril 37:593, 1982

Scott JR, Rote NS, Branch DW: Immunologic aspects of recurrent abortion and fetal death. Obstet Gynecol 70:645, 1987

Shirodkar VN: A new method of operative treatment for habitual abortions in the second trimester of pregnancy. Antiseptic 52:299, 1955

Simpson JL: Genes, chromosomes, and reproductive failure. Fertil Steril 33:107, 1980

Simpson JL: Genetics. CREOG Basic Science Monograph in Obstetrics and Gynecology. CREOG, Washington, DC, 1986

Simpson JL, Mills JL, Holmes LB, Ober CL, Aarons J, Jovanovic L, Knopp RH: Low fetal loss rates after ultrasound-proved viability in early pregnancy. JAMA 258:2555, 1987

Smith C, Gregori CA, Breen JL: Ultrasonography in threatened abortion. Obstet Gynecol 51:173, 1978

Stabile I, Campbell S, Grudzinskas JG: Ultrasonic assessment of complications during first trimester of pregnancy. Lancet 2:1237, 1987

Stein Z, Kline J, Susser E, Shrout P, Warburton D, Susser M: Maternal age and spontaneous abortion. In Porter IH, Hook EB (eds): Human Embryonic and Fetal Death. New York, Academic, 1980, p 129

Stray-Pedersen B, Eng J, Reikvan TM: Uterine T-mycoplasma colonization in reproductive failure. Am J Obstet Gynecol 130:307, 1978

Supreme Court of the United States Syllabus, *Roe et al. v. Wade,* District Attorney of Dallas County, January 22, 1973

Sutherland HW, Pritchard CW: Increased incidence of spontaneous abortion in pregnancies complicated by maternal diabetes mellitus. Am J Obstet Gynecol 155:135, 1986

Taylor PV, Hancock KW: Antigenicity of trophoblast and possible antigen masking effects during pregnancy. Immunology 28:973, 1975

Thomas ML, Harger JH, Wagener DK, Rabin BS, Gill TJ III: HLA sharing and spontaneous abortion in humans. Am J Obstet Gynecol 151:1053, 1985

Thomason JL, Sampson MB, Beckman CR, Spellacy WN: The incompetent cervix: A 1982 update. J Reprod Med 27:187, 1982

Tietze C: Introduction to the statistics of abortion. In Engle ET (ed): Pregnancy Wastage. Springfield, IL, Thomas, 1953, p 135

Tupper C, Weil RJ: The problem of spontaneous abortion. Am J Obstet Gynecol 83:421, 1962

United Nations, Department of Social Affairs, Foetal, Infant, and Early Childhood Mortality: I. The Statistics, New York, United Nations, 1954

Warburton D, Fraser FC: Spontaneous abortion risks in man: Data from reproductive histories collected in a medical genetics unit. Am J Hum Genet 16:1, 1964

Warburton D, Stein Z, Kline J, Susser M: Chromosome abnormalities in spontaneous abortion: Data from the New York City study. In Porter IH, Hook EB (eds): Human Embryonic and Fetal Death. New York, Academic, 1980, p 261

Whittaker PG, Taylor A, Lind T: Unsuspected pregnancy loss in healthy women. Lancet 1:1126, 1983

Wilson RD, Kendrick V, Wittmann BK, McGillivray B: Spontaneous abortion and pregnancy outcome after normal first-trimester ultrasound examination. Obstet Gynecol 67:352, 1986

Witter FR: Negative sonographic findings followed by rapid cervical dilatation due to cervical incompetence. Obstet Gynecol 64:136, 1984

Ectopic Pregnancy

Ectopic pregnancy is an unmitigated disaster of reproduction. The reproductive loss associated with this failure of proper nidation has increased steadily for the past 15 years, not only in the United States but also worldwide. Today, more than 1 in every 100 pregnancies in the United States is ectopic. The risk of death from an extrauterine pregnancy is 10 times greater than that for a vaginal delivery and 50 times greater than for an induced abortion (Dorfman, 1983). Moreover, the prognosis for a successful subsequent pregnancy is reduced significantly in these women, especially if they are primigravid and over the age of 30 years. Given the increasing incidence of ectopic pregnancies in all women, but especially those past 30, coupled with the tendency for women to delay childbearing until later in life, the tragedy of an ectopic pregnancy often is compounded. A clear understanding of the contributing factors responsible for ectopic pregnancies and of the effective and modern methods for their earlier diagnosis is essential. With earlier diagnosis both maternal survival and conservation of reproductive capacity will be enhanced.

GENERAL CONSIDERATIONS

DEFINITION

In a normal intrauterine pregnancy, the blastocyst implants in the endometrial lining the uterine cavity. Implantation anywhere else is referred to as an ectopic pregnancy. Although more than 95 percent of ectopic pregnancies involve the oviduct, tubal pregnancy is not synonymous with, but rather the most prevalent type of, ectopic gestation.

ETIOLOGY

The following have been implicated in the cause of ectopic pregnancy:

A. Mechanical factors that prevent or retard the passage of the fertilized ovum into the uterine cavity.
1. *Salpingitis,* especially endosalpingitis, which causes agglutination of the arborescent folds of the tubal mucosa with narrowing of the lumen or formation of blind pockets. Reduced ciliation of the tubal mucosa as the consequence of infection also may contribute to tubal implantation of the zygote (see Chap. 39, p. 852).
2. *Peritubal adhesions* subsequent to postabortal or puerperal infection, appendicitis, or endometriosis, which cause kinking of the tube and narrowing of the lumen.

3. *Developmental abnormalities of the tube,* especially diverticula, accessory ostia, and hypoplasia. Such abnormalities are extremely rare.
4. *Previous ectopic pregnancy,* and after one, the incidence of another is 7 percent to 15 percent (Breen and associates, 1970; Brenner and colleagues, 1980). The increased risk likely is due to previous salpingitis.
5. *Previous operations on the tube,* either to restore patency or, occasionally, the failure of a sterilization (Corson and Batzer, 1986; Tatum and Schmidt, 1977).
6. *Multiple previous induced abortions* increase the risk of ectopic pregnancy. The risk is unchanged after one induced abortion but doubled after two or more, likely due to small but significant increases in the incidence of salpingitis (Levin and associates, 1982).
7. *Tumors that distort the tube,* such as uterine myomas and adnexal masses.
8. Tubal pregnancies are not increased by abnormal embryos (Sopelak and Bates, 1987). Thus, this is not a significant etiological factor.
9. Current use of intrauterine devices increases the incidence (Marchbanks and associates, 1988).
B. Functional factors that delay the passage of the fertilized ovum into the uterine cavity.
1. External migration of the ovum is probably not an important factor except in cases of abnormal müllerian development resulting in a hemiuterus with an attached noncommunicating rudimentary uterine horn (Chap. 37, p. 733). There also may be a slightly increased risk of ectopic pregnancy for the woman with one oviduct whenever she ovulates from the contralateral ovary. The delay in transport of the fertilized ovum through the oviduct as the consequence of external migration increases invasive properties of the blastocyst while still within the oviduct. This is probably not an important factor in human ectopic gestation (Sopelak and Bates, 1987).
2. *Menstrual reflux* has been suggested as a cause. Delayed fertilization of the ovum with menstrual bleeding at the usual time theoretically could either prevent the ovum from entering the uterus or flush it back into the tube. There is little supporting evidence for this phenomenon.
3. *Altered tubal motility* may follow changes in serum levels of estrogens and progesterone. A change in the number and affinity of adrenergic receptors in uterine and tubal smooth muscle likely is responsible (Jacobson and associates, 1987). The practical aspect is that an increased incidence of ectopic pregnancies

has been reported after the use of *progestin-only oral contraceptives* (Ory, 1981; Tatum and Schmidt, 1977). Kaufman and co-workers (1984) and Herbst and associates (1981) reported a 4 to 13 percent increased incidence of ectopic pregnancies in women who were exposed in utero to *diethylstilbestrol* (DES), possibly as a consequence of altered tubal motality rather than structural abnormalities.

C. Increase in the receptivity of the tubal mucosa to the fertilized ovum. *Ectopic endometrial elements* may enhance tubal implantation. Although observers have reported foci of endometriosis in fallopian tubes, it is an uncommon finding.

Tubal pregnancy may rarely follow hysterectomy. Niebyl (1974) reviewed 21 such cases. In most instances, a very recently fertilized ovum was trapped in the oviduct at the time of hysterectomy, where it implanted and grew for a variable period. More rarely, an ovum was fertilized in the oviduct long after hysterectomy. In such cases, a fistula sufficient for passage of sperm had developed between the vagina and the severed end of the oviduct.

INCIDENCE

A marked increase in both the absolute number and rate of ectopic pregnancies has been documented in the United States in the past two decades. The actual number has increased out of proportion to population growth and it more than quadrupled, from 17,900 in 1970 to 78,400 in 1985. The numbers and rates of ectopic pregnancies reported in the United States are listed in Table 30–1. These rates are reported using three different methods:

1. Females 15 to 44 years: This rate refers to the number of ectopic pregnancies in women 15 to 44 years old per 10,000 females.

TABLE 30–1. NUMBERS AND RATES OF REPORTED ECTOPIC PREGNANCIES IN THE UNITED STATES, 1972–85

Year	No.	Rates		
		Females 15 to 44 years[a]	Livebirths[b]	Reported[c] Pregnancies
1972	24,500	5.5	7.5	6.3
1973	25,600	5.6	8.2	6.8
1974	26,400	5.7	8.4	6.7
1975	30,500	6.5	9.8	7.6
1976	34,600	7.2	11.0	8.3
1977	40,700	8.3	12.3	9.2
1978	42,400	8.5	12.8	9.4
1979	49,900	9.9	14.3	10.4
1980	52,200	9.9	14.5	10.5
1981	68,000	12.7	18.7	13.6
1982	61,800	11.5	17.0	12.3
1983	69,600	12.6	19.2	14.0
1984	75,400	13.6	20.6	14.9
1985	78,400	14.0	20.9	15.2
Total	717,000	9.0	13.0	10.0

[a] Rate per 10,000 females.
[b] Rate per 1,000 livebirths.
[c] Rate per 1,000 reported pregnancies (livebirths, legally induced abortions, and ectopic pregnancies).
From Centers for Disease Control: MMWR 37:637, 1988.

TABLE 30–2. NUMBERS AND RATES OF ECTOPIC PREGNANCY FOR THE UNITED STATES, 1970–78, EXPRESSED AS TWO CALCULATION METHODS

Age (Years)	No.	Rate per 1,000 Reported Pregnancies[a]	Rate per 10,000 Women Aged 15–44 Years
15–24	92,400	4.5	5.3
25–34	138,700	9.7	10.3
35–44	30,600	15.2	2.9
Total	261,600	7.1	6.3

[a] Reported pregnancies include livebirths, legally induced abortions, and ectopic pregnancies.
Modified from Rubin and co-workers: JAMA 249:1725, 1983.

2. Livebirths: This rate is the number of ectopic pregnancies per 1,000 livebirths.
3. Reported pregnancies: This rate is the number of ectopic pregnancies per 1,000 reported pregnancies, which includes livebirths, legally induced abortions, and ectopic pregnancies.

Unfortunately, none of these rates is totally accurate and the numerator may be falsely low for all calculations. For example, the number of ectopic pregnancies may be underestimated because the National Hospital Discharge Survey, from which these numbers are derived, does not include figures from federal hospitals. Also, an unknown number of ectopic pregnancies resolve spontaneously and thus are undiagnosed. Ectopic pregnancies certainly occur in women younger than 15 and older than 44. The denominator is falsely low in rates reported per livebirths since stillbirth rates are not considered. Finally, the rate per reported pregnancies is an underestimate because it does not include stillbirths, spontaneous abortions, and likely includes an incorrect estimate of legal abortions. Regardless of the method used to calculate rates, these all have increased three- to fourfold during the past two decades (Stock, 1988).

Care must be taken to insure that the rate method chosen to express a concept is not misinterpreted. For example, the ectopic pregnancy rate using women 15 to 44 years of age as a denominator can be used as a public health device to estimate the magnitude of the problem in reproductive age women. This method likely should not be used to ascertain risk factors for individual women since the denominator does not clearly define the population at risk. This is especially true when age as a risk factor is considered. For example, women 35 years and older are less likely to become pregnant than younger women. If the denominator includes women who will not become pregnant, the ectopic pregnancy rate must fall and the true effect of increasing age on the incidence of ectopic pregnancy is lost! This is illustrated in Table 30–2, where numbers and rates of ectopic pregnancies by age group using two different methods of calculation are listed. This increased incidence of ectopic pregnancy in older women also has been reported in Great Britain by Beral (1975) and in Sweden by Weström and associates (1981).

The incidence of ectopic pregnancy is increased in nonwhite compared to white women. Furthermore, rates for nonwhite women are higher in every age category than for whites, and similarly, this rate increases with age (Table 30–3). The combined factors of race and increasing age are at least additive. For example, nonwhite women 35 to 44 years were 5.4 times

TABLE 30–3. NUMBER AND RATE OF ECTOPIC PREGNANCIES BY AGE AND RACE IN THE UNITED STATES, 1970–80

Age (Years)	White No. (Rate)[a]	Nonwhite[b] No. (Rate)	Total No. (Rate)	Relative Risk (Nonwhite/White)
15–24	93,700 (4.8)	37,300 (6.1)	131,000 (5.1)	1.3
25–34	137,700 (9.1)	55,100 (17.6)	192,800 (10.5)	1.9
35–44	25,400 (13.2)	14,500 (26.0)	39,900 (16.0)	2.0
Total	256,800 (7.0)	106,900 (10.9)	363,700 (7.8)	1.6

[a] Rate is number of ectopics per 1,000 reported pregnancies, which includes livebirths, legally induced abortions, and ectopic pregnancies.
[b] Nonwhite includes all races other than white.
Modified from MacKay and co-workers: MMWR: 33:1SS, 1984.

more likely to have an ectopic pregnancy than a white woman aged 15 to 24 years. Overall, a nonwhite woman has a 1.6 times increased risk for ectopic pregnancy.

In summary, from 1970 through 1983, the rate of ectopic pregnancies in the United States tripled. This marked increase was greater for nonwhite than white women, and for both racial groups the incidence has increased with age. In 35- to 44-year-old white women, 1.3 of every 100 pregnancies was ectopic; however, this figure was 2.6 for nonwhite women. At Parkland Hospital, where the majority of obstetrical patients are less than 25 years old, the incidence of ectopic pregnancy almost doubled in the past decade. At Magee-Womens Hospital, the incidence increased 3.7 fold from 1965 through 1985 (Stock, 1988).

The reasons for these increases in the United States are not entirely clear; however, similarly increased incidences have been reported from Eastern Europe, Scandinavia, and Great Britain (Tuomivaara and associates, 1986; Weström and co-workers, 1981). Although the reasons for this internationally observed increase in ectopic pregnancies are multiple, some of the causes likely include the following: (1) increased prevalence of sexually transmitted tubal infection that damages tubal mucosa but not so severely as to cause complete occlusion, (2) popularity of contraception that prevents intrauterine but not extrauterine pregnancies, especially an intrauterine device and possibly low-dose progestational agents, (3) unsuccessful tubal sterilizations, (4) induced abortion followed by infection, (5) fertility induced by ovulatory agents, (6) previous pelvic surgery including salpingotomy for previous tubal pregnancy and tuboplasty, (7) exposure to stilbestrol in utero, and (8) better and earlier diagnostic techniques.

The reasons for the disparately increased incidence of ectopic pregnancies in nonwhite women also is not known. Possible explanations include (1) health care is less available or acceptable to nonwhite women compared to white women (Atrash and colleagues, 1987b) and (2) sexually transmitted disease are reported more frequently in nonwhite compared to white women (Darrow, 1976).

MORTALITY

Deaths from ectopic pregnancy in the United States decreased from 63 to 1970 to 46 in 1980 and 35 in 1983. Unfortunately, the percentage of all maternal deaths attributed to ectopic pregnancy increased from 8 percent in 1970 to 14 percent in 1980 (Atrash and colleagues, 1987b; Rubin and associates, 1983). **Ectopic pregnancy is now the second leading cause of maternal mortality in the United States.** The risk of death was increased in nonwhite compared to white women (Table 30–4); however,

increasing age was not associated with increased mortality (MacKay and associates, 1984). In both racial groups, a dramatic fall which has continued through 1983 has been documented in the death-to-case rate (Fig. 30–1). Because the incidence of ectopic pregnancy overall is 1.6 times greater in nonwhite than white women, the risk of dying from an ectopic pregnancy is six times greater in a nonwhite than a white woman.

The dramatic decrease in the death-to-case rate from 3.5 per 1,000 women in 1970 to 0.5 per 1,000 women in 1983 (see Fig. 30–1) is due most probably to improved diagnosis and management. Still, Dorfman and colleagues (1984) estimated that the death rate from ectopic pregnancies might be reduced another 50 percent by even more prompt diagnosis and treatment. They emphasized that another third of deaths might be prevented if the woman sought earlier care. In this carefully done analysis of ectopic mortalities in 1979 and 1980, they reported that 85 percent of women died from hemorrhage. Massive hemorrhage often was the result of abdominal and interstitial tubal pregnancies which were likely to become symptomatic later in gestation and consequently have increased blood supply. The remaining major causes of death were infection in 5 percent and anesthesia complications in 2 percent of women.

ANATOMICAL CONSIDERATIONS

The fertilized ovum may develop in any portion of the oviduct, giving rise to *ampullary, isthmic, and interstitial tubal pregnancies* (see Fig. 40–17). In rare instances, the fertilized ovum may be implanted in the fimbriated extremity and occasionally even on the fimbria ovarica. The ampulla is the most frequent site of implantation and the isthmus the next most common. Interstitial pregnancy is very uncommon, occurring in only about 3 percent of all tubal gestations. From these primary types, certain secondary forms of tubo-abdominal, tubo-ovarian, and broad ligament pregnancies occasionally develop.

Implantation of the Zygote
The fertilized ovum does not remain on the surface but promptly burrows through the epithelium. As the zygote penetrates the

TABLE 30–4. DEATH-TO-CASE RATE[a] FOR WOMEN WITH ECTOPIC PREGNANCIES, BY RACE AND YEAR, IN THE UNITED STATES, 1970–80

Year	White	Nonwhite	Total[b]	Relative Risk (Nonwhite/White)
1970	2.2	7.2	3.5	3.3
1971	1.5	7.5	3.2	5.0
1972	1.6	2.8	2.0	1.8
1973	1.5	2.2	1.8	1.5
1974	1.0	4.7	1.9	4.7
1975	0.9	3.5	1.6	3.9
1976	0.4	2.9	1.1	7.3
1977	0.5	2.4	1.1	4.8
1978	0.4	1.8	0.9	4.5
1979	0.5	1.6	0.8	3.2
1980	0.5	1.8	0.9	3.6
Total	0.8	2.9	1.4	3.6

[a] Deaths from ectopic pregnancy per 1,000 ectopic pregnancies.
[b] Race "unknown" was redistributed according to the known percentages for race.
Modified from MacKay and associates: MMWR 33:1SS, 1984.

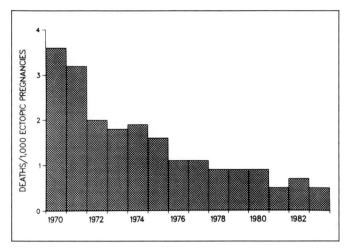

Figure 30–1. Mortality expressed as deaths per 1,000 ectopic pregnancies for women with ectopic pregnancies in the United States, 1970–83. (*From Centers for Disease Control: MMWR 35:290, 1986.*)

epithelium it comes to lie in the muscular wall, since the tube lacks a submucosa. At the periphery of the zygote is a capsule of rapidly proliferating trophoblast, which invades and erodes the subjacent muscularis of the tube. At the same time, maternal blood vessels are opened, and the blood pours out into the spaces of varying size, lying within the trophoblast or between it and the adjacent tissue, especially the covering tubal serosa.

The tube does not normally form an extensive decidua, although decidual cells can usually be recognized. The tubal wall in contact with the zygote offers but slight resistance to invasion by the trophoblast, which soon burrows through it, opening maternal vessels (Fig. 30–2).

The embryo or fetus in an ectopic pregnancy is often absent or stunted.

Uterine Changes

In ectopic pregnancies, the uterus undergoes some of the changes associated with early normal pregnancy, including softening of the cervix and isthmus and an increase in size. *These changes in the uterus do not, therefore, exclude an ectopic pregnancy.*

The degree to which the endometrium is converted to decidua is variable. The finding of uterine decidua without trophoblast certainly suggests ectopic pregnancy but is by no means an absolute indication. In 1954, Arias–Stella described, as had others before him, the following changes in the endometrium: The epithelial cells are enlarged and their nuclei are hypertrophic, hyperchromatic, lobular, and irregularly shaped. There is a loss of polarity, and the abnormal nuclei tend to occupy the luminal portion of the cells. The cytoplasm may be vacuolated and foamy, and occasional mitoses may be found. These endometrial changes have been collectively referred to as the *Arias–Stella reaction* (Fig. 30–3). The cellular changes in the Arias–Stella reaction are not specific for ectopic pregnancy but may occur with either intrauterine or extrauterine gestations.

The external bleeding seen commonly in cases of tubal pregnancy is uterine in origin and associated with degeneration and sloughing of the uterine decidua. Soon after the death of the fetus, the decidua degenerates and is usually shed in small pieces, but occasionally it is cast off intact, as a *decidual cast* of the uterine cavity. The absence of decidual tissue, however, does not exclude an ectopic pregnancy. Romney and co-workers (1950), for example, identified secretory endometrium in 40 percent of cases of ectopic pregnancy, proliferative in 30 percent, and menstrual in 6 percent, while decidua was present in only 20 percent.

NATURAL HISTORY OF TUBAL PREGNANCY

TUBAL ABORTION

A common termination of tubal pregnancy is separation of the products of conception from the implantation site and extrusion

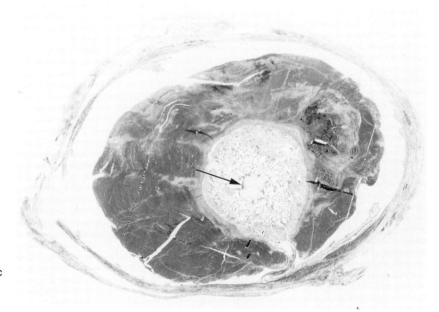

Figure 30–2. Early tubal pregnancy. The amnionic sac (*arrow*) is surrounded by chorionic villi, which, in turn, are encased in blood clot. (*Courtesy of Dr. Richard Voet.*)

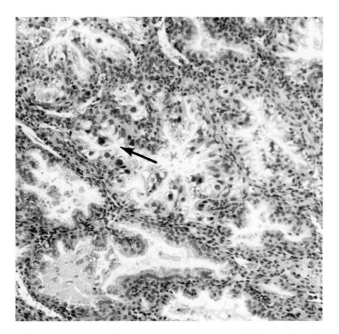

Figure 30–3. Arias–Stella reaction. Some of the nuclei are enlarged (*arrow*), hyperchromatic, and irregularly shaped. Some of the cytoplasm is vacuolated and foamy. (*Courtesy of Dr. Helen Graham.*)

of the abortus through the fimbriated end of the oviduct. The frequency of tubal abortion depends in great part upon the site of implantation of the zygote. In ampullary tubal pregnancy, it is common, whereas rupture of the tube is the usual outcome in isthmic pregnancy. The immediate consequence of the hemorrhage with tubal abortion is the further disruption of the connection between the placenta and membranes and the tubal wall, and if separation is complete, the entire products may be extruded through the fimbriated end into the peritoneal cavity. At that point, hemorrhage may cease and symptoms disappear.

In cases of complete tubal abortion, when the zygote is retained within the oviduct and hemorrhage is moderate, the abortus may become infiltrated with blood and converted into a structure analogous to the blood mole observed in uterine abortion. Some bleeding usually persists as long as the products of conception remain in the oviduct, and the blood slowly trickles from the fimbriated end into the peritoneal cavity and typically pools in the rectouterine cul-de-sac. If the fimbriated extremity is occluded, the fallopian tube may gradually become distended by blood, forming a *hematosalpinx.*

After incomplete tubal abortion, pieces of the placenta or membranes may remain attached to the tubal wall and, after becoming surrounded by fibrin, give rise to a *placental polyp,* as may occur in the uterus after an incomplete uterine abortion.

TUBAL RUPTURE

The invading, expanding products of conception may rupture the oviduct at any of several sites. Before sophisticated methods to measure chorionic gonadotropin were available, many cases of tubal pregnancy ended during the first trimester by intraperitoneal rupture. As a rule, whenever tubal rupture occurs in the first few weeks, the pregnancy is situated in the isthmic portion of the tube a short distance from the cornu of the uterus. When the fertilized ovum is implanted well within the interstitial portion of the tube, rupture usually does not occur until later.

The immediate cause of rupture may be trauma associated with coitus or a vigorous bimanual examination, although in the great majority of cases rupture occurs spontaneously. With intraperitoneal rupture, the entire products of conception may be extruded from the tube, or if the rent is small, profuse hemorrhage may occur without extrusion. In either event, commonly, the patient soon shows signs of collapse from hemorrhage and hypovolemia. If the woman is not operated upon and does not die from hemorrhage, the fate of the embryo or fetus will depend on the damage sustained by the products of conception during the rupture and on the duration of the gestation. If an early conceptus is expelled essentially undamaged into the peritoneal cavity, it may reimplant almost anywhere, establish adequate circulation, and survive and grow, but this outcome is most unlikely because of damage during the transition. The products of conception, if small, may be resorbed or, if larger, may remain in the cul-de-sac for years as an encapsulated mass or even become calcified to form a *lithopedion.*

Abdominal Pregnancy

If only the fetus is extruded at the time of rupture, the effect upon the pregnancy will vary depending on the extent of injury sustained by the placenta. If the placenta is damaged appreciably, death of the fetus and termination of the pregnancy are inevitable, but if the greater portion of the placenta still retains its attachment to the tube, further development is possible. The fetus may then survive for some time, giving rise to an *abdominal pregnancy.* Typically, in such cases, a portion of the placenta remains attached to the tubal wall and the periphery grows beyond the tube and implants on surrounding structures. Abdominal pregnancy is discussed on pp. 526–30.

Broad Ligament Pregnancy

When the original implantation of the zygote is toward the mesosalpinx, rupture may occur at the portion of the tube not immediately covered by peritoneum, and the contents of the gestational sac may be extruded into a space formed between the folds of the broad ligament. This condition is designated an intraligamentous or *broad ligament pregnancy.* It may terminate either in the death of the embryo or fetus and the formation of a *broad ligament hematoma* or in the further development of the pregnancy. Occasionally, the broad ligament sac ruptures at a later period, and the fetus is extruded into the peritoneal cavity while the placenta retains its position, forming an abdominal pregnancy.

INTERSTITIAL PREGNANCY

When the fertilized ovum implants within the segment of the tube that penetrates the uterine wall, an especially grave form of tubal gestation, *interstitial pregnancy,* results (Fig. 30–4). Implantation at this site has also been referred to as a *cornual pregnancy.* Interstitial tubal pregnancy accounts for about 3 percent of all tubal gestations. Because of the site of implantation, no adnexal mass is palpable, but rather, there is variable asymmetry of the uterus that often is difficult to distinguish from an intrauterine pregnancy. Hence, the early diagnosis is even more frequently overlooked than in other types of tubal implantation. Because of the greater distensibility of the myometrium covering the interstitial portion compared to tubal wall (not surrounded by myometrium), rupture of an interstitial pregnancy is likely to occur somewhat later, between the end of the 8th and 16th gestational week. Because of the abundant blood supply from branches of

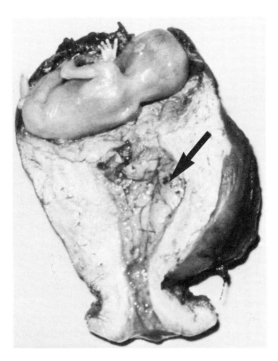

Figure 30–4. Right interstitial tubal pregnancy. The fetus weighed 55 g and measured 90 mm crown to rump (14 to 15 weeks gestational age). Note the abundant decidua (*arrow*) filling the uterine cavity. The patient sought medical help because of sudden severe abdominal pain with syncope following intercourse. Hysterectomy and blood transfusion (2,000 mL) were required.

both uterine and ovarian arteries immediately adjacent to the implantation site, the hemorrhage that attends the rupture may be rapidly fatal (Dorfman and associates, 1984). In fact, tubal pregnancies in which the woman dies before she can be brought to the hospital often fall into this group. Because of the large uterine defect, hysterectomy is commonly necessary. Very infrequently, an interstitial pregnancy may convert to a tubo-uterine pregnancy as described below.

MULTIFETAL ECTOPIC PREGNANCY

In rare instances, tubal pregnancy may be complicated by a coexisting intrauterine gestation, a condition designated as *combined pregnancy*. Combined pregnancy is quite difficult to diagnose clinically. Typically, laparotomy is performed because of a tubal pregnancy. At the same time, the uterus is congested, softened, and somewhat enlarged. Although these features are suggestive of intrauterine pregnancy, they are commonly induced by a tubal pregnancy alone. Gestational products are demonstrable ultrasonically within the uterine cavity in practically all instances of combined pregnancy. Aspiration of the uterus for amnionic fluid has been recommended, but amnionic fluid may be difficult to obtain, especially if the chorion and amnion have not yet fused. Moreover, a blind aspiration to try to confirm the presence of amnionic fluid may be traumatic to the products of conception.

Combined pregnancy is rare. Five cases were observed at Sloane Hospital for Women during which time 40,000 deliveries and 353 extrauterine gestations were cared for (Reece and associates, 1983). Simultaneous intrauterine and tubal pregnancy has followed induction of ovulation with either clomiphene therapy or menopausal gonadotropin.

The ultimate in combined pregnancies may have been reported by Funderburk (1974), who described a woman with a fetus in the right tube, a fetus in the left tube, and a fetus in the uterus. Since he preserved both oviducts, the potential for still another record persists.

Twin tubal pregnancy, at the same stage of development, has been reported with both embryos in the same tube, as well as with one in each tube. Arey (1923) considered the subject in detail and concluded that single-ovum twins form a far greater proportion of tubal than of uterine pregnancies. He postulated that difficulties in migration and implantation retarded the growth of the zygote, which was somehow stimulated to form two identical embryos. Simultaneous pregnancy in both fallopian tubes is the rarest form of double-ovum twinning.

Quadruplet tubal pregnancy in the same oviduct has been described by Fujii and associates (1981). The ruptured and hemorrhaging oviduct contained four amnionic sacs covered by a single chorion. Each of the sacs contained an embryo. There was appreciable difference in the size of the embryos, as is evident in Figures 30–5A and B, even though they arose almost certainly from a single fertilized ovum.

Tubal pregnancy with death of the conceptus without abortion or complete resorption may be followed by a tubal pregnancy in the opposite or the same oviduct or in the uterus.

TUBO-UTERINE, TUBO-ABDOMINAL, AND TUBO-OVARIAN PREGNANCIES

The so-called tubo-uterine pregnancy results from the gradual extension into the uterine cavity of products of conception that originally implanted in the interstitial portion of the tube. Tubo-abdominal pregnancy is derived from a tubal pregnancy in which the zygote, originally implanted in the neighborhood of the fimbriated end of the tube, gradually extends into the peritoneal cavity. In such circumstances, the portion of the fetal sac projecting into the peritoneal cavity may form troublesome adhesions to the surrounding organs. As a result, removal of the sac is much more difficult. Both of these conditions are very uncommon.

The term *tubo-ovarian* pregnancy is employed when the fetal sac is adherent partly to tubal and partly to ovarian tissue. Such cases arise from the development of the zygote in a tubo-ovarian cyst or in a tube, the fimbriated extremity of which was adherent to the ovary at the time of fertilization or became so soon thereafter. Rarely, the fetus and placenta may achieve appreciable size before a catastrophe befalls the mother and fetus (Fig. 30–6).

CLINICAL AND LABORATORY FEATURES OF TUBAL PREGNANCY

GENERAL CONSIDERATIONS

Before tubal rupture or abortion, the manifestations of a tubal pregnancy are diverse. Commonly the woman believes she is normally pregnant or believes she is aborting an intrauterine pregnancy. Less often, she does not even suspect that she is pregnant. In the so-called textbook case of ruptured tubal pregnancy, normal menstruation is replaced by variably delayed slight vaginal bleeding, which is usually referred to as "spotting." Suddenly, the woman is stricken with severe lower abdominal pain, frequently described as sharp, stabbing, or tearing in character. Vasomotor disturbances develop, ranging

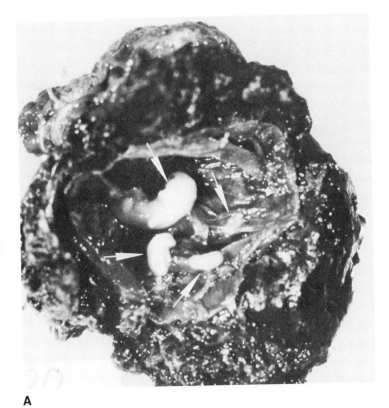

A

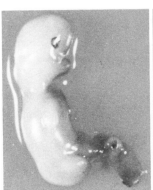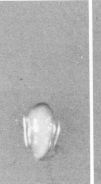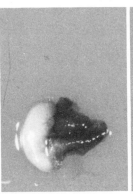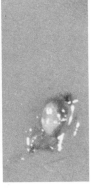

B

Figure 30–5. A. Ruptured, hemorrhaging oviduct containing four embryos (*arrows*), each in a separate amnionic sac, all enclosed by a single chorion. **B.** The four microscopically proven embryos arising from a single fertilized ovum differ markedly in size. (*From Fujii and Associates: Am J Obstet Gynecol 141:840, 1981.*)

from vertigo to syncope. Abdominal palpation discloses some tenderness, and vaginal examination, especially motion of the cervix, causes exquisite pain. The posterior fornix of the vagina may bulge because of blood in the cul-de-sac, or a tender, boggy mass may be felt to one side of the uterus. Symptoms of diaphragmatic irritation, characterized by pain in the neck or shoulder especially on inspiration, develop in perhaps 50 percent of women in whom there is sizable intraperitoneal hemorrhage. This is caused by intraperitoneal blood irritating the cervical sensory nerves that supply the inferior surface of the diaphragm, especially on inspiration. The woman may or may not be hypotensive while lying supine. If she is not hypotensive when supine, she may become so when placed in a sitting position.

In cases of tubal pregnancy that present the aforementioned clinical picture, the diagnosis is not difficult to make. Even though the symptoms and signs of ectopic pregnancy often range from indefinite to bizarre before rupture or abor-tion, increasing numbers of women are seeking medical care before the classical clinical picture develops. *The physician must make every reasonable effort to diagnose the condition before catastrophic events occur, but the task may not be simple.* The following symptoms, signs, and laboratory studies should be carefully evaluated.

SYMPTOMS AND SIGNS

Pain

The most frequently experienced symptoms of ectopic pregnancy are pelvic and abdominal pain (100 percent) and amenorrhea with some degree of vaginal spotting or bleeding (60 to 80 percent). Dorfman and associates (1984) also emphasized the importance of gastrointestinal symptoms (80 percent) and dizziness or light-headedness (58 percent). Of course, symptoms are variable in their incidence of appearance due to the rate and extent of hemorrhage as well as the delay of diagnosis.

Pain may be unilateral or bilateral, in the lower abdomen or generalized, or just in the upper abdomen. In the presence of hemoperitoneum, pain from diaphragmatic irritation may be experienced. It has been generally assumed that the abdominal pain, often excruciating, associated with rupture of an ectopic pregnancy is caused by the escape of blood into the peritoneal cavity. Since there may be considerable pain in instances in which there is little hemorrhage and little pain with considerable hemorrhage, it is obvious that blood is not the sole cause of the pain. Nonetheless, appreciable blood in the peritoneal cavity may lead to a degree of peritoneal irritation and varying degrees of discomfort. Pritchard and Adams (1957) observed that 500 mL of blood in the peritoneal cavity more often than not caused abdominal tenderness, moderate intestinal distention, and especially pain in the top of the shoulder and the side of the neck from diaphragmatic irritation.

Amenorrhea

The absence of a missed menstrual period by no means rules out tubal pregnancy. A history of amenorrhea is not obtained in a quarter or more of cases. One reason is that the woman mistakes the uterine bleeding that frequently occurs with tubal pregnancy for a true menstrual period and so gives an erroneous date for the last menses. This important source of diagnostic error can be eliminated in many cases by a carefully obtained menstrual history. It is extremely important that the character of the last menstrual period be elicited in detail with respect to time of onset, duration, and amount of bleeding, and it is advisable to ask whether it impressed her as abnormal in any way.

Vaginal Spotting or Bleeding

As long as placental endocrine function persists, uterine bleeding is usually absent, but when endocrine support of the endometrium becomes inadequate, the uterine mucosa bleeds.

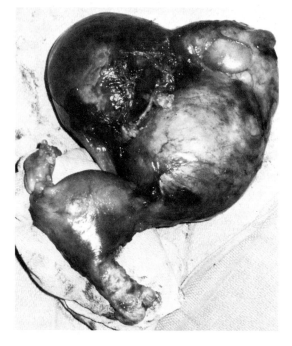

Figure 30–6. The markedly dilated left fallopian tube contains a recently dead fetus weighing 1,850 g.

The bleeding is usually scanty, dark brown, and may be intermittent or continuous. Although profuse vaginal bleeding is suggestive of an incomplete intrauterine abortion rather than an ectopic gestation, such bleeding can occur with tubal gestations.

Abdominal and Pelvic Pain

Exquisite tenderness on abdominal palpation and vaginal examination, especially on *motion of the cervix*, is demonstrable in over three quarters of women with ruptured or rupturing tubal pregnancies but occasionally may be absent prior to rupture.

Uterine Changes

Because of the action of placental hormones, the uterus grows during the first 3 months of a tubal gestation to nearly the same size as it would in an intrauterine pregnancy. Its consistency, too, is similar as long as the fetus is alive. The uterus may be pushed to one side by the ectopic mass. In broad ligament pregnancies or when the broad ligament is filled with blood, the uterus may be greatly displaced. Uterine casts (decidual casts) are passed by a small minority of patients, possibly 5 or 10 percent. Their passage may be accompanied by cramps similar to those with spontaneous expulsion of an abortus from the uterine cavity.

Blood Pressure and Pulse

The early response to moderate hemorrhage is no change in pulse and blood pressure or occasionally the same as that witnessed during the controlled phlebotomy of blood donation, namely, a slight rise in blood pressure (Fig. 36–2), or a vasovagal response with bradycardia and hypotension. In the otherwise healthy young woman with an extrauterine pregnancy, only if bleeding continues and hypovolemia becomes intense can the blood pressure be counted upon to fall and the pulse rate to rise appreciably.

Hypovolemia

There are two simple means for detecting significant hypovolemia before development of hypovolemic shock. (1) The blood pressure and pulse rates of the patient in the sitting and the supine positions are compared. A distinct decrease in blood pressure and rise in pulse rate in the sitting position are indicative most often of a sizable decrease in circulatory volume. Unfortunately, such changes may not develop until there is serious hypovolemia. Thus, the test is informative only if the blood pressure falls or pulse rate rises when the patient is moved from the supine to the sitting position. (2) Urine flow is monitored carefully, since hypovolemia (in the absence of potent diuretic treatment) often causes oliguria before overt hypotension develops. The diagnosis and treatment of obstetrical hemorrhage in general are considered in detail in Chapter 36.

Temperature

After acute hemorrhage, the temperature may be normal or even low. Temperatures up to 38°C, and perhaps related to hemoperitoneum, may develop, but higher temperatures are rare in the absence of infection. Fever is important, therefore, in distinguishing ruptured tubal pregnancy from acute salpingitis, in which the temperature is commonly above 38°C.

Pelvic Mass

A pelvic mass is palpable in about 20 percent of the patients. The mass varies in size, consistency, and position, ranging as a rule between 5 and 15 cm in diameter, and is often soft and elastic. With extensive infiltration of the tubal wall with blood, however, it may be firm. It is almost always either posterior or lateral to the uterus. Pain and tenderness often preclude identification of the mass by palpation.

Pelvic Hematocele

In many cases of ruptured tubal pregnancy, there is gradual disintegration of the tubal wall followed by a slow leakage of blood into the tubal lumen, the peritoneal cavity, or both. Signs of active hemorrhage are absent, and even the mild symptoms may subside, but gradually the trickling blood collects in the pelvis, more or less walled off by adhesions, and a pelvic hematocele results. In some cases, the hematocele is eventually absorbed, and the patient recovers without operation. In others, it may rupture into the peritoneal cavity, or it may become infected and form an abscess. Most commonly, however, the hematocele causes continued discomfort, and the physician is finally consulted weeks or even months after the original rupture. Such cases are atypical.

LABORATORY TESTS

Measurement of hemoglobin, hematocrit, and leucocyte count, as well as pregnancy tests, are useful in certain cases if their *limitations* are understood.

Hemoglobin and Hematocrit

After hemorrhage, the depleted blood volume is restored toward normal by hemodilution over the course of 1 or 2 days. Even after a substantive hemorrhage, therefore, the hemoglobin level or hematocrit reading may at first show only a slight reduction. For the first few hours after an acute hemorrhage, a decrease in the hemoglobin or hematocrit level while the patient is under observation is a more valuable index of blood loss than is the initial reading. This is true unless the initial reading is low and the anemia is normocytic and, therefore, characteristic of recent blood loss. If the bleeding stops and the shed erythrocytes are free in the peritoneal cavity, their absorption may help repair the anemia over several days. Hyperbilirubinemia usually does not develop (Pritchard and Adams, 1957).

Leucocyte Count

The leucocyte count varies considerably in ruptured ectopic pregnancy. In about half the patients, it is normal, but in the remainder, varying degrees of leucocytosis up to 30,000 per μL may be encountered.

Pregnancy Tests

Ectopic pregnancy cannot be diagnosed by a positive pregnancy test alone. However, the key issue when confronted with the possibility of an ectopic pregnancy is whether the woman is pregnant. In virtually all cases of ectopic gestation, chorionic gonadotropin will be detected in serum, but usually at a markedly reduced concentration compared to normal pregnancy (Olson and associates, 1983). The problem then is how to detect this marker of pregnancy in the most clinically efficacious manner.

Urinary pregnancy tests are most often latex agglutination inhibition slide tests with sensitivities for chorionic gonadotropin in the range of 500 to 800 mIU per mL. Their ease of use and rapidity is offset by their chance of being positive in a woman with an ectopic pregnancy of only 50 to 60 percent (Table 30–5). Even when the tube-type tests are used (hemagglutination inhibition or latex agglutination inhibition), detection of the β-subunit of human chorionic gonadotropin (β-hCG) is within the 150 to 250 mIU per mL range, and is positive only in 80 to 85 percent of ectopic pregnancies.

Tests using enzyme-linked immunosorbent assays (ELISA) are sensitive to 10 at 50 mIU per mL and are positive in 90 to 96 percent of women with ectopic pregnancies. This type of test also has the advantages of rapidity and easy performance.

Serum radioimmunoassay for β-hCG is the most precise method and virtually any pregnancy event can be detected with this. In all but one of the 10 tests cited in Table 30–5, the false-negative test was attributed to an assay technique not sensitive at the level of 5 to 10 mIU per milliliter (Olson and associates, 1983). In fact, because of the sensitivity of this assay, a pregnancy may be confirmed before there are pathological changes in the fallopian tube. Yaffe and associates (1979) reported such an event in a woman 5 days overdue for a menstrual period who developed pelvic pain and in whom serum chorionic gonadotropin was detected. At laparoscopy no lesion was seen; however, when laparoscopy was repeated 7 days later, there was an ampullary pregnancy.

For practical purposes, the absence of pregnancy can be established only when there is a negative test for serum chorionic gonadotropin in which an assay with a sensitivity of 5 to 10 mIU per mL is used.

TABLE 30–5. COMPARISON OF PREGNANCY TEST RESULTS IN WOMEN WITH ECTOPIC PREGNANCIES

Type Test	Test	No. Patients	Test Positive/Negative	Positive (%)	Sensitivity (mIU per mL)	Approximate Time Required
Radioimmunoassay	Serum β-hCG[a]	653	643/10	98.5	5–35	4–8 hr
ELISA	Tandem ICON[b]	27	26/1	96	10–50	3.5 min
ELISA	Tandem Visual hCG[c]	108	97/11	90	50	60 min
ELISA	Mod EI	108	97/11	90	50	75 min
Tube	Sensitex	108	92/16	85	250	90 min
Tube	UCG-Beta Stat	108	92/16	85	200	60 min
Tube	β-Neocyst	108	88/20	82	150	60 min
Slide	Sensislide	108	66/42	61	800	5 min
Slide	UCG-Beta Slide	106	54/52	51	500	5 min

ELISA = enzyme-linked immunosorbent assay.
[a] Combined values of β-hCG from Barnes (1985), Olson (1983), Forbes (1981), Hedges (1984), Milwidsky (1984), and all their co-workers.
[b] Study from Cartwright and co-workers: Ann Emerg Med 15:1198, 1986.
[c] This and following tests are from Barnes and associates: J Reprod Med 30:827, 1985.
Modified from Barnes and associates: J Reprod Med 30:827, 1985.

OTHER DIAGNOSTIC AIDS

Because of the difficulties in diagnosis of ruptured tubal pregnancy, a variety of diagnostic aids other than tests for chorionic gonadotropin have been utilized. These include sonography, the combination of sonography and serum β-hCG determinations, culdocentesis, curettage, colpotomy, laparoscopy, and laparotomy.

Sonography

In recent years, sonography has been applied to the diagnosis of tubal pregnancy. Identification of early products of conception in the fallopian tube by this means is difficult, but if a gestational sac is clearly identified within the cavity of the uterus, it is very unlikely that an ectopic pregnancy coexists. Moreover, the absence of any ultrasonic evidence of an intrauterine pregnancy but a positive pregnancy test, fluid in the cul-de-sac (Robinson and associates, 1985), and an abnormal pelvic mass are practically diagnostic of ectopic pregnancy (Romero and associates, 1988) (Table 30–6). Unfortunately, sonographic findings suggestive, at least, of early intrauterine pregnancy may be apparent in some cases of ectopic pregnancy. The sonographic appearance of a small sac (very early pregnancy) or a collapsed sac (dead products of conception) may actually be a blood clot or decidual cast (Coleman and colleagues, 1985). In fact, the presence of an intrauterine pregnancy usually is not recognized using real-time ultrasound until 5 to 6 menstrual weeks (Coleman and colleagues, 1985) or 28 days after timed ovulation (Batzer and co-workers, 1983). Conversely, demonstration of an adnexal or cul-de-sac mass by sonography is not necessarily helpful. Corpus luteum cysts and matted bowel can sometimes look like tubal pregnancies sonographically. However, the identification with real-time sonography of fetal heart action clearly outside the uterine cavity provides firm evidence of an ectopic pregnancy.

Quantitative β-hCG Values and Sonography

During the past decade, the clinical management of suspected ectopic pregnancy has changed remarkably. In essence, management is based upon the establishment or exclusion of pregnancy. If a sensitive urinary pregnancy test, such as ELISA (see p. 519) is positive, the diagnosis of pregnancy is established. A negative radioimmunoassay for serum β-hCG is required to exclude pregnancy.

When pregnancy is diagnosed in the hemodynamically stable women with no abdominal ultrasonic evidence for ectopic pregnancy and a negative culdocentesis, subsequent management is based upon serial quantitative serum β-hCG values and abdominal sonograms. Kadar and associates (1981a) described four clinical possibilities based upon quantitative β-hCG values:

1. When the β-hCG value is above 6,000 mIU per mL and an intrauterine gestational sac is seen using abdominal sonography, then normal pregnancy virtually is certain.
2. When the β-hCG value is above 6,000 mIU per mL and there is an empty uterine cavity, then an ectopic pregnancy is very likely. This observation has been confirmed by Batzer and co-workers (1983) and Holman and associates (1984), who found this situation to be uncommon in actual clinical practice.
3. When the β-hCG value is less than 6,000 mIU per mL and a definite intrauterine ring of pregnancy is visualized, then a spontaneous abortion is likely now or very soon. Ectopic pregnancy is still a possibility because of the degree of ultrasonic resolution available. A false diagnosis of a uterine gestational sac can be made when there are blood clots or decidual casts (Kadar and associates, 1981a).
4. When the β-hCG value is less than 6,000 mIU per mL and there is an empty uterus, no definitive diagnosis can be made. Failure to visualize a gestational sac within the uterus is not unusual using abdominal sonography prior to 5 weeks' gestation (Batzer and associates, 1983; Bryson, 1983; Coleman and colleagues, 1985). Unfortunately, precise gestational age often is unknown in the woman with a suspected ectopic pregnancy. In these instances, the woman may abort or she may continue pregnancy and develop a normal gestational sac (Fig. 30–7), or she may show evidence of an ectopic pregnancy. The methods of management in these circumstances are discussed below.

Some, but certainly not all, feel that with an empty uterus and any proof of pregnancy, laparoscopy or laparotomy is indicated (Bryson, 1983). Another approach is to admit these women to the hospital and perform serial hematocrits, frequent vital signs, and serial sonograms and β-hCG determinations. She will eventually continue with a normal pregnancy, abort, or develop clinical or ultrasonic evidence of an ectopic pregnancy.

Kadar and co-workers (1981b) proposed another plan. They observed that in women with normal pregnancies, the mean doubling time for β-hCG in serum was approximately 48 hours and the lowest normal value for this increase was 66 percent (Table 30–7). They calculated this number by subtracting the initial value for β-hCG from the 48-hour value and dividing the result by the initial value, which is multiplied by 100 to obtain a percentage:

$$\frac{\text{β-hCG at 48 hours } - \text{ initial β-hCG}}{\text{Initial β-hCG}} \times 100$$

TABLE 30–6. OUTCOME IN 94 WOMEN WITH POSSIBLE ECTOPIC PREGNANCY IN WHOM ULTRASONIC FINDINGS ARE CORRELATED WITH SERUM PREGNANCY TEST

| | Serum LH/hCG Assay[a] | | | |
| | Positive | | Negative | |
Ultrasonic Findings	Ectopic	No Ectopic	Ectopic	No Ectopic
Empty uterus alone	10	6	0	16
Empty uterus + adnexal mass	13	2	0	11
Empty uterus + free fluid in cul-de-sac	9	0	1	5
Empty uterus + free fluid in cul-de-sac + adnexal mass	19	0	0	2
Total	51	8	1[b]	34

[a] Three different radioimmunoassays for β-hCG were used in this series. One assay cross-reacted with human luteinizing hormone (LH).
[b] Although a negative pregnancy test was noted, the ectopic pregnancy had been aborted from the fallopian tube and was free in the hemoperitoneum.
Modified from Robinson and co-workers: Aust N Z J Obstet Gynaecol 25:49, 1985.

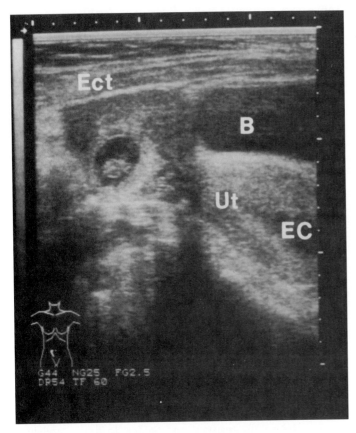

Figure 30–7. Longitudinal midline sonogram showing a well-defined ectopic pregnancy (*Ect*) overlying the uterus (*Ut*). B = bladder, EC = endometrial cavity (*Courtesy of Dr. Rigoberto Santos.*)

Kadar and colleagues (1981b) cautioned that both β-hCG determinations be performed simultaneously and that more reliable values could be obtained at 48-hour intervals. They concluded that a failure to maintain this rate of increased β-hCG production, along with an empty uterus, was strongly suggestive evidence for ectopic pregnancy. They further acknowledged that this plan would delay surgery at least 48 hours and that the test would still falsely identify 15 percent of normal women as likely to have an ectopic pregnancy and 13 percent of women with an ectopic pregnancy as normal. Although Pittaway and co-workers (1985) did not confirm these observations, Kadar and Romero (1987) subsequently reported a larger series of patients with evidence to support the concept.

Yet another approach to this problem is to predict when a gestational sac and fetal signs can be seen by sonography when these anatomical features are compared to quantitative serum β-hCG levels. At least two groups have constructed such nomograms (Batzer and colleagues, 1983; Kadar and Romero, 1982), but despite their use, a more accurate prediction of uterine versus ectopic pregnancy is not always obtained. Finally, vaginal sonography plus quantitative serum β-hCG values may prove to be an even more sensitive method of establishing the presence or absence of an early intrauterine gestation (Bernaschek and co-workers, 1988; Dashefsky and colleagues, 1988).

Culdocentesis

The simplest technique for identifying hemoperitoneum is culdocentesis, since it can be performed without hospitalization.

As the cervix is pulled toward the symphysis with a tenaculum, a long 16- or 18-gauge needle is inserted through the posterior vaginal fornix into the cul-de-sac, whence fluid can be aspirated. Failure to aspirate any fluid can be interpreted only as unsatisfactory entry into the cul-de-sac. Fluid containing fragments of old clots or bloody fluid that does not subsequently clot is compatible with the diagnosis of hemoperitoneum resulting from an ectopic pregnancy. If the blood subsequently clots, it may have been obtained from an adjacent perforated blood vessel rather than from a bleeding ectopic pregnancy. The very important exception to this generalization is brisk bleeding from the site of rupture, in which case the blood may be aspirated from the cul-de-sac before it has had time to clot. With bleeding of such intensity, culdocentesis is rarely necessary to establish the diagnosis of an intra-abdominal catastrophe. In most such instances, hypovolemic shock is or will be apparent rapidly so that immediate intravenous infusion of fluids, including whole blood, and prompt surgical intervention are required.

Culdocentesis may be unsatisfactory in women with previous salpingitis and pelvic peritonitis, since the cul-de-sac may have been obliterated. **Thus, the failure to obtain blood from the cul-de-sac does not exclude the diagnosis of hemoperitoneum and certainly is not proof against the presence of an ectopic pregnancy, either unruptured or ruptured.**

Curettage

Differentiation between threatened or incomplete abortion of an intrauterine pregnancy and a tubal pregnancy may also be accomplished in many instances by curettage. If embryo, fetus, or placenta are identified, a simultaneous tubal pregnancy is very unlikely. When none of these structures is identified, tubal pregnancy is a probability. The identification of decidua alone in the uterine curettings strongly implies extrauterine pregnancy, but decidua alone may be present following a complete abortion. The *Arias–Stella reaction* in the endometrium also is not diagnostic of an ectopic pregnancy. O'Connor and Kurman (1988) maintain, however, that intrauterine pregnancy can be diagnosed in the absence of villi by the presence of intermediate trophoblast associated with enlarged vessels replaced by hyaline or with fragments of fibrinoid matrix.

Colpotomy

Direct visualization of the oviducts and ovaries can be accomplished by use of colopotomy unless pelvic inflammation, recent or remote, has obliterated the cul-de-sac or the tubes are adherent to the broad ligaments or uterus to a degree that they cannot be mobilized sufficiently to be drawn into the field of vision. This procedure generally has been abandoned because more satisfactory results can be obtained using laparoscopy.

TABLE 30–7. LOWER NORMAL LIMITS FOR PERCENTAGE INCREASE OF SERUM β-HUMAN CHRONIC GONADOTROPIN DURING EARLY UTERINE PREGNANCY

Sampling Interval (days)	Percent Increase in β-hCG from Initial Value
1	29
2	66
3	114
4	175
5	255

Modified from Kadar and co-workers: Obstet Gynecol 58:162, 1981.

Laparoscopy

This technique provides a means of diagnosing disease of the pelvic viscera, including ectopic pregnancy. Refined optic and electronic systems have overcome most of the objections that arose in the course of previous attempts to utilize transabdominal intraperitoneal lighted probes for visualization of organs. Nonetheless, successful and safe laparoscopy demands refined equipment, an experienced operator, an operating room, and, usually, surgical anesthesia. Complete visualization of the pelvis may be impossible in the presence of pelvic inflammation or recent or remote bleeding. At times, identification of an early unruptured tubal pregnancy may be difficult using the laparoscope, even though the tube is fully visualized. Samuellson and Sjovall (1972) reported that four ectopic pregnancies out of 166 were not seen using the laparoscope, and that of 120 women with an intrauterine pregnancy, six were diagnosed as having an ectopic gestation. Such errors likely vary with the experience of the operator and the degree of anatomical distortion encountered. The tube may show little change in shape and minimal change in color if the pregnancy is early. Moreover, demonstration of tubal patency by the passage of dye through the tube does not exclude early tubal pregnancy (Yaffe and colleagues, 1976).

Laparotomy

If any doubt remains, laparotomy should be performed, since an unnecessary operation is far less tragic than death contributed to by indecision or delay. There is remarkably little morbidity associated with surgery that is limited to a carefully made and repaired suprapubic incision. At the same time, diagnosis is often enhanced appreciably by the direct visualization and palpation of the pelvic organs that laparotomy allows. **It is imperative that laparotomy not be delayed while laparoscopy is performed on the woman with an obvious pelvic or abdominal catastrophe that requires immediate definitive treatment.**

DIFFERENTIAL DIAGNOSIS

Prompt diagnosis of a ruptured tubal pregnancy may be lifesaving, and the earlier an unruptured tubal pregnancy is diagnosed, the greater will be the likelihood of a future successful pregnancy (p. 524). Unfortunately, there are few other disorders in obstetrics and gynecology that present so many diagnostic pitfalls. Brenner and associates (1980) reported findings from 300 women with an ectopic pregnancy and approximately a third had been seen once and 11 percent twice before the correct diagnosis was made. Dorfman and colleagues (1984), in an analysis of mortality from ectopic pregnancy in the United States in 1979 and 1980, concluded that more than half of the deaths might have been prevented had the woman or her physician(s) acted more expeditiously. The most commonly misdiagnosed conditions are listed in Table 30–8.

The conditions observed by us to be most frequently confused with tubal pregnancy are (1) acute or chronic salpingitis, (2) threatened or incomplete abortion of an intrauterine pregnancy, (3) rupture of a corpus luteum or follicular cyst with intraperitoneal bleeding, (4) torsion of an ovarian cyst, (5) appendicitis, (6) gastroenteritis, (7) discomfort from an intrauterine device, and (8) failure of a tubal sterilization.

Salpingitis

The disease most commonly mistaken for ruptured tubal pregnancy is salpingitis, in which there is often a history of similar

TABLE 30–8. MISDIAGNOSES FOR FATAL ECTOPIC PREGNANCIES IN THE UNITED STATES, 1979–80

Misdiagnosis	Occurrences	
	No.	%
Gastrointestinal disorder	14	25
Normal pregnancy	10	18
Pelvic inflammatory disease	8	14
Psychiatric disorder	5	9
Spontaneous abortion	5	9
Complication of induced abortion	4	7
Urinary tract infection	4	7
Adnexal cyst	2	4
Dysfunctional uterine bleeding	2	4
Fetal death	1	2
Placenta previa or abruption	1	2
Totals	56	100[a]

[a] Total exceeds 100% due to rounding figures.
Modified from Dorfman and associates: Obstet Gynecol 64:386, 1984.

attacks with usually no missed period. With salpingitis, abnormal bleeding is not nearly so common as the spotting characteristic of tubal gestation. Pain and tenderness are more likely to be bilateral in salpingitis. A pelvic mass in a tubal pregnancy, if palpable, is unilateral, whereas in salpingitis both fornices are likely to be equally resistant and tender. In fact, a unilateral mass with salpingitis should prompt consideration for an infected ectopic pregnancy. Dicker and associates (1984) reported a series of eight such women who presented with a clinical picture of unilateral tubo-ovarian or pelvic abscess. The correct preoperative diagnosis was made by a positive serum assay for chorionic gonadotropin.

The temperature in acute salpingitis usually exceeds 38°C. If there is any suspicion that there is an ectopic gestation, then a sensitive test for chorionic gonadotropin may be obtained rapidly (p. 519). A positive urinary pregnancy test is important information. A negative urinary pregnancy test does not exclude pregnancy and serum chorionic gonadotropin must be measured if pregnancy is to be excluded.

Abortion of Intrauterine Pregnancy

In threatened or incomplete abortion of an intrauterine pregnancy, the uterine bleeding is usually more profuse, and shock from hypovolemia, when present, is usually in proportion to the extent of vaginal hemorrhage. In tubal pregnancy, however, hypovolemic shock is almost always far in excess of what might be expected from the observed vaginal blood loss. The pain in uterine abortion is generally less severe, likely to be rhythmic, and located low in the midline of the abdomen, whereas in tubal pregnancy it is unilateral or generalized. If embryo or placenta is found in the vagina or at the external cervical os, the diagnosis of abortion of an intrauterine pregnancy is obvious. However, it should be remembered that shed decidua may be abundant with an ectopic pregnancy and might, unless carefully examined, be incorrectly considered products from an intrauterine pregnancy that is aborting. Moreover, combined extrauterine and intrauterine pregnancy may occur, albeit rarely. The marked histological variations in the endometrium in cases of ectopic pregnancy are such that endometrial biopsy provides an often unreliable diagnostic criterion as well as the likelihood of being disruptive if the pregnancy is intrauterine.

Rupture of a Corpus Luteum or Follicular Cyst

Intraperitoneal bleeding from an ovarian cyst may be difficult to distinguish from a ruptured tubal pregnancy. Even though the identification of chorionic gonadotropin will sometimes help to make the diagnosis preoperatively, frequently, the diagnosis is made at the time of exploratory laparotomy for hemoperitoneum (see Culdocentesis, p. 521).

Twisted Cyst or Appendicitis

In both torsion of an ovarian cyst and appendicitis, the signs and symptoms of pregnancy, including amenorrhea, are usually lacking and there is rarely a history of abnormal vaginal bleeding. The mass formed by a twisted ovarian cyst is more nearly discrete, whereas that of a tubal pregnancy is usually less well defined. With appendicitis, only rarely is there a mass found by vaginal examination, and pain on motion of the cervix is much less severe than in ruptured tubal pregnancy. The pain from appendicitis, furthermore, is often localized higher, over McBurney's point. If either appendicitis or a twisted ovarian cyst is mistaken for a tubal pregnancy, the error is not costly, since all three require prompt operation.

Gastrointestinal Disturbance

In some women with a ruptured ectopic pregnancy, the prominent symptoms are diarrhea, nausea, and vomiting, along with abdominal pain. The inappropriate diagnosis of gastroenteritis has led to death (Dorfman and associates, 1984).

Intrauterine Devices

Diagnosis of ectopic pregnancy is often more difficult in women who use an intrauterine device for contraception. The devices do not prevent ectopic pregnancies. Cramping pelvic pain and bleeding from the uterus, both common features of ectopic pregnancy, may be caused by an intrauterine device. Moreover, in some women the device predisposes to inflammation of the adnexa, which may be unilateral. The declining use of this contraceptive technique in the United States (Chap. 42, p. 930) likely will result in this being less of a problem in the differential diagnosis of tubal pregnancy.

Previous Tubal Sterilization

Such an operation does not absolutely preclude pregnancy. Tatum and Schmidt (1977) reported that approximately 16 percent of pregnancies conceived after a failed tubal sterilization were ectopic. Following laparoscopic tubal sterilization, as many as 50 percent of pregnancies are ectopic (McCausland, 1980).

TREATMENT AND PROGNOSIS

Treatment of tubal pregnancy most often has been salpingectomy to remove a shattered, bleeding oviduct with or without ipsilateral oophorectomy. The goal of such treatment was and should remain the preservation of the woman's life. Recently, treatment has changed from salpingectomy to procedures that favor tubal conservation. Such conservative management is made possible by the earlier diagnosis of ectopic pregnancy using ultrasound and serum β-hCG determinations. The traditionally more radical surgical approaches are presented first, followed by newer techniques designed to conserve fallopian tube function.

Salpingectomy

In removing the oviduct, it is advisable to excise as a wedge certainly no more than the outer third of the interstitial portion of the tube (so-called cornual resection) in an effort to minimize the rare recurrence of pregnancy in the tubal stump but not weaken the myometrium at that site of excision. Resection so extensive as to reach the cavity of the uterus must be avoided, lest the defect created lead to uterine rupture in a subsequent intrauterine pregnancy. Even with a cornual resection, a subsequent interstital pregnancy may not be prevented (Kalchman and Meltzer, 1966).

Ipsilateral Oophorectomy

Removal of the adjacent ovary at the time of salpingectomy, as demonstrated in Figure 30–8 has been suggested as a possible means for both improving fertility and decreasing the likelihood of a subsequent ectopic pregnancy (Jeffcoate, 1967). Ovulation would thus always occur from the ovary immediately adjacent to the remaining oviduct. This should facilitate the pickup of the ovum by that tube and avoid the possibility of external migration of the ovum and the ectopic pregnancy that might result from such a peripatetic egg. The important of this phenomenon in the genesis of ectopic pregnancy is not clear, although Hallatt (1975) identified the corpus luteum on the opposite ovary and, therefore, almost certainly, external migration of the ovum, in about one of every five tubal pregnancies. Even so, removal of an otherwise normal-appearing ovary on these grounds seems hardly justifiable. Most gynecologists leave the ovary when possible and, to minimize ovarian dysfunction and cyst formation, preserve all the blood supply possible by clamping the vessels in the mesosalpinx as close to the oviduct as possible.

Sterilization

It is important that before surgical exploration for a suspected ectopic pregnancy the woman be asked about her wishes for future pregnancies. If the woman has completed her childbearing and the ectopic pregnancy is the consequence of failed contraception, the decision usually is in favor of sterilization. If so, and her condition is good, hysterectomy may be considered. Otherwise, tubal sterilization usually can be performed very quickly without increased risk. Conversely, all organs possible should be conserved in the woman of low parity with a strong desire for future pregnancies in spite of the increased risk that she faces of a subsequent ectopic pregnancy.

Conservation of the Fallopian Tube

Because of the strong likelihood of infertility following tubal pregnancy treated by salpingectomy, an alternative to removing the oviduct should be considered. The cumulative experiences in seven reports concerned with 352 women with ectopic pregnancies, on whom procedures to remove the pregnancy but preserve the tube had been performed, were that 119, or one third, subsequently became pregnant in utero. Moreover, 15 percent of those who conceived again, had a repeat ectopic pregnancy (Hallatt, 1975). These outcomes have improved since this earlier report; however, many factors must be considered in evaluating the success or failure of subsequent attempts at pregnancy. These include, but are not limited to, age, parity, bilateral tubal disease, and whether the fallopian tube was ruptured. In general, women under age 30 and those of higher parity have significantly higher fertility rates and successful outcomes in

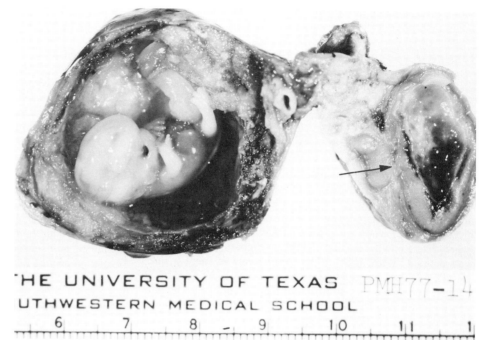

Figure 30–8. Right oviduct containing a fetus and placenta in the ampullary portion, and right ovary with corpus luteum of pregnancy (*arrow*). The woman had experienced vaginal spotting and intermittent dull pain for nearly a month. As she was refusing hospitalization the lower abdominal pain suddenly worsened and she became overtly hypotensive. At emergency laparotomy 1,100 mL of free blood and clots were removed from the peritoneal cavity!

subsequent pregnancies than older women of lower parity (Sherman and co-workers, 1982). A history of salpingitis and evidence of bilateral tubal disease are extremely bad prognostic signs. Finally, Sherman and co-workers (1982) reported that **subsequent pregnancy and lower recurrent ectopic pregnancy rates were observed in women in whom surgery was performed prior to rupture of the ectopic pregnancy.**

If the woman has no history of infertility and no gross evidence of previous salpingitis, then salpingotomy and salpingostomy result in equally favorable outcomes. Sherman and associates (1982) reported intrauterine pregnancy rates for both groups to be more than 85 percent (Table 30–9). If there is evidence for bilateral tubal disease, then salpingostomy is clearly superior to salpingotomy with subsequent intrauterine conception rates of 76 percent versus 44 percent, respectively (see Table 30–9). Similar results have been reported by DeCherney and Jones (1985) and Reyniak (1985).

Use of newer diagnostic techniques and surgical procedures to conserve damaged tubes will result in higher subsequent successful pregnancy outcomes. Several of the surgical approaches for tubal reconstruction are discussed below.

Salpingostomy

This technique is used to remove a small pregnancy that is usually less than 2 cm in length and located in the distal one third of the fallopian tube (Fig. 30–9). A linear incision, 2 cm in length or less, is made on the antimesenteric border immediately over the ectopic pregnancy. The ectopic usually will extrude from the incision and can be carefully removed. Small bleeding sites are controlled with needle point electrocautery or laser and the incision is left unsutured to heal by secondary intention. Sherman and associates (1982) and Timonen and Neiminen (1967) reported that salpingostomy is associated with a higher subsequent pregnancy rate than salpingectomy.

Salpingotomy

This procedure was first described by Stromme in 1953. A longitudinal incision is made on the antimesenteric border of the fallopian tube directly over the ectopic (Fig. 30–10). The products of conception are removed with forceps or gentle suction and the opened tube irrigated with lactated Ringer's solutions (not isotonic saline) so that bleeding sites are identified and controlled as described above. Most recommend one-layer closure with 7-0 interrupted vicryl sutures (DeCherney and Jones, 1985; Reyniak, 1985). Reyniak (1985) reports improved anatomical results with the use of optic magnification and microsurgical

TABLE 30–9. SURGICAL TREATMENTS AND SUBSEQUENT FERTILITY AMONG 151 WOMEN WITH A FIRST-EPISODE ECTOPIC PREGNANCY

Surgical Treatment[a]	No. Patients	(Subsequent Pregnancies %)		
		Intrauterine	Repeat Ectopic	Sterility
Conservative	21	16 (76)	1 (5)	4 (19)
Radical[b]	32	14 (44)	3 (9)	15 (47)
Conservative	26	23 (88)	2 (8)	1 (4)
Radical[c]	72	61 (85)	3 (4)	8 (11)
Totals[d]				
Conservative	47	39 (83)	3 (6)	5 (11)
Radical	104	75 (72)	6 (6)	23 (22)

[a] Radical surgery is salpingectomy and conservative surgery is conservation of the fallopian tube.
[b] These women had a history or operative findings consistent with coexisting sterility factors. The difference between conservative and radical were significant (*p* = 0.04).
[c] These women had a normal reproductive history and their other reproductive organs were normal at surgery. The difference between these groups was not significant (*p* = 0.9).
[d] All patients, conservative versus radical surgery, *p* = 0.2.
Modified from Sherman and co-workers: Fertil Steril 37:497, 1982.

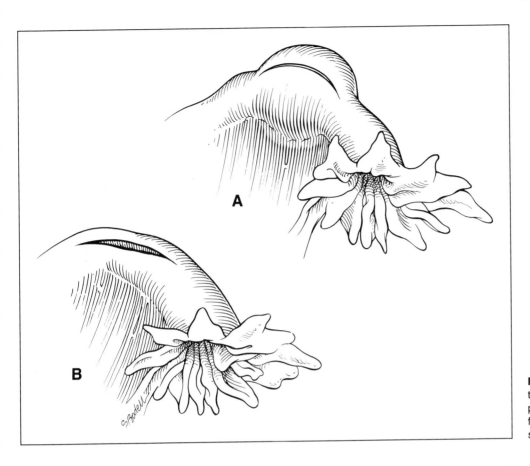

Figure 30–9. A. Linear salpingostomy for removal of a small tubal pregnancy in the distal third of the fallopian tube. **B.** The incision is not sutured.

techniques. He also recommends that, when possible, the incision not be extended through the end of the tube into the ampulla.

Segmental Resection and Anastomosis

This procedure is recommended for an unruptured ectopic in the isthmic portion of the tube since salpingotomy or salpingostomy likely would cause scarring and subsequent narrowing of this small lumen (Stangel and associates, 1976). After the segment of the tube is exposed, the mesosalpinx beneath the tube is incised, and the tubal isthmus containing the ectopic is resected (Fig. 30–11). The mesosalpinx is sutured, thus reapproximating the tubal stumps. The segments of the tube then are anastomosed to one another in layers with interrupted 7-0 vicryl sutures, preferably using magnification. Three sutures are used in the muscularis and three in the serosa with strict attention to avoid the tubal lumen. Suturing the serosal layer adds strength to the first layer.

Fimbrial Evacuation

There is a temptation with distally implanted tubal pregnancies to evacuate the conceptual products by "milking" or "suctioning" the ectopic from the tubal lumen. **This is not recommended** since this practice is associated with an ectopic recurrence rate twice that of salpingotomy (Sherman and co-workers, 1982; Stromme, 1953). There is also a high rate of surgical reexploration for recurrent bleeding from persistent trophoblastic tissue (Bell and colleagues, 1987).

Other Techniques

Fallopian tube reimplantation into the uterine cornu and the *Gepfert procedure* of everting the distal end of damaged fimbria or tubal

mucosa are associated with very poor pregnancy outcomes and are not recommended by DeCherney and Jones (1985).

All of the above techniques can be done at a later time if the woman is in shock! The first rule must be that bleeding is rapidly arrested and cardiovascular resuscitation performed. If time and clinical circumstances warrant, the above procedures then can be considered.

If a second procedure is planned for a later time, it is logical to obtain hemostasis with the least amount of tubal damage. This obtains even when the opposite fallopian tube appears to be grossly normal. Unfortunately, many of the normal-appearing contralateral tubes also have been damaged by salpingitis, which characteristically is bilateral.

If a tubal reconstructive procedure is done, all blood and debris should be irrigated from the abdomen and pelvis using lactated Ringer's solution. Some recommend the use of high-molecular-weight dextran to decrease postoperative adhesion formation (Reyniak, 1985).

The risk of persistent tubal trophoblastic tissue following a tubal reconstructive procedure is real (DiMarchi and associates, 1987). Because of this risk, Bell and colleagues (1987) recommend that another chorionic gonadotropin determination be performed 2 weeks later to compare to the original and to insure that the value is falling. With persistent or increasing values, the choice of reexploration or chemotherapy with methotrexate (see below) must be made. Kamrava and co-workers (1983) reported that values for chorionic gonadotropin usually are negative by 12 days following resection of tubal pregnancies, but occasionally they are elevated even 3 weeks after surgery.

Obviously, none of these procedures guarantees subsequent

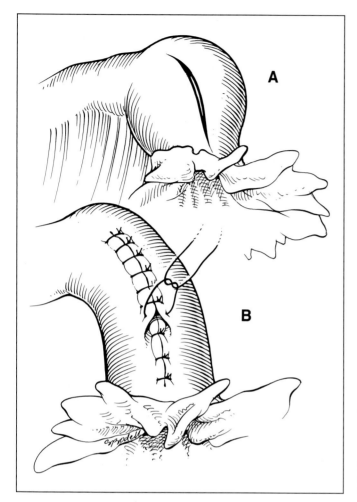

Figure 30–10. A. Linear salpingotomy for removal of an ectopic pregnancy larger than 2 cm in length from the distal third of the fallopian tube. **B.** The incision is sutured, usually with a single layer of 7–0 interrupted sutures.

tubal patency. Nonetheless, for women of low parity, these procedures should be considered unless the tube is destroyed beyond repair. The results obtained using such techniques were reported by Sherman and colleagues (1982) and are presented in Table 30–9.

> The intense desire of some women to procreate and the willingness of physicians to try to aid them in doing so is evident in a case reported by Kemmann and colleagues (1983). They outlined the obstetrical history of one woman in whom the first pregnancy was tubal and was treated by laparotomy and right salpingectomy plus cornual resection. The second pregnancy was tubal and treated by laparotomy and milking the tube to abort the pregnancy from the isthmic-ampullary region. The third pregnancy was tubal and at laparotomy was removed through a linear salpingostomy. The fourth pregnancy was tubal and at laparotomy was removed by midsegment resection followed by tubal anastomosis. The fifth pregnancy terminated with a normal spontaneous delivery of a healthy baby!

Nonsurgical Management

Since some tubal pregnancies either abort or resorb without causing the woman serious debility, some authors have sug-

gested that suspected early gestations may be simply watched closely to allow those that will terminate benignly to do so, especially those in whom the level of serum chorionic gonadotrophin appears not to be increasing (Mashiach and associates, 1982). Even methotrexate has been advocated to try to hasten resorption (Tanaka and associates, 1982). There is little advantage to most women from such an approach, since methotrexate is extremely toxic, quantitative assays for chorionic gonadotrophin are not always precise, and the expanding tubal pregnancy may severely damage the tube so that it becomes unsuitable for successful salpingotomy.

Autotransfusion

In the face of serious blood loss, retransfusion of blood collected from the abdomen at times has been advocated. Although this procedure is effective in an emergency, we do not advise it as a routine because of the frequency of adverse reactions. Merrill and associates (1980), however, were enthusiastic in their recommendation of autotransfusion in this circumstance.

Some workers have recommended that free blood be left in the abdomen to benefit the patient. Pritchard and Adams (1957) demonstrated by means of suitably labeled erythrocytes that absorption of erythrocytes from the adult peritoneal cavity occurs over a period of days and is much too slow to be of significant help in combating either hypovolemia or severe anemia. Moreover, free blood in the peritoneal cavity at the completion of surgery makes it difficult to ascertain that hemostasis has been accomplished satisfactorily. Finally, such blood is likely to serve as an excellent culture medium for bacteria!

Anti-D Immune Globulin

If the woman is D-negative but not yet sensitized to D-antigen and the potential for reproduction persists, anti-D immune globulin should be administered to protect against isoimmunization. Certainly, whenever D-positive blood is administered inadvertently to the previously unsensitized D-negative woman, sufficient immune globulin to protect her should be promptly administered. Moreover, if platelets were transfused, in all likelihood some contaminating D-positive red cells also were included. Therefore, the D-negative patient should also receive anti-D immune globulin soon after platelet transfusion.

Resumption of Ovulation

Spirtos and associates (1987) reported following resection of an ectopic pregnancy that approximately 14 percent of women ovulate by 19 days and 64 percent by 24 days. By the 30th postoperative day, almost three fourths of women have ovulated. Thus, contraception should be commenced at the time of discharge from the hospital.

ABDOMINAL PREGNANCY

FREQUENCY

The incidence of abdominal pregnancy is influenced by the frequency of ectopic gestation in the population being cared for, by the availability of care early in pregnancy, and by the degree of suspicion of ectopic pregnancy exercised by those providing care. Almost all cases of abdominal pregnancy follow early rupture or abortion of a tubal pregnancy into the peritoneal cavity. An incidence for abdominal pregnancy of 1 in 3,337 births at Charity Hospital in New Orleans was reported by Beacham and colleagues (1962), compared to 1 in 7,931 births at Indiana Uni-

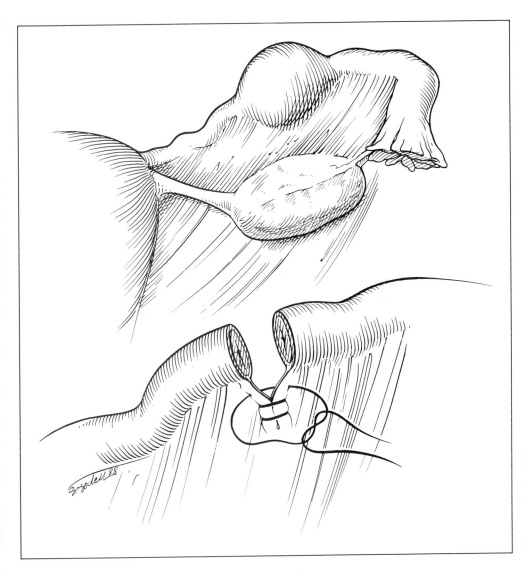

Figure 30–11. Segmental resection and anastomosis of the fallopian tube for an unruptured ectopic pregnancy. Closure of the mesosalpinx results in reapproximation of the tubal segments. Anastomosis is accomplished with interrupted 7–0 vicryl sutures (see text).

versity Hospital, noted by Strafford and Ragan (1977). The Center for Disease Control has estimated that the incidence of abdominal pregnancy is 1 in 10,000 livebirths (Atrash and coworkers, 1987a). At Parkland Hospital abdominal pregnancy is encountered in perhaps 1 in 25,000 births.

ETIOLOGY

Typically, the growing placenta, after penetrating the wall of the oviduct, maintains to a degree its tubal attachment but gradually encroaches upon and implants in the neighboring serosa. Meanwhile, the fetus, usually but not always surrounded by amnion, continues to grow within the peritoneal cavity. In such circumstances, the placenta is found in the general region of the oviduct, which eventually loses its identity as such, and over the posterior aspect of the broad ligament and uterus (Fig. 30–12). In rarer instances, the conceptus appears to have escaped from the tube after rupture to reimplant elsewhere in the peritoneal cavity. Primary implantation of the fertilized ovum on the peritoneum is so rare that many authors doubt its existence. Conclusive proof of a primary abdominal pregnancy, however, was provided by Studdiford's well-documented case (1942), which fulfills

the following criteria upon which proof of such a pregnancy must rest: (1) normal tubes and ovaries with no evidence of recent or remote injury, (2) absence of any evidence of uteroplacental fistula, and (3) presence of a pregnancy related exclusively to the peritoneal surface and young enough to eliminate the possibility of secondary implantation following primary nidation in the tube.

King (1932) directed attention to a rare cause of abdominal pregnancy, namely, postoperative separation of the uterine wound of a previous cesarean section. In three of his four reported cases, the ovum had implanted upon omentum, over the uterine defect, whereas in the fourth it had become attached to the abdominal wall. He believed that in each case the fertilized ovum escaped through the defect in the uterine wall and implanted as a primary abdominal pregnancy.

STATUS OF FETUS

The condition of the fetus in abdominal pregnancy is exceedingly precarious, and consequently the great majority have succumbed. In a review of the world's literature, Ware (1948) cited a perinatal loss of 75 percent, but that figure may have been falsely low because of the tendency to report cases with happy

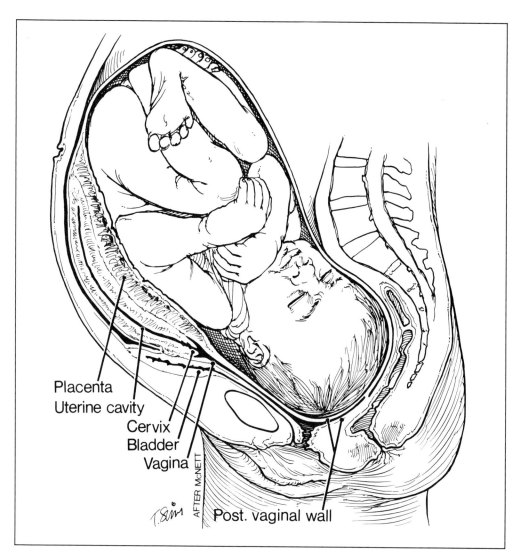

Placenta
Uterine cavity
Cervix
Bladder
Vagina
Post. vaginal wall

Figure 30–12. Abdominal pregnancy at term. The placenta is implanted on the posterior wall of the uterus and broad ligament. The enlarged, flattened uterus is located just beneath the anterior abdominal wall. The cervix and vagina are dislodged anteriorly and superiorly by the large fetal head in the cul-de-sac.

results. Beacham and co-workers (1962) reported a perinatal loss in their own series of about 95 percent. Some authors, moreover, report an incidence of congenital malformation in the infants as high as 50 percent.

If the fetus dies after reaching a size too large to be resorbed, it may undergo suppuration, mummification, calcification, or formation of an adipocere. Bacteria may gain access to the gestational products, particularly when they are adherent to the intestines, with suppuration of the products. Eventually, the abscess ruptures at the point of least resistance, and if the patient does not soon die of peritonitis and septicemia, fetal parts may be extruded through the abdominal wall or more commonly into the intestines or bladder. Mummification and the formation of a lithopedion occasionally ensue, and the calcified products of conception may be carried for years without producing symptoms until they cause dystocia in a subsequent pregnancy or symptoms from pressure. There are instances in which a period of 20 to 30 years elapsed before removal of a lithopedion at operation or autopsy. Much more rarely, the fetus is converted into a yellowish, greasy mass to which the term *adipocere* is applied. The various bizarre terminations of abdominal pregnancy have been well discussed, with illustrative cases graphically described by King (1954).

DIAGNOSIS

Since early rupture or abortion of a tubal pregnancy is the usual antecedent of an abdominal pregnancy, in retrospect, a history suggestive of the accident can usually be obtained. The abnormalities likely to be recalled include spotting or irregular bleeding and abdominal pain, which usually was most prominent in one or both lower quadrants. Unexplained transient anemia early in pregnancy may accompany the rupture or abortion.

Symptoms

Women with an abdominal pregnancy are likely to be uncomfortable but not sufficiently so to warrant thorough evaluation. Nausea, vomiting, flatulence, constipation, diarrhea, and abdominal pain may each be present in varying degrees. Multiparas may state that the pregnancy does not "feel right." Late in pregnancy, fetal movements may cause pain. Near term, the empty uterus has been alleged to go into spurious labor.

Physical Examination

By abdominal palpation, the abnormal position of the fetus, often a transverse or oblique lie, can frequently be confirmed. Ease of palpation of the fetal parts, however, is not a reliable sign, since they sometimes feel exceedingly close to the examining fingers in normal intrauterine pregnancies, especially in thin, multiparous women. *Massage of the abdomen over the pregnancy products does not stimulate the mass to become more firm, as it most always does with advanced intrauterine pregnancy.* The cervix is usually displaced (see Fig. 30–12), depending in part on the position of the fetus, and it may dilate somewhat, but appreciable effacement is lacking. The uterus may be outlined over the lower part of the pregnancy mass. By palpation of the fornices, small parts or the fetal head clearly outside the uterus may be identified occasionally.

Oxytocin Stimulation

Cross and co-workers (1951) emphasized that oxytocin stimulation could be a valuable aid in the diagnosis of abdominal pregnancy. If no evidence of uterine activity is detected using a sensitive strain gauge applied repeatedly to the maternal abdominal wall over the products of conception while oxytocin is infused intravenously in a sizable dose, the pregnancy almost certainly is extrauterine. Hertz and co-workers (1977) could detect no uterine activity while infusing oxytocin in excess of 50 milliunits per minute. In their case the empty uterus lay inferior and posterior to the fetus. If the uterus were anterior, as in Figure 30–12, it might contract in response to oxytocin and possibly lead to the false conclusion of intrauterine pregnancy.

In a case described by Orr and associates (1979), before the diagnosis of abdominal pregnancy was made, not only did the uterus presumably contract in response to oxytocin but also an oxytocin challenge test was interpreted as negative on two occasions. The growth-retarded fetus, which weighed 2,000 g, expired undelivered one week later. The relationship between the abdominal wall, the uterus, and the extrauterine fetus was very similar to that depicted in Figure 30–12.

Radiological Examination

A strong suspicion of abdominal pregnancy may be confirmed by x-ray with a probe or radiopaque material in the uterus. The fetus is then clearly shown to lie outside the uterine cavity. Unfortunately, such techniques are not safe diagnostic procedures if the fetus is intrauterine, especially if it is alive.

Sonography

In practice, sonographic findings with an abdominal pregnancy may not be so distinct as to allow an unequivocal diagnosis to be made. However, in some suspected cases, the sonographic findings may serve to identify the pregnancy as being extrauterine. For example, if the fetal head is seen to lie immediately adjacent to the maternal bladder with no interposed uterine tissue, a specific diagnosis of an abdominal pregnancy can be made, as in the case described by Kurtz and associates (1982). Magnetic resonance imaging has been used to confirm an abdominal pregnancy following a suspicious sonographic examination (Harris and associates, 1988).

TREATMENT

The operation for abdominal pregnancy may precipitate massive hemorrhage. Without massive blood transfusion, the outlook for many such patients is hopeless. Hence, it is mandatory that at least 2,000 mL of compatible blood be on hand in the operating room, with more readily available in the blood bank. Preoperatively, two intravenous infusion systems, each capable of delivering large volumes of fluid at a rapid rate, should be functioning. At the same time, techniques for monitoring the

adequacy of the circulation should be employed, as described in Chapter 36. Whenever time allows, the bowel should be prepared using both mechanical cleansing and antimicrobial agents, since the bowel is often intimately adherent to the placenta and membranes.

The massive hemorrhage that often occurs in the course of operations for abdominal pregnancy is related to the lack of constriction of hypertrophied opened blood vessels after placental separation. It has been recommended by some that the operation may be deferred until fetal viability is achieved (Hage and associates, 1988). However, procrastination may be dangerous and undesirable, since partial separation of the placenta with hemorrhage occasionally occurs spontaneously in the interval of waiting. Moreover, even though the fetus may have been dead several weeks, bleeding may still be torrential. For these reasons, operation is indicated as soon as the diagnosis has been established and the appropriate steps preparative for surgery have been completed.

Management of the Placenta

Since removal of the placenta in abdominal pregnancy always carries the risk of hemorrhage, one should be sure that the blood vessels supplying the placenta can be effectively ligated before attempting removal of the organ. Partial separation can develop spontaneously or, more likely, in the course of the operation from manipulation while attempting to locate the exact site of attachment of the placenta. Since massive hemorrhage can occur, it is, for the most part, best to avoid unnecessary exploration of the surrounding organs. In general, the infant should be delivered, the cord severed close to the placenta, and the abdomen closed.

Unfortunately, the placenta, if left in the abdominal cavity, commonly causes complications in the form of infection, abscesses, adhesions, intestinal obstruction, and wound dehiscence. In one case, evidence of consumptive coagulopathy, including overt hypofibrinogenemia, developed 2 months following laparotomy for delivery of the fetus but after leaving the placenta. The coagulation defects cleared spontaneously before the placenta was delivered surgically 3 weeks later. Removal of the placenta in that case was prompted by right ureteral obstruction, which was relieved. *Although the complications of leaving the placenta are troublesome and usually lead to subsequent laparotomy, they may be less grave than the hemorrhage that sometimes results from placental removal during the initial surgery.*

Selective Embolization of Bleeding Sites

Percutaneous femoral artery catheterization and pelvic angiography followed by embolization of specific placental bleeding sites has been lifesaving in instances of massive pelvic hemorrhage uncontrolled by conventional techniques. It also has been reported effective for massive bleeding from uterine atony, cervical and uterine lacerations, postabortion bleeding, uterine arteriovenous fistulas, gynecological malignancies, and abdominal pregnancy (Dehaeck, 1986; Haseltine, 1984; Kivikoski, 1988; Pais, 1980; Poppe, 1987, and their associates).

Briefly, the procedure consists of identification of the bleeding site(s) from the pelvic angiogram. The catheter tip then is advanced into the specific artery supplying the bleeding site and the artery is embolized using small pieces of shredded Gelfoam dissolved in saline or angiography dye. Microspheres have been injected and small pieces of wool have been pushed through the catheter to the bleeding site using a small steel wire. The last two methods result in permanent occlusion of the specific vessel(s) while the Gelfoam is believed to occlude the vessel for only 7 to 21 days.

The worst complication of the technique is that bleeding is not arrested. If bleeding is not arrested despite angiographic evidence of occlusion of the specific injured vessel(s), then a collateral vessel likely is the source of continued bleeding. Other complications include necrosis of tissues distal to the embolized site such as colon and gluteal muscle. Finally, any angiographic procedure involves the risk of an allergic reaction to the dye as well as vascular spasm and arterial thrombosis.

PROGNOSIS

Strafford and Ragan (1977) cite a 6 percent maternal mortality and a 91 percent perinatal mortality. Two of the 10 cases described by Rahman and associates (1982) proved fatal.

Abdominal pregnancy is still one of the most formidable of obstetrical complications. Detection and eradication of ectopic pregnancies during the first trimester continue to be the most effective means for avoiding these terrible risks!

OVARIAN PREGNANCY

In 1878, Spiegelberg formulated his criteria for diagnosis of ovarian pregnancy. He required that (1) the tube on the affected side be intact, (2) the fetal sac occupy the position of the ovary, (3) the ovary be connected to the uterus by the ovarian ligament, and (4) definite ovarian tissue be found in the sac wall.

Bobrow and Winkelstein (1956) were able to collect 154 cases from the literature and added 1 of their own that satisfied the criteria of Spiegelberg. Hallatt (1982) has described 25 cases of primary ovarian pregnancy, and Grimes and co-workers (1983) described 24 more. It is not clear whether the use of an intrauterine contraceptive device predisposes to ovarian pregnancy, as in Figure 30–13. Gray and Ruffolo (1978), for example, described four instances of ovarian pregnancy in which the women conceived with a Cu-7 intrauterine device in situ.

Although the ovary can accommodate itself more readily than the tube to the expanding pregnancy, rupture at an early period is the usual consequence. Nonetheless, there are recorded cases in which the ovarian pregnancy went to term, and a few produced infants that survived. For example, Williams and associates (1982), while attempting a cesarean delivery because of a transverse lie at 41 weeks' gestation, were surprised to find an ovarian pregnancy. The infant, who weighed nearly 8 pounds, survived. The ovary, placenta, and membranes were resected, and the severed right ureter was reimplanted in the bladder.

The products of conception may degenerate early without rupture and give rise to a tumor of varying size, consisting of a capsule of ovarian tissue enclosing a mass of blood, placental tissue, and possibly membranes. The absence of a distinct decidua leads to direct invasion of the ovarian stroma by the trophoblast (Fig. 30–13).

Symptoms and Signs

The symptoms and physical findings are likely to mimic those of a tubal pregnancy or a bleeding corpus luteum. At the time of operation, early ovarian pregnancies are likely to be considered to be corpus luteum cysts or a bleeding corpus luteum.

Management

Early ovarian pregnancies should be treated, when possible, by wedge resection or cystectomy; otherwise, oophorectomy is performed.

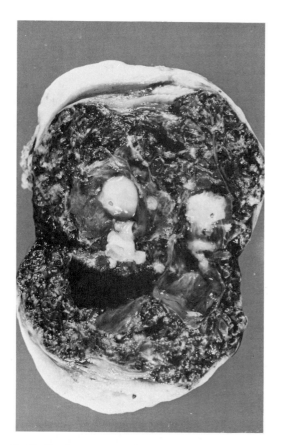

Figure 30–13. Ovarian pregnancy in a woman using an intrauterine device. There are twin embryos, each in a separate gestational sac. (*From Kalfayan and Gunderson: Obstet Gynecol 55:25 [Suppl] 1980.*)

CERVICAL PREGNANCY

Cervical pregnancy is a rare form of ectopic gestation in which the ovum implants within the cervix below the internal os. Dees (1966) estimated the incidence to be 1 in 18,000 pregnancies. In our experience, it is not nearly so common. The endocervix is eroded by the trophoblast, and the pregnancy proceeds to develop in the fibrous cervical wall, as illustrated in Figure 30–14.

SYMPTOMS AND SIGNS

Usually, painless bleeding appearing shortly after nidation is the first sign. As pregnancy progresses, a distended thin-wall cervix with the external os partially dilated may be evident. Bleeding without pain is the common clinical characteristic. Above the cervical mass, a slightly enlarged uterine fundus may be palpated. Gabbe and co-workers (1975) reported two cases of cervical pregnancy with high fever that initially was erroneously attributed to an infected intrauterine pregnancy. Cervical pregnancy rarely goes beyond the 20th week of gestation and is usually terminated surgically because of bleeding. Since attempts at removal of the placenta vaginally may result in profuse hemorrhage and even death of the patient, there should be little hesitation in performing hysterectomy to control the bleeding. Probably only in nulliparas very anxious to maintain fertility should conservative procedures be attempted. Bernstein and associates (1981) successfully managed two cases of early pregnancy implanted in the cervical canal

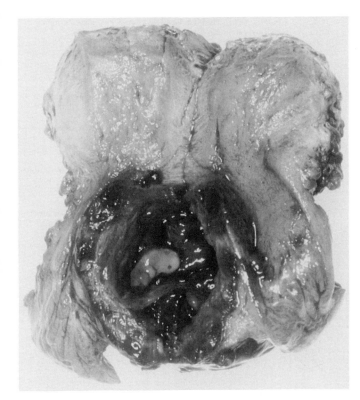

Figure 30–14. Cervical pregnancy in situ removed by hysterectomy nearly 3 months after last normal menstrual period and 1 month after onset of vaginal bleeding. (*Courtesy of Drs. D. Rubell and A. Brekken.*)

by placing a heavy silk ligature in and around the cervix above the implantation site similar to the McDonald cerclage technique (Chap. 29, p. 500), and then tying it quite snugly. The remaining products of pregnancy were then removed. Hemostasis was achieved, which persisted after removal of the ligature 8 and 10 days later.

OTHER SITES OF ECTOPIC PREGNANCY

A primary *splenic pregnancy* has been reported by Mankodi and associates (1977). The symptoms and signs that led to laparotomy included pain in the epigastrium and left shoulder, hypotension, tachycardia, syncope, and tenderness in the vaginal fornices. At laparotomy considerable hemoperitoneum but normal pelvic organs were found. A rent in the hilar surface of the spleen prompted splenectomy. Microscopically, chorionic villi were identified in the splenic rent. A similar case was reported by Yackel and associates (1988). A few cases of primary hepatic pregnancy have been described (Schlatter and colleagues, 1988), including one with lithopedion formation (Luwuliza-Kirunda, 1978).

REFERENCES

Arey LB: The cause of tubal pregnancy and tubal twinning. Am J Obstet Gynecol 5:163, 1923

Arias-Stella J: Atypical endometrial changes associated with the presence of chorionic tissue. Arch Pathol 58:112, 1954

Atrash HK, Friede A, Hogue CJR: Abdominal pregnancy in the United States: Frequency and maternal mortality. Obstet Gynecol 69:333, 1987a

Atrash HK, Friede A, Hogue CJR: Ectopic pregnancy mortality in the United States, 1970–1983. Obstet Gynecol 70:817, 1987b

Barnes RB, Roy S, Yee B, Duda MJ, Mishell DR Jr: Reliability of urinary pregnancy tests in the diagnosis of ectopic pregnancy. J Reprod Med 30:827, 1985

Batzer FR, Weiner S, Corson SL, Schlaff S, Otis C: Landmarks during the first forty-two days of gestation demonstrated by the β-subunit of human chorionic gonadotropin and ultrasound. Am J Obstet Gynecol 146:973, 1983

Beacham WD, Hernquist WC, Beacham DW, Webster HD: Abdominal pregnancy at Charity Hospital in New Orleans. Am J Obstet Gynecol 84:1257, 1962 (184 references cited)

Bell OR, Awadalla SG, Mattox JH: Persistent ectopic syndrome: A case report and literature review. Obstet Gynecol 69:521, 1987

Beral V: An epidemiological study of recent trends in ectopic pregnancy. Br J Obstet Gynaecol 82:775, 1975

Bernaschek G, Rudelstorfer R, Csaicsich P: Vaginal sonography versus serum human chorionic gonadotropin in early detection of pregnancy. Am J Obstet Gynecol 158:608, 1988

Bernstein D, Holzinger M, Ovadia J, Frishman B: Conservative treatment of cervical pregnancy. Obstet Gynecol 58:741, 1981

Bobrow ML, Winkelstein LB: Intrafollicular ovarian pregnancy. Am J Surg 91:991, 1956

Breen JL: A 21-year survey of 654 ectopic pregnancies. Am J Obstet Gynecol 106:1004, 1970

Brenner PF, Ray S, Mishell DR: Ectopic pregnancy: A study of 300 consecutive surgically treated cases. JAMA 243:673, 1980

Bryson SCP: β-Subunit of human chorionic gonadotropin, ultrasound, and ectopic pregnancy: A prospective study. Am J Obstet Gynecol 146:163, 1983

Centers for Disease Control: Ectopic pregnancy—United States, 1984 and 1985. MMWR 37:637, 1988

Coleman BG, Baron RL, Arger PH, Arenson RL, Axel L, Mayer DP, Costello P: Ectopic embryo detection using real-time sonography. J Clin Ultrasound 13:545, 1985

Corson SL, Batzer FR: Ectopic pregnancy: A review of the etiologic factors. J Reprod Med 31:78, 1986

Cross JB, Lester WM, McCain J: The diagnosis and management of abdominal pregnancy with a review of 19 cases. Am J Obstet Gynecol 62:303, 1951

Darrow WN: Venereal infections in three ethnic groups in Sacramento. Am J Public Health 66:446, 1976

Dashefsky SM, Lyons EA, Levi CS, Lindsay DJ: Suspected ectopic pregnancy: Endovaginal and transvesical US. Radiology 169:181, 1988

DeCherney AH, Jones EE: Ectopic pregnancy. Clin Obstet Gynecol 28:365, 1985

Dees HC: Cervical pregnancy associated with uterine leiomyomas. South Med J 59:900, 1966

Dehaeck CMC: Transcatheter embolization of pelvic vessels to stop intractable hemorrhage. Gynecol Oncol 24:9, 1986

Dicker D, Samuel N, Feldberg D, Goldman JA: Infected ectopic pregnancy presenting as unilateral tubo-ovarian abscess. Eur J Obstet Gynecol Reprod Biol 17:237, 1984

DiMarchi JM, Kosasa TS, Kobara TY, Hale RW: Persistent ectopic pregnancy. Obstet Gynecol 70:555, 1987

Dorfman SF, Grimes DA, Cates W Jr, Binkin NJ, Kafrissen ME, O'Reilly KR: Ectopic pregnancy mortality, United States, 1979 to 1980: Clinical aspects. Obstet Gynecol 64:386, 1984

Dorfman SF: Deaths from ectopic pregnancy, United States 1979 to 1980. Obstet Gynecol 62:344, 1983

Forbes K, Brennecke AM, Ho PC, Jones WR: Human chorionic gonadotrophin and pregnancy-specific β-1 glycoprotein (SP-1) in ectopic pregnancy. Aust N Z J Obstet Gynaecol 21:177, 1981

Fujii S, Ban C. Okamura H, Nishimura T: Unilateral tubal quadruplet pregnancy. Am J Obstet Gynecol 141:840, 1981

Funderburk AG: Bilateral ectopic pregnancy with simultaneous intrauterine pregnancy. Am J Obstet Gynecol 119:274, 1974

Gabbe SG, Kitzmiller JL, Kosasa TS, Driscoll SG: Cervical pregnancy presenting as septic abortion. Am J Obstet Gynecol 123:212, 1975

Gray CL, Ruffolo EH: Ovarian pregnancy associated with intrauterine contraceptive devices. Am J Obstet Gynecol 132:134, 1978

Grimes HG, Nosal RA, Gallagher JC: Ovarian pregnancy: A series of 24 cases. Obstet Gynecol 61:174, 1983

Hage MS, Wall LL, Killam A: Expectant management of abdominal pregnancy. A report of two cases. J Reprod Med 33:407, 1988

Hallatt JG: Repeat ectopic pregnancy: A study of 123 consecutive cases. Am J Obstet Gynecol 122:520, 1975

Hallatt JG: Primary ovarian pregnancy: A report of twenty-five cases. Am J Obstet Gynecol 143:55, 1982

Harris MB, Angtuaco T, Frazier CN, Mattison DR: Diagnosis of a viable abdominal pregnancy by magnetic resonance imaging. Am J Obstet Gynecol 159:150, 1988

Haseltine FP, Glickman MG, Marchesi S, Spitz R, D'Lugi A, DeCherney AA: Uterine embolization in a patient with postabortal hemorrhage. Obstet Gynecol 63:78S, 1984

Hedges JR, Kaib JJ, Armao JC: Detection of ectopic pregnancy in an outpatient population: The role of the beta-hCG level. J Emerg Med 2:85, 1984

Herbst AL, Hubby MM, Azizi F, Makii MM: Reproductive and gynecologic surgical experience in diethylstilbestrol-exposed daughters. Am J Obstet Gynecol 141:1019, 1981

Hertz RH, Timor-Tritch I, Sokol RJ, Zador I: Diagnostic studies and fetal assessment in advanced extrauterine pregnancy. Obstet Gynecol (Suppl) 50:63, 1977

Holman JF, Tyrey EL, Hammond CB: A contemporary approach to suspected ectopic pregnancy with use of quantitative and qualitative assays for the β-subunit of human chorionic gonadotropin and sonography. Am J Obstet Gynecol 150:151, 1984

Jacobson L, Riemer RK, Goldfien AC, Lykins D, Siiteri PK, Roberts JM: Rabbit myometrial oxytocin and alpha 2-adrenergic receptors are increased by estrogen but are differentially regulated by progesterone. Endocrinology 120:184, 1987

Jeffcoate TNA: Principles of Gynaecology, 3rd ed. New York, Appleton-Century-Crofts, 1967

Kadar N, DeVore G, Romero R: The discriminatory hCG zone: Its use in the sonographic evaluation for ectopic pregnancy. Obstet Gynecol 58:156, 1981a

Kadar N, Caldwell BR, Romero R: A method of screening for ectopic pregnancy and its indications. Obstet Gynecol 58:162, 1981b

Kadar N, Romero R: The timing of a repeat ultrasound examination in the evaluation for ectopic pregnancy. J Clin Ultrasound 10:211, 1982

Kadar N, Romero R: Observations on the log human chorionic gonadotropin-time relationship in early pregnancy and its practical implications. Am J Obstet Gynecol 157:73, 1987

Kalchman GG, Meltzer RM: Interstitial pregnancy following homolateral salpingectomy: Report of 2 cases and a review of the literature. Am J Obstet Gynecol 96:1139, 1966

Kamrava MM, Taymor ML, Berger MJ, Thompson IE, Seibel MM: Disappearance of human chorionic gonadotropin following removal of ectopic pregnancy. Obstet Gynecol 62:486, 1983

Kaufman RH, Noller K, Adam E, Irwin J, Gray M, Jefferies JA, Hilton T: Upper genital tract abnormalities and pregnancy outcome in diethylstilbestrol-exposed progeny. Am J Obstet Gynecol 148:973, 1984

Kemmann E, Grochmal SA, Harrigan JT: Term uterine pregnancy after four successive tubal pregnancies. JAMA 250:2673, 1983

King EL: Postoperative separation of the cesarean section wound, with subsequent abdominal pregnancy. Am J Obstet Gynecol 24:421, 1932

King G: Advanced extrauterine pregnancy. Am J Obstet Gynecol 67:712, 1954

Kivikoski AI, Martin C, Weyman P, Picus D, Giudice L: Angiographic arterial embolization to control hemorrhage in abdominal pregnancy: A case report. Obstet Gynecol 71:456, 1988

Kurtz AB, Dubbins PA, Wapner RJ, Goldberg BB: Problem of abnormal fetal position. JAMA 247:3251, 1982

Levin AA, Schoenbaum SC, Stubblefield PG, Zimicki S, Monson RR, Ryan KJ: Ectopic pregnancy and prior induced abortion. Am J Public Health 72:253, 1982

Luwuliza-Kirunda JMM: Primary hepatic pregnancy. Br J Obstet Gynaecol 85:311, 1978

MacKay HT, Hughes JM, Hogue CR: Ectopic pregnancy in the United States, 1979–1980. MMWR 33:1SS, 1984

Mankodi RC, Sankari K, Bhatt SM: Primary splenic pregnancy. Br J Obstet Gynaecol 84:634, 1977

Marchbanks PA, Annegers JF, Coulam CB, Strathy JH, Kurland LT: Risk factors for ectopic pregnancy. A population-based study. JAMA 259:1823, 1988

Mashiach S, Carp JHA, Serr DM: Nonoperative management of ectopic pregnancy: A preliminary report. J Reprod Med 27:127, 1982

McCausland A: High rate of ectopic pregnancy following laparoscopic tubal coagulation failures. Am J Obstet Gynecol 136:97, 1980

Merrill BS, Mitts DL, Rogers W, Weinberg PC: Autotransfusion. Intraoperative use in ruptured ectopic pregnancy. J Reprod Med 24:14, 1980

Milwidsky A, Segal S, Menashe M, Adoni A, Palti Z: Corpus luteum function in ectopic pregnancy. Int J Fertil 29:244, 1984

Niebyl JR: Pregnancy following total hysterectomy. Am J Obstet Gynecol 119:512, 1974

O'Connor DM, Kurman RJ: Intermediate trophoblast in uterine currettings in the diagnosis of ectopic pregnancy. Obstet Gynecol 72:665, 1988

Olson CM, Holt JA, Alenghat E, Greco S, Lumpkin JR, Geanon GD: Limitations of qualitative serum beta-hCG assays in the diagnosis of ectopic pregnancy. J Reprod Med 28:838, 1983

Orr JW Jr, Huddleston JF, Knox GE, Goldenberg RL, Davis RO: False negative oxytocin challenge test associated with abdominal pregnancy. Am J Obstet Gynecol 133:108, 1979

Ory HW: The woman's health study: Ectopic pregnancy and intrauterine contraceptive devices: New perspectives. Obstet Gynecol 57:137, 1981

Pais SO, Glickman M, Schwartz P, Pingoud E, Berkowitz R: Embolization of pelvic arteries for control of postpartum hemorrhage. Obstet Gynecol 55:754, 1980

Pittaway DE, Reish RL, Wentz AC: Doubling times of human chorionic gonadotropin increase in early viable intrauterine pregnancies. Am J Obstet Gynecol 152:299, 1985

Poppe W, Van Assche FA, Wilms G, Favril A, Baert A: Pregnancy after transcatheter embolization of a uterine arteriovenous malformation. Am J Obstet Gynecol 156:1179, 1987

Pritchard JA, Adams RH: The fate of blood in the peritoneal cavity. Surg Gynecol Obstet 105:621, 1957

Rahman MS, Al-Suleiman SA, Rahman J, Al-Sibai MH: Advanced abdominal pregnancy—observations in 10 cases. Obstet Gynecol 59:366, 1982

Reece EA, Petrie RH, Sirmans MF, Finster M, Todd WD: Combined intrauterine and extrauterine gestations: A review. Am J Obstet Gynecol 146:323, 1983

Reyniak JV: Conservative microsurgical management of gestation. Wiener Klinisch Wochenschrift 97:481, 1985

Robinson HP, deCrespigny LJC, Harvey J, Hay DL: Ectopic pregnancy—Potentials for diagnosis using ultrasound and urine and serum pregnancy tests. Aust N Z J Obstet Gynaecol 25:49, 1985

Romero R, Kadar N, Castro D, Jeanty P, Hobbins JC, DeCherney AH: The value of adnexal sonographic findings in the diagnosis of ectopic pregnancy. Am J Obstet Gynecol 158:52, 1988

Romney SL, Hertig AT, Reid DE: The endometria associated with ectopic pregnancy. Surg Gynecol Obstet 91:605, 1950

Rubin GL, Peterson HB, Dorfman SF, Layde PM, Maze JM, Ory HW, Cates W Jr: Ectopic pregnancy in the United States: 1970 through 1978. JAMA 249:1725, 1983

Samuellson S, Sjovall A: Laparoscopy in suspected ectopic pregnancy. Acta Obstet Gynecol Scand 51:31, 1972

Schlatter MC, DePree B, Vanderkolk KJ: Hepatic abdominal pregnancy: A case report. J Reprod Med 33:921, 1988

Sherman D, Langer R, Sadovsky G, Bukovsky I, Caspi E: Improved fertility following ectopic pregnancy. Fertil Steril 37:497, 1982

Sopelak VM, Bates GB: Role of transmigration and abnormal embryogenesis in ectopic pregnancy. Clin Obstet Gynecol 30:210, 1987

Spiegelberg O: Casuistry in ovarian pregnancy. Arch Gynaekol 13:73, 1978

Spirtos NM, Spirtos TW, Inouye C, Mishell DR Jr: Resumption of ovulation after ectopic pregnancy. Obstet Gynecol 69:933, 1987

Stangel JJ, Reyniak V, Stone ML: Conservative surgical management of tubal pregnancy. Obstet Gynecol 48:241, 1976

Stock RJ: The changing spectrum of ectopic pregnancy. Obstet Gynecol 71:885, 1988

Strafford JC, Ragan WD: Abdominal pregnancy: Review of current management. Obstet Gynecol 50:548, 1977

Stromme WB: Salpingotomy for tubal pregnancy. Obstet Gynecol 1:473, 1953

Studdiford WD: Primary peritoneal pregnancy. Am J Obstet Gynecol 44:487, 1942

Tanaka T, Hayashi H, Kutsuzawa T, Fujimoto S, Ichinoe K: Treatment of interstitial ectopic pregnancy with methotrexate: Report of a successful case. Fertil Steril 37:851, 1982

Tatum HJ, Schmidt FH: Contraceptive and sterilization practices and extrauterine pregnancy: A realistic perspective. Fertil Steril 28:407, 1977

Timonen S, Nieminen U: Tubal pregnancy, choice of operative method of treatment. Acta Obstet Gynecol Scand 46:327, 1967

Tuomivaara L, Kauppila A, Puolakka J: Ectopic pregnancy—an analysis of the etiology, diagnosis and treatment in 552 cases. Arch Gynecol 237:135, 1986

Ware HH: Observations on thirteen cases of late extrauterine pregnancy. Am J Obstet Gynecol 55:561, 1948

Weström L, Bengtsson LPH, Mårdh P-A: Incidence, trends, and risks of ectopic pregnancy in a population of women. Br Med J: 282:15, 1981

Williams PC, Malvar TC, Kraft JR: Term ovarian pregnancy with delivery of a live female infant. Am J Obstet Gynecol 142:589, 1982

Yackel DB, Panton ONM, Martin DJ, Lee D: Splenic pregnancy - case report. Obstet Gynecol 71:471, 1988

Yaffe H, Navot D, Laufer N: Pitfalls in early detection of ectopic pregnancy. Lancet 1:277, 1979

Yaffe H, Sadovsky E, Beyth Y: Tubal pregnancy and tubal patency. Int J Gynaecol Obstet 14:265, 1976

Diseases and Abnormalities of the Placenta and Fetal Membranes

ABNORMALITIES OF PLACENTATION

MULTIPLE PLACENTAS WITH A SINGLE FETUS

Occasionally, the placenta may be separated into lobes, most frequently two. When the division is incomplete and the vessels of fetal origin extend from one lobe to the other before uniting to form the umbilical cord, the condition is termed *placenta bipartita* or *bilobed placenta* (Fig. 31–1). The reported incidence of this anomaly varies widely, and Fox (1978) cited it at about 1 of 350 deliveries. If the two lobes are entirely separated and the vessels remain distinct, not uniting until just before entering the cord, the condition is designated *placenta duplex*. Sometimes both features are present. Occasionally, there is *placenta triplex* with three distinct lobes, and rarely, more than three lobes are present.

SUCCENTURIATE PLACENTA

An important anomaly is *placenta succenturiata*, in which one or more small accessory lobes are developed in the membranes at a distance from the periphery of the main placenta, to which they usually have vascular connections of fetal origin (see Chap. 4, Figs. 4–26 and 4–27). Accessory lobes are common, and their incidence is about 3 percent. They are of considerable clinical importance because this accessory lobe is sometimes retained in the uterus after expulsion of the main placenta, and when it separates subsequently, it may give rise to serious maternal hemorrhage. If, on examination of the placenta, the physician notes defects in the membranes a short distance from the placental margin, retention of a succenturiate lobe should be suspected. The suspicion is confirmed if vessels extend from the placenta to the margins of the tear. In such cases, even if there is no hemorrhage at the moment, the retained lobe should be removed manually.

RING-SHAPED PLACENTA

Ring-shaped placenta is a rare anomaly that is seen in fewer than 1 in 6,000 deliveries. The placenta is annular in shape and sometimes a complete ring of placental tissue is present, but because of atrophy of a portion of the tissue of the ring, a horseshoe shape is more common. These abnormalities appear to be associated with a greater likelihood of antepartum and postpartum bleeding and fetal growth retardation. Fox (1978) considers this anomaly to be a variant of membranaceous placenta.

MEMBRANACEOUS PLACENTA

In rare circumstances, all of the fetal membranes are covered by functioning villi, and the placenta develops as a thin membranous structure occupying the entire periphery of the chorion. *Placenta membranacea* is also referred to as *placenta diffusa*. Although this abnormality seldom, if ever, interferes with fetal nutrition, it occcasionally gives rise to serious hemorrhage. Diagnosis can be made using sonography (Fig. 31–2). Bleeding resembles that seen in central placenta previa, increasing in severity to necessitate pregnancy interruption by cesarean section, possibly followed by hysterectomy to control bleeding from the large area of implantation. During the third stage of labor, the placenta may not separate readily from its attachment, and manual removal is sometimes very difficult in such cases. An interesting example was described by Las Heras and associates (1982).

FENESTRATED PLACENTA

Fenestrated placenta is a rare anomaly in which the central portion of a discoidal placenta is missing. In some instances, there is an actual hole in the placenta, but more often the defect involves villous tissue only, and the chorionic plate is intact. The clinical significance of this anomaly is that it may be mistakenly considered to represent a missing portion that has been retained in the uterus.

EXTRACHORIAL PLACENTA

In *extrachorial placenta*, the chorionic plate, which is on the fetal side of the placenta, is smaller than the basal plate, which is located on the maternal side. If the fetal surface of such a placenta presents a central depression surrounded by a thickened, grayish-white ring, which is situated at a varying distance from the margins, it is called a *circumvallate placenta*. When the ring coincides with the placental margin, the condition is sometimes described as a marginate or *circummarginate placenta*. Within the ring, the fetal surface presents the usual appearance, gives attachment to the umbilical cord, and shows the usual large vessels that instead of coursing over the entire fetal surface, terminate abruptly at the margin of the ring. In a circumvallate placenta, the ring is composed of a double fold of amnion and chorion, with degenerated decidua and fibrin in between. In a marginate placenta, the chorion and amnion are raised at the margin by interposed decidua and fibrin, without folding of the membranes. These relations

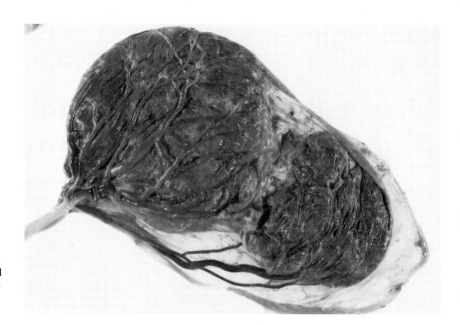

Figure 31–1. Placenta demonstrating bilobed structure, marginal insertion of umbilical cord, and partial velamentous insertion of cord (fetal vessels traversing membranes to reach smaller placental lobe on right).

are illustrated in Figure 31–3. The cause of circumvallate and circummarginate placentation is not understood. Antepartum hemorrhage, prematurity, perinatal deaths, and fetal malformations were reported to be increased for pregnancies with circumvallate placentas (Benirschke, 1974; Lademacher and coworkers, 1981).

LARGE PLACENTAS

While the normal-term placenta weighs on the average about 500 g, in certain diseases, such as syphilis, the placenta may weigh one fourth, one third, or even one half as much as the fetus (see Fig. 33–11, p. 618). The largest placentas are usually encountered in cases of *erythroblastosis fetalis* (see Fig. 33–5, p. 604).

PLACENTAL POLYP

Occasionally, parts of a normal placenta or a succenturiate lobe may be retained after delivery. These may form polyps consisting of villi in varying stages of degeneration and be covered by regenerated endometrium. The clinical sequelae are often subinvolution of the uterus and late postpartum hemorrhage (see Chap. 28, p. 483).

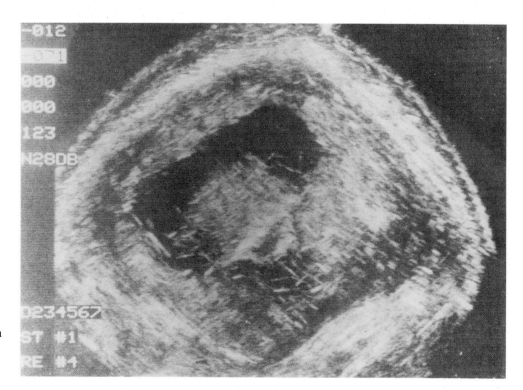

Figure 31–2. Transverse sonogram of 30-week pregnancy with placenta membranacea. (*From Hurley and Beischer: Br J Obstet Gynecol 94:798, 1987, with permission.*)

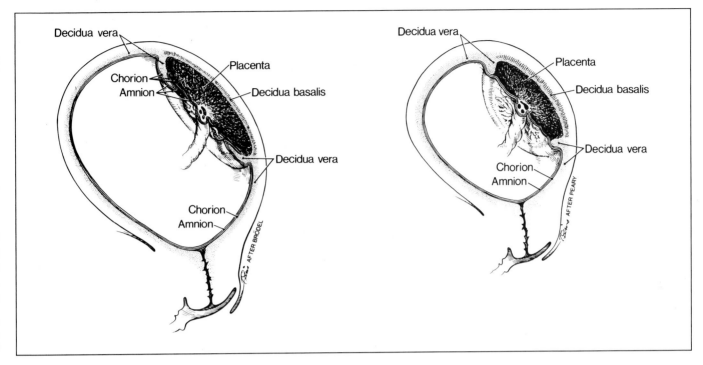

Figure 31–3. Circumvallate (*left*) and marginate (*right*) varieties of extrachorial placentas.

CIRCULATORY DISTURBANCES

PLACENTAL INFARCTS

The most common placental lesions, though of diverse origin, are referred to collectively as placental infarcts. The principal histopathological features include fibrinoid degeneration of the trophoblast, calcification, and ischemic infarction from occlusion of spiral arteries.

Overclassification of these infarcts has led to unnecessary confusion. Small subchorionic and marginal foci of degeneration are present in every placenta. These lesions are of clinical significance only when they are abundant, in which case they may interfere with the function of a sufficiently large portion of the placenta to hamper seriously fetal nutrition, and on occasion cause fetal death. In simplest terms, degenerative lesions of the placenta have two etiological factors in common: (1) changes associated with aging of the trophoblast and (2) impairment of the uteroplacental circulation causing infarction. Nutrition of the placental villi is derived more from the maternal than from the fetal circulation.

Although the placenta is by no means a dying organ at term (see Chap. 4, p. 52), there are morphologic indications of aging. During the latter half of pregnancy, syncytial degeneration begins and *syncytial knots* are formed. At the same time, the villous stroma usually undergoes hyalinization. The syncytium may then break away and float off, exposing the connective tissue directly to maternal blood. Clotting occurs as a result, and propagation of the clot may result in the incorporation of other villi. Macroscopically, such a focus resembles closely an ordinary blood clot, but if not seen until it has become thoroughly organized, on section a firm, white island of tissue is seen.

Around the edge of nearly every term placenta there is a dense yellowish-white fibrous ring representing a zone of degeneration and necrosis, which is usually termed a *marginal infarct*. It may be quite superficial in places, but occasionally it extends 1 to 2 cm into the substance of the placenta. Underneath the chorionic plate, there are nearly always similar lesions, most often pyramidal shaped, ranging from 0.2 cm to 2 or even 3 cm across the base, and extending downward with their apices in the intervillous space (*subchorionic infarcts*). Similar lesions are noted about the intercotyledonary septa, in which case the broadest portion rests upon the maternal surface and the apex points toward the chorionic plate. Occasionally, these lesions meet and form a column of cartilage-like material extending from the maternal surface to the fetal surface. Less frequently, round or oval islands of similar tissue occupy the central portions of the placenta (Fig. 31–4A, B).

The reported frequencies of placental infarction differ greatly for both normal and abnormal pregnancies. Fox (1978) found that about one fourth of placentas from uncomplicated term pregnancies have infarcts. In his experience, placentas in pregnancies complicated by severe hypertensive disease are infarcted in about two thirds of cases.

Calcification of the Placenta

Small calcareous nodules or plaques are observed frequently upon the maternal surface of the placenta and are occasionally so abundant that the organ feels like coarse sandpaper. In view of the widespread degenerative changes in the term placenta, calcification is not surprising. In fact, the conditions for calcium deposition in the aging placenta are almost ideal. Moderate degrees of calcification may be detected in at least half of all placentas examined radiographically. An extensive deposition of calcium is shown in Figure 31–5. Tindall and Scott (1965), in a study of placentas from 3,025 pregnancies, concluded that calcification in the placenta is a normal process, with the amount of calcium deposited increasing in amount throughout the third trimester. Placental calcification may be visualized using sonog-

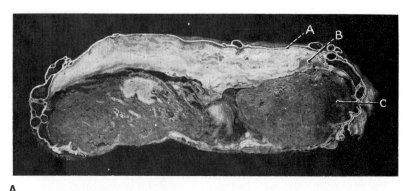

A

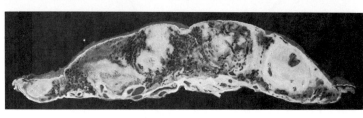

B

Figure 31–4. A. Placental infarcts: A = chorioamnionic membrane; B = fibrin deposited locally beneath the chorion; C = normal placental tissue. In this instance, the infarct was unusually extensive, most likely contributing to the death of the fetus. **B.** Generalized fibrin deposition with little normal tissue remaining.

raphy, and Spirit and colleagues (1982) reported that by 33 weeks more than half of placentas have some degree of calcification. As term approaches, the number of placentas involved, as well as the degree of calcification, increases substantively. Placental calcification graded ultrasonically correlates with fetal lung maturity (Grannum and co-workers, 1979).

CLINICAL SIGNIFICANCE OF DEGENERATIVE CHANGES IN THE PLACENTA

In general, placental infarcts caused either by local deposition of fibrin or by the more acute process of intervillous thrombosis, have little clinical significance, probably because of the relatively large margin of safety for most placental functions. Nonetheless, in certain maternal diseases, notably severe hypertension, the reduction in functioning placenta through infarction, especially when coupled with reduced blood flow to the uterus, may be sufficient to cause fetal death.

Villous (fetal) vessels may show endarteritic thickening and obliteration in association with fetal death. When the placental villi are excluded from their supply of maternal blood by fibrin deposits, hematomas, or direct blockage of the decidual circulation, they become infarcted and die. Histologically, the compromised villi are characterized by fibrosis, obliteration of fetal vessels, and gradual disappearance of the syncytium. Shen-Schwarz and associates (1988) have described hemorrhagic endovasculitis in less than 1 percent of placentas.

VILLOUS (FETAL) ARTERY THROMBOSIS

Thrombosis of a fetal villous stem artery produces a sharply demarcated area of avascularity. Fox (1978) found a single artery thrombosis in 4.5 percent of placentas from normal pregnancies and in 10 percent of those involving diabetic women. Benirschke and Driscoll (1974) observed an association between fetal artery thrombosis and antiplatelet antibodies in maternal serum. Fox (1978) estimated that thrombosis of a single fetal stem artery will deprive only 5 percent of the villi of their blood supply. However, he also observed a few placentas from recent stillbirths in which 40 to 50 percent of the villi were so deprived.

HYPERTROPHIC LESIONS OF THE CHORIONIC VILLI

Striking enlargement of the chorionic villi is seen commonly in association with severe erythroblastosis and fetal hydrops. It has also been described in diabetes and occasionally in severe fetal congestive heart failure.

PLACENTAL ABNORMALITIES DETECTED BY MICROSCOPIC EXAMINATION

Beginning after the 32nd week of gestation, clumps of syncytial nuclei are found to project into the intervillous space, and these are called *syncytial knots*. By term, up to 30 percent of villi may be involved; however, formation of knots by more than a third of villi is considered abnormal (Fox, 1978). In prolonged pregnancies there are marked increases in syncytial knots and avascular villi as the consequence of fetal artery thrombosis. Generally, increased numbers of syncytial knots are found in placentas in which reduced uteroplacental blood flow may have existed—for example, maternal hypertension. However, fetal hypoperfusion of villi appears to be more important in the pathogenesis of this lesion.

It is well recognized that the number of *cytotrophoblastic cells* becomes progressively reduced as pregnancy advances. In a normal mature placenta, cytotrophoblastic cells are found in about 20 percent of the villi (Fox, 1978). Most often, at this stage of pregnancy such cells are few and inconspicuous. However, numerous cytotrophoblastic cells are found in placentas of pregnant women with diabetes mellitus and erythroblastosis fetalis. Increased numbers of cytotrophoblasts have also been observed in placentas from women with pregnancy-induced hypertension, and the number seems to increase progressively with the severity and duration of preeclampsia.

Inflammation of the Placenta

Changes that are now recognized as various forms of degeneration and necrosis were formerly described under the term *placentitis*. For example, small placental cysts with grumous contents were formerly thought to be abscesses. Nonetheless, especially in cases of prolonged rupture of the membranes,

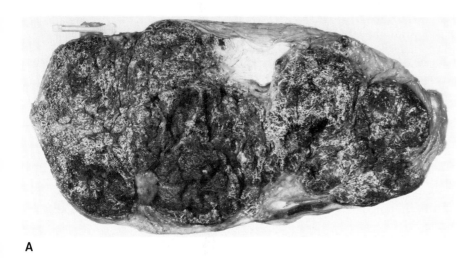

A

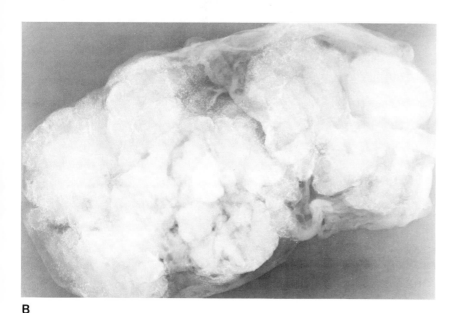

B

Figure 31–5. A. Placental calcification is evident as gray plaques on the maternal surface of the placenta, a common finding at term. **B.** A radiograph of the same placenta emphasizes the extensive calcification.

pyogenic bacteria do invade the fetal surface of the placenta and, after gaining access to the chorionic vessels, give rise to generalized infection of the fetus.

ABNORMALITIES OF THE UMBILICAL CORD (FUNIS)

ABNORMALITIES IN CORD LENGTH

Umbilical cord length varies appreciably, with the mean length being about 55 cm (Rayburn and associates, 1981). Extremes in cord length in abnormal instances range from apparently no cord (achordia) to lengths up to 300 cm. Vascular occlusion by thrombi and true knots are more common in excessively long cords, and they are more likely to prolapse through the cervix. Rarely, excessively short umbilical cords may be instrumental in abruptio placenta and uterine inversion. They may rupture with intrafunicular hemorrhage, which can cause fetal death from exsanguination.

An intriguing question is, "What factors determine the length of the umbilical cord?" Studies performed on animals and experiments of nature in human pregnancy support the concept that the length of the cord is influenced positively by the volume of amnionic fluid and by the mobility of the fetus. Miller and associates (1981) identified the human umbilical cord to be appreciably shortened when there had been either chronic fetal constraint from oligohydramnios or decreased fetal movement because of limb dysfunction. Excessive cord length may be the consequence of entanglement of cord and fetus and stretching of the cord during fetal movement. Soernes and Bakke (1986) reported that the mean cord length in fetuses presenting as breech was about 5 cm shorter than those with vertex presentations. They interpreted this as consistent with the theory that less mobile fetuses more frequently assumed the breech position.

ABSENCE OF ONE UMBILICAL ARTERY

Benirschke and Brown (1955) were principally responsible for drawing attention to the single umbilical artery and its frequent linkage with fetal malformation. The absence of one umbilical artery, according to Benirschke and Dodds (1967), characterized

0.85 percent of all cords in singletons and 5 percent of the cords of at least one twin. About 30 percent of all infants with one umbilical artery missing had associated congenital anomalies.

Bryan and Kohler (1974) identified the umbilical cords of 143 infants, or 0.72 percent, to have a single artery out of nearly 20,000 examined. Infants with a single-artery cord had an 18 percent incidence of major malformations, 34 percent were growth-retarded, and 17 percent delivered preterm. In the studies of Froehlich and Fujikura (1973), mortality was very high (14 percent) among infants with a single umbilical artery; but of those who survived infancy, serious anomalies were not much more common than in the control group. However, Bryan and Kohler (1974) followed beyond infancy 90 infants with a single umbilical artery and found previously unrecognized malformations in 10.

Peckham and Yerushalmy (1965) demonstrated that a single umbilical artery occurred twice as often in newborns of white women than in those of black women. The incidence is considerably increased in newborns of women with diabetes mellitus, a condition associated with a threefold increase in anomalous fetuses. Based on the finding of a high incidence of fetal malformations when a single umbilical artery exists, each umbilical cord should be examined carefully to ascertain the number of umbilical arteries present.

As expected, two-vessel cords are more frequently identified in fetuses aborted spontaneously, and Benirschke and Brown (1955) reported this to be 2.5 percent. Byrne and Blanc (1986) studied 879 consecutively aborted fetuses and identified a single umbilical artery in 1.5 percent. Eight of these 13 fetuses had serious malformations, most associated with chromosomal abnormalities.

FOUR-VESSEL CORD

Additional umbilical vessels are rarely apparent on casual examination; however, careful examination may disclose a venous remnant in 5 percent of cases (Fox, 1978). Four-vessel cords with an obvious extra umbilical vein were reported (Painter and Russell, 1977), but it is difficult to say whether the condition is associated with an increased incidence of fetal anomalies.

ABNORMALITIES OF CORD INSERTION

The umbilical cord usually, but not always, is inserted at or near the center of the fetal surface of the placenta.

Marginal Insertion

Insertion of the cord at the placental margin is sometimes referred to as a *battledore placenta*. Some have reported that such an insertion is more common in instances of preterm labor, but this opinion is not widely held (Robinson and co-workers, 1983).

Velamentous Insertion of Cord

Of considerable practical importance is velamentous insertion of the cord, since the umbilical vessels separate in the membranes at a distance from the placental margin, which they reach surrounded only by a fold of amnion (Figs. 31–1 and 31–6). This mode of insertion is noted in a little over 1 percent of singleton deliveries but much more frequently with twins, and it is almost the rule with triplets. With velamentous insertion of the cord the likelihood of fetal deformity is increased (Robinson and co-workers, 1983).

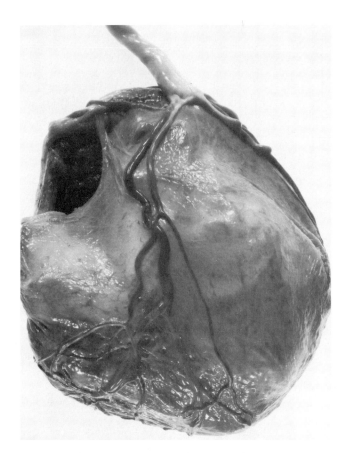

Figure 31–6. Velamentous insertion of cord. The placenta (*bottom*) and membranes have been inverted to expose the amnion. Note the large fetal vessels within membranes (*top*) and their proximity to the site of rupture of the membranes.

Vasa Previa

When with velamentous insertion, some of the fetal vessels in the membranes cross the region of the internal os and occupy a position ahead of the presenting part of the fetus, the condition is termed *vasa previa*. At times, the careful examiner will be able to palpate a tubular fetal vessel in the membranes overlying the presenting part. Compression of the vessels between the examining finger and the presenting part is likely to induce changes in the fetal heart rate. At times, the vessels may be visualized directly by employing amnioscopy, or they may be seen on ultrasonic examination (Fig. 31–7).

With vasa previa, there is considerable potential danger to the fetus, for rupture of the membranes may be accompanied by rupture of a fetal vessel with subsequent exsanguination of the infant.

Whenever there is hemorrhage antepartum or intrapartum, the possibility of vasa previa and a ruptured fetal vessel exists. Unfortunately, the amount of fetal blood that can be shed without killing the fetus is relatively small compared to the volumes of blood that usually cause concern with antepartum or intrapartum hemorrhage of maternal origin. Blood can be ascertained to be of fetal origin by demonstrating resistance of hemoglobin to denaturation with alkali. A quick, readily available approach is to smear the blood on glass slides, stain the smears with Wright's stain, and examine for nucleated red cells. Nucleated red cells are normally present in cord blood but are rarely so in maternal blood. Messer and colleagues (1987) re-

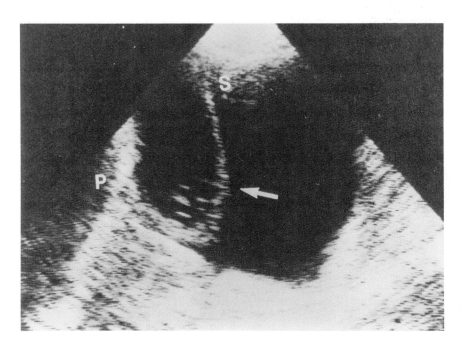

Figure 31–7. Sonogram showing placenta (*P*), succenturiate lobe (*S*), and leading fetal vessels in *vasa previa* (*arrow*). (*From Gianopoulos and colleagues: Obstet Gynecol 69:488, 1987.*)

ported that of 107 obstetricians at medical schools and 52 at community hospitals who returned a survey questionnaire, only about 15 percent routinely tested for fetal blood in late pregnancy bleeding.

The pessimism expressed by Kouyoumdjian (1980) for improving fetal salvage once a vessel is ruptured is probably justified. The likelihood of a poor fetal outcome in spite of vigorous therapy is made evident by the following case of vasa previa and fetal hemorrhage with prompt intervention:

Spontaneous premature rupture of the membranes at 36 weeks gestation was not soon followed by spontaneous labor. In preparation for oxytocin stimulation, an electrode was applied to the fetal scalp through a cervix dilated 2 cm. This was followed immediately by bleeding through the cervix into the vagina. There had been no bleeding before this. The previously normal fetal heart rate dropped to 70 per minute. Delivery of the fetus by cesarean section was performed less than 10 minutes after the application of the electrode. The infant was treated intensively but unsuccessfully with cardiopulmonary resuscitation, saline, sodium bicarbonate, and O negative blood.

CORD ABNORMALITIES CAPABLE OF IMPEDING BLOOD FLOW

Several mechanical and vascular abnormalities of the umbilical cord are capable of impairing fetal-placental blood flow.

Knots of the Cord
False knots, which result from kinking of the vessels to accommodate to the length of the cord, should be distinguished from *true knots*, which result from active movements of the fetus. In nearly 17,000 deliveries in the Collaborative Study on Cerebral Palsy, Spellacy and co-workers (1966) found an incidence of true knots of 1.1 percent. Perinatal loss was 6.1 percent in the presence of true knots. The incidence of true knots is especially high in monoamnionic twins.

Loops of the Cord
The cord frequently becomes coiled around portions of the fetus, usually the neck. In 1,000 consecutive deliveries studied by

Kan and Eastman (1957), the incidence of the umbilical cord around the neck ranged from one loop in 21 percent to three loops in 0.2 percent. Fortunately, coiling of the cord around the neck is an uncommon cause of fetal death. Typically, as labor progresses and the fetus descends the birth canal, contractions compress the cord vessels, which cause fetal heart-rate deceleration that persists until the contraction ceases. Hankins and colleagues (1987) reported 110 pregnancies in which labor at term was complicated by a nuchal cord. Compared to control infants, those with a nuchal cord had more moderate or severe variable fetal heart-rate decelerations in labor (19 versus 5 percent) and were more likely to be acidemic (20 versus 12 percent). With unrelenting occlusion, recognition and prompt delivery minimize the risk of fetal death or severe morbidity. In monoamnionic twinning, a significant fraction of the high perinatal mortality rate is attributed to entwining of the umbilical cords before labor (see Fig. 34–639).

Torsion of the Cord
As a result of fetal movements, the cord normally becomes twisted. Occasionally, the torsion is so marked that fetal circulation is compromised. Extreme degrees of torsion probably occur only after the death of the fetus by a mechanism that is not understood.

Stricture of the Cord
Most, but not all, infants with cord stricture are stillborns, and it seems that the stricture plays a role in producing fetal death (Fig. 31–8). Cord stricture, for unknown reasons, is associated with an extreme focal deficiency in Wharton's jelly. Stricture is commonly associated, causally, with torsion.

Hematoma of the Cord
Hematomas occasionally result from the rupture of a varix, usually of the umbilical vein, with effusion of blood into the cord (Fig. 31–9). More recently, cord hematomas have been described as resulting from ultrasound-directed umbilical vessel venipuncture. Sonographic visualization of a large cord he-

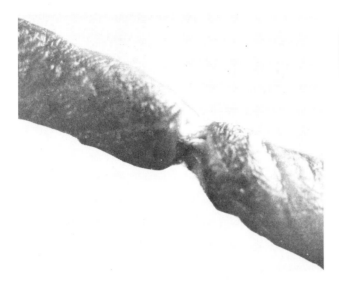

Figure 31–8. A sharply localized stricture in a cord from a stillborn infant. (*From Fox: Pathology of the Placenta, Philadelphia, Saunders, 1978, Volume 7, p. 442.*)

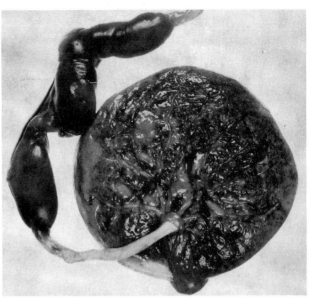

Figure 31–9. Hematoma of the umbilical cord.

matoma and a dead fetus was described (Ruvinsky and associates, 1981). Fox (1978), who reviewed the subject carefully, believes it unwise to attribute fetal death to a cord hematoma until other causes have been excluded.

Cysts of the Cord

Cysts occasionally are found along the course of the cord and are designated true and false, according to their origin. True cysts are quite small and may be derived from remnants of the umbilical vesicle or of the allantois. False cysts, which may attain considerable size, result from liquefaction of Wharton's jelly. Such cysts may be detected by sonography but are difficult to identify precisely. For example, the cord cyst demonstrated in Figures 31–10 A, B was thought possibly to be a meningocele when detected by sonography, since the cyst maintained a close and constant relationship over time with the lower spine of the fetus.

Edema of the Cord

Cord edema rarely occurs by itself but is frequently associated with edema of the fetus. It is very common with macerated fetuses.

GESTATIONAL TROPHOBLASTIC DISEASE

Gestational trophoblastic disease refers to a spectrum of pregnancy-related trophoblastic proliferative abnormalities, the classification of which for many years was based principally on histological criteria and included hydatidiform mole, chorioadenoma destruens, and choriocarcinoma. In 1973, Hammond and colleagues proposed a clinical diagnostic spectrum for gestational trophoblastic diseases based principally upon clinical findings and serial determinations of chorionic gonadotropin, which is secreted by the abnormal tissue. Although these two classifications have caused some confusion, the clinical one is now accepted.

Hydatidiform mole, also commonly referred to as molar pregnancy, is diagnosed when hydropic villi are identified grossly. The terms invasive mole and chorioadenoma destruens were once used to describe trophoblastic overgrowth with penetration into or through the myometrium. To make this diagnosis, however, required either deep curettings or a hysterectomy specimen, and the terms now are seldom used. The histological term choriocarcinoma still is used to describe the extremely malignant variant of trophoblastic disease that frequently metastasizes and formerly was almost invariably fatal.

The classification currently used is shown in Table 31–1. These diagnostic categories are arrived at by clinical examination that includes an assessment for extrauterine metastases. Initial evaluation of molar pregnancy includes chest x-ray, and classification is based upon trends in serum levels of chorionic gonadotropin measured by sensitive assay of the β-subunit. If metastatic disease is suspected, either because of clinical or x-ray findings or persistently elevated or rising serum chorionic gonadotropin levels, then a more thorough work-up is pursued. More recently, computed tomography has been used to evaluate the liver and brain, which are common sites of metastases. Thus, the term *gestational trophoblastic neoplasia* refers to persistent trophoblastic tissue that is presumably malignant and is identified by its continued secretion of chorionic gonadotropin. By clinical evaluation, the tissue may be confined to the uterus, and thus nonmetastatic, or it may have metastasized to any of several other organs.

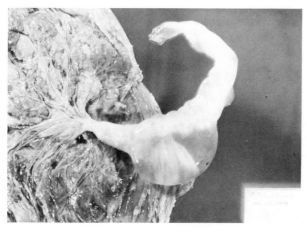

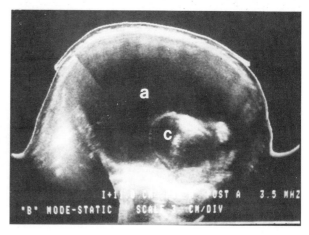

A   **B**

Figure 31–10. A. Cyst of umbilical cord at 27 weeks gestation in a monoamnionic twin pregnancy, further complicated by symptomatic acute hydramnios and marked discordance in the size of the fetuses. (*Courtesy of Dr. K. Leveno.*) **B.** Sonogram from the same case demonstrating the cyst of the cord (*c*) and marked hydramnios (*a*). The possibility that the cyst was a meningocele was considered originally. In spite of removal of fluid by amniocentesis and intravenous ritodrine, labor progressed. (*Courtesy of Dr. R. Santos.*)

HYDATIDIFORM MOLE (MOLAR PREGNANCY)

Histologically, hydatidiform moles are characterized by abnormalities of the chorionic villi, consisting of varying degrees of trophoblastic proliferation and edema of villous stroma. Moles usually occupy the uterine cavity; however, they may rarely be located in the oviduct and even the ovary (Stanhope and associates, 1983). The development of these trophoblastic diseases is interesting, and the presence or absence of fetal tissue has been used to classify them into *complete (classic)* and *partial (incomplete)* moles (Table 31–2).

COMPLETE (CLASSIC) HYDATIDIFORM MOLE

The chorionic villi are converted into a mass of clear vesicles (Fig. 31–11). The vesicles vary in size from barely visible to a few cm in diameter and often hang in clusters from thin pedicles. The mass may grow large enough to fill the uterus to the size occupied by an advanced normal pregnancy.

The histological structure demonstrated in Figure 31–12 is characterized by (1) hydropic degeneration and swelling of the villous stroma, (2) absence of blood vessels in the swollen villi,

(3) proliferation of the trophoblastic epithelium to a varying degree, and (4) absence of fetus and amnion.

Cytogenetic studies of complete molar pregnancies have identified the chromosomal composition most often, but not always, to be 46,XX, with the chromosomes completely of paternal origin. This phenomenon is referred to as *androgenesis.* Typically, the ovum has been fertilized by a haploid sperm, which then duplicates its own chromosomes after meiosis. The chromosomes of the ovum are either absent or inactivated. However, all complete hydatidiform moles are not so characterized, and infrequently, the chromosomal pattern in a complete mole may be 46,XY (Bagshawe and Lawler, 1982; Dodson, 1983).

TABLE 31–1. CLINICAL CLASSIFICATION OF GESTATIONAL TROPHOBLASTIC DISEASE

Hydatidiform mole (molar pregnancy)
Complete, or classic
Incomplete, or partial

Gestational trophoblastic neoplasia
Nonmetastatic
Metastatic
  Low risk (good prognosis)
  High risk (poor prognosis)

TABLE 31–2. CHARACTERISTICS OF PARTIAL AND COMPLETE HYDATIDIFORM MOLES

Feature	Partial (Incomplete) Mole	Complete (Classic) Mole
Embryonic or fetal tissue	Present	Absent
Hydatidiform swelling of villi	Focal	Diffuse
Trophoblastic hyperplasia	Focal	Diffuse
Stromal inclusions	Present	Absent
Villous scalloping	Present	Absent
Karyotype	Paternal and Maternal 69,XXY or 69,XYY	Paternal 46,XX (96%) 46,XY (4%)
Trophoblastic neoplasia	~5% (choriocarcinoma rare)	~20%

From Berkowitz and co-workers: Contemp Ob/Gyn, 27:77, 1986.

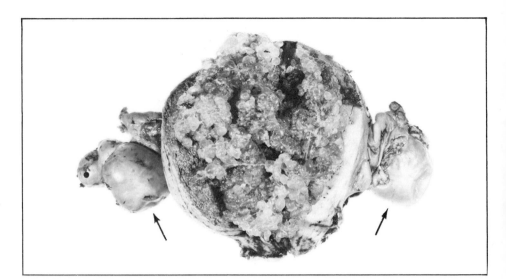

Figure 31–11. A complete (classic) hydatidiform mole characterized grossly by abundance of edematous enlarged chorionic villi but no fetus or fetal membranes. Note theca-lutein cysts in each ovary (*arrows*).

In this circumstance, two sperm have fertilized an ovum lacking chromosomes. Other variations also have been described—for example, 45,X. Thus, a morphologically complete hydatidiform mole can result from a variety of chromosomal patterns.

The risk of trophoblastic neoplasia developing from a complete mole is approximately 20 percent.

PARTIAL (INCOMPLETE) HYDATIDIFORM MOLE

When the hydatidiform changes are focal and less advanced, and there is a fetus or at least an amnionic sac, the condition has been classified as a partial hydatidiform mole. There is slowly progressing hydatidiform swelling of some usually avascular villi, while other vascular villi with a functioning fetal-placental circulation are spared (Fig. 31–13). Trophoblastic hyperplasia is focal rather than generalized. The karyotype typically is triploid,

either 69,XXY or 69,XYY, with one maternal but usually two paternal haploid complements (Berkowitz and colleagues, 1986). The fetus typically has stigmata of triploidy, which includes multiple congential malformations and growth retardation.

The risk of choriocarcinoma arising from a partial hydatidiform mole is slight; however, nonmetastatic gestational trophoblastic neoplasia may follow in 4 to 8 percent of partial moles, according to Szulman and Surti (1982), Czernobilisky and colleagues (1982), and Berkowitz and colleagues (1986).

Molar Degeneration

Difference of opinion remains as to when gross or histological hydatid villous changes warrant the term partial hydatidiform mole and when they are simply molar degeneration. Hertig and Edmonds (1940) found that two thirds of aborted pathological ova had early molar degeneration.

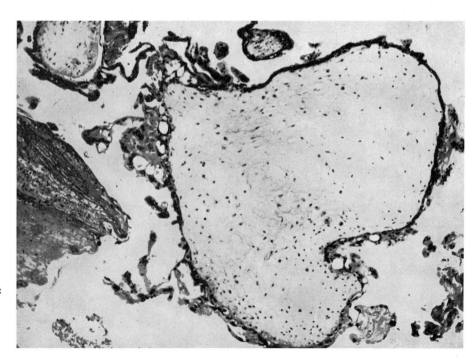

Figure 31–12. Photomicrograph of a hydatidiform mole with slight to moderate trophoblastic hyperplasia, confined to the syncytium and considered as probably benign. (*From Smalbraak:* Trophoblastic Growths. *Haarlem, Netherlands, Elsevier, 1957.*)

HISTOLOGICAL DIAGNOSIS

Attempts to relate the histological structure of individual complete hydatidiform moles to their subsequent malignant tendencies generally have been disappointing. Novak and Seah (1954), for example, were unable to establish precisely such a relation in 120 cases of hydatidiform mole or in the molar tissue in 26 cases of choriocarcinoma following hydatidiform mole.

OVARIAN THECA-LUTEIN CYSTS

In many cases of hydatidiform mole, the ovaries contain multiple theca-lutein cysts (Fig. 31–11), which may vary from microscopic size to 10 cm or more in diameter. The surfaces of the cysts are smooth, often yellowish, and lined with lutein cells. The incidence of obvious cysts in association with a mole is reported to be from 25 percent to as high as 60 percent.

Theca-lutein cysts of the ovaries are thought to result from overstimulation of lutein elements by large amounts of chorionic gonadotropin secreted by proliferating trophoblast. In general, extensive cystic change is usually associated with larger hydatidiform moles and a long period of stimulation. Montz and colleagues (1988) reported that persistent trophoblastic disease was more likely in women with theca-lutein cysts, especially if bilateral. Theca-lutein cysts are not limited to cases of hydatidiform mole, and they may be associated with placental hypertrophy with fetal hydrops or multifetal pregnancy.

Very large cysts especially may undergo torsion, infarction, and hemorrhage. However, oophorectomy should not be performed because of theca-lutein cysts; after delivery of the mole, the cysts eventually regress. At times, after evacuation of a mole, paradoxically, the cystic ovaries enlarge before they regress.

INCIDENCE

Hydatidiform mole develops in approximately 1 of about 2,000 pregnancies in the United States and Europe, but it is much more frequent in other countries, especially in parts of Asia where the frequency is at least 10 times that of the United States. A surprisingly high incidence also has been identified in Mexico and among native Alaskans. Grimes (1984) recently provided a review on the epidemiology of trophoblastic disease.

Age

There is a relatively high frequency of hydatidiform mole among pregnancies toward the beginning or end of the childbearing period. The most pronounced effect of age is seen in women older than 45, when the relative frequency of the lesion is more than 10 times greater than at ages 20 to 40. There are numerous authenticated cases of hydatidiform mole in women 50 years old and older, whereas normal pregnancy at such advanced ages is practically unknown (Jequier and Winterton, 1975).

Previous Mole

Recurrence of hydatidiform mole is uncommon, but it is seen in about 2 percent of cases. Wu (1973) described a woman who had nine consecutive molar pregnancies!

CLINICAL COURSE

In the very early stages of development of the mole, there are few characteristics to distinguish it from normal pregnancy, but later in the first trimester and during the second trimester the following changes are often evident. Symptoms are more likely to be dramatic with a classic, or complete, mole. Schlaerth and colleagues (1988) reported complications in two thirds of 381 women with molar pregnancies.

Bleeding

Uterine bleeding is the outstanding sign and may vary from spotting to profuse hemorrhage. It may begin just before abortion or, more often, it occurs intermittently for weeks or even months. As the consequence of such bleeding, anemia is rather

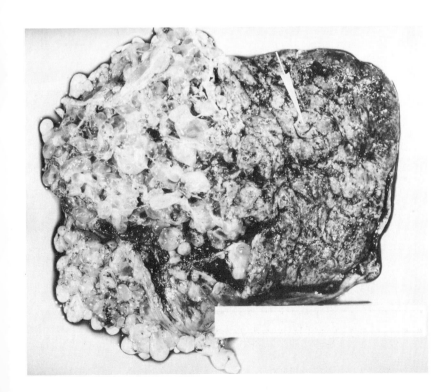

Figure 31–13. Molar placenta on the left and normal placenta (*white arrow*) on the right. The molar placenta was identified by sonography late in pregnancy when the mother developed preeclampsia. A healthy fetus was delivered near term by cesarean section. Most likely, this is a case of twins consisting of a placenta with a fetus from one ovum and a complete mole developing from the other ovum.

common. Moreover, a dilutional effect from appreciable hypervolemia has been demonstrated in some women with larger moles. At times, there may be considerable hemorrhage concealed within the uterus. Iron-deficiency anemia is a common finding and infrequently megaloblastic erythropoiesis is evident, presumably as a result of poor dietary intake because of nausea and vomiting coupled with increased folate requirement imposed by rapidly proliferating trophoblast.

Uterine Size
The growing uterus often, but not always, enlarges more rapidly than usual. In about half of the cases, uterine size clearly exceeds that expected from the duration of gestation. The uterus may be difficult to identify precisely by palpation in the nulliparous woman especially, because of its soft consistency beneath a firm abdominal wall. At times ovaries appreciably enlarged by multiple theca-lutein cysts may be difficult to distinguish from the enlarged uterus. The ovaries are likely to be tender.

Fetal Activity
Even though the uterus is enlarged sufficiently to reach well above the symphysis, typically no fetal heart action is detected even with sensitive instruments. Rarely, there may be twin placentas with a complete molar pregnancy developing in one, while the other placenta and its fetus appear normal. Also, very infrequently there may be extensive but incomplete molar change in the placenta accompanied by a living fetus (Fig. 31–14). Six cases of a fetus with either an incomplete hydatidiform mole for a placenta or with a normal placenta plus a "twin" hydatidiform mole were described by Block and Merrill (1982).

Pregnancy-Induced Hypertension
Of special importance is the frequent association of preeclampsia with molar pregnancies that persist into the second trimester. Since pregnancy-induced hypertension is rarely seen before 24 weeks, preeclampsia that develops before this time strongly suggests hydatidiform mole or extensive molar change.

Embolization
Variable amounts of trophoblast with or without villous stroma escape from the uterus in the venous outflow. The volume may be such as to produce signs and symptoms of acute pulmonary embolism and even a fatal outcome (Fig. 31–15). Such fatalities are rare. Hankins and colleagues (1987) obtained hemodynamic measurements using a pulmonary-artery catheter in six women with large molar pregnancies cared for at Parkland Hospital. They also searched for evidence of trophoblastic deportation before and during molar evacuation. Only small numbers of multinucleated giant cells and mononuclear cells, presumably trophoblasts, were identified. They found no evidence for acute cardiorespiratory changes, and concluded that massive trophoblastic embolization with molar evacuation was probably infrequent. Schlaerth and co-workers (1988) identified respiratory complications in 15 percent of women with a mole larger than 20-weeks' size.

Even though trophoblast, with or without villous stroma, embolizes to the lungs in volumes too small to produce overt blockade of the pulmonary vasculature, these subsequently can invade the pulmonary parenchyma to establish metastases that are evident radiographically. The lesions may consist of trophoblast alone (metastatic choriocarcinoma) or trophoblast with villous stroma (metastatic hydatidiform mole). The subsequent course of such lesions is unpredictable, and some have been observed to disappear spontaneously either soon after uterine evacuation or even weeks to months later, while others proliferate and kill the woman unless she is effectively treated.

Thyroid Dysfunction
Plasma thyroxine levels in women with molar pregnancy are usually elevated appreciably, but clinically apparent hyperthyroidism is less common. Amir and colleagues (1984) and Curry and associates (1975) identified hyperthyroidism in about 2 percent of cases. Plasma thyroxine elevation may be the effect primarily of estrogen, as in normal pregnancy, in which case free thyroxine levels are not elevated and the percentage of triiodothyronine bound by resin is increased. It remains controversial whether free thyroxine can be elevated as the consequence of the thyrotropin-like effect of chorionic gonadotropin, or whether variants of this hormone produce these effects (Amir and co-workers, 1984; Mann and colleagues, 1986).

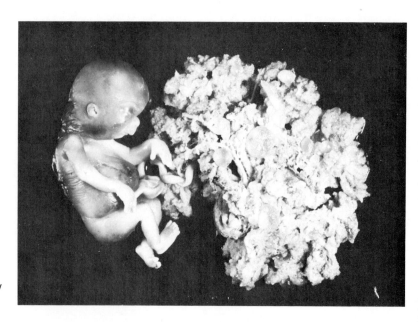

Figure 31–14. Extensive molar change and a fetus of 20 weeks gestation. The pregnancy was complicated further by eclampsia.

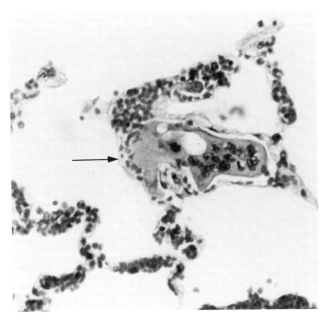

Figure 31–15. An embolus of trophoblast within a small pulmonary vein (*arrow*). The woman died from trophoblastic embolization complicated further by massive hemorrhage soon after hysterotomy to evacuate a large hydatidiform mole.

Spontaneous Expulsion

Occasionally, hydatid vesicles, or grapes, are passed before the mole is aborted spontaneously or removed by operation. Spontaneous expulsion is most likely around 16 weeks and is rarely delayed beyond 28 weeks.

DIAGNOSTIC FEATURES

Persistent bleeding and a uterus larger than the expected size arouse suspicion of a mole (Fig. 31–16A, B). Consideration must be given to an error in menstrual data or a pregnant uterus further enlarged by myomas, hydramnios, or especially multiple fetuses.

Ultrasound

The greatest diagnostic accuracy is obtained from the characteristic ultrasonic appearance of hydatidiform mole (Fig. 31–17A, B). The safety and precision of sonography make it the technique of choice. However, it must be kept in mind that some other structures may have an appearance similar to that of a mole, including uterine myoma with early pregnancy and pregnancies with multiple fetuses. A careful review of the history, coupled with careful sonar evaluation repeated in a week or two when necessary, should serve to avoid the incorrect sonographic diagnosis of hydatidiform mole when the pregnancy is actually normal.

Amniogram

Transabdominal intrauterine instillation of a radiopaque substance produces a characteristic radiograph in cases of hydatidiform mole. The uterine cavity is penetrated with the needle as for amniocentesis, 20 mL of Hypaque is injected quickly, and 5 to 10 minutes later an anteroposterior radiograph is made. A characteristic honeycombed x-ray pattern is produced by contrast material surrounding the chorionic vesicles. With a normal pregnancy, there is a

slight risk of abortion from the intra-amnionic injection of hypertonic contrast material. With the widespread availability of sonography this technique is seldom used now.

Chorionic Gonadotropin Measurements

Serum chorionic gonadotropin assay is sometimes used for diagnosis if a reliable quantitative method of measurements is available and the considerable variation in gonadotropin secretion in normal pregnancy is appreciated, especially the elevated levels that sometimes accompany pregnancy with multiple fetuses (see Chap. 5, p. 68). For the most part, however, these assays are no longer used for diagnosis, having been replaced by ultrasound evaluation. As discussed subsequently, serial determinations of chorionic gonadotropin are used to detect persistent gestational trophoblastic disease following molar evacuation.

In summary, the clinical and diagnostic features of a complete hydatidiform mole are:

1. Continuous or intermittent bloody discharge evident by about 12 weeks of pregnancy, usually not profuse, and often more nearly brown rather than red.
2. Uterine enlargement out of proportion to the duration of pregnancy in about half of the cases.
3. Absence of fetal parts on palpation and of fetal heart sounds even though the uterus may be enlarged to the level of the umbilicus or higher.
4. Characteristic ultrasonic appearance.
5. A very high serum chorionic gonadotropin level 100 days or more after the last menstrual period.
6. Preeclampsia–eclampsia developing before 24 weeks of gestation.

PROGNOSIS

In a collective review of 576 cases, Mathieu in 1939 found an immediate mortality rate of 1.4 percent. Since this report, mortality has been reduced practically to zero by more prompt diagnosis and appropriate therapy. With advanced molar pregnancies, these women usually are anemic and bleeding acutely. Intrauterine infection and sepsis in these cases may cause serious morbidity (Schlaerth and colleagues, 1988).

Nearly 20 percent of complete moles progress to gestational trophoblastic neoplasia. Rarely, years may intervene between molar pregnancy and the development of choriocarcinoma; and Natsume and Takada (1961) reported a woman in whom choriocarcinoma developed nine years after hysterectomy for invasive mole. From the subsequent course of 181 patients (Table 31–3) followed before the use of chemotherapy, it is evident that only a very small percentage of cases developed a lethal malignant tumor. A sizable proportion regressed spontaneously or were cured by surgical procedures, including curettage. It is precisely this spectrum of lesions, ranging from completely benign to highly malignant, with a rather unpredictable intermediate group, that has produced dilemmas in diagnosis unmatched by few other tumors.

TREATMENT

The treatment for hydatidiform mole consists of two phases, including the immediate evacuation of the mole and the later follow-up for detection of persistent trophoblastic proliferation

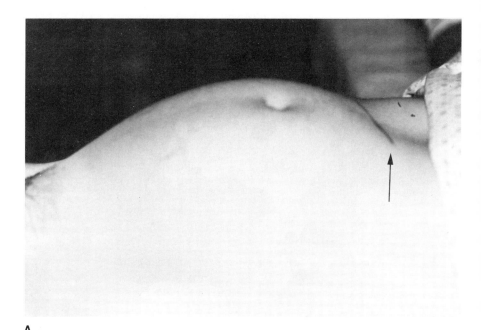

A

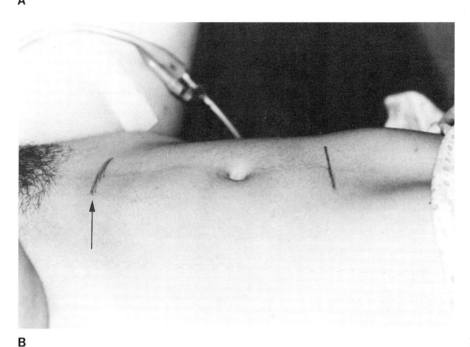

Figure 31–16. A. The uterine fundus (*arrow*) rises 27 cm above the symphysis in a woman with a complete hydatidiform mole 17 weeks after her last menstrual period. **B.** The uterine fundus (*arrow*) has decreased markedly immediately after evacuating the large hydatidiform mole by suction.

B

or malignant change. Initial evaluation prior to evacuation or hysterectomy includes at least a cursory search for metastatic disease. A chest radiograph should be done to look for pulmonary lesions. Although Mutch and colleagues (1986) showed that using computed tomography increased the likelihood of detecting metastatic disease, its routine use has not been evaluated. Unless there is other evidence of extrauterine disease, routine computed tomography or magnetic resonance imaging to evaluate the liver or brain is not routinely done.

In the rare circumstance of twinning with a complete hydatidiform mole plus a fetus and placenta, the possibility of allowing the fetus to mature in utero must be considered. Neither the risks to the mother nor the likelihood of a healthy offspring have been established. Suzuki and associates (1980) reported a case in which the outcome was a healthy infant and healthy mother, and cited several other previously reported instances. We have managed such pregnancies to favorable outcomes for both mother and fetus (Fig. 31–13).

Termination of Molar Pregnancy

Because of greater awareness, and certainly because of better technique for diagnosis, especially sonography, moles now are terminated more often when they are likely still to be small, and under controlled circumstances rather than the chaos commonly associated with their spontaneous abortion. Thus there is time for adequate evaluation of the woman who may be anemic, hypertensive, or fluid-depleted, or who shows any combination of these.

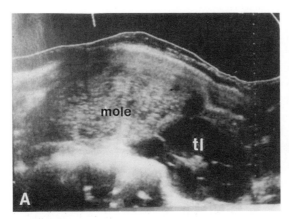
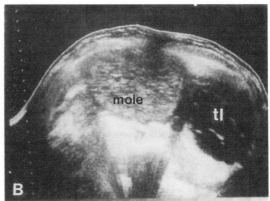

Figure 31–17. A. Longitudinal sonogram demonstrating a complete hydatidiform mole that fills a uterus enlarged to well above the umbilicus. A large theca-lutein cyst (*tl*) is seen above the uterus. **B.** Transverse sonogram of the same patient. (*Courtesy of Dr. R. Santos.*)

Prophylactic Chemotherapy

Although some advocate prophylactic chemotherapy before evacuation, this is questioned because of the complications that accompany molar evacuation. These include hemorrhage, uterine perforation, and infection. At times, evacuation initiated vaginally eventuates in hysterectomy. In these circumstances, the chemotherapeutic agents may contribute to morbidity and even mortality.

Goldstein (1974) and others earlier questioned the wisdom and necessity of administering toxic chemotherapeutic agents to women who, in the great majority of instances, will have a benign course subsequent to evacuation. The minority of women who will demonstrate persistent trophoblastic neoplasia may then be treated quite successfully. Moreover, it is essential that women treated prophylactically be followed just as closely as if they had not been treated, since there is failure of prophylactic chemotherapy, albeit infrequent. Curry and associates (1975) concurred with Goldstein that the benefits from prophylactic chemotherapy so administered to women with moles do not justify the additional risks. They noted two deaths caused by toxicity from prophylactic chemotherapy. Kim and colleagues (1986) recently reported a randomized study in which they gave prophylactic methotrexate to high-risk patients, and this reduced the incidence of persistent trophoblastic disease from 47 to 14 percent.

TABLE 31–3. SUBSEQUENT COURSE OF 181 WOMEN WITH HYDATIDIFORM MOLE FOLLOWED PRIOR TO 1947 AND GIVEN NO CHEMOTHERAPY

Outcome	Percent
Spontaneous resolution	73.0
Chorioepithelioma in situ [a]	3.5
Syncytial endometritis [b]	4.5
Chorioadenoma destruens	16.0
Choriocarcinoma	2.5

[a] Chorioepithelioma in situ: small, discrete mass of superficially invasive, apparently malignant trophoblast without villi found in uterine curettings usually in association with molar pregnancy.
[b] Syncytial endometritis: benign—the endometrium and myometrium are infiltrated by trophoblastic cells with varying degrees of inflammation.
Modified from Hertig and Mansell: Tumors of the Female Sex Organs. Armed Forces Institute of Pathology, 1957.

Vacuum Aspiration

For large moles, at least two and preferably four units of compatible whole blood are made ready and an intravenous system is established for rapid infusion of blood, if needed. Unless the cervix is long, very firm, and closed, which is very unlikely, dilatation can be safely accomplished under general anesthesia to a diameter sufficient to allow insertion of a plastic suction curette (Fig. 31–18A, B). Anesthetic agents that relax the uterus, such as halothane, should be avoided. Throughout the procedure, oxytocin is infused to contract the uterus as its contents are being evacuated. This decreases bleeding from the implantation site and, as the myometrium retracts, it thickens the uterine wall and thereby reduces the risk of perforating the uterus.

After the great bulk of the mole has been removed by aspiration and the myometrium has contracted and retracted, *thorough but gentle* curettage with a large sharp curette is usually performed. The tissue obtained by sharp curettage may be so labeled and submitted separately for histological examination. Although controversial, Driscoll (1987) maintains that this specimen may allow a better assessment of the malignant predisposition of the trophoblast and the subsequent biological behavior of any tissue that persists in the uterus. Care must be taken neither to perforate the uterus nor to scrape so vigorously with the sharp curette as to invade deeply the myometrium and thereby weaken it. Facilities and personnel for immediate laparotomy are mandatory in case there is uncontrollable hemorrhage or serious trauma to the uterus.

Evacuation of all the contents of a large mole is not always easily accomplished, and intraoperative ultrasonic examination may be helpful to establish that the uterine cavity is empty.

Oxytocin, Prostaglandins, and Hypertonic Saline

Use of oxytocin without suction curettage to expel a large mole may prove unsatisfactory because either the uterus is not sufficiently stimulated to contract effectively or, more likely, during the time the cervix is dilating and the mole is being extruded, hemorrhage becomes profuse. Prostaglandin E_2 has been used rather than oxytocin, but the same reservations apply. Intrauterine instillation of hypertonic saline is mentioned only to condemn its use.

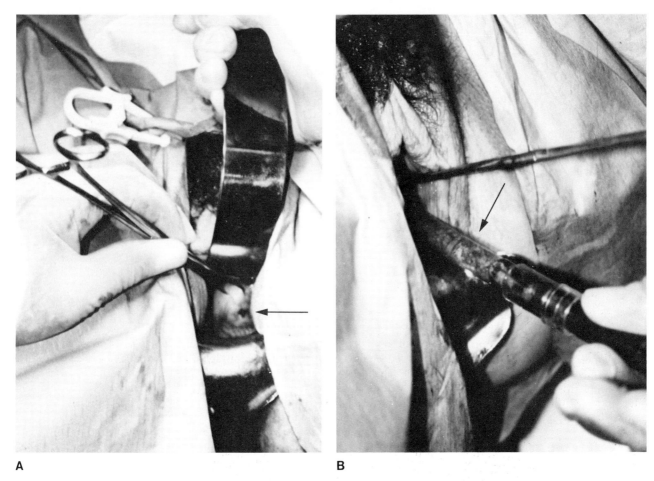

A   **B**

Figure 31–18. A. In the same case presented in Figure 31–16, the cervix (*arrow*) has been exposed and grasped with a tenaculum in preparation for dilatation and insertion of a suction curette. **B.** Molar tissue (*arrow*) is being rapidly removed from the uterine cavity by suction through the plastic curette.

Hysterotomy

Seldom is hysterotomy necessary for molar evacuation. If for some unusual reason suction curettage is not to be used to evacuate the large mole and the uterus is to be conserved, then hysterotomy is the alternative. The uterine incision should be large enough to evacuate the mole promptly, but no larger. Oxytocin is infused and, after evacuating the mole, sharp curettage is performed through the incision.

Hysterectomy

If the parity of the woman or her age are such that no further pregnancies are desired, then hysterectomy may be preferred to suction curettage. Hysterectomy is a logical procedure in women of 40 or over, because of the frequency with which malignant trophoblastic disease ensues in this age group. For example, Tow (1966) reported that 37 percent of women over age 40 with a complete mole went on to develop persistent disease. While hysterectomy does not eliminate trophoblastic neoplasia, it does reduce appreciably the likelihood of such disease developing subsequently.

In 69 cases of hydatidiform mole reported by Chun and associates (1964), in which initial hysterectomy was performed because of advanced age or parity, two women developed choriocarcinoma 2 to 3 years later, an incidence of 2.8 percent. In contrast, in 166 cases

treated by evacuation with conservation of the uterus, 14 women subsequently developed choriocarcinoma, a frequency of 8.4 percent. Thus, hysterectomy does not eliminate the necessity for careful follow-up.

FOLLOW-UP PROCEDURES

If the following extremely important procedures are not adhered to carefully, some women will die needlessly of malignant trophoblastic neoplasia. The prime objective of follow-up is prompt detection of any change suggestive of malignancy. A general method of follow-up is described:

1. Prevent pregnancy during the follow-up period—at minimum, 1 year.
2. Measure serum chorionic gonadotropin levels every 2 weeks using a specific radioimmunoassay. Although weekly assays are recommended by some, no distinct benefit from so frequent assay has been demonstrated.
3. Withhold therapy as long as the serum chorionic gonadotropin levels continue to regress. A rise or persistent plateau in the serum level demands evacuation and usually treatment.
4. Once the level is normal—that is, it has reached the lower limit of measurement—then test monthly for

6 months, and then every 2 months for a total of 1 year.

5. Follow-up may be discontinued and pregnancy allowed after 1 year.

Current follow-up and management centers on serial measurement of serum chorionic gonadotropin values to detect persistent trophoblastic neoplasia. Thus, any test must be sufficiently sensitive and specific to detect very low levels. As shown in Figure 31–19, chorionic gonadotropin levels should fall progressively to undetectable levels, otherwise trophoblast persists. An increase signifies proliferation of trophoblast that is most likely malignant unless the woman is again pregnant. Treatment of suspected persistent trophoblastic disease is discussed subsequently.

An initial chest radiograph is obtained at the first follow-up examination to compare with the pre-evacuation film and serve as a baseline should future x-ray studies become necessary.

Estrogen-progestin contraceptives have been used commonly to prevent a subsequent pregnancy and to suppress pituitary luteinizing hormone that cross-reacts with some tests for chorionic gonadotropin. Stone and co-workers (1976), however, observed that the need for chemotherapy for trophoblastic tumor was increased significantly among women who took oral contraceptives starting shortly after evacuation of a hydatidiform mole. Moreover, oral contraceptives appeared to delay the fall in chorionic gonadotropin levels in women who did not require treatment with chemotherapy. Subsequently, Yuen and Burch (1983) reported that neither the duration that chorionic gonado-

tropin persisted nor the frequency of invasive complications was increased in women after molar evacuation and who used an oral contraceptive that contained 50 μg of estrogen or less.

Although spontaneous disappearance of retained trophoblast is well known, the effectiveness of chemotherapeutic agents in the treatment of trophoblastic neoplasia has led to the use of these drugs in women with molar pregnancy to preclude the development of malignancy and to hasten the disappearance of the retained trophoblast. Since chemotherapeutic agents such as methotrexate are highly toxic and potentially lethal, the risk of chemotherapy must be weighed carefully against the chance of spontaneous regression.

TREATMENT OF PERSISTENT TROPHOBLASTIC DISEASE

Today, following evacuation of a hydatidiform mole, about 20 percent of women subsequently undergo further treatment for suspected persistent gestational trophoblastic disease (Lurain and co-workers, 1983). If serum chorionic gonadotropin values have plateaued or are rising, and there is no evidence for disease beyond the uterus, then if the uterus is not important for future reproduction, hysterectomy will effect a cure in some cases. Often chorionic gonadotropin will disappear and the woman will remain well. However, if the uterus is to be preserved or if there is radiographic evidence of lung lesions, or if there are vaginal metastases, chemotherapy is started at this time with or without curettage. Therapy with methotrexate or actinomycin D, singly or in combination with other chemotherapeutic agents, most often has been successful in these circumstances.

Very small amounts of viable trophoblastic tumor can be detected by assaying for the β-subunit of chorionic gonadotropin. Once gonadotropin activity has decreased to the limit of measurement, therapy can be stopped safely without likelihood of recurrence. Treatment is best carried out by experienced individuals in centers with appropriate facilities for monitoring precisely chorionic gonadotropin levels as well as bone marrow, hepatic, and renal function.

GESTATIONAL TROPHOBLASTIC NEOPLASIA

Gestational trophoblastic neoplasia is persistent trophoblastic proliferation that is considered malignant. It may follow molar pregnancy or normal pregnancy, or develop after abortive outcomes, including ectopic pregnancy. As shown in Table 31–4, gestational trophoblastic neoplasms are divided into two clinical categories, nonmetastatic and metastatic; the latter is further divided into those women with good and poor prognoses. As previously discussed, this clinical classification has largely replaced those based on histological descriptive terms that included choriocarcinoma, chorioadenoma destruens, and invasive mole.

ETIOLOGY

Malignant trophoblastic disease most always develops with or follows some form of pregnancy. Very rarely, choriocarcinoma may arise from a teratoma. Approximately half of malignant cases follow a hydatidiform mole, 25 percent follow an abortion, and 25 percent develop after a normal pregnancy. Of 48 fatal cases from the Brewer Trophoblastic Disease Center, only 14 (29 percent) developed in association with a hydatidiform mole (Lurain and co-workers, 1982). The remainder were associated

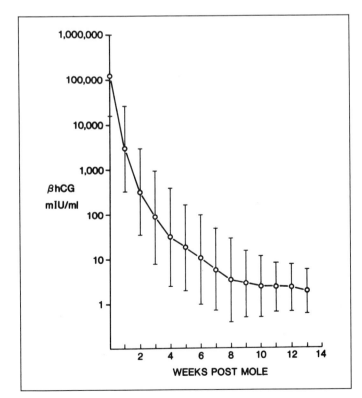

Figure 31–19. The mean value and 95 percent confidence limits describing the normal postmolar β-subunit chorionic gonadotropin regression curve. (*From Schlaerth and associates: Obstet Gynecol 58:478, 1981, with permission.*)

TABLE 31–4. CLASSIFICATION OF GESTATIONAL TROPHOBLASTIC NEOPLASIA

Nonmetastatic—Disease confined to the uterus

Metastatic—Disease has spread outside the uterus
  Good Prognosis—low risk
  1. Short duration—disease present less than 4 months
  2. Pretreatment chorionic gonadotropin less than 40,000 mIU/mL
  3. No prior chemotherapy
  Poor Prognosis—high risk; any of the following
  1. Long duration—disease present more than 4 months
  2. Pretreatment chorionic gonadotropin greater than 40,000 mIU/mL
  3. Brain or liver metastases
  4. Failure of prior chemotherapy
  5. Disease following term pregnancy

From American College of Obstetricians and Gynecologists: Management of Gestational Trophoblastic Neoplasia, Technical Bulletin No. 59, December 1980.

with term or near-term pregnancies, abortions, or ectopic pregnancies.

Malignancy has been identified rarely in the placenta of a seemingly normal pregnancy. In a case described by Brewer and Mazur (1981), widespread malignant trophoblast was evident at 18 weeks gestation, and a primary choriocarcinoma of the placenta was detected. A case in which malignant trophoblast metastasized to the fetus has also been described (Kruseman and colleagues, 1977).

PATHOLOGY

It is emphasized that clinical management is no longer dictated by histological findings. In most cases of gestational trophoblastic neoplasia, the diagnosis is made primarily by persistent chorionic gonadotropin. In most cases, no tissue is submitted for pathological study. In those cases with tissue submitted, either choriocarcinoma or invasive mole most often are found.

Choriocarcinoma

This extremely malignant form of trophoblastic neoplasia may be considered a carcinoma of the chorionic epithelium, although in its growth and metastasis it often behaves like a sarcoma. Factors involved in malignant transformation of the chorion are unknown. In choriocarcinoma, the predisposition of normal trophoblast to invasive growth and erosion of blood vessels is greatly exaggerated. The characteristic gross picture is that of a rapidly growing mass invading both uterine muscle and blood vessels, causing hemorrhage and necrosis (Fig. 31–20A). The tumor is dark red or purple and ragged or friable. If it involves the endometrium, then bleeding, sloughing, and infection of the surface usually occur early. Masses of tissue buried in the myometrium may extend outward, appearing on the uterus as dark, irregular nodules that eventually penetrate the peritoneum.

Microscopically, columns and sheets of trophoblast penetrate the muscle and blood vessels, sometimes in plexiform arrangement and at other times in complete disorganization, interspersed with clotted blood (Fig. 31–20B). An important diagnostic feature of choriocarcinoma, in contrast to hydatid mole or invasive mole, is absence of a villous pattern. Both cytotrophoblast and syncytial elements are involved, although one or the other may predominate. Cellular anaplasia exists, often in marked degrees, but is less valuable as a criterion of trophoblastic malignancy than in other tumors. The difficulty of cytologic evaluation is one of the factors leading to error in the diagnosis of choriocarcinoma from examination of uterine curettings. Cells of normal trophoblast at the placental site have been diagnosed erroneously as choriocarcinoma.

Metastases often develop early and generally are bloodborne because of the affinity of trophoblast for blood vessels. The most common site of metastasis is the lungs (over 75 percent), and the vagina is next most common (about 50 percent). The vulva, kidneys, liver, ovaries, brain, and bowel also contain metastases in many cases. Theca-lutein cysts of the ovary are identified in over one third of the cases.

Invasive Mole

The distinguishing features of invasive mole or chorioadenoma destruens are excessive trophoblastic overgrowth and extensive penetration by the trophoblastic elements, including whole villi,

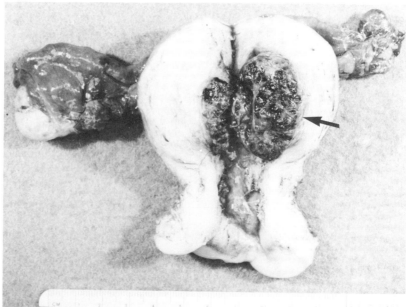

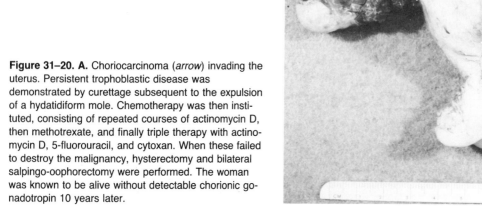

Figure 31–20. A. Choriocarcinoma (*arrow*) invading the uterus. Persistent trophoblastic disease was demonstrated by curettage subsequent to the expulsion of a hydatidiform mole. Chemotherapy was then instituted, consisting of repeated courses of actinomycin D, then methotrexate, and finally triple therapy with actinomycin D, 5-fluorouracil, and cytoxan. When these failed to destroy the malignancy, hysterectomy and bilateral salpingo-oophorectomy were performed. The woman was known to be alive without detectable chorionic gonadotropin 10 years later.

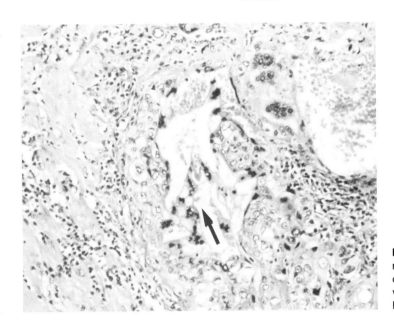

Figure 31–20. B. Histological characteristics of the choriocarcinoma demonstrated in Figure 31–20A. Malignant syncytio- and cytotrophoblast without villous stroma invade the myometrium and vascular spaces (*arrow*) accompanied by necrosis and hemorrhage.

into the depths of the myometrium, sometimes to involve the peritoneum or the adjacent parametrium or vaginal vault (Fig. 31–21). Such moles are locally invasive, but generally lack the pronounced tendency to widespread metastasis that is characteristic of choriocarcinoma. As contrasted microscopically with the typically benign hydatidiform mole, in invasive mole, large fields of trophoblast are usually found but accompanied by some villous stroma.

CLINICAL HISTORY

Malignant trophoblastic disease may follow hydatidiform mole, abortion, ectopic pregnancy, or normal pregnancy. The most common, though not constant, sign is irregular bleeding after the immediate puerperium in association with uterine subinvolution. The bleeding may be continuous or intermittent, with sudden and sometimes massive hemorrhages. Perforation of the uterus by the growth may cause intraperitoneal hemorrhage. Extension into the parametrium may cause pain and fixation that is suggestive of inflammatory disease.

In many cases, the first indication of the condition may be the metastatic lesions. Vaginal or vulvar tumors may be found. The woman may complain of cough and have bloody sputum from pulmonary metastases. In a few cases it has been impossible to find choriocarcinoma in the uterus or pelvis, the original lesion having disappeared, leaving only distant metastases growing actively.

If unmodified by treatment, the course of choriocarcinoma is rapidly progressive, and death usually follows within a few months in the majority of cases. The most common cause of death is hemorrhage in various locations.

DIAGNOSIS

Recognition of the possibility of the lesion is the most important factor in diagnosis. All women with a hydatidiform mole are at risk and need to be followed as described. Any case of unusual bleeding after term pregnancy or abortion should be investigated by curettage, but especially by measurements of chorionic gonadotropin, since absolute reliance cannot be placed on the findings of examination of curettings. Malignant tissue may be

buried within the myometrium, inaccessible to the curette, or hidden in a distant metastasis.

Solitary or multiple nodules present in the chest radiograph that cannot be otherwise explained are suggestive of the possibility of choriocarcinoma and warrant an assay for chorionic gonadotropin. It should be kept in mind, however, that some nontrophoblastic tumors secrete small amounts of chorionic gonadotropin (Shane and Naftolin, 1975).

Persistent or rising gonadotropin titers in the absence of pregnancy are indicative of trophoblastic neoplasia. Results of assays should be confirmed before beginning medical or surgical therapy.

Other evaluation before treatment is given includes computed tomography to evaluate the brain, lungs, liver, and pelvis. Hricak and colleagues (1986) reported the use of magnetic resonance imaging in nine women with malignant trophoblastic disease and concluded that this method was superior to sonography and computed tomography to evaluate the degree of uterine involvement.

TREATMENT

Current treatment for gestational trophoblastic neoplasia is much more successful than that used in the past. Formerly, the only hope for cure was hysterectomy or, even more remote, resection of a metastatic lesion. In 1956, Li and associates successfully treated a woman with metastatic gestational trophoblastic neoplasia by employing methotrexate. Since then, methotrexate and other agents effective against malignant tumors, especially actinomycin D, have been widely used with considerable success.

The pharmacology and clinical use of methotrexate have been reviewed extensively by Jolivet and colleagues (1983). The overall cure rate in recent years for persistent gestational trophoblastic neoplasia of all severities has been about 90 percent (Lewis, 1980). Patients classified as having a good prognosis have been cured virtually 100 percent of the time. As shown in Table 31–4, this category includes those women with duration of disease less than 4 months, serum chorionic gonadotropin levels less than 40,000 mIU per mL, no prior chemotherapy, and

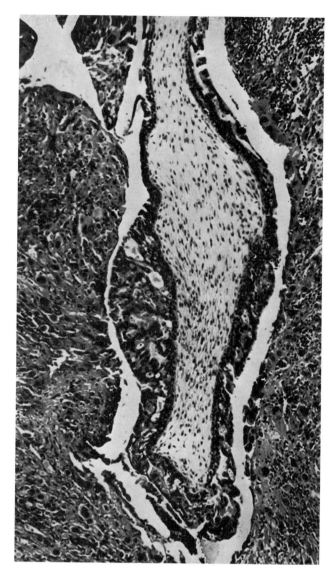

Figure 31–21. Invasive hydatidiform mole (chorioadenoma destruens), showing molar villus with hyperplastic trophoblast penetrating deeply into myometrium. (*Courtesy of Dr. Ralph M. Wynn.*)

tion chemotherapy, in spite of increased toxicity, has produced the highest cure rate. The regimen usually includes methotrexate, actinomycin D, and cyclophosphamide along with brain or liver irradiation if metastases are documented.

PROGNOSIS

Women with nonmetastatic trophoblastic neoplasia have an extremely good prognosis if single-agent chemotherapy is started as soon as persistent disease is identified, using serial chorionic gonadotropin levels. Lurain and colleagues (1983) reported their remarkable results from the Brewer Trophoblastic Disease Center of Northwestern University. From 1962 to 1978, 738 women with molar pregnancy were managed as generally outlined above. Chemotherapy was given for persistent disease in 19 percent, and all were living and disease-free 4 to 18 years later.

Women with low-risk metastatic gestational neoplasia who are treated aggressively with single- or multiagent chemotherapy in general do almost as well as those with nonmetastatic disease (DuBeshter and associates, 1987; Hammond and colleagues, 1980; Jones, 1987). Women with high-risk metastatic disease have appreciable mortality that depends on what factors were considered "high risk" (Soper and associates, 1988). Remission rates have been reported to vary from about 45 to 65 percent. Lurain (1987) recently analyzed 53 deaths from the Brewer Trophoblastic Center and concluded that the three factors primarily responsible were: (1) extensive choriocarcinoma at initial diagnosis, (2) lack of appropriately aggressive initial treatment, and (3) failure of currently used chemotherapy.

PREGNANCY AFTER TROPHOBLASTIC DISEASE

After gestational trophoblastic disease, women are at increased risk of developing trophoblastic disease in a subsequent pregnancy. Berkowitz and colleagues (1987) reported that 1.3 percent of 1,048 women treated at the New England Trophoblastic Disease Center for gestational trophoblastic disease had a recurrent molar pregnancy. Importantly, women who have been given chemotherapy do not have an increased risk for anomalous fetuses in subsequent pregnancies (Rustin and colleagues, 1984; Song and associates, 1988).

OTHER TUMORS OF THE PLACENTA

CHORIOANGIOMA (HEMANGIOMA)

Various angiomatous tumors of the placenta ranging widely in size have been described, and because of the resemblance of their components to the blood vessels and stroma of the chorionic villus, the term *chorioangioma*, or *chorangioma*, has been considered the most appropriate designation. The tumors are most likely hamartomas of primitive chorionic mesenchyme. Their incidence has been reported to be about 1 percent. Larger chorioangiomas may be strongly suspected on the basis of sonographic changes within the placenta. A dramatic example is provided in Figure 31–22A and B.

Small growths are essentially asymptomatic, but large tumors may be associated with hydramnios or antepartum hemorrhage. Fetal death and malformations are uncommon complications, although there may be a positive correlation with low birthweight. Stiller and Skafish (1986) described a case with multiple placental chorioangiomas in which a blood group A fetus bled acutely into her O group mother. The mother showed evidence of acute hemolysis without anemia, and the fetus de-

no brain or liver metastases. Cure usually has been achieved for these so-called low-risk patients following single-agent chemotherapy. Such treatment obviously reduces serious toxicity. Recently, Barter and associates (1987) reported success with methotrexate given orally; Homesley and associates (1988) reported similar results with weekly intramuscular methotrexate; and Petrilli and colleagues (1987) found that single-dose actinomycin D given every 2 weeks was highly effective in women with nonmetastatic disease. Fortunately, in those instances in which single-agent therapy proved ineffective, prompt treatment with combination chemotherapy, with or without radiotherapy, most often will provide a cure.

Patients classified as high risk because of their poorer prognosis for cure have disease for more than 4 months, their serum gonadotropin levels are greater than 40,000 mIU per mL, or they have liver or brain metastases or have had previous chemotherapy without success. Some authorities, but not all, include choriocarcinoma developing in association with term pregnancy as having a poor prognosis. In these high-risk women, combina-

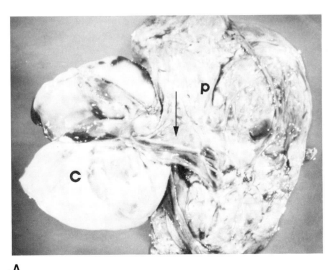
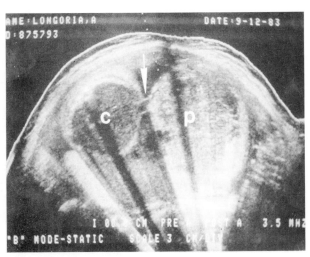

A   **B**

Figure 31–22. A. Placenta (*p*) and discrete very large (450 g) chorioangioma (*c*) connected to the placenta by a vascular stalk (*arrow*). The 34-week fetus was identified by sonography to have marked hydrothorax. Demonstrated in cord blood were severe hypofibrinogenemia, thrombocytopenia, hypoprothrombinemia, and microangiopathic hemolysis. The infant had cardiomegaly, heart failure, pleural effusion, and hepatomegaly. After several cardiac arrests the infant succumbed 3 days after birth. **B.** Sonogram of the same placenta (*p*) and chorioangioma (*c*) connected by a short pedicle (*arrow*). (*Courtesy of Dr. R. Santos.*)

veloped the sinusoidal heart rate pattern frequently seen in severe anemia. We have identified severe iron-deficiency anemia in the neonate as the consequence of chronic fetal to maternal hemorrhage associated with multiple small chorioangiomas (Cunningham and Pritchard, unpublished). Large chorioangiomas provide an arteriovenous shunt in the fetal circulation that can lead to heart failure with all of its complications (see Chap. 33, p. 609). With a large chorioangioma, consumptive coagulopathy and microangiopathic hemolytic anemia have also been observed in the fetus-infant. Figure 31–22A and B shows a placenta and a very large, discrete chorioangioma that led to heart failure, consumptive coagulopathy, and microangiopathic hemolysis in the fetus.

TUMORS METASTATIC TO THE PLACENTA

Metastases of malignant tumors are rare, and the subject was reviewed by Read and Platzer (1981). They reported that malignant melanoma is the most common malignancy metastatic to the placenta, and it makes up nearly a third of reported cases. Leukemias and lymphomas comprise another third. Interestingly, the fetus is involved with malignant tumor in about a fourth of reported cases. Any tumor with hematogenous spread is a potential source of placental metastases, as evidenced by the case of large-cell undifferentiated lung carcinoma metastatic to the placenta shown in Figure 31–23. The mother succumbed but the child remained healthy by 16 months.

DISORDERS OF THE AMNION AND AMNIONIC FLUID

DISEASES OF THE AMNION

MECONIUM STAINING

The brownish-green discoloration of the fetal membranes from meconium staining is characteristic. The amnion may be slippery from mucus discharged in the meconium. Meconium staining is relatively common, and Benirschke (1974) identified it in 13 percent of 2,000 consecutive placentas examined. He reported that in the majority of cases no other evidence of fetal distress was identified and the subsequent course of the newborn was normal. Fujikura and Klionsky (1975) identified meconium staining of the membranes or fetus in about 10 percent of 43,000 live-born infants in the Collaborative Study of Cerebral Palsy. The neonatal mortality rate was 3.3 percent in the group with neconium-stained membranes compared to 1.7 percent in the nonstained group.

Meconium staining of amnionic fluid is more common than meconium-stained membranes; at Parkland Hospital, this has been remarkably constant over the past 4 years. Of more than 50,000 women delivered during this period, 19 percent had amnionic fluid that contained some meconium identified during labor or at delivery (K. Leveno, unpublished).

INFLAMMATION OF THE AMNION

In some cases, amnionitis is a manifestation of an intrauterine infection, and it is associated frequently with prolonged membrane rupture and long labors (Fox, 1978). When mononuclear and polymorphonuclear leucocytes infiltrate the chorion, the resulting microscopic finding is properly designated *chorioamnionitis*. These findings, however, may be nonspecific and are not always associated with other evidence for fetal or maternal infection. When organisms are isolated from amnionic fluid or

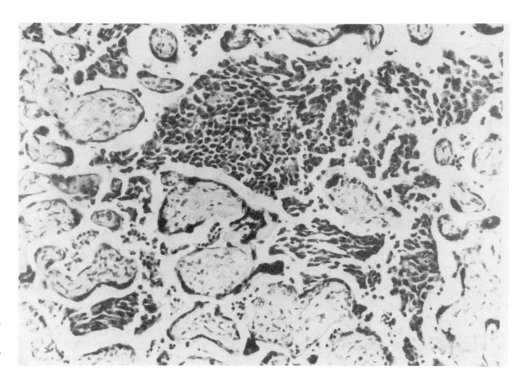

Figure 31–23. Lung carcinoma metastatic to the placenta. (*From Read and Platzer: Obstet Gynecol 58:387, 1981, with permission.*)

membranes, they invariably are the same as those that normally colonize in the vagina and cervix.

Clinically occult chorioamnionic infection caused by a wide variety of microorganisms has emerged recently as a possible explanation for many heretofore unexplained cases of ruptured membranes, preterm labor (see Chap. 38, p. 749), or both.

CYSTS OF THE AMNION

Small cysts lined by typical amnionic epithelium are formed occasionally. The common variety results from fusion of amnionic folds, with subsequent retention of fluid.

AMNION NODOSUM

These nodules in the amnion are sometimes called *squamous metaplasia* of the amnion or *amnionic caruncles.* They are seen most commonly in the amnion in contact with the chorionic plate, but they may also be found elsewhere. They usually appear near the insertion of the cord as elevations that are multiple, rounded or oval, and shiny, grayish-yellow opaque; they vary from less than 1 mm to 5 mm in diameter. Bartman and Driscoll (1968) reported an association between amnion nodosum and multiple congenital abnormalities, especially hypoplastic kidneys with oligohydramnios. The nodules most likely are made up of fetal ectodermal debris, including vernix caseosa.

AMNIONIC BANDS

Disruption of the amnion may lead to formation of bands or strings of amnion that adhere to the fetus and impair growth and development of the involved structure. Some of the conditions that appear to be the consequence of this phenomenon, including intrauterine amputations, are considered in Chapter 33 (p. 623).

DISORDERS OF THE AMNIONIC FLUID

HYDRAMNIOS

Hydramnios, sometimes called *polyhydramnios,* is excessive amnionic fluid. Normally, the volume of amnionic fluid increases to about 1 L, or somewhat more by 36 weeks, but decreases thereafter. Postterm, there may be only a few hundred mL or even less. Somewhat arbitrarily, more than 2,000 mL of amnionic fluid is considered excessive, or hydramnios. In rare instances, the uterus may contain an enormous quantity of fluid, with reports of as much as 15 L. In most instances, the increase in amnionic fluid is gradual, or *chronic hydramnios.* In *acute hydramnios,* the volume increases very suddenly and the uterus may become markedly distended within a few days. The fluid in hydramnios is usually similar in appearance and composition to the amnionic fluid in normal conditions.

Incidence

Minor to moderate degrees of hydramnios (2 to 3 L), are rather common, but the more marked grades are not. Because of the difficulty of complete collection of amnionic fluid, the diagnosis is usually based on clinical impression or, more recently, sonographic estimation (Fig. 31–24). Therefore, the frequency of the diagnosis varies appreciably with different observers, and it is not surprising that published data on the incidence have varied from 1 in about 60 deliveries to 1 in 750.

The carefully done studies of Hill and associates (1987) from the Mayo Clinic provide an accurate estimate of the incidence of hydramnios using ultrasound measurements. More than 9,000 regularly booked prenatal patients underwent routine ultrasonic evaluation near the end of the second or the beginning of the third trimester. These investigators defined mild hydramnios as pockets of amnionic fluid measuring 8 to 11 cm in vertical dimension. Hydramnios was classified as moderate if a pocket of fluid containing only small parts measured 12 to 15 cm deep.

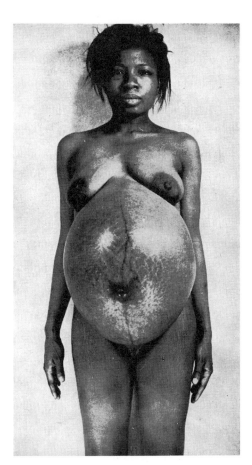

Figure 31–24. Advanced degree of hydramnios—5,500 mL of amnionic fluid was measured at delivery.

Finally, severe hydramnios was considered when a free-floating fetus was found in pockets of fluid of 16 cm or greater. Using these definitions, the overall incidence of hydramnios was 0.9 percent. The majority, almost 80 percent of these 85 cases, were mild; 17 percent were moderate; and in only 5 percent was hydramnios judged as severe.

Hydramnios is frequently associated with fetal malformations, especially of the central nervous system and the gastrointestinal tract. For example, hydramnios accompanies about half of the cases of anencephaly and esophageal atresia. According to Hill and colleagues (1987), the cause of mild hydramnios was identified in only about 15 percent of cases, whereas in cases with moderately or severely increased amnionic fluid, the cause was identified in more than 90 percent (Table 31–5). In almost half of those cases with moderate and severe hydramnios, a fetal anomaly was identified.

Landy and associates (1987) used ultrasound to quantify amnionic fluid and described in detail 59 pregnancies with subjective hydramnios but without other obvious abnormal findings. Subsequently, 15 percent of these infants were identified to have structural anomalies, the most common of which were gastrointestinal. One infant was found to have trisomy 18, and they recommended that consideration be given to fetal karyotyping if careful ultrasonic evacuation does not provide an explanation for hydramnios.

The incidence of hydramnios also is increased in pregnancies complicated by diabetes and in *immune* and *nonimmune*

hydrops (see Chap. 33, p. 609). Excessive amnionic fluid in one of the amnionic sacs is common in twin pregnancies and is more frequent and usually more intense in monozygotic than in dizygotic twinning.

Etiology

The volume of amnionic fluid is controlled in a number of ways. Early in pregnancy, the amnionic cavity is filled with fluid very similar in composition to extracellular fluid. During the first half of pregnancy, transfer of water and other small molecules takes place not only across the amnion but through the fetal skin. Lind and Hytten (1970) considered amnionic fluid to be an extension of the fetal extracellular fluid space during the first half of pregnancy.

During the second trimester, the fetus begins to urinate, to swallow, and to inspire amnionic fluid (Abramovich and colleagues, 1979; Duenhoelter and Pritchard, 1976; Pritchard, 1966). These processes almost certainly have a significant modulating role in the control of amnionic fluid volume. Although the major source of amnionic fluid in hydramnios most often has been assumed to be the amnionic epithelium, no histological changes in amnion or chemical changes in amnionic fluid have been found.

Since the fetus normally swallows amnionic fluid, it has been assumed that this mechanism is one of the ways by which the volume of the fluid is controlled. The theory gains validity by the nearly constant presence of hydramnios when swallowing is inhibited as, for example, in cases of esophageal atresia. Fetal swallowing is by no means the only mechanism for preventing hydramnios. Both Pritchard (1966) and Abramovich (1970) quantified amnionic-fluid swallowing and found in some instances of gross hydramnios appreciable volumes of fluid being swallowed.

In cases of anencephaly and spina bifida, increased transudation of fluid from the exposed meninges into the amnionic cavity may be an etiological factor. Another possible explanation of hydramnios in anencephaly when swallowing is not impaired is excessive urination caused by either stimulation of cerebrospinal centers deprived of their protective coverings or possibly the lack of antidiuretic hormone. The converse is well established that fetal defects that cause anuria nearly always are associated with oligohydramnios.

In hydramnios associated with monozygotic twin pregnancy, the hypothesis has been advanced that one fetus usurps the greater part of the circulation common to both twins and develops cardiac hypertrophy, which, in turn, results in increased urine output. Naeye and Blanc (1972) identified in this

TABLE 31–5. ASSOCIATED FACTORS WITH 102 CASES OF HYDRAMNIOS ACCORDING TO SEVERITY

Associated Factor	Number	Degree of Hydramnios		
		Mild	*Moderate*	*Severe*
Fetal anomalies	13	2	9	2
Overt diabetes	8	3	5	—
Gestational diabetes	7	7	—	—
Multifetal gestation	5	1	2	2
Idiopathic	68	66	2	—
Total	102	79	19	4

Modified from Hill and associates: Obstet Gynecol 69:21, 1987.

syndrome dilated renal tubules, enlarged bladder, and an increased urinary output in the early neonatal period, suggesting that increased fetal urine production is responsible for the hydramnios. Conversely, donor members of parabiotic transplacental transfusion pairs had contracted renal tubules with oligohydramnios.

Hydramnios that rather commonly develops with maternal diabetes during the third trimester remains unexplained. Wladimiroff and co-workers (1975) identified sonographically the rate of fetal urine formation in such a case to be in the normal range.

Naeye and Blanc (1972) described hypoplastic lungs commonly in neonates with hydramnios and questioned their role in the genesis of the hydramnios. The observations of Duenhoelter and Pritchard (1976) on both monkey and human fetuses establish that normal fetal lungs have the potential for the exchange of relatively large volumes of fluid as the consequence of amnionic fluid inspiration. Hypoplastic lungs may compromise this pathway for removal of amnionic fluid.

The weight of the placenta tends to be high in some cases of hydramnios. The enlarged placenta may contribute to the increase in amnionic fluid. Prolactin also has been suspected to have a role in the control of amnionic fluid volume. The concentration of prolactin in amnionic fluid is normally increased compared to that of maternal plasma, and prolactin receptors have been identified in chorion laeve. Healy and associates (1985) found that prolactin-receptor binding was less than normal in cases of idiopathic hydramnios, and they hypothesized that prolactin resistance owing to receptor deficiency may be the underlying cause of chronic hydramnios.

Symptoms

The major symptoms accompanying hydramnios arise from purely mechanical causes and result principally from the pressure exerted within and around the overdistended uterus upon adjacent organs. The effects on maternal respiratory functions may be striking. When distension is excessive, the mother may suffer from severe dyspnea and, in extreme cases, she may be able to breathe only when upright. Edema, the consequence of compression of major venous systems by the very large uterus, is common, especially in the lower extremities, the vulva, and the abdominal wall. Rarely, severe oliguria may result from ureteral obstruction by the very large uterus. With *chronic hydramnios*, the accumulation of fluid takes place gradually and the woman may tolerate the excessive abdominal distension with relatively little discomfort. In *acute hydramnios*, however, the distension may lead to disturbances sufficiently serious to be threatening. Acute hydramnios tends to develop earlier in pregnancy than does the chronic form, often as early as 16 to 20 weeks, and it may rapidly expand the hypertonic uterus to enormous size. Without treatment, pain is likely to become intense and the dyspnea so severe that the woman is unable to lie flat. As a rule, acute hydramnios leads to labor before the 28th week, or the symptoms become so severe that intervention is mandatory. In the majority of cases of chronic hydramnios, and thus differing from acute hydramnios, the amnionic fluid pressure is not appreciably higher than in normal pregnancy.

Diagnosis

Uterine enlargement in association with difficulty in palpating fetal small parts and in hearing fetal heart tones usually is the main diagnostic sign of hydramnios. In severe cases, the uterine wall may be so tense that it is impossible to palpate any part of the fetus (Fig. 31–24). Such findings call for prompt ultrasonic examination to better quantify amnionic fluid and to identify multiple fetuses or fetal abnormalities.

Sonography

The differentiation among hydramnios, ascites, and a large ovarian cyst usually can be made without difficulty by ultrasonic evaluation. Large amounts of amnionic fluid nearly always can be readily demonstrated as an abnormally large echo-free space

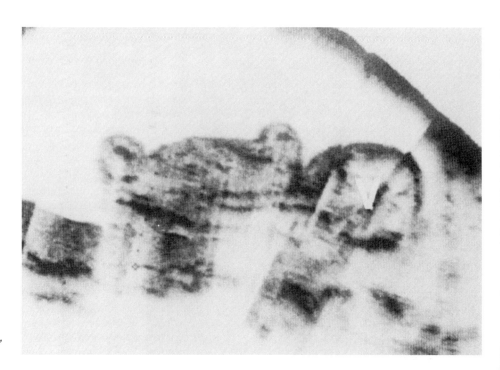

Figure 31–25. Longitudinal ultrasound scan showing moderate hydramnios at 28 weeks gestation (V = fetal vertex). (*From Hill and colleagues: Obstet Gynecol 69:21, 1987.*)

between the fetus and the uterine wall or placenta (Fig. 31–25). At times, a fetal abnormality such as anencephaly or other neural tube defects, or an anomaly of the gastrointestinal tract, may be seen.

Radiography

A large radiolucent area around the fetal skeleton suggests hydramnios, although a soft tissue mass such as a sacrococcygeal tumor may do the same. Most often, anencephaly and other gross skeletal defects are easily diagnosed. *Amniography*, using contrast material such as Hypaque, may help identify excess amnionic fluid, soft tissue tumors projecting from the fetus, and the presence or absence of fetal swallowing.

Prognosis

In general, the more severe the degree of hydramnios, the higher the perinatal mortality rate, so that the outlook for the infant in pregnancies with major degrees of hydramnios is poor. In the studies of Hill and co-workers (1987), almost 80 percent of women with mild hydramnios were delivered of normal, healthy, term infants. Conversely, half of those with moderate to severe hydramnios had anomalous fetuses. Even when the sonograph and radiograph show an apparently normal fetus, the prognosis is still guarded, since the incidence of fetal malformations is 15 to 20 percent (Landy and colleagues, 1987; Queenan and Gadow, 1970). There is a further increase in perinatal mortality from prematurity, since the frequency of preterm delivery even with a normal fetus was reported to be about 20 percent (Hill and colleagues, 1987). Erythroblastosis, difficulties encountered by infants of diabetic mothers, prolapse of the umbilical cord when the membranes rupture, and placental abruption as the uterus rapidly decreases in size add still further to the death rate.

The hazards imposed on the mother by hydramnios are significant but usually can be managed without serious threat to her life. The most frequent maternal complications are placental abruption, uterine dysfunction, and postpartum hemorrhage. Extensive premature separation of the placenta sometimes follows escape of massive quantities of amnionic fluid because of the decrease in the area of the emptying uterus beneath the placenta. Uterine dysfunction and postpartum hemorrhage are the result of uterine atony consequent to overdistention. Abnormal presentations are more common and operative intervention more frequently is required.

Treatment

Minor degrees of hydramnios rarely require treatment. Even moderate degrees, including cases in which there is some discomfort, usually can be managed without intervention until labor ensues or until the membranes rupture spontaneously. If there is dyspnea or abdominal pain, or if ambulation is difficult, hospitalization becomes necessary. There is no satisfactory treatment for symptomatic hydramnios other than removal of some of the amnionic fluid. Bed rest with sedation may make the situation endurable, but it rarely has any effect on fluid. Diuretics and water and salt restriction are likewise ineffective and potentially dangerous.

Amniocentesis

The principal purpose of amniocentesis is to relieve maternal distress, and to that end it is successful transiently. At times, amniocentesis appears to initiate labor even though only a part of the fluid is removed; hence, relief of distress may not allow continuation of pregnancy. The volume of fluid removed at one time appears to be critical. Queenan (1970) and Pitkin (1976) described cases of recurrent severe hydramnios treated by amniocentesis. Whereas removal of a large volume of fluid at one time during the first pregnancy was soon followed by delivery of a very immature infant that succumbed, repeated amniocenteses with the frequent removal of smaller volumes during the next pregnancy resulted in delivery of an infant sufficiently mature to survive.

The disadvantages inherent in rupture of the membranes through the cervix is the possibility of prolapse of the cord and especially of placental abruption. Very slow removal of the fluid helps to obviate these dangers, but it is very difficult to accomplish through the cervical canal, since even a small nick in the membranes is usually quickly converted into a large rent. Uncommon complications of abdominal amniocentesis in the presence of hydramnios are puncture of a fetal vessel and bacterial infection. Sonography is useful not only to identify hydramnios and associated fetal anomalies but also to locate the placenta and thereby allow performance of amniocentesis in a site distant from the placenta. Careful aseptic technique should minimize the risk of infection.

Technique

To remove amnionic fluid, a commercially available plastic catheter that tightly covers an 18-gauge needle (Angiocath) is inserted through the locally anesthetized abdominal wall into the amnionic sac, the needle is withdrawn, and an intravenous infusion set is connected to the catheter hub. The opposite end of the tubing is dropped into a graduated cylinder placed at floor level, and the rate of flow of amnionic fluid is controlled with the screw clamp so that about 500 mL per hour is withdrawn. After about 1,500 to 2,000 mL has been collected, the uterus usually has decreased in size sufficiently so that the plastic catheter may be withdrawn from the amnionic sac. At the same time, maternal relief is dramatic and the danger of placental separation from decompression is very slight. Using strict aseptic technique, this procedure can be repeated as necessary to make the woman comfortable.

OLIGOHYDRAMNIOS

In rare instances, the volume of amnionic fluid may fall far below the normal limits and occasionally be reduced to only a few mL of viscid fluid. The cause of this condition is not completely understood. Healy and colleagues (1985) reported that prolactin receptors in chorion laeve were normal in number in such cases. Very small amounts of amnionic fluid may be found relatively often with pregnancies that have continued for weeks beyond term. The risk of cord compression and, in turn, fetal distress is increased as the consequence of the scant volume of fluid (Leveno and colleagues, 1984). Oligohydramnios is practically always evident when there is either obstruction of the fetal urinary tract or renal agenesis. Therefore, anuria almost certainly has an etiological role in such cases of oligohydramnios. A chronic leak from a defect in the membranes may reduce the volume of amnionic fluid appreciably, but most often labor soon ensues.

Oligohydramnios early in pregnancy is generally associated with poor fetal outcome, owing both to cause as well as effect. Mercer and Brown (1986) described 34 middle-trimester pregnancies complicated by oligohydramnios diagnosed ultrasonically by the absence of amnionic-fluid pockets greater than 1 cm in any vertical plane. Nine of these fetuses (26 percent) had anomalies, and 10 of the 25 who were phenotypically normal were either aborted spontaneously or stillborn because of severe maternal hypertension, retarded fetal growth, or placental abruption. Of the 14 liveborns, 8 were preterm and 7 died. The 6 infants who were delivered at term did well. Thus, there were only 7 surviving infants born to the 34 women with severe early onset oligohydramnios.

Otherwise normal infants may suffer the consequences of severely diminished amnionic fluid since adhesions between the amnion and parts of the fetus may cause serious deformities including amputation. Moreover, subjected to pressure from all sides, the fetus assumes a peculiar appearance, and musculoskeletal deformities such as clubfoot are frequently observed. Typically in cases of oligohydramnios, the skin of the fetus appears dry, leathery, and wrinkled.

When amnionic fluid is scant, *pulmonary hypoplasia* is very common. The possibilities to account for the hypoplasia are (1) compression of the thorax by the uterus in the absence of amnionic fluid, which prevents chest wall excursion and lung expansion; (2) lack of fluid to be inhaled into the terminal air sacs of the lung and, as a consequence, inhibition of lung growth; and (3) an intrinsic lung defect with failure of the lung to excrete fluid essential to maintenance of amnionic fluid volume. The appreciable volumes of amnionic fluid demonstrated by Duenhoelter and Pritchard (1976) to be inhaled by the fetus normally is suggestive of a role for the inspired fluid in expansion and, in turn, the growth of the lung.

REFERENCES

Abramovich DR: Fetal factors influencing the volume and composition of liquor amnii. J Obstet Gynaecol Br Commonw 77:865, 1970

Abramovich DR, Garden A, Jandial L, Page KR: Fetal swallowing and voiding in relation to hydramnios. Obstet Gynecol 54:15, 1979

Amir SM, Osathanondh R, Berkowitz RS, Goldstein DP: Human chorionic gonadotropin and thyroid function in patients with hydatidiform mole. Am J Obstet Gynecol 150:723, 1984

Bagshawe KD, Lawler SD: Commentary: Unmasking moles. Br J Obstet Gynaecol 89:255, 1982

Barter JF, Soong SJ, Hatch KD, Orr JW Jr, Partridge EC, Austin JM Jr, Shingleton HM: Treatment of nonmetastatic gestational trophoblastic disease with oral methotrexate. Am J Obstet Gynecol 157:1166, 1987

Bartman J, Driscoll SG: Amnion nodosum and hypoplastic cystic kidneys. Obstet Gynecol 32:700, 1968

Benirschke K: Disease of the placenta. In Gluck L (ed): Modern Perinatal Medicine. Chicago, Year Book, 1974, p 99

Benirschke K, Brown WH: A vascular anomaly of the umbilical cord: The absence of one umbilical artery in the umbilical cords of normal and abnormal fetuses. Obstet Gynecol 6:399, 1955

Benirschke K, Dodds JP: Angiomyxoma of the umbilical cord with atrophy of an umbilical artery. Obstet Gynecol 30:99, 1967

Benirschke K, Driscoll SG (eds): The Pathology of the Human Placenta. New York, Springer-Verlag, 1974

Berkowitz RS, Goldstein DP, Bernstein MR: Management of partial molar pregnancy. Contemp Ob/Gyn 27:77, 1986

Berkowitz RS, Goldstein DP, Bernstein MR, Sablinska B: Subsequent pregnancy outcome in patients with molar pregnancy and gestational trophoblastic tumors. J Reprod Med 32:680, 1987

Block MF, Merrill JA: Hydatidiform mole with coexistent fetus. Obstet Gynecol 60:129, 1982

Brewer JI, Mazur MT: Gestational choriocarcinoma: Its origin in the placenta during a seemingly normal pregnancy. Am J Surg Pathol 5:267, 1981

Bryan EM, Kohler HG: The missing umbilical artery: II. Paediatric follow-up. Arch Dis Child 50:714, 1975

Byrne J, Blanc WA: Malformations and chromosome anomalies in spontaneously aborted fetuses with single umbilical artery. Am J Obstet Gynecol 151:340, 1985

Chun D, Braga C, Chow C, Lok L: Clinical observations on some aspects of hydatidiform moles. Br J Obstet Gynaecol 71:180, 1964

Curry SL, Hammond CB, Tyrey L, Creasman WT, Parker RT: Hydatidiform mole: Diagnosis, management, and long-time follow-up of 347 patients. Obstet Gynecol 45:1, 1975

Czernobilsky B, Barash A, Lancet M: Partial moles: A clinicopathology study of 25 cases. Obstet Gynecol 59:75, 1982

Dodson MG: New concepts and questions in gestational trophoblastic disease. J Reprod Med 28:741, 1988

Driscoll SG: Problems and pitfalls in the histopathologic diagnosis of gestational trophoblastic lesions. J Reprod Med 32:623, 1987

DuBeshter B, Berkowitz RS, Goldstein DP, Cramer DW, Bernstein MR: Metastatic gestational trophoblastic disease: Experience at the New England Trophoblastic Disease Center, 1965 to 1985. Obstet Gynecol 69:390, 1987

Duenhoelter JH, Pritchard JA: Fetal respiration: Quantitative measurements of amnionic fluid inspired near term by human rhesus fetuses. Am J Obstet Gynecol 125:306, 1976

Fox H: Pathology of the placenta. Monograph, Vol 7. Philadelphia, Saunders, 1987

Froehlich LA, Fujikura T: Follow-up of infants with single umbilical artery. Pediatrics 52:22, 1973

Fujikura T, Klionsky B: The significance of meconium staining. Am J Obstet Gynecol 121:45, 1975

Goldstein DP: Prevention of gestational trophoblastic disease by use of actinomycin D in molar pregnancy. Obstet Gynecol 43:475, 1974

Grannum PAT, Berkowitz RL, Hobbins JC: The ultrasonic changes in the maturing placenta and their relation to fetal pulmonic maturity. Am J Obstet Gynecol 133:915, 1979

Grimes DA: Epidemiology of gestational trophoblastic disease. Am J Obstet Gynecol 150:309, 1984

Hammond CB, Borchert I, Tyrey I, Creasman WT, Parker RT: Treatment of metastatic trophoblastic disease: Good and poor prognosis. Am J Obstet Gynecol 115:451, 1973

Hammond CB, Weed JC, Currie JL: The role of operation in the current therapy of gestational trophoblastic disease. Am J Obstet Gynecol 136:844, 1980

Hankins GDV, Snyder RR, Hauth JC, Gilstrap LC III, Hammond T: Nuchal cords and neonatal outcome. Obstet Gynecol 70:687, 1987

Hankins GDV, Wendel GW, Snyder RR, Cunningham FG: Trophoblastic embolization during molar evacuation: Central hemodynamic observations. Obstet Gynecol 69:368, 1987

Healy DL, Herington AC, O'Herlihy C: Chronic polyhydramnios is a syndrome with a lactogen receptor defect in the chorion laeve. Br J Obstet Gynaecol 92:461, 1985

Hertig AT, Edmonds HW: Genesis of hydatidiform mole. Arch Pathol 30:260, 1940

Hertig AT, Mansell H: Tumors of the Female Sex Organs: I. Hydatidiform Mole and Choriocarcinoma. Washington, DC, Armed Forces Institute of Pathology, 1957

Hertig AT, Sheldon WH: Hydatidiform mole: A pathologico-clinical correlation of 200 cases. Am J Obstet Gynecol 53:1, 1947

Hill LM, Breckle R, Thomas ML, Fries JK: Polyhydramnios: Ultrasonically detected prevalence and neonatal outcome. Obstet Gynecol 69:21, 1987

Homesley HD, Blessing JA, Rettenmaier M, Capizzi RL, Major FJ, Twiggs LB: Weekly intramuscular methotrexate for nonmetastatic gestational trophoblastic disease. Obstet Gynecol 72:413, 1988

Hricak H, Demas BE, Braga CA, Fisher MR, Winkler ML: Gestational trophoblastic neoplasm of the uterus: MR assessment. Radiology 161:11, 1986

Jequier AM, Winterton WR: Diagnostic problems of trophoblastic disease in women age 50 or more: Obstet Gynecol 42:378, 1975

Jolivet J, Cowan KH, Curt GA, Clendeninn NH, Chaber BA: The pharmacology and clinical use of methotrexate. N Engl J Med 309:1094, 1983

Jones WB: Current management of low-risk metastatic gestational trophoblastic disease. J Reprod Med 32:655, 1987

Kan PS, Eastman NJ: Coiling of the umbilical cord around the foetal neck. Br J Obstet Gynaecol 64:227, 1957

Kim DS, Moon H, Kim KT, Moon YJ, Hwang YY: Effects of prophylactic chemotherapy for persistent trophoblastic disease in patients with complete hydatidiform mole. Obstet Gynecol 67:690, 1986

Kouyoumdjian A: Velamentous insertion of the umbilical cord. Obstet Gynecol 56:737, 1980

Kruseman AC, Lent MV, Blom AH, Lauw GP: Choriocarcinoma in mother and child, identified by immunoenzyme histochemistry. Am J Clin Pathol 67:279, 1977

Lademacher DS, Vermeulen RCW, Harten JJVD, Arts NFT: Circumvallate placenta and congenital malformation. Lancet 1:732, 1981

Landy JH, Isada NB, Larsen JW: Genetic implications of idiopathic hydramnios. Am J Obstet Gynecol 157:114, 1987

Las Heras J, Harding PG, Haust MD: Recurrent bleeding associated with placenta membranacea partialis: Report of a case. Am J Obstet Gynecol 144:480, 1982

Leveno KJ, Quirk JG Jr, Cunningham FG, Nelson SD, Santos-Ramos R, Toofanian A, DePalma RT: Prolonged pregnancy: I. Observations concerning the causes of fetal distress. Am J Obstet Gynecol 150:465, 1984

Lewis JL Jr: Treatment of metastatic gestational trophoblastic neoplasms. Am J Obstet Gynecol 136:163, 1980

Li MC, Hertz R, Spencer DB: Effect of methotrexate therapy upon choriocarcinoma and chorioadenoma. Proc Soc Exp Biol Med 93:361, 1956

Lind T, Hytten FE: Relation of amnionic fluid volume to fetal weight in the first half of pregnancy. Lancet 1:1147, 1970

Lurain JR: Causes of treatment failure in gestational trophoblasic disease. J Reprod Med 32:677, 1987

Lurain JR, Brewer JI, Mazur MT, Torok EE: Fatal gestational trophoblastic disease: An analysis of treatment failures. Am J Obstet Gynecol 144:391, 1982

Lurain JR, Brewer JI, Torek EE, Halpern B: Natural history of hydatidiform mole after primary evacuation. Am J Obstet Gynecol 145:591, 1983

Mann K, Schneider N, Hoermann R: Thyrotropic activity of acidic isoelectric variants of human chorionic gonadotropin and trophoblastic tumors. Endocrinology 118:1558, 1986

Mathieu A: Hydatidiform mole and chorio-epithelioma: Collective review of literature for years 1935, 1936, and 1937. Int Abstr Surg 68:52,181, 1939

Mercer LJ, Brown LB: Fetal outcome with oligohydramnios in the second trimester. Obstet Gynecol 67:840, 1986

Messer RH, Gomez AR, Yambao TJ: Antepartum testing for vasa previa: Current standard of care. Am J Obstet Gynecol 156:1459, 1987

Miller ME, Higginbottom M, Smith DW: Short umbilical cord: Its origin and relevance. Pediatrics 67:618, 1981

Montz FJ, Schlaerth JB, Morrow CP: The natural history of theca lutein cysts. Obstet Gynecol 72:247, 1988

Mutch DG, Soper JT, Baker ME, Bandy LC, Cox EB, Clarke-Pearson DL, Hammond CB: Role of computed axial tomography of the chest in staging patients with nonmetastatic gestational trophoblastic disease. Obstet Gynecol 68:348, 1986

Naeye RL, Blanc WA: Fetal renal structure and the genesis of amniotic fluid disorders. Am J Pathol 67:95, 1972

Natsume M, Takada J: Choriocarcinoma: An unusual case recurring nine years after subtotal hysterectomy and followed by spontaneous regression of pulmonary metastases. Am J Obstet Gynecol 82:654, 1961

Novak E, Seah CS: Choriocarcinoma of the uterus. Am J Obstet Gynecol 67:933, 1954

Painter D, Russell P: Four-vessel umbilical cord associated with multiple congenital anomalies. Obstet Gynecol 50:505, 1977

Peckham CH, Yerushalmy J: Aplasia of one umbilical artery: Incidence by race and certain obstetric factors. Obstet Gynecol 26:359, 1965

Petrilli ES, Twiggs LB, Blessing JA, Teng NNH, Curry S: Single-dose actinomycin-D treatment for nonmetastatic gestational trophoblastic disease: A prospective Phase II trial of the Gynecologic Oncology Group. Cancer 60:2173, 1987

Pitkin RM: Acute polyhydramnios recurrent in successive pregnancies. Obstet Gynecol 48:425, 1976

Pritchard JA: Fetal swallowing and amniotic fluid volume. Obstet Gynecol 28:606, 1966

Queenan JT: Recurrent acute polyhydramnios. Am J Obstet Gynecol 106:625, 1970

Queenan JT, Gadow EC: Polyhydramnios: Chronic versus acute. Am J Obstet Gynecol 108:349, 1970

Rayburn WF, Beynen A, Brinkman DL: Umbilical cord length and intrapartum complications. Obstet Gynecol 57:450, 1981

Read EJ, Platzer PB: Placental metastasis from material carcinoma of the lung. Obstet Gynecol 58:387, 1981

Robinson LK, Jones KL, Benirschke K: The nature and structural defects associated with velamentous and marginal insertion of the umbilical cord. Am J Obstet Gynecol 146:191, 1983

Rustin GJ, Booth M, Dent J, Salt S, Rustin F, Bagshawe KD: Pregnancy after cytotoxic chemotherapy for gestational trophoblastic tumours. Br Med J 288:103, 1984

Ruvinsky ED, Wiley TL, Morrison JC, Blake PG: In utero diagnosis of umbilical cord hematoma by ultrasonography. Am J Obstet Gynecol 140:833, 1981

Schlaerth JB, Morrow CP, Montz FJ: Initial management of hydatidiform mole. Am J Obstet Gynecol 158:1299, 1988

Schlaerth JB, Morrow CP, Montz F, d'Ablaing G: Initial management of hydatidiform mole. Am J Obstet Gynecol 158:1299, 1988

Schlaerth JB, Morrow CP, Kletzky OA, Nalick RH, D'Ablaing GA: Prognostic characteristics of serum human chorionic gonadotropin titer regression following molar pregnancy. Obstet Gynecol 58:478, 1981

Shane JM, Naftolin F: Aberant hormone activity by tumors of gynecologic importance. Am J Obstet Gynecol 121:133, 1975

Shen-Schwarz S, Macpherson TA, Mueller-Heubach E: The clinical significance of hemorrhagic endovasculitis of the placenta. Am J Obstet Gynecol 159:48, 1988

Soernes T, Bakke T: The length of the human umbilical cord in vertex and breech presentations. Am J Obstet Gynecol 154:1086, 1986

Song HZ, Wu PC, Wang YE, Yang XE, Dong SY: Pregnancy outcomes after successful chemotherapy for choriocarcinoma and invasive mole: Long-term follow-up. Am J Obstet Gynecol 158:538, 1988

Soper JT, Clarke-Pearson D, Hammond CB: Metastatic gestational trophoblastic disease: Prognostic factors in previously untreated patients. Obstet Gynecol 71:338, 1988

Spellacy WN, Gravem H, Fisch RO: The umbilical cord complications of true knots, nuchal coils and cords around the body. Am J Obstet Gynecol 94:1136, 1966

Spirit BA, Cohen WN, Weinstein HM: The incidence of placental calcification in normal pregnancies. Radiology 142:707, 1982

Stanhope CR, Stuart GCE, Curtis KL: Primary ovarian hydatidiform mole: Review of the literature and report of a case. Am J Obstet Gynecol 145:886, 1983

Stiller AG, Skafish PR: Placental chorioangioma: A rare cause of fetomaternal transfusion with maternal hemolysis and fetal distress. Obstet Gynecol 67:296, 1986

Stone M, Dent J, Kardana A, Bogshawe KD: Relationship of oral contraception to development of trophoblastic tumour after evacuation of a hydatidiform mole. Br J Obstet Gynaecol 83:913, 1976

Suzuki M, Matsunobu A, Wakita K, Nishijima M, Osanai K: Hydatidiform mole with a surviving coexisting fetus. Obstet Gynecol 56:384, 1980

Szulman AE, Surti U: The clinicopathologic profile of the partial hydatidiform mole. Obstet Gynecol 59:597, 1982

Tindall R, Scott JS: Placenta calcification: A study of 3025 singleton and multiple pregnancies. Br J Obstet Gynaecol 72:356, 1965

Tow WSH: The classification of malignant growths of the chorion. Br J Obstet Gynaecol 73:1000, 1966

Wladimiroff JW, Barentsen R, Wallenburg HCS, Drogendijk AC: Fetal urine production in a case of diabetes associated with polyhydramnios. Obstet Gynecol 46:100, 1975

Wu FY: Recurrent hydatidiform mole: A case report of nine consecutive molar pregnancies. Obstet Gynecol 41:2000, 1973

Yuen BH, Burch P: Relationship of oral contraceptives and the intrauterine contraceptive devices to the regression of concentrations of the beta subunits of human chorionic gonadotropin and invasive complications after molar pregnancy. Am J Obstet Gynecol 145:214, 1983

Congenital Malformations and Inherited Disorders

Infants commonly are born with obvious structural aberrations, and Shepard (1986) estimates that 3 to 5 percent of all newborns have a recognizable anomaly. Unfortunately, the causes of these anomalies are myriad and frequently not identifiable. Beckman and Brent (1986) suggested the following etiological categories and the estimated contribution of each to fetal damage:

Genetic—chromosomal and single-gene defects	20–25%
Fetal Infections—cytomegalovirus, syphilis, rubella, toxoplasmosis, and others	3–5%
Maternal Diseases—diabetes, alcohol abuse, seizure disorders, and others	~ 4%
Drugs and Medications	< 1%
Multifactorial or unknown	65–75%

Importantly, detection of functional congenital aberrations increases with age, and the overall incidence increases to 6 or 7 percent in later childhood. The incidence of anomalies is increased in obstetrically abnormal pregnancies, and perhaps 50 percent of spontaneously aborted fetuses have a chromosomal abnormality (see Chap. 29, p. 490). Preterm and stillborn infants more commonly have major malformations, and performance of routine autopsies increases their detection. Birth defects are the leading cause of infant deaths before age 1, and they account for 20 percent of such deaths (Oakley, 1986). According to the Centers for Disease Control (1988), in 1986 congenital anomalies were the fifth leading cause of potential life lost before age 65.

GENETICS AND ENVIRONMENT

As emphasized by Fraser (1959), only a few congenital malformations appear to have a major environmental or genetic cause, and most probably result from interactions between genetic predisposition and subtle factors in the intrauterine environment. Perhaps the most dramatic example in past years of a major environmental cause of human malformation was maternal rubella infection (see Chap. 33, p. 615). When the fetus was infected during the first 8 to 10 weeks of pregnancy, rubella invariably caused a variety of malformations, including cataracts, cardiac defects, deafness, microcephaly, and mental retardation.

In experimental animals, chiefly rodents, fetal malformations have been produced by withdrawing various vitamins from the maternal diet and adding their chemical analogs; by injecting certain chemicals at specific stages in pregnancy, by cortisone administration, irradiation, and hyperthermia; and by other means. Although in many respects the results of these investigations may not be applicable to humans, such research has served to emphasize certain principles underlying induced malformations that bear on the etiology of many human deformities. They have been outlined by Wilson (1959) as follows:

1. The susceptibility of an embryo to a teratogen depends upon the developmental stage at which the agent is applied. The real determinant is the degree of differentiation within a susceptible tissue. Generally, all organs and systems seem to have a susceptible period early in primordial differentiation. Susceptibility to teratogens, in general, decreases as organ formation advances and usually becomes negligible after organogenesis is substantively completed.
2. Each teratogen acts on a particular aspect of cellular metabolism. Different teratogenic agents, therefore, tend to produce different effects, although acting at the same period of embryonic development and on the same system. The same agent, moreover, may produce different effects when acting at different stages of embryonic development.
3. The genotype influences to a degree the reaction to a teratogen. In many malformations, therefore, both a genetic predisposition and a teratogen are required to produce an anomaly.
4. An agent capable of causing malformations also usually causes an increase in embryonic mortality. This concept provides one explanation for early abortions.
5. A teratogen need not be deleterious to the maternal organism. Subclinical maternal rubella, for instance, may lead to congenital malformations.

The influences of purely genetic factors in the causation of congenital malformations is demonstrable in experimental animals and human beings. In certain strains of mice, for instance, about 15 percent of newborn young have cleft palate, but none has microphthalmia. However, in another strain, about 8 percent of the young have microphthalmia, but none has cleft palate (Fraser, 1959). These two examples are consistent with the observations that genetic composition predisposes one variety of embryo to cleft palate and the other to microphthalmia. In humans, the high frequency of supernumerary digits in black infants compared to white infants, not only in this country but throughout the world, also is consistent with this explanation.

TERATOLOGY

A teratogen is any agent or factor to which fetal exposure produces a permanent alteration in form or function of the offspring (Shepard, 1986). When considering whether a given chemical, drug, or physical force may be teratogenic by causing a specific malformation, several crucial factors are involved. Of premier importance is the time period in pregnancy during which there was fetal exposure. For these purposes, gestation is divided into three periods: (1) the *ovum*, from fertilization to implantation; (2) the *embryonic period*, from the 2nd through the 8th week; and (3) the *fetal period*, from after 8 completed weeks until term. The embryonic period is the most critical with regard to malformations since it encompasses organogenesis. By way of example, maternal rubella infection results in fetal infection early in pregnancy and frequently causes multiple congenital defects, while chronic but nondebilitating viral shedding less often follows late-pregnancy infection. Alternatively, a drug ingested during late pregnancy cannot cause malformations such as limb reduction defects. Although uncommon, certain drugs do have adverse effects when taken during the second half of pregnancy. For example, tetracyclines may cause yellow or brown discoloration of deciduous teeth. There is virtually no information regarding possible long-term effects, such as learning or behavioral problems, that might result from chronic prenatal medication ingestion.

Whether a chemical or a drug and its metabolites have fetal access in quantities sufficient to cause developmental anomalies is important. Maternal absorption and metabolism, protein binding and storage, molecular size, electrical charge, and lipid solubility are factors that may determine the degree of placental transfer. Important also is the concept that some agents are harmful only if given in sufficient amounts over prolonged periods.

In some instances, teratogenicity may not be apparent for years. For example, fetal rubella virus infection has been linked to progressive subacute sclerosing panencephalitis and diabetes in the second or third decade. Similarly, diethylstilbestrol may cause müllerian anomalies, as well as vaginal adenosis and carcinoma—problems which do not become apparent until reproductive age.

Given the plethora of drugs and medications available, as well as these complex factors, it is understandable that there is a paucity of information regarding the majority of drugs and their potential detrimental effects.

KNOWN TERATOGENS

The number of strongly suspected or proven human teratogens is surprisingly small, and these are listed in Table 32–1. Included are alcohol, thalidomide, certain folic acid antagonists (such as aminopterin), the vitamin A isomer isoretinoin, and some of the sex steroids such as diethylstilbestrol. Other drugs or medications considered by either some authorities or the manufacturer to have substantive fetal risk include oral contraceptives, valproic acid, some live-virus vaccines such as rubella, radioactive iodine, trimethadione, and some synthetic estrogens. Although there is no consensus regarding the teratogenicity of some of these latter medications, they obviously should be avoided during pregnancy when possible. For example, there

TABLE 32–1. STRONGLY SUSPECTED OR KNOWN HUMAN TERATOGENS

Drugs and chemicals	Infections
Aminopterin	Cytomegalovirus
Androgenic hormones	Rubella virus
Busulfan	Syphilis
Chlorbiphenyls	Toxoplasmosis
Coumarins	Venezuelan equine virus
Cyclophosphamide	**Maternal disorders**
Diethylstilbesterol	Alcoholism
Goitrogens (antithyroid drugs)	Connective tissue diseases
Isoretinoin	Diabetes
Lithium	Endemic cretinism
Organic mercury	Hyperthermia
Penicillamine	Virilizing tumors
Phenytoin	**Radiation**
Tetracyclines	Atomic weapons
Thalidomide	Radioiodine
Trimethadione	Radiotherapy
Valproic acid	

Adapted from Shepard: Adv Pediatr 33:225, 1986.

is good evidence that steroidal oral contraceptives and rubella vaccine do not cause birth defects, but they are never given intentionally during pregnancy. Fortunately, if inadvertently taken during pregnancy, fetal outcome is usually favorable with no significant adverse effects or malformations. **It is emphasized that this list is not all-inclusive, and the number of agents likely will increase as more information becomes available.**

DRUGS AND MEDICATIONS DURING PREGNANCY

Women commonly ingest medications or drugs while pregnant. The Centers for Disease Control (1987) surveyed 492 pregnant women in New York State and found that 90 percent took either prescription or over-the-counter drugs from 48 different classes. The average woman takes 3.8 medications during pregnancy. This may be less common in indigent women, and in a recent survey of several hundred women at Parkland Hospital, 46 percent took some type of drug or medication (other than iron or vitamins) during their pregnancy (Bertis Little, unpublished). These practices apparently are less common in the United Kingdom, where Rubin (1986), in a prospective survey, reported that only 35 percent of pregnant women took drugs or medications.

Besides prenatal vitamin and mineral supplements, commonly used drugs include antiemetics, antacids, antihistamines, analgesics, antimicrobials, tranquilizers, hypnotics, and diuretics. Although some of these are prescribed, many are taken either without physician advice or prior to realization of pregnancy. Thus, physicians providing prenatal care are frequently faced with the dilemma of whether a medication or drug might be harmful to the woman or, usually of more concern, to her fetus. **With rare exception, any drug that exerts a systemic effect in the mother will cross the placenta to reach the embryo or fetus.**

FOOD AND DRUG ADMINISTRATION CLASSIFICATION

The Food and Drug Administration, in 1979, established five categories for drugs and medications with regard to possible adverse fetal effects, and although not perfect, this classification certainly has removed some anxieties, for both patient and physician, concerning drug prescription during pregnancy.

Category A

Drugs for which controlled studies in humans have demonstrated no fetal risks. There are few category A drugs, and examples include multivitamins or prenatal vitamins but not "megavitamins."

Category B

Drugs for which animal or human studies have not demonstrated a significant risk. This category includes those drugs for which animal studies indicate no fetal risks but there are no human studies, or adverse effects have been demonstrated in animals with the drug but not in well-controlled human studies. Several classes of commonly used drugs, an example of which is the penicillins, are in this category.

Category C

Drugs for which there are no adequate studies, either animal or human, or drugs in which there are adverse fetal effects in animal studies but no available human data. Many drugs or medications commonly taken during pregnancy are in this category; therefore, it presents the most difficulty for the physician both with respect to clinical use and from a medicolegal standpoint.

Category D

Drugs for which there is evidence of fetal risk but benefits are thought to outweigh these risks. Anticonvulsants are examples, except for valproic acid.

Category X

Drugs with proven fetal risks that clearly outweigh any benefits. The acne medication, isoretinoin, which apparently causes multiple central nervous system, facial, and cardiovascular anomalies, is an example of a category X drug widely used in nonpregnant women.

No drug or medication should be taken during pregnancy unless clearly indicated, and it seems prudent to advise the woman of the specific indications. Obviously, this must be put into perspective. If there is no known fetal risk, and there is reasonable experience that a drug does not increase the baseline 3 to 5 percent malformation rate, then the woman should be reassured. As with genetic counseling, it is imperative to remind parents of this base malformation rate (see page 580). Alternatively, if the woman has taken category D or X drugs, she should be informed of potential fetal risks and options available. Not all drugs and medications have a Food and Drug Administration classification, and Briggs and colleagues (1986) have cataloged commonly used drugs according to this scheme (Table 32–2).

ANIMAL STUDIES

Although studies of teratogenic effects of drugs in animals must be conducted before prescribing during human pregnancy, there unfortunately is not always an obvious one-to-one relationship. The best example is the hypnotic drug thalidomide, which causes very few malformations in animals but is now one of the best-documented and potent human teratogens. The converse is more likely, and most small laboratory animals commonly employed for these experiments are generally very susceptible to teratogenic effects. Shepard (1986) emphasized that of nearly 1,600 drugs tested in animals, probably half cause teratogenic effects, although there are only approximately 30 documented human teratogens. Study animals also are susceptible to teratogenicity from environmental factors—for example, starvation—and the importance of controls is obvious.

TABLE 32–2. CLASSIFICATION BY INDICATION OF SOME DRUGS AND MEDICATIONS USED DURING PREGNANCY

Asthma	Cardiovascular disease	Hormones	Miscellaneous	Pain and inflammation
Albuterol C	β-blockers C	Clomiphene X	Antihistamines B/C	Acetaminophen B
Corticosteroids B,C,D	Coumarins D/X	Contraceptives X	Barbituates D	Aspirin C/D
Cromolyn B	Digoxin B/C	Estrogens X	Cocaine C	Codeine C/D
Ephedrine C	Furosemide C	Progestins D	Dextroamphetamine D/C	Ibuprofen B/D
Epinephrine C	Heparin B		Ethanol D/X	Indomethacin B/D
Metaproterenol C	Hydrochlorothiazide D	**Infections**	Guaifenesin C	Meperidine B/D
Terbutaline B	Methyldopa C	Acyclovir C	Heroin B/D	Morphine B/D
Theophylline C	Procainamide C	Amphotericin B	Insulin B	
	Quinidine C	Cephalosporins B	Isoretinoin X	**Psychiatric disorders**
Cancer	Verapamil C	Chloroquine B	Thioureas D	Amitriptyline D
Azathioprine D		Erythromycin B		Chlordiazepoxide D
Chlorambucil D	**Convulsive disorders**	Lindane B	**Nausea and vomiting**	Diazepam D
Cisplatin D	Carbamazepine C	Metronidazole B	Chlorpromazine C	Imipramine D
Cyclophosphamide D	Phenobarbital D/X	Miconazole B	Cyclizine B	Lithium D
Fluorouracil D	Phenytoin D	Nitrofurantoin B	Meclizine B	Nortriptyline D
Melphalan D	Trimethadione D/X	Nyastatin B	Promethazine C	Phenothiazines C
Methotrexate D	Valproic acid D/X	Penicillins B	Trimethobenzamide C	
Procarbazine D		Quinine D		
Vincristine D		Sulfonamides B		
		Tetracyclines D		
		Trimetroprim C		
		Zidovudine C		

Categories according to Food and Drug Administration guidelines, either by manufacturer or according to Briggs, Freeman and Yaffee: Drugs in Pregnancy and Lactations, 2nd ed. Baltimore, Williams & Wilkins, 1986.

POTENTIAL LITIGATION

The escalation of personal-injury suits has included those directed against physicians and pharmaceutical companies, alleging that medications taken during pregnancy caused malformations. Unfortunately, while not validated by scientific evidence, legal declarations of teratogenicity have prompted cessation of manufacture of some very useful drugs. An example is Bendectin, which was safe and effective for treatment of nausea and vomiting in early pregnancy. It is estimated that more than 30 million women used this drug worldwide (Brent, 1983). Despite contrary scientific evidence (Holmes, 1983), Bendectin was declared a "legal teratogen" by the court, and manufacture has ceased. More recently, a federal jury awarded an 8-year-old boy $95 million, presumably because the plaintiff's attorney convinced its members that the boy's deformed arms were the result of maternal ingestion of Bendectin (*Dallas Times Herald*, 15 July 1987).

Another worrisome example of judicial disregard for scientific proof lies in the *Wells v. Ortho* decision in which a judge-directed $5.1 million verdict was upheld by an appellate court. As summarized by Mills and Alexander (1986), the court rules that a spermicidal jelly was a teratogen, despite "the overwhelming body of evidence to the contrary," as well as the Food and Drug Administration's decision that no warning label concerning possible teratogenicity was necessary. The case prompted Brent (1985) to classify the spermicide as a *litogen*—a drug that does not cause malformations but does cause lawsuits!

SPECIFIC CONDITIONS

Not uncommonly, pregnant women have associated conditions or complications for which specific drug therapy is indicated. These women should be counseled about the possible teratogenic risks from the condition itself—for example, diabetes, epilepsy, or alcoholism—as well as any known fetal risks from specific drug therapy. Ideally, they should be counseled before attempting pregnancy; in actual practice, however, they frequently already have taken medications chronically during the critical period of organogenesis by the time they are seen first for prenatal care. Fortunately, but with a few notable exceptions, most drugs and medications prescribed for common medical and surgical complications of pregnancy can be used with relative safety. Moreover, in most cases the untreated condition poses more serious risks to both mother and fetus than any theoretical risks from these medications.

INFECTIONS

Infections, both minor as well as severe and life threatening, often complicate pregnancy. Some of the more commonly prescribed drugs for these infections are listed in Table 32–2.

Antibacterial Drugs

The most common bacterial infections complicating pregnancy are those of the urinary tract, and they include asymptomatic bacteriuria, cystitis, and acute pyelonephritis. Oral antimicrobials commonly given for these include penicillins, cephalosporins, sulfonamides, and nitrofurantoin. Beta-lactam antimicrobials have a long-established record of safety for use during pregnancy, and there are now a considerable number of oral and parenteral penicillins and cephalosporins for treatment of common and serious bacterial infections. While there have been very few studies, the majority of these drugs are listed as category B.

Nitrofurantoin is used widely and is in class B, as are sulfonamides, which may increase unbound bilirubin in the newborn if given very near delivery. Trimethoprim is in category C because it is a folic acid antagonist; however, Brumfitt and Pursell (1973) reported that congenital malformations were not increased in infants born to women given trimethoprim and sulfamethoxazole when compared to a placebo.

Erythromycin is a category B drug often used for penicillin-allergic patients, especially for treatment of syphilis and community-acquired pneumonias. Only small amounts gain fetal access, and this probably explains why the fetus is not always effectively treated when erythromycin is given for maternal syphilis (Fenton and Light, 1976).

The tetracyclines are in category D because they may cause discoloration of developing fetal deciduous tooth buds. Since there are several safe alternatives, tetracyclines should be avoided. A possible exception may be treatment for maternal syphilis in the penicillin-allergic woman for whom desensitization is impractical (see Chap. 33, p. 618).

Gentamicin is a widely used aminoglycoside that is in category C. While streptomycin and kanamycin are category D drugs because of an association with congenital hearing defects (Donald and Sellars, 1981), these effects are uncommon. Because of the latter association, the manufacturer of tobramycin has placed it in category D. Most pregnant women with pyelonephritis respond clinically to treatment with ampicillin or a cephalosporin; however, gentamicin or tobramycin are appropriate for treatment failures or resistant organisms (see Chap. 39, p. 809).

Antifungal Drugs

Symptomatic vaginal candidiasis is common during pregnancy, and three frequently used drugs for its treatment are clotrimazole, miconazole, and nystatin, all of which are usually classified as category B. In a recent report, Rosa and colleagues (1987a) found no increased frequency of birth defects in women given any of these for vaginitis in early pregnancy. Butoconazole, a relatively new imidazole derivative, is in category C.

Griseofulvin is given orally for ringworm infections of the skin, hair, and nails, and since there is little experience regarding its use during pregnancy, it is listed in category C by the manufacturer. Recently, concern was raised over a possible association of griseofulvin with conjoined twins (Rosa and colleagues, 1987b).

There is little information regarding the safety of amphotericin B given parenterally for systemic histoplasmosis, coccidioidomycosis, cryptococcosis, or candidosis. However, there are several case reports of its use during early pregnancy without adverse fetal effects, and it is classified as category B (Briggs and co-workers, 1986). Obviously, benefits of treatment for life-threatening systemic fungal infections, which rarely complicate pregnancy, outweigh any risks.

Antiparasitic Drugs

Parasitic infestations during pregnancy are probably much more common than appreciated; however, they are usually asymptomatic. As a general guideline, most do not need to be treated unless they cause symptoms. Metronidazole has received the most attention and controversy with regard to pregnancy, since it is the only truly effective agent for trichomoniasis, which commonly complicates pregnancy. A major concern is that it is mutagenic in bacteria and carcinogenic in some animals; however, it has been used with apparent safety for decades, and there are no substantive studies that implicate it as a teratogen. Rosa and colleagues (1987a) found no increased frequency of birth defects in offspring of 1,020 women given metronidazole during the first trimester. The drug is listed in category B.

Lindane is effective against *Sarcoptes scabiei* when topically applied, and although there are no large studies during pregnancy, it is classified as category B by the manufacturer. Mebendazole, a category C drug, is effective against a variety of helminths that includes pinworms, whipworms, roundworms, and hookworms.

Malaria is endemic in many parts of the world and is encountered in this country in refugees from Southeast Asia and Central America. Chloroquine is a valuable first-line antimalarial for which there is little published information regarding safety during pregnancy. Although best classified as category C, its benefits outweigh any theoretical risks in the woman with malaria. It is given for chemoprophylaxis in nonimmune pregnant women who must travel in malaria-endemic countries, but travel is not recommended if chloroquine-resistant strains are common (Centers for Disease Control, 1985b). Quinine is widely used for chloroquine-resistant falciparum malaria, but there are no large studies documenting its safety during pregnancy. Increased malformations were reported when large doses were used in attempts to induce abortion (Nishimura, 1976), and this prompted one manufacturer to classify its quinine sulfate tablets—utilized for leg cramps—as category X. While unproven for relief of muscle cramps, quinine should not be withheld in the woman ill with chloroquine-resistant malaria.

Antiviral Drugs

Acyclovir is an antiviral agent that has inhibitory activity against some herpesviruses that include simplex, varicella-zoster, and cytomegalovirus. It can be given topically, orally, or parenterally. There is virtually no information regarding its use in early pregnancy, although there are case reports of use in later pregnancy without adverse effects (Grover and colleagues, 1985; Hankins and co-workers, 1987). Burroughs Wellcome Company has established a registry to analyze effects of prenatal exposure, but by mid-1986 numbers were insufficient to draw definitive conclusions. Because of uncertainties of the mechanisms of action of antiviral agents, acyclovir should not be used to treat uncomplicated mucocutaneous herpes during pregnancy, but it should be given for life-threatening disseminated infections. It is listed as category C by the manufacturer.

Zidovudine, formerly called azidothymidine, was released in 1987 for treatment of retroviral infections, specifically human immunodeficiency virus, the causative agent of acquired immunodeficiency syndrome. It is teratogenic in rats at many times the usual adult human dose, but there are no data for human pregnancy. While listed as category C, owing to the universally fatal outcome of the condition for which the drug is given, it seems logical to treat afflicted pregnant women.

CARDIOVASCULAR DISEASE

Rheumatic cardiac valvar disease is the most common form of symptomatic heart disease encountered during pregnancy; however, improved techniques in cardiovascular surgery have resulted in an increasing number of women with clinically relevant congenital heart lesions becoming pregnant. These women often are given a myriad of drugs and medications, but fortunately, the majority can be used safely during pregnancy. Some of these commonly prescribed drugs are listed in Table 32–2, and an extensive review was provided by Rotmensch and colleagues (1983).

Heart Failure and Arrythmias

Cardiac glycosides are commonly prescribed, although their use is declining. They are used for heart failure, atrial fibrillation or flutter, as well as other supraventricular tachycardias. Digoxin is the most commonly used digitalis preparation, and while it rapidly crosses the placenta, there is no convincing evidence that it causes adverse fetal effects. Digoxin, as well as other antiarrhythmic drugs, have been maternally administered in attempts to control fetal tachycardias (Harrigan and co-workers, 1981).

Quinidine is used commonly for supraventricular tachycardias, as well as some ventricular arrhythmias. There is rapid placental transfer, but Hill and Malkasian (1979) reported no adverse fetal effects. Similarly, there is no evidence that procainamide used during early pregnancy has adverse fetal effects (Rotmensch and colleagues, 1983).

Propranolol is a β-adrenergic blocker used to treat both supraventricular and ventricular tachycardias during pregnancy, as well as hypertension and hyperthyroidism. There is no evidence that it causes fetal malformations, and the bulk of evidence indicates that it is not associated with fetal growth retardation (Briggs and colleagues, 1986). Neonatal side effects include possibly bradycardia and hypoglycemia.

Verapamil is an antiarrhythmic slow-channel calcium inhibitor with which there is limited experience during pregnancy (Klein and Repke, 1984). Nifedepine is used for treatment of hypertension. Both drugs have been used to forestall preterm labor, and ironically, concern has been raised, primarily from animal studies, that these drugs cause diminished uteroplacental perfusion (Besinger and Niebyl, 1988).

Chronic Hypertension

Methyldopa is widely used for chronic hypertension in pregnancy, and it is in category C. The newer β-adrenergic blocking agents, such as labetalol, metoprolol, and atenolol, are used widely in the United Kingdom for treatment of hypertension complicating pregnancy (Rubin and co-workers, 1983). Diuretics are prescribed by some, and they also are given acutely or chronically for pulmonary edema caused by heart failure. For the latter, furosemide often is used and is classified as category C by its manufacturer. The thiazide diuretics—hydrochlorothiazide and chlorothiazide—are listed in category D because of questionably increased malformations from first trimester exposure (Briggs and colleagues, 1986). They are widely used for chronic hypertension in the United States, and in many women treatment is continued throughout pregnancy.

Thromboembolism

Heparin is the drug of choice for either deep venous thrombosis or pulmonary embolism. It is a large, highly charged molecule that has minimal transplacental access. Its protracted use may cause maternal osteoporosis and thrombocytopenia, but there are no data that indicate heparin causes congenital anomalies.

Coumarin derivatives are of much smaller molecular weight and readily gain fetal access, where they may cause significant adverse effects. The genesis of these anomalies is probably from hemorrhages into any of several organs—for example, the brain. According to Hall (1980) and Stevenson (1980) and their colleagues, the *fetal warfarin syndrome* is identified in 15 to 25 percent of fetuses exposed during early pregnancy. The two most consistent findings reported are nasal hypoplasia and stippling of vertebral and femoral epiphyses seen on radiographs. Other adverse fetal effects that may follow second or third trimester exposure include optic atrophy, cataracts, microcephaly, microphthalmia, blindness, mental retardation, and skeletal abnormalities. These anomalies apparently arise as the result of hemorrhage from coumarin-induced coagulopathy. In addition, spontaneous abortions, stillbirths, and neonatal deaths are increased when coumadin therapy is given; therefore, it is not recommended for treatment of pregnant women except in the very few for whom heparin is absolutely contraindicated.

ASTHMA

Asthma complicates pregnancy in up to 1 percent of women (Hernandez and colleagues, 1980), and most medications for its treatment can be used with apparent safety during pregnancy. Those prescribed more commonly are listed in Table 32–2.

Theophylline salts are widely used bronchodilators, but there have been no large studies documenting their safety during pregnancy. Because of many years of use without observed teratogenicity, most are in category C. Aminophylline is the only salt available for parenteral use, but there are numerous oral forms, many of which contain other bronchodilators, such as ephedrine.

During an acute asthmatic attack, epinephrine may be given subcutaneously. While there is little evidence that epinephrine used in this manner causes adverse fetal effects, Heinonen and colleagues (1977) reported increased fetal malformations with first trimester use. These effects may have been related to the maternal illness itself, and it seems unlikely that an endogenously produced substance is a teratogen.

Terbutaline is a β-sympathomimetic drug that is a potent bronchodilator. There is no evidence that terbutaline given during pregnancy causes fetal anomalies, and Wallace and colleagues (1978) reported no increased adverse effects in a long-term study of infants exposed in utero. Two other β-mimetics—metaproterenol and albuterol—may be self-administered by inhalation, but there is little information regarding their safety.

For resistant cases, including women requiring hospitalization, any of several adrenal glucocorticoids usually are given. These agents are available in oral, parenteral, or inhaled forms. Interestingly, they are classified in categories B through D. For example, prednisone is listed in category B by Briggs and colleagues (1986), who list cortisone in category D. Severe asthma is dangerous to both mother and fetus, and if indicated, glucocorticoids should be given (see Chap. 39, p. 806).

SEIZURE DISORDERS

Epilepsy commonly coexists with pregnancy, and these women are at increased risk for giving birth to infants with congenital anomalies. It is unclear, however, whether epilepsy, per se, causes increased malformations or it is drug teratogenicity—or perhaps, the combination. According to Kelly (1984), women with epilepsy who take anticonvulsant medications chronically have a two- to threefold increased risk of malformed fetuses compared to nonepileptics. Some commonly prescribed anticonvulsants are listed in Table 32–2.

Phenytoin, previously called diphenylhydantoin, is the most commonly prescribed anticonvulsant; in 1975, Hanson and Smith described a clinical syndrome owing to the drugs. The *fetal hydantoin syndrome* is characterized by craniofacial and limb malformations accompanied by mental deficiency. In a prospective study of 468 women taking anticonvulsants, Kelly and associates (1984) reported that 30 percent of infants exposed to phenytoin in utero had minor craniofacial and digital anomalies, but that there was no increased frequency of major malformations or mental retardation. Gaily and colleagues (1988) described minor typical anomalies as genetically linked. Although it is unclear whether epilepsy itself or treatment with phenytoin causes these malformations, the drug usually is classified in category D.

Phenobarbital was once commonly used along with phenytoin for seizure control. While there is no firm scientific evidence that it is a human teratogen, many phenobarbital-containing compounds are listed as category X by manufacturers. Most of these latter drugs are for conditions other than epilepsy.

Trimethadione is used principally for petit mal seizures, and it is thought to be teratogenic, causing a syndrome similar to the hydantoin syndrome. There appears to be a phenotypic predisposition, since in nine families the incidence of congenital malformations was 69 percent (Briggs and colleagues, 1986). Valproic acid also is used for treatment of petit mal seizures and is associated with neural tube defects and microcephaly (Dalens and co-workers, 1980; Gomez, 1981). The Centers for Disease Control (1983) estimated that the risk of neural tube defects in exposed offspring may be as high as 2 percent. Trimethadione and valproic acid should be avoided during pregnancy.

Perhaps because of possible adverse effects of other anticonvulsants, carbamazepine now is used more frequently for grand mal epilepsy; in fact, some recommend it for new-onset epilepsy in pregnancy (Paulson and Paulson, 1981). Whether or not it is teratogenic still is unclear, and the manufacturer has listed it in category C.

Although several investigations have linked anticonvulsants with fetal malformations, the benefits of phenytoin, phenobarbital, and carbamazepine outweigh potential risks if such medications are necessary for seizure control.

HYPEREMESIS

Nausea and vomiting are common complaints, especially in early pregnancy, and until recently, antiemetics were probably the most widely prescribed drugs. Bendectin probably has received more attention, especially from a litigation standpoint, than any other drug given during pregnancy (see p. 561). The drug, a combination of doxylamine and pyridoxine, is no longer available in the United States—not because it was a proven teratogen but, rather, because it is a "popular litogen" (Brent, 1985). Indeed, numerous epidemiological studies, as well as animal studies, are consistent with the view that Bendectin is not associated with increased congenital malformations (Holmes, 1983).

Commonly prescribed antiemetics are listed in Table 32–2. In a prospective study of 543 women exposed to phenothiazines during early pregnancy, there was no evidence for increased malformations (Milkovich and colleagues, 1975). These investigators also reported no evidence for teratogenicity with Bendectin, meclizine, or cyclizine.

SOCIAL AND ILLICIT DRUGS

Social, or so-called recreational, drug use is virtually epidemic in the United States, and women of childbearing age also abuse these drugs. They have in common an addictive potential, and studies to determine their causality for almost any medical disorder are difficult to interpret, since the use of one frequently is accompanied by the use of others. For example, illicit drugs are usually admixed with alcohol or other legally obtained prescription drugs, such as minor tranquilizers.

Alcohol

Of the legal social drugs, alcohol is the most frequently used during pregnancy, and it is estimated that 1 to 2 percent of women of childbearing age are alcoholics (Golbus, 1980). Excessive and chronic ingestion of alcohol by the pregnant woman is likely to produce fetal maldevelopment, commonly referred to as the *fetal alcohol syndrome*. **Alcohol is now recognized as the leading known teratogen in the Western world** (Abel and Sokol, 1988a). In 1973 and 1974, Jones and associates described a common pattern of prenatal and postnatal growth retardation with characteristic cardiovascular, limb, and craniofacial defects in the offspring of alcoholic mothers. The facial characteristics included short palpebral fissures, short and upturned nose, flattened maxilla, and thinned upper vermillion of the mouth (Fig. 32–1). The children subsequently demonstrated impaired fine and gross motor function and impaired speech. The perinatal mortality rate was 17 percent. At 7 years of age, 44 percent of the survivors had an intelligence quotient below 80, compared to 9 percent in a control group. A 10-year follow-up of these infants subsequently was reported by Streissguth and colleagues (1985). Two of the 11 had died, and all of the 8 available for follow-up had growth deficiencies and dysmorphic features. Four children were described as being of borderline intelligence, whereas the other four were severely handicapped intellectually. The investigators further described new features of the syndrome that included dental malalignments, malocclusions, and eustachian tube dysfunction, which they hypothesize are related embryologically to midfacial hypoplasia.

While there is no doubt that heavy drinking causes fetal anomalies, differences of opinion persist in regard to possible adverse fetal effects from social drinking (Mills and Graubard, 1987; Sulaiman and colleagues, 1988). This is because the threshold dose varies with each patient. Rosett and co-workers (1983) found no differences in the frequency of abnormalities in offspring born to nondrinkers compared to rare and moderate drinkers. Binge drinking, however, is associated with malformations. The Council on Scientific Affairs of the American Medical Association (1983) estimated that between 1 in 300 and 1 in 2,000 liveborn infants are stigmatized by the syndrome. Moreover, the likelihood of fetal damage from even moderate drinking appears to be enhanced appreciably by the simultaneous use of a variety of drugs, including illicit drugs.

Women with chronic and severe drinking problems must be discouraged from becoming pregnant until they have been successfully treated, since as many as 30 to 40 percent of their offspring may be visibly affected. Consideration should be given to early pregnancy termination in alcoholic women. Although the more graphic examples of fetal alcohol syndrome usually are seen in infants of "alcoholic" mothers, it is certainly possible that isolated effects, such as learning or behavioral disorders, result from lesser exposure. **Alcohol ingestion is the most commonly identifiable cause of mental retardation** (Clarren and Smith, 1978). Therefore, the best advice to the woman pregnant or about to become pregnant is to abstain from all alcohol. It is hoped that the adverse effects of alcohol on pregnancy do not linger after the woman stops drinking.

Illicit Drugs

Chronic use by pregnant women of some illicit drugs, including opiates, barbituates, and amphetamines in large doses, is harmful to the fetus. Growth retardation and serious compromise as the consequence of drug withdrawal have been well documented. Often the mother who uses these drugs does not seek prenatal care and, even if she does, she may not admit to the use of such substances. As emphasized in Chapter 33 (page 613), the management of pregnancy and delivery, and successful care of the newborn, may be extremely difficult. Early abortion should be considered for addicted women.

Heroin is a commonly used illicit narcotic, and the principal adverse fetal effect of maternal addiction is drug withdrawal, which is associated with neonatal mortality of 3 to 5 percent (Madden, 1977). No increased frequency of congenital malformations has been reported in most studies; however, Ostrea and Chavez (1979) reported these to be increased in 830 heroin addicts. It is currently unclear whether heroin, per se, is associated with increased congenital malformations, since most users have atrocious dietary habits and commonly ingest a variety

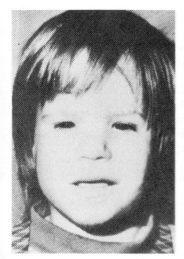
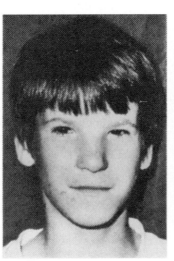
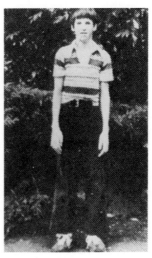

Figure 32–1. Fetal alcohol syndrome. Male child. **A.** At 2 years 6 months. **B, C.** At 12 years. Note persistence of short palpebral fissures, epicanthial folds, flat midface, hypoplastic philtrum, and thin upper vermillion border. He also has the short, lean prepubertal stature characteristic of young adolescent males with fetal alcohol syndrome. (*From Streissguth and colleagues: Lancet 1:85, 1985, with permission.*)

of other drugs and illicit substances, including, for example, alcohol. Methadone often is used as a narcotic substitute for treatment of heroin addiction, and although not associated with increased malformations, it may result in neonatal withdrawal symptoms worse than those from heroin (Newman and co-workers, 1975). Since 88 percent of women enrolled in a methadone program continued polydrug use, Edelin and colleagues (1988) rightfully questioned its use.

Because of its current popularity and news coverage, cocaine commonly is cited with regard to pregnancy. Bingol and associates (1987) and Little and co-workers (1989) reported significantly increased congenital malformations, stillbirths, and low birthweight infants born to cocaine users. Oro and Dixon (1987) and McGregor and colleagues (1987) reported increased preterm delivery and growth retardation associated with cocaine use. Placental hemorrhages were amplified if methamphetamines were used concurrently. Stillborns usually are related to placental abruptions, which likely are caused by the vasoconstrictor effects of cocaine taken intravenously or by nasal application (Acker and colleagues, 1983; Chasnoff and co-workers, 1985). Woods and colleagues (1987) reported a dose-dependent increase in maternal blood pressure and decreased uterine blood flow of as much as 200 percent in pregnant ewes given cocaine intravenously in doses similar to those taken "recreationally."

Marijuana is used by nearly 15 percent of pregnant women (Abel and Sokol, 1988b). While Δ9-tetrahydrocannabinol in high doses is teratogenic for animals, there is no evidence that marijuana is associated with any adverse human fetal effects (Greenland and colleagues, 1982). Likewise, it is unclear whether lysergic acid diethylamide (LSD) is teratogenic for the human fetus; while there have been reports of limb deformities, most infants exposed are normal (Stenchever and colleagues, 1970). Phencyclidine (PCP) is another popular hallucinogen, and it has been associated with fetal facial abnormalities (Strauss and colleagues, 1981). Methamphetamine is currently popular, especially the new form called *crank* that is smoked or snorted. While there is no evidence that amphetamines are teratogenic, their use is associated with increased preterm delivery and retarded fetal growth (Little and co-workers, 1988; Oro and Dixon, 1987).

PSYCHOTROPIC DRUGS

Major psychiatric illness is relatively uncommon during pregnancy; however, so-called minor tranquilizers are some of the more commonly ingested drugs. Diazepam is the prototype, and it is controversial as to whether it causes an increased incidence of cleft lip and palate (Entman and Vaughn, 1984; Rosenberg and co-workers, 1983). Another widely used benzodiazepine derivative, chlordiazepoxide, was associated with a fourfold increase in severe congenital anomalies (Milkovich and Van Den Berg, 1974). These two drugs are in category D, but others are listed in C, and they should not be used without appropriate indications (Table 32–2).

Meprobamate possibly is associated with increased defects. It is listed in category D and should be avoided. The barbituates are generally classified in category D because of the possible role of teratogenicity of phenobarbital when given to epileptic women, usually along with phenytoin.

Phenothiazines are used during pregnancy for major psychiatric illness, as well as for their antiemetic effects. Many have been in use for over 20 years, and experience with them generally has been good. The prototype, chlorpromazine, has been used extensively and is classified in category C, but no adverse affects were reported from the Collaborative Perinatal Project (Slone and colleagues, 1977). Other phenothiazines commonly used include fluphenazine, haloperidol, perphenazine, prochlorperazine, promazine, and thioridazine—all of which are in category C (Briggs and colleagues, 1986).

Lithium is uniquely used for manic-depressive illness, and its effects have been monitored by the Denmark-based Lithium Baby Register, which by 1977 reported an 11 percent congenital malformation rate when the drug was given in early pregnancy (Weinstein, 1977). Heart lesions are the most common, and the rare *Ebstein's anomaly* has occurred in a disparate number of exposed fetuses. Newborns also frequently suffer from acute lithium toxicity symptoms. The drug is listed in category D, and it should be reserved for women in whom the benefits are judged to outweigh the substantial risks.

Antidepressants are generally classified in category D, although epidemiological analysis of more than a half-million births indicate that the first trimester exposure to amitriptyline, nortriptyline, or imipramine was not associated with an increased number of birth defects (Briggs and colleagues, 1986).

OVER-THE-COUNTER MEDICATIONS

Aspirin

In eight surveys totaling nearly 55,000 women, over 60 percent said they took aspirin during pregnancy (Briggs and colleagues, 1986). Maternal use has been demonstrated to cause a variety of adverse effects, including some degree of platelet dysfunction and diminished factor XII activity (Bleyer and Breckenridge, 1970; Corby and Schulman, 1971). Shapiro and associates (1976) found no evidence that the use of aspirin during pregnancy caused perinatal death or reduced birthweight; moreover, aspirin does not appear to be teratogenic (Slone and co-workers, 1976). However, Australian workers reported that persistent ingestion of analgesic compounds containing salicylates, in combination with caffeine or phenacetin or both, was associated with an increased incidence of anemia, hemorrhage, prolonged gestation, perinatal mortality, and low birthweight (Collins and Turner, 1975). Aspirin is listed as category C, and because of its potentially adverse effects on the hemostatic mechanism and its displacement of bilirubin from protein-binding sites, its use from habit should be discouraged, especially late in pregnancy. Niebyl and Lietman (1988) suggest that acetaminophen is a better choice for antipyretic and analgesic use during pregnancy. Although acetaminophen is a category B drug, we have observed both severe maternal hepatic and renal failure as well as fetal death from acetaminophen toxicity.

Nonsteroidal Anti-inflammatory Drugs

Prostaglandin synthase inhibitors such as indomethacin have been used to arrest preterm labor, but they also may cause closure of the fetal ductus arteriosus. There are no reports, however, to suggest that these drugs are teratogenic in early pregnancy (Briggs and colleagues, 1986).

Antihistamines and Decongestants

Several drugs commonly are taken to provide symptomatic relief from mild upper respiratory illnesses, although they have no salutary effect on the course of the disease. Most such antihistamines and decongestants are classified in categories B or C, and while they are apparently harmless, they should be avoided, at least in early pregnancy.

CANCER

In general, most antineoplastic drugs should be considered capable of inducing teratogenic changes in the fetus, especially if given in the first trimester. Surprisingly, many are given without obvious adverse effects after this time. Long-term effects, however, have not been thoroughly evaluated. These drugs should not be withheld from the pregnant woman for whom cancer treatment is indicated. As expected, antineoplastic drugs are classified in category D (Table 32–2).

Another concern is the exposure of health-care workers to these agents. Selevan and colleagues (1985) reported a twofold increased risk of fetal loss in nurses exposed to antineoplastic drugs in the first trimester. They recommended that caution be exercised in mixing and administering these drugs. The long-term effects of cancer therapy, including chemotherapy and radiation, on infertility and birth defects also has been of concern. For example, treatment of advanced Hodgkin disease with multiple-drug regimens results in azospermia in many men, but a few recover to have oligospermia (Waxman, 1985). These regimens may induce amenorrhea, and if fertility is not lost, or if it returns, there appears to be no increase in abortions, fetal chromosomal damage, or fetal anomalies (Rustin and colleagues, 1984).

HORMONES

Before they are aware that they might be pregnant, many women take oral steroidal contraceptives during early pregnancy. In the past, a number of other sex steroids were given for various indications throughout early pregnancy, the foremost example being diethylstilbestrol. Although initial data from the Collaborative Perinatal Project indicated that oral contraceptives were associated with an increased fetal risk for cardiovascular defects, subsequent analysis has shown no difference when compared to control women who did not ingest these drugs (Wiseman and Dodds-Smith, 1984). Because of the former findings, however, estrogens, including oral contraceptives, usually are placed in category X.

Clomiphene is used for ovulation induction. There are isolated case reports of congenital malformations associated with its use; however, Kurachi and co-workers (1983) found no such association in 1,034 pregnancies in which ovulation was induced by clomiphene. The drug is classified in category X and should not be given until pregnancy is excluded.

ENVIRONMENTAL TERATOGENS

A variety of environmental hazards are associated with teratogenicity (Table 32–1). For example, several viruses and bacteria that cause fetal infections result in morphological and functional derangement, and these are considered in Chapter 33.

Excessively high levels of lead may be embryotoxic, and the Centers for Disease Control (1985a) recommends that maternal serum levels not exceed 25 μg per dL. This level was determined by studying the effects of lead on schoolchildren; and

recently, Bellinger and colleagues (1987) reported that cord lead levels in excess of 10 μg per dL were associated with subnormal infant development.

CHEMICALS

Methylmercury causes cerebral palsy and microcephaly in as many as 6 percent of children born to women who ingested fish from waters polluted with the chemical (Beckman and Brent, 1986). The syndrome is referred to as *Minamata disease,* after the Japanese village in which it was described.

Yusho is a syndrome caused by the ingestion by pregnant women of cooking oil contaminated with polychlorinated biphenyl. Characteristically, infants have low birthweight; pigmented gums, nails, and groins; hypoplastic nails; conjunctivitis with hypertrophied eyelid sebaceous glands; skull calcifications; rocker bottom heels; and possibly alterations of calcium metabolism (Beckman and Brent, 1986).

Herbicides, particularly Agent Orange, recently have received much publicity since millions of Vietnam veterans were exposed to this defoliant in the 1960s. The herbicide 2,4,5-trichlorophenoxyacetic acid is contaminated with variable concentrations of dioxin. To date, there are no studies that support a causal role between either of these chemicals and human malformation (Beckman and Brent, 1986; Shepard, 1986).

Paul and Himmelstein (1988) provided a review concerning chemical exposure in the workplace.

RADIATION

Radiation can cause cell death due to chromatin damage, which, in turn, may cause gross malformations, growth retardation, or embryonic death, depending on the dose (Beckman and Brent, 1986). The characteristic malformations seen with high-dose radiation from atomic bomb exposure are microcephaly and mental retardation. The risk of major malformations is not increased by in utero exposure to 5 rads or less (Shepard, 1986), and some studies suggest that the threshold for radiation effects may be 15 to 20 rads (Brent, 1987). The National Council on Radiation Protection and Measurements concluded that exposure of the embryo to less than 5 rads is associated with negligible risk, and it recommends against pregnancy termination (Brent, 1987). Children born to pregnant women who were exposed to the atomic bomb explosion had a 2.4 percent incidence of mental retardation with 10 to 49 rads exposure, and this increased to nearly 18 percent if exposure was 50 to 99 rads (Otake, 1984). The time most critical appeared to be between 8 to 15 weeks.

Most commonly used diagnostic procedures cause only low-level fetal x-ray exposure. For example, skull, chest, cervical and thoracic spine films, as well as mammography and computed cranial tomography, result in less than a 100 mrad fetal dose (Wagner and colleagues, 1985). Computed tomography of the chest or upper abdomen provides 1 to 3 rads exposure, and pelvic tomography is greater. For most procedures in which fluoroscopy is used—for example, a barium enema—a radiation dose can be calculated provided the time of exposure is known.

The potential of developing a malignancy during childhood following in utero radiation exposure is considered in Chapter 8 (p. 171).

INHERITED DISORDERS

As indicated on page 561, at least 20 to 25 percent of congenital malformations are the result of chromosomal abnormalities or single-gene defects. The majority, perhaps 65 to 75 percent, of birth defects are due to unidentifiable causes; however, because of their patterns of inheritance, they are presumed to be the consequence of a complex interaction between genetic predisposition and intrauterine environmental factors.

CHROMOSOMAL ABNORMALITIES

The incidence of chromosomal abnormalities in liveborn infants has been established in six studies to be between 1 in 50 and 1 in 200, and averages 1 in 178, or 0.56 percent (Boué and Boué, 1978). The frequency among stillbirths and infants who die during the neonatal period is 6 to 7 percent. The incidence of various chromosomal abnormalities among liveborn infants is presented in Table 32–3; and among stillbirths and neonatal deaths, in Table 32–4. As pointed out in Chapter 29, chromosomal abnormalities are identified in at least 50 percent of early spontaneous abortions.

Whether the involved chromosome is an autosome or a sex chromosome, the pathogenetic mechanism seems to be the same. During meiotic division in the gonad, a chromosome may "drop out" of the dividing cell (anaphase lagging) and thus be lost. Fertilization of such a gamete results in a zygote with one chromosome too few. In trisomies, one of the explanations of a chromosomal gain is *nondisjunction*, or failure of the gamete to split equally at meiotic division. If the cell with the extra chromosome is fertilized, the zygote becomes *trisomic*. These errors of meiotic division produce individuals whose cells are chromosomally equal but with an abnormal increase in chromosomal number. If nondisjunction occurs during mitosis after fertilization, however, the result is an individual with cells of two, and rarely even more, different chromosomal constitutions, or a chromosomal *mosaic*. In mosaicism, appraisal is more difficult, since the major phenotypic defects may be much less obvious and karyotypes may be misleading unless many cells are examined.

AUTOSOMAL TRISOMIES

Down Syndrome

This is the most common chromosomal defect reliably detected by amniocentesis early in the second trimester. In the past it also was referred to as mongolism and affected individuals were termed mongoloid. Most cases of Down syndrome result from an extra chromosome, and the most common trisomy is that of chromosome 21, which is identified in approximately 1 of every 800 liveborns. Trisomies of chromosomes 13 and 18 are less common. Also less common is a chromosomal *translocation*, which is the transfer of a segment of one chromosome to a different site on the same chromosome or to a different chromosome. In Down syndrome, such translocations are recog-

TABLE 32–3. MAJOR FINDINGS IN ESTABLISHED CHROMOSOMAL ANOMALIES IN MAN (FREQUENCY PER 1,000)

Syndrome	Chromosomal Complement	Sex Chromatin	Newborn Babies	Institution Populations	Signs Recognizable at Birth	Mean Parental Age[a]	
						Maternal	*Paternal*
Turner	45/X	Negative[b]	0.4		Lymphangiectatic edema of hands and feet Webbed neck	27.5	30.3
Klinefelter	47/XXY	Positive	2.0	10–30	None	33.6	37.7
Triple X	47/XXX	Double	0.6	4–7	None	32.5	35.8
YY	47/XYY	Negative	1.4–4[c]	10–30[d]	None		
Down trisomy 21	47	Depends on sex; ordinarily not abnormal	1.6	100	Mongoloid facies Simian line	36.7	
Translocation	46		Rare	Rare	Same		
Trisomy 13–15	47		Rare	Rare	Cleft palate Harelip Eye defects Polydactyly		
Trisomy 16–18	47		Rare	Rare	Finger flexion Lowset ears Digital arches	32.8	35.2
Cat cry	46 (Deletion B 5)		Rare	Rare	Cat cry Moon face		

[a] Data from Hamerton (ed.): Chromosomes in Medicine, London, Heinemann Medical Books Ltd., and from Rohde RA, Hodgeman JE, Cleland RS: Pediatrics 33:258, 1964.
[b] May be positive with iso-X complement.
[c] Ratcliffe and associates: Lancet 1:121, 1970; Sergovich and associates: N Engl J Med 280:851, 1969.
[d] Court Brown: J Med Genet 5:341, 1968. Refers to penal institutions.
Data from Maclean and associates: Lancet 1:286, 1964.

TABLE 32–4. INCIDENCE OF VARIOUS CHROMOSOMAL ABNORMALITIES AMONG STILLBIRTHS AND NEONATAL DEATHS

Abnormality	Percent
Sex chromosome	1.2
Autosomal trisomies	
Trisomy 21	0.7
Trisomy 18	1.8
Trisomy 13	0.5
Structural anomalies	
Balanced	0.35
Unbalanced	0.5
Others	0.7
Triploidy	0.35
Total	6.1

Adapted from Boué and Boué: In Shrimgeout (ed.): Towards the Prevention of Fetal Malformation. Edinburgh, Edinburgh University Press, 1978.

nized by study of karyotype. The important translocations are 13-15/21, 21/21, and 21/22. A female carrier with a 13-15/21 translocation has about a 20 percent chance of producing a Down infant. If either parent is a 21/21 carrier, 100 percent of the children will be affected; however, if any normal children have been produced or if one of the carrier's parents has the same balanced translocation, the carrier almost certainly has a 21/22 defect. The rate of recurrence of this specific type of translocation is reported to be low. A 21/21 translocation cannot be distinguished from 21/22 except by the birth of a normal child, which rules out the 21/21 translocation.

Down syndrome presents a striking clinical picture that may be recognizable at birth (Fig. 32–2). The facies of the infants are distinct, with narrow, slanting, closely set palpebral fissures. The tongue is thick and fissured, and the palatal arch is often high. Fingers are stubby and the hands present clear-cut dermatoglyphic patterns, particularly a simian line. Mental retardation subsequently becomes apparent. Associated heart le-

sions are common. Some infants have characteristic findings on chest radiographs (Edwards and colleagues, 1988).

Whereas in mothers up to the age of 30, the risk of birth of a liveborn infant with Down syndrome is less than 1 in 800, this risk increases to about 1 in 100 by age 40, and to 1 in 32 by age 45 (Table 32–5). The frequency of Down syndrome among conceptuses is higher than this, but a sizable fraction—perhaps twice as many—are lost as abortuses or stillborns (Hook, 1978).

Often, but not always, an experienced individual can accurately diagnose Down syndrome from the general appearance of the newborn (Fig. 32–2). Ideally, the capability for confirmation by chromosomal analysis should be available immediately for those instances in which other major complications are detected. Using bone marrow aspirate direct analysis, a karyotype can be obtained within a few hours. Thus, a decision as to the extent of treatment can be made promptly after informed consent for such treatment is obtained from the parents (Francke and colleagues, 1979).

Bovicelli and associates (1982) reviewed the pregnancy experiences of 26 affected mothers. Pregnancy in a woman with Down syndrome is rare and is associated with a high incidence of Down offspring. No male with Down syndrome is known definitely to have fathered a child.

Effect of Paternal Age

Paternal age does not appear to be an important risk factor for Down syndrome, but the age of the father does play a role in the development of autosomal dominant genetic diseases. The relative frequency of new autosomal dominant mutations in offspring increases logarithmically with paternal age during the usual period of fatherhood (Friedman, 1981). The absolute frequency of autosomal dominant disease as the consequence of new mutations among newborns whose fathers are 40 years of age or older is at least 0.3 percent.

Other Trisomies

Chromosomes 13 and 18 trisomies are less common than trisomy 21, and they are associated with much higher fetal and perinatal mortality, as well as decreased life expectancy.

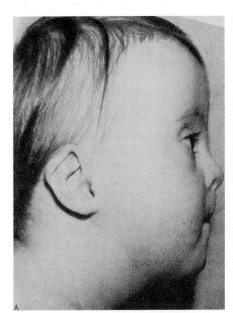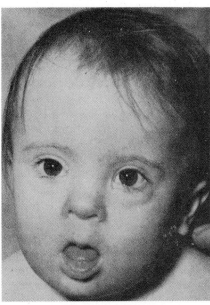

Figure 32–2. Young infant with Down syndrome (trisomy 21). (*From Smith and Jones: Recognizable Patterns of Human Malformation: Genetic, Embryologic and Clinical Aspects, Third Edition. Philadelphia, Saunders, 1982.*)

TABLE 32–5. RISK OF GIVING BIRTH TO A DOWN SYNDROME INFANT BY MATERNAL AGE

Maternal Age	Frequency of Down Syndrome Infants Among Births
30	1/885
31	1/826
32	1/725
33	1/592
34	1/465
35	1/365
36	1/287
37	1/225
38	1/176
39	1/139
40	1/109
41	1/85
42	1/67
43	1/53
44	1/41
45	1/32
46	1/25
47	1/20
48	1/16
49	1/12

From Hook and Lindsjo: Am J Hum Genet 30:19, 1978.

AUTOSOMAL DELETIONS

Loss of any appreciable amounts of autosomal genetic material, in most cases, is associated with fetal death. Rarely, some of these fetuses survive, but they are usually severely malformed and mentally retarded. One of the more common deletions results in the *cri-du-chat syndrome*, caused by deletion of a portion of the short arm of chromosome 5.

SEX CHROMOSOMAL ANOMALIES

Abnormalities of the sex chromosomes are relatively common, and they may result from either monosomies or polysomies. McKusick (1986) lists 124 X-linked defects.

Turner Syndrome (45,X)
Most sex monosomies result in early pregnancy loss, and nearly 20 percent of early spontaneous abortions are sex monosomies. Loss of the long arm of the X chromosome results in streaked ovaries and amenorrhea. In 70 percent of cases, the paternal X is missing. The short arm of X controls height, and phenotypic females with 45,X monosomy have normal intelligence and gonadal dysgenesis along with short stature and other physical stigmata, including a high incidence of cardiac and renal anomalies. Interestingly, these babies are born with a normal number of ovarian follicles, but by age 10 the ovaries are streaked. Occasionally, some follicles persist until puberty and pregnancy has been reported. These syndromes account for about half of the cases of gonadal dysgenesis, while other sex chromosome anomalies make up most of the rest.

Klinefelter Syndrome (47,XXY)
Additional X chromosomes to the normal male XY karyotype are relatively common polysomies, and are seen in 1 in 1,000 male infants. Males with 47,XXY constitute the most frequent abnormality of sexual differentiation and, except for some mo-

saics, are invariably infertile. They have testicular atrophy, azospermia, and elevated gonadotropins; usually there are associated somatic abnormalities, especially gynecomastia and obesity. Mild mental deficiency is common, and in syndromes caused by more than two X chromosomes, these abnormalities are greatly magnified.

Fragile X Syndrome
This X chromosome abnormality is the most commonly inherited cause of mental impairment, and it is second only to Down syndrome as a chromosomal cause of retardation (Chudley and Hagerman, 1987). The prevalence in the general population is estimated at 1 in 2,000 males, with a heterozygous prevalence in females of 1 in 1,000. The prevalence in severely mentally retarded populations varies from 2 to 6 percent.

The male patient with fragile X syndrome typically has before puberty a triangular face, prominent ears, and macroorchidism. Other organ system abnormalities are common and apparently are due to connective tissue dysplasia—for example, aortic dilation and mitral valve prolapse. A number of behavioral and speech patterns are present, and the degree of mental retardation is variable. Autism is common, and about 8 percent of autistic males are found to have fragile X syndrome (Brown and colleagues, 1986).

The cause of the disorder, which determines the phenotype described above, is the only known phenotype caused by an anomaly of the *fragile sites,* which are specific chromosome regions that fail to condense normally during mitosis. On karyotyping, these chromosomes are characterized by a nonstaining gap or constriction. Interestingly, only 5 to 50 percent (average 20 percent) of cells from affected males will have a demonstrable fragile site (Chudley and Hagerman, 1987).

The gene is not completely penetrant, and only about half of affected males have the obvious syndrome. Female heterozygotes also may be affected clinically, and approximately one third have varying degrees of mental retardation. There is a positive correlation between the proportion of cells containing fragile X chromosomes seen in females and mental impairment, consistent with the Lyon hypothesis of random X inactivation.

Prenatal diagnosis is possible through karyotyping of chromosomes obtained by either amniocentesis or chorionic villus biopsy. As emphasized by Jenkins and colleagues (1986), these tests are technically very difficult to perform.

SINGLE-GENE DEFECTS

Single-gene mutations cause defects that are manifest clinically by Mendelian inheritance patterns, which cause phenotypic abnormalities in 1 percent of all newborns. Individual disorders are rare, but the number so far catalogued—nearly 4,000—underscores the complexity of these mutations. As with any Mendelian inheritance, their clinical presentation can be classified into autosomal dominant, autosomal recessive, or X-linked. Some of the more common Mendelian disorders are shown in Table 32–6.

MODES OF INHERITANCE

Dominant Inheritance
A mutant gene producing its effects when present on one or both chromosomes of a given pair is referred to as a dominant gene, and nearly 1,200 have been identified (McKusick, 1986).

TABLE 32–6. SOME RELATIVELY FREQUENT MENDELIAN DISORDERS AFFECTING ADULTS

Autosomal dominant
Achondroplasia
Acute intermittent porphyria
Adult polycystic kidney disease
Familial hypercholesterolemia
Hereditary hemorrhagic telangiectasia
Hereditary spherocytosis
Huntington chorea
Idiopathic hypertrophic subaortic stenosis
Marfan syndrome
Myotonic dystrophy
Neurofibromatosis
Noonan syndrome
Osteogenesis imperfecta tarda
Polydactyly
Tuberous sclerosis
von Willebrand disease

Autosomal recessive
α-Thalassemia
Albanism
β-Thalassemia
Congenital adrenal hyperplasia
Cystic fibrosis
Deafness
Familial mediterranean fever
Friedrich ataxia
Hemochromatosis
Hereditary emphysema
Homocystinuria
Sickle cell anemia
Phenylketonuria
Tay-Sach disease
Wilson disease

X-Linked
Chronic granulomatous disease
Color blindness
Fabry disease
Glucose-6-phosphatase deficiency
Hemophilia A
Hypophosphatemic rickets
Ocular albinism
Testicular feminization

Modified from Goldstein and Brown: Genetic Aspects of Disease. Chapter 57 in Harrison's Principles of Internal Medicine, 11th Edition, New York, McGraw-Hill, 1987, p 290.

Some of those that are more common are listed in Table 32–6. A dominantly inherited disease caused by a single gene is transmitted from one generation to the next in a direct line so that each affected individual has an affected parent and there are no skipped generations. There is a 50 percent chance that the child of an affected parent with an unaffected mate will inherit the condition. The affected child will in turn transmit the defect to half of his or her offspring.

A dominant trait may be sex-lined or autosomal. If the trait is dominant and linked to the X-sex chromosome, all of the daughters of an affected father but normal mother will inherit the gene, and none of the sons will affected. If, however, the mother is heterozygous and affected and the father normal, she will transmit the condition to half of her daughters and half of her sons. If the mother is homozygous and affected, she will transmit the condition to all her children.

Nongenetic factors may mimic inherited determinants in the production of disease, but these *phenocopies* often can be detected by detailed history, appropriate clinical examination, and studies in the laboratory. Familial recurrence is unlikely with phenocopies.

Most autosomal disorders, unlike recessive ones, characteristically have a delayed age of onset and show variability in clinical expression.

Penetrance
A dominant gene with phenotypic expression in all individuals who carry the gene is said to have 100 percent penetrance. If not expressed in some individuals even though they have the gene, the gene is not completely penetrant. The degree of penetrance may be quantitatively expressed as the ratio of carriers who show the factor in question to the total number of individuals who have the gene. A gene that is 80 percent penetrant is expressed in only 80 percent of people who have that gene. The term penetrant is applicable not only to heterozygous dominant genes but also to homozygous genes, whether dominant or recessive.

Expressivity
The same gene may express itself in a variety of ways in different people. This characteristic is known as the expressivity of the condition. The expressivity of a gene varies from complete manifestation of the condition to complete absence.

Recessive Inheritance
A child with an inherited disease that requires for its clinical expression the contribution of a duplicate mutant gene from each of its parents—as, for example sickle cell anemia—is affected by a recessively inherited disease. More than 600 disorders have been described (McKusick, 1986), and some that are more common are shown in Table 32–6. Most inherited enzyme defects are recessive. The parents in these circumstances may be either heterozygous carriers of the mutant gene or homozygous and therefore affected. The clinical picture in these syndromes is more uniform than with autosomal dominant disorders and, in general, manifests at an early age.

If the recessively inherited disease is autosomal, either sex may be similarly affected, and the parents and more remote ancestors are usually unaffected. The probability of a subsequent child being affected in such a family is one in four. The likelihood that a normal sibling of an affected child is a carrier of the defect is two chances out of three. The carrier child will not produce affected children, however, except by mating with another carrier or an affected individual. If a recessive gene is rare, there is only a remote chance that unrelated carriers will procreate.

In sex-linked recessive inheritance, the affected individuals are nearly always males, since the female must have mutations in both X chromosomes to manifest disease. Red-green color blindness and hemophilia A and B are well-known examples of sex-linked recessive inheritance. The mothers of the affected males are the carriers and, as with all sex-linked inheritance, male-to-male transmission does not occur. Positive information in this type of inheritance comes from the maternal side of the family pedigree, whereas the paternal history is of little consequence.

INBORN ERRORS OF METABOLISM

There are several rare but heritable inborn errors of metabolism, most of which result from the absence of crucial enzymes, with resulting incomplete metabolism of proteins, sugars, or fats. In some cases, there are consequently high levels of toxic metabolites in the blood, causing mental retardation and other defects. These metabolic errors are true congenital defects, which are inherited most often as autosomal recessives.

Phenylketonuria

The inability to metabolize phenylalanine appropriately to tyrosine because of diminished *phenylalanine hydroxylase* activity is an example of an inborn error of metabolism that is inherited in an autosomal recessive manner. It has been reported in 1 in 10,000 to 1 in 15,000 white infants, but much less often in black infants. Early diagnosis is important, since optimal early treatment with limitation of phenylalanine consumption will result in normal levels of intelligence (Williamson and associates, 1981). Many states now require that a screening test for phenylketonuria be applied to all newborn infants. About 10 cases are identified annually by the Texas Newborn Screening program, which was begun in 1983.

Women with phenylketonuria adequately managed by diet during childhood may still have poor pregnancy outcomes, including high frequencies of spontaneous abortion, microcephaly, and mental retardation. These abnormalities are induced by excessive maternal phenylalanine concentrations, and women who wish to conceive should be advised to adhere to a diet low in phenylalanine before conception (Ghavami and associates, 1986; Rohr and colleagues, 1987). Even then, a normal outcome cannot be guaranteed (Lenke and Levy, 1982).

MULTIFACTORIAL OR POLYGENIC INHERITANCE

The largest source of genetic variability comes from the combined actions of a number of genes, each with a very small individual effect. The great range of effects so produced is thought to be responsible for the continuous variation seen among normal human beings, as expressed in stature, intelligence, blood pressure, and quite likely the susceptibility to a number of common diseases.

Many of the more common congenital malformations have a genetic factor in their causation. In multifactoral genetic diseases, there is a *polygenic* component that describes a series of genes interacting to produce a cumulative effect. The increased incidence in relatives, compared to the incidence in the general population, is difficult to explain in terms of any known environmental factors and is much below that found in single-gene transmission. Common congenital malformations with an incidence at birth of at least 1 in 1,000—such as cleft lip, pyloric stenosis, talipes equinovarus, congenital hip dislocations, spina bifida, anencephaly, and congenital heart defects—are polygenically inherited with varying degrees of environmental modification. Overall, these abnormalities are identified in about 1 percent of newborn infants.

EMPIRICAL RISKS

In the majority of cases, a simple pattern of inheritance cannot be demonstrated. In such patients, prognosis is derived from data on empirical risk, based on the pooled experience of many investigators. Such pooled data may be inapplicable to the individual case and occasionally misleading because they include high-risk and low-risk families. The average so obtained may thus either over- or underestimate the true risk. In many instances, however, such average data represent the only estimates available. As a rule of thumb, the risk of a significant malformation in any pregnancy is approximately 1 to 2 percent. The risk of a second malformed child is about 5 percent, and the risk increases with subsequent malformed children.

CONSANGUINITY

The risks of recurrence of affected offspring is greater for related than for nonrelated parents, and the closer the relationship, the greater is the risk. Even for closely related couples such as first cousins, however, the chance of having a significantly abnormal child, although twice that expected for children of nonrelatives, has been estimated by Motulsky and Hecht (1964) not to exceed 2 percent. Thus, there is no compelling genetic reason to discourage cousin marriage unless there is familial evidence of recessive disease. Reed (1963) reported a risk of malformation of about 10 percent in a child resulting from a brother-sister union.

DIAGNOSIS

Some fetal anomalies can be visualized by careful ultrasonic examination. In many cases, attention is called to a problem because of lack of fetal growth or abnormal amounts of amnionic fluid, or both (see Chap. 38, p. 767). Some cases are detected during level 2 ultrasound evaluation in women at high risk. Finally, many are detected at routine ultrasonic examination to determine gestational age, to verify suspected multifetal gestation, or perhaps to confirm fetal viability. Sabbagha and colleagues (1985) reported their results from the Northwestern Perinatal Center, to which 615 pregnant women at high risk for birth defects had been referred for targeted imaging. They found 81 fetal anomalies, or 14 percent, and importantly, the predictive values of abnormal and normal ultrasonic imaging were 95 to 99 percent, respectively. (Ultrasound screening is discussed in Chapter 15.)

In dealing with an anatomically abnormal fetus, it must be remembered that isolated defects are unusual, and that other anomalies frequently coexist. Sometimes these aberrations result from chromosomal abnormalities, and many are incompatible with extrauterine life. Therefore, and as emphasized by Vintzileos and colleagues (1987), reasonable management decisions can be made only if there is accurate prenatal ultrasonic anatomical assessment. In some cases, especially those at risk for cardiovascular anomalies, fetal echocardiography is done.

In some cases, fetal cells may be obtained for karyotyping, from either amnionic fluid or fetal blood obtained by ultrasonic guidance from the umbilical cord or placental vessels (see Chap. 15, p. 282). Platt (1986), Nicolaides (1986), and Williamson (1987) and their many colleagues have performed such studies in sonographically abnormal fetuses, and approximately a third of these were found to have a chromosomal anomaly.

NEURAL-TUBE DEFECTS

Neural-tube defects result from the tube's failure to close by day 26 to 28. This produces a spectrum of cranial and spinal canal defects that range from anencephaly to very slight defects of the vertebra. Some of the more common neural-tube anomalies are listed in Table 32–7. The incidence of neural-tube defects appears to be decreasing for unknown reasons (Owens and associates, 1981; Stein and colleagues, 1982). Lemire (1988) recently reviewed these defects in detail.

TABLE 32–7. INCIDENCE OF VARIOUS NEURAL-TUBE DEFECTS IN THE UNITED STATES

Type	Incidence per 1,000 Births	Neonatal Deaths (percent)	Long-Term Disability[a] (percent)
Anencephaly	0.6–0.8	100	0
Open spina bifida	0.5–0.8	33	65
Closed spina bifida	0.1–0.14	7	10
Total	1.2–1.7	60	60

[a] Includes lower limb paralysis, sensory loss, bladder and bowel problems, clubfoot, scoliosis, meningitis, hydrocephalus, and mental retardation.
From The American College of Obstetricians and Gynecologists: Prenatal Detection of Neural Tube Defects. Technical Bulletin No 99, December 1986.

Anencephaly

Anencephaly is a malformation characterized by absence of the skull and cerebral hemispheres that are either rudimentary or absent (Fig. 32–3). Most often the pituitary gland also is either absent or markedly hypoplastic. The absence of the cranial vault renders the face very prominent and somewhat extended, the eyes often bulge from their sockets, and the tongue hangs from the mouth. About 70 percent of anencephalic fetuses are females.

In addition to the virtual absence of brain tissue in anencephalic fetuses, typically there is extreme diminution in the size of the adrenal glands, the combined weight of which may be well under 1 g, in contrast to the normal weight of 5 g. The small size of the gland reflects the absence of fetal, or provisional, cortex, and it is commonly believed but not proved that the adrenal hypoplasia is secondary to the absence of the pituitary gland.

Nothing definite is known about the cause of anencephaly, but it appears that both genetic and environmental factors are involved. The possible role of folic acid in the genesis of neural-tube defects is considered in Chapter 14 (page 266). A genetic factor is suggested by the high frequency with which this malformation recurs in subsequent pregnancies. Yen and MacMahon (1968) emphasized, however, that the relatively small increase (about 5 percent) in sibship risk over the rate in the general population furnishes a strong argument against a single-gene hypothesis. A polygenic predisposition is possible, but the very rare occurrence of concordance in twins is difficult to reconcile with either genetic or environmental causes.

Extreme examples of recurrence in siblings have been reported, in which women have produced four successive anencephalic infants (Horne, 1958). The reported geographic differences in the incidence of anencephaly, however, have led to the belief that different environmental conditions in these several areas, notably differences in diet, predispose to the anomaly.

Inability to palpate a fetal head abdominally is suggestive of anencephaly, but sonographic or radiological examination provide for definitive diagnosis (Fig. 32–4). Since accompanying hydramnios occurs in the majority of cases, it too suggests anencephaly or, perhaps, another malformation. Anencephaly is probably the most common cause of gross hydramnios, which may occasionally be sufficiently massive to require therapeutic amniocentesis (see Chap. 31, p. 557). Because of the diminutive size and abnormal shape of the fetal head, breech and face presentations are common.

The most frequent practical question posed by pregnancies complicated by anencephaly is whether to initiate labor as soon as the diagnosis is confirmed. The uterus containing an anen-cephalic fetus may be refractory to oxytocin. Late in pregnancy, when severe hydramnios is almost the rule, the slow aspiration of 2 to 3 L of excess amnionic fluid usually will reduce the risk of placental abruption following spontaneous rupture of the membranes with sudden loss of amnionic fluid and marked uterine decomposition. Moreover, the myometrium appears to contract more effectively after slow removal of some of the fluid. The insertion of laminaria tents (see Chap. 29, p. 502), followed by vaginal administration of prostaglandin compounds to terminate the pregnancy, has proved ultimately to be effective in cases of anencephaly so managed by Osathanondh and associates (1980).

Holzgreve and colleagues (1987) reported that two anencephalic infants served as kidney donors for three recipients. From one anencephalic infant, two kidneys were transplanted, one each to a 4- and a 9-year-old. From the other anencephalic infant, both kidneys were placed in a 25-year-old recipient. The donors thrived and the kidneys were demonstrated to grow! These successes have caused considerable ethical debate regarding the potential of any abnormal fetus serving as an organ donor (Arras and Shinnar, 1988).

The duration of anencephalic pregnancies, especially in the absence of hydramnios, may be remarkably long and can exceed that reported in any other form of gestation with a living fetus. In the well-authenticated case of Higgins (1954), for example, the duration of pregnancy was 1 year and 24 days after the last menstrual period, with fetal movements perceived until the moment of delivery.

Elevated levels of α-fetoprotein (see p. 584) in amnionic fluid or maternal serum reliably predict the majority of cases of larger open neural-tube defects, including anencephaly. Closed or very small open neural-tube abnormalities may not be detected.

Spina Bifida and Meningomyelocele

Spina bifida consists of a hiatus, usually in the lumbosacral vertebrae, through which a meningeal sac may protrude, forming a *meningocele*. If the sac contains the spinal cord as well, the anomaly is called *meningomyelocele* (Fig. 32–5). In the presence of complete rachischisis, the spinal cord is represented by a ribbon

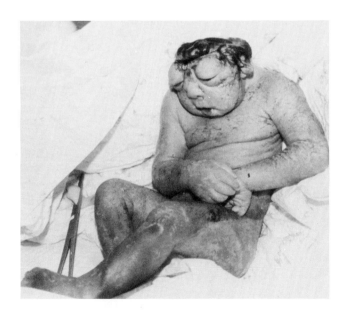

Figure 32–3. Anencephalic infant.

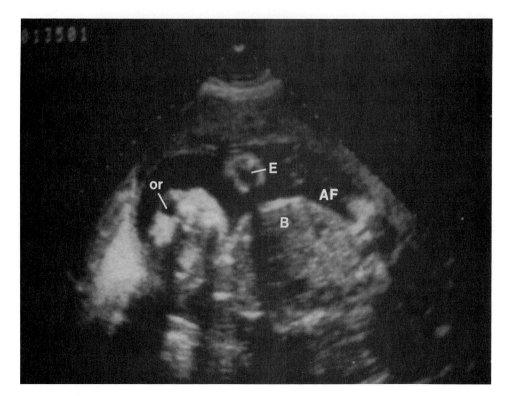

Figure 32–4. Longitudinal sonogram of an anencephalic fetus. The rudimentary head without a calvarium is apparent when the size of the orbit (*or*) of the eye is compared to it. The fetal body (*B*) and an extremity (*E*) are seen also. Amnionic fluid (*AF*) is not excessive. (*Courtesy of Dr. R. Santos.*)

of spongy, red tissue lying in a deep groove. In these circumstances, the infant dies soon after birth. In other instances, the defect may be very slight, as in *spina bifida occulta*. Associated malformations, particularly hydrocephaly, anencephaly, and clubfoot, are common. If part of the brain protrudes into the sac, a *meningoencephalocele* results. In case of open neural-tube defects, α-fetoprotein near midpregnancy is likely to be unusually high in both maternal plasma and in amnionic fluid (see p. 584).

Hydrocephaly

Because of the clinical importance of hydrocephaly as a cause of dystocia and rupture of the uterus, and the difficulties in decision making concerning route of delivery, this malformation is considered also in Chapter 19, (p. 371), together with other fetal causes of dystocia.

The characteristic ultrasonic finding is dilatation of the lateral ventricles (Fig. 32–6). Associated anomalies, including spina bifida, are fairly common. Hydrocephaly is seldom identified at or

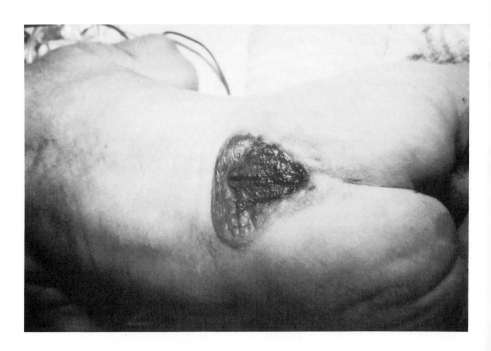

Figure 32–5. Large meningomyelocele. (*Courtesy of Dr. Victor Klein.*)

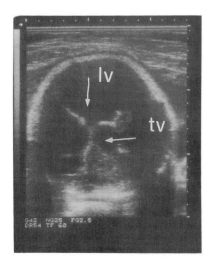
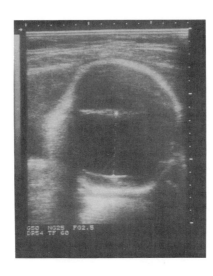

Figure 32–6. Fetal head showing marked dilatation of lateral ventricles (*lv*) and the third ventricle (*tv*). **B.** Same case showing marked dilatation of the lateral ventricle. (*Courtesy of Dr. Rigoberto Santos.*)

before midpregnancy, but if so, pregnancy termination is an option.

Because of the bleak outlook for normal intellectual development in fetuses with substantive degrees of ventricular distension, considerable enthusiasm developed among several groups of investigators to perform in utero shunts for cerebrospinal fluid. Emphasizing a team approach, and taking careful steps to first exclude fetuses with other anomalies by careful ultrasonic imaging and fetal karyotyping, most groups planned to surgically place shunts in those fetuses with isolated progressive ventriculomegaly (Harrison and colleagues, 1982). The results of such procedures, unfortunately, have been discouraging. Manning and co-workers (1986) described the results obtained in the first 44 cases so managed and reported to the International Fetal Surgery Registry. Although 83 percent of the fetuses survived, the procedure-related death rate was 10 percent. Of the survivors, more than half had severe neurological handicaps, and only 35 percent are developing normally.

A protocol for management of congenital hydrocephaly, including incidence, epidemiology, embryology, pathophysiology, and genetic counseling, has been provided by Vintzileos and associates (1983).

URINARY TRACT ANOMALIES

Renal Agenesis
The incidence of complete absence of the kidneys is about 1 in 4,000 births (Potter, 1965). This malformation is more frequent in male infants and is characteristically accompanied by oligohydramnios. Renal agenesis and the associated changes commonly are referred to as the *Potter syndrome*. The infant has prominent epicanthal folds; a flattened nose; and large, low-set ears. The skin is loose and the hands often seem large. Cardiac malformations are common, and one third of the infants are stillborn. The longest reported survival is 48 hours, since pulmonary hypoplasia is found almost invariably. Renal agenesis should be suspected when sonographic evidence of scant to absent amnionic fluid is observed and neither kidneys nor a filled bladder is observed.

Urinary Tract Obstruction
Persistent obstruction of the fetal urinary collecting system will destroy the kidneys unless relieved. Therefore, when obstruction of the lower urinary tract has been detected, relief may be accomplished in some circumstances by providing drainage from the bladder. Persistent obstruction almost certainly is accompanied by oligohydramnios. With normal amounts of amnionic fluid, obstruction most likely is intermittent and probably does not warrant attempts at drainage in utero. Results with urinary diversion for obstructive uropathy have been more encouraging than shunts done for hydrocephaly. Evaluation is similar for both procedures, and careful examination is done to look for other congenital anomalies as well as pulmonary hypoplasia from oligohydramnios. Determination of amnionic fluid α-fetoprotein and fetal karyotyping should be performed. In those fetuses with lower tract obstruction from a posterior uretheral valve, a catheter is guided transabdominally, as shown in Figure 32–7. Manning and colleagues (1986), described the results obtained in the first 73 shunt procedures done for obstructive uropathy and reported to the International Fetal Surgery Registry. The procedure-related death rate was 5 percent, and 41 percent of fetuses survived, with most of deaths due to pulmonary hypoplasia. **Importantly, 8 percent of fetuses had a karyotype abnormality and 7 percent had a renal dysplasia.**

Elder and associates (1987) reviewed 57 reported cases of fetal urinary tract drainage and found a 44 percent complication rate. Only 6 or 28 fetuses survived when there was associated oligohydramnios. They concluded that a prospective, randomized trial should be carried out.

CONGENITAL HEART DISEASE

Because of the inconsistency with which cases of congenital heart disease are reported, the frequency of these malformations cannot be stated precisely, but they are among the more common abnormalities. Cardiac malformations include such conditions as patent ductus arteriosus, coarctation of the aorta, septal defects, pulmonary stenosis, and tetralogy of Fallot. Cardiac anomalies also commonly occur as parts of other syndromes, such as Marfan, Ellis–van Creveld, Down, and a variety of chromosomal disorders. Half of cases diagnosed prenatally have associated extracardiac or chromosomal anomalies (Crawford and colleagues, 1988). Isolated ventricular septal defects are common and may close spontaneously by 2 years of age.

Whittemore and colleagues (1982) studied 372 liveborns of 233 women with congenital heart defects, and reported that 16 percent of infants had congenital heart disease. In half of these, the anomaly was concordant with the maternal defect. Others have not reported inheritance rates this high.

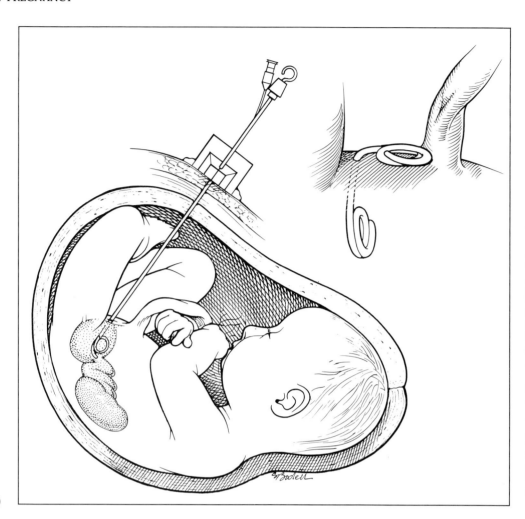

Figure 32–7. Intrauterine catheter placement to relieve fetal urinary obstruction. (*Redrawn from Williamson: Contemp Ob/Gyn 30:77, 1987.*)

Infants with severe congenital heart disease may look and react quite normally at birth, only to become symptomatic later. Therefore, the possibility of a cardiovascular defect should be considered for the mature infant who appears normal at birth and then develops tachypnea, cyanosis, marked tachycardia, and hepatomegaly in the early hours or days after birth.

ORTHOPEDIC ANOMALIES

Clubfoot (Talipes Equinovarus)

The extremities are involved in a large number of congenital defects, most of which are rare. Clubfoot is the most common, and is observed in about 1 in 1,000 births. Since the borderline between the normal and the pathological is not sharp in this malformation, early orthopedic consultation is essential.

Congenital Hip Dislocation

Hip dislocation is a fairly common malformation, more frequent in females and more common in breech than in vertex deliveries. It shows geographic variations, having been noted with unusual frequency in northern Italy, for example. It is rarely seen in black infants. The cause is a defective formation of the acetabulum, particularly its upper lip. As a result, the head of the femur may migrate upward and backward. In most cases, the displacement probably does not begin until after birth, developing gradually during the early weeks or months of life. From an obstetrical point of view, this is important because it is

sometimes alleged that these malformations were overlooked in the neonatal period. Carter (1963), reviewing the genetic aspects of the disease, found concordance in 40 percent of monozygous twins with congenital dislocation of the hip but in only 3 percent of dizygous twins. One percent of subsequent male siblings and 5 percent of later female siblings were affected.

Polydactylism

Supernumerary digits are occasionally seen, especially in black newborns. They usually consist of a small amount of skin and cartilage attached by a fine pedicle to the base of the fourth finger or fifth toe. Simple ligation of the stalk with a silk suture is generally sufficient treatment. If the base is broad and the digit is well developed, however, surgical removal may be required.

CLEFT LIP AND CLEFT PALATE

A cleft in the lip, either unilateral or bilateral, may or may not be associated with a cleft in the alveolar arch—that is, a cleft palate. It is one of the most frequent congenital deformities, with an incidence of 1.3 per 1,000 births. Khoury and colleagues (1987) reported that women who smoke cigarettes during pregnancy have a twofold increased incidence of infants with these lesions. Because of difficulties in feeding, it is advisable to surgically correct a cleft lip as soon as the infant's condition permits. Cleft palate may represent even greater difficulties in feeding, requiring the use of a prosthesis until around age 2 years.

While the risk of the first child of unaffected parents having a cleft lip is about 1 per 1,000, or 0.1 percent, the risk of cleft lip in the second child is about 40 times greater, or 4 percent. If both children are affected, the risk of the third child having a cleft lip is 10 percent. If a parent has a cleft lip, the risk of the first child being affected is about 4 percent and when the first child is affected, the risk to the second child is about 10 percent (Habib, 1978). Identification of cleft lip and cleft palate have been made at or before midpregnancy using real-time ultrasonography (Seeds and Cefalo, 1983).

ABDOMINAL-WALL DEFECTS

Omphalocele and gastroschisis are relatively common ventral-wall defects that may be confused on ultrasonic examination. While antepartum detection has increased, these defects commonly still are overlooked. An omphalocele is a defect in the umbilical ring from which protrudes a sac, covered with amnion and peritoneum, and into which abdominal contents have typically herniated (Fig. 32–8). It is the more common of the two, and is seen in about 1 in 4,000 livebirths. Gastroschisis is intestinal herniation through a defect in the anterior abdominal wall, usually to the right of the umbilicus. There is no sac and the intestines are covered with a thickened inflammatory exudate. This anomaly is identified in perhaps 1 in 10,000 births.

Associated congenital anomalies contribute to a high mortality rate for either condition (Hasan and Hermansen, 1986; Sermer and colleagues, 1987). Chromosomal aberrations also are common. Omphalocele is associated with other anomalies in up to 70 percent of cases. Gilbert and Nicolaides (1987) performed karyotyping in 35 fetuses with an omphalocele at 16 to 36 weeks, and they reported that 54 percent had chromosomal abnormalities. Anomalies are less common with gastroschisis and usually less than 30 percent of affected fetuses have them. Associated anomalies include those of the genitourinary, cardiac, musculoskeletal, and gastrointestinal systems. Preterm labor and delivery complicate over half of these pregnancies and the corresponding mortality rate is 60 percent for omphalocele and 40 percent for gastroschisis. The prognosis is good for the fetus born weighing more than 1,500 g with no associated anomalies, provided surgical correction is achieved rapidly. There is no evidence that delivery by cesarean section improves survival (Hasan and Hermansen, 1986), however, Fitzsimmons and colleagues (1988) point out that elective delivery optimizes surgical care of the neonate.

Congenital diaphragmatic hernia is associated with a poor outcome. Benacerraf and Adzick (1987) reported findings from 19 cases, and the overall survival rate was only 10 percent. Half of these fetuses had associated malformations.

UMBILICAL AND INGUINAL HERNIA

Umbilical hernias are common, especially in black infants. They are rarely serious, and strangulation of the bowel is almost unknown. Most small umbilical hernias disappear spontane-

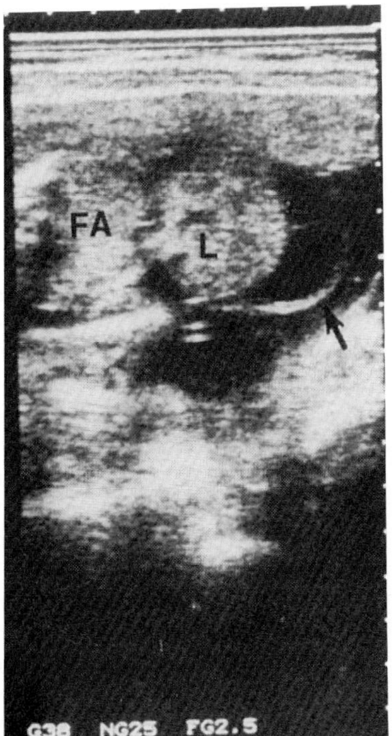

Figure 32–8. Transverse sonogram of an 18-week fetus demonstrating a large hepato-omphalocele and the covering amnioperitoneal membrane (*black arrows*). FA = fetal abdomen; L = fetal liver. (*From Vintzileos and colleagues: Obstet Gynecol 69:640, 1987, with permission.*)

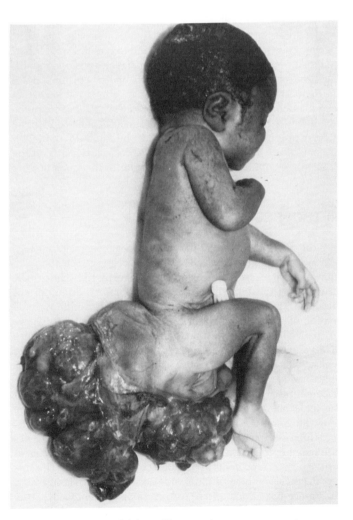

Figure 32–9. A 29-week infant with a massive sacrococcygeal teratoma. (*Courtesy of Dr. Victor Klein.*)

ously within a few months, whereas the larger varieties generally are treated successfully by simple mechanical measures, such as strapping the surrounding skin with a band of adhesive tape. Inguinal hernias may become incarcerated, however, especially in preterm infants. Most often, these cause no problems and resolve spontaneously during the first year of life.

IMPERFORATE ANUS

This uncommon abnormality, seen in perhaps 1 in 20,000 newborns, is caused by atresia of the anus, and the rectum ends in a blind pouch. Examination of the newborn in the delivery room usually will disclose the condition. More commonly, it is discovered on the first attempt to record the rectal temperature, or because there has been no bowel movement. Surgical intervention is imperative.

SACROCOCCYGEAL TERATOMA

These tumors are located over and under the coccyx, and large ones fill the sacrum and buttocks. Malignancies have been re-

ported but are uncommon. A preterm newborn infant with a very large sacrococcygeal tumor is shown in Figure 32–9. The mass ruptured during vaginal delivery with considerable bleeding and the infant expired.

Gross and colleagues (1987) reported their experiences with 10 sacrococcygeal tumors. Nine were in females, and none was malignant. Preterm labor was common, and they emphasized that individualization of the delivery route is done with consideration given for tumor size, since larger tumors may rupture during vaginal delivery, as in the case shown in Figure 32–9.

Musci and associates (1983) described an intriguing case in which all of the fetus except the 2,120 g teratoma was delivered vaginally; however, the tumor could not be extricated from the birth canal. The infant was intubated and resuscitated until cesarean delivery 10 minutes later, during which the fetus-infant was guided as a breech delivery back through the birth canal and through the uterine incision. The infant with tumor weighed 5,060 g. The "born again" infant underwent excision of the tumor mass 24 hours later and at 3 years of age was described as normal.

GENETIC COUNSELING

Along with the current trend for smaller families is the concern that children be born healthy and free of inherited diseases. Genetic counseling supplies information to families with inherited disorders, helping them make intelligent decisions regarding future childbearing. A malformed child often precipitates the request for such guidance, although other problems that lead frequently to consultation include inheritable disease in the family and advanced maternal age. Human genetic counseling is becoming increasingly complex with the rapid accumulation of new information, and amateurish advice, particularly of the unjustifiably optimistic variety, may produce tragic results.

RETROSPECTIVE COUNSELING

Birth of an affected child or disease in a near relative often calls attention to a genetic disorder. In other cases, couples may be unaware that a condition is genetically transmitted. Thus, forecasting the probability of an inherited disorder is an important step, but it requires a precise medical history. In addition to the routine history obtained from all pregnant women (see Chap. 14, p. 259), specific questions such as those listed in Figure 32–10 should be asked to help identify the expectant mother whose fetus is at unusual risk of having or subsequently acquiring a serious disability. The completed record also serves to document that the mother was informed of any unusual risk of the fetus being abnormal, or that referral for further genetic counseling was advised.

Upon completion of the history, it often is possible to decide whether the disease follows an easily recognized pattern of inheritance or represents an isolated congenital defect. The correct diagnosis is integral to provide accurate advice concerning recurrence risks. Most often, further steps to identify the fetus at risk of a serious disorder and to counsel the expectant parents are best handled through a specialized genetics center with

established expertise in counseling and quality control of the variety of laboratory procedures that may be employed. The Council on Accreditation and Certification of the American Society of Human Genetics has established standards of accreditation for genetic counselors. Techniques for intrauterine diagnosis of inherited fetal defects are considered under Prenatal Diagnosis.

In addition to supplying positive information, appropriate genetic studies and subsequent counseling help dispel many misapprehensions and ill-founded rumors concerning congenital malformations. They also help relieve the guilt feelings that frequently follow the birth of a child with a malformation.

EVALUATION OF MALFORMED INFANTS WHO DIE IN THE PERINATAL PERIOD

A *detailed history* of events from before the time of conception through delivery should be obtained. Times of exposure to potential teratogens are especially important. *Photographs* should be made of the face, body, and all anomalies. A *radiographic skeletal survey* may prove valuable. *Chromosomal analysis* is carried out either on 2 to 3 mL of blood collected aseptically from a large vessel or the heart, or on sterile skin, umbilical cord, amnion, or lung. A *complete autopsy* during which all malformations, both external and internal, are carefully examined, should be described in detail. Histological sections should be made of any tissue that appears abnormal.

The value of routine autopsy for all perinates recently has been encouraged. For example, Pitkin (1987) emphasized that only half of fetal deaths are caused by known or suspected conditions. Mueller and associates (1983) performed autopsies in 124 cases of stillborns or early neonatal deaths, and found that 35 percent had structural anomalies. Almost 80 percent of these were due to inherited disorders. Meier and colleagues (1986) reported that in 26 percent of cases, the autopsy was the sole means of establishing the cause of death. In a third of all

Sample Prenatal Genetic Screen*

Name_____ Patient#_____   Date_____

1. Will you be 35 years or older when the baby is due?   Yes_____ No_____
2. Have you, the baby's father, or anyone in either of your families ever had any of the following disorders?   Yes_____ No_____
   - Down syndrome (mongolism)   Yes_____ No_____
   - Other chromosomal abnormality   Yes_____ No_____
   - Neural tube defect, ie, spina bifida (meningomyelocele or open spine), anencephaly   Yes_____ No_____
   - Hemophilia   Yes_____ No_____
   - Muscular dystrophy   Yes_____ No_____
   - Cystic fibrosis   Yes_____ No_____
   If yes, indicate the relationship of the affected person to you or to the baby's father: _____
3. Do you or the baby's father have a birth defect?   Yes_____ No_____
   If yes, who has the defect and what is it?_____
4. In any previous marriages, have you or the baby's father had a child, born dead or alive, with a birth defect not listed in question 2 above?   Yes_____ No_____
   If yes, what was the defect and who had it? _____
5. Do you or the baby's father have any close relatives with mental retardation?   Yes_____ No_____
   If yes, indicate the relationship of the affected person to you or to the baby's father: _____
   Indicate the cause, if known: _____
6. Do you, the baby's father, or a close relative in either of your families have a birth defect, any familial disorder, or a chromosomal abnormality not listed above?   Yes_____ No_____
   If yes, indicate the condition and the relationship of the affected person to you or to the baby's father: _____
   _____
7. In any previous marriages, have you or the baby's father had a stillborn child or three or more first-trimester spontaneous pregnancy losses?   Yes_____ No_____
   Have either of you had a chromosomal study?   Yes_____ No_____
   If yes, indicate who and the results: _____
8. If you or the baby's father are of Jewish ancestry, have either of you been screened for Tay-Sachs disease?   Yes_____ No_____
   If yes, indicate who and the results: _____
9. If you or the baby's father are black, have either of you been screened for sickle cell trait?   Yes_____ No_____
   If yes, indicate who and the results: _____
10. If you or the baby's father are of Italian, Greek, or Mediterranean background, have either of you been tested for β-thalassemia?   Yes_____ No_____
    If yes, indicate who and the results: _____
11. If you or the baby's father are of Philippine or Southeast Asian ancestry, have either of you been tested for α-thalassemia?   Yes_____ No_____
    If yes, indicate who and the results: _____
12. Excluding iron and vitamins, have you taken any medications or recreational drugs since being pregnant or since your last menstrual period? (include nonprescription drugs.)   Yes_____ No_____
    If yes, give name of medication and time taken during pregnancy:_____
    _____

*Any patient replying "YES" to questions should be offered appropriate counseling. If the patient declines further counseling or testing, this should be noted in the chart. Given that genetics is a field in a state of flux, alterations or updates to this form will be required periodically.

Figure 32–10. Sample questionnaire used in screening for inherited disorders. (*From American College of Obstetricians and Gynecologists: Antenatal Diagnosis of Genetic Disorders. Technical Bulletin No 108, September 1987.*)

deaths, a need for specific genetic counseling was identified, and half of these were ascertained by autopsy findings.

PROSPECTIVE COUNSELING

In prospective counseling, advice is provided to possible carriers of recessive genes before birth or, ideally, before conception. First, there is identification of heterozygotes by population-screening procedures. The individual then is advised of the risk of an affected child if conception is with another carrier. Finally, the heterozygote couple is counseled concerning the possibility of pregnancy interruption if the disease can be diagnosed in utero.

SCREENING PROGRAMS

There are screening programs to identify some of the more common autosomal recessive disorders, and examples include

sickle cell anemia, Tay-Sachs disease, and thalassemia major. These programs raise many social, ethical, economic, and legal questions, not to mention many possible psychological stigmata of carrying "bad genes." Equally important to the success of such screening programs is an intensive education program for persons undergoing testing, and this, unfortunately, is where many programs typically have failed. As the worst example, such a program may cause more harm than good.

Because of problems inherent with testing the entire population, several screening programs have been developed for the pregnant woman. Examples that are discussed in detail below include maternal serum α-fetoprotein screening for neural-tube defects and cytogenetic studies on fetal cells obtained by amniocentesis or chorionic villus sampling in women over 35.

Neonatal screening programs are also popular, and many states have laws for newborn screening for certain disorders. Texas law, for example, mandates neonatal screening be performed for phenylketonuria, congenital hypothyroidism, sickle cell disease, and galactosemia.

PRENATAL DIAGNOSIS

No other area in clinical obstetrics has experienced more intensive application of rapid technological expansion than the area of prenatal diagnosis. In the past 20 years there has been incredible advancement in techniques that allow for early and accurate diagnosis of a myriad of fetal disorders. Beginning with simple cytogenetic techniques to determine gross chromosomal abnormalities, there are now methods that permit rapid detection using minute quantities of fetally derived DNA, obtained by direct sampling of chorionic tissue. This, coupled with the techniques of molecular genetics, allows detection of a large number of inherited conditions. The list of these conditions is expanding daily.

SONOGRAPHY

The role of ultrasound in detection of fetal anomalies cannot be overestimated. Moreover, its value as a guide to obtaining fetal tissue for analysis has become indispensable as older and less precise fetoscopic techniques have been replaced by sonar-directed chorionic villus sampling, amniocentesis, and fetal blood and tissue sampling.

As technical resolution has improved with development of more sophisticated equipment, it is now possible to detect anatomical anomalies that have far-reaching clinical impact. Some examples are various heart lesions. Another is identification of the Down syndrome fetus by thickened nuchal folds and relatively short femurs (Benacerraf and colleagues, 1987; Perrella and associates, 1988). The experiences of Sabbagha and colleagues (1985), from the Northwestern Perinatal Center, were cited earlier. Of 615 women at high risk for birth defects referred to them for targeted ultrasound imaging (see Chap. 15, p. 283),

they found 81 fetal anomalies, or 14 percent, and reported predictive values of abnormal and normal studies to be 95 and 99 percent, respectively.

AMNIOCENTESIS

Easy and safe accessibility of amnionic fluid undoubtedly has influenced obstetrical care tremendously. Amniocentesis allows access to fetal somatic cells and fluid that can be used to identify the cytogenetic constitution of the fetus or to assess a variety of abnormal biochemical processes that are listed in Table 32–8. **This list is by no means complete, and its length is increasing rapidly.**

To identify several genetic disorders in the fetus, chromosomal or other laboratory analysis can be employed. It is most often of value in the following circumstances:

1. Pregnancies in women 35 years of age or older
2. A previous pregnancy that resulted in the birth of a chromosomally abnormal offspring
3. Chromosomal abnormality in either parent, including
   a. balanced translocation carrier
   b. aneuploidy
   c. mosaicism
4. Down syndrome or other chromosomal abnormality in a close family member
5. Biochemical studies in pregnancies at risk of a serious autosomal or X-linked recessive disorder
6. A previous child or a parent with a neural-tube defect or an abnormally low or high maternal serum α-fetoprotein level obtained during routine screening

TABLE 32–8. A PARTIAL LIST OF INHERITED DISORDERS FOR WHICH PRENATAL DIAGNOSIS IS FEASIBLE

Carbohydrate metabolism
Galactosemia
Galactokinase deficiency
Glycogen storage diseases—
    Types II, III, IV
Pyruvate decarboxylase deficiency
 	
Amino acid metabolism
Argininosuccinicaciduria
Citrullinemia
Homocystinuria
Ketotic hyperglycemia
Maple syrup urine disease
Methylmalonic aciduria
Isovaleric acidemia
 	
Lipoproteins and lipid metabolism
Homozygous familial
    hypercholesterolemia
Refsum syndrome
 	
Steroid metabolism
21-Hydroxylase deficiency
Steroid sulfatase deficiency
	Lysosomal enzymes
	Farber disease (lipogranulomatosis)
	Fucosidosis
	Fabry disease
	Generalized gangliosidosis
	Gaucher disease
	Krabbe disease (globoid cell leukodystrophy)
	I-cell disease
	Juvenile gangliosidosis
	Lysosomal acid phosphatase deficiency
	Mannosidosis
	Mucopolysaccharidosis, type I (Hurler),
	    II (Hunter), III (Sanfillipo),
	    VI (Maroteaux-Lamay), VII (β-glucuronidase
	    deficiency)
	Niemann-Pick disease
	Sandhoff disease
	Tay-Sach disease
	Wolman syndrome and cholesteryl
	    ester storage disease
		Purine and pyrimidine metabolism
		Adenosine deminase deficiency (combined
		    immunodeficiency)
		Hereditary orotic aciduria
		Lesch–Nyhan syndrome
		Xeroderma pigmentosum
		
		Metal metabolism
		Menke syndrome
		
		Porphyrin and heme metabolism
		Acute intermittent porphyria
		
		Connective tissue
		Hypophosphatasia (some types)
		
		Hematopoietic
		Glucose-6-phosphate dehydrogenase
		    deficiency
		Sickle cell anemia
		α-Thalassemia
		β-Thalassemia
		
		Transport
		Cystinosis

From Goldstein and Brown: *Prevention and Treatment of Genetic Disorders*. Chapter 61 in *Harrison's Principles of Internal Medicine*, 11th Edition. New York, McGraw-Hill, 1987, p 327.

7. Abnormal fetus identified by sonographic examination (this is not always done)
8. A previous infant with multiple major malformations in whom no cytogenetic study was performed (this is not always done)
9. Fetal sex determination in pregnancies at risk of a serious X-linked hereditary disorder (this is better accomplished using the new DNA techniques to identify Y chromosomal material)

Technical considerations, including maternal and fetal risks, are considered in Chapter 15 (p. 277). For prenatal diagnosis, amnionic fluid most often is aspirated at 16 to 18 weeks gestation, when it is likely that there are sufficient fetal cells to allow successful cell culture. There is the possibility that the fluid collected at this time is maternal urine rather than amnionic fluid. The two fluids usually can be quickly differentiated by the presence of crystallization when amnionic fluid is dried on a glass slide and examined microscopically under low power. Moreover, amnionic fluid contains glucose and protein, whereas urine usually does not.

More recently, there has been a trend to perform amniocentesis earlier. Hanson and colleagues (1987) described their experiences with 541 procedures performed before 15 weeks and reported a pregnancy loss of 1.7 percent within 2 weeks of the procedure. Drugan and co-workers (1988a) reported normal amnionic fluid values for α-fetoprotein and acetylcholinesterase in 476 samples obtained between 10 and 15 weeks.

The frequencies of the more common significant cytogenetic abnormalities in newborn infants in the United States are listed in Table 32–3. The National Institutes of Health (1979) estimated that, without cytogenetic studies, each year in the United States at least 15,000 infants would be born with a chromosomal abnormality. There are probably 175,000 spontaneous abortions of chromosomally abnormal fetuses annually.

The most common abnormality in the liveborn infant is trisomy 21, or Down syndrome, even though it is estimated that two thirds of conceptuses with trisomy 21 do not survive the pregnancy. Whereas the risk of a liveborn with Down syndrome is 1 in 885 at maternal age 30, this risk increases progressively with maternal age (Table 32–5). The frequencies of most other trisomies and sex chromosome aneuploidies also increase with maternal age.

Cytogenetic studies are recommended for all women 35 years or older, although any age limit is selected arbitrarily rather than being decided on the basis of sudden biological difference between women immediately above or below a certain age. The magnitude of the problem created by attempting to provide genetic counseling and cytogenetic screening of fetuses of all women who are 35 or older becomes readily apparent when it is appreciated that in one recent year there were 142,000 births to women 35 or older, compared to only 25,000 to women who were 40 or older. Moreover, it has been predicted that soon the number of births to women 35 or older will exceed 200,000 annually.

As discussed on page 570, when a parent is the carrier of a balanced chromosomal translocation, there is a 4 to 20 percent risk that the fetus will be abnormal.

With X-linked recessive diseases for which no specific prenatal diagnostic test is readily available to differentiate affected male fetuses, at least the sex of the fetus can be identified accurately. When the fetus is female and the father is not affected, the risk of the offspring being affected is eliminated.

As discussed on page 574, approximately a third of sonographically abnormal fetuses have chromosomal anomalies.

FETAL SEX

At 15 to 18 weeks gestation, the sex of the fetus can be determined cytologically by demonstrating the nuclear sex chromatin mass (Barr body) and by Y chromosome staining of cells obtained from amnionic fluid, or more accurately by cell culture and karyotyping. With very careful studies to identify the presence or absence of nuclear sex chromatin in uncultivated, directly stained amnionic fluid cells, the overall accuracy is about 95 percent (Milunsky, 1973). Staining for the Y chromosome in uncultured cells from amnionic fluid, Valenti and co-workers (1972) reported an accuracy of about 97 percent. Thus, the test did not improve the accuracy significantly over the sex chromatin method, and when the prediction of sex is crucial, they recommend that confirmation be derived by karyotyping cultured amnionic fluid cells.

Identification of the sex of the fetus has been attempted by measuring testosterone and follicle-stimulating hormone in amnionic fluid. In one study, overlap of values for female and male fetuses was so great that in 7 percent neither determination was indicative of fetal sex (Belisle and colleagues, 1977).

High-resolution sonography can be used for identification of fetal sex by visualizing the external genitalia, especially the penis (Fig. 32–11). Birnholz (1983) reported that sonographic views were obtained sufficient to allow an attempt at diagnosis in 69 percent of fetuses at 15 or more gestational weeks. For 590 fetuses, sex was determined correctly 99 percent of the time. After 20 weeks gestation, the genitalia were visualized in more than 90 percent of all fetuses examined. Reece and colleagues (1987) studied fetuses between 16 and 20 weeks and were able to visualize genitalia in 83 percent; however, accuracy of identification was only 93 percent.

OTHER INHERITABLE DISORDERS

A great variety of inheritable disorders have been detected by appropriate study of amnionic fluid contents. Some of these are included in Table 32–8.

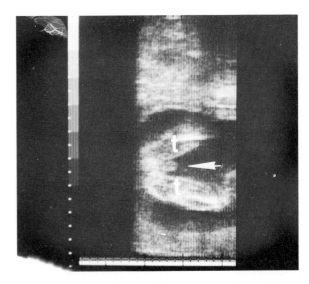

Figure 32–11. Sonographic caudal view of a male fetus at 24 weeks gestation. The arrow points to the penis and the thigh is marked by the t. (*Courtesy of Dr. R. Santos.*)

Approximately 75 recessively inherited X chromosome-linked or autosomal metabolic disorders are now detectable in tissue culture systems, and therefore are approachable in the fetus through amniocentesis or chorionic villus sampling. It is emphasized that this list is expanding rapidly. The risk of an autosomal recessive disorder in the fetus may have become apparent either from the previous birth of an affected infant or from screening of the parents for the carrier state, or by family history. If both parents are carriers, the risk of the fetus being homozygous and therefore seriously affected is 25 percent, whereas for X-linked disease, if the mother is a carrier, the risk of male offspring being affected is 50 percent, but for female offspring it is zero, unless the father is affected.

Unfortunately, the carrier state for several recessive conditions cannot be detected except by birth of an affected infant. One recessive condition that can be detected, however, is Tay-Sachs disease, for which screening programs have been established. Tay-Sachs disease is 100 times more frequent in Jews, and routine screening for heterozygotes is considered standard practice (American College of Obstetricians and Gynecologists, 1987). Serum hexosaminidase A decreases in pregnancy, and this may incorrectly suggest that some women are carriers. The affected fetus of heterozygous parents can be detected by measuring hexosaminidase A levels in fetal cells cultured from amnionic fluid.

Parents who are heterozygous for the gene for abnormal hemoglobin production or for β-thalassemia can be identified readily and the potential for an affected offspring thereby recognized. The fetus destined to develop a serious hemoglobinopathy or thalassemia major can now be identified in utero through appropriate analysis of DNA from amniocytes taken from amnionic fluid or from chorionic villi.

ELEVATED α-FETOPROTEIN

The value of measurement of α-fetoprotein in amnionic fluid between 16 and 20 weeks gestation to detect fetal abnormalities, especially open neural-tube defects, is now established.

The site of production of most, if not all, of the increased α-fetoprotein is the fetus. It is the major protein in the serum of the embryo and early fetus. Initially, it is produced in the yolk sac, but by the end of the first trimester it is nearly all of hepatic origin. In both fetal serum and amnionic fluid the concentration of α-fetoprotein is highest around the 13th week of gestation (Fig. 32–12). The concentration in fetal serum is about 150 times that in amnionic fluid. The normal source of the protein in amnionic fluid is fetal urine. Some of that protein, in turn, crosses the fetal membranes to enter the maternal circulation. The concentration of α-fetoprotein levels in maternal serum are only 1/100th to 1/1,000th those of fetal serum. After 13 weeks the levels in both fetal serum and amnionic fluid normally decrease rapidly in essentially parallel fashion while those in maternal serum continue to rise until late in pregnancy. **Since fetal serum and amnionic fluid levels decrease sharply, correct interpretation of its concentration requires precise knowledge of gestational age.**

The α-fetoprotein level in amnionic fluid, maternal serum, or both, may be elevated in a great variety of circumstances in which fetal integument is not intact and the protein leaks from the capillaries into the amnionic fluid. Levels also are increased in circumstances in which the amount leaked by the fetal kidney is increased, and whenever the placenta contains increased numbers of thin-walled vessels that contain fetal blood. Some

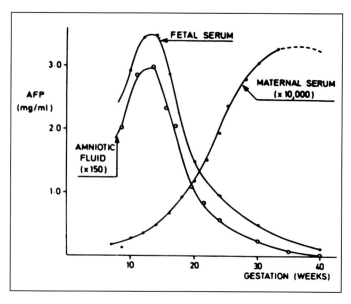

Figure 32–12. Maternal and fetal serum and amnionic fluid α-fetoprotein (AFP) levels corresponding with gestational age. (*From Roberts and Dunn: J Repro Med 28:167, 1983, with permission.*)

conditions associated with abnormally elevated or low levels of α-fetoprotein in maternal serum and amnionic fluid are shown in Table 32–9.

Open Neural-Tube Defects

Experiences with screening for open neural-tube defects are now extensive, especially in Great Britain where neural-tube defects are much more common. As one consequence, consid-

TABLE 32–9. SOME CONDITIONS ASSOCIATED WITH ABNORMAL MATERNAL SERUM α-FETOPROTEIN CONCENTRATIONS

Elevated levels
Neural tube defects
Pilonidal cysts
Esophageal or intestinal obstructions
Liver necrosis
Cystic hygroma
Sacrococcygeal teratoma
Abdominal wall defects—omphalocoele, gastroschisis
Urinary obstruction
Renal anomalies—polycystic or absent kidneys
Congenital nephrosis
Osteogenesis imperfecta
Congenital skin defects
Cloacal exstrophy
Low birthweight
Oligohydramnios
Multifetal gestation
Decreased maternal weight
Underestimated gestational age

Low levels
Chromosomal trisomies
Gestational trophoblastic disease
Fetal death
Increased maternal weight
Overestimated gestational age

erable enthusiasm has been generated for measuring near mid-pregnancy the level of serum α-fetoprotein of most women. When levels are sufficiently elevated to suspect the possibility of a neural-tube defect, then amniocentesis is performed to look for distinctly elevated levels in amnionic fluid. Moreover, the fetus is usually carefully visualized ultrasonically for evidence of abnormality, especially anencephaly and spina bifida.

The level of α-fetoprotein at which amniocentesis is performed is based on statistical possibilities whether a fetus will be affected at that level. It is customary to report values as *multiples of the median* since serum α-fetoprotein levels do not follow a Gaussian distribution. Shown in Figure 32–13 is a schematic of this concept. Additionally, tables have been compiled that forecast the risk using a combination of α-fetoprotein concentration and maternal age (Palomaki and Haddow, 1987). **Regardless of the cutoff point chosen as "abnormal," there will always be false-positive and false-negative results.**

Most laboratories routinely test for α-fetoprotein levels in all midtrimester amnionic fluid samples, regardless of the indication for which the fluid was obtained.

Congenital Nephrosis

Children with congenital nephrosis, although severely handicapped, may live for as long as 2 or 3 years. The abnormality is inherited as an autosomal recessive trait. In the case of a previous infant born with congenital nephrosis, or a strong family history, an affected fetus may be identified through measurements of α-fetoprotein in maternal serum and especially in amnionic fluid (Aula and colleagues, 1978).

Amnionic Fluid Acetylcholinesterase Activity

Elevated levels of acetylcholinesterase in amnionic fluid accompany most open neural-tube defects. By demonstrating the absence of an acetylcholinesterase band in amnionic fluid using the technique of slab gel electrophoresis, Milunsky and Sapirstein (1982) were able to reclassify correctly 89 percent of the

normal pregnancies in which they had found spuriously high α-fetoprotein levels in the amnionic fluid. Acetylcholinesterase in amnionic fluid most likely comes from fetal neural tissue—for example, an open neural-tube lesion—however, it has been found to be elevated at times in the absence of such a defect.

MATERNAL SERUM α-FETOPROTEIN SCREENING

Routine screening for neural-tube defects by measuring α-fetoprotein levels in maternal serum currently is widely employed in the United States as it has been now for some time in many European countries. Indeed, some states mandate that it be made available to all prenatal patients. After initial controversy surrounding its implementation, primarily because of numerous technical problems, the American College of Obstetricians and Gynecologists (1986) now recommends that such screening programs be established, but only within a coordinated system that includes quality control, counseling, follow-up, and level 2 sonographic facilities. These guidelines also were emphasized in the policy statement of the American Society of Human Genetics (1987). **They emphasized that screening should be voluntary and that screening tests are not perfect and that there will be false positives as well as false negatives.**

If the procedure is accepted after informed consent is obtained, initial serum screening is done at 16 to 18 weeks gestation. About 5 percent of all women will have abnormally high levels, defined by most as greater than 2.5 multiples of the median determined for the population under study. Repeat serum testing eliminates 2 percent of the total, and ultrasound evaluation is performed for the remaining 3 percent. In 1 percent of the total, multiple gestation, inaccurate gestational age estimation, or missed abortion are identified. Thus, 2 percent of all women screened will need to undergo amniocentesis so that amnionic fluid α-fetoprotein concentration can be measured as described above, and only a small fraction of these will be found to have abnormally elevated levels. Richards and colleagues (1988) recently reported that the likelihood of a neural-tube defect associated with an abnormal serum screening value is decreased by 90 percent if the ultrasound examination is normal. Conversely, Drugan and co-workers (1988b) emphasized that a fourth of fetal malformations will be missed if amniocentesis is not performed routinely for elevated maternal serum levels accompanied by a normal ultrasonic examination.

It also is important to emphasize that a growing number of conditions other than neural-tube defects have been recognized as associated with both abnormally elevated and low serum α-fetoprotein concentrations. Some of these are shown in Table 32–9. Nelson and associates (1987a) reported that if serum values are greater than 5 multiples of the median, then 66 percent of pregnancies had a diagnosis that affected pregnancy outcome, compared to 18 percent if the serum value was 2.5 to 4.9 multiples of the median. Adverse outcomes included fetal anomalies, fetal death, and obstetrical complications.

Abnormally Low α-Fetoprotein Values

Following the observations of Merkatz (1984) and Cuckle (1984) and their colleagues that serum α-fetoprotein concentrations were abnormally low in women bearing chromosomally abnormal fetuses, it is now appreciated that the value of screening is greatly enhanced. Simpson and colleagues (1986) reported results from screening of over 1,400 women, of which 9 percent had serum levels abnormally low, defined as less than 0.4 multiples of the median. Half of these women still had low values when repeated, and 3 of 49 who underwent amniocentesis had

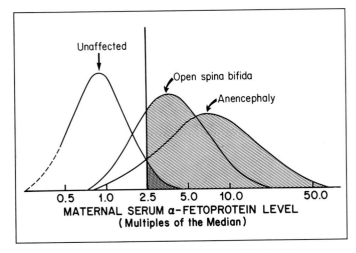

Figure 32–13. Maternal serum α-fetoprotein levels in singleton gestations at 16 to 18 weeks. The cutoff value of 2.5 multiples of the median results in both false-positive and false-negative diagnosis. However, any cutoff point chosen would result in false-positive (cross-hatched area) and false-negative rates. (*Redrawn from American College of Obstetricians and Gynecologists: Prenatal Detection of Neural Tube Defects. Technical Bulletin No 99, December 1986.*)

a chromosomally triploid fetus. These workers appropriately emphasized that the yield of 6 percent was much greater than that for routine amniocentesis in women who were 35 to 36 years old. Similarly, Nelson and associates (1987b) screened over 28,000 pregnancies and reported that maternal serum levels less than 0.2 multiples of the median yielded a positive finding in 83 percent of cases. The most common finding was less advanced gestational age (60 percent), followed by fetal demise (17 percent) and nonpregnancy (5 percent); only 17 percent had normal ultrasound findings. Unfortunately, low serum α-fetoprotein levels will detect only one third of Down fetuses (DiMaio and co-workers, 1987), and the number of normal fetuses lost because of amniocentesis will exceed the number of abnormal fetuses detected.

Although reported by others, Simpson and co-workers (1987) found no association with low maternal serum α-fetoprotein levels and adverse perinatal outcomes—specifically, fetal losses. Thus, if the serum level of α-fetoprotein was low but fetal viability was confirmed and the karyotype normal, they found the fetus to be normal.

CHORIONIC VILLUS BIOPSY

Since its development beginning in the early 1970s, biopsy— or sampling of the chorion, either transvaginally or trans-

abdominally—has become a widely accepted first-trimester alternative to amniocentesis for prenatal diagnosis. The chorion is of fetal origin, and thus cells obtained by villus biopsy can be examined using the same techniques as for amniocytes obtained by amniocentesis. The primary difference is that amniocentesis must be used for assays for which amnionic fluid is integral, an example being α-fetoprotein concentration. The major advantage of villus biopsy is that fetal cells are obtained earlier and lengthy culture procedures are unnecessary, since chorion cells divide very rapidly. Thus, a diagnosis is made earlier and pregnancy can be terminated sooner and with greater safety.

As described by Liu (1983), Rodeck (1983), and Simoni (1983) and their many colleagues, much of the earlier work with chorion biopsy was done in Europe. To further assess the safety and efficacy of the technique, the National Institutes of Health has funded an ongoing multicenter study conducted in seven American academic institutions. By early 1988, more than 41,000 chorionic biopsies had been done by the transcervical route. The technique is shown in Figure 32–14. The immediate loss of a sonographically normal pregnancy was 3.5 percent, compared to a 2 percent spontaneous loss; therefore, the procedure-related loss is around 2 percent (Jackson, 1988).

The San Francisco group reported their experiences with the first 1,000 transvaginal chorion biopsies (Hogge and colleagues, 1986). As expected, since sampling was performed before 12 weeks, the 4.2 percent incidence of chromosomal

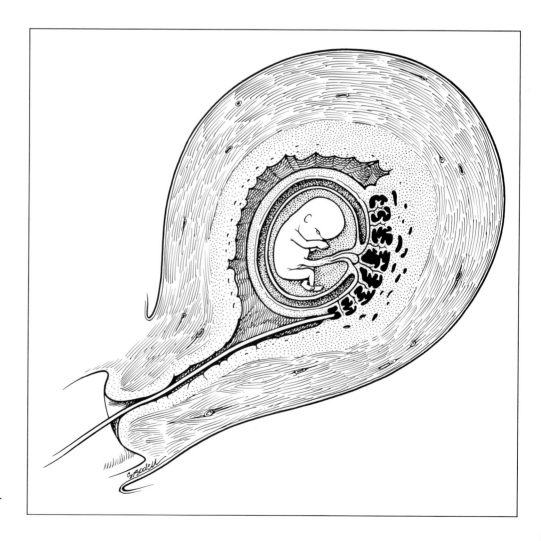

Figure 32–14. Transcervical chorionic villus sampling.

abnormalities was higher than 2.5 percent reported with second-trimester studies (Golbus, 1980). Importantly, there was a 1.7 percent incidence of discrepancy between the apparent karyotype of the chorionic tissue and that of the fetus. Some of these were ascribed to maternal cell contamination; however, a fourth of all chromosomal aberrations were mosaicisms that were not confirmed by amniocentesis or fetal tissue studies. It was concluded that they represented true placental mosaicism, and although their significance is unknown, Kalousek and Dill (1983) suggested an association with fetal growth retardation. Hogge and associates (1986) reported an abortion rate of 3.8 percent following villus sampling, which was not in excess of that predicted in ultrasonically normal pregnancies between 9 and 11 weeks. Complications, while infrequent, were quite worrisome. They identified severe oligohydramnios that followed sampling in six cases, and three other women developed chorioamnionitis shortly after the procedure. From the same group, Barela and colleagues (1986) reported a woman who developed septicemia with shock and renal failure from infection 4 days following chorion biopsy at 11 weeks gestation.

Green and colleagues (1988) reported similar results from over 1,000 patients referred to the Genetics and IVF Institute. Of 940 women undergoing biopsy, two developed chorioamnionitis. The total fetal loss was 2.4 percent and the procedure-related loss was 0.6 percent. Trophoblastic mosaicism was identified in 1.7 percent, and in all of these amniocentesis confirmed a karyotypically normal fetus.

Experience with transabdominal chorionic villus sampling is less extensive, but preliminary reports indicate that it is a potentially useful technique (Lilford and colleagues, 1987).

MOLECULAR GENETICS

Until recently, the only method available to investigate the molecular basis for a genetic disorder was isolation of the end-result gene product, either an enzyme or another protein. In the past decade, techniques have been developed that allow for sophisticated analysis of the structure of human genes, and these changes resulted in the *New Genetics*, so adequately christened by David Comings in 1979 (Weatherall, 1985). The following is meant to be a cursory review of molecular genetics as it relates to obstetrics; for detailed descriptions, the reader is referred to any of a number of authoritative works.

TRANSMISSION OF GENETIC MATERIAL

Enzymes and other biologically important proteins are composed of one or more polypeptide chains that are genetically transmitted through inheritance of specific DNA molecules. A *gene* represents the total sequence combinations of four purine and pyrimidine bases in DNA that specify the amino-acid sequence for a single polypeptide chain of a protein molecule (Goldstein and Brown, 1987). It is estimated that there are as many as 100,000 genes in each human cell nucleus, and these are tightly intertwined in the DNA of the 23 pairs of chromosomes. Their complexity is emphasized by Weatherall (1985), who noted that the DNA from each cell nucleus, if uncoiled, would stretch 2 meters!

In the nucleus, genetic information is transcribed onto *messenger RNA*, which in the cytoplasm translates this information by forming a template for ribosomal protein synthesis. Informa-

tion is expressed by a two-stage process. *Transcription* generates a single-stranded RNA identical in sequence with one of the strands of the DNA helix. *Translation* converts the RNA-nucleotide sequence into the amino-acid sequence that constitutes a protein.

A *mutation* is an alteration of DNA sequencing that is passed on to future progeny. These can be visible alterations of chromosomes, such as deletions, or they may involve a single change in just one of the purine or pyrimidine bases of a single gene, resulting in a *point* or *single-gene mutation*, such as that causing sickle cell anemia.

ANALYTICAL TECHNIQUES

Complementary DNA

Reverse transcriptases are enzymes isolated from tumor viruses, which are used to synthesize a DNA copy from messenger RNA isolated from human cell nuclei. These copies, called *complementary DNA* or *cDNA*, are labeled by inserting radioactive bases into the sequences, and the probe is used to look for complementary sequences of DNA on nitrocelluose filters. It is now possible to clone cDNA sequences in bacterial plasmids. These probes are very specific in combining with their complementary single-stranded DNA from the cell nucleus to be analyzed, and the radioactive label allows for detection of this binding.

Restriction Endonucleases

DNA fractionation became possible with isolation of bacterial enzymes termed *restriction endonucleases*, which cleave a specific sequence of base pairs. More than 200 restriction enzymes have been identified. As shown in Figure 32–15, some enzymes recognize sequences of four nucleotides, some six, and others seven. Depending on the types and numbers of enzymes used, hundreds of thousands of fragments are produced with varying numbers of nucleotides. These DNA fragments are then separated, using the technique known as *Southern blotting*, into single strands and hybridized with their radiolabeled complementary DNA probe, which can be identified by autoradiography (Fig. 32–16). Known sequences, or probes, are used to determine if these same sequences are present in the patient's genome, and in this way, abnormal sequences (mutations) can be verified.

An example of an exciting aspect of prenatal diagnosis using the new molecular technology involves sickle cell anemia. In 1972, Kan and colleagues reported a method of detection of the types of globin chains synthesized by the fetus, using umbilical vessel blood from

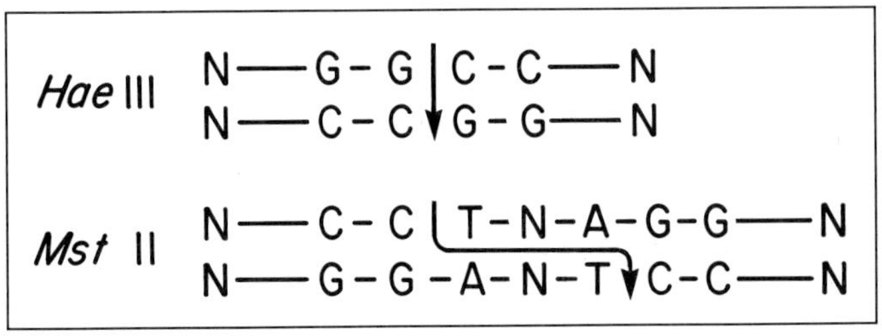

Figure 32–15. Restriction endonucleases. Hae III (*H. influenzae III*) cleaves a four-base sequence. Mst II (*Microcoleus*) cleaves a seven-base sequence, the center of which is a nonspecific nucleotide, shown here as N.

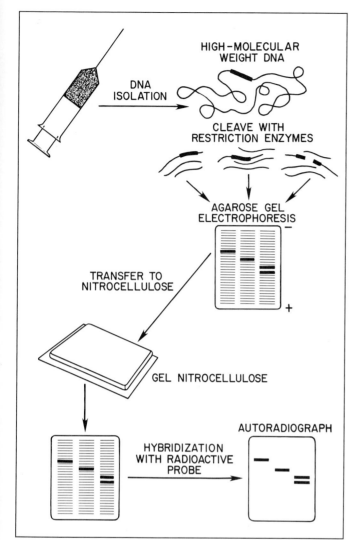

Figure 32–16. Southern blotting analysis. Genomic DNA is isolated from leucocytes or amniocytes and digested with a restriction enzyme. This yields a series of reproducible fragments that are separated by agarose gel electrophoresis. DNA is then transferred to a nitrocellulose membrane that binds DNA. The membrane is treated with a solution containing a radioactive single-stranded nucleic acid probe, which forms a double-stranded nucleic acid complex at membrane sites when homologous DNA is present. These regions are then detected using x-ray film.

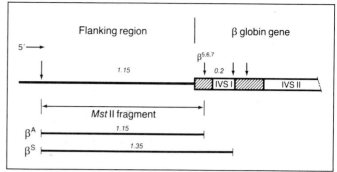

Figure 32–17. Mst II restriction enzyme used to identify hemoglobin A and S. Arrows indicate the Mst II restriction sites, including the one corresponding to amino acids 5, 6, and 7. Using the ^{32}P-labeled 1.15 kilobase Mst II fragment probe indicated in the diagram, the 1.15 kilobase fragment was seen as DNA from hemoglobin A, and the 1.35 kilobase fragment was seen in sickle hemoglobin DNA. Southern blotting analysis using the appropriate β-globin fragment as a DNA probe then allows for identification of AS, AA, and SS genotypes. (*From Chang and colleagues: N Engl J Med 307:30, 1982.*)

Restriction Fragment Length Polymorphisms

Another advantage of restriction endonucleases is use of the technique called *linkage analysis,* an extremely valuable method of analyzing genetic diversity. Obviously, not all abnormal genes are associated with an identifiable alteration in a restriction endonuclease cleavage site. Prenatal diagnosis may still be possible, however, since mutations are frequently linked to other DNA sequences that vary from person to person. Consequently, digested pieces of DNA generated by restriction endonucleases differ so often in a population that it is frequently possible to associate a mutant gene with a nearby restriction enzyme site. While the abnormal gene is not identified, a *marker gene* is found closely linked to the mutant gene. Such *restriction fragment length polymorphisms (RFLPs)* are inherited in a Mendelian fashion. A change in DNA sequence that affects or changes a restriction site is detected by a difference in restriction fragments. It is through such linkage analysis that many hereditary conditions, heretofore not amenable to prenatal detection, have become identifiable. Examples include α-1-antitrypsin defi-

fetuses removed at hysterotomy. Kan and Dozy (1978) subsequently reported an indirect approach to the diagnosis of sickle cell based on linkage analysis and restriction fragment length polymorphisms. Chang and Kan (1982) then described an assay with the restriction enzyme Mst II for direct prenatal diagnosis of sickle cell mutations. This technique, which provides accurate diagnosis of sickle cell anemia, can be performed on chorionic villus specimens or amnionic fluid. The normal β-globin gene is separated into two fragments by Mst II, 1.15 kb and 0.2 kb long (Fig. 32–17). The sickle mutation at the sixth amino acid changes the amino acid from glutamic acid to valine with a corresponding change in DNA sequence. This causes a loss of the Mst II recognition site and results in a single 1.35 kb fragment. By using Southern blotting analysis and the 1.15 kb Mst II fragment as a probe, they found 1.15 kb fragments in the AA genotype, the 1.35 kb fragment with SS, and both fragments in patients with AS.

TABLE 32–10. PARTIAL LIST OF GENE PROBES AVAILABLE FOR PRENATAL DIAGNOSIS OF INHERITED CONDITIONS

Disease	Gene Probe
Adult polycystic kidney disease	HVR region 3' to α-globin
Alpha-1-antitrypsin deficiency	Synthetic oligonucleotide
Cystic fibrosis	Chromosome 4 or 19 DNA segments
Hemophilia A and B	Cloned factor VIII, IX
Huntington disease	G8 (D4S10)
Hypercholesterolemia	LDL receptor
Marfan syndrome	α2 (I) Collagen (RFLP)
Neurofibromatosis	Complement C$_3$
	Apolipoprotein C$_2$
Phenylketonuria	Phenylalanine hydroxylase
Sickle cell disease	β-globin
Thalassemia syndromes	α- and β-globins

Modified from Cooper and Schmidtke: Hum Genet 77:66, 1987.

ciency (Hejtmancik and co-workers, 1986), carriers of hemophilia A (Antonarakis and colleagues, 1985), and Huntington disease (Quarrell and colleagues, 1987). Conversely, Darras and co-workers (1987) reported serious pitfalls caused by chromosomal crossover events in using this technology for prenatal diagnosis of Duchenne muscular dystrophy.

PRACTICAL APPLICATIONS

The power of such techniques for studying inherited disease is indeed extraordinary. A partial list of some available gene probes is given in Table 32–10. Thus, with a small amount of fetal DNA, obtained either by amniocentesis or by chorion biopsy, the limits of diagnosis of fetal disease are those imposed by the number of gene probes to which this DNA may be exposed. It is readily apparent that obstetricians cannot be expected to keep current on all aspects of this complex technology; however, a working knowledge, with appropriate consultation from a clinical geneticist, provides significant contributions to prenatal diagnosis of many inherited disorders.

REFERENCES

Abel EL, Sokol RJ; Alcohol use in pregnancy. In Niebyl JR (ed): Drug Use in Pregnancy, 2nd ed. Philadelphia, Lea & Febiger, 1988a, p 193

Abel EL, Sokol RJ: Marijuana and cocaine use during pregnancy. In Niebyl JR (ed): Drug Use in Pregnancy, 2nd ed. Philadelphia, Lea & Febiger, 1988b, p 223

Acker D, Sachs BP, Tracey KJ, Wise WE: Abruptio placentae associated with cocaine use. Am J Obstet Gynecol 146:220, 1983

American College of Obstetricians and Gynecologists: Antenatal diagnosis of genetic disorders. Tech Bull, No 108, September 1987

American College of Obstetricians and Gynecologists: Prenatal detection of neural tube defects. Tech Bull, No 99, December 1986

American Medical Association Council on Scientific Affairs: Fetal effects of maternal alcohol use. JAMA 249:2517, 1983

American Society of Human Genetics: Policy statement for maternal serum alpha-fetoprotein screening programs and quality control for laboratories performing maternal serum and amnionic fluid alpha-fetoprotein assays. Am J Hum Genet 40:75, 1987

Antonarakis SE, Waber PG, Kittur SD, Patei AS, Kazazian HH Jr, Mellis MA, Counts RB, Stamatoyannopoulos G, Bowie EJ, Fass DN, Pittman DD, Wozney JM, Toole JJ: Hemophilia A: Detection of molecular defects and of carriers by DNA analysis. N Engl J Med 313:842, 1985

Arras JD, Shinnar S: Anencephalic newborns as organ donors: A critique. JAMA 259:2284, 1988

Aula P, Rapola J, Karjalainen O, Lindgren J, Hartikainen AL, Seppälä M: Prenatal diagnosis of congenital nephrosis in 23 high-risk families. Am J Dis Child 132:984, 1978

Barela AI, Kleinman GE, Golditch IM, Menke DJ, Hogge WA, Golbus MS: Septic shock with renal failure after chorionic villus sampling. Am J Obstet Gynecol 154:1100, 1986

Beckman DA, Brent RL: Mechanism of known environmental teratogens: Drugs and chemicals. Clin Perinatol 13:649, 1986

Bellinger D, Leviton A, Waternaux C, Needleman H, Rabinowitz M: Longitudinal analyses of prenatal and postnatal lead exposure and early cognitive development. N Engl J Med 316:1037, 1987

Benacerraf BR, Adzick NS: Fetal diaphragmatic hernia: Ultrasound diagnosis and clinical outcome in 19 cases. Am J Obstet Gynecol 156:573, 1987

Benacerraf BR, Gelman R, Frigoletto FD Jr: Sonographic identification of second-trimester fetuses with Down's syndrome. N Engl J Med 317:1371, 1987

Besinger RE, Niebyl JR: Tocolytic agents for the treatment of preterm labor. In Niebyl JR (ed): Drug Use in Pregnancy, 2nd ed. Philadelphia, Lea & Febiger, 1988, p 127

Beslisle S, Fencl MD, Tulchinsky D: Amniotic fluid testosterone and follicle-stimulating hormone in the determination of fetal sex. Am J Obstet Gynecol 128:514, 1977

Bingol N, Fuchs M, Diaz V, Stone RK, Gromisch DS: Teratogenicity of cocaine in humans. J Pediatr 110:93, 1987

Birnholz JC: Determination of fetal sex. N Engl J Med 309:942, 1983

Bleyer WA, Breckenridge RT: Studies on the detection of adverse drug reactions in the newborn. JAMA 213:2049, 1970

Boué A, Boué J: Chromosomal abnormalities associated with fetal malformations. In Schrimgeout J (ed): Towards the Prevention of Fetal Malformation. Edinburgh, Edinburgh University Press, 1978

Bovicelli L, Orsini LF, Rizzo N, Montacuti V, Bacchetta M: Reproduction in Down's syndrome. Obset Gynecol 59:13S, 1982

Brent RL: The Bendectin saga: Another American tragedy [editorial comments]. Teratology 27:283, 1983

Brent RL: Teratogen update: Bendectin [editorial comments]. Teratology 31:429, 1985

Brent RL: Ionizing radiation. Contemp Ob/Gyn 30:20, 1987

Briggs GG, Freeman RK, Yaffe SJ: Drugs in Pregnancy and Lactation, 2nd ed. Baltimore, Williams & Wilkins, 1986

Brown WT, Jenkins EC, Cohen IL, Fisch GS, Wolf-Schein EG, Gross A, Waterhouse L, Fein D, Mason-Brothers A, Ritvo E: Fragile X and autism: A multicenter survey. Am J Med Genet 23:341, 1986

Brumfitt W, Pursell R: Trimethoprim/sulfamethoxazole in the treatment of bacteriuria in women. J Infect Dis 128S:657, 1973

Carter CO: Genetic factors in congenital dislocation of the hip. Proc R Soc Med 56:803, 1963

Centers for Disease Control: Premature mortality due to congenital anomalies—United States. MMWR 37:505, 1988

Centers for Disease Control: Preventing lead poisoning in young children. MMWR 34:66, 1985a

Centers for Disease Control: Revised recommendations for preventing malaria in travelers to areas with chloroquine-resistant Plasmodium falciparum. MMWR 34:185, 1985b

Centers for Disease Control: Use of supplements containing high-dose vitamin A—New York. MMWR 36:80, 1987

Centers for Disease Control: Valproate: A new cause of birth defects—Report from Italy and follow-up from France. MMWR 32:439, 1983

Chang JC, Kan YW: A sensitive new prenatal test for sickle cell anemia. N Engl J Med 307:30, 1982

Chasnoff LJ, Burns WJ, Schnoll SH, Burns KA: Cocaine use in pregnancy. N Engl J Med 313:666, 1985

Chudley AE, Hagerman RJ: Fragile X syndrome. J Pediatr 110:821, 1987

Clarren SK, Smith DW: The fetal alcohol syndrome. N Engl J Med 298:1063, 1978

Collins E, Turner G: Maternal effects of regular salicylate ingestion in pregnancy. Lancet 2:335, 1975

Corby DG, Shylman I: The effect of antenatal drug administration on aggregation of platelets of newborn infants. J Pediatr 79:307, 1971

Crawford DC, Chita SK, Allan LD: Prenatal detection of congenital heart disease: Factors affecting obstetric management and survival. Am J Obstet Gynecol 159:352, 1988

Cuckle HS, Wald NJ: Maternal serum alpha-fetoprotein measurement: A screening test for Down's syndrome. Lancet 1:926, 1984

Dalens B, Raymond EJ, Gaulme J: Teratogenicity of valproic acid. J Pediatr 97:332, 1980

Darras BT, Harper JF, Francke U: Prenatal diagnosis and detection of carriers with DNA probes in Duchenne's muscular dystrophy. N Engl J Med 316:985, 1987

DiMaio MS, Baumgarten A, Greenstein RM, Saal HM, Mahoney MJ: Screening for fetal Down's syndrome in pregnancy by measuring maternal serum alpha-fetoprotein levels. N Engl J Med 317:342, 1987

Donald PR, Sellars SL: Streptomycin ototoxicity in the unborn child. S Afr Med J 60:316, 1981

Drugan A, Syner FN, Greb A, Evans MI: Amniotic fluid alpha-getoprotein and acetylcholinesterase in early genetic amniocentesis. Obstet Gynecol 72:35, 1988a

Drugan A, Zador IE, Syner FN, Sokol RJ, Sacks AJ, Evans MI: A normal ultrasound does not obviate the need for amniocentesis in patients with elevated serum alpha-fetoprotein. Obstet Gynecol 72:627, 1988b

Edelin KC, Gurganious L, Golar K, Oellerich D, Kyei-Aboagye K, Hamid MA: Methadone maintenance in pregnancy. Consequences to care and outcome. Obstet Gynecol 71:399, 1988

Edwards DK III, Berry CC, Hilton SVW: Trisomy 21 in newborn infants: Chest radiographic diagnosis. Radiology 167:317, 1988

Elder JS, Duckett JW Jr, Snyder HM: Intervention for fetal obstructive uropathy: Has it been effective? Lancet 2:1007, 1987

Entman SS, Vaughn WK: Lack of relation of oral clefts to diazepam use in pregnancy [letter]. N Engl J Med 310:1121, 1984

FDA Drug Bulletin: Pregnancy categories for prescription drugs. September 1979

Fenton LG, Light LJ: Congenital syphilis after maternal treatment with erythromycin. Obstet Gynecol 47:492, 1976

Fitzsimmons J, Nyberg DA, Cyr DR, Hatch E: Perinatal management of gastroschisis. Obstet Gynecol 71:910, 1988

Francke U, Brown MG, Jones KL: Immediate chromosome diagnosis on bone marrow cells: An aid to management of the malformed newborn infant. J Pediatr 94:289, 1979

Fraser FC: Causes of congenital malformations in human beings. J Chron Dis 10:97, 1959

Friedman JM: Genetic disease in the offspring of older fathers. Obstet Gynecol 57:745, 1981

Gaily E, Granström M-L, Hiilesmaa V, Bardy A: Minor anomalies in offspring of epileptic mothers. J Pediatr 112:520, 1988

Ghavami M, Levy HL, Erbe RW: Prevention of fetal damage through dietary control of maternal hyperphenylalaninemia. Clin Obstet Gynecol 29:580, 1986

Gilbert WM, Nicolaides KH: Fetal omphalocele: Associated malformations and chromosomal defects. Obstet Gynecol 70:633, 1987

Golbus MS: Teratology for the obstetrician: Current status. Obstet Gynecol 55:269, 1980

Goldstein JC, Brown MS: Genetics aspects of disease. In Braunwald E, Isselbacher KJ, Petersdorf RG, Wilson JD, Martin JB, Fauci AS (eds): Harrison's Principles of Internal Medicine, 11th ed. New York, McGraw-Hill, 1987, p 285

Gomez MR: Possible teratogenicity of valproic acid. J Pediatr 98:508, 1981

Green JE, Dorfmann A, Jones SL, Bender S, Patton L, Schulman JD: Chorionic villus sampling: Experience with an initial 940 cases. Obstet Gynecol 71:208, 1988

Greenland S, Staisch KJ, Brown N, Gross SJ: The effect of marijuana use during pregnancy: A preliminary epidemiology study. Am J Obstet Gynecol 143:408, 1982

Gross SJ, Benzie RJ, Sermer M, Skidmore MB, Wilson SR: Sacrococcygeal teratoma: Prenatal diagnosis and management. Am J Obstet Gynecol 156:393, 1987

Grover L, Kane J, Kravitz J, Cruz A: Systemic acyclovir in pregnancy: A case report. Obstet Gynecol 65:284, 1985

Habib Z: Genetic counselling and genetics of cleft lip and cleft palate. Obstet Gynecol Surv 33:44, 1978

Hall JG, Pauli RM, Wilson K: Maternal and fetal sequelae of anticoagulation during pregnancy. Am J Med 68:122, 1980

Hankins GDV, Gilstrap LC, Patterson A: Acyclovir treatment of varicella pneumonia in pregnancy. Crit Care Med 15:336, 1987

Hanson JW, Smith DW: The fetal hydantoin syndrome. J Pediatr 87:285, 1975

Hanson FW, Zorn FM, Tennant FR, Marioanos S, Samuels S: Amniocentesis before 15 weeks' gestation: Outcome, risks and technical problems. Am J Obstet Gynecol 156:1574, 1987

Harrigan JT, Kangos JJ, Sikka KR, Spisso KR, Natarajan N, Rosenfeld D, Leimans S, Korn D: Successful treatment of fetal congestive failure secondary to tachycardia. N Engl J Med 304:1527, 1981

Harrison MR, Golbus MS, Filly RA, Callen PW, Katz M, de Lorimier AA, Rosen M, Jonsen AR: Fetal surgery for congenital hydronephrosis. N Engl J Med 306:591, 1982

Hasan S, Hermansen MC: The prenatal diagnosis of ventral abdominal wall defects. Am J Obstet Gynecol 155:842, 1986

Heinonen OP, Slone D, Shapiro S: Birth Defects and Drugs in Pregnancy. Littleton, MA, Publishing Sciences Group, 1977

Hejtmancik JF, Ward PA, Mansfield T, Sifers RN, Harris S, Cox DW: Prenatal diagnosis of α_1-antitrypsin deficiency by restriction fragment length polymorphisms, and comparison with oligonucleotide probe analysis. Lancet 2:767, 1986

Hernandez E, Angell CS, Johnson JWC: Asthma in pregnancy: Current concepts. Obstet Gynecol 55:739, 1980

Higgins LG: Prolonged pregnancy. Lancet 2:1154, 1954

Hill LM, Malkasian GD: The use of quinidine sulfate throughout pregnancy. Obstet Gynecol 54:366, 1979

Hogge WA, Schonberg SA, Golbus MS: Chorionic villus sampling: Experience of the first 1000 cases. Am J Obstet Gynecol 154:1249, 1986

Holmes LB: Teratogen update: Bendectin. Teratology 27:277, 1983

Holzgreve W, Beller FK, Buchholz B, Hansmann M, Köhler K: Kidney transplantation from anencephalic donors. N Engl J Med 316:1069, 1987

Hook EB: Spontaneous deaths of fetuses with chromosomal abnormalities diagnosed prenatally. N Engl J Med 299:1036, 1978

Horne HW: Anencephaly in four consecutive pregnancies. Fertil Steril 9:67, 1958

Illingworth RS: Why blame the obstetrician?: A review. Br Med J 1:797, 1979

Jackson L: CVS Newsletter No 24, February 14, 1988

Jenkins EC, Brown WT, Wilson MG, Lin MS, Alfi OS, Wassman ER, Brooks J, Duncan CJ, Masia A, Krawczun MS: The prenatal detection of the fragile X chromosome: Review of recent experience. Am J Med Genet 23:297, 1986

Jones KL, Smith DW, Streissguth AP, Myrianthopoulos NC: Incidence of fetal alcohol syndrome in offspring of chronically alcoholic women. Pediatr Res 8:440, 1974

Jones KL, Smith DW, Ulleland CN, Streissguth P: Patterns of malformations in offspring of chronic alcoholic mothers. Lancet 1:1267, 1973

Kalousek DK, Dill FJ: Chromosomal mosaicism confined to the placenta in human conceptions. Science 221:665, 1983

Kan YW, Dozy AM: Antenatal diagnosis of sickle-cell anemia by DNA analysis of amniotic fluid cells. Lancet 2:910, 1978

Kan YW, Dozy AM, Alter BP, Frigoletto FD, Nathan DG: Detection of the sickle gene in the human fetus. N Engl J Med 287:1, 1972

Kelly TE: Teratogenicity of anticonvulsant drugs: I. Review of the literature. Am J Med Genet 19:413, 1984

Kelly TE, Edwards P, Rein M, Miller JQ, Dreifuss FE: Teratogenicity of anticonvulsant drugs: II. A prospective study. Am J Med Genet 19:435, 1984

Khoury MJ, Weinstein A, Panny S, Holtzman NA, Lindsay PK, Farrel K, Eisenberg M: Maternal cigarette smoking and oral clefts: A population-based study. Am J Public Health 77:623, 1987

Klein V, Repke JT: Supraventricular tachycardia in pregnancy: Cardioversion with verapamil. Obstet Gynecol 63:16S, 1984

Kurachi K, Aorp T, Minagawa J, Miyake A: Congenital malformations of newborn infants after clomiphene-induced ovulation. Fertil Seril 40:187, 1983

Lemire RJ: Neural tube defects. JAMA 259:558, 1988

Lenke RR, Levy HL: Maternal phenylketonuria—Results of dietary therapy. Am J Obstet Gynecol 142:548, 1982

Lilford RJ, Linton G, Irving HC, Mason MK: Transabdominal chorion villus biopsy: 100 consecutive cases. Lancet 2:1415, 1987

Little BB, Snell LM, Gilstrap LC III: Methamphetamine abuse during pregnancy: Outcome and fetal effects. Obstet Gynecol 72:541, 1988

Little BB, Snell LM, Klein VR, Gilstrap LC III: Cocaine abuse during pregnancy: Maternal and fetal implications. Obstet Gynecol (in press), 1989

Liu DTY, Mitchell J, Johnson J, Wass DM: Trophoblast sampling by blind transcervical aspiration. Brit J Obstet Gynaecol 90:1119, 1983

MacGregor SN, Keith LG, Chasnoff IJ, Rosner MA, Chisum GM, Shaw P, Minogue JP: Cocaine use during pregnancy: Adverse perinatal outcome. Am J Obstet Gynecol 157:686, 1987

Madden JD, Chappel JN, Zuspan F, Gumpel J, Mejia A, Davis R: Observation and treatment of neonatal narcotic withdrawal. Am J Obstet Gynecol 127:199, 1977

Manning FA, Harrison MR, Rodeck C, and Members of the International Fetal Medicine and Surgery Society: Catheter shunts for fetal hydronephrosis and hydrocephalus—Report of the International Fetal Surgery Registry. N Engl J Med 315:336, 1986

McKusick VA: Mendelian Inheritance in Man: Catalogs of Autosomal Dominant, Autosomal Recessive, and X-linked Phenotypes, 7th ed. Baltimore, Johns Hopkins University Press, 1986

Meier PR, Manchester DK, Shikes RH, Clewell WH, Steward M: Perinatal autopsy: Its clinical value. Obstet Gynecol 67:349, 1986

Merkatz IR, Nitowsky HM, Macri JN, Johnson WE: An association between low maternal serum α-fetoprotein and fetal chromosome abnormalities. Am J Obstet Gynecol 148:886, 1984

Milkovich L, Van Den Berg BJ: An evaluation of the teratogenicity of certain antinauseant drugs. Am J Obstet Gynecol 125:245, 1975

Milkovich L, Van Den Berg BJ: Effects of prenatal meprobamate and chlordiazepoxide hydrochloride on human embryonic and fetal development. N Engl J Med 291:1268, 1974

Mills JL, Alexander D: Teratogens and "litogens." N Engl J Med 315:1234, 1986

Mills JL, Graubard BI: Is moderate drinking during pregnancy associated with an increased risk for malformations? Pediatrics 80:309, 1987

Milunsky A: The Prenatal Diagnosis of Hereditary Disorders. Springfield, IL, Thomas, 1973

Milunsky A, Sapirstein VS: Prenatal diagnosis of open neural tube defects using the amniotic fluid acetylcholinesterase assay. Obstet Gynecol 59:1, 1982

Motulsky A, Hecht F: Genetic prognosis and counseling. Am J Obstet Gynecol 90:1227, 1964

Mueller RF, Sybert VP, Johnson J, Brown ZA, Chen WJ: Evaluation of a protocol for post-mortem examination of stillbirths. N Engl J Med 309:586, 1983

Musci MN Jr, Clark MJ, Ayres RE, Finkel MA: Management of dystocia caused by a large sacrococcygeal teratoma. Obstet Gynecol 62S:10, 1983

National Institute of Child Health and Human Development: Antenatal Diagnosis. Report of a Consensus Development Conference. NIH Publication No 79, 1973. Washington, DC, GPO, 1979

Nelson LH, Bensen J, Burton BK: Outcomes in patients with unusually high maternal serum α-fetoprotein levels. Am J Obstet Gynecol 157:572, 1987a

Nelson LH, Burton BK, Sowers S: Ultrasonography in patients with low maternal serum α-fetoprotein. J Ultrasound Med 6:59, 1987b

Newman RG, Bashkow S, Calko D: Results of 313 consecutive live births of infants delivered in patients in the New York City methadone maintenance program. Am J Obstet Gynecol 121:233, 1975

Nicolaides KH, Rodeck CH, Gosden CM: Rapid karyotyping in non-lethal fetal malformations. Lancet 1:283, 1986

Niebyl JR, Lietman PS: The use of mild analgesics in pregnancy. In Niebyl JR (ed): Drug Use in Pregnancy, 2nd ed. Philadelphia, Lea & Febiger, 1988, p 21

Nishimura H, Tanimura T: Clinical aspects of the teratogenicity of drugs. Amsterdam, Excerpta Medica, 1976, p 140

Oakley GP: Frequency of human congenital malformation. Clin Perinatol 13:545, 1986

Oro AS, Dixon SD: Perinatal cocaine and methamphetamine exposure: Maternal and neonatal correlates. J Pediatr 111:571, 1987

Osathanondh R, Donnenfeld AE, Frigoletto FD, Driscoll SG, Ryan KJ: Induction of labor with anencephalic fetus. Obstet Gynecol 56:655, 1980

Ostrea EM, Chavez CJ: Perinatal problems (excluding neonatal withdrawal) in maternal drug addiction: A study of 830 cases. J Pediatr 94:292, 1979

Otake M, Schull WJ: In utero exposure to A-bomb radiation and mental retardation: A reassessment. Br J Radiol 57:409, 1984

Owens JR, McAllister E, Harris F, West L: 19-year incidence of neural tube defects in area under constant surveillance. Lancet 2:1032, 1981

Palomaki GE, Haddow JE: Maternal serum α-fetoprotein, age and Down syndrome risk. Am J Obstet Gynecol 156:460, 1987

Paul M, Himmelstein J: Reproductive hazards in the workplace: What the practitioner needs to know about chemical exposures. Obstet Gynecol 71:921, 1988

Paulson GW, Paulson RB: Teratogenic effects of anticonvulsants. Arch Neurol 38:140, 1981

Perrella R, Duerinckx AJ, Grant EG, Tessler F, Tabsh K, Crandall BF: Second-trimester sonographic diagnosis of Down syndrome: Role of femur-length shortening and nuchal-fold thickening. AJR 151:981, 1988

Pitkin RM: Fetal death: Diagnosis and management. Am J Obstet Gynecol 157:583, 1987

Platt LD, DeVore GR, Lopez E, Herbert W, Falk R, Alfi O: Role of amniocentesis in ultrasound-detected fetal malformations. Obstet Gynecol 68:153, 1986

Potter EL: Bilateral absence of ureters and kidneys: A report of 50 cases. Obstet Gynecol 25:3, 1965

Quarrell OWJ, Meredith AL, Tyler A, Youngman S, Upadhyaya M, Harper PS: Exclusion testing for Huntington's disease in pregnancy with a closely linked DNA marker. Lancet 2:1281, 1987

Reece EA, Winn HN, Wan M, Burdine C, Green J, Hobbins JC: Can ultrasonography replace amniocentesis in fetal gender determination during the early second trimester? Am J Obstet Gynecol 156:579, 1987

Reed SC: Counseling in Medical Genetics, 2nd ed. Philadelphia, Saunders, 1963

Richards DS, Seeds JW, Katz VL, Lingley LH, Albright SG, Cefalo RC: Elevated maternal serum alpha-fetoprotein with normal ultrasound: Is amniocentesis always appropriate? A review of 26,069 screened patients. Obstet Gynecol 71:203, 1988

Rodeck CH, Gosden CM, Gosden JR: Development of an improved technique for first-trimester microsampling of chorion. Br J Obstet Gynaecol 90:1113, 1983

Rohr FJ, Doherty LB, Waisbren SE, Bailey IV, Ampola MG, Benacerraf B, Levy HL: New England Maternal PKU Project: Prospective study of untreated and treated pregnancies and their outcomes. J Pediatr 110:391, 1987

Rosa FW, Baum C, Shaw M: Pregnancy outcomes after first trimester vaginitis drug therapy. Obstet Gynecol 69:751, 1987a

Rosa FW, Hernandez C, Carlo WA: Griseofulvin teratology, including two thoracopagus conjoined twins. Lancet 1:71, 1987b

Rosenberg L, Mitchell AA, Parsells JL, Pashayan H, Louik C, Shapiro S: Lack of relation of oral clefts to diazepam use during pregnancy. N Engl J Med 309:1282, 1983

Rosett HL, Weiner L, Lee A, Zuckerman B, Dowling E, Oppenheimer E: Patterns of alcohol consumption and fetal development. Obstet Gynecol 61:539, 1983

Rotmensch HH, Elkayam U, Frishman W: Antiarrhythmic drug therapy during pregnancy. Ann Int Med 98:487, 1983

Rubin PC: Prescribing in pregnancy. Br Med J 293:1415, 1986

Rubin PC, Butters L, Clark DM, Reynolds B, Summer DJ, Steedman D, Low RA, Reid JL: Placebo-controlled trial of atenolol in treatment of pregnancy-induced hypertension. Lancet 1:431, 1983

Rustin GJ, Booth M, Dent J, Salt S, Rustin F, Bagshawe KD: Pregnancy after chemotherapy for gestational trophoblastic tumours. Br Med J 288:103, 1984

Sabbagha RE, Sheikh Z, Tamura RK, DalCompo S, Simpson JL, Depp R, Gerbie A: Predictive value, sensitivity, and specificity of ultrasonic targeted imaging for fetal anomalies in gravid women at high risk for birth defects. Am J Obstet Gynecol 152:822, 1985

Seeds JW, Cefalo RC: Technique of early sonographic diagnosis of bilateral cleft lip and palate. Obstet Gynecol 62S:2, 1983

Selevan SG, Lindbohm M-L, Hornung RW, Hemminki K: A study of occupational exposure to antineoplastic drugs and fetal loss in nurses. N Engl J Med 313:1173, 1985

Sermer M, Benzie RJ, Pitson L, Carr M, Skidmore M: Prenatal diagnosis and management of congenital defects of the anterior abdominal wall. Am J Obstet Gynecol 156:308, 1987

Shapiro S, Monson RR, Kaufman DW, Siskind V, Heinonen OP, Slone D: Perinatal mortality and birth-weight in relation to aspirin taken during pregnancy. Lancet 1:1375, 1976

Shepard TH: Human teratogenicity. Adv Pediatr 33:225, 1986

Simoni G, Brambati B, Danesino C, Rosella F, Terzoli GL, Ferrari M, Fraccaro M: Efficient direct chromosome analyses and enzyme determinations from chorionic villi samples in the first trimester of pregnancy. Hum Genet 63:349, 1983

Simpson JL, Baum LD, Depp R, Elias S, Somes G, Marder R: Low maternal serum α-fetoprotein and perinatal outcome. Am J Obstet Gynecol 156:852, 1987

Simpson JL, Baum LD, Marder R, Elias S, Ober C, Martin AO: Maternal serum α-fetoprotein screening: Low and high values for detection of genetic abnormalities. Am J Obstet Gynecol 155:593, 1986

Slone D, Heinonen OP, Kaufman DW, Siskind V, Monson RR, Shapiro S: Aspirin and congenital malformations. Lancet 1:1373, 1976

Slone D, Siskine V, Heinonen OP, Monson RR, Kaufman DW, Shaprio S: Antenatal exposure to the phenothiazines in relation to congenital malformations, perinatal mortality rate, birth weight, and intelligence quotient score. Am J Obstet Gynecol 128:486, 1977

Stein SC, Feldman JG, Friedlander M, Klein RJ: Is myelomeningocele a disappearing disease? Pediatrics 69:511, 1982

Stenchever MA, Javris JA: Lysergic acid diethylamide (LSD): Effect on human chromosomes in vivo. Am J Obstet Gynecol 106:485, 1970

Stevenson RE, Burton M, Ferlauto GJ, Taylor HA: Hazards of oral anticoagulants during pregnancy. JAMA 243:1549, 1980

Strauss AA, Mondanlou HD, Bosu SK: Neonatal manifestations of maternal phencyclidine (PCP) abuse. Pediatrics 68:550, 1981

Streissgurth AP, Clarren SK, Jones KL: Natural history of the fetal alcohol syndrome: A 10-year follow-up of eleven patients. Lancet 2:85–91, 1985

Sulaiman ND, Florey CDV, Taylor DJ, Ogston SA: Alcohol consumption in Dundee primigravidas and its effects on outcome of pregnancy. Br Med J 296:1500, 1988

Valenti C, Lin CC, Baum A, Masobrio M: Prenatal sex determination. Am J Obstet Gynecol 112:890, 1972

Vintzileos AM, Ingardia CJ, Nochimson DJ: Congenital hydrocephalus: A review and protocol for perinatal management. Obstet Gynecol 62:529, 1983

Vintzileos AM, Ingardia CJ, Nochimson DJ, Weinbaum PJ: Antenatal evaluation and management of ultrasonically defected fetal anomalies. Obstet Gynecol 69:640, 1987

Wagner LK, Lester RG, Saldana LR: Exposure of the pregnant patient to diagnostic radiations: A guide to medical management. Philadelphia, J B Lippincott, 1985

Wallace R, Caldwell D, Ansbacher R, Otterson W: Inhibition of premature labor by terbutaline. Obstet Gynecol 51:387, 1978

Waxman J: Cancer, chemotherapy and fertility. Br Med J 290:1096, 1985

Weatherall DJ: The New Genetics and Clinical Practice, 2nd ed. Oxford, Oxford University Press, 1985

Weinstein MR: Recent advances in clinical psychopharmacology: I. Lithium carbonate. Hosp Formul 12:759, 1977

Whittemore R, Hobbins JC, Engle MA: Pregnancy and its outcome in women with and without surgical treatment of congenital heart disease. Am J Cardiol 50:641, 1982

Williamson RA, Pringle KC: Correcting hydrocephalus and fetal uropathy: How good are the prospects? Contemp Ob/Gyn 30:77, 1987

Williamson RA, Weiner CP, Patil S, Benda J, Varner MW, Abu-Yousef MM: Abnormal pregnancy sonogram: Selective indication for fetal karyotype. Obstet Gynecol 69:15, 1987

Williamson JL, Kock R, Azen C, Chang C: Correlates of intelligence test results in treated phenylketonuric children. Pediatrics 68:161, 1981

Wilson JG: Experimental studies on congenital malformations. J Chron Dis 10:111, 1959

Wiseman RA, Dodds-Smith IC: Cardiovascular birth defects and antenatal exposure to female sex hormones: A reevaluation of some basic data. Teratology 30:359, 1984

Woods JR Jr, Plessinger MA, Clark KE: Effect of cocaine on uterine blood flow and fetal oxygenation. JAMA 257:957, 1987

Yen S, MacMahon B: Genetics of anencephaly and spina bifida? Lancet 2:623, 1968

Diseases, Infections, and Injuries of the Fetus and Newborn Infant

The fetus and newborn infant are subject to a great variety of diseases, some of which are the direct consequence of maternal disease, which has been considered along with the maternal illness, especially in Chapter 39. This chapter provides an introduction to other fetal and neonatal diseases and injuries of major clinical importance. Congenital malformations are considered in Chapter 32.

DISEASES OF THE FETUS AND NEWBORN

HYALINE MEMBRANE DISEASE

To provide prompt blood-gas exchange after birth, the infant must rapidly fill his lungs with air while clearing them of fluid, and he simultaneously must increase remarkably the volume of blood that perfuses his lungs. Some of the fluid usually is expressed as the chest is compressed during vaginal delivery, and the remainder is absorbed especially through the pulmonary lymphatics. Of great importance is the presence of appropriate surfactant synthesized by the type II pneumonocytes to stabilize the air-expanded alveoli by lowering surface tension and thereby preventing lung collapse during expiration.

About two decades ago, the development of *idiopathic respiratory distress syndrome*, also termed *hyaline membrane disease*, was found to be due to deficiency of pulmonary surfactant (see Chap. 6, p. 106). If the alveoli cannot be maintained in an expanded state because of inappropriate surfactant action, obvious respiratory distress develops that is characterized by the formation of hyaline membranes in the distal bronchioles and alveoli, considerable cardiopulmonary shunting of blood, and the likelihood of death from hypoxemia and acidosis unless treatment is prompt and appropriate.

Hyaline membrane disease has decreased as a cause of neonatal deaths in the United States. According to Malloy and colleagues (1987), from 1969 to 1973, 19 in 1,000 liveborns died from respiratory distress, but from 1979 to 1983, this number was 12 in 1,000. Boys are more prone than girls to develop these problems, and white infants appear to be more often and more severely affected than are black infants.

DIAGNOSIS

The atelectatic lungs are stiff with substantively decreased compliance, and thus the work of breathing is increased remarkably. Progressive shunting of blood through nonventilated areas of the lung contributes to the hypoxemia and to both metabolic and respiratory acidosis. Clinically these infants exhibit an increased respiratory rate accompanied by severe retraction of the chest wall during inspiration. Expiration is often accompanied by a whimper and grunt. Grunting is common in the newborn whenever there is uneven expansion of the lungs or lower airway obstruction. Finally, poor peripheral circulation and systemic hypotension may be evident.

Other forms of respiratory insufficiency may be confused with idiopathic respiratory distress syndrome. These include respiratory insufficiency as the consequence of sepsis, pneumonia, aspiration, pneumothorax, diaphragmatic hernia, and heart failure. Common causes of cardiac decompensation in the early newborn period are patent ductus arteriosus and primary myocardial disease. The chest radiograph, coupled with careful physical examination, is likely to be of considerable aid in differential diagnosis. In case of idiopathic respiratory distress, the chest x-ray shows a diffuse reticulogranular infiltrate throughout the lung fields with an air-filled tracheobronchial tree (air bronchogram).

PATHOLOGY

In the fatal case, the atelectatic lungs on gross examination resemble liver. Histologically, many alveoli are collapsed while some are dilated widely, hyaline membranes of fibrin-rich protein and cellular debris line the dilated alveoli and terminal bronchioles, and the epithelium underlying the membrane is necrotic.

TREATMENT

The establishment of appropriately staffed and equipped neonatal intensive-care units has served to reduce dramatically the number of deaths from idiopathic respiratory distress, even in very small infants. Similarly, advances in respiratory therapy and ventilatory support have been crucial. An arterial Po_2 below 40 mm Hg is indicative of the need for effective oxygen therapy. Anaerobically collected blood is required to assess Po_2, Pco_2, and pH. The blood may be obtained from a peripheral artery, but more easily from a catheter in an umbilical artery that also may be used for fluid infusion. The concentration of oxygen administered to these infants should be sufficient to relieve hypoxia and acidosis, but not higher. Arterial oxygen tensions of 50 to 70 mm Hg are adequate. Humidification of inspired air also is important. During recovery, careful blood gas monitoring allows P_{O_2} to be maintained with progressively lower concentrations of inspired oxygen. The infant from the time of birth must be kept warm, since chilling increases oxygen consumption.

The use of oxygen-enriched air under pressure to prevent the collapse of unstable alveoli, or *continuous positive airway pressure*, has brought about an appreciable reduction in the mortality rate from respiratory distress syndrome. In order to be successful, any technique to augment ventilation requires continuous observation by skilled personnel. Successful ventilation usually allows reduction of high inspired oxygen concentrations that are otherwise required, and thereby reduces pulmonary and retinal oxygen toxicity. Disadvantages are that venous return to the heart may be impaired, causing a fall in cardiac output, and there is always the possibility of barotrauma, characterized by rupture of the lung with interstitial emphysema and pneumothorax or pneumomediastinum. These complications are not always the consequence of overzealous resuscitation and ventilation, and are encountered even with low ventilatory pressures. While vigorous mechanical ventilation has undoubtedly improved survival, it is probably an important factor in the genesis of bronchopulmonary dysplasia, as pointed out below.

Treatment with Surfactant

Since the early 1980s, when Fujiwara and colleagues (1980) demonstrated that aerosolized surfactant treatment appeared to ameliorate the severity of the respiratory distress syndrome, there have been a number of clinical trials to study its efficacy. Preparations that have been used include animal lung extracts, human amnionic fluid extracts, and artificial surfactants.

Merritt and colleagues (1986) performed a randomized trial in which they instilled endotracheally human surfactant extracted from sterile amnionic fluid obtained from other women at elective cesarean section. Infants in the study, born between 24 and 29 weeks gestation, had proven pulmonary immaturity, and surfactant prophylaxis was associated with significantly decreased mortality (16 versus 52 percent), bronchopulmonary dysplasia among survivors (16 versus 31 percent), and pneumothorax (7 versus 31 percent). They observed no protection from intraventricular hemorrhage.

The Ten Centre Study Group (1987) from the United Kingdom reported similar findings from its large collaborative trial in which artificial surfactant was instilled into infants born at 24 to 29 weeks gestation. This crystalline suspension of phospholipids was placed into the pharynx or trachea at birth, and its use significantly reduced mortality and periventricular hemorrhages, as well as the incidence and severity of respiratory distress. Using bovine surfactant, Raju and colleagues (1987) had similar experiences, and reported decreased bronchopulmonary dysplasia with surfactant treatment.

As emphasized by Avery and colleagues (1986), these results are certainly encouraging, and it will be interesting to see if surfactant therapy, either human or artificial, will reduce appreciably the morbidity from respiratory insufficiency from other causes—for example, neonatal sepsis.

Long-term benefits of surfactant therapy remain undefined. Dunn and colleagues (1988) performed a 2-year follow-up of 55 survivors from their randomized trial. They reported that neurodevelopmental handicaps were not lessened by surfactant

therapy. Vaucher and associates (1988) reported similar findings in 46 survivors evaluated at 12 to 24 months of age.

OTHER COMPLICATIONS

Oxygen therapy is not innocuous. Persistent hypoxia is likely in itself to injure the lung, especially the alveoli and capillaries. If hyperoxemia is produced, the infant is at risk of developing *retrolental fibroplasia*. Therefore, the concentration of oxygen administered must be reduced appropriately as the arterial P_{O_2} rises. Endotracheal tubes after prolonged use cause erosion and serious infection of the upper airway, and they must be removed as soon as possible. *Bronchopulmonary dysplasia*, or oxygen toxicity lung disease, may develop in infants treated for severe respiratory distress with high concentrations of oxygen at high pressures. This is a chronic lung condition characterized by hypoxia, hypercarbia, and oxygen dependence as the consequence of alveolar and bronchiolar epithelial damage followed by peribronchial and interstitial fibrosis. Pulmonary hypertension is also a frequent complication. In a preliminary study, administration of vitamin E during the acute phase of the respiratory distress syndrome appeared to modify the development of bronchopulmonary dysplasia; however, in a subsequent randomized double-blind study, Ehrenkranz and co-workers (1979) were unable to confirm their earlier observations.

SURVIVAL

Death from the respiratory distress syndrome formerly was quite common, especially among very small infants. In recent years, the mortality rate, even for very small infants, has decreased remarkably (see Chap. 38, p. 745). Overt lung disease did persist or reappear following hyaline membrane disease, but it was not a frequent occurrence in a group of children evaluated by Stahlman and co-workers (1982).

RETROLENTAL FIBROPLASIA

Retrolental fibroplasia had become by 1950 the largest single cause of blindness in this country. After the discovery that the etiology of the disease was hyperoxemia, its frequency decreased remarkably.

PATHOLOGY

The retina vascularizes centrifugally from the optic nerve starting about the fourth month of gestation and continuing until shortly after birth. During the time of vascularization, the retinal vessels are very sensitive to, and thus are easily damaged by, excessive oxygen. The temporal portion of the retina, which is the last to be vascularized, is most vulnerable. Oxygen induces severe vasoconstriction, endothelial damage, and obliteration of the affected vessel. When the oxygen level is reduced, there is new vessel formation at the site of previous vascular damage. The new vessels penetrate the retina and extend intravitreally, where they are prone to leak proteinaceous material or actually burst with subsequent hemorrhage. Adhesions then form which detach the retina.

PREVENTION

The precise levels of hyperoxemia that can be sustained without causing retrolental fibroplasia are not known. Unfortunately, a cooperative study did not provide answers to many difficult but important questions concerning arterial P_{O_2} levels and retrolental fibroplasia (Kinsey and colleagues, 1977). It is felt by many pediatricians that the inhalation of air enriched with oxygen to no more than 40 percent will not cause retrolental fibroplasia. Some believe, however, that whenever oxygen-enriched air is provided the blood P_{O_2} must be monitored.

Very small infants born remote from term and who develop respiratory distress are most likely to require ventilation with high concentrations of oxygen to maintain life until the respiratory distress clears. During this period, it is important that overzealous treatment not lead to dangerous hyperoxemia and, in turn, retrolental fibroplasia. Frequent measurements of P_{O_2}, therefore, may be necessary first to assure adequate oxygen and then to prevent hyperoxemia.

Vitamin E has been administered to very low birthweight infants to try to prevent or minimize the development of retrolental fibroplasia. Hittner and co-workers (1983) are of the opinion that its use has merit and have provided a description as to how the vitamin might work.

MECONIUM ASPIRATION

The aspiration of some amnionic fluid before birth is most likely a physiological event (see Chap. 6, p. 106). Unfortunately, this normal process can be the cause of inhalation by the fetus of amnionic fluid containing thick meconium, which, in some cases, leads to subsequent respiratory distress and hypoxia with many complications described above. On the other hand, some neonates inhale meconium at birth. Thus, *meconium aspiration syndrome* may follow delivery in otherwise normal labor, but it more often is encountered in postterm pregnancy or in those complicated by fetal growth retardation. The common feature of these pregnancy complications appears to be reduced amnionic fluid volume into which the fetus defecates copious amounts of meconium. From the work of Leveno and colleagues (1984) on prolonged pregnancy, these events likely follow transient episodes of umbilical-cord compression in the otherwise healthy fetus, an event more likely if there is oligohydramnios.

Dooley and co-workers (1985) conducted a study to determine if intrapartum meconium aspiration was more common in labors complicated by evidence of fetal hypercarbia or hypoxia. They used meconium visualized beneath the vocal cords as being indicative of aspiration, and they found that 21 percent of fetuses from 272 pregnancies with meconium-stained amnionic fluid had aspirated some meconium. This incidence was not predicted by variable, saltatory, or late fetal heart decelerations during labor. Importantly, these investigators reported that liberal cesarean section (60 percent) for labors complicated by meconium and fetal heart rate abnormalities did not alter the frequency of meconium found beneath the cords. The single death was not prevented by aggressive pulmonary toilet described below.

Yeomans and associates (1988) showed that labors complicated by meconium-stained amnionic fluid were more likely to be associated with fetal-neonatal acidosis, arbitrarily defined as an umbilical artery pH of less than 7.2. They reported that 22 percent of 203 newborns had an umbilical artery pH of less than 7.2 if there was meconium-stained fluid. Persistent moderate to severe variable fetal heart rate decelerations, late decelerations, or baseline bradycardia during labor increased the likelihood of acidosis.

PATHOLOGY

Aspiration of meconium is likely to cause both mechanical obstruction of the airways and chemical pneumonitis. There is also evidence that the free fatty acids in meconium strip away alveolar surfactant (Clark and colleagues, 1987). Atelectasis, consolidation, and pneumothorax and pneumomediastinum may prove rapidly fatal unless vigorously treated. Even with prompt and appropriate therapy, seriously affected infants frequently die. Yeh and co-workers (1979) emphasized that the initial chest roentgenogram is useful for predicting outcome in these infants, and consolidation of atelectasis, most commonly associated with aspiration of thick meconium, is indicative of a poor outcome.

Marshall and associates (1978) found no evidence of persistent chronic lung disease among survivors of meconium aspiration; however, two of three infants who developed seizures while acutely ill subsequently demonstrated psychomotor retardation.

DIAGNOSIS AND MANAGEMENT

At Parkland Hospital, whenever meconium has been identified in amnionic fluid before or during delivery, someone skilled in resuscitative techniques is present at the delivery. To prevent further aspiration, the mouth and nares are carefully suctioned by the obstetrician before the shoulders are delivered from the vagina, or as the mouth is visualized through the uterine incision at cesarean delivery (see Chap. 26, p. 450). As soon as possible after delivery, all meconium-stained fluid that remains above the vocal cords is aspirated and the cords are visualized. Tracheal intubation and suction are then performed and as much meconium as possible is aspirated from the trachea. It is essential to perform these procedures swiftly. The stomach is emptied to avoid the possibility of further meconium aspiration. **It is emphasized that ventilation of the lungs must not be delayed unduly while these procedures are carried out.**

These practices have been questioned recently. Falciglia (1988) and Linder and colleagues (1988) reported that tracheal suctioning of meconium did not reduce the incidence or severity of respiratory distress from aspiration.

Suction Bulb Versus DeLee Trap

Locus and colleagues (1988) studied 80 women whose labors were complicated by moderate to thick meconium-stained amnionic fluid. Fetus-infants were randomly assigned to undergo suction at delivery of the head by either bulb or DeLee trap. They quantified meconium recovered from below the cords at tracheal suctioning and found that both methods were equally efficacious. Importantly, even with careful suctioning, 5 percent of these infants developed meconium aspiration syndrome, but none died.

INTRAVENTRICULAR HEMORRHAGE

Intraventricular hemorrhage, or hemorrhage into the germinal-matrix tissues, which then may extend into the ventricular system and brain parenchyma, is a common problem in preterm neonates. While these lesions are usually seen in infants born at less than 34 weeks, they may develop later and even are seen in term neonates. Most hemorrhages will develop within 72 hours of birth; however, they have been observed as late as 24 days (Perlman and Volpe, 1986). While external perinatal and postnatal influences undoubtedly alter the incidence and severity of these lesions, the greatest impact is that of prematurity. Unfortunately, since their onset is usually within three days of delivery, their genesis often is attributed erroneously to birth events.

PATHOLOGY

Central to the pathological process is damage to the germinal-matrix capillary network that predisposes to subsequent extravasation of blood into the surrounding tissue. Hemorrhage usually develops within 72 hours after delivery, and this may be influenced by several factors. One that seems to be of primary importance is fluctuation in velocity of cerebral blood flow (Hambleton and Wigglesworth, 1976).

If death does not follow from extensive hemorrhage, or from other complications of prematurity, these lesions are sometimes, but not always, associated with major neurodevelopmental handicaps (Morales, 1987; Papile and co-workers, 1983). Interestingly, DeVries and colleagues (1985) attribute long-term sequelae to cystic areas, or *periventricular leucomalacia*, that develop more commonly as a result of ischemic lesions, and less commonly to hemorrhages per se.

INCIDENCE AND SEVERITY

The incidence undoubtedly depends upon the level of immaturity, and about half of all neonates born before 34 weeks will have evidence of some hemorrhage. Interestingly, Hayden and colleagues (1985) reported that 4 percent of asymptomatic term neonates have sonographic evidence of subependymal hemorrhage. Perlman and Volpe (1986) have shown that very low birthweight infants have the earliest onset of hemorrhage, the greatest likelihood for progression into parenchymal tissue, and the highest mortality rate. Morales and Koerten (1986) reported similar experiences with 488 infants born weighing between 500 and 1,500 g, and the incidence of associated mortality and intraventricular hemorrhage is shown in Figure 33–1.

The severity of intraventricular hemorrhage can be assessed by ultrasound and computed tomography, and various grading schemes are used to quantify the extent of the lesion. The following scheme was proposed by Papile and colleagues (1978) and is used commonly:

Grade I   Hemorrhage limited to the germinal-matrix
Grade II   Intraventricular hemorrhage
Grade III Hemorrhage with ventricular dilatation
Grave IV   Parenchymal extension

It is emphasized that events that predispose to germinal-matrix hemorrhage are multifactorial and complex. Factors other than immaturity itself that predispose low birthweight infants to such hemorrhages appear to be those events that lead to hypoxia. Strauss and colleagues (1985) suggested that intrapartum fetal distress and acidosis at birth were significant predictive factors. Morales and Koerten (1986) showed that an umbilical cord pH of less than 7.2 and severe respiratory distress were associated with significantly increased severe hemorrhages. Luthy and co-workers (1987) reported a threefold increased risk for grade III or IV hemorrhage when the cord arterial pH was less than 7.2. Respiratory distress syndrome and mechanical ventilation are commonly associated factors. Finally, Lesko and colleagues (1986) reported that heparin used to maintain vascular catheter patency in intensive-care units was associated with a fourfold increased risk of germinal-matrix

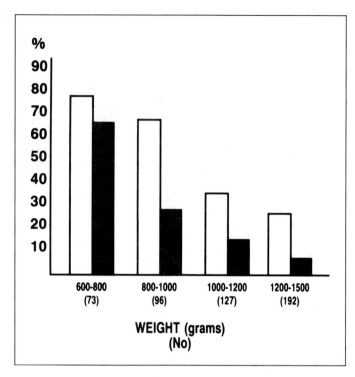

Figure 33–1. Incidence of intraventricular hemorrhage (white bars) and mortality (black bars) according to birthweight groupings. (*From Morales and Koerten: Obstet Gynecol 68:37, 1986, with permission.*)

hemorrhage. Obviously, other factors that cause hypoxia and acidosis, a prime example being sepsis, must be important.

PREVENTION AND TREATMENT

Attention to those intrapartum events that lead to hypoxia should help decrease the incidence of neonatal acidosis and thus lessen the risk of intraventricular hemorrhage. Intrapartum care given preterm fetuses during labor is discussed in Chapter 38. There is no evidence that routine cesarean delivery for the preterm fetus presenting vertex will decrease the incidence of periventricular hemorrhage (Morales and Koerten, 1986; Newton and colleagues, 1986; Tejani and co-workers, 1987; Welch and Bottoms, 1986). Moreover, Strauss and colleagues (1985) found no association with the presence of labor or its duration.

Avoiding hypoxic episodes after delivery is also of paramount importance, and these are considered under Hyaline Membrane Disease, above. Administration of muscle relaxants appears to diminish some of the cerebral blood-flow fluctuations, and thus hemorrhage (Perlman and colleagues, 1985). Phenobarbital, administered either to the neonate or to the mother during labor, has been shown to diminish the frequency and severity of these hemorrhages (Donn and colleagues, 1981; Morales and Koerten, 1986). Similarly, vitamin K_1 given intramuscularly to women with preterm labor improved neonatal prothrombin activity and significantly decreased the frequency of intraventricular hemorrhage (Pomerance and colleagues, 1987). Vitamin E injections given to these neonates may have decreased the incidence and severity of hemorrhage, but it did not decrease mortality (Sinha and colleagues, 1987). Conversely, indomethacin given to neonates weighing less than 1,000 g had a similar incidence of hemorrhage but a higher mortality rate than untreated controls (Hanigan and colleagues, 1988).

BRAIN DISORDERS

In 1862, a London orthopedist, William Little, described 47 children with spastic rigidity, and he concluded that virtually nothing other than abnormalities of birth could cause this clinical picture. Although others have suggested that prenatal events may be causal factors, Paneth (1986) stated that the *presumed* birth-injury etiology for cerebral palsy has endured and has influenced the opinions and practices of countless obstetricians and pediatricians. Unfortunately, this presumption likely accounts in part for the high malpractice premiums among those who deliver and care for newborns.

In 1985, a report was published by a panel of experts assembled by the National Institutes of Child Health and Human Development and the National Institute of Neurologic and Communicative Disorders and Stroke (Freeman, 1985). This information has done much to enhance our knowledge of brain disorders that previously were assumed due to intrapartum factors. Importantly, the report set some guidelines that are crucial to resolving some medicolegal issues that invariably surround children with brain disorders that includes cerebral palsy, mental retardation, learning disabilities, and seizure disorders. The term *newborn hypoxic ischemic encephalopathy* is used frequently by pediatricians to designate clinical and neuropathological findings thought to develop in the term infant following either intrapartum or neonatal asphyxia. Unfortunately, "asphyxia" itself is an imprecise term, and its diagnosis is frequently based on low Apgar scores alone, which may be caused by other factors such as prematurity, maternal sedation, or anesthesia (see Chap. 12, p. 237). Perhaps the increasing use of umbilical vessel acid-base studies will provide some answers to these important questions.

CEREBRAL PALSY

The National Institutes panel defined cerebral palsy as a nonprogressive motor disorder of early infant onset, involving one or more limbs, with resulting muscular spasticity or paralysis. This is a common disorder of children, and according to Paneth (1986), it affects at least 1 of every 500 school-age children. While affected children may have associated mental retardation or epilepsy, many often have neither, and 70 percent of cerebral palsy victims are of normal intelligence.

In many cases, cerebral palsy is erroneously attributed to perinatal events. Contrary to earlier teachings, and as shown in Table 33–1, perinatal asphyxia, again a poorly defined term, is identified in only about a third of cases of cerebral palsy. This has been examined extensively by Nelson and Ellenberg (1984, 1986a, 1986b), who described findings from the Collaborative Perinatal Project. They reported that maternal mental retarda-

tion, birthweight less than 2,000 g, and fetal malformations were leading predictors of cerebral palsy, while obstetrical complications were not strongly predictive. Only 21 percent of affected children had markers for perinatal asphyxia, and over half of these had associated congenital malformations, low birthweight, microcephaly, or another explanation for the brain disorder. **They concluded that the causes of most cases of cerebral palsy are unknown.** Importantly, studies from humans (Bejar and colleagues, 1988) and animals (Clapp and associates, 1988) have focused on *prenatal* causes of brain lesions.

Intraventricular hemorrhage is a risk factor for cerebral palsy. Luthy and colleagues (1987) reported that more than 40 percent of low birthweight infants with cerebral palsy had grade III or IV hemorrhages. They computed a sixteenfold increased risk for cerebral palsy when these infants were compared to those with no hemorrhage or those with grade I or II hemorrhage. Graham and associates (1987) reported that multiple cystic areas following periventricular hemorrhage were strongly associated with subsequent cerebral impairment.

Apgar Scores

Nelson and Ellenberg (1984) studied the interaction of obstetrical complications and a low Apgar score as a predictor of poor neurological outcome. A variety of late pregnancy complications were identified in 62 percent of pregnancies, and when considered alone, they were not strongly associated with cerebral palsy. However, in infants with complicated births who also had 5-minute Apgar scores of 3 or less, the incidences of mortality and cerebral palsy were appreciably increased. In the absence of complications, low Apgar scores alone were not associated with a high level of risk. Dijxhoorn and colleagues (1986) reported similar findings and concluded that most neonatal neurological abnormalities were due to factors other than perinatal hypoxia. Luthy and associates (1987) reported that in low birthweight infants with 1-minute Apgar scores of 3 or less, the incidence of death was increased fivefold and the incidence was increased threefold for cerebral palsy.

The American College of Obstetricians and Gynecologists (1986a) has summarized the use and misuse of the Apgar score to assess asphyxia and to predict future neurological deficit (see Chap. 12, p. 237). It was concluded that low scores at 1 and 5 minutes are excellent indicators for identification of those infants who need resuscitation. Although low scores may be caused by hypoxia, they are influenced by many other factors that affect tone, responsiveness, and respiration. Prematurity is the outstanding example of these factors. It was further concluded that low Apgar scores alone are not evidence for sufficient hypoxia to result in neurological damage. In a child found to have cerebral palsy, low 1- or 5-minute Apgar scores provide insufficient evidence that the damage was due to hypoxia. To substantiate that hypoxia led to neurological deficit, the following three additional perinatal adverse factors are required: 10-minute Apgar scores of 0 to 3, early neonatal seizures, and prolonged hypotonia. One of these alone is considered insufficient evidence for severe asphyxia, and in the absence of such evidence, subsequent neurological deficit cannot be ascribed to perinatal asphyxia. Data reported from the Collaborative Perinatal Project (Ellenberg and Nelson, 1988) support these contentions.

Neonatal Encephalopathy

Seizures and recurrent apnea are important predictors of cerebral palsy and future cognitive defects. Low and colleagues (1985) studied 303 high-risk preterm and term neonates, 30

TABLE 33–1. FACTORS CONTRIBUTING TO CEREBRAL PALSY

Factor	Percent[a]
Prenatal causes—preeclampsia, bleeding, diabetes, dysmaturity	30
Preterm birth	35
Fetal growth retardation	10
Perinatal asphyxia—5-minute Apgar score less than 6	40
Other perinatal causes—trauma and others	5

[a] Exceeds 100 percent since overlap of risks not removed.
Modified from Rosen and Hobel: Obstet Gynecol 68:416, 1986.

percent of whom had newborn encephalopathy. *Mild* encephalopathy was defined as hyperalertness, irritability, jitteriness, and hyper- and hypotonia. *Moderate* encephalopathy included lethargy, severe hypertonia, and occasional seizures. *Severe* encephalopathy was defined by coma, multiple seizures, and recurrent apnea. Cognitive and motor deficits were more likely in infants with mild or moderate (25 percent) or severe (55 percent) encephalopathy, compared to those without neonatal seizures (17 percent). Neonatal respiratory complications were the most commonly identifiable risk factor, but in 72 percent of those with mild to moderate encephalopathy, there were no risk factors identified (Fig. 33–2). Perinatal hypoxia was associated with, or contributed to, 26 percent of cases of mild to moderate encephalopathy and 66 percent of those with severe encephalopathy.

MENTAL RETARDATION

Etiological factors for severe mental retardation, which has a prevalence of 3 per 1,000 children, are shown in Table 33–2. In the National Institutes of Health report, the panel ascertained that isolated mental retardation—that is, mental retardation without epilepsy or cerebral palsy—was associated with perinatal hypoxia in only 5 percent of cases. Alternatively, mental

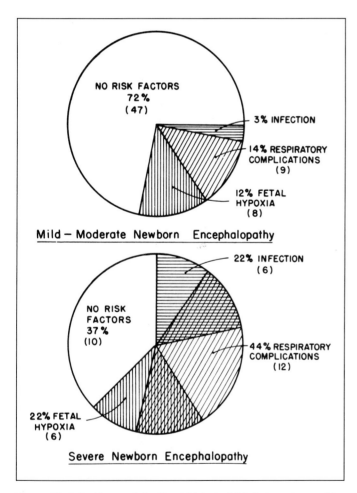

Figure 33–2. Incidence of significant biological risk factors observed in high-risk preterm and term neonates with mild-to-moderate and severe neonatal encephalopathy. (*From Low and colleagues: Am J Obstet Gynecol 152:256, 1985, with permission.*)

TABLE 33–2. SOME ETIOLOGICAL FACTORS FOR SEVERE MENTAL RETARDATION

Factor	Percent
Prenatal	**73**
Chromosomal	36
Mutant genes	7
Multiple congenital anomalies	20
Acquired—infections, diabetes, dysmaturity	10
Perinatal	**10**
Asphyxia/hypoxia	5
Unidentified causes	5
Postnatal	**11**
Unknown	**6**

Modified from Rosen and Hobel: Obstet Gynecol 68:416, 1986.

retardation coinidental with cerebral palsy is strongly associated with evidence for perinatal asphyxia or hypoxia (Rosen and Hobel, 1986).

SEIZURE DISORDERS

Unless manifest in association with cerebral palsy, seizure disorders or epilepsy are not related to perinatal hypoxia. Nelson and Ellenberg (1986b) determined that the major predictors of seizure disorders were congenital fetal malformations (cerebral and noncerebral), family history of seizure disorders, and neonatal seizures.

ANEMIA

DIAGNOSIS

The diagnosis of anemia in the newborn infant is not always simple. After 35 weeks gestation, the mean cord hemoglobin concentration is about 17 g per dL and values much below 14 g per dL may be regarded as pathologically low. During the first several hours of life, the hemoglobin value may rise by as much as 20 percent, especially when cord clamping was delayed, and as the consequence, an appreciable volume of blood was expressed from the placenta through the cord into the infant. Alternatively, if the placenta was cut or torn, a fetal vessel was perforated or lacerated, or the infant was held well above the level of the placenta for some time before cord clamping, the hemoglobin concentration is more likely to fall during the hours after delivery.

FETAL-TO-MATERNAL HEMORRHAGE

The presence of fetal red cells in the maternal circulation may be identified by use of the acid elution principle first described by Kleihauer, Brown, and Betke, or any of several modifications. Very small volumes of red cells commonly escape from the fetal intravascular compartment across the generally intact placental barrier into the maternal intervillous space. Large bleeds are uncommon, and Bowman (1985) reported that only 21 of 9,000 women had fetal hemorrhage at delivery exceeding 30 mL. Although the bleed is usually small, it may incite maternal isoimmunization, as discussed later. Stedman and colleagues (1986), using the erythrocyte rosette test, reported hemorrhage of this magnitude in only 6 of 1,000 women. Interestingly, evidence of maternal-to-fetal bleeding is much less common (Bernard and co-workers, 1977), and presumably a pressure gradient that is higher on the fetal than on the maternal side persists across the placenta.

Rarely, fetal-to-maternal hemorrhage may be so severe as to kill the fetus (Fig. 33–3). The hypovolemic or severely anemic fetus-infant may be salvaged if the condition is recognized and treatment with blood, red cells, or both, is promptly initiated. The fetus who is severely anemic is more likely to demonstrate one or more ominous heart rate patterns (see Chap. 15, p. 299). On occasion, the hemorrhage may have been chronic and so severe as to produce evidence of iron deficiency in the fetus. Maternal iron deficiency, however, even when severe, is not accompanied by anemia in the fetus, and the same is true for maternal megaloblastic anemia due to folate deficiency.

With larger fetal-to-maternal hemorrhages, a placental lesion—for example, a chorioangioma—is likely the cause. We know of two instances of severe fetal-to-maternal hemorrhage in which the mothers were later found to have choriocarcinoma. While neither placenta was studied, the subsequent recognition of choriocarcinoma in the mothers suggests that a placental lesion was the site of transfer of blood from the fetus to the mother. Placental abruption, in our experience, does not commonly cause appreciable fetal-to-maternal hemorrhage.

At Parkland Hospital, for some time maternal blood has been studied for fetal red cells in each instance of stillbirth whenever a cause was not readily apparent, and massive bleeds have been found in only a small minority of stillborn infants. Laube and Schauberger (1982) identified massive fetal-to-maternal bleeding in 4 of 29 otherwise unexplained antepartum fetal deaths.

Large fetal-to-maternal hemorrhages also may prove dangerous to the mother. It is possible for up to 400 mL of fetal blood to be transferred from the fetoplacental circulation into the maternal circulation. A transfusion reaction may then develop in the mother whenever A or B antigens are present in fetal, but not maternal, erythrocytes. Bergin and associates (1978) described many of the characteristic features of a transfusion reaction developing in a blood type O mother immediately after delivery of an infant who was blood type B.

HEMOLYSIS FROM ISOIMMUNIZATION

In 1892, Ballantyne established clinicopathological criteria for the diagnosis of *hydrops fetalis*. In 1932, Diamond, Blackfan, and Baty reported that fetal anemia characterized by numerous circulating erythroblasts was associated with this syndrome. Certainly ranking as a major contribution to medicine is the subsequent delineation of the pathogenesis of most cases of hemolytic disease in the fetus and newborn, including the related discovery of the rhesus factor by Landsteiner and Weiner in 1940. In 1941, Levine and associates confirmed that erythroblastosis was due to maternal isoimmunization with paternally inherited fetal factors, and the subsequent development of effective maternal prophylaxis was attributed to Finn and associates (1961) in England, and Freda and co-workers (1963) in the United States.

ISOIMMUNIZATION

Originally, the Rh concept was extremely simple, defined by one antiserum and two blood group factors, namely Rh-positive and Rh-negative. The Rh factors, however, have become increasingly complex, and more than 400 other red cell antigens have since been identified. Although some of them are immunologically and genetically important, fortunately many are so rare as to be of little clinical significance in the genesis of erythroblastosis fetalis.

Any person who lacks a specific red cell antigen can potentially produce an antibody when exposed to that antigen. The antibody may prove harmful to the individual in case of a blood transfusion or to a fetus when a woman conceives. The vast majority of humans have at least one such factor inherited from their father and lacking in their mother. In these cases, the mother could be sensitized if enough erythrocytes from the fetus were to reach her circulation to elicit an immune response. In these terms, hemolytic disease is a possibility in nearly every pregnancy. That the disease is identified in very few pregnancies is a result of several circumstances. These include (1) the varying rates of occurrence of the offending red cell antigens, (2) their variable antigenicity, (3) insufficient transplacental passage of antigen from fetus to mother, (4) the variability of maternal response to the antigen, (5) protection from isoimmunization by ABO incompatibility of fetus and mother, and (6) lack of transfer of antibody across the placenta from mother to fetus in amounts sufficient to affect the fetus.

To best illustrate the likelihood of Rh or D isoimmunization, the report of Bowman (1985) is cited. A D-negative woman delivered of a D-positive, ABO-compatible infant has a likelihood of isoimmunization of 16 percent. About 2 percent of such women will be immunized by the time of delivery, another 7 percent will have anti-D by 6 months postpartum, and the remaining 7 percent will demonstrate D isoimmunization when challenged in a subsequent pregnancy by another D-positive fetus. ABO incompatibility confers some protection against D

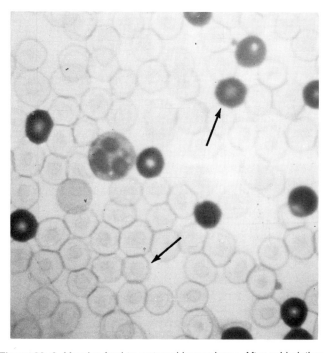

Figure 33–3. Massive fetal-to-maternal hemorrhage. After acid-elution treatment, fetal red cells rich in hemoglobin F stain darkly (*upper arrow*), whereas maternal red cells with only very small amounts of hemoglobin F stain lightly (*lower arrow*).

isoimmunization as well as other antigens, since fetal red cells entering the mother are usually rapidly destroyed before they elicit an antigenic response. The D-negative woman delivered of a D-positive, but ABO-incompatible, infant has only a 2 percent chance of D isoimmunization by 6 months postpartum.

CDE (RHESUS) BLOOD GROUP SYSTEM

The CDE, or rhesus, blood group system is of considerable clinical importance because the majority of individuals who lack its major antigentic determinant, D or Rho, become immunized after a single exposure to erythrocyte antigen. Several nomenclature systems are currently used; however, the CDE grouping system seems best, especially to describe the non-D antigens and their respective antibodies, anti-C, anti-c, anti-E, and anti-e.

The CDE antigens are inherited independent of other blood group antigens and are located on the short arm of chromosome 1. There is apparently no difference in the distribution of the CDE antigens with regard to sex; however, there are important racial differences. American Indians and Chinese and other Asiatic peoples are almost all D-positive (99 percent). Among black Americans there is a lesser incidence of D-negative individuals (7 to 8 percent) than among white Americans (13 percent). Of all racial and ethnic groups studied thus far, the Basques show the highest incidence of D-negativity (34 percent).

Rhesus antigens, other than D, have low immunogenicity and are typically ignored unless the pregnant woman has already formed an antibody to them, which, in turn, is detected by an antibody screening test. **All pregnant women should be routinely tested for the presence or absence of D (Rho) antigen on their erythrocytes and for other irregular antibodies in their serum.** Barss and colleagues (1988) have argued convincingly that this be only done once in D-positive women.

ABO BLOOD GROUP SYSTEM

The major blood group antigens A and B are the most common, but are not the most serious cause of hemolytic disease in the newborn. For example, group O women may from early life have anti-A and anti-B isoagglutinins, which may be augmented by pregnancy, particularly if the fetus is a secretor. Athough about 20 percent of all infants have an ABO maternal blood group incompatibility, only 5 percent of them show overt signs of hemolytic disease. Moreover, when they do, the disease is usually much milder than that with D isoimmunization. **Unlike Rh hemolytic disease, the incidence of stillbirths among ABO-incompatible pregnancies is not increased.**

Thus, ABO isoimmunization will cause hemolytic disease of the newborn, but seldom if ever will it cause hydrops fetalis as subsequently described. The reasons for this are probably at least twofold. First, most species of isoantibodies to A and B antigens are immunoglobulin M, and thus not likely to substantively gain access to fetal erythrocytes. Second, fetal red cells have a diminished number of A and B antigenic sites, at least when compared to later in life. Thus, there is no need for amnionic fluid analysis with presumed ABO isoimmunization.

Black infants are more likely to develop ABO disease than are white infants (Kirkman, 1977); however, it does not appear to be any more severe (Peevy and Wiseman, 1978). Desjardins and co-workers (1979) studied a large number of infants of blood group O mothers to try to identify a relationship between the degree of red cell sensitization by antibody and the cord blood hemoglobin and bilirubin concentrations. They found that when the infant blood type was A or B, the bilirubin was higher and hemoglobin was lower than in cord blood from blood group O infants, even when no antibody was identified on the type A or B red cells. They concluded that ABO incompatibility represents a spectrum of hemolytic disease that ranges from those with little laboratory evidence of red cell sensitization, but some evidence of hemolysis, to those with severe hemolytic disease in which red cell sensitization is readily demonstrable.

The usual criteria for diagnosis of hemolysis due to ABO incompatibility include the following: (1) The mother is major blood group O, with anti-A and anti-B in her serum, while the fetus is group A, B, or AB; (2) there is onset of jaundice within the first 24 hours; (3) there are varying degrees of anemia, reticulocytosis, and erythroblastosis; (4) there has been careful exclusion of other causes of hemolysis. Unlike the result in rhesus hemolytic disease, the Coombs' antiglobulin test in ABO incompatibility may be negative, although it is usually positive.

Since there is no adequate method of antenatal diagnosis, careful observation is essential in the neonatal period if cases are to be detected. Although the infants with ABO hemolytic disease most often are less severely affected than are those with rhesus hemolytic disease, they are equally incompetent in coping with excess bilirubin and its toxic effects on the central nervous system. Unlike Rh hemolytic disease, ABO disease frequently is seen in infants of primigravidas, and it is likely, but not absolutely certain, to recur in subsequent pregnancies. Katz and co-workers (1982) identified a recurrence rate of 87 percent, and 62 percent of the affected infants required treatment, but most often this was limited to phototherapy for hyperbilirubinemia.

The principles of management of the newborn infant with ABO hemolytic disease are similar to those for the infant born with Rhesus isoimmunization, particularly with reference to the behavior of hemoglobin and bilirubin. For simple transfusion or exchange transfusion, group O blood is used. Since the incidence of stillbirths among ABO-incompatible pregnancies is not increased, there is seldom justification for early labor induction, or for performing an amniocentesis except in the rare situation in which the previous infant was hydropic and no other cause was found.

OTHER BLOOD GROUP INCOMPATIBILITIES

D antigen incompatibility and ABO heterospecificity account for approximately 98 percent of all cases of hemolytic disease. For each red cell antigen there is the potential for hemolytic disease in the fetus and infant if the fetus has the antigen but the mother does not, the antigen has reached the mother and she has responded with antibody formation, the antibody is of IgG type and can cross the placenta, and the antibody does so in amounts sufficient to cause hemolysis.

The possibility of hemolytic disease from rarer blood groups may be suspected from the results of the indirect Coombs' test done to screen for abnormal antibodies in maternal serum. Listed in Table 33–3 are a number of red cell antigens and their capacity for causing hemolytic disease when the fetus possesses that antigen and the mother is isoimmunized.

An idea of the frequency of some of these antibodies comes from the report of Bowell and colleagues (1986a), who screened 70,000 pregnant women from the Oxford region over a 2-year period. They identified 677 pregnancies with atypical red cell antibodies, for an incidence of nearly 1 percent. A fourth of these were from the Lewis system, which do not cause fetal hemolysis since the antigens do not develop on erythrocytes

TABLE 33–3. SOME RED CELL ANTIGENS AND THEIR PROPENSITY TO CAUSE HEMOLYTIC DISEASE IN THE FETUS-INFANT WHOSE MOTHER IS ISOIMMUNIZED

Blood Group System	Antigen	Severity of Hemolytic Disease	Proposed Management
Rh(CDE)	D	Mild to severe with hydrops fetalis	Amnionic fluid studies
	C	Mild to moderate	Amnionic fluid studies
	c	Mild to severe	Amnionic fluid studies
	E	Mild to severe	Amnionic fluid studies
	e	Mild to moderate	Amnionic fluid studies
I		Not a proven cause of hemolytic disease	
Lewis		Not a proven cause of hemolytic disease	
Kell	K	Mild to severe with hydrops fetalis	Amnionic fluid studies
	k	Mild to severe	Amnionic fluid studies
Duffy	Fy^a	Mild to severe with hydrops fetalis	Amnionic fluid studies
	Fy^b	Not a cause of hemolytic disease	
Kidd	Jk^a	Mild to severe	Amnionic fluid studies
	Jk^b	Mild to severe	Amnionic fluid studies
MNSs	M	Mild to severe	Amnionic fluid studies
	N	Mild	Expectant
	S	Mild to severe	Amnionic fluid studies
	s	Mild to severe	Amnionic fluid studies
	U	Mild to severe	Amnionic fluid studies
Lutheran	Lu^a	Mild	Expectant
	Lu^b	Mild	Expectant
Diego	Di^a	Mild to severe	Amnionic fluid studies
	Di^b	Mild to severe	Amnionic fluid studies
Xg	Xg^a	Mild	Expectant
P	$PP_1P^k(Tj^a)$	Mild to severe	Amnionic fluid studies
Public Antigens	Yt^a	Moderate to severe	Amnionic fluid studies
	Yt^b	Mild	Expectant
	Lan	Mild	Expectant
	En^a	Moderate	Amnionic fluid studies
	Ge	Mild	Expectant
	Jr^a	Mild	Expectant
	Co^a	Severe	Amnionic fluid studies
Private Antigens	Co^{a-b}	Mild	Expectant
	Batty	Mild	Expectant
	Becker	Mild	Expectant
	Berrens	Mild	Expectant
	Biles	Moderate	Amnionic fluid studies
	Evans	Mild	Expectant
	Gonzales	Mild	Expectant
	Good	Severe	Amnionic fluid studies
	Heibel	Moderate	Amnionic fluid studies
	Hunt	Mild	Expectant
	Jobbins	Mild	Expectant
	Radin	Moderate	Amnionic fluid studies
	Rm	Mild	Expectant
	Ven	Mild	Expectant
	$Wright^a$	Severe	Amnionic fluid studies
	$Wright^b$	Mild	Expectant
	Zd	Moderate	Amnionic fluid studies

Modified from American College of Obstetricians and Gynecologists, Technical Bulletin No 90: Management of Isoimmunization in Pregnancy, January 1986.

until a few weeks after birth. Of the remaining 544 antibodies, 72 percent were of the CDE group, and anti-D was most common (158), followed by anti-E (130), anti-c (49), and anti-C (19). Antibodies to the Kell system antigens also were common (76).

The clinical importance of anti-c isoimmunization has recently been emphasized by Wenk (1986) and Bowell (1986b) and their colleagues. In their experiences, this antibody was the next most common cause of clinically significant isoimmunization

following anti-D. Although anti-c isoimmunization most commonly resulted from previous pregnancies, those fetuses whose mothers had been transfused were more likely to have moderate to severe hemolysis.

Mother as Provider of Rare Type Red Cells
Following isoimmunization of the mother who has a rare blood type, the possibility exists of hemolytic disease in the fetus and

neonate. This could create a need for red cells devoid of the antigen or antigens to which the mother is isoimmunized. Moreover, the mother herself may require red cells—for example, because of a complication of hemorrhage at delivery. For such circumstances, usually even while pregnant, she can successfully donate her own red cells, which are then appropriately frozen for subsequent use, as demonstrated by the following case:

> G.D., a 17-year-old gravida 2, P1, lacked immunological evidence of all Rhesus antigens except D, and had acquired antibodies during the previous pregnancy to C, c, E, and e. Compatible red cells available in the United States were limited to two units frozen in Portland, Oregon. Therefore, repeated phlebotomies, according to the schedule provided in Table 33–4, were performed during pregnancy and the red cells promptly frozen for possible subsequent use. In spite of her small size (67 inches tall and 109 pounds, nonpregnant), she tolerated quite well the removal of 6 units (3 L total) of blood at the rate of 500 mL every 3 to 5 weeks. Iron was provided orally and parenterally along with supplementary folic acid. Oral iron alone, if taken regularly, would have provided sufficient iron (see Chap. 14, p. 264).
>
> Repeat cesarean delivery was accomplished without incident. Hemolytic disease in the newborn was treated with exchange transfusions using all of the red cells harvested and stored from the six phlebotomies plus the two frozen units from Portland (Pritchard and Cunningham, unpublished).

PATHOLOGICAL CHANGES IN HEMOLYTIC DISEASE

Maternal antibodies gain access to the fetal circulation. In D-positive fetuses, such antibodies are both adsorbed to the D-positive erythrocytes and exist unbound in fetal serum. The adsorbed antibodies act as hemolysins, leading to an accelerated rate of red cell destruction. The earlier this process begins in utero and the greater its intensity, the more severe will be the effects upon the fetus.

Maternal antibodies detectable at birth gradually disappear from the infant's circulation over a period of 1 to 4 months. Their rate of disappearance is influenced to some extent by exchange transfusion. Detection of adsorbed antibodies is best accomplished by the direct Coombs' test. If D red cells coated with anti-D antibody are typed with an anti-D saline agglutinin, they may be reported incorrectly as D-negative because of the blocking effect produced by the adsorbed antibody. Therefore, erythrocytes reported to be D-negative from an infant whose mother may be isoimmunized must always be checked by the direct Coombs' test.

Immune Hydrops

The pathological changes in the organs of the fetus and newborn infant vary with the severity of the process. The severely affected fetus or infant may show considerable subcutaneous edema as well as effusion into the serous cavities (*hydrops fetalis*). At times, the edema is so severe that the diagnosis can be easily identified using sonography (Fig. 33–4). In these cases, the placenta also is markedly edematous, appreciably enlarged and boggy, with large, prominent cotyledons and edematous villi. Excessive and prolonged hemolysis serves to stimulate marked erythroid hyperplasia of the bone marrow as well as large areas of *extramedullary hematopoiesis*, particularly in the spleen and liver. Histological examination of the liver may also disclose fatty degenerative parenchymal changes as well as deposition of hemosiderin and engorgement of hepatic canaliculi with bile. There may be cardiac enlargement and pulmonary hemorrhages. The ascites, and to a lesser degree hepatomegaly and splenomegaly, may be so massive as to lead to severe dystocia as the consequence of the greatly enlarged abdomen. Hydrothorax may be so severe as to compromise respirations after birth.

The pathophysiology of hydrops remains obscure. Theories of its causation include heart failure from profound anemia, capillary leakage caused by hypoxia from severe anemia, portal and umbilical venous hypertension from hepatic parenchymal disruption by extramedullary hematopoiesis, and decreased colloid oncotic pressure from hypoproteinemia caused by liver dysfunction. To study this, Nicolaides and colleagues (1985) performed percutaneous umbilical artery blood sampling in 17 severely D-isoimmunized fetuses at 18 to 25 weeks gestation. All fetuses with hydrops had hemoglobin values of less than 3.8 g per dL as well as plasma protein concentrations less than 2 standard deviations from the mean for normal fetuses of the same age. The hydropic fetuses also had substantive protein concentrations in ascitic fluid collected at fetoscopy. Conversely, all nonhydropic fetuses had hemoglobin values that exceeded 4 g per dL; however, 6 of 10 had hypoproteinemia of the same magnitude as the hydropic fetuses. These investigators concluded that the degree and duration of anemia influence the severity of ascites, and this is made worse by hypoproteinemia. They also hypothesized that severe chronic anemia causes tissue hypoxia with resultant capillary endothelial leakage with protein loss.

Fetuses with hydrops may die in utero from profound anemia and circulatory failure (Fig. 33–5). A sign of severe anemia

TABLE 33–4. PATIENT GD, ISOIMMUNIZED AGAINST MOST RHESUS ANTIGENS EXCEPT D

Gestation (wk)	Hemoglobin (g/dL)	MCV (μ^3)	Phlebotomy (mL)	Iron-Dextran
14	12.0		500	500 mg
19			500	
24	11.4		500	500 mg
28			500	500 mg
31	11.1	95	500	500 mg
35			500	
36	11.1	Blood Volume 3,826 mL (47% above nonpregnant)		
37	11.5	95		Cesarean Section—3,060 g boy; Apgar score 9/9; hemolytic anemia; 4 exchange transfusions, subsequently thriving

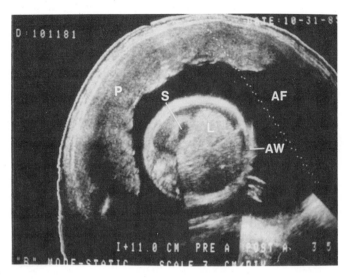

Figure 33–4. Transverse sonogram of a hydropic fetus. Illustrated are the edematous fetal abdominal wall (*AW*) and the fetal liver (*L*) and stomach (*S*). Increased amnionic fluid (*AF*) is apparent, and there is also a large placenta (*P*). (*Courtesy of Dr. R. Santos.*)

and impending death is a *sinusoidal fetal heart rate* pattern (see Chap. 15, p. 299). The liveborn hydropic infant appears pale, edematous, and limp at birth, often requiring resuscitation. The spleen and liver are enlarged, and there may be widespread ecchymoses or scattered petechiae. Dyspnea and circulatory collapse are common. Death may occur within a few hours in spite of transfusions.

Hyperbilirubinemia

Less severely affected infants may appear well at birth, only to become jaundiced within a few hours. Marked hyperbilirubinemia, if untreated, may lead to central nervous system damage, especially to the basal ganglia or to *kernicterus*. This is characterized clinically by lethargy, stiffness of the extremities, retraction of the head, squinting, a high-pitched cry, poor feeding, and convulsions. In such cases, death usually occurs within the first week of life. Surviving infants may be physically helpless, unable to support their heads or sit. Ability to walk is delayed or never acquired. In less severe forms, there may be varying degrees of motor incoordination, whereas some infants demonstrate residual nerve deafness as the only manifestation of neurological injury.

Anemia, in part resulting from impaired erythropoiesis, may persist for many weeks to months in the infant who had demonstrated hemolytic disease at birth. In the absence of hypoxia, erythrocyte production normally falls after birth, especially in the preterm infant. The observations of McIntosh (1975) implicate low production of erythropoietin in this phenomenon.

MORTALITY

The number of perinatal deaths from hemolytic disease caused by D isoimmunization has dropped dramatically for the following reasons:

1. Pregnant women who are D-negative and who are isoimmunized can be identified readily.

2. Hemolysis in the fetus of the sensitized D-negative woman can be predicted with considerable accuracy by the identification of abnormally high levels of bilirubin in the amnionic fluid or by sonographically directed umbilical vessel sampling.

3. The fetus who is most likely to be affected seriously can be treated by intraperitoneal or direct intravascular transfusions of D-negative red cells, or be delivered preterm before expiring in utero, or both.

4. The appropriate administration to the D-negative mother of D immune globulin during or immediately after pregnancy has eradicated most, but not all, D isoimmunization.

The favorable impact on reducing perinatal mortality as the consequence of these procedures is exemplified by experiences in Manitoba. In that Canadian province, the number of perinatal deaths from hemolytic disease decreased from 29 in 1964 to 0 in 1974 and only 1 in 1975 (Bowman and colleagues, 1977).

IMMUNE GLOBULIN PROPHYLAXIS FOR THE D-NEGATIVE, NONSENSITIZED MOTHER

The incidence of hemolytic disease of the fetus and newborn from D isoimmunization has become much less common because of passive immunization of D-negative women delivered of D-positive infants. Anti-D immune globulin is a 7S immune globulin G extracted by cold alcohol fractionation from plasma containing high-titer D antibody. Each dose provides not less than 300 µg of D-antibody as determined by radioimmunoassay.

Freda and co-workers (1975) summarized their 10 years of clinical experience with D immune globulin, confirming their original observations that such globulin given to the previously unsensitized D-negative woman within 72 hours of delivery is highly protective, although not absolutely so. D-negative women undergoing abortion should be treated, since up to 2 percent having spontaneous abortions and 5 percent having elective terminations will become isoimmunized without D immune globulin. Likewise, women with ectopic pregnancies or hydatidiform moles should be treated, as well as those who bleed vaginally during pregnancy. The observation of Blajchman and co-workers (1974) of detectable fetal-maternal hemorrhage after 6 percent of amniocenteses has provided support for a policy that all unsensitized D-negative women suspected of having a D-positive fetus should receive D immune globulin following such a procedure.

D-negative women who receive blood or blood fractions are at risk of becoming sensitized. Red cells can supply massive amounts of foreign antigen if the cells are D-positive and their recipient is D-negative. Moreover, platelet transfusions and plasmapheresis can provide sufficient D antigen to cause sensitization, which can be prevented by an injection of D antiglobulin. **Freda (1973), as well as Bowman (1985), emphasize that when in doubt whether to give anti-D immune globulin, then it should be given.**

While adherence to the above guidelines, including the administration of D immune globulin to the apparently nonsensitized mother within the first 72 hours after delivery of an D-positive infant, has decreased dramatically the risk of maternal isoimmunization, the problem has not been eliminated. For example, Bowman and Pollock (1978) identified 1.8 percent of women who became isoimmunized in spite of adherence to the

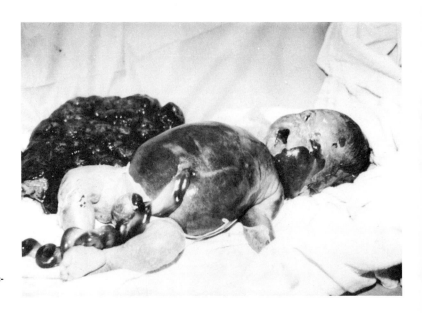

Figure 33–5. Severe erythroblastosis fetalis. Hydropic macerated stillborn infant and characteristically large placenta.

above recommendations. They and their colleagues deduced that most often the failures were the consequence of spontaneous silent fetal-maternal bleeds before delivery and before the administration postpartum of D immune globulin. Therefore, to try to avoid isoimmunization from fetal-maternal bleeds remote from term, 300 µg of antibody was routinely administered intramuscularly to all nonsensitized D-negative women at 28 weeks, again at 34 weeks gestation, as well as at the time of amniocentesis or uterine bleeding. If the infant was D-positive, a third dose of the immunoglobulin was administered to the mother after delivery. This program was followed by a reduction in the incidence of D isoimmunization during pregnancy from 1.8 percent to 0.07 percent. A single dose at about 28 weeks proved to be almost as effective as were the two doses antepartum, and only 2 of 1,799 D-negative women developed D isoimmunization despite antenatal prophylaxis.

The small amount of antibody that crosses the placenta results at times in a weakly positive direct Coombs' test in cord and infant blood; however, none of the infants showed evidence of anemia or exaggerated hyperbilirubinemia.

Appropriate concern has been raised for the possibility that the human immunodeficiency virus may be transmitted by plasma-derived products such as D immunoglobulin. Fortunately, there is overwhelming evidence to the contrary. Each year, more than 350,000 women are given 500,000 doses of D immune globulin, and there has been no verified case of immunodeficiency transmission (Centers for Disease Control, 1987a). The reasons for its safety is at least twofold: (1) The globulin is prepared using Cohn-Oncley fractionation, which is effective in removing human immunodeficiency viral particles, and (2) since 1985, all plasma lots used for D immunoglobulin production are tested for the virus. Thus, there is no evidence to implicate this product as a source of immunodeficiency virus infection.

Recommendations

A single intramuscular dose of 300 µg of D immunoglobulin is administered routinely to all D-negative, *nonimmunized* women at 28 to 32 weeks gestation and again within 72 hours of the birth of a D-positive infant. A similar dose also is given at the time of amniocentesis and whenever there is uterine bleeding, unless the routine dose at 28 to 32 weeks had been given very

recently. If a massive fetal-maternal hemorrhage is recognized, more immune globulin should be given, as described below. One dose of 300 µg will protect the mother against a bleed of up to 15 mL of D-positive red cells, or 30 mL of fetal blood. Adoption of these dosage schedules will reduce the incidence of maternal isoimmunization to essentially zero.

The report by Ness and colleagues (1987) provided data for the incidence of excessive fetal-maternal hemorrhage that may cause isoimmunization despite postpartum immune globulin administration. Using the enzyme-linked antiglobulin test, they studied 789 D-negative mothers giving birth to D-positive infants, and found evidence in 1 percent of the mothers for fetal whole blood in excess of 30 mL. Another 5.6 percent of these pregnancies had fetal-maternal bleeds of between 11 and 30 mL. Thus, at least 1 percent, and perhaps more, of susceptible mothers would have been given insufficient immune globulin if not tested. Importantly, they identified no risk factors that predicted excess bleeding, and recommended that all women be tested at delivery. Stedman and co-workers (1986) used the erythrocyte rosette test and reported similar results, except that intermediate levels of hemorrhage were found in only about 1 percent.

At Parkland Hospital, for many years the policy has been to verify free circulating D antibody, using the indirect Coombs' test, 24 hours after immune globulin is given postpartum. If excessive antibody is identified, then it is unlikely that persisting fetal erythrocytes will incite immunization.

Rarely, a woman who is classified as *D^u-positive* may, when challenged with D antigen, develop antibodies that can hemolyze D-positive red cells (Lacey and associates, 1983; White and associates, 1983). Whether to provide routinely D antiglobulin prophylaxis for D^u-positive women is controversial. Bowman (1985) cites 5 instances in 750,000 pregnancies in which a D^u-negative mother produced anti-D antibody. Fortunately, in none of these was the fetus severely affected. If there is any doubt about D antigen status, then globulin should be given.

Large Fetal to Maternal Bleed

In the case of a larger fetal-maternal hemorrhage, the D-positive erythrocytes may, by careful examination, be identified at times as clumps in the crossmatch of the erythrocytes from maternal blood and the D immune globulin. However, the acid-elution technique for identifying erythrocytes that contain appreciable hemoglobin is best used to identify a major bleed and to approximate its magnitude.

When the acid-elution test is performed, red cells rich in fetal hemoglobin are easy to identify (Fig. 33–3). A careful differential count will serve to approximate closely the percentage of fetal cells in the maternal blood. From this value, multiplied by maternal hematocrit and by maternal blood volume, an estimate of the volume of fetal red cells in the maternal circulation can be made. (Maternal blood volume will average about 5 L before delivery and 4 L shortly afterwards.) The volume of fetal red cells so calculated is then divided by 15 (volume of red cells effectively neutralized by 300 μg of antibody), and this provides a reasonable estimate of the number of 300 μg ampules of D immune globulin required for protection. If the estimate is doubled, almost certainly more than adequate protection would be afforded the mother. In practice, in cases of fetal-maternal hemorrhage, sensitization of the mother can be prevented by injecting sufficient D immune globulin intramuscularly to provide demonstrable free antibody in the maternal serum.

In a case of massive fetal-maternal hemorrhage successfully treated at Parkland Hospital, 14 vials of D immune globulin (4,200 μg at least) were injected intramuscularly over 48 hours to maintain a clearly demonstrable excess of antibody after delivery of a recently exsanguinated, very large infant. From the differential count of erythrocytes of maternal and fetal origin identified by acid-elution treatment of maternal blood and measurements of maternal hematocrit and apparent blood volume, at least 150 mL of type O, D-positive fetal erythrocytes were demonstrated to have entered the maternal circulation (Fig. 33–3). The mother subsequently gave birth to three unaffected type O, D-positive infants, including a set of twins. She remains free from evidence of D sensitization.

Maternal-Fetal Bleed

Rarely, the D-negative woman will have been exposed in utero to D antigen from her mother and become sensitized as the consequence. For this to occur, the woman's mother must have been D-positive and there must have been a maternal-fetal bleed. As with fetal-maternal bleeds, a major blood group (ABO) incompatibility offers appreciable protection against D sensitization. Jennings and Clauss (1978), in a study of 105 D-negative infants born to D-positive mothers, identified a maternal-fetal bleed in only two instances, or 1.9 percent—a value in very close agreement with that found by Cohen and Zuelzer (1965). Jennings and Clauss (1978) and Bowman (1985), on the basis of their extensive studies, do not believe that D immune globulin prophylaxis is warranted for D-negative babies born to D-positive mothers. We do not test for this situation at Parkland Hospital.

MANAGEMENT

The management of isoimmunization, except for ABO incompatibility, is similar regardless of the inciting antigen. Since D isoimmunization is most common, general management for this clinical situation is discussed.

The mother who is sufficiently immunized to produce enough antibody to cause overt hemolytic disease in the fetus and newborn will have demonstrable D antibody in her serum by 36 weeks gestation. Most often, if appropriate techniques are used, the antibody will be demonstrable much earlier. According to Freda (1973), if nothing is done in the way of interference

with the pregnancy of a sensitized D-negative woman with a D-positive fetus, the perinatal mortality rate can be anticipated to be about 30 percent. With aggressive management, including diagnostic amniocenteses or studies performed on fetal blood obtained by ultrasonically directed percutaneous sampling of umbilical cord blood, repeated ultrasound examinations, intrauterine transfusions in selected cases, and early delivery in most cases, the perinatal mortality rate can be lowered remarkably (Harman and co-workers, 1983; Queenan and King, 1987).

For optimal outcome, management is individualized and aided by the following information:

1. Past obstetrical history, with emphasis on fetal outcome and how that outcome was achieved
2. Accurate knowledge of fetal age
3. The paternal D antigen status, since if he is negative the fetus cannot be affected
4. Maternal antibody determinations repeated throughout pregnancy
5. Spectrophotometric analyses of amnionic fluid, or sonographically directed fetal blood sampling (see Chap. 15, p. 281)
6. Identification of other pregnancy complications

An antibody titer, performed using the indirect Coombs' test, that goes no higher than 1:16 almost always means that the fetus will not die in utero from hemolytic disease and that with appropriate care after birth he will survive. A titer higher than this indicates the *possibility* of severe hemolytic disease. It is emphasized that the titer in the previously sensitized woman may, during a subsequent pregnancy, rise infrequently to high levels even though her fetus is D-negative, the so-called *amnestic response.*

Whenever the antibody titer is sufficiently elevated to be clinically significant, fetal evaluation is warranted. In most institutions this *critical titer* is considered to be 1:16 or greater; however, in some laboratories, if the titer remains below 1:32, then a good fetal outcome is anticipated.

Until recently, indirect evaluation of fetal hemolytic disease was accomplished by determining the amount of bilirubin pigment in amnionic fluid by spectrophotometric analysis. This area of fetal medicine is evolving rapidly, and there is now reasonable experience with sonographically directed fetal blood sampling to assess the degree of hemolysis and anemia. Both methods are discussed.

Amniocentesis

If use of intrauterine transfusion is being considered, amniocentesis may be initiated as early as 22 weeks gestation. The technique for amniocentesis is described in Chapter 15 (p. 278). The absorbance of breakdown pigments, mostly bilirubin, in the supernatant of amnionic fluid, when measured in a continuously recording spectrophotometer, is demonstrable as a hump with maximum absorbance at 450 nm wavelength (ΔOD_{450}), as shown in Figure 33–6. The magnitude of the increase in optical density above baseline at 450 nm most often, but not always, correlates well for any gestational age with the intensity of the hemolytic disease.

Liley (1964) constructed a graph that provides for reasonably precise prediction of the severity of hemolysis, a modification of which is demonstrated in Figure 33–7. Depending on the severity of disease, amniocenteses are repeated at 1- to 3-week

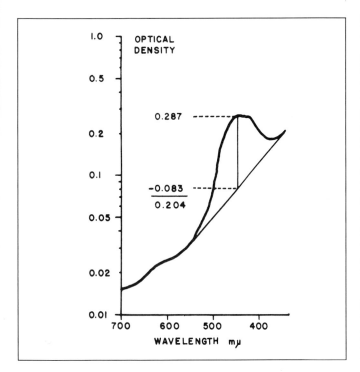

Figure 33–6. Spectral absorption curve of amnionic fluid in hemolytic disease. (*From Liley: In Greenhill (ed): Yearbook of Obstetrics and Gynecology, 1964–1965. Chicago, Year Book, 1964, p. 156.*)

intervals, as recommended by the American College of Obstetricians and Gynecologists (1986b):

1. If the increase in optical density falls in zone 1, then the fetus is D-negative, or will be unaffected, or will have mild hemolytic disease. Repeat the amniocentesis in 2 or 3 weeks, and deliver close to term.
2. In zone 2, the prognosis is less accurate, but the fetus is at moderate to severe risk and repeated amniocenteses may be required to establish a trend. In lower zone 2, the infant's expected hemoglobin is between 11.0 and 13.9 g per dL, whereas in upper zone 2, the anticipated hemoglobin will range from 8.0 to 10.9 g per dL. Trends and time of gestation will indicate the necessity for early delivery or intrauterine transfusions.
3. Values in zone 3 indicate a severely affected infant, and fetal death within 1 week to 10 days may be expected. Transfusions are indicated, and whether these are best accomplished after prompt delivery or by fetal transfusion depends on gestational age.

Fetal Blood Sampling

Nicolaides and colleagues (1986) studied 59 D-isoimmunized pregnancies at 18 to 25 weeks, and reported poor correlation in nonhydropic fetuses between the degree of fetal anemia and the trend in amnionic fluid analysis using the Liley graph. They concluded that the only reliable method to determine severity in the second trimester is direct measurement of fetal hemoglobin. Nicolaides and co-workers (1988a) recommend that transfusions be commenced when the hemoglobin deficit exceeds 2 g per dL from the mean for normal fetuses of corresponding gestational age.

INTRAPERITONEAL FETAL TRANSFUSIONS

The refinement in prognostic precision furnished by the analysis of amnionic fluid led Liley (1963) to try, in apparently hopeless cases, intrauterine transfusion of blood into the fetal peritoneal cavity. The procedure, in general, should be limited to cases in which, between 23 and 32 weeks, the spectrophotometric tracings and history forecast, in all likelihood, death of the fetus. Thirty-two weeks represents about the earliest gestational age at which the nontransfused affected fetus, if delivered, has a reasonable likelihood of surviving the adverse effects of prematurity, hemolytic disease, and exchange transfusion. For reasons that are not clear, the preterm infant with hemolytic disease from maternal D isoimmunization is at increased risk of developing severe hyaline membrane disease. Bowman (1978) emphasized that, in his hands, mortality following fetal transperitoneal transfusions at 32 weeks gestation and delayed delivery is appreciably lower than with delivery at 32 weeks. This is certainly not true in centers with less experience.

With fetal transfusion, the overall survival rate in more recent years probably has been about 50 percent. However, the team in Winnipeg has been much more successful. They reported 100 percent survival of nonhydropic fetuses and 75 percent survival of hydropic fetuses when treated with intrauterine transfusion, or an overall survival rate of 22 out of 24, or 92 percent (Harman and co-workers, 1983). Watts and colleagues (1988) reported similar results. Both groups emphasized improved fetal evaluation through the use of real-time sonography before, during, and after fetal transfusion.

At Winnipeg Center, 731 fetal transfusions have been carried out on 302 fetuses since the first transfusion was attempted in 1964. Mortality has decreased progressively as follows: 1964 to 1968, 55 percent; 1968 to 1972, 34 percent; 1972 to 1976, 34 percent; 1976 to 1980, 29 percent; and the recent study cited above, 8 percent. Importantly, the publicly funded anti-D prophylaxis program in Manitoba has lowered the risk of sensitization of mothers in that province from 13 percent to 0.18 percent, and, in turn, has virtually eliminated the need for intrauterine transfusions among pregnant Manitoba residents.

INTRAVASCULAR FETAL TRANSFUSIONS

In 1981, the group from Lewisham Hospital in London described a technique for direct intravascular blood transfusion using fetoscopy (Rodeck and colleagues, 1981). Subsequent to this (1984), they reported results from 25 severely D-isoimmunized fetuses, including 15 with hydrops who were given intravascular transfusions between 19 and 32 weeks. They again used fetoscopy, but some of these transfusions have now been accomplished using sonographically directed needle placements. Those fetuses in whom treatment was begun before 25 weeks had a remarkable 84 percent survival. Since this time, investigators from Yale (Grannum and colleagues, 1986, 1988) and Mount Sinai in New York (Berkowitz and co-workers, 1988) also have reported their successes with the method, which is depicted in Figure 33–8.

Fetuses chosen for such treatment generally have been severely affected, with amnionic fluid studies plotted in Liley zone 3, or sonographic evidence of hydrops, or both. Obviously, if there is sonographic evidence of hydrops, then treatment is warranted. Indeed, Frigoletto and colleagues (1986) have shown that careful ultrasonic fetal surveillance, combined with amnionic fluid analysis, will obviate the need for many intrauterine procedures. However, Nicolaides and associates (1988b) showed that, in the absence of fetal hydrops, a number of ultrasonic

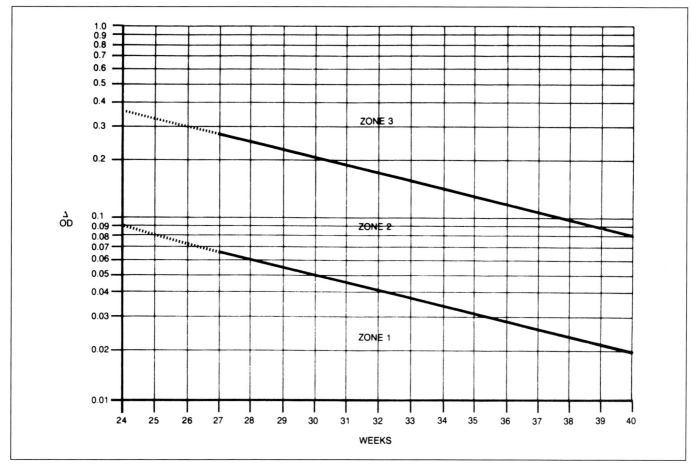

Figure 33–7. Modified Liley graph used to detect severity of fetal hemolysis. The dotted line represents a linear extrapolation from the original Liley data shown in the solid line. (*From American College of Obstetricians and Gynecologists, Technical Bulletin No 90: Management of Isoimmunization in Pregnancy, January 1986, with permission.*)

determinations did not distinguish reliably mild from severe fetal hemolytic disease.

Subsequent Child Development

In Bowman's experience (1978), the great majority of fetal transfusion survivors developed normally; 74 of 89 tested when 18 months of age or older were completely normal, 4 were abnormal, while development in 11 appeared to be delayed somewhat, perhaps because of preterm birth.

OTHER METHODS TO TRY TO MINIMIZE FETAL HEMOLYSIS

In an attempt to prevent D antibody formation, to remove antibody already formed, or to block the action of the antibody on the red cell, a number of techniques have been tried without consistent success. *Plasmapheresis* does not appear to provide benefits that outweigh the risks and the costs. *Promethazine* in large doses has been cited by some as being beneficial (Charles and Blumenthal, 1982); however, this is unproven. D-positive *erythrocyte membrane* in enteric coated capsules has been administered orally to sensitized women throughout pregnancy on the basis that such treatment might induce T-suppressor cell formation that would, in turn, reduce antibody response to

challenges by the antigen, but it does not appear to provide any benefit (Gold and co-workers, 1983). Attempts at immunosuppression with corticosteroids once were considered by some to be beneficial, but subsequently were proven to be of no benefit.

DELIVERY BEFORE TERM

In many circumstances, as alluded to above, delivery somewhat before term is advantageous. Obviously, when it is considered necessary to utilize fetal transfusions, delivery rather than further attempts at fetal transfusion is desirable once sufficient maturity has been achieved to provide an excellent chance of survival.

Sinusoidal fetal heart rate and repetitive decelerations have been identified in a number of circumstances, including erythroblastosis fetalis. These changes in the presence of D isoimmunization serve to imply, at least, that there is severe fetal anemia. Thus, their message is ominous and should stimulate strong consideration for prompt delivery (Lowe and colleagues, 1984).

Whenever a decision is reached to terminate pregnancy before term, adequate facilities for care of preterm infants must be available, as well as the necessary equipment for carrying out exchange transfusion. The neonatologist is consulted well in advance of delivery, so that skilled personnel, blood, and equipment can be immediately available in or adjacent to the delivery

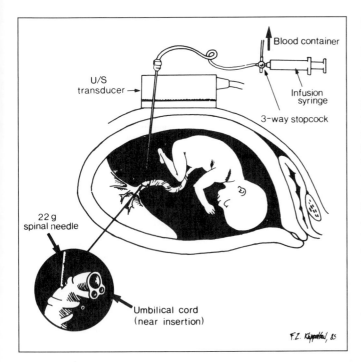

Figure 33–8. Diagrammatic view of direct fetal intravascular transfusion. U/S = ultrasound. (*From Grannum and colleagues: N Engl J Med 314:1431, 1986, with permission.*)

room. The need for immediate transfusion is determined by the hemoglobin concentration. Subsequently, the plasma bilirubin concentration is the important determinant.

Method of Delivery

The fetus who is to be delivered remote from term because of evidence of hemolytic disease will sometimes benefit from cesarean section. By so doing, the time of birth is set and the most experienced of neonatologists and laboratory personnel can be assembled to provide for precise evaluation of the infant at birth and optimal treatment at that critical time, as well as subsequently. Moreover, the likelihood of a difficult, prolonged, or unsatisfactory induction of labor is avoided. In any event, the fetus-infant must be protected from hypoxia, acidosis, and sepsis.

EXCHANGE TRANSFUSION IN THE NEWBORN

Examination of cord blood should be carried out immediately for any pregnancy in which the D-negative mother is known to be sensitized. The cord blood hemoglobin concentration and the direct Coombs' test are of considerable importance when the infant is D-positive. If the infant is overtly anemic, it is often best to carry out the initial exchange promptly to correct the anemia using recently collected, packed, type O, D-negative red cells.

For infants who are not overtly anemic, exchange transfusion is determined by the rate of increase in bilirubin concentration, the maturity of the infant, and the presence or absence of other complications. While exchange transfusion is not an innocuous procedure, if moribund, hydropic, and kernicteric infants are excluded, the mortality rate is 1 percent or less.

HYPERBILIRUBINEMIA

DISPOSAL OF BILIRUBIN

Bilirubin metabolism in the fetus is complex and not completely understood. Before birth, unconjugated or free bilirubin is readily transferred across the placenta from the fetal to the maternal circulation (and vice versa, if the maternal plasma level of unconjugated bilirubin is high). Whereas bilirubin glucuronide is water soluble and is normally excreted into the bile by the liver and by the kidney when the plasma level is elevated, unconjugated bilirubin is not excreted in the urine or to any extent in the bile. Glucuronic acid is made available for this reaction by transfer from uridine diphosphoglucuronic acid catalyzed by the microsomal enzyme uridine diphosphoglucuronyl transferase. Conjugated bilirubin is secreted from the hepatocytes through the canalicular apparatus into the biliary tree and then into the small intestine.

KERNICTERUS

The great concern over unconjugated hyperbilirubinemia in the newborn is its association with *kernicterus*. This complication occurs with greater frequency in preterm infants. The yellow staining of the basal ganglia and hippocampus is indicative of profound degeneration in these regions. Surviving infants show spasticity, muscular incoordination, and varying degrees of mental retardation. There is a positive correlation between kernicterus and unconjugated bilirubin levels above 18 to 20 mg per dL, although kernicterus may develop at lower concentrations, especially in very premature infants.

Factors other than the serum bilirubin concentration contribute to the development of kernicterus. Hypoxia and acidosis enhance bilirubin toxicity. Both hypothermia and hypoglycemia predispose the infant to kernicterus by raising the level of non-esterified fatty acids, which compete with bilirubin for the binding sites on albumin and inhibit bilirubin conjugation. Sepsis contributes to kernicterus, although the mechanism of action is not clear. Sulfonamides and salicylates such as aspirin may increase the incidence of kernicterus because they compete with unconjugated bilirubin for protein-binding sites. Sodium benzoate, in injectable diazepam, furosemide, and gentamicin, displaces bilirubin from albumin. Excessive doses of vitamin K analogues may be associated with hyperbilirubinemia. The importance of the serum albumin concentration and the binding sites so provided is obvious.

BREAST MILK JAUNDICE

Breast feeding can cause nonphysiological jaundice in the otherwise normal newborn. The jaundice has been attributed to the excretion of pregnane-3α,20β-diol into breast milk by some mothers. This steroid was reported by Arias and colleagues (1964) to block bilirubin conjugation by inhibiting glucuronyl transferase activity. Breast milk samples from mothers of infants with hyperbilirubinemia have been described to have an unusually high lipolytic activity and can liberate large quantities of fatty acids that could inhibit bilirubin conjugation (Foliot and co-workers, 1976). Another explanation is that bilirubin is broken down in the intestine to form free bilirubin, which can be reabsorbed. Usually, cow's milk and human milk appear to block the reabsorption of free bilirubin, whereas the milk of mothers with jaundiced offspring does not, and may even enhance its reabsorption.

With breast milk jaundice the serum bilirubin level rises from about the fourth day after birth to a maximum by 15 days. If breast feeding is continued, the high levels persist for another 10 to 14 days and decline slowly over the next several weeks. No cases of overt bilirubin encephalopathy have been reported owing to this phenomenon, according to Maisels (1979), who also emphasizes that there have been no prospective studies of the problem. One obvious solution to severe jaundice as the consequence of breast milk is to discontinue breast feeding and substitute an appropriate formula.

PHYSIOLOGICAL JAUNDICE

By far the most common form of unconjugated nonhemolytic jaundice is so-called *physiological jaundice.* In the mature infant, the serum bilirubin increases for 3 to 4 days to achieve serum levels up to 10 mg per dL or so and then falls rapidly. In preterm infants, the rise is more prolonged and may be more intense. The mechanisms involved in physiological jaundice include, when compared to older children and adults, (1) a normally increased rate of erythrocyte destruction and, therefore, of bilirubin production; (2) probably a decreased rate of uptake of free bilirubin by hepatic cells because of lower levels of Y and Z anion-binding proteins; (3) a decreased rate of hepatic bilirubin conjugation; and (4) a reduced conversion of bilirubin to urobilinogen by intestinal bacteria, which, in turn, allows a greater fraction of excreted bilirubin to be reabsorbed (enterohepatic circulation). Thus, almost every phase of bilirubin metabolism has been implicated.

Jaundice in the newborn infant should not be ignored as being physiological in the following circumstances:

1. The infant is visibly jaundiced in the first 24 hours after birth.
2. The total bilirubin concentration in serum is increasing daily by more than 5 mg per dL.
3. The total bilirubin concentration is above 15 mg per dL.
4. Jaundice is visible for more than 1 week in a term infant or 2 weeks in a preterm infant.

TREATMENT

Exchange transfusion for severe hyperbilirubinemia, discussed earlier (p. 608), is not an innocuous procedure, but the mortality rate is less than 1 percent when moribund, hydropic, and kernicteric infants are excluded from analysis.

Phototherapy is now widely used to treat hyperbilirubinemia. In most instances, its use leads to a lower bilirubin level from oxidation of the compound. Light that penetrates the skin also increases peripheral blood flow, which enhances photooxidation. By some unknown mechanism, light seems to promote hepatic excretion of unconjugated bilirubin. Moreover, intestinal transit time may be shortened, thereby reducing reabsorption of bilirubin. A common situation in which phototherapy is justified, besides that of the infant with hemolytic disease, is the jaundiced low birthweight infant who appears otherwise well.

As much of the infant's surface as possible should be exposed, and he should be turned every 2 hours. His eyelids should be closed and completely shielded from the light. Temperature must be closely monitored and dehydration from excessive heat should be avoided. Effective photodecomposition requires that the fluorescent bulbs be carefully selected and monitored for appropriate wavelength. The serum bilirubin concentration needs to be monitored for at least 24 hours after phototherapy has been stopped.

Phenobarbital has been shown to induce microsomal enzymes and thereby increase hepatic bilirubin conjugation and excretion.

NONIMMUNE HYDROPS FETALIS

Hydrops fetalis need not always have an immunological basis. Anderson and co-workers (1983) found nonimmune hydrops to be more common in recent years than that from isoimmunization. Hutchison and associates (1982) reported an incidence of nonimmune hydrops of 1 in 3,700 pregnancies. Undoubtedly, hydrops is identified in utero much more frequently since high-resolution sonography has become available, and these cases most often come under scrutiny because of increased intrauterine volume, almost always associated with hydramnios.

The formation and the accumulation of serous fluid in body cavities and subcutaneous edema have been attributed to a great variety of causes, many of which were tabulated by Holzgreve and associates (1984) and are presented in Table 33–5. There also appears to be a category of transient idiopathic hydrops, and we, as well as Mueller–Heubach and Mazer (1983), have observed sonographic evidence of fetal hydrops, especially ascites, remote from term, only to have the ascites resolve and the fetus be normal at birth.

The precise incidence of these various causes of hydrops is unclear and there are definite population biases. For example, the San Francisco group reported a 10 percent incidence of hydrops caused by α-thalassemia (Holzgreve and colleagues, 1984). From their data, as well as those of Allan (1986), Gough (1986), and Castillo (1986), and their many co-workers, cardiac abnormalities, either structural or rhythm related, or both, are associated with 20 to 45 percent of cases of nonimmune hydrops. Approximately 35 percent are due to chromosomal anomalies or other malformations, and 10 percent are associated with twin-twin transfusions. Those cases previously labeled idiopathic are less common, and Holzgreve and colleagues (1984) were able to identify the cause in 42 of 50 affected fetuses. Previously unknown causes are being reported. For example, Anand and colleagues (1987) and Maeda and associates (1988) documented hydrops from maternal-fetal *parvovirus* infection.

Mortality of nonimmune hydrops depends on the cause, but in general, the prognosis is poor, and less than 10 to 20 percent of affected fetuses survive.

DIAGNOSIS

Ultrasonic evaluation is the most useful method for evaluating pregnancy complicated by fetal hydrops; however, there are other noninvasive steps that may be taken (Gough and co-workers, 1986; Holzgreve and colleagues, 1984). After immunological hydrops has been excluded, hematological, chemical, and serological studies are done to look for maternal causes such as severe anemia, diabetes, or syphilis. A Kleihauer–Betke stain of maternal blood may disclose evidence for significant fetomaternal hemorrhage. If these and detailed sonar evaluation fail to disclose the apparent cause, then fetal echocardiography is done to search again for cardiac abnormalities. If still no cause is found, then some recommend amniocentesis or sono-

TABLE 33–5. CAUSES OF NONIMMUNE HYDROPS FETALIS AND ASSOCIATED CLINICAL CONDITIONS

Category	Condition	Category	Condition
Cardiovascular	Tachyarrhythmia	Urinary	Urethral stenosis or atresia
	Congenital heart block		Posterior urethral valves
	Anatomical defects (atrial septal defect, ventricular defect, hypoplastic left heart, pulmonary valve insufficiency, Ebstein's subaortic stenosis, aortic valve stenosis, subaortic stenosis, dilated heart, atrioventricular canal defect, single ventricle, tetralogy of Fallot, premature closure of foramen ovale, subendocardial fibroelastosis, dextrocardia in combination with pulmonic stenosis)		Bladder neck obstruction
			Spontaneous bladder perforation
			Neurogenic bladder with reflux
			Ureterocele
		Gastrointestinal	Jejunal atresia
			Midgut volvulus
			Malrotation of intestines
			Duplication of intestinal tract
			Meconium peritonitis
	Calcified aortic valve	Liver	Hepatic calcifications
	Coronary artery embolus		Hepatic fibrosis
	Myocarditis (coxsackie virus)		Cholestasis
	Atrial hemangioma		Polycystic disease of liver
	Intracardial rhabdomyoma		Biliary atresia
	Endocardial teratoma		Hepatic vascular malformations
			Familial cirrhosis
Chromosomal	Down syndrome (trisomy 21)	Maternal	Severe diabetes mellitus
	Other trisomies		Severe anemia
	Turner syndrome		Hypoproteinemia
	Triploidy	Medications	Antepartum indomethacin (taken to stop preterm labor, causing fetal ductus closure and secondary non-immune hydrops fetalis)
Malformation syndromes	Thanatophoric dwarfism		
	Arthrogryposis multiplex congenita		
	Asphyxiating thoracic dystrophy		
	Hypophosphatasia	Placenta-umbilical cord	Chorioangioma
	Osteogenesis imperfecta		Chorionic vein thrombosis
	Achondrogenesis		Fetal–maternal transfusion
	Neu-Laxova syndrome		Placental and umbilical vein thrombosis
	Recessive cystic hygroma		Umbilical cord torsion
	Saldino-Noonan syndrome		True cord knots
	Pena-Shokeir type I syndrome		Angiomyxoma of umbilical cord
			Aneurysm of umbilical artery
Hematological	α-Thalassemia	Infections	Cytomegalovirus
	Arteriovenous shunts (vascular tumors)		Toxoplasmosis
	Kasabach-Merritt syndrome		Syphilis
	In utero closed-space hemorrhage		Congenital hepatitis
	Caval, portal, or femoral thrombosis		Rubella
			Leptospirosis
			Chaga's disease
Twin pregnancy	Twin-twin transfusion syndrome	Miscellaneous	Congenital lymphedema
	Parabiotic (acardiac) twin syndrome		Congenital hydrothorax or chylothorax
Respiratory	Diaphragmatic hernia		Polysplenia syndrome
	Cystic adenoma of lung		Congenital neuroblastoma
	Hamartoma of lung		Tuberous sclerosis
	Mediastinal teratoma		Torsion of ovarian cyst
			Fetal trauma
			Sacrococcygeal teratoma

From Holzgreve and co-workers: Am J Obstet Gynecol, 150:805, 1984.

graphically directed fetal blood sampling for karyotyping or other tests appropriate for the specific cause. Appelman and colleagues (1988) have detected bilirubin in Liley zone 3 in three pregnancies with nonimmune hydrops.

TREATMENT

Treatment will vary considerably and is dependent upon the cause of the hydrops. Since most lesions that are associated with these syndromes ultimately prove fatal for the fetus or newborn, knowledge of the cause is important in planning the route of delivery. In general, when the hydrops persists and the fetus is mature enough that survival is likely, then delivery should be accomplished. When hydrops appears to be the consequence of heart failure from supraventricular tachyarrhythmia, then conversion is attempted by maternal administration of digoxin, a beta-blocker, or verapamil. If heart failure is due to structural lesions, reversal of failure is less likely, and the prognosis is much worse.

Maternal complications include an increased incidence of preeclampsia, which may develop early and necessitate delivery. Preterm labor is common since about half the cases are complicated by polyhydramnios. Finally, postpartum hemorrhage is common and is related to uterine overdistension as well as retained placenta.

FETAL CARDIAC ARRHYTHMIAS

Recognition of fetal cardiac rhythm disturbances has become more common because of extensive use of Doppler ultrasound technology. While most of these arrhythmias are transient and benign, and usually are isolated extrasystoles, some tachyarrhythmias, if sustained, result in congestive heart failure, nonimmune hydrops, and fetal death. Sustained bradycardia, while less often associated with hydrops, may signify underlying cardiac pathology that includes structural lesions or autoimmune myocarditis.

Kleinman and associates (1985) summarized their experiences with fetal arrhythmias, which are shown in Table 33–6. They emphasize that sustained supraventricular tachycardia, usually more than 200 beats per minute, is most likely to cause cardiac failure, and they have documented fetal ascites developing after only 36 hours. Treatment, usually with digoxin, is almost always successful if there are no underlying heart lesions.

The prognosis for the fetus with bradycardia resulting from heart block is less promising. Taylor and colleagues (1986) demonstrated that half the mothers of children with congenital heart block have antibodies to fetal myocardial tissue. Many of these women have, or subsequently develop, lupus erythematosus or another connective-tissue disease (see Chap. 39, p. 839). A serological marker for congenital myocarditis is the anti-SS-A (anti-Ro) antibody, and as many as 1 in 20 fetuses born to women positive for this have cardiac disease (Ramsey-Goldman and colleagues, 1986). Fetal cardiac antigens to which anti-SS-A affixes are not confined to the conduction system as once thought, and if there is extensive carditis, the prognosis is poor. Of seven infants described by Ramsey-Goldman and colleagues (1986), three died within 9 months, two required permanent pacemaking, and two underwent cardiac surgery. Only one infant had no problems.

Cameron and associates (1988) and Shenker and colleagues (1987) recently reported that fetal cardiac anomalies are common with heart block in the absence of connective-tissue disease. Their recommended work-up includes fetal echocardiography and consideration for karyotyping.

TABLE 33–6. TYPES OF ARRHYTHMIAS IN 198 FETUSES FROM PREGNANCIES REFERRED TO YALE UNIVERSITY

Arrhythmias (Number)
Isolated extrasystoles (164)
Atrial (145)
Ventricular (19)
Sustained arrhythmias (34)
Supraventricular tachycardia (15)
Complete heart block (8)
Atrial flutter or fibrillation (5)
Ventricular tachycardia (2)
Second-degree heart block (2)
Sinus bradycardia (2)

From Kleinman and colleagues: Semin Perinatol, 9:113, 1985.

HEMORRHAGIC DISEASE OF THE NEWBORN

Hemorrhagic disease of the newborn is a syndrome characterized by spontaneous internal or external bleeding accompanied by hypoprothrombinemia and very low levels of other vitamin K–dependent coagulation factors (V, VII, IX, and X). Bleeding may begin any time after birth but typically is delayed for a day or two. The infant may be mature and healthy in appearance, although a greater incidence of the disease has been noted in preterm infants.

The prothrombin and partial thromboplastin times are greatly prolonged. The coagulation changes of vitamin K deficiency, especially if accompanied by a lowered platelet count, might lead to an erroneous diagnosis of disseminated intravascular coagulation, which has a much poorer prognosis (Lane and Hathaway, 1985). Moreover, the treatment of disseminated intravascular coagulation with anticoagulants, as recommended by some but not all, would intensify hemorrhagic disease of the newborn. In the differential diagnosis, hemophilia, congenital syphilis, bacterial sepsis, thrombocytopenic purpura, erythroblastosis, and intracranial hemorrhage all must be considered.

Hypoprothrombinemia in the neonate appears to be the consequence of poor placental transport of vitamin K_1 to the fetus. Plasma vitamin K_1 levels are somewhat lower in pregnant women than in nonpregnant adults, and the vitamin is undetectable in cord plasma (Shearer and associates, 1982). When 1 mg of vitamin K_1 was administered intravenously to mothers shortly before delivery, maternal plasma levels were remarkably raised, but cord plasma levels were still very low. However, Pomerance and colleagues (1987) reported that prothrombin activity was improved in preterm neonates whose mothers were given intramuscular vitamin K_1 during labor. Interestingly, benefits were greater for female infants.

The main cause of hemorrhagic disease of the newborn from vitamin K deficiency appears to be a dietary deficiency of vitamin K as the consequence of small amounts of the vitamin in breast milk in an infant already depleted at birth. The prothrombin time 24 hours after the start of feedings with cow's milk is comparable to that found 24 hours after vitamin K administration, whereas in infants fed with breast milk it remains prolonged (Keenan and colleagues, 1971).

Serious reduction of vitamin K–dependent clotting factors during the first week after birth in infants of women with epilepsy treated with anticonvulsant drugs has been described by Mountain and associates (1970). These drugs apparently have a mechanism similar to warfarin and act by depressing hepatic synthesis of several coagulation factors (VII, IX, and X).

PROPHYLAXIS

As prophylaxis against hemorrhagic disease of the newborn, the intramuscular injection of 1 mg of vitamin K_1 has proved very efficacious. Although controversial in other countries, this practice is almost universal in the United States (Lane and Hathaway, 1985). For treatment of active bleeding, the vitamin is injected intravenously. Abnormalities in clotting are usually corrected over several hours.

The toxic effects of menadione, a synthetic vitamin K, and its derivatives in causing hyperbilirubinemia were the consequence of unnecessarily large doses, particularly to preterm infants. There is no evidence that the small but effective dose of 1 mg of vitamin K_1 (phytonadione) to the infant, or 2.5 to 5 mg given to the mother before delivery, are associated with significant hyperbilirubinemia.

THROMBOCYTOPENIA

A number of diseases or conditions are associated with neonatal thrombocytopenia of varying degrees. It tends to be more severe in preterm fetuses, especially those with respiratory distress and hypoxia or sepsis.

Antiplatelet IgG antibody transferred from mother to fetus and causing thrombocytopenia in the fetus-neonate can be suspected when the mother has thrombocytopenia from an autoimmune disease, especially *immunological thrombocytopenic purpura*. Avoidance of traumatic delivery and appropriate corticosteroid therapy to try to improve hemostasis are important to a successful outcome (see Chap. 39, p. 791). Maternally produced antibody most often is directed against almost all platelets; thus donor platelet transfusions are of little benefit. Corticosteroids or intravenous immune globulin given to the infant may be helpful; in desperation, exchange transfusion and platelet replacement may be tried. Blood transfusions may be necessary if hemorrhage develops.

Neonatal thrombocytopenia as the result of *preeclampsia–eclampsia* has been suggested by some. However, in a large number of infants born to women with pregnancy-induced hypertension at Parkland Hospital, we identified no case where neonatal thrombocytopenia correlated with maternal thrombocytopenia (Pritchard and colleagues, 1987). Instead, thrombocytopenia commonly developed after delivery in low birthweight infants who were hypoxic or who had evidence for sepsis (see Chap. 35, p. 664).

Isoimmune thrombocytopenia may develop in a manner similar to D antigen isoimmunization. In this condition, thrombocytopenia follows maternal isoimmunization against fetal platelet antigens, usually PL^{A1}, which is found in 98 percent of the population. Thus, the mother lacks the common platelet antigen and becomes immunized when exposed to the antigen by fetal platelets that enter the maternal circulation. Even though diagnostic tests to type platelet antigens are not commonly available, the diagnosis can most often be made correctly on clinical grounds: (1) The mother has a normal platelet count and there is no evidence of a disorder which causes autoimmune thrombocytopenia; (2) the infant has thrombocytopenia without evidence of other disease. In the case of active bleeding, treatment ideally includes transfusion with platelets compatible with those of the mother. Unfortunately, most of the donor population will have the platelet antigen to which the maternal antibody is directed. However, maternal platelets are appropriate since they lack the inciting antigen, and platelets collected from the mother by plasmapheresis and differential centrifugation are likely to be of greatest benefit. When one infant has been affected, there is appreciable likelihood that subsequent infants also will be affected. Cesarean section to minimize birth trauma is likely to be advantageous to the affected fetus-infant yet of little added risk to the mother, since she is not thrombocytopenic. This is not always protective, and Morales and Stroup (1985) described a case in which the fetus apparently suffered massive spontaneous intraventricular hemorrhage in utero at 34 weeks. Kaplan and colleagues (1988) have described treatment with fetal platelet transfusions using sonographically directed umbilical vein catheterization. Bussel and co-workers (1988) reported that maternal intravenous gamma globulin increased fetal platelet counts in seven cases.

POLYCYTHEMIA AND HYPERVISCOSITY

Several conditions predispose to polycythemia and hyperviscosity of blood in the neonate. These include *chronic hypoxia* in utero and *placental transfusion* from a twin or, much more rarely, from the mother. As the hematocrit rises above 65, blood viscosity increases markedly. Signs and symptoms include plethora, cyanosis, and neurological aberrations. Laboratory findings include hyperbilirubinemia, thrombocytopenia, fragmented erythrocytes, and hypoglycemia. Treatment consists of prompt recognition and lowering of the hematocrit by partial exchange transfusion with plasma.

NECROTIZING ENTEROCOLITIS

This condition commonly presents with clinical findings of abdominal distension, ileus, and bloody stools, and with radiological evidence of *pneumotosis intestinalis*, caused by intestinal wall gas as the consequence of invasion by gas-forming bacteria and bowel perforation (Fig. 33–9).

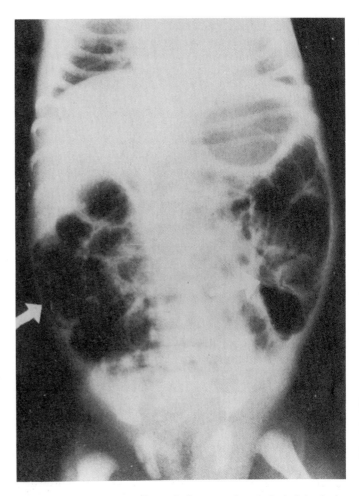

Figure 33–9. Abdominal radiograph demonstrating marked abdominal distention and the classical linear markings along the bowel surface characteristic of pneumatosis intestinalis. (*From Walsh and Kliegman: Ped Clin N Amer 33:179, 1986, with permission.*)

The disease is seen primarily in low birthweight infants, but is occasionally encountered in larger, more mature neonates. Various causes have been suggested for necrotizing enterocolitis, including perinatal hypotension, hypoxia, or sepsis, as well as umbilical catheters, exchange transfusions, and the feeding of cow's milk and hypertonic solutions (Kliegman and Fanaroff, 1984). The disease tends to occur in clusters, and coronaviruses have been suspected of having an etiological role. Kanto and colleagues (1987) reported that 5.7 percent of 2,123 preterm infants developed necrotizing enterocolitis. They reported that incidence of the disease was related to birthweight, but not to other perinatal factors. They concluded that gastrointestinal immaturity, and not ischemia, is the major causative factor for necrotizing enterocolitis. Orally administered immunoglobulin was shown to prevent enterocolitis when given to preterm infants (Eibl and associates, 1988).

Abdominal distension or blood in the stools may signal developing enterocolitis. Usually, further oral feeding is withheld until the condition clears, although at times it is so severe that bowel resection is necessary. The prognosis appears to be improving with such management (Walsh and Kliegman, 1986).

DRUG ADDICTION

An unfortunately large number of women use *heroin* and other highly addictive drugs during pregnancy. These women and their offspring suffer not only from the direct effects of the drug or drugs but also are at appreciably increased risk of coincidental infections and varying degrees of malnutrition. Pelosi and co-workers (1975) observed the risks of the following pregnancy complications to be increased two to six times among pregnant women who used heroin: birthweight less than 2,500 g from preterm delivery, growth retardation, or both; pregnancy-induced hypertension; late pregnancy bleeding; malpresentation; and puerperal morbidity. Interestingly, accelerated fetal lung maturation, manifested by a high lecithin-spingomyelin ratio in amnionic fluid and a low incidence of idiopathic respiratory distress in the newborn, is characteristic of pregnancies complicated by maternal heroin addiction.

At least half of newborn infants of heroin addicts develop withdrawal symptoms. Without treatment, an appreciable number of them will die. The newborn infant must be closely watched during the first week of life for irritability, convulsions, nasal congestion, vomiting, diarrhea, tachypnea, and fever. Treatment has included paregoric, phenobarbital, chlorpromazine, and diazepam. Therapy may be required for many days to weeks, and is slowly withdrawn but reinstituted if symptoms recur.

Methadone treatment programs have commonly included pregnant women. Even though the drug is deleterious to the fetus-infant, it is probably less so than heroin. The newborn of the methadone-treated mother also is very likely to demonstrate withdrawal symptoms, and Newman and co-workers (1975) reported an incidence of 80 percent, while Harper and associates (1974) cited 94 percent. Whereas withdrawal symptoms in the infant of a heroin-addicted mother usually develop within 24 hours of delivery, the infant whose mother has been using methadone may not demonstrate signs of withdrawal for a week or so after birth. Thus, withdrawal from methadone while the woman is still pregnant is ideal, but must be done carefully. Moreover, citing that 88 percent of women continue other drug use, Edelin and colleagues (1988) rightfully have questioned the efficacy of methadone maintenance during pregnancy.

The mother's ability to care for her infant after discharge from the hospital should be assessed by frequent observations, including home visits.

INFECTIONS OF THE FETUS AND NEWBORN

The active immunological capacity of the fetus and neonate is compromised compared to that of older children and adults. Passive immunity is provided by the mother principally by IgG transferred across the placenta; however, the degree of passive immunity is much lower in preterm infants. Infection, especially in its early stages, may be difficult to diagnose because of the newborn's failure to respond in classic fashion. The signs of infection can be vague, nonspecific, and certainly not dramatic until the infant becomes moribund. If infected in utero, he may have been depressed and acidotic at birth for no apparent reason. The infant may suck poorly, vomit, or develop abdominal distension. He may develop respiratory insufficiency, which is similar in many ways to the idiopathic respiratory distress syndrome. He may be lethargic or jittery. The response to sepsis may be hypothermia rather than hyperthermia, and the total leucocyte count and the neutrophil count may be depressed or not influenced by sepsis, although the band count is likely to be increased.

As shown in Table 33–7, bacteria, viruses, or parasites may cross the placenta from the mother, or they may cross the membranes even though unruptured, but most commonly after they rupture. Fetal infections may develop early in pregnancy to produce obvious stigmata at birth. Conversely, the organisms may colonize and infect the fetus during delivery; and thus, preterm rupture of membranes, prolonged labor, and digital cervical examinations and manipulations may increase appreciably the risk of neonatal infection. Infection at less than 72 hours of age is usually but not always caused by bacteria acquired in utero or during delivery, while infections after that time are most likely to have been acquired after birth.

A major mechanism for inducing infection subsequent to birth is the transfer of pathogens from those caring for the infant, who may be colonized with the organism or may passively transfer it from another infected infant. The use of indwelling venous and arterial umbilical catheters demands scrupulous care to prevent infection. Ventilatory life-support systems that involve moisture quickly become contaminated with bacteria and can be the source of life-threatening infection. It is apparent that the very low birthweight infant who survives the first few days is at considerable risk of dying later from infection that he acquires in the intensive-care nursery (LaGamma and co-workers, 1983).

Any infant who appears ill should be suspected of having an infection. If infection is suspected at vaginal delivery, some recommend that cultures of a swabbing from the ear or of gastric aspirate be taken, or amnionic fluid can be collected at cesarean section and promptly cultured. Since bacteria from the normal maternal flora almost always are found, the pragmatic

TABLE 33–7. SOME CAUSES OF FETAL AND NEONATAL INFECTIONS

Intrauterine
Transplacental—Rubella, cytomegalovirus, syphilis, toxoplasmosis, varicella-zoster, listeriosis, coxsackie and parvovirus, other viruses
Ascending chorioamnionitis—Bacteria associated with:
Preterm rupture of membranes
Preterm labor with intact membranes

Intrapartum
Maternal exposure—Gonorrhea, herpesvirus, chlamydia, papillomavirus, group B streptococcus, hepatitis B, human immunodeficiency virus
External contamination—Staphylococcus, coliforms, others

Neonatal
Human transmission—Staphylococcus, coliforms, viruses
Respiratory equipment and catheters—Staphylococcus, coliforms

use of such cultures is unproven. Subsequently, cultures of blood and cerebrospinal fluid of the infant may be essential for appropriate evaluation.

Bacteria most often responsible for sepsis in the newborn in the United States have varied remarkably during the past several decades. For example, in the 1930s and 1940s, group A β-hemolytic streptococci were principally involved. With the widespread use of penicillin, these infections were reduced remarkably, and next came the staphylococcus in the 1950s and coliforms and group B streptococcus in the 1970s. At similar times elsewhere in the world other pathogens were likely to have been more prominent in causing neonatal sepsis (Siegal and McCracken, 1981). Recently, Waites and colleagues (1988) reported that *Ureaplasma urealyticum* and *Mycoplasma hominis* were isolated from the spinal fluid of 13 percent of preterm infants with suspected sepsis.

ANAEROBIC INFECTIONS

Infections with anaerobic pathogens also have been recognized more frequently, in part because of better culture techniques and increased awareness of their importance. Considering their importance in maternal infections, it is perplexing that they do not have a more important role in neonatal infections. Anaerobic bacteremia may be self-limited with a favorable prognosis, regardless of antimicrobial therapy, but can be associated with serious perinatal morbidity.

EPIDEMIC DIARRHEA OF THE NEWBORN

Outbreaks of epidemic diarrhea in the nursery may occur at any time, and many have been reported. Although it is unlikely that a single pathogen is responsible for all epidemics, certain pathogenic strains of *Escherichia coli* have been isolated in many outbreaks. It is probable that many epidemics are caused by these bacteria and that the organism is brought into the nursery either by infected personnel, with or without symptomatic disease, or by an already infected infant.

The clinical symptoms are diarrhea with loose, watery, greenish stools, along with lethargy, dehydration, unstable temperature, and anorexia. The mortality rate varies, at times ranging as high as 6 percent in term infants and 35 percent in low birthweight infants. To halt the epidemic, nursery admissions are stopped and affected infants are isolated, after which the unit is evacuated followed by rigid cleansing of all equipment

and of the nursery itself. A stool culture should be obtained from all exposed infants to identify carriers and potentially ill babies.

STAPHYLOCOCCUS

In the 1950s, penicillin-resistant staphylococcal disease was observed in epidemic proportions. Reemphasis on hand washing, screening for carriers of unusually virulent staphylococci, and newer antibiotics controlled the epidemics.

Currently recommended procedures to control staphylococcal disease in newborn nurseries include the following: (1) close attention to each staff member's technique for handling infants and frequent, careful hand washing; (2) routine umbilical care given by applying triple dye or bacitracin; (3) a program of continuous epidemiological surveillance.

GROUP B STREPTOCOCCUS

Neonatal infections with group B β-hemolytic streptococci are almost as prevalent as those from coliform organisms, which are the most common pathogens that cause neonatal septicemia. During the 1970s, group B streptococcal infections in the newborn increased remarkably in frequency, but then in many institutions the frequency decreased. The reasons for either the marked increase or the subsequent decrease are not clearly understood.

It is clear that intrapartum transmission to the fetus of group B streptococci from a colonized maternal genital tract may lead to severe sepsis in the infant soon after birth. Depending on the population studied, as many as 10 to 40 percent of women during late pregnancy are colonized with group B streptococci in the lower genital tract, and half of newborn infants exposed become colonized. Maternally transmitted antibodies protect most of these infants; however, 1 to 2 percent develop clinical disease. Preterm or low birthweight infants are at highest risk, but more than half of the cases of neonatal streptococcal sepsis are in term neonates. For infants with infection the mortality rate is nearly 25 percent.

With septicemia from group B streptococci that characterizes *early onset disease*, signs of serious illness usually develop within 48 hours of birth. Typically, membranes have been ruptured for some time before delivery, or there has been preterm labor. The low birthweight infant is more likely to develop serious clinical infection. The signs of early onset infection include respiratory distress, apnea, and shock. At the outset, therefore, the physician must be astute to differentiate the illness from idiopathic respiratory distress or transient tachypnea of the newborn. Immediate treatment with antimicrobials, as well as treatment for respiratory problems, is mandatory for survival. The mortality rate with early onset disease has varied from 30 percent to as high as 90 percent, and preterm infants fare less well.

Late onset disease usually becomes evident as meningitis a week or more after birth. Whereas the serotype with early onset disease varies from infant to infant, most often it is the same for organisms in the maternal vagina and in the infant. However, cases of meningitis most often are caused by serotype III. The mortality rate, while appreciable, is less for late onset meningitis than for early onset sepsis.

TREATMENT AND PREVENTION

There is no universal agreement whether to screen for or to treat maternal group B streptococcal carriers. Evidence has accrued that women colonized with the organism may have excess preterm labor and prematurely ruptured membranes, as discussed in Chapter 38. The earliest studies showed the futility of attempts to rid the genital tract of these bacteria remote from term, since recurrences almost invariably were demonstrated. More recently, treatment schemes designed to prevent neonatal colonization, and thus sepsis, have been more productive.

Steigman and associates (1978) reported an absence of early onset group B streptococcal sepsis in 130,000 newborn infants given 50,000 units of aqueous penicillin G intramuscularly at birth as prophylaxis against ophthalmia neonatorum. A prospective study of 18,738 infants was then carried out by Siegal and co-workers (1980) at Parkland Hospital. Aqueous procaine penicillin G—50,000 units for infants who weighed 2,000 g or more and 25,000 units for those who were smaller—was administered intramuscularly within 1 hour of birth as prophylaxis against ophthalmia neonatorum and also to evaluate its impact on group B streptococcal infections. The incidence of group B streptococcal disease was appreciably less, but not absent, in those given penicillin. It was worrisome that the incidence of infection and mortality caused by penicillin-resistant nonstreptococcal organisms increased.

Pyati and co-workers (1983) subsequently reported that such penicillin prophylaxis was of little benefit in preventing early onset group B streptococcal disease in low birthweight neonates. Many of these infants who did poorly were found subsequently to have cord blood cultures positive for streptococci, and single-dose prophylaxis failed to prevent ongoing neonatal infection. These findings also served to emphasize the important association of group B streptococci in preterm delivery.

The recent emphasis has been on intrapartum treatment of mothers found to be colonized near the time of delivery. Boyer and Gotoff (1986) randomized intrapartum and neonatal ampicillin treatment of colonized mothers and reported decreased neonatal colonization (9 versus 51 percent) and early onset sepsis (none versus 6 percent) in infants born to treated women. They estimated that universal screening with intrapartum treatment of colonized mothers would be cost-effective. While these data suggest that screening for streptococcal carriage in women at high risk for preterm delivery, with subsequent intrapartum penicillin administration, might decrease the prevalence of neonatal infections, unfortunately labor or ruptured membranes are frequently the first signs of impending preterm delivery. Morales and Lim (1987) subsequently showed that rapid streptococcal identification using coagglutination methods in women with preterm prematurely ruptured membranes, along with treatment given for those positive, reduced the incidence of chorioamnionitis and neonatal group B streptococcal sepsis.

Since protection against serious neonatal infection is conferred by maternal antibody, it is logical that vaccination with capsular polysaccharide antigen may ultimately prove efficacious. From preliminary findings, Baker and colleagues (1988) reported that maternal immunization to Type III antigen may provide passive neonatal immunity.

RUBELLA

Rubella, or German measles, a disease usually of minor import in the absence of pregnancy, has been directly responsible for inestimable pregnancy wastage, and even more serious, for severe congenital malformations. The relation between maternal rubella and grave congenital malformations was first recognized by Gregg (1942), an Australian ophthalmologist.

PREVENTION

Although large epidemics of rubella have virtually disappeared in the United States because of immunization, the disease, with its horrible teratogenic potential, still prevails. For example, the Centers for Disease Control (1986b) reported at least seven outbreaks in New York City in 1985; five of these were in hospitals and 91 percent of those infected were 20 years or older. Increased reporting of congenital rubella syndrome followed 8 to 10 months after the peak of the outbreak. To eradicate the disease completely, the following approach is recommended for immunizing the adult population, particularly women of childbearing age:

1. Education of health-care providers and the general public on the dangers of rubella infection
2. Vaccination of susceptible women as part of routine medical and gynecological care
3. Vaccination of all women visiting family planning clinics
4. Identification and vaccination of unimmunized women immediately after childbirth or abortion
5. Vaccination of nonpregnant susceptible women identified by premarital serology
6. Immunity assurance for all hospital personnel who might be exposed to patients with rubella or who might have contact with pregnant women

It is advised that rubella vaccination be avoided shortly before or during pregnancy since the vaccine is an attenuated live virus. The Centers for Disease Control (1987b) have maintained a registry since 1971 to monitor the fetal effects of vaccination. Through 1986, 1,176 susceptible women were immunized within 3 months of conception, and fortunately, there is no evidence that the vaccine induces malformations in the embryo or fetus. Cases in which susceptible women were immunized during pregnancy should be reported to this registry (Centers for Disease Control, Atlanta, Georgia, 404-329-1870).

DIAGNOSIS

The diagnosis of rubella is at times difficult. Not only are the clinical features of other illnesses quite similar, but subclinical cases with viremia and infection of the embryo and fetus do not occur. Absence of rubella antibody indicates lack of immunity. The presence of antibody denotes an immune response to rubella viremia that may have been acquired anywhere from a few weeks to many years earlier. If maternal rubella antibody is demonstrated at the time of exposure to rubella or before, the mother can be assured that it is exceedingly unlikely her fetus will be affected.

The nonimmune person who acquires rubella viremia demonstrates peak antibody titers 1 to 2 weeks after the onset of the rash, or 2 to 3 weeks after the onset of viremia, since the viremia precedes clinically evident disease by about 1 week. The promptness of the antibody response, therefore, may complicate serodiagnosis unless serum is collected initially within a very few days after the onset of the rash. If, for example, the first specimen was obtained 10 days after the rash, detection of antibodies would fail to differentiate between two possibilities: (1) that the very recent disease was actually rubella; or (2) that it was not rubella, but the person was already immune to rubella. The demonstration of specific IgM in the pregnant woman indicates a primary infection within several months or so.

There is no chemotherapeutic or antibiotic agent that will prevent viremia in nonimmune subjects exposed to rubella. The use of gamma globulin for this purpose is not recommended.

CONGENITAL RUBELLA SYNDROME

With rubella as with any fetal infection, the concept of an *infected* **versus an affected infant must be understood.** Rubella is a potent teratogen, and 80 percent of women with rubella infection and a rash during the first 12 weeks have a fetus with congenital infection (Miller and colleagues, 1982). At 13 to 14 weeks this incidence was 54 percent, and it was 25 percent at the end of the second trimester. As the duration of pregnancy increases, infections are less likely to cause congenital malformations. For example, rubella defects were seen in *all* infants with evidence of intrauterine infections before 11 weeks, but only in 35 percent of those infected at 13 to 16 weeks. While no defects were found in 63 children infected after 16 weeks, they were followed only 2 years, and the *extended rubella syndrome* with progressive panencephalitis and type I diabetes may not develop clinically until the second or third decade of life. Perhaps as many as a third of infants who are asymptomatic at birth may manifest such developmental injury (American College of Obstetricians and Gynecologists, 1988).

Infants whose mothers contract the disease after the first trimester will not necessarily be healthy, as demonstrated by Hardy and associates (1969). Their long-term prospective epidemiological inquiry to assess the impact of the extensive 1964 rubella epidemic in this country revealed 24 instances of serological evidence of rubella infection after the first trimester. Of the 22 liveborn infants, only 7 could be considered completely normal when followed for periods of up to 4 years.

The syndrome of congenital rubella includes one or more of the following abnormalities:

1. Eye lesions, including cataracts, glaucoma, microphthalmia, and various other abnormalities
2. Heart disease, including patent ductus arteriosus, septal defects, and pulmonary artery stenosis
3. Auditory defects
4. Central nervous system defects including meningoencephalitis
5. Retarded fetal growth
6. Thrombocytopenia and anemia
7. Hepatosplenomegaly and jaundice
8. Chronic diffuse interstitial pneumonitis
9. Osseous changes
10. Chromosomal abnormalities

Infants born with congenital rubella may shed the virus for many months and thus be a threat to other infants, as well as to susceptible adults who come in contact with them.

CYTOMEGALOVIRUS

Cytomegalovirus is an ubiquitous organism that eventually infects the majority of humans, and evidence for fetal infection is found in from 0.5 to 2 percent of all neonates. Following primary infection, which is usually asymptomatic, the virus becomes latent and there is periodic reactivation with viral shedding despite the presence of serum antibody. Humoral antibody is produced, but cell-mediated immunity appears to be the primary mechanism for recovery, and immunosuppressed states, whether naturally acquired or drug induced, increase the propensity for serious cytomegalovirus infection. Presumably, it is decreased cell-mediated immune surveillence that places the fetus-infant at high risk for sequelae of these infections.

MATERNAL INFECTION

There is no evidence that pregnancy increases the risk of maternal cytomegalovirus infection (Stagno and colleagues, 1982). As shown in Figure 33–10, the risk of seroconversion among susceptible women during pregnancy is from 1 to 4 percent. Immunity from previous infection can be demonstrated in up to 85 percent of pregnant women from lower socioeconomic backgrounds, whereas the seropositivity rate for women in higher income groups is only about 50 percent. Women who are not immune at conception constitute the major reservoir of those who give birth to infants with clinically apparent infection. Thus, primary infection, which is transmitted to the fetus in approximately 40 percent of cases, is more often associated with severe morbidity (Stagno and co-workers, 1986). Although transplacental infection is not universal, an infected fetus is more likely with maternal infection during the first half of pregnancy.

As with other herpesviruses, maternal immunity to cytomegalovirus does not prevent recurrence (reactivation), nor does it prevent congenital infection. In fact, since most infections during pregnancy are recurrent, the majority of congenitally infected neonates are born to these women. Fortunately, congenital infections that result from recurrent infection are less often associated with clinically apparent sequelae than are those from primary infections.

CONGENITAL INFECTION

Congenital cytomegalovirus infection, termed *cytomegalic inclusion disease*, causes a syndrome that includes low birthweight, microcephaly, intracranial calcifications, chorioretinitis, mental and motor retardation, sensorineural deficits, hepatosplenomegaly, jaundice, hemolytic anemia, and thrombocytopenic purpura. Fortunately, of the estimated 33,000 infants born infected in the United States each year, only approximately 10 percent demonstrate this syndrome, which, as discussed above, is more prevalent in neonates born to women with primary infection during the first half of pregnancy. The mortality among these congenitally infected infants may be as high as 20 to 30 percent, and more than 90 percent of the survivors have mental retardation, hearing loss, impaired psychomotor development, seizures, or other central nervous system impairment (Pass and colleagues, 1980).

The outcome is much better for the 90 percent of infants without obvious clinical disease at birth, and only 5 to 15 percent of these are at risk for similar developmental abnormalities within 2 years of birth (Saigal and co-workers, 1982). Sensorineural hearing deficits are the most important late sequelae, and these may be progressive.

MANAGEMENT

There is no effective therapy for maternal infection, and since the risk of fetal morbidity is low, serological screening during

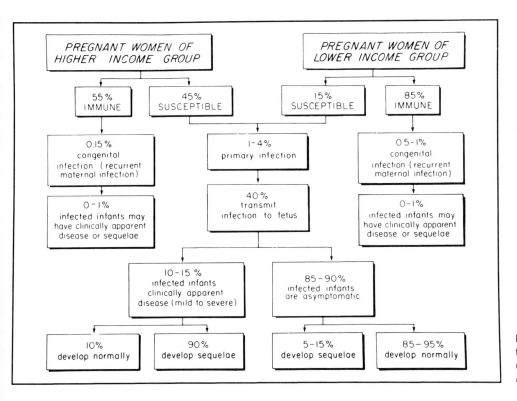

Figure 33–10. Characteristics of cytomegalovirus infection in pregnancy. (*From Stagno and Whitley: N Engl J Med 313:1271, 1985, with permission.*)

pregnancy has limited value (Peckham and co-workers, 1983; Sever, 1985). This is true since (1) current knowledge does not allow accurate predictability of the sequelae of primary infection, (2) knowledge of immune status at conception serves no purpose since there is no vaccine, and (3) 1 to 2 percent of all infants excrete cytomegalovirus in the urine, and attempts to identify and isolate them are expensive and impractical.

The predictive value of a positive maternal genitourinary culture or cervical cytology in assessing fetal risk for infection is likewise minimal. Asymptomatic cytomegalovirus excretion can be shown in up to 10 percent of pregnant women, and most of these have low-risk recurrent infections. Primary infection is diagnosed by fourfold increased IgG titers in paired acute and convalescent sera measured simultaneously, or by detecting IgM antibody to cytomegalovirus in maternal serum. Unfortunately, neither of these methods is totally accurate in confirming maternal infection. Counselling regarding fetal outcome must be individualized and it depends on the stage of gestation during which primary infection is documented. Unfortunately, there are no reliable methods to assess the effects of fetal infection, including sonography or amnionic fluid cultures for cytomegalovirus.

SYPHILIS

In the past, syphilis accounted for nearly a third of stillborns, and indeed, delivery of a macerated fetus was considered diagnostic of infection with *Treponema pallidum*. Today, syphilis has a smaller but persistent role in the genesis of fetal deaths, and as emphasized by the Centers for Disease Control (1986a), the number of cases of congenital infection increased by 150 percent from 1978 through 1985. As shown in Table 33–8, half of the mothers had inadequate prenatal care, and thus infection was not diagnosed. **Half of congenitally in-**fected infants were born to women who received prenatal care but in whom serological screening was not done, and thus maternal syphilis was not treated.** Predictably, the rise in congenital infection paralleled a similar increase in adult primary and secondary syphilis.

PATHOLOGY

Syphilis is a chronic infection, and the spirochete causes lesions in the internal organs that include interstitial changes in the lungs (*pneumonia alba of Virchow*), liver (*hypertrophic cirrhosis*), spleen, and pancreas. It causes *osteochondritis* in the long bones, which is most readily recognizable radiographically at the lower ends of the femur, tibia, and radius.

Under the influence of syphilitic infection, the placenta becomes large and pale. Microscopically, the villi appear to have lost their characteristic aborescent appearance and to have become thicker and club shaped. There is a marked decrease in the number of blood vessels, which in advanced cases almost en-

TABLE 33–8. FACTORS ASSOCIATED WITH CONGENITAL SYPHILIS AMONG 437 INFANTS—UNITED STATES, 1983–85

Factor	Number of Infants
Prenatal care	229 (52%)
No serological testing	18
Positive serology, not treated	32
Negative early serology, not repeated	58
Prenatal treatment failure	81
3rd trimester benzathine penicillin (55%)	
2nd trimester benzathine penicillin (14%)	
Erythromycin (14%)	
No prenatal care	208 (48%)

From Centers for Disease Control: MMWR 35:275, 1986a.

tirely disappear as a result of endarteritis and proliferation of the stromal cells. Spirochetes are only sparsely scattered throughout the placenta even when they are present in large numbers in the fetal organs. They may be demonstrated by examination under the darkfield microscope of scrapings from the intima of the vessels of the fresh cord. Cox and colleagues (1988) have shown, especially with primary or secondary syphilis, that motile spirochetes are frequently seen in amnionic fluid obtained transabdominally.

Shown in Figure 33–11A is an infant with congenital lues who has a large abdomen owing mostly to marked hepatosplenomegaly. His placenta is seen in Figure 33–11B. It weighed almost as much as the infant!

TREATMENT AND FAILURES

Maternal treatment for syphilis is described in Chapter 39 (p. 851). There is concern that despite recommended treatment during pregnancy, almost 20 percent of newborns have obvious clinical stigmata of congenital syphilis (Centers for Disease Control, 1986a). As shown in Table 33–8, half of these method failures were identified in mothers not given treatment until the third trimester. This also has been our experience at Parkland

Hospital, and it seems likely that these fetal infections are of such duration and severity that there is irreversible damage (Maberry and colleagues, 1988). Importantly, in about half of these women penicillin treatment is followed by the *Jarisch–Herxheimer reaction* and uterine contractions frequently develop followed by evidence for fetal distress manifested as late fetal heart rate declerations (Cox and colleagues, 1987). Obvious fetal involvement, characterized by ultrasonic evidence for ascites, is associated with almost universally bad fetal outcome, despite therapy.

Alternative treatment with erythromycin given to women with presumed penicillin allergy has been linked to treatment failures (Fenton and Light, 1976; Hashisaki and colleagues, 1983). Erythromycin therapy was associated with about 15 percent of cases of congenital syphilis that were identified despite completion of recommended maternal treatment (Table 38–8). Therefore, for the pregnant women with penicillin allergy, desensitization followed by benzathine penicillin G is recommended (Wendel and co-workers, 1985). If this is not feasible, then we agree with Fiumara (1984) and Holmes and Lukehart (1987) that tetracycline should be given. The risk is for staining of deciduous, not permanent, teeth.

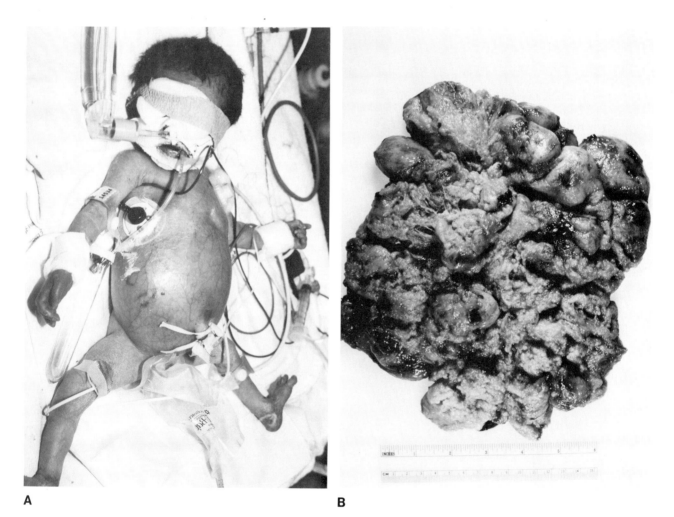

A   **B**

Figure 33–11. A. An infant born at 29 weeks gestation and gravely ill with congenital lues. Note the enlarged abdomen caused by marked hepatosplenomegaly plus ascites. **B.** The large syphilitic placenta of the infant in A. The placenta weighed 1,200 g, almost the birthweight of the infant. (*Photographs courtesy of Dr. G. Wendel.*)

CHLAMYDIAL INFECTIONS

Chlamydia trachomatis is an obligate intracellular bacterium considered to be the most prevalent cause of sexually transmitted disease in the United States. There are several serovars (serotypes), but those important in neonatal infection are the same that cause cervical infection near delivery. Maternal infections with chlamydiae are considered in Chapter 39 (p. 853).

PATHOGENESIS

Depending upon epidemiological variables, the prevalence of maternal cervical carriage ranges from 3 to 26 percent (Eschenbach, 1985). Seldom is the fetus infected, despite the fact that neonatal disease is acquired by contact with the infected cervix at delivery.

Conjunctivitis

Ophthalmic chlamydial infections are one of the most common causes of preventable blindness in undeveloped countries. Inclusion conjunctivitis develops in as many as a third of neonates born to mothers with cervical infection, and there is some preliminary evidence that erythromycin ointment applied topically for gonococcal ophthalmia may substantively decrease this attack rate (Centers for Disease Control, 1985). Symptomatic conjunctivitis tends to appear later than disease caused by *N. gonorrhoeae*, and the two must be differentiated using culture or Gram and Giemsa staiing, since treatment is not the same.

Pneumonitis

Approximately 10 percent of infants born through an infected cervix develop chlamydial pneumonitis within 1 to 3 months (American College of Obstetricians and Gynecologists, 1985). These infections are characteristic of chlamydiae by their long latency periods and indolence. Clinically, bilateral pulmonary infiltrates and chronic cough are often associated with poor weight gain. As in their incubation, these infections resolve slowly, even with therapy.

TREATMENT

Oral erythromycin is given for both conjunctivitis and pneumonitis. Schachter and colleagues (1986) demonstrated that treatment of maternal cervical infection at 36 weeks with erythromycin ethylsuccinate, 400 mg four times daily for 7 days, eradicated cervical chlamydiae in 92 percent of women. In infants of treated women there was substantively decreased incidence of neonatal chlamydial infections, compared to infants born to women with untreated infection (7 versus 50 percent).

TOXOPLASMOSIS

Toxoplasmosis is a protozoal infection caused by *Toxoplasma gondii*. Infection is transmitted through encysted organisms by eating infected raw or undercooked meat or through contact with infected cat feces, or it can be congenitally acquired by transplacental transfer.

PATHOGENESIS

Maternal immunity appears to protect against intrauterine transmission of the parasite; therefore, for congenital toxoplasmosis to develop, the mother must have acquired the infection during pregnancy. About a third of American women acquire protective antibody before pregnancy, and this is higher in those keeping cats as pets.

Fatigue, muscle pains, and sometimes lymphadenopathy are identified in the infected mother, but most often the maternal infection is subclinical. Infection in pregnancy may cause abortion or result in a liveborn infant with evidence of disease. The risk of infection increases with duration of pregnancy and is approximately 15, 30, and 60 percent in the first, second, and third trimesters (Remington and Desmonts, 1983).

Virulence of fetal infection is greatest when maternal infection is acquired early in pregnancy—fortunately the time least common. Less than 10 percent of newborns with congenital toxoplasmosis have signs of clinical illness at birth. Affected infants usually have evidence of generalized disease with low birthweight, hepatosplenomegaly, icterus, and anemia. Some infants primarily have neurological disease with convulsions, intracranial calcifications, and hydrocephaly or microcephaly. Both groups of infants eventually develop chorioretinitis.

SCREENING AND MANAGEMENT

Although Remington and Desmonts (1983) made a credible argument for prenatal toxoplasmosis serum screening, this is done uncommonly because of the technical difficulty in interpreting the tests (Sever, 1985). Some women, usually those who own cats, will request serological testing. Perhaps, as suggested by the American College of Obstetricians and Gynecologists (1988), preconceptual screening may be reasonable.

If antibody, usually determined by indirect fluorescence on enzyme-linked immunosorbent assay, is present in low titers, it probably represents previously acquired immunity; however, it could be IgM from recent infection, although IgM may persist for years and false positive results may be due to rheumatoid factor (Fuccillo and associates, 1987). Unfortunately, differentiation between the two is difficult, and consultation from a state reference laboratory, the Centers for Disease Control, or the National Institutes of Health is advised.

The most accurate confirmation of active infection is a rise in IgG titer in two appropriately spaced but simultaneously tested serum samples. Very high titers—that is, greater than 1:512—more likely indicate recent or current illness. Sever and colleagues (1988) reported increased microcephaly, deafness, and mental retardation in women whose titers were 1:256 or higher.

For the woman thought to have active disease, treatment is recommended by Remington and Desmonts (1983). There is good evidence that spiramycin, used widely in Europe, reduces the incidence of fetal infection, but it may not modify its severity. Desmonts and colleagues (1985) employed amnionic fluid and fetal blood sampling in 183 women with proven first-trimester infection. These women were given spiramycin, 3 g daily when serological diagnosis was made, and then fetal samples were taken at 20 to 24 weeks. Only 4 percent of fetuses were *possibly* infected, suggesting that spiramycin was effective.

Subsequently, Daffos and co-workers (1988) reported the French group's experiences with 746 pregnancies in which maternal infection was diagnosed by toxoplasma-specific IgM antibody. All women with presumed infection were treated with spiramycin. Only 6 percent of their fetuses were found to have infection, and 39 of these 42 were diagnosed by demonstrating IgM-specific antibody in serum obtained by umbilical vessel sampling. For these women, pyrimethamine and either sulfadoxine or sulfadiazine were added to the spiramycin regime. In

TABLE 33–9. UNNECESSARY USE OF TORCH TESTING

Test	Unnecessary Use	Reason
Toxoplasma	Routine screening of women Routine tests of paired sera during pregnancy	Clinical laboratory tests unreliable Outcome data for similarly tested women in United States limited
Cytomegalovirus	Routine screening of women Routine paired sera during pregnancy	Reliability of clinical laboratories uncertain No outcome data on similarly tested women in United States Recurrent shedding of virus occurs in presence of antibody Virus isolation best method for documenting active infection
Herpes simplex	Routine screening of women	Most antibody tests cross-react with HSV-1 and HSV-2; some cross with other herpesviruses
	Documentation of clinical herpes	Recurrent shedding of virus occurs in presence of antibody Antibody frequently does not increase with recurrence of infection Virus isolation best method for documenting active infection

From Sever: Contemp Ob/Gyn 18:175, 1981.

the United States, spiramycin is currently not available, and treatment is given with pyrimethamine plus sulfadiazine; however, the efficacy of such management has not been established.

TORCH TESTS

In recent years, TORCH (*Toxoplasmosis, Other, Rubella, Cytomegalovirus, Herpesvirus*) serum screening has become popular in the United States, even though on careful analysis the information obtained often has not proved to be of any value

and the cost is appreciable. Sever (1985) analyzed results obtained from TORCH package testing and recommended that only rubella serology be used routinely (Table 33–9). The results from a significant number of large laboratories were unreliable. Moreover, the presence of antibody does not exclude the presence of the pathogen in the case of cytomegalovirus or herpes simplex. Sever urged that such tests, when ordered, be selected on an individual basis. Specific serological confirmation is recommended for suspected toxoplasmosis and rubella, whereas virus isolation is employed for herpesvirus and cytomegalovirus.

INJURIES OF THE FETUS AND NEWBORN

Considered here are several varieties of birth injuries. Others are described elsewhere in connection with specific obstetrical complications that led to or contributed to the injury.

INTRACRANIAL HEMORRHAGE

Hemorrhage within the head of the fetus-infant may be located at any of several sites: subdural, subarachnoid, cortical, white matter, cerebellar, intraventricular, and periventricular. Intraventricular hemorrhage into the germinal matrix is the most common type of intracranial hemorrhage encountered, and as previously discussed (p. 595), it usually is a result of prematurity and not a traumatic injury. Hayden and colleagues (1985) reported that nearly 4 percent of otherwise normal newborns at term have sonographic evidence for subependymal germinal matrix hemorrhages unrelated to obstetrical factors.

Sachs and associates (1987) identified the incidence of symptomatic intracranial hemorrhage to be 5.9 per 10,000 births at the Beth Israel and Brigham and Women's Hospitals in 1982 and 1983. Risk factors included precipitate delivery, prolonged second stage of labor, oxytocin use, and forceps delivery.

Birth trauma may cause intracranial hemorrhage, but it is no longer a common cause. The head of the fetus may undergo appreciable molding during passage through the birth canal. The skull bones, the dura mater, and the brain itself permit considerable alteration in the shape of the fetal head without untoward results. The dimensions of the head are changed, with lengthening especially of the occipitofrontal diameter of the skull (Fig. 33–12). Bridging veins from the cerebral cortex to the sagittal sinus may tear as the consequence of severe molding and marked overlap of the parietal bones or of difficult forceps delivery. Less common are rupture of the internal cerebral veins, the vein of Galen at its junction with the straight sinus, or the tentorium itself. Compression of the skull can stretch the tenorium cerebelli and may tear the vein of Galen or its tributaries. The common types and locations of intracranial hemorrhages are illustrated in Figure 33–13. Wigglesworth and Pape (1980) have provided lucid descriptions of the pathophysiology of intracranial hemorrhages in the newborn.

Illingworth (1979), an English pediatrician, rightfully contended that because of superficial thinking, obstetricians have been blamed unjustifiably for causing brain damage and other injuries, the genesis of which was not limited just to difficulties

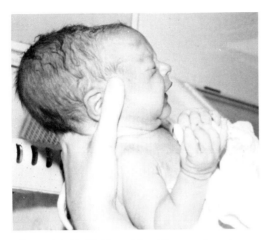

Figure 33–12. Molding of head in normal newborn.

during labor and delivery, but involved prenatal factors, including those that were genetic and environmental in nature. Nonetheless, the elimination of difficult forceps operations, the use of cesarean section when there was cephalopelvic disproportion, the correct management of breech delivery, and the virtual eradication of internal version and extraction have all contributed significantly to a reduction in the incidence of all birth injuries, including intracranial hemorrhage.

CLINICAL FINDINGS

Commonly, infants suffering intracranial hemorrhage from mechanical injury are born depressed but their conditions appear to improve until about 12 hours of age. Then drowsiness, apathy, feeble cry, pallor, failure to nurse, dyspnea, cyanosis, vomiting, and convulsions may become evident. Atelectasis, hypoxia, acidosis, meconium aspiration, and forceps trauma may be associated findings. To help rule out diaphragmatic hernia, congenital heart disease, atelectasis, idiopathic respiratory distress, and pneumonia, prompt radiographic examination of the chest is useful. In recent years, head scanning using sonography and computed tomography not only has proved of diagnostic value but also has contributed appreciably to an understanding of the etiology of some forms of intracranial hemorrhage and the frequency with which they occur. For example, periventricular and intraventricular hemorrhages occur often in infants born quite preterm and these hemorrhages usually develop without birth trauma.

TREATMENT

Therapy includes oxygen when there is dyspnea and cyanosis as well as sedation to control convulsions. The blood can be removed from some subdural hematomas by careful needle aspiration. In other instances, surgical intervention may be required. The value of administering plasma clotting factors to infants with intracranial hemorrhage is not clear; however, prompt intramuscular administration of vitamin K to all newborn infants is indicated (p. 611).

Surviving infants subsequently may develop functional disturbances, incuding cerebral palsy and mental deficiency. Certain cases of idiopathic epilepsy also may be caused by intracranial injury sustained at birth.

CEPHALOHEMATOMA

A cephalohematoma (Figs. 33–14 and 33–15) is usually caused by injury to the periosteum of the skull during labor and delivery, although it may develop in the absence of birth trauma when hemostasis is defective. The incidence is 2.5 percent according to the 10-year review by Thacker and colleagues (1987). The subperiosteal hemorrhages may develop over one or both parietal bones. The periosteal limitations with definite palpable edges differentiate the cephalohematoma from *caput succedaneum*. The latter lesion consists of a focal swelling of the scalp from edema fluid that overlies the periosteum (Fig. 33–14). Furthermore, a cephalohematoma may not appear for hours after delivery, often growing larger and disappearing only after weeks or even months (Fig. 33–15). In contrast, caput succedaneum is maximal at birth, grows smaller, and disappears usually within a few hours if small and within a few days even when very large.

Increasing size of the hematoma and other evidence of extensive hemorrhage are indications for additional investigation, including radiographic studies of the skull and assessment of coagulation factors, since the infant may have defective blood clotting, as exemplified by the infant with severe thrombocytopenia illustrated in Figure 39–5 (p. 792).

NERVE INJURIES

SPINAL INJURY

Overstretching the spinal cord and associated hemorrhage may follow excessive traction during a breech delivery, and there may be actual fracture or dislocation of the vertebrae. Complete data on such lesions are lacking, since even the most careful autopsy seldom includes thorough examination of the spine.

BRACHIAL PLEXUS INJURY

Brachial plexus injuries are common and encountered in nearly 1 in 500 term births (Levine and colleagues, 1984). The injury usually follows a difficult delivery, but in rare cases after an apparently easy one, the infant is born with a paralyzed arm. *Duchenne's*, or *Erb's*, *paralysis* involves paralysis of the deltoid and infraspinatus muscles, as well as the flexor muscles of the forearm, causing the entire arm to fall limply close to the side of the body with the forearm extended and internally rotated. The function of the fingers is usually retained.

The lesion results from stretching or tearing of the upper roots of the brachial plexus, which is readily subjected to extreme tension as a result of pulling laterally upon the head, thus sharply flexing it toward one of the shoulders. Since traction in this direction is employed frequently to effect delivery of the shoulders in normal vertex presentations, Erb's paralysis may result without the delivery appearing to be difficult. In extracting the shoulders, therefore, care should be taken not to impose excessive lateral flexion of the neck. Most often, in the case of cephalic presentations, the afflicted fetus is unusually large, typically weighing 4,000 g or more. Other risk factors reported by Levine and co-workers (1984) and McFarland and associates (1986) are prolonged labor, forceps delivery, and shoulder dystocia, which is discussed in Chapter 19 (p. 365).

In breech extractions, particular attention should be devoted to preventing the extension of the arms over the head. Extended arms not only materially delay breech delivery but also

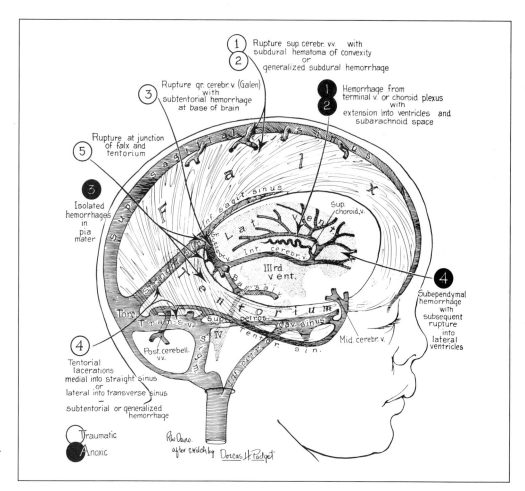

Figure 33–13. The common types and locations of intracranial hemorrhage in the fetus-infant. (*From Haller and colleagues: Obstet Gynecol Surv 11:179, 1956, with permission.*)

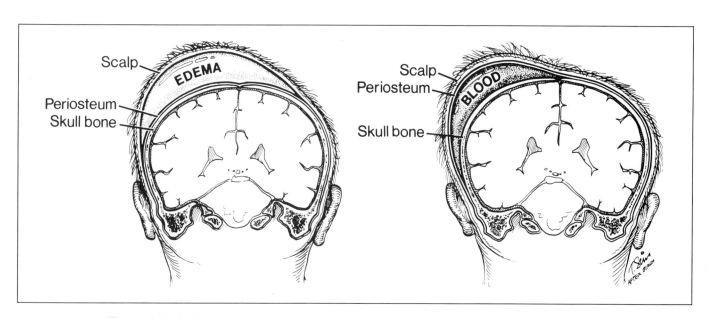

Figure 33–14. Difference between a large caput succedaneum (*left*) and cephalohematoma (*right*). In a caput succedaneum, the effusion overlies the periosteum and consists of edema fluid; in a cephalohematoma, it lies under the periosteum and consists of blood.

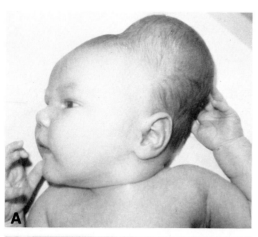

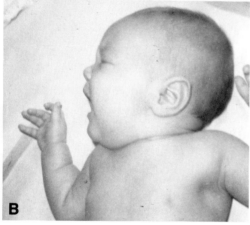

Figure 33–15. A. A very large cephalohematoma photographed 2 weeks after delivery. **B.** The same infant 4 weeks later. (*Courtesy of Dr. William Austin.*)

increase the risk of paralysis. The prognosis is usually good with prompt, appropriate physiotherapy. Occasionally, however, a case may resist all treatment, and the arm may remain permanently paralyzed.

Less frequently, trauma is limited to the lower nerves of the brachial plexus, which leads to paralysis of the hand, or *Klumpke's paralysis.*

FACIAL PARALYSIS

According to Levine and colleagues (1984), the incidence of facial nerve injury was 7.5 per 1,000 term births; however, this has decreased recently. The child may be born with *facial paralysis*, a condition that also may develop shortly after birth (Fig. 33–16). It usually is seen with delivery of an infant in which the head has been seized obliquely with forceps. The injury is caused by pressure exerted by the posterior blade of the forceps on the stylomastoid foramen, through which the facial nerve emerges. Very often, facial lacerations from the forceps are quite obvious (Fig. 33–17). Not every case of facial paralysis following delivery of forceps should be attributed to the operation, however, since the condition is also encountered after spontaneous delivery. In fact, Levine and co-workers (1984) reported that a third of cases of facial palsy followed spontaneous delivery. Spontaneous recovery within a few days is the rule (Fig. 33–16).

SKELETAL AND MUSCLE INJURIES

FRACTURES

Fractures of the clavicle were identified in 2 per 1,000 term births by Levine and colleagues (1984). They further reported a significant reduction in its incidence over an 8-year period. Humeral fractures are less common. Difficulty encountered in the delivery of the shoulders in cephalic deliveries and extended arms in breech deliveries are the main factors in the production of such fractures. A fractured femur is relatively uncommon and is usually associated with breech delivery. Upper extremity fractures associated with delivery are often of the greenstick type, although complete fracture with overriding of the bones may occur. Palpation of the clavicles and long bones should be performed on all newborns when a fracture is suspected, and any crepitation or unusual irregularity should prompt radiographic examination. It also is important to seek evidence of brachial palsy so that treatment can be instituted.

Fracture of the skull usually follows forcible attempts at delivery, especially with forceps, although it may follow spontaneous delivery or even cesarean section (Saunders and colleagues, 1979; Skajaa and associates, 1987). In the radiograph presented in Figure 33–18, a focal, but marked, depressed skull fracture is apparent. Labor was characterized by vigorous contractions, full dilatation of the cervix, and arrest of descent of the head, which was tightly wedged in the pelvis. The fracture was the consequence of compression of the skull against the sacral promontory of the mother, or perhaps from pressure from an assistant's hand in the vagina or as the head was pushed upwards out of the birth canal at cesarean delivery. Surgical decompression was successful. Saunders and colleagues (1979) reported successful use of the obstetrical vacuum extractor to apply negative pressure to reduce these fractures.

MUSCULAR INJURIES

Injury to the sternocleidomastoid muscle may occur, particularly during a breech delivery. There may be a tear of the muscle or possibly of the fascial sheath, leading to a hematoma and gradual cicatricial contraction. As the neck lengthens in the process of normal growth, the child's head is gradually turned toward the side of the injury, since the damaged muscle is less elastic and does not elongate at the same rate as its normal contralateral counterpart, thus producing the deformity of *torticollis*. Roemer (1954) reported that 27 of 44 infants showing this deformity had been delivered by breech or internal podalic version. He postulated that lateral hyperextension sufficient to rupture the sternocleidomastoid may occur as the aftercoming head passes over the sacral promontory.

CONGENITAL INJURIES

AMNIONIC BAND SYNDROME

Focal ring constrictions of the extremities and actual loss of a digit or a limb are rare complications. Their genesis is debated. Streeter (1930), and others since, maintain that localized failure of germ plasm usually is responsible for the abnormalities. Torpin (1968) and others contend that the lesions are the consequence of early rupture of the amnion, which then forms adherent tough bands that constrict and, at times, actually amputate an extremity of the fetus. Occasionally, the amputated

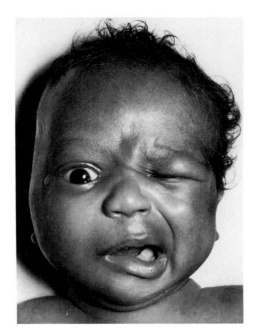
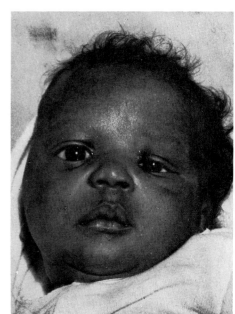

Figure 33–16. A. Paralysis of left side of face 15 minutes after forceps delivery. **B.** Same infant 24 hours later. Recovery was complete in another 24 hours.

part may be found within the uterus. Although this mechanism is favored currently, Hunter and Carpenter (1986) recently reported four cases with associated anomalies not explicable entirely by band disruptions.

An unusual fetal fatality from cord vessel occlusion by "strings" of amnion is demonstrated in Figure 33–19.

CONGENITAL POSTURAL DEFORMITIES

Mechanical factors arising from chronically low volumes of amnionic fluid and restrictions imposed by the small size and inappropriate shape of the uterine cavity may mold the growing fetus into distinct patterns of deformity, including talipes (clubfoot), scoliosis, hip dislocation, limb reduction, and body wall deficiency (Miller and co-workers, 1981). Hypoplastic lungs also can result from oligohydramnios.

COINCIDENTAL INJURIES

Experience at Parkland Hospital, with a very large trauma service, has been that trauma to the fetus inflicted at the time of severe trauma to the mother is less common than might be expected. Since the fetus is floating in amnionic fluid, he is likely to be shielded from forces that cause serious injury to adjacent maternal structures. Even so, as emphasized by Buchsbaum (1979), the fetus is not completely immune to external trauma. Moreover, fetal well-being may be jeopardized indirectly by injuries to the mother that lead to inadequate maternal oxygenation and, in turn, inadequate fetal oxygenation, or to maternal cardiac output insufficient for adequate perfusion of vital organs, including the placenta.

It is important that in case of accident, the readily measurable vital sign of the fetus—the heart rate—should be moni-

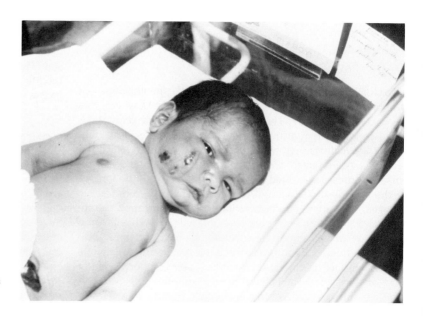

Figure 33–17. Healing abrasions and lacerations from a difficult forceps delivery. Palsy of the right facial nerve has nearly cleared.

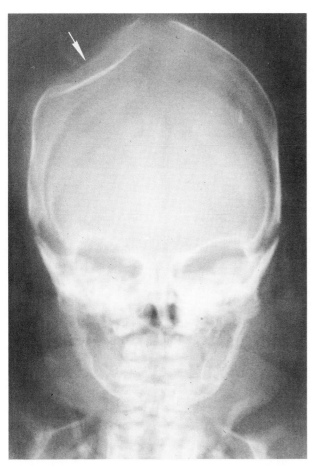

Figure 33–18. Depressed skull fracture evident immediately after birth. Delivery followed vigorous but obstructed labor and dislodgement upward of the fetal head from the birth canal by an assistant's hand in the vagina at the time of cesarean section.

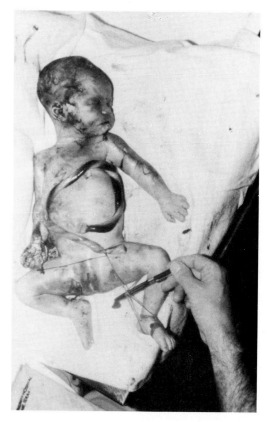

Figure 33–19. Death of a fetus at term from an amnionic band that formed after premature rupture of the amnion. A tough string of rolled amnion was wrapped centrally around the cord and at each end was adherent to the right thigh and the left foot and ankle. Movements of these extremities tightened the amnionic string and constricted the cord. (*Courtesy of Dr. Allan Dutton.*)

tored, especially in the third trimester, since the fetus has considerable potential for survival. At times, however, the fetus may expire before delivery can be safely accomplished. Such an instance is illustrated in Figures 36–5A and B (p. 704). The placenta was partially separated and grossly lacerated as the consequence of the mother's lower abdomen forcibly striking the steering wheel during an auto accident. The cause of fetal death was massive fetomaternal hemorrhage as the consequence of the gross laceration of the placenta. The fetus was not injured otherwise, and the uterus was intact. Stafford and colleagues (1988) emphasized that lethal placental or fetal injury can occur even if maternal injuries are mild or insignificant.

An unusual case was described by Buchsbaum and Caruso (1969) in which a pregnant woman was shot in the abdomen. A radiograph showed that the bullet was lodged most likely somewhere in the fetus, and at laparotomy an entrance wound was evident in the large pregnant uterus. However, a liveborn, apparently uninjured infant was delivered and no bullet was found in the uterus or elsewhere in the mother. It then was discovered that the rapidly decelerating bullet had entered the mouth of the fetus and been swallowed. It was subsequently expelled per rectum!

REFERENCES

Allan LD, Crawford DC, Sheridan R, Chapman MG: Aetiology of non-immune hydrops: The value of echocardiography. Br J Obstet Gynaecol 93:223, 1986

American College of Obstetricians and Gynecologists: Committee Statement—Use and misuse of the Apgar score. November 1986a

American College of Obstetricians and Gynecologists: Management of Isoimmunization in Pregnancy. Technical Bulletin No 90, January 1986b

American College of Obstetricians and Gynecologists: Gonorrhea and Chlamydial Infections. Technical Bulletin No 89, November 1985

American College of Obstetricians and Gynecologists: Perinatal Viral and Parasitic Infections. Technical Bulletin No 114, March 1988

Anand A, Gray ES, Brown T, Clewley JP, Cohen BJ: Human parvovirus infection in pregnancy and hydrops fetalis. N Engl J Med 316:183, 1987

Anderson HM, Hutchison AA, Fortune DW: Non-immune hydrops fetalis: A changing contribution to perinatal mortality. Br J Obstet Gynaecol 90:636, 1983

Appelman Z, Blumberg BD, Golabi M, Golbus MS: Nonimmune hydrops fetalis may be associated with an elevated ΔOD_{450} in the amniotic fluid. Obstet Gynecol 71:1005, 1988

Arias IM, Gartner LM, Seifter S, Furman M: Prolonged neonatal unconjugated hyperbilirubinemia associated with breast feeding and steroid, pregnane-3(alpha),20(beta)-diol in maternal milk that inhibits glucuronide formation in vitro. J Clin Invest 43:2037, 1964

Avery ME, Taeusch HW, Floros J: Surfactant replacement. N Engl J Med 315:825, 1986

Baker CJ, Rench MA, Edwards MS, Carpenter RJ, Hays BM, Kasper DL: Immunization of pregnant women with a polysaccharide vaccine of group b streptococcus. N Engl J Med 319:1180, 1988

Barss VA, Frigoletto FD, Konugres A: The cost of irregular antibody screening. Am J Obstet Gynecol 159:428, 1988

Bejar R, Wozniak P, Allard M, Benirschke K, Vaucher Y, Coen R, Berry C, Schragg P, Villegas I, Resnik R: Antenatal origin of neurologic damage in newborn infants. Am J Obstet Gynecol 159:357, 1988

Bergin FT, Cefalo RC, Lewis PE: Self-limited hemolytic transfusion reaction in an ABO-incompatible maternal-fetal unit. Am J Obstet Gynecol 132:116, 1978

Berkowitz RL, Chitkara U, Wilkins IA, Lynch L, Plosker H, Bernstein HH: Intravascular monitoring and management of erythroblastosis fetalis. Am J Obstet Gynecol 158:783, 1988

Bernard B, Presley M, Caudillo G, Clauss B, Rouault CL, McGregor J, Jennings ER: Maternal-fetal hemorrhage: Incidence and sensitization. Pediatr Res 11:467, 1977

Blajchman MA, Maudsley RF, Uchida I, Zipursky A: Diagnostic amniocentesis and fetal-maternal bleeding. Lancet 1:993, 1974

Bowell PJ, Allen DL, Entwistle CC: Blood group antibody screening tests during pregnancy. Br J Obstet Gynaecol 93:1038, 1986a

Bowell PJ, Brown SE, Dike AE, Inskip MJ: The significance of anti-c alloimmunization. Br J Obstet Gynaecol 93:1044, 1986b

Bowman JM: Controversies in Rh prophylaxis: Who needs Rh immune globulin and when should it be given? Am J Obstet Gynecol 151:289, 1985

Bowman JM: The management of Rh-isoimmunization. Obstet Gynecol 52:1, 1978

Bowman JM, Chown B, Lewis M, Pollock J: Rh isoimmunization, Manitoba, 1963–1975. Can Med Assoc J 116:282, 1977

Bowman JM, Pollock JM: Antenatal Rh prophylaxis: 28 week gestation service program. Can Med Assoc J 118:622, 1978

Boyer KM, Gotoff SP: Prevention of early-onset neonatal Group B streptococcal disease with selective intrapartum chemoprophylaxis. N Engl J Med 314:1665, 1986

Buchsbaum HJ: Trauma in Pregnancy. Philadelphia, Saunders, 1979

Buchsbaum HJ, Caruso PA: Gunshot wound of the pregnant uterus. Obstet Gynecol 3:673, 1969

Bussel JB, Berkowitz RL, McFarland JG, Lynch L, Chitkara U: Antenatal treatment of neonatal alloimmune thrombocytopenia. N Engl J Med 319:1374, 1988

Cameron A, Nicholson S, Nimrod C, Harder J, Davies D, Fritzler M: Evaluation of fetal cardiac dysrhythmias with two-dimensional, M-mode, and pulsed Doppler ultrasonography. Am J Obstet Gynecol 158:286, 1988

Castillo RA, Devoe LD, Hadi HA, Martin S, Giest D: Nonimmune hydrops fetalis: Clinical experience and factors related to a poor outcome. Am J Obstet Gynecol 155:812, 1986

Centers for Disease Control: *Chlamydia trachomatis* infections: Policy guidelines for prevention and control. Publication 00-4770, August 1985

Centers for Disease Control: Congenital syphilis—United States, 1983–1985. MMWR 35:275, 1986a

Centers for Disease Control: Lack of transmission of human immunodeficiency virus through Rh$_o$(D) immune globulin (human). MMWR 36:728, 1987a

Centers for Disease Control: Rubella and congenital rubella syndrome—New York City. MMWR 35:50, 1986b

Centers for Disease Control: Rubella vaccination during pregnancy—United States, 1971–1985. MMWR 36:457, 1987b

Charles AG, Blumenthal LS: Promethazine hydrochloride therapy in severe Rh-sensitized pregnancies. Obstet Gynecol 60:627, 1982

Clapp III JF, Peress NS, Wesley M, Mann LI: Brain damage after intermittent partial cord occlusion in the chronically instrumented fetal lamb. Am J Obstet Gynecol 159:504, 1988

Clark DA, Nieman GF, Thompson JE, Paskanik AM, Rokhar JE, Bredenberg CE: Surfactant displacement by meconium free fatty acids: An alternative explanation for atelectasis in meconium aspiration syndrome. J Pediatr 110:765, 1987

Cohen F, Zuelzer WW: The transplacental passage of maternal erythrocytes into the fetus. Am J Obstet Gynecol 93:566, 1965

Cox SM, Maberry MC, Casey ML, MacDonald PC, Wendel GD: Characterization of amniotic fluid from pregnancies complicated by syphilis. Presented at the Society of Perinatal Obstetricians, Las Vegas [Abstract No 165], 1988

Cox SM, Klein VR, Wendel GD: The Jarisch–Herxheimer reaction in pregnancy. Presented at the Society of Perinatal Obstetricians, Lake Buena Vista, Florida [Abstract No 106], 1987

Daffos F, Forestier F, Capella-Pavlovsky M, Thulliez P, Aufrant C, Valenti D, Cox W: Prenatal management of 746 pregnancies at risk for congenital toxoplasmosis. N Engl J Med 381:271, 1988

Desjardins L, Blajchman MA, Chintu G, Gent M, Zipursky A: The spectrum of ABO hemolytic disease of the newborn infant. J Pediatr 74:247, 1979

Desmonts G, Daffos F, Forestier F, Capella-Pavlovsky M, Thulliez PH, Chartier M: Prenatal diagnosis of congenital toxoplasmosis. Lancet 1:500, 1985

De Vries LS, Dubowitz V, Lary S, Whitelaw A, Dubowitz LMS, Kaiser A, Silverman M, Wigglesworth JS: Predictive value of cranial ultrasound in the newborn baby: A reappraisal. Lancet 2:137, 1985

Dijxhoorn MJ, Visser GHA, Fidler VJ, Touwen BCL, Huisjes HJ: Apgar score, meconium and acidaemia at birth in relation to neonatal neurological morbidity in term infants. Br J Obstet Gynaecol 86:217, 1986

Donn SM, Roloff DW, Goldstein GW: Prevention of intraventricular hemorrhage in preterm infants by phenobarbitone. Lancet 2:215, 1981

Dooley SL, Pesavento DJ, Depp R, Socol ML, Tamura RK, Wiringa KS: Meconium below the vocal cords at delivery: Correlation with intrapartum events. Am J Obstet Gynecol 153:767, 1985

Dunn MS, Shennan AT, Hoskins EM, Lennox K, Enhorning G: Two-year follow-up of infants enrolled in a randomized trial of surfactant replacement therapy for prevention of neonatal respiratory distress syndrome. Pediatrics 82:543, 1988

Edelin KC, Gurganious L, Golar K, Oellerich D, Kyei-Aboagye K, Hamid MA: Methadone maintenance in pregnancy: Consequences to care and outcome. Obstet Gynecol 71:399, 1988

Ehrenkranz RA, Ablow RC, Warshaw JB: Prevention of bronchopulmonary dysplasia with vitamin E administration during the acute stages of respiratory distress syndrome. J Pediatr 95:873, 1979

Eibl MM, Wolf HM, Fürnkranz H, Rosenkranz A: Prevention of necrotizing enterocolitis in low-birth-weight infants by IgA-IgG feeding. N Engl J Med 319:1, 1988

Ellenberg JH, Nelson KB: Cluster of perinatal events identifying infants at high risk for death or disability. J Pediatr 113:546, 1988

Eschenbach DA: Contending with the problem of chlamydial infection. Contemp Ob/Gyn 27:125, 1985

Falciglia HS: Failure to prevent meconium aspiration syndrome. Obstet Gynecol 71:349, 1988

Fenton LJ, Light IJ: Congenital syphilis after maternal treatment with erythromycin. Obstet Gynecol 47:492, 1976

Finn R, Clarke CA, Donohoe W, McConnell RB, Sheppard PM, Lehane D, Kulke W: Experimental studies on the prevention of Rh haemolytic disease. Br Med J 1:1486, 1961

Fiumara NJ: Letters to the editor. Sex Transm Dis 11:49, 1984

Foliot A, Ploussard JP, Housset E, Christoforov B: Breast milk jaundice: In vitro inhibition of rat liver bilirubin-uridine diphosphate glucuronyltransferase activity and Z protein-bromosulfonphthalein binding by human breast milk. Pediatr Res 10:594, 1976

Freda V: Hemolytic disease. Clin Obstet Gynecol 16:72, 1973

Freda VJ, Gorman JG, Pollack W: Successful prevention of sensitization to Rh with an experimental anti-Rh gamma$_2$ globulin antibody preparation. Fed Proc 22:374, 1963

Freda VJ, Gorman JG, Pollack W, Bowe E: Prevention of Rh hemolytic disease: Ten years' clinical experience with Rh immune globulin. N Engl J Med 292:1014, 1975

Freeman J (ed): Prenatal and Perinatal Factors Associated with Brain Disorders. US Department of Health and Human Services, Public Health Service, National Institutes of Health, NIH Publication No 85-1149, 1985

Frigoletto FD, Greene MF, Benacerraf BR, Barrs VA, Saltzman DH: Ultrasonographic fetal surveillance in the management of the isoimmunized pregnancy. N Engl J Med 315:430, 1986

Fuccillo DA, Madden DL, Tzan N, Sever JL: Difficulties associated with serological diagnosis of *Toxoplasma gondii* infections. Diagn Clin Immunol 5:8, 1987

Fujiwara T, Maeta H, Shida S, Morita T, Watabe Y, Abe T: Artificial surfactant therapy in hyaline-membrane disease. Lancet 1:55, 1980

Gold WR Jr, Queenan JT, Woody J, Sacher RA: Oral desensitization in Rh disease. Am J Obstet Gynecol 146:980, 1983

Gough JD, Keeling JW, Castle B, Iliff PJ: The obstetric management of nonimmunological hydrops. Br J Obstet Gynaecol 93:226, 1986

Graham M, Trounce JQ, Levene MI, Rutter N: Prediction of cerebral palsy in very low birthweight infants: Prospective ultrasound study. Lancet 2:593, 1987

Grannum PA, Copel JA, Moya FR, Scioscia AL, Robert JA, Winn HN, Coster BC, Burdine CB, Hobbins JC: The reversal of fetal hydrops by intravascular intrauterine transfusion in severe isoimmune fetal anemia. Am J Obstet Gynecol 158:914, 1988

Grannum PA, Copel JA, Plaxe SC, Scioscia AL, Hobbins JC: In utero exchange transfusion by direct intravascular injection in severe erythroblastosis fetalis. N Engl J Med 314:1431, 1986

Gregg NM: Congenital cataract following German measles in the mother. Trans Ophthalmol Soc Aust 3:35, 1942

Hambleton G, Wigglesworth JS: Origin of intraventricular haemorrhage in the preterm infant. Arch Dis Child 51:651, 1976

Hanigan WC, Kennedy G, Roemisch F, Anderson R, Cusack T, Powers W: Administration of indomethacin for the prevention of periventricular-intraventricular hemorrhage in high-risk neonates. J Pediatr 112:941, 1988

Hardy JB, McCracken GH Jr, Gilkeson MB, Sever J: Adverse fetal outcome following maternal rubella after the first trimester of pregnancy. JAMA 207:2414, 1969

Harman CR, Manning FA, Bowman JM, Lange IR: Severe Rh disease—Poor outcome is not inevitable. Am J Obstet Gynecol 145:823, 1983

Harper RG, Solish GI, Purow HM, Sang E, Panepinto WC: The effect of a methadone treatment program upon pregnant heroin addicts and their newborn infants. Pediatrics 54:300, 1974

Hashisaki P, Wertzberger GG, Conrad GL, Nichols CR: Erythromycin failure in the treatment of syphilis in a pregnant woman. Sex Transm Dis 10:36, 1983

Hayden CK, Shattuck KE, Richardson CJ, Ahrendt DK, House R, Swischuk LE: Subependymal germinal matrix hemorrhage in full-term neonates. Pediatrics 75:714, 1985

Hittner HM, Godio LB, Speer ME, Rudolph AJ, Taylor MM, Blifeld C, Kretzer FL: Retrolental fibroplasia: Further clinical evidence and ultrastructural support for efficacy of vitamin E in the preterm infant. Pediatrics 71:423, 1983

Holmes KK, Lukehart SA: Syphilis. In Braunwald E, Isselbacher KJ, Petersdorf RG, Wilson JD, Martin JB, Fauci AS (eds): Harrison's Principles of Internal Medicine, 11th ed. New York, McGraw-Hill, 1987, p 639

Holzgreve W, Curry CJR, Golbus MS, Callen PW, Filly RA, Smith JC: Investigation of nonimmune hydrops fetalis. Am J Obstet Gynecol 150:805, 1984

Hunter AGW, Carpenter BF: Implications of malformations not due to amniotic bands in the amniotic band sequence. Am J Med Genet 24:691, 1986

Hutchison AA, Drew JH, Yu VYH, Williams ML, Fortune DW, Beischer NA: Nonimmunologic hydrops fetalis: A review of 61 cases. Obstet Gynecol 59:347, 1982

Illingworth RS: Why blame the obstetrician?: A review. Br Med J 1:797, 1979

Jennings ER, Clauss B: Maternal-fetal hemorrhage: Its incidence and sensitizing effects. Am J Obstet Gynecol 131:725, 1978

Kanto WP Jr, Wilson R, Breart GL, Zierler S, Purohit DM, Peckham GJ, Ellison RC: Perinatal events and necrotizing enterocolitis in premature infants. Am J Dis Child 141:167, 1987

Kaplan C, Daffos F, Forestier F, Cox WL, Lyon-Caen D, Dupuy-Montbrun MC, Salmon CH: Management of alloimmune thrombocytopenia: Antenatal diagnosis and in utero transfusion of maternal platelets. Blood 72:340, 1988

Katz MA, Kanto WP Jr, Korotkein JH: Recurrence rate of ABO hemolytic disease of the newborn. Obstet Gynecol 59:611, 1982

Keenan WJ, Jewitt T, Glueck HI: Role of feeding and vitamin K in hypoprothrombinemia of the newborn. Am J Dis Child 121:271, 1971

Kinsey VE, Arnold HJ, Kalina RE, Stern L, Stahlman M, Odell G, Driscoll J, Elliott J, Payne J, Patz A: Pao2 levels and retrolental fibroplasia: A report of the cooperative study. Pediatrics 60:655, 1977

Kirkman HN Jr: Further evidence for a racial difference in the frequency of ABO hemolytic disease. J Pediatr 90:717, 1977

Kleinman CS, Copel JA, Weinstein EM, Santulli TV, Hobbins JC: In utero diagnosis and treatment of fetal supraventricular tachycardia. Semin Perinatol 9:113, 1985

Kliegman RM, Fanaroff AA: Necrotizing enterocolitis. N Engl J Med 310:1093, 1984

Lacey PA, Caskey CR, Werner DJ, Moulds JJ: Fatal hemolytic disease of a newborn due to anti-D in an Rh-positive Du variant mother. Transfusion 23:91, 1983

LaGamma EF, Drusin LM, Mackles AW, Machalek S, Auld PAM: Neonatal infections. Am J Dis Child 137:838, 1983

Lane PA, Hathaway WE: Vitamin K in infancy. J Pediatr 106:351, 1985

Laube DW, Schauberger CW: Fetomaternal bleeding as a cause for "unexplained" fetal death. Obstet Gynecol 60:649, 1982

Lesko SM, Mitchell AA, Epstein MF, Louik C, Giacoia GP, Shapiro S: Heparin use as a risk factor for intraventricular hemorrhage in low-birth-weight infants. N Engl J Med 314:1156, 1986

Levine MG, Holroyde J, Woods JR, Siddiqi TA, Scott M, Miodovnik M: Birth trauma: Incidence and predisposing factors. Obstet Gynecol 63:792, 1984

Leveno KJ, Quirk JG, Cunningham FG, Nelson SD, Santo-Ramos R, Toofanian A, DePalma RT: Prolonged pregnancy: I. Observations concerning the causes of fetal distress. Am J Obstet Gynecol 150:465, 1984

Liley AW: Intrauterine transfusion of foetus in hemolytic disease. Br Med J 2:1107, 1963

Liley AW: Amniocentesis and amniography in hemolytic disease. In Greenhill JP (ed): Yearbook of Obstetrics & Gynecology, 1964–1965 Series. Chicago, Year Book, 1964, p 256

Linder N, Aranda JV, Tsur M, Matoth I, Yatsiv I, Mandelberg H, Rottem M, Feigenbaum D, Ezra Y, Tamir I: Need for endotracheal intubation and suction in meconium-stained neonates. J Pediatr 112:613, 1988

Locus P, Yeomans E, Crosby U: The efficacy of bulb versus DeLee suction at deliveries complicated by meconium-stained amniotic fluid. Presented at District VII, American College of Obstetricians and Gynecologists, October 1987

Low JA, Galbraith RS, Muir DW, Killen HL, Karchmar EJ: The relationship between perinatal hypoxia and newborn encephalopathy. Am J Obstet Gynecol 152:256, 1985

Lowe TW, Leveno KJ, Quirk JG Jr, Santos-Ramos R, Williams ML: Sinusoidal fetal heart rate pattern after intrauterine transfusion. Obstet Gynecol 64:21S, 1984

Luthy DA, Shy KK, Strickland D, Wilson J, Bennett FC, Brown ZA, Benedetti TJ: Status of infants at birth and risk for adverse neonatal events and long-term sequelae: A study in low birthweight infants. Am J Obstet Gynecol 157:676, 1987

Maberry M, Theriot S, Wendel G: Syphilis treatment failures in pregnancy. Society of Perinatal Obstetricians, Las Vegas [Abstract No 165], January 1988

Maeda H, Shimokawa H, Satoh S, Nakano H, Nunoue T: Nonimmunologic hydrops fetalis resulting from intrauterine human parvovirus B-19 infection: Report of two cases. Obstet Gynecol 72:482, 1988

Maisels MJ: Neonattal jaundice: III. Breast feeding and jaundice. Perinat Press 3:19, 1979

Malloy MH, Hartford RB, Kleinman JC: Trends in mortality caused by respiratory distress syndrome in the United States, 1969–83. Am J Public Health 77:1511, 1987

Marshall R, Tyrala E, McAlister W, Sheehan M: Meconium aspiration syndrome: Neonatal and follow-up study. Am J Obstet Gynecol 131:672, 1978

McFarland LV, Raskin M, Daling JR, Benedetti TJ: Erb/duchenne's palsy: A consequence of fetal macrosomia and method of delivery. Obstet Gynecol 68:784, 1986

McIntosh S: Erythropoietin excretion in the premature infant. J Pediatr 86:202, 1975

Merrit TA, Hallman M, Bloom BT, Berry C, Benirschke K, Sahn D, Key T, Edwards D, Jarvenaa A-L, Pohjavuori M, Kankaanpaa K, Kunnas M, Paatero H, Rapola J, Jaaskelainen J: Prophylactic treatment of very premature infants with human surfactant. N Engl J Med 315:785, 1986

Miller E, Cradock-Watson JE, Pollock TM: Consequences of confirmed maternal rubella at successive stages of pregnancy. Lancet 2:781, 1982

Miller ME, Graham JM Jr, Higginbottom MC, Smith DW: Compression-related defects from early amnion rupture: Evidence for mechanical teratogenesis. J Pediatr 98:292, 1981

Morales WJ: Effect of intraventricular hemorrhage on the one-year mental and neurologic handicaps of the very low birth weight infant. Obstet Gynecol 70:111, 1987

Morales WJ, Koerten J: Prevention of intraventricular hemorrhage in very low birth weight infants by maternally administered phenobarbital. Obstet Gynecol 68:295, 1986

Morales WJ, Lim D: Reduction of Group B streptococcal maternal and neonatal infections in preterm pregnancies with premature rupture of membranes through a rapid identification test. Am J Obstet Gynecol 157:13, 1987

Morales WJ, Stroup M: Intracranial hemorrhage in utero due to isoimmune neonatal thrombocytopenia. Obstet Gynecol 65:20S, 1985

Mountain K, Hirsh J, Gallus AS: Neonatal coagulation defect and maternal anticonvulsant treatment. Lancet 1:265, 1970

Mueller-Huebach E, Mazer J: Sonographically documented disappearance of fetal ascites. Obstet Gynecol 61:253, 1983

Nelson KB, Ellenberg JH: Obstetric complications as risk factors for cerebral palsy or seizure disorders. JAMA 251:1843, 1984

Nelson KB, Ellenberg JH: Antecedents of cerebral palsy: Multivariate analysis of risk. N Engl J Med 315:81, 1986a

Nelson KB, Ellenberg JH: Antecedents of seizure disorders in early childhood. Am J Dis Child 140:1053, 1986b

Ness PM, Baldwin ML, Niebyl JR: Clinical high-risk designation does not predict excess fetal-maternal hemorrhage. Am J Obstet Gynecol 156:154, 1987

Newman RG, Bashkow S, Calko D: Results of 313 consecutive live births of infants delivered to patients in the New York City methadone maintenance treatment program. Am J Obstet Gynecol 121:233, 1975

Newton ER, Haering WA, Kennedy JL, Herschel M, Cetrulo C, Feingold M: Effect of mode of delivery on morbidity and mortality of infants at early gestational age. Obstet Gynecol 67:507, 1986

Nicolaides KH, Clewell WH, Mibashan RS, Soothill PW, Rodeck CH, Campbell S: Fetal haemoglobin measurement in the assessment of red cell isoimmunisation. Lancet 1:1073, 1988a

Nicolaides KH, Fontanarosa M, Gabbe SG, Rodeck CH: Failure of ultrasonographic parameters to predict the severity of fetal anemia in rhesus isoimmunization. Am J Obstet Gynecol 158:920, 1988b

Nicolaides KH, Rodeck CH, Mibashan RS, Kemp JR: Have Liley charts outlived their usefulness? Am J Obstet Gynecol 155:90, 1986

Nicolaides KH, Warenski JC, Rodeck CH: The relationship of fetal plasma protein concentration and hemoglobin level to the development of hydrops in rhesus isoimmunization. Am J Obstet Gynecol 152:341, 1985

Paneth N: Birth and the origins of cerebral palsy. N Engl J Med 315:124, 1986

Papile L-A, Burstein J, Burstein R, Koffler H: Incidence and evolution of subependymal and intraventricular hemorrhage: A study of infants with birth weights less than 1500 gm. J Pediatr 92:529, 1978

Papile L-A, Munsick-Bruno G, Schaefer A: Relationship of cerebral intraventricular hemorrhage and early childhood neurologic handicaps. J Pediatr 103:273, 1983

Pass RF, Stagno S, Myers GJ, Alford CA: Outcome of symptomatic congenital cytomegalovirus infection: Results of a long-term longitudinal follow-up. Pediatrics 66:758, 1980

Peckham CS, Chin KS, Coleman JC, Henderson K, Hurley R, Preece PM: Cytomegalovirus infection in pregnancy: Preliminary findings from a prospective study. Lancet 1:1352, 1983

Peevy KJ, Wiseman HJ: ABO hemolytic disease of the newborn: Evaluation of management and identification of racial and antigenic factors. Pediatrics 61:475, 1978

Pelosi MA, Frattarola M, Apuzzio J, Langer A, Hung CT, Oleske JM, Bai J, Harrigan JT: Pregnancy complicated by heroin addiction. Obstet Gynecol 45:512, 1975

Perlman JM, Goodman S, Kreusser KL, Volpe JJ: Reduction in intraventricular hemorrhage by elimination of fluctuating cerebral blood-flow velocity in preterm infants with respiratory distress syndrome. N Engl J Med 312:1353, 1985

Perlman JM, Volpe JJ: Intraventricular hemorrhage in extremely small premature infants. Am J Dis Child 140:1122, 1986

Pomerance JJ, Jeal JG, Gogolok JF, Brown S, Stewart ME: Maternally administered antenatal vitamin K1: Effect on neonatal prothrombin activity, partial thromboplastin time and intraventricular hemorrhage. Obstet Gynecol 70:235, 1987

Pritchard JA, Cunningham FG, Pritchard SA, Mason RA: How often does maternal preeclampsia-eclampsia incite thrombocytopenia in the fetus? Obstet Gynecol 69:292, 1987

Pyati SP, Pildes RS, Jacobs NM, Ramamurthy RS, Yeh TF, Raval DS, Lilien LD, Amma P, Metzger WI: Penicillin in infants weighing two kilograms or less with early-onset Group B streptococcal disease. N Engl J Med 308:1383, 1983

Queenan JT, King JC: Intrauterine transfusion for severe Rh-EBF—Past and future. Contemp Ob/Gyn 30:51, 1987

Raju TNK, Vidyasgar D, Bhat R, Sobel D, McCulloch KM, Anderson M, Maeta H, Levy PS, Furner S: Double-blind controlled trial of single-dose treatment with bovine surfactant in severe hyaline membrane disease. Lancet 1:651, 1987

Ramsey-Goldman R, Hom D, Deng J, Ziegler GC, Kahl LE, Steen VD, LaPorte RE, Medsger TA Jr: Anti-SS-A antibodies and fetal outcome in maternal systemic lupus erythematosus. Arthritis Rheum 29:1269, 1986

Remington JS, Desmonts G: Toxoplasmosis. In Remington JS, Klein JO (eds): Infectious Diseases of the Fetus and Newborn Infant. Philadelphia, Saunders, 1983, pp 143–263

Rodeck CH, Holman CA, Karicki J, Kemp JR, Whitmore DN, Austin MA: Direct intravascular fetal blood transfusion by fetoscopy in severe rhesus isoimmunization. Lancet 1:625, 1981

Rodeck CH, Nicolaides KH, Warsof SL, Fysh WJ, Gamsu HR, Kemp JR: The management of severe rhesus isoimmunization by fetoscopic intravascular transfusions. Am J Obstet Gynecol 150:769, 1984

Roemer RJ: Relation of torticollis to breech delivery. Am J Obstet Gyncol 67:1146, 1954

Rosen MG, Hobel CJ: Prenatal and perinatal factors associated with brain disorders. Obstet Gynecol 68:416, 1986

Sachs BP, Acker D, Tuomala R, Brown E: The incidence of symptomatic intracranial hemorrhage in term appropriate-for-gestation-age infants. Clin Pediatr 26:355, 1987

Saigal S, Lunyk O, Larke RPB, Chernesky MA: The outcome in children with congenital cytomegalovirus infection: A longitudinal follow-up study. Am J Dis Child 136:896, 1982

Saunders BS, Lazoritz S, McArtor RD, Marshall P, Bason WM: Depressed skull fracture in the neonate. J Neurosurg 50:512, 1979

Schachter J, Sweet RL, Grossman M, Landers D, Robbie M, Bishop E: Experience with the routine use of erythromycin for chlamydial infections in pregnancy. N Engl J Med 314:276, 1986

Sever JL: TORCH tests and what they mean. Am J Obstet Gynecol 152:495, 1985

Sever JL, Ellenberg JH, Ley AC, Madden DL, Fuccillo DA, Tzan NR, Edmonds DM: Toxoplasmosis: Maternal and pediatric findings in 23,000 pregnancies. Pediatrics 82:181, 1988

Shearer MJ, Barkhan P, Rahim S, Stimmler L: Plasma vitamin K_1 in mothers and their newborn babies. Lancet 2:460, 1982

Shenker L, Reed KL, Anderson CF, Marx GR, Sobonya RE, Graham AR: Congenital heart block and cardiac anomalies in the absence of maternal connective tissue disease. Am J Obstet Gynecol 157:248, 1987

Siegal JD, McCracken GH Jr: Sepsis neonatorum. N Engl J Med 304:642, 1981

Siegal JD, McCracken GH Jr, Threlkeld N, Milvenan B, Rosenfeld CR: Single-dose penicillin prophylaxis against neonatal Group B streptococcal infections. N Engl J Med 303:769, 1980

Sinha S, Davies J, Toner N, Bogle S: Vitamin E supplementation reduces frequency of periventricular hemorrhage in very preterm babies. Lancet 1:466, 1987

Skajaa K, Hansen ES, Bendix J: Depressed fracture of the skull in a child born by cesarean section. Acta Obstet Gynecol Scand 66:275, 1987

Stafford PA, Biddinger PW, Zumwalt RE: Lethal intrauterine fetal trauma. Am J Obstet Gynecol 159:485, 1988

Stagno S, Pass RF, Cloud G, Britt WJ, Henderson RE, Walton PD, Veren DA, Page F, Alford CA: Primary cytomegalovirus infection in pregnancy. JAMA 256:1904, 1986

Stagno S, Pass RF, Dworsky ME, Henderson RE, Moore EG, Walton PD, Alford CA: Congenital cytomegalovirus infection: The relative importance of primary and recurrent maternal infection. N Engl J Med 306:945, 1982

Stahlman M, Hedvall G, Linstrom D, Snell J: Role of hyaline membrane disease in production of later childhood lung abnormalities. Pediatrics 69:572, 1982

Stedman CM, Baudin JC, White CA, Cooper ES: Use of the erythrocyte rosette test to screen for excessive fetomaternal hemorrhage in Rh-negative women. Am J Obstet Gynecol 154:1363, 1986

Steigman AJ, Bottone EJ, Hanna BA: Control of perinatal Group B streptococcal sepsis: Efficacy of single injection of aqueous penicillin at birth. Mt Sinai J Med 45:685, 1978

Strauss A, Kirz D, Modanlou HD, Freeman RK: Perinatal events and intraventricular/subependymal hemorrhage in the very low-birth weight infant. Am J Obstet Gynecol 151:1022, 1985

Streeter GL: Contrib Embryol 22:1, 1930

Taylor PV, Scott JS, Gerlis LM, Esscher E, Scott O: Maternal antibodies against fetal cardiac antigens in congenital complete heart block. N Engl J Med 315:667, 1986

Tejani N, Verma U, Hameed C, Chayen B: Method and route of delivery in the low birth weight vertex presentation correlated with early periventricular/intraventricular hemorrhage. Obstet Gynecol 69:1, 1987

Ten Centre Study Group: Ten centre trial of artificial surfactant (artificial lung expanding compound) in very premature babies. Br Med J 294:991, 1987

Thacker KE, Lim T, Drew JH: Cephalhaematoma: A 10-year review. Aust NZ J Obstet Gynaecol 27:210, 1987

Torpin R: Fetal malformations caused by amnion rupture during gestation. Springfield, IL, Thomas, 1968

Vaucher YE, Merritt TA, Hallman M, Jarvenpaa A, Telsey AM, Jones BL: Neurodevelopmental and respiratory outcome in early childhood after human surfactant treatment. AJDC 142:927, 1988

Waites KB, Crouse DT, Nelson KG, Rudd PT, Canupp KC, Ramsey C, Cassell GH: Chronic ureaplasma urealyticum and mycoplasma hominis infections of central nervous system in preterm infants. Lancet 1:17, 1988

Walsh MC, Kliegman RM: Necrotizing enterocolitis: Treatment based on staging criteria. Pediatr Clin North Am 33:179, 1986

Watts DH, Luthy DA, Benedetti TJ, Cyr DR, Easterling TR, Hickok D: Intraperitoneal fetal transfusion under direct ultrasound guidance. Obstet Gynecol 71:84, 1988

Welch RA, Bottoms SF: Reconsideration of head compression and intraventricular hemorrhage in the vertex very-low-birth-weight fetus. Obstet Gynecol 68:29, 1986

Wendel GD Jr, Stark BJ, Jamison RB, Molina RD, Sullivan TJ: Penicillin allergy and desensitization in serious infections during pregnancy. N Engl J Med 312:1229, 1985

Wenk RE, Goldstein P, Felix JK: Alloimmunization by hr' (c), hemolytic disease of newborns, and perinatal management. Obstet Gynecol 67:623, 1986

White CA, Stedman CM, Frank S: Anti-D antibodies in D- and D^u-positive women: A cause of hemolytic disease of the newborns. Am J Obstet Gynecol 145:1069, 1983

Wigglesworth JS, Pape KE: Pathophysiology of intracranial hemorrhage in the newborn. J Perinat Med 8:119, 1980

Yeh TF, Harris V, Srinvasin G, Lilien L, Pyati S, Pildes RS: Roentgenographic findings in infants with meconium aspiration syndrome. JAMA 242:60, 1979

Yeomans E, Gilstrap LC, Leveno KJ, Burris JS: Meconium-stained amniotic fluid and neonatal acid-base status. Obstet Gynecol 73:175, 1989

Multifetal Pregnancy

Morbidity and mortality are increased appreciably in pregnancies with multiple fetuses. It is not an overstatement, therefore, to consider a pregnancy with multiple fetuses to be a complicated pregnancy. Many of the complications that occur more commonly with multiple fetuses and are of obvious clinical significance are listed below:

1. Abortion
2. Perinatal mortality
3. Low birthweight
   Preterm delivery
   Fetal growth retardation
4. Malformations
5. Fetal–fetal hemorrhage
   Hypovolemia and anemia
   Hypervolemia and hyperviscosity
6. Pregnancy-induced or aggravated hypertension
7. Maternal anemia
   Acute blood loss
   Iron deficiency
   Folate deficiency
8. Placental accidents
   Placental abruption
   Placenta previa
9. Other maternal hemorrhage
   Uterine atony
10. Cord accidents
    Prolapse
    Entwinement
    Vasa previa
11. Hydramnios
12. Complicated labor
    Preterm labor
    Ineffective labor
13. Abnormal fetal presentation

ETIOLOGY OF MULTIPLE FETUSES

Twin fetuses more commonly result from fertilization of two separate ova (double-ovum, dizygotic, or "fraternal" twins). About one third as often, twins arise from a single fertilized ovum that subsequently divides into two similar structures, each with the potential for developing into a separate individual (single-ovum, monozygotic, or "identical" twins). Either or both processes may be involved in the formation of higher numbers of fetuses. Quadruplets, for example, may arise from one, two, three, or four ova.

FRATERNAL VERSUS IDENTICAL TWINS

Dizygotic twins are not in a strict sense true twins, since they result from the maturation and fertilization of two ova during a single ovulatory cycle. Newman (1923) wrote: *"Strictly speaking, twainning is twinning or twoing—the division of an individual into two equivalent and more or less completely separate individuals."* Also, monozygotic or identical twins are not always identical. As is pointed out below, the process of division of one fertilized zygote into two does not necessarily result in equal sharing of protoplasmic materials. In fact, dizygotic, or fraternal twins of the same sex, may *appear* more nearly identical at birth than do monozygotic twins; growth of monozygotic twin fetuses may be discordant and at times dramatically so.

GENESIS OF MONOZYGOTIC TWINS

Valid hypotheses to explain single-ovum, or monozygotic, twinning, are lacking. Monozygotic twins arise from division of the fertilized ovum at various early stages of development as follows:

1. If division occurs before the inner cell mass is formed and the outer layer of blastocyst is not yet committed to become chorion—that is, within the first 72 hours after fertilization—two embryos, two amnions, and two chorions will develop. There will evolve a *diamnionic, dichorionic*, monozygotic twin pregnancy. The frequency of two chorions with monozygotic twinning in various reports has ranged from 18 to 36 percent (MacGillivray, 1978). There may be two distinct placentas or a single fused placenta, as depicted in Figure 34–1A and 34–1B respectively.
2. If division occurs between the fourth and eighth day, after the inner cell mass is formed and cells destined to become chorion have already differentiated but those of the amnion have not, two embryos will develop, each in separate amnionic sacs. The two amnionic sacs will eventually be covered by a common chorion, thus giving rise to *diamnionic, monochorionic*, monozygotic twin pregnancy (Fig. 34–1C).
3. If, however, the amnion has already become established, which occurs about 8 days fertilization, division will result in two embryos within a common amnionic sac, or *a monoamnionic, monochorionic*, monozygotic twin pregnancy.
4. If division is initiated even later—that is, after the embryonic disk is formed—cleavage is incomplete and conjoined twins are formed.

Figure 34–1. Placenta and membranes in twin pregnancies. **A.** Two placentas, two amnions, two chorions (from either dizygotic twins or monozygotic twins with cleavage of zygote during first 3 days after fertilization). **B.** Single placenta, two amnions, and two chorions (from either dizygotic twins or monozygotic twins with cleavage of zygote during first 3 days). **C.** One placenta, one chorion, two amnions (monozygotic twins with cleavage of zygote from the fourth to the eighth day after fertilization).

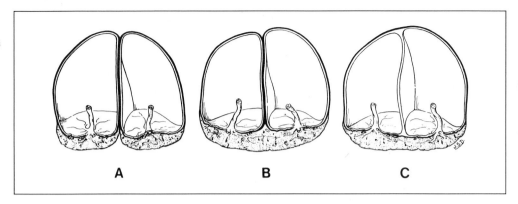

FREQUENCY OF TWINS

The frequency of *monozygotic twinning* is relatively constant worldwide at approximately one set per 250 births and is largely independent of race, heredity, age, and parity. Until recently, the frequency was thought to be independent of therapy for infertility; however, there is now evidence that the incidence of zygotic splitting is doubled following ovulation induction (Derom and colleagues, 1987). The incidence of delivery of *dizygotic twins* is influenced remarkably by race, heredity, maternal age, parity, and especially, fertility drugs. The epidemiology of multifetal pregnancy was recently reviewed by MacGillivray (1986).

It is now apparent through the use of ultrasound early in pregnancy that the incidence of twin conceptions is much higher than indicated by figures based on the delivery of two fetuses. Robinson and Caines (1977), for example, by means of ultrasound performed during the first trimester, identified twin conceptions in 30 women, only 14 of whom eventually gave birth to two infants. Eleven of the 16 women who did not do so were delivered of a single fetus and a blighted ovum. Four more were diagnosed as having twin blighted ova, and one a blighted ovum and a missed abortion. Varma (1979) and others have provided similar data. Undoubtedly, some "threatened" abortions have resulted in actual abortion of one embryo from an unrecognized twin gestation while the other embryo continued its growth and development.

Remarkably, fetal death as late as the end of the first trimester can be followed by complete resorption of the fetus, leaving no gross evidence at delivery near term that twins ever existed. Sonographic demonstration of such a case is presented in Figure 34–2A–D.

Multiple embryos and fetuses may develop in varying degrees ectopically—that is, outside the uterus. Such multiple ectopic pregnancies, as well as *combined pregnancies* in which there are one or more embryos or fetuses extrauterine as well as one or more intrauterine, are considered in Chapter 30 (p. 516).

Race

The frequency of birth of multiple fetuses varies significantly among different races (Table 34–1). For example, Myrianthopoulos (1970) identified in the Collaborative Cerebral Palsy Study the birth of twins in 1 out of every 100 pregnancies among white women, compared to 1 out of 79 pregnancies for black women. In some areas of Africa the frequency of twinning is

very high. Knox and Morley (1960), in a survey of one rural community in Nigeria, found that twinning occurred once in every 19 births! Twinning among Orientals is less common. In Japan, for example, among more than 10 million pregnancies analyzed, twinning was identified only once in every 155 births. These marked racial differences are the consequence of variations in the frequency of dizygotic twinning.

Heredity

As a determinant of twinning, the genotype of the mother is much more important than that of the father. White and Wyshak (1964), in a study of 4,000 records of the General Society of the Church of Jesus Christ of Latter-day Saints, noted that women who themselves were a dizygotic twin gave birth to twins at the rate of 1 set per 58 births. However, women not a twin but whose husbands were a dizygotic twin, gave birth to twins at the rate of 1 set per 126 pregnancies. Moreover, in Bulmer's (1960) analysis of twins, 1 out of 25 (4 percent) of their mothers was also a twin but only 1 out of 60 (1.7 percent) of their fathers was a twin.

Maternal Age and Parity

The positive effects of increasing maternal age and parity on the incidence of twinning have been well demonstrated by Waterhouse (1950). For any increase in age up to about 40, or parity up to 7, the frequency of twinning increased. Twin pregnancies were less than one third as common in women under 20 years of age with no previous children than in women 35 to 40 years of age with four or more previous children. In Sweden, Pettersson and associates (1976) confirmed the remarkable increase in multiple birth rate associated with increased parity. In first

TABLE 34–1. TWINNING RATES (PER 1,000 BIRTHS) BY ZYGOSITY IN FIVE COUNTRIES

Country	Monozygotic	Dizygotic	Total
Nigeria	5.0	49	54
United States			
Black	4.7	11.1	15.8
White	4.2	7.1	11.3
England and Wales	3.5	8.8	12.3
India (Calcutta)	3.3	8.1	11.4
Japan	3.0	1.3	4.3

From MacGillivray: Semin Perinatol 10:4, 1986.

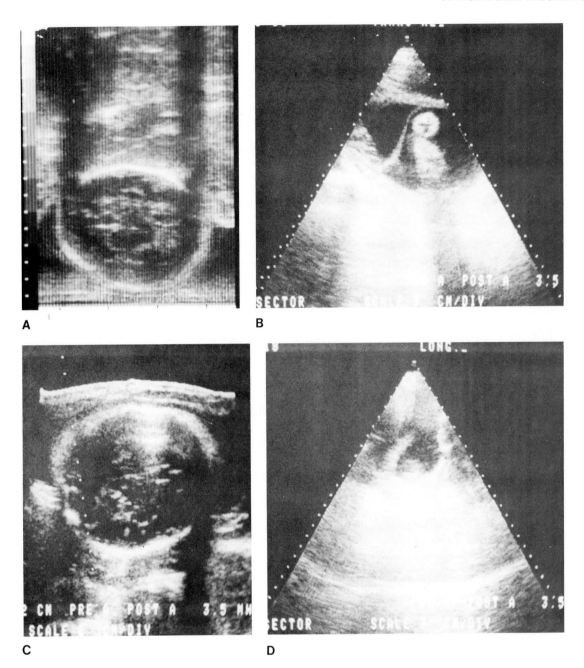

Figure 34–2. A. Sonography at 27 weeks gestation identified an appropriately grown fetus whose head is demonstrated in **A,** accompanied by **B,** a gestational sac containing a dead fetus of 12 weeks gestational age as estimated by crown–rump length. Four weeks later appropriate growth of one fetal head, **C,** was ascertained and now resorption of the dead fetus, **D,** had occurred leaving an empty gestational sac. Three weeks later that sac was no longer visible sonographically and at delivery by repeat cesarean section 1 week later no gross evidence of twins was found. (*Courtesy of Dr. R. Santos.*)

pregnancies, the frequency of multiple fetuses was 1.27 percent, compared to 2.67 percent in the fourth birth order.

In Nigeria, Azubuike (1982) identified the frequency of twinning to increase from 1 in 50 (2 percent) pregnancies among women pregnant for the first time to 1 in 15 (6.6 percent) for women pregnant six or more times!

Since the likelihood of twins increases with both parity and maternal age, it is not altogether surprising that a woman who, at the age of 50, conceived for the ninth time and had twins. The remarkable feature is that the pregnancy was completed successfully, with one infant weighing 8 pounds, 3 ounces at birth, and the other 7 pounds, 6 ounces (*Dallas Times Herald*, 1982).

Maternal Size

Dizygotic twinning is more common in large and tall women than in small women (MacGillivray, 1986). For example, in Aberdeen, the incidence of dizygous twinning in thin women was much less than in normal-size or obese women. This may be related more to nutrition than to just body size. During World War II, the incidence of dizygous twinning decreased in Europe when food deprivation was common. Even so, those women who had twins apparently did not consume more calories than those with singletons (Bulmer, 1959).

Endogenous Gonadotropin

Benirschke and Kim (1973), in their excellent review, presented intriguing reasons for implicating elevated levels of endogenous follicle-stimulating hormone in the genesis of spontaneous dizygous twinning. A higher rate of dizygous twinning has been described for women who conceive within 1 month after stopping use of oral contraceptives, but not during subsequent months (Rothman, 1977). One possibility to account for the apparent increase is release of pituitary gonadotropin in amounts greater than usual during the first spontaneous cycle after stopping contraception. Another is increased fecundity among very recent users of oral contraceptives.

Infertility Agents

The induction of ovulation by use of gonadotropins (follicle-stimulating hormone plus chorionic gonadotropin) or of clomiphene enhances remarkably the likelihood of ovulations of multiple ova. Multiple fetuses are common in pregnancies of women in whom ovulation was induced by injections of gonadotropins. The incidence of multiple fetuses following gonadotropin therapy is 20 to 40 percent, and in one instance as many as 11 fetuses were aborted (Jewelewicz, Vande Wiele, 1975). Nonuplet pregnancy with spontaneous labor 27 weeks after induction of ovulation with human pituitary gonadotropin has been described by Garrett and associates (1976). None of the nine infants survived. Two of octuplets survived in Italy. Sextuplets after gonadotropin therapy survived in South Africa, as did five of the sextuplets born in Denver.

With clomiphene therapy, the likelihood of multiple fetuses is somewhat less than with human menopausal gonadotropin. Even so, among 2,369 pregnancies following clomiphene, 165 (6.9 percent) were known to be twin, 11 (0.5 percent) triplet, 7 (0.3 percent) quadruplet, and 3 (0.13 percent) quintuplet (Merrell-National Laboratories Product Information Bulletin, 1972.) Harlap (1976) identified in smaller groups in Israel the frequency of multiple fetuses following clomiphene treatment to be 13 percent.

Ovulation induction likely increases both dizygotic and monozygotic twinning. Derom and colleagues (1987) studied the incidence of monozygotic twinning in 972 twin pairs delivered in East Flanders, Belgium, and reported that the incidence of zygotic splitting was doubled after induced ovulation. They also reported an alarming increase in monochorionic twinning in monozygotes conceived following induced ovulation.

In Vitro Fertilization

Twinning is more common in pregnancies that result from in vitro fertilization, and several sets of triplets after in vitro fertilization have now been delivered. The practice of some groups of attempting fertilization of all the ova collected after inducing superovulation and then depositing in utero more than one blastocyst when available accounts, in part, at least, for the increased frequency of multifetal pregnancies. Liveborn quadruplets have been delivered in Australia and elsewhere following in vitro fertilization!

Andrews and colleagues (1986) described their experiences with pregnancies resulting from in vitro fertilization performed at the Jones Institute for Reproductive Medicine. The average number of conceptuses transferred was three and there were 125 consecutive pregnancies that resulted. Excluding 30 preclinical pregnancies and 23 early abortions, 37 percent of pregnancies were multiple before 12 weeks, but by delivery, only 22 percent were multiple. Thus, only about half of multiple pregnancies progressed to viability. In 10 of these 12 cases, reduction was accompanied by vaginal bleeding.

SEX RATIOS WITH MULTIPLE FETUSES

The percentage of male conceptuses in the human species decreases as the number of fetuses per pregnancy increases. Strandskov and co-workers (1946) found the sex ratio, or percentage of males, for 31 million singleton births in the United States to be 51.59 percent. For twins, it was 50.85 percent; for triplets, 49.54 percent; and for quadruplets, 46.48 percent. Two explanations have been offered: First, the differential fetal mortality between the sexes is well known, as it is for the newborn infant, child, and adult. Survival is always in favor of the female and against the male. The "population pressure" with multiple fetuses in utero may exaggerate the biological tendency noted in singleton pregnancies. A second possible explanation is that the female-producing zygote has a greater tendency to divide into twins, triplets, and quadruplets.

DETERMINATION OF ZYGOSITY

With the advent of organ transplantation, the zygosity of multiple fetuses from a single pregnancy has assumed more than theoretical importance.

EXAMINATION OF PLACENTA

A knowledgeably performed examination of the placenta and membranes serves to establish zygosity promptly in about two thirds of cases (Benirschke and Kim, 1973). Moreover, appropriate examination of the placenta and membranes often serves to identify the zygosity of fetuses more firmly than do subsequent studies, which yield less precise information at considerable inconvenience and expense.

The following system for examination is recommended: As the first infant is delivered, one clamp is placed on the portion of the cord coming from the placenta. As the second infant is delivered, two clamps are placed on the cord toward the placental side. Three clamps are used to mark the cord of a third infant, and so on as necessary. Until the delivery of the last fetus is completed, it is important that each segment of cord attached to the placenta remain clamped lest fetal hemorrhage occur through anastomosed fetal vessels in the placenta.

Delivery of the placenta should be accomplished with care to preserve the attachment of the amnion and chorion to the placenta, since identification of the relationship of the membranes to each other is critical. With one common amnionic sac, which is a rare finding, or with juxtaposed amnions not separated by chorion arising between the fetuses, the infants are monozygotic. If adjacent amnions are separated by chorion, the fetuses may be monozygotic, but more often are dizygotic (Figs. 34–1, 34–3, 34–4). If the infants are of the same sex, blood group studies to identify zygosity may be initiated at this time on samples of blood obtained from the umbilical cords. A difference in major blood groups is indicative of dizygosity. If these simple procedures fail to identify zygosity, more complicated

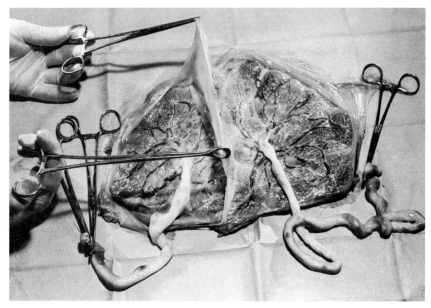

A

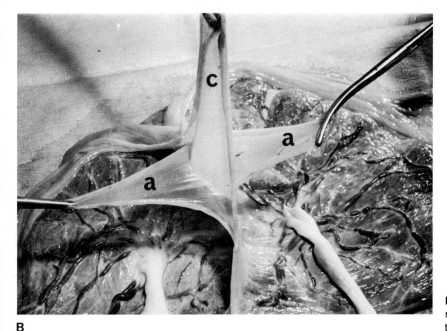

B

Figure 34–3. A. The membrane partition that separated twin fetuses is elevated. **B.** The membrane partition consists of chorion (**c**) between two amnions (**a**).

techniques, such as extensive blood and tissue antigen typing of the twins and their parents, may have to be used to look for differences.

SEX AND ZYGOSITY

Although twins of opposite sex are almost always dizygotic, monozygotic twins rarely may be discordant for phenotypic sex. Schmidt and co-workers (1974), for example, described adolescent twins in whom concordance for 22 blood groups and other biochemical markers was demonstrated. The proband demonstrated classic features of Turner syndrome, including a single sex chromosome (karyotype 45, X), in tissue cultures from streak gonads. The karyotype of the other twin, a normal-appearing male, was 46,XY. Pedersen and associates (1980) summarized

the salient features of 16 cases of monozygotic twins in whom one or both twins had gonadal dysgenesis and a 45,X karyotype, at least in some cells.

CONJOINED TWINS

In the United States, united or conjoined twins are commonly referred to as Siamese twins, after Chang and Eng Bunker of Siam (Thailand), who were displayed worldwide by P. T. Barnum. If twinning is initiated after the embryonic disc and the rudimentary amnionic sac have been formed, and if division of the embryonic disc is incomplete, conjoined twins result. When each of the joined twins is nearly complete, the commonly shared body site may be (1) anterior (*thoracopagus*),

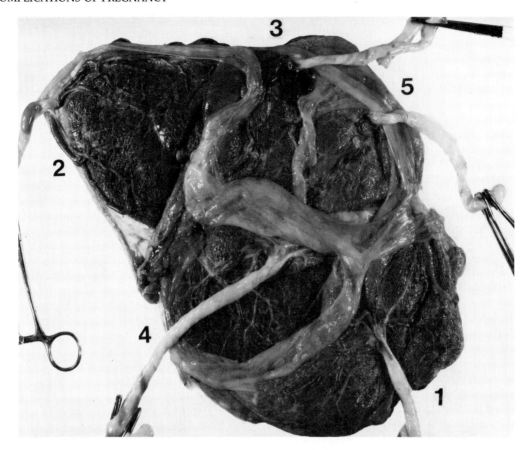

Figure 34–4. Quintuplet placenta with five separate amnionic sacs delivered at 32 weeks gestation. Amnionic sacs no. 3 and 5 were not separated by chorion and therefore those infants are identical. Infant birthweights ranged from a high of 1,530 g (no. 1) to 860 g (no. 5). All of the infants survived.

(2) posterior (*pyopagus*), (3) cephalic (*craniopagus*), or (4) caudal (*ischiopagus*). The majority are of the thoracopagus variety (Figs. 34–5, 34–6).

When the bodies are only partly duplicated, the attachment is more often lateral. The incomplete division of the embryonic disc may begin at either or both poles and produce two heads; two, three, or four arms; two, three, or four legs; or some combination thereof. The frequency of conjoined twins is not well established. At Kandang Kerbau Hospital in Singapore, Tan and co-workers (1971) identfied seven cases of conjoined twins among somewhat more than 400,000 deliveries (1 in 60,000).

The diagnosis of conjoined twins at midpregnancy by sonography is demonstrated in Figure 34–6. The use of sonography to detect conjoined twins has been considered in some depth by Koontz and associates (1983).

Vaginal delivery of conjoined twins is possible, since the union most often is somewhat pliable, although dystocia is common. However, if mature, vaginal delivery may be traumatic. Surgical separation of conjoined twins may be successful when organs essential for life are not intimately shared.

HYDATIDIFORM MOLE

At times, twinning is expressed as a single fetus from one ovum plus a hydatidiform mole from another. The development of a hydatidform mole is described in Chapter 31. Severe pregnancy-

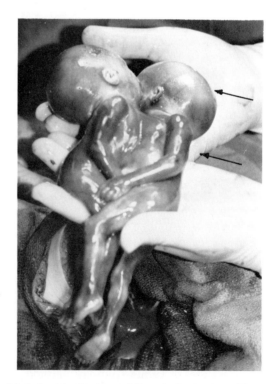

Figure 34–5. Conjoined twins at delivery by hysterotomy. The arrows indicate the approximate levels of transverse sonograms depicted in Figure 34–6.

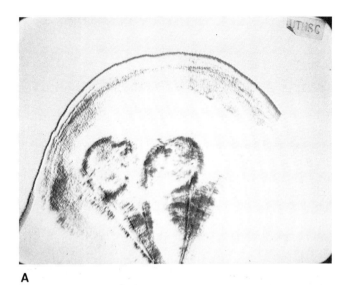

A

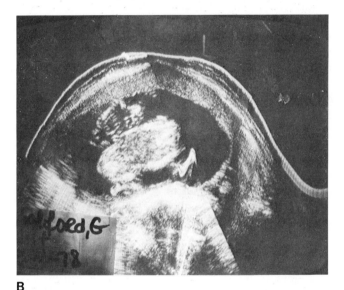

B

Figure 34–6. Transverse sonograms of the conjoined twins shown in Figure 34–5. Two fetal heads are seen in sonogram **A**. In sonogram **B**, made parallel to **A** but 5 cm below, the fused thoraces are evident. Below the thoraces are extremities and above are the umbilical cords. (*Courtesy of Dr. R. Santos.*)

induced hypertension may develop at times before the 24th week, but this is about as early as preeclampsia–eclampsia develops in the absence of a hydatidiform mole. The presence of a fetal heart and hypertension earlier in pregnancy may cloud the etiology of the hypertension until the unsuspected mole is identified either by sonography or at delivery (see Chap. 35, p. 656).

VASCULAR COMMUNICATIONS BETWEEN FETUSES

Frequently demonstrable in monochorionic placentas are vascular anastomoses, either artery to artery, artery to vein (arteries are recognized as crossing over veins), or vein to vein (Fig. 34–7). The most troublesome interfetal vascular connection is

artery to vein. Anastomoses are rarely demonstrable in dichorionic placentas (Robertson and Neer, 1983). Arteriovenous anastomoses may develop quite early in pregnancy and may vary appreciably in number and in size. As emphasized by Benirschke and Kim (1973), the arteriovenous communication often proceeds through the capillary bed of a placental cotyledon. As the consequence of such anastomoses blood is pumped from artery to vein, out of one fetus into the other.

EFFECTS OF ANASTOMOTIC CIRCULATIONS

The effects from the arteriovenous anastomoses can be profound. One monozygous twin may be very much smaller than the other as the consequence of chronic intrauterine malnutrition. The anatomic changes described by Naeye (1965), for example, in the underperfused twin resemble those found in growth-retarded singletons whose placentas were extensively infarcted. In monozygotic twins with anastomosed circulations, the hemoglobin concentration may be 8 g per dL or less in the hypoperfused twin and as much as 27 g per dL in the other! Hypotension, microcardia, and generalized runting characterize the overtly affected hypovolemic "identical" donor twin, in contrast to hypertension and cardiac hypertrophy in the hypertransfused twin. Hydramnios, perhaps the consequence of increased renal perfusion and, in turn, increased urine formation, may accompany the hypervolemia and polycythemia in the typically larger recipient twin. At the same time, amnionic fluid may be scant to absent in the other sac, possibly as a result of marked oliguria in the underperfused donor twin. Death of one monozygotic fetus has been reported to precipitate serious consumption coagulopathy in the other fetus (p. 639).

The neonatal period may be complicated by dangerous circulatory overload with heart failure if severe hypervolemia and

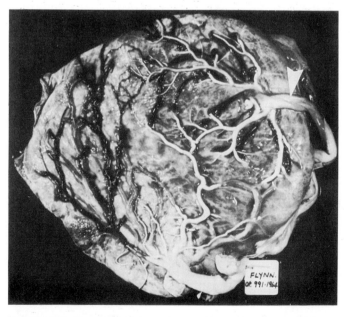

Figure 34–7. Monochorionic twin placenta from which the amnion has been stripped. The arteries of cord 1 (*arrow*) have been injected with barium solution and a direct communication with an artery from cord 2 (*label*) is apparent. A major artery of cord 2 was injected with India ink and a communication with veins in placenta 1 is evident, indicating a deep vascular communication. (*From Fox: Pathology of the Placenta, London, Saunders, 1978, p. 77.*)

blood hyperviscosity at birth are not promptly identified and treated by phlebotomy. Occlusive thrombosis is also much more likely to develop in this setting. Polycythemia may lead during the neonatal period to severe hyperbilirubinemia and, in turn, kernicterus (see Chap. 33, p. 608).

Viewed from the maternal side, one portion of the placenta often appears quite pale compared to the rest of the placenta when there is anemia in one twin and polycythemia in the other. The vascular anastomoses can usually be visualized directly after the overlying amnion is removed, especially after injecting milk into an umbilical artery (Fig. 34–7).

CHIMERISM

A chimera is an individual with a mixture of genotypes from more than one ovum and sperm. Possible mechanisms include double fertilization of one ovum, and, in case of nonidentical fetuses, the transfer of genetic material from one across chorionic vascular anastomoses to the other. For example, the transfer of primitive blood cells from one dizygotic twin fetus through a vascular anastomosis to the other twin can lead to the production in the recipient of two populations of blood cells of quite dissimilar blood types, or *blood chimerism*. The transposed cells are not destroyed, since exposure of the recipient twin to the dissimilar antigens of the donor twin early in fetal development renders the recipient twin tolerant to the donor twin's tissues. Most commonly, blood chimerism has been discovered at the time of blood typing when discordant blood types are found (Benirschke, 1974).

Chimerism, in which cell lines are derived from different zygotes, is to be distinguished from *mosaicism*, in which two or more cell lines of different chromosomal composition arise from the same zygote as the consequence of nondisjunction during meiotic division.

DIAGNOSIS OF MULTIPLE FETUSES

It is unfortunate that the diagnosis of twins frequently has not been made until late in pregnancy, often as late as the time of parturition. Powers (1973), in his analysis of complications and treatment in twin pregnancy, ascertained from various reports that from 5 percent to more than 50 percent of the time twins were not diagnosed before labor. The identification of pregnancy complicated by multiple fetuses is missed not so much because it is unusually difficult but because the examiner fails to keep the possibility in mind.

HISTORY AND PHYSICAL EXAMINATION

A familial history of twins by itself provides only a weak clue, but knowledge of recent administration of either clomiphene or pituitary gonadotropin provides a strong one.

Physical examination with accurate measurement of fundal height, as described in Chapter 14 (p. 260), is essential. **During the second trimester, a discrepancy develops between gestational age determined from menstrual data and that from uterine size. The uterus that contains two or more fetuses clearly becomes larger than one with a single fetus!** In the case of the uterus that appears large for gestational age the obstetrician must carefully consider the following possibilities: (1) multiple fetuses, (2) the elevation of the uterus by a distended bladder, (3) inaccurate menstrual history, (4) hydramnios, (5) hydatidiform mole, (6) uterine myomas or adenomyosis, (7) a closely

attached adnexal mass, and (8) fetal macrosomia late in pregnancy.

DIAGNOSTIC AIDS

A variety of techniques are utilized to identify a multifetal pregnancy.

Fetal Parts

Before the third trimester, it is difficult to diagnose twins by palpation of fetal parts. It is apparent in Figure 34–8 that even late in pregnancy it may not always be possible to identify twins by transabdominal palpation, especially if one twin overlies the other, if the woman is obese, or if hydramnios is present.

Fetal Heart Sounds

Late in the first trimester fetal heart action may be detected with generally available Doppler ultrasonic equipment (see Chap. 2, p. 18). Sometime thereafter it becomes possible to identify the separate contractions of two fetal hearts if their rates are clearly distinct from each other as well as from that of the mother. It is possible by careful examination to identify fetal heart sounds with the usual aural fetal stethoscopes at 18 to 20 weeks gestation.

Sonography

By careful ultrasonic examination, separate gestational sacs can be identified very early in twin pregnancy (Fig. 34–9). Subse-

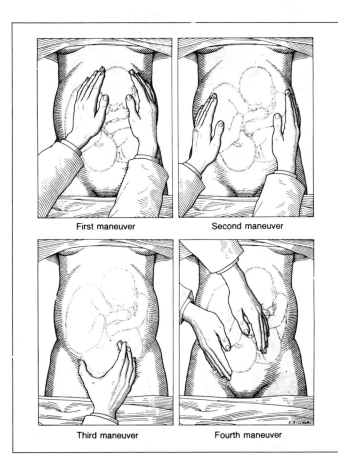

Figure 34–8. Abdominal palpation in twin pregnancy. Cephalic presentation on the mother's right and frank breech on the left.

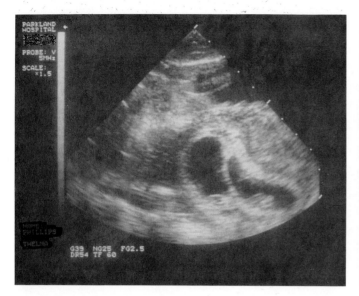

Figure 34–9. Longitudinal sonogram demonstrating two gestational sacs, each containing a fetus, at 7 weeks menstrual age. (*Courtesy of J. and J. Ackerman and Dr. R. Santos.*)

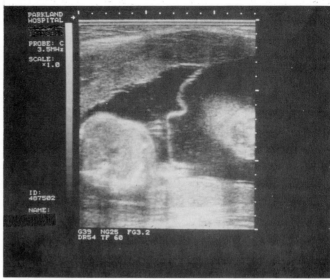

Figure 34–10. Sonogram of twins at 18 weeks gestational age. Two fetal poles are separated by intervening membranes that divide the amnionic sacs. (*Courtesy of Dr. R. Santos.*)

quently, the identification of each fetal head should be made in two perpendicular planes so as not to mistake a cross section of the fetal trunk for a second fetal head. A cross section of the fetal head remains nearly round in both planes, whereas the trunk does not. Carefully performed sonographic scanning should detect practically all sets of twins and even the presence of one amnionic sac or two (Fig. 34–10).

As the number of fetuses increases, the accuracy of diagnosis, both as to the number of fetuses and to the biparietal diameter of each head, decreases. In the case of quintuplets, demonstrated in the radiograph in Figure 34–11, only four fetuses were identified with certainty either by sonography or by radiography. It is not surprising that in the case of nonuplets studied by Kossoff and associates (1976), at 25 weeks gestation, only six of the nine fetuses were identified by sonography.

At times, sonographic examination will serve to identify conjoining of twins, as demonstrated in Figure 34–6A and B.

In multifetal pregnancies, there is a general slowing of the rate of fetal growth compared to singleton pregnancies. Moreover, individual growth in the same multifetal gestation may be discordant. Significant discordance can usually be detected by careful ultrasonic measurement of the abdominal circumference as well as the biparietal diameter. Measurements of the biparietal diameters solely may provide misleading information, since dolichocephaly in one fetal head may suggest erroneously growth discordance.

Radiographic Examination

The indiscriminate use of x-ray should be avoided during pregnancy. Moreover, a radiograph of the maternal abdomen to try to demonstrate multiple fetuses in the following circumstances will provide no useful information and may be responsible for an incorrect diagnosis: (1) when taken during the first 18 weeks of pregnancy since the fetal skeletons are insufficiently radiopaque; (2) if the film is of poor quality from inappropriate exposure time or from malposition of the mother, so that her upper abdomen and the fetus beneath are excluded from the x-ray; (3) when the mother is obese; (4) when there is hydramnios; and (5) if one fetus moves during the exposure. There are times, however, when the importance of diagnosing the presence of multiple fetuses surely overrides the minimal risk associated with a carefully obtained and interpreted radiograph.

Biochemical Tests

The amounts of *chorionic gonadotropin* in plasma and in urine, on the average, are higher than those found with a singleton pregnancy but not so high as to allow a definite diagnosis (Thiery and co-workers, 1976). Neither are the amounts of chorionic gonadotropin so low as to differentiate clearly between a twin pregnancy and a hydatidiform mole. *Placental lactogen* levels in maternal plasma average somewhat higher in a twin pregnancy than in a singleton pregnancy. Measurement of placental lactogen at 29 to 30 weeks gestation to screen for twins has been proposed in the past by Mägiste (1976) and Spellacy (1978) and their colleagues; however, this scheme has not been widely adopted. Ideally, diagnosis of twins should be made somewhat before 29 to 30 weeks. Moreover, if the gestational age is known, clinical acumen alone should lead the obstetrician to suspect twins and to employ a technique for diagnosis that is far more precise than is the measurement of placental lactogen. The α-*fetoprotein level* in maternal plasma is commonly higher in pregnancies with twins than in those with a single fetus. Even though Keilani and co-workers (1978) found that in 40 percent of twin pregnancies the level was above the 95th percentile of the normal range for singleton gestations, the measurement provides little help in diagnosing twins over that provided by careful clinical evaluation. There are also somewhat higher maternal plasma levels on the average for *estrogens, alkaline phosphatase,* and *leucine aminopeptidase* ("oxytocinase"), and in urine for *estriol* and *pregnanediol*. So far, however, there is no biochemical test that in any individual case will clearly differentiate between the presence of one and more than one fetus.

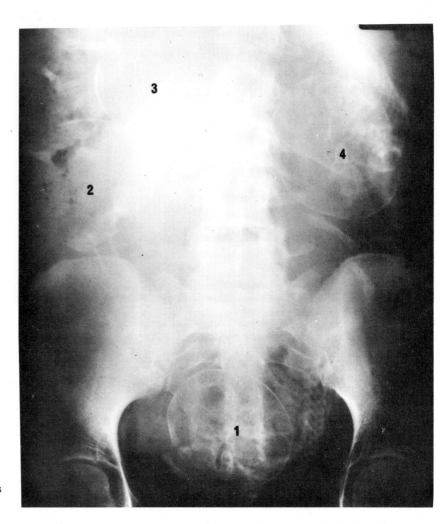

Figure 34–11. Radiograph at 27 weeks gestation that clearly demonstrates four fetal heads. A fifth fetus, not identifiable in this radiograph, weighed but 860 g when delivered 5 weeks later. (The placenta is demonstrated in Figure 34–4.)

PREGNANCY OUTCOME

ABORTION

Abortion is more likely with multiple fetuses than with a single fetus. The demonstration sonographically of two gestational sacs with the subsequent disappearance of one or even both sacs is evidence that silent early abortion or resorption of one embryo is fairly common (p. 630). Both spontaneous abortion and surgically induced abortion have, on occasion, served to remove one embryo or fetus, with the pregnancy nevertheless continuing until the birth of another fetus who survives.

DEATH OF ONE FETUS

On occasion, one fetus succumbs remote from term, but the pregnancy continues with one living fetus. At delivery, the dead fetus with placenta and membranes may be readily identified but may be appreciably compressed (*fetus compressus*) or may be remarkably flattened through loss of fluid and most of the soft tissue except skin (*fetus papyraceous*). A striking example is presented in Figure 34–12, in which the papyraceous fetus died at midpregnancy while the other fetus and placenta thrived. Sometimes the dead fetus will undergo complete resorption even though the conceptus had advanced well beyond

the status of an embryo before succumbing, as demonstrated by serial sonography in Figure 34–2.

Theoretically, at least, acquired coagulation defects (disseminated intravascular coagulation, consumptive coagulopathy) could be triggered in the mother by the death of one of multiple fetuses. However, there is documented dangerous maternal hypofibrinogenemia and troublesome hemorrhage at delivery only when both of twin fetuses were dead in utero for a prolonged period (Chap. 36, p. 718 and Fig. 36–18A and B). We have observed transient, spontaneously corrected consumptive coagulopathy when one fetus died and was retained in utero along with the other who was alive. As concern mounted over the well-being of the mothers and their surviving fetuses, the fibrinogen concentration rose spontaneously and the level of serum fibrinogen–fibrin degradation products fell to normal. At delivery the portions of the placenta that supplied the living fetus appeared quite normal, whereas that which had once provided for the dead fetus was the site of massive deposition of fibrin. The fibrin deposition may have accounted directly for the fall in maternal fibrinogen and, in turn, an increase in fibrin degradation products; or it may have served to block the escape of thromboplastin from fetus and placenta into the maternal circulation and thereby prevented disseminated intravascular coagulation; or both mechanisms may have been operational

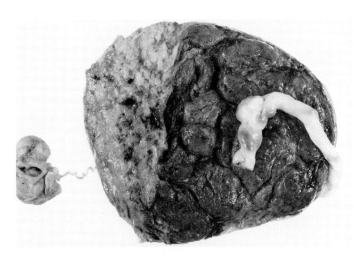

Figure 34–12. To the left are a papyraceous fetus that died at mid-pregnancy, its cord, and its pale placenta. To the right are the normal placenta and cord of the healthy 3,200 g twin.

until the extensive fibrosis had been achieved. The fetuses who were alive at the time of demise of the womb-mate continued to thrive in utero as they did after birth. At birth their plasma fibrinogen levels, serum fibrinogen–fibrin degradation products, and platelet counts were normal.

Romero and co-workers (1984) observed maternal hypofibrinogenemia to develop sometimes after death of one of twin fetuses. The hypofibrinogenemia was soon corrected in the mother by heparin infusion. The first time heparin therapy was discontinued the hypofibrinogenemia recurred, but the next time heparin was stopped hypofibrinogenemia did not recur. Presumably, by the second time consumption coagulopathy in the mother was arrested by the sealing off of the maternal vascular bed with the fibrin. The liveborn infant appeared normal at 14 months of age.

The risk to a surviving fetus of developing serious consumptive coagulopathy may be enhanced if there are anastomoses between the fetal circulations, commonly found with monoamnionic twins, as emphasized by Benirschke and Kim (1973). So far, however, we have not identified consumptive coagulopathy in cord blood of the living monozygotic twin when the other had been long dead.

PERINATAL MORTALITY

The perinatal mortality rate for pregnancies complicated by twin fetuses has been remarkably higher than for single fetuses. Perinatal loss with twins at many centers in the United States commonly has in the recent past ranged from 10 to 15 percent. For example, Kohl and Casey (1975) identified at several collaborative obstetrical units in the United States a perinatal death rate of 10.9 percent (109 per 1,000) for twins who weighed at least 500 g at birth. For twins who weighed 1,000 g or more, the perinatal death rate was 6.2 percent, or three times that for singletons. Naeye and co-workers (1978), from data compiled through a prospective collaborative study in the United States, found that the perinatal death rate was 13.9 percent for twins compared to 3.3 percent for singletons.

The perinatal death rate for monozygotic twins was 2.5 times that for dizygotic twins. There is an extremely high fetal death rate with the relatively rare variety of monozygous twinning in which both fetuses occupy the same amnionic sac—that is, *monoamnionic twins*. A common cause of death is intertwining of their umbilical cords, which has been estimated to complicate 50 percent or more of cases (Benirschke, 1983). An example is provided in Figure 34–13.

When only one amnionic sac can be identified sonographically, because of the likelihood of death of one or both monoamnionic twins from cord entanglement, the destruction of one to try to protect the other has been considered by some. Following the death of the other twin, the possibility of an adverse effect on the "protected" twin, as a consequence of severe consumptive coagulopathy, has been raised (Benirschke, 1983).

We have observed a case of monozygous, monoamnionic twins in which at 31 weeks gestation one twin was confirmed to be dead by real-time sonography while the other appeared to be thriving. Four weeks later, after spontaneous labor, an apparently healthy infant was delivered whose Apgar score was 9 at 5 minutes. In cord

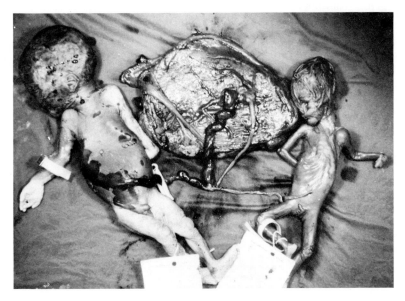

Figure 34–13. Monozygotic twins in a single amnionic sac; the smaller fetus apparently died first and the second subsequently succumbed when the umbilical cords entwined.

blood the levels of fibrinogen, fibrin degradation products, and platelets were normal. The other fetus, badly decomposed and obviously dead in utero for more than 4 weeks, weighed 770 g. The two umbilical cords were in close proximity at their insertions into the single placenta. The cords were entwined for nine complete turns!

In one recorded instance the cord of the twin who was delivered second was around the neck of the first-born. The cord was clamped and divided to facilitate vaginal delivery. Fortunately, the second twin whose cord had been severed was soon delivered and did survive (McLeod and McCoy, 1981).

DURATION OF GESTATION

As the number of fetuses increases, the duration of gestation and birthweight decrease. McKeown and Record (1952) identified the mean duration of gestation for twins to be 260 days (37 weeks), and for triplets 247 days (35 weeks), compared to 281 days (40 weeks) for single fetuses. Caspi and associates (1976) ascertained precisely the time of ovulation for 111 pregnancies in women in whom ovulation was induced with pituitary plus chorionic gonadotropins. As shown in Table 34–2, the average duration of gestation decreased dramatically as the number of fetuses increased.

BIRTHWEIGHT

Powers (1973), in the several reports from the United States and Europe that he surveyed, noted the birthweight to be less than 2,501 g in from 43 to 63 percent of twin infants. Retarded fetal growth, as well as preterm delivery, is important in the genesis of low birthweight in multifetal gestations. After the second trimester, growth of the multiple fetuses, as determined either by sonographic measurements or by birthweight, is likely to be impaired somewhat compared to that of the singleton fetus. In general, the larger the number of fetuses, the greater the degree of growth retardation. Moreover, when two or more fetuses are derived from a single ovum, the degree of growth retardation is likely to be greater than when each fetus is derived from a different ovum. The differences in birthweight were dramatic in the Davis quintuplets presented in Figure 34–14. When delivered at 31½ weeks gestation, the three infants from separate ova weighed 1,420, 1,530, and 1,440 g, whereas the two derived from the same ovum weighed 990 and 860 g. Although the birthweights of these two monozygotic infants were nearly the same, remarkable differences have been observed. Marked discordance in size may also complicate pregnancies in which each fetus arose from a separate ovum. For example, dizygotic twins, one of whom weighed 2,300 and the other 785 g, were delivered

at Parkland Hospital (Fig. 34–15). Both survived but one remains appreciably smaller than the other.

MALFORMATIONS

Kohl and Casey (1975) identified major malformations in 2.12 percent of twin infants, compared to 1.05 percent of singletons delivered during the same times and in the same institutions. The frequency of minor malformation was 4.13 percent in twins, compared to 2.45 percent in singletons. It appears, on the basis of the studies of Kohl and Casey, and others, that the frequency of malformations is nearly twice as great in twins as in singletons. Malformations are more common among monozygotic than dizygotic twins.

Persistent or chronic hydramnios is more likely to be associated with fetal anomalies of one or both twins. Hashimoto and colleagues (1986) identified subjectively increased amnionic fluid in a fourth of twin pregnancies. In half, hydramnios at midpregnancy was transient and all of these fetuses were normal. In the 10 pregnancies in which hydramnios persisted, 9 fetuses had anomalies.

Genetic Amniocentesis

Several debilities are best detected by examination of amnionic fluid. Most often there are two amnionic sacs and ideally fluid should be obtained separately from each. The use of real-time sonography is recommended to identify a site for penetration into one amnionic sac adjacent to one fetus. After fluid is obtained a marker consisting of a few milliliters of dilute indigo carmine is injected. After a few minutes the second fetus is located by ultrasonic examination, and the procedure is repeated. The fluid, if from the second sac, should not be discolored by indigo carmine. The complication rate of amniocentesis in one series appeared to be minimal (Elias and co-workers, 1980).

SUBSEQUENT DEVELOPMENT

Nilsen and associates (1984) in Norway evaluated the physical and intellectual development of male twins at 18 years of age. Compared to singletons, twice as many twins were found to be physically unfit for military service. They attributed this to preterm delivery rather than twinning per se. General intelligence did not appear to differ between twins and singletons.

The pattern of subsequent development of the growth-retarded infant from a multifetal pregnancy varies. Babson and Phillips (1973), for example, reported that in monozygotic twins whose birthweights differed on the average by 36 percent, the twin who was smaller at birth remained so into adulthood. In their experience, height, weight, head circumference, and apparently intelligence often remained superior in the twin who weighed more at birth. Fujikura and Froelich (1974), however, failed to confirm a significant difference in mental and motor scores.

Baigts and co-workers (1982) studied monozygotic twins who, at age 17, had body frames that were quite similar but who were remarkably dissimilar in bodyweight, as they were at birth. The investigators documented hyperplasia of adipocytes in the heavier twin compared to her lighter sister. Their investigations excluded genetic differences (through identity of the HLA system and eight other genetic markers) and nutritional differences except for intrauterine nutrition. They suggested that perhaps, in human beings, early (intrauterine) nutritional status helps to determine adipocyte numbers and the way the body evolves.

TABLE 34–2. AVERAGE LENGTH OF GESTATION FOR PREGNANCIES WITH KNOWN TIME OF OVULATION AND 20 OR MORE WEEKS GESTATION

No. of Fetuses	No. of Pregnancies	Weeks Completed[a]
Singleton	82	39
Twins	21	35
Triplets	5	33
Quadruplets	3	29

[a] Calculated from 2 weeks before ovulation.
From Caspi and co-workers: Br J Obstet Gynaecol 83:967, 1976.

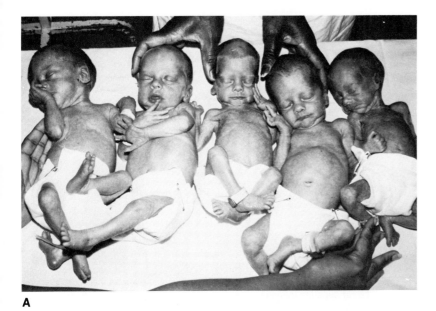

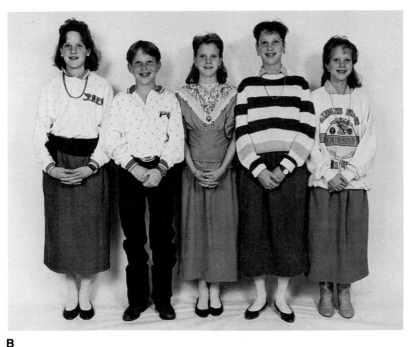

Figure 34–14. A. Davis quintuplets at 3 weeks of age. The first, second, and fourth infants from the left each arose from separate ova, while the third and fifth infants are from the same ovum. **B.** Davis quintuplets at 12½ years of age.

It seems reasonable to summarize that each fetus involved in a multifetal pregnancy is at some disadvantage from the outset compared to the fetus who is the sole occupant of the uterus. Those who do survive the newborn period may suffer some form of physical, intellectual, or psychological handicap, with the smaller usually at greater risk. Fortunately, in most instances their handicap will be minimal.

SUPERFETATION AND SUPERFECUNDATION

In superfetation, an interval as long as or longer than an ovulatory cycle intervenes between fertilizations. Superfetation has not been unequivocally demonstrated in women, although it is theoretically possible until the uterine cavity is obliterated by the fusion of the decidua capsularis to the decidua vera. Thus, superfetation requires ovulation during the course of an established pregnancy, as yet unproven in humans though known to occur in mares. Most authorities believe that the alleged cases of human superfetation result from marked inequality in growth and development of fetuses of the same gestational age, as described above.

Superfecundation refers to the fertilization of two ova within a short period of time but not at the same coitus, nor necessarily by sperm from the same man. It may be that, in many cases, twin ova are not fertilized by sperm from the same ejaculate, but the fact can be demonstrated only in exceptional circumstances.

It is interesting that John Archer, the first physician to receive a medical degree in America, related in 1810 that a white woman after intercourse with both a white and a black man

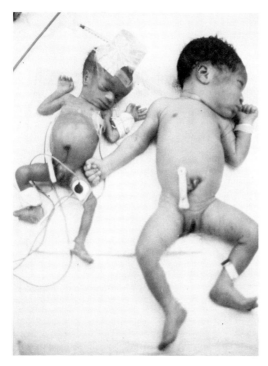

Figure 34–15. Marked discordance in dizygotic twins. The larger infant weighed 2,300 g, appropriate for gestational age. The markedly growth-retarded smaller infant weighed only 785 g. Both thrived.

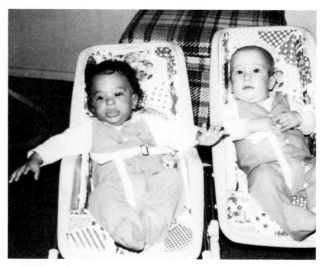

Figure 34–16. An example of dizygotic twin boys as the consequence of superfecundation. (*Courtesy of Dr. David Harris.*)

within a short period was delivered of twins, one of whom was white and the other mulatto. A similar instance of superfecundation, documented by Harris (1982), is demonstrated in Figure 34–16. The mother was raped on the tenth day of her menstrual cycle and had intercourse one week later with her husband. She went into labor very near term and was delivered vaginally of a mulatto infant whose blood type was A and a white infant whose blood type was O. The blood type of both the mother and her husband was O. HLA typing was not done. Terasaki and co-workers (1978) have described the use of HLA typing to establish that dizygotic twins were sired by different fathers.

MATERNAL ADAPTATION

In general, the degree of maternal physiological change is greater with multiple fetuses than when there is a single fetus. For example, the average increase in maternal blood volume induced during pregnancy with twin fetuses is significantly larger (Pritchard, 1965; Rovinsky and Jaffin, 1966). Whereas the average increase in late pregnancy is about 40 to 50 percent with a single fetus, the mean increase amounts to about 50 to 60 percent with twins. Measurements in the same woman late in one pregnancy with a single fetus and at the same time in another pregnancy with twins are indicative that, typically, the maternal blood volume is about 500 mL greater with twins (Pritchard and Chase, unpublished). Interestingly, the average blood loss with vaginal delivery of 25 sets of twins averaged 935 mL, or nearly 500 mL more than with the delivery of a single fetus. Both the remarkable increase in maternal blood volume and the increased iron and folate requirements imposed by a second fetus predisposed to a greater prevalence of maternal anemia.

Veille and associates (1985) used M-mode echocardiography to assess cardiac function in women with twin pregnancies. As expected, cardiac output was increased compared to singleton pregnancy; however, end-diastolic ventricular dimensions were the same. During the third trimester, cardiac output was increased as a result of both increased pulse rate and increased stroke volume. Stroke volume was higher by virtue of an increased shortening fraction, which suggests increased contractility.

The larger size of the uterus with multiple fetuses intensifies the variety of mechanical effects that occur during pregnancy. The uterus and its contents may achieve a volume of 10 L or more and weigh in excess of 20 pounds! Especially with monozygotic twins, rapid accumulation of grossly excessive amounts of amnionic fluid—that is, *acute hydramnios*—may develop. In these circumstances, it is easy to envision appreciable compression and displacement of many of the abdominal viscera as well as the lungs by the elevated diaphragm. The size and weight of the very large uterus may preclude more than a very sedentary existence for the woman pregnant with multiple fetuses.

At times, in pregnancies with multiple fetuses further complicated by hydramnios, maternal renal function may become seriously impaired, most likely as the consequence of obstructive uropathy. Quigley and Cruikshank (1977), for example, described two pregnancies with twin fetuses plus acute and severe hydramnios in which oliguria and azotemia developed. Maternal urine output and plasma creatinine levels promptly returned to normal after delivery. In the case of gross hydramnios, transabdominal amniocentesis may be employed to provide relief for the mother and, it is hoped, to allow the pregnancy to continue (see Chap. 31, p. 554). Unfortunately, the hydramnios is often characterized by acute onset remote from term and by rapid reaccumulation following amniocentesis.

The various stresses of pregnancy on the mother and the likelihood of serious maternal complications almost invariably will be greater with multiple fetuses than with a singleton. This should be taken into account, especially when counseling the women whose health is compromised and who is recognized early in pregnancy to have multiple fetuses, or, for that matter, who is not pregnant but is considering treatment with agents used to induce ovulation.

MANAGEMENT OF PREGNANCIES WITH MULTIPLE FETUSES

To reduce perinatal mortality and morbidity significantly in pregnancies complicated by twins, it is imperative that (1) delivery of markedly preterm infants be prevented, (2) failure of one or both fetuses to thrive be identified and fetuses so afflicted be delivered before they become moribund, (3) fetal trauma during labor and delivery be eliminated, and (4) expert neonatal care be provided continuously from the time of birth. The first major step in fulfilling these goals is to identify early the pregnancy complicated by multiple fetuses. As soon as multiple fetuses (or embryos) are identified, meaningful efforts should be directed toward providing the fetuses with the best intrauterine environment possible.

DIET

The requirements for calories, protein, minerals, vitamins, and essential fatty acids are further increased in women with multiple fetuses. The Recommended Dietary Allowances made by the Food and Nutrition Board of the National Research Council for uncomplicated pregnancy should not only be met but in most instances exceeded (see Chap. 14, p. 263). Therefore, consumption of energy sources should be increased by another 300 kcal per day. Failure of the mother to gain weight equal at least to the weight of the pregnancy products, both fetal and maternal, is clear proof that the diet being consumed is inadequate. Iron supplementation is essential; 60 to 100 mg per day is recommended. Folic acid, 1 mg per day, may prove beneficial, although a diet adequate in protein provided from a variety of sources should supply adequate amounts of folate. Rigid sodium restriction is not beneficial.

MATERNAL HYPERTENSION

Pregnancy-induced and pregnancy-aggravated hypertension are much more likely to develop in pregnancies with multiple fetuses (see Chap. 35, p. 654). Hypertension not only develops more often but tends to develop earlier and be more severe. In their analysis of 341 twin pregnancies at the University of Colorado, Thompson and associates (1987) reported that 18 percent were complicated by pregnancy-induced hypertension. Long and Oats (1987) reported this complication in 26 percent of 642 twin pregnancies: 35 percent in nulliparas and 20 percent in multiparas. Importantly, of those developing preeclampsia, it was identified before 37 weeks in nearly 70 percent of twin pregnancies, whereas it was found in only 25 percent of women with singleton pregnancies. In 284 twin pregnancies cared for at Parkland Hospital over a 22-month period, the incidence of pregnancy-induced hypertension was 17 percent compared to 11 percent in 25,579 women with a singleton fetus (K. Leveno, unpublished).

In singleton pregnancies, pregnancy-induced hypertension occurs less commonly in parous than in nulliparous women. This is not true, however, in multifetal pregnancies. At Parkland Hospital, pregnancy-induced hypertension developed in 10 percent of 204 multiparious women with twins, compared to 6 percent of 15,412 multiparas women with singleton gestations.

ANTEPARTUM SURVEILLANCE OF FETAL GROWTH

As discussed earlier (p. 640), fetal growth is slower in multifetal pregnancies than in singleton gestations. Leveno and colleagues (1979) reported an average difference of 3.5 mm in biparietal diameters between 16 and 40 weeks gestation. An important aspect of ultrasonic assessment of fetal growth is to identify *discordancy* between twin-pairs. This most often is defined by using the larger twin as the index. Brown and colleagues (1987) chose a 15 percent or greater birthweight difference and reported a 25 percent incidence of discordancy. Erkkola (1985) described outcomes in 460 twin pregnancies, and by defining discordancy as a 25 percent difference in birthweight, reported an incidence of 9 percent. **The perinatal mortality rate with discordancy of this magnitude was 97 per 1,000 compared to 37 per 1,000 for nondiscordant twin-pairs.**

Although some investigators have claimed that discordancy can be identified by disparity between biparietal diameters in twin-pairs, more recent evidence is consistent with the view that measurement of abdominal circumference is a more sensitive marker. Using an intrapair difference in abdominal circumference of 20 mm or greater to predict 20 percent discordant growth, Storlazzi and colleagues (1987) reported a sensitivity of 80 percent, specificity of 85 percent, positive predictive value of 62 percent, and negative predictive value of 93 percent. When the abdominal circumference was correlated with the biparietal diameter to estimate fetal weight, the positive predictive value was now 80 percent while the negative predictive remained 93 percent. Brown and colleagues (1987) found that the abdominal circumference was superior to the biparietal diameter to predict discordancy; however, they emphasized that more experience was needed before these techniques can be used alone to make clinical decisions. They also encouraged the liberal use of tests to establish fetal pulmonary maturation before effecting preterm delivery for suspected growth discordancy.

Doppler Velocimetry

Differences of vascular resistance estimated by blood flow velocity using continuous-wave Doppler ultrasound have been used to assess well-being in twin fetuses (Farmakides and colleagues, 1985; Giles and associates, 1985). Gerson and co-workers (1988) reported that the relationship between the systolic/diastolic ratio and gestational age is the same in singleton and twin pregnancies. As discussed in Chapter 15 (p. 288), increased vascular resistance with diminished diastolic blood flow velocity may accompany retarded fetal growth. Gerson and co-workers (1987) used duplex Doppler ultrasound to measure umbilical venous blood flow and arterial systolic-diastolic velocity ratios. Normal studies correctly predicted 44 of 45 concordant twin-pairs, and abnormal values, especially of the umbilical artery, correctly predicted 9 of 11 sets of discordant twins. These techniques need more extensive evaluation before they are applied routinely in clinical settings.

PREVENTION OF PRETERM DELIVERY

Several techniques have been applied to try to prolong gestation in multifetal pregnancy. These include considerable bed rest, especially through hospitalization, prophylactic administration of β-mimetic drugs, prophylactic cervical cerclage, and repeated injections of progestins.

Bed Rest

Several authors, but certainly not all, have claimed bed rest to be beneficial to twin fetuses, presumably by enhancing uterine perfusion and perhaps by reducing the physical forces that might act deleteriously on the cervix to hasten effacement and dilatation. Unfortunately, the benefits from bed rest are difficult to evaluate. Several of the experiences are summarized below:

Laursen (1973) concluded from his study of 315 pregnancies with twins that rest in the hospital will prolong pregnancy, increase birthweights significantly, and reduce perinatal mortality. Komáromy and Lampé (1977), on the basis of a large study in Hungary, reached the same conclusions as Laursen. They identified the following differences between their hospitalized and nonhospitalized groups, respectively: mean gestational age at delivery 37.4 weeks compared to 35.0 weeks; mean birthweight 2,580 g compared to 1,970 g; and a frequency of weights below 2,500 g of 43 percent compared to 77 percent. At any gestational age, the birthweights of twins whose mothers had been hospitalized averaged appreciably more than did the birthweights of those whose mothers were not hospitalized. Finally, perinatal mortality was 6 percent for twins in the hospitalized group compared to 22 percent in the nonhospitalized group.

In Malmö, Sweden, during a 4-year period 88 percent of all twin pregnancies were identified by routine ultrasonic scanning during the second trimester. For those with twins, rest at home was prescribed until 28 weeks, at which time hospitalization was urged. The average hospital stay for the 86 women who participated was 55 days. If undelivered at 36 weeks, they were discharged from the hospital, provided that the course of pregnancy was completely normal. With few exceptions, the pregnancies were not allowed to go beyond 38 weeks gestation. The perinatal mortality rate was 0.6 percent, the same as for singleton pregnancies, whereas for twin gestations not so managed the perinatal mortality rate was 10.5 percent (Persson and colleagues, 1979). Similar decreases in perinatal mortality have been reported by Hartikainen-Sorri and co-workers (1983). They favor hospitalization by the 28th week at least and doubt if it is of much value begun after the 34th week.

Gilstrap and colleagues (1987) reported salutary effects of prophylactic hospitalization in 132 twin pregnancies born to military dependents and personnel at Wilford Hall USAF Medical Center from 1977 through 1985. Half of the women agreed to recommended hospitalization before 28 weeks gestation, and their pregnancy outcomes were compared to those of women who declined early admission and who were hospitalized after 28 weeks or if a complication was identified. Perinatal mortality was significantly lower in the hospitalized group (2.2 percent) compared to that in nonhospitalized women (8.5 percent). This difference was attributed principally to the increased incidence of very low birthweight infants (less than 1,000 g) born to women who were not routinely hospitalized at 28 weeks (0 versus 12 percent).

O'Connor and co-workers (1981) reported their experiences with twin pregnancies in which routine hospitalization during the last trimester was replaced by "intensive antenatal care" provided in a special clinic. The abolition of routine hospitalization was not followed by an increase in perinatal mortality, which was 4 percent, or preterm delivery or fetal growth retardation. Their program of intensive antenatal care did emphasize the importance of rest at home throughout pregnancy (at least 10 hours at night and 2 hours in the afternoon!) Moreover, "routine" hospitalization during the third trimester averaged only about 2 weeks per pregnancy, usually for pregnancy-induced or pregnancy-aggravated hypertension.

Saunders and associates (1985) randomized routine admission at 32 weeks of 212 women with multifetal pregnancies. They reported that preterm delivery actually was more common in the hospitalized group (30 versus 19 percent); however, perinatal mortality was less for the women who were hospitalized (2.3 versus 3.8 percent).

In recent years at Parkland Hospital, women with twins have been offered hospitalization on the High-Risk Pregnancy Unit as early as the onset of the third trimester. Although women so hospitalized lead a very sedentary life, they are not strictly confined to bed. In a preliminary audit, 144 of 166 women so admitted stayed either until delivery or until they had completed 38 weeks gestation. The duration of stay was 2 weeks or more for 90 percent and 4 weeks or more for 68 percent. Perinatal mortality for the 288 fetuses was 2.8 percent. Of the eight perinatal deaths, five were stillborn. Four of the five stillbirths were the consequence of fetal death or at very near 40 weeks gestation. The fifth dead fetus had expired remote from term before admittance to the hospital. Of the three neonatal deaths, only one was the consequence of prematurity. Another infant delivered at term died from a malformation incompatible with life (sirenomelia). The third infant born at 39 weeks died soon after birth with intracranial hemorrhage and renal cortical necrosis. The co-twin had died in utero some time before delivery, which may have triggered the apparent consumptive coagulopathy.

The fetal outcome was much worse in the 22 instances in which the undelivered mothers soon left the High-Risk Pregnancy Unit, against medical advice. Seven of the 44 fetuses, or 15.9 percent, died!

It is our impression that especially for the typically socioeconomically deprived women cared for at Parkland Hospital, the benefits to be derived from hospitalization during the third trimester of twin gestation include increased birthweight, decreased frequency of severe preeclampsia, and lowered perinatal mortality.

β-Mimetics

At least two double-blind trials of β-mimetics in twin pregnancies failed to demonstrate a significant reduction in the rates of preterm delivery (Marivate and associates, 1977, O'Connor and co-workers, 1979). However, Skjaerris and Åberg (1982) claimed a reduction in the frequency of threatened preterm labor among pregnant women with twins who were given oral terbutaline prophylactically. Six of 25 so treated were subsequently treated intravenously with terbutaline, compared to 15 to 25 who had not received any oral terbutaline.

Cerclage

No significant reduction in preterm delivery or perinatal deaths has been demonstrated from prophylactic cervical cerclage (Weekes, 1977; Dor and associates, 1982).

Progestin Administration

Serial injections of 17-hydroxyprogesterone caproate (Delalutin) to prevent premature delivery has been advocated by some. However, Hartikainen-Sorri and co-workers (1980) identified no benefits from its administration throughout the third trimester of pregnancy to women with twins. The length of gestation, birthweight, and neonatal outcomes were quite similar in the treated and the control groups.

Pulmonary Maturation

According to Leveno and associates (1984), pulmonary maturation measured by determination of the lecithin-sphingomyelin ratio is usually synchronous in twins. Moreover, while this ratio usually exceeds 2 by 36 weeks in singleton pregnancies, it often does so by about 32 weeks in multifetal pregnancy. In some cases, however, there may be marked disparity of pulmonary function. We observed the L/S ratio with quintuplets to vary from less than 2 for the largest infant, who weighed 1,530 g at 32 weeks gestation and was of appropriate size for his gestational age, to greater than 5 for the severely growth-retarded smallest infant, who weighed 860 g. The largest infant developed appreciable respiratory distress, whereas the smallest infant did not.

Prolonged Gestation

Experiences at Malmö, Sweden, and at Parkland Hospital cited above under the section on Bed Rest suggest, at least, that twin fetuses may fail to thrive in utero when the pregnancy persists for 40 weeks or more. Unfortunately, there are not sufficient data to identify clearly the risks versus possible benefits from allowing a twin pregnancy to continue beyond 39 weeks.

DELIVERY OF MULTIPLE FETUSES

LABOR

Many complications of labor and delivery, including preterm labor, uterine dysfunction, abnormal presentations, prolapse of the umbilical cord, premature separation of the placenta, and immediate postpartum hemorrhage, are encountered much more often with multiple fetuses. Therefore, the conduct of labor and delivery with multiple fetuses is an excellent test of the skills of the obstetrical team that provides care for the woman and her fetuses.

For women pregnant with multiple fetuses, to date the capability is limited for safely arresting preterm labor once labor is established. Pulmonary edema associated with the use of β-mimetic agents, for example, has been observed much more frequently in twin gestations. Bed rest, if not already being used, should be instituted. The problems of preterm labor and attempts to arrest it and of lack of fetal lung maturity and possible modification by corticosteroid therapy are considered elsewhere (see Chap. 38, p. 756).

As soon as it is apparent that labor has been established, a number of steps are immediately taken to help assure a satisfactory outcome:

1. An appropriately trained obstetrical attendant remains with the mother throughout labor. The fetal heart rates are monitored frequently, using any system of monitoring that, in that particular situation, will promptly identify significant changes in fetal heart rates. At times, continuous external electronic monitoring or, if the membranes are ruptured and the cervix dilated, evaluation of both fetuses by simultaneous internal and external electronic monitoring may prove quite satisfactory.
2. One liter of compatible whole blood or its equivalent in blood fractions is readily available.
3. A well-functioning intravenous infusion system capable of delivering fluid rapidly into the mother is established. In the absence of hemorrhage or metabolic disturbance during labor, lactated Ringer's with aqueous dextrose solution is infused at a rate of 60 to 120 mL per hour.
4. Two obstetricians are immediately available and both are scrubbed and gowned at delivery. At least one should be skilled in intrauterine identification of fetal parts and intrauterine manipulation of the fetus.
5. An experienced anesthesiologist is immediately available in the event that intrauterine manipulation or cesarean section is necessary.
6. For *each* fetus, two people, one of whom is skilled in resuscitation and care of newborn infants, are appropriately informed of the case and remain immediately available.
7. The delivery area is immediately operational and provides adequate space for all members of the team to work effectively. Moreover, the site is appropriately equipped to take care of all possible maternal problems plus resuscitation and maintenance of each infant.

Presentation and Position

With twins, all possible combinations of fetal positions may be encountered. Either or both fetuses may present by the vertex, breech, or shoulder. Compound, face, brow, and footling breech presentation are relatively common, especially when the fetuses are quite small or there is excess amnionic fluid, or maternal parity is high. Prolapse of the cord is fairly common in these circumstances.

Often the presentation can be ascertained by real-time sonography. However, if any confusion about the relationship of the twins to each other or to the maternal pelvis persists, a single anteroposterior x-ray of the abdomen may be very helpful.

Induction or Stimulation of Labor

Even though labor, in general, is shorter with twins, both rupture of the membranes without effective labor and prolonged inefficient labor with or without previous rupture of the membranes do develop. These problems are often better handled by cesarean section unless there is little hope of salvaging the infants because of their gross immaturity. Occasionally, termination of pregnancy is desirable before the spontaneous onset of labor, as, for example, with severe pregnancy-induced hypertension. In these circumstances if the presenting part is well fixed in the pelvis and the cervix dilated somewhat, amniotomy often will initiate labor and effect delivery. There is no reluctance by some obstetricians to give oxytocin by dilute intravenous infusion to initiate or to stimulate labor in pregnancies complicated by multiple fetuses. The risks compared to the benefits to mother and fetuses of oxytocin to initiate and maintain labor and delivery, compared with cesarean section, have not yet been adequately delineated in this circumstance.

Analgesia and Anesthesia

During labor and delivery of multiple fetuses, deciding what to use for analgesia and for anesthesia is unusually difficult because of the frequency of and, in turn, the problems imposed by (1) prematurity, (2) maternal hypertension, (3) desultory labor, (4) need for intrauterine manipulation, and (5) uterine atony and hemorrhage after delivery. There are undesirable effects from most forms of analgesia and anesthesia. Continuous epidural or caudal analgesia in hypertensive women, or those who have hemorrhaged, may cause hypotension, with inadequate perfusion of vital organs, especially the placenta, which is dangerous to both the mother and her fetuses. The woman pregnant with multiple fetuses is even less tolerant of the supine position during labor and delivery. Moreover, conduction analgesia may cause or further aggravate desultory or prolonged labor and will not provide adequate uterine relaxation for intrauterine manipulation when such is necessary.

Epidural analgesia for vaginal delivery of twins has been described by Crawford (1987). In his series of 130 women with twins delivered vaginally, 105 who were given epidural analgesia had a significantly prolonged interval from complete dilatation until delivery. For women with epidural analgesia, the mean was about 90 minutes compared to 30 minutes for those without epidural analgesia. Interestingly, the mean delivery intervals between delivery of the first and second twins were not altered by epidural analgesia.

Use of narcotics, sedatives, and tranquilizers may lead to undue fetal depression if the fetuses are premature. Most forms of general anesthesia used for delivery will also depress the fetuses unless the anesthetic agents are carefully selected and skillfully administered, with little delay between induction of anesthesia and delivery. Paracervical block may cause transient fetal bradycardia.

The combination of thiopental, nitrous oxide plus oxygen, and succinylcholine, appropriately timed and in appropriate doses, has proved satisfactory at Parkland Hospital for cesarean section to deliver twins. Pudendal block skillfully administered along with nitrous oxide plus oxygen provides appreciable relief of pain for spontaneous vaginal delivery. When intrauterine manipulation is necessary, as with internal podalic version, uterine relaxation is probably best accomplished with halothane or one of the other halogenated hydrocarbons. Although halothane provides effective relaxation for intrauterine manipulation, it also commonly leads to an increase in blood loss during the third stage of labor until the uterus regains its ability to contract (see Chap. 17, p. 329).

VAGINAL DELIVERY

In a study of 341 twin pregnancies, Thompson and associates (1987) reported a cephalic presentation in the first twin in 72 percent of cases (Figure 34–17). In only about half of their cases was the presenting fetus the larger of the twin-pair. Typically, this twin bears the major brunt of dilating the cervix and the remaining soft tissues of the birth canal. Seldom with cephalic presentations are there unusual problems with delivery of the first infant. After appropriate episiotomy, spontaneous delivery, or delivery assisted by the use of outlet forceps, usually proves to be quite satisfactory.

When the first fetus presents as a breech, major problems are most likely to develop if (1) the fetus is unusually large and the aftercoming head taxes the capacity of the birth canal, (2) the fetus is quite small so that the extremities and trunk are delivered through a cervix inadequately effaced and dilated for the head to escape easily, or (3) the umbilical cord prolapses. When

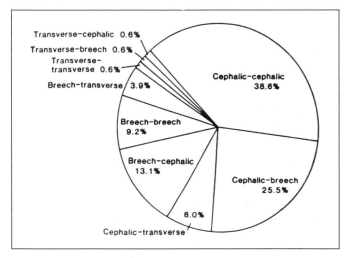

Figure 34–17. Presentation of 341 twin-pairs at delivery. (*From Thompson and colleagues: J Reprod Med 32:328, 1987, with permission.*)

these problems are anticipated or identified, cesarean section will often be the better way to effect delivery, except in those instances in which the fetuses are so immature that they will not survive. Otherwise, breech delivery may be accomplished as described in Chapter 22 (p. 393).

The safety of vaginal delivery for the second nonvertex twin has been reported by Acker (1982), Blickstein (1987), Chervenak (1985), and Rabinovici (1987) and their associates, and by Laros and Dattel (1988). They all stress that vaginal delivery for the second twin presenting as breech and weighing less than 1,500 g has not been studied adequately to warrant its routine application. Unfortunately, cesarean section does not guarantee an atraumatic delivery. Chervenak and co-workers (1985) described a neonatal death caused by trauma during cesarean delivery of a 1,000 g breech second twin through a low vertical uterine incision.

The phenomenon of *locked twins* is rare (once in 817 twin gestations, according to Cohen and co-workers, 1965). In order for locking to occur, the first fetus must present by the breech and the second by the vertex. With descent of the breech through the birth canal, the chin of the first fetus locks in the neck and chin of the second cephalic fetus. If unlocking cannot be effected, either cesarean section before the body is delivered or decapitation must be performed.

DELIVERY OF SECOND TWIN

This demands experience that includes for some cases intrauterine manual dexterity. As soon as the first twin has been delivered, the presenting part of the second twin, his size, and relationship to the birth canal are quickly determined by careful combined abdominal, vaginal, and, at times, intrauterine examination. Intrapartum real-time sonography has proved quite valuable in some cases. If the vertex or the breech is fixed in the birth canal, moderate fundal pressure is applied and the membranes are ruptured. Immediately afterward, the examination is repeated to identify prolapse of the cord or other abnormality. Labor is allowed to resume while the fetal heart rate is monitored closely. With reestablishment of labor there is no need to hasten delivery, unless there is ominous deceleration of the fetal heart rate or persistent bradycardia, or bleeding from the uterus. Bleeding from the uterus indicates placental separation, which can be deleterious to both the fetus and the mother. If contractions do not resume within 10 minutes or so, then dilute oxytocin may be used to stimulate appropriate myometrial activity, which will lead to spontaneous delivery or delivery assisted by outlet forceps.

If the occiput or the breech presents immediately over the pelvic inlet but is not fixed in the birth canal, the presenting part can often be guided into the pelvis with the vaginal hand while a hand on the uterine fundus exerts moderate pressure. More recently, intrapartum external version of the nonvertex second twin has become popular. Using the method shown in Figure 34–18, the fetus who presents with breech or shoulder may be gently converted into a vertex presentation. Once the presenting part is fixed in the pelvic inlet, the membranes are ruptured and delivery is carried out as described above. Chervenak and colleagues (1983) recommend that this be done using epidural analgesia, which is placed before delivery of the first twin. They reported a 71 percent success with attempted versions of transverse presentations and a 73 percent success with breech presentations.

If the occiput or the breech is not over the pelvic inlet and cannot be so positioned by gentle pressure on the presenting

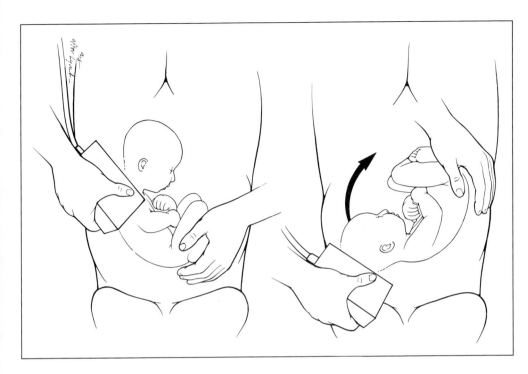

Figure 34–18. External version of second breech twin fetus. Ultrasound transducer is being used to help guide vertex into pelvis. (*Redrawn from Chervenak and colleagues: Obstet Gynecol 62:160, 1983, with permission.*)

part, or if appreciable uterine bleeding develops, the problem of delivery of the second twin assumes serious dimensions. So as to take maximum advantage of the very recently dilated cervix before the uterus contracts and the cervix retracts, procrastination must be avoided. An obstetrician skilled in intrauterine manipulation of the fetus and an anesthesiologist skilled in providing anesthesia that will effectively relax the uterus are essential for vaginal delivery with a favorable outcome. Prompt delivery of the second fetus by cesarean section is the better choice if there is no one present who is skilled in the performance of internal podalic version (described below) or if anesthesia that will provide effective uterine relaxation is not immediately available.

In the past, the interval between delivery of the first and second twins was commonly cited to be safest if less than 15 to 30 minutes. Subsequently, as shown by Rayburn and colleagues (1984), as well as others, if continuous fetal monitoring is employed, there is a good outcome even if this interval is longer. Of 115 twin-pairs at 34 weeks or more gestation, the mean interval between delivery of twins was 21 minutes, but it ranged from 1 to 134 minutes. In 61 percent, the interval was 15 minutes or less. Importantly, there was no excess trauma or evidence for fetal depression in those born after the 15-minute interval. As expected, the cesarean section rate was much higher if the interval was more than 15 minutes (18 percent) than if the interval was less than 15 minutes (3 percent).

Rarely, in the circumstances where one of the fetuses has been expelled very preterm and uterine activity then ceased, the pregnancy has been allowed to continue with delivery of another fetus days to even many weeks later. Cardwell and associates (1988) described delivery of triplets at 24, 24½, and 26 weeks. Most observations indicate that procrastination in the delivery of the second fetus has rarely proved advantageous to that fetus.

Regardless of the route of delivery, respiratory distress is more common in the second twin. Although suspected, the reason never has been proved to be depression of the second twin at birth. Arnold and colleagues (1987) studied 221 twin-pairs delivered between 27 and 36 weeks, and confirmed the higher incidence of respiratory distress in the second twin. They documented this to be independent of malpresentation or depression at birth. Since the incidence was identical in twin-pairs delivered by cesarean section without labor, they hypothesized that the first twin benefited disproportionately from the salutary effects of labor if delivered vaginally.

INTERNAL PODALIC VERSION

Through careful abdominal, vaginal, and intrauterine examinations, the various parts of the fetus are located. (Typically, if the buttocks and legs are toward the left side of the mother, or right side of the obstetrician, a sterile intrauterine examining glove that covers the gown to above the elbow is drawn over the right hand and arm.) The membranes are ruptured, both feet are accurately identified and grasped, and only then are they gently pulled toward the birth canal (Fig. 34–19). With the other hand applied to the abdomen, the vertex is simultaneously gently elevated toward the mother's sternum (Fig. 34–20). An episiotomy is made or extended whenever more room is needed for uterine and vaginal manipulation. The legs of the fetus are slowly drawn through the birth canal until the buttocks are visible anteriorly just beyond the maternal symphysis. A moist, warm towel is applied to the buttocks and gentle traction is continued until the lower thirds of both scapulas are visible. Next, the trunk is slowly rotated with gentle traction until the shoulder and arm on one side of the fetus are delivered. The rotation of the fetal trunk is now gently reversed to deliver the other arm and shoulder into the vagina. The after-coming head may now be delivered either by simultaneous suprapubic external pressure to flex the head and gentle traction applied to the trunk, or by use of Piper forceps (see Chap. 22, p. 397).

The cord is clamped promptly with two clamps on the placental side to identify it as the cord of the second infant. The

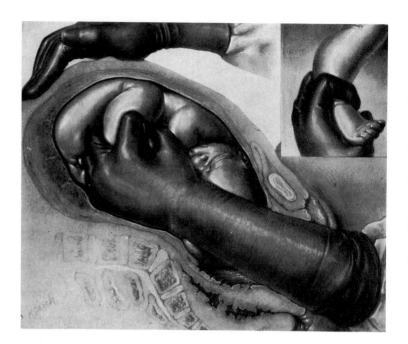

Figure 34–19. Internal podalic version. Note the use of the long version gloves, which, unfortunately, are not currently available.

placenta or placentas are immediately delivered by manual removal, if necessary. The uterus is promptly explored for defects and for retained pregnancy products. As these steps are being carried out, the uterine-relaxing anesthetic agent is discontinued, and just as soon as uterine exploration has been completed, oxytocin is administered through the intravenous infusion system. Fundal massage or, preferably, manual compression of the uterus with one hand in the vagina against the lower uterine segment and the other transabdominally over the uterine fundus, is applied to hasten and enhance myometrial contraction and retraction.

The cervix, vagina, periurethral region, vulva, and peri-

neum are carefully inspected. Lacerations likely to bleed are repaired along with the episiotomy.

CESAREAN SECTION

There has been a trend recently for delivery of multiple fetuses by cesarean section. For example, Chervenak and colleagues (1985) reported a rate of 36 percent while Thompson and associates (1987) delivered 46 percent of both twins by cesarean section and another 9 percent of second twins by this route. At Parkland Hospital recently, 47 percent of the twins cared for in the High-Risk Pregnancy Unit, as cited previously, were deliv-

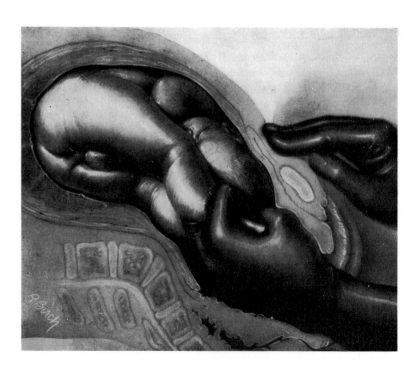

Figure 34–20. Internal podalic version. Upward pressure on head is applied as downward traction is exerted on feet.

ered by cesarean section. The most common indication was presentation other than cephalic by one or both fetuses. Other major indications were hypotonic uterine dysfunction, hypertension induced or aggravated by the pregnancy, fetal distress, gross discordance in the size of the fetuses, with the smaller fetus the first candidate for vaginal delivery, and prolapsed cord.

The use of cesarean delivery has been recommended by Barrett and associates (1982) for any twin expected to have a birthweight of less than 1,500 g. However, not enough cesarean deliveries were performed among the pregnancy outcomes reviewed by them to verify unequivocally benefits from cesarean delivery. Welch and co-workers (1983) could demonstrate no improvement in neonatal outcome from cesarean section for delivery of infants who weighed less than 2,000 g. Unfortunately, nearly one half of the cases were previously undiagnosed and overall twin mortality was 16 percent.

Twin fetuses create other unusual problems. The mother is likely to be even less tolerant of the supine position and therefore it is important to rotate her position so as to move the uterus and its contents to one side (see Chap. 7, p. 147). A vertical incision in the lower uterine segment may be advantageous. If a fetus lies traversely and the arms are inadvertently delivered first, it is much easier and safer to extend upward the vertical uterine incision than to extend a transverse incision.

It is important that the uterus be well contracted during completion of the cesarean section and thereafter. Remarkable blood loss from the uterus may be concealed within the uterus and vagina and beneath the operating drapes during the time taken to close the incisions.

At times, attempts to deliver the second twin vaginally, after vaginal delivery of first twin, may be not only unwise but even impossible, as, for instance, when the second fetus is much larger than the first and in the breech position or in a transverse lie; or, even more perplexing, when the cervix promptly contracts and thickens after delivery of the first infant and does not subsequently dilate. Prompt cesarean section may be performed in these circumstances and the infant saved. The Colorado group (Thompson and colleagues, 1987) reported that 16 percent of second twins were delivered by cesarean section following vaginal delivery of the first twin. Of 29 such operations, 19 were for malpresentation, 5 for fetal distress, 4 for prolapsed cord, and 1 for arrested labor. Undoubtedly, maternal and perinatal morbidity and mortality would be appreciably less if in these circumstances cesarean section had been used at the outset.

THREE OR MORE FETUSES

All of the problems of twin gestation are intensified remarkably by the presence of even more fetuses. With vaginal delivery, the first infant is commonly born spontaneously or with little manipulation. However, subsequent infants are delivered according to the presenting part and may require complicated obstetrical maneuvers, such as total breech extraction or internal podalic version, followed by breech extraction, or may necessitate the addition of cesarean delivery. Associated with malposition of the fetuses is an increased incidence of cord prolapse and fetal collision. Moreover, reduced placental perfusion and hemorrhage from separating placentas are likely during the intrapartum period. Therefore, speed of delivery is very important.

Holcberg and associates (1982) reported outcomes in 31 triplet gestations. The overall perinatal mortality rate was 312 per 1,000 and common complications included preterm labor (97 percent), pregnancy-induced hypertension (46 percent), anemia (29 percent), and postpartum hemorrhage (13 percent). They attributed improved perinatal outcome over recent years to early diagnosis, prolonged hospitalization, and planned delivery by cesarean section. Loucopoulos and Jewelewicz (1982) also reported salutary results under these circumstances and recommend routine administration of betamethasone at 26 to 28 weeks to induce fetal pulmonary maturation. They cautioned against vaginal delivery if the operator is inexperienced.

For all of the above reasons, we believe that delivery of pregnancies complicated by the presence of three or more fetuses is probably better accomplished by cesarean section, reserving vaginal delivery for those circumstances in which the fetuses are markedly immature or maternal complications make cesarean section hazardous to the mother.

POSTPARTUM

The kinds of puerperal complications following the birth of multiple fetuses are not different from those after the birth of a single infant; their frequency and intensity, however, are often enhanced. The mother may be troubled by considerable physical fatigue and at times emotional depression from the increased physical work and other responsibilities associated with the care of two or more infants.

Troublesome uterine bleeding later in the puerperium seems to be increased. Perhaps this is the consequence of impairment of involution and of reepithelialization of the larger placental implantation site. In general, supplemental iron should be continued for some weeks after delivery.

SELECTIVE TERMINATION

With high-resolution sonography, three and more fetuses can be identified at very early stages of pregnancy and fetal structural anomalies may be visualized precisely in many instances. With such diagnostic capabilities, it is not surprising that investigators have considered reducing the number of fetuses in some multifetal pregnancies in order to prevent many of the maternal and fetal complications described above. Certainly, the possibility of preventing the birth of one grossly abnormal fetus of a twin pair has been considered since Bang and co-workers (1975) reported the first successful karyotyping of twin fetuses. In fact, they predicted the inevitable medical and ethical dilemmas created by finding one abnormal and one normal fetus.

TWINS DISCORDANT FOR ABNORMALITIES

With the identification of twin pregnancy discordant for structural or genetic abnormalities, three options are available: (1) abortion of both fetuses, (2) selective termination of the abnormal fetus, or (3) continuation of the pregnancy. Continuing the pregnancy most often results in delivery of a normal infant along with an abnormal one who may require tremendous familial and societal support. In other cases, the abnormal twin may jeopardize the normal one—for example, by pathological hydramnios developing around an anencephalic twin.

Identification of the Abnormal Fetus

Amnionic fluid can be obtained from each sac at the time of genetic amniocentesis (see Chap. 15, p. 278). This may be accomplished by injecting dye into the first sac sampled. Additionally, careful mapping of uterine structure, placental location, and fetal relationships are established so that if no dye is found later, the two fetuses still can be identified.

Maternal and Fetal Outcome

When selective termination is performed, maternal morbidity is uncommon. However, outcome of the surviving normal fetus is not universally good. Of 14 twin pregnancies in which selective reduction was attempted, only 6 of 13 normal fetuses went to term, 1 was aborted, and 6 were delivered preterm with 3 survivors (Table 34–3).

GRAND MULTIFETAL PREGNANCIES

The incidence of multifetal pregnancies with extremely large numbers of fetuses has increased during the past two decades because of newer techniques for ovulation induction and the placement of multiple embryos during in vitro fertilization (Evans and associates, 1988; Levene, 1986). Those with four or more embryos are referred to commonly as *grand multifetal pregnancies*. Unfortunately, pregnancy often is desperately desired and a successful outcome may be impossible. In contrast to one abnormal fetus of a twin pair, the fetuses most often are normal, but their number likely precludes successful pregnancy outcome unless selective termination is performed.

Maternal and Fetal Outcome

Selective reduction of quadruplet, quintuplet, and octuplet pregnancies to either twin or triplet pregnancies has been reported (Berkowitz, 1988; Brandes, 1987; Evans, 1988; Kanhai, 1986, and their colleagues). There were no maternal complications. Twenty-four out of a possible 45 infants survived to be delivered at or after 30 weeks gestation. In one case reported by Evans and co-workers (1988), one fetus of the remaining pair was anephric (Potter syndrome), and the associated oliguria may have caused spontaneous abortion at 20 weeks.

INFORMED CONSENT FOR SELECTIVE TERMINATION

With twin pregnancies, there is always the risk of identifying one abnormal fetus. Prior to any attempt at prenatal diagnosis, genetic counseling should be conducted with this information provided to the couple (see Chap. 32, p. 580). Specific risks that are common to selective termination include, but are not limited to, (1) abortion of the remaining fetus(es), (2) abortion of the wrong (normal) fetus in twins, (3) retention of genetic or structurally abnormal fetuses after a reduction in number, (4) damage without death to a fetus, (5) preterm labor complicating pregnancies with the remaining fetus(es), (6) development of discordant twins or growth-retarded fetuses, or (7) maternal infection, hemorrhage, or possible disseminated intravascular coagulopathy owing to retained products of conception.

TECHNIQUES FOR SELECTIVE TERMINATION

Many of the techniques that have been used are presented in Table 34–3. These procedures are not easily performed, and the

TABLE 34–3. SELECTIVE TERMINATION IN TWIN PREGNANCIES DISCORDANT FOR STRUCTURAL AND GENETIC ABNORMALITIES

Author	Disorder	Technique	Maternal Morbidity	Outcome of Normal Fetus
Åberg (1978)	Hurler syndrome	Cardiac puncture	None	Preterm labor and delivery at 33 weeks—survived
Antsaklis (1984)	Thalassemia major	Cardiac puncture—exsanguination plus calcium gluconate	None	Preterm labor and delivery at 34 weeks—survived
Beck (1980)	Trisomy 21	Hysterotomy	None	Liveborn at 38 weeks
Berg (1984)	Trisomy 21	Cardiac puncture and injection	None	Preterm labor and delivery at 28 weeks—survived
Kerenyi (1981)	Trisomy 21	Cardiac puncture—exsanguination	None	Liveborn at 40 weeks
Mulcahy (1984)	Hemophilia A	Amnionic fluid and tissue removal	None	Not reported
Petres (1981)	Tay-Sachs	Cardiac puncture—air embolism	None	Preterm labor and delivery at 28 weeks—neonatal death
Redwine (1984)	Tay-Sachs	Cardiac puncture—air embolism	None	Liveborn at 37 weeks
Redwine (1986)	Trisomy 21	Cardiac puncture—air embolism	None	Liveborn at 37 weeks
	Trisomy 21	As above	None	Preterm labor and delivery at 27 weeks—neonatal death
Rodeck (1982)	Microcephaly	Air embolism of umbilical vein using fetoscope	None	Liveborn at 36 weeks
	Hemophilia A	As above	None	Preterm labor and delivery at 30 weeks—neonatal death
	Spina bifida	As above	None	Liveborn at 38 weeks—survived
Totals	14 pregnancies		None	9 of 13 survivors: term (6); preterm, viable (3); preterm, neonatal death (3); spontaneous abortion (1); unreported (1)

technical skills and equipment required are formidable. They should be attempted only by those experienced in amniocentesis and high-resolution sonography. In addition, Dumez and Oury (1986) reported a transcervical suction technique to remove selectively any fetuses with a crown–rump length of up to 40 mm, or about 11 weeks. They reported that 9 of 11 pregnancies had gone to term. Berkowitz and colleagues (1988) described 11 women with 12 multifetal pregnancies and 32 embryos. Selective reduction was performed by transcervical aspiration or by fetal thoracic injection with potassium chloride. Three women spontaneously aborted but a total of 15 fetuses born after 30 weeks survived.

ETHICS OF SELECTIVE TERMINATION

The confusion surrounding the ethical dilemmas associated with selective termination is best illustrated by listing its various names: (1) selective termination, (2) selective reduction, (3) selective fetocide, (4) selective embryocide, (5) selective abortion, and (6) selective birth. The ethical problems associated with these techniques are almost limitless and the interested reader is referred to the excellent review by Evans and co-workers (1988). In two earlier publications, the ethical problems associated with selective termination of one abnormal fetus of a twin pair was discussed (Motulsky and Murray, 1983; Silber, 1981).

REFERENCES

Abert A, Mitelman F, Cantz M, Gehler J: Cardiac puncture of fetus with Hurler's disease avoiding abortion of unaffected co-twin. Lancet 2:991, 1978

Acker D, Lieberman M, Holbrook H, James O, Phillippe M, Edelin KC: Delivery of second twin. Obstet Gynecol 59:710, 1982

Andrews MC, Muasher SJ, Levy DL, Jones HW Jr, Garcia JE, Rosenwaks Z, Jones GS, Acosta AA: An analysis of the obstetric outcome of 125 consecutive pregnancies conceived in vitro and resulting in 100 deliveries. Am J Obstet Gynecol 154:848, 1986

Antsaklis A, Politis J, Karagiannopoulos C, Kaskarelis D: Selective survival of only the healthy fetus following prenatal diagnosis of thalassemia major in binovular twin gestation. Prenat Diagn 4:289, 1984

Archer J: Observations showing that a white woman, by intercourse with a white man and a Negro man, may conceive twins, one of which shall be white and the other mulatto. Medical Repository, 3d Hexade 1:319, 1810

Arnold C, McLean FH, Kramer MS, Usher RH: Respiratory distress syndrome in second-born versus first-born twins: A matched case-control analysis. N Engl J Med 317:1121, 1987

Azubuike JC: Multiple births in Igbo women. Br J Obstet Gynaecol 89:77, 1982

Babson SG, Phillips DS: Growth and development of twins dissimilar in size at birth. N Engl J Med 289:937, 1973

Baigts F, Dunica S, Fumeron F, Apfelbaum M: Birthweight difference in monozygous twins followed by differences in development of body weight. Lancet 2:274, 1982

Bang J, Nielsen H, Philip J: Prenatal karyotyping of twins by ultrasonically guided amniocentesis. Am J Obstet Gynecol 123:695, 1975

Barrett JM, Staggs SM, Van Hooydonk JE, Growdon JH, Killam AP, Boehm FM: The effect of type of delivery upon neonatal outcome in premature twins. Am J Obstet Gynecol 143:360, 1982

Beck L, Terinde R, Dolff M: Zwillingsschwangerschaft mit frier trisomie 21 eines kindes: Sectio parva mit entfernung des kracken und spätere guburt des gesunden kindes. Gerburts Frauenheilk 40:397, 1980

Benirschke K: Personal communication, 1983

Benirschke K: Chimerism and mosaicism—Two different entities. In Wynn RM (ed): Obstetrics and Gynecology Annual, New York, Appleton, 1974, p 33

Benirschke K, Kim CK: Multiple pregnancy. N Engl J Med 288:1276, 1329, 1973

Berg D, Baumgärtner M, Köring K, Lohe KJ, Zander J: Selektive entfernung eines zwillings mit trisomie 21 durch sectio parva in der 21: Schwangerschaftswoche und spätere spontangebrut des gesunden zweiten zwillings. Gerburts Frauenheilk 44:563, 1984

Berkowitz RL, Lynch L, Chitkara U, Wilkins IA, Mehalek KE, Alvarez E: Selective reduction of multifetal pregnancies in the first trimester. N Engl J Med 318:1043, 1988

Blickstein I, Schwartz-Shoham Z, Lancet M, Borenstein R: Vaginal delivery of the second twin in breech presentation. Obstet Gynecol 68:774, 1987

Brandes JM, Itskovitz J, Timor-Tritsch IE, Drugan A, Frydman R: Reduction of the number of embryos in a multiple pregnancy: Quintuplet to triplet. Fertil Steril 48:326, 1987

Brown CEL, Guzick DS, Leveno KJ, Santos-Ramos R, Whalley PJ: Prediction of discordant twins using ultrasound measurement of biparietal diameter and abdominal perimeter. Obstet Gynecol 70:667, 1987

Bulmer MG: The effect of parental age, parity, and duration of marriage on the twinning rate. Ann Hum Genet 23:454, 1959

Bulmer MG: The familial incidence of twinning. Ann Hum Genet 24:1, 1960

Cardwell MS, Caple P, Baker CL: Triplet pregnancy with delivery on three separate days. Obstet Gynecol 71:448, 1988

Caspi E, Ronen J, Schreyer P, Goldberg MD: The outcome of pregnancy after gonadotropin therapy. Br J Obstet Gynaecol 83:967, 1976

Chervenak FA, Johnson RE, Berkowitz RL, Hobbins JC: Intrapartum external version of the second twin. Obstet Gynecol 62:160, 1983

Chervenak FA, Johnson RE, Youcha S, Hobbins JC, Berkowitz RL: Intrapartum management of twin gestation. Obstet Gynecol 65:119, 1985

Cohen M, Kohl SG, Rosenthal AH: Fetal interlocking complicating twin gestation. Am J Obstet Gynecol 91:407, 1965

Crawford JS: A prospective study of 200 consecutive twin deliveries. Anaesthesia 42:33, 1987

Dallas Times Herald: 50-year-old Michigan woman thrilled by unexpected twins. January 6, 1982

Derom C, Derom R, Vlietinck R, Van den Berghe H, Thiery M: Increased monozygotic twinning rate after ovulation induction. Lancet 1:1237, 1987

Dor J, Shalev J, Masiach J, Blankstein J, Serr DM: Elective cervical suture of twin pregnancies diagnosed ultrasonically in the first trimester following induced ovulation. Gynecol Obstet Invest 13:55, 1982

Dumez Y, Oury JF: Method for first trimester selective abortion in multiple pregnancy. Contrib Gynecol Obstet 15:50, 1986

Elias S, Gerbie AB, Simpson JL, Nadler HL, Sabagha RE, Shkolnik A: Genetic amniocentesis in twin gestations. Am J Obstet Gynecol 138:169, 1980

Erkkola R, Ala-Mello S, Piiroinen O, Kero P, Sillanpää M: Growth discordancy in twin pregnancies: A risk factor not detected by measurements of biparietal diameter. Obstet Gynecol 66:203, 1985

Evans MI, Fletcher JC, Zador IE, Newton BW, Quigg MH, Struyk CD: Selective first-trimester termination in octuplet and quadruplet pregnancies: Clinical and ethical issues. Obstet Gynecol 71:289, 1988

Farmakides G, Schulman H, Saldana LR, Bracero LA, Fleischer A, Rochelson B: Surveillance of twin pregnancy with umbilical aterial velocimetry. Am J Obstet Gynecol 153:789, 1985

Fujikura T, Froelich LA: Mental and motor development in monozygotic co-twins with dissimilar birth weights. Pediatrics 53:884, 1974

Garrett WJ, Carey HM, Steven LM, Climie CR, Osborn RA: A case of nonuplet pregnancy. Aust N Z J Obstet Gynaecol 16:93, 1976

Gerson A, Johnson A, Wallace D, Bottalico J, Weiner S, Bolognese R: Umbilical arterial systolic/diastolic values in normal twin gestation. Obstet Gynecol 72:205, 1988

Gerson AG, Wallace DM, Bridgens NK, Ashmead GG, Weiner S, Bolognese RJ: Duplex Doppler ultrasound in the evaluation of growth in twin pregnancies. Obstet Gynecol 70:419, 1987

Giles WB, Trudinger BJ, Cook CM: Fetal umbilical artery flow velocity-time waveforms in twin pregnancies. Br J Obstet Gynaecol 92:490, 1985

Gilstrap LC III, Hauth JC, Hankins GDV, Beck A: Twins: Prophylactic hospitalization and ward rest at early gestational age. Obstet Gynecol 69:578, 1987

Harlap S: Ovulation induction and congenital malformations. Lancet 2:961, 1976

Harris DW: Letter to the editors. J Reprod Med 27:39, 1982

Hartikainen-Sorri AL, Kauppila A, Risto T: Inefficacy of 17α-hydroxyprogesterone caproate in the prevention of prematurity in twin pregnancy. Obstet Gynecol 56:692, 1980

Hartikainen-Sorri AL, Kauppila A, Tuimala R, Koivisto M: Factors related to improved outcomes for twins. Acta Obstet Gynecol Scand 62:23, 1983

Hashimoto B, Callen PW, Filly RA, Laros RK: Ultrasound evaluation of polyhydramnios and twin pregnancy. Am J Obstet Gynecol 154:1069, 1986

Holcberg G, Biale Y, Lewenthal H, Insler V: Outcome of pregnancy in 31 triplet gestations. Obstet Gynecol 59:472, 1982

Jewelewicz R, Vande Wiele RL: Management of multifetal gestation. Contemp Ob/Gyn 6:59, 1975

Kanhai HHH, Van Rijssel EJC, Meerman RJ, Bennebroek-Gravenhorst J: Selective termination in quintuplet pregnancy during first trimester. Lancet 2:1447, 1986

Keilani Z, Clarke PC, Kitau MJ: The significance of raised maternal plasma alphafetoprotein in twin pregnancy. Br J Obstet Gynaecol 85:510, 1978

Kerehyi TD, Chitkara U: Selective birth in twin pregnancy with discordancy for Down's syndrome. N Engl J Med 304:1525, 1981

Knox G, Morley D: Twinning in Yoruba women. J Obstet Gynaecol Br Emp 67:981, 1960

Kohl SG, Casey G: Twin gestation. Mt Sinai J Med 42:523, 1975

Komaromy B, Lampe L: The value of bed rest in twin pregnancies. Int J Gynaecol Obstet 15:262, 1977

Koontz WL, Herbert WNP, Seeds JW, Cefalo RC: Ultrasonography in the antepartum diagnosis of conjoined twins. J Reprod Med 28:627, 1983

Kossoff G, Garrett WJ, Radovanovich G: Ultrasonic examination of a nonuplet pregnancy. Aust N Z J Obstet Gynaecol 16:203, 1976

Laros RK, Dattel BJ: Management of twin pregnancy: The vaginal route is still safe. Am J Obstet Gynecol 158:1330, 1988

Laursen B: Twin pregnancy: The value of prophylactic rest in bed and the risk involved. Acta Obstet Gynecol Scand 52:367, 1973

Levene MI: Grand multiple pregnancies and demand for neonatal intensive care. Lancet 2:347, 1986

Leveno KJ, Quirk JG, Whalley PJ, Herbert WNP, Trubey R: Fetal lung maturation in twin gestation. Am J Obstet Gynecol 148:405, 1984

Leveno KJ, Santos-Ramos R, Duenhoelter JH, Reisch JS, Whalley PJ: Sonar cephalometry in twins: A table of biparietal diameters for normal twin fetuses and a comparison with singletons. Am J Obstet Gynecol 135:727, 1979

Long PA, Oats JN: Preeclampsia in twin pregnancy—Severity and pathogenesis. Aust NZ J Obstet Gynaecol 27:1, 1987

Loucopoulos A, Jewelewicz R: Management of multifetal pregnancies: Sixteen years' experience at the Sloane Hospital for Women. Am J Obstet Gynecol 143:902, 1982

MacGillivray I: Epidemiology of twin pregnancy. Semin Perinatol 10:4, 1986

MacGillivray I: Twin pregnancies. In Wynn RM (ed): Obstetrics and Gynecology Annual. New York, Appleton, 1978 p 135

Mägiste M, Von Schenck H, Sjöberg NO, Thorell JI, Åberg A: Screening for detecting twins. Am J Obstet Gynecol 126:697, 1976

Marivate M, De Villiers KO, Fairbrother P: Effect of prophylactic outpatient administration of fenoterol on the time of onset of spontaneous labour and fetal growth rate in twin pregnancy. Am J Obstet Gynecol 128:707, 1977

Mashiach S, Ben-Rafael Z, Dor J, Serr DM: Triplet pregnancy in uterus didelphys with delivery interval of 72 days. Obstet Gynecol 58:519, 1981

McKeown T, Record RG: Observations on foetal growth in multiple pregnancy in man. J Endocrinol 5:387, 1952

McLeod FN, McCoy DR: Monoamniotic twins with an unusual cord complication. Br J Obstet Gynaecol 88:774, 1981

Motulsky AG, Murray J: Will prenatal diagnosis with selective abortion affect society's attitude toward the handicapped? Prog Clin Biol Res 128:277, 1983

Mulcahy MT, Roberman B: Chorion biopsy, cytogenetic diagnosis and selective termination in a twin pregnancy at risk of haemophilia. Lancet 2:866, 1984

Myrianthopoulos NC: An epidemiologic survey of twins in a large prospectively studied population. Am J Hum Genet 22:611, 1970

Naeye RL: Organ abnormalities in a human parabiotic syndrome. Am J Pathol 46:829, 1965

Naeye RL, Tafari N, Judge D, Marboe CC: Twins: Causes of perinatal death in 12 United States cities and one African city. Am J Obstet Gynecol 31:267, 1978

Newman HH: The Physiology of Twinning. Chicago, Chicago University Press, 1923

Nilsen ST, Bergsjø P, Nome S: Male twins at birth and 18 years later. Br J Obstet Gynaecol 91:122, 1984

O'Connor MC, Arias E, Royston JP, Dalrymple IJ: The merits of special antenatal care for twin pregnancies. Br J Obstet Gynaecol 88:222, 1981

O'Connor MC, Murphy H, Dalrymple IJ: Double blind trial of ritodrine and placebo in twin pregnancy. Br J Obstet Gynaecol 86:706, 1979

Pedersen IK, Philips J, Sele V, Starup J: Monozygotic twins with dissimilar phenotypes and chromosome complements. Acta Obstet Gynecol Scand 59:459, 1980

Persson P-H, Grennert L, Gennser G, Kullander S: On improved outcome of twin pregnancies. Acta Obstet Gynecol Scand 58:3, 1979

Petres RE, Redwine FO: Selective birth in twin pregnancy. N Engl J Med 305:1218, 1981

Pettersson F, Smedby B, Lindmark G: Outcome of twin birth: Review of 1636 children born in twin birth. Acta Paediatr Scand 64:473, 1976

Powers WF: Twin pregnancy: Complications and treatment. Obstet Gynecol 42:795, 1973

Pritchard JA: Changes in blood volume during pregnancy. Anesthesiology 26:393, 1965

Quigley MM, Cruikshank DP: Polyhydramnios and acute renal failure. J Reprod Med 19:92, 1977

Rabinovici J, Barkai G, Reichman B, Serr DM, Mashiach S: Randomized management of the second nonvertex twin: Vaginal delivery or cesarean section. Am J Obstet Gynecol 156:52, 1987

Rayburn WF, Lavin JP Jr, Miodovnik M, Varner MW: Multiple gestation: Time interval between delivery of the first and second twins. Obstet Gynecol 63:502, 1984

Recommended Dietary Allowances, 9th rev ed: National Research Council, National Academy of Sciences, 1979

Redwine FO, Hays PM: Selective birth. Semin Perinatol 10:73, 1986

Redwine FO, Petres RE: Selective birth in a case of twins discordant for Tay-Sachs disease. Acta Genet Med Gemellol 33:35, 1984

Robertson EG, Neer KJ: Placental injection studies in twin gestation. Am J Obstet Gynecol 147:170, 1983

Robinson HP, Caines JS: Sonar evidence of early pregnancy failure in patients with twin conceptions. Br J Obstet Gynaecol 84:22, 1977

Rodeck CH, Mibashan RS, Abramowicz T, Campbell S: Selective feticide of the affected twin by fetoscopic air embolism. Prenat Diagn 2:189, 1982

Romero R, Duffy TP, Berkowitz RL, Chang E, Hobbins JC: Prolongation of a preterm pregnancy complicated by death of a single twin in utero and disseminated intravascular coagulation: Effects of treatment with heparin. N Engl J Med 310:772, 1984

Rothman KJ: Fetal loss, twinning and birthweight after oral-contraceptive use. N Engl J Med 297:468, 1977

Rovinsky JJ, Jaffin H: Cardiovascular hemodynamics in pregnancy: III. Cardiac rate, stroke volume, total peripheral resistance, and central blood volume in multiple pregnancy: Synthesis of results. Am J Obstet Gynecol 95:787, 1966

Saunders MC, Dick JS, Brown IM: The effects of hospital admission for bed rest on the duration of twin pregnancy: A randomised trial. Lancet 2:793, 1985

Schmidt R, Nitowsky HM, Sobel EH: Monozygotic twins discordant for sex. Pediatr Res 8:395, 1974

Silber TJ: Amniocentesis and selective abortion. Pediatr Ann 10:31, 1981

Skjaerris J, Åberg A: Prevention of prematurity in twin pregnancy by orally administered terbutaline. Acta Obstet Gynecol Scand Suppl 108:39, 1982

Spellacy WN, Buhi WC, Birk SA: Human placental lactogen levels in multiple pregnancies. Obstet Gynecol 52:210, 1978

Storlazzi E, Vintzileos AM, Campbell WA, Nochimson DJ, Weinbaum PJ: Ultrasonic diagnosis of discordant fetal growth in twin gestations. Obstet Gynecol 69:363, 1987

Strandskov HH, Edelen EW, Siemens GJ: Analysis of the sex ratios among single and plural births in the total "white" and "colored" U.S. populations. Am J Phys Anthropol 4:491, 1946

Tan KL, Goon SM, Salmon Y, Wee JH: Conjoined twins. Acta Obstet Gynecol Scand 50:373, 1971

Terasaki PI, Gjertson D, Bernoco D, Perdue S, Mickey MR, Bond J: Twins with two different fathers identified by HLA. N Engl J Med 299:590, 1978

Thiery M, Dhont M, Vandekerckhove D: Serum HCG and HPL in twin pregnancies. Acta Obstet Gynecol Scand 56:495, 1976

Thompson SA, Lyons TL, Makowski EL: Outcomes of twin gestations at the University of Colorado Health Sciences Center, 1973–1983. J Reprod Med 32:328, 1987

Varma TR: Ultrasound evidence of early pregnancy failure in patients with multiple conceptions. Br J Obstet Gynaecol 86:290, 1979

Veille JC, Morton MJ, Burry KJ: Maternal cardiovascular adaptations to twin pregnancy. Am J Obstet Gynecol 153:261, 1985

Waterhouse JAH: Twinning in twin pedigrees. Br J Soc Med 4:197, 1950

Weekes AR, Menzies DN, deBoer CH: The relative efficacy of bed rest, cervical suture, and no treatment in the management of twin pregnancy. Br J Obstet Gynaecol 84:161, 1977

Welch R, Mariona FC, Agronow SJ: Obstetrical outcome of very low and low birthweight twins. Proceedings of the Third Annual Scientific Meeting of the Society of Perinatal Obstetricians, San Antonio, TX. January, 1983

White C, Wyshak G: Inheritance in human dizgotic twinning. N Engl J Med 271:1003, 1964

Hypertensive Disorders in Pregnancy

In some mysterious way the presence of chorionic villi in certain women incites vasospasm and hypertension. Moreover, to effect a cure the chorionic villi must be expelled or surgically removed. The vasospastic hypertensive state and related pathological changes somehow induced by the presence of chorionic villi may not be so great that pregnancy need be terminated prematurely. (Pritchard, 1978)

Pregnancy may induce hypertension in previously normotensive women or aggravate hypertension in women who have underlying hypertension. Generalized edema, proteinuria, or both, often accompany hypertension induced or aggravated by pregnancy. Convulsions also may develop in association with hypertension, especially if hypertension is ignored.

Hypertensive disorders complicating pregnancy are common and form one of the great triad, along with hemorrhage and infection, that continues to be responsible for a large number of maternal deaths in the United States. Kaunitz and colleagues (1985) reported that 20 percent of 2,067 maternal deaths from 1974 to 1978 were caused by hypertensive diseases. With improved prenatal care and a rational approach to the management of hypertensive disorders complicating pregnancy, dramatic declines in maternal mortality rates have been reported more recently (Lehmann and colleagues, 1987; Rochat and coworkers, 1988; Sachs and associates, 1987). Hypertensive disorders are also an important cause of perinatal mortality and severe morbidity.

How pregnancy per se incites or aggravates hypertensive vascular disease remains unsolved despite decades of intensive research, and these disorders remain among the most important unsolved problems in obstetrics. The large toll of maternal and infant lives that may be taken by hypertension induced or aggravated by pregnancy is most often preventable. Good prenatal supervision followed by appropriate treatment will ameliorate many cases sufficiently that the outcomes for both fetus-infant and mother are satisfactory.

GENERAL CONSIDERATIONS

CLASSIFICATION AND DIFFERENTIAL DIAGNOSIS

TERMINOLOGY

The unsatisfactory term *toxemia of pregnancy* has been applied variably to any or all disorders in which hypertension, proteinuria, or edema was present during pregnancy or the puerperium, and to other disorders, as well. The American College of Obstetricians and Gynecologists (1986) proposed the following definitions and classification of hypertension that develop during pregnancy or the puerperium. *Hypertension* is defined as a diastolic blood pressure of at least 90 mm Hg or a systolic pressure of at least 140 mm Hg, or a rise in diastolic pressure of at least 15 mm Hg or in systolic pressure of 30 mm Hg. The blood pressure readings cited must be obtained on at least two occasions 6 hours or more apart. *Preeclampsia* is the development of hypertension with proteinuria, edema, or both, induced by pregnancy after the 20th week of gestation, and sometimes earlier when there are extensive hydatidiform changes in the chorionic villi (see Chap. 31, p. 544). *Eclampsia* is diagnosed when convulsions, not caused by any coincidental neurological disease such as epilepsy, develop in a woman who also has clinical criteria for preeclampsia. *Superimposed preeclampsia or eclampsia* is defined as preeclampsia or eclampsia that develops in a woman with chronic hypertensive vascular or renal disease. *Chronic hypertensive disease* is defined as persistent hypertension, of whatever cause, antedating pregnancy or detected before the 20th week of gestation in the absence of hydatidiform mole or extensive molar change, or hypertension that persists beyond 6 weeks postpartum.

Unfortunately, not all women can be categorized neatly as having one of these syndromes. Earlier, the Committee on Terminology of the American College of Obstetricians and Gynecologists (Hughes, 1972) sought to improve the diagnosis of preeclampsia. It defined *gestational hypertension* as elevated blood pressure that develops during the latter half of pregnancy or during the first 24 hours following delivery. It is not accompanied by other evidence for preeclampsia or chronic underlying hypertension, and it disappears within 10 days of delivery. It is unclear whether this is mild or incipient preeclampsia forestalled by delivery or if it is a marker for latent chronic hypertension, but we agree with Chesley (1985) that it is probably the latter. If so, then it is certainly inappropriately classified. *Gestational edema* is characterized by abnormal fluid retention that regresses after delivery, hypertension never developing. Rarely, so-called *gestational proteinuria* exceeds 300 mg per day in the absence of hypertension, edema, renal infection, or other known renovascular disease. These terms are not used by many teaching centers in the United States.

Because of the confusion that has arisen from these classifications of hypertensive disorders complicating pregnancy, we have made the modifications shown in Table 35–1. Our principal reason was to separate hypertension that is in some way induced by pregnancy from hypertension that merely coexists with it. At the same time it needs to be emphasized that chronic underlying hypertension will increase the frequency and intensity of superimposed preeclampsia.

PREGNANCY-INDUCED HYPERTENSION

As shown in Table 35–1, pregnancy-induced hypertension is divided into three categories: (1) hypertension alone, (2) preeclampsia, and (3) eclampsia. The diagnosis of *preeclampsia* is based on the development of hypertension plus proteinuria or of edema that is generalized and overt, or both. *Eclampsia* is characterized typically by the abnormalities just cited with the addition of convulsions that are precipitated by the pregnancy-induced hypertension. Only rarely does preeclampsia develop earlier than 20 weeks gestation, and then usually in cases of hydatidiform mole or appreciable molar degeneration (see Chap. 31, p. 544). As emphasized by Chesley (1985), preeclampsia is almost exclusively a disease of nulliparous women. Although it more commonly affects the woman who is at the extremes of reproductive age, that is, teenagers or those older than 35 years, preeclampsia in the latter usually reflects pregnancy-aggravated hypertension. Pregnancy-induced hypertension is occasionally seen in the multipara with multifetal pregnancy or fetal hydrops. Pregnancy-aggravated hypertension is common in multiparas with vascular diseases, including chronic essential hypertension and diabetes mellitus, or those with coexisting renal disease.

DIAGNOSIS

The diagnosis of pregnancy-induced hypertension is usually straightforward and made when the *blood pressure* is 140/90 mm Hg or greater. Although it has been accepted in the past that an increase of 30 mm Hg systolic or 15 mm Hg diastolic over baseline values on at least two occasions 6 or more hours apart be considered as possibly diagnostic for pregnancy-induced hypertension, these vague criteria have little clinical value. Such findings, however, may increase the risk for pregnancy-induced

hypertension. Villar and colleagues (1988) reported that 31 percent of young primigravidas with a 15 mm Hg rise in diastolic blood pressure developed pregnancy-induced hypertension. For those without such a rise, the incidence was 15 percent. For women in whom the systolic pressure rose 30 mm Hg or more, 42 percent developed pregnancy-induced hypertension, compared to an incidence of 17 percent in women without such a rise. If both systolic and diastolic pressure increased as defined, then 56 percent developed pregnancy-induced hypertension, compared to only 15 percent if there had not been a preceding elevation. Midpregnancy blood pressure elevations more likely forecast future chronic hypertension (Chesley and Sibai, 1988).

Although the diagnosis of preeclampsia has traditionally required the identification of pregnancy-induced hypertension plus proteinuria *or* generalized edema, many authorities concur that edema, even of the hands and face, is such a common finding in pregnant women that its presence should not validate the diagnosis of preeclampsia any more than its absence should preclude the diagnosis. Indeed, Robertson (1971) reported that one third of women developed generalized edema by the 38th week of pregnancy, and he was unable to show a significant statistical correlation between edema and hypertension. In another study, Friedman and Neff (1976) identified perinatal mortality for women with edema alone to be 30 percent lower than for the general population. Thus, the edema of preeclampsia is pathological and not dependent, and it usually involves the face and hands and persists even after arising. A useful indicator of nondependent edema is the woman's complaint that her rings have become too tight.

Proteinuria is an important sign of preeclampsia and Chesley (1985) rightfully concluded that the diagnosis is questionable in its absence. Proteinuria is defined as 300 mg or more of urinary protein during a 24-hour period or 100 mg per dL or more in at least two random urine specimens collected 6 hours or more apart. The degree of proteinuria may fluctuate widely over any 24-hour period, even in severe cases. Therefore, a single random sample may fail to detect significant proteinuria.

The combination of proteinuria and hypertension during pregnancy markedly increases the risk of perinatal mortality. McCartney and co-workers (1971), in their extensive study of renal biopsy specimens obtained from hypertensive pregnant women, invariably found that proteinuria was present when the glomerular lesion considered to be characteristic of preeclampsia was evident. It is important to recognize, however, that both proteinuria and alterations of glomerular histology develop late in the course of pregnancy-induced hypertension. Actually, preeclampsia becomes evident clinically only near the end of an often protracted, covert pathophysiological process that may begin 3 to 4 months before hypertension develops.

The fact that *perinatal mortality* is increased by maternal hypertension is evident from an analysis of data collected from the Collaborative Perinatal Project conducted by the National Institute of Neurologic and Communicative Disorders and Stroke (Friedman and Neff, 1976). From this 13-year prospective study, 38,636 pregnancies were selected for analysis because they satisfied the following criteria: (1) antepartum care before the 28th week of pregnancy, (2) singleton fetus, (3) four or more antepartum visits, and (4) date of last menstrual period known. In Table 35–2 the fetal death rate for these pregnancies is presented in relation to the presence or absence of hypertension, proteinuria, or both. Hypertension alone, defined by diastolic blood pressure of 95 mm Hg or greater, was associated with a threefold rise in the fetal death rate. Worsening hypertension,

---

TABLE 35–1. CLASSIFICATION OF HYPERTENSIVE DISORDERS COMPLICATING PREGNANCY

Pregnancy-induced hypertension
Hypertension that develops as a consequence of pregnancy, and regresses postpartum
1. Hypertension without proteinuria or pathological edema
2. Preeclampsia—with proteinuria and/or pathological edema
   a. Mild
   b. Severe
3. Eclampsia—proteinuria and/or pathological edema along with convulsions

Pregnancy-aggravated hypertension
Underlying hypertension worsened by pregnancy
1. Superimposed preeclampsia
2. Superimposed eclampsia

Coincidental hypertension
Chronic underlying hypertension that antecedes pregnancy or persists postpartum

TABLE 35–2. FETAL DEATH RATE PER 1,000 BIRTHS ANALYZED ACCORDING TO DIASTOLIC PRESSURE AND PROTEINURIA COMBINATIONS

Diastolic Blood Pressure (mm Hg)	Proteinuria						
	None	*Trace*	*1+*	*2+*	*3+*	*4+*	*Total*
< 65	15.5[a]	13.6	6.2	—	—	—	13.6
65–74	9.3	8.1	5.6	32.9[a]	41.5	—	8.8
75–84	6.2	7.4	6.2	19.2[a]	—	—	6.8
85–94	8.7	9.3	23.6[a]	—	22.3	—	10.2
95–104	19.2[a]	17.4[a]	26.7[a]	55.8[a]	115.3[a]	143[a]	25.2
105 +	20.5[a]	27.9[a]	62.6[a]	68.8[a]	125.2[a]	111[a]	41.5[a]
Total	8.6	9.5	12.9	23.2[a]	42.0[a]	57[a]	

[a] $P < 0.01$.

Modified from Friedman and Neff: In Lindheimer, Katz, and Zuspan (eds): Hypertension in Pregnancy. New York, Wiley, 1976.

TABLE 35–3. INDICATORS OF SEVERITY OF PREGNANCY-INDUCED HYPERTENSION

Abnormality	Mild	Severe
Diastolic blood pressure	< 100 mg Hg	110 mm Hg or higher
Proteinuria	Trace to 1+	Persistent 2+ or more
Headache	Absent	Present
Visual disturbances	Absent	Present
Upper abdominal pain	Absent	Present
Oliguria	Absent	Present
Convulsions	Absent	Present (eclampsia)
Serum creatinine	Normal	Elevated
Thrombocytopenia	Absent	Present
Hyperbilirubinemia	Absent	Present
Liver enzyme elevation	Minimal	Marked
Fetal growth retardation	Absent	Obvious
Pulmonary edema	Absent	Present

especially if accompanied by proteinuria, was more ominous. Conversely, proteinuria without hypertension had little overall influence on the frequency of fetal death.

In an evaluation of the causes of perinatal deaths in this same study population, Naeye and Friedman (1979) concluded that 70 percent of the excess deaths were due to three disorders: large placental infarcts, markedly small placental size, and abruptio placentae. They further stated, "All three [disorders] display microscopic placental lesions [that] are the consequence of reduced uteroplacental perfusion. . . ." Uteroplacental perfusion is considered in detail on page 671.

When the blood pressure rises appreciably during the latter half of pregnancy it is dangerous, to the fetus especially, not to take action simply because proteinuria has not yet developed. As Chesley (1985) emphasizes, 10 percent of eclamptic seizures develop before overt proteinuria. Thus, from pathophysiological and epidemiological perspectives it is clear that hypertension is the *sine qua non* of preeclampsia and that from the moment blood pressure begins to rise, both mother and fetus are at increased risk. Once the blood pressure exceeds 140/90 mm Hg, pregnancy-induced hypertension is diagnosed and the woman treated accordingly. Proteinuria is a sign of worsening hypertensive disease, specifically preeclampsia, and when it is overt and persistent, the maternal and fetal risks are increased even more.

SEVERITY OF PREGNANCY-INDUCED HYPERTENSION

The severity of pregnancy-induced hypertension is assessed by the frequency and intensity of those abnormalities shown in Table 35–3. At the ouset it is appreciated that many women have clinical syndromes that are somewhere between those two extremes. **Importantly, the differentiation between mild and severe preeclampsia cannot be rigidly pursued since apparently mild disease may rapidly become severe.**

Blood pressure alone is not always a dependable indicator of severity. For example, an adolescent woman may have 3+ proteinuria and convulsions while her blood pressure is 140/85 mm Hg, whereas most women with blood pressures as high as 180/120 mm Hg do not have seizures. Convulsions usually are preceded by an unrelenting severe headache or visual disturbances; thus, these symptoms are considered ominous.

Proteinuria is an important indicator of severity, since, as discussed, it usually develops late in the course of the disease. Certainly, persistent proteinuria of 2+ or more, or 24-hour urinary excretion of 4 g or more, is indicative of severe preeclampsia. With severe renal involvement, glomerular filtration may be impaired and the plasma creatinine concentration become abnormally high, or it may begin to rise.

Epigastric or right upper quadrant pain is presumed to result from hepatocelluar necrosis and edema that stretches Glisson's capsule. The characteristic pain frequently is accompanied by elevation of serum liver enzymes, and usually prompts definitive therapy. Rarely, the pain presages liver rupture, or more correctly, catastrophic rupture of an hepatic subcapsular hematoma.

Thrombocytopenia is characteristic of worsening preeclampsia and is probably caused by microangiopathic hemolysis engendered by severe vasospasm. Whatever the cause, evidence of gross hemolysis from hemoglobinemia, hemoglobinuria, or hyperbilirubinemia is indicative of severe disease.

Other factors indicative of severe hypertension most often are seen in association with pregnancy-aggravated hypertension. These factors include cardiac dysfunction with pulmonary edema as well as fetal growth retardation.

The more profound the frequency and intensity of these aberrations, the more severe the disease and the greater the need for pregnancy termination.

ECLAMPSIA

In neglected or, less often, fulminant cases of pregnancy-induced hypertension, eclampsia may develop. The seizures are grand mal and may first appear before labor, during labor, or postpartum. Any seizure that develops more than 48 hours postpartum is more likely to be the consequence of some other lesion of the central nervous system. However, we have encountered otherwise typical eclampsia up to 10 days postpartum (Brown and colleagues, 1987).

COINCIDENTAL (CHRONIC) HYPERTENSION

All *chronic hypertensive disorders*, regardless of their cause, predispose to the development of superimposed preeclampsia or eclampsia. These disorders can create a difficult problem of diagnosis and management in women who are not seen for prenatal care until after midpregnancy. The diagnosis of coincidental or chronic underlying hypertension is suggested by the following: (1) hypertension (140/90 mm Hg or greater) antecedent to pregnancy, (2) hypertension (140/90 mm Hg or greater) detected before the 20th week of pregnancy (unless there is gestational trophoblastic disease), or (3) persistent hypertension long after delivery. Additional historical factors that help support the diagnosis of coincidental hypertension are multiparity and hypertension complicating a previous pregnancy other than the first one.

When the woman is not seen until the latter half of pregnancy, the diagnosis of chronic hypertension may be difficult to make, because blood pressure usually decreases during the second and early third trimester in chronically hypertensive women. Thus, a woman with chronic vascular disease who is seen for the first time at 20 weeks frequently will have a normal blood pressure. During the third trimester, however, the blood pressure returns to its former hypertensive level, presenting a diagnostic problem: is this chronic (coexistent) hypertensive disease or is it pregnancy-induced hypertension?

There are many diseases and syndromes associated with underlying hypertension that may be encountered during pregnancy. Sims (1970) proposed the modified classification presented in Table 35–4. As is true for the general population of the same age group, essential hypertension is the cause of underlying vascular disease in more than 90 percent of pregnant women. McCartney (1964) studied renal biopsies from women with "clinical preeclampsia," and found chronic glomerulonephritis in 21 percent of the nulliparas and in nearly 70 percent of the multiparas. Fisher and co-workers (1969), however, did not confirm a high prevalence of chronic glomerulonephritis in their own patients.

It must be remembered that chronic hypertension causes morbidity whether the woman is pregnant or not. Specifically, chronic hypertension may lead to premature cardiovascular deterioration and cause cardiac decompensation and cerebrovascular accidents. Intrinsic renal damage also may result from chronic hypertensive disease, but more commonly in young women, hypertension develops as the result of underlying renal parenchymal disease. Dangers specific to pregnancy complicated by chronic hypertension include the risk of pregnancy-aggravated hypertension, which may develop in as many as 20 percent of these women. Additionally, the risk of abruptio placentae is increased substantively, and may be as high as 5 to 10 percent. Moreover, the fetus of the woman with chronic hypertension is at increased risk for growth retardation and intrauterine death.

PREGNANCY-AGGRAVATED HYPERTENSION

In some women with preexisting chronic hypertension there is worsening of hypertension, typically in later pregnancy. Such pregnancy-aggravated hypertension may be accompanied by proteinuria or pathological edema and is then termed *superimposed preeclampsia*. Frequently, superimposed preeclampsia has an onset earlier in pregnancy than pure preeclampsia, and it tends to be quite severe in many cases. Fetal growth retardation commonly accompanies these syndromes.

Diagnosis includes documentation of chronic underlying hypertension. Pregnancy-aggravated hypertension is characterized by at least a 15 mm Hg increase in diastolic or a 30 mm Hg rise in systolic blood pressure, and preeclampsia is accompanied by proteinuria or pathological edema, or both. Indicators of severity shown in Table 35–3 also are used to further characterize these disorders.

INCIDENCE OF PREGNANCY-INDUCED HYPERTENSION

Pregnancy-induced hypertension most often affects nulliparous women. Older women, who accrue an increasing incidence of chronic hypertension with advancing age, are at greater risk of pregnancy-aggravated hypertension or superimposed preeclampsia. Thus, women at either end of the reproductive age in the past have been considered more susceptible. For example, Duenhoelter and colleagues (1975) observed that very young teenage nulligravidas were at appreciably greater risk for preeclampsia. This traditional view is not supported by Guzick and associates (1987) who reported that younger-age women did not have a higher incidence of pregnancy-induced hypertension when parity was considered. Spellacy and associates (1986) reported that women over 40 had a threefold (9.6 versus 2.7 percent) increased incidence of hypertension compared to control women aged 20 to 30 years. Hansen (1986) reviewed several studies and reported a two- to threefold increase in the incidence of preeclampsia in nulliparas over 40 compared to those 25 to 29 years old.

The incidence of preeclampsia is commonly cited to be about 5 percent, although remarkable variations are reported. The incidence is influenced by parity, it is related to racial—and thus to genetic—predisposition, and environmental factors may have a role. From 1983 through 1986, 13 percent of 49,992 women who were delivered at Parkland Hospital were identified as having pregnancy-induced or aggravated hypertension (Cunningham and Leveno, 1987). Almost 70 percent were nulliparous, but only half of these had proteinuria and thus preeclampsia according to Chesley. The effects of parity were striking, since nearly 20 percent of nulliparas had hypertension

TABLE 35–4. UNDERLYING CHRONIC HYPERTENSIVE DISORDERS UPON WHICH PREECLAMPSIA MAY BE SUPERIMPOSED

Hypertensive diseases
Essential familial hypertension
(hypertensive vascular disease)
Renovascular hypertension
Coarctation of the aorta
Primary aldosteronism
Pheochromocytoma

Renal and urinary tract disease
Glomerulonephritis (acute and chronic)
Nephrotic syndrome
Chronic renal insufficiency
Pyelonephritis
Lupus erythematosus
Scleroderma
Periarteritis nodosa
Acute renal failure
Tubuler necrosis
Cortical necrosis
Polycystic kidney disease
Diabetic nephropathy

Modified from Sims: Am J Obstet Gynecol 107:154, 1970.

antepartum, intrapartum, or in the puerperium, compared to an incidence of 7 percent in multiparas.

Racial and genetic factors are important since they contribute to the incidence of underlying chronic hypertension. We analyzed pregnancy outcomes of 5,622 nulliparas delivered at Parkland Hospital in 1986, and 18 percent of white, 20 percent of Hispanic, and 22 percent of black women had hypertension complicating pregnancy (Cunningham and Leveno, 1987). Again, about half of these women had preeclampsia defined as proteinuric hypertension. The incidence of hypertension in multiparas during pregnancy was 6.2 percent in white, 6.6 in Hispanic, and 8.5 percent in black women, reflecting the increased incidence of underlying hypertension in blacks. Slightly more than half of these multiparous women with hypertension also had proteinuria and thus superimposed preeclampsia.

The tendency for preeclampsia–eclampsia is inherited. Chesley and Cooper (1986) studied the sisters, daughters, granddaughters, and daughters-in-law of eclamptic women delivered at the Margaret Hague Maternity Hospital during the 49-year period 1935 to 1984. They concluded that preeclampsia–eclampsia is highly heritable and that the single-gene model, with a frequency of 0.25, best explained their observations; however, multifactorial inheritance also was considered possible (see Chap. 32, p. 574).

Although Chesley (1974) disagrees, some have concluded that socioeconomically advantaged women have a lesser incidence of preeclampsia, even after racial factors are controlled. Regardless, when a socially affluent woman develops preeclampsia, it can be as severe and life-threatening as preeclampsia in a ghetto teenager.

In general, eclampsia is preventable, and it has become less common in the United States, since most women now receive prenatal care. For example, in the seventeenth edition of *Williams Obstetrics*, the incidence of eclampsia at Parkland Hospital was cited to be 1 in 700 deliveries for the past 25-year period. For the 4-year period 1983–1986 the incidence was 1 in 1,150 deliveries. During this same time, there were proportionally more nulliparous women delivered at our hospital, and this should favor an increased incidence of eclampsia rather than the decrease noted.

THEORIES ABOUT THE CAUSE OF PREGNANCY-INDUCED HYPERTENSION

Any satisfactory theory must take into account the following observations: pregnancy-induced or -aggravated hypertension is very much more likely to develop in the woman who (1) is exposed to chorionic villi for the first time, (2) is exposed to a superabundance of chorionic villi, as with twins or hydatidiform mole, (3) has preexisting vascular disease, or (4) is genetically predisposed to hypertension developing during pregnancy. While chorionic villi are essential, they need not support a fetus nor be located within the uterus.

The possibility that immunological as well as endocrine and genetic mechanisms are involved in the genesis of preeclampsia is intriguing. The risk of pregnancy-induced hypertension is enhanced appreciably in circumstances where formation of blocking antibodies to antigenic sites on the placenta *might* be impaired, such as during immunosuppressive therapy to protect a renal transplant during pregnancy; where effective immunization by a previous pregnancy is lacking, as in first pregnancies;

or where the number of antigenic sites provided by the placenta is unusually great compared to the amount of antibody, an example of which is multiple fetuses (Beer, 1978). Strickland and associates (1986) provided data that do not lend strong support to "immunization" by a previous pregnancy. They analyzed the outcomes of 29,484 pregnancies at Parkland Hospital and reported that pregnancy-induced hypertension was only slightly decreased (22.3 versus 25.4 percent) in women who had previously aborted and now were having their first baby. However, supporting the immunization concept is the observation that preeclampsia develops in multiparous women impregnated by a new consort (Feeney and Scott, 1980) or in those pregnant as the result of donor insemination (Need and colleagues, 1983).

As summarized by Chesley (1974), everyone from allergist to zoologist has proposed a theory and suggested "rational therapy" based upon that theory. Some schemes proposed included mastectomy, oophorectomy, renal decapsulation, trephination, alignment of the woman with the earth's magnetic field, and a myriad of medical regimens. Everything from watermelon season to infestation with a worm (*Hydatoxi lualba*) has been claimed to be of importance. The interested reader is urged to examine the scholarly and entertaining review of various theories provided by Chesley (1978) in his elegant book, *Hypertensive Disorders in Pregnancy*.

As discussed above, the tendency to develop preeclampsia is inherited. Cooper and Liston (1979) examined the possibility that susceptibility to preeclampsia is dependent upon a single recessive gene. They calculated the expected first-pregnancy frequencies of daughters of women with eclampsia; daughters-in-law served as controls. The frequencies calculated by them and those actually observed by Chesley and co-workers (1968) in daughters and daughters-in-law of women with eclampsia are in remarkably close agreement. Subsequently, Chesley and Cooper (1986) reanalyzed Chesley's extensive data and concluded that the single-gene hypothesis fits well, but multifactorial inheritance cannot be excluded.

Preeclampsia may be more common among indigent women; however, in the early 1900s eclampsia was believed to be most common in middle- and upper-class women. Indeed, that observation led to the ready acceptance of the hypothesis that dietary restriction of protein accounted for the reduction in the incidence of eclampsia in Germany during World War I. Although there are suggestions that dietary deficiencies might cause preeclampsia, this hypothesis also lacks supportive data. Since pregnancy "depletes" a woman nutritionally, preeclampsia might be expected to be more common in multiparous women compared to nulliparas; however, the opposite is true. Moreover, in a number of studies in which dietary supplementation was provided, no reduction in the frequency of hypertension was demonstrated (see Chap. 14, p. 263). Zlatnik and Burmeister (1983) provided convincing evidence that the incidence of preeclampsia is *not* related to the level of dietary protein. Calcium deficiency has been implicated by some; however, appropriate clinical trials have not been done to test this hypothesis (Belizán and colleagues, 1988).

Carefully controlled epidemiological studies of pregnancy have been conducted in Aberdeen, Scotland, where for many years the relevant data have been available for most deliveries. Baird (1969) found that the incidence of preeclampsia did not differ significantly among the five social classes ranging from the professional and well-to-do (class I) through the unskilled laborers (class V), except for some slight increase in class III (skilled manual occupations).

PATHOPHYSIOLOGY OF PREECLAMPSIA–ECLAMPSIA

VASOSPASM

Vasospasm is basic to the pathophysiology of preeclampsia–eclampsia. This concept, first advanced by Volhard (1918), is based upon direct observation of small blood vessels in the nail beds, ocular fundi, and bulbar conjunctivae, and it has been surmised from histological changes that are seen in various affected organs. In preeclampsia, Hinselmann (1924), and later several others, noted alterations in the size of the arterioles in the nail bed, with evidence of segmental spasm that produced alternate regions of constriction and dilatation. Landesman and co-workers (1954) described marked arteriolar constriction in the bulbar conjunctivae, even to the extent that capillary circulation was intermittently abolished. Further evidence that vascular changes play an important role in preeclampsia–eclampsia is afforded by the frequency with which spasm of the retinal arterioles, commonly segmental, is found.

Vascular constriction causes a resistance to blood flow and accounts for the development of arterial hypertension. It is likely that vasospasm also exerts a noxious effect on the vessels themselves as circulation in the vasa vasorum is impaired, leading to vascular damage. Alternating segmental dilatation, which commonly accompanies the segmental arteriolar spasm, probably contributes further to the development of vascular damage, since endothelial integrity may be compromised by the stretched dilated segments. Moreover, angiotensin II appears to have a direct action on endothelial cells, causing them to contract. These factors could lead to interendothelial cell leaks through which blood constituents, including platelets and fibrinogen, are deposited subendothelially (Brunner and Gavras, 1975). The vascular changes, together with local hypoxia of the surrounding tissues, presumably lead to hemorrhage, necrosis, and other end-organ disturbances that have been observed at times with severe preeclampsia. With this scheme, fibrin deposition is then likely to be prominent, as seen in fatal cases (McKay, 1965).

INCREASED PRESSOR RESPONSES

Normally pregnant women develop refractoriness to the pressor effects of infused angiotensin II (Abdul-Karim and Assali, 1961). Increased vascular reactivity to this and other pressor hormones in women with early preeclampsia has been identified by Raab and co-workers (1956) and Talledo and associates (1968) using either angiotensin II or norepinephrine, and by Dieckmann and Michel (1937) and Browne (1946) using vasopressin. Subsequently, Gant and co-workers (1973) demonstrated that increased vascular sensitivity to angiotensin II clearly preceded the onset of pregnancy-induced hypertension. Normal nulliparas who remained normotensive were refractory to the pressor effect of infused angiotensin II (Fig. 35–1). However, women who subsequently became hypertensive lost this normal pregnancy refractoriness to angiotensin II weeks before the onset of hypertension. Of women studied at 28 to 32 weeks gestation who required more than 8 ng per kg per minute of angiotensin II to provoke a standardized pressor response, 91 percent remained normotensive throughout pregnancy. Conversely, among normotensive primigravidas who required for a pressor response less than 8 ng per kg per minute at 28 to 32 weeks, 90 percent subsequently developed overt hypertension.

Similar results from 231 women subsequently were reported from Germany by Öney and Kaulhausen (1982).

> A pressor response induced by having the woman assume the supine position after lying laterally recumbent has been demonstrated in some pregnant women by Gant and co-workers (1974b). The majority of nulliparous women at 28 to 32 weeks who demonstrated increased diastolic blood pressure of at least 20 mm Hg when the maneuver was performed later developed pregnancy-induced hypertension. Conversely, most women whose blood pressure did not become elevated when this was done did not later become hypertensive. As perhaps expected, those women who demonstrated a *supine pressor response* were also abnormally sensitive to infused angiotensin II, while those without a hypertensive response were normally refractory. The mechanism by which assuming the supine position incites a rise in blood pressure is not clear, but it is likely to be a manifestation of increased vascular responsivity of those who will later develop pregnancy-induced hypertension.

Women with chronic underlying hypertension have similar responses. An identically performed study of angiotensin II pressor responsiveness was conducted in women whose pregnancies were complicated by coexistent (chronic) hypertension (Gant and colleagues, 1977). Two groups were identified on the basis of clinical outcome and serial determinations of vascular reactivity to infused angiotensin II. All women were refractory to angiotensin II between 21 and 25 weeks; however, women who subsequently developed pregnancy-aggravated hypertension began to lose this refractoriness after 27 weeks (Fig. 35–2). The pattern of angiotensin II responsiveness observed in these two groups of women with chronic hypertension is similar to that seen in primigravidas, shown in Figure 35–1. Thus, it seems that the basic pathophysiology of preeclampsia, whether in a

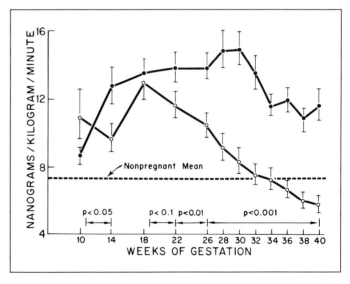

Figure 35–1. Comparison of the mean angiotensin II infusion doses required to evoke a pressor response in 120 nulliparous women who remained normotensive (solid circles) and 72 who subsequently developed pregnancy-induced hypertension (open circles). (*From Gant and co-workers: J Clin Invest 52:2682, 1973.*)

nullipara or superimposed upon chronic hypertension in a multipara, has a similar pregression.

Other factors may be operative in the refractoriness to angiotensin II. For example, aldosterone secretion is strikingly increased in pregnant women (Chap. 7, p. 155), and this is modulated by the effects of angiotensin II on the zona glomerulosa of the adrenal cortex. However, based on the findings of a number of studies—Gant and co-workers (1974a), Cunningham and associates (1975), and Everett and colleagues (1978a, 1978b)—it was concluded that the blunted pressor response to angiotensin II was specifically due to decreased vascular responsiveness. Angiotensin II refractoriness is likely to be mediated by vascular endothelial synthesis of prostaglandins or prostaglandin-like substance, for example, prostacyclin or prostaglandin E₂. For example, the refractoriness to angiotensin II in pregnant women is abolished by large doses of the prostaglandin inhibitors indomethacin and aspirin (Everett and colleagues, 1978a). In some tissues, angiotensin II action is mediated, at least in part, by promoting either accelerated synthesis or prostaglandin release, or both. It is interesting to speculate that pregnancy normally causes an increased capacity for endothelial prostaglandin synthesis with relatively greater synthesis of vasodilator than of vasoconstricting prostaglandins.

The exact mechanism by which prostaglandin(s) or related substances mediate vascular reactivity during pregnancy is unknown, but recent findings have served to elucidate these, at least in part. Goodman and colleagues (1982) reported increased concentrations of vasodilating prostaglandins during normal pregnancy. Everett and colleagues (1978a) demonstrated that indomethacin and aspirin diminished vascular responsivity to

infused angiotensin II, and they postulated that vasoconstrictor prostaglandin(s) synthesis was preferentially suppressed compared to that of vasodilator prostaglandins. Sanchez-Ramos and colleagues (1987) documented similarly diminished vascular response within 2 hours of ingestion of 40 mg of aspirin.

Walsh (1985) reported that, compared to normal pregnancy, placental production of prostacyclin is significantly decreased and thromboxane A₂ significantly increased in preeclampsia. He subsequently reported (1988) that placental progesterone production is increased in vitro in placentas taken from preeclamptic pregnancies, and hypothesized that increased progesterone concentrations may inhibit prostacyclin production. Preliminary work by Spitz and colleagues (1988) indicates that 81 mg of aspirin given daily suppresses synthesis of both prostacyclin and platelet-derived thromboxane A₂. However, prostacylin synthesis, estimated by measuring its stable metabolite, was decreased by 21 percent. Similarly, prostaglandin E levels decreased only 29 percent, whereas simultaneously the synthesis of thromboxane A₂ was diminished by 75 percent. Brown and associates (1989) reported similar findings in angiotensin-sensitive women rendered "resistant" by low-dose aspirin; however, in those remaining sensitive despite aspirin, all three prostaglandins were reduced significantly by aspirin ingestion. These observations indicate that vessel reactivity may be mediated through a delicate balance of production and metabolism of at least these three vasoactive prostaglandins. In this scheme, preeclampsia may follow inappropriately increased production or destruction of one prostaglandin or diminished synthesis or release of the other, or perhaps both. Indeed, Beaufils (1985) and Wallenburg (1986) and their colleagues have reported that chronic low-dose aspirin ingestion may prevent pregnancy-induced hypertension.

Friedman (1988) has provided an extensive review of the role of prostaglandins in preeclampsia.

MATERNAL AND FETAL CONSEQUENCES OF PREECLAMPSIA–ECLAMPSIA

Deterioration of function in a number of organs and systems, presumably in large part as the consequence of vasospasm, has been identified in severe preeclampsia and eclampsia. For descriptive purposes, these effects are separated into maternal and fetal consequences; however, it is emphasized that these aberrations often occur simultaneously in both patients.

While there are many possible maternal consequences of pregnancy-induced hypertension, for simplicity, these effects are considered by analysis of cardiovascular, hematological, endocrine and metabolic, and regional blood flow changes with subsequent end-organ derangements. The major cause of fetal compromise is from changes in uteroplacental perfusion.

CARDIOVASCULAR CHANGES

The hemodynamic changes that accompany severe preeclampsia and eclampsia have been studied recently by a number of investigators. Key issues addressed include the cardiovascular status of these women before treatment, as well as attempts to relieve vasospasm by pharmacological manipulation or by intravascular volume loading. Elucidation of the mechanisms that cause heart failure and pulmonary edema complicating the course of some of these women has also been sought. Before

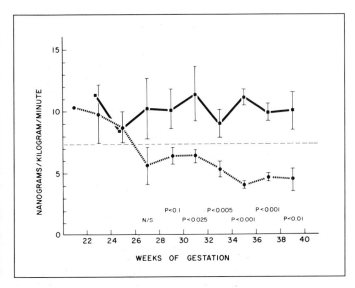

Figure 35–2. Comparison of angiotensin II responsiveness in 29 women with essential hypertension who remained normotensive to responsiveness in 34 women with essential hypertension who subsequently developed pregnancy-aggravated hypertension. The dose of angiotensin II needed to elevate diastolic blood pressure by 20 mm Hg is shown on the vertical axis and is plotted as a function of weeks of gestation. The results obtained in women with chronic hypertension alone are indicated by squares connected by a solid line. The results obtained in women with chronic hypertension destined to develop superimposed preeclampsia are shown as dots connected by a broken line. The vertical bars represent the standard error of the mean. (*From Gant and co-workers: Am J Obstet Gynecol 127:369, 1977.*)

discussing these alterations, a basic review of cardiovascular physiology follows.

CLINICAL ASSESSMENT OF CARDIAC FUNCTION

In assessing cardiac function, four areas must be addressed: (1) preload—end-diastolic pressure and chamber volume, (2) afterload—intramyocardial systolic tension or resistance to ejection, (3) contractile or inotropic state of the myocardium, and (4) heart rate. An informative review of this subject was provided recently by Hankins (1986).

Preload

Preload is determined by intraventricular pressure and volume, thus setting the initial myocardial muscle fiber length. Clinically, the right and left ventricular end-diastolic filling pressures are assessed by central venous pressure and pulmonary capillary wedge pressure, respectively. By plotting cardiac output against these filling pressures, a *cardiac function curve* can be developed for the right and left heart chambers. As illustrated in Figure 35–3, the failing heart requires a higher preload or filling pressure to achieve the same output as the normally functioning heart. Preload can be increased by intravenously administered crystalloid, colloid, or blood, and it can be decreased by diuretics, vasodilators (especially of the capacitance system), or phlebotomy, including blood loss at delivery.

Afterload

Afterload is defined as the ventricular wall tension during systole and is dependent on the end-diastolic radius of the ventricle, the aortic diastolic pressure, and ventricular wall thickness. The extent to which the left intraventricular pressure will rise during systole depends primarily on the total systemic vascular resistance (Fig. 35–4). For clinical purposes, the aortic or mean arterial pressure is a direct reflection of afterload. In the presence of heart failure, increases in afterload worsen the degree of failure by decreasing both the stroke volume and the cardiac output.

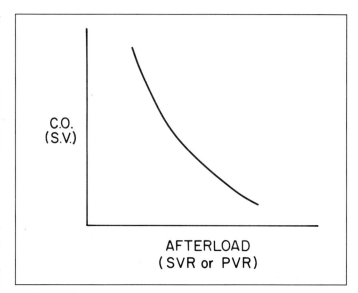

Figure 35–4. Relationship of afterload [systemic vascular resistance (SVR) or pulmonary vascular resistance (PVR)] to cardiac output (C.O.) or stroke volume (S.V.) at a constant preload. (*Adapted from Hankins and associates: Perinatol Neonatol 7:29, 1983.*)

As with preload, afterload can be increased or decreased therapeutically as indicated by the clinical setting. Increases in afterload are mediated through modulation of the α-adrenergic system. Decreases in afterload, or systemic vascular resistance, best estimated by arterial pressure, can be achieved with a number of drugs, an example of which is hydralazine.

Contractile State of the Heart

The third variable in the assessment of cardiac function is the contractile, or inotropic, state of the heart, defined as the force and velocity of ventricular contraction when preload and afterload are held constant. While cardiac output can be measured directly, the adequacy of cardiac output may be assessed indirectly by acid-base status, arteriovenous oxygen differences, and urinary output. In low-output cardiac failure, both preload and afterload should be optimized through previously mentioned therapeutic regimens. If these fail to restore the cardiac output to acceptable levels, then attention should be directed to improving myocardial contractility. β-sympathomimetics, such as dopamine and isoproterenol, usually improve cardiac output acutely. Depending on the cause of myocardial failure, either short- or long-term therapy may be necessary.

Heart Rate

The final determinant of myocardial function is heart rate. Although heart block is rare in pregnant women, cardiac output can be compromised by heart rates too slow to maintain adequate output. In this setting, treatment with either atropine or cardiac pacing is indicated. Alternatively, sustained tachycardia can lead to heart failure due to shortened systolic ejection and diastolic filling time or to myocardial ischemia. The cause of tachycardia, for example, fever, hypovolemia, pain, or hyperthyroidism, should be determined and corrected. Treatment with propranolol, digoxin, or calcium channel blockers, such as verapamil, is seldom required in obstetrical patients.

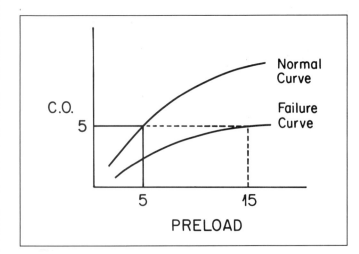

Figure 35–3. Ventricular function curve for heart failure. In order to maintain cardiac output (C.O.), the failing heart is required to function at higher preload or filling pressures (either pulmonary capillary wedge or central venous pressure). (*Adapted from Hankins and associates: Perinatol Neonatol 7:29, 1983.*)

HEMODYNAMIC CHANGES

Values obtained by invasive cardiovascular monitoring in a number of studies of women with severe preeclampsia and eclampsia are listed in Table 35–5. The differences in reported values for variables that define cardiovascular status range from high cardiac output with low vascular resistance to low cardiac output with high vascular resistance. Similarly, left ventricular filling pressures, estimated by pulmonary capillary wedge pressure determination, range from low to pathologically high. There are at least three factors that may explain these differences: (1) women with preeclampsia might present with a spectrum of cardiovascular findings dependent upon both the severity and duration of pregnancy-induced hypertension, (2) chronic underlying disease may modulate the clinical presentation, or (3) therapeutic interventions may significantly alter these findings. It is likely that in many of these women, more than one of these is operative.

The women in the studies listed in Table 35–5 were separated into three groups, based upon clinical managment prior to initial hemodynamic observations: (1) no therapy for preeclampsia, (2) magnesium sulfate and hydralazine without infusing a large volume of intravenous fluid, or (3) magnesium sulfate and hydralazine plus intravenous volume loading. Ventricular function from the six studies listed in Table 35–5 is plotted in Figure 35–5. In all, cardiac function is hyperdynamic, but filling pressures vary markedly.

Hemodynamic data obtained prior to active treatment of preeclampsia has been reported by Groenendijk (1984) and Cotton (1984) and their colleagues. They identified normal left ventricular filling pressures, high systemic vascular resistances, and hyperdynamic ventricular function. Benedetti (1984) and Hankins (1984) and their associates reported similar findings in women with severe preeclampsia or eclampsia who were being treated with magnesium sulfate, hydralazine, and intravenous crystalloid given at 75 to 100 mL per hour. Cardiac function in these women was appropriate, and the lower systemic vascular resistance most likely reflected the effects of hydralazine treatment.

By comparison, women similarly treated with magnesium sulfate and hydralazine, but in whom more aggressive intravenous therapy or volume expansion was employed, have the lowest systemic vascular resistances and highest cardiac outputs. As shown in Figure 35–6, although there is evidence of hyperdynamic ventricular function in both groups, a comparison of women managed with volume restriction to those hydrated aggressively shows two responses with respect to left ventricular stroke work index and pulmonary capillary wedge pressure. All women managed with fluid restriction had wedge pressures less than 10 mm Hg, and most were less than 5 mm Hg. Thus, hyperdynamic ventricular function was largely a re-

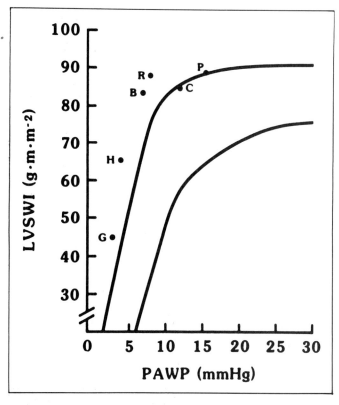

Figure 35–5. Ventricular function in severe preeclampsia–eclampsia. Data plotted represent mean values obtained in each of six studies cited in Table 35–5. Left ventricular stroke work index (LVSWI) and pulmonary artery wedge pressure (PAWP) are plotted on a standard ventricular function curve. Points falling within the two solid lines represent normal function, while those below represent depressed function. Points above the solid lines represent hyperdynamic ventricular function. Each letter adjacent to the data points is the first initial of the last name of the investigator who reported this value.

TABLE 35–5. HEMODYNAMIC MEASUREMENT MADE IN WOMEN WITH SEVERE PREECLAMPSIA AND ECLAMPSIA

Therapy	No.	Cardiac Output (L/min)	Pulmonary Capillary Wedge Pressure (mm Hg)	Left Ventricular Stroke Work Index $(g/m/m^{-2})$	Systemic Vascular Resistance $(dynes/sec/cm^{-5})$
No therapy					
Cotton and associates (1984)	5	7.56	12.0	83	2256
Groenendijk and co-workers (1984)	10	4.66	3.3	44	1943
Magnesium, hydralazine, and fluid restriction					
Benedetti and colleagues (1980)	10	7.4	6.0	82	1322
Hankins and associates (1984)	8	6.7	3.9	66	1357
Magnesium, hydralazine, and volume expansion					
Rafferty and Berkowitz (1980)	3	11.0	7.0	89	780
Phelan and Yurth (1982)	10	9.3	16.0	89	1042

Values are those reported soon after pulmonary artery catheterization was performed, and are the means for each study.

sult of the low wedge pressures, and not because of augmented left ventricular stroke work index, which more directly measures myocardial contractility. By comparison, women given appreciably larger volumes of fluid commonly had pulmonary capillary wedge pressures that exceeded normal; however, ventricular function remained hyperdynamic because of increased cardiac output. Subsequently, Cotton and co-workers (1988) reported findings from 45 women with severe preeclampsia or eclampsia and described high systemic vascular resistance and hyperdynamic ventricular function in most. It is reasonable to conclude that aggressive fluid administration given to women with severe preeclampsia causes normal left-sided filling pressures to become substantively elevated, while increasing an already normal cardiac output to supranormal levels.

SUMMARY OF HEMODYNAMIC CHANGES

Five general observations can be made. (1) Before treatment, at least, myocardial contractility rarely is impaired and ventricular function is usually within the normal to hyperdynamic range. (2) Cardiac afterload, measured as systemic vascular resistance, is elevated in the absence of therapeutic interventions. (3) Cardiac output predictably varies inversely with vascular resistance, and as blood pressure and systemic vascular resistance increase, cardiac output falls. (4) Medications that reduce vascular resistance, for example, hydralazine, result in increased cardiac output. (5) Ventricular preload, measured by central venous and pulmonary capillary wedge pressures, is usually normal or even low in severe preeclampsia and eclampsia, unless substantial volumes of fluids are administered.

BLOOD VOLUME

Hemoconcentration in women with eclampsia was emphasized by Dieckmann (1952) in his monograph, *The Toxemias of Pregnancy.*

More recently, Pritchard and co-workers (1984) reported blood volume measurements of women with eclampsia. Their findings are consistent with the view that in eclampsia pregnancy hypervolemia most often is scant to absent (Table 35–6). The woman of average size can be expected to have a blood volume of nearly 5,000 mL during the last several weeks of a normal pregnancy, compared to about 3,500 mL when nonpregnant. With eclampsia, however, much or all of the added 1,500 mL of blood normally present late in pregnancy can be anticipated to be missing.

The virtual absence of pregnancy-induced hypervolemia is very likely the consequence of generalized vasoconstriction, or it could result from increased vascular permeability, which would account for the classic features, when compared to normal pregnancy, of too little fluid intravascularly but a marked excess extravascularly. Both mechanisms could be involved.

It was taught by Dieckmann (1952), and more recently by others, that clinical improvement is characterized by hemodilution manifested by a fall in hematocrit. In our experience, however, a significant fall in hematocrit occurs most often only with delivery. Moreover, rather than directly reflecting clinical improvement, the fall, at least acutely, is usually the consequence of blood loss at delivery in the absence of normal pregnancy hypervolemia. Occasionally, an acutely decreased hematocrit results from intense erythrocyte destruction, as described below.

In the absence of hemorrhage, the intravascular compartment in eclamptic women usually is not underfilled. Vasospasm has contracted the space to be filled; the reduction persists until hours to a few days after delivery, when typically the vascular system dilates, the blood volume increases, and the hematocrit falls. **The woman with eclampsia, therefore, is unduly sensitive to vigorous fluid therapy administered in an attempt to expand the contracted blood volume to normal pregnancy**

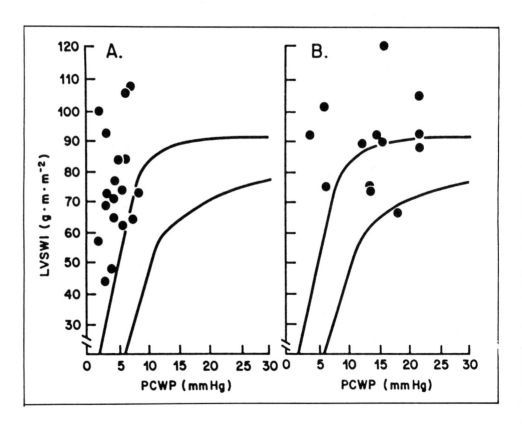

Figure 35–6. Ventricular function in women with severe preeclampsia–eclampsia. Left ventricular stroke work index (LVSWI) and pulmonary capillary wedge pressure (PCWP) are plotted. **A.** Restricted intravenous fluids (Benedetti and colleagues, 1980; Hankins and co-workers, 1984). **B.** Aggressive fluid therapy (Rafferty and Berkowitz, 1980; Phelan and Yurth, 1982) (*From Hankins and colleagues: Am J Obstet Gynecol, 150:506, 1984.*)

TABLE 35–6. BLOOD VOLUMES IN FIVE WOMEN MEASURED WITH ^{51}Cr-TAGGED ERYTHROCYTES DURING ANTEPARTUM ECLAMPSIA, AGAIN WHEN NONPREGNANT, AND FINALLY AT A COMPARABLE TIME IN A SECOND NORMOTENSIVE PREGNANCY

	Eclampsia	Nonpregnant	Normal Pregnant
Blood volume (mL)	3,530	3,035	4,425
Change (percent)	+16		+47
Hematocrit	40.5	38.2	34.7

From Pritchard, Cunningham, and Pritchard: Am J Obstet Gynecol 148:951, 1984.

levels. She is likewise sensitive as well to even normal blood loss at delivery. Management of blood loss in these circumstances is considered in Chapter 36 (p. 695).

HEMATOLOGICAL CHANGES

The following hematological abnormalities may develop in some women, but certainly not all, who demonstrate pregnancy-induced or pregnancy-aggravated hypertension. (1) Thrombocytopenia may develop and, at times, become so severe as to be life threatening. (2) The level of some plasma clotting factors may be decreased. (3) Erythrocytes may be so traumatized that they display bizarre shapes and undergo rapid hemolysis.

These hematological changes have been considered by some to be the genesis of preeclampsia–eclampsia, that is, a hypercoagulable state that, if arrested, might provide effective therapy. Unfortunately, during the past half-century, attempts to induce remissions in women with preeclampsia by giving heparin have been unsuccessful.

COAGULATION

Hematological changes consistent with intravascular coagulation, and less often erythrocyte destruction, may further complicate cases of pregnancy-induced hypertension, especially eclampsia (Pritchard and colleagues, 1954a, 1954b; Stahnke, 1922). In recent years, renewed interest in these changes has led to the concept by some investigators that disseminated intravascular coagulation is not only a characteristic feature of preeclampsia, but it also plays a dominant role in the pathogenesis of the syndrome. For example, Page (1972) theorized that many of the changes of preeclampsia were the consequence of fibrin deposited in vital organs as a product of slow disseminated intravascular coagulation initiated by thromboplastin entering the maternal circulation from the placenta, while rapid disseminated intravascular coagulation and fibrin so formed caused cerebral vascular occlusion and the convulsions of eclampsia.

Since the early reports by Pritchard and co-workers (1954a, 1954b), we have continued to search for evidence of coagulopathy in eclamptic women. The results of some of these studies are presented in Table 35–7. Thrombocytopenia, infrequently severe, was the most common finding. Elevated levels of fibrin degradation products in serum were elevated only occasionally. Unless some degree of placental abruption had developed, plasma fibrinogen did not differ remarkably from levels found late in normal pregnancy. Interestingly, the thrombin time was somewhat prolonged in one third of the cases of eclampsia even when elevated levels of fibrin degradation products were not identified (Pritchard and colleagues, 1976). The reason for this

TABLE 35–7. CHANGES IN COAGULATION FACTORS THAT IMPLY DISSEMINATED INTRAVASCULAR COAGULATION

	Intrapartum Primigravidas Normally Pregnant	Most Abnormal Value for Each Case of Eclampsia
Platelets[a]		
Mean (per μL)	278,000	206,000
− 2 standard deviations	150,000	—
< 150,000	0/20	24/91
< 100,000	0/20	14/91
< 50,000	0/20	3/91
Fibrin degradation products[b]		
8 μg per mL or less	17/20	51/59
16 μg per mL	3/20	6/59
> 16 μg per mL	0/20	2/59
Plasma fibrinogen[a]		
Mean (mg per dL)	415	413
− 2 standard deviations	285	—
< 285 mg per dL	0/20	7/89
Fibrin monomer		
Positive	1/20	1/14

[a] Lowest value identified for each case of eclampsia.
[b] Highest value identified for each case of eclampsia.
From Pritchard, Cunningham, and Mason: Am J Obstet Gynecol 124:855, 1976.

elevation is not known, but we have attributed it to hepatic derangements discussed subsequently. The various coagulation changes just described are also identified in women with severe preeclampsia but are certainly no more common. Our observations on eclampsia, as well as those reported by Kitzmiller and associates (1974) for preeclampsia, are most consistent with the concept that the coagulation changes are the consequence of preeclampsia–eclampsia, rather than the cause.

THROMBOCYTOPENIA

It clearly has been established that maternal thrombocytopenia can be induced acutely by preeclampsia–eclampsia. Moreover, once the products of conception have been expelled, the platelet count will increase progressively to reach a normal level within a few days after delivery. The frequency and the intensity of maternal thrombocytopenia vary in different studies, apparently dependent upon the intensity of the disease process, the length of delay between the onset of preeclampsia–eclampsia and delivery, and the frequency with which platelet counts are performed.

Most workers consider the development of overt thrombocytopenia, that is, a platelet count less than 100,000 per μL, to be an ominous sign in women with preeclampsia, and they recommend delivery. Otherwise, the platelet count most often continues to decrease and may reach levels that can result in excessive blood loss during and after delivery, especially by cesarean section. The risk of maternal intracranial hemorrhage is also increased appreciably by thrombocytopenia.

The cause of the thrombocytopenia is not firmly established. We, for example, have vacillated between favoring an immunological process and simply ascribing it to platelet deposition at sites of endothelial damage (Pritchard and colleagues, 1954, 1976). Samuels and colleagues (1987) performed direct and indirect antiglobulin tests and found that platelet-bound and circulating platelet-bindable immunoglobulin were increased in preeclamptic women and their neonates. They interpreted these findings to suggest platelet surface alterations. Burrows and colleagues (1987) reported that platelets from women with preeclampsia were more likely to have platelet-associated IgG, even if thrombocytopenia did not develop (Fig. 35–7). Although they considered that this mechanism might imply an autoimmune process, they noted that IgG also could be bound to platelets damaged by any mechanism.

These same investigators amplified their previous work (Kelton and colleagues, 1985) and again showed that thrombocytopenia with preeclampsia frequently was associated with a prolonged bleeding time. Moreover, they identified this even with normal platelet levels, and they attributed it to impaired thromboxane synthesis.

Neonatal Thrombocytopenia

Several investigators have described thrombocytopenia in the newborn of mothers with preeclampsia–eclampsia. Thiagaraiah and co-workers (1984) reported severe thrombocytopenia in 2 of 10 neonates whose mothers had preeclampsia and emphasized that these findings should be a consideration in selecting the mode of delivery. They found no correlation between the maternal platelet count at delivery and the fetal platelet count. Weinstein (1985) later reported initial platelet counts to have been less than 150,000 per μL in 11 of the 46 infants whose mothers were thrombocytopenic as the consequence of preeclampsia–eclampsia. The exact times that the thrombocytopenia was identified after delivery were not stated, nor was the intensity of the thrombocytopenia described. While our experience with maternal thrombocytopenia complicating preeclampsia–eclampsia began more than three decades ago, we have *not* observed severe thrombocytopenia in the fetus-infant when measured at or very soon after delivery (Pritchard and colleagues, 1987). As shown in Figure 35–8, in no case was fetal-neonatal thrombocytopenia identified, despite severe maternal thrombocytopenia. Alternatively, thrombocytopenia that developed in some of these infants *later* was attributed to hypoxia, acidosis, and sepsis. **Hence, maternal thrombocytopenia is not a fetal indication for cesarean delivery.**

FRAGMENTATION HEMOLYSIS

Thrombocytopenia that accompanies severe preeclampsia and eclampsia may be accompanied by evidence of erythrocyte destruction characterized by hemolysis, schizocytosis, spherocytosis, reticulocytosis, hemoglobinuria, and occasionally, hemoglobinemia (Pritchard and colleagues 1954, 1976). These derangements result in part from microangiopathic hemolysis; human and animal studies have shown that intense vasospasm causes endothelial disruption, with platelet adherence and fibrin deposition. More recently, erythrocyte morphological characteristics have been described in hypertension using scanning electron microscopy (Cunningham and associates, 1985).

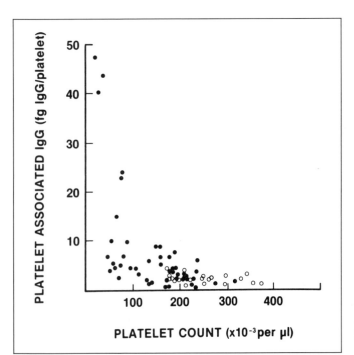

Figure 35–7. The relationship of platelet-associated IgG to the platelet count in preeclamptic and in control women. The level of platelet-associated IgG is shown along the ordinate, and the platelet count along the abscissa. Women with preeclampsia are shown by solid dots and normally pregnant women by circles. (*From Burrows and colleagues: Obstet Gynecol 70:334, 1987.*)

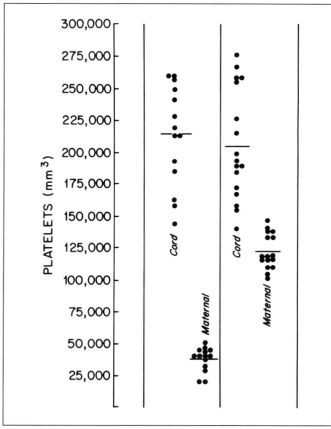

Figure 35–8. Umbilical cord platelet counts in newborns of 14 eclamptic or severely preeclamptic mothers with platelet counts less than 50,000 per mm³ are compared to those from 16 eclamptic or severely preeclamptic mothers with platelet counts of 100,000 to 150,000 per mm³. The severity of the maternal thrombocytopenia had no demonstrable impact on the 31 cord platelet counts. (*From Pritchard and associates: Obstet Gynecol 69:292, 1987.*)

Women with eclampsia, and to a lesser degree, those with severe preeclampsia, demonstrated schizocytosis and echinocytosis, but not spherocytosis, when compared to normally pregnant women. It is likely that plasma-erythrocyte membrane lipid changes that accompany preeclampsia are magnified by decreased serum albumin concentration, and that these serve even more to intensify fragmentation hemolysis.

OTHER CLOTTING FACTORS

A severe deficiency of any of the soluble coagulation factors is very uncommon in severe preeclampsia–eclampsia unless another event coexists that predisposes to consumptive coagulopathy, examples being placental abruption and ruptured liver.

Antithrombin III has been reported to be lower in women with preeclampsia compared to normally pregnant women and those with chronic hypertension (Saleh and associates, 1987; Weenik and colleagues, 1983; Weiner and Brandt, 1982). *Fibronectin*, a glycoprotein associated with vascular endothelial cell basement membrane is elevated in women with preeclampsia (Saleh and colleagues, 1987; Stubb and associates, 1984). These observations are consistent with those described above, that preeclampsia causes vascular endothelial injury with subsequent hematological aberrations. The clinical utility of serial antithrombin III or fibronectin measurements for the diagnosis and management of preeclampsia awaits further evaluation.

ENDOCRINE AND METABOLIC CHANGES

ENDOCRINE CHANGES

During normal pregnancy, plasma levels of *renin, angiotensin II,* and *aldosterone* are increased. Paradoxically, with pregnancy-induced hypertension, these substances commonly decrease toward the normal nonpregnant range (Weir and colleagues, 1973). With the development of sodium retention, hypertension, or both, the rate of renin release by the juxtaglomerular apparatus decreases. Since renin is the enzyme that catalyzes the conversion of angiotensinogen to angiotensin I (which is then transformed into angiotensin II by converting enzyme), angiotensin II levels decline, and thus, aldosterone secretion decreases. Despite this, women with preeclampsia avidly retain infused sodium (Brown and colleagues, 1988).

Another potent mineralocorticoid, *deoxycorticosterone* (DOC), is strikingly increased in the plasma of women during the third trimester (see Chap. 7, p. 156). Importantly, its increase does not appear to be the consequence of increased secretion of DOC by the maternal adrenal glands. Treatment of pregnant women with the potent adrenal glucocorticoid dexamethasone to reduce corticotropin secretion does not decrease plasma levels of DOC, and neither does corticotropin treatment of near-term pregnant women cause an increase in plasma DOC levels. Since plasma progesterone is converted to DOC in nonadrenal tissues, it is reasonable to conclude that this pathway is not subject to control by angiotensin II. Thus, the amount of DOC formed from plasma progesterone is not reduced by sodium retention or hypertension, and it may play a role in the pathogenesis or perpetuation of preeclampsia.

Winkel and co-workers (1980) found that the fractional conversion of plasma progesterone to DOC varied widely among individuals (0.002 to 0.22). This is very intriguing, since ordinarily, the fractional conversion of one steroid hormone to another seldom varies among normal persons. Thus, in near-term pregnant women producing 250 mg of progesterone per day, the amount of DOC produced from plasma progesterone could vary from 0.5 mg to 11 mg per 24 hours. Nonpregnant women produce, on average, 0.15 mg DOC per day. Given the progesterone produced in women who are prone to develop preeclampsia, for example, women with diabetes, multiple fetuses, fetal hydrops, and hydatidiform mole, the amount of DOC produced from plasma progesterone could be enormous.

DOC production cannot be the only factor in the development of pregnancy-induced hypertension. Brown and co-workers (1972) reported that levels of this hormone in pregnant women who were already hypertensive were not greater than were those in normotensive controls. Parker and colleagues (1980) measured the hormone throughout pregnancy and found that plasma DOC concentrations in the plasma of a group of primigravidas who ultimately developed preeclampsia were not greater than its concentrations in primigravidas who remained normotensive. However, Winkel and co-workers (1983) subsequently reported that the conversion of progesterone into DOC was significantly increased in women who later developed pregnancy-induced hypertension. It may be that DOC has a local effect and that it is produced and metabolized within the kidney such that its plasma concentration need not be different in hypertensive women. The possibility of a yet unidentified pressor hormone certainly persists.

Increased *antidiuretic hormone* activity to account for oliguria has been previously suggested. In fact, normal (Elias and colleagues, 1988) or even low levels have been identified (J. Pritchard and J. Porter, unpublished). *Chorionic gonadotropin* levels in plasma have been found inconstantly to be elevated; conversely, *placental lactogen* has been found inconstantly to be reduced.

Necrosis of the adrenal and the pituitary has been identified in some fatal cases of eclampsia (McKay, 1965). In our experience, which is limited to nonfatal cases, compromised adrenal or pituitary function is rare.

Atrial natriuretic peptide is released upon atrial wall stretching from blood volume expansion, and it acts upon the kidney to promote sodium and water excretion. Thomsen and colleagues (1987), but not Hirai and associates (1988), reported that this peptide is increased in normal pregnancy. However, both groups reported that the atrial natriuretic peptide substantively increased in women with preeclampsia (Fig. 35–9). Since blood volume is substantively decreased in preeclamptic women, they concluded that factors other than volume expansion must play a role in release of this peptide.

FLUID AND ELECTROLYTE CHANGES

Commonly, the volume of *extracellular fluid* in women with severe preeclampsia–eclampsia has expanded appreciably beyond the increased volume that characterizes normal pregnancy. The mechanism responsible for the pathological expansion is not clear. Edema is evident at a time when, paradoxically, aldosterone levels are reduced compared to the remarkably elevated levels of normal pregnancy. As noted above, however, plasma DOC levels remain elevated, but are not consistently greater than those in normotensive women. The electrolyte concentrations do not differ appreciably from those of normal pregnancy unless there has been vigorous diuretic therapy, dietary sodium restriction, or the administration of water with sufficient oxytocin to produce antidiuresis. Edema, by itself, is not indicative of a poor prognosis, nor does lack of appreciable edema guarantee a favorable outcome for pregnancies complicated by preeclampsia–eclampsia.

Following an eclamptic convulsion, the *bicarbonate* concen-

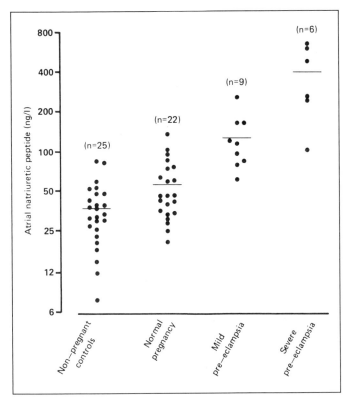

Figure 35–9. Plasma immunoreactive atrial natriuretic peptide concentrations in normal nonpregnant and pregnant women, and preeclamptic women. Horizontal bars represent group means. (*From Thomsen and colleagues: Br Med J 294:1508, 1987.*)

tration is lowered as the consequence of lactic acidosis and compensatory loss of carbon dioxide from plasma through the lungs. The intensity of the acidosis will relate to the amount of lactic acid produced and its rate of metabolism, as well as the rate at which carbon dioxide is exhaled.

THE KIDNEY

During normal pregnancy, renal blood flow and glomerular filtration rate are increased appreciably above nonpregnant levels (see Chap. 7, p. 148). With the development of pregnancy-induced hypertension, renal perfusion and glomerular filtration are variably reduced. Levels that are much below normal nonpregnant levels are the consequence of severe disease. Therefore, in milder cases the plasma creatinine or urea concentration is seldom elevated appreciably above normal nonpregnant values. The plasma uric acid concentration typically is elevated, especially in women with more severe disease. The elevation is a result primarily of decreased renal clearance of uric acid, a decrease that exceeds the reduction in glomerular filtration rate and creatinine clearance (Chesley and Williams, 1945). Thiazide diuretics contribute to increased plasma uric acid. In our experience, measurements of plasma uric acid concentration is generally of little practical value for diagnosis or prognosis.

In the majority of women with preeclampsia, mild to moderately diminished glomerular filtration appears to be the consequence of reduced plasma volume; thus, plasma creatinine is seldom below normal nonpregnant levels. However, in some

cases of severe preeclampsia and eclampsia, but certainly not all, renal involvement is profound and plasma creatinine may be elevated two to three times over nonpregnant normal values. We have speculated that this is due to intrinsic renal changes most likely caused by severe vasospasm (Pritchard and colleagues, 1984). Subsequently, Lee and associates (1987) reported normal ventricular filling pressures in seven severely preeclamptic women with oliguria and concluded that this was consistent with our hypothesis. In most of these latter women, urine sodium concentration was abnormally elevated, which suggested intrinsic renal pathology. However, urine osmolality, urine–plasma creatinine ratio, and fractional excretion of sodium were consistent with the view that a prerenal mechanism also might be contributory. Importantly, as discussed later, their conclusion was that intensive intravenous fluid therapy was not indicated for these women with oliguria. Subsequently, the same group (Kirshon and co-workers, 1988) infused dopamine into oliguric preeclampsit women. This renal vasodilator caused increased urine output, fractional sodium excretion, and free water clearance.

Taufield and associates (1987) reported that preeclampsia is associated with diminished urinary excretion of calcium because of increased tubular reabsorption.

The experience at Parkland Hospital has been that after delivery, in the absence of underlying chronic renovascular disease, complete recovery of renal function can be anticipated. This would not be the case, of course, if *renal cortical necrosis*, an irreversible but rare lesion, had developed.

PROTEINURIA

The pregnant hypertensive woman must have some degree of proteinuria for the diagnosis of preeclampsia–eclampsia to be accurate (Chesley, 1985). However, since proteinuria usually develops late in the course of the disease, some women may be delivered before it appears and thus have true preeclampsia without proteinuria.

Use of the term *albuminuria* to describe proteinuria of preeclampsia is incorrect. As with any other glomerulopathy, there is increased permeability to most large molecular weight proteins; thus, abnormal albumin excretion is accompanied by that of other proteins, for example, hemoglobin, globulins, and transferrin. Normally, these large protein molecules are not filtered by the glomerulus, and thus their appearance in urine signifies a glomerulopathic process. Some of the smaller proteins that are usually filtered but reabsorbed also are detected in the urine.

Because of the similarity with other renal diseases thought to be caused by immune-complex glomerulonephritis, it is tempting to regard these renal changes of preeclampsia as induced by immunological mechanisms, and indeed, as discussed on page 657, this is regarded by many as a probable inciting cause. Certainly, if there is not underlying chronic renal disease, proteinuria gradually recedes following delivery and resolution of hypertension. This usually occurs within a week or so, even with heavy proteinuria and severe preeclampsia.

MICROSCOPIC CHANGES

Changes identifiable by light and electron microscopy are usually found in the kidney. Sheehan (1950) observed that the glomeruli were enlarged by about 20 percent, often pouting into the neck of the tubule. The capillary loops are variably dilated and contracted. The endothelial cells are swollen, and deposited within and beneath them are fibrils that have been mistaken for thickening and reduplication of the basement membrane.

Sheehan's interpretations have been confirmed by electron microscopic studies of renal biopsies taken from women with preeclampsia. Most, but not all, of these studies are consistent with the view that the characteristic changes are glomerular capillary endothelial swelling. These changes, accompanied by subendothelial deposits of protein material, are called *glomerular capillary endotheliosis* by Spargo and associates (1959). The endothelial cells are so swollen as to block partially, or even completely, the capillary lumens. Homogeneous deposits of an electron-dense substance are found between the basal lamina and the endothelial cell and within the cells themselves (Figs. 35–10 and 35–11). Vassalli and co-workers (1963), on the basis of immunofluorescent staining, considered the material to be a fibrinogen derivative and regarded its presence as characteristic of preeclampsia. This observation, in part, led to a theory that the renal lesions of preeclampsia are the result of intravascular coagulation initiated by something, presumably thromboplastin, released from the placenta (Page, 1972). Lichtig and co-workers (1975), however, were able to identify fibrinogen or its derivatives so deposited in only 13 of 30 renal biopsy specimens from women with preeclampsia, and in only 2 of the 30 was the amount of fibrin graded as more than a trace. An alternative explanation for the renal lesion has been proposed by Petrucco and colleagues (1974), who detected IgM and IgG, and sometimes complement, in the glomeruli of preeclamptic women in proportion to the severity of the disease. They suggested that an immunological mechanism was active in the production of the glomerular lesion.

The renal changes identified by electron microscopy have been held out by some as being pathognomonic of preeclampsia. The uncertainties of clinical diagnosis are so great, however, as to preclude acceptance of such a one-to-one relation, except as an act of faith. The history of pathognomonic lesions in eclampsia engenders such skepticism.

Renal tubular lesions are common in women with eclampsia, but what has been interpreted as degenerative changes may represent only an accumulation within the cells of protein reabsorbed from the glomerular filtrate. The collecting tubules may appear obstructed by casts from derivatives of protein, including, at times, hemoglobin.

Acute renal failure from *tubular necrosis* may develop. Although this is more common in neglected cases, in our experiences it is most often induced by hemorrhage, usually associated with delivery, for which adequate blood replacement is not given. Rarely, *renal cortical necrosis* develops when the major portion of the cortex of both kidneys undergoes necrosis. Both cause acute renal failure characterized clinically by oliguria or anuria and rapidly developing azotemia. Renal cortical necrosis is irreversible, and although it develops in nonpregnant women and in men, in many institutions the lesion has been associated most often with pregnancy.

THE LIVER

With severe preeclampsia, there are, at times, alterations in tests of hepatic function and integrity, including delayed excretion of bromosulfophthalein and elevation of serum aspartate aminotransferase levels (Combes and Adams, 1972). Severe hyperbilirubinemia is uncommon with preeclampsia, and in our report of 134 women, including 45 with eclampsia, only 3 had a serum bilirubin greater than 1.2 mg per dL, with 2.3 mg per dL as the highest value (Pritchard and colleagues, 1976). Much of the increase in serum alkaline phosphatase is usually in the form of heat-stable alkaline phosphatase, which most likely is of placental origin.

The most likely lesion that accounts for serum liver enzyme elevation is *periportal hemorrhagic necrosis* in the periphery of the liver lobule. In the past, this was commonly identified at autopsy and was long considered to be the characteristic lesion of eclampsia (Fig. 35–12). Fortunately, changes this extensive sel-

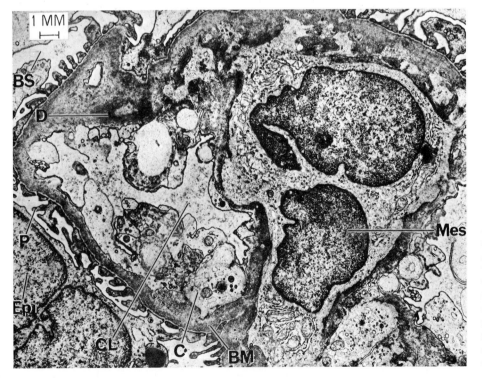

Figure 35–10. The glomerular capillary lesion of preeclampsia. BS = Bowman's space. D = electrodense deposit, probably a derivative of fibrinogen. P = podocytes, or foot processes of epithelial cell. Epi = epithelial cell nucleus. CL = lumen of glomerular capillary. C = markedly swollen endothelial cytoplasm. BM = basement membrane (normal). Mes = mesothelial cell nucleus. (*From Chesley: Hypertensive Disorders of Pregnancy. New York, Appleton-Century-Crofts, 1978.*)

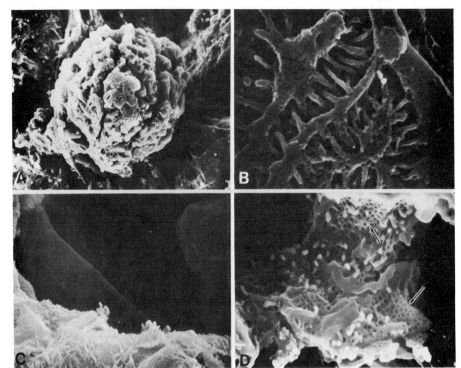

Figure 35–11. Scanning electron micrographs of kidneys. **A.** Enlarged, swollen glomerulus x 500. **B.** Branching and interdigitation of terminal epithelial foot processes, usually normal in preeclampsia x 20,000. **C.** Interior of glomerular capillary. Endothelial fenestrae are not seen because of severe swelling of the cytoplasm x 5,000. **D.** Normal glomerulus for comparison; note polygonal endothelial fenestrae (arrows) x 5,000. (*Photographs by N. G. Ordóñoz, from Lindheimer and Katz: Renal Function and Disease in Pregnancy. Philadelphia, Lea and Febiger, 1977.*)

dom are identified in liver biopsies from nonfatal cases. In our experiences from Parkland Hospital, liver histology was normal in biopsies from 6 preeclamptic and 12 eclamptic women (Combes and Adams, 1972). Since the specimen taken was small, and since appreciable thrombocytopenia was considered exclusionary, it is likely that women with some hepatocellular necrosis were missed. In our experiences, as well as those of Sibai and colleagues (1986), abnormally elevated serum liver enzymes, and thus liver damage, are likely to be accompanied by thrombocytopenia.

Bleeding from these lesions may extend beneath the hepatic capsule and form a *subcapsular hematoma*. Actually, such hemorrhages without rupture may be more common than previously suspected. Manas and colleagues (1985) described seven

women with preeclampsia and upper abdominal pain, and using computed tomography, showed that five had hepatic hemorrhage (Fig. 35–13). Surgical repair was not necessary in any of these women, but six required blood and component transfusions. In rare instances, subcapsular hemorrhage may be so extensive as to cause rupture of the capsule, with bleeding into the peritoneal cavity, which at times may be massive and fatal. With rupture, prompt surgical intervention may be lifesaving. One woman at Parkland Hospital survived after receiving blood and blood products from more than 200 donors.

Liver involvement in preeclampsia–eclampsia is serious and is frequently accompanied by evidence for involvement of other organs, especially the kidney and brain, along with hemolysis and thrombocytopenia (Pritchard and colleagues, 1954a; Sibai

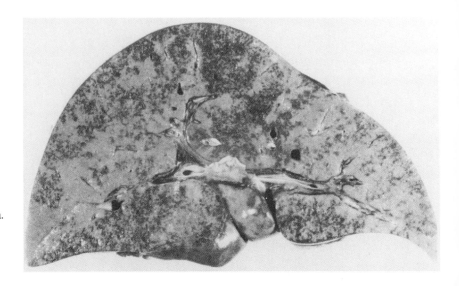

Figure 35–12. Hepatic involvement in preeclampsia. The liver has a grossly mottled appearance due to areas of widespread hemorrhage and necrosis. (*From Rolfes and Ishak: Am J Gastroenterol 81:1140, 1986.*)

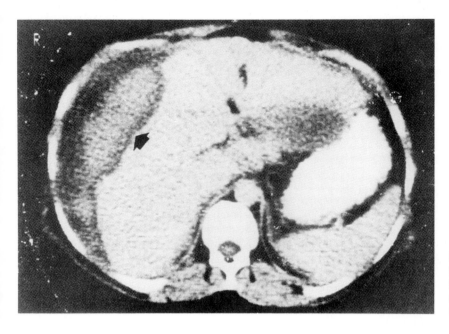

Figure 35–13. Computed tomographic scan of liver showing a subcapsular hematoma (*arrow*) along the right margin of the liver. (*From Manas and colleagues: N Engl J Med 312:426, 1985, with permission.*)

and colleagues, 1986a; Weinstein, 1985). Workers from the University of Tennessee identified this constellation in almost 10 percent of women with severe preeclampsia or eclampsia and reported that it was more common in white multiparas (Sibai and co-workers, 1986a). Other complications also were common, and these included placental abruption (20 percent), acute renal failure (8 percent), and pulmonary edema (5 percent). Two of the 112 women died.

THE BRAIN

McCall (1953) reported that cerebral blood flow, oxygen consumption, and vascular resistance were not altered in women with preeclampsia, eclampsia, or essential hypertension; however, the possibility of focal cerebral hypoperfusion or hyperperfusion could not be excluded.

Nonspecific abnormalities in the electroencephalogram usually can be demonstrated for some time after eclamptic convulsions. Sibai and colleagues (1985a) observed that 75 percent of 65 eclamptic women had abnormal electroencephalograms within 48 hours of seizures. Half of these persisted past 1 week, but most were normal by 3 months. An increased incidence of electroencephalographic abnormalities has been described for members of families of women with eclampsia, a finding that suggests that some women who convulse as the consequence of pregnancy-induced hypertension are by inheritance predisposed to do so (Rosenbaum and Maltby, 1943).

The principal postmortem lesions that have been described in the brain of women who died with eclampsia are edema, hyperemia, focal anemia, thrombosis, and hemorrhage. Sheehan (1950) examined the brains of 48 eclamptic women very soon after their death, and hemorrhages, ranging from petechiae to gross bleeding, were found in 56 percent. According to Sheehan, if the brain is examined within an hour after death, most often it is as firm as normal and there is no obvious edema. Govan (1961) investigated the cause of death in 110 fatal cases of eclampsia and concluded that cerebral hemorrhage was responsible in 39. Of 47 women who died of cardiorespiratory failure,

small cerebral hemorrhagic lesions were found in 85 percent. He further described as a regular finding fibrinoid changes in the walls of cerebral vessels. The lesions sometimes appeared to have been present for some time, as judged from the surrounding leucocytic response and hemosiderin-pigmented macrophages, a finding that suggested that the prodromal neurological symptoms and the convulsions may be related to these lesions.

Until recently, cranial computed tomographic scans usually were reported to be normal in women with otherwise uncomplicated eclampsia. Sibai and colleagues (1985a) evaluated 20 eclamptic women who had persistent seizures despite magnesium sulfate therapy, seizures late postpartum, or neurological deficits, and they found no radiographic abnormalities. However, in a later investigation with more advanced equipment, Brown and colleagues (1988) found that nearly half of eclamptic women studied at Parkland Hospital had abnormal radiographic findings. The most common of these findings, shown in Figure 35–14, were hypodense areas, frequently seen in the cortical areas. These hypodense areas corresponded to the areas of petechial hemorrhage and infarction reported at autopsy by Sheehan and Lynch (1973).

These findings may provide some explanation why some women with preeclampsia convulse but others do not. It seems reasonable that the brain, like the liver and kidney, may be involved in some women more than in others, and that the extent of ischemic and petechial subcortical lesions perhaps further altered by an inherent seizure threshold influences the incidence of eclampsia.

BLINDNESS

While visual disturbances are common with severe preeclampsia, blindness, either alone, or accompanying convulsions, is uncommon. We have cared for several such women whose clinical courses were complicated by *amaurosis* of varying degrees (Cunningham and Pritchard, unpublished). Many of these women were found to have radiographic evidence for extensive occipital lobe hypodensities, and we concluded that this was an

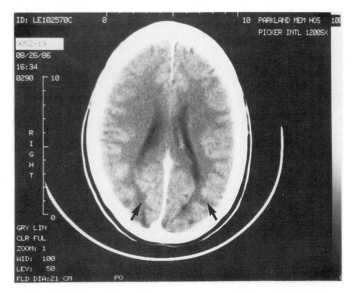

Figure 35–14. Cranial computed tomograph of a woman with eclampsia. Radiographic hypodensities (*arrows*) are seen in the occipital and parietal areas. (*From Brown and co-workers: Am J Obstet Gynecol 159:915, 1988.*)

exaggeration of the lesions described above and shown in Figure 35–14. The prognosis is good, and all women completely recovered within a week.

Retinal detachment also may cause altered vision, although it is usually one sided and seldom causes total visual loss as in some women with cortical blindness. In our experiences, seldom is surgical treatment indicated, the prognosis is good, and vision returns to normal within a week or so.

COMA

It is rare that a woman with eclampsia does not awaken after a seizure or that a woman with severe preeclampsia becomes comatose without antecedent seizure activity. We have encountered only a few such women, and their outcomes have been good. In two of these we documented extensive cerebral edema by computed tomography, and radiographic findings from one woman are shown in Figures 35–15A and B. From these limited experiences, it does not appear that this is from an extension of the ischemic and hemorrhagic lesions described above, since eclamptic women without coma have minimal cerebral edema (Brown and colleagues, 1988). More likely, since coma usually followed sudden and severe blood pressure elevations, this phenomen probably represents an inability to autoregulate cerebral blood flow with severe acute hypertension, and the result is generalized cerebral edema.

Another cause of coma is *intracranial hemorrhage* from a ruptured intracerebral vessel, an arteriovenous malformation, or a berry aneurysm. Sheehan and Lynch (1973) reported that 6 of 76 women with fatal eclampsia had massive white matter hemorrhage that caused coma and death. They also reported a high mortality rate with bleeding into the basal ganglia or pons. These lesions have a much poorer prognosis than coma from cerebral edema, and the two should be differentiated by computed tomography. Treatment is the same as for the nonpregnant patient.

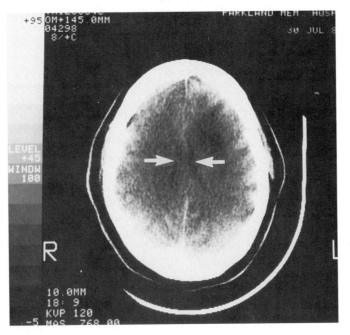

A

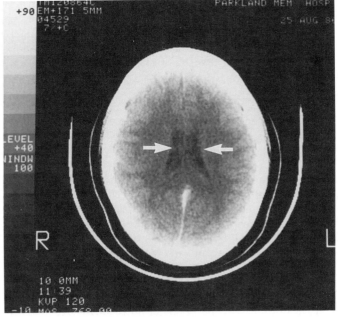

B

Figure 35–15. Cranial computed tomographs of an eclamptic woman who was also comatose. **A.** July 30, 1986: Cerebral edema is characterized by loss of gyral configuration, as well as by much-narrowed lateral ventricles (*arrows*). **B.** August 25,1986: After complete neurological recovery, gyral architecture is better seen and ventricles are normal in size. (*From Brown and colleagues: Am J Obstet Gynecol 159:915, 1988.*)

UTEROPLACENTAL PERFUSION

Compromised placental perfusion from uterine vasospasm is almost certainly a major culprit in the genesis of increased perinatal morbidity and mortality associated with pregnancy-induced or pregnancy-aggravated hypertension.

MEASUREMENTS OF PLACENTAL PERFUSION

Attempts to measure human maternal placental blood flow have been hampered by several obstacles, including inaccessibility of the placenta, the complexity of its venous effluent, and the unsuitability of certain investigative techniques for humans.

Despite the formidable problems encountered in attempts to measure uterine blood flow, Assali and associates (1953), Browne and Veall (1953), and Metcalfe and co-workers (1955) measured uterine blood flow in pregnant women and obtained reasonably consistent results. Both Assali and Metcalfe and their associates used a nitrous oxide method, a technique that is based on the Fick principle and required cannulation of a uterine vein. Total uterine perfusion was estimated, rather than maternal placental blood flow. Browne and Veall estimated changes in maternal placental flow through the use of a [24]Na clearance technique. This method required the insertion of a needle into the intervillous space. Both of these methods required technical proficiency and the use of invasive techniques in stressed subjects and threatened some risk to the mother and fetus. These investigators concluded from their studies that uterine blood flow in the normal-term pregnant woman was approximately 500 to 700 mL per minute.

Browne and Veall (1953), Morris and colleagues (1956), Johnson and Clayton (1957), and Weis and associates (1958), observed that [24]Na, when injected into the intervillous space, was cleared 2 to 3 times more rapidly in normotensive pregnant women than in preeclamptic women, implying a two- to three-fold decrease in uteroplacental perfusion in hypertensive women compared to normotensive gravidas.

INDIRECT METHODS

The consistent results and conclusions from these early studies continue to be supported by more recent studies using other methods of investigation. For instance, Brosens and associates (1972) reported that the mean diameter of myometrial spiral arterioles of 50 normal pregnant women was 500 μm. The same measurement in 36 women with preeclampsia was 200 μm.

Dehydroisoandrosterone Sulfate Clearance

Everett and colleagues (1980) presented evidence that the rate of clearance of dehydroisoandrosterone sulfate through placental conversion to estradiol-17β was an accurate reflection of maternal placental perfusion. Normally, as pregnancy advances, the placental clearance rate of maternal plasma dehydroisoandrosterone sulfate through placental estradiol-17β formation increases greatly. Moreover, in women destined to develop pregnancy-induced hypertension, the placental clearance rate of dehydroisoandrosterone sulfate is greater before the onset of hypertension than in control subjects, an intriguing observation in itself (Chap. 5, p. 73). The placental clearance rate decreases before the onset of overt hypertension (Worley and associates, 1975).

This placental clearance technique has been shown by Fritz and colleagues (1985) to parallel uteroplacental perfusion in primates.

The placental clearance rate of dehydroisoandrosterone sulfate has been measured in a study of the effect of *thiazide diuretics* on placental function and perfusion (Shoemaker and co-workers, 1973). The placental clearance rate of dehydroisoandrosterone sulfate was computed for one woman with preeclampsia, another with chronic hypertension complicating pregnancy, and a third woman who had been hospitalized at 36 weeks gestation simply because of excessive weight gain. The placental clearance rate of dehydroisoandrosterone sulfate was markedly lowered during diuretic therapy in all three women. A similar reduction in uteroplacental perfusion was noted following furosemide (Gant and co-workers, 1976).

Gant and co-workers (1976) reported that the intravenous administration of hydralazine to eight chronically hypertensive women near term was followed by a decrease in the metabolic clearance rate of dehydroisoandrosterone sulfate by a mean of nearly 25 percent, apparently as the result of the 37 percent decrease in diastolic blood pressure and presumably reduced small vessel perfusion. Thus, even the intermittent administration of intravenous hydralazine, as described below, may decrease uteroplacental perfusion. While the fetus in most normal pregnancies tolerates an appreciable decrease in placental perfusion without suffering profoundly, the fetus in a pregnancy complicated by severe preeclampsia or eclampsia, especially if growth-retarded, may not tolerate such reductions, since uteroplacental perfusion is most likely already compromised.

Doppler Velocimetry

Measurement of velocity of blood flowing through the uterine arteries has been used to estimate uteroplacental blood flow (see Chap. 15, p. 286). Using arterial velocity waveforms obtained by Doppler ultrasound, vascular resistance is estimated by comparing systolic and diastolic waveforms. Normally, the uterine vascular bed is a low-resistance circuit and flow continues throughout diastole. As resistance increases, diastolic velocity diminishes in relation to systolic velocity and this relationship has been used to estimate decreased flow. Fleischer (1986) and Trudinger (1985) and their colleagues have reported an increased systolic–diastolic ratio in uterine arteries of women with preeclampsia. Conversely, Hanretty and colleagues (1988) reported that technical factors severely limited data analysis obtained by using these methods.

Ducey and associates (1987) described systolic–diastolic velocity ratios from both uterine and umbilical arteries in 136 pregnancies complicated by hypertension. Among 51 women considered to have preeclampsia, 20 percent had normal umbilical artery velocity ratios, 16 percent had normal umbilical but abnormal uterine artery ratios, and in 41 percent both ratios were abnormal.

From our preliminary experiences, there seldom is evidence for diminished uterine artery flow velocity in *uncomplicated* preeclampsia. This is so even with dangerously elevated blood pressures. However, if there is associated fetal growth retardation, as reported by Cameron and colleagues (1988), the fetuses frequently will show aberrant flow velocity both in the umbilical and in the aortic vessels. In many previous reports, for example, that of Trudinger and colleagues (1985), women were studied *because of* growth retardation. Thus, it appears from these preliminary studies that pure preeclampsia may not be associated with significant changes in uterine artery systolic—diastolic ratios. Aberrations in fetal blood flow velocity can be detected, and these are much more likely if there is retarded fetal growth.

HISTOLOGICAL CHANGES IN THE PLACENTAL BED

Hertig (1945) identified in preeclamptic pregnancies a lesion of the uteroplacental arteries characterized by prominent lipid-rich foam cells. Zeek and Assali (1950) extended these observations and concluded that in preeclampsia there is a pathognomonic lesion of the uteroplacental vessels that they termed *acute atherosis*. Most investigators are now in accord that there is a lesion, but they do not necessarily agree on its precise nature. Using electron microscopic studies of arteries at the uteroplacental implantation site, DeWolf and co-workers (1975) reported that early preeclamptic changes include endothelial damage, insudation of plasma constituents into the vessel wall, proliferation of myointimal cells, and medial necrosis. They also found that lipid accumulates first in the myointimal cells and then in macrophages. Robertson and colleagues (1986) recently provided a careful review of these microscopic vascular findings.

CLINICAL ASPECTS OF PREECLAMPSIA

CLINICAL FINDINGS

The two especially important signs of preeclampsia—hypertension and proteinuria—are abnormalities of which the pregnant woman is usually unaware. By the time symptoms such as headache, visual disturbances, or epigastric pain develop, the disorder is most always severe. Hence, the importance of prenatal care in the early detection and management of preeclampsia becomes obvious.

BLOOD PRESSURE

The basic derangement in preeclampsia is arteriolar vasospasm, and it is not surprising, therefore, that the most dependable warning sign is an increase in blood pressure. The diastolic pressure is probably a more reliable prognostic sign than the systolic, and any diastolic pressure of 90 mm Hg or more that persists is abnormal. The fifth Korotkoff sound is used.

WEIGHT GAIN

A sudden increase in weight may precede the development of preeclampsia, and indeed, excessive weight gain in some women is the first sign. Weight increase of about 1 pound per week is normal, but when weight gain exceeds much more than 2 pounds in any given week, or 6 pounds in a month, developing preeclampsia must be suspected. Characteristic of preeclampsia is the suddenness of the excessive weight gain rather than an increase distributed throughout gestation. Sudden and excessive weight gain is attributable almost entirely to abnormal fluid retention and is demonstrable, as a rule, before visible signs of nondependent edema, such as, swollen eyelids and puffiness of the fingers. In cases of fulminating preeclampsia or eclampsia, fluid retention may be extreme, and in such women a weight gain of 10 pounds or more within a week is not unusual.

PROTEINURIA

The degree of proteinuria varies greatly in preeclampsia, not only from case to case but also in the same woman from hour to hour. The variability points to a functional (vasospasm) rather than an organic cause. In early preeclampsia, proteinuria may be minimal or entirely lacking. In the most severe forms proteinuria is usually demonstrable and may be as much as 10 g per L. Proteinuria almost always develops later than hypertension and usually later than excessive weight gain.

HEADACHE

Headache is unusual in milder cases but is increasingly frequent in more severe disease. It is often frontal but may be occipital, and it is resistant to relief from ordinary analgesics. **In women who develop eclampsia, severe headache almost invariably precedes the first convulsion.**

EPIGASTRIC PAIN

Epigastric or right upper quadrant pain often is a symptom of severe preeclampsia and may be indicative of imminent convulsions. It may be the result of stretching of the hepatic capsule, possibly by edema and hemorrhage (p. 667).

VISUAL DISTURBANCES

A spectrum of visual disturbances, ranging from slight blurring of vision to scotomata to partial or complete blindness, may accompany preeclampsia. These probably develop as the result of vasospasm, ischemia, and petechial hemorrhages within the occipital cortex (Brown and colleagues, 1988). In some women, visual symptoms may arise from retinal arteriolar spasm, ischemia, and edema, and in rare cases, retinal detachment (p. 670). In general, the prognosis for such detachments is good, and the retina usually reattaches spontaneously within a few weeks after delivery. Hemorrhages and exudates are extremely rare in preeclampsia and when present, are almost invariably due to underlying chronic hypertensive vascular disease.

IMMEDIATE PROGNOSIS

The prognosis for the mother and fetus is dependent to a considerable extent on the gestational age of the fetus, whether improvement follows hospitalization, when and how delivery is accomplished, and whether eclampsia supervenes.

The perinatal mortality rate is variably increased for pregnancies complicated by pregnancy-induced hypertension, as with the other hypertensive disorders. It is dependent primarily upon the time of onset and the severity of the disease. Much of the loss is the consequence of prematurity, either from spontaneous labor or because of induced preterm delivery necessitated by severe preeclampsia.

PROPHYLAXIS AND EARLY TREATMENT

EARLY DETECTION

Because women are usually asymptomatic and seldom notice the signs of incipient preeclampsia, its early detection demands careful observation at appropriate intervals, especially in women known to be predisposed to preeclampsia. Major predisposing factors are (1) nulliparity, (2) familial history of preeclampsia–eclampsia, (3) multiple fetuses, (4) diabetes, (5) chronic vascular disease, (6) renal disease, (7) hydatidiform mole, and (8) fetal hydrops.

Rapid weight gain any time during the latter half of pregnancy, or an upward trend in the diastolic blood pressure, even while still in the normal range, is worrisome. Every woman should be examined at least weekly during the last month of pregnancy and every 2 weeks during the previous 2 months. At these visits, the woman is weighed and careful blood pressure measurements made. Furthermore, all women should be advised verbally and preferably also by means of suitable printed instructions to report immediately any of the well-known symptoms or signs of preeclampsia, such as headache, visual disturbances, and puffiness of hands or face. The reporting of any such symptoms calls for an immediate examination to confirm or exclude preeclampsia.

Weight Gain

Obstetricians in the past often attempted to limit maternal weight gain to about 20 pounds, or even less, in the belief that preeclampsia could thereby be prevented. The total weight gained during pregnancy, however, probably has no relation to preeclampsia unless a large component of the gain is edema. Stringent restriction of weight gain is more likely to be detrimental rather than beneficial to both mother and fetus. The physician's scale, unfortunately, does not distinguish between the accumulation of edema fluid and the normal deposition of fetal and maternal tissue.

DIURETICS AND SODIUM RESTRICTION

Natriuretic drugs, such as chlorothiazide and its congeners, have been severely overused in the past. Although diuretics have been alleged to prevent the development of preeclampsia, the results of several studies cast doubt on their real value. The women studied by Kraus and associates (1966) took either a placebo or 50 mg of hydrochlorothiazide daily during at least the last 16 weeks of gestation. The incidence of preeclampsia was 6.67 percent in primigravid women given hydrochlorothiazide, as well as in those who took the placebo. Moreover, the frequency of hypertension was not altered in multiparous women. Collins and colleagues (1985) reviewed the results of nine such studies that included more than 7,000 women, and they concluded that perinatal mortality was not improved when diuretics were given to prevent preeclampsia. The failure of natriuretic drugs in the prevention of preeclampsia also raises serious doubt about the efficacy of rigid dietary sodium restriction.

Thiazide diuretics and similar compounds are not used in the treatment or prophylaxis of preeclampsia at Parkland Hospital. While there is no clear evidence that they are of any value, there is evidence that these drugs can reduce renal perfusion as measured by creatinine clearance and more importantly, probably reduce uteroplacental perfusion as cited above (Gant and colleagues, 1975). Thiazides can induce serious sodium and potassium depletion, hemorrhagic pancreatitis, and severe thrombocytopenia in some newborns.

OTHER DRUGS

Wallenburg and co-workers (1986) reported their experiences in which they gave either 60 mg of aspirin or placebo to primigravid women at 28 weeks gestation. These women were judged to be at high risk for developing preeclampsia because they were abnormally sensitive to infused angiotensin II. The reduced incidence of preeclampsia in the treated group was attributed to suppression of thromboxane synthesis by platelets,

with subsequent endothelial prostacyclin dominance. In a group of women with prior bad pregnancy outcomes due to hypertension and placental insufficiency, Beaufils and colleagues (1985) reported that early prophylactic treatment with dipyridamole and aspirin reduced their recurrence. They also attributed these results to the antiplatelet actions of these drugs. Although these reports seem encouraging, more extensive investigations to confirm these observations are necessary before they can be recommended for clinical practice. Currently the National Institutes of Health is sponsoring a multicenter study designed to investigate this hypothesis.

OBJECTIVES OF TREATMENT

The basic management objectives for any pregnancy complicated by pregnancy-induced hypertension are (1) termination of the pregnancy with the least possible trauma to the mother and the fetus, (2) birth of an infant who subsequently thrives, and (3) complete restoration of the health of the mother. In certain cases of preeclampsia, especially in women at or near term, these three objectives may be served equally well by careful induction of labor. **Therefore, the most important information that the obstetrician has for the successful management of pregnancy, and especially pregnancy that becomes complicated by hypertension, is precise knowledge of the age of the fetus (see Chap. 14, p. 260).**

AMBULATORY TREATMENT

Ambulatory treatment has no place in the management of pregnancy-induced or pregnancy-aggravated hypertension. Excluding young nulliparas, some women whose systolic blood pressure does not exceed 135 mm Hg and whose diastolic pressure does not exceed 85 mm Hg, and in whom proteinuria is absent, may be managed tentatively at home as long as the disease does not become more severe and fetal growth retardation is not suspected. Bed rest throughout the greater part of the day is essential. Moreover, these women should be examined twice weekly rather than once weekly, and they should be instructed in detail about reporting symptoms. With minor elevations of blood pressure, the response to this regimen is often immediate, but the woman must be cooperative and the obstetrician wary.

HOSPITAL MANAGEMENT

The indication for hospitalization of women with pregnancy-induced hypertension is a sustained elevation in systolic blood pressure of 140 mm Hg or above or a diastolic pressure of 90 mm Hg or above. For an intelligent continuing appraisal of the severity of the disease, upon admittance to the hospital, a systematic study should be instituted that includes the following:

1. An appropriate history and general physical examination followed by daily search for the development of signs and symptoms such as headache, visual disturbances, epigastric pain, and rapid weight gain
2. Weight measurement on admittance and every 2 days thereafter
3. Urine test for protein on admittance and subsequently at least every 2 days

4. Blood pressure readings with an appropriate-size cuff every 4 hours, except between midnight and morning, unless the midnight pressure has increased
5. Measurements of plasma creatinine, hematocrit, platelets, and serum liver enzymes, the frequency to be determined by the severity of hypertension
6. Frequent evaluation of fetal size and amnionic fluid volume by the same experienced examiner and by serial sonography if remote from term

Whenever these observations serve to establish a diagnosis of severe preeclampsia (Table 35–3), further management is the same as described for eclampsia (p. 679).

Bed rest, or at least reduced physical activity, throughout much of the day is beneficial. Ample, but not excessive, protein and calories should be included in the diet (Chap. 14, p. 263). Sodium and fluid intakes should be neither limited nor forced. Phenobarbital or other sedatives or tranquilizers have been used routinely by some; we do not use them or recommend their use.

The further management of a pregnancy complicated by preeclampsia will depend upon (1) its severity, determined by the presence or absence of the conditions cited in Table 35–3, (2) the duration of gestation, and (3) the condition of the cervix. Fortunately, many cases prove to be sufficiently mild and near enough to term that they can be managed conservatively until labor commences spontaneously or until the cervix becomes favorable for labor induction. Complete abatement of all signs and symptoms, however, is uncommon until after delivery. *Almost certainly, the underlying disease persists until after delivery!*

DRUG THERAPY

The use of antihypertensive drugs in an attempt to prolong pregnancy or modify perinatal outcomes in pregnancies complicated by various types and severities of hypertensive disorders has been of considerable interest, primarily in Western Europe, since Redman and colleagues (1976) first published their experiences with methyldopa. Theoretically, such antihypertensive therapy has potential usefulness when preeclampsia severe enough to warrant termination of pregnancy develops early enough so that neonatal survival is precluded. Unfortunately, such management, based upon control of maternal hypertension with agents such as methyldopa and hydralazine may be catastrophic. Sibai and colleagues (1985b) attempted to prolong pregnancy because of fetal immaturity in 60 women with severe preeclampsia diagnosed between 18 and 27 weeks gestation. **The total perinatal mortality rate was 87 percent, and although no mothers died, 13 suffered placental abruption, 10 eclampsia, 5 consumptive coagulopathy, 3 renal failure, 2 hypertensive encephalopathy, 1 intracerebral hemorrhage, and 1 a ruptured hepatic hematoma.**

The development of β-blocker drugs has stimulated renewed interest in controlling maternal blood pressure in the interest of improving perinatal outcomes. Gallery and colleagues (1979) compared methyldopa and oxyprenolol and suggested that the latter offered a specific advantage since pregnancies treated with oxyprenolol resulted in infants of greater birthweight. Rubin and colleagues (1983) randomized 120 women of mixed parity who were mildly to moderately hypertensive during the last trimester, to be given atenolol or placebo. A total of 85 women completed the trial, and those given atenolol had significantly reduced blood pressures, less frequently developed proteinuria, and had fewer hospital admissions. There were no advantages found for infants born to mothers who completed the trial, and indeed, *the perinatal mortality was 35 per 1,000.* Nevertheless, these investigators concluded that atenolol was more effective than conventional obstetrical management and does not adversely affect mother or baby. Constantine and co-workers (1987) reported that if nifedipine was added because of a poor response to atenolol then the perinatal mortality rate was 130 per 1,000. Similar results were obtained by Högstedt and associates (1985) who used metoprolol plus hydralazine versus nonpharmacological management, but they concluded that drug treatment was not mandatory for good outcome of pregnancy in cases of mild and moderate hypertension. Fidler and co-workers (1983) found no significant fetal benefits of either oxyprenolol or methyldopa in maternal treatment. Plouin and colleagues (1988) reported that labetalol and methyldopa produced similar pregnancy outcomes, but they did not include a control group.

Recently, Sibai and associates (1987a) reported their results from a well-designed randomized, comparative study done to evaluate the effectiveness of labetalol and hospitalization alone for 200 nulliparous women with proteinuric hypertension diagnosed between 26 and 35 weeks. Although women given labetalol had significantly lower mean blood pressures, there were no differences between the groups for mean pregnancy prolongation, gestational age at delivery, or birthweight (Table 35–8). The cesarean section rates were similar, as were the number of infants admitted to the special care nurseries. **Importantly, growth-retarded infants were twice as frequent in the women given labetalol, compared to those treated by hospitalization alone (19 versus 9 percent).**

There have been no studies published that convince us to attempt pharmacological control of pregnancy-induced hypertension in an effort to prolong gestation. In most investigations no effort has been made to distinguish pregnancy-induced hypertension from chronic underlying hypertension. Specifically, seldom was preeclampsia in the nullipara considered separately from chronic hypertension in the multipara. Importantly, antihypertensive therapy and nonintervention in pregnancies complicated by severe preeclampsia before fetal maturity benefits neither the fetus nor the mother, and indeed, it places both in dire jeopardy. Thus, those pregnancies most in need of prolongation appear to be least served by the pharmacological attempt.

SEVERE PREECLAMPSIA

Occasionally, fulminant or neglected preeclampsia is encountered, with blood pressure recordings in excess of 160/110 mm Hg, edema, and proteinuria. Headache, visual disturbances, or epigastric pain are indicative that convulsions are imminent, and oliguria is another ominous sign. Severe preeclampsia demands anticonvulsant and usually antihypertensive therapy followed by delivery. Treatment is identical to that described below for eclampsia (p. 679). The prime objectives are to forestall convulsions, to prevent intracranial hemorrhage and serious damage to other vital organs, and to deliver a healthy infant.

In a more severe case of preeclampsia, as well as eclampsia, magnesium sulfate administered parenterally is a most valuable anticonvulsant agent, as attested by the experience of many clinics over many years. Magnesium sulfate may be given intramuscularly by intermittent injection or intravenously by continuous infusion. The dosage schedule for severe preeclampsia is the same as for eclampsia (p. 679). Since the period of labor and delivery is a more likely time for convulsions to develop, all women suspected to have pregnancy-induced hypertension are

TABLE 35–8. MILD PREECLAMPSIA IN 200 NULLIPAROUS WOMEN: RESULTS OF TREATMENT WITH HOSPITALIZATION ALONE OR HOSPITALIZATION WITH LABETALOL TREATMENT

Factor	Hospitalization Alone (N = 100)	Hospitalization Plus Labetalol (N = 100)	Significance
Entry (weeks)	32.4 ± 2.4	32.6 ± 2.4	NS
Delivery (weeks)	35.5 ± 3.0	35.4 ± 3.0	NS
Prolongation (days)	21.3 ± 13	20.1 ± 14	NS
Blood Pressure (means)			
Systolic (initial/treatment)	144/141	142/132[a]	[a]$P < 0.0005$
Diastolic (initial/treatment)	95/95	90/82[a]	[a]$P < 0.005$
Proteinuria (mg per day)			
Initial	565 ± 305	541 ± 303	NS
At Delivery	1,555 ± 1,941	2,032 ± 3,135	NS
Increased excretion	58%	57%	NS
Decreased excretion	26%	20%	NS
Severe hypertension	15%	5%	$P < 0.05$
Placental abruption	0	2	NS
Cesarean section	32%	36%	NS
Stillbirths	0	0	NS
Neonatal death	0	1	NS
Birthweight (mean)	2,258 ± 762 g	2,204 ± 756 g	NS
Fetal growth retardation	9%	19%	$P < .005$

From Sibai and colleagues: Obstet Gynecol 70:323, 1987a.

treated at Parkland Hospital with intramuscular magnesium sulfate during labor and for 24 hours postpartum. Hydralazine, administered intravenously in appropriate doses intermittently, has proven to be an effective and safe antihypertensive agent. Its use is discussed in more detail below (p. 683).

Conservative Management

It is again emphasized that development of severe preeclampsia warrants consideration for prompt delivery, regardless of fetal age. To allow pregnancy to continue under these circumstances is dangerous for the mother at least, as well as for the fetus, assuming the fetus has reached viability. Cited above were the experiences of Sibai and colleagues (1985b), who reported pregnancy outcomes for 60 women with severe preeclampsia who, because of extreme fetal immaturity, were managed conservatively with hospitalization, bed rest, and antihypertensive therapy. Complications were common and included placental abruption (22 percent), eclampsia (17 percent), renal failure (5 percent), as well as hypertensive encephalopathy, stroke, and ruptured hepatic hematoma. Fortunately, none of the mothers died; however, in more than half of the pregnancies, the infant was stillborn, and only eight infants survived, giving a perinatal mortality of 87 percent.

Glucocorticoids

To try to enhance fetal lung maturation, glucocorticoids have been administered by some to severely hypertensive pregnant women who are to be delivered remote from term. Several reports have appeared in which such treatment seemed not to worsen maternal hypertension, and a decrease in the incidence of respiratory distress and improved fetal survival have been claimed. For example, Nochimson and Petrie (1979) administered betamethasone to 20 severely hypertensive women and observed no untoward effect. Perinatal survival was 86 percent.

Similar results have been reported by Semchyshyn and associates (1983) and Ruvinsky and colleagues (1984).

We do not use corticosteroids in these circumstances for two reasons: (1) their administration poses potential risks to the mother and the fetus-infant, and (2) when the mother has severe preeclampsia requiring delivery, severe respiratory distress is uncommon even when the neonate is born preterm.

TERMINATION OF PREGNANCY

The cure for preeclampsia is delivery. However, when the fetus is known or suspected to be preterm, the tendency is widespread to temporize in the hope that a few more weeks in utero will reduce the risk to the infant of death or serious morbidity. Such a policy is justified in milder cases, but in severe preeclampsia, procrastination can prove to be ill advised, since the preeclampsia itself may kill the fetus. Even for the fetus remote from term, the probability of fetal survival may be greater in a well-operated neonatal intensive care unit than when the fetus is left in utero.

Assessments of fetal well-being and placental function have been attempted especially when there is hesitation to deliver the fetus because of prematurity. The use of serial measurements of plasma or urinary estriol, or of placental lactogen, have been abandoned by most. Some recommend frequent performance of various tests used currently to assess fetal well-being, for example, the *oxytocin challenge or contraction stress test*, or the *nonstress test* (Chap. 15 p. 290). Even more popular now is the *biophysical profile*, which includes performance of the nonstress test. While they have not been clearly demonstrated to provide valuable information otherwise unavailable for management of pregnancy complicated by preeclampsia, some of these are helpful to verify appropriate fetal growth and amnionic fluid volume.

Failure of the fetus to grow or diminution of amnionic fluid volume, as estimated clinically and by sonography, are ominous signs of fetal jeopardy. Measurement of the lecithin-sphingomyelin ratio in amnionic fluid may provide evidence of lung maturity, but it should be kept in mind during management of more severe cases that even when this ratio is less than 2.0, respiratory distress may not develop, and when it does, most often it does not prove fatal (see Chap. 15, p. 279, and Chap. 33, p. 593).

With moderate or severe preeclampsia that does not improve after a few days of hospitalization as outlined above, termination of pregnancy usually is advisable for the welfare of both the mother and the fetus. Labor may be induced by intravenous oxytocin (see Chap. 18, p. 343). In severe cases this procedure is often successful, even when the cervix is judged unfavorable for induction. Whenever it appears that labor induction almost certainly will not succeed, or attempts at induction of labor are not fruitful, cesarean delivery is accomplished for the more severe cases. In women with severe preeclampsia and eclampsia, subarachnoid or epidural block performed to provide analgesia may induce hypotension detrimental to the fetus, as well as to the mother (see Chap. 17, p. 338). Spinal analgesia is felt to be contraindicated by most authorities, and if epidural analgesia is to be used, it should be administered by a physician with special expertise in obstetrical analgesia.

For a woman near term, with a soft, partially effaced cervix, even milder degrees of preeclampsia probably carry more risk to the mother and her fetus-infant than does induction of labor by carefully monitored oxytocin stimulation. This is not likely to be the case, however, if the preeclampsia is mild but the cervix is firm and closed, indicating that abdominal delivery might be necessary if pregnancy is to be terminated. The hazard of cesarean delivery may be greater than that of allowing the pregnancy to continue *under close observation* in the hospital until the cervix is more suitable for induction.

HIGH-RISK PREGNANCY UNIT

A high-risk pregnancy unit was established at Parkland Hospital in 1973 to provide care as just described; the results were described by Hauth (1976) and Gilstrap (1978) and their colleagues. In the latter report 576 nulliparous women, usually teenage and often black, were admitted to the unit because of hypertension remote from term. In the 545 women who remained for care until delivery, the perinatal mortality rate was 9 per 1,000. In the 31 who left the unit before delivery, although advised not to, the perinatal mortality was 130 per 1,000. The mean birthweight of the infants whose mothers remained on the unit was 2,975 g, with 83 percent weighing 2,500 or more.

The majority of such women hospitalized will have a salutary response characterized by disappearance or improvement of hypertension (Table 35–9). **It is emphasized that these women are not "cured," and thus they are not discharged. Indeed, nearly 90 percent of women who subsequently became normotensive after hospitalization had recurrent hypertension before or during labor.** Whalley and colleagues (1983) reported that although these women became normotensive following hospitalization, they remained abnormally sensitive to infused angiotensin II. Moreover, using the placental clearance rate of dehydroisoandrosterone to estradiol-17β, Gant and colleagues (1976) showed evidence for persistently decreased uteroplacental perfusion despite amelioration of hypertension.

Through 1988, more than 2,500 nulliparous women with mild to moderate early-onset pregnancy-induced hypertension

TABLE 35–9. BLOOD PRESSURE RESPONSE IN 545 NULLIPAROUS WOMEN WITH PREGNANCY-INDUCED HYPERTENSION HOSPITALIZED ON THE HIGH-RISK PREGNANCY UNIT AT PARKLAND HOSPITAL

Initial Response	No.	%
Good		
Diastolic pressure decreased to < 90 mm Hg	441	81
Hypertension[a] recurred before labor	183	41
Hypertension recurred during labor	199	45
Remained normotensive through delivery	59	13
Moderate		
Hypertensive[a] intermittently until delivery	70	13
Poor		
Hypertension[a] persisted until delivery	34	6

[a] Diastolic blood pressure 90 mm Hg or greater.
Modified from Gilstrap and colleagues: Semin Perinatol 2:73, 1978.

have now been managed as described above and with equally good results (K. Leveno, personal communication). The costs of providing the relatively simple physical facility, modest nursing care, no drugs other than iron supplement, and the very few laboratory tests that are essential are slight compared to the cost of neonatal intensive care for the infant delivered preterm.

Some have argued that this approach to management of the woman with mild pregnancy-induced hypertension is overly cautious and that further hospitalization is not warranted if hypertension abates within a few days. Unfortunately, many third-party payors even refuse hospital reimbursement under these circumstances. Indeed, many of the results cited above include single teenagers, and perhaps a couple would be better motivated to have the woman follow instructions regarding limited activity at home. **If this approach is elected, it is emphasized that careful and frequent outpatient visits are mandatory to detect evidence of worsening of hypertension.** Unfortunately, such an approach has never been studied in a systematic fashion; therefore, its impact on maternal and fetal morbidity and mortality are only speculative.

POSTPARTUM

After delivery, there is usually rapid improvement, although at times hypertension may worsen transiently. If eclampsia develops, it most likely will do so during the first 24 hours after delivery, although we have described typical eclampsia in six primiparous women with its onset as late as 10 days postpartum (Brown and colleagues, 1987). At Parkland Hospital, magnesium sulfate therapy instituted before or during parturition is continued for 24 hours postpartum, and intravenous hydralazine is given intermittently, if needed, to lower diastolic blood pressures of 110 mm Hg or higher.

The woman may be discharged, even though still hypertensive, if there is evidence that severe hypertension has abated and she is otherwise well. Unless hypertension persists at dangerous levels during the puerperium, antihypertensive drugs are not prescribed; instead, the woman is reevaluated in 2 weeks. Typically, but not always, hypertension induced by pregnancy will have dissipated during this period. If so, the episode of preeclampsia does not mitigate against the use of oral contraceptives (see Chap. 42, p. 927). Conversely, hypertension persisting at this time usually signifies chronic vascular disease, often essential hypertension, and close follow-up is necessary to determine if treatment is indicated.

CLINICAL ASPECTS OF ECLAMPSIA

Eclampsia is characterized by generalized tonic–clonic convulsions that develop in some women with hypertension induced or aggravated by pregnancy. Coma without convulsions has also been called eclampsia; however, it is better to limit the diagnosis to women with convulsions and to regard fatal nonconvulsive cases as due to severe preeclampsia. As shown in Table 35–3, convulsions caused by cerebral involvement in pregnancy-induced hypertension are but one manifestation of severe preeclampsia, however, due to associated high mortality, eclampsia is regarded with particular fear.

CLINICAL COURSE

Depending on whether convulsions first appear before labor, during labor, or in the puerperium, eclampsia is designated as antepartum, intrapartum, or postpartum. Eclampsia is most common in the last trimester and becomes increasingly more frequent as term approaches. Nearly all cases of postpartum eclampsia develop within 24 hours of delivery, but we have seen typical cases up to 10 days postpartum (Brown and colleagues, 1987). Certainly, in women in whom the convulsions first appear more than 48 hours postpartum, another diagnosis should be considered.

Almost without exception, preeclampsia precedes the onset of eclamptic convulsions. Isolated cases are occasionally cited in which an eclamptic convulsion is said to have developed without warning in women who were apparently in good health. Usually such a woman had not been examined by her physician for some days or—more likely—weeks previously, and she had neglected to report symptoms of preeclampsia. Headache, visual disturbance, and epigastric or right upper quadrant pain are symptoms that should incite grave concern.

The convulsive movements usually begin about the mouth in the form of facial twitchings. After a few seconds the entire body becomes rigid in a generalized muscular contraction. The face is distorted, the eyes protrude, the arms are flexed, the hands are clenched, and the legs are inverted. All muscles are now in a state of tonic contraction. This phase may persist for 15 to 20 seconds. Suddenly the jaws begin to open and close violently, and soon after, the eyelids as well. The other facial muscles and then all muscles alternately contract and relax in rapid succession. So forceful are the muscular movements that the woman may throw herself out of her bed, and almost invariably, unless protected, the tongue is bitten by the violent action of the jaws (Fig. 35–16). Foam, often blood tinged, exudes from the mouth. The face is congested and the conjuctivae are injected. This phase, in which the muscles alternately contract and relax, may last about a minute. Gradually, the muscular movements become smaller and less frequent, and finally the woman lies motionless. Throughout the seizure the diaphragm has been fixed, with respiration halted. For a few seconds the woman appears to be dying from respiratory arrest, but just when a fatal outcome seems almost inevitable, she takes a long, deep, stertorous inhalation, and breathing is resumed. Coma then ensues. She will not remember the convulsion or, in all probability, events immediately before and afterward.

Most often the first convulsion is the forerunner of other convulsions, which may vary in number from 1 or 2 in mild cases to 10 to 20, or even 100 or more, in untreated severe cases. In rare instances, they follow one another so rapidly that the woman appears to be in a prolonged, almost continuous convulsion.

The duration of coma after a convulsion is variable. When the convulsions are infrequent, the woman usually recovers some degree of consciousness after each attack. As the woman arouses, a semiconscious combative state may ensue. In very severe cases, the coma persists from one convulsion to another, and death may result before she awakens. In rare instances, a single convulsion may be followed by coma from which the woman may never emerge, although, as a rule, death does not occur until after frequent repetitions of the convulsive attacks.

Respiration after an eclamptic convulsion usually is increased in rate and may be stertorous. The rate may reach 50 or more per minute, in response presumably to hypercarbia from lactic acidemia, as well as to varying intensities of hypoxia. Cyanosis may be observed in severe cases. Temperatures of 39°C or more are a very grave sign since the fever probably is the consequence of a central nervous system hemorrhage.

Proteinuria almost always is present and frequently is pronounced. Urine output is likely to be diminished appreciably, and occasionally anuria develops. Hemoglobinuria is common, but hemoglobinemia is observed only rarely.

Some degree of edema is probably present in all women with eclampsia. Often, as shown in Figure 35–17A, the edema is pronounced, (at times, massive), but it also may be occult.

As with severe preeclampsia, after delivery an increase in urinary output is usually an early sign of improvement. Proteinuria and edema ordinarily disappear within a week (Fig. 35–17B). In most cases, but certainly not all, the blood pressure returns to normal within 2 weeks after delivery. The longer

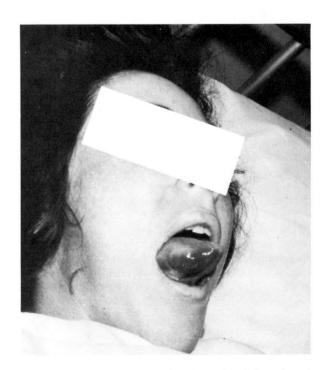

Figure 35–16. Hematoma of tongue from laceration during eclamptic convulsion. Thrombocytopenia may have contributed to the bleeding.

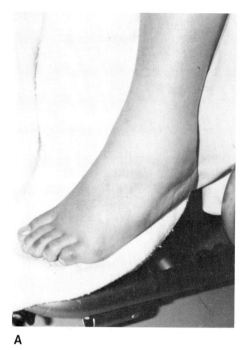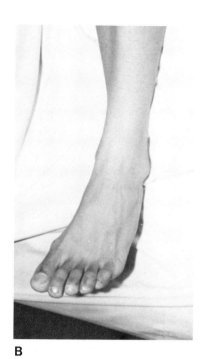

Figure 35–17. A. Severe edema in a young primigravida with antepartum eclampsia and a markedly reduced blood volume compared to normal pregnancy. **B.** The same woman as depicted in A, 3 days after delivery. The remarkable clearance of pedal edema, accompanied by diuresis and a 28-pound weight loss was spontaneous and unprovoked by any diuretic drug therapy. (*From Cunningham and Pritchard: Med Clin North Amer 68:505, 1984.*)

A   **B**

hypertension persists postpartum, the more likely it is the consequence of chronic vascular or renal disease.

In antepartum eclampsia, labor may begin spontaneously shortly after convulsions ensue, and progress rapidly to completion, sometimes before the attendants are aware that the unconscious or stuporous woman is having effective uterine contractions. If the attack occurs during labor, the contractions may increase in frequency and intensity and the duration of labor may be shortened. Because of maternal hypoxemia and lactic acidosis caused by convulsions, it is not unusual for fetal bradycardia to follow a seizure. This usually recovers within 3 to 5 minutes; if it persists more than 10 minutes, another cause must be considered, for example, rapid labor or placental abruption.

> Very uncommonly, convulsions cease, the coma disappears, labor does not commence, and the woman becomes completely oriented. This improved state may continue for several days or longer, a condition known as *intercurrent eclampsia*. It has been claimed that such pregnancies may return entirely to normal with complete regression of hypertension and proteinuria, but such an event appears to be rare. Although convulsions and coma may subside entirely and the blood pressure and proteinuria may decrease somewhat, most women continue to show substantial evidence of disease and are likely to convulse again unless given treatment, including delivery. This second attack may be much more severe.

Pulmonary edema, which is a grave prognostic sign, may follow eclamptic convulsions. There are at least two sources. (1) Aspiration pneumonitis may follow inhalation of gastric contents if simultaneous vomiting accompanies convulsions. (2) Cardiac failure may be the result of a combination of severe hypertension and vigorous intravenous fluid administration.

In some women with eclampsia, sudden death occurs synchronously with a convulsion or follows shortly thereafter, as the result of a massive cerebral hemorrhage (Fig. 35–18). Hemiplegia may result from sublethal hemorrhage. Cerebral hemorrhages are more likely in older women with underlying chronic

hypertension; more rarely they may be due to a ruptured berry aneurysm or arteriovenous malformation. Rarely, coma or substantively altered consciousness follows a seizure, or may even accompany preeclampsia without convulsions. At least in some cases, and as shown in Figure 35–15, this is due to extensive cerebral edema (Brown and colleagues, 1989). The prognosis in our limited experience has been quite good, provided that a ruptured vessel is not the cause of the coma and appropriate supportive care is given until the woman regains consciousness.

Blindness may follow a seizure, or it may arise spontaneously with preeclampsia. There are at least two causes. (1) Varying degrees of retinal detachment cause visual disturbances and, if bilateral, blindness. (2) In some women, ophthalmoscopic evaluation is normal and occipital lobe radiographic densities are seen using computed tomography. These probably represent areas of ischemia, infarction, and hemorrhage described by Sheehan and Lynch (1973). Whether due to cerebral or retinal pathology, the prognosis for return of normal vision is good and usually complete within a week.

Rarely, eclampsia is followed by psychosis in which the woman becomes violent. This usually lasts for 1 or 2 weeks, and the prognosis for return to normal is good, provided there is no preexisting mental illness. Chlorpromazine in carefully titrated doses has proved effective in the few cases of posteclampsia psychosis treated at Parkland Hospital.

DIFFERENTIAL DIAGNOSIS

Generally, eclampsia is much more likely to be diagnosed too frequently rather than overlooked, because epilepsy, encephalitis, meningitis, cerebral tumor, ruptured cerebral aneurysm, and even hysteria during late pregnancy and the puerperium may simulate it. Consequently, such conditions should be borne in mind whenever convulsions or coma develop during pregnancy, labor, or the puerperium, and they should be excluded before a tentative diagnosis of eclampsia is confirmed. **Until other causes are excluded, all pregnant women with convulsions should be considered to be eclamptic.**

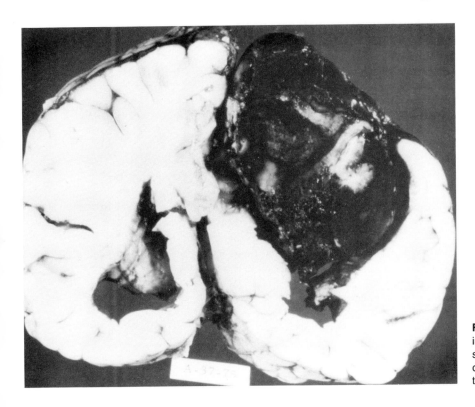

Figure 35–18. Massive fatal cerebral hemorrhage in a primigravid woman with eclampsia. Magnesium sulfate had been given appropriately, but diastolic blood pressures of 120 mm Hg were not treated. (*Courtesy of Dr. K. Leveno.*)

TREATMENT OF ECLAMPSIA

The basic treatment of eclampsia consists of (1) control of convulsions, (2) correction of hypoxia and acidosis, (3) lowering blood pressure when markedly elevated, and (4) steps to effect delivery once the mother is free of convulsions and hopefully is conscious. Once delivery is accomplished, the pathological changes of eclampsia soon ameliorate and eventually are completely reversed. This generalization holds true for dysfunctions of the central nervous system, liver, and kidneys, for hematological abnormalities, including thrombocytopenia and intense hemolysis, and usually for subsequent pregnancies.

PROGNOSIS

The prognosis is always serious, for eclampsia is one of the most dangerous conditions with which those caring for the pregnant woman and her fetus must deal. Fortunately, the maternal mortality rate in eclampsia has fallen in the past three decades. The maternal mortality rate reported since World War II for various methods of treatment applied in several countries is summarized in Table 35–10. In these reports, the maternal mortality has ranged from less than 1 percent to as much as 17.5 percent. At the same time, the perinatal mortality rate has ranged from 130 to 300 per 1,000. Precise comparisons of perinatal mortality rates are difficult to make because of different definitions of stillbirths and neonatal deaths in different countries.

HISTORICAL CONSIDERATIONS

As the consequence of very poor outcomes from immediate delivery without medical stabilization, by the late 1920s the slogan had become *"Treat the eclampsia medically and ignore the pregnancy."* From this time, almost every drug suspected of having a sedative, hypotensive, or diuretic effect has been ad-ministered to the woman (and her fetus) with eclampsia. Usually a large combination of drugs was employed simultaneously. Often the convulsions were controlled, but coma persisted, because of the medications rather than the disease. As the consequence of such empirical therapy, women with eclampsia have been, and perhaps still are, treated in a variety of ways, especially in institutions where eclampsia is uncommon.

PARKLAND HOSPITAL ECLAMPSIA REGIMEN

In 1955 Pritchard initiated a standardized treatment regimen at Parkland Hospital and this has since been used to manage women with eclampsia. The carefully analyzed results of treatment of 245 cases of eclampsia, typically the severest form of pregnancy-induced or -aggravated hypertension, were reported by Pritchard and associates in 1984. The specific plan of management is summarized:

1. Control of convulsions with magnesium sulfate, using an intravenously administered loading dose and periodic intramuscular injections standardized in the amount injected and the frequency of injections.
2. Control of severe hypertension with intermittent intravenous injections of hydralazine to lower the blood pressure whenever the diastolic pressure is 110 mm Hg or higher.
3. Avoidance of diuretics and hyperosmotic agents.
4. Limitation of intravenous fluid administration unless fluid loss is excessive.
5. Initiation of steps to effect delivery.

MAGNESIUM SULFATE TO CONTROL CONVULSIONS

Magnesium sulfate is used to arrest and prevent the convulsions of eclampsia without producing generalized central ner-

TABLE 35–10. RESULTS OF SOME REPORTS OF MATERNAL MORTALITY FROM ECLAMPSIA

Authors	Treatment	Patients	Maternal Deaths (Percent)
Dewar and Morris (1947)	Tribromethanol	44	4.5
Browne (1950)	Thiopental	26	7.6
Shears (1957)	Lytic cocktail	124	8.8
Menon (1961)	Lytic cocktail[a]	402	2.2
Llewellyn-Jones (1961)	Lytic cocktail	150	6.6
Bryant and Fleming (1962)	Magnesium sulfate and veratrum alkaloids	253	1.6
Zuspan and Ward (1964)	Magnesium sulfate	59	3.4
López-Llera (1982)			
A(1967)	Lytic cocktail	108	10.2
B(1970)	Lytic cocktail	120	11.7
C(1973)	Diazepam + reserpine	137	17.5
D(1976)	Furosemide, reserpine + volume expansion (albumin) + antithrombotic	160	12.5
E(1979)	Barbiturates + magnesium sulfate + reserpine and/or isoxsuprine	179	16.2
Total: A–E (1967–79)	Those listed in A–E	704	13.9
Lean and co-workers (1968)	Chlordiazepoxide	90[b]	3.3
	Diazepam	60	5.0
Kawathekar and associates (1973)	Diazepam	16	6.3
Mojadidi and Thompson (1973)	Morphine + magnesium sulfate	30	6.7
Gedekoh and colleagues (1981)	Magnesium sulfate + hydralazine	52	5.8
Pritchard and associates (1984)	Magnesium sulfate + hydralazine + standardized regimen	245	0.4
Sibai and associates (1985b)	Magnesium sulfate + hydralazine	186	0.5

[a] Chlorpromazine, diethazine and meperidine.
[b] Includes postpartum eclampsia (up to 14 days).
[c] Excludes postpartum eclampsia.

vous system depression in either the mother or the fetus-infant. **Magnesium sulfate is not given to treat hypertension.** Based on the studies of Borges and Gücer (1978) cited below, as well as extensive clinical observations, the drug most likely exerts a rather specific anticonvulsant action on the cerebral cortex. Typically, the mother stops convulsing after the initial administration of magnesium sulfate, and within an hour or two regains consciousness sufficiently to be oriented as to place and time.

The magnesium sulfate dosage schedule is presented in Table 35–11, and the response in plasma magnesium levels is illustrated in Figures 35–19A and B. Using this regimen, there has been no evidence of neonatal depression due to magnesium intoxication.

In the unusual case in which magnesium sulfate in the initial dose of 4 g intravenously plus 10 g intramuscularly has not arrested eclamptic convulsions, 2 g more, as a 20 percent solution, have been administered slowly intravenously. In a small woman, an additional 2 g dose may be used once, and twice if needed in a larger woman. In only 5 of the 245 women with eclampsia was it necessary to use supplementary medication to control the convulsions. Then the slow intravenous administration of sodium amobarbital in doses up to 250 mg was effective. Maintenance magnesium sulfate therapy for eclampsia is continued intramuscularly every 4 hours for 24 hours after delivery. For eclampsia that develops postpartum, magnesium sulfate is administered for 24 hours after the onset of convulsions.

Parenterally administered magnesium is cleared almost to-

tally by renal excretion, and magnesium intoxication is avoided by demonstrating before administering the next dose that (1) urine flow was at least 100 mL during the previous 4 hours, (2) the patellar reflex is present, and (3) there is no respiratory depression. Eclamptic convulsions almost always are prevented by plasma magnesium levels maintained at 4 to 7 mEq per L. As discussed below, loss of the patellar reflex begins with plasma

TABLE 35–11. MAGNESIUM SULFATE DOSAGE SCHEDULE FOR SEVERE PREECLAMPSIA AND ECLAMPSIA

1. Give 4 g of magnesium sulfate (MgSO₄· 7H₂O, USP) as a 20 percent solution intravenously at a rate not to exceed 1 g per minute.

2. Follow promptly with 10 g of 50 percent magnesium sulfate solution, one half (5 g) injected deeply in the upper outer quadrant of both buttocks through a 3-inch-long 20-guage needle. (Addition of 1.0 mL of 2 percent lidocaine minimizes discomfort.)

   If convulsions persist after 15 minutes, give up to 2 g more intravenously as a 20 percent solution at a rate not to exceed 1 g per minute. If the woman is large, up to 4 g may be given slowly.

3. Every 4 hours thereafter give 5 g of a 50 percent solution of magnesium sulfate injected deeply in the upper outer quadrant of alternate buttocks, but only after assuring that
   a. The patellar reflex is present.
   b. Respirations are not depressed.
   c. Urine output the previous 4 hours exceeded 100 mL.

4. Magnesium sulfate is discontinued 24 hours after delivery.

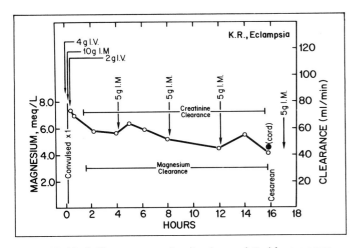

Figure 35–19. A. Plasma magnesium levels are plotted for a woman with antepartum eclampsia in whom 4 g of magnesium sulfate intravenously and 10 g intramuscularly were administered at the outset. When she soon convulsed again, 2 g more were injected slowly followed by 5 g intramuscularly every 4 hours, as described in Table 35–11. She did not convulse again.

Figure 35–19. B. The same woman as in A. Maternal magnesium levels during the first 28 hours postpartum and 4 days after magnesium sulfate was discontinued are plotted. Before and the day after delivery the renal clearance of magnesium remained relatively constant at about 35 percent of the somewhat depressed creatinine clearance. The mother recovered fully and the baby thrived. (*From Pritchard and associates: Am J Obstet Gynecol 148:951, 1984.*)

levels of 8 to 10 mEq per L and, importantly, severe respiratory depression and arrest at levels of 12 mEq per L or more. Calcium gluconate, 1 g **administered slowly** intravenously, plus oxygen usually suffices for the treatment of respiratory depression. If respiratory arrest occurs, prompt tracheal intubation and ventilation are lifesaving (McCubbin and associates, 1981).

Impaired Renal Function

Since magnesium is cleared almost exclusively by renal excretion, when glomerular filtration is substantively decreased, plasma magnesium concentration will be excessive using the doses described above. Renal function is estimated by measuring the plasma creatinine, and whenever it is 1.3 mg per dL or higher, we routinely give half of the maintenance magnesium sulfate dose outlined in Table 35–11. Thus, the woman with eclampsia who has impaired renal function is given a loading dose of 4 g intravenously in addition to the 10 g intramuscular dose, to be followed by 2.5 g intramuscularly every 4 hours. As shown in Figure 35–20, plasma magnesium levels obtained usually are within the desired range of 4 to 6 mEq per L. Some prefer in these circumstances to give magnesium sulfate intravenously by continuous infusion. **With either method, when there is renal insufficiency, plasma magnesium levels must be checked periodically.**

Pharmacology and Toxicology of Magnesium Sulfate

Even though magnesium sulfate continues to be widely used by most obstetricians in the United States, probably no drug is so misunderstood and underrated by physicians who do not have personal clinical experience with its efficacy. Magnesium sulfate has been condemned primarily because its mechanism of action in controlling convulsions has not been clearly understood, a problem that has also existed with other anticonvulsant agents, including phenytoin.

Magnesium sulfate USP is $MgSO_4 \cdot 7H_2O$ and not $MgSO_4$. When administered as described, the drug will practically always arrest eclamptic convulsions and prevent their recurrence. The initial in-

travenous injection of 4 g is used to establish promptly a therapeutic level that is then maintained by the nearly simultaneous intramuscular administration of 10 g of the compound, followed by 5 g intramuscularly every 4 hours, as long as there is no evidence of potentially dangerous hypermagnesemia. With this dosage schedule, the plasma levels for magnesium that are achieved are therapeutically effective and range from 4 to 7 mEq per L, compared to pretreatment plasma levels of less than 2.0 mEq per L (Chesley and Tepper, 1957; Stone and Pritchard, 1970). Magnesium sulfate injected deeply into the upper outer quadrant of the buttocks, as described above, has not resulted in erratic absorption and, in turn, erratic plasma levels.

Sibai and co-workers (1984) performed a prospective study in which they compared continuous intravenous magnesium sulfate and intramuscular magnesium sulfate. There was no significant difference between the mean magnesium levels observed after intramuscular magnesium sulfate and those observed following the

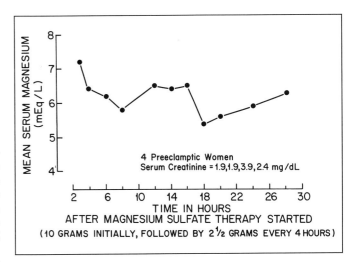

Figure 35–20. Plasma magnesium levels with chronic renal insufficiency.

intravenous regimen using a maintenance dose of 2 g per hour. However, the intramuscular regimen resulted in serum magnesium levels that were significantly higher than those obtained with a continuous intravenous maintenance dose of 1 g per hour (Fig. 35–21). It was concluded that there was no therapeutic advantage to the intravenous route of administration except for the avoidance of discomfort at the intramuscular injection site. When given intravenously, magnesium should be delivered by an infusion pump, and careful attention must be given to the solution concentration rate of delivery. Most recommend that 2 g per hour be given, to be followed by serial magnesium level determinations to detect toxicity. We favor the intramuscular route because of its safety.

The patellar reflex disappears by the time the plasma magnesium level reaches 10 mEq per L, presumably as the consequence of a curariform action. This sign serves to warn of impending magnesium toxicity, since a further increase will lead to respiratory depression. Plasma cholinesterase activity is substantively decreased in preeclamptic women, but this is not altered further by magnesium therapy (Kambam and associates, 1988).

When the plasma levels rise above 10 mEq per L, respiratory depression develops, and at 12 mEq per L or more, respiratory paralysis and arrest follow. Treatment with calcium gluconate, 1 g intravenously, along with the withholding of magnesium sulfate usually will reverse mild to moderate respiratory depression. For severe respiratory depression and arrest, prompt tracheal intubation and mechanical ventilation are lifesaving. Direct toxic effects on the myocardium from high levels of magnesium have been claimed; however, in humans it appears that a major cause of cardiac dysfunction must be hypoxia, the consequence of respiratory arrest, rather than a direct effect of the magnesium. With appropriate ventilation, cardiac action can be satisfactory even when plasma levels are very high (McCubbin and associates, 1981).

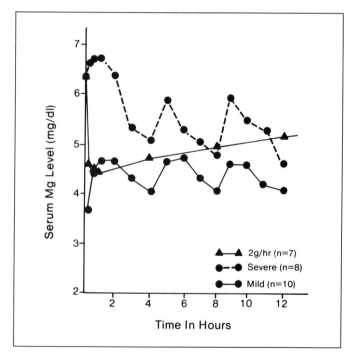

Figure 35–21. Comparison of serum magnesium levels following (1) mild preeclampsia—10-g intramuscular loading dose of magnesium sulfate and a 5-g maintenance dose every 4 hours (● — ●), (2) severe preeclampsia—4-g intravenous loading dose followed by the same regimen as in (1) (● --●), compared with (3) 4-g intravenous loading dose followed by a continuous infusion of 2 g per hour (▲—▲). (*From Sibai and co-workers: Am J Obstet Gynecol, 150:728, 1984, with permission.*)

Parenterally injected magnesium is filtered through the glomerulus and variably reabsorbed by the tubule. As the plasma magnesium concentration increases, more magnesium is filtered and less is reabsorbed. Nonetheless, when glomerular filtration is impaired, so is magnesium clearance. Therefore, an appreciably elevated plasma creatinine level serves to warn of diminished capacity of the kidney to excrete magnesium (Fig. 35–20). Despite its antidiuretic action, concomitant oxytocin administration does not alter plasma magnesium levels (Bloss and colleagues, 1987). A fraction of the injected magnesium is deposited reversibly in surface bone.

The acute cardiovascular effects of parenteral magnesium ion in women with severe preeclampsia have been studied by Cotton and associates (1984), who obtained data using pulmonary and radial artery catheterization. Following a 4-g intravenous dose given over 15 minutes, mean arterial blood pressure fell slightly, and this was accompanied by a 13 percent increase in cardiac index. Thus, magnesium decreased systemic vascular resistance and mean arterial pressure, and at the same time it increased cardiac output with no evidence for myocardial depression. These findings were coincidental with transient nausea and flushing, and the cardiovascular effects persisted for only 15 minutes despite continued infusion of magnesium sulfate at 1.5 g per hour.

In monkeys with angiotensin-induced hypertension late in pregnancy, Harbert and co-workers (1969) demonstrated slightly increased uterine blood flow in response to the infusion of magnesium sulfate. At the same time, arterial blood pressure decreased minimally. Thiagarajah and colleagues (1985) infused magnesium into nonpregnant monkeys and found that while cardiac output was unchanged, uterine blood flow increased by 20 percent. They concluded that this was due to selectively decreased uterine vascular resistance.

Altura and colleagues (1983) observed that when isolated umbilical arteries and veins obtained from normal term infants were incubated with 0 to 9.6 mmol per L of magnesium, basal tension of the vessels increased in the absence of magnesium and decreased as the concentration of magnesium increased. They also observed that the absence of magnesium potentiated the contractile response of the vessels to bradykinin, angiotensin II, serotonin, and prostaglandin $F_{2\alpha}$. Watson and colleagues (1986) reported the effects of magnesium on cultured human umbilical vein endothelial cells. In concentrations similar to those achieved in plasma with therapeutic doses described above, magnesium stimulated prostacyclin release in a dose-dependent fashion. Plasma from women given magnesium sulfate therapy stimulated a two- to fivefold increase in prostacyclin production, compared to pretherapy plasma. Presumably also mediated by prostacyclin, magnesium enhanced the platelet aggregation inhibition characteristic of endothelial cells.

Somjen and co-workers (1966) induced in themselves, by intravenous infusion, marked hypermagnesemia, achieving plasma levels up to 15 mEq per L. **Predictably, at such high plasma levels, respiratory depression developed that necessitated mechanical ventilation, but depression of the sensorium was not dramatic as long as hypoxia was prevented.** Thurnau and colleagues (1987) showed that there was a small, but highly significant increase in cerebrospinal fluid magnesium concentration after magnesium therapy for preeclampsia. The magnitude of the increase was directly proportional to the corresponding serum concentration. Borges and Gücer (1978) provided convincing evidence that the magnesium ion exerts an effect on the central nervous system much more specific than generalized depression. They measured the actions of parenterally administered magnesium sulfate on epileptic neural activity induced in awake, unmedicated subhuman primates. The infused magnesium sulfate suppressed neuronal burst firing and interictal electroencephalographic spike generation in neuronal populations rendered epileptic by topically applied penicillin G. The degree of suppression increased as the plasma magnesium concentration increased and decreased as it fell. Therefore, even though elevated concentrations of plasma magnesium do inhibit acetylcholine release in response to motor nerve impulses, reduce motor end-plate sensitivity to acetylcholine, and decrease the motor end-plate potential, these actions do not account for, nor should they necessarily be implicated in, the explanation of the beneficial effects of magnesium sulfate in controlling the convulsions of eclampsia. Goldman and Finkbeiner (1988) attribute therapeutic effects to neuronal calcium influx blocking through the glutamate channel.

Interestingly—indeed, amazingly—Donaldson (1978, 1986) and other neurologists, for reasons that are hard to discern, erroneously have emphasized that magnesium sulfate is a peripherally acting anticonvulsant and therefore "bad medicine." They imply that the drug works only in concentrations that cause paralysis and that consequently, the woman with eclampsia so treated is *"quiet on the outside but still convulsing on the inside."* This conclusion obviously was not based on any direct experience with eclampsia and its control with parenterally administered magnesium! At the same time, Donaldson has urged other forms of anticonvulsant therapy, but cites no data. Most other drugs that effectively arrest and prevent eclamptic convulsions do cause appreciable general depression of the central nervous system in both the mother and the newborn. Most recently, Donaldson (1986) concluded that convulsions result from inability of cerebral blood flow autoregulation and that nitroprusside, diazoxide, or hydralazine will prevent most seizures. While dangerous hypertension most certainly must be treated, we have prevented further convulsions in more than 300 women with eclampsia by using magnesium sulfate as described, but perhaps only a third or so were given hydralazine to lower dangerously elevated blood pressure.

Magnesium ions in relatively high concentration will depress myometrial contractility both in vivo and in vitro. With the regimen described above and the plasma levels that have resulted, no evidence of depression of myometrial function has been observed beyond a transient decrease in activity during and immediately after the initial intravenous loading dose. Typically, as the cutaneous flushing from the intravenous dose disappeared, uterine activity returned to preinjection intensity.

Magnesium ions administered parenterally to the mother cross the placenta promptly to achieve equilibrium between mother and fetus. Given as a large single dose intravenously, but not with smaller doses, magnesium sulfate may transiently cause a loss of beat-to-beat variability in the fetal heart rate (Pritchard, 1979).

The newborn infant may be depressed by magnesium only if *severe* hypermagnesemia exists at delivery. The kind of compromises described by Lipsitz and English (1967) to develop at times in the newborn after maternal continuous intravenous therapy with magnesium sulfate have not been observed by us (Stone and Pritchard, 1970; Cunningham and Pritchard, 1984) nor by Green and associates (1983). The regimen used at Parkland Hospital, coupled with the safeguards observed before each injection, have effectively prevented worrisome adverse effects from hypermagnesemia in newborns. Indeed, Lipsitz (1971) found in a subsequent study that infants were unlikely to be compromised when the mother had received magnesium sulfate according to the protocol that we have used for over 30 years.

HYDRALAZINE TO CONTROL SEVERE HYPERTENSION

At the time that this treatment regime for eclampsia was formulated, it was appreciated that severe acute hypertension increased the maternal risk of intracranial hemorrhage (Fig. 35–18). Moreover, contrary to much of the teaching at that time, it also was apparent that severe hypertension frequently persisted or promptly recurred after parenteral administration of magnesium sulfate in doses that effectively arrested convulsions and prevented their recurrence. The likelihood that maternal hypertension helped maintain placental perfusion also was recognized. Thus there was concern, which since has proven to be

appropriate, that aggressive treatment that promptly lowered the blood pressure to strictly normotensive levels might further compromise placental perfusion to the detriment of the fetus. From the outset, the regimen provided for intravenous injections of hydralazine whenever the diastolic blood pressure was 110 mm Hg or higher, to be administered in 5 to 10 mg doses at 15- to 20-minute intervals until a satisfactory reponse was achieved. A satisfactory response antepartum or intrapartum was defined as a decrease in diastolic blood pressure to 90 to 100 mm Hg, but not much lower lest placental perfusion be compromised.

Hydralazine so administered has proven remarkably effective, and importantly, cerebral hemorrhage has been avoided. At Parkland Hospital approximately 8 percent of all women with pregnancy-induced hypertension are given hydralazine as described; at this writing, we have administered this drug to more than 2,000 women to control acute peripartum hypertension. In none of these women was another antihypertensive agent needed because of poor response to hydralazine. In most European centers, too, by virtue of extensive experiences with the regimen, hydralazine is favored (Naden and Redman, 1985).

An example of very severe hypertension in a woman with chronic hypertension complicated by superimposed eclampsia that responded to repeated intravenous injections of hydralazine is shown in Table 35–12. Hydralazine was injected more frequently than recommended in the protocol, and the blood pressure decreased in less than 1 hour from 240–270/130–150 mm Hg to 110/80 mm Hg. Ominous fetal heart rate decelerations were evident when the pressure fell to 110/80 mm Hg and persisted until the maternal blood pressure increased.

The tendency to give a larger initial dose of hydralazine when the blood pressure is higher must be avoided. The response to even 5- to 10-mg doses cannot be predicted by the level of hypertension; thus we always give 5 mg as the initial dose.

Other Antihypertensive Agents

Intravenously administered diazoxide has been championed by some for use in preeclampsia–eclampsia because of its very

TABLE 35–12. INTRAVENOUS HYDRALAZINE FOR ACUTE CONTROL OF SEVERE HYPERTENSION

Time	Blood Pressure (mm Hg)
1140	240/150
1145	Magnesium sulfate, 4 g IV and 10 g IM
1155	270/130
1156	Hydralazine, 5 mg IV bolus
1200	200/120
1201	Hydralazine, 5 mg IV bolus
1205	230/130
1206	Hydralazine, 10 mg IV bolus
1210	185/120
1220	180/120
1221	Hydralazine, 5 mg IV bolus
1230	150/105
1235	150/105
1250	110/80—fetal distress
1310	130/90
1345	130/100–return to normal
1430	150/105 of fetal heart
1500	150/90 rate

potent antihypertensive action. Unfortunately, intravenous diazoxide therapy is accompanied by many adverse side effects.
For example, it is likely to arrest labor. It causes retention of
sodium, water, and uric acid. It causes serious hyperglycemia in
the mother and newborn infant. Importantly, it may produce
irreversible, and therefore lethal, hypotension when administered with or after other antihypertensive agents. Diazoxide is
seldom used in the United States, although some nonobstetri-
cians continue to recommend it. The drug is used in the United
Kingdom for blood pressure control, although it is reserved for
the most extreme situations (Naden and Redman, 1985; Rubin,
1986). Undoubtedly many of the serious adverse reactions reported as being due to diazoxide were associated with the standard 300-mg bolus dose recommended for nonpregnant
patients, and titration by intermittent administration of small
boluses of 30 to 60 mg apparently is safer. In our experience, as
well as that of most obstetricians in academic centers, diazoxide
has not been needed since hydralazine, given as described
above, has proved to be effective.

A variety of other agents, for example, nitroglycerin, pra-
zosin, and some β-blockers, have been used for acute hypertension control (Cotton and colleagues, 1986; Rubin, 1986).
Mabie and assoicates (1987) compared intravenous hydralazine
to labetalol for blood pressure control in 60 peripartum women
with severe pregnancy-associated hypertension. Labetalol lowered blood pressure more rapidly, and associated tachycardia
was minimal, but hydralazine more effectively lowered mean
arterial pressure to safe levels. Subsequently, Mabie and colleagues (1988) evaluated nifedipine administered sublingually
to 34 women with peripartum hypertension. Although its antihypertensive effects were potent and rapid, two women developed worrisome hypotension, and they caution against
antepartum use. Toppozada and co-workers (1988) infused
prostaglandin A_1 to lower blood pressure. Since experience with
agents other than hydralazine is limited, we do not currently
recommend any of them.

Hypertension Persisting Postpartum
The potential problem of serious compromise of placental perfusion and, in turn, fetal well-being that can be induced by
antihypertensive agents is obviated by delivery. If there is a
problem after delivery in controlling severe hypertension and
the intravenous hydralazine regime described above is being
used repeatedly early in the puerperium to control persisting
severe hypertension, hydralazine is then administered intramuscularly, usually in 10 mg doses at 4 to 6 hour intervals.
Rarely are larger doses needed. Once repeated blood pressure
readings remain near normal, the hydralazine is stopped. If
hypertension of appreciable intensity recurs, oral antihypertensive drugs are then given for as long as necessary.

AVOIDANCE OF DIURETICS AND HYPEROSMOTIC AGENTS

At the time of formulation of this regimen, expansion of the
extravascular component of the extracellular fluid compartment,
that is, generalized edema, had long been recognized as a common feature of severe preeclampsia and eclampsia. Most treatment regimens included liberal use of diuretics to try to clear the
edema, but most of the diuretic agents that were then available
were not very potent. There were also strong suspicions at that
time, which subsequently have been amply verified, that the
maternal blood volume in women with severe preeclampsia and

eclampsia typically is constricted appreciably, compared to normal pregnancy (Table 35–6).

It was reasoned at the outset that potent diuretics could
further compromise placental perfusion, since their immediate
effects would include further depletion of intravascular volume,
which most often is already reduced compared to normal pregnancy. Therefore, diuretics were not used to lower blood pressure lest they enhance the intensity of the maternal hemoconcentration and its adverse effects on the mother and the fetus.

Once delivery is accomplished, in almost all cases of severe
preeclampsia and eclampsia there is a spontaneous diuresis that
usually begins within 24 hours and results in the disappearance
of excessive extravascular extracellular fluid over the next 3 to 4
days, as demonstrated in Figures 35–17A and B.

With infusion of hyperosmotic agents the potential exists
for an appreciable intravascular influx of fluid and, in turn, the
subsequent escape of intravascular fluid in the form of edema
into vital organs, especially the lungs and brain. Moreover, an
oncotically active agent that leaks through capillaries into the
lungs and brain would promote the accumulation of edema at
these sites. Finally, a sustained beneficial effect from their use
has not been demonstrated. For all of these reasons, hyperosmotic agents have not been administered, and the use of furosemide or similar drugs has been limited to the rare instance in
which pulmonary edema was identified or strongly suspected.

FLUID THERAPY

Fluid, primarily lactated Ringer's solution containing 5 percent
dextrose, has been administered routinely at the rate of 60 mL to
no more than 125 mL per hour unless there was unusual fluid
loss from vomiting, diarrhea, diaphoresis, or, more likely, excessive blood loss at delivery. Oliguria, which is common in
cases of severe preeclampsia and eclampsia, coupled with the
knowledge that the maternal blood volume is very likely to be
constricted compared to normal pregnancy, makes it tempting
to administer intravenous fluids more vigorously. The rationale
for controlled, conservative fluid administration is that the typical eclamptic woman already has a considerable excess of extracellular fluid that, for reasons that remain unclear, is
inappropriately distributed between the intravascular and extravascular spaces of the extracellular fluid compartment. The
infusion of large volumes of fluid could and does enhance the
maldistribution of extracellular fluid and thereby increases appreciably the risk of pulmonary and cerebral edema (Benedetti
and Quilligan, 1980; Gedekoh and associates, 1981; Sibai and
co-workers, 1981, 1987b).

Pulmonary Edema
Women with severe preeclampsia–eclampsia who develop pulmonary edema most often do so postpartum (Benedetti and
colleagues, 1985; Cunningham and associates, 1986; Sibai and
co-workers, 1987b). Aspiration of gastric contents, the result of
convulsions or perhaps from anesthesia, should be excluded;
however, the majority of these women have cardiac failure.
Some normal pregnancy changes, magnified by preeclampsia,
predispose to pulmonary edema. Plasma oncotic pressure, for
example, decreases appreciably in normal term pregnancy,
since serum albumin decreases, and it falls even more with
preeclampsia (Benedetti and Carlson, 1979). Moreover, Oian
and colleagues (1986) described increased extravascular fluid
oncotic pressure in preeclamptic women, and this favors capillary fluid extravasation. It is suspected but has not been proved
that there is a capillary endothelial leak in preeclampsia. Bhatia

and associates (1987) reported a correlation between plasma colloid osmotic pressure and fibronectin concentration, which suggested to them that protein loss was from increased permeability caused by vessel injury.

The frequent findings of hemoconcentration and more recently the identification of reduced central venous and pulmonary capillary wedge pressures in women with severe preeclampsia have tempted some obstetricians to infuse vigorously various fluids or albumin concentrates, or both, to try to expand the blood volume and thereby somehow to relieve vasospasm and reverse organ deterioration. So far, clear-cut evidence of benefits from this approach is lacking; however, serious complications, especially pulmonary edema, have been reported. López-Llera (1982) reported that vigorous volume expansion was associated with the highest incidence of pulmonary edema in his series of more than 700 eclamptic women. Benedetti and colleagues (1985) described pulmonary edema in 7 of 10 severely preeclamptic women who were given colloid therapy. Sibai and colleagues (1987b) cited excessive colloid and crystalloid infusions as causing most of 37 cases of pulmonary edema associated with severe preeclampsia–eclampsia. Finally, Lehmann and co-workers (1987) reported that pulmonary edema caused nearly a third of maternal deaths due to pregnancy-associated hypertension at Charity Hospital.

For these reasons, until it is understood how to contain more fluid within the intravsacular compartment and, at the same time, less fluid outside the intravascular compartment, we remain convinced that, in the absence of marked fluid loss, fluids can be administered safely only in moderation. To date, no serious adverse effects have been observed from such a policy. Importantly, dialysis for renal failure had never been required for any of the 245 cases of eclampsia so managed and previously reported (Pritchard and colleagues, 1984). By way of comparison, in one large European renal dialysis center, eclampsia was identified to be the leading associated cause of acute renal failure among women (Silke and co-workers, 1980). Finally, in the great majority of women with eclampsia that we have managed, sufficient follow-up has been achieved to ascertain that either normal renal function returned, or in those women with preexisting impaired renal function, subsequent plasma creatinine levels were no higher than before.

Invasive Hemodynamic Monitoring

As summarized in Table 35–3, much of what has been learned within the past decade about the cardiovascular and hemodynamic pathophysiological alterations associated with severe preeclampsia–eclampsia has been made possible by invasive hemodynamic monitoring using a flow-directed pulmonary artery catheter. The need for clinical implementation of such technology for the woman with preeclampsia–eclampsia, however, has not been established. The subject has been reviewed recently by Hankins (1986), Wasserstrum and Cotton (1986), and Clark and Cotton (1988). Two conditions that frequently are cited as indications for such monitoring are preeclampsia associated with oliguria and preeclampsia associated with pulmonary edema. Perhaps somewhat paradoxically, it is usually vigorous treatment of the former that results in most cases of the latter! The American College of Obstetricians and Gynecologists (1988a) does not list severe preeclampsia–eclampsia as an indication for pulmonary artery catheterization.

Since, as described in detail above, it is our policy at Parkland Hospital to avoid vigorous intravenous hydration and osmotically active agents in women with severe preeclampsia and

eclampsia, we have not utilized invasive hemodynamic monitoring for the vast majority of these women. Oliguria associated with preeclampsia, unless also associated with blood loss, will improve after delivery, and thus, vigorous hydration antepartum is unnecessary and potentially dangerous.

The routine use of such monitoring even if pulmonary edema develops is questionable. Most women who develop pulmonary edema from ventricular failure respond quickly to furosemide given intravenously. Afterload reduction with intermittent doses of intravenous hydralazine to lower blood pressure, as described above, also may be necessary, since in our experiences, women with chronic hypertension and severe superimposed preeclampsia are more likely to develop heart failure (Cunningham and associates, 1986). Our observations, as well as those of Mabie and colleagues (1988a), indicate that obese women in these circumstances are even more likely to develop heart failure.

Invasive monitoring should be considered for those women with multiple clinical factors that might cause pulmonary edema by more than one mechanism. This is particularly relevant if pulmonary edema is inexplicable or refractory to treatment. Still, in most of these cases we have not found it necessary to perform pulmonary catheterization for clinical management. Finally, pulmonary artery catheterization may be associated with serious morbidity and even with mortality. In a review, Robin (1985) cited a major complication rate of 20 to 33 percent, with associated mortality of up to 4 percent.

DELIVERY

When this treatment regimen was formulated in the 1950s, the identification of eclampsia immediately caused appropriate concern for the welfare of the mother. Therefore, to avoid risks to the mother from cesarean delivery, steps to effect vaginal delivery were employed even in some circumstances in which it appeared that the fetus might have been better served by cesarean section. It became apparent early on that labor often ensued spontaneously or could be induced successfully even remote from term without subjecting the fetus to appreciably greater risk. It also became apparent early on that a magic cure did not immediately follow delivery by any route, but serious morbidity was less common in the puerperium among women delivered vaginally. For these reasons, we continue to try to effect vaginal delivery, and quite often we have been successful. For example, labor culminating in vaginal delivery was accomplished in nearly 75 percent of 209 women with antepartum eclampsia (Cunningham and Pritchard, 1984). Moreover, labor often was induced successfully and vaginal delivery of a fetus in good condition was accomplished even when remote from term, for example, in 16 of the last 20 instances in which the fetuses weighed 1,500 g or less.

Although it has been stated that labor is impaired by magnesium sulfate, this claim is not supported by the successes obtained in delivering eclamptic women vaginally (Pritchard, 1955; Stallworth and co-workers, 1981).

Blood Loss at Delivery

Hemoconcentration, or lack of normal pregnancy-induced hypervolemia, is an almost predictable feature of severe preeclampsia. **The woman with severe preeclampsia or eclampsia who consequently lacks normal pregnancy hypervolemia is much less tolerant to blood loss than is the normally pregnant woman.** It is of great importance to recognize that an appreciable fall in blood pressure very soon after delivery most often means excessive blood loss and not sudden dissolution of the vasospasm. When oliguria follows delivery, the hematocrit is evaluated frequently to help detect excessive blood loss that, when identified, is treated by careful blood transfusion.

The average-sized normally pregnant woman can shed in the course of delivery almost all of the 1,500 mL or so of blood that she had added to her nonpregnant volume without suffering an appreciable fall in hematocrit. The impact of comparable blood loss when pregnancy hypervolemia is seriously restricted is evident in the woman with eclampsia present in Figure 35–22. Associated with her delivery was the loss of 405 mL of red blood cells, equivalent to 1,100 mL of predelivery blood, primarily from uterine atony. Blood volume was restored by careful infusion of lactated Ringer's solution. The hematocrit fell from 38 to 23, whereas if the blood volume had been normal for late pregnancy (about 45 percent greater than the non-pregnant volume, rather than 16 percent), it is anticipated that there would have been no decrease in hematocrit. In fact, that was just the sequence of events with her second pregnancy: an increase of blood volume of 43 percent followed by blood loss of a liter at delivery, but no fall in hematocrit.

ANALGESIA AND ANESTHESIA

Intravenous or intramuscular meperidine, usually with promethazine, is given in moderation for discomforts of labor and after cesarean delivery. For women with severe preeclampsia and eclampsia we continue to use local or pudendal analgesia for nearly all vaginal deliveries. General anesthesia, using thiopental, succinylcholine, nitrous oxide, and oxygen, is administered for cesarean section and indicated forceps deliveries. Hodgkinson and colleagues (1980) described a transient but severe hypertensive reponse to tracheal intubation and extubation in women with severe preeclampsia in whom general anesthesia was used. We, too, have noted this reponse, and while it is worrisome, we have not seen serious sequelae from it. The hypertensive reponse often may be prevented by the intravenous administration of 5 mg of hydralazine just prior to the induction of anesthesia. Ramanathan and colleagues (1988) like-

wise attenuated this response by administering labetalol intra venously.

Conduction analgesia has been avoided in women with severe preeclampsia and eclampsia because of concern for sudden, severe hypotension induced by splanchnic blockade and in turn, the dangers from pressor agents or large volumes o intravenous fluid given to try to correct the hypotension sc induced. In many other centers, conduction analgesia is used tc ameliorate vasospasm and thus to lower pressure. There is nc doubt that lumbar epidural analgesia decreases peripheral vas cular resistance and thus mean arterial blood pressure (New some and colleagues, 1986). However, since such vasodilatatior results in hypovolemia that dangerously lowers uteroplacenta perfusion, variable volumes of crystalloid must be infused ei ther prior to or coincidentally with epidural injection to main tain cardiac output. This results in increased filling pressure: that, as previously discussed, predispose to pulmonary anc cerebral edema. Finally, even in the most experienced hands and even with preload crystalloid, epidural analgesia still re sults occasionally in hypotension (see Chap. 17, p. 338). At tempts to restore blood pressure pharmacologically with vasopressors must be approached cautiously because these women are exquisitely sensitive to these agents. As cautionec by the American College of Obstetricians and Gynecologists (1988b) and Moore and associates (1985), if epidural analgesia is to be used, it should be entrusted to the most experienced obstetrical anesthesiologists.

OTHER TREATMENT AGENTS

Although widely used to control convulsions from a variety o causes in nonpregnant individuals, diazepam therapy remain unproven as a substitute for magnesium sulfate. Our experience has been limited to a few women with eclampsia brought to the Obstetrics Emergency Room after receiving a modest dose of to 10 mg of diazepam elsewhere. Apparently, larger doses o diazepam alone are often required to control eclamptic convul sions. Moreover, Cree and co-workers (1973) documented ir

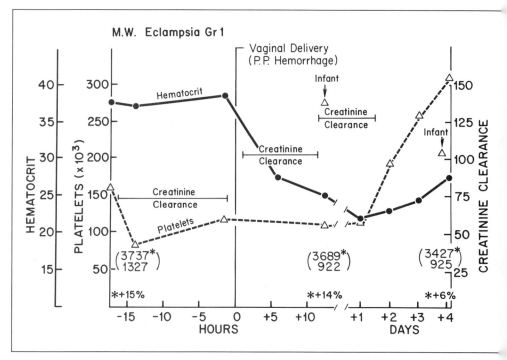

Figure 35–22. Changes in maternal hematocrit, blood, and red cell volumes, determined using ^{51}Cr-labeled erythrocytes (numbers in parentheses), maternal and infant platelet counts, and maternal creatinine clearance in a woman with eclampsia who was delivered vaginally. Her blood volume was expanded only 15 percent over that when nonpregnant, and modest documented blood loss of only 1,100 mL was followed by a fall in the hematocrit from 38 to 23. The creatinine clearance returned to normal soon after delivery, the maternal platelet count was normal by 2 days, and the newborn's platelet count was always normal.

newborns low Apgar scores, apnea persisting several hours after birth, hypotonia, drowsiness, and impaired metabolic response to cooling as a consequence of the intrapartum administration of diazepam to their mothers. We have observed one case of respiratory arrest in which diazepam was given repeatedly to a hypertensive woman postpartum to try to arrest convulsions so that computer tomography could be performed. She was then successfully managed with magnesium sulfate, given as previously described.

Surprisingly, there are few published observations that describe phenytoin given to prevent or treat seizures of eclampsia. Slater and colleagues (1987) recently reported their experiences with a limited number of women with preeclampsia–eclampsia given intravenous phenytoin. Although the drug appeared to be effective for controlling convulsions, 6 of the 26 infants had 5-minute Apgar scores of 4 or less.

Morphine and most sedatives will control convulsions only in doses that render the woman nearly unconscious. Such intense generalized central nervous depression in the mother and her fetus should be avoided. Some other drugs of the great variety that have been used in the treatment of eclampsia and severe preeclampsia are presented in Table 35–10. We have had little personal experience with most of them, and for further information the interested reader is referred to the various reports that are listed.

It should be pointed out that a tendency persists among some medical experts to group together for the purpose of treatment of a variety of disease states that appear to have a common functional disturbance. So-called *hypertensive encephalopathy* is one that from time to time attracts interest and, in turn, incites recommendations for treatment broad in scope, without full appreciation of all the problems created by the disease or evoked by the proposed treatment. Too often, when eclampsia is included under the category of hypertensive encephalopathy, lack of concern for the impact of the recommended therapy on the fetus is apparent. Moreover, it is not unusual for the recommendations to have been based on little or no data (Anonymous, 1979).

The recurrent recognition of thrombocytopenia occasionally and of other changes in the coagulation mechanism rarely, with or without evidence of abnormal erythrocyte destruction (microangiopathic hemolysis), has led to the recommendation for treatment with heparin, fresh whole blood, fresh frozen plasma, platelets, fibrinogen, and other specific clotting factors. Merit, if any, from heparin treatment remains to be established. In two reports it was concluded that heparin was not effective in ameliorating the clinical course of established preeclampsia (Bonnar and associates, 1976; Howie and co-workers, 1975). These experiences with heparin treatment appear similar to those reported by Butler and associates in 1950. We never have used heparin in these circumstances because of fear of enhancing intracranial hemorrhage, on the one hand, and an appreciation that spontaneous correction of the hematological defects promptly follows delivery, on the other. The outcomes have been satisfactory, as already described. The safety of deliberate anticoagulation with heparin in the presence of severe hypertension is dangerous and cannot be recommended.

LONG-TERM CONSEQUENCES OF ECLAMPSIA

REPRODUCTION AFTER ECLAMPSIA

Because of the catastrophic implications of eclampsia, women so affected and their families often are quite concerned over the prognosis for future pregnancies. Chesley and co-workers (1962), through meticulous, long-term follow-up of women with eclampsia at the Margaret Hague Maternity Hospital between 1931 and 1952 have provided us with most useful information. For example, of 466 subsequent pregnancies in 189 of the eclamptic women, the fetal salvage was 76 percent, but much of the loss was from early abortion. Of the pregnancies that continued to 28 weeks or more, 93 percent resulted in infants who survived. Of subsequent pregnancies in the 189 previously eclamptic women, 25 percent were complicated by hypertension (Chesley, 1964). The hypertension, however, was severe in only 5 percent, while 2 percent were again eclamptic. Our observations on previously eclamptic women are very similar.

Chesley emphasized that many cases of recurrent pregnancy-associated hypertension represent nothing more than chronic hypertension. Some women have normal blood pressures between pregnancies and at follow-up, but in general, pregnancies following eclampsia are an excellent screening test for latent hypertensive disease. A large percentage of women who develop recurrent hypertension during subsequent pregnancies will become hypertensive, whereas the prevalence of ultimate hypertension is extremely low in those who are normotensive in later pregnancies.

Chesley and co-workers (1976) obtained follow-up to 1974 in all but three of the 270 women who survived eclampsia at the Margaret Hague Maternity Hospital in the period 1931 through 1952. Nulliparous women in whom eclampsia complicated pregnancy after 28 weeks or more had no increase over the expected number of deaths. In sharp contrast, multiparous women who were eclamptic, the majority of whom undoubtedly had underlying chronic vascular disease, had three times the expected number of deaths.

Racial factors are important regarding the incidence of chronic hypertension and thus pregnancy-aggravated hypertension or superimposed preeclampsia. Sibai and colleagues (1986c) reported on the subsequent pregnancy outcomes of 406 young women whose first pregnancy was complicated by severe preeclampsia or eclampsia. Compared to a group of normotensive women matched for age, race, and gestational age at delivery, the women with preeclampsia had a much higher incidence of pregnancy-induced hypertension in their second pregnancy (47 versus 8 percent), as well as in pregnancies subsequent to that (21 versus 8 percent). These investigators also reported that the 15 percent incidence of subsequent chronic hypertension was increased threefold over that which occurred in women who were normotensive during their first pregnancy. More than 85 percent of these women were black, and their increased incidence of chronic hypertension undoubtedly influenced the incidence of preeclampsia. These observations are in agreement with those of Chesley that pregnancies subsequent to one complicated by eclampsia are an excellent screening test for latent hypertensive disease.

RELATION OF PREECLAMPSIA–ECLAMPSIA TO SUBSEQUENT HYPERTENSION

Whether preeclampsia and eclampsia actually cause ensuing chronic hypertension has been a subject of considerable debate. One point of view has been that preeclampsia and eclampsia represent an acute vascular disorder in the form of arteriolar muscle spasm that, if allowed to continue for several weeks, would result in a permanent structural injury to the vascular wall through hypoxia. This view led some to teach that permanent hypertension might be avoided by delivery of women within 3 weeks fter the onset of preeclampsia. For some time, Chesley (1978) was of this school, but reappraisal of his data led him to reverse his conclusions. The problem has been confused by the erroneous diagnosis of pure preeclampsia in primigravid women who had underlying chronic renal disease or essential hypertension. Another problem was that in some studies a substantial proportion of multiparas were included, and only a few of these actually had pure preeclampsia. To contribute to the confusion, at least 40 percent of women with essential hypertension have substantial decreases in blood pressure during much of pregnancy, and in most, these normal pressures are observed beginning early in gestation. Typically, the blood pressure rises again early in the third trimester, and some edema, and perhaps minimal proteinuria, may follow. Inasmuch as blood pressures before pregnancy were seldom known, the erroneous diagnosis of preeclampsia was likely to have been made.

The results of the long-term follow-up studies of Chesley and associates (1976), who have reexamined women repeatedly for up to 44 years after eclampsia in the first pregnancy, indicate that the prevalence of hypertension is not increased over that in women matched for age and race. Tillman (1955) accumulated a series of 377 women whose blood pressures were recorded before, during, and at intervals after pregnancy. He could find no indication that normal, preeclamptic, or hypertensive pregnancies had any effect on the blood pressure at follow-up examination and concluded that preeclampsia neither causes residual hypertension nor aggravates preexisting hypertension. Conversely, Sibai and associates (1986c), in the study discussed above, reported that young, predominately black primigravidas with severe preeclampsia–eclampsia have a threefold incidence of subsequent chronic hypertension. Like Chesley, they concluded that pregnancy was a screening test for chronic hypertension, rather than that pregnancy was a cause of chronic hypertension.

CHRONIC HYPERTENSION

Hypertension that antedates pregnancy is one of the most common medical complications encountered during pregnancy. Its variable incidence and severity, along with the well-known proclivity for pregnancy to induce or aggravate hypertension, has caused much confusion concerning the management of the pregnant hypertensive woman. For example, and as previously discussed, the majority of pregnant women with underlying chronic hypertension demonstrate improved blood pressure control and have largely uneventful pregnancies. However, some experience dangerous worsening of hypertension that frequently is accompanied by proteinuria, pathological edema, and convulsions, and except that chronic hypertension antedated pregnancy, they are indistinguishable from an otherwise healthy young nullipara with severe preeclampsia–eclampsia.

DIAGNOSIS

A diagnosis of chronic hypertension complicating pregnancy is made whenever there is evidence that hypertension preceded pregnancy, or when a woman is hypertensive before 20 weeks (see p. 655). In addition to obvious chronic hypertension, there are instances of repeated pregnancies during which hypertension appears late in pregnancy, but the blood pressure is normal between pregnancies. Many authors, notably Dieckmann (1952), regarded these recurrent episodes as evidence of latent hypertensive vascular disease. Others, however, concluded that they are repeated attacks of preeclampsia, and still others regarded recurrent hypertension as a separate entity. The results of the long-term follow-up studies of Chesley and co-workers (1976), as well as those of Sibai and colleagues (1986c), are supportive of Dieckmann's view.

In most women with chronic hypertensive vascular disease, increased blood pressure is the only demonstrable finding. A few women, however, have complications that are often grave in relation not only to pregnancy but also to life expectancy. These include hypertensive heart disease, ischemic heart disease, renal insufficiency, and retinal hemorrhages and exudates. Moreover, the blood pressure may vary from levels scarcely

above normal to extremes of 300 mm Hg systolic and 160 mm Hg or more diastolic.

Hypertensive vascular disease in pregnancy is encountered more frequently in older women. Obesity is another important predisposing factor; for example, 7 percent of pregnant women who weigh more than 200 pounds have chronic hypertension (Kleigman and Gross, 1985). As perhaps expected in these older and commonly obese women, diabetes is also prevalent. Finally, heredity, which includes racial factors, has an important role in the development of chronic hypertension; it is common in blacks, and frequently many members of a single family are hypertensive.

As discussed above, in most women with chronic hypertension the blood pressure falls by the second trimester, but the decrement is usually temporary. In most cases the blood pressure rises during the third trimester to levels somewhat above those in early pregnancy. Adverse outcomes in these women are largely dependent on whether superimposed preeclampsia develops. As discussed on page 658, most of these women destined to develop superimposed preeclampsia become abnormally sensitive to infused angiotensin II sometime after midpregnancy but before they are clinically hypertensive (Gant and colleagues, 1977). The incidence of pregnancy-aggravated hypertension or superimposed preeclampsia averages about 15 to 25 percent, and estimates are influenced largely by criteria used in making the diagnosis. Other factors that impact on its incidence are the severity of underlying disease, whether there is renal involvement, and whether other conditions coexist, notably, diabetes and obesity. Although adverse pregnancy outcomes are more likely in chronically hypertensive women who develop superimposed preeclampsia, they also are increased in those who remain normotensive throughout pregnancy. Some of the more common complications include hypertensive encephalopathy, heart failure, worsening of renal insufficiency, placental abruption, fetal growth retardation, and fetal death.

TREATMENT DURING PREGNANCY

The value of continued administration of antihypertensive drugs to pregnant women with chronic hypertension is debated. For example, although it may be of benefit to the hypertensive mother to lower her blood pressure, the lower pressure may reduce uteroplacental perfusion and thereby jeopardize the fetus. While it is not generally agreed whether antihypertensive therapy, as usually prescribed in the absence of pregnancy, is beneficial or detrimental to pregnancy outcome, there are now a few studies that might be used as a clinical guide (Table 35–13).

REVIEW OF SOME STUDIES

Redman and associates (1976) treated one group of hypertensive women with α-methyldopa and compared outcomes with those of a group of untreated women. They selected patients with blood pressures at or above 140/90 mm Hg but less than 170/100 mm Hg and who were less than 28 weeks gestation. Women with blood pressures of 170/100 mm Hg or higher were treated but not included in the study. A total of 101 women received α-methyldopa, and 107 did not. No diuretics were given, and both groups of women underwent early delivery at 37 to 38 weeks gestation. In the control group there was one stillbirth in a pregnancy complicated by superimposed preeclampsia and one neonatal death that was likely due to birth asphyxia and trauma. In the treatment group there was one stillbirth in a pregnancy complicated by superimposed preeclampsia. The average birthweight and laboratory values were essentially the same for both groups. There were four abortions in the control group but none in the treatment group.

Sibai and colleagues (1983) reported their experiences with chronic hypertension in 211 consecutive women whose diastolic blood pressure was 90 to 110 mm Hg. Antihypertensive drugs were discontinued at the first prenatal visit, or they were not given, and all women were followed closely. Only 13 percent required antihypertensive therapy later in pregnancy for diastolic pressures exceeding 110 mm Hg, and the perinatal mortality was 28 per 1,000. They concluded that factors other than chronic hypertension might be responsible for poor perinatal outcomes reported by others in such pregnancies.

Mabie and colleagues (1986) reported their experiences with pregnancies complicated by chronic hypertension at Charity Hospital of New Orleans. They stressed commonly associated conditions, which included obesity in a third and diabetes in a fifth. Antihypertensive drugs, usually methyldopa, with or without a thiazide, were given to 82 women in whom diastolic pressure exceeded 90 mm Hg, while 82 women whose diastolic pressures remained less than 90 mm Hg were given no treatment. The perinatal mortality in each group was similar, but fetal growth retardation was increased fourfold in the treated group, presumably because of worse hypertension. Superimposed preeclampsia, defined as hypertension with either nondependent edema or proteinuria, developed in a third, but was more common in those women who were given treatment. The authors concluded that aggressive treatment did not improve perinatal outcome and that blood pressure control was but one aspect of management of these women.

A summary of some of these studies is presented in Table

TABLE 35–13. CHRONIC HYPERTENSION AND SUPERIMPOSED PREECLAMPSIA—METHOD OF TREATMENT AND PERINATAL OUTCOME

Study and Treatment	No.	Superimposed Preeclampsia (%)	Perinatal Mortality (per 1,000)
Chesley (1978)			
Chronic hypertension[a]			
(1972–74) No antihypertensives	593	6	32
Superimposed preeclampsia[b]			
(1960–74) Hydralazine + α-methyldopa	196	—	214
Redman (1980)[c]			
Chronic hypertension			
α-methyldopa and/or hydralazine	184	25	16
Superimposed preeclampsia			
α-methyldopa + others	69	—	145
Sibai and associates (1983)			
Chronic hypertension			
No antihypertensives	193	10	5
Superimposed preeclampsia			
α-methyldopa and/or hydralazine	22		227
Mabie and associates (1986)			
Chronic hypertension, diastolic pressure			
< 90 mm Hg; no treatment	137	29	29
Chronic hypertension, diastolic pressure			
90–100 mm Hg; α-methyldopa	26	46	0
Sibai and associates (1986d)			
Severe chronic hypertension, 170/110 mm			
Hg or greater; α-methyldopa			
+ hydralazine	44	52	250

[a] Three maternal deaths due to stroke, pulmonary embolus, and aspiration pneumonia.

[b] Two deaths due to stroke and postoperative infection.

[c] Data extracted from Table 1 from Ounsted and associates (1983), reporting on long term follow-up of children from the original and continuing study of treatment of chronic hypertension in pregnancy by Redman (1980).

35–13. All investigators reported that superimposed pre-eclampsia or pregnancy-aggravated hypertension was a bad complication. It appears unlikely that treatment with antihypertensive medications decreases the incidence of this complication (Redman and co-workers, 1976; Redman, 1980; Sibai and colleagues, 1983). Importantly, most pregnancy outcomes were good for these women with chronic hypertension, whether or not antihypertensive treatment was given. The uncorrected perinatal mortality rates were acceptable unless superimposed preeclampsia developed. Three maternal deaths reported in detail by Chesley warrant careful analysis. Death from stroke followed in a woman who was transferred from another hospital. She was in coma and died within 20 minutes of arrival. A second woman died of a pulmonary embolus after cesarean delivery of a 5,000-g infant, followed by a complicated postoperative course and wound evisceration. The other death was the result of aspiration during anesthesia for a cesarean delivery.

Severe Chronic Hypertension

The prognosis for pregnancy outcome with antecedent hypertension is related to the severity of disease before pregnancy. Many women with severe hypertension also have underlying renal disease. Sibai and co-workers (1986d) described 44 pregnancies in women whose blood pressure at 6 to 11 weeks was 170/110 mm Hg or higher (Table 35–13). They were given treatment with α-methyldopa and oral hydralazine to maintain blood pressures less than 160/110 mm Hg, and they were hospitalized for treatment with parenteral hydralazine if blood pressures exceeded 180/120 mm Hg. Half developed superimposed preeclampsia, and all adverse perinatal outcomes were in this group: all infants were born prematurely, nearly 80 percent were growth retarded, and the perinatal mortality rate was 48 percent. By contrast, in the women with severe hypertension who did not develop superimposed preeclampsia, only 5 percent of fetuses were growth retarded and all survived.

The use of α-methyldopa during early pregnancy has been questioned because of smaller head circumferences observed in male infants of women who received the drug between 16 and 20 weeks gestation (Redman, 1980). However, the long-term follow-up of the infants in Redman's 1976 and 1980 studies are reassuring. There have been no major adverse effects noted in the infants or children for up to 7½ years of life (Cockburn and associates, 1982; Ounsted and co-workers, 1983).

ANTIHYPERTENSIVE DRUG SELECTION

Despite the relatively good results obtained with α-methyldopa (Redman, 1980), and the comparable results obtained without antihypertensive drugs (Chesley, 1978; Sibai and colleagues, 1983), adrenergic blocking drugs are being tested extensively in England, Scotland, and Australia (Michael, 1982; Redman, 1982; Rubin, 1983; Walker and associates, 1983). The early results of treatment with labetalol, a combined α- and β-adrenergic blocker, are consistent with the view that the drug offers no advantages over α-methyldopa. Rubin and colleagues (1983) reported salutary results from a double-blind prospective study in which they compared placebo to the β-blocker atenolol given to 120 women with hypertension first apparent early in the third trimester. Since nearly 60 percent of their subjects were nulliparous, it was difficult to separate women with chronic hypertension from those with preeclampsia, and indeed, although the placebo group had worse perinatal outcomes, there were more nulliparas assigned (67 versus 50 percent), and thus pre-sumably more had preeclampsia at the outset. As discussed earlier (p. 674), antihypertensive drugs are not recommended for treatment of preeclampsia.

Captopril, the angiotensin I converting enzyme inhibitor, has been shown to reduce uteroplacental perfusion and often kill the fetuses of experimental animals (Broughton-Pipkin and associates, 1982; Ferris and Weir, 1983).

At Parkland Hospital, pregnancy complicated by chronic hypertension has not been treated with antihypertensive drugs or diuretics unless (1) blood pressure is above 150/110 mm Hg or (2) the woman was receiving antihypertensive medications prior to the pregnancy and her hypertension is well controlled. If the blood pressure increases rapidly and persists above 110 mm Hg diastolic, if significant proteinuria develops, if renal function deteriorates, or if fetal growth retardation is suspected, for the reasons that follow, the pregnancy is terminated as recommended above for severe preeclampsia and eclampsia.

PREGNANCY-AGGRAVATED HYPERTENSION

DIAGNOSIS

The most common hazard faced by pregnant women with chronic hypertensive vascular disease is the superimposition of preeclampsia. The frequency of pregnancy-aggravated hypertension is difficult to specify precisely, for the incidence varies with the diagnostic criteria employed. If the diagnosis is made only on the basis of (1) significant aggravation of the hypertension, (2) sustained proteinuria, and (3) generalized edema, then the incidence will be relatively low since delivery is often accomplished before intense superimposed preeclampsia or eclampsia has developed. If, however, the diagnosis is made on the basis of a modest rise in blood pressure and minimal to modest proteinuria, the incidence will be much higher. For example, with mild chronic hypertension, the incidence of superimposed preeclampsia cited in studies in Table 35–13 varied from 6 to 46 percent!

Pregnancy-aggravated hypertension typically becomes manifest by a sudden rise in blood pressure that almost always is eventually complicated by substantive proteinuria. In neglected cases especially, extreme hypertension (systolic pressure greater than 200 mm Hg and diastolic pressure of 130 mm Hg or more), oliguria, and impaired renal clearance may rapidly ensue; the retina may contain extensive hemorrhages and cottonwool exudates; and convulsions and coma are likely. Therefore, in its most severe form, the resultant syndrome is similar to hypertensive encephalopathy. With the development of superimposed preeclampsia or eclampsia, the outlook for both the infant and the mother is grave unless the pregnancy is rapidly terminated. The frequency of fetal growth retardation and preterm delivery is increased appreciably because of its relatively early onset in pregnancy, as well as the marked severity of the process itself (López-Llera and associates, 1972; Redman, 1980). However, if the infant is liveborn and survives the perinatal period, the long-term prognosis is good (Ounsted and colleagues, 1983).

REFERENCES

Abdul-Karim R, Assali NS: Pressor reponse to angiotonin in pregnant and non-pregnant women. Am J Obstet Gynecol 82:246, 1961
Altura BM, Altura BT, Carella A: Magnesium deficiency-induced spasms of umbilical vessels: Relation to preeclampsia, hypertension, growth retardation. Science 221:376, 1983

American College of Obstetricians and Gynecologists: Invasive hemodynamic monitoring in obstetrics and gynecology. Technical Bulletin No 121, 1988a

American College of Obstetricians and Gynecologists: Management of preeclampsia. Technical Bulletin No 91, February 1986

American College of Obstetricians and Gynecologists: Obstetric Anesthesia and Analgesia. Technical Bulletin No 112, January 1988

Anonymous: Hypertensive encephalopathy. Br Med J 2:1387, 1979

Assali NS, Douglas RA, Baird WW: Measurement of uterine blood flow and uterine metabolism. Am J Obstet Gynecol 66:248, 1953

Baird D: Combined Textbook of Obstetrics and Gynaecology for Students and Practitioners. Edinburgh and London, Livingston, 1969, p 631

Beaufils M, Uzan S, Donsimoni R, Colau JC: Prevention of preeclampsia by early antiplatelet therapy. Lancet 1:840, 1985

Beer AE: Possible immunologic bases of preeclampsia/eclampsia. Semin Perinatol 2:39, 1978

Belizán JM, Villar J, Repke J: The relationship between calcium intake and pregnancy-induced hypertension: Up-to-date evidence. Am J Obstet Gynecol 158:898, 1988

Benedetti TJ, Cotton DB, Read JC, Miller FC: Hemodynamic observations in severe preeclampsia with a flow-directed pulmonary artery catheter. Am J. Obstet Gynecol 136:465, 1980

Benedetti TJ, Carlson RW: Studies of colloid osmotic pressure on pregnancy-induced hypertension. Am J Obstet Gynecol 135:308, 1979

Benedetti TJ, Kates R, Williams V: Hemodynamic observations in severe pre-eclampsia complicated by pulmonary edema. Am J Obstet Gynecol 152:330, 1985

Benedetti TJ, Quilligan EJ: Cerebral edema in severe pregnancy-induced hypertension. Am J Obstet Gynecol 137:860, 1980

Bhatia RK, Bottoms SF, Saleh AA, Norman GS, Mammen EF, Sokol RJ: Mechanisms for reduced colloid osmotic pressure in preeclampsia. Am J Obstet Gynecol 157:106, 1987

Bloss JD, Hankins GDV, Hauth JC, Gilstrap LC: The effect of oxytocin infusion on the pharmacokinetics of intramuscular magnesium sulfate therapy. Am J Obstet Gynecol 157:156, 1987

Bonnar J, Redman CWG, Denson KW: The role of coagulation and fibrinolysis in preeclampsia. In Lindheimer MD, Katz AI, Zuspan FP (eds): Hypertension in Pregnancy. New York, Wiley, 1976

Borges LF, Gücer G: Effect of magnesium on epileptic foci. Epilepsia 19:81, 1978

Brosens IA, Robertson WB, Dixon HG: The role of the spiral arteries in the pathogenesis of preeclampsia. Obstet Gynecol Ann 1:177, 1972

Broughton-Pipkin F, Symonds EM, Turner SR: The effect of captopril upon mothers and fetuses in the chronically cannulated ewe and in the pregnant rabbit. J Physiol 323:415, 1982

Brown CEL, Cunningham FG, Pritchard JA: Convulsions in hypertensive, proteinuric primiparas more than 24 hours after delivery: Eclampsia or some other cause? J Reprod Med 32:499, 1987

Brown CEL, Gant NF, Rosenfeld CR, Magness RR: Effect of low dose aspirin on circulating prostaglandins (PG) in angiotensin II (AII) sensitive and nonsensitive women. Presented at the Society for Gynecological Investigation, San Diego, California, March 1989

Brown CEL, Purdy PD, Cunningham FG: Head computed tomographic scans in women with eclampsia. Am J Obstet Gynecol 159:915, 1988

Brown MA, Gallery EDM, Ross MR, Esber RP: Sodium excretion in normal and hypertensive pregnancy: A prospective study. Am J Obstet Gynecol 159:297, 1988

Brown RD, Strott CA, Liddle GW: Plasma deoxycorticosterone in normal and abnormal human pregnancy. J Clin Endocrinol Metab 35:736, 1972

Browne FJ: Sensitization of the vascular system in pre-eclamptic toxaemia and eclampsia. Br J Obstet Gynecol 53:510, 1946

Browne JCM, Veall N: The maternal placental blood flow in normotensive and hypertensive women. J Obstet Gynaecol Br Emp 60:141, 1953

Browne O: The treatment of eclampsia. Br J Obstet Gynaecol 57:573, 1950

Brunner HR, Gavras H: Vascular damage in hypertension. Hosp Pract 10:97, 1975

Bryant RD, Fleming JG: Veratrum viride in the treatment of eclampsia. Obstet Gynecol 19:372, 1962

Burrows RF, Hunter DJS, Andrew M, Kelton JG: A prospective study investigating the mechanism of thrombocytopenia in preeclampsia. Obstet Gynecol 70:334, 1987

Butler BC, Taylor HC, Graff S: The relationship of disorders of the blood-clotting mechanism to toxemia of pregnancy and the value of heparin in therapy. Am J Obstet Gynecol 60:564, 1950

Cameron AD, Nicholson SF, Nimrod CA, Harder JR, Davies DM: Doppler waveforms in the fetal aorta and umbilical artery in patients with hypertension in pregnancy. Am J Obstet Gynecol 158:339, 1988

Chesley LC: A short history of eclampsia. Obstet Gynecol 43:599, 1974

Chesley LC: Diagnosis of preeclampsia. Obstet Gynecol 65:423, 1985

Chesley LC: Superimposed preeclampsia or eclampsia. In Chesley LC(ed): Hypertensive Disorders in Pregnancy. New York, Appleton, 1978, pp 14, 302, 482

Chesley LC, Annitto JE, Cosgrove RA: Long-term follow-up study of eclamptic women: Sixth periodic report. Am J Obstet Gynecol 124:446, 1976

Chesley, LC, Annitto JE, Cosgrove RA: Prognostic significance of recurrent toxemia of pregnancy. Obstet Gynecol 23:874, 1964

Chesley LC, Annitto JE, Cosgrove RA: The familial factor in toxemia of pregnancy. Obstet Gynecol 32:303, 1968

Chesley LC, Cooper DW: Genetics of hypertension in pregnancy: Possible single gene control of pre-eclampsia and eclampsia in the descendants of eclamptic women. Br J Obstet Gynaecol 93:898, 1986

Chesley LC, Cosgrove RA, Annitto JE: A follow-up study of eclamptic women: Fourth periodic report. Am J Obstet Gynecol 83:1360, 1962

Chesley LC, Sibai BM: Clinical significance of elevated mean arterial pressure in the second trimester. Am J Obstet Gynecol 159:275, 1988

Chesley LC, Tepper I: Plasma levels of magnesium attained in magnesium sulfate therapy for preeclampsia and eclampsia. Surg Clin North Am, April 1957, p 353

Chesley LC, Williams LO: Renal glomerular and tubular function in relation to the hyperuricemia of pre-eclampsia and eclampsia. Am J Obstet Gynecol 50:367, 1945

Clark SL, Cotton DB: Clinical indications for pulmonary artery catheterization in the patient with severe preeclampsia. Am J Obstet Gynecol 158:453, 1988

Cockburn J, Moar VA, Ounsted M, Redman CWG: Final report of study on hypertension during pregnancy: The effects of specific treatment on the growth and development of the children. Lancet 1:647, 1982

Collins R, Yusuf S, Peto R: Overview of randomised trials of diuretics in pregnancy. Br Med J 290:17, 1985

Combes B, Adams RH: Disorders of the liver in pregnancy. In Assali NS (ed): Pathophysiology of Gestation, Vol I. New York, Academic, 1972

Constantine G, Beevers DG, Reynolds AL, Luesley DM: Nifedipine as a second line antihypertensive drug in pregnancy. Br J Obstet Gynaecol 984:1136, 1987

Cooper DW, Liston WA: Genetic control of severe preeclampsia. J Med Genet 16:409, 1979

Cotton DB, Gonik B, Dorman KF: Cardiovascular alterations in severe pregnancy-induced hypertension: Acute effects of intravenous magnesium sulfate. Am J Obstet Gynecol 148:152, 1984

Cotton DB, Jones MM, Longmire S, Korman KF, Tessem J, Joyce TH: Role of intravenous nitroglycerine in the treatment of severe pregnancy-induced hypertension complicated by pulmonary edema. Am J Obstet Gynecol 154:91, 1986

Cotton DB, Lee W, Huhta JC, Dorman KF: Hemodynamic profile of severe pregnancy-induced hyptertension. Am J Obstet Gynecol 158:523, 1988

Cree JE, Meyer J, Hailey DM: Diazepam in labour: Its metabolism and effect on the clinical condition and thermogenesis of the newborn. Br Med J 4:251, 1973

Cruikshank DP, Pitkin RM, Reynolds WA, Williams GA, Hargis GK: Effects of magnesium sulfate treatment on perinatal calcium metabolism: I. Maternal and fetal responses. Am J Obstet Gynecol 134:243, 1979

Cunningham FG, Cox K, Gant NF: Further observations on the nature of pressor responsivity to angiotensin II in human pregnancy. Obstet Gynecol 146:581, 1975

Cunningham FG, Leveno KJ: Management of pregnancy-induced hypertension. Chapter 16 in Rubin PC (ed): Handbook of Hypertension. Vol 10: Hypertension in Pregnancy. Amsterdam, Elsevier Science, 1988, p290

Cunningham FG, Lowe T, Guss S, Mason R: Erythrocyte morphology in women with severe preeclampsia and eclampsia. Am J Obstet Gynecol 153:358, 1985

Cunningham FG, Pritchard JA: How should hypertension during pregnancy be managed?: Experience at Parkland Memorial Hospital. Med Clin North Am 68:505, 1984

Cunningham FG, Pritchard JA, Hankins GDV, Anderson PL, Lucas MK, Armstrong KF: Idiopathic cardiomyopathy or compounding cardiovascular events? Obstet Gynecol 67:157, 1986

Dewar JB, Morris WIC: Sedation with rectal tribromethanol (Avertin Bromethol) in the management of eclampsia. J Obstet Gynaecol Br Emp 54:417, 1947

DeWolf F, Robertson WB, Brosen I: The ultrastructure of acute atherosis in hypertensive pregnancy. Am J Obstet Gynecol 123:164, 1975

Dieckmann WJ: The Toxemias of Pregnancy, 2nd ed. St Louis, Mosby, 1952

Dieckmann WJ, Michel HL: Vascular-renal effects of posterior pituitary extracts in pregnant women. Am J Obstet Gynecol 33:131, 1937

Donaldson JO: Does magnesium sulfate treat eclamptic convulsions? Clin Neuropharmacol 9:37, 1986

Donaldson JO: Neurology in Pregnancy. Philadelphia, Saunders, 1978

Ducey J, Schulman H, Farmakides G, Rochelson B, Bracero L, Fleischer A, Guzman E, Winter D, Penny B: A classification of hypertension in pregnancy based on Doppler velocimetry. Am J Obstet Gynecol 157:680, 1987

Duenhoelter JH, Jimenez JM, Baumann G: Pregnancy performance in patients under fifteen years of age. Obstet Gynecol 46:49, 1975

Elias AN, Vaziri ND, Pandian MR, Powers DR, Domurat E: Atrial natriuretic peptide and arginine vasopressin in pregnancy and pregnancy-induced hypertension. Nephron 49:140, 1988

Everett RB, Porter JC, MacDonald PC, Gant NF: Relationship of maternal placental blood flow to the placental clearance of maternal plasma dehydroisoandrosterone sulfate through placental estriol formation. Am J Obstet Gynecol 136:435, 1980

Everett RB, Worley RJ, MacDonald PC, Gant NF: Effect of prostaglandin synthetase inhibitors on pressor response to angiotensin II in human pregnancy. J Clin Endocrinol Metab 46:1007, 1978a

Everett RB, Worley RJ, MacDonald PC, Gant NF; Modification of vascular reponsiveness to angiotensin II in pregnant women by intravenously infused 5α-dihydroprogesterone. Am J Obstet Gynecol 131:352, 1978b

Feeney JG, Scott JS: Pre-eclampsia and changed paternity. Eur J Obstet Gynaecol Reprod Biol 11:35, 1980

Ferris TF: How should hypertension during pregnancy be managed?: An internist's approach. Med Clin North Am 68:491, 1984

Ferris TF, Weir EK: Effect of captopril on uterine blood flow and prostaglandin E synthesis in the pregnant rabbit. J Clin Invest 71:809, 1983

Fidler J, Smith V, Fayers P, DeSwiet M: Randomised controlled comparative study of methyldopa and oxyprenolol in treatment of hypertension in pregnancy. Br Med J 286:1927, 1983

Fisher ER, Pardo V, Paul R, Hayashi TT: Ultrastructural studies in hypertension: IV. Toxemia of pregnancy. Am J Pathol 55:901, 1969

Fleischer A, Schulman H, Farmakides G, Bracero L, Grunfeld L, Rochelson B, Koenigsberg M: Uterine artery Doppler velocimetry in pregnant women with hypertension. Am J. Obstet Gynecol 154:806, 1986

Friedman EA, Neff RK: Pregnancy outcome as related to hypertension, edema, and proteinuria. In Lindheimer MD, Katz AI, Zuspan FP (eds): Hypertension in Pregnancy. New York, Wiley, 1976, p 13

Friedman SA: Preeclampsia: A review of the role of prostaglandins. Obstet Gynecol 71:122, 1988

Fritz MA, Stanczyk FZ, Novy MJ: Relationship of uteroplacental blood flow to the placental clearance of maternal dehydroepiandrosterone through estradiol formation in the pregnant baboon. J Clin Endocrinol Metab 61:1023, 1985

Gallery EDM, Saunders DM, Hunyor SN, Gyory AZ: Randomized comparison of methyldopa and oxyprenolol for treatment of hypertension in pregnancy. Br Med J 1:1591, 1979

Gant NF, Chand S, Whalley PJ, MacDonald PC: The nature of pressor responsiveness to angiotensin II in human pregnancy. Obstet Gynecol 43:854, 1974a

Gant NF, Chand S, Worley RJ, Whalley PJ, Crosby UD, MacDonald PC: A clinical test useful for predicting the development of acute hypertension in pregnancy. Am J Obstet Gynecol 120:1, 1974b

Gant NF, Daley GL, Chand S, Whalley PJ, MacDonald PC: A study of angiotensin II pressor response throughout primigravid pregnancy. J Clin Invest 52:2682, 1973

Gant NF, Jimenez JM, Whalley PJ, Chand S, MacDonald PC: A prospective study of angiotensin II pressor responsiveness in pregnancies complicated by chronic essential hypertension. Am J Obstet Gynecol 127:369, 1977

Gant NF, Madden JD, Siiteri PK, MacDonald PC: The metabolic clearance rate of dehydroisoandrosterone sulfate: III. The effect of thiazide diuretics in normal and future preeclamptic pregnancies. Am J Obstet Gynecol 123:159, 1975

Gant NF, Madden JD, Siiteri PK, MacDonald PC: The metabolic clearance rate of dehydroisoandrosterone sulfate: IV. Acute effect of induced hypertension, hypotension, and naturesis in normal and hypertensive pregnancies. Am J Obstet Gynecol 124:143, 1976

Gedekoh RH, Hayashi TT, MacDonald HM: Eclampsia at Magee-Womens Hospital, 1970–1980. Am J Obstet Gynecol 140:860, 1981

Gilstrap LC, Cunningham FG, Whalley PJ: Management of pregnancy-induced hypertension in the nulliparous patient remote from term. Semin Perinatol 2:73, 1978

Goldman RS, Finkbeiner SM: Therapeutic use of magnesium sulfate in selected case of cerebral ischemia and seizure. N Engl J Med 319:1224, 1988

Goodman RP, Killam AP, Brush AR, Branch RA: Prostacyclin production during pregnancy: Comparison of production during normal pregnancy and pregnancy complicated by hypertension. Am J Obstet Gynecol 142:817, 1982

Govan ADT: The pathogenesis of eclamptic lesions. Pathol Microbiol 24:561, 1961

Green KW Key TC, Coen R, Resnik R: The effects of maternally administered magnesium sulfate on the neonate. Am J Obstet Gynecol 146:29, 1983

Groenendijk R, Trimbros JBM, Wallenburg HCS: Hemodynamic measurements in preeclampsia: Preliminary observations. Am J Obstet Gynecol 150:232, 1984

Guzick DS, Klein VR, Tyson JE, Lasky RE, Gant NF, Rosenfeld CR: Risk factors for the occurrence of pregnancy-induced hypertension. Clin Exp Hyper-Hyper Preg B6:281, 1987

Hankins GDV: Principles of invasive hemodynamic monitoring. Clin Perinatol 13:765, 1986

Hankins GDV, Wendel GW Jr, Cunningham FG, Leveno KJ: Longitudinal evaluation of hemodynamic changes in eclampsia. Am J Obstet Gynecol 150:506, 1984

Hankins GDV, Wendel GW Jr, Whalley PJ, Quirk JG Jr: Cardiovascular monitoring in the high risk pregnancy. Perinatol Neonatol 7:29, 1983

Hanrexty KP, Whittle MJ: Doppler uteroplacental waveforms in pregnancy-induced hypertension: A re-appraisal. Lancet 1:850, 1988

Hansen JP: Older maternal age and pregnancy outcome: A review of the literature. Obstet Gynecol Surv 41:726,1986

Harbert GM Jr, Cornell GW, Thornton WN Jr: Effect of toxemia therapy on uterine dynamics. Am J Obstet Gynecol 105:94, 1969

Hauth JC, Cunningham FG, Whalley PJ: Management of pregnancy-induced hypertension in the nullipara. Obstet Gynecol 48:253, 1976

Heller PJ, Scheider EP, Marx GF: Pharyngolaryngeal edema as a presenting symptom in eclampsia. Obstet Gynecol 62:523, 1983

Hertig AT: Vascular pathology in the hypertensive albuminuric toxemias of pregnancy. Clinics 4:602, 1945

Hinselmann H: Die Eklampsie. Bonn, F Cohen, 1924

Hirai N, Yanaihara T, Nakayama T, Ishibashi M, Yamaji T: Plasma levels of atrial natriuretic peptide during normal pregnancy and in pregnancy complicated by hypertension. Am J Obstet Gynecol 159:27, 1988

Hodgkinson R, Husain FJ, Hayashi RH: Systemic and pulmonary blood pressure during cesarean section in parturients with gestational hypertension. Can Anaesth Soc J 27:389, 1980

Högstedt S, Lindeberg S, Axelsson O, Lindmark G, Rane A, Sandström B, Lindberg BS: A prospective controlled trial of metoprolol-hydralazine treatment in hypertension during pregnancy. Acta Obstet Gynecol Scand 64:505, 1985

Howie PW, Prentice CRM, Forbes CD: Failure of heparin therapy to affect the clinical course of severe preeclampsia. Br J Obstet Gynaecol 82:711, 1975

Hughes EC (ed): Obstetric-Gynecologic Terminology. Philadelphia, Davis, 1972

Johnson T, Clayton CG: Diffusion of radioactive sodium in normotensive and preeclamptic pregnancies. Br Med J 1:312, 1957

Kambam JR, Perry SM, Entman S, Smith BE: Effect of magnesium on plasma cholinesterase activity. Am J Obstet Gynecol 159:309, 1988

Kaunitz AM, Hughes MJ, Grimes DA, Smith JC, Rochat RW, Kafrissen ME: Causes of maternal mortality in the United States. Obstet Gynecol 65:605, 1985

Kawathekar P, Anusuya SR, Sriniwas P, Lagali S: Diazepam (Calmpose) in eclampsia: A preliminary report of 16 cases. Curr Ther Res 15:845, 1973

Kelton JG, Hunter DJS, Naeme PB: A platelet function defect in preeclampsia. Obstet Gynecol 65:107, 1985

Kirshon B, Lee W, Mauer MB, Cotton DB: Effects of low-dose dopamine therapy in the oliguric patient with preeclampsia. Am J Obstet Gynecol 159:604, 1988

Kitzmiller JL, Lang JE, Yelonosky PF, Lucas WE: Hematologic assays in preeclampsia. Am J Obstet Gynecol 118:362, 1974

Kliegman RM, Gross T: Perinatal problems of the obese mother and her infant. Obstet Gynecol 66:299, 1985

Kraus GW, Marchese JR, Yen SSC: Prophylactic use of hydrochlorothiazide in pregnancy. JAMA 198:1150, 1966

Landesman R, Douglas RG, Holze E: The bulbar conjunctival vascular bed in the toxemias of pregnancy. Am J Obstet Gynecol 68:170, 1954

Lean, TH, Ratnam SS, Sivasamboo R: Use of benzodiazepines in the management of eclampsia. J Obstet Gynaecol Br Commonw 75:856, 1968

Lee W, Gonik B, Cotton DB: Urinary diagnostic indices in preeclampsia-associated oliguria: Correlation with invasive hemodynamic monitoring. Am J Obstet Gynecol 156:100, 1987

Lehmann DK, Mabie WC, Miller JM, Pernoll ML: The epidemiology and pathology of maternal mortality: Charity Hosptial of Louisiana in New Orleans, 1965–1984. Obstet Gynecol 69:833, 1987

Levine B, Coburn JW: Magnesium, the mimic/antagonist of calcium. N Engl J Med 310:1253, 1984

Lichtig C, Luger AM, Spargo BH, Lindheimer MD: Renal immunofluorescence and ultrastructural findings in preeclampsia. Clin Res 23:368A,1975

Lipsitz PJ: The clinical and biochemical effects of excess magnesium in the newborn. Pediatrics 47:501, 1971

Lipsitz PJ, English IC: Hypermagnesemia in the newborn infant. Pediatrics 40:856, 1967

Llewellyn-Jones D: The treatment of eclampsia. Br J Obstet Gynecol 68:33, 1961

Lopez-Espinoza I, Dhar H, Humphreys S, Redman CWG: Urinary albumin excretion in pregnancy. Br J Obstet Gynaecol 93:176, 1986

López-Llera M: Complicated eclampsia: Fifteen years' experience in a referral medical center. Am J Obstet Gynecol 142:28, 1982

López-Llera M, Hernandez-Horta JL, Huttich FC: Retarded fetal growth in eclampsia. J Reprod Med 9:229, 1972

Mabie WC, Gonzalez AR, Sibai BM, Amon E: A comparative trial of labetalol and hydralazine in the acute management of severe hypertension complicating pregnancy. Obstet Hynecol 70:328, 1987

Mabie WC, Pernoll ML, Biswas MK: Chronic hypertension in pregnancy. Obstet Gynecol 67:197, 1986

Mabie WC, Ratts TE, Ramanathan KB, Sibai BM: Circulatory congestion in obese hypertensive women. A subset of pulmonary edema in pregnancy. Obstet Gynecol 72:553, 1988a

Mabie WC, Sibai BM, Anderson GD, Gonzalez-Ruiz AR, Moretti ML, Harvey CJ: Nifedipine in the treatment of severe peripartum hypertension. Abstract No 87 presented at the eighth annual meeting of The Society of Perinatal Obstetricians, Las Vegas, February 1988b

Manas KJ, Welsh JD, Rankin RA, Miller DD: Hepatic hemorrhage without rupture in preeclampsia. N Engl J Med 312:426, 1985

McCall ML: Cerebral circulation and metabolism in toxemia of pregnancy: Observations on the effects of veratrum viride and apresoline (1-hydrazinophthalazine). Am J Obstet Gynecol 66:1015, 1953

McCartney CP: Pathological anatomy of acute hypertension of pregnancy. Circulation (Suppl 2) 30:37, 1964

McCartney CP, Schumacher GFB, Spargo BH: Serum proteins in patients with toxemic glomerular lesion. Am J Obstet Gynecol 111:580, 1971

McCubbin JH, Sibai BM, Abdella TN, Anderson GD: Cardiopulmonary arrest due to acute maternal hypermagnesemia. Lancet 1:1058, 1981

McKay DG: Disseminated Intravascular Coagulation. New York, Harper & Row, 1965

Menon MKK: The evolution of the treatment of eclampsia. J Obstet Gynaecol Br Commonw 68:417, 1961

Metcalfe J, Romney SL, Ramsey LH, Reid DE, Burwell CS: Estimation of uterine blood flow in normal human pregnancy at term. J Clin Invest 34:1632, 1955

Michael CA: The evaluation of labetalol in the treatment of hypertension complicating pregnancy. Br J Clin Pharmacol (Suppl 1) 127:127A, 1982

Mojadidi Q, Thompson RJ: Five years' experience with eclampsia. South Med J 66:414, 1973

Moore TR, Key TC, Reisner LS, Renick RR: Evaluation of the use of continuous lumbar epidural anesthesia for hypertensive pregnant women in labor. Am J Obstet Gynecol 152:104, 1985

Morris N, Osborn SB, Wright HP, Hart A: Effective uterine bloodflow during exercise in normal and pre-eclamptic pregnancies. Lancet 2:481, 1956

Naden RP, Redman CW: Antihypertensive drugs in pregnancy. Clin Perinatol 12:521, 1985

Naeye RL, Friedman EA: Causes of perinatal death associated with gestational hypertension and proteinuria. Am J Obstet Gynecol 133:8, 1979

Need JA, Bell B, Meffin E, Jones WR: Pre-eclampsia in pregnancies from donor inseminations. J Reprod Immunol 5:329, 1983

Newsome LR, Bramwell RS, Curling PE: Severe preeclampsia: Hemodynamic effects of lumbar epidural anesthesia. Anesth Analg 65:31, 1986

Nishimura RN, Koller R: Isolated cortical blindness in pregnancy. West J Med 137:335, 1982

Nochimson DJ, Petrie RH: Glucocorticoid therapy for the induction of pulmonary maturity in severely hypertensive gravid women. Am J Obstet Gynecol 133:449, 1979

Oian P, Maltau Jm, Noddleland H, Fadnes HO: Oedema-preventing mechanisms in subcutaneous tissue of normal pregnant women. Br J Obstet Gynaecol 92:1113, 1985

Oian P, Maltau JM, Noddleland H, Fadnes HO: Transcapillary fluid balance in preeclampsia. Br J Obstet Gynaecol 93:235, 1986

Öney T, Kaulhausen H: The value of the angiotensin sensitivity test in the early diagnosis of hypertensive disorders of pregnancy. Am J Obstet Gynecol 142:17, 1982

Ounsted M, Cockburn J, Moar VA, Redman CW: Maternal hypertension with superimposed pre-eclampsia: Effects on child development at 7½ years. Br J Obstet Gynaecol 90:644, 1983

Page EW: On the pathogenesis of pre-eclampsia and eclampsia. J Obstet Gynaecol Br Commonw 79:883, 1972

Parker CR, Everett RB, Quirk JG, Whalley PJ, Gant NF, MacDonald PC: Hormone production during pregnancy in the primigravida: II. Plasma levels of deoxycorticosterone throughout pregnancy in normal women and women who developed pregnancy-induced hypertension. Am J Obstet Gynecol 138:626, 1980

Petrucco OM, Thomson NM, Lawrence JR, Weldon MW: Immunofluorescent studies in renal biopsies in pre-eclampsia. Br Med J 1:473, 1974

Phelan JP, Yurth DA: Severe preeclampsia: I. Peripartum hemodynamic observations. Am J Obstet Gynecol 144:17, 1982

Plouin P-F, Breart G, Maillard F, Papierrnik E, Relier J-P, The Labetalol Methyldopa Study Group: Comparison of antihypertensive efficacy and perinatal safety of labetalol and methyldopa in the treatment of hypertension in pregnancy: A randomized controlled trial. Br J Obstet Gynaecol 95:868, 1988

Pritchard JA: Management of severe preeclampsia and eclampsia. Semin Perinatol 2:83, 1978

Pritchard JA: The use of the magnesium ion in the management of eclamptogenic toxemias. Surg Gynecol Obstet 100:131, 1955

Pritchard JA: The use of magnesium sulfate in preeclampsia-eclampsia. J Reprod Med 23:107, 1979

Pritchard JA, Cunningham FG, Mason RA: Coagulation changes in eclampsia: Their frequency and pathogenesis. Am J Obstet Gynecol 124:855, 1976

Pritchard JA, Cunningham FG, Pritchard SA: The Parkland Memorial Hospital protocol for treatment of eclampsia: Evaluation of 245 cases. Am J Obstet Gynecol 148:951, 1984

Pritchard JA, Cunningham FG, Pritchard SA, Mason RA: How often does maternal preeclampsia–eclampsia incite thrombocytopenia in the fetus? Obstet Gynecol 69:292, 1987

Pritchard JA, Ratnoff OD, Weismann R Jr: Hemostatic defects and increased red cell destruction in preeclampsia and eclampsia. Obstet Gynecol 4:159, 1954b

Pritchard JA, Weisman R Jr, Ratnoff OD, Vosburgh G: Intravascular hemolysis, thrombocytopenia and other hematologic abnormalities associated with severe toxemia of pregnancy. N Engl J Med 250:87, 1954a

Raab W, Schroeder G, Wagner R, Gigee W: Vascular reactivity and electrolytes in normal and toxemic pregnancy. J Clin Endocrinol 16:1196, 1956

Rafferty TD, Berkowitz RL: Hemodynamics in patients with severe toxemia during labor and delivery. Am J Obstet Gynecol 138:263, 1980

Ramanathan J, Sibai BM, Mabie WC, Chauhan D, Ruiz AG: The use of labetalol for attenuation of the hypertensive response to endotracheal intubation in preeclampsia. Am J Obstet Gynecol 159:650, 1988

Redman CWG: Controlled trials of treatment of hypertension during pregnancy. Obstet Gynecol Surv 37:523, 1982

Redman CWG: Treatment of hypertension in pregnancy. Kidney Int 18:267, 1980

Redman CWG, Beilin LJ, Bonnar J, Ounsted MK: Fetal outcome in a trial of antihypertensive treatment in pregnancy. Lancet 2:753, 1976

Robertson AL, Khairallah PA: Effects of angiotensin II and some analogues on vascular permeability in the rabbit. Circ Res 31:923, 1972

Robertson EG: The natural history of oedema during pregnancy. J Obstet Gynaecol Br Commonw 78:520, 1971

Robertson WB, Khong TY, Brosens I, DeWolf F, Sheppard BL, Bonnar J: The placental bed biopsy: Review from three European centers. Am J Obstet Gynecol 155:401, 1986

Robin ED: The cult of the Swan-Ganz catheter. Ann Intern Med 103:445, 1985

Rochat RW, Koonin LM, Atrash HK, Jewett JF, The Maternal Mortality Collaborative: Maternal mortality in the United States: Report from the Maternal Mortality Collaborative. Obstet Gynecol 72:91, 1988

Rolfes DB, Ishak KG: Liver disease in toxemia of pregnancy. Am J Gastroenterol 81:1140, 1986

Rosenbaum M, Maltby G: Cerebral dysrhythmia in relation to eclampsia. Arch Neurol Psychiatr 49:204, 1943

Rubin PC: Treatment of hypertension in pregnancy. Clin Obstet Gynaecol 13:307, 1986

Rubin PC, Butters L, Clark DM, Reynolds B, Summer DJ, Steedman D, Low RA, Reid JL: Placebo-controlled trial of atenolol in treatment of pregnancy-associated hypertension. Lancet 1:431, 1983

Ruvinsky ED, Douvas SG, Roberts WE, Martin JN Jr, Palmer SM, Rhodes PG, Morrison JC: Maternal administration of dexamethasone in severe pregnancy-induced hypertension. Am J Obstet Gynecol 149:722, 1984

Sachs BP, Brown DAJ, Driscoll SG, Schulman E, Acker D, Ransil BJ, Jewett JF: Maternal mortality in Massachusetts—Trends and prevention. N Engl J Med 316:667, 1987

Saleh AA, Bottoms SF, Welch RA, Ali AM, Mariona FG, Mammen EF: Preeclampsia, delivery and the hemostatic system. Am J Obstet Gynecol 157:331, 1987

Samuels P, Main EK, Tomaski A, Mennuti MT, Gabbe SG, Cines DB: Abnormalities in platelet antiglobulin tests in preeclamptic mothers and their neonates. Am J Obstet Gynecol 157:109, 1987

Sanchez-Ramos L, O'Sullivan MJ, Garrido-Calderone J: Effect of low-dose aspirin on angiotensin II pressor response in human pregnancy. Am J Obstet Gynecol 156:193, 1987

Semchyshyn S, Zuspan F, Cordero L: Cardiovascular response and complications of glucocorticoid therapy in hypertensive pregnancies. Am J Obstet Gynecol 145:530, 1983

Shears BH: Combination of chlorpromazine, promethazine, and pethidine in treatment of eclampsia. Br Med J 2:75, 1957

Sheehan HL: Pathological lesions in the hypertensive toxaemias of pregnancy. In Hammond J, Browne FJ, Wolstenholme GEW (eds): Toxaemias of Pregnancy, Human and Veterinary. Philadelphia, Blakiston, 1950

Sheehan HL, Lynch JB (eds): Cerebral lesions. In: Pathology of Toxaemia of Pregnancy, Baltimore, Williams & Wilkins, 1973

Shoemaker ES, Gant NF, Madden JD, MacDonald PC: The effect of thiazide diuretics on placental function. Tex Med 69:109, 1973

Sibai BM, Abdella TN, Anderson GD: Pregnancy outcome in 211 patients with mild chronic hypertension. Obstet Gynecol 61:571, 1983

Sibai BM, Anderson GD: Pregnancy outcome of intensive therapy in severe hypertension in first trimester. Obstet Gynecol 67:517, 1986d

Sibai BM, El-Nazer A, Gonzalez-Ruiz A: Severe preeclampsia-eclampsia in young primigravid women: Subsequent pregnancy outcome and remote prognosis. Am J Obstet Gynecol 155:1011, 1986c

Sibai BM, Gonzalez AR, Mabie WC, Moretti M: A comparison of labetalol plus hospitalization versus hospitalization alone in the management of preeclampsia remote from term. Obstet Gynecol 70:323, 1987a

Sibai BM, Graham JM, McCubbin JH: A comparison of intravenous and intramuscular magnesium sulfate regimens in preeclampsia. Am J Obstet Gynecol 150:728, 1984

Sibai BM, Mabie BC, Harvey CJ, Gonzalez AR: Pulmonary edema in severe preeclampsia-eclampsia: Analysis of thirty-seven consecutive cases. Am J Obstet Gynecol 156:1174, 1987b

Sibai BM, McCubbin JH, Anderson GD, Lipshitz J, Dilts PV Jr: Eclampsia: I. Observations from 67 recent cases. Obstet Gynecol 58:609, 1981

Sibai BM, Spinnato JA, Watson DL, Lewis JA, Anderson GA: Eclampsia: IV. Neurological findings and future outcome. Am J Obstet Gynecol 152:184, 1985a

Sibai BM, Taslimi M, Abdella TN, Brooks TF, Spinnato JA, Anderson GD: Maternal and perinatal outcome of conservative management of severe preeclampsia in midtrimester. Am J Obstet Gynecol 152:32, 1985b

Sibai BM, Taslimi MM, El-Nazer A, Amon E, Mabie BC, Ryan GM: Maternal-perinatal outcome associated with the syndrome of hemolysis, elevated liver enzymes, and low platelets in severe preeclampsia-eclampsia. Am J Obstet Gynecol 155:501, 1986a

Silke B, Carmody M, O'Swyer WF: Acute renal failure in pregnancy. In Bonnar J, MacGillivray I, Symonds EM (eds): Pregnancy Hypertension. Baltimore, University Park Press, 1980, p 511

Sims EAH: Pre-eclampsia and related complications of pregnancy. Am J Obstet Gynecol 107:154, 1970

Slater RM, Wilcos FL, Smith WD, Donnai P, Patrick J, Richardson T, Mawer GE, D'Souza SW, Anderton JM: Phenytoin infusion in severe preeclampsia. Lancet 2:1417, 1987

Somjen G, Hilmy M, Stephen CR: Failure to anesthetize human subjects by intravenous administration of magnesium sulfate. J Pharmacol Exp Ther 154:652, 1966

Spargo B, McCartney CP, Winemiller R: Glomerular capillary endotheliosis in toxemia of pregnancy. Arch Pathol 68:593, 1959

Spellacy WN, Miller SJ, Winegar A: Pregnancy after 40 years of age. Obstet Gynecol 68:452, 1986

Spitz B, Magness RR, Cox SM, Brown CEL, Rosenfeld CR, Gant NF: Low-dose aspirin: I. Effect on angiotensin II pressor responses and blood prostaglandin concentrations in pregnant women sensitive to angiotensin II. Am J Obstet Gynecol 159:1035, 1988

Stahnke E: Über das Verhalten der Blutplättchen bei Eklampsie. Zentralbl Gynaekol 46:391, 1922

Stallworth JC, Yeh S-Y, Petrie RH: The effect of magnesium sulfate on fetal heart rate variability and uterine activity. Am J Obstet Gynecol 140:702, 1981

Stone SR, Pritchard JA: Effect of maternally administered magnesium sulfate on the neonate. Obstet Gynecol 35:574, 1970

Strickland DM, Guzick DS, Cox K, Gant NF, Rosenfeld CR: The relationship between abortion in the first pregnancy and the development of pregnancy-induced hypertension in the subsequent pregnancy. Am J Obstet Gynecol 154:146, 1986

Stubbs TM, Lazarchick J, Horger EO: Plasma fibronectin levels in preeclampsia: A possible biochemical marker for vascular endothelial damage. Am J Obstet Gynecol 150:885, 1984

Talledo OE, Chesley LC, Zuspan FP: Renin-angiotensin system in normal and toxemic pregnancies: III. Differential sensitivity to angiotensin II and norepinephrine in toxemia of pregnancy. Am J Obstet Gynecol 100:218, 1968

Taufield PA, Ales KL, Resnick LM, Druzin ML, Gertner JM, Laragh JH: Hypocalcuria in preeclampsia. N Engl J Med 316:715, 1987

Thiagarajah S, Bourgeois FJ, Harbert GM, Caudle MR: Thrombocytopenia in preeclampsia: Associated abnormalities and management principles. Am J Obstet Gynecol 150:1, 1984

Thiagarajah S, Harbert GM, Bourgeois FJ: Magnesium sulfate and ritodrine hydrochloride: Systemic and uterine hemodynamic effects. Am J Obstet Gynecol 153:666, 1985

Thomsen JK, Storm T, Thamsborg G, de Nully M, Bodker B, Skouby S: Atrial natriuretic peptide concentrations in preeclampsia. Br Med J 294:1508, 1987

Thurnau GR, Kemp DB, Jarvis A: Cerebrospinal fluid levels of magnesium in patients with preeclampsia after treatment with intravenous magnesium sulfate: A preliminary report. Am J Obstet Gynecol 157:1435, 1987

Tillman AJB: The effect of normal and toxemic pregnancy on blood pressure. Am J Obstet Gynecol 70:589, 1955

Toppozada MK, Ismail AAA, Hegab HM, Kamel MA: Treatment of preeclampsia with prostaglandin A_1. Am J Obstet Gynecol 159:160, 1988

Trudinger BJ, Giles WB, Cook CM: Flow velocity waveforms in the maternal uteroplacental and fetal umbilical placental circulations. Am J Obstet Gynecol 152:155, 1985

Valenzuela G, Hayashia R, Johns A: Effects of magnesium sulfate upon uterine contractility in humans. Magnesium 2:120, 1983

Vassalli P, Morris RH, McCluskey RT: The pathogenic role of fibrin deposition in the glomerular lesions of toxemia of pregnancy. J Exp Med 118:467, 1963

Villar MA, Sibai BM, Moretti ML, Mundy DC, Tabb TN, Anderson GD: The clinical significance of elevated mean arterial blood pressure in the second trimester and a threshold increase in systolic and diastolic blood pressures during the third trimester. Abstract No 92 presented at the eighth annual meeting of The Society of Perinatal Obstetricians, Las Vegas, February 1988

Volhard F: Die Doppelseitigen Haematogenen Nierenerkrankungen. Berlin, Springer, 1918

Walker JJ, Bonduelle M, Greer I, Calder AA: Antihypertensive therapy in pregnancy. Lancet 1:932, 1983

Wallenburg HCS, Dekker GA, Makovitz JW, Rotmans P: Low-dose aspirin prevents pregnancy-induced hypertension and preeclampsia in angiotensin-sensitive primigravidae. Lancet 1:1, 1986

Walsh SW: Preeclampsia: An imbalance in placental prostacyclin and thromboxane production. Am J Obstet Gynecol 152:335, 1985

Walsh SW: Progesterone and estradiol production by normal and preeclamptic placentas. Obstet Gynecol 71:222, 1988

Wasserstrum N, Cotton DB: Hemodynamic monitoring in severe pregnancy-induced hypertension. Clin Perinatol 13:781, 1986

Watson KV, Moldow CF, Ogburn PL, Jacob JS: Magnesium sulfate: Rationale for its use in preeclampsia. Proc Natl Acad Sci USA 83:1075, 1986

Weenik GH, Borm JJ, Ten Cate JW, Treffers PE: Antithrombin III levels in normotensive and hypertensive pregnancy. Gynecol Obstet Invest 16:230, 1983

Weiner CP, Brandt J: Plasma antithrombin III activity: An aid in the diagnosis of preeclampsia-eclampsia. Am J Obstet Gynecol 142:275, 1982

Weiner CP, Kwaan HC, Xu C, Paul M, Burmeister L, Hauck W: Antithrombin III activity in women with hypertension during pregnancy. Obstet Gynecol 65:301, 1985

Weinstein L: Preeclampsia-eclampsia with hemolysis, elevated liver enzymes, and thrombocytopenia. Obstet Gynecol 66:657, 1985

Weir, RJ, Fraser R, Lever AF, Morton JJ, Brown JJ, Kraszewski A, McIlevine GM, Robertson JIS, Tree M: Plasma renin, renin substrate, angiotensin II, and aldosterone in hypertensive disease of pregnancy. Lancet 1:291, 1973

Weis EB Jr, Bruns PD, Taylor ES: A comparative study of the disappearance of radioactive sodium from human uterine muscle in normal and abnormal pregnancy. Am J Obstet Gynecol 76:340, 1958

Wellen I: Specific "toxemia," essential hypertension, and glomerulonephritis associated with pregnancy. Am J Obstet Gynecol 39:16, 1940

Whalley PJ, Everett RB, Gant NF, Cox K, MacDonald PC: Pressor responsiveness to angiotensin II in hospitalized primigravid women with pregnancy-induced hypertension. Am J Obstet Gynecol 145:481, 1983

Winkel CA, Casey ML, Guerami A, Rawlins SC, Cox K, MacDonald SC, Parker CR: Ratio of plasma deoxycorticosterone (DOC) levels to plasma progesterone (P) levels in pregnant women who did not develop pregnancy-induced hypertension (PIH). Presented at the Society for Gynecologic Investigation, 30th annual meeting. [Abstract 341], Washington, DC, March 17–20, 1983

Winkel CA, Milewich L, Parker CR Jr, Gant NF, Simpson ER, MacDonald PC: Conversion of plasma progesterone to deoxycorticosterone in men, nonpregnant and pregnant women, and adrenalectomized subjects: Evidence for steroid 21-hydroxylase activity in non-adrenal tissues. J Clin Invest 66:803, 1980

Winkler AW, Smith PK, Hoff HE: Intravenous magnesium sulfate in the treatment of nephritic convulsions in adults. J Clin Invest 21:207, 1942

Worley RJ, Everett RB, MacDonald PC, Gant NF: Placental clearance of dehydroisoandrosterone sulfate and pregnancy outcome in three categories of hospitalized patients with pregnancy-induced hypertension. Gynecol Obstet Invest 6:28, 1975

Zeek PM, Assali NS: Vascular changes in decidua associated with eclamptogenic toxemia of pregnancy. Am J Clin Pathol 20:1099, 1950

Zlatnik FJ, Burmeister LF: Dietary protein and preeclampsia. Am J Obstet Gynecol 147:345, 1983

Zuspan FP, Ward MC: Treatment of eclampsia. South Med J 57:954, 1964

Obstetrical Hemorrhage

GENERAL CONSIDERATIONS

MORTALITY FROM HEMORRHAGE

Obstetrics is "bloody business." Even though the maternal mortality rate has been reduced dramatically by hospitalization for delivery and the availability of blood for transfusion, death from hemorrhage remains prominent in the majority of mortality reports. The Centers for Disease Control recently surveyed 2,067 nonabortion-related maternal deaths in the United States from 1974 through 1978 and reported that hemorrhage was a direct cause in at least 13 percent (Kaunitz and colleagues, 1985). There is evidence that great improvement in mortality from hemorrhage has followed modernization of American obstetrics (Rochat and co-workers, 1988). Sachs and associates (1987, 1988) reported that maternal deaths from obstetrical hemorrhage in Massachusetts decreased tenfold from the mid-1950s to the mid-1980s. Obstetrical hemorrhage is most likely to be fatal to the mother in circumstances in which whole blood or blood components are not immediately available. The establishment and maintenance of facilities that allow prompt administration of blood are absolute requirements for acceptable obstetrical care. Bleeding from the maternal reproductive tract, including those cases in which the cause is unclear, is also dangerous to the fetus. For pregnancies complicated by bleeding during the second and third trimesters, the rate of preterm delivery and perinatal mortality are at least quadrupled (Jouppilla, 1979).

BLOOD LOSS AT PARTURITION

Loss of 500 mL or more of blood after completion of the third stage of labor has persisted as the definition of postpartum hemorrhage (Hughes, 1972). Nonetheless, nearly one half of all women who are delivered vaginally and almost all who undergo cesarean delivery shed that amount of blood or more, when measured quantitatively, as emphasized by Newton (1966), by Pritchard and co-workers (1962) (Fig. 36–1A), and more recently by others.

The woman who develops a normal degree of pregnancy hypervolemia usually increases her blood volume by 30 to 60 percent, which for an individual of average size amounts to 1,000 to as much as 2,000 mL (Pritchard, 1965). Consequently, she will tolerate, without any remarkable decrease in postpartum hematocrit, blood loss at delivery that approaches the volume of blood she added during pregnancy (Fig. 36–1B). Data from a specific case that serve to illustrate the protective nature of pregnancy hypervolemia are presented in Table 36–1, and a brief case summary follows.

In spite of a blood loss of 2,200 mL, incited by cesarean delivery plus radical hysterectomy and pelvic lymphadenectomy performed on an otherwise normally pregnant woman, hypovolemia was effectively combatted with only 500 mL of blood augmented by sufficient lactated Ringer's solution to maintain urine output. Total blood loss was not much greater than the sum of the 500 mL of blood transfused plus the 1,700 mL of blood she had added as pregnancy-induced hypovolemia. Instead of the hematocrit falling, the blood volume promptly did so to approximate closely her normal nonpregnant volume.

The tolerance to hemorrhage at parturition that is normally induced by pregnancy undoubtedly allowed the human race to survive before the era of hospitalization and blood banks. Nonetheless, deaths from hemorrhage were common because of the number of obstetrical complications that predisposed to severe hemorrhage and, in turn, death in the absence of expert management, including appropriate blood replacement therapy.

CONDITIONS THAT PREDISPOSE TO OBSTETRICAL HEMORRHAGE

Listed in Table 36-2 are the many clinical circumstances in which risk of obstetrical hemorrhage is appreciably increased. It is apparent that serious obstetrical hemorrhage may occur at any time throughout pregnancy and the puerperium. Moreover, more than one of the conditions listed may contribute either simultaneously or in sequence to the perpetuation of the hemorrhage.

The time of bleeding in pregnancy is widely used to classify obstetrical hemorrhage, especially bleeding during the third trimester. The term *third trimester bleeding* serves only one useful purpose and that is to warn people *not* to proceed in routine fashion with pelvic examination on the bleeding woman, which could incite severe hemorrhage if there was a placenta previa. The term otherwise is so imprecise for describing gestational (fetal) age and, in turn, intelligent management of the pregnancy that it ought to be abandoned.

UTERINE BLEEDING BEFORE DELIVERY

Slight bleeding through the vagina is common during active labor. This bleeding, or bloody show, is the consequence of effacement and dilatation of the cervix with tearing of small veins and, in turn, slight shedding of blood.

Uterine bleeding from a site above the cervix before delivery of the fetus is cause for concern! The bleeding may be the consequence of some separation of a placenta implanted in the immediate vicinity of the cervical canal, i.e., *placenta previa*, or from separation of a placenta located elsewhere in the uterine cavity, i.e., *abruptio placentae*. Rarely, the bleeding may be the consequence of velamentous insertion of the umbilical cord with rupture of a fetal blood vessel at the time of rupture of the

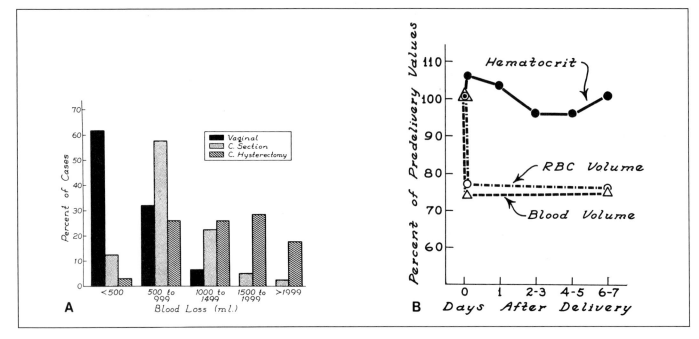

Figure 36–1. A. Blood loss associated with vaginal delivery, repeat cesarean section, and repeat cesarean section plus total hysterectomy. **B.** In a group of women undergoing cesarean section, the hematocrit postpartum changed insignificantly from the predelivery value in spite of an average blood loss of 1,000 mL. At the same time, the blood volume and total erythrocyte volume dropped nearly 25 percent. (*From Pritchard and co-workers: Am J Obstet Gynecol 84:1271, 1962.*)

membranes, i.e., *vasa previa*, with fetal hemorrhage (Chap. 31, Fig. 31–6, p. 538).

In actual practice, the source of uterine bleeding that originates above the level of the cervix is not always identified. In that circumstance, typically the bleeding occurs with little or no other symptomatology, then stops, and at delivery, days, weeks, or months later, no anatomical cause is identified. Almost always the bleeding must have been the consequence of slight marginal separation of the placenta that did not expand. It is emphasized that the pregnancy in which such bleeding occurs remains at increased risk for a poor outcome even though the bleeding soon stops and placenta previa appears to have been excluded by sonography.

ETIOLOGY OF OBSTETRICAL HEMORRHAGE

Obstetrical hemorrhage is the consequence of excessive bleeding from the placental implantation site or trauma to the genital tract and adjacent structures, or both.

Bleeding from Placental Site

Near term, it is estimated that approximately 600 mL per minute of blood flows through the intervillous spaces that make up the maternal blood compartment of the placenta. With separation of the placenta, the many arteries and veins of the uterus that carry blood to and from the maternal compartment of the placenta are severed abruptly. Effective hemostasis demands that the patency of these vessels be quickly obliterated.

Elsewhere in the body hemostasis in the absence of surgical ligation depends upon intrinsic vasospasm and formation of blood clot locally. At the placental implantation site, most important for achieving hemostasis are contraction and retraction of the myometrium to compress the vessels and obliterate their lumens. Adherent pieces of placenta or large blood clots, and especially a hypotonic myometrium, will prevent effective contraction and retraction of the myometrium and thereby impair hemostasis at the implanation site. Fatal postpartum hemorrhage can occur from a hypotonic uterus while the maternal

TABLE 36–1. PATIENT 37 WEEKS PREGNANT. CARCINOMA OF CERVIX, RADICAL HYSTERECTOMY AND PELVIC LYMPHADENECTOMY

| Day | Hematocrit | Volume (mL) | | Loss (mL) | |
		Blood	RBC	RBC	Blood
− 1	34.0	5,444	1,850		
Surgery		Transfused 500 mL blood			
+ 1	34.0	3,835	1,304	746[a]	2,200
+ 2	30.5				
+ 4	30.5				
+ 6	29.0				
+ 8	31.0	4,023	1,247	813[a]	2,400
+84	42.0	3,755	1,577		

[a] Includes 200 mL of transfused RBC.

TABLE 36–2. CONDITIONS THAT PREDISPOSE TO OR WORSEN OBSTETRICAL HEMORRHAGE

Abnormal placentation	**Uterine atony**
Placental previa	Overdistended uterus
Abruptio placentae	1. Multiple fetuses
Placenta accreta	2. Hydramnios
Ectopic pregnancy	3. Distension with clots
Hydatidiform mole	Anesthesia or analgesia
	1. Halogenated agents
Trauma during labor and delivery	2. Conduction analgesia with hypotension
Complicated vaginal delivery	Exhausted myometrium
Cesarean section or hysterectomy	1. Rapid labor
Uterine rupture; risk increased by:	2. Prolonged labor
1. Previously scarred uterus	3. Oxytocin or prostaglandin stimulation
2. High parity	Previous uterine atony
3. Hyperstimulation	**Coagulation defects—intensifies other causes**
4. Obstructed labor	Placental abruption
5. Intrauterine manipulation	Prolonged retention of dead fetus
	Amnionic fluid embolism
Small maternal blood volume	Saline-induced abortion
Small woman	Sepsis with endotoxemia
Pregnancy hypervolemia not yet maximal	Severe intravascular hemolysis
Pregnancy hypervolemia constricted	Massive transfusions
1. Severe preeclampsia	Severe preeclampsia and eclampsia
2. Eclampsia	Congenital coagulopathies

blood coagulation mechanism is quite normal. Conversely, if the myometrium at and adjacent to the denuded implantation site contracts and retracts vigorously, fatal hemorrhage *from the placental implantation site* is unlikely even though the blood coagulation mechanism may be severely impaired.

Bleeding from Sites of Trauma

Lacerated or incised blood vessels in the reproductive tract other than those in the body of the uterus lack the unique mechanism for obliterating vessel patency that is provided by a vigorously contracting and retracting myometrium. Consequently, oxytocic drugs and uterine massage to stimulate vigorous myometrial contractility are ineffective in controlling hemorrhage if the hemorrhage is not of uterine origin. Therefore, following delivery of an intact placenta, hemorrhage from the genital tract that persists with the uterus firmly contracted and retracted is indicative almost certainly of bleeding from lacerations of the genital tract.

MANAGEMENT OF HEMORRHAGE

Whenever there is any suggestion of excessive blood loss from the genital tract, irrespective of apparent cause, it is essential that steps be taken immediately to identify the presence of uterine atony, retained placental fragments, and trauma to the genital tract. It is imperative that at least one and, in the presence of frank hemorrhage, two intravenous infusion systems of large caliber be established immediately to allow rapid administration of aqueous electrolyte solutions and blood as one or both are needed. An operating room and surgical team, including an anesthesiologist, must be immediately available.

ESTIMATION OF EXCESSIVE BLOOD LOSS

A number of techniques are employed to estimate the magnitude of the hemorrhage, most of which by themselves may yield grossly erroneous values, especially when hemorrhage is exter-

nal but brisk or when hemorrhage is concealed, as with placental abruption or hemoperitoneum.

Visual Estimate

Visual inspection is resorted to most often but is notoriously inaccurate. In several reports the amount of blood estimated by inspection to have been lost was on average about one half the actual measured loss. The estimates may be greatly excessive but are more likely to be dangerously low. Furthermore, part of all of the hemorrhage may be concealed.

Blood Pressure and Pulse

Overt hypotension and tachycardia are, of course, signs of dangerous hypovolemia that cannot be ignored, but the converse is not necessarily true. Vital signs, if apparently normal, can be quite misleading. **A blood pressure reading in the normal range, or even hypertension, does not preclude imminently dangerous hypovolemia.** Hypertension, either pregnancy-induced or chronic, is not unusual in pregnant women, and therefore serious hemorrhage and the resultant hypovolemia may in this circumstance result in a fall in blood pressure only to normotensive levels. The normotensive reading may create a false sense of security, with delay in identification of compromised perfusion of vital organs.

The pulse rate may be equally misleading, since it may be elevated in circumstances in which the degree of hemorrhage is negligible, and normal, or even slow, in the presence of severe hypovolemia (Jansen, 1978).

"Tilt Test"

The woman who has bled appreciably but whose blood pressure and pulse rate are normal when recumbent may, when placed in the sitting position, become hypotensive or develop tachycardia, or do both. This so-called tilt test should be applied and interpreted with caution for the following reasons. (1) For the woman who is already hypotensive when recumbent, the tilt test is needless and potentially dangerous. (2) The parturient who has not yet fully recovered from the sympathetic blockade of conduction analgesia, especially spinal, may become hypotensive when placed in the sitting position, without necessarily having suffered serious hemorrhage. (3) The normally hypervolemic pregnant woman may lose a large amount of blood before demonstrating orthostatic hypotension, as demonstrated in Figure 36–2.

> The immediate effects from appreciable hemorrhage demonstrated in Figure 36–2 seem paradoxical. The woman with sickle cell–hemoglobin C disease near term underwent phlebotomy for exchange transfusion. Her measured blood volume was 6 L and hematocrit 38. One L of blood was removed over a period of 8 minutes while she was very carefully observed lying on her side. Her blood pressure and pulse, as well as the fetal heart rate, were monitored continuously. During the 20 minutes following hemorrhage, until infusion of packed erythrocytes was begun, she was observed, first, laterally recumbent, then supine, and finally sitting. Her blood pressure was unchanged until she sat up, when it rose moderately, as did the maternal and fetal heart rates. Thus, the initial response to appreciable hemorrhage in the pregnant woman may be a rise in blood pressure similar to that observed at times in normal nonpregnant individuals.

Urine Flow

When carefully measured, the rate of urine formation *in the absence of potent diuretics* reflects the adequacy of renal perfusion and, in turn, the perfusion of other vital organs, since renal blood flow is especially sensitive to changes in blood volume. With potentially serious hemorrhage, an indwelling catheter should be inserted promptly, first, to empty the bladder completely and then to collect quantitatively all urine formed and thereby monitor its rate of formation. *Whenever*

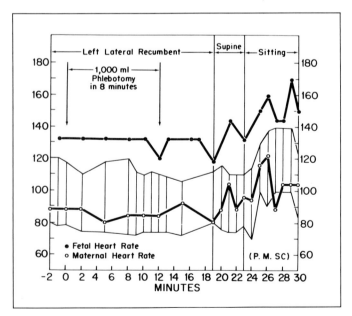

Figure 36–2. Responses late in pregnancy to phlebotomy and changes in posture following phlebotomy. Partial exchange transfusion was being carried out in a woman with sickle cell–hemoglobin C disease; her pregnancy-induced hypervolemia amounted to 1,400 mL. Systolic and diastolic blood pressures are plotted as light lines and each reading is interconnected. The open circles connected by a heavy line demonstrate the maternal pulse rate, and the solid dots so connected are the fetal heart rates.

urine flow through the catheter is very low to absent, the patency of the catheter must be investigated. Blood clots in the bladder may plug the catheter!

Unfortunately, a potent diuretic, such as furosemide, is very likely to invalidate the relationship between urine flow and renal perfusion. This need not be a problem in the management of the woman who is hemorrhaging, however, since there are no proven benefits to be derived from the use of furosemide in this setting. Actually, the reverse is more likely true in that there is great potential for deleterious effects. An almost immediate effect of furosemide is venodilatation, which would further reduce venous return of blood to the heart and thereby further compromise cardiac output. The other dangerous effect is "renal diarrhea," with loss of fluid and electrolyte from the already seriously depleted intravascular compartment.

The antidiuretic agent to which the hemorrhaging woman is likely to be exposed is oxytocin. However, with the infusion of isotonic electrolyte solution, such as lactated Ringer's solution, the amount of free water that is reabsorbed by the renal tubules is not greatly enhanced, and therefore, *severe* oliguria does not develop as the consequence of oxytocin per se.

FLUID REPLACEMENT FOR HEMORRHAGE

Treatment of serious hemorrhage demands prompt and adequate refilling of the intravascular compartment. Two general guidelines have proven to be most valuable for determining the amounts and kinds of fluids that are needed to combat hypovolemia from obstetrical hemorrhage irrespective of cause: **Lactated Ringer's solution and whole blood are given in such amounts and in such proportions that (1) urine flow is at least 30 mL per hour and ideally approaches 60 mL per hour and (2) the hematocrit reading is maintained at 30 percent.**

Further support for the recommendation noted above that the hematocrit be raised to and kept at about 30 has been provided by Czer and Shoemaker (1978). In their series of 94 critically ill postoperative patients, mortality rates were lowest wth hematocrit values maintained between 27 and 33.

Two precautions require emphasis. (1) Urine flow after administration of a potent diuretic does not necessarily bear any precise relationship to the level of renal perfusion. Therefore, if the rate of urine flow is to be used successfully to identify adequate perfusion of the kidney and, in turn, other vital organs, such diuretic agents as furosemide should not be given. (2) Insertion of catheters for monitoring central blood pressures may lead to troublesome bleeding at the site of venipuncture if significant coagulation defects exist. Hence, in circumstances where there may be coagulation defects, rather than insert a central pressure catheter into the subclavian vein, a vein in the antecubital fossa is preferable, since bleeding can be controlled by pressure and a dangerous hemorrhage avoided.

BLOOD AND COMPONENT REPLACEMENT

Whole Blood

Fresh compatible whole blood, rather than stored blood, would appear to be more nearly ideal for treatment of hypovolemia from serious acute hemorrhage, since stored blood soon suffers from loss of functional platelets especially. In spite of this disadvantage, the policy of the Obstetrics Service and the Blood Bank at Parkland Hospital, dictated by the practicalities of blood banking, is to treat hypovolemia from severe hemorrhage with any readily available whole blood that is compatible based on identification of the recipient's blood group and the absence of abnormal red cell antibodies in the recipient's plasma. The panel of red cells used to identify antibodies has been enzyme treated, and all incubations are performed at 37° C. Clinically significant antibodies have been detected only in 1 to 2 percent of cases. To date this so-called *group and screen* technique has been used in more than 133,000 obstetrical and surgical cases at Parkland Hospital (Dr. E. Steane, personal communication). In all cases in which transfusions were given, follow-up crossmatch disclosed no serious incompatibilities and there were no transfusion reactions. **Clinical errors resulting in mislabeled tubes and administration of incompatible ABO blood group transfusions are potentially life-threatening complications.**

Because of the practices of many blood banks for fractionation of donor units to provide component therapy, the availability of whole blood, whether fresh or stored, has diminished remarkably in the past decade. Along with this nonavailability of whole blood, use of fresh-frozen plasma has increased tenfold within the past 10 years and is nearly 2 million units annually. Since there is little justification for the use of fresh-frozen plasma alone as a volume expander, and since each unit exposes the recipient to another additional source of transfusion-related infection, justifiable concerns have been raised over its use. A Consensus Development Conference to consider these issues was called by the National Institutes of Health and the Food and Drug Administration (Consensus Conference, 1985). Unfortunately, while condemning the use of fresh-frozen plasma as a volume expander given for treatment of severe life-threatening hemorrhage and massive transfusion, the committee did not stress the need for whole blood replacement for treatment of massive hemorrhage. Obstetrics notwithstanding, there appears to be a great need for availability of whole blood (Miller, 1985), and it is reasonable to hope that such conferences will stimulate more blood banks to provide whole blood. However, if whole blood is lacking, packed red cells plus recently thawed fresh-frozen plasma are administered. Under some circumstances, autologous blood storage for transfusion seems worthwhile (Herbert and associates, 1988).

Blood Fractions

Fractionation of donor blood by blood banks to provide for component therapy is very common. One drawback to the use of blood component therapy in the treatment of severe obstetrical hemorrhage is lack of prompt availability of reconstituted blood. Infusion of large volumes of packed red cells plus normal saline is not an appropriate substitute for the whole blood that is being rapidly shed in large quantity. The deleterious effects of saline infused in large volume on coagulation factors, plasma proteins, and, in turn, plasma oncotic pressure are shown in Table 36–3. In normally pregnant women the colloid oncotic pressure is already reduced, since the concentration of albumin

in plasma is about 25 percent lower than when nonpregnant. Typically, with reconstituted blood the risk to the recipient of infection transmitted in the blood is increased, since the likelihood of the red cells and plasma coming from the same donor is extremely remote.

At times, after the infusion of many units of stored whole blood, generalized bleeding may develop as a consequence of intense thrombocytopenia. To treat hemorrhage believed to be the direct consequence of severe thrombocytopenia, platelets should be administered from 6 to 10 U of blood that has been obtained very recently from donors of the same blood type as the recipient. If the platelets from an Rh(D) positive donor are given to an $Rh_o(D)$ negative recipient who might conceive again, immune globulin containing $Rh_o(D)$ antibody should be administered promptly. Even with massive hemorrhage and blood replacement, it is highly unlikely that levels of factors V and VIII are sufficiently depressed to be clinically significant (Counts and associates, 1979). If these are identified, however, they can be readily corrected by infusion of fresh-frozen plasma.

Transfusion-Related Infections

With each unit of blood or its component, the donor is exposed to the risk of bloodborne infections. Fortunately, the most feared, infection with human immunodeficiency virus that causes acquired immunodeficiency syndrome, is the most rare. Bove (1987) has estimated that with donor screening for immunodeficiency virus antibody, the risk is 1 in 250,000 transfusions. Ward and colleagues (1988) estimate this risk to be about 1 in 40,000. Much more common is non-A, non-B hepatitis, which may complicate 1 percent of all transfusions. Most cases are undetected since they are anicteric, but chronic hepatitis may result (see Chap. 39, p. 831).

CONSUMPTIVE COAGULOPATHY

Gross derangement of the coagulation mechanism as the direct consequence of a variety of obstetrical accidents, or less commonly as the result of a coincidental disease, may incite or enhance obstetrical hemorrhage.

Pregnancy normally induces appreciable increases in the concentrations of coagulation factors I (fibrinogen), VII, VIII, IX, and X. Other plasma factors and platelets do not change so remarkably. Plasminogen levels are increased considerably, yet plasmin activity during the antepartum period is normally decreased compared to the nonpregnant state. Various stimuli act to incite the conversion of plasminogen to plasmin, and one of the most potent is activation of coagulation.

Observations that extensive placental abruption, as well as other accidents of pregnancy, was frequently associated with hypofibrinogenemia served to stimulate much interest in this as a cause of intense intravascular coagulation. In fact, these observations were initially confined almost totally to obstetrical accidents but subsequently were made for almost all areas of

TABLE 36–3. RUPTURED UTERUS WITH MASSIVE FATAL HEMORRHAGE TREATED VIGOROUSLY WITH ELECTROLYTE SOLUTION, CAUSING MARKED LOWERING OF COAGULATION FACTORS AND COLLOID ONCOTIC PRESSURE

	Plasma Proteins		Fibrinogen (mg/dL)	Platelets (μL)	Prothrombin Time (sec)	Partial Thromboplastin Time (sec)
	Total (g/dL)	Albumin (g/dL)				
Initial	6.4	3.4	324	187,000	11.3	28.3
Terminal	2.3	1.2	104	67,000	17.0	76.3

medicine. These syndromes are now commonly termed *consumptive coagulopathy* or *disseminated intravascular coagulation*.

PATHOLOGICAL ACTIVATION OF COAGULATION

Appreciable continuous physiological intravascular coagulation does not occur, probably because there is limited exposure of circulating blood to stimuli capable of initiating clotting, as well as a preponderance of effective cellular mechanisms to remove traces of activated procoagulants, especially by the liver. In pathological states, however, coagulation may be activated via the extrinsic pathway by thromboplastin from tissue destruction and perhaps via the intrinsic pathway by collagen and other tissue components to which plasma is exposed when there is loss of endothelial integrity. Another mechanism is by direct activation of factor X by proteases, for example, as produced by certain neoplasms, or induction of procoagulant activity in lymphocytes or neutrophils, or stimulation with bacterial toxins.

Consumptive coagulopathy almost always is seen as a complication of an identifiable, underlying pathological process against which treatment must be directed to reverse defibrination. With pathological activation of procoagulants that trigger disseminated intravascular coagulation, there is consumption of platelets and coagulation factors in variable quantities, probably dictated by the degree of the stimulus. As a consequence, fibrin may be deposited in small vessels of virtually every organ system. Typically, coagulation incites the activation of plasminogen to plasmin, which can lyse fibrinogen, fibrin monomer, and fibrin polymers to form a series of fibrinogen–fibrin degradation products or split products. Some of these degradation products, depending upon their size, further contribute to defective hemostasis by delaying fibrin polymerization (prolonged thrombin time) and by causing defective fibrin polymerization as a consequence of their incorporation into fibrin polymer (impaired clot retraction and stability).

SIGNIFICANCE OF CONSUMPTIVE COAGULOPATHY

There are three possible clinical consequences of consumptive coagulopathy (Rappaport, 1977):

1. A bleeding tendency is created by consumption of platelets and clotting factors, potentiated by anticoagulant effects of fibrin degradation products.
2. Ischemic tissue damage may result from fibrin deposition and microcirculatory blockage. The prototype organ for which this event is best described and most commonly cited is the kidney with resultant tubular necrosis or irreversible cortical necrosis. Since, at least in obstetrics, these two conditions are usually encountered in clinical situations in which massive bleeding is encountered, there is undoubtedly a profound contribution from ischemia engendered by hypotension and hypovolemia. Besides the kidney, other organs that may be affected include the adrenals, pituitary, lungs, and liver. Of critical interest is the development of the *adult respiratory distress syndrome*, which is frequently associated with clinical syndromes that also cause disseminated intravascular coagulation (see Chap. 39, p. 807). Although this syndrome is usually prominently featured as a complication of septicemia, bacterial endotoxins are also potent stimulators of intravascular coagulation, and there is evidence that such activation initiates or contrib-

utes to the severity of pulmonary insufficiency incited by alveolar-capillary disruption.
3. Consumptive coagulopathy may be associated with microangiopathic hemolysis, caused by mechanical disruption of the erythrocyte membrane within small vessels in which fibrin has been deposited. Varying degrees of hemolysis with anemia, hemoglobinemia, hemoglobinuria, and erythrocyte morphological changes are produced. It remains uncertain whether or not this syndrome arises de novo as a result of disseminated intravascular coagulation, or if it represents endothelial damage incited by stimuli that caused defibrination, or both.

As the recognition of consumptive coagulopathy in nonobstetrical conditions advanced, so did undue emphasis of certain recommendations for management. These included (1) heroic attempts to replace the deficient clotting factors, especially fibrinogen, (2) injection of heparin in the hope of blocking further intravascular coagulation, (3) administration of ε-aminocaproic acid to try to block fibrinolysis, or (4) some combination of these. Not infrequently, the precise nature of the underlying disease has not been considered thoroughly or has even been ignored. The use of heparin, for example, has been urged by some in circumstances in which the likelihood of benefit would appear to be slight but the risk of potentiating hemorrhage great. More specifically, a disease such as placental abruption, in which the process of intravascular coagulation ceases at delivery, if not before, rarely if ever justifies the use of heparin. It is perplexing that recommendations for treatment of obstetrical hemorrhage with heparin have commonly been made in general medical textbooks and journals, as well as in those works concerned primarily with obstetrics, by authors who cite no significant data either personally accumulated or gleaned from the publications of others. This has been particularly true for placental abruption.

While the injection of coagulation factors, the blocking of fibrin formation with heparin, and the use of drugs to inhibit fibrinolytic activity have been unduly stressed, the value of vigorous restoration and maintenance of the circulation to combat intravascular coagulation has not received appropriate attention. With adequate perfusion of vital organs, activated coagulation factors and circulating fibrin and fibrin degradation products are much more promptly removed by the reticuloendothelial system. At the same time, synthesis of procoagulants is promoted, especially by the liver.

The likelihood of life-threatening hemorrhage in obstetrical situations complicated by defective coagulation will depend not only on the extent of the coagulation defects but—of great importance—on whether or not the vasculature is intact or disrupted and, when it is disrupted, the magnitude of the disruption. With gross derangement of blood coagulation, there may be fatal hemorrhage when vascular integrity is disrupted, yet no hemorrhage as long as all blood vessels remain intact. Moreover, each category of disease must be considered separately, and for each case in any category the intensity of the intravascular coagulation and the dangers therefrom must be carefully measured before a decision is made to employ a therapy as potentially dangerous as heparin, fibrinogen, or ε-aminocaproic acid. It cannot be overemphasized that the laboratory identification of possible stigmas of intravascular coagulation, such as thrombocytopenia, fibrin degradation products in serum, or distorted erythrocytes in a blood smear suggesting microangiopathic hemolytic anemia, should *not* in themselves serve as indications for the prompt use of heparin, fibrinogen, or ε-aminocaproic acid. It also must be kept in mind that impaired synthesis or even dilution by vigorous treatment with electrolyte solutions, rather than abnormal consumption, may be the cause of pathologically low levels of some procoagulants.

CLINICAL AND LABORATORY EVIDENCE OF DEFECTIVE HEMOSTASIS

Excessive bleeding at sites of modest trauma characterizes defective hemostasis. Persistent bleeding from venipuncture sites, nicks incurred from shaving the perineum or abdomen, trauma from insertion of a catheter, and spontaneous bleeding from the gums or nose are signs of possible coagulation defects. Purpuric areas at pressure sites may indicate incoagulable blood, or more commonly, troublesome thrombocytopenia. Finally, a surgical incision provides the ultimate "bioassay" for intactness of coagulation. The presence of continuous generalized oozing from the skin, subcutaneous, and fascial tissues, as well as the vascular retroperitoneal space, should suggest that there is a coagulopathy. Such evidence also may be gained by observing continuous oozing from episiotomy incisions or perineal lacerations.

Hypofibrinogenemia

If serious *hypofibrinogenemia* is present, the clot formed from whole blood in a glass tube may be soft initially but not necessarily remarkably reduced in volume. Then, over the next half hour or so, it becomes quite small, so that many of the erythrocytes are extruded and the volume of liquid clearly exceeds that of the clot. The addition of a drop of topical thrombin to hasten the conversion of circulating fibrinogen to fibrin has practical utility.

Thrombin Clot Test

One drop of fresh bovine thrombin, 5,000 units per mL, is placed into each of a series of clean, small, plain glass tubes, which are then stoppered and promptly frozen. As needed, a frozen thrombin tube is obtained, and about 2 mL of venous blood (a column about 1 inch high) is promptly ejected from a syringe into the tube without foam. The time is marked on the tube, which is then taped upright and inspected at intervals of 5 to 10 minutes over the next half hour or so. The important feature is the size of the clot that evolves and persists and not the rate at which the clot forms.

Thrombocytopenia

Serious thrombocytopenia is likely if petechiae are abundant or clotted blood fails to retract over a period of an hour or so, or if platelets are rare in a stained blood smear. Confirmation is provided by actual platelet count.

Prothrombin and Partial Thromboplastin Times

Prolonged partial thromboplastin time or prothrombin time may be the consequence, singly or in combination, of appreciable reductions in those coagulants essential for generating thrombin, of a fibrinogen concentration below a critical level of about 100 mg per dL, of appreciable amounts of circulating fibrinogen–fibrin degradation products, or of all three. Moreover, prolongation of the prothrombin time and partial thromboplastin time need not be the consequence of disseminated intravascular coagulation. For example, sepsis can derange vitamin K metabolism sufficiently that vitamin K-dependent coagulation factors are reduced appreciably (Corrigan, 1984).

Thrombin Time

A long thrombin time may be the consequence of low fibrinogen, of appreciable amounts of fibrinogen–fibrin products, or of both. Moreover, in some cases of severe preeclampsia, and especially in cases of eclampsia, the thrombin time may be prolonged for reasons not readily apparent (Pritchard and coworkers, 1976).

PLACENTAL ABRUPTION

NOMENCLATURE

The separation of the placenta from its site of implantation in the uterus before the delivery of the fetus has been called variously placental abruption, abruptio placentae, ablatio placentae, accidental hemorrhage, and premature separation of the normally implanted placenta.

The term *premature separation of the normally implanted placenta* is most descriptive, since it differentiates the placenta that separates prematurely but is implanted some distance beyond the cervical internal os from one that is implanted over the cervical internal os, i.e., placenta previa. It is cumbersome, however, and hence the shorter term *abruptio placentae*, or *placental abruption*, has been employed. The Latin *abruptio placentae*, which means "rending asunder of the placenta," denotes a sudden accident, a clinical characteristic of most cases of this complication. *Ablatio placentae* means "a carrying away of the placenta," analogous to *ablatio retinae*; this term is not extensively used. The term frequently employed in Great Britain for this complication is *accidental hemorrhage*. The rationale for its use is that the condition is an accident in the sense of an event that takes place without expectation, in contrast to the unavoidable hemorrhage of placenta previa, in which bleeding is inevitable because of the anatomical relations between the placenta and dilating cervix. Since the term *accidental hemorrhage* may suggest an element of trauma, which is rarely a factor in these cases, it may be misleading and is seldom used in the United States.

Some of the bleeding of placental abruption usually insinuates itself between the membranes and uterus, then escapes through the cervix, and appears externally, causing an *external hemorrhage* (Fig. 36–3). Less often, the blood does not escape externally but is retained between the detached placenta and the uterus, leading to *concealed hemorrhage* (Figs. 36–3 and 36–4). Placental abruption with concealed hemorrhage carries with it much greater maternal hazards, not only because the likelihood of intense consumptive coagulopathy is increased, but also because the extent of the hemorrhage is not appreciated.

FREQUENCY, INTENSITY, AND SIGNIFICANCE

The frequency with which abruptio placentae is diagnosed will vary, since criteria employed for diagnosis differ. For example, especially during the second stage of labor as the fetus is slowly extruded from the uterus into the vagina, the placenta may separate partially and be diagnosed as placental abruption by

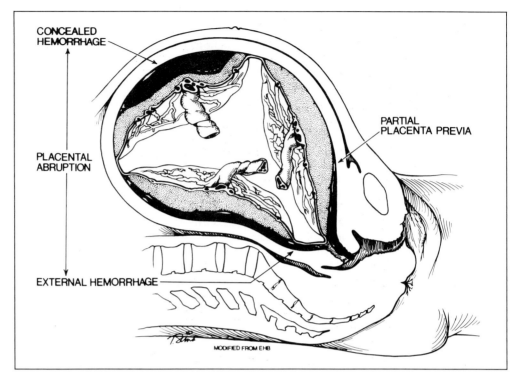

Figure 36–3. Hemorrhage from premature placental separation. *Upper left:* Extensive placental abruption but with the periphery of the placenta and the membranes still adherent, resulting in completely concealed hemorrhage. *Lower:* Placental abruption with the placenta detached peripherally and with the membranes between the placenta and cervical canal stripped from underlying decidua, allowing external hemorrhage. *Right:* Partial placenta previa with placental separation and external hemorrhage.

some but not all obstetrical units. This event alone will appreciably alter the recorded frequency. The intensity of the abruption often will vary depending on how fast the woman seeks and receives care following the onset of abdominal pain or vaginal bleeding or both. With delay, the likelihood of extensive separation causing death of the fetus is increased remarkably.

The reported frequency for placental abruption is 1 in 75 to 90 deliveries (Abdella and associates, 1984; Hurd and colleagues, 1983; Pritchard and Brekken, 1967). Käregärd and Gennser (1986) surveyed 849,619 births in Sweden from 1973 to l982 and reported that 3,959 (0.44 percent, or 1 in 225) were complicated by abruptio placentae. In recent years at Parkland Hospital the frequency of diagnosis of abruption is about 1 in 200 deliveries. Applying the criterion of placental separation so extensive as to kill the fetus, the incidence at Parkland Hospital was 1 in 500 deliveries (Pritchard and Brekken, 1967). However, as the frequency of high parity in women cared for has decreased in more recent years and community-wide availability of emergency transportation has increased, the frequency of placental abruption fatal to the fetus has dropped to about 1 in 850 deliveries.

Even so, as stillbirths from other causes have decreased appreciably, examples being maternal diabetes and maternal isoimmunization causing hydrops fetalis, stillbirth from abruptio placentae has become especially prominent. Of all third-trimester stillbirths at Parkland Hospital during 1985 and l986, 12 percent were the consequence of placental abruption, the same frequency as found by Hovatta and associates (1983).

At the University of Tennessee the frequency of placental abruption in recent years has been about 1 in 90 deliveries (Abdella and associates, 1984). The perinatal mortality rate was about 35 percent for all cases and 25 percent for infants who weighed 1,000 g or more.

Hurd and co-workers (1983) in Cincinnati have observed a frequency for abruptio placentae of about 1 per 75 deliveries,

with a perinatal mortality rate of 30 percent, about equally divided between stillbirths and neonatal deaths. Paterson (1979) in Birmingham, England, identified the perinatal mortality rate associated with placental abruption to be 35 percent. More recently, Krohn and associates (1987) reported that the perinatal mortality was 21 percent in 884 pregnancies complicated by placental abruption in Washington state. Similarly, Käregärd and Gennser (1986) reported a 20 percent perinatal mortality among 3,959 pregnancies complicated by abruption in Sweden.

It is quite obvious that placental abruption is a common obstetrical problem that is especially dangerous to the fetus and newborn infant. Even though the fetus survives, the newborn infant may succumb. If the infant survives, he or she may be compromised. For example, of the 182 infants who survived placental abruption in the study by Abdella and associates (1984), 25 were identified to have significant neurological deficits within the first year of life! While maternal mortality is now uncommon (none in the experiences cited above), morbidity is common and may be severe for reasons to be considered below.

ETIOLOGY

The primary cause of placental abruption is unknown, but the following conditions have been suggested as etiological factors: trauma, shortness of the umbilical cord, sudden decompression of the uterus, uterine anomaly or tumor, pregnancy-induced or chronic hypertension, pressure by the enlarged uterus on the inferior vena cava, and dietary deficiency. Recently, O'Brien and colleagues (1987) reported that there is diminished inhibitory activity of platelet aggregation by adenosine diphosphate in extracts of placentas that have separated prematurely.

In the Parkland Hospital study of 201 cases of placental abruption so severe as to kill the fetus, maternal *hypertension* was apparent in nearly half of the cases once the depleted intravascular compartment was adequately refilled (Pritchard and co-workers, 1970). One half of the hypertensive women had chronic vascular disease; in the remainder, the hypertension appeared to be pregnancy induced. The high frequency of maternal hypertension in pregnancies complicated by placental abruption has been observed by some others (Abdella and co-workers, 1984) but not by all (Paterson, 1979). It appears that there is not an increased incidence of hypertension in pregnancies with lesser degrees of placental abruption (Sholl, 1987), whereas severe placental abruption is much more likely to be associated with maternal hypertension.

External trauma, an unusually short cord, or a uterine anomaly or tumor could be implicated only rarely in cases of severe placental abruption cared for at Parkland Hospital. Moreover, our experiences are similar to those of Kettel (1988) and Stafford (1988) and their co-workers who stress that abruption caused by relatively minor maternal trauma may cause fetal jeopardy that is not always associated with obvious clinical evidence for placental separation. Hydramnios with sudden uterine decompression causing placental abruption is also uncommon (Pritchard and co-workers, 1970).

Lesser degrees of abruption may occur shortly before delivery of a singleton fetus when the amnionic fluid has drained from the uterus and the fetus has descended until the head is on the perineum. With twins, decompression following delivery of the first fetus may lead to premature separation of the placenta that endangers the second fetus (Chap. 34, p. 646).

Experimental obstruction of the inferior vena cava and ovarian veins was reported to produce placental abruption. There are, however, several recorded instances of ligation of ovarian veins and the inferior vena cava during the third trimester without subsequent placental abruption (Stone and colleagues, 1968).

Hibbard and Jeffcoate (1966) and some others contended that folic acid deficiency played an etiological role in placental abruption (Chap. 14, p. 266). The hypothesis has been carefully examined by Whalley and associates (1969) and Alperin and colleagues (1969), and these investigators found no evidence to support such a relationship.

Marbury and colleagues (1983) suggest that maternal ethanol consumption (14 or more drinks per week), but not smoking, predisposes to placental abruption.

RECURRENCE

Of considerable importance to the prognosis in women with a previous placental abruption, the risk of recurrence in a subsequent pregnancy is much higher than for the general population. Paterson (1979) noted a recurrence rate of 1 in 18 pregnancies, Pritchard and co-workers (1970) identified a recurrence rate of 1 in 10 pregnancies, and Hibbard and Jeffcoate (1966) observed the remarkably high rate of 1 in 6 pregnancies. Käregärd and Gennser (1986) reported that the recurrent placental abruption risk was increased tenfold, from 0.4 to 4 percent, or 1 in 25.

Indeed the likelihood of recurrence makes a subsequent pregnancy a high-risk pregnancy. Management of the subsequent pregnancy is made difficult by the fact that the placental separation may occur suddenly at any time, even remote from term. Beischer and associates (1970) found that normal levels of urinary estriol provided no assurance against imminent severe placental abruption. Moreover, Seski and Compton (1976) documented both normal acceleration of the fetal heart rate with fetal movement (normal nonstress test) and no abnormal deceleration of the fetal heart rate in response to uterine contractions (normal contraction stress test) when the test were employed 4 hours before the onset of placental abruption so severe that it promptly killed the fetus.

PATHOLOGY

Placental abruption is initiated by hemorrhage into the decidua basalis. The decidua then splits, leaving a thin layer adherent to the myometrium. Consequently, the process in its earliest stages consists of the development of a decidual hematoma that leads to separation, compression, and the ultimate destruction of the placenta adjacent to it. In its early stage, there may be no clinical symptoms. The condition is discovered only upon examination of the freshly delivered organ, which will present on its maternal surface a circumscribed depression measuring a few centimeters in diameter, covered by dark, clotted blood. Undoubtedly, it takes several minutes for these anatomical changes to materialize. Thus, a very recently abrupted placenta may appear no different from a normal placenta at delivery.

In some instances, a decidual spiral artery ruptures to cause a retroplacental hematoma, which, as it expands, disrupts more vessels to separate more placenta with more bleeding and, in turn, more separation. The area of separation rapidly becomes more extensive and reaches the margin of the placenta. Since the uterus is still distended by the products of conception, it is unable to contract sufficiently to compress the torn vessels that supply the placental site. The escaping blood may dissect the membranes from the uterine wall and eventually appear externally (Fig. 36–3) or may be completely retained within the uterus (Fig. 36–4).

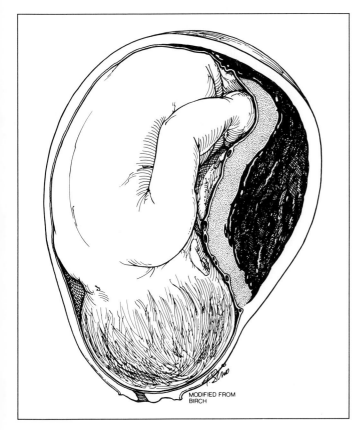

MODIFIED FROM BIRCH

Figure 36–4. Total placental abruption with concealed hemorrhage. The fetus is now dead.

Concealed Hemorrhage

Retained, or concealed, hemorrhage is likely to occur when (1) there is an effusion of blood behind the placenta but its margins still remain adherent, (2) the placenta is completely separated, yet the membranes retain their attachment to the uterine wall, (3) the blood gains access to the amnionic cavity after breaking through the membranes, and (4) the fetal head is so closely applied to the lower uterine segment that the blood cannot make its way past it. In the majority of such cases, however, the membranes are gradually dissected off the uterine wall, and blood sooner or later escapes from the cervix.

Chronic Placental Abruption

Most often, hemorrhage from the placental implantation site persists either until delivery, following which the blood vessels can be successfully constricted by the contracting and retracting myometrium, or until the woman dies. In a small minority of cases, however, hemorrhage with retroplacental hematoma for

mation is somehow completely arrested without delivery having taken place. We have been able to document this phenomenon by labeling maternal red cells with a chromium isotope. This technique served to demonstrate that red blood cells concealed as clot within the uterus at delivery some days later contained no chromium and therefore were shed long before, even though separation at the time of introduction of labeled red cells had been so massive as to kill the fetus (Cunningham, Pritchard, unpublished data).

Fetal-to-Maternal Hemorrhage

Severe fetal-to-maternal hemorrhage associated with placental abruption has been very uncommon in our experience, but it does occur. An example of massive bleeding from the fetus into the maternal circulation as the consequence of placental abruption is provided in Figures 36–5A and B.

At 33 weeks gestation, the mother was forcefully thrown against the steering wheel during an auto accident even though she was

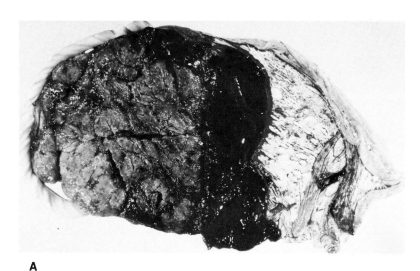

A

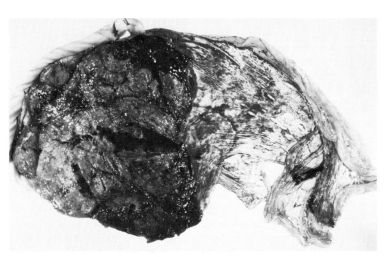

B

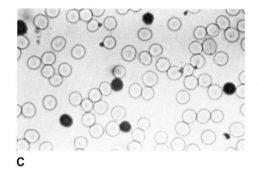

C

Figure 36–5. A. Partial placental abruption with adherent blood clot. The fetus died from massive hemorrhage, chiefly into the maternal circulation. **B.** The adherent blood clot has been removed. Note the laceration of the placenta. **C.** Smear of maternal blood after fetal death. The dark cells are fetal red cells, whereas the empty cells are maternal in origin. Hemoglobin A has been eluted from the maternal cells by treatment with acid, while hemoglobin F remains in the red cells of fetal origin.

wearing an over-the-shoulder seat belt. The fetal heart was not heard when listened for 20 minutes later. Spontaneous labor developed 22 hours after the accident. At that time, the maternal blood contained at least 75 mL of fetal erythrocytes, or 115 mL of fetal blood, calculated from the percentage of red cells rich in fetal hemoglobin found in maternal blood (4.5 percent, as demonstrated in Fig. 36–5C), the maternal blood volume, and hematocrit. The macerated fetus weighed 2,140 g. The placenta contained a long rent that extended to the chorionic plate. The clot adherent to the placenta at the site of partial placental abruption contained nearly all maternal red cells. Moreover, these red cells had been shed before the onset of labor, since they contained none of the labeled chromium usd to measure the maternal blood volume at the onset of labor.

CLINICAL DIAGNOSIS

It is emphasized that the signs and symptoms with abruptio placentae can vary considerably. For example, external bleeding can be profuse, yet placental separation not so extensive as to compromise the fetus directly, or there may be no external bleeding but the placenta is completely sheared off and the fetus dead as the direct consequence.

> In one very unusual case, a multiparous Hispanic woman presented to the Parkland Hospital obstetrical emergency room because of nosebleed. She complained of no abdominal or uterine pain, and there was no tenderness or vaginal bleeding. Her fetus, which had moved the evening before, was dead, and her blood did not clot when placed in a tube containing thrombin. The plasma fibrinogen level was less than 25 mg per dL and fibrin–fibrinogen degradation products in serum were greater than 1,000 µg per mL. Oxytocin induction was successful, and at delivery a total placental abruption with fresh clots was found.

Abruption with concealed hemorrhage carries with it much greater maternal hazards, not only because the likelihood of consumptive coagulopathy is higher, but also because the extent of hemorrhage is not appreciated, and consequently blood replacement has commonly been too little and too late.

Hurd and co-workers (1983), in a relatively small but impressive prospective study of abruptio placentae in which placenta previa was excluded by sonography, identified the frequency of a variety of pertinent signs and symptoms (Table 36–4). Note that in 22 percent of cases idiopathic preterm labor was considered to be the diagnosis until subsequent fetal distress, including fetal death, serious bleeding, back pain, uterine tenderness, rapid uterine contractions, or persistent uterine hypertonus, were detected singly or more often in combination.

TABLE 36–4. SIGNS AND SYMPTOMS WITH ABRUPTIO PLACENTAE (59 PROSPECTIVE CASES)

Sign or Symptom	Frequency (%)
Vaginal bleeding	78
Uterine tenderness or back pain	66
Fetal distress	60
High frequency contractions (17%) Hypertonus (17%)	34
Idiopathic preterm labor[a]	22
Dead fetus	15

[a] All treated with tocolytic agents.
From Hurd and associates: Obstet Gynecol 61:467, 1983.

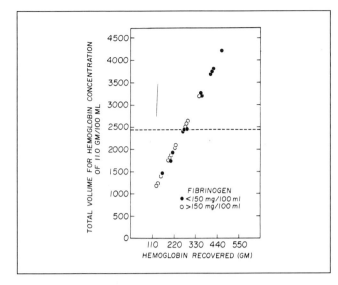

Figure 36–6. Volumes of hemorrhage concealed within the uterus until delivery in women with extensive placental abruption. The dotted line identifies the median value; the open circles represent cases with severe hypofibrinogenemia. (*From Pritchard and Brekken: Am J Obstet Gynecol 97:681, 1967.*)

They were able to recognize a retroplacental hematoma sonographically in only 1 of 59 cases. Using sonography, Sholl (1987) confirmed the clinical diagnosis of abruption in only 25 percent of women and concluded that its principal utility is to rule out placenta previa. **Importantly, negative findings with ultrasound examination do not exclude life-threatening placental abruption.**

SHOCK

It was long held that the shock sometimes seen in placental abruption was out of proportion to the amount of hemorrhage. An explanation proposed for this disparity was that thromboplastin from decidua and placenta entered the maternal circulation at the site of placental separation and incited intravascular coagulation and, in turn, acute cor pulmonale. Admittedly, the sudden intravenous injection of large doses of thromboplastic material into experimental animals can cause profound shock, as shown by Schneider (1954), but the weight of evidence is that the intensity of shock is seldom out of proportion to the maternal blood loss. Pritchard and Brekken (1967), for example, studied the blood loss in 141 gravidas with placental abruption so severe as to kill the fetus and found blood loss often to amount to one half of the pregnant blood volume (Fig. 36–6).

Neither hypotension nor anemia is obligatory in cases of concealed hemorrhage even when the acute hemorrhage has achieved considerable magnitude. An example is cited:

> P.P., 34 weeks pregnant, experienced continuous lower abdominal pain that became progressively more severe. When first seen 4 hours after the onset of the pain, fetal heart action was lacking, there was no external bleeding, her blood pressure was 150/100 mm Hg, and the hematocrit was 42, compared to 38 recorded 4 weeks before. She subsequently expelled spontaneously a dead fetus, placenta, and blood clots, plus liquid equivalent to 2 L of blood! Along with total placental abruption, preeclampsia causing severe hypertension and hemoconcentration complicated the pregnancy and

accounted for the hypertension and rise in hematocrit in spite of serious concealed hemorrhage. Prompt refilling of the intravascular compartment was accompanied by a rise in blood pressure, reestablishment of urine flow, and preservation of vital organ functions.

Oliguria caused by inadequate renal perfusion but responsive to vigorous treatment of hypovolemia is frequently observed in these circumstances. Fortunately, in this case the hypertension and high hematocrit initially were not misinterpreted as excluding serious concealed hemorrhage, and appropriate fluid replacement was initiated promptly.

DIFFERENTIAL DIAGNOSIS

The severe case of placental abruption is usually, but not always, marked by such classic signs and symptoms that the diagnosis is at once obvious, but the milder and more common forms are difficult to recognize with certainty, and the diagnosis is often made by exclusion. Therefore, with vaginal bleeding in the last trimester, it often becomes necessary to rule out placenta previa and other causes of bleeding by clinical inspection and ultrasound evaluation. It has long been taught, perhaps with some justification, that painful uterine bleeding means abruptio placentae, while painless uterine bleeding is indicative of placenta previa. Unfortunately, the differential diagnosis is not that simple. Labor accompanying placenta previa may cause pain suggestive of abruptio placentae. On the other hand, abruptio placentae may mimic normal labor.

Unfortunately, there are neither laboratory tests nor diagnostic methods that will accurately detect lesser degrees of separation of the placenta. The cause of the vaginal bleeding at times remains obscure even after delivery.

Classic placental abruption with pain, shock, uterine rigidity, and absent fetal heart sounds may develop in the middle trimester of pregnancy. Oláh and colleagues (1988) described a woman with severe coagulopathy from abruption at 19 weeks. The fetus remained alive, the coagulopathy reversed, and delivery ensued at 26 weeks. From our experiences, these women present the same complications as do more advanced pregnancies and may cause the death of the woman unless she is appropriately treated.

CONSUMPTIVE COAGULOPATHY

The most common cause of consumptive coagulopathy in pregnancy is placental abruption. Overt *hypofibrinogenemia* (less than 150 mg per dL of plasma), along with elevated levels of fibrinogen–fibrin degradation products and variable decreases in other coagulation factors, can be demonstrated in about 30 percent of women with placental abruption severe enough to kill the fetus. Such coagulation defects may be found but are very uncommon in those cases in which the fetus survives. The experience at Parkland Hospital has been that serious coagulopathy, when it develops, usually is evident by the time the symptomatic woman is hospitalized.

The major mechanism in the genesis of the coagulation defects of placental abruption almost certainly is the induction of coagulation intravascularly and, to a lesser degree, retroplacentally. Although an appreciable amount of fibrin is commonly deposited within the uterine cavity in cases of severe placental abruption and hypofibrinogenemia, the amounts are insufficient to account for all of the fibrinogen missing from the circulation (Pritchard and Brekken, 1967). Moreover, Bonnar and co-workers (1969) have observed, and we have confirmed, the

levels of fibrin degradation products to be higher in serum from peripheral blood than in serum from blood contained in the uterine cavity. The reverse would be anticipated in the absence of significant intravascular coagulation.

An important consequence of intravascular coagulation is the activation of plasminogen to plasmin, which lyses microemboli of fibrin, thereby maintaining patency of the microcirculation. In every instance of placental abruption severe enough to kill the fetus, we have identified clearly pathological levels (greater than 100 µg per mL) of fibrinogen–fibrin degradation products in maternal serum. At the outset, severe hypofibrinogenemia may or may not be accompanied by overt thrombocytopenia. After repeated blood transfusions, however, thrombocytopenia is common.

RENAL FAILURE

Acute renal failure that persists for any length of time is rare with lesser degrees of placental abruption but is seen in the severe forms when there is delayed or incomplete treatment of hypovolemia (see Chap. 39, p. 813). Renal failure, usually renal cortical necrosis, was identified in 6 of 10 fatal cases of placental abruption reported by Krupp and associates (1970). However, the renal lesion more commonly encountered is that of acute tubular necrosis (Silke and associates, 1980). The precise cause of the renal damage that may be associated with placental abruption is not clear, but the major factors very likely are seriously impaired renal perfusion from both reduced cardiac output and intrarenal vasospasm as the consequence of massive hemorrhage and, at times, coexisting acute or chronic hypertensive disorders. Even when placental abruption is complicated by severe intravascular coagulation, prompt and vigorous treatment of hemorrhage with blood and electrolyte solution nearly always will prevent life-threatening renal dysfunction.

During nearly 35 years at Parkland Hospital, more than 400 cases of placental abruption so severe as to kill the fetus have received fluid replacement therapy consisting of whole blood and lactated Ringer's solution, as discussed throughout this chapter. In only one instance has dialysis for renal failure been necessary, and in this woman, at least in retrospect, blood and crystalloid replacement were inadequate following delivery by cesarean section, which was further complicated postoperatively by occult intra-abdominal hemorrhage. Even among women who unfortunately suffered severe placental abruption and intense consumptive coagulopathy more than once, impaired renal function has not been a consequence.

Proteinuria is common, especially with more severe forms of placental abruption, but it usually clears soon after delivery.

UTEROPLACENTAL APOPLEXY (COUVELAIRE UTERUS)

In the more severe forms of placental abruption, widespread extravasation of blood into the uterine musculature and beneath the uterine serosa often occurs (Fig. 36–7). Such effusions of blood are also seen occasionally beneath the tubal serosa, in the connective tissue of the broad ligaments, and in the substance of the ovaries, as well as free in the peritoneal cavity, presumably from uterine bleeding through the oviducts.

The phenomenon of *uteroplacental apoplexy*, first described by Couvelaire early in this century and now frequently called *Couvelaire uterus*, was thought at one time to impair uterine contractility after delivery, with severe postpartum uterine hemorrhage as the consequence. These myometrial hematomas seldom interfere with uterine contractions sufficiently to produce

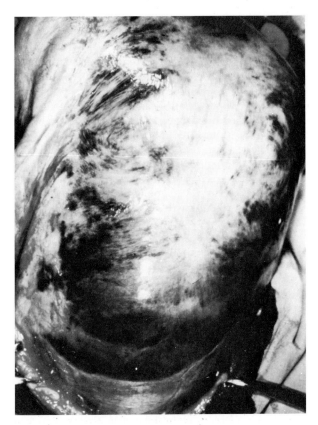

Figure 36–7. Couvelaire uterus with total placental abruption before being emptied by cesarean section. Blood had markedly infiltrated much of the myometrium to reach the serosa. After the infant was delivered and the uterus closed, the uterus remained well contracted despite extensive extravasation of blood into the uterine wall.

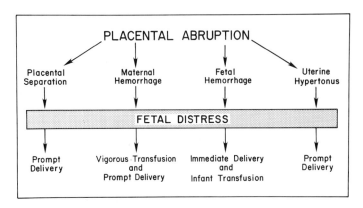

Figure 36–8. Various causes of fetal distress from placental abruption and their treatment.

severe postpartum hemorrhage. Shown in Figure 36–7 is an example of Couvelaire uterus just before cesarean section early in the third trimester. The uterus remained well contracted after being emptied, appropriately sutured, and stimulated to contract with intravenous oxytocin. The infiltration of blood characteristic of Couvelaire uterus, therefore, is not an indication for hysterectomy. It is impossible to give a precise frequency of the incidence of Couvelaire uterus because the condition can only be demonstrated conclusively at laparotomy.

MANAGEMENT

Treatment will vary depending upon the status of the mother and of the fetus. With the development of massive external bleeding, intense therapy with whole blood plus electrolyte solution and prompt delivery to try to control the hemorrhage together are life-saving for the mother and, hopefully, for the fetus. In this circumstance the bleeding is more likely to be the consequence of placenta previa, but it may be from premature separation of a placenta that is located away from the cervical canal, i.e., abruptio placentae.

With blood loss occurring at a much slower rate, management will be influenced considerably by the status of the fetus. If the fetus is alive and there is no evidence of fetal distress, i.e., persistent bradycardia, ominous decelerations, or a sinusoidal heart rate pattern, and if maternal hemorrhage is not causing

serious hypovolemia or anemia, procrastination with very close observation, coupled with facilities for immediate intervention, can be practiced. This is likely to prove most beneficial when the fetus is immature.

Sholl (1987) recently presented data from 130 women with clinically diagnosed placental abruption. Of the 72 women with pregnancies between 26 and 37 weeks, half were delivered within 3 days of admission because of progression to serious hemorrhage or fetal distress, or both. Interestingly, the cesarean section rate was about 50 percent for those delivered soon after admission, as well as those in whom delivery was postponed for at least 3 days.

Sonography has served in some cases to identify a blood clot in the uterine cavity formed there as the consequence of placental abruption. **As emphasized earlier, failure to so identify such a clot does not exclude serious placental abruption.**

If the degree of separation is extensive, ominous decelerations in fetal heart rate are likely, especially when the myometrium contracts. Lack of ominous decelerations, however, does not guarantee the safety of the intrauterine environment for any period of time. The placenta may separate further at any instant and very soon seriously compromise the fetus and even kill the fetus unless delivery is performed immediately.

Some of the immediate causes of fetal distress from abruptio placentae are presented in Figure 36–8. It is very important for the welfare of the distressed fetus that steps be initiated immediately to correct maternal hypovolemia, anemia, and hypoxia so as to restore and maintain the function of any placenta that is still implanted and therefore capable of functioning. Little can be done to modify favorably the other causes that contribute to fetal distress except to remove the fetus promptly from the very unfavorable environment. For example serious fetal hemorrhage, as demonstrated in Figure 36–5, cannot be treated effectively until the fetus is delivered. Moreover, we have not been able to decrease uterine hypertonicity significantly with parenterally administered magnesium sulfate in doses given for preeclampsia (Hauth and Pritchard, unpublished). Ritodrine and other β-receptor agonists are not recommended, since they are likely to cause vasodilatation of the underfilled vascular system, as well as to adversely affect the maternal heart.

Åstedt (1982) emphasized another potential risk from the use of β-receptor agonists to try to inhibit labor. In his experience the agonist can minimize the pain and uterine hypertonicity that typifies more extensive placental abruption, and the abruption may go unrecognized for a dangerously long period, especially in the absence of external hemorrhage. Hurd and associates (1983) have also encountered this problem. Sholl (1987), on the other hand, provided data that ritodrine tocolysis may have marginally improved outcome in a highly selected group of preterm pregnancies complicated by partial abruption. He concluded that at least there was no evidence that tocolysis increased the hazards of fetal distress or hemorrhage or that it increased the incidence of cesarean delivery.

Because of these many uncertainties, and because of their marginal efficacy (see Chap. 38, p. 756), we do not use tocolytic drugs for women with suspected placental separation.

CESAREAN DELIVERY

Rapid delivery of the fetus who is alive but in distress practically always means cesarean section. It is emphasized that an electrode applied directly to the fetus to record the fetal EKG may provide misleading information, as in the case of severe placental abruption illustrated in Figure 36–9. At first impression at least, fetal bradycardia of 80 to 90 beats per minute with a degree of beat-to-beat variability seemed evident. The fetus, however, was dead. There were no audible fetal heart sounds, and the maternal pulse rate was identical to that recorded through the fetal scalp electrode. Emergency cesarean section at this time might have proved especially dangerous to the mother, since she was profoundly hypovolemic despite the absence of tachycardia and she had developed severe hypofibrinogenemia. Moreover, because of a potentially dangerous antibody in her blood, compatible blood was not immediately available.

If the fetus is alive but cesarean delivery is not carried out promptly, the fetus must be monitored closely for evidence of distress and be delivered immediately whenever distress is detected. Therefore, appropriate facilities and staff for cesarean section must be continuously available whenever placental abruption is suspected.

VAGINAL DELIVERY

If the separation is so severe that there is no evidence of fetal life, vaginal delivery is preferred unless hemorrhage is so brisk that it cannot be successfully managed even by vigorous blood replacement or there are other obstetrical complications that prevent vaginal delivery.

Why vaginal delivery? The presence of serious coagulation defects is likely to prove especially troublesome when delivery is accomplished transabdominally for reasons that do not apply to vaginal delivery. Vessels incised in the abdominal wall and the uterine incision are prone to bleed excessively when coagulation is seriously impaired. Avoidance of these incisions by vaginal delivery obviates this problem. Hemostasis at the placental implantation site depends primarily upon myometrial contraction and retraction to obstruct the many vessels that transport blood within the myometrium to and from the placental implantation site. Therefore, with vaginal delivery, stimulation of the myometrium pharmacologically and by uterine massage will cause these vessels to be constricted sufficiently that serious hemorrhage can be avoided even though defects in the coagulation mechanism persist. Moreover, bleeding that does occur is shed through the vagina, whereas with the incisions imposed by cesarean delivery, the blood is likely to accumulate as troublesome large hematomas. An example of an indication for abdominal delivery despite a documented fetal demise is illustrated by the following case:

> Since the rupture of a prior cesarean section incision could not be reliably excluded, a 26-week stillborn fetus was delivered by repeat cesarean section (Fig. 36–10). Serious bleeding was encountered from all surgical incisions, undoubtedly the results of consumptive coagulopathy caused by the total abruption. Hysterectomy followed by hypogastric artery ligation was performed to achieve hemostasis. Ringer's lactate solution was given along with 17 U of blood, 8 U of plasma, and 10 platelet packs to maintain perfusion and treat the coagulopathy, which finally resolved intraoperatively.

Amniotomy

Rupture of the membranes as early as possible has long been championed in the management of placental abruption. The rationale for amniotomy is that the escape of amnionic fluid might both decrease bleeding from the implantation site and reduce the entry into the maternal circulation of thromboplastin and perhaps activated coagulation factors from the retroplacen-

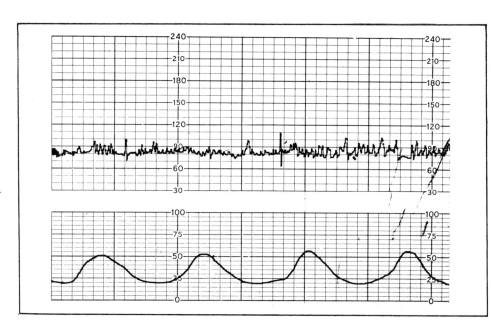

Figure 36–9. A recording of uterine pressures and presumed fetal heart rate in a case of placental abruption so severe as to have killed the fetus. The scalp electrode conducted the maternal ECG signal. Note the increased uterine basal tone. Commonly, in cases of severe placental abruption both the basal tone and the maximum uterine pressure are greater than illustrated here.

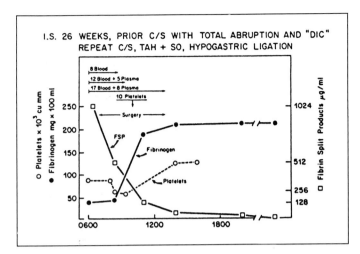

Figure 36–10. Total placental abruption with severe consumptive coagulopathy at 26 weeks. (C/S = cesarean section; TAH + SO = total abdominal hysterectomy, salpingo-oophorectomy; FSP = fibrin split products.)

tal clot. There is no evidence, however, that either is accomplished by amniotomy. If the fetus is reasonably mature, rupture of the membranes may hasten delivery. If the fetus is immature, the intact sac may be more efficient in promoting cervical dilatation than will a small fetal part poorly applied to the cervix.

LABOR

With slight degrees of placental separation, uterine contractions usually are of normal frequency, duration, and intensity, and uterine tone between contractions is low. With extensive placental abruption, the uterus is likely to be persistently hypertonic. The baseline intra-amnionic pressure may be 25 to 50 mm Hg or higher, with rhythmic increases up to 75 to 100 mm Hg. Because of persistent hypertonus, it is difficult at times to determine by palpation if the uterus is contracting and relaxing to any degree, although periodic complaints by the woman of increased pain often signal cyclic increases in uterine activity.

Sher (1977, 1978) has emphasized that in his experience hypotonic uterine dysfunction refractory to the usual therapy develops in about one of five cases of placental abruption complicated by severe consumptive coagulopathy. He claimed that in this circumstance the administration of Trasylol resulted in rapid recovery of uterine activity. Trasylol is an inhibitor of proteases, such as plasmin, and also possesses antithromboplastin and antikallikrein effects. In our extensive experiences with severe placental abruption, as well as those of many others, **hypertonicity** has characterized myometrial function in women with placental abruption complicated by gross disruption of the coagulation mechanism. Therefore, the need for Trasylol (which is not available for clinical use in the United States) is questioned. In fact, we and others have been looking for an agent that will safely decrease myometrial activity somewhat in these circumstances.

If severe placental abruption develops before cervical effacement and dilatation, the subsequent pattern of change in the cervix typically is one of progressive effacement with little dilatation until effacement is complete. Dilatation is then usu-

ally rapid. Therefore, failure of the cervix to dilate while obviously effacing should not be considered lack of progress.

Oxytocin

Uterine stimulation with oxytocin to effect vaginal delivery appears to provide benefits that override the risks. Care must be exercised not to provoke the uterus into self-destruction, especially in women of high parity or with fetopelvic disproportion. The use of oxytocin has been challenged on the basis that it might enhance the escape of thromboplastin into the maternal circulation and thereby initiate or enhance consumptive coagulopathy. There is no evidence to support this fear (Pritchard and Brekken, 1967).

TIMING OF DELIVERY AFTER SEVERE PLACENTAL ABRUPTION

In some of the earlier editions of this book, delivery within 6 hours was advocated. This recommendation arose from the general clinical impression that maternal morbidity and mortality were less when delivery was thus accomplished. Experiences at both the University of Virginia and Parkland Hospitals indicate that the outcome depends upon the diligence with which adequate fluid replacement therapy, especially blood, is pursued, rather than upon the time to delivery (Brame and associates, 1968; Pritchard and Brekken, 1967). At the University of Virginia Hospital, women with severe placental abruption, who were transfused for 18 hours or more before delivery, experienced complications that were neither more numerous nor greater in severity than did the group in which delivery was accomplished sooner. Serial observations at Parkland Hospital on one of the most severe cases in terms of the prolonged interval between the onset of symptoms and delivery and the necessity of transfusing a large volume of blood are summarized in Figure 36–11. She recovered rapidly after spontaneous delivery!

HEMORRHAGE AND HYPOVOLEMIA

To combat hypovolemia successfully, blood must be available in large quantities, as demonstrated in Figure 36–11. More than 10 L of blood were administered to another woman with severe placental abruption who recovered at Parkland Hospital.

The basic rule for treating obstetrical hemorrhage is applied. Blood and balanced salt solution (lactated Ringer's solution) are infused in such proportions that the hematocrit is maintained at 30 percent or slightly higher and urine flow precisely measured is at least 30 mL per hour, and preferably 60 mL per hour. For the oliguric patient, the dangers from furosemide outweigh any advantages, actual or theoretical, that might result from its use. If *vigorous* fluid therapy does not relieve oliguria, the central venous pressure should be monitored as more fluids are administered. Since central venous pressure measurement might not detect early pulmonary congestion, the woman must simultaneously be observed for other signs, especially dyspnea, cough, and rales. If pulmonary congestion were to develop, furosemide then would be beneficial!

COAGULATION DEFECTS

Much concern has been expressed over the rate of development of coagulation defects, as well as their intensity. The extensive experiences at Parkland Hospital have been that coagulation defects most often develop within the first few hours, and perhaps even minutes, after the onset of pain or bleeding and

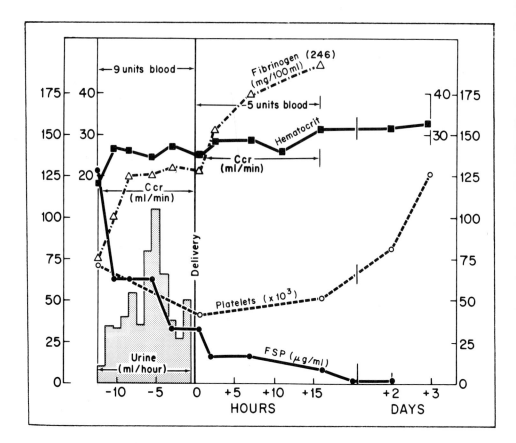

Figure 36–11. Serial data from a case of placental abruption so extensive as to kill the fetus and induce serious consumptive coagulopathy, as well as severe anemia. Symptoms of abruption began 2 hours before hospitalization and 14 hours before delivery. Ccr = creatinine clearance; FSP = fibrin degradation products. Note the normal creatinine clearances. The patient left the hospital on the third postpartum day.

usually do not worsen subsequently, except for dilutional effects from vigorous transfusion with stored whole blood and lactated Ringer's solution. We have observed a fibrinogen level of only 40 mg per dL less than 3 hours after the onset of intermittent pain thought to be labor and less than 2 hours after the onset of constant pain. Moreover, sufficient placenta remained attached that the infant survived immediate delivery by cesarean section performed to try to save the distressed fetus (Table 36–5).

If the clot observation test yields a small or absent clot, the usual coagulation studies will be grossly abnormal and will provide very little immediately useful information, with the possible exception of a platelet count. Even though *platelet counts* have been recommended to identify disseminated intravascular coagulation, low *fibrinogen* levels may develop with placental abruption, yet the platelet count simultaneously may be above 100,000 per μL, as occurred in the case shown in Table 36–5. With extensive placental abruption, elevated *fibrin degradation products* are so

TABLE 36–5. PARTIAL ABRUPTIO PLACENTAE WITH RAPID SEVERE DEFIBRINATION YET DELIVERY OF AN INFANT WHO SURVIVED

Time	Hematocrit	Fibrinogen (mg/dL)	Fibrin Split Products (μg/mL)	Platelets (μL)	Plasma Creatinine (mg/dL)
10/9					
0530		Onset of labor			
0630		Constant pain			
0805	34	43	1,024	151,000	1.1
		Cesarean delivery at 0808			
0930	30	(Units 1 and 2 of whole blood started)			
1150	29	91	512		
		(Units 3 and 4 of whole blood infused)			
1425	32	166	128	87,000	1.6
1700	32	178	64	85,000	
10/10					
0500	26	263	8	95,000	2.2
10/11	25	—	—	124,000	2.1
10/12	24	—	—	198,000	1.8
10/16	24	—	—	638,000	1.1

common as to be anticipated; therefore, their measurement provides little immediate help in clinical management. Erythrocyte distortion or fragmentation characteristic of *fragmentation* or *microangiopathic hemolysis* is very uncommon unless renal failure supervenes.

Fibrinogen and Cryoprecipitate

Lyophilized fibrinogen was used in cases of placental abruption with severe hypofibrinogenemia for years. Then, concern, mostly theoretical in origin, was expressed that the use of fibrinogen simply added fuel to the fire of disseminated intravascular coagulation, with the dire consequences of fibrin deposition and obstruction of the microcirculation in vital organs, especially the kidneys, adrenals, pituitary, and brain. There is no good evidence, however, that effective doses of 4 to 8 g of fibrinogen did so. For example, after 4 g of fibrinogen administered intravenously in less than 10 minutes to a woman with severe hypofibrinogenemia very soon before cesarean section, we observed no changes in central venous pressure, arterial blood pressure, pulse rate, or respiratory rate. Moreover, apprehension, a common occurrence with embolization to the lungs, did not develop. Typically, 4 g of fibrinogen proved to be an effective dose, raising the fibrinogen concentration in plasma by about 100 mg per dL.

Cryoprecipitate has replaced lyophilized fibrinogen. The risk of fatal hepatitis from the latter was significant, since each lot was prepared from plasma pooled from thousands of donors. Conversely, each unit or bag of cryoprecipitate carries a one-donor risk of hepatitis or other bloodborne infections. To supply 4 g of fibrinogen, 15 to 20 bags or units must be given. Ness and Perkins (1979) reported an average fibrinogen content of 270 mg per bag of cryoprecipitate; however, the range was from 60 to 420 mg.

For many years at Parkland Hospital, fibrinogen and cryoprecipitate have been used very infrequently. To avoid their use, trauma to the genital tract has been kept to a minimum through simple vaginal delivery, most often spontaneous. No episiotomy was made if the fetus was small or the perineum was relaxed; otherwise, a midline episiotomy was made and carefully repaired. The emptied and intact uterus was immediately stimulated with oxytocin, 100 to 200 mU per minute intravenously at the outset, and the uterine fundus was continuously monitored and massaged when not firmly contracted.

Uterine Massage

Effective uterine massage necessitates that the fundus of the uterus be clearly identified. If abnormally enlarged, the uterus is compressed to evacuate blood clots. Next a hand is placed over the anterior surface of the uterus with the fingers extending over the top of the fundus, and the uterus is now firmly rubbed to induce and maintain a contracted myometrium. An effective analgesic, such as meperidine, improves the mother's tolerance to this procedure.

Blood loss immediately postpartum may have been somewhat greater with this approach than if fibrinogen or cryoprecipitate had been given, but the overall risks and costs very likely were reduced.

Even with cesarean delivery, fibrinogen or cryoprecipitate has been given only if there was gross evidence of disruption of the coagulation mechanism, including uncontrolled bleeding from all sites of trauma. With lesser amounts of bleeding, ligation of all bleeding points with, at times, drainage of the abdominal incision subfascially with Penrose drains has proved satisfactory. Most often, however, delivery of the woman with severe placental abruption and a dead fetus has been accomplished vaginally.

Other Coagulation Factors

As indicated earlier, massive transfusions using stored whole blood may occasionally result in lack of hemostasis from factor V and VIII deficiency. More often, thrombocytopenia is the likely cause and, if the platelet count is less than 50,000 per μL, there may be troublesome oozing from surgical incisions. In these cases, 10 platelet packs are transfused rapidly in order to raise the platelet count well above 50,000 per μL.

Following delivery, the coagulation defects repair spontaneously within 24 hours or so, except for platelets that, if very low, take 2 to 4 days to reach normal range (Fig. 36–11, Table 36–5).

Fibronectin

This opsonic protein normally present in plasma influences clearance of bloodborne particulate material that arises from intravascular coagulation. Fibronectin stimulates clearance of such debris from the blood by macrophages. Transfusion with blood should help replenish fibronectin, whose actions probably protect from ischemia vital organs of women suffering from intravascular coagulation. Cryoprecipitate is enriched with fibronectin.

Heparin

The infusion of heparin to try to block disseminated intravascular coagulation associated with placental abruption is mentioned only to condemn its use. Heparin should not be used for the following reasons. (1) No one has reported more than a few anecdotal experiences in which heparin did not appear to make hemorrhage worse. (2) The stimulus to active intravascular coagulation ceases after delivery. In fact, the intense phase of intravascular coagulation occurs most often during and very soon after the placental separation. (3) Heparin is a potent anticoagulant that can be predicted to aggravate hemorrhage when there has been gross disruption of the vasculature. (4) Excellent results have been achieved with the plan of management described above. For example, more than 400 cases so severe as to kill the fetus have been managed without permanent renal impairment.

ε-Aminocaproic Acid

This agent has been administered apparently to try to control fibrinolysis by inhibiting the conversion of plasminogen to plasmin and the proteolytic action of plasmin on fibrinogen, fibrin monomer, and fibrin polymer (clot). Failure to clear fibrin polymer from the microcirculation especially could result in organ ischemia and infarction, for example, renal cortical necrosis. Its use is *not* recommended.

Hysterectomy

In the presence of coagulation defects, the more extensive the surgery, the more likely the hemorrhage is to intensify (Fig. 36–10). Therefore, hysterectomy to attempt prophylactically to minimize blood loss is unwise. At times, fortunately uncommon, the procedure must be performed because the uterus has been severely lacerated or simply will not contract to effect hemostasis at the implantation site. Supracervical hysterectomy, if the cervix is intact, will result in less blood loss than will total hysterectomy. For reasons already considered, the bruised Couvelaire uterus is of itself not an indication for hysterectomy.

Consumptive Coagulopathy in the Infant
Although we have never observed the phenomenon, changes in the coagulation mechanism of the newborn infant characteristic of those of intravascular coagulation have been described as accompanying placental abruption (Edson and colleagues, 1968; Nielsen, 1970). However, a variety of conditions predispose to the development of disseminated intravascular coagulation in the newborn in the absence of placental abruption. These include trauma, prematurity, hypoxia, and sepsis.

PLACENTA PREVIA

DEFINITION

In placenta previa, the placenta, instead of being implanted in the body of the uterus well away from the cervical internal os, is located over or very near the internal os. Four degrees of the abnormality have been recognized:

1. Total placenta previa. The cervical internal os is covered completely by placenta (Fig. 36–12).
2. Partial placenta previa. The internal os is partially covered by placenta (Figs. 36–3 and 36–13).
3. Marginal placenta previa. The edge of the placenta is at the margin of the internal os.
4. Low-lying placenta. The placenta is implanted in the lower uterine segment such that the placental edge does not actually reach the internal os but is in close proximity to it.

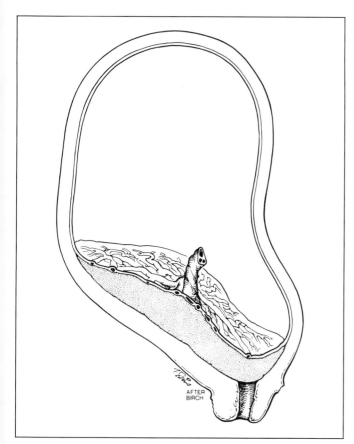

Figure 36–12. Total placental previa. Even with the modest cervical dilatation illustrated, copious hemorrhage would be anticipated.

The degree of placenta previa will depend in large measure on the cervical dilatation at the time of examination. For example, a low-lying placenta at 2 cm dilatation may become a partial placenta previa at 8 cm dilatation because the dilating cervix has uncovered placenta. Conversely, a placenta previa that appears to be total before cervical dilatation may become partial at 4 cm dilatation because the cervix dilates beyond the edge of the placenta (Figs. 36–13A and B). **It is emphasized that digital palpation to try to ascertain these changing relations between the edge of the placenta and the internal os as the cervix dilates can incite severe hemorrhage!**

In both the total and partial varieties, a certain degree of spontaneous separation of the placenta is an inevitable consequence of the formation of the lower uterine segment and the dilatation of the cervix. Such separation is associated with hemorrhage from blood vessels so disrupted.

Frequency
The zygote that implants very low in the uterine cavity is likely to form a placenta that at the outset lies in very close proximity to the internal os of the cervix. The placenta so located may then be aborted, it may (and frequently does) migrate toward the fundus, or it may remain in situ, giving rise to placenta previa. Ultrasonic investigations of early pregnancies that subsequently aborted have disclosed an unexpectedly large number of low-lying embryos. Not all that do not abort eventuate in placenta previa, however. As the placenta and uterus both grow, the placental site is likely to be pulled further up into the uterus, and the placenta eventually becomes located some distance from the cervix.

Placenta previa that becomes apparent clinically is a serious but uncommon complication. In the Dallas community, in recent years, placenta previa was diagnosed once in every 260 deliveries, or 0.4 percent. Brenner and co-workers (1978) identified during the latter half of pregnancy an incidence of placenta previa of 0.6 percent, or 1 per 167 pregnancies; 20 percent were of the complete, or total, variety. Contradictory statistics on the incidence of the various degrees of placenta previa reflect mostly the lack of precision in definition and identification for the reasons discussed above. A question difficult to answer is "Should painless bleeding from focal separation of a placenta implanted in the lower uterine segment but away from a partially dilated cervical os be classified as placenta previa or placental abruption?" Obviously it is both.

ETIOLOGY

Multiparity, advancing age, and previous cesarean delivery increase the risk of placenta previa. Singh and associates (1981), for example, identified placenta previa in 3.9 percent of women who had undergone cesarean delivery, compared to 1.9 percent for the whole obstetrical population. One factor in the develop-

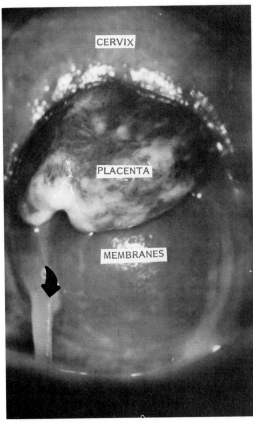

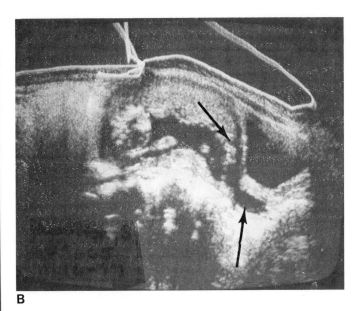

Figure 36–13. A. Partial placenta previa seen through a cervix 3 to 4 cm dilated at 22 weeks gestation. The arrow points to mucus dropping from the cervix. Uterine cramping was evident, but earlier intermittent bleeding had stopped 1 month before. The fetus weighed 410 g when delivered vaginally the next day. Blood loss was not massive. **B.** Gray scale longitudinal midline sonogram obtained the day after the photograph in Figure 36–13A. The upper arrow points to a partial placenta previa from an anteriorly implanted placenta. The lower arrow points to the amnionic sac bulging through the cervix. (*Courtesy of Dr. R. Santos.*)

ment of placenta previa is said to be defective vascularization of the decidua, the possible result of inflammatory or atrophic changes. Another is a large placenta, which spreads over a large area of the uterus, as seen with fetal erythrobastosis and with multiple fetuses. In such spreading, the lower portion of the placenta occasionally approaches the region of the internal os, completely or partially overlapping it.

Uncommonly, placenta previa is associated with *placenta accreta* or one of its more advanced forms, *placenta increta* or *percreta* (Chap. 24, p. 419). Such abnormally firm attachment of the placenta might be anticipated because of poorly developed decidua in the lower uterine segment.

CLINICAL FINDINGS

SIGNS AND SYMPTOMS

The most characteristic event in placenta previa is painless hemorrhage, which usually does not appear until near the end of the second trimester or after. Many abortions, however, probably result from such an abnormal location of the developing placenta.

Character of the Hemorrhage

Frequently, the hemorrhage from placenta previa occurs without warning in a pregnant woman who appeared previously in perfect health. Occasionally, it makes its first appearance while she is asleep, and on awakening, she is surprised to find herself in a pool of blood. Fortunately, the initial bleeding is rarely so profuse as to prove fatal. It usually, but certainly not always, ceases spontaneously, only to recur when least expected. In some cases, particularly with placentas implanted near but not over the cervical os, bleeding does not appear until the onset of labor, when it may vary from slight to profuse hemorrhage.

The cause of the hemorrhage is reemphasized. When the placenta is located over the internal os, the formation of the lower uterine segment and the dilatation of the internal os result inevitably in tearing of placental attachments, followed by hemorrhage from the uterine vessels. The bleeding is augmented by the inability of the myometrial fibers of the lower uterine segment to contract and retract and thereby compress the torn vessels, as occurs normally when the placenta separates from the otherwise empty uterus during the third stage of labor.

As the result of abnormal adherence, such as is seen with placenta accreta, or an excessively large area of attachment, the process of placental separation is sometimes impeded, and then excessive hemorrhage is likely after the birth of the infant. Hemorrhage from the placental implantation site in the lower uterine segment may continue after delivery of the placenta, since the lower uterine segment is more prone to contract poorly than is the body of the uterus, and as a consequence, there is less compression of the maternal vessels that traverse the lower segment. Bleeding may also result from lacerations in the friable cervix and lower uterine segment, especially with attempts at manual removal of a somewhat adherent placenta.

Coagulation Defects

Whereas coagulation defects characteristic of consumptive co-agulopathy are rather common with placental abruption, they are rare with placenta previa even when extensive separation of the placenta from the implantation site has occurred. Presumably the incitors of intravascular coagulation that commonly characterize extensive abruptio placentae escape readily through the cervical canal rather than being forced into the maternal circulation. Of course, when very large volumes of stored donor blood have been transfused, thrombocytopenia and, less commonly, clinically significant deficiencies of factors V and VIII can be anticipated, since donor blood is variably deficient in these components (see p. 699).

DIAGNOSIS

In women with uterine bleeding during the latter half of pregnancy, placenta previa or abruptio placentae should always be suspected. The possibility of placenta previa should not be dismissed until appropriate evaluation, including sonography, has clearly proved its absence, in which case the diagnosis of placental abruption must be considered. The diagnosis of placenta previa seldom can be firmly established by clinical examination unless a finger is passed through the cervix and the placenta is palpated. **Such examination of the cervix is never permissible unless the woman is in an operating room with all the preparations for immediate cesarean section, since even the gentlest examination of this sort can cause torrential hemorrhage.** Furthermore, such an examination should not be made unless delivery is planned, for the trauma may cause bleeding of such a degree that immediate delivery becomes necessary even though the fetus is immature.

After the fetus has reached a gestational age of 37 weeks, the neonatal mortality rate is not greatly improved by further intrauterine development. In such cases, the cause of vaginal bleeding may be ascertained by pelvic examination but only under those conditions emphasized above. If placenta previa is identified, delivery should be accomplished forthwith.

Direct examination is withheld in women with preterm fetuses for whom delay of delivery is advisable. In such instances, location of the placenta may be useful information, and it often can be obtained by careful sonography (Table 36–6). Such information does not alter management remarkably, since those women who have bled must be carefully watched in any event. With proof that the placenta is normally located, the obstetrician may be more willing to discharge the mother. Whether at home or hospitalized, all women who have bled from the uterus are to be followed closely until delivery.

Localization by Sonography

The simplest, most precise, and safest method of placental localization is provided by sonography, which can locate the placenta with considerable accuracy (Figs. 36–13B, 36–14, 36–15, and 36–16). Accuracies of as high as 98 percent have been obtained (Table 36–6). **The false positive results very likely were contributed to by bladder distention. Therefore, the ultrasonic scans in apparently positive cases should be repeated after nearly emptying the bladder.** An uncommon source of error has been identification of abundant placenta implanted in the uterine fundus but failure to appreciate that the placenta was large and extended downward all the way to the internal os of the cervix. Farine and associates (1988) reported that transvaginal ultrasonic examination substantively improved diagnostic accuracy.

TABLE 36–6. ACCURACY OF PLACENTAL LOCALIZATION BY ULTRASOUND

Authors	Year	Results
Gottesfeld et al. (Denver)	1966	112 cases: accuracy rate 97% 18 cesarean sections, 2 wrong predictions
Donald and Abdulla (Glasgow)	1968	613 cases: accuracy rate 94% 107 cesarean sections
Campbell and Kohorn (London)	1968	72 cases: accuracy rate 94% 9 cesarean sections 38 patients, no confirmation obtained 29 exploration of the uterus
Kobayashi et al. (Brooklyn)	1970	100 cases: accuracy rate 95% 92 cesarean sections, 4 errors 8 hysterotomies, 1 error
Sunden (Sweden)	1970	107 cases: accuracy rate 95% 45 cesarean sections, 2 wrong predictions
Santos et al. (Dallas)	1978	100 cases: accuracy rate 98% at cesarean section
Bowie et al. (Chicago)	1978	164 cases: accuracy rate 93% Missed 1 of 13 proven placenta previas

Placental Migration

Since the report of King (1973), the peripatetic nature of the placenta has come to be generally appreciated. Wexler and Gottesfeld (1977), for example, demonstrated sonographically that before the third trimester, up to one half of pregnancies were characterized by low-lying placenta. Young (1978) reached a similar conclusion upon localizing the placenta by means of arteriography. Therefore, placentas that lie close to the internal cervical os during the second trimester or even early in the third trimester are very likely to migrate subsequently toward the fundus, with avoidance of the morbidity and mortality imposed by placenta previa. The low frequency with which placenta previa persists when it has been identified sonographically be-

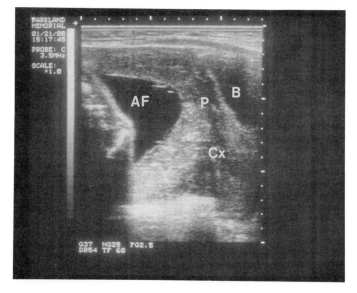

Figure 36–14. Total placenta previa at 34 weeks gestation. Placenta (P) completely overlies cervix (Cx). Bladder (B) and amnionic fluid (AF) are also visualized clearly.

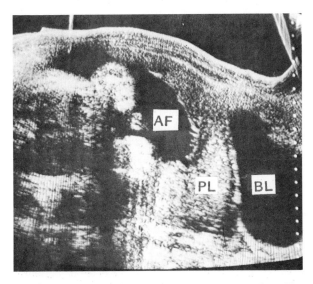

Figure 36–15. Gray scale sonogram of total placenta previa at 33 weeks gestation. (BL = maternal bladder; PL = total placenta previa; AF = amnionic fluid.) (*Courtesy of Dr. R. Santos.*)

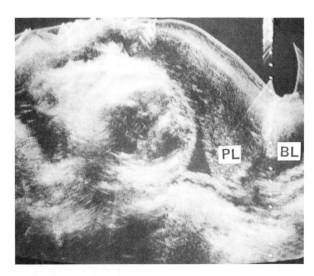

Figure 36–16. Gray scale sonogram of partial placenta previa at 37 weeks gestation. (BL = partly filled maternal bladder; PL = partial placenta previa.) (*Courtesy of Dr. R. Santos.*)

fore the 30th week of gestation is shown in Table 36–7. It is apparent from these data, collected by Comeau and associates (1983), that in the absence of any other abnormality, sonography need not be repeated frequently simply to follow the migration of the placenta away from the cervix. Since the great majority of cases of asymptomatic placenta previa found early are cured by placental migration, restriction of activity need not be practiced unless the placenta previa persists beyond 30 weeks or becomes clinically apparent before that time.

MANAGEMENT

Women with placenta previa may be assigned to the following groups: (1) those in whom the fetus is preterm but there is no pressing need for delivery, (2) those in whom the fetus is within 3 weeks of term, (3) those in whom labor is in progress, and (4) those in whom hemorrhage is so severe as to necessitate evacuation of the uterus despite the immaturity of the fetus.

Management of the pregnancy known to be complicated by placenta previa and a preterm fetus, but with no active bleeding, consists of procrastination in an environment that provides the greatest safety for both mother and fetus. Hospitalization, which provides close observation, a very sedentary life-style, avoidance of any intravaginal manipulation, and immediate availability of appropriate therapy, is ideal. Such therapy includes intravenous electrolyte solution, blood, cesarean delivery, and expert neonatal care from the time of delivery. However, in this practical world, compromises in care must be made at times and the mother and fetus not hospitalized. In this instance, the mother and her family must fully appreciate the problems of placenta previa and be prepared to transport her to the hospital immediately, where, in turn, her problem will be recognized immediately by hospital staff.

With delay of delivery, one of the benefits that may occur sometimes even relatively late in pregnancy is sufficient migration of the placenta away from the cervix so that placenta previa is no longer a major problem. Arias (1988) described outstanding results from cervical cerclage done between 24 and 30 weeks in women with bleeding caused by placenta previa.

Procedures available for delivery fall into two categories of cesarean or vaginal delivery. The rationale for cesarean delivery is twofold: first, immediate delivery of the fetus and placenta allows the uterus to contract and to stop the bleeding, and second, cesarean delivery forestalls the possibility of cervical lacerations, a serious potential complication of vaginal delivery in total and partial placenta previa. The rationale for vaginal delivery is, hopefully, to be able to press the detached placenta against the bleeding implantation site during labor and thereby tamponade the bleeding vessels sufficiently to prevent severe hemorrhage.

DELIVERY

Cesarean Section
This is the accepted method of delivery in practically all cases of placenta previa. In justifying cesarean section in the presence of a dead fetus, it is again necessary to understand that abdominal delivery is done for the welfare of the mother.

When the placenta lies far enough posteriorly that the lower uterine segment can be incised transversely without encountering placenta, and when the fetus is cephalic, the transverse incision is preferred. If, however, such an incision were to be made through the placenta, bleeding, both maternal and fetal, could be severe, and extension of the incision to involve one or

TABLE 36–7. SONOGRAPHIC IDENTIFICATION OF PLACENTA PREVIA AND SUBSEQUENT CLINICAL DISEASE

Gestational Age at Time of Sonography (wk)	Placenta Previa or Hemorrhage at Delivery (%)
< 20	2.3
20 to 25	3.2
25 to 30	5.2
30 to 35	23.9

Adapted from Comeau and associates: Obstet Gynecol 61:577, 1983.

both uterine arteries could occur with surprising ease. Therefore, with anterior placenta previa, a vertical uterine incision may be safer. When placenta previa is complicated by degrees of placenta accreta that render control of bleeding from the placental bed difficult by conservative means, total hysterectomy may be the procedure of necessity (Chap. 24, p. 419). For women whose placenta is implanted anteriorly in the site of a prior cesarean section incision, the likelihood is increased for an associated placenta accreta and need for hysterectomy to control hemorrhage (Read and colleagues, 1980).

Vaginal Methods

There are four compression, or tamponade, methods for vaginal delivery, although only simple rupture of the membranes in cases of partial or marginal placenta previa is now in general use. Willett forceps, insertion of a Voorhees bag, and Braxton Hicks version have all but disappeared from modern practice for a variety of good reasons that have been described in previous editions of this book.

PROGNOSIS

A marked reduction in maternal mortality has been achieved, a trend that began in 1927 when Arthur Bill advocated adequate transfusion and cesarean section in the treatment of placenta previa. Since 1945, when Macafee and Johnson independently suggested expectant therapy for patients remote from term, a similar trend has been evident in perinatal loss. Half the patients are already near term when bleeding occurs, but preterm delivery still poses a formidable problem for the remainder, since not all women with placenta previa and a preterm fetus can be treated expectantly. Delivery is forced by profuse hemorrhage in many instances and by labor in some.

Prematurity is a major cause of perinatal death even though expectant management of placenta previa is practiced. Moreover, for any fetal weight, perinatal mortality is likely to be somewhat greater with placenta previa than in the general population. Brar and colleagues (1988) reported that the incidence of retarded fetal growth was nearly 20 percent. Serious fetal malformations are also somewhat more common.

FETAL DEATH AND DELAYED DELIVERY

In general, during the past two decades, the management for the woman whose fetus has died and who fails to go into labor spontaneously has changed from watchful waiting to more active intervention. Although most women will eventually go into labor spontaneously, the psychological stress imposed upon the mother carrying a dead fetus, the dangers of blood coagulation defects that may develop, and the advent of more effective methods of induction of labor have increased the desirability of early delivery. With the widespread availability of real-time ultrasound equipment, any doubts about fetal death can be resolved quickly and reliably. Still, since the majority of women enter spontaneous labor within 2 weeks of fetal death (Goldstein and Reid, 1963; Tricomi and Kohl, 1957), and in the absence of other complications, attempts to evacuate the uterus may be delayed for this interval.

COAGULATION CHANGES

Weiner and associates reported in 1950 that some isoimmunized Rh-negative women who carried a dead fetus developed coagulation defects. A prospective study indicated that gross disruption of the maternal coagulation mechanism rarely developed in less than 1 month after fetal death (Pritchard, 1959, 1973). If the fetus was retained for longer periods of time, however, about 25 percent of the women developed significant changes in the coagulation mechanism. Thus the old wives' tale that the dead baby would poison the mother, although scoffed at by physicians for many generations, proved to be true. Maternal isoimmunization with fetomaternal blood incompatibility is not essential to the development of the coagulation changes, as originally thought by Weiner and associates (1950). Extrauterine pregnancy with fetal death and delayed delivery may also be complicated by acquired hypofibrinogenemia (Dehner, 1972).

A few cases have been described with abrupt alterations in the plasma fibrinogen concentration, the values vacillating repeatedly between normal and very low over the course of a few days (Goldstein and Reid, 1963). Our experiences, however, have been that typically the fibrinogen concentration falls from

levels that are normal for pregnancy to levels that are normal for the nonpregnant state, and in some cases the decrease continues to reach potentially dangerous concentrations of 100 mg per dL or less (Pritchard, 1973). The rate of decrease that was commonly found is demonstrated in Figure 36–17. Simultaneously, fibrin degradation products are elevated in serum. The platelet count tends to be reduced in these instances, but in our experience, severe thrombocytopenia does not necessarily develop, even though the fibrinogen level is quite low (Fig. 36–18A). Spontaneous correction of the coagulation defects can eventu-

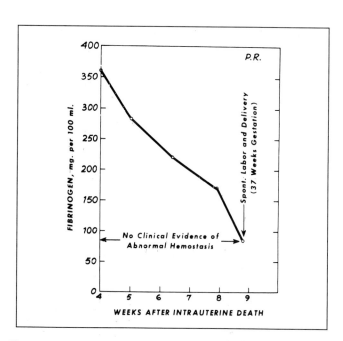

Figure 36–17. Slow development of maternal hypofibrinogenemia following fetal death and delayed delivery. (*From Pritchard: Obstet Gynecol 14:574, 1959.*)

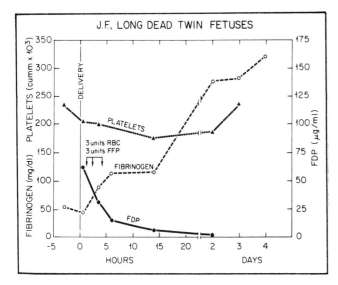

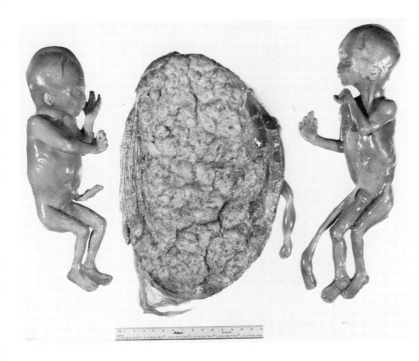

Figure 36–18. A. Data from a case of fetal death and delayed delivery treated on an emergency basis at Parkland Hospital. The twin fetuses had been dead for 8 weeks or more. Spontaneous delivery after spontaneous labor was followed by appreciable bleeding, which was treated with intravenous oxytocin, uterine massage, and blood transfusion. (Blood fractions were used because of nonavailability of type-specific blood.) Initially there was marked hypofibrinogenemia and elevation of fibrin degradation products without thrombocytopenia. Recovery was uneventful; the hematocrit at discharge was 29. In retrospect, hypofibrinogenemia was apparent from the very small clot in blood drawn for serology upon admittance to the hospital. (FDP = fibrin degradation products in maternal serum.)

plantation site is sealed eventually by fibrin deposited in the attached placenta (Figs. 36–18B and 36–20B).

PATHOGENESIS

A series of reports clearly establish that consumptive coagulopathy, presumably mediated by thromboplastin from the dead products of conception, is operational in these cases (Jimenez and Pritchard, 1968; Lerner and associates, 1967; Sherman and Middleton, 1958). As shown in Figure 36–19, heparin infused alone over a few days corrected the coagulation defects, but ε-aminocaproic acid did not. While these observations serve to establish the cause, they do not precisely identify the site where fibrinogen is converted to fibrin. The placenta from such a case commonly contains much insoluble protein (Fig. 36–18B) that can be made soluble by treatment with bovine fibrinolysin (Pritchard, 1973), but most likely, considerably more fibrinogen has been converted to fibrin, presumably intravascularly, than can be recovered from the placenta.

Use of Heparin

Correction of coagulation defects has been accomplished using heparin under carefully controlled conditions *in women with an intact circulation*. Heparin appropriately administered can block further pathological consumption of fibrinogen and other clotting factors and thereby allow the coagulation mechanism to repair spontaneously. Once correction has been accomplished and the heparin infusion is stopped, steps can be taken promptly to evacuate the dead products of conception (Jimenez and Pritchard, 1968). **It is emphasized that for heparin to be used safely to block the consumptive coagulopathy, and thereby allow spontaneous repair of the coagulation mechanism, it is essential that the maternal circulatory system be intact.** Otherwise, heparin most likely will incite or enhance hemorrhage. Importantly, as soon as the dead products of conception have been evacuated, if not before, spontaneous repair

ally occur before evacuation of the dead products of conception, but this happens quite slowly (Jennison and Walker, 1956; Pritchard, 1959). Apparently the access route for thromboplastin from the uterine contents through the vasculature of the im-

Figure 36–18. B. Long-dead twin fetuses from case described in Figure 36–18A. The placenta contains much fibrin.

will follow, so there is no good reason to give heparin at that time.

Fetal Death in Multifetal Pregnancy

As demonstrated in Figure 36–18, twin fetuses with death of both can cause severe hypofibrinogenemia. However, there is a paucity of reports in which an obvious derangement in coagulation has been detected in a mother pregnant with multiple fetuses, some alive and some dead. Potentially dangerous coagulation defects have been described for one mother in the following circumstances: one of three fetuses died remote from term, and later a second fetus succumbed in utero, while a third fetus was born alive (Skelly and co-workers, 1982). In this case, following the first fetal death shortly after midpregnancy, consumptive coagulopathy was identified. Treatment with heparin intravenously reversed the hypofibrinogenemia. Even so, a second fetus died near 35 weeks of gestation. Cesarean section was performed very soon thereafter, and the third fetus survived.

We have observed, following death of one of twin fetuses and delayed delivery, a progressive but transient fall in maternal fibrinogen concentration and rise in fibrin split products. However, in the absence of therapy, these changes ceased spontaneously with normalization of the coagulation mechanism (Fig. 36–20A). The surviving fetus, when delivered near term, was healthy. The placenta of the long-dead fetus was filled with fibrin (Fig. 36–20B).

Romero and colleagues (1984) reported that heparin administration resulted in prompt reversal of consumptive coagulopathy in a woman with one dead twin. Since it is unlikely that heparin will reverse any coagulopathy in the surviving fetus, more data carefully obtained in these circumstances are needed, especially concerning the benefits versus the risks from chronically administered heparin, as well as the optimal time and route of delivery.

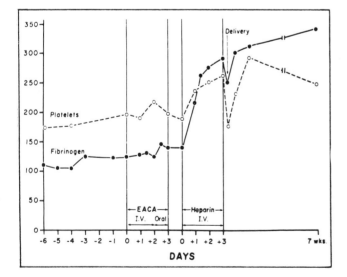

Figure 36–19. Coagulation defects with prolonged retention of a dead fetus. Fibrinogen concentration rose during intravenous infusion of heparin, 1,500 units per hour, but not during administration of ε-aminocaproic acid (EACA). (*From Jimenez and Pritchard: Obstet Gynecol 32:449, 1968.*)

Treatment of Active Hemorrhage

If serious hemorrhage is encountered as the products of conception are being expelled or surgically removed and overt hypofibrinogenemia and associated coagulation defects are identified, treatment with heparin almost certainly will enhance the bleeding. In this circumstance, effective primary treatment is blood and lactated Ringer's solution, according to the guidelines for treatment of hemorrhage described under Fluid Replacement Therapy. The consumptive coagulopathy stops once the products of conception are expelled, and repair soon takes place. If there is excessive bleeding from lacerations or incisions, cryoprecipitate, fresh-frozen plasma, and platelet packs, alone or in combination, coupled with careful ligation of all severed blood vessels, will prove effective in arresting hemorrhage.

To raise the fibrinogen concentration 100 mg per dL usually requires 15 to 20 bags or units of cryoprecipitate. (Such treatment also provides fibronectin, which may provide a beneficial effect by stimulating macrophages to clear fibrin-containing debris from the maternal circulation.) Fresh-frozen plasma provides labile coagulation factors, especially factors V and VIII. If severe thrombocytopenia is documented or suspected, 10 platelet packs should prove to be sufficient for adequate platelet function and effective hemostasis.

Hatch and associates (1985) reported that 5 of 10 women whose fetuses were dead bled from a coagulopathy that developed acutely during (or very soon after) dilatation and evacuation, which had been preceded by intracervical laminaria insertion. Of concern, the plasma fibrinogen levels recorded by them and implicated as the culprits in a genesis of the postevacuation hemorrhage were 155 mg per dL or higher in 4 of the 5 women. It is difficult to ascribe hemorrhage to hypofibrinogenemia with fibrinogen levels of this magnitude.

PREGNANCY TERMINATION WITH DEAD FETUS

Near term, intravenously administered oxytocin usually is effective when given in a dose that stimulates uterine activity, although induction may have to be repeated. Remote from term, however, it is less likely to prove effective unless given in high concentration and on more than one occasion. It is not unusual for the infused oxytocin to initiate some palpable contractions, which then abate even when the amount infused is increased. The oxytocin appears at times to influence the uterus to spontaneously contract subsequently, since during the next 24 hours or so after oxytocin infusion, it is not rare, especially late in pregnancy, for spontaneous evacuation to take place. One or more laminaria tents placed in the cervical canal before the use of oxytocin may enhance expulsion of the dead products. The magnitude of risk of infection from use of laminaria in the presence of dead products of conception has not yet been quantified.

Water intoxication as a consequence of the antidiuretic effect of oxytocin administered with large volumes of aqueous dextrose has been documented repeatedly since first described in these circumstances by Liggins (1962) and Whalley and Pritchard (1963). Administration of small volumes of lactated Ringer's solution, rather than large volumes of aqueous dextrose solution, minimizes this risk.

Prostaglandin E₂ given as a 20-mg suppository to induce labor in pregnancy complicated by fetal death is one option recommended by the American College of Obstetricians and Gynecologists (1986). Since after 28 weeks there is greater likelihood of hyperstimulation, the possibility of uterine rupture

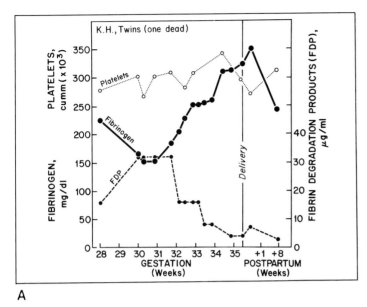

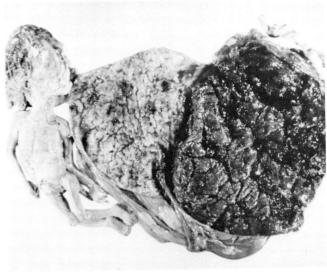

A   B

Figure 36–20. A. Death of one twin was confirmed sonographically at 28 weeks gestation. Coagulation studies initiated then demonstrated a somewhat low plasma fibrinogen concentration and distinctly abnormal amounts of fibrin degradation products (FDP) in maternal serum. The abnormalities in both became more intense 2 weeks later. Then, spontaneously, the fibrinogen concentration rose, and the fibrin degradation products fell in mirror fashion. The liveborn infant was healthy, and coagulation studies on cord plasma and serum were normal. **B.** The fibrin-filled placenta of the long-dead fetus is apparent. Presumably, the fibrin curtailed the escape of thromboplastin from the dead products into the maternal circulation.

increases and special cautions must be used. These are presumed to include careful clinical monitoring of the woman in labor. Almost all women develop nausea, vomiting, and diarrhea after prostaglandin suppositories are inserted intravaginally; fever is also common (Phelan and Cefalo, 1978). Apparently rare complications that have been reported include uterine rupture (Schulman and associates, 1979) and myocardial infarction (Patterson and colleagues, 1979).

Orr and co-workers (1979) have emphasized that failure of prostaglandin E₂ suppositories to expel the dead products of conception must raise the question of extrauterine fetal death, and they cite four such experiences. **Fetal death with delayed delivery should always provide the stimulus for asking the question, "Is the pregnancy extrauterine?"**

The intra-amnionic injection of hypertonic saline is not recommended for evacuation of dead products of conception, since the volume of amnionic fluid is often reduced and the potentially highly toxic salt solution, therefore, is difficult to inject quantitatively into the sac. Coagulation defects may be induced or enhanced by intra-amnionic hypertonic saline. In addition, the risk to the mother of inadvertent intravenous injection of hypertonic saline solution with subsequent death or serious morbidity is increased appreciably in instances of fetal demise.

AMNIONIC FLUID EMBOLISM

PATHOGENESIS

Entry of amnionic fluid into the maternal circulation in some circumstances may prove fatal. Essential to the development of amnionic fluid embolism are (1) a rent through the amnion and chorion, (2) opened uterine or endocervical veins, and (3) a pressure gradient sufficient to force the fluid into the venous circulation. Marginal separation of the placenta or laceration of the uterus or cervix serves to create an opening into the maternal circulation. Vigorous labor, including that induced with overdosage of oxytocin, is more likely to provide the pressure. These events may also distress the fetus, leading to defecation of meconium in utero, thereby markedly potentiating the toxic

nature of amnionic fluid if it should enter the maternal circulation.

In the typical case of amnionic fluid embolism, the woman is laboring vigorously, or has just done so, and is in the process of being delivered when she develops varying degrees of respiratory distress and circulatory collapse. If the woman does not die immediately, serious hemorrhage with severe coagulation defects is soon evident from the genital tract and all other sites of trauma.

TOXICITY OF AMNIONIC FLUID

The lethality of intravenously infused amnionic fluid appears to vary remarkably, depending especially upon the particulate

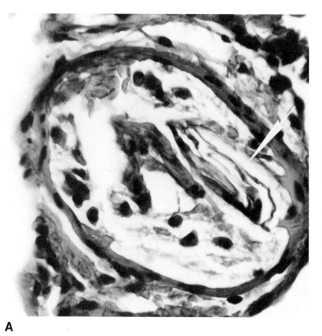

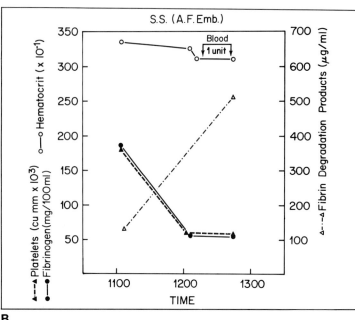

A   **B**

Figure 36–21. A. Fetal squames (arrow) packed into a small pulmonary artery from a fatal case of amnionic fluid embolism. Most of the empty spaces within the vessel were demonstrated by appropriate staining for lipid to have been filled with vernix caseosa. **B.** Levels of fibrinogen, fibrinogen–fibrin degradation products, and platelets during fatal amnionic fluid embolism.

matter it contains. The suddenness and the intensity of cardio-respiratory problems that develop in many cases of amnionic fluid embolism and the histological findings in the pulmonary vessels at autopsy strongly suggest, at least, that the likelihood of infused amnionic fluid proving lethal is greatest when it has been appreciably enriched with particulate debris, especially thick meconium.

Schneider (1955) showed that the lethal nature of human amnionic fluid infused intravenously into dogs was enhanced very greatly by the addition of meconium. Under these circumstances, it is envisioned that the particulate matter shed previously into the amnionic fluid or contained in the meconium, including shed fetal squamous cells (squames) (Fig. 36–21A), fetal hairs (lanugo), vernix caseosa, and mucin, is pumped by a vigorous contraction from the disrupted amnionic sac into a maternal vein that drains the uterus. Severe pulmonary vascular obstruction from the particulate matter and possibly from fibrin formed intravascularly leads to *acute cor pulmonale* (Schneider and Henry, 1968). Abruptly, hypoxia and reduced cardiac output develop, and if they are not immediately fatal, hemorrhage from coagulation defects is soon evident from disrupted blood vessels. Severe thrombocytopenia develops and the blood typically clots poorly when treated with thrombin, or, at most, there is formed a small, mushy clot that soon lyses completely. Plasma from such a patient, mixed with normal plasma and recalcified or with thrombin added to form a clot, has been observed by us to lyse rapidly, whereas the clotted normal plasma alone did not do so for days. Moreover, when fibrinogen was injected into the circulation, the thrombin–clottable protein promptly disappeared. These observations implicate intense fibrinolytic and even fibrinogenolytic activity, in some cases at least, as well as consumptive coagulopathy.

Coagulation Initiated by Amnionic Fluid

The clot-accelerating activity of amnionic fluid is greater at term than early in the third trimester, an observation that led Hastwell (1974) to suggest its measurement as an index of fetal maturity. Even at term, however, the activity normally is not great. The clot accelerator principle appears to behave more like Russell's viper venom than tissue thromboplastin, in that factor VII is not essential for the clot-accelerating action of amnionic fluid (Courtney and Allington, 1972; Phillips and Davidson, 1972). Of significance, amnionic fluid at times contains appreciable amounts of mucus, which, in case of amnionic fluid embolism, might incite or aggravate intravascular coagulation. Extracts of human mucus have been shown in vitro and in vivo to induce coagulation, apparently by activation of factor X (Pineo and co-workers, 1973).

Amnionic fluid contaminated with bacterial products, especially endotoxin, would almost certainly prove toxic if it were to enter the maternal circulation. The same is very likely to be true for amnionic fluid enriched with cytolytic products from a dead fetus.

Experimental Amnionic Fluid Embolism

Studies by Hanzlik and Karsner (1924) indicated that the intravenous injection of finely divided particulate matter, such as suspensions of charcoal particles or India ink, produced not only altered coagulability of the blood but also dramatic systemic phenomena, such as restlessness, tremors, marked dyspnea, convulsions, and often death. In the experiments of Halmagyi and co-workers (1962), after human amnionic fluid was injected into sheep, pulmonary hypertension, arterial hypoxia, and a marked fall in pulmonary compliance were noted. These changes, however, are similar to those found in pulmonary embolism of other causes, and, importantly, they failed to occur when the amnionic fluid was filtered. Moreover, they were not completely prevented by heparin. Adamson and associates (1971) and Stolte and co-workers (1967) could not produce the syndrome in monkeys, nor could Spence and Mason (1974) do so in rabbits. Attwood (1964) caused the death of only 5 of 15 dogs by the intravenous injection of 50 mL of amnionic fluid, and Pritchard and Capps (unpublished observations) noted an even lower mortality rate in dogs when sterile human amnionic fluid obtained at repeat cesarean section at or very near term was used. However, a suspension of human meconium injected into dogs has been shown to be highly lethal (Schneider, 1955).

DIAGNOSIS

Fatal amnionic fluid embolism can be confirmed by the appearance of amnionic fluid debris, especially squames, vernix, mucin, and lanugo, widespread in small pulmonary blood vessels. Fatal amnionic fluid embolism has been encountered rarely at Parkland Hospital. A fairly typical case follows.

S.S., a young primigravida at term, felt no fetal movement for 12 hours before the onset of discomforts of labor. When first evaluated 2 hours later, no fetal heart sounds were heard, but regular uterine contractions without uterine hypertonus or tenderness were identified clinically and electronically. The cervix was 2 cm dilated and 90 percent effaced. Neither amnionic fluid nor blood was visualized coming through the cervical canal until amniotomy, when brown meconium-laden fluid escaped. She was moderately hypertensive and received magnesium sulfate prophylactically. The hematocrit was 34, and a blood clot of appreciable size formed in a thrombin tube. The platelet count, prothrombin time, and partial thromboplastin time were normal. Two hours after admittance, her blood pressure began to fluctuate between 135/105 and 90/60 mm Hg. The hematocrit was now 29. She received 2 U of whole blood for presumed abruptio placentae, although uterine hypertonus and tenderness were lacking, there was no vaginal bleeding, and urine flow the previous hour was 60 mL per hour. She suddenly became very quiet and then unresponsive; her blood pressure was undetectable, and the apical pulse dropped to 60 and then to zero. Endotracheal intubation and cardiopulmonary resuscitation were initiated as a heavily meconium-stained, slightly macerated infant was delivered. The flattened placenta with the maternal surface covered with clot followed promptly.

The uterus contracted poorly and attempts at ventilation were thwarted by lack of pulmonary compliance. Cardiac function was maintained by closed chest compression, and hemorrhage from the flaccid uterus was combatted with blood transfusions. However, oxygenation was inadequate in spite of endotracheal intubation and mechanical ventilation. She was pronounced dead.

Histologically, small blood vessels in the lungs were plugged by debris, including squames, mucin, and vernix caseosa, which accounted for the inability to oxygenate the patient (Fig. 36–21A). Serial values for plasma fibrinogen, serum fibrinogen–fibrin degradation products, and platelets are presented in Figure 36–21B. Abnormalities suggestive of modest consumptive coagulopathy were present when she was hospitalized. These changes had become severe when she demonstrated loss of consciousness, hypotension, and bradycardia, and they persisted until death.

An unusual feature of this case is the presence of much meconium presumably from fetal distress associated with abruptio placentae. In our considerable experience, meconium is rarely found with extensive placental abruption, even when severe enough to kill the fetus.

There almost certainly have been women who survived amnionic fluid embolism, although the diagnosis is always open to question without definite identification of obvious amnionic fluid debris within blood vessels in histological sections of lung or at least in the buffy coat of blood from the right side of the heart (Clark and associates, 1988).

Intriguing but in some ways troublesome observations have been reported in recent years in which the buffy coat of blood drawn from the right side of the maternal heart or pulmonary artery has been identified morphologically to contain amnionic fluid debris—typically squames or vernix caseosa— many hours to even days after suspected amnionic fluid embolism. Studies are needed to evaluate blood so collected and processed in the absence of suspicion of embolization. Tuck (1972) has described the identification of squames presumed to be from amnionic fluid in sputum stained with Nile blue sulfate. Confirmatory experiences with this technique are needed.

TREATMENT

Successful treatment for amnionic fluid embolism probably relates to its severity. From the observations reported above, it is reasonable to conclude that the clinical spectrum is varied and the incidence of amnionic fluid embolism is probably underestimated. If complicated by thick meconium, embolism seems to cause acute hypoxia, diminished pulmonary compliance, and rapid death. Vigorous and prompt treatment is mandatory and usually necessitates mechanical ventilation and blood replacement (Price and associates, 1985; Resnik and co-workers, 1976). The patient with cor pulmonale, however, tolerates any deficit or excess in blood volume very poorly.

With lesser degrees of meconium contamination, and probably to some extent with large amounts of mucus-containing but clear amnionic fluid, the pulmonary insult is subacute, resulting in oxygen desaturation, which is amenable to treatment. Simultaneously, intravascular coagulation is incited and may cause death from hemorrhage, but survival usually will follow if bleeding is arrested and subsequent infection promptly treated.

When amnionic fluid embolism is strongly suspected, use of a flow-directed pulmonary artery catheter, an arterial line to facilitate measurement of blood pressure and obtain blood samples, and instrumentation to record systemic, pulmonary artery and wedge pressures, cardiac output, and blood oxygenation are likely to prove beneficial. Invasion of large vessels in the presence of grossly defective hemostasis may in itself lead to dangerous hemorrhage. Clark and associates (1985, 1988) reported the use of such instrumentation in women with amnionic-fluid embolism and concluded that there was little evidence for pulmonary circulatory obstruction. It is possible that their findings of isolated left-ventricular failure resulted from end-stage hypoxia, since these studies were performed after the acute events. Quance (1988) described a fatal case in a woman whose first finding was intraoperative oxygen desaturation detected by routine oximetry. Silent pulmonary edema soon followed, and 3 hours after delivery cardiac arrest ensued.

Use of fibrinogen or cryoprecipitate and other blood-component therapy, heparin, fibrinolytic agents, and antifibrinolytic agents have been described in case reports, but their efficacy is difficult to evaluate (Price and colleagues, 1985).

OTHER CAUSES OF OBSTETRICAL COAGULOPATHIES

The most common causes of serious obstetrical hemorrhage seldom are associated with consumptive coagulopathy. For example, hemorrhage is common from postpartum uterine atony or lacerations with either vaginal or cesarean delivery. In these instances, coagulation is usually intact; however, nonclotting blood intensifies hemorrhage from both of these, and especially from the latter. Placental abruption, as discussed above, is the prototype of consumptive coagulopathy, and at least one third of those severe enough to kill the fetus also cause clinically significant coagulopathy. Considered now are other conditions that may be associated with disseminated intravascular coagulation.

COAGULATION DEFECTS POSSIBLY INDUCED BY HEMORRHAGE

Rarely, severe hemorrhage with overt disruption of the coagulation mechanism may develop in a woman without recognized evidence of any disease known to incite consumptive coagulopathy, for example, in an apparently uncomplicated repeated cesarean section. The experimental observations of Turpini and Stefanini (1959) support the thesis that severe hemorrhage of itself can induce consumptive coagulopathy. Animal studies by some other investigators, however, have not confirmed their observations (Herman and associates, 1972; Karayalcin and colleagues, 1973). In the case of massive fatal hemorrhage from rupture of the uterus considered in Table 36–3, the marked decrease in coagulation factors was primarily the consequence of hemodilution by electrolyte solution rather than of intense intravascular coagulopathy. Prompt treatment with blood and lactated Ringer's solution and, at times, a concentrated source of fibrinogen (cryoprecipitate), fresh frozen plasma, and platelet packs, as described earlier in this chapter for placental abruption, has been effective in cases treated at Parkland Hospital.

SEPTICEMIA

Infections that lead to bacteremia and septic shock in obstetrics are most commonly due to septic abortion, antepartum pyelonephritis, or puerperal sepsis. The last is more commonly seen with infections following cesarean delivery.

PATHOGENESIS

Septic shock is a life-threatening syndrome characterized by hypotension that is associated with pooling of blood in the microcirculation and inadequate tissue perfusion, resulting in hypoxia and metabolic acidosis. The microvascular instability, with extracellular fluid extravasation, endothelial damage, and consumption of procoagulants, results in reduced effective blood volume and cardiac output. These latter factors are discussed in Chapter 27 (p. 472).

COAGULOPATHY

The lethal properties of bacterial toxins, and especially endotoxins, undoubtedly are mediated largely by destruction of vascular endothelium. However, it is unclear whether this is the major mechanism that initiates consumptive coagulopathy. For example, in experimental animals endothelial damage is greatest 24 hours after endotoxin is given, but intravascular coagulation usually occurs during the first few hours. More likely, endotoxin initiates intrinsic clotting through activation of factor XII or extrinsic clotting through release of thromboplastic activity from leucocytes (Lerner and associates, 1968). Whether the pregnant woman is more susceptible to these effects is not clear.

As with any situation in which the blood is rendered incoagulable, surgical procedures become more hazardous. An example follows.

> A 31-year-old primigravida was delivered by cesarean section for fetopelvic disproportion further complicated by chorioamnionitis (Fig. 36–22). Blood loss was massive from uterine atony plus incisional hemorrhages that resulted from severe hypofibrinogenemia, marked elevation of fibrin split products, and some degree of thrombocytopenia engendered by sepsis. During supracervical hysterectomy, blood, fresh-frozen plasma, and cryoprecipitate were given to maintain perfusion and to help correct the deficiencies in the coagulation mechanism. At the completion of the second surgical procedure, generalized bleeding from the various surfaces had abated.

MANAGEMENT

Therapy for women with septicemia from any cause is outlined in Chapter 27 (p. 473). In general, treatment of the inciting cause will be followed by reversal of the coagulopathy. If bleeding is encountered with surgical incisions or lacerations, then whole blood and lactated Ringer's solution are given to maintain blood volume, as previously outlined. In some cases, especially if surgical procedures are performed before sepsis is controlled and the coagulopathy is reversed, treatment with fresh-frozen plasma, cryoprecipitate, and platelet packs usually will arrest such bleeding.

Heparin therapy is dangerous and should not be given. As alluded to above, the genesis of the coagulation abnormalities is extremely complex and difficult to pinpoint in clinical studies. The concept that intravascular coagulation occludes the microcirculation in septic shock, and also consumes coagulation factors and thereby causes hemorrhage, led to the recommendation by some that heparin be used in these circumstances. To date, no adequate clinical trial has been reported identifying benefits from heparin that outweighed the risks of enhanced hemorrhage. Moreover, animal studies of gram-negative sepsis are consistent with the view that inhibition of intravascular coagulation by heparin does not necessarily lower mortality (Corrigan and associates, 1974). **Control of disseminated intravascular coagulation is dependent upon control of the inciting disease, which in this circumstance is sepsis.**

HEMORRHAGE WITH ABORTION

ETIOLOGY OF HEMORRHAGE

Remarkable blood loss, especially acute hemorrhage but sometimes chronic, may occur as the consequence of abortion. Hemorrhage during the first trimester is less likely to be severe unless the abortion was induced and the procedure was trau-

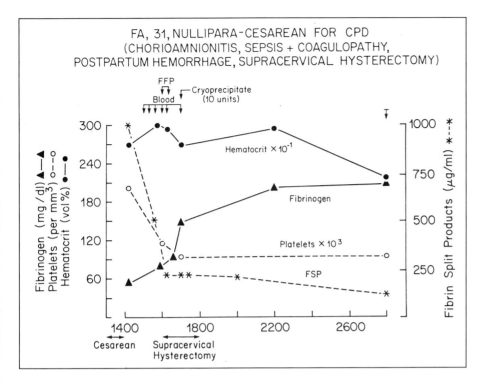

Figure 36–22. Uterine atony with severe hemorrhage complicating cesarean section worsened by consumptive coagulopathy, the consequence of chorioamnionitis and sepsis. (CPD = cephalopelvic disproportion; FFP = fresh-frozen plasma; FSP = fibrin split products.)

matic. However, when the pregnancy is more advanced, the mechanisms responsible for the hemorrhage most often are the same as those described for placental abruption and placenta previa, i.e., the disruption of a large number of maternal blood vessels at the site of placental implantation without myometrial contraction and retraction appropriate for mechanical constriction of these vessels. At times, appreciable changes in the coagulation mechanism complicate abortion.

COAGULATION DEFECTS

Serious disruption of the coagulation mechanism as the consequence of abortion may develop in the following circumstances: (1) prolonged retention of a dead fetus, as described above, (2) sepsis, a notorious cause, (3) the intrauterine instillation of hypertonic saline or urea solutions, (4) medical induction with a prostaglandin, and (5) during instrumental termination of the pregnancy.

The kinds of changes in coagulation that have been identified with abortion induced with markedly *hypertonic solutions* imply at least that thromboplastin is released from placenta, fetus, decidua, or all three by the necrobiotic effect of the hypertonic solutions, which then initiates coagulation within the maternal circulation (Burkman and associates, 1977). Coagulation defects have been observed to develop rarely during induction of abortion with prostaglandin.

Gross disruption of the coagulation mechanism has been an uncommon but serious complication among women with *septic abortion* cared for at Parkland Hospital. The incidence of coagulation defects has been highest in those with *Clostridium perfringens* sepsis and intense intravascular hemolysis (Pritchard and Whalley, 1971). In the presence of gross intravascular hemolysis, plasma fibrinogen concentrations ranged from normal to low, as did the platelet counts, while fibrin degradation products in serum were variably elevated. It has long been recognized that intense intravascular hemolysis is capable of inciting

disseminated intravascular coagulation, which, if the circulatory system is not intact, contributes significantly to serious hemorrhage.

Severe disruption of the coagulation mechanism, presumably by endotoxin, can develop with abortion complicated by gram-negative sepsis even in the absence of intense intravascular hemolysis.

Prompt restoration and maintenance of the circulation and appropriate steps to control the infection, including evacuation of the infected products of conception, are most important for a successful outcome. There is no good evidence that routine hysterectomy, rather than prompt curettage to remove infected products of conception in an intact uterus, improves the outcome. Management is described further in Chapter 29, p. 507.

Midtrimester abortion induced by *dilatation and evacuation* has also served to induce severe consumptive coagulopathy. There has been an array of cases reported, especially in the 1970s, in which midpregnancy abortions without prolonged fetal death have been complicated by severe consumptive coagulopathy (Guidotti and co-workers, 1981; White and colleagues, 1983). Usually the etiology has been ascribed to amnionic fluid embolism, although it has been our experience that amnionic fluid at or near midpregnancy contains very little particulate matter to obstruct the pulmonary microcirculation, and its capability for activating the coagulation mechanism is weak, at least in vitro.

We have observed four patients in whom dilatation of the cervix and mechanical evacuation of the pregnancy at 15 to 21 weeks gestation somehow induced severe consumptive coagulopathy with fibrinogen levels that were low to undetectable and accompanied by high levels of fibrin degradation products. Three of the women were treated as described above for placental abruption and survived. One woman, described below, died:

During attempts at dilatation and evacuation at an abortion clinic, she convulsed and suffered apparent cardiac arrest, which was treated immediately with closed chest cardiac compression and artificial ventilation. Spontaneous cardiac activity was soon evident, and she regained consciousness once vigorous therapy with lactated Ringer's solution and whole blood was instituted and maintained. Intense hypofibrinogenemia and markedly elevated levels of fibrinogen–fibrin degradation products were identified. However, pulmonary function was not impaired; arterial blood Po_2 was 151 mm Hg while receiving oxygen by mask. Severe hemorrhage from the superior portion of the liver and a torn hepatic vein, apparently traumatized during cardiopulmonary resuscitation, proved fatal. While this case has been ascribed to amnionic fluid embolism (Cates and associates, 1981), the results of histological examinations of the lungs are equivocal (Pritchard, unpublished).

It seems plausible that in some of these cases, at least, rather than amnionic fluid debris being the culprit, mechanical separation of the placenta during the course of the abortion allowed thromboplastic materials from injured placenta and decidua to enter the maternal circulation at the implantation site, therby triggering intense consumptive coagulopathy.

It seems unlikely that amnionic fluid per se is the major culprit, for reasons considered in the section on Amnionic Fluid Embolism. In our experience, the coagulation defects are soon repaired and recovery is uneventful if perfusion of vital organs is maintained by appropriate refilling of the intravascular compartment, as described above for placental abruption, and the products of conception are removed from the uterine cavity.

OTHER COAGULATION DEFECTS

Coagulation defects caused by *eclampsia* or *severe preeclampsia* are discussed in Chapter 35. Rarely, a hemophilia-like state may be acquired during the postpartum period as a consequence of development of antibody to factor VIII. Treatment may require massive amounts of blood and cryoprecipitate. Attempts at immunosuppression with corticosteroids and plasmapheresis to try to remove antibody to factor VIII do not seem to have been of benefit.

Coagulation defects that coincide with pregnancy are considered in Chapter 39.

REFERENCES

Abdella TN, Sibae BM, Hays JM Jr, Anderson GD: Perinatal outcome in abruptio placentae. Obstet Gynecol, 63:365, 1984

Adamsons K, Mueller-Heuback E, Myers RE: The innocuousness of amniotic fluid infusion in the pregnant rhesus monkey. Am J Obstet Gynecol 109:988, 1971

Alperin JB, Haggard ME, McGanity WJ: Folic acid, pregnancy, and abruptio placentae. Am J Clin Nutr 22:1354, 1969

American College of Obstetricians and Gynecologists: Diagnosis and management of fetal death. Technical Bulletin No 98, November 1986

Arias F: Cervical cerclage for temporary treatment of patients with placenta previa. Obstet Gynecol 71:545, 1988

Åstedt B: Risk of β-receptor agonists delaying diagnosis of abruptio placentae. Acta Obstet Gynecol Scand [Suppl] 108:35, 1982

Attwood HD: A histological study of experimental amniotic-fluid and meconium embolism in dogs. J Pathol Bacteriol 88:285, 1964

Beischer NA, Brown JB, Macafee J: Urinary estriol excretion before severe placental abruption. Obstet Gynecol 36:697, 1970

Bill AH: The treatment of placenta previa by prophylactic blood transfusion and cesarean section. Am J Obstet Gynecol 14:523, 1927

Bonnar J, McNicol GP, Douglas AS: The behavior of the coagulation and fibrinolytic mechanism in abruptio placentae. J Obstet Gynaecol Br Commonw 76:799, 1969

Bove JR: Transfusion-associated hepatitis and AIDS: What is the risk: N Engl J Med 317:242, 1987

Bowie JD, Rochester D, Cadkin AV, Cooke WT, Kunzman A: Accuracy of placental localization by ultrasound. Radiology 128:177, 1978

Brame RG, Harbert GM Jr, McGaughey HS Jr, Thornton WN Jr: Maternal risk in abruption. Obstet Gynecol 31:224, 1968

Brar HS, Platt DL, DeVore GR, Horenstein J: Fetal umbilical velocimetry for the surveillance of pregnancies complicated by placenta previa. J Repro Med 33:741, 1988

Brenner WE, Edelman DA, Hendricks CH: Characteristics of patients with placenta previa and results of expectant management. Am J Obstet Gynecol 132:180, 1978

Burkman RT, Bell WR, Atienza MF, King TM: Coagulopathy with midtrimester induced abortion: Association with hyperosmolar urea administration. Am J Obstet Gynecol 127:533, 1977

Campbell S, Kohorn E: Placental localization by ultrasonic compound scanning. J Obstet Gynaecol Br Commonw 75:1007, 1968

Cates W Jr, Boyd C, Halvorson-Boyd G, Holck S, Gilchrest TF: Death from amniotic fluid embolism and disseminated intravascular coagulation after a curettage abortion. Am J Obstet Gynecol 141:346, 1981

Clark SL, Cotton DB, Gonik B, Greenspoon J, Phelan JP: Central hemodynamic alterations in amniotic fluid embolism. Am J Obstet Gynecol 158:1124, 1988

Clark SL, Montz FJ, Phelan JP: Hemodynamic alterations associated with amniotic fluid embolism: A reappraisal. Am J Obstet Gynecol 151:617, 1985

Comeau J, Shaw L, Marcell CC, Lavery JP: Early placenta previa and delivery outcome. Obstet Gynecol 61:577, 1983

Consensus Conference: Fresh-frozen plasma: Indications and risks. JAMA 253:551, 1985

Corrigan Jr JJ: Vitamin K-dependent coagulation factors in gram-negative septicemia. Am J Dis Child 138:240, 1984

Corrigan JJ, Kiornat JF, Pagel CJ: Experimental gram-negative sepsis: Effect of heparin. Pediatr Res 8:399, 1974

Counts RB, Haisch C, Simon TL, Maxwell NG, Heimbach DM, Carrico CJ: Hemostasis in massively transfused trauma patients. Ann Surg 190:91, 1979

Courtney LD, Allington M: Effect of amniotic fluid on blood coagulation. Br J Haematol 22:353, 1972

Czer LSC, Shoemaker WC: Optimal hematocrit value in critically ill postoperative patients. Surg Gynecol Obstet 147:363, 1978

Dehner LP: Advanced extrauterine pregnancy and the fetal death syndrome. Obstet Gynecol 40:525, 1972

Donald I, Abdulla U: Placentography by sonar. J Obstet Gynaecol Br Commonw 75:993, 1968

Edson JR, Blaese RM, White JG, Krivit W: Defibrination syndrome in an infant born after abruptio placentae. Pediatrics 72:342, 1968

Farine D, Fox HE, Jakobson S, Timor-Tritsch IE: Vaginal ultrasound for diagnosis of placenta previa. Am J Obstet Gynecol 159:566, 1988

Goldstein DP, Reid DE: Circulating fibrinolytic activity: A precursor of hypofibrinogenemia following fetal death in utero. Obstet Gynecol 22:174, 1963

Gottesfeld KR, Thompson HE, Holmes JH, Taylor ES: Ultrasound placentography: A new method for placental localization. Am J Obstet Gynecol 96:538, 1966

Guidotti RJ, Grimes DA, Cates W Jr: Fatal amniotic fluid embolism during legally induced abortion, United States 1972 to 1978. Am J Obstet Gynecol 141:257, 1981

Halmagyi DR, Starzecki B, Shearman RP: Experimental amniotic fluid embolism: Mechanism and treatment. Am J Obstet Gynecol 84:251, 1962

Hanzlik PJ, Karsner HT: Anaphylactoid phenomena from the intravenous administration of various colloids, arsenicals and other agents. J Pharmacol Exp Ther 14:379, 1920; 23:173, 1924

Hastwell GB: Amniotic fluid thromboplastic activity as an index of fetal maturity: A preliminary report. Aust NZ J Obstet Gynecol 14:196, 1974

Hatch RI, Barke JI, Barke MW: Coagulopathy associated with dilatation and evacuation for intrauterine fetal death. Obstet Gynecol 66:463, 1985

Herbert WNP, Owen HG, Collins ML: Autologous blood storage in obstetrics. Obstet Gynecol 72:166, 1988

Herman CM, Moquin RB, Horwitz DL: Coagulation changes of hemorrhagic shock in baboons. Ann Surg 175:197, 1972

Hibbard BM, Jeffcoate TNA: Abruptio placentae. Obstet Gynecol 27:155, 1966

Hovatta O, Lipasti A, Rapola J, Karjalainen O: Causes of stillbirth: A clinicopathological study of 243 patients. Acta Obstet Gynecol Scand 90:691, 1983

Hughes EC (ed): Obstetric-Gynecologic Terminology. Philadelphia, David, 1972, p 417

Hurd WW, Miodovnik M, Hertzberg V, Lavin JP: Selective management of abruptio placentae: A prospective study. Obstet Gynecol 61:467, 1983

Jansen RPS: Relative bradycardia: A sign of acute intraperitoneal bleeding. Aust NZ J Obstet Gynaecol 18:206, 1978

Jennison RF, Walker AC: Foetal death in utero with hypofibrinogenemia managed conservatively. Lancet 2:607, 1956

Jimenez JM, Pritchard JA: Pathogenesis and treatment of coagulation defects resulting from fetal death. Obstet Gynecol 32:449, 1968

Johnson HW: The conservative management of some varieties of placenta previa. Am J Obstet Gynecol 50:248, 1945

Jouppilla P: Vaginal bleeding in the last two trimesters of pregnancy: A clinical and ultrasonic study. Acta Obstet Gynecol Scand 58:461, 1979

Karayalcin G, Kim KY, Aballi AJ: Coagulation changes after acute blood loss. Pediatr Res 7:357, 1973

Käregård M, Gennser G: Incidence and recurrence rate of abruptio placentae in Sweden. Obstet Gynecol 67:523, 1986

Kaunitz AM, Hughes JM, Grimes DA, Smith JC, Rochat RW, Kafrissen ME: Causes of maternal mortality in the United States. Obstet Gynecol 65:605, 1985

Kettel LM, Branch DW, Scott JR: Occult placental abruption after maternal trauma. Obstet Gynecol 71:449, 1988

King DL: Placental migration demonstrated by ultrasonography. Radiology 109:163, 1973

Kobayashi M, Hellman L, Fillisti L: Placenta localization by ultrasound. Am J Obstet Gynecol 106:279, 1970

Krohn M, Voigt L, McKnight B, Daling JR, Starzyk P, Benedetti TJ: Correlates of placental abruption. Br J Obstet Gynaecol 94:333, 1987

Krupp PJ Jr, Barclay DL Roeling WM, Wegener G: Maternal mortality: A 20-year study of Tulane Department of Obstetrics and Gynecology at Charity Hospital. Obstet Gynecol 35:823, 1970

Lerner R, Margolin M, Slate WG: Heparin in the treatment of hypofibrinogenemia complicating fetal death in utero. Am J Obstet Gynecol 97:373, 1967

Lerner RG, Rappaport SI, Siemsen KJ, Spitzer JM: Disappearance of fibrinogen ^{131}I after endotoxin: Effects of a first and second injection. Am J Physiol 214:532, 1968

Liggins GC: Treatment of missed abortion by high dosage syntocinon intravenous infusion. J Obstet Gynaecol Br Commonw 69:277, 1962

Macafee CHG: Placenta previa: A study of 174 cases. J Obstet Gynaecol Br Emp 52:313, 1945

Marbury MC, Linn S, Monson R, Schoenbaum S, Stubblefield PG, Ryan KJ: The association of alcohol consumption with outcome of pregnancy. Am J Public Health 73:1165, 1983

Miller RD: The National Institutes of Health Consensus Development Conference on fresh-frozen plasma: Indications and risks. Anesthesiology 62:379, 1985

Ness PM, Perkins HA: Cryoprecipitate as a reliable source of fibrinogen replacement. JAMA 241:1690, 1979

Newton M: Postpartum hemorrhage. Am J Obstet Gynecol 94:711, 1966

Nielsen NC: Coagulation and fibrinolysis in mothers and their newborn infants following premature separation of the placenta. Acta Obstet Gynecol Scand 49:77, 1970

O'Brien WF, Knuppel RA, Saba HI, Angel JL, Benoit R, Bruce A: Platelet inhibitory activity in placentas from normal and abnormal pregnancies. Obstet Gynecol 70:597, 1987

Oláh KS, Gee HY, Needham PG: The management of severe disseminated intravascular coagulopathy complicating placental abruption in the second trimester of pregnancy. Br J Obstet Gynaecol 95:419, 1988

Orr JW Jr, Huddleston JF, Goldenberg RL, Knox GE, Davis RO: Association of extrauterine fetal death with failure of prostaglandin E₂ suppositories. Obstet Gynecol (Suppl) 53:57, 1979

Paterson MEL: The aetiology and outcome of abruptio placentae. Acta Obstet Gynecol Scand 58:31, 1979

Patterson SP, White JH, Reaves EM: A maternal death associated with prostaglandin E₂. Obstet Gynecol 54:123, 1979

Phelan JP, Cefalo RC: A better approach to fetal demise—PGE₂ suppository. Contemp Ob/Gyn ll:93, 1978

Phillips LL, Davidson EC Jr: Procoagulant properties of amniotic fluid. Am J Obstet Gynecol 113:911, 1972

Pineo GF, Recoeczi E, Hatton MWC, Brain MC: The activation of coagulation by extracts of mucus: A possible pathway of intravascular coagulation accompanying adenocarcinomas. J Lab Clin Med 82:255, 1973

Price TM, Baker VV, Cefalo RC: Amniotic fluid embolism: Three case reports with a review of the literature. Obstet Gynecol Surv 40:462, 1985

Pritchard JA: Changes in the blood volume during pregnancy and delivery. Anesthesiology 26:393, 1965

Pritchard JA: Fetal death in utero. Obstet Gynecol 14:573, 1959

Pritchard JA: Haematological problems associated with delivery, placental abruption, retained dead fetus, and amniotic fluid embolism. Clin Haematol 2:563, 1973

Pritchard JA, Baldwin RM, Dickey JC, Wiggins KM: Blood volume changes in pregnancy and the puerperium: II. Red blood cell loss and changes in apparent blood volume during and following vaginal delivery, cesarean section, and cesarean section plus total hysterectomy. Am J Obstet Gynecol 84:1271, 1962

Pritchard JA, Brekken AL: Clincal and laboratory studies on severe abruptio placentae. Am J Obstet Gynecol 97:681, 1967

Pritchard JA, Cunningham FG, Mason RA: Coagulation changes in eclampsia: Their frequency and pathogenesis. Am J Obstet Gynecol 124:855, 1976

Pritchard JA, Mason R, Corley M, Pritchard S: Genesis of severe placental abruption. Am J Obstet Gynecol 108:22, 1970

Pritchard JA, Ratnoff OD: Studies of fibrinogen and other hemostatic factors in women with intrauterine death and delayed delivery. Surg Gynecol Obstet 101:467, 1955

Pritchard JA, Whalley PJ: Abortion complicated by Clostridium perfringens infection. Am J Obstet Gynecol 11:484, 1971

Quance D: Amniotic fluid embolism: Detection by pulse oximetry. Anesthesiology 68:951, 1988

Rappaport SI: Defibrination syndromes. In Williams WJ, Beutler E, Erslev AJ, Rundles RW (eds): Hematology. New York, McGraw-Hill, 1977, p 1454

Read JA, Cotton DB, Miller FC: Placenta accreta: Changing clinical aspects and outcome. Obstet Gynecol 56:31, 1980

Resnick R, Swartz WH, Plumer MH, Benirschke K, Stratthaus ME: Amniotic fluid embolism with survival. Obstet Gynecol 47:295, 1976

Rochat RW, Koonin LM, Atrash HK, Jewett JF, The Maternal Mortality Collaborative: Maternal mortality in the United States: Report from the Maternal Mortality Collaborative. Obstet Gynec 72:91, 1988

Romero R, Duffy TP, Berkowitz RL, Chang E, Hobbins JC: Prolongation of a preterm pregnancy complicated by death of a single twin in utero and disseminated intravascular coagulation: Effects of treatment with heparin. N Engl J Med 310:772, 1984

Sachs BP, Brown DAJ, Driscoll SG, Schulman E, Acker D, Ransil BJ, Jewett JF: Hemorrhage, infection, toxemia, and cardiac disease, 1954–85: Causes for their declining role in maternal mortality. Am J Public Health 78:671, 1988

Sachs BP, Brown DAJ, Driscoll SG, Schulman E, Acker D, Ransil BJ, Jewett JF: Maternal mortality in Massachusetts: Trends and prevention. N Engl J Med 316:667, 1987

Santos R, Jimenez J, Duenhoelter J: Unpublished observations, 1978

Schneider CL: Coagulation defects in obstetric shock: Meconium embolism and heparin; fibrin embolism and defibrination. Am J Obstet Gynecol 69:758, 1955

Schneider CL: Obstetric shock: Some interdependent problems of coagulation. Obstet Gynecol 4:273, 1954

Schneider CL, Henry MM: Meconium embolism in vivo. Am J Obstet Gynecol 101:909, 1968

Schulman H, Saldana L, Lin C-C, Randolph G: Mechanism of failed labor after fetal death and its treatment with prostaglandin E₂. Am J Obstet Gynecol 133:742, 1979

Seski JC, Compton AA: Abruptio placentae following a negative oxytocin challenge test. Am J Obstet Gynecol 125:276, 1976

Sher G: A rational basis for the management of abruptio placentae, J Reprod Med 21:123, 1978

Sher G: Pathogenesis and management of uterine inertia complicating abruptio placentae with consumption coagulopathy. Am J Obstet Gynecol 129:164, 1977

Sherman E, Middleton EH: The management of missed abortion with hypofibrinogenemia. Maryland State Med J 7:300, 1958

Sholl JS: Abruptio placentae: Clinical management in nonacute cases. Am J Obstet Gynecol 156:40, 1987

Silke B, Carmody M, O'Dwyer WF: Acute renal failure in pregnancy. In Bonnar J, MacGillivray I, Symonds EM (eds): Pregnancy Hypertension. Baltimore, University Park Press, 1980

Singh PM, Rodrigues C, Gupta AN: Placenta previa and previous cesarean section. Acta Obstet Gynecol Scand 60:367, 1981

Skelly H, Marivate M, Norman R, Kenoyer G, Martin R: Consumptive coagulopathy following fetal death in a triplet pregnancy. Am J Obstet Gynecol 142:595, 1982

Spence MR, Mason KG: Experimental amniotic fluid embolism in rabbits. Am J Obstet Gynecol 119:1073, 1974

Stafford PA, Biddinger PW, Zumwalt RE: Lethal intrauterine fetal trauma. Am J Obstet Gynecol 159:485, 1988

Stolte L, Seelen J, Eskes T, Wagatsuma T: Failure to produce the syndrome of amniotic fluid embolism by infusion of amniotic fluid and meconium into monkeys. Am J Obstet Gynecol 98:694, 1967

Stone SR, Whalley PJ, Pritchard JA: Inferior vena cava and ovarian vein ligation during late pregnancy. Obstet Gynecol 32:267, 1968

Sunden B: Placentography by ultrasound. Acta Obstet Gynecol Scand 49:179, 1970

Tricomi V, Kohl SG: Fetal death in utero. Am J Obstet Gynecol 74:1092, 1957

Tuck CS: Amniotic fluid embolism. Proc R Soc Med 65:2, 1972

Turpini R, Stefanini M: The nature and mechanism of the hemostatic breakdown in the course of experimental hemorrhagic shock. J Clin Invest 38:53, 1959

Ward JW, Holmbert DS, Allen JR, Cohn DL, Critchley SE, Kleinman SH, Lenes BA, Ravenholt O, Davis JR, Quinn MG, Jaffee HW: Transmission of human immunodeficiency virus (HIV) by blood transfusions screened as negative for HIV antibody. N Engl J Med 318:473, 1988

Weiner AE, Reid DE, Roby CC, Diamond LK: Coagulation defects with intrauterine death from Rh sensitization. Am J Obstet Gynecol 60:1015, 1950

Wexler P, Gottesfeld KR: Second trimester placenta previa: An apparently normal placentation. Obstet Gynecol 50:706, 1977

Whalley PJ, Pritchard JA: Oxytocin and water intoxication. JAMA 186:601, 1963

Whalley PJ, Scott DE, Pritchard JA: Maternal folate deficiency and pregnancy wastage: I. Placental abruption. Am J Obstet Gynecol 105:670, 1969

White PF, Coe V, Dworsky WA, Margolis A: Disseminated intravascular coagulation following midtrimester abortions. Anesthesiology 58:99, 1983

Young GB: The peripatetic placenta. Radiology 128:183, 1978

Abnormalities of the Reproductive Tract

DISEASES OF THE VULVA AND VAGINA

INFLAMMATION OF THE BARTHOLIN GLANDS

Gonococci or other pathogenic organisms may gain access to Bartholin glands and form abscesses. The labium majus on the side affected becomes swollen and painful at and surrounding the collection of pus. Aside from causing pain and discomfort, such abscesses may be the starting point of a puerperal infection. For these reasons, drainage must be established whenever an abscess develops during pregnancy. After the contents have escaped, the cut edge of the abscess cavity, if actively bleeding, is sutured with fine chromic catgut. A gauze wick is inserted to keep the ostium open until granulation is complete. McCoy and Cunningham (unpublished observations) found in pus from Bartholin abscesses both aerobic and anaerobic bacteria in nearly 90 percent of cases. *Neisseria gonorrhoeae* was identified in only 4 of 53 cases. A broad-spectrum antibiotic to which *N. gonorrhoeae* is sensitive should be administered for 7 to 10 days.

The treatment of asymptomatic *Bartholin duct cysts*, which are frequently the sequelae of Bartholin gland abscesses, is best postponed until after delivery. Rarely is a labial cyst of sufficient size to cause difficulty at delivery. If this should occur, aspiration with a syringe and small needle will suffice as a temporary measure. Because of the hyperemia induced by pregnancy, excision should not be attempted. Definitive surgery, if necessary, should be postponed until later.

URETHRAL DIVERTICULAE, CYSTS, AND ABSCESSES

Trauma to the urethra or infection of the periurethral glands may be followed by the formation of periurethral abscesses, cysts, and diverticulae. Abscesses usually resolve spontaneously, with, at times, cyst formation as a sequela. Most often, periurethral cysts are asymptomatic and are best not disturbed during pregnancy. A urethral diverticulum may fill with debris that empties intermittently through the urethra to give rise to proteinuria of obscure etiology until the diverticulum is recognized as the source. In general, an attempt at surgical excision should not be made during pregnancy.

CONDYLOMA ACUMINATA

Condyloma acuminata, sometimes called *venereal warts*, are caused by papillomaviruses. These are sexually transmitted and are discussed in Chapter 39 (p. 858). There is a strong association between several types of papillomaviruses and squamous carcinoma of the cervix and vulva, discussed below.

VULVAR VARICES

Varicosities sometimes appear in the lower part of the vagina but are more common around the vulva. There they may attain considerable size and cause a sensation of weight and discomfort. Vulvar varices may rupture during labor or be torn or cut by lacerations or episiotomy. Unless so traumatized, the varicosities in most instances become asymptomatic and decrease remarkably, or even disappear, after delivery. Vulvar varices are considered further in Chapter 14 (p. 271).

CYSTOCELE AND RECTOCELE

Attenuation of the fascial support that is normally interposed between the vagina and the bladder leads to prolapse into the vagina of the bladder, or cystocele. Attenuation between the vagina and the rectum results in a rectocele. In former years, a vaginal delivery after a prolonged labor of a large infant without episiotomy, but with appreciable tearing of the lower genital tract, predisposed to the development of a cystocele and a rectocele. The more liberal use of cesarean section in cases of less than absolute cephalopelvic disproportion and of episiotomies for vaginal deliveries, especially when the fetus is large, coupled with generally lower parity, have made large symptomatic cystoceles and rectoceles very uncommon.

Urinary stasis associated with a large cystocele predisposes to urinary tract infection. A large rectocele may fill with feces that, at times, can only be evacuated manually. Both lesions can block the normal descent of the fetus through the birth canal, unless they are emptied and pushed out of the way. Surgical repair of either should not be attempted during the antepartum or intrapartum periods. Rather, definitive repair, often with vaginal hysterectomy for associated uterine prolapse and sterilization, should be carried out after pregnancy-induced pelvic hyperemia has completely subsided.

URINARY STRESS INCONTINENCE

Infrequently, women may develop stress incontinence during pregnancy. Iosif and Ulmsten (1981), who studied a group of such pregnant women, identified low urethral closing pressure that did not increase sufficiently to compensate for the progressive increase in bladder pressure induced by the enlarging uterus. Moreover, at the outset the urethra was shorter, and it did not increase in length during pregnancy in the group with stress incontinence, thereby differing from pregnant women who remained continent.

VAGINAL TUMORS

Vaginal cysts, the most frequent of benign vaginal tumors, may be discovered during pregnancy or sometimes not until the time of labor. Such cysts, usually embryological rests (Gartner or müllerian duct), may be of sufficient size to cause dystocia. Treatment depends upon the size and location of the cyst, as well as the time at which it is first recognized. Rarely, drainage may be necessary to allow vaginal delivery to be completed. It is advisable to postpone surgical excision until after delivery and the puerperium when pelvic hyperemia has subsided.

CERVICAL NEOPLASIA

The effects of pregnancy and delivery on premalignant and malignant epithelial lesions of the cervix are not completely understood, and disagreements persist in spite of the considerable interest displayed by numerous investigators for many years. In one study at least, pregnancy did not seem to be a potent stimulus for progression of epithelial change from dysplasia to invasive neoplasia (Kiguchi and associates, 1981). The progression rate from dysplasia to invasive carcinoma (0.4 percent) after delivery was almost half that in the nonpregnant state (1 percent). Moreover, the regression rates of moderate and marked dysplasia within the 6-month period after delivery seemed much higher than those of dysplasia in the general population.

While not proven, these conflicting viewpoints are likely to be the consequence of failure to identify the specific type of human papillomavirus associated with the reported observations. Human papillomavirus types 6 and 11 are likely to be associated with mild dysplasia, which usually undergoes spontaneous regression, whereas types 16, 18, and 31 are associated with more severe cervical neoplasia (Syrajanen, 1985).

HUMAN PAPILLOMAVIRUS AND CERVICAL CANCER

The association between cervical cancer and the human papillomavirus seems well established (American College of Obstetricians and Gynecologists, 1987). Syrajanen (1985) reported that types 16 and 18 were associated with the development of invasive carcinoma within 3 years of detection. McCance and co-workers (1985) identified type 16 papillomavirus in more than 90 percent of squamous cell cervical carcinomas. Finally, there is growing evidence that identification of papillomavirus types 16, 18, and 31 in dysplastic lesions is associated with a greater likelihood of developing cervical carcinoma and at a more rapid rate (Reid and Fu, 1986).

While standard laboratories cannot presently identify the specific type of papillomavirus in a biopsy or cervical smear, it is likely that such techniques will become available. Thus, dysplastic lesions most likely to advance to cervical or vulvar cancer may be identified and definitive therapy applied.

SCREENING FOR CERVICAL CANCER

As described in Chapter 14 (p. 259), all pregnant women should undergo an examination that includes evaluation of the cervix cytologically as well as by visual inspection and palpation, ex-

cept when there is active bleeding late in the second trimester or beyond and placenta previa is a possibility (Chap. 36, p. 712). Any visible fungating or ulcerating lesion should be evaluated by colposcopy or direct biopsy, since cytological screening at times may not detect a frankly invasive carcinoma.

ABNORMAL CERVICAL CYTOLOGY

If cytological changes of mild dysplasia are identified and confirmed subsequently in another set of smears, further follow-up during pregnancy may consist of colposcopic evaluation. Simply repeating the cervical smears later in pregnancy to identify more serious cytological changes, if any, should prove quite satisfactory. Cytological changes in cervical smears compatible with severe dysplasia or neoplasia require confirmation and colposcopic evaluation to identify the responsible lesion. The cervix is examined and colposcopically directed biopsies made of any suspicious lesion. Multiple biopsies need not all be made on one occasion. Instead, the squamocolumnar junction can be "mapped" and biopsies obtained systematically over a period of time without hospitalization. Bleeding from biopsy sites usually can be controlled by a vaginal pack well applied to the cervix for a few hours. Occasionally, during pregnancy the cervix may bleed to the extent that a suture about the biopsy site must be used to effect hemostasis. Colposcopy and directed focal biopsy during pregnancy has proved to be safe and reliable, thereby, in most cases, eliminating the need for conization.

Conization of the cervix is less satisfactory during pregnancy than in its absence, for three reasons. (1) The epithelium and underlying stroma within the cervical canal cannot be so extensively excised because of the risk to the fetal membranes adjacent to the internal os. (2) Blood loss from the cervix during and after conization is appreciable in pregnant women and at times may be severe. (3) There is some increased risk of abortion or preterm delivery in the current pregnancy (Hannigan and associates, 1982), and probably subsequent ones as well (Larsson and co-workers, 1982). Fortunately, it has been the experience of most workers that colposcopically directed biopsies of the squamocolumnar junction are an effective means of identifying invasive carcinoma.

Because of the risks of hemorrhage and rupture of the membranes, endocervical curettage should not be performed during pregnancy.

DYSPLASIA AND CARCINOMA IN SITU

These epithelial lesions need no immediate treatment when detected during pregnancy. The pregnancy should be allowed to continue and delivery to be accomplished without regard to the presence of either lesion. In general, the cervix should be reevaluated for neoplastic disease after the puerperium. Appropriate therapy ranges from periodic reevaluation to hysterectomy, depending upon the lesion that persists and the parity. In general, cesarean hysterectomy to terminate the pregnancy and remove the affected cervix should be avoided unless there are other compelling indications for performing cesarean section. At times, it is difficult to be sure that all the cervix has been removed by cesarean hysterectomy.

INVASIVE CARCINOMA

Pregnancy coexisting with invasive carcinoma of the cervix complicates both staging and treatment. Accurate identification of the extent of the cancer may be more difficult during pregnancy since induration of the base of the broad ligaments, which in nonpregnant women characterizes spread of tumor beyond the cervix, may be less prominent in the pregnant woman. Consequently, the extent of the tumor is more likely to be underestimated in the pregnant woman. Moreover, the decision between immediate interruption of the pregnancy and allowing the fetus to achieve several more weeks of maturity before interruption almost always is difficult.

Although few, if any, institutions have had great experience with the treatment of carcinoma of the cervix complicated by pregnancy, some generalizations can be made on the basis of some reports, as well as from the cumulative experiences at Parkland Hospital. Interestingly, the survival rate for invasive carcinoma of the cervix has not been profoundly different for pregnant and nonpregnant women within a given stage of disease. Moreover, the mode of delivery has not been shown to affect maternal survival significantly (Hacker and associates, 1982). Nonetheless, when frankly invasive carcinoma is known to exist, most clinicians favor hysterotomy or cesarean section for terminating pregnancy, rather than labor and vaginal delivery, if for no other reason than that the cervix would not lacerate during dilatation.

Sufficient experience has accumulated to establish that for stage I invasive carcinoma complicated by pregnancy, extensive (radical) hysterectomy plus pelvic lymphadenectomy is often the procedure of choice (Hacker and associates, 1982). Dissection is facilitated by the softening of uterine supportive structures induced by pregnancy, although blood loss is usually somewhat greater than in a nonpregnant woman, as is evident from Table 36–1.

For more extensive invasive cervical cancer, radiation therapy should be used. Early in pregnancy, external irradiation may be started. The pregnancy products usually will be expelled spontaneously or, if not, they can be removed by curettage. Sources of radiation are subsequently applied in standard fashion to the cervix and adjacent parts. If the uterus is enlarged sufficiently to be easily palpated above the symphysis (beyond the first trimester), hysterotomy with the uterine incision made remote from the cervix is performed to remove the pregnancy products. Care is taken to try to minimize adhesions, especially of the bowel. After a week or so, external irradiation is started, followed by intracavitary application of radiation sources.

There are no data with which to establish, with any degree of confidence, the risk to the mother from delay in treatment of frankly invasive carcinoma for many weeks while the fetus matures. In general, during the first half of pregnancy, at least, immediate treatment should be advised.

OTHER TUMORS

Adenocarcinoma of the Endometrium

This malignancy associated with pregnancy is rare. Sandstrom and associates (1979) described a case and reviewed the few others reported. The most common lesion found was adenoacanthoma.

Uterine Myomas

These are relatively common during pregnancy and are discussed in Chapter 21 (p. 387).

Carcinoma of the Oviduct

This malignancy has rarely been found complicating pregnancy. Schinfeld and Winston (1980) reported such a lesion encountered at the time of cesarean delivery for a breech presentation.

Carapeto and associates (1978) reported an ectopic pregnancy associated with a primary carcinoma of the fallopian tube, and Starr and colleagues (1978) reported a case discovered at the time of puerperal tubal ligation.

Ovarian Tumors

Such tumors, if large, may cause or contribute to dystocia and are considered in Chapter 21 (p. 391).

SPONTANEOUS DEVELOPMENTAL ABNORMALITIES OF THE REPRODUCTIVE TRACT; MÜLLERIAN ANOMALIES

Developmental anomalies of the female genital tract are uncommonly encountered in obstetrics. However, even minor defects may result in an increased incidence of threatened abortion and abnormal fetal lie (Sorensen and Trauelsen, 1987). More serious defects often result in significant fetal and maternal hazards. There is little familial tendency associated with these defects that at most may be polygenic or multifactorial traits (Elias and associates, 1984).

These genitourinary defects result from abnormalities in the embryological process. In order to understand their etiology, it is necessary to know how the structures are formed and where and when an interruption in these processes takes place. Briefly, development begins when the metanephric ducts emerge and connect with the cloaca between the third and fifth gestational weeks. Between the fourth and fifth weeks, two ureteric buds develop distally from the mesonephric ducts and begin to grow upward (cephalad) toward the mesonephros. Müllerian (paramesonephric) ducts form bilaterally between the developing gonad and the mesonephros. The müllerian ducts extend downward and laterally to the mesonephric ducts and finally turn medially to meet and fuse together in the midline. The fused müllerian duct descends to the urogenital sinus to join the müllerian tubercle. **The close association between the müllerian and mesonephric ducts has clinical relevance, because damage to either duct system most often will be associated with damage to both (uterine horn, kidney, and ureter).**

The uterus is formed by the union of the two müllerian ducts at about the 10th week. The fusion begins in the middle of what will become the uterus, and then extends caudally and cephalad. The characteristic shape of the uterus is now formed with cellular proliferation at the upper portion of the uterus and a simultaneous dissolution of cells at the lower pole, thus establishing the first uterine cavity. This cavity is at the lower pole with a thick wedge of tissue above. The upper thick wedge of tissue (septum) is slowly dissolved, creating the uterine cavity. This process usually is completed by the 20th week. It is reasonable to envision that any failure to fuse the two müllerian ducts or failure to resorb the cavity between them would result in separate uterine horns or some degree of persistence of the uterine septum.

The vagina forms between the urogenital sinus and the müllerian tubercle by a dissolution of the cell mass (cord) between the two structures. It is believed that this dissolution starts at the hymen and moves upward toward the cervix, which is also being canalized. A failure of this process will be associated with persistence of the cell cord, and agenesis of the vagina or lesser abnormalities of this process will result in varying degrees of vaginal septum formation.

GENESIS AND CLASSIFICATION OF MÜLLERIAN ABNORMALITIES

Because fusion of the two müllerian ducts forms the vagina, cervix, and uterine body, the principal groups of deformities arising from three types of embryological defects can be classified as follows:

1. There may be defective canalization of the vagina, resulting in a transverse vaginal septum, or in the most extreme form, absence of the vagina.
2. There may be unilateral maturation of the müllerian duct with incomplete or absent development of the opposite duct. The resulting defects often are associated with abnormalities of the upper urinary tract.
3. The most common abnormality is absent or faulty midline fusion of the müllerian ducts. If there is complete lack of fusion, the result is two entirely separate uteri, cervices, and vaginas. With incomplete resorption of the tissue between the two fused müllerian ducts, a uterine septum results.

Various classifications of these anomalies have been proposed, but none is completely satisfactory. The terminology often is so complicated and replete with Latin words that their relative obstetrical significance is obscured. One classification for müllerian duct abnormalities suggested by Buttram and Gibbons (1979) is based upon the failure of normal development. The classification separates a diversity of anomalies into groups with similar clinical characteristics, prognosis for pregnancy, and treatment (Table 37–1 and Fig. 37–1). The classification includes a category for abnormalities associated with in utero exposure to diethylstilbestrol (DES). The authors stressed that vaginal anomalies may exist alone or in association with other müllerian anomalies but vaginal anomalies were not classified because they are not associated with fetal loss. Vaginal anomalies using their scheme most often were associated with classes III and IV.

There is, in fact, no simplified classification for uterine, cervical, and vaginal abnormalities. Toaff and co-workers (1984) proposed another classification, but it is complicated and further burdened with Latin titles and subtitles. They did, however, provide an excellent and complete set of anatomical drawings with their classification. We prefer the simplified classification for cervical and vaginal abnormalities outlined below.

Types of cervices

1. *Single.* The normal cervix.
2. *Septate.* A cervix consisting of a single muscular ring partitioned by a septum. The septum may be confined to the cervix, or, more often, may be the downward continuation of a uterine septum or the upward extension of a vaginal septum.
3. *Double.* Two distinct cervices, each resulting from separate müllerian duct maturation. Both a septate and a true double cervix are frequently associated with a longitudinal vaginal septum, the result being that many septate cervices are erroneously classified as double. The diagnosis depends on careful visual and digital examination of the cervix and is of clinical importance.
4. *Single hemicervix.* Arises from unilateral müllerian maturation.

TABLE 37–1. CLASSIFICATION OF MÜLLERIAN ANOMALIES

I. Segmental müllerian agenesis or hypoplasia
  A. Vaginal
  B. Cervical
  C. Fundal
  D. Combined anomalies

II. Unicornuate uterus
  A. With rudimentary horn
    1. With endometrial cavity
      a. Communicating
      b. Noncommunicating
    2. Without endometrial cavity
  B. Without rudimentary horn

III. Uterine didelphys

IV. Bicornuate uterus
  A. Complete (division down to internal os)
  B. Partial
  C. Arcuate

V. Septate uterus
  A. Complete (septum to internal os)
  B. Partial

VI. Diethylstilbestrol-related

Modified from Buttram and Gibbons: Fertil Steril 32:40, 1979.

Types of vaginas

1. *Single.* The normal vagina
2. *Longitudinally septate.* More or less complete longitudinal septum.
3. *Double.* It is often difficult to distinguish the double from the completely septate vagina. The true double vagina includes a double introitus and resembles a double-barreled shotgun, with each passage terminating in a distinct, separate cervix. At times with double vaginas, one may end blindly.
4. *Transversely septate.* Transverse vaginal septa are of different developmental origin, resulting from faulty canalization of the united müllerian anlage, rather than faulty longitudinal fusion.

DIAGNOSIS

Vaginal septa usually are discovered during routine examinations by the physician or by the woman who notices that vaginal tampons are not always effective in absorbing menses.

Uterine malformations are discovered by simple inspection or during bimanual examination. They occasionally are discovered at cesarean section or during manual exploration of the uterine cavity after vaginal delivery. Fundal notching, palpated abdominally, most often is indicative of a malformed uterus and the clinical impression can be confirmed by laparoscopy. Without radiological examination, high-resolution sonography, or direct visualization of the uterine cavity, and often laparoscopic examination, it is difficult to distinguish the septate from the bicornuate uterus. *Hysteroscopic examination* and *hysterography* are of value in ascertaining the configuration of the uterine cavity. When combined with a laparoscopic confirmation of the absence or presence of an external division of the uterus and the presence or absence of a rudimentary uterine horn, virtually all uterine abnormalities can be accurately described and classified.

A high index of suspicion is important for detection. Green and Harris (1976) identified 80 uterine developmental anomalies during the course of 31,836 deliveries. They emphasized that detection was greatest during a period when one especially interested staff member espoused uterine exploration at delivery, and when an anomaly was suspected, suggested that hysterosalpingography be performed 6 to 8 weeks postpartum.

Sonography may be used to identify abnormal uterine development, although it lacks the precision of diagnosis provided by hysteroscopy and hysterosalpingography. During actual or suspected pregnancy, however, sonographic examination can be quite informative.

UROLOGICAL EVALUATION

When asymmetrical development of the reproductive tract is found, urological evaluation is indicated because of the frequent association of urinary tract anomalies. When there is uterine atresia on one side or when one side of a double vagina terminates blindly, an ipsilateral urological anomaly is common (Fedele and associates, 1987; Heinonen, 1983, 1984; Toaff, 1974; Wiersma and colleagues, 1976; Wolf and Allen, 1953).

OBSTETRICAL SIGNIFICANCE

Müllerian Hypoplasia or Agenesis (Buttram and Gibbons Class I)

The significance of these defects can be anticipated. Vaginal hypoplasia or agenesis renders pregnancy virtually impossible, and even in those rare cases where a uterus is sugically attached to a neovagina, successful pregnancy is extremely rare. The various types of vaginal septa are easily dilated, displaced, or surgically divided. The septate cervix functions remarkably well, but during labor there is possible danger of rupture and hemorrhage.

Buttram and Gibbons Classes II through V

The major obstetrical difficulties arise from uterine anomalies. The uterus must dilate and hypertrophy sufficiently to accommodate a term-sized fetus in a longitudinal lie; and at the proper time, it must contract efficiently to expel the fetus. The uterine defects that result from maturation of only one müllerian duct or from lack of fusion often give rise to a hemiuterus that fails to dilate and hypertrophy resulting in a host of possible difficulties, including abortion, ectopic pregnancy, rudimentary horn pregnancy, preterm delivery, fetal growth retardation, abnormal fetal lie, uterine dysfunction, and even uterine rupture. Surprisingly, even in those conditions in which only a uterine septum is present, there is an appreciable increase in the incidence of abortion (Buttram and Gibbons, 1979). Because of these obstetrical problems, each uterine defect will be discussed within the classification suggested by Buttram and Gibbons (1979) and outlined in Table 37–1.

Reproductive Performance of Women with Unicornuate Uterus (Buttram and Gibbons, Class II).

The incidence of unicornuate uterus in a series of 1,160 uterine anomalies was 14 percent (Zanetti and associates, 1978). It is likely that this is an underestimate, because the major diagnostic technique used was hysterosalpingography. In fact, in their series from the literature of 328 cases of pregnancy in rudimentary horns, O'Leary and O'Leary (1963) estimated that in 90 percent of unicornuate uteri with rudimentary horns there was no communication between the horns. This information has both gynecological and obstetrical significance. Specifically, the increased incidence of infertility, endometriosis, and dysmenorrhea in such cases is certainly a more easily understood concept (Buttram and Gibbons, 1979; Fedele and Associates, 1987; Heinonen, 1983).

As illustrated in Table 37–2, pregnancy outcome is poor. The reproductive failure is likely to be due to anatomical defects. For example, the increased incidence of abortion may be explained partially by the smaller uterine size and the possible implantation of the zygote in a communicating rudimentary horn. The smaller hemiuterine size almost certainly is an explanation for the increased rates of preterm delivery, fetal growth retardation (Andrews and Jones, 1982), breech presentation (Fedele and associates, 1987; Heinonen, 1983), abnormal uterine function in labor, and the increased incidence of cesarean section.

Tubal pregnancies and pregnancies in the rudimentary horn are special problems associated with a noncommunicating rudimentary horn (Heinonen, 1983). Rolen and associates (1966) reported that in 70 pregnancies with implantations in rudimentary horns, uterine rupture usually occurred prior to 20 weeks gestation. Intraperitoneal hemorrhage may be massive and life threatening.

TABLE 37–2. PREGNANCY OUTCOME IN WOMEN WITH A UNICORNUATE UTERUS

	Semmens 1962	Beernink 1976	Andrews 1982	Heinonen 1982	Buttram[a] 1983	Fedele 1987
Patients	5	5	5	13	31	20
Conceiving	4	4	5	10	?	13
Pregnancies	11	8	13	15	60	29
Horn pregnancy	1	—	—	—	—	1
Abortion (%)	4	1	7	7	29	17
	(36)	(12)	(54)	(47)	(48)	(59)
Premature labor (%)	?	3	2	3	10	3
		(37)[b]	(15)	(20)	(17)	(10)
Term delivery	?	4	4	5	21	8
Live birth rate (%)	(63)	(75)	(45.1)	(40)	(40)	(38)

[a] Partly personal data.
[b] One twin pregnancy.
Modified from Fedele and co-workers: Fertil Steril 47:416, 1987.

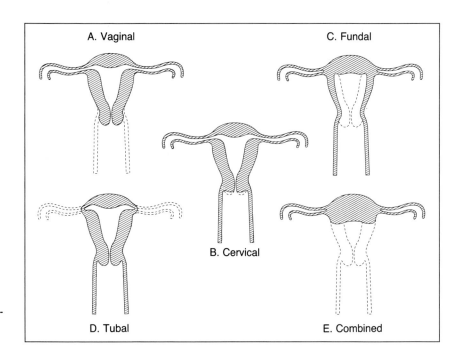

Figure 37–1–I. Class I: Segmental müllerian agenesis or hypoplasia with subdivisions: I-A, vaginal through I-E, combined.

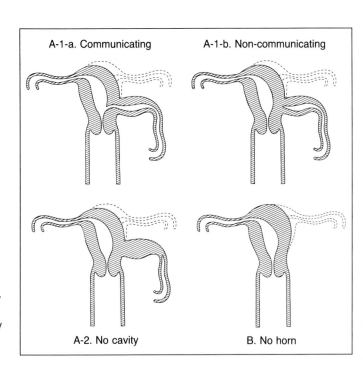

Figure 37–1–II. Class II: Unicornuate uterus either with rudimentary horn (II-A) or without rudimentary horn (II-B). Those with a rudimentary horn (II-A) are divided into those with an endometrial cavity (II-A-1) or without an endometrial cavity (II-A-2). Those with an endometrial cavity either have a communication with the opposite uterine horn (II-A-1-a) or do not have a communication with the opposite horn (II-A-1-b).

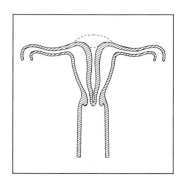

Figure 37–1–III. Class III: Uterine didelphys.

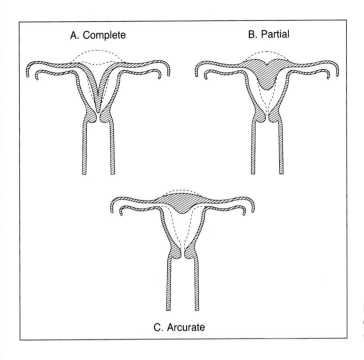

Figure 37–1–IV. Class IV: Bicornuate uterus in which the septum is complete down to the internal os (IV-A), partial (IV-B), or arcuate (IV-C).

A. Complete

B. Partial

C. Arcurate

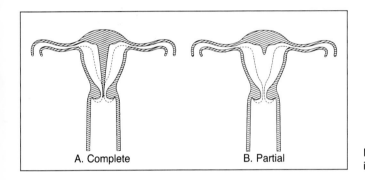

A. Complete

B. Partial

Figure 37–1–V. Class V: Septate uterus with complete septum to the internal or external os (V-A) or partial septum (V-B).

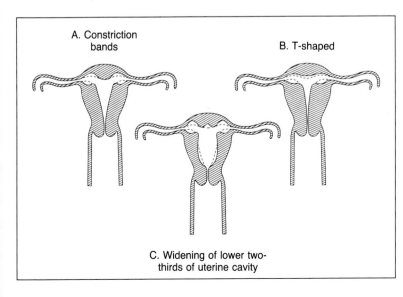

A. Constriction bands

B. T-shaped

C. Widening of lower two-thirds of uterine cavity

Figure 37–1–VI. Class VI: DES anomalies, including uterus with luminal changes, such as constriction bands in the uterine cavity (VI-A), T-shaped cavity (VI-B), and widening of the lower two-thirds of the uterine cavity (VI-C). (*Modified from Buttram and Gibbons: Fertil Steril 32:40, 1979.*)

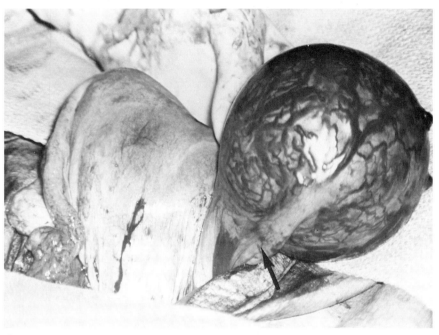

A

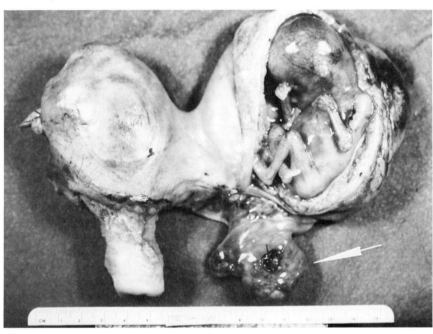

Figure 37–2. A. Pregnancy of 15 weeks gestational age in left rudimentary hemiuterus as seen at laparotomy. The tense, vascular rudimentary uterus was bleeding from veins over its extremely vascular surface. The attached oviduct (*arrow*) was patent and the adjacent left ovary contained the corpus luteum of pregnancy. **B.** Hysterectomy specimen from Figure 37–2A, now with left hemiuterus opened to display the fetus and placenta. The inferior mass (*arrow*) consists of left tube and ovary. There is no cervix on the left and no communication with the right hemiuterus, which does have a cervix that communicated freely with the vagina.

B

Pregnancy in a rudimentary uterine horn 15 weeks after the last menstrual period is shown in Figure 37–2. There was no connection between the rudimentary horn and the opposite uterine horn or the vagina. The fertilizing sperm had to migrate out the oviduct attached to the patent uterine horn and cross transperitoneally to enter the oviduct attached to the rudimentary uterine horn. After the patient had missed three menstrual periods, she complained of sudden, severe, cramping lower abdominal pain. A tender mass was felt to the left of a somewhat enlarged uterus. Fetal heart action was identified in this mass with Doppler ultrasound. At laparotomy, about 200 mL of blood was found free in the peritoneal cavity. A total hysterectomy and left salpingo-oophorectomy were performed. Her three previous pregnancies, all breech presentations,

terminated with delivery of infants who weighed 750 g (expired), 1,220 g (lived), and 2,815 g (lived). The 2,815-g infant was delivered by cesarean section. Although a rudimentary horn was identified at that time, tubal patency to that horn was not interrupted.

Reproductive Performance in Women with Uterine Didelphys (Buttram and Gibbons, Class III). Uterine didelphys is distinguished from bicornuate and septate uteri by the presence of complete reduplication of cervices and hemiuterine cavities (Fig. 37–1–III). In a series of 26 such women, Heinonen (1984) reported that all had longitudinal vaginal septums as well. Although the problems associated with uterine didelphys are similar to those seen with a unicornuate uterus (except for ectopic and rudimentary horn pregnancies), Heinonen (1984) reported a better pregnancy outcome. For example, overall successful pregnancy outcome was 68 percent, with a 30 percent abortion rate and a perinatal mortality rate of only 4 percent.

A uterine didelphys is not without significant problems, however. In addition to the 30 percent abortion rate noted above, Heinonen (1984) observed a preterm delivery rate of 21 percent, fetal growth retardation in 11 percent, breech presentation in 43 percent, and a cesarean section rate of 82 percent! The following case is illustrative of these complications.

A sonogram was obtained in a woman whose uterus was too large for dates (Fig. 37–3A and B). Two separate uterine cavities were seen. A gestational ring, probably abnormal, was first identified in the left cavity. It subsequently degenerated, but tissue was not expelled. Ninety days later, a pregnancy ring was identified in the right uterine cavity (Fig. 37–3C). The interpretation was a missed abortion in the left hemiuterus and a normal-appearing early pregnancy in the right hemiuterus. The latter conception produced a normal fetus who presented as a breech and was delivered at 38 weeks early in labor by cesarean section. The infant weighed 2,900 g and thrived. At the time of surgery, the left kidney was absent. She conceived again, this time in the left hemiuterus and delivered

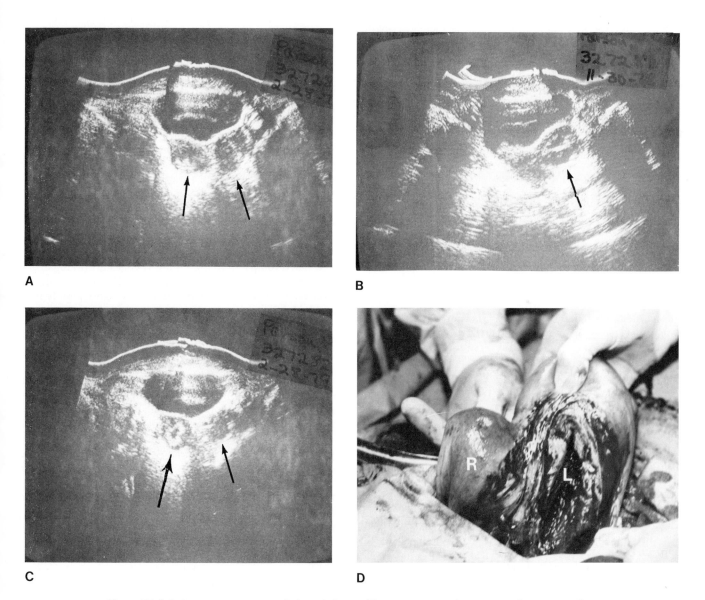

Figure 37–3. In transverse sonogram **A,** two uterine cavities are apparent above arrows. In sonogram **B,** a pregnancy ring, probably abnormal, is seen in the *left* uterine cavity above the arrow. In sonogram **C,** made 90 days later, a normal pregnancy ring is seen in the *right* uterine cavity above the larger arrow but not in the left uterine cavity above the smaller arrow. After seven abortions, a 2,900-g infant was delivered from the right uterus as a double footling breech by cesarean section at 38 weeks gestation. Necrotic placental villi from the missed abortion were expelled from the left uterus 2 days postpartum. **D.** Mother in Figure 37–3A–C conceived again 3 years later in the left uterus (L). A growth-retarded fetus who thrived after cesarean birth was delivered at 37 weeks through a vertical uterine incision. The small right uterus (R) is larger than when nonpregnant.

a severely growth-retarded infant weighing 1,690 g at 37-week gestation. The hemiuteri as they appeared immediately after cesarean delivery are shown in Figure 37–3D.

It is unusual but not rare for twin pregnancies to occur in women with uterine didelphys (Heinonen, 1984; Hochner-Celnikier and colleagues, 1983; Leiberman and co-workers, 1980). Mashiach and associates (1981) even reported a case of triplets with a delivery interval of 72 days! Leiberman and co-workers (1980) also reported a delayed interval between delivery of fetuses from each hemiuterus.

Reproductive Performance in Women with Bicornuate and Septate Uteri (Buttram and Gibbons Classes IV and V). In both these categories, there is a marked increase in abortion rate except for the arcuate uterus, which is merely a slight deviation from normal state. Pregnancy losses in the first 20 weeks were observed by Buttram and Gibbons (1979) to be 88 percent for septate and 70 percent for bicornuate uteri. The etiology of this extraordinarily high pregnancy wastage is thought to be due to partial or complete implantation on the largely avascular septum and the ultimate failure of the conceptus to acquire an adequate blood supply. Once pregnancy is well established, overall outcome is associated with an increased incidence of preterm delivery, abnormal fetal lie, and cesarean section rate.

A hysterosalpingogram usually cannot be used alone to differentiate the septate and bicornuate uterus because of the difficulty of establishing the presence or absence of an external division of the uterus. Buttram and Gibbons (1979) stressed the necessity of laparoscopy to establish the presence of an external uterine division.

TREATMENT

Abnormal fetal presentations, which are commonly seen with an abnormal uterus, generally are treated in the same way as when they are encountered in a normal uterus. Attempts at external podalic version, however, are less likely to be successful and may prove dangerous. If uterine dysfunction develops, it is unwise to stimulate these defective uteri with oxytocin. Cesarean section is safer, but unfortunately the diagnosis often is unexpected.

Cerclage has been attempted in some cases in which cervical incompetence was suspected, and it may be indicated in unicornuate, didelphys, bicornuate, and septate uteri. The question of whether to place a suture in both cervices of a uterus didelphys is unresolved (Heinonen, 1984). There appears to be no reason for cerclage with the arcuate uterus. If active labor supervenes, procrastination in severing a cerclage ligature must be avoided because of the increased risk of uterine rupture (Chap. 29, p. 499).

Progestational agents and β-mimetic drugs administered either acutely or chronically have been used in attempts to prolong gestation. Their efficacy has not been established.

A woman with a uterine anomaly and a poor obstetrical history, for example, repeated abortions not ascribable to some other cause, may benefit from **metroplasty** or plastic repair. Musich and Behrman (1978) and Heinonen and associates (1982) concluded that women with septate or bicornuate anomalies and poor previous obstetrical outcomes are very likely to have good outcomes after repair. In bicornuate uteri (Class IVA and IVB, Fig. 37–1–IV), the method of repair is usually a transab-

dominal metroplasty involving resection of the septum and recombination of the uterine fundus (Kessler and co-workers, 1986). With uterine septa (Class V, Fig. 37–1–V), the management of choice appears to be a transcervical intrauterine resection of the septum accomplished by scissors passed through a hysteroscope (Israel and March, 1984; Fayez, 1986).

INDUCED DEVELOPMENTAL ABNORMALITIES OF THE REPRODUCTIVE TRACT; DIETHYLSTILBESTROL EXPOSURE IN UTERO

For nearly a quarter of a century, until the early 1970s, diethylstilbestrol, a synthetic, nonsteroidal estrogen, was prescribed for an estimated 3 million women in the United States. The enthusiastic endorsements provided in early uncontrolled reports from prestigious medical centers soon established it as the obstetrician's "magic bullet." It was claimed to be highly efficacious in the prevention of most forms of pregnancy wastage, including those resulting from abortion, preeclampsia and other hypertensive disorders, diabetes, and preterm labor!

The first serious problem to be linked to the use of stilbestrol (other than it provided none of the miraculous powers attributed to it initially) was the identification of clear cell adenocarcinoma of the vagina in some daughters who were exposed in utero to stilbestrol (Herbst and co-workers, 1971). It has been established subsequently that the risk of malignancy is slight but real (from 0.14 to 1.4 per 1,000 exposed daughters observed through the age of 24 years).

More recently, the reproductive performances of daughters exposed in utero to stilbestrol have been recognized to be impaired when compared to their unexposed sisters (Mangan and associates, 1982). Moreover, a variety of deformities of the reproductive tract of women exposed in utero subsequently have been identified.

STRUCTURAL ABNORMALITIES

One fourth to one half of women exposed in utero to stilbestrol demonstrate structural variations in the cervix and vagina, including transverse or circumferential ridges involving the vagina and cervix and the presence of hoods and collars over the cervix. The cervix also may be hypoplastic.

Anomalies of the uterine cavity are evident on hysterography in perhaps two thirds of exposed women (Kaufman and associates, 1980). Significantly smaller uterine cavities, shortened upper uterine segments, and T-shaped uterine cavities have been described (Figs. 37–1–VI and 37–4). About one half of those with uterine defects also have cervical defects, especially a hypoplastic cervix. In at least one study, cervical intraepithelial neoplasia has been more common among women exposed to stilbestrol in utero (Fowler and associates, 1981). Finally, a variety of abnormalities of the oviduct have been described, including shortening, narrowing, and absence of fimbriae.

REPRODUCTIVE PERFORMANCE

Lower conception rates are reported for women who were exposed to stilbestrol in utero (Senekjian and co-workers, 1988). Of those who conceive, spontaneous abortions, ectopic pregnancies, and preterm births are increased (Herbst and co-workers, 1981; Kaufman and associates, 1984). The risk is greatest for women with demonstrated structural abnormalities.

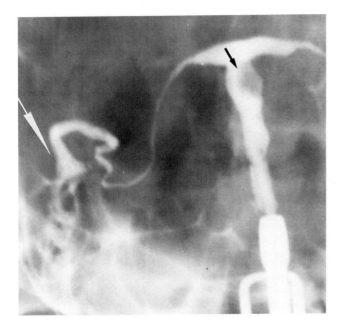

Figure 37–4. Hysterosalpingogram from a woman who was exposed in utero to stilbestrol. Note the T-shaped uterine cavity filled with contrast material that has also spilled from the end of the right oviduct (*white arrow*), demonstrating tubal patency. The filling defect within the uterine cavity (*black arrow*) probably is hyperplastic myometrium, the consequence of the stilbestrol exposure. She has since been pregnant successfully. (*Courtesy of Dr. Bruce R. Carr*.).

TREATMENT

The treatment of clear cell carcinoma of the vagina is gruesome, involving irradiation or radical extirpation. A case of clear cell carcinoma further complicated by pregnancy has been described. The mother was delivered by cesarean section followed immediately by radical hysterectomy, vaginectomy, and pelvic node dissection (Jones and co-workers, 1981).

Management of pregnancies in the presence of structural defects is empirical. The value of cervical cerclage for an incompetent cervix and of tocolytic therapy for preterm labor are not known. Cerclage did not prove to be beneficial in the experiences of Kaufman and colleagues (1984). Conversely, Ludmir and associates (1987) reported that prophylactic cerclage in women with a hypoplastic cervix or a prior second-trimester loss improved prenatal outcome substantively.

Fortunately, these problems from in utero exposure to stilbestrol should eventually disappear since, hopefully, no one has been providing stilbestrol for pregnant women.

UTERINE MALPOSITION

ANTEFLEXION

Exaggerated degrees of anteflexion are frequently observed in the early months of pregnancy, but are without significance. In later months, particularly when the abdominal walls are very lax, the uterus may fall forward. The sagging occasionally is so exaggerated that the fundus lies considerably below the lower margin of the symphysis pubis. Even in less striking instances of so-called *pendulous abdomen*, the pregnant woman may complain of various annoying symptoms, especially dragging pains

in the back and lower abdomen. Amelioration of symptoms is effected by wearing a properly fitted abdominal support.

RETRODISPLACEMENT

Retroversion of the uterus is occasionally encountered during the first trimester, occurring in about 11 percent of women, according to Weekes and associates (1976). They noted not only a higher frequency of bleeding early in pregnancy in women with a retroverted uterus, but also an abortion rate of 16 percent, compared to 9 percent in women whose uterus was not retroverted. In their survey, perinatal mortality was slightly less, however, among women with a retroverted uterus. The biological significance of these observations is not clear. Most authorities no longer regard the retroverted uterus per se to be a pathological finding. Thus, it needs no treatment during pregnancy, except in the rare circumstance in which the growing retroverted uterus does not rise out of the pelvis by the end of the first trimester, but rather remains incarcerated in the hollow of the sacrum, as shown in Figure 37–5. Women with a retroverted uterus should be evaluated frequently early in the second trimester, to make sure that the uterus is not incarcerated. If the uterus cannot be readily identified abdominally above the symphysis, pelvic examination is indicated.

The woman who becomes symptomatic with an incarcerated pregnant uterus is usually first seen complaining of abdominal discomfort and inability to void. As pressure from the full bladder increases, small amounts of urine are passed involuntarily, but the bladder never empties entirely (*paradoxical incontinence*). After the bladder has been emptied by catheterization, the uterus can usually be pushed out of the pelvis when the woman is placed in the knee–chest position; anesthesia is seldom necessary. A retention catheter should be left in place until bladder tone returns. Insertion of a soft pessary usually will prevent reincarceration.

The urinary obstruction from an incarcerated gravid uterus can be so severe as to cause azotemia. With relief of the obstruction, there may be a marked diuresis with the loss of large amounts of sodium and potassium. Swartz and Komins (1977) have described such a case.

SACCULATION OF THE UTERUS

This condition usually arises as a consequence of the pregnant uterus being persistently entrapped in the pelvis by old inflammatory disease or endometriosis. This often will result in the development of an anterior uterine sacculation. Friedman and associates (1986) reported a new version of this complication with the development of a posterior uterine sacculation following aggressive treatment of intrauterine adhesions (Asherman syndrome).

Rarely, the persistently entrapped retroverted uterus produces few symptoms, and yet extensive dilatation of the lower portion of the body of the uterus takes place to accommodate the fetus (Jackson and associates, 1988). In one case at Parkland Hospital, at the time of cesarean section, the Foley catheter bulb just above the urethra in the bladder lay at the level of the umbilicus. The cervix was at an equally high level. Most of the fetus (who was alive and weighed 2,500 g), the amnionic fluid, and the fetal membranes were contained in a remarkably thin sacculation of the anterior wall of the lower segment. The fetal head was entrapped in the most superior part of the saccula-

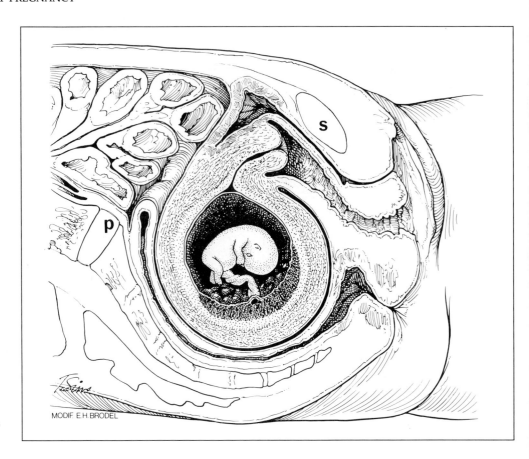

Figure 37–5. Incarceration of retro-flexed pregnant uterus.

MODIF E.H. BRODEL

tion, along with three loops of cord, by a constricting ring of myometrium. The fundus of the uterus and the placenta were contained in the true pelvis beneath a sharp sacral promontory. After delivery, the uterus soon contracted and retracted to assume a more normal shape.

Spearing (1978) stressed the importance of the extremely distorted anatomy just described, and suggested that the finding of an elongated vagina passing above the level of a fetal head deeply placed into the pelvis is suggestive of a sacculation or an abdominal pregnancy. He recommended extension of the abdominal incision to above the umbilicus and delivery of the gravid uterus from the abdomen before an attempt was made to incise it. This simple procedure will restore anatomy to the correct relationships and prevent inadvertent incisions into and through the vagina and bladder. Weissberg and Gall (1972) reviewed the relatively few published reports of sacculation of the pregnant uterus, and Engel and Rushovich (1984) reported the rare possibility of a true uterine diverticulum being confused with sacculation.

PROLAPSE OF THE PREGNANT UTERUS

Impregnation in a totally prolapsed uterus is very rare because of the difficulty of successful coitus, but impregnation when the uterus is only partially prolapsed is more common. In such cases, the cervix, and occasionally a portion of the body of the uterus, may protrude to a variable extent from the vulva during the early months of pregnancy. As pregnancy progresses, however, the body of the uterus usually rises gradually above the pelvis, and may draw the cervix up with it. If the uterus persists in its prolapsed position, symptoms of incarceration may appear during the third or fourth month of pregnancy.

For treatment of uterine prolapse during early pregnancy, the uterus should be replaced and held in position with a suitable pessary. If, however, the pelvic floor is too relaxed to permit retention of the pessary, the woman should be kept recumbent as long as possible until after the fourth month of pregnancy. When the cervix reaches or slightly protrudes from the vulva, scrupulous hygiene is mandatory. If much of the cervix persists outside the vulva and cannot be replaced, the pregnancy should be terminated.

When the vaginal outlet is markedly relaxed, the congested anterior or posterior vaginal walls may prolapse during pregnancy, usually along with bladder (cystocele) and rectum (rectocele), although the uterus may still remain in its normal position. This condition may give rise to considerable discomfort and interfere with locomotion, and it is not amenable to definitive treatment until after delivery. During labor, these structures may be forced down in front of the presenting part and interfere with its descent. In that event, they should be carefully cleansed and pushed back over the descending fetal presenting part.

MISCELLANEOUS CONDITIONS

ACUTE EDEMA OF THE CERVIX

In rare instances, the cervix, particularly its anterior lip, may become so acutely edematous and enlarged during pregnancy that it protrudes from the vulva. This condition, if not associated with preexisting hypertrophy, may disappear with bed rest almost as suddenly as it developed.

ENTEROCELE

In rare instances, an enterocele of considerable size filled with loops of intestine may complicate pregnancy. If this condition occurs during pregnancy, the protrusion should be replaced and the woman kept in the recumbent position. During labor, the mass may interfere with the advance of the fetal head. In such cases, it should be pushed up or held out of the way as well as possible, to allow delivery of the head past the mass.

TORSION OF THE PREGNANT UTERUS

Rotation of the pregnant uterus, most often to the right, is very common during pregnancy. However, torsion of the pregnant uterus of sufficient degree to arrest the uterine circulation and produce an acute abdominal catastrophe is a rare accident of human gestation. We have encountered this situation only rarely in Parkland Hospital.

Bakos and Axelsson (1987) reported a case of severe levotorsion associated with repeated fetal heart rate decelerations to the range of 60 to 70 beats per minute, lasting up to 4 minutes. Because of fetal bradycardia, a cesarean section was performed. As a consequence of the extreme torsion of the uterus, the uterine incision inadvertently was made in the posterior side of the uterus! Both mother and infant survived and no anatomical explanation was found to explain the torsion.

SALPINGITIS AND TUBO-OVARIAN ABSCESS

Gonococcal salpingitis, salpingo-oophoritis, and pelvic peritonitis may develop during the first trimester of pregnancy by ascent of bacteria from the cervix to the endosalpinx, Once the chorion fuses with the decidua to obliterate completely the uterine cavity early in the second trimester, this pathway for ascending bacterial spread by way of the uterine mucosa is interrupted. Thereafter, primary acute inflammation of the tubes and ovaries is rarely, if ever, seen, although tubo-ovarian abscesses may form in previously damaged structures. Presumably, the organisms reach the previously damaged oviduct and ovary through lymphatics or the bloodstream. Jafari and associates (1977) described the successful outcome of a term pregnancy complicated by a tubo-ovarian abscess, as well as the few experiences of others that have been reported.

> In one of two instances of tubo-ovarian abscess complicating midpregnancy treated at Parkland Hospital during the past three decades, hysterectomy, as well as bilateral salpingo-oophorectomy, was carried out. The woman recovered after a very complicated postoperative course. In the other instance, the tubo-ovarian abscess was smaller and was mobilized intact. Therefore, only the affected tube and ovary were removed. The pregnancy subsequently proceeded normally, terminating in spontaneous vaginal delivery of a normal infant.

Even with extensive pelvic adhesions from previous pelvic infection, women usually suffer no adverse effects during pregnancy.

HYDRORRHEA GRAVIDARUM

Rarely, pregnant women may lose clear fluid from the uterus throughout much of pregnancy. The cause of this condition is not always obvious but may represent persistent *amniorrhea* following rupture of the membranes. Gregersen (1976) described a case with loss of fluid beginning about the 10th week

of pregnancy and continuing until delivery at 31 weeks. Up to 20 mL of fluid per day was collected. The ruptured membranes may retract to such an extent as to create an *extramembranous* pregnancy, with the fetus no longer contained within the amnionic sac. Extramembranous pregnancy involving a twin has also been described (Panayiotis and Grunstein, 1979). The membranes were diamnionic and dichorionic, with a single placenta in which there was appreciable circumvallate involvement on the side of the extramembranous fetus. That newborn quickly succumbed from anoxia. Pulmonary hypoplasia, presumably due to lack of amnionic fluid and the inability to inspire in utero, was evident at autopsy. In an era of frequent amniocentesis, this rare complication, fortunately, does not appear to have increased, although Vago and Chaukin (1980) described such a case.

ENDOMETRIOSIS

Severe, active endometriosis is an uncommon complication of pregnancy. As emphasized in Scott's early report (1944), however, women with endometriosis do become pregnant and, in the course of gestation, sometimes exhibit bizarre and vexing clinical symptoms.

A rare complication of ovarian endometriosis in pregnancy is rupture of an endometrial cyst, with clinical features that are suggestive of pyelonephritis, acute appendicitis, or tubal pregnancy (Rossman and associates, 1983). Another is an enlarging pelvic endometrioma that causes dystocia in labor. Most women with unrecognized endometriosis, however, doubtless do go through pregnancy and labor without complications.

ADENOMYOSIS

Azziz (1986) reviewed the literature published for the past 80 years and reported that the incidence of adenomyosis was approximately 17 percent in women over 35 years of age. The condition therefore occurs frequently in pregnancy, but it is rarely associated with obstetrical or surgical problems. In fact, only 29 complications were reported over the 80-year period. These complications consisted of uterine rupture, ectopic pregnancy, uterine atony, and placenta previa.

REFERENCES

American College of Obstetricians and Gynecologists: Genital human papillomavirus infections. Technical Bulletin No 105, June 1987

Andrews MC, Jones HW Jr: Impaired reproductive performance of unicornuate uterus: Intrauterine growth retardation, infertility and recurrent abortion in five cases. Am J Obstet Gynecol 144:173, 1982

Azziz R: Adenomyosis in pregnancy: A review. J Reprod Med 31:223, 1986

Bakos O, Axelsson O: Pathologic torsion of the pregnant uterus. Acta Obstet Gynecol Scand 66:85, 1987

Beernink FJ, Beernink HE, Chinn A: Uterus unicornis with uterus solidaris. Obstet Gynecol 47:651, 1976

Buttram VC, Gibbons WE: Müllerian anomalies: A proposed classification (an analysis of 144 cases). Fertil Steril 32:40, 1979

Carapeto R, Nogales F Jr, Matilla A: Ectopic pregnancy coexisting with a primary carcinoma of the fallopian tube: A case report. Int J Gynaecol Obstet 16:263, 1978

Elias S, Simpson JL, Carson SA, Malinak LR, Buttram VC Jr: Genetic studies in incomplete Müllerian fusion. Obstet Gynecol 63:276, 1984

Engel G, Rushovich AM: True uterine diverticulum: A partial Müllerian duct duplication? Arch Pathol Lab Med 108:734, 1984

Fayez JA: Comparison between abdominal and hysteroscopic metroplasty. Obstet Gynecol 68:399, 1986

Fedele L, Zamberletti D, Vercellini P, Dorta M, Candiani GB: Reproductive performance of women with unicornuate uterus. Fertil Steril 47:416, 1987

Fowler WC Jr, Schmidt G, Edelman DA, Kaugman DG, Fenoglio CM: Risks of cervical intraepithelial neoplasia among DES exposed women. Obstet Gynecol 58:720, 1981

Friedman A, DeFazio J, DeCherney A: Severe obstetric complications after aggressive treatment of Asherman syndrome. Obstet Gynecol 67:864, 1986

Green LK, Harris RE: Uterine anomalies: Frequency of diagnosis and associated obstetric complications. Obstet Gynecol 47:427, 1976

Gregersen E: Extramembranous pregnancy with amniorrhoea. Acta Obstet Gynecol Scand 55:69, 1976

Hacker NF, Berek JS, Lagasse LD, Charles EH, Moore JG: Carcinoma of the cervix associated with pregnancy. Obstet Gynecol 59:735, 1982

Hannigan EV, Whitehouse HH III, Atkinson WD, Becker SN: Cone biopsy during pregnancy. Obstet Gynecol 60:450, 1982

Heinonen PK: Clinical implications of the unicornuate uterus with rudimentary horn. Int J Gynaecol Obstet 21:145, 1983

Heinonen PK: Uterus didelphys: A report of 26 cases. Eur J Obstet Gynecol Reprod Biol 17:345, 1984

Heinonen PK, Saarikoski S, Pystynen P: Reproductive performance of women with uterine anomalies: An evaluation of 182 cases. Acta Obstet Gynecol Scand 61:157, 1982

Herbst AL, Hubby MM, Azizi F, Makii MM: Reproductive and gynecologic surgical experiences in diethylstilbestrol-exposed daughters. Am J Obstet Gynecol 141:1019, 1981

Herbst AL, Ulfelder H, Poskanzer DC: Adenocarcinoma of the vagina, N Engl J Med 284:878, 1971

Hochner-Celnikier D, Yagel S, Beller U, Milwidsky A: Simultaneous pregnancy in each cavity of a double uterus: A case report. Int J Gynaecol Obstet 21:51, 1983

Iosif S, Ulmsten U: Comparative urodynamic studies of continent and stress incontinent women in pregnancy and in the puerperium. Am J Obstet Gynecol 140:645, 1981

Israel R, March CM: Hysteroscopic incision of the septate uterus. Am J Obstet Gynecol 149:66, 1984

Jackson D, Elliott JP, Pearson M: Asymptomatic uterine retroversion at 36 weeks gestation. Obstet Gynecol 71:466, 1988

Jafari K, Vilovic-Kos J, Webster A, Steptoe R: Tubo-ovarian abscess in pregnancy. Acta Obstet Gynecol Scand 56:1, 1977

Jones WB, Woodruff JM, Erlandson RA, Lewis JL Jr: DES-related clear cell adenocarcinoma of the vagina in pregnancy. Obstet Gynecol 57:775, 1981

Kaufman RH, Adam E, Binder GL, Gerthoffer E: Upper genital tract changes and pregnancy outcome in offspring exposed in utero to diethylstilbestrol. Am J Obstet Gynecol 137:299, 1980

Kaufman RH, Noller K, Adam E, Irvine J, Gray M, Jeffries JJ, Hilton J: Upper genital tract abnormalities and pregnancy outcome in DES-exposed progeny. Am J Obstet Gynecol 148:973, 1984

Kessler I, Lancet M, Appelman Z, Borenstein R: Indications and results of metroplasty in uterine malformations. Int J Gynaecol Obstet 24:137, 1986

Kiguchi K, Bibbo M, Hasegawa T, Tsutsui F, Wied GL: Dysplasia during pregnancy: A cytologic follow-up study. J Reprod Med 26:66, 1981

Larsson G, Grundsell H, Gullberg B, Svennerud S: Outcome of pregnancy after conization. Acta Obstet Gynecol Scand 61:461, 1982

Leiberman JR, Schuster M, Piura B, Chaim W, Cohen A: Müllerian malformations and simultaneous pregnancies in didelphys uteri: Review and report of a case. Acta Obstet Gynecol Scand 59:89, 1980

Ludmir J, Landon MB, Gabbe SG, Samuels P, Mannuti MT: Management of the diethylstilbestrol-exposed pregnant patient: A prospective study. Am J Obstet Gynecol 157:665, 1987

Managan CE, Borow L, Burtnett-Rubin MM, Egan V, Giuntoli RL, Mikuta JJ: Pregnancy outcome in 98 women exposed to diethylstilbestrol in utero, their mothers, and unexposed siblings. Obstet Gynecol 59:315, 1982

Mashiach S, Ben-Rafael Z, Dor J, Serr DM: Triplet pregnancy in uterus didelphys with delivery interval of 72 days. Obstet Gynecol 58:519, 1981

McCance DJ, Campion MJ, Clarkson PK, Chesters PM, Jenkins D, Singer A: Prevalence of human papillomavirus type 16 DNA sequences in cervical intraepithelial neoplasia and invasive carcinoma of the cervix. Br J Obstet Gynaecol 92:1101, 1985

McCoy C, Cunningham FG: Unpublished observations

Musich J Jr, Behrman SJ: Obstetric outcomes before and after metroplasty in women with uterine anomalies. Obstet Gynecol 52:63, 1978

O'Leary JL, O'Leary JA: Rudimentary horn pregnancy. Obstet Gynecol 22:371, 1963

Panayiotis G, Grunstein S: Extramembranous pregnancy in twin gestation. Obstet Gynecol (Suppl) 53:34S, 1979

Reid R, Fu YS: Is there a morphologic spectrum linking condyloma to cervical cancer? In Banbury Report 21: Viral Etiology of Cervical Cancer. Cold Spring Harbor, NY, Cold Spring Harbor Laboratory, 1986

Rolen AC, Choquette AJ, Semmens JP: Rudimentary uterine horn: Obstetric and gynecologic implications. Obstet Gynecol 27:806, 1966

Rossman F, D'Ablaing G III, Marrs RP: Pregnancy complicated by ruptured endometrioma. Obstet Gynecol 62:519, 1983

Sandstrom RE, Welch WR, Green TH: Adenocarcinoma of the endometrium in pregnancy. Obstet Gynecol (Suppl) 53:73S, 1979

Scott RB: Endometriosis and pregnancy. Am J Obstet Gynecol 47:608, 1944

Schinfeld JS, Winston HG: Primary tubal carcinoma in pregnancy. Am J Obstet Gynecol 137:512, 1980

Semmens JP: Congenital anomalies of female genital tract: Functional classification based on review of 56 personal cases and 500 reported cases. Obstet Gynecol 19:328, 1962

Senekjian EK, Potkul RK, Frey K, Herbst AL: Infertility among daughters either exposed or not exposed to diethylstilbestrol. Am J Obstet Gynecol 158:493, 1988

Sorensen SS, Trauelsen AGH: Obstetric implications of minor Müllerian anomalies in oligomenorrheic women. Am J Obstet Gynecol 156:1112, 1987

Spearing GJ: Uterine sacculation. Obstet Gynecol 51:11(S), 1978

Starr AJ, Ruffolo EH, Shenoy BV, Marston BR: Primary carcinoma of the fallopian tube: A surprise finding in a postpartum tubal ligation. Am J Obstet Gynecol 132:344, 1978

Swartz EM, Komins JI: Postobstructive diuresis after reduction of an incarcerated gravid uterus. J Reprod Med 19:262, 1977

Syrajanen K: Cervical papillomavirus infection progressing to invasive cancer in less than three years. Lancet l:510, 1985

Toaff ME, Lev-Toaff AS, Toaff S: Communicating uteri: Review and classification with introduction of two previously unrecorded types. Fertil Steril 41:661, 1984

Toaff R: A major malformation—Communicating uteri. Obstet Gynecol 43:221, 1974

Vago T, Chavkin J: Extramembranous pregnancy: An unusual complication of amniocentesis. Am J Obstet Gynecol 137:511, 1980

Weekes ARL, Atlay RD, Brown VA, Jordan EC, Murray SM: The retroverted gravid uterus and its effect on the outcome of pregnancy. Br Med J 1:622, 1976

Weissberg SM, Gall SA: Sacculation of the pregnant uterus. Obstet Gynecol 39:691, 1972

Wiersma AF, Peterson LF, Justema EJ: Uterine anomalies associated with renal agenesis. Obstet Gynecol 47:654, 1976

Woolf RB, Allen WM: Concomitant malformations: Frequent simultaneous occurrence of congenital malformations of the reproductive and urinary tracts. Obstet Gynecol 2:236, 1953

Zanetti E, Ferrari LR, Rossi G: Classification and radiographic features of uterine malformations: Hysterosalpingographic study. Br J Radiol 51:161, 1978

Preterm and Postterm Pregnancy and Inappropriate Fetal Growth

A fetus or newborn infant whose weight is appreciably above or below normal is at increased risk of dying or, if he or she survives, at increased risk of physical and intellectual impairment. Two distinct mechanisms are responsible for these increased risks; these are altered gestational age and inappropriate fetal growth. In the low-birthweight neonate, gestational age may have been shortened or the fetus may have failed to maintain a normal growth rate. In the excessively large neonate, the gestational time may have been prolonged or the fetus may have exceeded the normal growth rate.

In any pregnancy it is essential to have a precise knowledge of the gestational age of the fetus; this knowledge is exceedingly important when the pregnancy is complicated. Gestational age must be known before any diagnosis of inappropriate fetal growth can be made. Unfortunately, for a variety of reasons, gestational age may be unknown or, worse, in error. It may be unknown as a consequence of the woman not obtaining prenatal care until long after events important for the identification of fetal age have passed or been forgotten. An error may result from an unrecognized ovulation delay, for example, following menses induced by withdrawal of an oral contraceptive. Regardless, without an accurate gestational age, the appropriateness of fetal growth *cannot* be established, and serious errors in patient management may result.

ESTABLISHMENT OF GESTATIONAL AGE

It is customary to estimate the time of delivery by adding 7 days to the date of the first day of the last normal spontaneous menses and subtracting 3 months (Naegele's Rule, Chap. 14, p. 258). It is essential to establish that previous spontaneous menses were cyclically predictable and normal in length and that the last bleeding episode was *not* the consequence of oral contraceptive withdrawal.

Additional objective evidence can be established. A urinary pregnancy test (Chap. 30, p. 519) is useful to help document an early pregnancy if the test is positive during the first 6 weeks after the last normal menstrual bleeding began. The time of quickening as well as the detection of fetal heart sounds with a DeLee fetoscope between 17 and 19 weeks gestation (Jimenez and co-workers, 1983) may be used as reliable landmarks of gestational age when they coincide with menstrual history. Measurement of fetal size by ultrasound before the 26th week provides reliable gestational age within days (Sholl and Sabbagha, 1984). Robinson and Fleming (1975) reported that fetal

crown–rump measurements between 7 and 14 weeks gestation had an error of only ±1.2 mm and a range in gestational age of ±4.7 days. O'Brien and associates (1981) reported that measurements of femur length between 12 and 22 weeks gestation varied by only ±1.6 mm and gestational age by ±6.7 days. Biparietal diameter measurements between 17 and 26 weeks gestation were reported to have an error in measurements of only ±0.8 mm but a range of ±10 days (Crane and colleagues, 1977; Hughey and Sabbagha, 1978). After 26 weeks gestation, gestational age assessment by ultrasound has a range of ±14 to 21 days.

Other information is helpful, but does not narrow the gestational age estimate to less than 2 weeks. For example, the height of the uterine fundus corresponds in centimeters to weeks gestation between the 22nd and 30th weeks *when the bladder is empty* (Belizan and associates, 1978; Calvert and associates, 1982; Jimenez and co-workers, 1983; Quaranta and colleagues, 1981). For practical purposes, if the uterine height in centimeters between 22 and 30 weeks is within 2 weeks of the estimated gestational age, based upon an accurate last normal spontaneous menstrual period, then there is sufficient evidence to establish a reasonable but not exact gestational age.

When the last spontaneous menses is known precisely and any one or more of these clinical landmarks—fundal height between 22 and 30 weeks, time of onset of fetal heart sounds, positive pregnancy test at or before 6 weeks—correlate with the estimated age, then assignment of gestational age is possible to within 2 weeks. If the information is unknown or, worse, if it is disparate or appears contradictory, gestational age must be considered uncertain. An exception can be made with the use of sonography during the first half of gestation. If gestational age cannot be assigned accurately, a realistic approach to management of the pregnancy must be based upon the acceptance of this fact (Yeh and Read, 1982; Leveno and associates, 1985b).

DEFINITIONS

The fetus or newborn infant is referred to as a *fetus at term* or an *infant at term* during the interval from the 38th to the 42nd week after the onset of a menstrual period that was followed 2 weeks later by ovulation. The critical date for determining the age of the fetus is the date of ovulation or of fertilization. *The date of onset of the last normal menstrual period is of clinical importance for determining fetal age because it is usually known rather precisely, and when menstrual bleeding is spontaneous and previously regular, it most often is followed by ovulation and fertilization 2 weeks later.* Before the 38th week, *preterm* is the word best applied to categorize the fetus and the pregnancy; at 42 completed weeks and thereafter *postterm* is appropriate. Gestational (menstrual) age should be cited in weeks rather than months or trimesters.

In 1935 the American Academy of Pediatrics defined prematurity as a liveborn infant weighing 2,500 g or less (Cone, 1985). These criteria were used widely until it became apparent that there were discrepancies between gestational age and birthweight because of retarded fetal growth. The World Health Organization in 1961 added gestational age as a criterion for prematurity and defined premature infants as those born at 37 weeks gestation or less. A distinction was made between *low birthweight* (2,500 g or less) and *prematurity* (37 weeks gestation or less).

With continued improved care of the preterm infant, other definitions have been developed. For example, the Collaborative Group on Antenatal Steroid Therapy (1981) reported that the great preponderance of mortality and serious morbidity from preterm birth is prior to 34 weeks. Hence, low birthweight, defined as less than 2,500 g, has been modified now to describe *very low birthweight* (infants weighing 1,500 g or less) and *extremely low birthweight* (those who weigh 1,000 g or less).

Although the term *premature* was used to designate the fetus or infant before the 38th week of gestational age, *premature* should be used to describe function. For example, an infant at birth may have a gestational age of 32 weeks and thus be chronologically preterm, yet from the standpoint of pulmonary function, the infant may demonstrate no respiratory difficulties because pulmonary function is mature. Such an infant probably should be described as preterm with mature pulmonary function. Thus, it seems more appropriate to designate *preterm and postterm to refer to age* and *maturity to refer to function.* We now recognize, as in the example cited above, that time and function are not synchronous, much less synonymous.

Postterm describes the fetus or newborn infant whose gestational age has exceeded 42 weeks. *Postdates* is another term that has achieved considerable usage although the word seems to defy a precise definition as to the "dates" involved, other than perhaps the last menstrual period. Presumably, if the term *postdates* is acceptable, "predates" and "dates" are eligible for incorporation into the medical lexicon.

With respect to gestational age, a fetus or infant may be **preterm, term,** or **postterm.** With respect to size, the fetus or infant may be normally grown or *appropriate for gestational age,* small in size or *small for gestational age,* or overgrown and consequently *large for gestational age.* In recent years, the term *small for gestational age* has been used widely, especially by neonatologists, to categorize an infant whose birthweight is clearly below average and usually below the 10th percentile for its gestational age. Obstetricians more often have used the terms *fetal growth retardation* or the less precise term *intrauterine growth retardation.* The infant whose birthweight is above the 90th percentile has been categorized as *large for gestational age,* and the infant whose weight is between the 10th and 90th percentiles is designated *appropriate for gestational age* (Fig. 38–1).

Typically, the fetus continues to grow after 36 weeks but at a slower rate (Fig. 38–2). When gestation is prolonged beyond term, some fetuses, perhaps the majority, continue to grow and some may achieve a remarkably large size. Those infants who do so have been referred to by some as *postmature* as well as *postterm.* Fetuses who become undernourished and demonstrate evidence of chronic distress in utero have been classified by

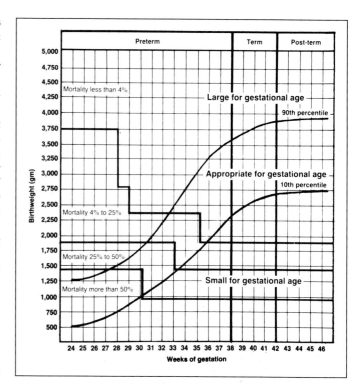

Figure 38–1. Perinatal mortality in relation to birthweight plotted as a function of gestational age. A significant increase in mortality is observed in growth-retarded fetuses below 1,500 g. (*Reproduced with permission from Queenan: Contemp Ob/Gyn 19:197, 1982.*)

some as *dysmature.* Unfortunately, some obstetricians and pediatricians use "postmature" to designate all fetuses and infants in which the pregnancy is postterm, while others apply it only to the macrosomic "overgrown" postterm fetus or infant, and still others designate only the undernourished, chronically distressed, postterm newborn infant as postmature. The term *postmature* literally means "after maturity." For this reason alone, the term *postmature* should be discarded, since the fetus-infant faces many years of growth and development before "maturity" is reached.

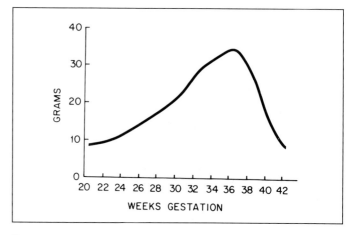

Figure 38–2. Mean daily fetal growth (in grams) during previous week of gestation. (*Adapted from Hendricks: Obstet Gynecol 24:357, 1964.*)

It is more logical to consider time, size, and function as three distinctly different and frequently separate entities. With respect to size, a small for gestational age infant may be *constitutionally* small for genetic reasons, such as small parents, or small as the consequence of an abnormality in function, that is, *growth retarded*. Therefore, *small for gestational age* is a descriptive term for *size* plotted as a function of *time*. *Constitutional* and *growth retardation* are functional terms used to describe the reasons for the small size. *Constitutional* implies a normal, nonpathological course and *growth retardation* implies an abnormal process. Fetal growth retardation then may be further subdivided into *symmetrical* and *asymmetrical* (Fig. 38–3). Similarly, large for gestational age infants may be *constitutionally large* because of large parents or they may be *macrosomic* as a consequence of a pathological process, such as diabetes mellitus. Finally, a neonate whose weight is appropriate for gestational age, that is, between the 10th and 90th percentiles, may still be growth retarded or macrosomic. Put another way, the neonate may be within a normal weight range but appear obese or too thin.

SIGNIFICANCE

These descriptions are shown in Figure 38–3, and the implications are immediately apparent. For example, an infant may be preterm and appropriately grown, or small or large for gestational age. If small for gestational age, the infant may be constitutionally small or may be growth-retarded from a variety of problems. If symmetrically growth-retarded, the fetus may have a chromosomal abnormality. If asymmetrically growth retarded, the fetus may be small because its mother is suffering from any one of a variety of disorders known to reduce maternal-placental perfusion. The preterm constitutionally small for gestational age infant and the symmetrically growth-retarded infant might be expected to have normal amnionic fluid volume. Conversely, the asymmetrically growth-retarded infant likely would have a reduced amnionic fluid volume with intrapartum problems more likely due to umbilical cord compression or placental insufficiency arising from the vascular problems that caused the growth retardation.

Problems in these neonates at birth might then be reversed. For example, the preterm, constitutionally or symmetrically small infant would more likely have respiratory distress than the asymmetrically growth-retarded fetus (Gluck and associates, 1973, 1974). Certainly, there would be more problems if the cause were a chromosomal abnormality. Although the preterm, asymmetrically growth-retarded infant is less likely to have respiratory distress, such an outcome is not assured, and this fetus is more likely to have meconium aspiration and hypoglycemia (Klaus and Fanaroff, 1979; Lubchenco and Bard, 1971).

SUMMARY

The concepts of time, size, and function working as independent or multiple variables must be understood. As cited above, these concepts have immediate obstetrical and pediatric significance. Thus, in the screening, diagnosis, and management of fetuses with different gestational ages and sizes, the use of a common terminology will be likely to result in more appropriate care for these women and their fetuses-infants. There is no perfect classification for comparing the length of gestation to function and fetal or infant size, but the foregoing suggestions are based upon descriptive criteria that can be established, easily understood, and communicated.

STANDARDS FOR NORMAL FETAL GROWTH AND DEVELOPMENT

By now the practice of equating fetal size or maturation with fetal age, which unfortunately has been firmly ingrained into obstetrical and pediatric practices, should have been abandoned. For normal pregnancies there is a strong correlation among these, but at times the fetus-infant who is very small at birth may be chronologically and functionally mature. This phenomenon is likely to be most dramatic when maternal

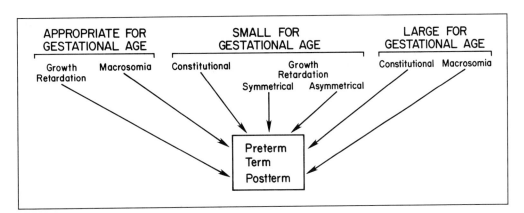

Figure 38–3. Fetal-neonatal age compared to birthweight and functional growth. *Preterm* describes a neonate delivered prior to 38 weeks gestation, and *postterm* after 42 weeks gestation. A term neonate is one delivered between 38 and 42 weeks gestation. A small for gestational age fetus-neonate is below the 10th percentile for weight, while a large for gestational age fetus-neonate is above the 90th percentile. An appropriate for gestational age fetus-neonate is between the 10th and 90th percentiles. A fetus-neonate destined to be either large or small may be described as constitutionally large or small; that is, normal growth potential was reached for that infant. A pathological process results in a growth-retarded or macrosomic fetus-neonate.

chronic vascular disease complicates pregnancy (Figs. 38–4A and B). Conversely, the infant of normal term size may be precariously preterm, as in some pregnancies complicated by gestational diabetes.

FETAL WEIGHTS AT VARIOUS GESTATIONAL AGES

It is difficult to obtain precise standards for determining appropriate or inappropriate growth of the human fetus who is remote from term. In order to determine fetal weight directly, the fetus obviously must have been delivered and weighed, but the fetus of known gestational age who is born preterm often is not the product of a normal pregnancy. Persson and co-workers (1978a and b) reported that fetal growth rate, as measured by serial ultrasonic determination of biparietal diameters, was somewhat retarded before preterm delivery when compared with measurements obtained in fetuses born at term. The differences increased during the third trimester, reaching 3 to 4 mm at 36 weeks. Nonetheless, several investigators have tabulated birthweights at various gestational ages, even though the data are not likely to be as precise as desired (Brenner and colleagues, 1976; Lubchenco and co-workers, 1963).

There is general agreement that the following factors influence birthweight, at least in term pregnancies: (1) *sex:* boys weigh more than girls; (2) *parity:* birthweight increases with parity at least through para 2; and (3) *race:* white babies at term weigh more than black babies. Ideally the standardization of birthweight for gestational age also should take into account maternal height and weight, since they both may influence birthweight.

In four different studies in the United States, the mean birthweights identified at 40 weeks gestation were similar for liveborn infants (Brenner and colleagues, 1976; Hoffman and co-workers, 1974, Lubchenco and associates, 1963; Naeye and Dixon, 1978). The mean birthweight at 40 weeks gestation was 3,335 g and ranged from 3,280 to 3,400 g. As gestational age decreased, however, the relative differences in mean birthweights increased more markedly, mostly because of the large weights recorded by Hoffman compared to the other three groups. Fetal weights throughout pregnancy, including the 10th, 25th, 50th, 75th, and 90th percentiles, with correction factors for parity, race, and sex, as detemined by Brenner and co-workers (1976), are presented in Figure 38–5. The tabulation provided by Lubchenco and associates (1963) appears to be more widely used, despite the fact that these values were obtained in Denver at an altitude of 5,280 feet. The information provided by Brenner and colleagues is likely to be more appropriate for sea level.

PHYSICAL CHARACTERISTICS AT VARIOUS GESTATIONAL AGES

A reasonably precise approximation of gestational age may be obtained in the delivery room or nursery by evaluating the infant's physical and neurological development. Examination of the sole creases, breast nodule size, scalp hair, earlobe formation, posture, and in the male size of the testes and scrotal rugae is performed (Fig. 38–6A). A neurological examination done the day after delivery may be helpful as well (Fig. 38–6B).

Just as fetal or infant size cannot always be equated with age, neither can assessments of physical characteristics be used to assign in all neonates an accurate gestational age. At term there is, indeed, a strong correlation between gestational age and physical characteristics; however, a preterm, small for gestational age infant may exhibit accelerated lung maturation as well as physical characteristics that appear earlier than usually expected. An excellent example of this was seen in the case of the Davis quintuplets (Chap. 34, p. 641). The delivery was by cesarean section at 31.5 weeks gestation. The three largest infants were from separate ova, with the male infant being the heaviest at 1,530 g and the two female infants weighing 1,440 and 1,420 g. The two female infants derived from a single ovum weighed 990 and 860 g. Only the largest infant, the male, developed respiratory distress. Interestingly, in all the neonates, including the male, physical characteristics

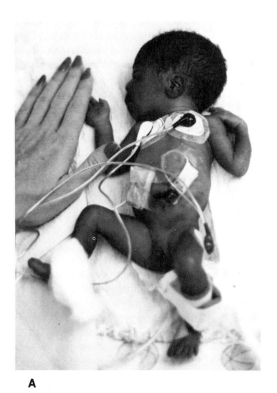

A

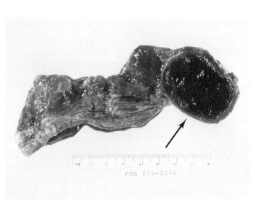

B

Figure 38–4. A. The infant weighed 650 g when delivered at 29 to 30 weeks gestation. The mother had become severely hypertensive. At delivery by cesarean section, there was a subchorial hematoma of many days' duration in the placenta. The infant thrived with no evidence of respiratory distress. **B.** Cross-sectional view of the subchorial hematoma (*arrow*) contained in the placenta of the severely asymmetrically growth-retarded, preterm infant.

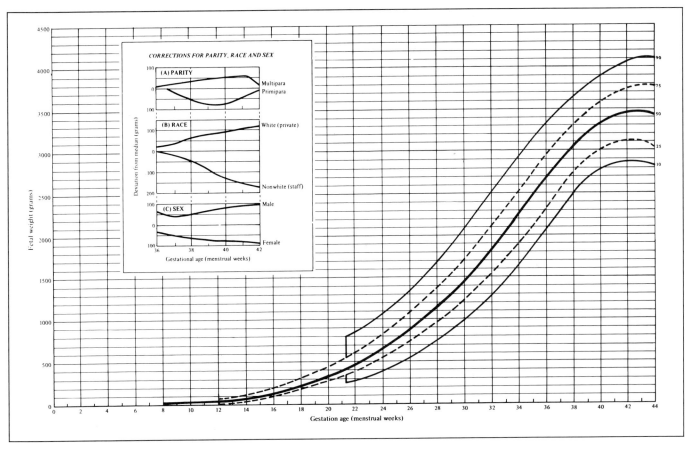

Figure 38–5. Fetal weight. The 10th, 25th, 50th, 75th, and 90th percentiles of fetal weight in grams throughout pregnancy and correction factors for parity, race (socioeconomic status), and sex are graphed. Data obtained from 31,202 prostaglandin-induced abortions and spontaneous deliveries. (*From Brenner and colleagues: Am J Obstet Gynecol 126:555, 1976.*)

were advanced by 2 to 4 weeks beyond what was expected. Moreover, these characteristics varied appreciably from infant to infant by as much as 3 weeks gestational age. The time of conception was known precisely since the pregnancy was the result of induced ovulation. Thus, these five infants were certainly the same age, yet their physical characteristics were quite disparate!

Physical and neurological data used to correlate gestational ages in infants less than 34 weeks necessarily are de-rived from infants whose preterm status may not have been the result of a "normal process," otherwise they would not have been delivered preterm. Physical and neurological evaluations at or shortly after birth can be used to provide reasonable estimates of gestational age but only in a broad sense, similar to that for weight. It does appear, however, that the use of these techniques may narrow the range of gestational age estimates when these methods are compared with size and weight measurements.

PRETERM BIRTH

Obstetrical aproaches to preterm labor and delivery are guided in large part by expectations the obstetrician has for survival of the premature or immature neonate, as well as the therapeutic alternatives available for management of preterm labor. That some very small infants do survive when provided with prolonged, very expensive intensive care has created serious problems in decision making for the obstetrician (Table 38–1). The obstetrician faces the challenge of effecting delivery in such a way as to optimize the status of the fetus-infant at birth, in the event that intensive care will be applied. The neonatologist in turn must make a judgmental decision as how best to dispense the finite resources for medical care provided by the insurance carrier, the family, governmental agencies, the hospital, and by the health care team.

Aside from the survival, another important issue is the quality of life achieved by quite immature, extremely low-birthweight infants. It is apparent that appreciable compromise, both physical and intellectual, afflicts many such children. Given these concerns, at what time in gestation should obstetrical interventions be practiced? Although it is impossible to set precisely the earliest limit for neonatal survival, certain factors inevitably have an impact on the clinical decision-making pro-

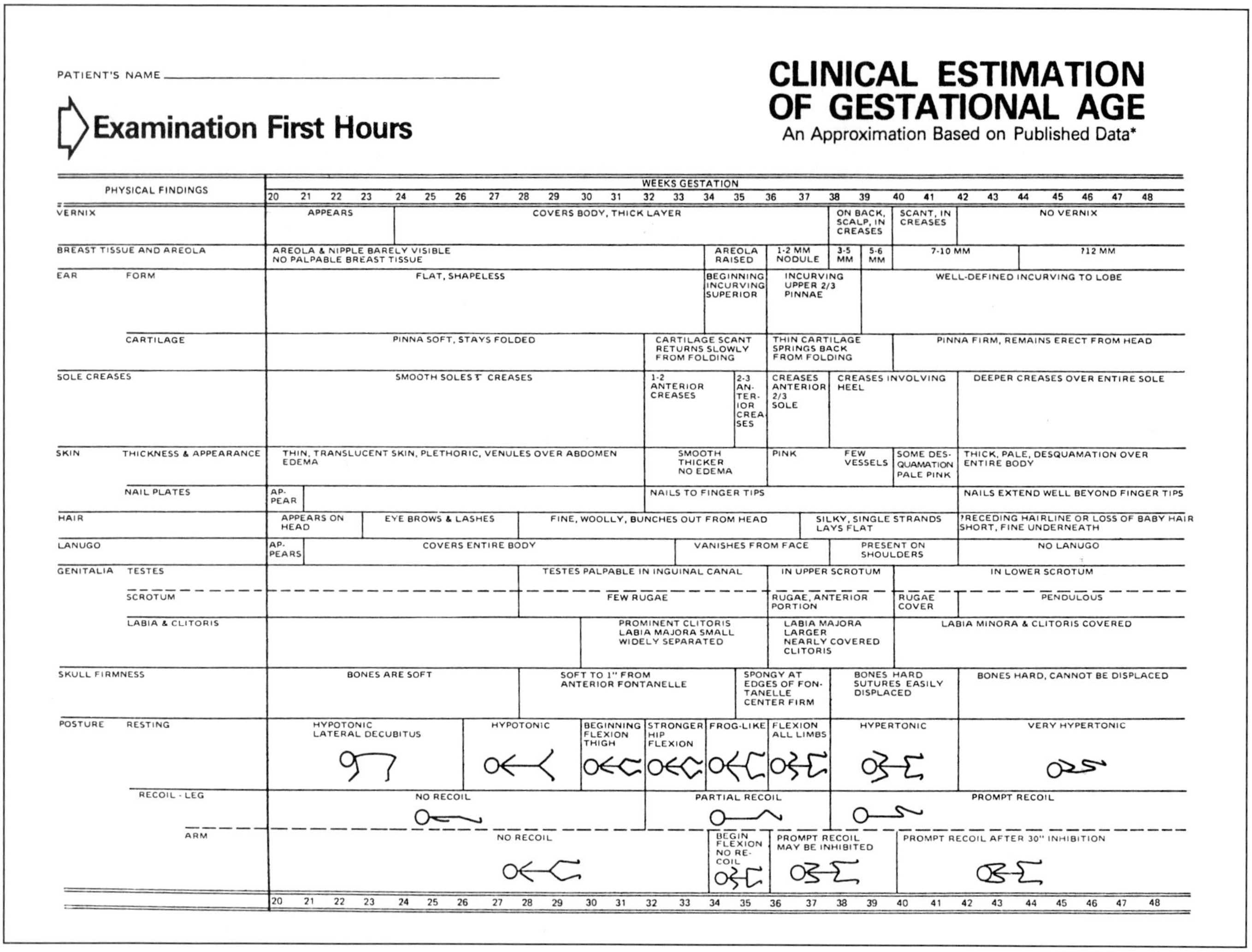

Figure 38–6. A. Clinical estimation of gestational age. (*Reproduced with permission from Brazle and Lubchenco: In Kenipe, Silver, and O'Brien [eds]: Current Pediatric Diagnosis and Treatment, 3rd ed., Lange Medical Publications, 1974, Chap. 3.*)

cess. For example, the obstetrical perception of viability probably influences survival of extremely-low-birthweight infants. Goldenberg and colleagues (1982) surveyed physicians in Alabama in 1978 concerning their perceptions of survival for infants weighing 1,500 g or less or who were at less than 32 weeks, and they found that the physicians tended to underestimate the

TABLE 38–1. MORTALITY AND COST OF MEDICAL CARE FOR 247 INFANTS WEIGHING 500 TO 999 g AND DELIVERED BETWEEN 1977 AND 1981 AT PROVIDENCE, RHODE ISLAND

Birthweight (g)	Number of Infants	Mortality (%)	Cost of Care per Survivor
500–599	15	100	No survivors
600–699	38	97	$363,000
700–799	79	76	$116,000
800–899	50	62	$101,000
900–999	65	40	$ 41,000
Total	247	68	

From Walker and associates: Pediatrics 74:20, 1984.

potential for survival. Importantly, these estimations correlated with their management decisions.

Perceptions of the potential for survival are inevitably confused by difficulties incurred by imprecisely known gestational age, as previously discussed. Most survival data are based upon birthweight rather than fetal age, and individual birthweights vary appreciably between 24 and 26 weeks. For example, infants born between 24 and 26 weeks gestation can vary in weight from 420 to 1,320 g (Brenner and colleagues 1976).

The birthweight-linked survival rates for livebirths during 1985 at Parkland Hospital are shown in Table 38–2. Chances for survival appreciably increase at or above 1,000-g birthweight, whereas this likelihood decreases substantially for those weighing less. These data are consistent with the view that survival, albeit only 13 percent, is possible for infants weighing 500 to 750 g. **In careful review of these extremely low-birthweight surviving infants, it was observed that they were typically growth retarded and therefore of more advanced maturity** (Fig. 38–7). Moreover, they experienced substantial morbidity in the nursery, and the developmental prognosis for several is decidedly guarded. Clearly, expectations for neonatal survival are

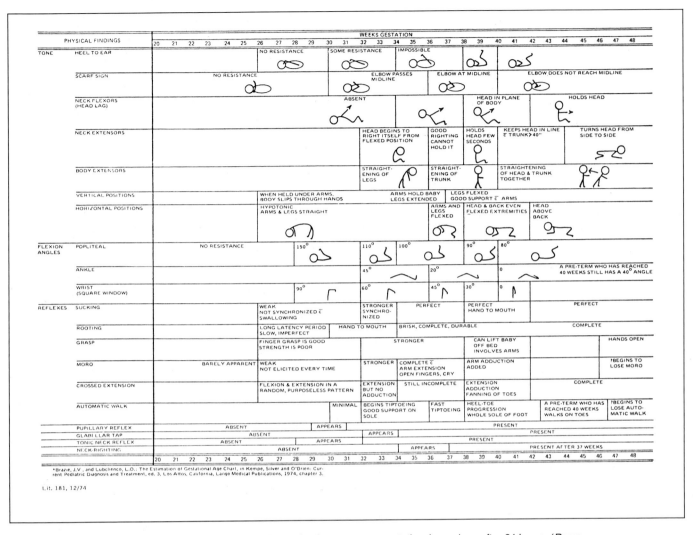

Figure 38–6 (cont.). B. Neurological examination to access gestational age done after 24 hours. (*Reproduced with permission from Brazle and Lubcheneo: In Kenipe, Silver, and O'Brien [eds]: Current Pediatric Diagnosis and Treatment, 3rd ed., Lange Medical Publications, 1974, Chap. 3.*)

TABLE 38–2. SURVIVAL RATES BY BIRTHWEIGHT FOR 13,055 INFANTS BORN DURING 1985 AT PARKLAND HOSPITAL

Birthweight (g)	Number of Livebirths	Number of Neonatal Deaths	Percent Survival
500–750	45	39	13
751–1,000	45	16	64
1,001–1,250	59	7	88
1,251–1,500	73	4	95
1,501–1,750	100	3	97
1,751–2,000	145	4	97
2,001–2,250	318	6	98
2,251–2,500	586	5	99.1
2,501–3,000	3,121	3	99.9
3,001–3,500	5,081	4	99.9
3,501–4,000	2,738	3	99.9
>4,000	746	1	99.9
Total	13,055	95	

Data courtesy of Drs. K. Leveno and C. Rosenfeld.

influenced by gestational age and maturity rather than simply by birthweight.

Unfortunately, there are few studies of neonatal survival according to careful obstetrically determined gestational ages. Gilstrap and co-workers (1985) in San Antonio described survival and short-term morbidity for 105 infants born at 23 to 32 weeks and delivered between 1979 and 1984. The survival rates by gestation are shown in Table 38–3; it appears that survival is possible at 24 but not at 23 weeks. Unfortunately, most survivors born between 24 and 26 weeks had serious morbidity, viz., eight of nine had mild to severe intracranial hemorrhages and seven also suffered retrolental fibroplasia of varying severity.

Yu and colleagues (1986a and b) in Melbourne described their extensive experiences for extremely low-birthweight infants born between 1977 and 1984. They analyzed these outcomes both according to gestational age and to birthweight; their results are shown in Tables 38–4 and 38–5. From their data, it appears that survival as early as 23 weeks is possible;

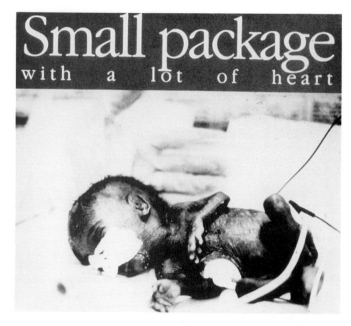

Figure 38–7. Photograph from Parkland Hospital's bimonthly publication, *Highlights*, showing the smallest infant to survive at this institution. The severely asymmetrically growth-retarded infant weighed 520 g when delivered at 28 weeks gestation because of severe maternal hypertension.

however, the prospects for survival without long-term sequelae are remote. At best, no more than 6 or 7 of 100 surviving infants born at 23 to 25 weeks were free of subsequent impairment. *They emphasized that growth-retarded infants had significantly greater survival, but higher disability rates.*

Hack and Fanaroff (1986) in Cleveland reported their results with infants who weighed less than 750 g at birth. They observed that intensive support was being applied to progressively smaller infants, and that such practices had evolved without specific policy. While there were no survivors among 56 infants who received no intensive care, 11 of 41 of these very small infants admitted to the intensive care unit survived to be discharged. Unfortunately, one third of these had moderate to severe neurosensory impairment. Nwaesei and associates (1987) reported that active obstetrical management of preterm delivery at 24 to 26 weeks improved neonatal survival. Although they reported much higher mortality for infants born at 24 to 26

TABLE 38–3. SURVIVAL OF 105 LIVEBORN INFANTS AT WILFORD HALL USAF MEDICAL CENTER ACCORDING TO GESTATIONAL AGE

Gestational Age (wk)	Livebirths	Survivors (%)
23	4	None
24	6	3 (50)
25	7	2 (29)
26	6	4 (67)
27	3	3 (100)
28	17	15 (88)
29	7	7 (100)
30–32	55	52 (95)
Total	105	86 (82)

From Gilstrap and associates: Obstet Gynecol 65:37, 1985.

TABLE 38–4. NEONATAL SURVIVAL BY GESTATIONAL AGE IN 342 EXTREMELY-LOW-BIRTHWEIGHT INFANTS BORN AT ROYAL VICTORIA MEDICAL CENTER, MELBOURNE, AUSTRALIA, 1977–84

Gestational Age[a] (wk)	Inborn Without Malformations	1-Year Survival (%)	Impairment[b] at 2 years (%)	Intact Survivors Calculated per 100 Livebirths
23	27	7	50	3.5
24	40	33	15	4.9
25	39	26	45	11.7
26	58	60	26	15.6
27	83	76	14	10.6
28	91	75	15	11.3

[a] Gestational age based on menstrual data or sonar examination of gestational sac, or both.
[b] Based on 192 infants—includes cerebral palsy (58 percent), developmental delay, blindness, and neurosensory deafness.
From Yu and associates: Br Med J 293:1200, 1986a.

weeks (72 percent), compared to those born at 27 weeks (24 percent), there was similar long-term morbidity for each group at 2 to 4 years of age. This included bronchopulmonary dysplasia, cerebral palsy, blindness, and deafness.

Based on these results from San Antonio, Melbourne, Cleveland, and Halifax, as well as from our experiences in Dallas, it appears that survival between 24 and 26 weeks gestation is possible, but that the long-term prognosis is decidedly guarded. Experiences such as these make it reasonable to set the gestational age for survival at 26 or 27 weeks gestation, which is the current practice at Parkland Hospital.

CAUSES OF PRETERM LABOR

In the majority of instances, the precise cause or causes of labor before term are not known. Listed below are some conditions that predispose to preterm labor and delivery:

1. *Spontaneous rupture of membranes.* Spontaneous labor remote from term commonly is preceded by spontaneous rupture of the membranes. Seldom is the cause of membrane rupture known, but local infection has been implicated more frequently in recent years.
2. *Amnionic fluid infection.* Although its exact incidence in the genesis of preterm labor is not known, there is mounting evidence that perhaps one third of the cases of preterm delivery are associated with chorioamnionic membrane infection. These cases are linked with preterm rupture of membranes, as well as with idiopathic preterm labor.
3. *Anomalies of conception.* Malformations of the fetus or of the placenta not only predispose to fetal growth retardation, but also increase the likelihood of preterm labor as well.
4. *Previous preterm delivery or late abortion.* The woman who previously gave birth remote from term is more likely to do so again, even when no other predisposing factor is identified.
5. *Overdistended uterus.* Hydramnios, especially when acute and marked, or the presence of two or more fetuses, increases the risk of preterm labor, presumably as the consequence of uterine overdistension.
6. *Fetal death.* Death of a fetus remote from term commonly, but not always, is followed by spontaneous preterm labor.
7. *Cervical incompetency.* In a small percentage of women remote from term, an incompetent cervix effaces and dilates not as the result of increased uterine activity, but rather because of an intrinsic cervical weakness.

TABLE 38–5. NEONATAL SURVIVAL BY BIRTHWEIGHT IN 210 EXTREMELY-LOW-BIRTHWEIGHT INFANTS BORN AT ROYAL VICTORIA MEDICAL CENTER, MELBOURNE, AUSTRALIA, 1977–82

Birthweight (g)	Inborn Without Malformations (N = 210)	1-Year Survival (%)	Disability at 2 years[a] (%)	Intact Survivors Calculated per 100 Livebirths
500–599	35	11	33	3.6
600–699	37	27	29	7.8
700–799	34	50	27	13.5
800–899	56	63	24	15.1
900–999	48	67	30	20.1

[a] Based on 108 infants, and includes cerebral palsy (16 percent), blindness (3 percent), sensorineural deficiencies (3 percent), and developmental delay (14 percent).

From Yu and associates: *Br J Obstet Gynaecol* 93:162, 1986b.

8. *Uterine anomalies.* Very uncommonly, anomalies of the uterus are identified in cases of preterm labor and delivery.
9. *Faulty placentation.* Abruptio placentae and placenta previa are more likely to be associated with preterm labor.
10. *Retained intrauterine device.* The likelihood of a preterm labor is increased appreciably when pregnancy and an intrauterine device coexist.
11. *Serious maternal disease.* Systemic disease in the mother, when it is severe, may cause preterm labor and delivery.
12. *Elective labor induction.* Incorrect estimation of gestational age can create undue concern over presumed prolonged gestation, or it leads to considerable patient pressure for intervention. Induction of labor in some instances has been performed primarily for convenience, but the use of oxytocin specifically for **elective** induction has been disapproved by the Food and Drug Administration.
13. *Unknown causes.* Unfortunately, too many cases have to be so categorized.

Arias and Tomich (1982), in their study of 355 liveborn infants weighing between 600 and 2,500 g, reported the following causes of preterm birth: prematurely ruptured membranes (35 percent), preterm labor (30 percent), and other maternal fetal complications (35 percent). The latter included multifetal pregnancy, hypertensive disorders, congenital malformations, placental abruption, and placenta previa. Thus, approximately two thirds of preterm births are the result of either idiopathic preterm labor or preterm rupture of membranes. Leveno and associates (1985a) described a similar distribution of causes for preterm births before 34 weeks gestation at Parkland Hospital.

AMNIONIC FLUID INFECTION

Chorioamnionic infection caused by a variety of microorganisms has emerged as a possible explanation for many heretofore unexplained cases of ruptured membranes and/or preterm labor. Although group B streptococcal cervical infection was associated with prematurity more than 25 years ago, there was renewed interest when Bobbitt and Ledger (1977) implicated subclinical amnionic fluid infection as a cause of preterm labor. The list of putative microorganisms has become extensive (Hiller and associates, 1988). The possibilities include many of the organisms that commonly comprise normal cervicovaginal flora, such as aeorbic and anaerobic bacteria, mycoplasmas, chlamydiae, and yeast. This extensive list is consistent with the view that a common mechanism may exist. Schwarz and co-workers

(1976) suggested that term labor is initiated by activation of phospholipase A_2, which cleaves arachidonic acid from within fetal membranes, thereby making free arachidonic acid available for prostaglandin synthesis. Subsequently, Bejar and colleagues (1981) reported that many microorganisms produce phospholipase A_2, and thus, potentially at least, may initiate preterm labor. More recently, Cox and associates (1989) provided data that are consistent with the view that bacterial endotoxin (lipopolysaccharide) in amnionic fluid stimulates decidual cells to produce cytokines and prostaglandins that may initiate labor. Romero and co-workers (1987 and 1988) and Cox and associates (1988a) reported that the *Limulus* amebocyte lysate assay for endotoxin may be of clinical use in detecting intra-amnionic infections caused by gram-negative bacteria.

PRETERM LABOR WITH RUPTURED MEMBRANES

An intense inflammatory reaction at the site of prematurely ruptured membranes was noted as early as 1950, and this suggested infection. More recently, McGregor and colleagues (1987) demonstrated that in vitro exposure to bacterial proteases reduced the bursting load of fetal membranes. Thus, microorganisms given access to fetal membranes may be capable of causing membrane rupture, preterm labor, or both.

The renewed interest in a possible microbial pathogenesis of preterm labor has prompted many investigators to evaluate amniocentesis for management of women with preterm labor or prematurely ruptured membranes. Garite and colleagues (1979) successfully performed sonar-directed amniocentesis in 30 of 59 women with ruptured membranes between 28 and 35 weeks. As none had clinical infection, their purpose was to establish fetal lung maturity while evaluating Gram stain and culture of amnionic fluid. Surprisingly, the fluids from nine women (30 percent) contained bacteria; six of these women developed chorioamnionitis, and two neonates developed infection. They suggested that this approach might be reasonable when management choices included a substantial delay in delivery.

Several authors now have reported that bacteria, but not leucocytes, seen on stained amnionic fluid reliably correlate with infection. Moreover, mature lecithin:sphingomyelin ratios were found by Cotton and associates (1984a) in 62 percent of cases. Amniocentesis seems quite safe, although Broekhuizen and co-workers (1985) reported one case of heavy vaginal bleeding in 79 attempts. More recently, Gonik and colleagues (1985) reported that oligohydramnios identified by ultrasound was linked to antepartum clinical chorioamnionitis. Vintzileos and colleagues (1986) reported a similar association between oligohydramnios and bacterial colonization of amnionic fluid collected at amniocentesis.

Despite these reports, it has not been shown that amniocentesis in the management of preterm rupture of the membranes is associated with improved pregnancy outcomes. For example, Feinstein and colleagues (1986) compared 73 cases of preterm ruptured membranes managed with the aid of amniocentesis to 73 matched historical controls. There were no differences in fetal condition at delivery, incidence of neonatal infection, or perinatal mortality.

PRETERM LABOR WITH INTACT MEMBRANES

In 8 of 31 pregnancies (25 percent) with preterm labor and intact membranes, amnionic fluid bacterial colonization was identified without clinical evidence of infection (Bobbitt and colleagues, 1981). Women from whom bacteria were identified almost always delivered within 48 hours despite tocolysis, in contrast to those with sterile amnionic fluids. Others since have confirmed "silent amnionitis" in some cases of preterm labor and have suggested that amniocentesis might be useful. Leigh and Garite (1986) observed that women with membrane rupture following amniocentesis were encountered only when amnionic fluid was colonized, and they suggested a bacterial pathogenesis for membrane rupture following the onset of preterm labor. As previously discussed, the efficacy of the routine use of amniocentesis in preterm labor has not been established.

Other approaches to defining a role for microorganisms include studies of the vaginal flora during pregnancy. Colonizations versus **possible** infection with *Trichomonas vaginalis*, *Bacteroides* species (Minkoff and associates, 1984), *Chlamydia trachomatis* (Alger, 1988; Gravett, 1986, and their co-workers), and mycoplasma (McCormack and colleagues, 1987) have been implicated as causes of preterm birth or low-birthweight infants. These observations led some to give antimicrobial treatment, and McCormack and colleagues (1987) reported that erythromycin given after midpregnancy prevented most low-birthweight deliveries in mycoplasma-colonized women. The Infectious and Prematurity Study Group (Eschenbach and associates, 1988) subsequently presented data that erythromycin given beginning at 23 to 26 weeks and continued until 36 weeks had no impact on pregnancy outcome in women colonized with *Ureaplasma urealyticum*. McGregor and associates (1988) reported that a 1-week course of erythromycin therapy given at 26 to 29 weeks to 200 women at high risk for preterm birth showed a trend to greater birthweight and gestational age, as well as reduced preterm ruptured membranes and preterm birth. Further investigation is warranted before adopting widespread screening and treatment to eradicate these genital tract microorganisms.

PRETERM RUPTURE OF MEMBRANES

Rupture of the membranes remote from term is better referred to as *preterm rupture of the membranes* rather than *premature rupture of the membranes*. Premature rupture of the membranes has been applied most commonly to rupture of the membranes at any time before the onset of labor irrespective of whether the duration of gestation at the time of rupture was 24 weeks or 44 weeks.

Preterm rupture of the membranes is defined as rupture of the membranes before 38 weeks gestation and is an important cause of maternal and perinatal morbidity and mortality. Most often, rupture is spontaneous and for unknown reasons. At times, unfortunately, the cause is iatrogenic, as the consequence of an ill-timed attempt to induce labor. Techniques for identification of rupture of the membranes are discussed in Chapter 16 (p. 308).

NATURAL HISTORY OF PRETERM MEMBRANE RUPTURE

Cox and associates (1988b) described the pregnancy outcomes of 298 consecutive women delivered following spontaneously ruptured membranes between 24 and 34 weeks gestation. Although this complication was identified in only 1.7 percent of pregnancies, it contributed to 20 percent of all perinatal deaths during that time period.

Preterm membrane rupture was found to be associated with other obstetrical complications that impact perinatal out-

come, including multifetal gestation, breech presentation, chorioamnionitis, and fetal distress in labor. As a consequence of these complications, cesarean sections were done in nearly 40 percent of the women. The most striking finding was the apparent inevitability of labor within a short time following membrane rupture. At admission, 76 percent of the women were already in labor, 5 percent were delivered for other complications, and another 11 percent were delivered following spontaneous labor within 48 hours. Thus, in only 7 percent was delivery delayed 48 hours or more after membrane rupture. This latter subgroup, however, appeared to benefit from delayed delivery, since no neonatal deaths occurred. This was in contrast to a neonatal death rate of 80 per 1,000 in infants delivered within 48 hours of membrane rupture.

Unfortunately, perinatal outcome in surviving infants in whom labor is delayed is not always satisfactory (Moretti and Sibai, 1988). In a previous study from Parkland Hospital, Hankins and associates (1984) reported that 30 percent of 176 such infants required ventilator therapy. Overall, 13 percent died in the neonatal period and another 3 percent died before age 1. Care of these infants born preterm required 5,104 newborn hospital days (almost 14 years) and cost $2.3 million just for bed space. Importantly, follow-up to 4 years of age was carried out for 105 of these infants, and neurological abnormalities of varying degrees were found in 17. Based upon these experiences, it seems that of infants born to women with preterm ruptured membranes, and in whom labor was delayed, at least 30 percent either died or were neurologically damaged.

MANAGEMENT

Attempts to avoid delivery when there is preterm ruptured membranes is of two primary forms: (1) nonintervention or *expectant management*, in which nothing is done and spontaneous labor is simply awaited, and (2) intervention that may include corticosteroids, given with or without tocolytic agents to arrest preterm labor in order that the corticosteroids have sufficient time to induce pulmonary maturation. Simple expectant management, apparently widely practiced in the 1950s, was again adopted during the 1970s, and most obstetricians today elect such management. Capeless and Mead (1987) conducted a national survey of management practices for preterm ruptured membranes and reported that 97 percent of respondents recommended expectant management. There was no consensus regarding use of corticosteroids for inducing lung maturation or tocolytics to forestall labor.

Despite an extensive literature on the management of preterm ruptured membranes, few prospective randomized studies have been performed. An exception, however, is the study by Garite and colleagues (1981), who studied 160 pregnancies with preterm ruptured membranes between 28 and 34 weeks gestation. The women were divided into two groups: (1) expectant management only or (2) corticosteriods plus tocolysis with either intravenous ethanol or magnesium sulfate. The authors concluded that active interventions did not improve perinatal outcomes and may have aggravated certain infection-related complications, such as maternal pelvic infections. Subsequent randomized studies by Garite and associates (1987) and Nelson and colleagues (1985) failed to show benefits for tocolysis, either with or without steroid therapy.

Thus, current data are consistent with a view that favors hospitalization with simple expectant management that includes close observation for evidence of maternal or fetal infection. At Parkland Hospital, pregnancy complicated by preterm rupture of the membranes is managed as follows:

1. One sterile speculum examination is performed to identify fluid coming from the cervix or pooled in the vagina. Demonstration of visible fluid or a positive Nitrazine test is indicative of ruptured membranes. Attempts are made to visualize the extent of cervical effacement and dilatation, but a digital examination is not performed.
2. Ultrasound examination is performed to help confirm gestational age, identify the presenting part, and assess amnionic fluid volume.
3. If the gestational age is 33 completed weeks or less and there are no other maternal or fetal indications for delivery, the woman is observed closely in Labor and Delivery, with continuous fetal heart rate monitoring to look for evidence for cord compression, especially if labor supervenes.
4. If there is no evidence of fetal jeopardy, or if labor does not begin, the woman is transferred to the High-Risk Pregnancy Unit for close observation for signs of labor, infection, or fetal jeopardy.
5. If the gestational age is greater than 33 completed weeks and if labor has not begun spontaneously in 12 hours, a time period that provides for adequate evaluation, labor is induced carefully with an intravenous infusion of dilute oxytocin, avoiding hyperstimulation. A breech presentation or transverse lie are contraindications for induction. If induction fails, cesarean section is performed. At this and many other institutions, neonatal mortality is now very low for infants born after 33 weeks gestation.
6. Labor and delivery are managed so as to minimize maternal hypotension and fetal hypoxia and acidosis, as well as infection, since these events are known to increase the likelihood of fatal respiratory distress.

CHORIOAMNIONITIS

Assuming that no untoward perinatal outcome results from an entangled or prolapsed cord or perhaps from placental abruption associated with oligohydramnios (Vintzileos and associates, 1987), the greatest concern of prolonged membrane rupture is for maternal and fetal infection. If chorioamnionitis is diagnosed, prompt efforts to effect delivery, preferably vaginally, are initiated. Unfortunately, fever is the only reliable indicator for making this diagnosis; a temperature of 38°C or higher accompanying ruptured membranes implies infection. Leucocytosis has been found to be unreliable, at least by most investigators, and this has also been our experience.

With chorioamnionitis, fetal and neonatal morbidity are substantively increased. In a prospective study of 698 women between 26 and 34 weeks with preterm ruptured membranes, Morales (1987) reported that 13 percent developed chorioamnionitis diagnosed by oral temperatures of 38°C and no other cause for fever. As shown in Table 38-6, infants born to women with chorioamnionitis had a fourfold increased neonatal mortality and a threefold increase in the incidence of respiratory distress, neonatal sepsis, and intraventricular hemorrhage. Antibiotic therapy prior to overt chorioamnionitis appears to reduce these complications and may prolong the time interval from membrane rupture to delivery (Amon and co-workers, 1988; Gilstrap and colleagues, 1988).

ACCELERATED MATURATION OF PULMONARY FUNCTION

The infant who is born long before term is a candidate for the development of severe idiopathic *respiratory distress syndrome* (Chap. 33, p. 593). The intense hypoxia and acidosis that ensue as the consequence of inadequate alveolar-capillary exchange of oxygen and carbon dioxide may prove fatal. Moreover, some infants who survive severe respiratory distress may suffer lifelong physical or functional impairment. Since a major factor in the development of the respiratory distress syndrome is inadequate production of pulmonary surfactant, intense interest persists concerning those phenomena involved in surfactant production (Chap. 6, p. 107).

A variety of clinical events, some well defined and others that are not, predispose to accelerated maturation of surfactant production sufficient to protect against the development of respiratory distress. Gluck (1979) emphasized that surfactant production is likely to be accelerated remote from term in pregnancies complicated by the following conditions:

1. *Maternal:* Chronic renal or cardiovascular disease, long-standing pregnancy-induced hypertension, sickle cell disease, heroin addiction, or hyperthyroidism.
2. *Placenta and membranes:* Placental infarction, chronic focal retroplacental hemorrhage, chorioamnionitis, or ruptured membranes.
3. *Fetal:* The anemic member of parabiotic twins or the smaller member of nonparabiotic twins.

TABLE 38-6. PRETERM RUPTURED MEMBRANES—EFFECT OF CHORIOAMNIONITIS ON NEONATAL OUTCOME

Infection	Gestational Age (wk)	Respiratory Distress (%)	Intraventricular Hemorrhage (%)		Sepsis (%)	1-Minute Apgar < 7 (%)	Mortality
			Total	Severe			
Not identified (N = 606)	31.2	35	22	8	11	16	60/1,000
Chorioamnionitis (N = 92)	30.2	62[a]	56[a]	24[a]	28[a]	49[a]	250/1,000[a]
Diagnosis to delivery Interval							
< 6 hr	30.2	67	58	25	27	50	250/1,000
> 6 hr	30.1	57	55	23	30	50	250/1,000

[a] P < 0.01 for chorioamnionitis group compared to group with no infection.
Adapted from Morales: Obstet Gynecol 70:183, 1987.

RUPTURE OF THE MEMBRANES

Of those conditions listed above, ruptured membranes remote from term is of exceptional importance. This is true not only because of its frequency but also because of the possibility that delay in delivery may soon be followed by lung maturation, either spontaneous or pharmacologically induced, that would more than offset the risk of infection imposed by delay in delivery. In some reports, but not all, a remarkable decrease in the incidence of respiratory distress has been reported for the grossly preterm infant who was delivered more than 24 hours after gross rupture of the membranes. Yoon and Harper (1973), for example, in a retrospective study of infants whose birthweights were 1,000 g to 2,165 g, noted a frequency of respiratory distress of only 3 percent if membranes were ruptured more than 24 hours before delivery, compared to 21 percent if ruptured less than 12 hours. Other investigators have provided—at most—only partial confirmation, while some have failed to provide any confirmation. Interestingly, removal of most of the amnionic fluid does not appear to accelerate pulmonary maturation in the fetal lamb.

GLUCOCORTICOID THERAPY

The observations by Liggins and Howie of the effects of glucocorticoids on lung maturation rightfully have received considerable attention (Howie and Liggins, 1977; Liggins and Howie, 1974). On the basis of their previous observations that corticosteroids administered to the ewe accelerated lung maturation in the preterm fetus, they performed a well-designed study to evaluate the effects of maternally administered betamethasone to prevent respiratory distress in the subsequently delivered preterm infant. Infants born before 34 weeks had a significantly lowered incidence of respiratory distress and neonatal mortality from hyaline membrane disease if birth was delayed for at least 24 hours and up to 7 days after completion of steroid therapy.

The mechanism by which betamethasone or other corticosteroids reduces the frequency of respiratory distress is not clear. Interestingly, the protective action is likely to be transient. Liggins and Howie (1974) noted that the frequency of respiratory distress increased when the infant was born more than 7 days after treatment with betamethasone, compared to that for infants delivered 1 to 7 days after completion of therapy. Moreover, Brown and associates (1979) observed in chronically catheterized fetal lambs that the increase in surfactant that followed dexamethasone administration was transient, with surfactant levels falling to pretreatment values within 8 to 10 days. Therefore, if such compounds are used, retreatment must be considered whenever delivery has not occurred within 7 days of the initial treatment and the risk of early delivery persists.

Not all workers have reported salutary effects from corticosteroid administration. Quirk and co-workers (1979) identified no difference in fetal outcomes with and without the use of betamethasone. The incidence of respiratory distress (about 15 percent) and survival (about 87 percent) was similar in both groups of infants whose mothers were or were not given betamethasone. Subsequently, Simpson and Harbert (1985) reported that respiratory distress was significantly more frequent following the use of glucocorticoids in women with preterm ruptured membranes if the fetus was delivered after 48 hours.

Collaborative Study on Antenatal Steroid Therapy (1981)

A trial of corticosteroid therapy, funded by the National Institutes of Health, was initiated in 1976, and the results published in 1981.

This double-blind collaborative trial was conducted at five centers, and of 7,893 women identified to be in preterm labor, 696 women at risk for preterm birth between 26 and 37 weeks were entered. Women randomized to steroid therapy were given intramuscular dexamethasone, 5 mg every 12 hours for a total of up to four doses. A total of 720 infants were available for analysis. A smaller number of infants, but significantly fewer, whose mothers were given dexamethasone, developed respiratory distress (13 versus 18 percent). Importantly, more than 80 percent in each study group did not develop respiratory distress.

In September 1985 a workshop on approaches for preventing neonatal respiratory distress was held in Washington, DC, to review the results of the Collaborative Study (Avery and colleagues, 1986). The group agreed that no difference in terms of cognitive, motor, or neurological function were found when 406 of the study infants were followed to 36 months of age, suggesting that steroid treatment did not adversely effect the subsequent short-term neurological development (Collaborative Group, 1984). They further concluded that dexamethasone appeared beneficial only to a female fetus of more than 30 weeks gestation who was delivered within 24 hours. Thus it is apparent that there are still many unresolved issues regarding the efficacy of antenatal steroid treatment for the prevention of respiratory distress.

The decision whether or not to use potent glucocorticoids to try to minimize the risk of severe respiratory distress in the preterm infant is a difficult one. There is evidence that some reduction in the frequency of this serious pulmonary disorder follows the use of glucocorticoids, but these compounds do not eradicate the disease. At the same time, there are risks, immediate and remote, from the use of agents as potent as betamethasone. From the standpoint of the mother, the metabolic derangements that characterize diabetes are likely to be intensified, and severe pregnancy-induced hypertension may be worsened, the risk of infection is increased, and wound healing may be impaired, especially so in cases of abdominal delivery. Moreover, the combination of a glucocorticoid to hasten lung maturation and and a tocolytic agent to try to delay delivery may induce maternal pulmonary edema. Pulmonary edema has developed during the course of therapy with betamethasone or dexamethasone plus the β-adrenergic stimulators terbutaline or ritodrine, the prostaglandin synthase inhibitor indomethacin, and magnesium sulfate (Elliott and colleagues, 1979; Rogge and co-workers, 1979).

From the standpoint of the fetus-infant there is an increased immediate risk from maternally administered steroids. These risks include deterioration in utero as a consequence of the maternal complications just described, as well as an increased risk of sepsis from the use of the steroids. Taeusch and associates (1979) identified serious infection in 13 percent of liveborn infants whose mothers had ruptured membranes and had received dexamethasone. In addition, 27 percent of the mothers also became infected. In the control group, 6 percent of the infants and 12 percent of the women became infected. While neonatal deaths due to respiratory distress were decreased in the steroid-treated group compared to the control group, the overall neonatal mortality in both groups was the same because of the increased number of fetal deaths due to sepsis in the steroid-treated group.

The long-term risks to the surviving infant from glucocorticoids so used are not yet known. The adverse effects to experimental animals that have been described following the administration of such steroids around the time of birth are discouraging. For example, in pregnant rats, following betamethasone administration, the fetal death rate was increased;

among survivors, growth was impaired, with total body weight and weights of the brain, heart, liver, kidneys, and adrenals reduced (Mosier and colleagues, 1979). In the rhesus monkey fetus, reduced fetal head circumference has been described (Johnson and co-workers, 1979). Liggins (1976, 1982), however, found no gross difference with regard to intelligence quotient and social adjustment among children at 4 years of age whose mothers had received betamethasone according to the protocol described. In the preliminary observations made by Brown and associates (1979), no delay in development was found following antenatal treatment with dexamethasone beyond that seen in infants not so exposed.

Opinion as to the efficacy of glucocorticoid prophylaxis remains sharply divided in major perinatal centers. If there has been a recent trend, it probably has been toward not using them. For all of these reasons, and especially because of their questionable benefits, at Parkland Hospital glucocorticoids have not been employed routinely in women remote from term to try to reduce the risk of respiratory distress.

IDENTIFICATION OF WOMEN AT RISK FOR PRETERM BIRTH

Obstetrical approaches to preterm birth traditionally have been focused primarily on treatment interventions rather than earlier identification of women at risk. Papiernik and Kaminski (1974) and Creasy and associates (1980), however, have emphasized the potential importance of identification, since many treatment interventions fail once labor is firmly established.

RISK-SCORING SYSTEMS

Application of the risk-scoring system devised by Papiernik and modified by Creasy has resulted in preliminary observations that such a system might be beneficial. The efficacy of this approach is currently being tested in a multicenter trial supported by the March of Dimes. In this system, scores of 1 through 10 are given to a variety of pregnancy factors, including socioeconomic status, reproductive history, daily habits, and current pregnancy complications (Creasy and associates, 1980). Women with scores of 10 or more are considered to be at high risk for preterm delivery. While Creasy (1980) and Covington and associates (1988) reported salutary results, the experiences of Main and associates (1985) in Philadelphia using this scoring system with indigent women was less satisfactory.

Certain features included in these scoring systems may be more useful than others in predicting the risk of preterm delivery and therefore warrant closer examination.

Prior Preterm Birth

A history of prior preterm delivery strongly correlates with subsequent preterm labor. Shown in Table 38–7 is the incidence of recurrent spontaneous preterm birth in 6,072 Scottish women (Carr-Hill and Hall, 1985). The risk of recurrent preterm delivery for those whose first delivery was preterm increased threefold compared to women whose first infant reached term. Strikingly, almost one third of women whose first two infants were preterm delivered preterm infants during their third pregnancies.

Cervical Dilatation

Asymptomatic cervical dilatation after midpregnancy recently has gained renewed attention as a risk factor for preterm deliv-

TABLE 38–7. RECURRENT SPONTANEOUS PRETERM BIRTH ACCORDING TO PRIOR OUTCOME IN 6,072 SCOTTISH WOMEN

First Birth	Second Birth	Next Birth Preterm (%)
Term	—	5
Preterm	—	15
Term	Preterm	24
Preterm	Preterm	32

From Carr-Hill and Hall: Br J Obstet Gynaecol 92:921, 1985.

ery. Some have considered such dilatation to be a normal anatomical variant, particularly in parous women; however, this is no longer universally accepted (Leveno, 1986a; Neilson, 1988; Papiernik, 1986; Stubbs, 1986, and their co-workers). Shown in Table 38–8 are the results of routine cervical examinations performed between 26 and 30 weeks gestation in 185 women cared for at Parkland Hospital (Leveno and co-workers, 1986a). Approximately one fourth whose cervix was dilated 2 or 3 cm delivered prior to 34 weeks, either from unexplained labor or from labor that followed preterm rupture of membranes. Many of these women had experienced the same complication in earlier pregnancies. Similarly, Papiernik and colleagues (1986), in a study of cervical status before 37 weeks in 4,430 women, found that precocious cervical dilatation increased the risk of preterm birth. Stubbs and colleagues (1986) performed cervical examinations in 191 women between 28 and 34 weeks and found that those with dilatation of 1 cm or more or effacement of more than 30 percent were at increased risk for preterm delivery.

AMBULATORY UTERINE CONTRACTION TESTING

The diagnosis of preterm labor before it is irreversibly established is a goal of management. To this end, uterine activity monitoring, using tocodynamometry, recently has received considerable interest. Subsequent development and application of a new technology for sensing uterine contractions prompted Zahn (1973), Bell (1983), Katz (1986a and b), and their co-workers to propose that ambulatory monitoring of uterine contractions might improve recognition of women destined to deliver preterm and thus lead to earlier and more effective interventions.

In 1957 Smyth described an external tocodynamometer with an innovative sensor that employed the so-called guard-ring principle. The abdominal wall is flattened by an outer ring, thus permitting the inner contraction-sensing transducer to be ap-

TABLE 38–8. CERVICAL DILATATION BETWEEN 26 AND 30 WEEKS GESTATION AND RISK OF DELIVERY BEFORE 34 WEEKS

	Total N = 185 (%)	Cervical Status at 26 to 30 Weeks		
		< 1 cm N = 170 (%)	2–3 cm N = 15 (%)	Comparison
Prior low birthweight[a]	9 (5)	6 (4)	3 (20)	p < 0.001
Current pregnancy low birthweight	7 (4)	3 (2)	4 (27)	p < 0.002

[a] Less than 2,200 g (50th percentile for 34 weeks).
From Leveno and associates: Obstet Gynecol 68:434, 1986a.

plied more directly to the underlying uterine wall. Several preterm birth-prevention programs incorporating a device using the guard-ring principle are now available for ambulatory uterine monitoring in women at risk for preterm labor. Patients wear the contraction sensor belted about their abdomens and connected to a small electronic recorder worn at the waist. This recorder is used to transmit uterine activity via phone on a daily basis to receiving centers. Patients are educated concerning signs and symptoms of preterm labor, and their attending physicians are kept apprised of their progress. The program is expensive; in Dallas in 1989 this service costs the patient $75 per day.

The group from San Francisco reported that maternal perception of contractions is improved using the Term-Guard sensor, and they found that only 10 percent of women correctly perceived their contractions more than 50 percent of the time (Newman and associates, 1986). In addition, as shown in Figure 38–8, they found that women who subsequently had a preterm delivery experienced increased uterine activity beginning about 30 weeks gestation (Katz and associates, 1986b). Subsequently, Katz and associates (1986a) reported outcomes in 60 women at risk for preterm birth who were managed using this system and compared them with 60 similar matched controls. Women with four or more contractions per hour were admitted for evaluation and given either ritodrine or terbutaline if cervical changes accompanied regular contractions. Although no ultimate prenatal outcomes are described, the investigators noted that significantly fewer women enrolled in the Term-Guard system (7 percent) failed tocolysis, compared with the controls (22 percent), and as a consequence, there were fewer births prior to 36 weeks.

The first randomized study conducted using ambulatory uterine contraction monitoring was reported by Morrison and co-workers (1987). Women at high risk for preterm birth were randomized to use the Term-Guard device; a control group of women used self-palpation to identify uterine activity. Both groups received similar education. Those not electronically monitored were contacted by phone at least twice weekly, and cervical examinations were performed every 2 weeks. Women who suspected preterm labor were admitted. If uterine activity was verified, accompanied by progressive cervical changes, tocolysis was initiated with either magnesium sulfate or ritodrine. Although preterm labor was identified with almost equal frequency in each group (71 percent and 67 percent), preterm labor was diagnosed earlier in women using Term-Guard. Fewer women so monitored had advanced cervical dilatation when labor was diagnosed, and therefore, presumably fewer failed tocolysis due to the earlier detection. Consequently, 85 percent of women using Term-Guard were delivered at 37 weeks or more, compared with only 55 percent of those using uterine activity self-palpation (Table 38–9). Unfortunately, details of perinatal mortality and morbidity, as well as of expenses of maternal and neonatal care, were not given.

Iams and colleagues (1987) challenged the value of the Term-Guard system. In their study, 157 women at increased risk for preterm labor were randomized to either the Term-Guard sensor or uterine self-palpation. Both groups were educated and given intensive nurse surveillance. A similar number of women (about 20 percent) in each group delivered before 35 weeks (Table 38–10). They concluded that advantages ascribed to electronic contraction monitoring were obtainable with frequent supportive nursing contact and self-assessment of uterine activity. An expansion of this original series resulted in no change in the initial conclusions (Iams and associates, 1988).

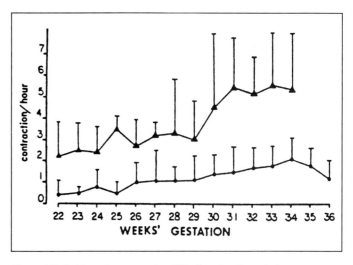

Figure 38–8. Mean frequency (± SD) of contractions during pregnancy in women having preterm labor (▲) compared with those with term labor (●). (*From Katz and colleagues: Am J Obstet Gynecol 154:44, 1986b, with permission*).

Similar observations were reported by Nageotte (1988) and Scioscia (1988) and their associates, who also questioned the cost-effectiveness. It is obvious that confirmatory data are necessary before ambulatory electronic uterine monitoring becomes a standard of care.

DIAGNOSIS OF PRETERM LABOR

Early differentiation between true and false labor often is difficult before there is demonstrable cervical effacement and dilatation. Progressive dilatation, of course, is indicative of labor. A frequently used criterion for labor is that of uterine contractions with a frequency of at least once every 10 minutes and a duration of 30 seconds or more. Uterine function often is evaluated further by means of external tocography to record the frequency and duration of contractions. Uterine contractions alone can be misleading however, because of *Braxton Hicks contractions*. These contractions, described as irregular, nonrhythmical, and painless, with intensities of approximately 10 to 15 mm Hg, can cause considerable confusion in the diagnosis of preterm labor. Not infrequently, women who deliver before term have uterine

TABLE 38–9. UNIVERSITY OF MISSISSIPPI RANDOMIZED STUDY OF AMBULATORY UTERINE CONTRACTION MONITORING (TERM-GUARD)

	Uterine Activity Monitored	
Factor	**Term-Guard (N = 34)**	**Self-Palpation (N = 33)**
Gestation at initial contact (mean)	18.6 wk	18.4 wk
Gestation at start of monitoring	25.9 wk	Not stated
Preterm labor diagnosed	24 (71%)	22 (67%)
Gestational age (mean)	27.9 wk	29.4 wk
Cervical dilatation ≥ 3 cm	2 (6%)	15 (45%)
Failed tocolysis	2 (6%)	13 (39%)
Delivery after 37 wk	29 (85%)	18 (55%)

From Morrison and colleagues: Am j Obstet Gynecol 156:536, 1987.

activity that is attributed to such Braxton Hicks contractions, prompting an incorrect diagnosis of false labor.

Because uterine contractions alone may be misleading, Herron and associates (1982) require the following criteria to document preterm labor: regular uterine contractions after 20 weeks gestation or before 37 weeks, which are 5 to 8 minutes apart or less, and accompanied by one or more of the following: (1) progressive change in the cervix, (2) cervical dilatation of 2 cm or more, or (3) cervical effacement of 80 percent or more.

As a consequence of the confusion and imprecision as to the diagnosis of preterm labor, there has been corresponding uncertainty about the effectiveness of most preterm labor treatment regimens. For example, most attempts to prevent preterm delivery in patients with ruptured membranes are less than satisfactory. This is likely to be due to the considerable certainty of preterm delivery that follows. In other words, ruptured membranes definitively establish a diagnosis of impending preterm delivery, whereas uterine contractions alone may not be so predictive.

Other signs and symptoms that may aid in the early diagnosis of women at risk for preterm delivery include (1) passage of cervical mucus, often slightly bloody, (2) low backache, (3) pelvic pressure due to descent of the fetus, (4) menstrual-like cramps, and (5) intestinal cramping with or without diarrhea (Herron and co-workers, 1982). Recently, Iams and associates (1987) interviewed 180 women with either preterm labor or ruptured membranes and found that approximately 30 to 50 percent of these women experienced one or more such premonitory symptoms. Diarrhea was not found to be a reliable sign of impending preterm birth, however.

MANAGEMENT OF PRETERM LABOR AND DELIVERY

In general, the more immature the fetus, the greater the risks from labor and delivery. This is well established for breech delivery, which is a common presentation for the preterm fetus (Chap. 19, p. 353), and undoubtedly also is true to a degree for all immature fetuses regardless of presentation.

LABOR

If labor is induced, it must not be unduly forceful (Chap. 18, p. 344). Whether labor is induced or spontaneous, abnormalities

TABLE 38–10. OHIO STATE UNIVERSITY RANDOMIZED STUDY OF AMBULATORY UTERINE CONTRACTION MONITORING (TERM-GUARD)

Factor	Uterine Activity Monitored	
	Term-Guard (N = 98)	Self-Palpation (N = 44)
Prior preterm delivery (%)	61	61
Twins (%)	25	34
Prophylactic tocolysis (%)	27	27
Preterm labor (%)	39	36
Delivery (%)		
< 35 weeks	23	20
< 37 weeks	43	52
Gestational age at delivery (mean)	35.7 wks	35.8 wks
Birthweight (mean)	2,722 g	2,718 g

From Iams and associates: Am J Obstet Gynecol 157:638, 1987.

of fetal heart rate and uterine contractions should be looked for, preferably by continuous electronic monitoring. If the fetal heart is not monitored continuously, it must be evaluated at very close intervals by adequately trained attendants (see Chap. 16, p. 310). Tachycardia, especially in the presence of ruptured membranes, is suggestive of sepsis. Periodic decelerations imply cord compression, which is rather common with preterm rupture of membranes and loss of amnionic fluid, but late decelerations also may occur and are suggestive of placental insufficiency. In either case, if an attempt is to be made to salvage the fetus, prompt cesarean section often is advisable. It is imperative that the uterine incision be large enough to allow for a nontraumatic delivery of the fetal head. Even though fetopelvic disproportion is not a problem, except when there is a transverse lie, the resistance of the cervix and of the lower genital tract to dilatation by the presenting part of the fetus may be formidable, especially in a nulliparous woman with a long, firm, and little dilated cervix.

At times, conduction analgesia may be precluded by the maternal disease that led to preterm delivery, for example, severe maternal hypertension, hemorrhage, or cyanotic heart disease. For the mother whose discomfort is too unpleasant, a mixture of nitrous oxide, 50 percent, and oxygen, administered during contractions, is likely to provide appreciable analgesia without depressing the fetus. The addition of pudendal or local nerve block provides adequate analgesia for delivery (Chap 17, p. 334).

Importantly, just as the markedly preterm infant is to be afforded special care in the neonatal intensive care unit, the mother and fetus should be very closely observed in the labor and delivery unit. That is, especially skilled physicians should monitor the labor and personally effect the delivery of the markedly preterm fetus.

DELIVERY

In the absence of a relaxed vaginal outlet, a liberal episiotomy for delivery is advantageous once the fetal head reaches the perineum. Argument persists as to the merits of spontaneous delivery versus forceps delivery to protect the more fragile preterm fetal head (Chap. 25, p. 427). It is doubtful whether use of forceps in most instances produces less trauma. Indeed, to compress and pull on the head of a grossly premature infant might be more traumatic than to push the fetus out by force applied to the buttocks. The use of outlet forceps of appropriate size may be of aid when conduction analgesia is used and voluntary expulsion efforts are obtunded. Forceps should not be employed to pull the fetus through a vagina that is resistant to dilation or over a firm perineum. Following the report of Bejar and colleagues (1980) that preterm infants frequently had germinal matrix bleeding that might extend to be more serious intraventricular hemorrhage, there was the idea that cesarean delivery to obviate trauma from labor and delivery might prevent these complications (see Chap. 33, p. 596). These initial observations have not been validated by all subsequent studies. From 1982 through 1987, 15 studies were published regarding the outcomes of preterm infants delivered from the cephalic presentation. In 12 of these reports the conclusion was reached that there was no advantage of delivery by cesarean section for prematurity, per se.

A physician proficient in resuscitative techniques who has been fully oriented to the specific problems of the case should be present at **delivery. The principles of resuscitation described in Chapter 12 are applicable, including prompt tracheal intubation and ventilation.**

METHODS USED TO ARREST PRETERM LABOR

As previously mentioned, early differentiation between true and false labor often is difficult before there is effacement and dilatation of the cervix. Unfortunately, by this time, attempts to arrest labor often are ineffective. Successful arrest of preterm labor appears to require early implementation.

Before an attempt is made to arrest preterm labor, the question must be asked and correctly answered, *"Is further intrauterine stay more likely to benefit or harm the fetus?"* In the past, the answer was no more than academic, but highly effective agents for inhibiting labor now are available. Many neonatal deaths continue to be the direct consequence of marked prematurity, and the number of such deaths could undoubtedly be reduced by delaying delivery. Not all fetuses, however, will benefit from a further intrauterine stay. This is borne out by an annual stillbirth rate in the United States that now exceeds the neonatal death rate. Obviously, some of these stillborn fetuses would have lived if only the fetus had been delivered earlier. For example, retarded fetal growth may be confused with a preterm fetus, and the malnourished fetus, to his or her detriment, may be left in a hostile uterine environment rather than a more favorable one provided by the nursery. Thus, the problem as to what is best for the fetus—as well as for the mother—is not so simple that the obstetrician can automatically attempt to delay delivery in all cases of presumed preterm labor. **The decision to attempt arrest of labor is made much easier if the gestational age is precisely known.**

BED REST

The treatment regimen that has been used most often is bed rest, with the mother lying more comfortably on her side. In the relatively few controlled studies of the effect of various treatment modalities, the control group most often was placed at bed rest and, at times, given a placebo. Satisfactory results in the prevention or arrest of preterm labor often was obtained in the control group. The success was attributable to bed rest and perhaps, in part, to the reassurance of the mother that she was being treated.

MAGNESIUM SULFATE

It has been recognized for some time that ionic magnesium in a sufficiently high concentration can alter myometrial contractility in vivo as well as in vitro. The role of magnesium presumably is that of an antagonist of calcium.

Steer and Petrie (1977) concluded that intravenously administered magnesium sulfate, 4 g given as a loading dose followed by a continuous infusion of 2 g per hour, usually will arrest labor. Subsequent studies have been reported, some favorable and some not so favorable. Elliott (1983), in a retrospective study, found tocolysis with magnesium sulfate to be successful, inexpensive, and relatively nontoxic. He reported 87 percent success when the cervix was dilated 2 cm or less, but the period of arrest was as short as 48 hours. Spisso and co-workers (1982) were favorably impressed by the efficacy of magnesium sulfate when given intravenously in relatively large doses to women with intact membranes who had

not begun the active phase of labor. They emphasized that for therapy to be effective it must be given in the early latent phase of labor. This seems to be true for all currently used tocolytic regimens.

Cotton and associates (1984b) compared magnesium sulfate to ritodrine as well as to a placebo, and they identified little difference in outcomes. Miller and associates (1982) compared magnesium sulfate and terbutaline, a β-adrenergic agonist, and on the basis of their small study, reported both drugs to be equally effective for controlling preterm labor. They identified less adverse side effects from the use of magnesium sulfate, however. Similarly, Hollander and colleagues (1987) used an unprecedented infusion dose of magnesium sulfate that averaged 4.5 g per hour. They reported that such therapy was equal to ritodrine. Semchyshyn and associates (1983) failed to stop labor in a woman who inadvertently was given 17.3 g of magnesium sulfate in 45 minutes!

In any event, the woman in labor must be monitored very closely for evidence of hypermagnesemia that might prove toxic to her and to her fetus-infant. It should be remembered that magnesium promptly crosses the placenta to produce concentrations in fetal plasma comparable to those in the mother. If magnesium intoxication is to be avoided, the patellar reflex should be present and certainly respirations should not be depressed. The pharmacology and toxicology of parenterally administered magnesium are considered in more detail in Chapter 35 (p. 681).

β-ADRENERGIC RECEPTOR AGONISTS

Earlier in this century, epinephrine in low doses was demonstrated to exert a depressant effect on the myometrium of the pregnant uterus. Its tocolytic effects, however, proved to be rather weak, quite transient, and likely to be accompanied by troublesome cardiovascular effects. More recently, several compounds capable of reacting predominantly with β-adrenergic receptors have been investigated. Some of these now are used extensively in obstetrics, but only ritodrine hydrochloride has been approved by the Food and Drug Administration for use in the treatment of preterm labor.

The adrenergic receptors are located on the outer surface of the smooth muscle cell membrane, where a specific agonist can couple with them. Adenylcyclase in the cell membrane is activated by the coupling of an agonist to the receptor. Adenylcyclase enhances the conversion of adenosine triphosphate to cyclic AMP, which in turn initiates a number of reactions that reduce the intracellular concentration of ionized calcium and thereby prevent activation of the contractile proteins, as described in Chapter 10 (p. 210).

There are two classes of β-adrenergic receptors; these commonly are referred to as $β_1$- and $β_2$-adrenergic receptors. The $β_1$ receptors are dominant in the heart and intestines, while $β_2$ receptors are dominant in the myometrium, blood vessels, and bronchioles.

A number of compounds generally similar in structure to epinephrine have been evaluated in the search for one that ideally would provide optimal stimulation of $β_2$-adrenergic receptors on myometrial cells and thus inhibit uterine contractions but, at the same time, cause little or no adverse effects from stimulation of adrenergic receptors elsewhere. Thus far, no compound has exhibited these utopian properties. Compounds that have been or are being employed in attempts to arrest preterm labor include the following:

Isoxuprine

This was one of the first compounds to be evaluated extensively for tocolytic action. It does not appear to be remarkably effective, at least in doses that do not produce potentially dangerous side effects, especially marked tachycardia and hypotension.

Ritodrine

This is the only drug whose specific indication is for arrest of preterm labor. In a multicenter study in the United States, infants whose mothers were treated with this drug for presumed preterm labor had a lower mortality rate, developed respiratory distress less often, and achieved a gestational age of 36 weeks or a birth weight of 2,500 g more often than did infants whose mothers were not so treated (Merkatz and colleagues, 1980). Hesseldahl (1979), however, in a multicenter controlled study in Denmark, did not find any of several ritodrine regimens tested to be more efficacious than standard treatment, which consisted of bed rest and glucose infusion plus placebo tablets.

Because of concerns for the efficacy and safety of ritodrine, Leveno and associates (1986b) evaluated the drug before we allowed its general use on the obstetrics service at Parkland Hospital. Preterm labor was rigidly defined to include cervical dilation plus regular uterine contractions, and 106 women between 24 and 33 weeks gestation were randomly allocated to receive either intravenous ritodrine or no tocolytic treatment. Although ritodrine treatment significantly delayed delivery for 24 hours or less, it did not modify significantly the ultimate perinatal outcomes following preterm labor.

The infusion of ritodrine, and the other β-adrenergic agonists cited, has resulted in frequent and, at times, serious side effects. In the mother, tachycardia, hypotension, apprehension, chest tightness or actual pain, electrocardiographic S-T segment depression, pulmonary edema, and death have been observed. Maternal metabolic effects include hyperglycemia, hyperinsulinemia (unless diabetic), hypokalemia, and lactic and ketoacidosis. Less serious, but nonetheless troublesome, side effects include emesis, headaches, tremulousness, fever, and hallucinations. The same derangements undoubtedly occur in the fetus. After birth, hypoglycemia, which may become profound, is frequent. Therefore, if these drugs are used and labor persists, they should be stopped so as to minimize these deleterious effects in the fetus before birth.

A single mechanism has not been identified to explain the development of pulmonary edema, but maternal infection appears to increase the risk (Hatjis and Swain, 1988). Certainly ventricular failure is a mechanism (Hadi and colleagues, 1987; Hauth and co-workers, 1983b). Increased cardiac demands imposed by pregnancy, especially with multiple fetuses, also can contribute, as can preexisting cardiac impairment. Ritodrine infusion causes a decrease in peripheral vascular resistance and sodium and water retention. Sodium and water retention apparently increase pulmonary capillary wedge pressure, and this seems to be a factor in the genesis of pulmonary edema, along with myocardial fatigue from high output. The simultaneous administration of potent glucocorticoids to try to hasten lung maturation also may contribute, although pulmonary edema has developed in their absence. Caritis and associates (1983) summarized the pharmacodynamics of ritodrine in women during preterm labor.

Terbutaline

This drug is used commonly to forestall preterm labor and has been claimed by some, but certainly not by all, to inhibit myometrial contractions effectively even when cervical dilatation is far advanced. Toxicity, especially maternal pulmonary edema, and glucose intolerance have been evident with use of the drug (Angel and associates, 1988).

Fenoterol

This drug structurally is very similar to ritodrine. It is not clear whether fenoterol is any more or less effective or causes more or less adverse reactions than do the other β-mimetic agents currently being used in several countries. Epstein and associates (1979) documented sustained hypoglycemia accompanied by elevated insulin levels in most infants who were delivered within 2 days after terminating the infusion of fenoterol to the mother. As mentioned above, a similar response has been documented for ritodrine and other β-adrenergic agonists.

The use of fenoterol has been extremely popular in West Germany. Kubli (1977), however, commented that, despite the use of at least 1 million ampules and 6 million tablets of fenoterol annually for a birth rate of about 6 million, there had been no remarkable decrease in the number of low-birthweight infants.

COMBINED THERAPY

To try to reduce the adverse effects of ritodrine while effectively arresting preterm labor, Ferguson and co-workers (1984) evaluated the response to magnesium sulfate and ritodrine administered together. They were forced to abandon the study because of the frequency and intensity of the maternal side effects that resulted from the use of this combination. Respiratory distress was troublesome, and both symptoms and EKG evidence of myocardial ischemia were common.

Hatjis and colleagues (1987) reported that ritodrine combined with magnesium sulfate was superior in arresting labor, compared to ritodrine alone, but Wilkins and associates (1988) could not confirm this observation. Ferguson and associates (1987) reported no differences in potassium, glucose, urea nitrogen, or hematocrit values in women given ritodrine alone or in combination with magnesium sulfate.

ANTIPROSTAGLANDINS

Antiprostaglandins have been the subject of considerable interest since it was appreciated that prostaglandins are intimately involved in the myometrial contractions that characterize labor (Chap. 10, p. 197). Antiprostaglandin agents may act by inhibiting the synthesis of prostaglandins or by blocking the action of prostaglandins on target organs.

A group of enzymes collectively called *prostaglandin synthase* are responsible for the conversion of free arachidonic acid to prostaglandins. Several drugs are known to block the prostaglandin synthase system, including aspirin and other salicylates, indomethacin, naproxen, and meclofenamic acid. Zuckerman and co-workers (1974) reported the successful treatment of preterm labor using indomethacin, but in their study no controls were used. Niebyl and colleagues (1980) also reported good results using indomethacin. Unfortunately, indomethacin and other such prostaglandin synthase inhibitors may adversely affect the fetus by inducing major cardiovascular changes, especially premature closure of the ductus arteriosus.

CALCIUM CHANNEL BLOCKING DRUGS

Smooth muscle activity, including myometrium, is directly related to free calcium within the cytoplasm, and a reduction in calcium concentration inhibits myometrial contraction. Calcium ions reach the cytoplasm through specific membrane portals or channels, and there is a new class of drugs known as *calcium channel blockers*, which act to inhibit, by a variety of different mechanisms, the entry of calcium through the cell membrane channels. Calcium entry blockers, because of their smooth muscle arteriolar relaxation effects, are currently being used for the treatment of coronary artery disease and hypertension.

The possibility that calcium channel blocking drugs might have applications in the treatment of preterm labor has been the subject of research in both animals and humans since the late 1970s. Forman and co-workers (1981) reported that nifedipine inhibited contractile activity in myometrial strips taken at cesarean section. Similarly, in women undergoing midtrimester abortion, nifedipine effectively inhibits uterine contractions induced by prostaglandin $F_{2\alpha}$. The first clinical trial in which nifedipine was given for preterm labor was reported from Denmark by Ulmsten and colleagues (1980). Nifedipine treatment postponed delivery at least 3 days in 10 women with preterm labor at 33 weeks gestation or less. No serious maternal or fetal side effects were noted. Similarly, Read and Wellby (1986) compared orally administered nifedipine to either intravenous ritodrine or no treatment for preterm labor before 36 weeks gestation. They concluded that nifedipine was more effective than ritodrine and was associated with fewer troublesome side effects.

As promising as calcium channel blocks may appear for treatment of preterm labor, some investigators caution that more research is needed to clarify the potential maternal or fetal dangers of such drugs. Parisi and colleagues (1986) reported that hypercapnia, acidosis, and possibly hypoxemia developed in fetuses of hypertensive ewes given nicardipine, another calcium channel blocker. Similarly, Lirette and colleagues (1987) observed a fall in uteroplacental blood flow in pregnant rabbits (also see Chap. 7, p. 131). Finally, Duscay and co-workers (1987) reported fetal acidosis and hypoxemia in rhesus monkeys infused with nicardipine in doses sufficient for tocolysis.

NARCOTICS AND SEDATIVES

Fear of arresting desirable labor by early administration of narcotics, such as meperidine and morphine, and by sedatives, such as secobarbital and pentobarbital, long has permeated the arena of clinical obstetrics. The evidence is weak, however, that the fear is justified (Chap. 17, p. 328). Certainly, there is no evidence that such drugs are effective in arresting preterm labor. There is good evidence, however, that narcotics and sedatives may depress the preterm infant when administered to the mother near the time of delivery. Moreover, if they are employed in conjunction with ethanol, maternal depression is likely to be profound. In fact, aspiration pneumonitis, with the death of both mother and fetus, has occurred in this circumstance.

Diazoxide

This very potent antihypertensive agent also can inhibit contractions of the pregnant uterus. Side effects from diazoxide administration include maternal hypotension, tachycardia, increased cardiac output, hyperglycemia, hyperuricemia, and the retention of water, sodium, potassium, chloride, and bicarbonate. It appears likely that these multiple detrimental side effects outweigh any favorable effects on the prevention of preterm labor. The drug is neither approved nor recommended for the treatment of preterm labor.

Progestational Agents

Historically, with the recognition that parenterally administered progesterone would prolong pregnancy in rabbits, progesterone and subsequently synthetic progestins were employed to try to prevent preterm labor. Most of the evidence to date is not very convincing that such agents are clinically effective (Hauth and associates, 1983a).

Ethanol

The use of intravenously administered ethanol to try to arrest preterm labor became popular following the favorable report by Fuchs and co-workers (1967). Initially, ethanol was thought to block the release of oxytocin from the neurohypophysis. The role, if any, of endogenous oxytocin in the initiation of human labor now is questioned (Chap. 10, p. 195). Ethanol, however, may have a direct depressant action on the myometrium. It also is apparent that ethanol induces inebriation of the mother and fetus-infant and induces deleterious metabolic derangements in both. Hopefully, its use has been abandoned.

SUMMARY

Benefits derived from the use of the above agents are not profound. The same cannot be said for complications from their use.

If β-adrenergic agonists are to be used, certain precautions must be taken to avoid misuse. The woman considered to be in preterm labor must be carefully evaluated for pregnancy complications that may not be readily apparent but nonetheless may be dangerous. Examples are placental abruption or intrauterine sepsis. The use of tocolytic agents, therefore, should be considered only after it is decided that the uterine contractions are not a consequence of or associated with a complication potentially dangerous to the woman, to her fetus, or to both. Certainly, the possibility of underlying maternal disease that would contraindicate the use of tocolytics must be considered. These diseases include many forms of heart disease, diabetes, pregnancy-induced or aggravated hypertension, hyperthyroidism, and severe anemia. The status of the fetus also must be considered, and unless the intrauterine environment is normal, his or her interests may be served better by prompt delivery. This is true for the overtly growth-retarded fetus or when there is intrauterine infection. Finally, if the fetus has achieved reasonable maturity, delivery is more advantageous than are attempts at pharmacological intervention. For all of these reasons, we do not attempt pharmacological tocolysis at Parkland Hospital.

POSTTERM PREGNANCY

A postterm pregnancy is one that persists for 42 weeks or more from the onset of a menstrual period that was followed by ovulation 2 weeks later. Although this includes perhaps 10 percent of pregnancies, some may not be actually postterm but rather the result of an error in the estimation of gestational age.

Once again the value of precise knowledge of the duration of gestation is evident, since in general the longer the truly postterm fetus stays in utero, the greater the risk of a severely compromised fetus and newborn infant (Shime and co-workers, 1984). Eden and associates (1987) compared 3,457 postterm pregnancies to 8,135 infants delivered at 40 weeks and reported that several adverse pregnancy outcomes were significantly increased (Table 38–11).

CAUSES

Some rare conditions associated with prolonged pregnancy include *anencephaly, fetal adrenal hypoplasia, absence of the fetal pituitary, placental sulfatase deficiency,* and *extrauterine pregnancy.* Although the etiology of prolonged pregnancy is not understood completely, these clinical conditions share a common feature: the lack of the usually high estrogen levels that characterize normal pregnancy (Chap. 5). In the case of fetal pituitary or adrenal insufficiency, the precursor hormone, dehydroisoandrosterone sulfate, is secreted in insufficient amounts for conversion to estradiol and indirectly to estriol in the placenta (see Fig. 5–4 p. 75). A classic example of the deficiency of estrogen precursor is anencephaly (MacDonald and Siiteri, 1965).

Placental sulfatase deficiency is inherited as a sex-linked recessive trait (Ryan, 1980). In this condition, precursor hormone is produced by the fetal adrenal gland, but the placenta lacks the enzyme to cleave the sulfate from dehydroisoandrosterone sulfate, the initial enzymatic step in the conversion of this biologically weak androgen into estradiol and estriol (France and Liggins, 1969).

Reduced estrogen concentrations, which characterize these cases of prolonged pregnancy, are believed to be important, since there is insufficient estrogen to stimulate production and storage of glycerophospholipids in fetal membranes. With normal and continuously increasing amounts of estrogen, as pregnancy advances, the fetal membranes are especially enriched with two glycerophospholipids, phosphatidylinositol and phosphatidylethanolamine, both containing arachidonate in the *sn*-2 position (Fig. 10–9 p. 203). The human fetus apparently triggers labor by some as yet poorly defined mechanism that results in the cleaving of arachidonate from these two glycerophospholipids. The arachidonate then is available for conversion into prostaglandins E_2 and $F_2\alpha$, which in turn stimulate cervical effacement and the rhythmic uterine contractions that characterize normal labor (see Chap. 10).

It is easy to understand how relatively minor variations in this intricate chain of organ communications between the fetus and mother might result in a failure of labor to commence at the appropriate time. Labor normally begins during the 4-week period between 38 and 42 weeks gestation, and there appears to

be the usual biological variability. Certainly, women who have had a prolonged gestation with one pregnancy are at increased risk of recurrence in a subsequent pregnancy. Unfortunately, until less well-defined abnormalities are identified that result in prolonged gestation, the physician must remain alert and wary of this insidious cause of jeopardy for both the mother and her fetus-infant.

EFFECTS ON THE FETUS-INFANT

The postterm fetus may continue to gain weight in utero and thus be an unusually large infant at birth or *gain weight postterm and be large for gestational age.* The fact that the fetus continues to grow serves as an indication of uncompromised placental function, with the implication he or she should tolerate the rigors of normal labor without problems. This, however, *may not* be the result. For example, continued growth may have created a worrisome degree of fetopelvic disproportion, and consequently, labor may not progress normally. Moreover, as discussed below, oligohydramnios commonly develops as pregnancy advances past 42 weeks, and decreased amnionic fluid is associated with cord compression, which leads to fetal distress, including defecation and aspiration of thick meconium.

At the other extreme, the intrauterine environment may be so hostile that further fetal growth is arrested, and the fetus is *postterm and growth retarded* (Fig. 38–3). The fetus may appear at birth actually to have lost considerable weight, especially from loss of subcutaneous fat and muscle mass. In fact, some already growth-retarded infants may become postterm, and this pathological process may worsen. In the extreme case, the limbs appear long and very thin, there is severe epidermal desquamation, and the fingernails and amnion commonly are meconium stained.

ANTEPARTUM MANAGEMENT OF POSTTERM PREGNANCY

Even in the absence of any recognizable maternal complication, there remains little doubt that some fetuses who stay in utero much beyond 42 weeks are in progressively greater danger of sustaining serious morbidity or even death. Therefore, it would be advantageous to such fetuses to deliver them by 42 weeks. Unfortunately, at least five difficult problems persist that serve to discourage a policy of delivering all fetuses whose gestational age is merely **suspected** to be at least 42 weeks:

1. Gestational age is not always known precisely, and thus the fetus actually may be less mature than believed.
2. It is very difficult to identify with precision those fetuses who are likely to die or to develop serious morbidity if left in utero.
3. The great majority of these fetuses fare rather well.
4. Induction of labor is not always successful.
5. Delivery by cesarean section increases appreciably the risk of serious maternal morbidity not only in this pregnancy, but also to a degree in subsequent ones.

In view of this list of problems, a definite plan of management should be established for all cases of prolonged gestation. It seems reasonable to decide as a first step whether gestational age is firmly established or is uncertain (Leveno and co-workers, 1985b; Yeh and Read, 1982). Management is then directed at

TABLE 38–11. OUTCOMES IN POSTTERM PREGNANCIES COMPARED TO THOSE DELIVERED AT 40 WEEKS

Factor[a]	40 wks (N = 8,135) (%)	Postterm (N = 3,457) (%)
First pregnancy	33	38
Meconium	19	27
Oxytocin induction	3	14
Cesarean section	8	18
Shoulder dystocia	0.7	1.3
Macrosomia (>4,500 g)	0.8	2.8
Meconium aspiration	0.6	1.6
Congenital malformations	2	2.8

[a] For all comparisons between 40– and 42–week groups, $p < 0.05$.
From Eden and associates: Obstet Gynecol 69:296, 1987.

these two variations of postterm pregnancy. Finally, there must be equipment and personnel necessary to care for the patient in what may be a difficult labor and delivery. Pediatric personnel also should be present at delivery to render any necessary care required for the neonate.

GESTATIONAL AGE KNOWN

If gestational age is known, management by most includes delivery at the end of a fixed period of time, ranging from 42 to 44 weeks gestation, regardless of the condition of the cervix (Granados, 1984; Leveno and colleagues, 1985b; Shime and associates, 1984). If induction fails, many favor cesarean section. It is unclear as to the best method of fetal surveillance between 42 and 44 weeks in those pregnancies in which inductions are not done.

In many institutions, management between 42 and 44 weeks consists of serial evaluations directed especially at identifying fetal jeopardy (p. 759) while awaiting the onset of spontaneous labor. With documented or suspected fetal distress, the infant is delivered either by labor induction or by cesarean section, depending on obstetrical indications (Yeh and Read, 1982).

Leveno and associates (1985b) reported a more active approach in a prospective 3½-year study of 1,369 women with suspected prolonged pregnancy as the *only* complication. Definitely prolonged pregnancy (42 completed weeks) was diagnosed in 376 women, and 994 others were designated as uncertain. Fetal jeopardy or well-being was evaluated by clinical assessment of amnionic fluid volume and maternal perception of fetal movement. During the first 2½ years, labor was induced in all women who completed a definite 43 weeks gestation, and at the end of 42 weeks gestation during the last year of the study. Women with uncertain prolonged pregnancy were followed weekly, without intervention unless fetal jeopardy was identified by diminished amnionic fluid suspected clinically or by maternal perception of decreased fetal motion.

Induction of labor at 42 rather than 43 weeks in women with definitely prolonged pregnancy resulted in an increase in the number of inductions from 39 to 87 percent, but surprisingly, there was no increase in the cesarean section rate. By delivering all women at 42 weeks gestation, the perinatal mortality rate was reduced from 10 per 1,000 to zero. The perinatal mortality rate in the group of women with uncertain gestational age was 2 per 1,000. These investigators concluded that:

1. Patients with definite versus uncertain prolonged pregnancy represent two clinically separable groups with distinctly different perinatal risks.
2. Women with a definite prolonged pregnancy should be induced after 42 completed weeks.
3. More frequent induction attempts are not associated with an increased cesarean rate.

More recently, in some practices there has been a trend to begin labor induction or fetal surveillance at the end of 41, and even 40, completed weeks because of a small number of unexplained stillbirths (Bochner and co-workers, 1988). Whether or not this practice is associated with a higher cesarean section rate is unknown.

GESTATIONAL AGE UNKNOWN

In many medical centers, if gestational age is unknown, clinical, electronic, or biochemical surveillance techniques, or various combinations of these (Chap. 15), are used after the best esti-

mate of the 42nd week, and delivery is not induced unless there is evidence of fetal jeopardy. In these studies, because delivery dates most often are miscalculated, there is generally a favorable outcome. Leveno and associates (1985b) reported a perinatal mortality of 2 per 1,000 using only clinical methods of detecting fetal jeopardy (decreased amnionic fluid volume or decreased fetal movements perceived by the pregnant woman).

MEDICAL OR OBSTETRICAL COMPLICATIONS

In the event of a medical or another obstetrical complication, it generally is unwise to allow a pregnancy to continue past 42 weeks. Indeed, in many such instances *early* delivery is indicated. Timing of delivery will depend on the individual complication. Examples include pregnancy-induced hypertension, prior cesarean delivery, diabetes, and many others.

IDENTIFICATION OF FETAL JEOPARDY

It now is common practice in the management of postterm pregnancy to apply a variety of tests or procedures that have been championed to predict fetal well-being. These tests have included measurements from one to seven times weekly of either the amount of estriol excreted in the urine per 24 hours or its concentrations in plasma, or the evaluation one or more times each week of changes in fetal heart rate, either in response to fetal movement (nonstress test) or in response to uterine contractions, usually induced with oxytocin (contraction stress test), or both (Chap. 15). As long as these tests remain normal, the fetus is considered to be in minimal jeopardy and delivery most often is not attempted.

The major problems associated with the use of these tests, aside from costs and inconvenience, are the frequencies of false-positive and false-negative results that are unacceptable, at least to some obstetricians. Yeh and Read (1983) stated that because of the false-negative rate of 13 percent, plasma conjugated estriol determinations alone are inadequate to identify growth-retarded fetuses. Moreover, there is no convincing evidence that the use of estriol surveillance for postterm pregnancies has produced better results than has routine labor induction in all women who complete 42 weeks gestation (Devoe and Sholl, 1983; Leveno and co-workers, 1985b).

As emphasized by Kirschbaum (1979), some techniques commonly employed to assess fetal well-being with prolonged pregnancy were incorporated into clinical practice without vigorous objective proof of their value as measured by their predictive strength and prevention of perinatal morbidity and death. For example, Schneider and co-workers (1978) in their study of postterm pregnancies, found that thrice-weekly measurements of 24-hour urinary *estriol excretion* were of little value. Devoe and Sholl (1983) used plasma and urinary estriol determinations and weekly fetal heart rate tests for fetal surveillance in 248 documented postterm pregnancies and reported a fetal death rate of 8 per 1,000.

Benedetti and Easterling (1988) recently reviewed the use of antepartum tests in postterm pregnancy.

Nonstress Test
Miyazaki and Miyazaki (1981) were disappointed in fetal outcomes in which the *nonstress test* was used to ascertain fetal well-being. In their relatively small series, they reported four fetal deaths and one neonatal death (corrected fetal death rate, 61 per 1,000) despite a recently reactive nonstress test. Barss and co-workers (1985) reported similar outcomes in women with

a postterm pregnancy that was assessed weekly with nonstress testing. Small and colleagues (1987) reported that twice-weekly nonstress testing resulting in a corrected perinatal mortality rate of 4.3 per 1,000. Khouzami and associates (1983) reported that perinatal mortality in postterm pregnancies was 2.1 per 1,000 using *urinary estriol/creatinine ratios*, 6.5 per 1,000 using the *contraction stress test*, and 24 per 1,000 using the *nonstress test*. Others have reported similar experiences, and outcomes tend to be worse when the interval between tests was as long as 1 week. This is especially true with the nonstress test (Barrett and associates, 1982), but it also appears to be true when fetal biophysical profile testing is used.

It now is appreciated that *fetal heart rate decelerations* observed during nonstress testing are predictive of increased fetal and neonatal morbidity and mortality in postterm pregnancy (Benedetti and Easterling, 1988). Small and associates (1987), as well as many others, recommend induction in these instances, regardless of whether there are accompanying normal fetal heart accelerations. Divon and co-workers (1988) described similar findings using the biophysical profile described below. It seems likely that these decelerations are the result of diminished amnionic fluid that predisposes to cord compression.

Biophysical Profile

Manning and associates (1981a) reported a fetal death rate of 4.6 per 1,000 in postterm pregnancies when a *biophysical profile* was used weekly. Indeed, the only unexplained fetal death in their series occurred after a perfect score of 10 was observed 5 days before the fetal death. Manning and associates (1987) now recommend twice-weekly testing in postterm fetuses and delivery if there is oligohydramnios. Phelan and co-workers (1984) reported two similar episodes of fetal death following biophysical profiles of 8 and 10 using the method described by Manning and associates.

Contraction Stress Test

The *contraction stress test* also has been used to identify the suspected postterm fetus who is in jeopardy in utero. Freeman and associates (1981) reported excellent outcomes when this test was used at weekly intervals and without active intervention as long as the test result remained negative. The experiences of some others have not been so rewarding (Khouzami and co-workers, 1983; Knox and associates, 1979). An example of a bad outcome is shown in Figure 38–9. In this case, at 42-*plus* weeks gestational age, oxytocin induction of labor was done, during which time the fetal heart rate was recorded continuously. Throughout the 8-hour induction of labor, no evidence of fetal heart rate decelerations was observed and the fetal heart rate accelerated with fetal movement; that is, there was a *negative and reactive contraction stress test* (see Chap. 15, p. 290). Unfortunately, effective labor was not established, and 3 days later the procedure was repeated with the same result. After 3 more days, labor induction was attempted for the third time with the same result. Two days later the fetus died. Oxytocin subsequently proved effective for accomplishing labor and delivery, and thick meconium was present in the scant amnionic fluid. Careful pathological examination of the fetus and placenta disclosed no abnormality to account for the death, which was presumed to have been caused by cord entanglement.

Amnionic Fluid Volume

Several authors have suggested that the identification of *oligohydramnios* determined by various ultrasound methods may be

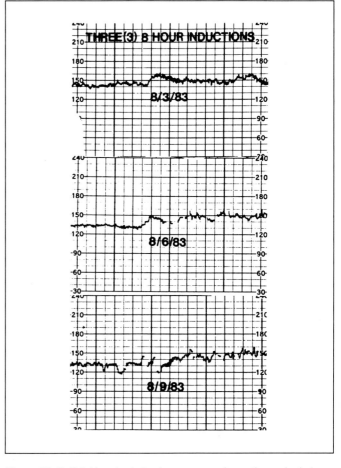

Figure 38–9. Fetal heart rate tracings were made continuously during three 8-hour intravenous oxytocin infusions to attempt labor induction in a woman between 42 and 43 weeks gestation. Even though there was no evidence of abnormality in fetal heart rate during or after uterine contractions, and despite fetal heart accelerations associated with fetal movements, the fetus died 2 days later.

used alone (Crowley and co-workers, 1984), with the nonstress test (Phelan and associates, 1984, 1985), or in conjunction with a fetal biophysical profile (Phelan and co-workers, 1984, 1985) to identify those postterm fetuses most at risk. While there is certainly an association between oligohydramnios and increased fetal risk, both before and during labor, the degree of risk has not been defined accurately.

The problem of assigning risk to a fetus based upon ultrasonic quantification of amnionic fluid is, in part, the consequence of different criteria used by various investigators. For example, Crowley and co-workers (1984) defined this as "no single vertical pool of amnionic fluid measured greater than 30 mm." Phelan and co-workers (1985) divided women into three groups based upon an amnionic fluid volume: (1) adequate—amnionic fluid throughout the cavity, with the largest pocket greater than 1 cm in its vertical diameter; (2) adequate but decreased—a vertical amnionic fluid pocket greater than 1 cm but with the "overall impression of the sonographer that fluid is decreased"; (3) decreased—absence of amnionic fluid throughout the cavity and a single pocket equal to or less than 1 cm.

The definitions for amnionic fluid volume in at least two different techniques for fetal biophysical profile testing also are different, as are the testing intervals. Manning and associates (1981a and b) define as adequate "a pocket of amnionic fluid that measures at least 1 cm in two perpendicular planes.'' They initially recommended testing weekly but now recommend twice-weekly testing. Shime and colleagues (1984) did not include fetal tone in their biophysical profile evaluation and used a different scoring system than did Manning and associates (see Chap. 15, p. 294). Shime recommends testing biweekly and defines amnionic fluid volume in three groups: adequate fluid is present when at least one vertical pocket greater than 2 cm is observed; a second group is identified by a vertical pocket of fluid 1 to 2 cm; the third group has less than 1 cm of fluid in the vertical pocket.

Despite the numerous variations cited above, there are several outcome factors that can be compared. Manning and associates (1981a) reported a fetal death rate of 4.6 per 1,000, and Phelan and co-workers (1985), 8.5 per 1,000. In the latter study, one fetal death was in a postterm pregnancy with adequate amnionic fluid, and in another death there was decreased fluid. They concluded that if amnionic fluid volume was decreased, regardless of nonstress tests results, a trial of labor should be considered. Manning and co-workers (1987) now recommend the same. No fetal deaths were reported by Crowley and associates (1984) or by Shime and colleagues (1984), with both groups performing twice-weekly testing but using different criteria. False-positive results were high, however, in both groups with respect to the accuracy of predicting postterm fetal dysmaturity.

Shime and co-workers (1984) reported that their fetal biophysical profile testing had a false-positive rate of 79 percent and a false-negative rate of 0.4 percent for dysmaturity. If the amnionic fluid pocket was between 1 and 2 cm, the false-positive rate was 86 percent and the false-negative rate zero. If amnionic fluid volume was less than 1 cm, the false-positive rate was still high (71 percent) and the false-negative rate was 2.6 percent. The false-positive rate in the group with decreased amnionic fluid reported by Phelan and associates (1985) was 86 percent.

There is no doubt that when amnionic fluid is decreased in a postterm pregnancy, or any pregnancy for that matter, the fetus is at increased risk. Besides fetal mortality, albeit uncommon, there is significant morbidity with oligohydramnios. For example, the incidence of meconium-stained amnionic fluid was reported to be 37 percent with adequate fluid, compared to 71 percent when there was decreased fluid volume (Phelan and colleagues, 1984). In addition, the cesarean section rate for fetal distress was 43 percent in women identified as having decreased amnionic fluid, and 1-minute Apgar scores of less than 7 were observed in 86 percent of newborns.

Leveno and associates (1984) reported that diminished amnionic fluid estimated clinically was associated with an increased incidence of intrapartum fetal distress and an increased cesarean section rate. More recently, Bochner and co-workers (1987) reported significantly increased cesarean delivery for intrapartum fetal distress (16 versus 0.8 percent) in women in whom an amnionic fluid volume pocket was less than 3 cm. They further concluded that nonstress testing added nothing to the predictive value of fluid volume assessment, a view also shared by Manning and colleagues (1987).

Thus, the use of any one of several different ultrasound techniques, applied once or twice weekly, to detect decreases in amnionic fluid volume, may be helpful in identifying a postterm fetus in jeopardy. *Although the false-positive rates associated with these techniques are quite high, and range from 50 to 86 percent, use of amnionic fluid volume assessments may result in fewer interventions than empirical induction at 42 weeks.* Until there is a comparative study of both methods, however, we will continue routinely to induce labor after 42 completed weeks.

Doppler Velocimetry

In a study of 25 pregnancies beyond 42 weeks, Rightmire and Campbell (1987) reported that while the umbilical artery waveform did not change, the Pourcelot index of the umbilical artery was higher in fetuses who had worse clinical outcomes. The descending fetal aorta velocities did decrease with increasing duration of pregnancy. However, Guidetti and colleagues (1987) found no significant changes in mean umbilical artery systolic-diastolic ratios in 46 postterm pregnancies. Farmakides and associates (1988) studied uterine and umbilical artery Doppler velocimetry in 149 women whose pregnancies exceeded 41 weeks and found no changes in flow velocity. This obtained even if there was other evidence for fetal compromise.

ETIOLOGY OF FETAL JEOPARDY

The reasons for the increased risks to postterm fetuses have been explained, at least partially, by Leveno and associates (1984). They reported that both antepartum fetal jeopardy and intrapartum fetal distress with postterm pregnancies was not due to placental insufficiency, but rather was the consequence of umbilical cord compression associated with oligohydramnios. This observation was confirmed subsequently by Phelan and co-workers (1984, 1985) and Bochner and associates (1987). More recently, Silver and colleagues (1987) reported that umbilical cord diameter, measured ultrasonically, was predictive of intrapartum fetal distress when decreased, and especially if further associated with oligohydramnios. **The exact role of placental insufficiency is unclear, but in our experience it has not been identified even in those fetuses who were obviously postterm and growth retarded.**

INTRAPARTUM MANAGEMENT OF POSTTERM PREGNANCY

Labor is a particularly dangerous time for the postterm fetus. Therefore, it is important that women whose pregnancies are known or suspected to be postterm come to the hospital as soon as they suspect they are in labor. Upon arrival, while being observed for possible labor, electronic fetal heart rate and uterine contractions should be monitored very closely for rate variations consistent with fetal distress (American College of Obstetricians and Gynecologists, 1987). Thus, electronic monitoring of the fetal heart rate and of uterine contractions throughout all of labor is advantageous and may be lifesaving for the fetus.

The question, *"When should the membranes be ruptured?"* is difficult to answer. Further reduction in amnionic fluid volume following amniotomy certainly can enhance the possibility of cord compression, but on the other hand, amniotomy is likely to identify the presence of thick meconium, which is dangerous to the fetus if aspirated during labor. Moreover, once the membranes are ruptured, a scalp electrode and intrauterine pressure catheter can be placed, the use of which usually provides more precise data concerning fetal heart rate and uterine contractions than does external electronic monitoring. With internal fetal monitoring, the woman is more likely to lie on her side, which should favor placental perfusion, whereas when wearing external fetal-monitoring equipment on her abdomen, she most often is inclined to stay on her back.

Identification of *thick meconium* in amnionic fluid is particularly worrisome. It is evidence of fairly recent fetal distress that may or may not persist. Miller and Read (1981) reported that postterm infants with thick meconium-stained amnionic fluid had significantly lower pH values in late labor than did those with thin meconium. They suggested that in a labor complicated with thick meconium, fetal scalp pH sampling was reasonable, even with normal fetal heart rate patterns.

Of great importance, *meconium* aspiration may cause severe pulmonary dysfunction and death during the newborn period (Chap. 33, p. 595). This may be minimized but not eliminated by effective suctioning of the pharynx as soon as the head is delivered but before the thorax is delivered. If meconium is identified, the trachea should be aspirated as soon as possible after delivery by someone skilled in this technique (Chap. 33, p. 595). Immediately thereafter, the infant should be ventilated as needed. The likelihood of successful vaginal delivery is reduced appreciably for the nulliparous woman who is in early labor with thick meconium-stained amnionic fluid. Therefore, when the woman is remote from delivery, strong consideration must be given to prompt cesarean section, especially when cephalopelvic disproportion is suspected or either hypotonic or hypertonic dysfunctional labor is evident. Certainly, oxytocin is to be avoided in these cases.

At times, the continued growth of the fetus postterm will result in a *postterm and large for gestational age* infant, and shoulder dystocia may develop following delivery of the head. Freeman and associates (1981) reported a 25 percent incidence of fetal macrosomia (more than 4,000 g) in their series of postterm pregnancies, and this was associated with a 2 percent incidence of shoulder dystocia. Likewise, Eden and colleagues (1987) reported that macrosomia of more than 4,500 g was increased threefold and shoulder dystocia increased twofold in postterm pregnancies, compared to women delivered at 40 weeks (Table 38–11). Therefore, an obstetrician who is experienced in managing shoulder dystocia should be available to effect delivery (Chap. 19, p. 368).

PEDIATRIC SUPPORT

At the time of delivery of an infant known or suspected to be postterm, a physician trained in neonatal resuscitation—including the skill to place umbilical artery and venous catheters—should be in attendance. Immediate tracheal suctioning of meconium, as well as the skill to manage immediate and long-term respiratory support if needed, may prove essential in the survival of such an infant. The management of neonatal hypoglycemia and hypocalcemia, which may further complicate the neonatal course, should be anticipated, and appropriate plans made for such contingencies prior to the delivery.

MANAGEMENT OF POSTTERM PREGNANCY AT PARKLAND HOSPITAL

Until better methods of assessing fetal well-being are available, an active approach to the management of postterm pregnancies is warranted, based upon the classification of definite or uncertain gestational age (Leveno and associates, 1985b). This approach is used in postterm pregnancies in which prolongation of pregnancy is the *only* complication identified.

In women with definitely established gestational age, labor is induced at the completion of 42 weeks, or sooner if amnionic fluid volume is judged to be decreased or if she reports a decrease in fetal activity. Almost 95 percent of women are induced successfully, or enter labor within 2 days of attempted induction. For those who do not deliver with the first induction, a second induction is performed within 3 days. Almost all women will be delivered by this plan of management, but in the unusual few who are not delivered, a cesarean section may be justified (Fig. 38–9). This approach is not as aggressive as it might first appear when one recalls that the use of ultrasound techniques to identify decreased amnionic fluid volume results in false-positive rates of up to 86 percent, in which cases induction is performed. Equally important, despite the use of various fetal surveillance techniques, including nonstress tests, contraction stress tests, and fetal biophysical profile testing, unpredicted fetal deaths continue to occur along with significant intrapartum and neonatal morbidity.

This plan of active intervention has not resulted in an increased cesarean section rate but has appreciably reduced fetal deaths (Leveno and co-workers, 1985b). The number of inductions has increased, however. Others also have reported that a comparable plan was beneficial for similar reasons (Barss and associates, 1985; Devoe and Sholl, 1983).

Women classified as having uncertain postterm pregnancies are followed on a weekly basis, without intervention unless fetal jeopardy is suspected. Fetal jeopardy is based upon the clinical or sonographic perception of decreased amnionic fluid volume. Currently we use sonar to assess fluid volume subjectively since, as discussed above, a more precise definition has not been validated. Equally worrisome is diminished fetal motion reported by the mother. If fetal jeopardy is suspected by either method, labor induction is carried out as described previously for the woman with a definite postterm gestation.

CONCLUSIONS

The risk to the fetus-infant increases substantively after 42 weeks gestation. Unfortunately, there are presently no antenatal tests of fetal well-being that can be used to provide a complete sense of security. All currently available methods and combinations of methods to assess fetal jeopardy have been associated with unpredictable fetal deaths. Equally important, the use of some of these tests may result in delay of delivery until more subtle forms of fetal compromise develop, which may increase intrapartum and neonatal risks.

Because of these problems, "the answer" for management of postterm pregnancy is not obvious. What is obvious, however, is the need for a specific clinical plan for the management of such pregnancies. An active intervention plan that does not rely upon antenatal hormonal tests, electronic fetal heart rate responses to stress or no stress, ultrasonic assessment of amnionic fluid volume, or biophysical profile testing has been used successfully at Parkland Hospital for several years. More recently we have used ultrasound to assess amnionic fluid subjectively along with clinical examination. Other plans of management that rely more heavily on such antenatal tests as a central point around which management is planned have been reported by others to be successful. There are advantages and disadvantages to both methods of management, and these must be accepted as the currently imprecise state-of-the-art. What must not be accepted is the lack of recognition of the problem and the failure to pursue any one of the definite and logical plans of management that have been discussed. **Finally, regardless of the management plan chosen, and no matter how diligently it is applied, inevitably there will be an unpredicted fetal death.**

INAPPROPRIATE FETAL GROWTH

Inappropriate fetal growth occurs whenever the fetus is either too large or too small for its age. The problems associated with macrosomic or constitutionally large fetuses have been or will be addressed in other areas of this book, especially under discussions of shoulder dystocia (Chap. 19, p. 365), postterm pregnancy (p. 759), and diabetes (Chap. 39, p. 817). This section is devoted to the problems associated with the fetus who is too small for his or her gestational age.

Each year in the United States approximately 250,000 babies are born weighing less than 2,500 g. The National Institutes of Health estimated that approximately 40,000 are at term but likely to be growth retarded (Frigoletto, 1986). The remaining infants include the preterm and the preterm who are also growth retarded, which results in even greater risks.

The actual number of growth-retarded neonates is unknown. In fact, it was not until 25 years ago that physicians first recognized that *runting*, or fetal growth retardation, was a human as well as an animal phenomenon. In 1961 Warkany and co-workers reported normal values for infant weights, lengths, and head circumferences and defined fetal growth retardation. Gruenwald (1963) reported that approximately one third of low-birthweight infants were *mature* and that their small size could be explained by *chronic fetal distress* due, it was likely, to *placental insufficiency.* Following these reports, the concept was accepted only slowly.

CLASSIFICATION OF SMALL FOR GESTATIONAL AGE FETUSES

With a detailed comparison of gestational ages to birthweights, Lubchenco and co-workers (1963) constructed fetal growth curves. Battaglia and Lubchenco (1967) then classified *small for gestational age* (SGA) infants as those whose weights were below the 10th percentile for their gestational age. *Large for gestational age* (LGA) infants had weights above the 90th percentile for their gestational ages. Infants between the 10th and 90th percentiles were classified as *appropriate for gestational age* (AGA). This simple but effective method of defining normal and abnormal fetal growth was followed by the recognition that small for gestational age infants, whether preterm or term, had significantly increased perinatal mortality (Lubchenco and co-workers, 1972).

As illustrated in Figure 38–3, a fetus may be small for gestational age due to a genetically predetermined reason (constitutionally small) or due to a pathological process (fetal growth retardation). Acceptance of *fetal growth retardation* as a reality has led to the understanding that it may be caused by many different diseases and conditions. In fact, because of these diverse etiologies, a simple solution to the problem of fetal growth retardation is not readily available. Significant advances have been made, however, in the establishment of etiologies, screening techniques, diagnoses, management, and follow-up of this complication. **It is emphasized again that before recognition and management of fetal growth retardation can be accomplished, gestational age must be established accurately.**

Fetal growth retardation is divided into two clinical types: *type I, or symmetrical,* and *type II, or asymmetrical.* These two types are likely to be the consequence of different times of onset and duration of the events that caused the retarded growth. For example, Winick (1971) described three phases of cellular growth in the placenta and fetus. The first consisted of an increase in cell numbers (hyperplasia), the second phase was an increase in number and size of the cells (hyperplasia and hypertrophy), and the third phase was further hypertrophy (Fig. 38–10).

Type I, symmetrical growth retardation, results, it is likely, from a noxious injury very early, that is, at a time when fetal growth is predominantly from hyperplasia. Injuries to the fetus at this time might be expected to produce profound effects. This is borne out clinically, because symmetrical forms of growth retardation most often are caused by structural or chromosomal abnormalities or early congenital infections, such as rubella (Creasy, 1982; Knox, 1978). This type of growth retardation is thus *intrinsic*, and perhaps 20 percent of cases of retarded fetal growth are symmetrical.

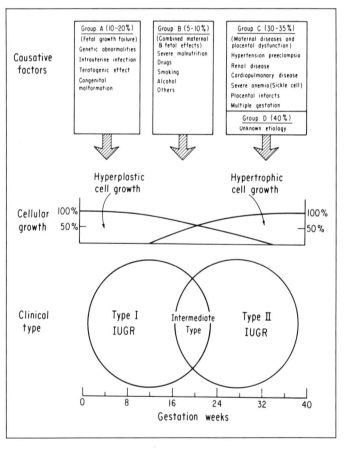

Figure 38–10. A schematic illustration of causative factors, timing of injury on placental and fetal cellular growth, and clinical type of fetal growth retardation (intrauterine growth retardation [IUGR]). Injuries to cellular growth early in pregnancy often will result in type I (symmetrical) fetal growth retardation, while injuries later in pregnancy most often will result in type II (asymmetrical) fetal growth retardation. (*Reproduced with permission from Lin and Evans [eds]: Intrauterine Growth Retardation. McGraw-Hill, 1984, p. 10.*)

Type II, asymmetrical growth retardation, most often results from adverse effects during the phase of cellular hypertrophy, that is, during later gestation. Thus, the majority of the asymmetrically growth-retarded fetuses have the *appropriate number* of cells but are smaller than normal. Fetal injury at this time would not be expected to cause damage as severe as an earlier insult, and this indeed has been observed clinically.

The cause of asymmetrical growth retardation cannot be explained merely by a reduction in the size of all cells; it is likely the consequence also of the sparing of selected cells, for example, those of the central nervous system. The pathological processes that most often result in asymmetrical growth retardation are maternal diseases that are *extrinsic* to the fetus. These diseases may alter fetal size by reducing uteroplacental blood flow, as with hypertensive disorders, or by restricting oxygen and nutrient transfer, as perhaps with sickle cell disease, or by reduced placental size with infarcts (Fig. 38–4). A combination of events may be seen with twins when blood supply and placental size both are reduced late in pregnancy as a consequence of "sharing."

These alterations in uteroplacental blood flow and transfer of oxygen and nutrients take place over a protracted period that, it is likely, allows the fetus to compensate by redirecting its blood flow to the brain and away from visceral organs such as the liver and kidneys (Cohn and colleagues, 1974; Reuss and co-workers, 1982). These compensatory mechanisms may result in normal head growth or *brain sparing;* however, the liver and other visceral organs including the intestine have reduced blood flow (p. 770), which results in a smaller liver and abdominal circumference caused by a reduction in hepatic glycogen stores. Reduced intestinal blood flow also may be a contributing factor for *necrotizing enterocolitis* (Hackett and colleagues, 1987; Kleigman and Fanaroff, 1984; Chap. 33, p. 612).

It is possible that combinations of these two types of clinical fetal growth retardation develop (Fig. 38–10). Such events are often consequences of combined maternal and fetal effects, as well as the time of onset and duration of the injury. Such classifications naturally are quite uncertain. Finally, some forms of retarded fetal growth cannot be given a probable cause and are classified as due to an unknown etiology.

ANIMAL STUDIES OF FETAL GROWTH RETARDATION

The assumptions, intuitive reasoning, and clinical observations used to support the etiological classifications listed above have been tested experimentally and support the concept. Specifically, caloric and protein restriction in the pregnant rat results in decreased total cell numbers of 15 to 20 percent in the offspring (Winick, 1971). This would be analogous to human symmetrical fetal growth retardation.

Asymmetrical fetal growth retardation has been produced in animals in a variety of ingenious ways. Uteroplacental blood flow has been reduced late in pregnancy in the rat by ligating the uterine artery to one horn of a bicornuate uterus. This Wigglesworth model (1964) results in asymmetrically runted pups from the uterine horn on the side of the vascular ligature and normal-size pups from the unligated side. Similar results have been obtained in the sheep by chronically embolizing the placenta with microspheres (Creasy and colleagues, 1972). Chronic hypoxia in rats results in a reduced litter size and a disparate reduction of fetal body weight compared to brain weight (van Geijn and associates, 1980). Finally, Evans and

associates (1981) produced typical asymmetrical fetal growth retardation in the mouse by superovulating the animals and increasing the litter size.

CLINICAL CAUSES OF SMALL FOR GESTATION AGE FETUSES

An etiological classification and brief description of some known clinical causes of small for gestational age fetuses follows. Symmetrical and asymmetrical categories just described are used, and the classification is as imperfect as any other. Furthermore, the list is not and cannot be precise or complete and hopefully soon will be rendered obsolete by a better understanding of the multiple etiologies of this clinical entity.

Constitutionally Small

Small women typically have smaller babies. If a woman begins pregnancy weighing less than 100 pounds, the risk of delivering a small for gestational age infant is increased, at least by a factor of two (Eastman and Jackson, 1968; Simpson and colleagues, 1975). In a small woman with a small pelvis, the birth of a small baby whose genetically determined weight is below the average for the entire population is not necessarily an undesirable event.

Growth Retardation
I. Symmetrical
  A. *Poor maternal weight gain.* In the woman of average or low weight, lack of weight gain throughout pregnancy or arrested weight gain after 28 weeks gestation often is associated with fetal growth retardation (Simpson and colleagues, 1975). If the mother is large and otherwise healthy, however, below-average maternal weight gain (Chaps. 7 and 14) without maternal disease is unlikely to be associated with appreciable fetal growth retardation. Marked restriction of weight gain during pregnancy should not be encouraged. During the last half of pregnancy, calories apparently have to be restricted to less than 1,500 per day to cause fetal growth retardation (Lechtig and co-workers, 1975).
  B. *Fetal infections.* Viral, bacterial, protozoan, and spirochetal infections all have been associated with fetal growth retardation (Chap. 33, p. 613). Certainly, the best known of these are infections caused by rubella (Lin and Evans, 1984) and cytomegalovirus (Hanshaw, 1971; Stagno and associates, 1977). Hepatitis A and B are associated with preterm delivery but also may cause retarded fetal growth (Schweitzer, 1975; Waterson, 1979). Varicella and influenza rarely cause congenital infection and growth retardation (Varner and Galask, 1984). Listeriosis, tuberculosis, and syphilis have been reported to cause fetal growth retardation. Paradoxically, in cases of syphilis, the placenta almost always is increased in weight and size due to edema and perivascular inflammation (Varner and Galask, 1984). The protozoan infection most often associated with fetal growth retardation is toxoplasmosis, but congenital malaria may produce the same result (Varner and Galask, 1984).
  C. *Congenital malformations.* In general, the more severe the malformation, the more likely the fetus is to be small for gestational age. This is especially evident in fetuses with chromosomal abnormalities or those with serious cardiovascular malformations. For example, the anencephalic fetus is often growth retarded even when considering the missing brain and cranium (Honnebier and Swaab, 1973). Retarded growth of this degree is not seen in infants with spina bifida, but those infants are smaller than controls (Wald and associates, 1980).

D. *Chromosomal abnormalities.* The most severe forms of fetal growth retardation caused by chromosomal defects are trisomies, especially of chromosomes 13 and 18 (Larsen and Evans, 1984). Fetal growth retardation caused by trisomy 21 is less severe. Most often, trisomy 18 is associated with severe and early symmetrical fetal growth retardation and hydramnios. Trisomy 13 and Turner syndrome (45,X or gonadal dysgenesis) also are associated with some degree of retarded fetal growth (Larsen and Evans, 1984). Barlow (1973) reported that extra X chromosomes are associated with minimally decreased fetal weight.

E. *Dwarf syndromes.* Numerous inherited syndromes such as osteogenesis imperfecta and other such abnormalities are associated with fetal growth retardation.

II. Combined Symmetrical and Asymmetrical
  A. *Teratogenic drugs.* Any drug that causes a teratogenic injury is capable of producing fetal growth retardation.
    1. Tobacco impairs fetal growth in a direct relationship with the number of cigarettes smoked (Dougherty and Jones, 1982; Meyer, 1978).
    2. Narcotics act by decreasing maternal food intake and fetal cell number (Stone and associates, 1971). Interestingly, it is likely that heroin accelerates fetal lung maturation (Glass and colleagues, 1971).
    3. Alcohol acts in a linear dose-related fashion, and 2 to 3 percent of the infants of moderate drinkers have the fetal alcohol syndrome even though their mothers are not alcoholics (Sokol and associates, 1980). There is an 11 percent incidence of the fetal alcohol syndrome in fetuses whose mothers are moderate drinkers (two to three drinks per day), and up to a 32 percent incidence in fetuses whose mothers are heavy drinkers (five or more drinks per day) (Hanson and co-workers, 1978)
    4. Some anticonvulsants, such as phenytoin (Dilantin) and trimethadione (Tridione), may produce specific and characteristic syndromes that include fetal growth retardation (Hanson and co-workers, 1976).
  B. *Severe malnutrition.* Most often, the fetus grows normally despite significantly decreased maternal caloric intake. The best-documented effect of famine on fetal growth was in the winter of 1944 in Holland when the German Army enforced a restriction of approximately 600 kcal per day for pregnant women. The famine persisted for 28 weeks and there was an average birthweight decrease of 250 g per infant (Stein and colleagues, 1975). Although this was a small **average** decrease, fetal mortality rates were increased significantly.

III. Asymmetrical
  A. *Vascular disease.* Chronic vascular disease, especially when further complicated by superimposed preeclampsia, commonly causes growth retardation. Conversely, pregnancy-induced hypertension without underlying vascular or renal disease is unlikely to be accompanied by fetal growth retardation (Robertson and associates, 1975).
  B. *Chronic renal disease.* Renal insufficiency commonly is accompanied by retarded fetal growth (Katz and associates, 1980).
  C. *Chronic hypoxia.* Fetuses of women who reside at high altitude usually weigh less than those born to women who live at a lower altitude. Fetuses of women with cyanotic heart disease are frequently growth retarded.
  D. *Maternal anemia.* Although maternal anemia has been implicated in the genesis of fetal growth retardation, in our experiences, this has been common only in fetuses of women with sickle cell disease or with other inherited anemias associated with serious maternal disease.
  E. *Placental and cord abnormalities.* Chronic focal placental abruption, extensive infarction, or chorioangioma are likely to cause retarded fetal growth (Fig. 38–4). A circumvallate placenta or a placenta previa may impair growth, but usu-

ally the fetus is not markedly smaller than normal. Marginal insertion of the cord and especially velamentous insertions are more likely to be accompanied by a growth-retarded fetus (Chap. 31).
  F. *Multiple fetuses.* Pregnancy with two or more fetuses is likely to be complicated by appreciable growth retardation of one or both fetuses, compared with normal singletons (Chap. 34).
  G. *Postterm pregnancy.* While the majority of postterm fetuses probably continue to gain weight, the longer pregnancy progresses past term, the greater the likelihood of the fetus appearing undernourished and chronically distressed. During this time the fetus not only may fail to gain weight but also may actually lose weight.
  H. *Extrauterine pregnancy.* Commonly, the fetus who has not been housed in the uterus is growth retarded.

SCREENING AND DIAGNOSIS OF FETAL GROWTH RETARDATION

IDENTIFICATION AFTER DELIVERY

Identification through history of any of the above factors, as well as *a history of a previously growth-retarded fetus or fetal or neonatal death* should alert the obstetrician to the possibility of growth retardation during the current pregnancy (Galbraith and associates, 1979). Early and meticulous establishment of gestational age and careful measurements of uterine height throughout pregnancy should serve to identify most instances of abnormal fetal growth; however, the *definitive diagnosis* cannot be made until delivery. Even then, minor degrees of fetal growth retardation often are overlooked if only the neonatal weight is considered. For example, in late-onset pregnancy-induced hypertension, a fetus destined to be born with a birthweight in the 70th percentile may, at least theoretically, have this reduced to the 50th percentile. Such weight reduction usually results in little or no morbidity or significant consequences. Thus, inappropriate fetal growth also occurs in fetuses below the 90th and above the 10th percentile for gestational age. Put another way, there may be abnormal growth even in normal-weight infants.

A variety of techniques have been developed in attempts to identify less obvious forms of fetal growth retardation. The majority are used to identify forms of inappropriate growth, such as macrosomia and asymmetrical fetal growth retardation. These techniques usually are based on a ratio of too much or too little weight, skin thickness measured at various sites, or chest or midarm circumference compared to body length or head or chest circumference. The advantage of such ratios is that each fetus serves as its own standard, that is, obese or lean, based upon his or her length or head or chest circumference.

The *ponderal index* has been used most often to identify such inappropriate forms of fetal growth. The index is calculated using the formula:

$$\text{Ponderal Index} = \frac{\text{weight (g)}}{(\text{length in cm})^3} \times 100$$

The technique can be used to identify the macrosomic as well as the asymmetrically growth-retarded infant, but it cannot be used to identify the constitutionally small for gestational age or symmetrically growth-retarded neonate.

The *midarm circumference: occipitofrontal head circumference (MAC/HC) ratio* is claimed by some to be a more sensitive and possibly more specific anthropometric method of identifying fetuses who are macrosomic and not just constitutionally large

(Georgieff and co-workers, 1986; Meadows and associates, 1986). The same claim has been made for fetuses who are small for gestational age. Specifically, babies who are constitutionally small for gestational age have a normal ratio, while it is abnormally low in those who have late-onset growth retardation and thus are at risk for hypoglycemia. Its inherent accuracy derives from the ratio being between the midarm circumference, which is an anthropometric measurement markedly affected by changes in nutritional status, and head circumference, which is the measurement least affected by nutritional conditions (Meadows and associates, 1986). Using this index, Georgieff and associates (1986), reported that symptomatic, small for gestational age infants with growth retardation were born to mothers who had chronic medical complications throughout pregnancy, while neonates of "normal weight" but with signs and symptoms of growth retardation were born to mothers whose pregnancy complications caused impaired fetal growth late in the third trimester (Fig. 38–11). Both pregnancy and neonatal complications were uncommon in apparently constitutionally small for gestational age infants.

ANTEPARTUM IDENTIFICATION

The challenge remains primarily with the obstetrician to identify the fetus who is inappropriately growing in utero. This difficulty is underscored by the fact that such identification is not always possible even in the nursery! Regardless, there are clinical techniques and high-technological equipment that may prove useful in helping to screen and hopefully to diagnose fetal growth retardation. Some of the widely used techniques, as well as those potentially useful, are described below.

Uterine Fundal Height

In 1977 Westin published a graph of symphysial-fundal height measurements from 100 normal Swedish women. Using this chart, he was able to predict 75 percent of neonates who were more than one standard deviation below and 65 percent of neonates who were one standard deviation above the mean weight for gestational age. In a subsequent prospective study from this same group (Wallin and colleagues, 1981), there was a reported sensitivity of 74 percent and a specificity of 84 percent in detecting small for gestational age infants. Unfortunately, predictive values for a positive or negative test were not reported. Wallin and associates (1981) identified four types of fetal growth curves: high, normal, static, and low. After 30 weeks gestation, the true predictive value of a low- or static-type growth curve (both considered to be abnormal) in identifying a small for gestational age infant was calculated at *approximately* 40 percent.

Belizan and co-workers (1978) were able to predict 38 out of 44 neonates with birthweights below the 10th percentile and 85 of 94 with adequate birthweights, using uterine fundal measurements. They failed to report true predictive values, but these are *estimated* to be 80 percent for a positive test and 93 percent for a negative test.

Calvert and associates (1982) reported that a single measurement below the 10th percentile identified 64 percent of women who ultimately delivered small for gestational age infants. Similar results were reported by Quaranta and associates (1981). However, Rosenberg and co-workers (1982) reported that uterine fundal height measurements were no better than the other clinical means for identifying small for gestational age infants. Cnattinguis and associates (1984) reported that low or catch-up growth patterns identified 79 percent (sensitivity) of neonates with birthweights less than two standard deviations for gestational age and 92 percent of normal-birthweight infants (specificity). The predictive value for a positive test was 21 percent; it was 99 percent for a negative test.

Carefully performed serial uterine fundal height measurements throughout gestation are a simple, safe, inexpensive, and reasonably accurate screening method that may be used to detect many small for gestational age fetuses. The principal prob-

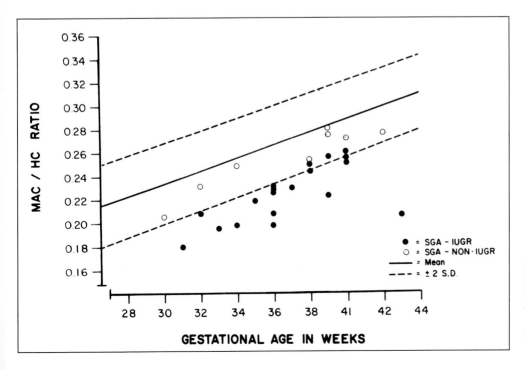

Figure 38–11. Comparison of MAC/HC in symptomatic (●) and non-symptomatic (○) SGA infants plotted on a standard curve. (*Reproduced with permission from Georgieff and co-workers: J Pediatr 109:316, 1986*).

lem is a high false-positive predictive value and the inability to differentiate between symmetrically or asymmetrically growth-retarded infants. These measurements are not applicable, however, in multifetal pregnancies, hydramnios, or for fetuses in a transverse lie.

The method used in Parkland Hospital prenatal clinics was reported by Jimenez and colleagues (1983). Briefly this consists of a tape calibrated in centimeters being applied over the abdominal curvature from the top of the symphysis to the top of the uterine fundus, which is identified by palpation or percussion. The measurement is made after the bladder is emptied, and the tape is applied with the markings away from the examiner to avoid prejudice. Between 20 and 34 weeks, the uterine fundal height in centimeters roughly coincides with weeks of gestation. If the measurement is more than 2 cm from the expected height, inappropriate fetal growth is suspected.

Ultrasonic Measurements

Evaluation and measurement by sonar for screening, diagnosis, and management of inappropriate fetal growth has become indispensable. Several techniques are used, and it is emphasized again that knowledge of accurate gestational age is paramount.

In 1971 Campbell and Dewhurst suggested that serial cephalometry of the *biparietal diameter* could be utilized to identify the growth-retarded fetus. This technique was used by Campbell (1972) to identify two patterns. In the *low-profile pattern*, head growth was continuously low throughout pregnancy, and this was associated with congenital abnormalities, infections, and chromosomal abnormalities. The *late-flattening pattern* was characterized by previously normal head growth followed by slowing or cessation of fetal head growth during the third trimester. This growth pattern was associated with placental and maternal factors, such as hypertension. Campbell and Dewhurst's initial observations have been confirmed by many others, but in most subsequent reports the authors have reported a failure to detect all cases of fetal growth retardation (Persson and associates, 1978a and b; Queenan and colleagues, 1976).

Campbell and Wilkin (1975) first described ultrasonic measurements of abdominal circumference made at the level of the umbilical vein. They defined an abnormal measurement as one at or less than the 5th percentile for gestational age. A variety of different techniques have been reported either to measure this circumference directly or to calculate it from measurements of anterior-posterior or transverse diameters.

Campbell and Thoms (1975) described a nomogram for the *ratio of head to abdominal circumference*. Normally, head circumference is larger than abdominal circumference until approximately 32 weeks. Between 32 and 36 weeks gestation the two circumferences are about equal. After 36 weeks gestation, the abdominal circumference usually exceeds head circumference. This technique was reported to improve identification of retarded fetal growth, as well as to distinguish symmetrical from asymmetrical growth patterns. The initial observations of Campbell and Thoms (1975) have been confirmed by others, including Sabbagha (1978) and Varma and colleagues (1979).

Estimates of total intrauterine volume include the fetus and amnionic fluid, both of which often are decreased with fetal growth retardation. Gohari and associates (1977) reported decreased total intrauterine volume was useful to diagnose fetal growth retardation. An excessively high false-positive rate (Grossman and co-workers, 1982) and the now widespread use of real-time sonography has resulted in the abandonment of this measurement, which is obtained using a static scanner.

Because of the association of oligohydramnios with retarded fetal growth, Manning and associates (1981b) suggested that a *qualitative estimation of amnionic fluid volume* could be used to identify fetal growth retardation. They defined as abnormal a fluid pocket of less than 1 cm. This correlated well with fetal growth retardation. This has been questioned by Hoddick and associates (1984) and by Philipson and colleagues (1983), who reported high false-positive rates. Basticle and co-workers (1986), however, emphasized that oligohydramnios is an ominous sign, and when severe, it is often an indication for delivery.

Different formulas based upon fetal diameters, circumferences and areas from all parts of the body have been used to calculate *fetal weight* at various stages of gestation (Campbell and Wilkin, 1975; Eik-Nes and associates, 1982). The formulas are complex and the tables created for fetal weights are awesome (Shepard and colleagues, 1987). The daily use and reliability of these techniques presently are not well established, but the techniques apparently result in a higher predictive value than many other methods (Benson and co-workers, 1986).

Cerebellar measurements appear promising, but the initial observations of Goldstein and associates (1987) must be confirmed.

Kazzi and colleagues (1983a and b) reported that a grade III placenta, in a preterm or small for gestational age fetus, defined by a biparietal diameter equal to or less than 87 mm, was associated with fetal growth retardation in a high percentage of cases. As yet, this has not been confirmed in singleton pregnancies, but accelerated placental aging has been reported when twin gestations were compared to singletons (Trudinger and Cook, 1985).

EVALUATION OF ULTRASONIC METHODS

Benson and associates (1986) critically analyzed a large series of published ultrasonic criteria for identifying fetal growth retardation to ascertain the positive and negative predictive values (Table 38–12). The study was drawn from 21 reports and included those from which sensitivity and specificity could be calculated. Predictive values were computed using Bayes theorem and based upon a 10 percent prevalence rate of fetal growth retardation. Seven of the nine techniques had positive predictive values of less than 50 percent. Thus, when one of these measurements was abnormal, a fetus was more likely to be normal than growth-retarded. The best predictive value, 62 percent, was obtained using the ratio of head to abdominal circumference. Benson and colleagues concluded that none of these methods allows for a confident antenatal diagnosis of fetal growth retardation.

Techniques used to identify low fetal weight can be expected to detect 88 percent of growth-retarded fetuses; however, 12 percent (specificity 88 percent) of normal fetuses will be included in the abnormal group. Because of this specificity and because few fetuses are actually growth retarded, only 45 percent of fetuses estimated to be small for gestational age will actually be small.

The only two methods with a predictive value above 50 percent were estimation of amnionic fluid volume and the head circumference/abdominal circumference ratio. However, amnionic fluid volume measurements have little practical use, since the technique detects only 24 percent (sensitivity) of the cases in which fetal growth retardation actually is present. The 62 percent predictive value of the head circumference/abdominal circumference ratio appears to be the best clinical tool, with a sensitivity of 82 percent.

TABLE 38–12. VALUE OF ULTRASONIC METHODS TO DETECT FETAL GROWTH RETARDATION

			Predictive Value	
Criterion	Sensitivity[a] (%)	Specificity[a] (%)	Positive (%)	Negative (%)
Advanced placental grade	62	64	16	94
Increased femur length/abdominal circumference ratio	34–49	78–83	18–20	92–93
Decreased total intrauterine volume	57–80	72–76	21–24	92–97
Small biparietal diameter	24–88	62–94	21–44	92–98
Small biparietal diameter plus advanced placental grade	59	86	32	95
Slow rate of biparietal diameter growth	75	84	35	97
Abnormally low estimated fetal weight	89	88	45	99
Decreased amnionic fluid volume	24	98	55	92
Elevated head circumference/abdominal circumference ratio	82	94	62	98

[a] A range of values is given for a criterion when different studies apply to that criterion in two or more ways.
In one study (Crane and colleagues, 1977), sensitivity and specificity were reported to be 100 %. This study was omitted since it included only four growth-retarded fetuses.
Modified from Benson and colleagues: Radiology 160:415, 1986.

The promise of an accurate prediction of fetal growth retardation using sonography has not been achieved. Despite these low predictive values, it has been claimed that a negative predictive value of 92 to 99 percent proves the value of these tests because the obstetrician can safely conclude that the risk of fetal growth retardation is small. The prevalence of fetal growth retardation in the general population, however, is 10 percent or less.

COMPARISON OF UTERINE FUNDAL HEIGHT AND ULTRASONIC MEASUREMENTS

Pearce and Campbell (1983) compared serial fundal height measurements with a single third-trimester measurement of abdominal circumference and reported that both methods had an almost equal sensitivity of 85 percent and a false-positive rate of 55 percent. Cnattinguis and associates (1985) compared serial fundal height measurements to two separately obtained biparietal diameters, the first obtained between 16 and 21 weeks, and the second at least 10 weeks after the first. They reported that fundal height measurements were more accurate than ultrasonic measurements for diagnosing fetal growth retardation. For every correct diagnosis obtained with the fundal height measurement there were three false positives (predictive value, 25 percent). However, for every correct diagnosis using the biparietal diameter, there were 10 false positives (predictive value, 9 percent).

From these two studies, Pearce and Campbell (1983) and Cnattinguis and colleagues (1985) concluded that either technique was an acceptable method to *screen* for fetal growth retardation. Once an abnormal result was obtained, they recommended complete anthropometric fetal assessment, ultrasonic examination to rule out fetal anomalies and to assess amnionic fluid volume, and appropriate tests to assess fetal well-being.

DOPPLER VELOCIMETRY

Detection and Diagnosis

The identification of abnormal umbilical artery waveforms (indices) appears to be useful in detecting some but not all fetuses who have or may develop fetal growth retardation (Fig. 38–12) (Berkowitz, 1988; Erskine, 1985; Fleisher, 1985; McCowan, 1987, 1988; Rochelson, 1987a and b; Whittle, 1987; Woo, 1987; and all

their associates). One possible explanation for this variability in diagnostic accuracy has been provided by Giles and co-workers (1985). In an elegant study, these workers counted the number of muscular arteries per high-power field in placental samples taken from 106 pregnancies in which antenatal Doppler studies had been performed. The number of arteries per high-power field were reduced significantly in placentas from fetuses with abnormally high umbilical artery S/D ratios; however, the absolute number of tertiary stem villi were not different in abnormal and control groups. These workers concluded that abnormal waveforms in the umbilical artery may identify a specific placental microvascular lesion that includes obliteration of small muscular arteries in the tertiary stem villi. **These findings, there-**

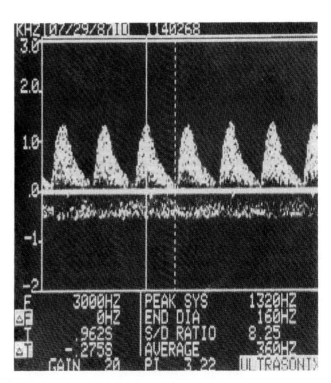

Figure 38–12. Umbilical artery velocimetry waveforms from a growth-retarded fetus at 35 weeks gestation. Note absence of end-diastolic flow. (*Courtesy of Drs. R. Santos and M. Lucas.*)

fore, are consistent with the view that if the fetus is constitutionally small, or if retarded growth is not due to obliterated placental vessels, it is likely that there will be no changes in the umbilical arterial waveforms.

It is likely that the ability to detect fetal growth retardation has varied for several other reasons as well. For example, studies to date have been hampered by the absence of reliable standards to diagnose growth retardation. In many studies, there are little data concerning the birthweight of the fetuses, and in others, ultrasound estimates of fetal weight have been used with 10 to 15 percent error rates. Another difficulty is the lack of well-controlled, prospective studies in which umbilical artery Doppler studies have been performed. Unfortunately, many reports have included pregnancies at risk for growth retardation or those in which the diagnosis already was suspected. Therefore, two pertinent clinical questions need to be answered. The first is, can Doppler studies be used to distinguish the small for gestational age fetus from the incorrectly dated gestation? The second is, can Doppler be used to predict which fetuses ultimately will be growth retarded?

Prediction of Fetal Growth Retardation

Campbell and colleagues (1986) screened 126 consecutive pregnancies for the development of fetal growth retardation, uteroplacental insufficiency, and pregnancy-induced hypertension. They used *uterine artery* waveform analysis (Chap. 15, p. 286) and reported that the identification of an abnormal waveform had a sensitivity of 68 percent, with a specificity of 69 percent, a positive predictive value of 42 percent, and a negative predictive value of 87 percent. Thus, while most complications were detected, a normal examination did not exclude the possibility of complications ultimately developing.

Trudinger and co-workers (1987) reported the results of a prospective, randomized trial in which *umbilical artery* waveform analysis was used in obstetrical decision making. In the study, 300 women whose fetuses were at risk for a variety of reasons, including fetal growth retardation, were randomized so that only half of the clinicians caring for the women were given results of the Doppler studies. Between the two groups, there were no differences in gestational age at delivery, birthweight, or elective cesarean delivery, but a higher frequency of cesarean section for fetal distress in labor was observed in the group of women in whom Doppler results were withheld. If Doppler studies were useful in decision making, a reciprocal increase in the frequency of elective cesarean would have been expected, but it was not found. In summary, to date the positive predictive value of an abnormal test has been disappointing (Berkowitz and associates, 1988a and b; McCowan and colleagues, 1987), but this, in part, is dependent upon the prevalence of fetal growth retardation.

Fetal Adaptation to Growth Retardation

Fetal adaptation to the stress of various causes of growth retardation has been studied. Reduced *umbilical vein* blood flow has been observed simultaneously with abnormal umbilical artery waveforms (Gill and co-workers, 1984; Laurin and associates, 1987). Abnormal fetal aortic waveforms also have been reported in growth-retarded fetuses by some (Griffin and associates, 1984; Jouppila and colleagues, 1986; Tonge and co-workers, 1986) but not all workers (Copel and associates, 1988). Decreased fetal aortic volume flow also has been reported (see Chap. 15, p. 286). For example, Laurin and co-workers (1987) reported that mean and peak aortic velocities,

as well as volume flow (normalized to estimated fetal weight), fell in direct relation to the weight percentile. Umbilical venous blood flow also was decreased in growth-retarded fetuses in this study.

The question of whether the growth-retarded human fetus has the ability to redistribute blood flow preferentially to the brain has been addressed by several groups of investigators using similar methods. Wladimiroff and associates (1987) compared the pulsatility index of the intracranial internal carotid artery with that of the umbilical artery. In growth-retarded fetuses, an increase in umbilical artery pulsatility index (abnormal value) was identified concomitantly with a reduced carotid artery index (possibly compensatory improved flow), and the ratio of the two indices was significantly different in pregnancies with retarded fetal growth. Arbeille and colleagues (1987) defined a *cerebral-placental ratio*, which is the Pourcelot index of the anterior cerebral artery compared to that of the umbilical artery. It was found to be less than one in all pregnancies studied, including 40 with normal fetuses and 21 with growth-retarded fetuses. Similar findings have been reported by others (Arduini, 1987; Kirkinen, 1987; Woo, 1987; and their co-workers).

Fetal Outcome and Treatment

Fetuses who have the most abnormal umbilical artery waveforms have been observed to have much more complicated neonatal courses than those of neonates without such findings (McCowan and colleagues, 1987; Rochelson and associates, 1987a; Trudinger and associates, 1985; Woo and co-workers, 1987). At first glance this suggests some value to Doppler studies to predict which growth-retarded fetuses might do better with delivery. Rochelson and associates (1987a) and Woo and colleagues (1987) reported that many of the fetuses with reversed diastolic flow also had classic cardiotocographic signs of fetal distress concurrently. Without careful observation of the natural course of such pregnancies, however, it may not be possible to determine the exact temporal development of these abnormalities. That is, what must be known is whether the abnormal Doppler findings precede abnormal cardiotocographic changes, or even whether the appearance of reversed diastolic flow represents a stage of fetal deterioration after which salvage is impossible or of dubious benefit.

The most intriguing studies of treatment for fetal growth retardation were conducted by Soothill and colleagues (1986a). They combined fetal aorta Doppler blood flow velocity determinations with percutaneous umbilical blood sampling to assess oxygenation and reported significant inverse relationships between fetal aortic mean blood velocity and severity of fetal hypoxia. They also reported a positive correlation with pH; that is, there was worsening acidosis in fetuses with lower mean aortic velocity measurements. When the mothers of these fetuses chronically inhaled high concentrations of oxygen (Nicolaides and co-workers, 1987), the fetuses demonstrated improved oxygenation and a concurrent return toward normal aortic blood flow velocity.

Wallenburg and Rotmans (1987) have presented preliminary data from 24 women who had idiopathic fetal growth retardation in previous pregnancies. Treatment with aspirin and dipyridamole, given daily from 16 to 31 weeks, reduced the incidence of retarded fetal growth (13 versus 60 percent) when compared to a nonrandomized but similar group of women who were not given antiplatelet drug therapy.

Biochemical Markers

In attempts to identify fetuses with growth retardation, a variety of placental enzymes, steroids, and protein hormones have been measured in amnionic fluid and in maternal plasma and urine. These include placental oxytocinase, placental lactogen, urinary or plasma estrogens, and pregnancy-specific glycoproteins. By and large, these have been abandoned by most clinics. Newer assays for a wide assortment of different compounds are currently under investigation, as well as studies of the clearance rates of estrogen precursors and glucose (Gross, 1981; Langer, 1986; Miodovinik, 1982; Sokol, 1982; and their co-workers). As yet, none of these tedious and expensive assays or methods has been shown to approach, much less surpass, the sensitivity, specificity, or predictive value of uterine fundal height measurements.

MANAGEMENT OF FETAL GROWTH RETARDATION

Clinical screening using carefully obtained gestational age and serial uterine fundal height measurements will detect many fetuses who are small for gestational age. Carefully obtained serial ultrasonic measurements done in high-risk groups such as women with chronic hypertension, diabetes, or those with renal or connective tissue diseases will identify even more fetuses at risk. *Even with intensive screening, not all fetuses can be identified.* Once a small for gestational age fetus is suspected, however, intensive efforts should be made to determine if growth retardation is present and, if so, the type of growth retardation and the etiology. The physician also should ensure delivery, when possible, of an infant who will subsequently thrive and grow to its normal potential. Finally, this must be done at the least cost to the patient in terms of finances and physical risk to herself and her fetus.

At Parkland Hospital, once a fetus is suspected of being growth retarded, an extensive sonographic survey is done to look for structural abnormalities. Anthropometric measurements are made, including head and abdominal circumferences, biparietal diameter, femur length, and the head circumference/abdominal circumference ratio. A clinical and ultrasonic assessment of amnionic fluid volume also is made. The gestational age is reconfirmed or, if not already known, established whenever possible. The condition of the cervix is assessed, and a decision is made as to whether or not to deliver the fetus.

GROWTH RETARDATION NEAR TERM

Prompt delivery is likely to afford the best outcome for the fetus who is suspected of being growth retarded at or near term. Here, as in the management of such fetuses who are remote from term, growth retardation should be identified as symmetrical or asymmetrical, and antepartum and intrapartum care provided as outlined below.

GROWTH RETARDATION REMOTE FROM TERM

Symmetrical Growth Retardation

If the fetus is symmetrically growth retarded, a meticulous search should be made for fetal anomalies, and consideration should be given to obtaining umbilical blood for karyotyping, especially if a chromosomal anomaly is suspected (Chap. 32). Umbilical venous blood can be obtained by ultrasonically directed percutaneous umbilical blood sampling (see Chap. 15, p. 282). Although some recommend that screening be done for toxoplasmosis, rubella, cytomegalovirus, herpes, and other viral agents (Pearce and Campbell, 1985), we have not found this to be productive.

Often a diagnosis of structural or chromosomal abnormality is established too late for therapeutic abortion, but even so, it is better that the parents, obstetrician, and pediatrician be forewarned. In some cases, such as with trisomy 13 or 18 fetuses who have multiple congenital anomalies and markedly attenuated life expectancies, cesarean section may be avoided.

Having excluded as nearly as possible structural, chromosomal, and possibly congenital infection, the woman is hospitalized, put at decreased physical activity, and given an adequate diet, and fetal surveillance is started. At a minimum, this includes fetal movement charts and clinical and sonographic assessment of fetal growth and amnionic fluid volume. Many recommend a battery of fetal surveillance tests, which includes, but certainly is not limited to, nonstress tests, contraction stress tests, biophysical profiles, serial Doppler velocity waveform measurements, and combinations thereof. We follow fetal well-being with daily clinical evaluations of the pregnant woman, daily fetal movement counts, and weekly fetal heart rate monitoring (see Chap. 15, p. 295). Most often, in the case of a seriously compromised fetus, the mother will notice decreased fetal activity or the physician will detect decreased amnionic fluid volume. In some cases, there may be a cessation of fetal growth detected by serial sonographic assessments.

Asymmetrical Fetal Growth Retardation

After diagnosis, the woman should be hospitalized and fetal surveillance, as described above, started. Since a number of asymmetrically growth-retarded fetuses are the consequence of abnormalities in uteroplacental perfusion, many chose to monitor these pregnancies with Doppler velocimetry (Fleisher, 1985; Hackett, 1987; McCowan, 1987; Soothill, 1987; Trudinger, 1987; and their associates). In most such reports, the fetus is already severely ill and often acidotic when these tests became ominous. However, there have been remarkable outcomes and sometimes spectacular rescues of apparently doomed fetuses (Nicolaides and colleagues, 1987; Soothill and associates, 1986a and b). At Parkland Hospital we follow selected fetuses in this manner, and our preliminary observations support to a lesser degree the glowing reports just cited. Importantly, the loss or reversal of end-diastolic flow in the umbilical artery and fetal descending aorta often identifies the fetus who is in imminent danger of dying (Brar and Platt, 1988) (Fig. 38–12).

Pearce and Campbell (1985) suggested that another reason for finding normal Doppler studies was that a small for gestational age fetus with normal uterine arcuate and fetal aortic velocity waveforms was probably not growth retarded, but instead was consitutionally small. If this observation is confirmed, constitutionally small fetuses can be separated from growth-retarded fetuses and intensive surveillance of the constitutionally small fetus eliminated.

In most instances of fetal growth retardation remote from term, there is no specific treatment that will ameliorate the condition. Possible exceptions are inadequate maternal nutrition, heavy smoking, use of street drugs, and possibly chronic alcoholism. Ideally, the use of tobacco, illicit drugs, and alcohol can be curtailed and ingestion of an adequate diet should favorably influence fetal growth. Very sedentary living that approaches full-time bed rest also may favorably influence fetal growth and, at the same time, possibly reduce the risk of preterm labor.

Occasionally, the overtly growth-retarded fetus is in serious jeopardy irrespective of whether he remains in utero or is delivered. For the fetus who is severely growth retarded but remote from term, the decision to proceed with delivery becomes a matter of trying to ascertain the degree of risk from further uterine stay compared to the risks from preterm delivery. Certainly, the loss or reversal of Doppler end-diastolic waveforms in fetal aorta or umbilical arteries favors delivery (Fig. 38–12). Fortunately, there frequently is accelerated lung maturation in these fetuses. Confirmation of a lecithin:sphingo-myelin (L/S) ratio of 2 or more or identification of phosphatidylglycerol in amnionic fluid is reassuring; however, a lower ratio or no detectable phosphatidylglycerol does not always predict that respiratory distress will develop (Chap. 15).

Generally, delivery of an obviously growth-retarded fetus under the conditions outlined below, rather than procrastination, with further fetal deterioration, offers the best chance for survival. By the time in gestation that fetal growth retardation has become severe, the fetus is usually mature enough to survive if (1) delivery is prompt rather than allowing the risk of further compromise, (2) there is close monitoring during labor to avoid further compromise or delivery is accomplished by cesarean section, and (3) excellent neonatal care begins immediately after delivery.

The presence of maternal disease that is worsening as a consequence of the pregnancy and thereby threatens the well-being of the mother as well as the fetus certainly should influence the decision to deliver the severely growth-retarded fetus. Almost any maternal disease falls into this category when it is characterized by vascular disease, renal involvement, or both, and decidedly so if preeclampsia supervenes (Chap. 35, p. 690). With prompt delivery, fetal and neonatal salvage is likely to be improved compared to unduly delayed delivery, even though the L/S ratio is considered immature (Fig. 38–4). At the same time, with prompt delivery, maternal deterioration is likely to be arrested.

LABOR AND DELIVERY

Throughout labor, spontaneous or induced, those fetuses who are suspected of being growth retarded should be monitored very closely for evidence of distress, including abnormalities of fetal heart rate and the presence of appreciable amounts of meconium in the amnionic fluid. The likelihood of severe fetal distress during labor is considerably increased. Fetal growth retardation commonly is the result of insufficient placental function occurring as a consequence of either faulty maternal perfusion or ablation of functional placenta, or both. These conditions are likely to be aggravated by vigorous labor. Importantly, lack of amnionic fluid predisposes to cord compression and its dangers. Consequently, the capabilities for immediate cesarean section should be available. Furthermore, it can be anticipated that the infant at birth may need expert assistance in making a successful transition to air breathing. The fetus is at risk of being born hypoxic and of having aspirated meconium

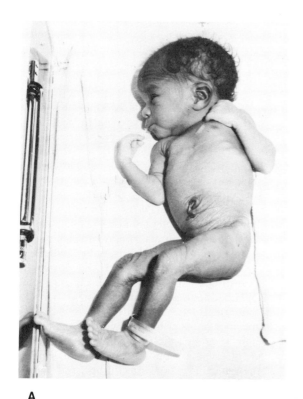

A

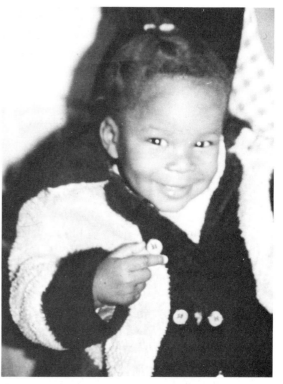

B

Figure 38–13. A. A severely asymmetrically growth-retarded infant at 38 weeks gestational age but with a birthweight of only 1,800 g. Delivery was by cesarean section. The chronically hypertensive mother had suffered two previous stillbirths. **B.** The same infant at 13 months of age. Physical and intellectual development was normal at that time.

into the lungs, thus compromising chances of successful ventilation. As soon as the head is delivered from the vagina, or from the uterus during a cesarean section, the mouth, pharynx, and nares should be aspirated quickly by the obstetrician. Moreover, it is essential that care for the newborn be provided immediately by someone who can skillfully clear the airway below the vocal cords, especially of meconium, and ventilate the infant as needed. The severely growth-retarded newborn infant is particularly susceptible to hypothermia and also may develop other metabolic derangements, especially serious hypoglycemia (Soothill and colleagues, 1987). Polycythemia and blood hyperviscosity occasionally may cause serious difficulty (Jones and Battaglia, 1977).

SUBSEQUENT DEVELOPMENT OF THE GROWTH RETARDED FETUS

Subsequent growth of the individual newborn who is growth retarded cannot be predicted reliably from anthropometric measurements obtained at birth (Philip, 1978). In general, prolonged symmetrical, or generalized, growth retardation in utero is likely to be followed by slow growth after birth, whereas the asymmetrically growth-retarded fetus is more likely to catch up after birth (Fig. 38–13). Specifically, the infant whose weight is reduced can be expected to grow normally, but if length also is compromised, he or she is likely to remain small (Brook, 1983). Finally, the infant's sex and parent's size play important roles in determining somatic size (Brook, 1983; Ounsted and associates, 1985).

The subsequent neurologial and intellectual capabilities of the infant who was growth retarded in utero cannot be predicted precisely. Fancourt and associates (1976) found, however, that in children with sonographic evidence of delayed head growth starting before the third trimester, subsequent neurological and intellectual development also was delayed. The overall outcome is not bleak, however, and Vohr and associates (1979) reported that preterm, small for gestational age infants had similar outcomes at 18 to 24 months, compared to appropriate for gestational age preterm infants. A longer follow-up of preterm small for gestational age infants also supports the view that a long-term favorable outcome may be expected (Vohr and Oh, 1983). Finally, the outcome is good for neurological and cognitive development, *but not for somatic growth in term nonasphyxiated* small for gestational age infants (Westwood and co-workers, 1983).

FETAL GROWTH RETARDATION IN SUBSEQUENT PREGNANCIES

The risk of repeat instances of fetal growth retardation is increased in women in lower socioeconomic circumstances (Bakketeig and colleagues, 1986). This is especially true in women with a previous history of fetal growth retardation and a current medical complication (Patterson and colleagues, 1986).

REFERENCES

Alger LS, Lovchik JC, Hebel JR, Blackmon LR, Crenshaw MC: The association of *Chlamydia trachomatis, Neisseria gonorrhoeae,* and group B streptococci with preterm rupture of the membranes and pregnancy outcome. Am J Obstet Gynecol 159:397, 1988

American College of Obstetricians and Gynecologists: Committee opinion: Postterm pregnancy. Committee on Obstetrics: Maternal and Fetal Medicine No 57, October 1987

Amon E, Lewis SV, Sibai BM, Villar MA, Arheart KL: Ampicillin prophylaxis in preterm premature rupture of the membranes: A prospective randomized study. Am J Obstet Gynecol 159:539, 1988

Angel JL, O'Brien WF, Knuppel RA, Morales WJ, Sims CJ: Carbohydrate intolerance in patients receiving oral tocolytics. Am J Obstet Gynecol 159:762, 1988

Arbeille P, Roncin A, Berson M, Patet F, Pourcelot L: Exploration of the fetal cerebral blood flow by duplex Doppler-linear array system in normal and pathological pregnancies. Ultrasound Med Biol 13:329, 1987

Arduini D, Rizzo G, Romanini C, Mancuso S: Fetal blood flow velocity waveforms as predictors of growth retardation. Obstet Gynecol 70:7, 1987

Arias F, Tomich P: Etiology and outcome of low birth weight and preterm infants. Obstet Gynecol 60:277, 1982

Avery ME, Aylward G, Creasy R, Little AB, Stripp B: Update on prenatal steroids for prevention of respiratory distress: Report of a conference—September 26–28, 1985. Am J Obstet Gynecol 155:2, 1986

Bakketeig LS, Bjerkedal T, Hoffman HJ: Small-for-gestational age births in successive pregnancy outcomes: Results from a longitudinal study of births in Norway. Early Hum Dev 14:187, 1986

Barlow P: The influence of inactive chromosomes on human development: Anomalous sex chromosome complements and the phenotype. Hum Genet 17:105, 1973

Barrett JM, Salyer SL, Boehm FH: Nonstress test: Evaluation of 1000 patients. Am J Obstet Gynecol 143:243, 1982

Barss VA, Frigoletto FD, Diamond F: Stillbirth after nonstress testing. Obstet Gynecol 65:541, 1985

Basticle A, Manning F, Harman C, Lange I, Morrison I: Ultrasound evaluation of amniotic fluid: Outcome of pregnancies with severe oligohydramnios. Am J Obstet Gynecol 154:895, 1986

Battaglia FC, Lubchenco LO: A practical classification of newborn infants by weight and gestational age. J Pediatr 71:159, 1967

Bejar R, Curbelo V, Coen RW, Leopold G, James H, Gluck L: Diagnosis and follow-up of intraventricular and intracerebral hemorrhages by ultrasound studies of infant's brain through the fontanelles and sutures. Pediatrics 66:661, 1980

Bejar R, Curbelo V, Davis C, Gluck L: Premature labor: II. Bacterial sources of phospholipase. Obstet Gynecol 57:479, 1981

Belizan JM, Villar J, Nardin JC, Malamud J, Sainz de Vicuna L: Diagnosis of intrauterine growth retardation by a simple clinical method: Measurement of uterine height. Am J Obstet Gynecol 131:643, 1978

Bell R: The prediction of preterm labour by recording spontaneous antenatal uterine activity. Br J Obstet Gynaecol 90:844, 1983

Benedetti TJ, Easterling T: Antepartum testing in postterm pregnancy. J Reprod Med 33:252, 1988

Benson CB, Doubilet PM, Saltzman DH: Intrauterine growth retardation: Predictive value of U.S. criteria for antenatal diagnosis. Radiology 160:415, 1986

Berkowitz GS, Chitkara U, Rosenberg J, Cogswell C, Walker B, Lahman EA, Mehalek KE, Berkowitz RL: Sonographic estimation of fetal weight and Doppler analysis of umbilical artery velocimetry in the prediction of intrauterine growth retardation: A prospective study. Am J Obstet Gynecol 158:1149, 1988a

Berkowitz GS, Mehalek KE, Chitkara U, Rosenberg J, Cogswell C, Berkowitz RL: Doppler umbilical velocimetry in the prediction of adverse outcome in pregnancies at risk for intrauterine growth retardation. Obstet Gynecol 71:742, 1988b

Bobbitt JR, Haslip CC, Damato JD: Amniotic fluid infection as determined by transabdominal amniocentesis in patients with intact membranes in premature labor. Am J Obstet Gynecol 140:947, 1981

Bobbitt JR, Ledger WJ: Unrecognized amnionitis and prematurity: A preliminary report. J Reprod Med 19:8, 1977

Bochner CJ, Medearis AL, Davis J, Oakes GK, Hobel CJ, Wade ME: Antepartum predictors of fetal distress in postterm pregnancy. Am J Obstet Gynecol 157:353, 1987

Bochner CJ, Williams J III, Castro L, Medearis A, Hobel CJ, Wade M: The efficacy of starting postterm antenatal testing at 41 weeks as compared with 42 weeks of gestational age. Am J Obstet Gynecol 159:550, 1988

Brar HS, Platt LD: Reverse end-diastolic flow velocity on umbilical artery velocimetry in high-risk pregnancies: An ominous finding with adverse pregnancy outcome. Am J Obstet Gynecol 159:559, 1988

Brazle JV, Lubchenco LO: The estimation of gestational age chart. In Kenipe CH, Silver HK, and O'Brien D: Current Pediatric Diagnosis and Treatment, 3rd ed. Los Altos, Calif., Lange Medical Publications, 1974

Brenner WE, Edelman DA, Hendricks CH: A standard of fetal growth for the United States of America. Am J Obstet Gynecol 126:555, 1976

Broekhuizen FF, Gilman M, Hamilton PR: Amniocentesis for Gram stain and culture in preterm premature rupture of the membranes. Obstet Gynecol 66:316, 1985

Brook CGD: Consequences of intrauterine growth retardation. Br Med J 286:164, 1983

Brown ER, Nielsen H, Torday JS, Tauesch HW: Reversible induction of surfactant production in fetal lambs treated with glucocorticoids. Pediatr Res 13:491, 1979

Calvert JP, Crean EE, Newcombe RG, Pearson JF: Antenatal screening by measurement of symphysis-fundus height. Br Med J 285:846, 1982

Campbell S: Fetal growth. Clin Obstet Gynecol 1:41, 1972

Campbell S, Dewhurst CJ: Diagnosis of the small-for-dates fetus by ultrasound cephalometry. Lancet 2:1002, 1971

Campbell S, Pearce JM, Hackett G, Cohen-Overbeek T, Hernandez C: Qualitative assessment of uteroplacental blood flow: Early screening test for high-risk pregnancies. Obstet Gynecol 68:649, 1986

Campbell S, Thoms A: Ultrasound measurement of the fetal head to abdominal ratio in the assessment of growth retardation. Br J Obstet Gynaecol 84:165, 1975

Campbell S, Wilkin D: Ultrasonic measurement of fetal abdominal circumference in the estimation of fetal weight. Br J Obstet Gynaecol 84:165, 1975

Capeless EL, Mead PB: Management of preterm premature rupture of membranes: Lack of a national census. Am J Obstet Gynecol 157:11, 1987

Caritis SN, Lin LS, Toig G, Wong LK: Pharmacodynamics of ritodrine in pregnant women during preterm labor. Am J Obstet Gynecol 147:752, 1983

Carr-Hill RA, Hall MH: The repetition of spontaneous preterm labour. Br J Obstet Gynaecol 92:921, 1985

Cnattingius S, Axelsson O, Lindmark G: Symphysis-fundus measurements and intrauterine growth retardation. Acta Obstet Gynecol Scand 63:335, 1984

Cnattingius S, Axelsson O, Lindmark G: The clinical value of measurements of the symphysis-fundus distance and ultrasonic measurements of the biparietal diameter in the diagnosis of intrauterine growth retardation. J Perinat Med 13:227, 1985

Cohn HE, Sacks EJ, Heymann MA, Rudolph AM: Cardiovascular responses to hypoxemia and acidemia in fetal lambs. Am J Obstet Gynecol 120:817, 1974

Collaborative Group on Antenatal Steroid Therapy: Effect of antenatal dexamethasone administration on the prevention of respiratory distress syndrome. Am J Obstet Gynecol 141:276–288, 1981

Collaborative Group on Antenatal Steroid Therapy: Effects of antenatal dexamethasone administration in the infant: Long-term follow-up. J Pediatr 104:259, 1984

Cone JE: History of the Care and Feeding of the Premature Infant. Boston, Little, Brown, & Co, 1985, p 180

Copel JA, Grannum PA, Hobbins JC, Cunningham FG: Doppler ultrasound in obstetrics. Williams Suppl No 16, Appleton & Lange, January/February, 1988

Cotton DB, Hill LM, Strassner HT, Platt LD, Ledger WJ: Use of amniocentesis in preterm gestation with ruptured membranes. Obstet Gynecol 63:38, 1984a

Cotton DB, Strasner HT, Hill LM, Schifrin BS, Paul RH: Comparison between magnesium sulfate, terbutaline and a placebo for inhibition of preterm labor: A randomized study. J Reprod Med 29:92, 1984b

Covington DL, Carl J, Daley JG, Cushing D, Churchill MP: Effects of the North Carolina Prematurity Program among public patients delivering at New Hanover Memorial Hospital. Am J Public Health 78:1493, 1988

Cox SM, MacDonald PC, Casey ML: Assay of bacterial endotoxin (lipopolysaccharide) in human amniotic fluid: Potential usefulness in diagnosis and management of preterm labor. Am J Obstet Gynecol 159:99, 1988a

Cox SM, MacDonald PC, Casey ML: Cytokines and protaglandins in amniotic fluid of preterm labor pregnancies: Decidual origin in response to bacterial toxins [lipopolysaccharide (LPS) and lipotechnoic acid (LTA)]. Presented at the 36th annual meeting of the Society of Gynecologic Investigation {Abstract}, San Diego, March 1989

Cox S, Williams ML, Leveno KJ: The natural history of preterm ruptured membranes: What to expect of expectant management. Obstet Gynecol 71:558, 1988b

Crane JP, Kopta MM, Welt SI: Abnormal fetal growth patterns: Ultrasonic diagnosis and management. Obstet Gynecol 50:205, 1977

Creasy RK: Intrauterine growth retardation related to research and clinical application. Presented at the 10th World Congress of Gynecology and Obstetrics. San Francisco, 1982

Creasy RK, Barrett CT, deSwiet M, Kahanpää KV, Rudolph AM: Experimental intrauterine growth retardation in sheep. Am J Obstet Gynecol 112:566, 1972

Creasy RK, Gummer BA, Liggins GC: System for predicting spontaneous preterm birth. Obstet Gynecol 55:692, 1980

Crowley P, O'Herlihy C, Boylan P: The value of ultrasound measurement of amniotic fluid volume in the management of prolonged pregnancies. Br J Obstet Gynaecol 91:444, 1984

Devoe LD, Sholl JS: Postdates pregnancy: Assessment of fetal risk and obstetric management. J Reprod Med 28:576, 1983

Divon MY, Guidetti DA, Cantu U, Sklar AJ, Lev-Gur M, Langer O, Merkatz IR: Fetal biophysical profile scoring: The significance of fetal heart rate late decelerations: Presented at the 35th annual meeting of the Society for Gynecologic Investigation, [Abstract 199], Baltimore, March 1988

Dougherty CR, Jones AD: The determinants of birth weight. Am J Obstet Gynecol 144:190, 1982

Duscay CA, Thompson JS, Wu AT, Novy MJ: Effects of calcium entry blocker (nicardipine) tocolysis in rhesus macaques: Fetal plasma concentrations and cardiorespiratory changes. Am J Obstet Gyecol 157:1482, 1987

Eastman NJ, Jackson E: Weight relationships in pregnancy: I. The bearing of maternal weight gain and prepregnancy weight on birthweight in full term pregnancies. Obstet Gynecol Surv 22:1003, 1968

Eden RD, Seifert LS, Winegar A, Spellacy WN: Perinatal characteristics of uncomplicated postdate pregnancies. Obstet Gynecol 69:296, 1987

Eik-Nes SH, Marsal K, Brubakk AO, Kristofferson K, Ulstein M: Ultrasonic measurement of human fetal blood flow. J Biomed Eng 4:28, 1982

Elliott JP: Magnesium sulfate as a tocolytic agent. Am J Obstet Gynecol 147:277, 1983

Elliott JP, O'Keeffe DF, Greenberg P, Freeman RK: Pulmonary edema associated with magnesium sulfate and betamethasone administration. Am J Obstet Gynecol 134:717, 1979

Epstein MF, Nicholls E, Stubblefield PG: Neonatal hypoglycemia after beta-sympathomimetic tocolytic therapy. J Pediatr 94:449, 1979

Erskine RLA, Ritchie JWK: Quantitative measurement of fetal blood flow using Doppler ultrasound. Br J Obstet Gynaecol 92:600, 1985

Eschenbach DA, Gibbs RS, Martin DA, Rettig P, Regan J, Rao AY: Infectious and Prematurity Study Group: A randomized, placebo-controlled trial of erythromycin in pregnancy to prevent prematurity. Presented at the 35th annual meeting of the Society for Gynecologic Investigation [Abstract], Baltimore, March 1988

Evans JI, Schulman JD, Golden L: Superovulation-induced intrauterine growth retardation in mice. Am J Obstet Gynecol 141:433, 1981

Fancourt R, Campbell S, Harvey D, Norman AP: Follow-up studies of small-for-dates babies. Br Med J 1:1435, 1976

Farmakides G, Schulman H, Ducey J, Guzman E, Saladana L, Penny B, Winter D: Uterine and umbilical artery Doppler velocimetry in postterm pregnancy. J Reprod Med 33:259, 1988

Feinstein SJ, Vintzileos AM, Lodiero JG, Campbell WA, Weinbaum PJ, Nochimson DJ: Amniocentesis with premature rupture of membranes. Obstet Gynecol 68:147, 1986

Ferguson JE II, Hensleigh PA, Kredenster D: Adjunctive use of magnesium sulfate with ritodrine for preterm labor tocolysis. Am J Obstet Gynecol 148:166, 1984

Ferguson JE II, Holbrook RH Jr, Stevenson DK, Hensleigh PA, Kredenster D: Adjunctive magnesium sulfate infusion does not alter metabolic changes associated with ritodrine tocolysis. Am J Obstet Gynecol 156:103, 1987

Fleisher A, Schulman H, Farmakides G, Bracero L, Blattner P, Randolph G: Umbilical artery velocity waveforms and intrauterine growth retardation. Am J Obstet Gynecol 151:502, 1985

Forman A, Andersson K-E, Ulmsten U: Inhibition of myometrial activity by calcium antagonists. Semin Perinatol 5:288, 1981

France JT, Liggins GC: Placental sulfatase deficiency. J Clin Endocrinol 29:138, 1969

Freeman RK, Garite TJ, Modanlou H, Dorchester W, Rommal C, Devaney M: Postdate pregnancy: Utilization of contraction stress testing for primary fetal surveillance. Am J Obstet Gynecol 140:128, 1981

Frigoletto F: Diagnostic Ultrasound Imaging in Pregnancy. US Department of Health and Human Services, Public Health Service, National Institutes of Health Publication No 84667, 1986

Fuchs F, Fuchs A-R, Poblete V, Resk A: Effect of alcohol on threatened premature labor. Am J Obstet Gynecol 99:627, 1967

Galbraith RS, Karchmar EJ, Piercy WN: The clinical prediction of intrauterine growth retardation. Am J Obstet Gynecol 133:281, 1979

Garite TJ, Freeman RK, Linzey EM, Braly PS, Dorchester WL: Prospective randomized study of corticosteroids in the management of premature rupture of the membranes and the premature gestation. Am J Obstet Gynecol 141:508, 1981

Garite TJ, Freeman RK, Linzey EM, Braly PS: The use of amniocentesis in patients with premature rupture of membranes. Obstet Gynecol 54:226, 1979

Garite TJ, Keegan KA, Freeman RK, Nageotte MP: A randomized trial of ritodrine tocolysis versus expectant management in patients with premature rupture of membranes at 24 to 30 weeks of gestation. Am J Obstet Gynecol 157:388, 1987

Georgieff MK, Sasnow SR, Mammel MC, Pereira GR: Mid-arm circumference/head circumference ratios for identification of symptomatic LGA, AGA, and SGA newborn infants. J Pediatr 109:316, 1986

Giles WB, Trudinger BJ, Baird PJ: Fetal umbilical artery flow velocity waveforms and placental resistance: Pathological correlation. Br J Obstet Gynaecol 92:31, 1985

Gill RW, Kossoff G, Warren PS, Garrett WJ: Umbilical venous flow in normal and complicated pregnancy. Ultrasound Med Biol 10:349:1984

Gilstrap LC, Hauth JC, Belle RE, Ackerman NB, Yoder BA, Delemos R: Survival and short-term morbidity of the premature neonate. Obstet Gynecol 65:37, 1985

Gilstrap LC III, Leveno KJ, Cox SM, Burris JS, Mashburn M, Rosenfeld CR: Intrapartum treatment of acute chorioamnionitis: Impact on neonatal sepsis. Am J Obstet Gynecol 159:579, 1988

Glass L, Rajegowda BK, Evans HE: Absence of respiratory distress syndrome in premature infants of heroin-addicted mothers. Lancet 3:685, 1971

Gluck L: Fetal lung maturity. Presented at the 78th Ross Conference on Pediatric Research, San Diego, May 30, 1979

Gluck L, Kulovich MV: Lecithin/sphingomyelin ratios in amniotic fluid in normal and abnormal pregnancy. Am J Obstet Gynecol 115:539, 1973

Gluck L, Kulovich MV, Borer RC Jr, Keidel WN: The interpretation and significance of the lecithin/sphingomyelin ratio in amniotic fluid. Am J Obstet Gynecol 120:142, 1974

Gohari P, Berkowitz RL, Hobbins JC: Prediction of intrauterine growth retardation by determination of total intrauterine volume. Am J Obstet Gynecol 127:255, 1977

Goldenberg RL, Nelson KG, Dyer RL, Wayne J: The variability of viability: The effect of physicians' perceptions of viability on the survival of very low-birth-weight infants. Am J Obstet Gynecol 143:678, 1982

Goldstein I, Reece A, Pilu G, Bovicelli L, Hobbins JC: Cerebellar measurements with ultrasonography in the evaluation of fetal growth and development. Am J Obstet Gyencol 1567:1065, 1987

Gonik B, Bottoms SF, Cotton DB: Amniotic fluid volume as a risk factor in preterm premature rupture of the membranes. Obstet Gynecol 65:456, 1985

Granados JL: Survey of the management of postterm pregnancy. Obstet Gynecol 63:651, 1984

Gravett MG, Nelson HP, DeRouen T, Critchlow C, Eschenbach DA, Holmes KK: Independent associations of bacterial vaginosis and Chlamydia trachomatis infection with adverse pregnancy outcome. JAMA 256:1899, 1986

Griffin D, Bilardo K, Masini L, Diaz-Recasens J, Pearce JM, Willson K, Campbell S: Doppler blood flow waveforms in the descending thoracic aorta of the human fetus. Br J Obstet Gynaecol 91:997, 1984

Gross TL, Sokol RJ, Wilson MV, Kuhnert PM, Hirsch V: Amniotic fluid phosphatidylglycerol: A potentially useful predictor of intrauterine growth retardation. Am J Obstet Gynecol 140:277, 1981

Grossman M, Flynn JJ, Aufrichtig D, Handler CR: Pitfalls in determination of total intrauterine volume. JCU 10:17, 1982

Gruenwald P: Chronic fetal distress and placental insufficiency. Biol Neonate 5:215, 1963

Guidetti DA, Divon MY, Cavalieri RL, Langer O, Merkatz IR: Fetal umiblical artery flow velocimetry in postdate pregnancies. Am J Obstet Gynecol 157:1521, 1987

Hack M, Fanaroff A: Changes in the delivery room care of the extremely small infant (<750 g): Effects on morbidity and outcome. N Engl J Med 314:660, 1986

Hackett GA, Campbell S, Gamsu H, Cohen-Overbeek T, Pearce JMF: Doppler studies in the growth retarded fetus and prediction of neonatal necrotizing enterocolitis, hemorrhage, and neonatal morbidity. Br Med J 294:15, 1987

Hadi HA, Abdulla AM, Fadel HE, Stefadouros MA, Metheny WP: Cardiovascular effects of ritodrine tocolysis: A new noninvasive method to measure pulmonary capillary pressure during pregnancy. Obstet Gynecol 70:608, 1987

Hankins GDV, Leveno KJ, Whalley PJ, DePalma RT, Williams ML, Nelson S: Maternal, fetal, neonatal, and infant outcomes with expectant management for preterm rupture of the membranes. Presented at the Society of Perinatal Obstetricians, San Antonio, Texas, February 2–4, 1984

Hanshaw JB: Congenital cytomegalovirus infection: A 15-year prospective study. J Infect Dis 123:555, 1971

Hanson JW, Myrianthopoulas NC, Harvey MAS, Smith DW: Risks to the offspring of women treated with hydantoin anticonvulsants, with emphasis on the fetal hydantoin syndrome. J Pediatr 89:662, 1976

Hanson JW, Streissguth AP, Smith DW: The effects of moderate alcohol consumption during pregnancy on fetal growth and morphogenesis. Pediatrics 92(3):457, 1978

Hatjis CG, Swain M: Systemic tocolysis for premature labor is associated with an increased incidence of pulmonary edema in the presence of maternal infection. Am J Obstet Gynecol 159:723, 1988

Hatjis CG, Swain M, Nelson LH, Meis PJ, Ernest JM: Efficacy of combined administration of magnesium sulfate and ritodrine in the treatment of premature labor. Obstet Gynecol 69:317, 1987

Hauth JC, Gilstrap LC, Brekken AL, Hauth JM: The effect of 17α-hydroxyprogesterone caproate on pregnancy outcome in an active-duty military population. Am J Obstet Gynecol 146:187, 1983a

Hauth JC, Hankins GD, Kuehl TJ, Pierson WP: Ritodrine hydrochloride infusion in pregnant baboons: I. Biophysical effects. Am J Obstet Gynecol 146:916, 1983b

Hendricks CH: Patterns of fetal and placental growth: The second half of normal pregnancy. Obstet Gynecol 24:357, 1964

Herron MA, Katz M, Creasy RK: Evaluation of a preterm birth prevention program: Preliminary report. Obstet Gynecol 59:452, 1982

Hesseldahl H: A Danish multicenter study of ritodrine in the treatment of pre-term labor. Danish Med Bull 25:126, 1979

Hillier SL, Martius J, Krohn M, Kiviat N, Holmes KK, Eschenbach DA: A case-control study of chorioamnionic infection and histologic chorioamnionitis in prematurity. N Engl J Med 319:972, 1988

Hoddick WK, Callen PW, Filly RA, Creasy RK: Ultrasonic determination of qualitative amniotic fluid volume in intrauterine growth retardation: Reassessment of the 1 cm rule. Am J Obstet Gynecol 149:758, 1984

Hoffman HJ, Stark CR, Lunden FE Jr, Ashbrook JD: Analyses of birth weight, gestational age, and fetal viability: U.S. births, 1968. Obstet Gynecol Surv 29:651, 1974

Hollander DI, Nagey DA, Pupkin MJ: Magnesium sulfate and ritodrine hydrochloride: A randomized comparison. Am J Obstet Gynecol 156:631, 1987

Honnebier WJ, Swaab DF: The influence of anencephaly upon intrauterine growth of fetus and placenta and upon gestational length. Br J Obstet Gynaecol 80:577, 1973

Howie RN, Liggins GC: Clinical trial of antepartum betamethasone therapy for prevention of respiratory distress in preterm infants: Proceedings of Fifth Study Group, Royal College of Obstetricians and Gynecologists, October 1977, p. 281

Hughey M, Sabbagha RE: Cephalometry by real time imaging: A critical evaluation. Am J Obstet Gynecol 131:825, 1978

Iams JD, Johnson FF, O'Shaughnessy RW: A prospective random trial of home uterine activity monitoring in pregnancies at increased risk of preterm labor. Part II. Am J Obstet Gynecol 159:595, 1988

Iams JD, Johnson FF, O'Shaughnessy RW, West LC: A prospective random trial of home uterine activity monitoring in pregnancies at increased risk of preterm labor. Am J Obstet Gynecol 157:638, 1987

Jimenez JM, Tyson JE, Reisch J: Clinical measurements of gestational age in normal pregnancies. Obstet Gynecol 61:438, 1983

Johnson JWC, Mitzner W, London WT, Palmer AE, Scott R: Betamethasone and the rhesus fetus: Multisystemic effects. Am J Obstet Gynecol 133:677, 1979

Jones MD Jr, Battaglia FC: Intrauterine growth retardation. Am J Obstet Gynecol 127:540, 1977

Jouppila P, Kirkinen P: Blood velocity waveforms of the fetal aorta in normal and hypertensive pregnancies. Obstet Gynecol 67:856, 1986

Katz AI, Davison JM, Hayslett JP, Singson E, Lindheimer MD: Pregnancy in women with kidney disease. Kidney Int 18:192, 1980

Katz M, Gill PJ, Newman RB: Detection of preterm labor by ambulatory monitoring of uterine activity for the management of oral tocolysis. Am J Obstet Gynecol 154:1253, 1986a

Katz M, Newman RB, Gill PJ: Assessment of uterine activity in ambulatory patients at high risk of preterm labor and delivery. Am J Obstet Gynecol 154:44, 1986b

Kazzi GM, Gross TL, Sokol RJ: Fetal biparietal diameter and placental grade: Predictors in intrauterine growth retardation. Obstet Gynecol 62:755, 1983a

Kazzi GM, Kazzi NJ, Gross TL, Sokol RJ: Detection of intrauterine growth retardation: New uses for sonographic placental grading. Am J Obstet Gynecol 145:733, 1983b

Khouzami VA, Johnson JWC, Diakoku NH, Rotmensch J, Hernandez E: Comparison of urinary estrogens, contraction stress tests and nonstress tests in the management of postterm pregnancy. J Reprod Med 28:189, 1983

Kirkinen P, Muller R, Huch R, Huch A: Blood flow velocity waveforms in human fetal intracranial arteries. Obstet Gynecol 70:613, 1987

Kirschbaum TH: Management of prolonged pregnancy: Result of a prospective randomized trial (Discussion of paper by Knox GE, Huddleston JF, Flowers CE). Am J Obstet Gynecol 134:376, 1979

Klaus MH, Fanaroff AA: Care of the High Risk Neonate, 2nd ed. Philadelphia, WB Saunders, 1979

Kleigman RM, Fanaroff AA: Necrotizing enterocolitis. N Engl J Med 310:1093, 1984

Knox GE: Influence of infection on fetal growth and development. J Reprod Med 21:352, 1978

Knox GE, Huddleston JF, Flowers CE: Management of prolonged pregnancy: Result of a prospective randomized trial. Am J Obstet Gynecol 134:376, 1979

Kubli F: In Anderson A, Beard R, Brudenell JM, Dunn PM (eds): Preterm Labor. London, Royal College of Obstetricians and Gynaecologists, 1977, p. 218

Langer OL, Damus K, Maiman M, Divon M, Levy J, Bauman W: A link between relative hypoglycemia-hypoinsulinemia during oral glucose tolerance tests and intrauterine growth retardation. Am J Obstet Gynecol 155:711, 1986

Larsen JW Jr, Evans MI: Genetic causes. In Lin C-C and Evans MI (eds): Intrauterine Growth Retardation. New York, McGraw-Hill, 1984, p. 10

Laurin J, Lingman G, Marsal K, Persson P: Fetal blood flow in pregnancies complicated by intrauterine growth retardation. Obstet Gynecol 69:895, 1987

Lechtig A, Delgado H, Lasky RE, Yarbrough C, Klein RE, Habicht JP, Behar M: Maternal nutrition and fetal growth in developing societies. Am J Dis Child 129:434, 1975

Leigh J, Garite TJ: Amniocentesis and the management of premature labor. Obstet Gynecol 67:500, 1986

Leveno KJ, Cox K, Roark ML: Cervical dilatation and prematurity revisited. Obstet Gynecol 68:434, 1986a

Leveno KJ, Cunningham FG, Roark ML, Nelson SD, Williams ML: Prenatal care and the low birth weight infant. Obstet Gynecol 66:599, 1985a

Leveno KJ, Klein VR, Guzick DS, Young DR, Hankins DV, Williams ML: Single-centre randomised trial of ritodrine hydrochloride for preterm labour. Lancet 1:1293, 1986b

Leveno KJ, Lowe TW, Cunningham FG, Wendel GD, Nelson S: Management of prolonged pregnancy at Parkland Hospital. Proceedings of the Society for Gynecologic Investigation, [Abstract 290P], March 1985b

Leveno KJ, Quirk JG, Cunningham FG, Nelson SD, Santos-Ramos R, Toofanian A, DePalma RT: Prolonged pregnancy: I. Observations concerning the causes of fetal distress. Am J Obstet Gynecol 150:465, 1984

Liggins GC: The prevention of RDS by maternal betamethasone administration. In Lung Maturation and the Prevention of Hyaline Membrane Disease. Report of the Seventieth Ross Conference on Pediatric Research, Columbus, Ohio, Ross Laboratories, 1976

Liggins GC: Report on children exposed to steroids in utero. Contemp Ob/Gyn 19:205, 1982

Liggins GC, Howie RN: The prevention of RDS by maternal steroid therapy. In Gluck L (ed): Modern Perinatal Medicine. Chicago, Year Book, 1974

Lin C-C, Evans MI: Introduction. In Lin C-C, Evans MI (eds): Intrauterine Growth Retardation. New York, McGraw-Hill, 1984

Lirette M, Holbrook RH, Katz M: Cardiovascular and uterine blood flow changes during nicardipine HC1 tocolysis in the rabbit. Obstet Gynecol 69:79, 1987

Lubchenco LO, Bard H: Incidence of hypoglycemia in newborn infants classified by birth weight and gestational age. Pediatrics 47:831, 1971

Lubchenco LO, Hansman C, Dressler M, Boyd E: Intrauterine growth as estimated from liveborn birth-weight data at 24 to 42 weeks of gestation. Pediatrics 32:793, 1963

Lubchenco LO, Searls DT, Brazie JV: Neonatal mortality rate: Relationship to birth weight and gestational age. J Pediatr 81:814, 1972

MacDonald PC, Siiteri PK: Origin of estrogen in women pregnant with an anencephalic fetus. J Clin Invest 44:465, 1965

Main DM, Gabbe SG, Richardson D, Strong S: Can preterm deliveries be prevented? Am J Obstet Gynecol 151:892, 1985

Manning FA, Baskett TF, Morrison I, Lange I: Fetal biophysical profile scoring: A prospective study in 1,184 high-risk patients. Am J Obstet Gynecol 140:289, 1981a

Manning FA, Hill LM, Platt LD: Quantitative amniotic fluid volume determined by ultrasound: Antepartum detection of intrauterine growth retardation. Am J Obstet Gynecol 139:254, 1981b

Manning FA, Morrison I, Harman CR, Lange IR, Menticoglou S: Fetal assessment based on fetal biophysical profile scoring: Experience in 19,221 referred high-risk pregnancies: II. An analysis of false-negative deaths. Am J Obstet Gynecol 157:880, 1987

McCormack WM, Rosner B, Lee Y-H, Munoz A, Charles D, Kass EH: Effect on birth weight of erythromycin treatment of pregnant woman. Obstet Gynecol 69:202, 1987

McCowan LM, Erskine LA, Ritchie K: Umbilical artery Doppler blood flow studies in the preterm, small for gestational age fetus. Am J Obstet Gynecol 156:655, 1987

McCowan LM, Ritchie K, Mo LY, Bascom PA, Sherret H: Uterine artery flow velocity waveforms in normal and growth-retarded pregnancies. Am J Obstet Gynecol 158:499, 1988

McGregor JA, French JI, Lawellin D, Franco-Buff A, Smith C, Todd JK: Bacterial protease-induced reduction of chorioamniotic membrane strength and elasticity. Obstet Gynecol 69:167, 1987

McGregor JA, French JI, Richter R, Vuchetich M, Bachus V, Franco-Buff A, Hillier S, Todd JK: Prospective, double-blinded, randomized, placebo-controlled trial of short-course erythromycin (E) base in women at high risk for preterm birth. Presented at the 35th annual meeting of the Society for Gynecologic Investigation [Abstract 62], Baltimore, March 1988

Meadows NJ, Till J, Leaf A, Hughes E, Jani B, Larcher V: Screening for intrauterine growth retardation using ratio of mid-arm circumference to occipitofrontal circumference. Br Med J 292:1039, 1986

Merkatz IR, Peter JB, Barden TP: Ritodrine hydrochloride: A betamimetic agent for use in preterm labor: II. Evidence of efficacy. Obstet Gynecol 56:7–12, 1980

Meyer MB: How does maternal smoking affect birth weight and maternal weight gain? Am J Obstet Gynecol 131:888, 1978

Miller FC, Read JA: Intrapartum assessment of the postdate fetus. Am J Obstet Gynecol 141:516, 1981

Miller JM, Keane MWD, Horger EO III: A comparison of magnesium sulfate and terbutaline for the arrest of premature labor. J Reprod Med 27:348, 1982

Minkoff H, Grunebaum AN, Schwarz RH, Feldman J, Cummings M, Crombleholme W, Clark L, Pringle G, McCormack WM: Risk factors for prematurity and premature rupture of membranes: A prospective study of the vaginal flora in pregnancy. Am J Obstet Gynecol 150:965, 1984

Miodovinik M, Lovin JP, Gimmon Z, Hill J, Fischer JE, Barden TP: The use of an amniotic fluid 3-methyl histidine to creatinine molar ratio for the diagnosis of intrauterine growth retardation. Obstet Gynecol 60:288, 1982

Miyazaki FS, Miyazaki BA: False reactive nonstress tests in postterm pregnancies. Am J Obstet Gynecol 140:269, 1981

Morales WJ: The effect of chorioamnionitis on the developmental outcome of preterm infants at one year. Obstet Gynecol 70:183, 1987

Moretti M, Sibai BM: Maternal and perinatal outcome of expectant management of premature rupture of membranes in the midtrimester. Am J Obstet Gynecol 159:390, 1988

Morrison JC, Martin JN Jr, Martin RW, Gookin KS, Wiser WL: Prevention of preterm birth by ambulatory assessment of uterine activity: A randomized study. Am J Obstet Gynecol 156:536, 1987

Mosier HD Jr, Dearden LC, Tanner SM, Jansons RA, Biggs CS: Disproportionate organ growth in the fetus after betamethasone administration. Pediatr Res 13:486, 1979

Naeye RL, Dixon JB: Distortions in fetal growth standards. Pediatr Res 12:987, 1978

Nageotte M, Porto M, Hill O, Dorchester W, Freeman RK: Cost effectiveness of home uterine activity monitoring. Presented at the 8th annual meeting of the Society of Perinatal Obstetricians. [Abstract 71], February 1988

Neilson JP, Verkuyl DAA, Crowther CA, Bannerman C: Preterm labor in twin pregnancies: Prediction by cervical assessment. Obstet Gynecol 72:719, 1988

Nelson LH, Meis PJ, Hatjis CG, Ernest JM, Dillard R, Schey HM: Premature rupture of membranes: A prospective, randomized evaluation of steroids, latent phase, and expectant management. Obstet Gynecol 66:55, 1985

Newman RB, Gill PJ, Wittreich P, Katz M: Maternal perception of prelabor uterine activity. Obstet Gynecol 68:765, 1986

Nicolaides KH, Campbell S, Bradely RJ, Bilardo CM, Soothill PW, Gibb D: Maternal oxygen therapy for intrauterine growth retardation. Lancet 1:942, 1987

Niebyl JR, Blake DA, White RD, Kumor KM, Dubin NH, Robinson D, Egner PG: The inhibition of premature labor with indomethacin. Am J Obstet Gynecol 136:1014, 1980

Nwaesei CG, Young DC, Byrne JM, Vincer JM, Sampson D, Evans JR, Allen AC, Stinson DA: Preterm birth at 23 to 26 weeks' gestation: Is active obstetric management justified? Am J Obstet Gynecol 157:890, 1987

O'Brien GD, Queenan JT, Campbell S: Assessment of gestational age in the second trimester by real-time ultrasound measurement of the femur length. Am J Obstet Gynecol 139:540, 1981

Ounsted M, Moar VA, Scott A: Children of deviant birthweight: The influence of genetic and other factors on size at seven years. Acta Paediatr Scand 74:707, 1985

Papiernik E, Bouyer J, Collin D, Winisdoerffer G, Dreyfus J: Precocious cervical ripening and preterm labor. Obstet Gynecol 67:238, 1986

Papiernik E, Kaminski M: Multifactorial study of the risk of prematurity at 32 weeks of gestation: A study for the frequency of 30 predictive characteristics. J Perinat Med 2:30, 1974

Parisi V, Salina J, Stockman E: Fetal cardiorespiratory responses to maternal administration of nicardipine in the hypertensive ewe. Proceedings of The Society of Perinatal Obstetricians. [Abstract], San Antonio, Texas. January 30–February 1, 1986

Patterson RM, Gibbs CE, Wood RC: Birthweight percentile and perinatal outcome: Recurrence of intrauterine growth retardation. Obstet Gynecol 68:464, 1986

Pearce JMF, Campbell S: Intrauterine growth retardation: Birth Defects 21:109, 1985

Pearce JMF, Campbell S: Ultrasonic monitoring of normal and abnormal fetal growth. In Laurensen NH (ed): Modern Management of High Risk Pregnancy. New York, Plenum Press, 1983, p 57

Persson PH, Grennert L, Gennser G: Diagnosis of intrauterine growth retardation by serial ultrasound cephalometry. Acta Obstet Gynaecol Scand (Suppl) 78:40, 1978b

Persson PH, Grennert L, Gennser G: Impact of fetal and maternal factors on the normal growth of biparietal diameter. Acta Obstet Gynecol Scand (Suppl) 78:21, 1978a

Phelan JP, Platt LD, Yeh SY, Boussard P, Paul RH: The role of ultrasound assessment of amniotic fluid volume in the management of the postdate pregnancy. Am J Obstet Gynecol 151:304, 1985

Phelan JP, Platt LD, Yeh SY, Trujillo M, Paul RH: Continuing role of the nonstress test in the management of postdates pregnancy. Obstet Gynecol 64:624, 1984

Philip AGS: Fetal growth retardation: Femurs, fontanels, and follow-up. Pediatrics 62:446, 1978

Philipson EH, Sokol RJ, Williams MA: Oligohydramnios: Clinical associations and predictive value for intrauterine growth retardation. Am J Obstet Gynecol 146:271, 1983

Quaranta P, Currell R, Redman CWG, Robinson JS: Prediction of small-for-date infants by measurements of symphysial-fundal height. Br J Obstet Gynaecol 88:115, 1981

Queenan JT: How to diagnose IUGR. Contemp Ob/Gyn 19:195, 1982

Queenan JT, Kubargch SF, Cook LN: Diagnostic ultrasound for detection of intrauterine growth retardation. Am J Obstet Gynecol 124:865:1976

Quirk JG, Raker RK, Petrie RH, Williams AM: The role of glucocorticoids, unstressful labor, and atraumatic delivery in the prevention of respiratory distress syndrome. Am J Obstet Gynecol 1134:768, 1979

Read MD, Wellby DE: The use of a calcium antagonist (nifedipine) to suppress preterm labor. Br J Obstet Gynaecol 93:933, 1986

Reuss ML, Parer JT, Harris JL, Krueger TR: Hemodynamic effects of alpha-adrenergic blockade during hypoxia in fetal sheep. Am J Obstet Gynecol 142:410, 1982

Rightmire DA, Campbell S: Fetal and maternal Doppler blood flow parameters in postterm pregnancies. Obstet Gynecol 69:891, 1987

Robertson WB, Brosens I, Dixon G: Maternal uterine vascular lesions in the hypertensive complications of pregnancy. In Lindheimer M, Katz A, Zuspan F (eds): Hypertension in Pregnancy. New York, Wiley, 1975

Robinson HP, Fleming JEE: A critical evaluation of sonar crown-rump length measurements. Br J Obstet Gynaecol 82:702, 1975

Rochelson B, Schulman H, Farmakides G, Bracero L, Ducey J, Fleisher A, Penny B, Winter D: The significance of absent end-diastolic velocity in umbilical artery velocity waveforms. Am J Obstet Gynecol 156:1213, 1987a

Rochelson B, Schulman H, Farmakides G, Bracero L, Ducey J, Fleisher A, Penny B, Winter D: The clinical significance of Doppler umbilical artery velocimetry in the small-for-gestational-age fetus. Am J Obstet Gynecol 156:1223, 1987b

Rogge P, Young S, Goodlin R: Post-partum pulmonary oedema associated with preventive therapy for premature labor. Lancet 1:1026, 1979

Romero R, Kadar N, Hobbins JC, Duff GW: Infection and labor: The detection of endotoxin in amniotic fluid. Am J Obstet Gynecol 157:815, 1987

Romero R, Roslansky P, Oyarzun E, Wan M, Emamian M, Novitsky TJ, Gould MJ, Hobbins JC: Labor and infection. II. Bacterial endotoxin in amniotic fluid and its relationship to the onset of preterm labor. Am J Obstet Gynecol 158:1044, 1988

Rosenberg K, Grant JM, Tweedie I, Aitchison T, Gallagher F: Measurement of fundal height as a screening test for fetal growth retardation. Br J Obstet Gynaecol 89:447, 1982

Ryan KJ: Placental synthesis of steroid hormones. In Tulchinsky D, Ryan KJ (eds): Maternal-Fetal Endocrinology. Philadelphia, Saunders, 1980

Sabbagha RE: Intrauterine growth retardation: Antenatal diagnosis by ultrasound. Obstet Gynecol 52:252, 1978

Schneider JM, Olson RW, Curet LB: Screening for fetal and neonatal risk in the postdate pregnancy. Am J Obstet Gynecol 131:473, 1978

Schwarz BE, Schultz FM, MacDonald PC: Initiation of human parturition: IV. Demonstration of phospholipase A_2 in the lysosomes of human fetal membranes. Am J Obstet Gynecol 125:1089, 1976

Schweitzer JL: Infection of neonates and infants with the hepatitis B virus. Prog Med Virol 20:27, 1975

Scioscia A, Nickless N, Hodgson P, Belanger K, Hobbins JC: A randomized clinical trial of outpatient monitoring of uterine contractions in women at risk for preterm delivery: Self-palpation versus tocodynamometer. Presented at the 8th annual meeting of the Society of Perinatal Obstetricians. [Abstract 72], February 1988

Semchyshyn S, Zuspan FP, O'Shaughnessy R: Pulmonary edema associated with the use of hydrocortisone and a tocolytic agent for the management of premature labor. J Reprod Med 28:47, 1983

Shepard MJ, Richards VA, Berkowitz RL, Warsof SL, Hobbins JC: An evaluation of two equations for predicting weight by ultrasound. Am J Obstet Gynecol 142:47, 1987

Shime J, Gare DJ, Andrews J, Bertrand M, Salgado J, Whillans G: Prolonged pregnancy: Surveillance of the fetus and the neonate and the course of labor and delivery. Am J Obstet Gynecol 148:547, 1984

Sholl JS, Sabbagha RE: Ultrasound detection. In Lin C-C, Evans MI (eds): Intrauterine Growth Retardation. New York, McGraw-Hill, 1984

Silver RK, Dooley SL, Tamura RK, Depp R: Umbilical cord size and amniotic fluid volume in prolonged pregnancy. Am J Obstet Gynecol 157:716, 1987

Simpson GF, Harbert GM Jr: Use of beta-methasone in management of preterm gestation with premature rupture of membranes. Am J Obstet Gynecol 66:168, 1985

Simpson JW, Lawless RW, Mitchell AC: Responsibility of the obstetrician to the fetus: II. Influence of prepregnancy weight and pregnancy weight gain on birth weight. Obstet Gynecol 45:481, 1975

Small JL, Phelan JP, Smith CV, Paul RH: An active management approach to the postdate fetus with a reactive nonstress test and fetal heart rate decelerations. Obstet Gynecol 70:636, 1987

Smyth CN: The guard-ring tocodynamometer: Absolute measurement of intra-amniotic pressure by a new instrument. J Obstet Gynaecol Br Commonw 64:59, 1957

Sokol RJ, Kazzi GM, Kalhan SC, Pillay SK: Identifying the pregnancy at risk for intrauterine growth retardation: Possible usefulness of the intravenous glucose tolerance test. Am J Obstet Gynecol 143:220, 1982

Sokol RJ, Miller SI, Reed G: Alcohol abuse during pregnancy: An epidemiologic study. Alcoholism 4:135, 1980

Soothill PW, Nicolaides KH, Bilardo CM, Campbell S: Relation of fetal hypoxia in growth retardation to mean blood velocity in the fetal aorta. Lancet 1:118, 1986a

Soothill PW, Nicolaides KH, Campbell S: Prenatal asphyxia, hyperlacticaemia, hypoglycaemia and erythroblastosis in growth retarded fetuses. Br Med J 294:1051, 1987

Soothill PW, Nicolaides KH, Rodeck CH, Campbell S: The effect of gestational age on blood gas and acid-base values in human pregnancy. Fetal Ther 1:166, 1986b

Spisso KR, Harbert GM Jr, Thiagarajah S: The use of magnesium sulfate as the primary tocolytic agent to prevent premature delivery. Am J Obstet Gynecol 142:840, 1982

Stagno S, Reynolds DW, Hwang ES: Congenital cytomegalovirus infection. N Engl J Med 296:1254, 1977

Steer CM, Petrie RH: A comparison of magnesium sulfate and alcohol for the prevention of premature labor. Am J Obstet Gynecol 129:1, 1977

Stein Z, Susser M, Saenger G, Marolla F: Famine and Human Development: The Dutch Hunger Winter of 1944–1945. New York, Oxford University Press, 1975

Stone ML, Salerno LJ, Greene M, Zelson C: Narcotic addiction in pregnancy. Am J Obstet Gynecol 109:716, 1971

Stubbs TM, Van Dorsten P, Miller MC: The preterm cervix and preterm labor: Relative risks, predictive values, and change over time. Am J Obstet Gynecol 155:829, 1986

Taeusch HW, Frigoletto F, Kitzmiller J, Avery ME, Hehne A, Fromm B, Lawson E, Neff RK: Risks of respiratory distress syndrome after prenatal dexamethasone treatment. Pediatrics 63:64, 1979

Tonge HM, Wladimiroff JW, Noordam MJ, Van Kooten C: Blood flow velocity waveforms in the descending fetal aorta: Comparison between normal and growth-retarded pregnancies. Obstet Gynecol 67:851, 1986

Trudinger BJ, Cook CM: Umbilical and uterine artery flow velocity wave forms in pregnancy associated with major fetal abnormality. Br J Obstet Gynaecol 92:666, 1985

Trudinger BJ, Cook CM, Giles WB, Connelly A, Thompson RS: Umbilical artery flow velocity waveforms in high-risk pregnancy: Randomized controlled trial. Lancet 1:188, 1987

Ulmsten U, Andersson K-E, Wingerup L: Treatment of premature labor with the calcium antagonist nifedipine. Arch Gynecol 229:1, 1980

van Geijn HP, Kaylor WM, Nicola KR: Induction of severe intrauterine growth retardation in the Sprague-Dawley rat. Am J Obstet Gynecol 137:43, 1980

Varma TR, Taylor H, Bridges C: Ultrasound assessment of fetal growth, Br J Obstet Gynaecol 86:633, 1979

Varner MW, Galask RP: Infectious causes. In Lin C-C and Evans MI (eds): Intrauterine Growth Retardation. New York, McGraw-Hill, 1984

Vintzileos AM, Campbell WA, Nochimson DJ, Weinbaum PJ: Preterm premature rupture of the membranes: A risk factor for the development of abruptio placentae. Am J Obstet Gynecol 156:1235, 1987

Vintzileos AM, Campbell WA, Nochimson DJ, Weinbaum PJ, Escoto DT, Mirochnick MH: Qualitative amniotic fluid volume versus amniocentesis in predicting infection in preterm premature rupture of the membranes. Obstet Gynecol 67:579, 1986

Vohr BR, Oh W: Growth and development in preterm infants small for gestational age. J Pediatr 103:941, 1983

Vohr BR, Oh W, Rosenfield AG, Cowett RM, Berstein J: The preterm small-for-gestational-age infant: A two-year follow-up study. Am J Obstet Gynecol 133:425, 1979

Wald NJ, Cuckle HS, Boreham J, Althouse R: Birthweight of infants with spina bifida cystica. Br J Obstet Gynaecol 87:578, 1980

Walker D-JB, Feldman A, Vohr BR, Oh W: Cost-benefit analysis of neonatal intensive care for infants weighing less than 1,000 grams at birth. Pediatrics 74:20–25, 1984

Wallenburg HCS, Rotmans N: Prevention of recurrent idiopathic fetal growth retardation by low-dose aspirin and dipyridamole. Am J Obstet Gynecol 157:1230, 1987

Wallin A, Gyllensward A, Westin B: Symphysis-fundus measurement in prediction of fetal growth disturbances. Acta Obstet Gynecol Scand 60:317, 1981

Warkany JB, Monroe B, Sutherland BS: Intrauterine growth retardation. Am J Dis Child 102:24, 1961

Waterson AP: Virus infections (other than rubella) during pregnancy. Br Med J 2:564, 1979

Westin B: Gravidogram and fetal growth. Acta Obstet Gynecol Scand 56:273, 1977

Westwood M, Kramer MS, Munz D, Lovett JM, Watters GV: Growth and development of full-term nonasphyxiated small-for-gestational-age newborns: Follow-up through adolescence. Pediatrics 71:376, 1983

Whittle MJ, Hanretty KP: Doppler studies in the growth retarded fetus. Br Med J 294:644, 1987

Wigglesworth JS: Experimental growth retardation in the foetal rat. J Path Bact 88:1, 1964

Wilkins IA, Lynch L, Mehalek KE, Berkowitz GS, Berkowitz RL: Efficacy and side effects of magnesium sulfate and ritodrine as tocolytic agents. Am J Obstet Gynecol 159:685, 1988

Winick M: Cellular changes during placental and fetal growth. Am J Obstet Gynecol 109:166, 1971

Wladimiroff JW, Wijngaard J, Degani S, Noordam MJ, van Eyck J, Tonge HM: Cerebral and umbilical arterial blood flow velocity waveforms in normal and growth-retarded pregnancies. Obstet Gynecol 69:705, 1987

Woo JSK, Liang ST, Lo RLS: Significance of an absent or reversed end diastolic flow in Doppler umbilical artery waveforms. J Ultrasound Med 6:291, 1987

Yeh SY, Read JA: Management of post-term pregnancy in a large obstetrics population. Obstet Gynecol 60:282, 1982

Yeh SY, Read JA: Plasma unconjugated estriol as an indicator of fetal dysmaturity in postterm pregnancy. Obstet Gynecol 62:22, 1983

Yoon JJ, Harper RG: Observations on the relationship between duration of rupture of the membranes and the development of idiopathic respiratory distress syndrome. Pediatrics 52:161, 1973

Yu VYH, Loke HL, Szymonowicz W, Orgill AA, Astbury J: Prognosis for infants born at 23 to 28 weeks gestation. Br Med J 293:1200, 1986a

Yu VYH, Wong PY, Bajuk B, Orgill AA, Astbury J: Outcome of extremely-low-birthweight infants. Br J Obstet Gynaecol 93:162, 1986b

Zahn V: Die kontrole der tokolyse durch ambulante wehenmessung. In Dudenhausen JW, Saling E (eds): Perinatale Medizin. Stuttgart, George Ghieme, Verlag, 1973, pp 57–58

Zuckerman H, Reiss U, Robenstin I: Inhibition of human premature labor by indomethacin. Obstet Gynecol 44:787, 1974

Part IX

MEDICAL AND SURGICAL ILLNESSES COMPLICATING PREGNANCY

Medical and Surgical Illnesses Complicating Pregnancy

Almost any disease that affects a childbearing-age nonpregnant woman may complicate pregnancy, and the majority of diseases in young women do not prevent conception. For many systemic illnesses, the physiological and anatomical changes inherent in normal pregnancy influence the symptoms, signs, and laboratory values to a considerable degree. As a consequence, the physician who is not aware of these normal pregnancy-induced changes may not be able to recognize a disease or may diagnose incorrectly some other disease, to the jeopardy of the mother and her fetus. Throughout this chapter, emphasis has been placed on the effect of interaction between the disease and the pregnancy as well as on the problems in diagnosis and treatment imposed by the gestational state. In practically all instances, the following questions are pertinent:

1. Is pregnancy likely to make the disease more serious, and if so, how?
2. Does the disease jeopardize the pregnancy, and if so, how and to what degree?

3. Should the pregnancy be terminated because of either serious risk to the mother or likelihood of grave damage to the fetus?
4. Should the pregnancy be allowed to continue under a very carefully defined regimen of therapy?
5. If the disease exists before pregnancy, is pregnancy contraindicated, and if so, what steps should be taken to protect the woman from pregnancy.

A woman should never be penalized *because* she is pregnant. Put differently, if a treatment regimen usually given a nonpregnant woman is altered because of pregnancy, then there must be strong justification for its modification. This approach allows individualization of care for most disorders that complicate pregnancy, and it should always be remembered, especially when dealing with the medical and surgical consultants who often are asked to see such patients.

HEMATOLOGICAL DISORDERS

Pregnancy normally induces appreciable changes that may complicate the diagnosis of hematological disorders and the assessment of treatment. This is true especially for anemia.

ANEMIA

DEFINITION OF ANEMIA

A precise definition of anemia in women is complicated by the normal differences in the concentrations of hemoglobin between women and men, between white and black women, between women who live at high altitude and those who live near sea level, between women who are pregnant and those who are not, and between pregnant women who receive iron supplements and those who do not. On the basis of data presented in

Table 39–1, anemia probably exists in women residing at lower altitudes if the hemoglobin is much below 12.0 g per dL in the nonpregnant state, or is less than 10.0 g per dL during pregnancy or the puerperium. However, early in pregnancy and again near term, the hemoglobin level of most healthy iron-sufficient women is usually 11.0 g per dL or higher. During the puerperium, the hemoglobin concentration, in the absence of excessive blood loss, is not appreciably less than predelivery. After delivery the hemoglobin level typically fluctuates to a modest degree around the predelivery value for a few days and then rises to a somewhat higher nonpregnant level. The rate and magnitude of increase early in the puerperium are to a considerable degree the result of the amount of hemoglobin added to the intravascular compartment during pregnancy and the amount lost by hemorrhage after delivery.

TABLE 39–1. HEMOGLOBIN CONCENTRATIONS IN HEALTHY WOMEN WITH PROVEN IRON STORES.

Hemoglobin	Nonpregnant	Midpregnancy	Late Pregnancy
Mean	**13.7 g/dL**	**11.5 g/dL**	**12.3 g/dL**
Less than 12.0			
	1%	72%	36%
Less than 11.0			
	None	29%	6%
Less than 10.0			
	None	4%	1%
Lowest	**11.7 g/dL**	**9.7 g/dL**	**9.8 g/dL**

From Scott and Pritchard: JAMA 199:147, 1967.

Extensive hematological measurements have been made in healthy nonpregnant women, none of whom were iron deficient since each had histochemically proven iron stores, and none were deficient in folic acid since marrow erythropoiesis remained normoblastic. As shown in Table 39–1, the hemoglobin concentration of 85 healthy iron-sufficient nonpregnant women averaged 13.7 g per dL and two standard deviations ranged from 12.0 to 15.0 g per dL. In healthy iron-sufficient women who were 16 to 22 weeks pregnant, the mean hemoglobin was only 11.5 g per dL, and in three of these it was 9.7 or 9.8 g per dL. The hemoglobin level at or very near term averaged 12.3 g per dL, and in only 7 of 95 was the hemoglobin less than 11.0 g per dL with the lowest value 9.8 g per dL.

The modest fall in hemoglobin levels observed during pregnancy in healthy women not deficient in iron or folate is caused by relatively greater expansion of plasma volume compared to the increase in hemoglobin mass and red cell volume. The disproportion between the rates at which plasma and erythrocytes are added to the maternal circulation normally is greatest during the second trimester. Late in pregnancy, plasma expansion essentially ceases while hemoglobin mass continues to increase (see Chap. 7, p. 141).

FREQUENCY OF ANEMIA

Although anemia is somewhat more common among indigent pregnant women, it is by no means restricted to them. The frequency of anemia during pregnancy varies considerably, depending primarily upon whether supplemental iron is taken during pregnancy. For example, at Parkland Hospital the hemoglobin levels at the time of delivery among women who took iron supplements averaged 12.4 g per dL whereas it was only 11.3 g per dL among those who received no iron. Moreover, in none of the group receiving iron supplements was the hemoglobin less than 10.0 g per dL, but it was below this level in 16 percent of those who took no supplements (see Chap. 14, p. 264). More recently, and confirming many previous observations, Taylor and associates (1982a) identified hemoglobin levels to average at term 12.7 g per dL among women who received supplemental iron compared to 11.2 g per dL for those who did not.

ETIOLOGY OF ANEMIA

The etiologies of anemia during pregnancy are the same as those encountered in the nonpregnant woman and all anemias common to childbearing age women may complicate pregnancy. A classification based primarily on etiology and including most of the common causes of anemia in pregnant women is shown in Table 39–2. Although laboratory error as a cause of apparent anemia has not been included, the results from clinical laboratories may sometimes be grossly inaccurate. A common source of error during pregnancy stems from the rapid erythrocyte sedimentation rate, which is induced by hyperfibrinogenemia of normal pregnancy. If the specimen of blood is not effectively mixed *immediately* before sampling, the results are likely to be inaccurate. Most automated devices used currently have constant mixing features that obviate this problem.

The observed differences between hemoglobin concentrations in pregnant and nonpregnant women, coupled with the well-recognized phenomenon of hypervolemia induced by normal pregnancy, have led to the use of the term *physiological anemia*. This is a poor term for describing a normal process and should be discarded since there is virtually no anemia during normal pregnancy if anemia is defined as a decrease in hemoglobin mass.

Screening for Anemia

A limited but practical hematological evaluation may be carried out quickly and rather easily at the time of the first prenatal visit. The equipment and reagents required are simple and inexpensive. A few mL of venous blood are anticoagulated with Versenate (EDTA). A centrifuge for performing microhematocrit measurements and a hematocrit reading device are employed to detect anemia. For normocytic, normochromic red cells, the hematocrit is almost 3 times the hemoglobin concentration.

The plasma in the hematocrit tube is examined for icterus, and the thickness of the buffy coat is noted. If icterus is observed, studies to detect hemolysis or hepatic dysfunction are initiated. For black patients, a sickle cell preparation is made using isotonic sodium metabisulfite solution or Sickledex, and if positive, hemoglobin electrophoresis is done. Whenever the hematocrit approaches 30 or less, or when there is icterus, or when sickling is demonstrated, a blood smear is stained and the blood cells evaluated morphologically. These rather simple studies not only detect anemia but also provide important etiological clues.

IRON-DEFICIENCY ANEMIA

The two most common causes of anemia during pregnancy and the puerperium are iron deficiency and acute blood loss. Not infrequently the two are intimately related, since excessive blood loss with its concomitant loss of hemoglobin iron and exhaustion of iron stores in one pregnancy can be an important cause of iron-deficiency anemia in the next pregnancy.

TABLE 39–2. CAUSES OF ANEMIA DURING PREGNANCY

Acquired
    Iron-deficiency anemia
    Anemia caused by acute blood loss
    Anemia of inflammation or malignancy
    Megaloblastic anemia
    Acquired hemolytic anemia
    Aplastic or hypoplastic anemia
Hereditary
    Thalassemias
    Sickle cell hemoglobinopathies
    Other hemoglobinopathies
    Hereditary hemolytic anemias

As discussed elsewhere (see Chap. 7, p. 141 and Chap. 14, p. 264) the iron requirements of pregnancy are considerable, but the majority of American women have small stores. In a typical gestation with a single fetus, the maternal need for iron induced by pregnancy averages close to 800 mg, of which about 300 mg go to the fetus and placenta whereas about 500 mg, if available, are used to expand the maternal hemoglobin mass. Approximately 200 mg more are shed through the gut, urine, and skin. This total amount—1,000 mg—exceeds considerably the iron stores of most women. Unless the difference between the amount of stored iron available to the mother and the iron requirements of normal pregnancy cited above is compensated for by absorption of iron from the gastrointestinal tract, iron-deficiency anemia develops.

With the rather rapid expansion of the blood volume during the second trimester, the lack of iron often manifests itself by an appreciable drop in the maternal hemoglobin concentration. Although the rate of expansion of the blood volume is not so great in the third trimester, the need for iron remains high because augmentation of the maternal hemoglobin mass continues and considerable iron is now transported across the placenta from mother to fetus. Since the amount of iron diverted to the fetus from an iron-deficient mother is not much different from the amount normally transferred, the newborn infant of a severely anemic mother does not suffer from iron-deficiency anemia (Murray and co-workers, 1978). Iron stores in the infant are influenced much more by when and how the cord is clamped rather than by maternal iron stores.

IDENTIFICATION

Classic morphological evidence of iron-deficiency anemia—erythrocyte hypochromia and microcytosis—is much less likely to be as prominent in the pregnant woman as in the nonpregnant woman with the same hemoglobin concentration. Less severe iron-deficiency anemia during pregnancy, for example, a hemoglobin concentration of 9 g per dL or so, is usually not accompanied by obvious morphological changes in the circulating erythrocytes. However, with this degree of anemia from iron deficiency, the serum ferritin levels are lower than normal, and there is no stainable iron in the bone marrow. The serum iron-binding capacity is elevated, but by itself is of little diagnostic value, since it is also elevated during normal pregnancy in the absence of iron deficiency. Moderate normoblastic hyperplasia of the bone marrow is also found to be similar to that in normal pregnancy. *Thus, iron-deficiency anemia during pregnancy is the consequence primarily of the expansion of the plasma volume without normal expansion of maternal hemoglobin mass.*

The initial evaluation of a pregnant woman with moderate anemia should include measurements of hemoglobin, hematocrit, and cell indices, careful examination of a well-prepared smear of the peripheral blood, a sickle cell preparation if the woman is black, and the measurement of the serum iron concentration, serum ferritin level, or both. Examination of the bone marrow at this point is seldom done, although the demonstration of hemosiderin rules out iron deficiency. The diagnosis of iron deficiency in moderately anemic pregnant women is usually presumptive and it is based largely on the exclusion of other causes of anemia.

When the pregnant woman with moderate iron-deficiency anemia is given adequate iron therapy, hematological response can be detected by seeing newly formed erythrocytes as well as an elevated reticulocyte count. The rate of increase of hemoglo-

bin concentration or hematocrit varies considerably but is usually slower than in nonpregnant women. The reason is related largely to the differences in blood volumes, and during the latter half of pregnancy newly-formed hemoglobin is added to the characteristically much larger volume (Fig. 39–1). There is no evidence that pregnancy per se depresses erythropoiesis to any degree.

In severe iron-deficiency anemia during pregnancy, the erythrocytes undergo the classic morphological changes of hypochromia and microcytosis, and the diagnosis is usually made from the red cell indices and confirmed by examination of a well-prepared smear of the peripheral blood. In our now extensive experience, spoon nails, changes in the appearance of the tongue (other than paleness), and other stigmata of the Plummer–Vinson syndrome are rarely found.

TREATMENT

There has been some disagreement regarding the best way to treat iron-deficiency anemia during pregnancy and the puerperium. The use of an effective parenteral iron medication guarantees that the woman receives the iron. Oral preparations are preferred, however, if she understands the importance of taking the medication regularly. If she will not or, much less likely, cannot take the oral doses of iron, parenteral therapy is an alternative. Whatever treatment is employed, the objectives are correction of the severe deficit in hemoglobin mass and eventually restitution of iron stores. Both of these objectives can be accomplished with orally administered, simple iron compounds—ferrous sulfate, fumarate, or gluconate—that pro-

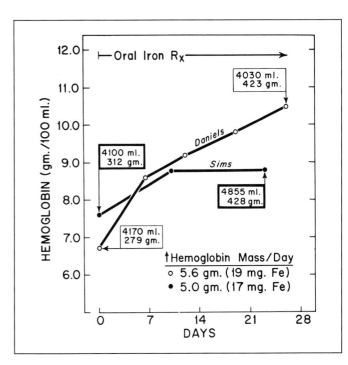

Figure 39–1. Two pregnant women with iron-deficiency anemia, when treated with the same simple iron compound, responded by increasing their hemoglobin mass at similar rates but not their hemoglobin levels. The excellent response in Sims treated late in the second trimester was masked by a simultaneous increase in blood volume of nearly 20 percent. The blood volume did not increase in Daniels who was treated late in the third trimester.

vide a daily dose of about 200 mg of *elemental iron*. There is no need to prescribe ascorbic acid or fruit juices or to withhold food to enhance iron absorption, nor is there any advantage from so-called delayed-release or sustained-release medication. To replenish iron stores, oral therapy should be continued for three months or so after the anemia has been corrected (Pritchard and Mason, 1964).

Iron preparations that provided significant amounts of iron when administered parenterally have been plagued by adverse reactions that are frequent and, at times, severe. Moreover, the rate of hemoglobin synthesis in response to parenterally administered iron is little, if any, faster than with oral iron taken in the dosage described above. An example of similarity in response is shown in Figure 39–2.

Folic acid may be given along with the iron as a safeguard against folate deficiency, although in our experience the response of pregnant women with iron-deficiency anemia treated with iron and folic acid is usually not appreciably better than when iron is given alone (Fig. 39–2). There is no good evidence that the addition of cobalt, copper, molybdenum, or ascorbic acid to the iron tablet is advantageous. Ascorbic acid does enhance iron absorption somewhat, so that less iron need be ingested to achieve a comparable level of absorption. However, there is no advantage from reducing the amount of iron ingested since any adverse gastrointestinal effects from oral iron relate primarily to the amount of iron absorbed rather than to the amount ingested. Iron preparations that contain significant amounts of iron but are totally free of any adverse effects are very poorly absorbed and consequently ineffective.

Transfusions of red cells or whole blood are seldom indicated for the treatment of iron-deficiency anemia unless hypovolemia from blood loss coexists or an operative procedure must be performed on a *severely* anemic woman. Whereas hypovolemia may be a prominent feature of anemia caused by acute blood loss, severe anemia from either failure of production of erythrocytes or their accelerated destruction may lead to patho-

logical hypervolemia and cardiac dysfunction. Therefore, the administration of packed red cells in the latter case must be done with meticulous care to prevent severe circulatory overloading, pulmonary edema, and even death. Exchange transfusion is an effective way to raise the hemoglobin concentration of severely anemic women without inducing or intensifying circulatory overload. Alternatively, the intravenous administration of furosemide shortly before slowly transfusing packed erythrocytes is of value in reducing plasma volume and thereby allowing the intravascular compartment to accommodate the added erythrocytes without causing circulatory overload.

ANEMIA FROM ACUTE BLOOD LOSS

Anemia resulting from recent hemorrhage is more likely to be evident during the puerperium. Both abruptio placentae and placenta previa may be sources of serious blood loss and of anemia before as well as after delivery. Earlier in pregnancy, anemia caused by acute blood loss is common in instances of abortion, ectopic pregnancy, and hydatidiform mole.

TREATMENT

Acute hemorrhage may have no immediate effect on the hemoglobin concentration even though the hemorrhage leads to hypovolemia so severe as to cause cardiovascular collapse. Massive hemorrhage demands immediate blood replacement with whole blood in amounts that restore and maintain adequate perfusion of vital organs (see Chap. 36, p. 698). Even though the amount of blood replaced commonly does not repair completely the hemoglobin deficit created by the hemorrhage, in general, once dangerous hypovolemia has been overcome and hemostasis has been achieved, the residual anemia should be treated with iron. The moderately anemic woman (hemoglobin more than 7.0 g per dL) whose condition is stable, who no longer faces the likelihood of further serious hemorrhage, who can ambulate without adverse symptoms, and who is not febrile is usually better treated with iron rather than blood transfusions.

ANEMIA ASSOCIATED WITH CHRONIC DISEASE

A large variety of disorders—chronic infections and neoplasms especially—may produce moderate and sometimes severe anemia, usually with normocytic or slightly microcytic erythrocytes (Lee, 1983). Typically, bone marrow cytology is not markedly altered. The serum iron concentration is decreased, and the serum iron-binding capacity, although lower than in normal pregnancy, is not necessarily much below the normal nonpregnant range. The anemia appears to result, at least in part, from alterations in reticuloendothelial function and iron metabolism. Iron released from senescent erythrocytes is retained rather than being returned promptly to the plasma to be reutilized by erythroblasts. The fate of iron administered in therapeutic doses is similar. The life span of the erythrocyte, furthermore, is usually slightly shortened. Anemia therefore results from decreased erythropoiesis coupled with slightly increased destruction.

Renal disease, suppuration, inflammatory bowel disease, systemic lupus erythematosus, granulomatous infections, malignant neoplasms, and rheumatoid arthritis also may cause anemia, presumably by these same mechanisms. At least some cases of so-called *refractory anemia of pregnancy* probably are the

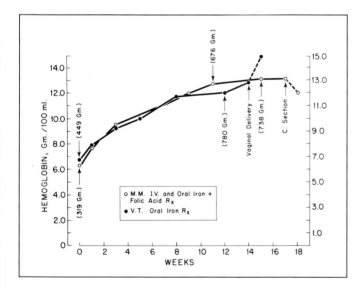

Figure 39–2. Excellent and nearly identical hematological responses in two pregnant women with severe iron-deficiency anemia. The response in one to oral iron alone (65 mg of iron three times a day) was as rapid as it was in the other, who received oral iron in the same dosage plus intravenous iron in excess as well as folic acid 3 mg per day.

consequence of one of these diseases which has gone unrecognized. The anemia of infection, renal disease, and malignancy is refractory in the sense that it is not corrected by treatment with iron, folic acid, vitamin B$_{12}$, or any other hematinic agent. Nonetheless, prophylaxis with iron and folic acid usually is desirable to offset any deficiency induced by pregnancy.

It has been our experience that women with severe *acute pyelonephritis,* but not those with asymptomatic bacteriuria or cystitis, often develop overt anemia. The genesis of the anemia appears to be increased red cell destruction, coupled with impaired production that may persist for some weeks (Cunningham, 1988).

MEGALOBLASTIC ANEMIA

The prevalence of megaloblastic anemia during pregnancy varies considerably throughout the world, and it is rare in the United States. In this country, megaloblastic anemia beginning during pregnancy almost always results from folic acid deficiency, and in the past was referred to as *pernicious anemia of pregnancy.* It is usually found in pregnant women who consume neither fresh vegetables, especially of the uncooked green leafy variety, nor foods with a high content of animal protein. Women with megaloblastic anemia may have developed troublesome nausea, vomiting, and anorexia during pregnancy. As the folate deficiency and anemia increases, the anorexia often becomes more intense, thus aggravating the dietary deficiency. In some instances, ethanol ingestion is either the cause or contributes to its development.

Deficiency of metabolically active forms of folic acid induces many biochemical and hematological changes. The sequence of changes from folate deficiency is probably unaltered by pregnancy. In the peripheral blood, the earliest biochemical evidence is low folic acid activity in plasma. The earliest morphological evidence of folic acid deficiency usually is hypersegmentation of some of the neutrophils. As anemia develops, the newly formed erythrocytes, now being produced in reduced numbers, are macrocytic, even when there has been previous iron deficiency with microcytosis. With preexisting iron deficiency, the more recently formed macrocytic erythrocytes would not be detected from the measurement of the mean corpuscular volume of the erythrocytes. Careful examination of a well-prepared smear of the peripheral blood, however, will usually demonstrate some macrocytes. As the anemia becomes more intense, an occasional nucleated erythrocyte appears in the peripheral blood. If smears of the buffy coat from peripheral blood are made in order to concentrate the nucleated erythrocytes, several such cells with the distinct features of megaloblasts are usually demonstrable. At the same time, examination of the bone marrow discloses megaloblastic erythropoiesis. As the maternal folate deficiency and, in turn, the anemia become severe, thrombocytopenia, leucopenia, or both also may develop.

Herbert and co-workers (1962) estimated that in normal nonpregnant women the daily folate requirements expressed as folic acid are in the range of 50 to 100 μg per day. During pregnancy, however, the requirements for folic acid are increased. The fetus and placenta extract folate from maternal circulation so effectively that the fetus is not anemic even when the mother is severely anemic from folate deficiency. Cases have been recorded in which the newborn hemoglobin levels were 18.0 g or more per dL, while the maternal values were as low as 3.6 g per dL (Pritchard and co-workers, 1970).

The treatment of megaloblastic anemia induced by pregnancy should include folic acid, a nutritious diet, and usually iron. As little as 1 mg of folic acid administered orally once a day produces a striking hematological response. By 4 to 7 days after the beginning of treatment, the reticulocyte count is appreciably increased, and leucopenia and thrombocytopenia are promptly corrected. Sometimes the rate of increase in hemoglobin concentration or hematocrit is disappointing, especially when compared with the usual exuberant reticulocytosis that starts soon after therapy has been initiated. Severe megaloblastic anemia during pregnancy is accompanied frequently by an appreciably smaller blood volume than that of a normal pregnancy, but soon after folic acid therapy has been started the blood volume usually increases considerably. Therefore, even though hemoglobin is being rapidly added to the circulation, the hemoglobin concentration does not precisely reflect the total amount of additional hemoglobin because of the simultaneous expansion of the blood volume.

Women who develop megaloblastic anemia during pregnancy commonly are also deficient in total body iron. Paradoxically, ineffective erythropoiesis resulting from the folate deficiency and, in turn, a decreased amount of iron being incorporated into hemoglobin induce a considerable elevation of the plasma iron and even some accumulation of storage iron. However, with the onset of effective erythropoiesis the concentration of iron in the plasma falls precipitously and any stored iron is rapidly exhausted. Iron may then become the limiting factor in production of hemoglobin.

Megaloblastic anemia recurs rather often in subsequent pregnancies, very likely because of persistence of dietary inadequacies and perhaps in part because of a peculiarity in absorption or utilization of folic acid. Congenital folate malabsorption has been identified (Poncz and associates, 1981).

A great deal of attention has been devoted to the frequency of maternal folate deficiency and megaloblastic anemia in pregnancy and the puerperium, the possible role of folate deficiency in various forms of reproductive failure, and the value of prophylactic administration of folic acid throughout pregnancy as discussed in some detail in Chapter 14 (p. 266). A good case can be made for supplemental folic acid in circumstances where folate requirements are unusually excessive, for example, multifetal pregnancy or hemolytic anemia. Whether to administer folic acid routinely to all pregnant women in the United States is debatable. If, however, prenatal vitamin supplements are prescribed, folic acid should be included, since there is more evidence that the pregnant woman might suffer from a deficiency of that vitamin than of the several others that are almost always included.

Megaloblastic anemia caused by lack of vitamin B$_{12}$ during pregnancy is quite rare. *Addisonian pernicious anemia,* in which there is failure to absorb vitamin B$_{12}$ because of lack of intrinsic factor, is extremely uncommon in women of reproductive age. Moreover, unless women with this disease are treated with vitamin B$_{12}$, infertility may be a complication (Ball and Giles, 1964). In our limited experiences, vitamin B$_{12}$ deficiency in pregnant women is more likely encountered following partial or total gastric resection. There is little reason for withholding folic acid during pregnancy simply out of fear of jeopardizing the neurological integrity of women who might be pregnant and simultaneously have unrecognized, and therefore untreated, Addisonian pernicious anemia.

Breast-fed infants of mothers who suffer vitamin B$_{12}$ deficiency, either as the consequence of lack of intrinsic factor or because of chronic ingestion of a strict vegetarian diet, may develop megaloblastic anemia during infancy (see Chap. 14, p. 266).

ACQUIRED HEMOLYTIC ANEMIAS

Women with *autoimmune acquired hemolytic anemia* sometimes demonstrate marked acceleration of the rate of hemolysis during pregnancy. Usually, prednisone and similar compounds seem to be nearly as effective as in the nonpregnant state. Thrombocytopenia, if present, also may be favorably affected by corticosteroid therapy. Pregnancy is not a contraindication to the use of these steroids, but since the underlying disease is chronic and progressive, repeated pregnancies are not advisable in women with hemolytic anemia caused by autoimmune disease.

With autoimmune hemolytic anemia typically both the direct and indirect antiglobulin (Coombs) tests are positive. Hemolysis and the positive antiglobulin tests may be the consequence of either IgM or IgG anti-erythrocyte antibodies. IgM antibodies readily agglutinate red cells suspended in saline whereas IgG antibodies do not do so and therefore have been referred to as incomplete antibodies. The antiglobulin test, appropriately performed, does identify IgG antibodies.

IgM antibodies do not cross the placenta and therefore the fetal red cells are not affected. However, IgG antibodies, especially subclasses IgG_1 and IgG_3, do cross the placenta. The most common example of the adverse fetal effects from maternally produced IgG antibodies is maternal D isoimmunization with hemolytic disease in the fetus and neonate. Whenever IgG antibodies are detected in the mother, the fetus should be considered at risk of serious hemolytic disease and appropriate steps should be taken to gauge its intensity (see Chap. 33, p. 605).

Transfusion of red cells for the mother with severe autoimmune hemolytic disease is complicated by the presence of circulating anti-erythrocyte antibodies. Warming the donor cells to body temperature decreases their destruction by cold agglutinins.

The clinical course of a woman with acquired hemolytic anemia and multiple problems cared for at Parkland Hospital is now summarized:

A 29-year-old gravida 6 para 5, was first seen in early labor with twin fetuses at 36 weeks gestation. She also complained of jaundice, pruritus, and malaise of 3 weeks duration. Her hematocrit was 15, MCV 121 fL, reticulocytes 13 percent, platelets 219,000 per µL, and serum bilirubin 5.4 mg per dL (3.5 mg direct). Direct and indirect Coombs tests were positive and a warm IgG autoantibody was identified. About 8 and 9 months before, or about the time of conception, she had been hospitalized elsewhere because of acquired hemolytic anemia with a hematocrit of 9 on one occasion and 13 on the other. At this time, she had been transfused with several units of packed red cells and treatment with prednisone was initiated.

Before red cell transfusions could be given, spontaneous vaginal delivery of twin A was followed by assisted breech delivery of twin B. Their size was appropriate for gestational age and 5-minute Apgar scores were 9 for both. Separate placentas were delivered. Blood loss at delivery was not excessive.

There was no clinical or laboratory evidence of hemolytic disease in either twin although the potential for such existed since IgG antibody was identified in the mother. In fact, the central hematocrit of the second twin soon after birth was 70 and exchange transfusion was performed to lower the hematocrit.

Even though the mother's hematocrit remained at 14, red cell transfusions were withheld because of difficulty in cross-matching her blood. Additionally, blood loss had not been excessive and she could ambulate without difficulty. Examination of bone marrow aspirate demonstrated marked erythroid hyperplasia with prominent megaloblastic changes and no storage iron. Prednisone, 100 mg per day, oral folic acid, 2 mg per day, and oral iron, 200 mg per day, coupled with delivery without excessive blood loss resulted in rapid hematological improvement. The reticulocyte count rose promptly to 20 percent and then to as high as 31 percent.

Nine days postpartum she experienced sudden, severe left-sided pleuritic pain which radiated to the left shoulder and arm. She had difficulty breathing. While breathing room air, arterial Po_2 was 80 mmHg. X-ray and lung scan were normal; however, two distinct infarcts in the enlarged spleen were detected by Technetium scanning. Since the hematocrit was only 16, a unit of packed red cells was slowly infused without problems. The signs and symptoms of splenic infarction cleared, the hematocrit rose to 29, and tubal sterilization was performed.

Six months later, severe hemolytic anemia recurred when she stopped taking prednisone. Since then she has maintained an adequate hematocrit on 10 mg of prednisone daily.

PREGNANCY-INDUCED HEMOLYTIC ANEMIA

Unexplained hemolytic anemia during pregnancy is a rare but apparently distinct entity in which severe hemolysis develops early in pregnancy and resolves within months after delivery. It is characterized by absence of evidence for an immune mechanism or of any intra- or extraerythrocytic defects (Starksen and associates, 1983). However, the fetus-infant also may demonstrate transient hemolysis, which at least suggests an antibody-mediated etiology. Maternal corticosteroid treatment is usually effective. We have observed one woman with recurrent hemolysis during several pregnancies, and in each instance, intense severe hemolytic anemia was controlled by prednisone given until delivery. Her children appear to be normal.

PAROXYSMAL NOCTURNAL HEMOGLOBINURIA

This is a rare, acquired hemolytic anemia of insidious onset and chronic course. The hemoglobinuria is not necessarily nocturnal. Hemolysis is the consequence of a defect in the erythrocyte and granulocyte membrane which makes them unusually susceptible to lysis by complement and in vitro by acid treatment. The defect is seen in discrete red cell populations and already exists in newly-formed cells rather than being acquired after entering the circulation.

Paroxysmal nocturnal hemoglobinuria is not familial. The disease may range from mild to lethal. Serious complications include marrow aplasia, infections, and thromboses. Except possibly for marrow transplantation, no definitive treatment exists. Heparin therapy, in general, has been disappointing, but corticosteroids sometimes may be of value. Transfusions should be limited to compatible, washed red cells. Iron loss from hemoglobinuria can be high and iron-deficiency anemia frequently co-exists.

Paroxysmal nocturnal hemoglobinuria is a serious and unpredictable disease and pregnancy may be dangerous. Hurd and associates (1982) reported a woman with severe anemia which was further complicated by skin lesions characteristic of purpura fulminans. Heparin proved to be of no benefit. Cesarean section was performed primarily because of maternal thrombocytopenia and demonstration of maternal platelet antibody which caused concern for the fetal status; however, his platelet count at birth was normal. After a stormy postpartum course, which included a splenectomy, the mother survived. Greene and colleagues (1983) analysed 31 reported cases during pregnancy and cited a maternal death rate of 10 percent. Only half of the pregnancies resulted in surviving infants.

DRUG-INDUCED HEMOLYTIC ANEMIA

These hemolytic reactions are encountered occasionally during pregnancy. Infrequently, the hemolysis results from an antibody that, in the presence of a drug such as quinine acting as a hapten, may cause lysis of erythrocytes. Especially in black women, drug-induced hemolysis may much more often be related to an *inherited* erythrocyte enzymatic defect, namely severe *glucose-6-phosphate dehydrogenase (G6PD) deficiency*. There are many variants of this enzyme and the erythrocytes of about 2 percent of American black women are markedly deficient in enzyme activity. In this the homozygous state, both X chromosomes are affected. The heterozygous state, with one deficient and one normal X chromosome, is identified in 10 to 15 percent of black women and results in a modest deficiency of enzyme activity. Several oxidant drugs may induce hemolysis in homozygous women.

Since young erythrocytes contain more G6PD activity than do older erythrocytes, in the absence of bone marrow depression, the anemia ultimately stabilizes and is corrected soon after the drug is discontinued.

OTHER ACQUIRED ANEMIAS

As described by Pritchard and associates (1976), overt fragmentation (microangiopathic) hemolysis with visible hemoglobinemia complicates *preeclampsia–eclampsia* very infrequently (see Chap. 35, p. 663). The most fulminant acquired hemolytic anemia encountered during pregnancy is caused by exotoxin of *Clostridium perfringens* and may prove fatal (see Chap. 29, p. 507). Bacterial endotoxin, especially with severe acute pyelonephritis, may be accompanied by evidence for hemolysis and mild to moderate anemia (Cunningham and colleagues, 1987).

APLASTIC OR HYPOPLASTIC ANEMIA

Although rarely encountered during pregnancy, aplastic anemia is a grave complication. The diagnosis is readily made when anemia, usually with thrombocytopenia, leucopenia, and markedly hypocellular bone marrow are demonstrated. Aplastic anemia may be congenital but is more commonly induced by drugs and other chemicals, infection, irradiation, leukemia, and immunological disorders. The basic functional defect appears to be a marked decrease in committed marrow stem cells. In most cases, aplastic anemia and pregnancy appear to have been a chance association. In a few women, however, aplastic anemia first has been identified during a pregnancy and then improved or even resolved when the pregnancy terminated, only to recur with a subsequent pregnancy.

None of the erythropoietic agents that produce remission in other anemias are effective. Corticosteroids such as prednisone are possibly of value, as are large doses of testosterone or other androgenic steroids. All of the effects from the administration of large doses of testosterone or other potent androgens during pregnancy are unknown. The women almost certainly would become virilized. The female fetus may develop the stigmata of androgen excess (pseudohermaphroditism) depending upon the compound, the dose, and the capacity of the placenta to aromatize the androgen. Liver toxicity has been a common complication of therapy with large doses of androgens.

The treatment for severe aplastic anemia that is most likely to be effective is *bone marrow transplantation*. This typically requires immunosuppressive therapy for some months after infusion of marrow obtained from a histocompatible donor. Unfortunately, previous blood transfusions enhance considerably the risk of marrow graft rejection. Acute and chronic graft-versus-host disease is a serious complication following marrow transfusion. *Antithymocyte globulin* is probably the best available therapy for patients who do not have a suitable marrow donor (Bayever and co-workers, 1984). We have followed only one woman in whom bone marrow transplantation was done at age 12 for hypoplastic anemia. When seen at 30 weeks, she had normal hemoglobin mass, platelets, and leucocytes and her reticulocyte count was 2.3 percent. She was delivered without complications at term of a normal infant.

The two great risks to the woman with aplastic anemia during pregnancy are hemorrhage and infection. A continuous search for infection should be made, and when found, specific antimicrobial therapy should be started promptly. Granulocyte transfusions are given only during actual infection. Red cell transfusions are likely to be required for symptomatic anemia and we routinely transfuse to maintain the hematocrit at about 20. If the platelet count is very low, platelet transfusions may be needed to control hemorrhage. Vaginal delivery performed so as to minimize incisions and lacerations will lessen blood loss if the uterus is stimulated to contract vigorously after delivery. Even when thrombocytopenia is intense, the risk of severe hemorrhage can be minimized by vaginal delivery performed so as to avoid lacerations and an extensive episiotomy.

We have managed throughout pregnancy and the puerperium two women with severe aplastic anemia characterized by intense pancytopenia. The mothers were transfused to maintain the maternal hemoglobin concentration between 4 and 6 g per dL and they were given large doses of prednisone throughout most of pregnancy. The pregnancies were terminated by vaginal delivery of healthy infants, one of whom has been followed now for 26 years, and continues to appear quite normal (J. Pritchard, personal communication).

An extensive review of aplastic anemia has been provided by Camitta and associates (1982). Experience with pregnancy following bone marrow transplanation or the use of antithymocyte globulin is too limited to make any recommendations at this time. Our experiences are limited to one woman who did well throughout pregnancy.

SICKLE CELL HEMOGLOBINOPATHIES

Sickle cell anemia (SS disease), sickle cell–hemoglobin C disease (SC disease), and sickle cell–β-thalassemia disease (S–β-thalassemia disease) are the most common of the sickle hemoglobinopathies. Maternal morbidity and mortality, abortion, and perinatal mortality are variably increased with each of these diseases and, therefore, the problems associated with each of the hemoglobinopathies and their management are considered separately.

SICKLE CELL ANEMIA

The inheritance of the gene for the production of sickle, or S, hemoglobin from each parent results in sickle cell anemia

(SS disease). In most communities in the United States, one out of every 12 black individuals has the sickle cell trait, which results from inheritance of one gene for the production of S hemoglobin and one for normal hemoglobin A. The theoretical incidence of sickle cell anemia among blacks is one out of every 576 ($\frac{1}{12} \times \frac{1}{12} \times \frac{1}{4} = 576$), but the disease is not so common among pregnant black women. A high death rate, especially during early childhood, and lower parity among women with SS disease account for this.

Pregnancy is a serious burden to the woman with SS disease, for the anemia often becomes more intense, vaso-occlusive episodes with severe pain—so-called *sickle cell crises*—usually become more frequent, and infections and pulmonary complications are more common. Maternal mortality has been excessive and nearly one-half of pregnancies have terminated in abortion, stillbirth, or neonatal death (Table 39–3). Powars and colleagues (1986), in an extensive review, compared maternal and perinatal outcomes before and after 1972, and they reported that maternal mortality fell from 6 to 1 percent.

Adequate care of women with sickle cell anemia or other sickle cell hemoglobinopathies in pregnancy necessitates close observation with careful evaluation of all symptoms, physical findings, and laboratory studies. One rather common danger is that the symptomatic woman may categorically be considered to be suffering from a sickle cell crisis. As a result, ectopic pregnancy, placental abruption, pyelonephritis, and other serious obstetrical problems that cause pain or anemia, or both, may be overlooked. **The term *sickle cell crisis*, if used, should be applied only after all other possible causes of pain or reduction in hemoglobin concentration have been excluded.**

In our experience, in the absence of infection or nutritional deficiency, the hemoglobin concentration does not fall much below 7 g per dL, a level at or above which pregnant women with sickle cell anemia usually have no symptoms attributable to anemia. Since these women maintain their hemoglobin concentration by intense erythropoiesis to compensate for the markedly shortened erythrocyte life span, any factor that impairs erythropoiesis, or increases destruction of erythrocytes, or both, aggravates the anemia. The folic acid requirements during pregnancy complicated by sickle cell anemia are considerable. Since the dietary intake of folic acid may be inadequate, especially during episodes of anorexia induced or enhanced by pain, supplementary folic acid is indicated and 1 mg per day is adequate.

There are special circumstances during pregnancy that increase appreciably the morbidity of these women. Covert bacteriuria and thus acute pyelonephritis are substantively increased, and careful surveillance for bacteriuria and its eradication is important to prevent most symptomatic renal infections. If pyelonephritis develops, these erythrocytes are extremely susceptible to endotoxin, which can cause dramatic and rapid destruction along with suppressed erythropoiesis. Pneumonia, especially due to *Streptococcus pneumoniae*, is common and the woman with advanced pregnancy may not tolerate severe pulmonary infections. Women with sickle cell disease seldom die of heart failure; however, the basal hemodynamic state is characterized by high cardiac output, which is further augmented by pregnancy (Falk and Hood, 1982). While most of these women tolerate the changes of normal pregnancy well, when severe preeclampsia or serious infection develops, then ventricular failure is more likely (Cunningham and associates, 1986).

Labor in women with hemoglobin SS disease should be managed the same way as for those with cardiac disease. The woman should be kept comfortable but not oversedated. Compatible blood should be readily available. If a difficult vaginal delivery or cesarean section is contemplated, the hemoglobin concentration should be raised by careful administration of packed erythrocytes. At the same time, care must be taken to prevent circulatory overload from ventricular failure and pulmonary edema. Oxygen therapy should be instituted during times of increased oxygen need.

Intense sequestration of sickled erythrocytes may develop acutely, especially late in pregnancy, during labor and delivery, and early in the puerperium. Rarely, dangerous anemia rapidly appears as a consequence of sequestration, but more likely it is due to increased hemolysis. Acute sequestration is usually accompanied by severe bone pain. Whenever the hemoglobin spontaneously dropped below 6.0 g per dL or decreased at a rate of 2 g or more per 24 hours, Hendrickse and Watson-Williams (1966) recommended exchange transfusion with donor red cells known to contain only hemoglobin A.

Hendrickse and Watson-Williams (1966) also advocated heparin therapy in patients with sickle cell anemia who developed severe bone pain during late pregnancy or the puerperium. The benefits derived from heparin in this circumstance have not been established, and from our observations, heparinization has no salutary effects. Dextran infusion was originally claimed to reduce bone pain and marrow infarction, but a well-controlled study subsequently failed to demonstrate any benefit over that provided by hydration with aqueous glucose solution (Barnes and co-workers, 1965). Liberal hydration may be of value to prophylactically reduce the frequency and intensity of attacks of pain.

For severe pain, use of potent analgesics, such as meperidine or morphine administered parenterally, is certainly indi-

TABLE 39–3. PREGNANCY OUTCOMES REPORTED SINCE 1956 FOR WOMEN WITH SICKLE CELL ANEMIA AND HEMOGLOBIN SC DISEASE NOT TRANSFUSED PROPHYLACTICALLY

Hemoglobin	Women	Pregnancies	Maternal Deaths (per 100,000)	Spontaneous Abortions (%)	Perinatal Mortality (per 1,000)
Sickle cell (SS) disease	607	1,331	2,704	18	191
Hemoglobin SC disease	211	605	2,311	16	75

Data from Carache and colleagues: Obstet Gynecol 55:407, 1980; Milner and associates: Am J Obstet Gynecol 138:239, 1980; Poddar and co-workers: Br J Obstet Gynaecol 93:727, 1986; Powars and colleagues: Obstet Gynecol 67:217, 1986.

cated. The risk of addiction under these circumstances is remarkably low. Red cell transfusions administered after the onset of severe pain, in our experience, have no dramatic effect on the intensity or the duration of the attack of pain whereas prophylactic red cell transfusions almost have eliminated pain by preventing these vaso-occlusive episodes.

Because of the chronic debility from sickle cell anemia, the further complications caused by pregnancy, and the predictably shortened life span of women with sickle cell anemia, sterilization, or at least a very effective means of contraception, is indicated, even for women of low parity. Oral contraceptives in the form of estrogen-progestin combinations probably are contraindicated in women with SS disease since erythrocyte sequestration and vascular occlusion inherent in the disease might be intensified. Infection as the consequence of an intrauterine device likely would prove much more dangerous than in an otherwise healthy woman.

SICKLE CELL–HEMOGLOBIN C DISEASE

About 1 in 40 American blacks has the gene for production of hemoglobin C. Therefore, the probability of hemoglobin SC in a black couple is about 1 in 500, and the probability of their child inheriting the gene for hemoglobin S and an allelic gene for hemoglobin C is 1 in 4. As the consequence of these genetic frequencies, about 1 out of every 2,000 ($\frac{1}{12} \times \frac{1}{40} \times \frac{1}{4}$) pregnant black women are expected to have sickle cell–hemoglobin C, or SC disease, barring any significant mortality either before or during the years of reproductivity or an appreciable reduction in parity compared to black women in general.

In nonpregnant women, morbidity and mortality from sickle cell–hemoglobin C disease are appreciably lower than from sickle cell anemia. Indeed, less than half of women with SC disease have ever been symptomatic prior to pregnancy. During pregnancy and the puerperium, however, morbidity and mortality are increased considerably (Cunningham and associates, 1983). Attacks of severe bone pain and episodes of pulmonary infarction and embolization are fairly common during these times. A particularly worrisome pulmonary complication appears to be related to embolization of necrotic bone marrow, both fat and cellular, and acute respiratory insufficiency may develop.

In an 18-year anterospective study at Parkland Hospital, the maternal mortality rate for a relatively large series of pregnancies in women with sickle cell–hemoglobin C disease was close to 2 percent, and one out of eight pregnancies resulted in abortion, stillbirth, or neonatal death (Pritchard and co-workers, 1973). Thus, the perinatal mortality rate was somewhat greater than that of the general population but nowhere as great as with sickle cell anemia. Similar experiences have been reported by others (Table 39–3). Powars and associates (1986) reported that maternal mortality decreased from 6 percent before 1972 to zero since that time.

As with other pregnancies complicated by overt hemolytic anemia, the need for folic acid in women with SC disease is increased, especially when anorexia is present. Iron deficiency develops occasionally, unless the mother has received transfusions previously. Therefore, supplementation not only with folic acid but also with iron is likely to be of benefit unless red cell transfusions have been used previously or are contemplated. Whenever the hemoglobin concentration drops below 8.0 g per dL, a thorough search for the cause or causes is essential. The guidelines used for blood transfusion in the absence of prophy-

lactic transfusion have been similar to those described above for sickle cell anemia.

The frequent morbidity and relatively high mortality rate during late pregnancy and the puerperium in women with sickle cell–hemoglobin C disease warrant limitation of family size.

SICKLE CELL–β-THALASSEMIA DISEASE

The inheritance of the gene for hemoglobin S from one parent and the allelic gene for β-thalassemia from the other results in sickle cell–β-thalassemia disease. Our experience with 37 pregnancies implies that the perinatal mortality and morbidity of this disease are similar to those of sickle cell–hemoglobin C disease (Pritchard and colleagues, 1973). The frequencies of maternal morbidity and mortality perhaps are somewhat less, although deaths have been observed during pregnancy (Morrison, 1972). Our recommendations for general prenatal care, labor and delivery, and the restriction on future pregnancies are similar for sickle cell–thalassemia, sickle cell–hemoglobin C disease, and sickle cell anemia.

PROPHYLACTIC RED CELL TRANSFUSIONS

Currently, we transfuse prophylactically during pregnancy women with sickle cell anemia, sickle cell–hemoglobin C disease, or sickle cell–β-thalassemia disease as outlined below:

At the outset, once the diagnoses of pregnancy and a sickle cell hemoglobinopathy are confirmed, recently collected packed red cells that contain no abnormal hemoglobin are transfused in amounts and frequencies sufficient to reduce and maintain the percentage of red cells that contain hemoglobin S to no more than 60 percent and to keep the hematocrit at 25 or higher as described in detail by Cunningham and Pritchard (1979). Essentially 100 percent of red cells that contain hemoglobin S will sickle when treated for at least 1 hour with fresh, isotonic sodium metabisulfite solution and sealed between a glass slide and coverslip. An alternative to differential counting of red cells by an experienced technologist is to separate electrophoretically the S hemoglobin and determine the percentage using a densitometer.

When the hematocrit is low, as is commonly the case with sickle cell anemia, most often simple transfusions of packed red cells are carefully administered. Since usually 2 or 3 units are given in close succession, the third unit is given after stimulating a brisk diuresis by administering 20 mg of furosemide intravenously. When the hematocrit is higher, as it usually was with SC or S–β-thalassemia disease, exchange transfusion was commonly employed. More recently, prophylactic transfusions have not been initiated in women with SC disease or S–β-thalassemia until the end of the second trimester since the mothers seldom develop serious debility before that time (Cunningham and associates, 1983).

Consideration should be given to a number of techniques that may reduce the adverse effects from transfusions. These include use of red cells that are (1) fresh from the donor, (2) compatible for troublesome minor blood groups, (3) obtained from volunteer donors to reduce the risk of hepatitis, (4) washed to reduce reactions, and (5) predominantly young and therefore capable of surviving longer in the recipient. Young red cells are readily provided by a donor who undergoes frequent phlebotomy and takes iron.

Among the nearly 100 pregnancies complicated by sickle hemoglobinopathy so managed at Parkland Hospital, maternal mortality has been zero and maternal morbidity from the sickle hemoglobinopathy has been minimal. The degree of relief from chronically debilitating sickle cell anemia provided one woman by transfusion during pregnancy is illustrated in Figure 39–3.

The most dramatic impact of prophylactic erythrocyte transfusion is on maternal morbidity. Although perinatal outcome has been substantively improved, it has been appropriately emphasized that other management advances contributed significantly to this. Even though there was at times worrisome evidence of a compromised intrauterine environment in the form of fetal growth retardation, meconium staining of amnionic fluid, and during labor ominous decelerations of the fetal heart rate, perinatal mortality was remarkably low when compared to previous experiences. Koshy and colleagues randomized 72 pregnant women with sickle cell disease to be given prophylactic red cell transfusions. They too cited significantly decreased maternal morbidity in women transfused, however, they reported no improved perinatal outcomes, and concluded that omission of transfusion therapy was justified.

Morbidity from the transfusions has proved troublesome, especially isoimmunization and hepatitis. We calculated recently that the incidence of isoimmunization per unit of blood transfused was 3 percent (J. Cox and associates, 1988). The spectre of iron overload and transfusion hemochromatosis is worrisome; however, in the nearly 50 liver biopsies performed to date, no evidence for substantive liver disease has been found. Since further transfusion can be anticipated to enhance these complications, we have concluded tentatively that during one pregnancy the mother with sickle cell hemoglobinopathy and her fetus are likely to benefit from prophylactic transfusions of normal donor red cells administered according to the protocol employed. Most recently published data support this conclusion.

The following biophysical and physiological changes induced in blood by substituting normal red cells for red cells of sickle cell anemia are of interest: When subjected to reduced oxygen tension, the viscosity of blood containing mixtures of normal red cells and those of sickle cell anemia increases but not nearly so much as in blood that has only hemoglobin S-containing cells (Murphy and co-workers, 1976). In vivo this phenomenon would likely affect the microcirculation in a deleterious way. Miller and associates (1980) have studied exercise performance in subjects with sickle cell anemia before and after exchange transfusion and describe appreciable improvement in work performance following replacement of 50 percent of the abnormal cells by normal red cells even though the degree of anemia remained essentially unchanged.

SICKLE CELL TRAIT

The inheritance of the gene for the production of S hemoglobin from one parent and for A hemoglobin from the other results in sickle cell trait. In this circumstance, the amount of S hemoglobin produced is distinctly less than the amount of A hemoglobin. The frequency of red cell sickling among black individuals is about 1 in 12 or about 8 percent (Schneider and co-workers, 1976). Erythrocytes in smears of blood from women with sickle cell trait usually appear normal unless the blood previously has been markedly depleted of oxygen to produce sickled forms.

Extensive studies of the effect, or lack of effect, of sickle cell trait on pregnancy have been reported (Pritchard and associates, 1973; Tuck and co-workers, 1983; Whalley and associates, 1965). Sickle cell trait did not influence unfavorably the frequency of abortion, perinatal mortality, low birthweight, or pregnancy-induced hypertension. Urinary infection, however, was about twice as common in the group with sickle cell trait. Subsequent investigations disclosed that twice as many pregnant women with sickle cell trait had asymptomatic bacteriuria as did black women whose erythrocytes did not sickle.

Sickle cell trait should not be considered a deterrent to pregnancy on the basis of increased risks to the mother. However, the probability for a debilitating sickle cell hemoglobinopathy in her offspring is 1 in 4 whenever the father carries a gene for an abnormal hemoglobin or for β-thalassemia.

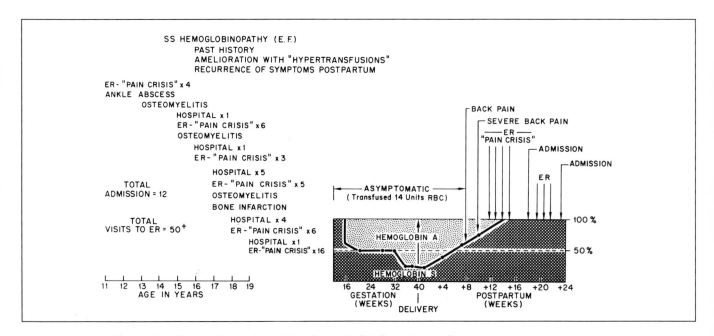

Figure 39–3. Patient E.F who has sickle cell anemia. Debility before her first pregnancy is summarized on the left. To the right, the reduction in hemoglobin S level as the consequence of transfusion of 14 units of packed red cells, and the recurrence of severe pain 9 weeks after delivery are emphasized (ER = Emergency Room). (*From Cunningham and Pritchard: Am J Obstet Gynecol 135:994, 1979.*)

OTHER HEMOGLOBINOPATHIES

HEMOGLOBIN C AND C-THALASSEMIA

About 2 to 3 percent of the black population has the mutant gene for hemoglobin C. Hemoglobin C trait does not cause anemia, nor does it predispose to pathological pregnancies in our experience. Pregnancy and homozygous hemoglobin C disease or hemoglobin C–β–thalassemia appear also to be rather benign associations (Cunningham and Pritchard, unpublished; Smith and Krevans, 1959). The degree of anemia is usually mild or moderate. We occasionally see women with homozygous CC disease whose hematocrit is less than 20. When severe anemia is identified, then iron or folic acid deficiency or some other superimposed cause should be explored. Supplementation with folic acid and iron, unless blood is transfused, is likely to prove of value in pregnant women with any hemoglobinopathy.

HEMOGLOBIN E

Substitution of a single specific amino acid in both β-globin chains gives rise to hemoglobin E. This hemoglobin has become more prevalent in the United States since the influx of a large number of Southeast Asians. Hurst and co-workers (1983), for example, identified homozygous hemoglobin E, hemoglobin E plus α-thalassemia, or hemoglobin E trait in 36 percent of Cambodian children and 25 percent of Laotians, but in only 1 percent of Vietnamese, whereas α- and β-thalassemia traits were prevalent in all groups.

The homozygous state for hemoglobin E is characterized by mild anemia even though red cell microcytosis is marked and targeting is common. Pregnancies in women homozygous for hemoglobin E do not appear to be at increased risk as the consequence of this clinically mild hemoglobinopathy. However, hemoglobin E-β–thalassemia has been reported to cause severe anemia that may require transfusion during pregnancy (Ferguson and Reilly, 1985). It is not clear whether sickle cell–hemoglobin E disease is as ominous during pregnancy as sickle cell–hemoglobin C disease.

Iron-deficiency anemia as the consequence of intestinal parasites, repeated pregnancies, or both, may coexist with E hemoglobinopathy. We are providing supplements of folic acid as well as iron for pregnant women identified to have homozygous hemoglobin E or hemoglobin E-thalassemia diseases.

HEMOGLOBINOPATHY IN THE NEWBORN

Hemolytic anemias characteristic of hemoglobinopathies are not operational in utero or at birth since most of the hemoglobin in the red cells is fetal (F) hemoglobin. After birth, as more newly synthesized red cells contain more abnormal hemoglobin, the disease becomes clinically apparent. Newborn infants with sickle cell anemia, sickle cell–hemoglobin C disease, and homozygous hemoglobin C disease can be accurately identified at birth by electrophoresis performed on hemoglobin obtained from uncontaminated cord blood using cellulose acetate support medium and buffer at pH 8.4 plus citrate agar gel and buffer at pH 6.0 (Nussbaum and colleagues, 1984). In many states, including Texas, such screening is performed routinely on blood submitted for phenylketonuria and hypothyroidism screening (Chap. 32, p. 586). Vichinsky and colleagues (1988) described recently the benefits of early diagnosis of sickle cell disease provided by screening of nearly 85,000 newborns in California.

GENETIC COUNSELING

Identification of the common hemoglobinopathies and their traits involves relatively simple laboratory procedures, and the genetic aspects of these diseases are straightforward. Therefore, genetic counseling can be readily provided. One out of every four children, on the average, will be afflicted with the disease whenever both parents have a trait form, as pointed out above. If one parent has the hemoglobinopathy and the other only the trait form, half of their children can be expected to inherit the hemoglobinopathy and the other half the trait form. If both parents have a hemoglobinopathy, so will all their children.

Remarkable technical advances have been made for identifying the fetus who is genetically destined to develop sickle cell disease, especially sickle cell anemia. Early procedures required the collection of fetal red cells whose capabilities for synthesizing abnormal β-globin chains were then measured in vitro. It was next demonstrated that amniocytes cultured from amnionic fluid could be treated with a *restriction endonuclease* enzyme that would cleave DNA into fragments which, at first by linkage analysis and subsequently by direct analysis of the fragments, could serve to identify prenatally most or all fetuses who were destined to develop sickle cell anemia. A new assay has been developed which is so sensitive that restriction endonuclease MstII can be applied immediately to cells obtained from 10 to 20 mL of amnionic fluid without prior culture and thereby avoid the delay which had been imposed by need for cell culture (Chang and Kan, 1982; Orkin and co-workers, 1982).

Hemoglobin C cannot be identified using the MstII enzyme, but hemoglobin C and most instances of β-thalassemia can be identified by analysis of DNA polymorphism or by identifying in vitro the kinds of globin chains synthesized by fetal red cells obtained from the fetus or placenta. The usefulness of DNA polymorphisms in circumstances where the inheritance of these diseases cannot be determined directly is borne out by the experiences of Boehm and associates (1983).

Chorionic villus biopsy during the first trimester has been used to identify fetal sickle cell anemia or β-thalassemia (Chap. 32, p. 586). DNA extracted from the trophoblast without prior culture is treated with an appropriate restriction enzyme and oligonucleotide analysis is performed (Monni and colleagues, 1987; Old and co-workers, 1986).

THALASSEMIAS

The genetically determined hematological disorders that are classified as thalassemias are characterized by an impaired rate of production of one or more of the peptide chains that are normal components of globin. The various forms of thalassemia are classified according to the globin chain which is deficient in amount compared to its partner chain. The two major forms of thalassemias involve either impaired production of alpha peptide chains causing α-thalassemia, or of beta chains to cause β-thalassemia. The incidence of traits during pregnancy for all races is probably 1 in 300 to 500 (Gehlbach and Morgenstern, 1988).

α-THALASSEMIAS

Four clinical syndromes, the consequence of impaired α-globin chain synthesis, have been identified. For each syndrome a close correlation has been established between clinical severity and the degree of impairment of synthesis of α-globin chains. In most propulations the α-globin chain gene loci are duplicated on chromosome 16 and thus the normal genotype for diploid cells can be expressed as αα/αα. There are two α-thalassemia genotypes: $α_1$-thalassemia is characterized by the deletion of both loci from one chromosome (– –/αα), whereas $α_2$-thalassemia is characterized by the loss of a single locus from one chromosome (–α/αα, heterozygote) or both (–α/–α, homozygote).

The deletion of all four α-globin chain genes (––/––) characterizes homozygous α-thalassemia. Without α-globin chains, hemoglobin Bart ($γ_4$) and hemoglobin H ($β_4$) are formed as abnormal tetramers. Deletion of three of the four genes (––/–α), leaving only one functional α-globin gene per diploid genome typifies hemoglobin H ($β_4$) disease. Clinically, α-thalassemia minor is the consequence of deletion of any two of the four α-chain genes (–α/–α or ––/αα), while the deletion of a single α-chain gene (–α/αα) is responsible for the silent carrier state.

In the homozygous form of α-thalassemia, no α-chains are produced. The hemoglobin in the fetus consists chiefly of hemoglobin Bart, the globin of which is made up of four gamma chains rather than the two alpha and two gamma chains which characterize normal hemoglobin F. Hemoglobin Bart has an appreciably increased affinity for oxygen. The fetus dies either in utero or very soon after birth and demonstrates the typical clinical features of nonimmune hydrops fetalis (see Chap. 33, p. 609).

The deletion of three genes is compatible with extrauterine life and the condition is referred to as hemoglobin H disease. The abnormal red cells at birth contain a mixture of hemoglobin Bart ($γ_4$), hemoglobin H ($β_4$), and hemoglobin A. Hemoglobin H disease is characterized by hemolytic anemia of varying severity and is usually worsened during pregnancy. The neonate appears well at birth, but as early infancy passes he develops a hemolytic anemia. Most, if not all, of the 20 to 40 percent of hemoglobin Bart present at birth is replaced by hemoglobin H postnatally.

A deletion of two genes results in α-thalassemia minor which is characterized by minimal to moderate hypochromic microcytic anemia. Because there is no associated clinical abnormality with α-thalassemia minor, it is often unrecognized. Red cells are hypochromic and microcytic and the hemoglobin concentration is normal to slightly depressed. Women with α-thalassemia minor appear to tolerate pregnancy quite well.

No clinical abnormality is evident in the individual with a single gene deletion.

The relative frequency of α-thalassemia minor, hemoglobin H disease, and hemoglobin Bart disease varies remarkably among racial groups. All of these variants are encountered in Orientals. However, in individuals of African descent, even though α-thalassemia minor is demonstrated in about 2 percent, hemoglobin H disease is extremely rare and hemoglobin Bart disease is unreported. The reason for the discrepancy is that Orientals usually have with $α_1$-thalassemia minor with both gene deletions typically from the same chromosome (––/αα), whereas in blacks with $α_2$-thalassemia minor one gene is deleted from each chromosome (–α/–α). The α-thalassemia syndromes appear sporadically in other racial and ethnic groups.

β-THALASSEMIAS

The β-thalassemias are also the consequence of impaired globin chain synthesis. The specific defect is impaired production of β-globin chains rather than α-globin chains. The molecular pathology for the defective production is complex. Kazazian and Boehm (1988) describe 51 point mutations in the β-globin gene.

Most are single nucleotide substitutions which produce transcription defects, RNA splicing or modification, translation, or highly unstable hemoglobins. The Δ–γ–β gene cluster is on chromosome 11.

A deficiency in globin chain synthesis has two important consequences: (1) There is a decreased rate of hemoglobin production and (2) when there is globin chain imbalance, precipitation of the excess globin chain damages the cell membrane which leads to intense hemolysis. These basic defects lead to the panorama of pathology that characterizes homozygous β-thalassemia (β-thalassemia major or Cooley's anemia). With the heterozygous β-thalassemia minor, hypochromia, microcytosis, and slight to moderate anemia develop without the intense hemolysis that characterizes the homozygous state.

In the typical case of thalassemia major, the infant appears healthy at birth, but as the hemoglobin F level falls he becomes severely anemic and fails to thrive. Those females who do survive beyond childhood are usually sterile.

With β-thalassemia minor, A_2 hemoglobin (comprised of two α- and two Δ-globin chains) is increased more than 3.5 percent and hemoglobin F (two α- and two γ-globin chains) may be somewhat elevated (more than 2 percent). The red cells are hypochromic and microcytic but the anemia is mild. The hemoglobin concentration is typically 8 to 10 g per dL late in the second trimester, with an increase to between 9 and 11 g per dL near term, as compared with a hemoglobin level of 10 to 12 g per dL in the nonpregnant state (Alger and colleagues, 1979; Freedman, 1969; Pritchard, 1962a). There is usually augmentation of erythropoiesis during pregnancy, as in normal women.

There is no specific therapy for β-thalassemia minor during pregnancy. Most often, the outcome for the mother and fetus is satisfactory (Pritchard, 1962a; Smith and associates, 1975). Blood transfusions are seldom indicated except for hemorrhage. Iron and folic acid in prophylactic daily doses of about 30 mg and 1 mg, respectively, are given. Any disease that depresses the function of the bone marrow or increases destruction of erythrocytes naturally intensifies the anemia. Infections, therefore, should be promptly identified and treated. The modest anemia, when not correctly diagnosed, has led to overzealous treatment especially with parenteral iron and at times with blood transfusions. The potential exists, of course, for the fetus to have inherited the serious problem of β-thalassemia major or a sickle hemoglobinopathy. Techniques for prenatal diagnosis of β-thalassemia may be difficult and are successful in only 80 percent of cases. Techniques include a combination of site-specific restriction endonuclease analysis, restriction fragment polymorphism linkage, and oligionucleotide probes (Old and colleagues, 1986)

The term β-*thalassemia intermedia* has been applied commonly to the clinical condition of individuals whose disease was nowhere near as intense as in β-thalassemia major but obviously more severe than that of β-thalassemia minor. Weatherall and co-workers (1981) identified in some such individuals, at least, the loss of a single α-globin gene which appeared to have favorably modified homozygous β-thalassemia from a severe transfusion-dependent state into the much milder thalassemia intermedia.

OTHER HEREDITARY HEMOLYTIC ANEMIAS

HEREDITARY SPHEROCYTOSIS

This disorder is characterized clinically by varying degrees of anemia and jaundice as the consequence of hemolysis of microspherocytic red cells. The molecular defect is within the proteins of the erythrocyte cytoskeleton and is associated with spectrin deficiency (Chasis and co-workers, 1988). The resultant membrane defect causes the spherocytic contour. Hereditary spherocytosis is considered to be transmitted as an autosomal dominant trait with variable penetrance, or possibly, multiple closely linked genes are essential for clinically apparent gene expression. Severe, recessively inherited spherocytosis has been described (Agre and co-workers, 1982).

Hemolysis and thus anemia are dependent upon an intact spleen which is usually enlarged. Splenectomy, while not correcting the membrane defect, spherocytosis, or increased osmotic fragility, does greatly reduce hemolysis, anemia, and jaundice. So-called *crises*, characterized by severe anemia from accelerated red cell destruction or more likely failure of production, or both, may develop in the woman with a functioning spleen. Infection must be vigorously searched for and treated. A previously normal pregnancy does not rule out the sudden development of severe anemia in a subsequent pregnancy (Ventura, 1982). Folic acid supplementation avoids the risk of megaloblastic erythropoiesis and impaired red cell production.

The newborn infant who has inherited hereditary spherocytosis may or may not demonstrate hyperbilirubinemia and anemia during the neonatal period. We have observed the hemoglobin level to fall to as low as 5.0 g per dL by 5 weeks of age in the daughter of a woman with hereditary spherocytosis who became symptomatic during pregnancy.

RED CELL ENZYME DEFICIENCIES

A number of erythrocyte enzymes are necessary for its anaerobic utilization of glucose. A deficiency of many, but certainly not all, of these enzymes may cause *hereditary nonspherocytic anemia*. As expected, most of these are inherited as autosomal recessive traits. Glucose-6-phosphate dehydrogenase deficiency, by far the most commonly identified enzyme deficiency, is a well-known exception that is X-linked. Pyruvate kinase deficiency, probably next most common, is an autosomal recessive trait. Although the degree of chronic hemolysis varies, most episodes of severe anemia with these deficiencies are induced by drugs or infections as previously discussed (p. 785).

During pregnancy, we routinely prescribe iron and folic acid for these women. Transfusions with red cells are given only if the hematocrit falls below 20, unless there is evidence for heart failure or hypoxia. Oxidant drugs are avoided, and bacterial infections are treated promptly.

POLYCYTHEMIA

Erythrocytosis during pregnancy is usually of the secondary type and related to chronic hypoxia, most often from congenital cardiac disease or a pulmonary disorder. Occasionally it follows heavy cigarette smoking. If polycythemia is severe, the probability of a successful pregnancy outcome is remote.

Polycythemia vera and pregnancy rarely coexist. Ruch and Klein (1964) described a case in which the hematocrit in the nonpregnant state was as high as 63. During each of two pregnancies, however, the hematocrit ranged from a low of about 35 during the second trimester to about 44 at term. Fetal loss seems to be high in women with polycythemia vera.

Koeffler and Goldwasser (1981) reported that measurement of serum erythropoietin by radioimmunoassay will differentiate polycythemia vera (low values) from secondary polycythemia (high values). No experiences during pregnancy were noted.

THROMBOCYTOPENIAS

Thrombocytopenia may appear clinically to be idiopathic or, more often, to be associated with one of the following disorders: acquired hemolytic anemia, severe preeclampsia or eclampsia, severe obstetrical hemorrhage with blood transfusions, consumptive coagulopathy from placental abruption or similar hypofibrinogenemic states, septicemia, lupus erythematosus, antiphospholipid antibodies, megaloblastic anemia caused by severe folate deficiency, drugs, viral infections, allergies, aplastic anemia, or excessive irradiation. **Burrows and Kelton (1988) recently reported that 8 percent of otherwise healthy women at term had mild thrombocytopenia (platelet count 97,000 to 150,000 per μL) that had no apparent adverse sequelae.**

IMMUNOLOGIC THROMBOCYTOPENIC PURPURA

The entity long referred to as *idiopathic thrombocytopenic purpura* is the consequence most often of an immune process in which antibodies against platelets are the culprits. Antibody-coated platelets are destroyed prematurely in the reticuloendothelial system, especially the spleen. The mechanism of production of antibodies is not known, and although unproven it usually is considered to be an autoantibody. Familial occurrence is rare.

Splenectomy performed on women with symptomatic immune thrombocytopenia often results in substantive improvement as the consequence of decreased removal of platelets by the spleen and reduced antibody production. Corticosteroid therapy often proves beneficial by increasing the platelet count and decreasing capillary fragility. Immunosuppressive drugs, including cyclophosphamide, vinca alkaloids, and azathioprine, also have been used with some success in cases refractory to corticosteroids and splenectomy as has intravenously administered polyvalent immunoglobulin therapy (see p. 793).

Pregnancy is especially challenging to women with immune thrombocytopenia and to their fetuses and newborn infants. Some feel that pregnancy may increase the risk of relapse in women previously in remission and to make the condition worse in women with active disease. It is certainly not unusual for women who have been in clinical remission for several years to relapse during pregnancy; however, this may be because of closer surveillance during pregnancy. The reason or reasons for possible deleterious effects from pregnancy are unknown but hyperestrogenemia has been suspected.

There is no strong contraindication to the use of corticosteroids such as prednisone during pregnancy. Large doses may be required for improvement and most likely treatment will have to be continued for the rest of the pregnancy. In our experiences, it is the unusual patient in whom corticosteroid therapy fails to achieve adequate amelioration, but if so, splenectomy can be performed. Late in pregnancy the procedure is technically more difficult and cesarean section may be necessary to improve exposure. At the same time, the fetus who may be severely thrombocytopenic avoids vaginal delivery trauma.

IgG antibodies are formed in immune thrombocytopenia, and these can cross the placenta and cause thrombocytopenia in the fetus and neonate. In our experience, this is more likely in the mother who previously had undergone splenectomy. The severely thrombocytopenic fetus is at increased risk of serious hemorrhage, especially intracranial hemorrhage, as the consequence of labor and delivery.

Considerable attention has been given to the problem of identifying the fetus with potentially dangerous thrombocytopenia. It is evident, as shown in Figure 39–4, that there is not a strong correlation between fetal and maternal platelet counts. Unfortunately, the conclusion of Karpatkin and associates (1981) that the administration of corticosteroids to the mother assures a platelet count in the fetus-infant adequate for hemostasis during labor and delivery is incorrect. It cannot be substantiated by either the findings demonstrated in the infant shown in Figure 39–5 and described below, or by observations of others (Cines and associates, 1982; Kelton and colleagues, 1982; Scott and co-workers, 1983). These latter investigators also have investigated the relationship between the levels of maternal IgG circulating platelet antibody, platelet-associated antibody, and the fetal platelet count. Cines and associates (1982) reported that monitoring circulating platelet antibody, but not platelet associated antibody, may help identify a fetus with severe thrombocytopenia. However, Kelton and colleagues (1982) reported that measurement of platelet-associated antibody could be used to predict thrombocytopenia in the fetus. Scott and co-workers (1983) found neither to be of special value and concluded that no antepartum maternal clinical characteristic or laboratory test tried so far would accurately predict the fetal platlet count. They urge the use of intrapartum platelet counts made on blood obtained from the fetal scalp once the cervix is 2 to 3 cm dilated and the membranes are ruptured (see Chap. 15). Whenever the platelet count in scalp blood was identified to be less than 50,000 per μL, they performed immediate cesarean section.

Daffos and colleagues (1985) and Hobbins and co-workers (1985) have done direct umbilical cord blood sampling and platelet counts in fetuses whose mothers have immune thrombocytopenia and are in labor. With documented fetal thrombo-

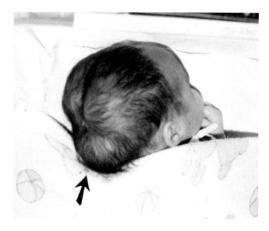

Figure 39–5. Newborn with extensive cephalohematomas, especially over the occipital bone (arrow). The mother had chronic immunological thrombocytopenic purpura, which was treated with prednisone. Her platelet count at the time of cesarean section was 115,000 per μL and the newborn's platelet count was as low as 3,000 per μL.

cytopenia, Daffos and co-workers (1984) have administered platelets to the fetus via the umbilical cord (Chap. 15, p. 282). Treatment of the mother and direct fetal transfusion with polyvalent immunoglobulin prior to labor might be attempted in a case with both mother and fetus affected (Dr. J. Scott, personal communication, 1988; also see p. 793).

Unfortunately, neither an acceptable maternal platelet count nor cesarean section provides absolute assurance that the fetus-infant will not hemorrhage as the consequence of severe thrombocytopenia as exemplified by the infant shown in Figure 39–5 and described now:

> This gravida 2 para 1 woman was troubled intermittently for many years by thrombocytopenia even though she had undergone splenectomy. Her first infant bled profusely following circumcision after which he was documented to be severely thrombocytopenic. The mother again became severely thrombocytopenic during this pregnancy but this was corrected as long as she took prednisone. Her platelet count exceeded 100,000 per μL at the time of delivery, but because of the possibility that the fetus might be thrombocytopenic and her desire for sterilization, it was elected to perform a cesarean section. This was accomplished with no serious problems for the mother, however, the infant demonstrated cephalohematomas over the occipital bone and both parietal bones—the region of the infant's head which had been manipulated by the surgeon to deliver the head. The platelet count was 17,000 per μL in cord blood and dropped promptly to as low as 3,000 per μL. The newborn was treated with corticosteroids, platelet transfusions, and exchange transfusions to attempt removal of platelet antibody. The infant survived the hemorrhage and the treatment.

For the mother with an adequate stable platelet count and who is not taking corticosteroids, cesarean section is unlikely to be any more a risk than for the normal woman. The administration of larger doses of steroids increases the risks somewhat of poor wound healing and infection. The obstetrician faces the dilemma that the route of delivery that may be best for the fetus–infant is likely to be bad for the mother if the mother has severe thrombocytopenia at the time of the operation. Unfortunately, the mother with severe thrombocytopenia who undergoes cesarean section is at appreciably increased risk for serious

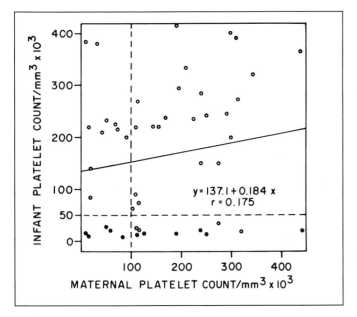

Figure 39–4. Pregnancies complicated by immune thrombocytopenic purpura. Lack of a strong correlation between maternal and newborn platelet counts is apparent. (*From Scott and co-workers: Am J Obstet Gynecol 145:932, 1983.*)

morbidity and even mortality. It can be anticipated with cesarean section that blood loss commonly will be severe. Moreover, troublesome hematomas prone to infection are common. However, blood loss at and after vaginal delivery will not be massive when delivery is managed so as to avoid lacerations and to minimize episiotomy size and maximize myometrial contraction and retraction. Platelet transfusions most often prove ineffective since donor platelets are attacked by antibody and rapidly cleared from the circulation.

In some instances where other accepted treatment modalities had failed to correct dangerous thrombocytopenia, yet life-threatening hemorrhage had developed or extensive surgery needed to be performed, high-dose intravenous *polyvalent immunoglobulin therapy* has been cited by some as being beneficial. The responses noted have varied from a marked increase in the platelet count within a few days after the start of a several day course of treatment, with the increase persisting after treatment was stopped, to little or no change in platelet count (Bierling and co-workers, 1982; Carroll and associates, 1983; Fehr and associates, 1982). Blanchette and co-workers (1983) cite evidence which supports reticuloendothelial blockade as the mechanism by which intravenous IgG therapy increases platelet counts. The efficacy, if any, of high-dose immunoglobulin for correcting severe thrombocytopenia in pregnancy is not known. It is possible that the risk from thrombocytopenia to the fetus-infant, as well as the mother, could be reduced appreciably by maternal administration of this maternal and placental transfer of IgG to the fetus. Such therapy is expensive, and is more than $4,000 for one course in 1988.

Effective contraception is often desirable. Tubal sterilization meticulously performed at the time of cesarean section should not increase blood loss appreciably. When done postpartum or remote from pregnancy the risk of morbidity relates to the platelet count. Since immunological thrombocytopenia is most common in women of reproductive age and may intensify during pregnancy, estrogen has been implicated in its pathogenesis. Even so this theoretical possibility would not appear to outweigh the advantages of highly effective contraception and reduced menstrual blood loss that can be achieved with estrogen plus progestin oral contraceptives. An intrauterine device in the presence of thrombocytopenia is likely to enhance appreciably bleeding from the uterus.

Martin and colleagues (1984) and Patriarco and Yeh (1986) have provided detailed reviews of immunological thrombocytopenia complicating pregnancy.

ISOIMMUNE THROMBOCYTOPENIA

Platelet isoimmunization can develop in a manner identical to erythrocyte antigen isoimmunization. If fetal platelet antigens for which maternal platelets are negative gain access to her circulation, the mother then may produce antibodies in subsequent pregnancies that will destroy fetal platelets that have this antigen. This disorder was recently reviewed by Deaver and colleagues (1986) and is discussed in Chapter 33 (p. 612).

THROMBOTIC MICROANGIOPATHIES

The original description in 1925 by Moschcowitz of *thrombotic thrombocytopenic purpura* was characterized by the pentad of thrombocytopenia, fever, neurological abnormalities, renal impairment, and hemolytic anemia. In 1955, Gasser and colleagues described the *hemolytic uremic syndrome*, which was similar to thrombotic thrombocytopenic purpura but with more profound renal involvement and fewer neurological aberrations. In 1968, Robson and Wagoner and their colleagues described *postpartum renal failure* characterized by uremia associated with microangiopathic hemolytic anemia and thrombocytopenia. Subsequently, attempts have been made to establish the existence of a variant of postpartum renal failure that occurs antepartum, which, in turn, led to the term *peripartal renal failure*.

Although it is likely that there are different etiologies to account for the variable findings within these syndromes, at this time it usually is impossible to separate them at least clinically (Hayslett, 1985). That a pure form of the hemolytic uremic syndrome incited by viral or bacterial infection exists in children seems indisputable; however, its sporadic adult form differs little from thrombotic thrombocytopenic purpura except for the severity of renal involvement. Moreover, there is no evidence that postpartum renal failure differs remarkably from the hemolytic uremic syndrome other than that the woman had been recently pregnant.

PATHOGENESIS

These syndromes are characterized by microthrombi within arterioles and capillaries consisting of a hyaline material made up of platelets plus small amounts of fibrin. The general consensus is that intravascular platelet aggregation stimulates the cascade of events leading to end-organ failure, and although there is evidence for endothelial damage, this is thought to be a consequence rather than a cause. Neither the precise pathogenesis of the disease nor the mechanisms by which cure is now often achieved are understood at this time. One hypothesis is that a plasma factor, which somehow inhibits platelet aggregation, is deficient. One such suspected factor is prostacyclin (prostaglandin I_2), although an excess of its natural antagonist, thromboxane A_2, also has been implicated as an inciting factor.

COAGULOPATHY

Thrombocytopenia is usually severe. Fortunately, even with very low platelet counts, spontaneous severe hemorrhage is uncommon. Microangiopathic hemolysis is associated with moderate to marked anemia. The blood smear is characterized by erythrocyte fragmentation with schizocytosis. The reticulocyte count is usually high, and nucleated red blood cells are frequent. Consumptive coagulopathy, however, is subtle, and increased levels of fibrin split products in serum are usually found only in low concentrations.

TREATMENT

Treatment of these syndromes until recently has been controversial. Early enthusiasm for heparin was followed by concern for its efficacy and safety, especially in hypertensive and thrombocytopenic patients. Antiplatelet agents have been tried with variable success. More recently, exchange transfusion with normal plasma and plasmapheresis, usually in combination, has improved remarkably the outcome for these formerly commonly fatal diseases. In many of these cases, however, preceding therapy with corticosteroids and antiplatelet agents, especially aspirin and dipyridamole, has obfuscated the exact utility of these other agents. Vincristine or splenectomy, alone or in combination, may cause amelioration of disease that does not respond to plasma exchange. It is generally agreed that heparin administration is of no benefit, and platelet transfusions may even worsen the disease.

Transfusions with red blood cells are imperative to counteract life-threatening anemia. Unless surgery is contemplated, in the normovolemic woman the hematocrit is maintained at about 20 or somewhat higher. Hemodialysis may be necessary, and placement of an arteriovenous shunt for this procedure also greatly facilitates repeated plasmaphereses.

PREGNANCY

In the past three decades, we have identified only a few pregnant women with these syndromes, or their presumed variants, among the large number of women cared for at Parkland Hospital. Since their frequency has not been greater than that in our general hospital, the question persists concerning the role, if any, of pregnancy and puerperium in the genesis of these syndromes. Our experiences support the thesis that they are coincidental and thus represent another example of sporadic idiopathic hemolytic uremic syndrome or thrombotic thrombocytopenic purpura that developed during pregnancy. It is possible that some pregnancy-related event may contribute to their development, such as bacterial sepsis, viral infections, and possibly some drugs, for example ergot alkaloids. As discussed above, the concept of faulty endothelial prostacyclin production is currently popular, and in this respect there is a similarity to severe preeclampsia-eclampsia (Chap. 35, p. 658). It is not surprising that severe preeclampsia and eclampsia complicated further by thrombocytopenia and overt hemolysis have been confused with thrombotic thrombocytopenic purpura and vice versa (Schwartz and colleagues, 1985; Vandekerckhove and associates, 1984). However, as described below and in Chapter 35, delivery with supportive care appropriate for severe preeclampsia and eclampsia soon results in the disappearance of both severe thrombocytopenia and the evidence of hemolysis, and is followed by complete recovery. Otherwise, the disease process is not preeclampsia–eclampsia.

It is not established whether pregnancy worsens the prognosis for these syndromes characterized by thrombocytopenic microangiopathy, or whether termination of the pregnancy improves the prognosis. Unless the diagnosis is unequivocally one of these thrombotic microangiopathies, rather than severe preeclampsia or eclampsia, the response to prompt termination of the pregnancy should be evaluated before resorting to exchange transfusion, plasmapheresis, and antiplatelet drug therapy. **Most certainly, in our extensive experiences, plasmapheresis is not indicated for preeclampsia–eclampsia complicated by hemolysis and thrombocytopenia.**

In a few instances, thrombotic thrombocytopenic purpura has developed so early in pregnancy that preeclampsia could be excluded. In five cases summarized by Ambrose and colleagues (1985), a variety of therapeutic regimens allowed prolongation of pregnancy until fetal viability. However, in at least one other woman, termination of early pregnancy was followed by amelioration of the disease on two occasions (Natelson and White, 1985). In one woman managed at Parkland Hospital, recurrent hemolysis and thrombocytopenia developed peripartum in two successive pregnancies, but delivery had no ameliorative effect. Repeated plasmapheresis, and ultimately splenectomy after the second pregnancy were necessary to induce remission. In the one woman cared for at Parkland Hospital in whom the syndrome was identified in early pregnancy, termination did not reverse the disease process as now illustrated:

This 28-year-old white gravida 2 para 1 developed hemolytic anemia at 7 weeks. Peripheral smear was consistent with microangiopathic hemolysis and the platelet count was 20,000 per μL. Her blood pressure was 160/90 mmHg, there was 3+ proteinuria and the serum cretinine was 1.5 mg per dL. She was given prednisone; however, her anemia was transfusion-dependent and she was transferred to Parkland Hospital at 15 weeks (Table 39–4). Thrombotic thrombocytopenia puerpura was diagnosed, and over the next 2 weeks she underwent plasmapheresis nine times, following which 10 to 14 units of fresh-frozen plasma were infused. Prednisone, aspirin, and dipyridamole were given and she received two

TABLE 39–4. THROMBOTIC MICROANGIOPATHY COMPLICATING EARLY PREGNANCY

	Hematocrit	Platelets	Reticulocytes	Creatinine	Comments
7 weeks	18	75,000	4%	0.9	Normotensive; 2 RBC[a] transfusions
8 weeks	12	60,000	—	—	RBC transfusions; prednisone; BP 160/90, 3+ proteinuria; total of 10 RBC transfused
Transferred to Parkland Hospital					
15 weeks	20	13,000	11%	1.3	Plasmapheresis + 10–15 U FFP[b] transfusions 9 times over 14 days. RBC transfusions continued.
17 weeks	20	10,000	10%	1.4	Therapeutic abortion. RBC transfusions continued
Postabortion					
1 week	20	11,000	13%	1.4	Plasmapheresis + cryoprecipitate-poor plasma infusions
2 weeks	18	18,000	16%		Splenectomy
3 weeks	30	55,000	5%	1.5	Discharged. Given total of 17 RBC and 150 FFP
Discharged					
1 month	27	110,000		1.5	No transfusions since discharge; severe hypertension; no proteinuria
1 year	37	250,000	1.0	1.6	Severe hypertension

[a] RBC = packed red blood cells
[b] FFP = fresh-frozen plasma

courses of vincristine therapy. Neither thrombocytopenia nor anemia improved, and during this time she was given 13 units of packed erythrocytes to maintain the hematocrit at about 20.

Because of the poor prognosis and because it was thought by some that pregnancy termination might reverse whatever process was operative, at 17 weeks she underwent therapeutic termination induced by prostaglandin suppositories followed by intravenous oxytocin. There was no improvement and she remained transfusion-dependent. Plasmapheresis was performed using cryoprecipitate-poor plasma without salutary effects, so approximately 3 weeks after termination, splenectomy was performed. Following this hemolysis became compensated and the platelet count reached about 60,000 per μL.

After discharge, and 1 month after splenectomy, the platelet count was 110,000 per μL and the hemoglobin was stable at 9 grams per dL. Proteinuria had cleared; however, the serum creatinine was still 1.5 mg per dL and severe hypertension persisted. Hemolysis and thrombocytopenia continued to improve and by 6 months these had resolved completely. Two years later she continues to have hypertension and mild renal insufficiency.

INHERITED COAGULATION DEFECTS

Obstetrical hemorrhage, a common event, is rarely the consequence of an inherited defect in the coagulation mechanism.

HEMOPHILIA A

Hemophilia A is characterized by a marked deficiency of small component antihemophilic factor (factor VIII:C). It is rare among women compared to men. With few exceptions, the homozygous state that results from the inheritance of two abnormal X chromosomes is the requisite for classic hemophilia A in women, whereas one affected X chromosome, the homozygous state, is responsible for the disease in men. In a few instances hemophilia A appears to have developed in women spontaneously, presumably as the consequence of a newly mutant gene.

The degree of risk is influenced markedly by the level of circulating factor VIII:C. If the level is at or very close to zero, the risk is major, but if the level is higher, the risk is reduced. Factor VIII:C activity increases appreciably during normal pregnancy. Some increase is likely in hemophiliacs who can synthesize some factor VIII:C. The obstetrician can reduce the risk of grave hemorrhage at and after delivery by avoiding lacerations, minimizing episiotomy, and maximizing myometrial contractions and retraction.

Vaginal delivery of a fetus who inherited hemophilia A usually has not resulted in birth of an infant who has bled seriously. After delivery the risk of hemorrhage in the neonate increases, especially if circumcision is attempted. Why labor and vaginal delivery do not commonly incite serious bleeding in the fetus and neonate is not clear since maternal factor VIII:C does not cross the placenta.

Whenever the mother has hemophilia A, so will all of her sons and all of her daughters will be carriers. If she is a carrier, one half of her sons will inherit the disease and one half of her daughters will be carriers.

Prenatal diagnosis of hemophilia A is now possible in some families using chorionic villus biopsy (Chap. 32, p. 586). The identification of fetal sex identifies those at risk of inheriting hemophilia A, namely, male fetuses.

Factor VIII Inhibitor

Rarely, antibodies directed against factor VIII are acquired and may lead to life-threatening hemorrhage. This phemonenon has been identified in women during the puerperium. The prominent clinical feature is severe, protracted, repetitive hemorrhage from the reproductive tract starting a week or so after an apparently uncomplicated delivery (Reece and associates, 1982). The activated partial thromboplastin time is markedly prolonged. Treatment has included many transfusions of whole blood and plasma, huge doses of cryoprecipitate, large volumes of an admixture of activated coagulation factors (Autoplex), immunosuppressive therapy, and attempts at various surgical procedures especially curettage and hysterectomy.

HEMOPHILIA B

The genetic and clinical features of severe deficiency of factor IX (Christmas disease or hemophilia B) are quite similar to those for hemophilia A. The homozygous state, essential for severe disease in women, is rare. Pregnancy, with a favorable outcome from vaginal delivery and not requiring replacement therapy, even though factor IX actively remained quite low, has been described in detail by Rust and associates (1975). The male newborn infant appeared to tolerate labor and vaginal delivery without hemorrhage.

VON WILLEBRAND DISEASE

The larger component of factor VIII complex, namely factor VIII-related von Willebrand factor (VIII:vWF), is essential for adhesion of platelets to subendothelial collagen and formation of a primary hemostatic plug at the site of blood vessel injury. The factor is synthesized by endothelium and megakaryocytes under the control of autosomal genes on chromosome 12. The factor is present in platelets as well as plasma.

Clinically, von Willebrand disease is a heterogenous group of functional disorders involving aberrations of factor VIII complex and platelet dysfunctions. Most variants of von Willebrand disease are inherited as autosomal dominant traits, but type III, which is the most severe, is phenotypically recessive. These diseases are the most common inherited bleeding disorders and may be identified in 1 in 1,000 patients. The possibility of von Willebrand disease is usually considered most often in women with bleeding suggestive of a chronic disorder of coagulation. The classic autosomal dominant form is usually symptomatic in the heterozygous state. The less common but clinically more severe autosomal recessive form is manifest when inherited from both parents, both of whom demonstrate little or no disease. Von Willebrand disease is characterized clinically by easy bruising, mucosal hemorrhage, and excessive bleeding with trauma, including surgery. Its laboratory features are a prolonged bleeding time, prolonged partial thromboplastin time, decreased factor VIII (immunological activity as well as coagulation-promoting activity), and inability of platelets in plasma from an affected person to react to a variety of stimuli.

Conti and associates (1986) summarized 38 cases, including five of their own, of pregnancy complicated by von Willebrand disease. In a fourth of these women, bleeding was reported at the time of abortion, delivery, or the puerperium. Characteristically, the hemostatic defects improve during pregnancy, but if factor VIII activity is very low, the administration of factor VIII-rich cryoprecipitate at delivery is recommended. Factor VIII concentrate does not contain some multimers of VIII:vWF and thus is ineffective. With significant bleeding, 15 or 20 units of cryoprecipitate must be given every 12 hours. However, as reported by Chediak and colleagues (1986), worrisome hemorrhage may still be encountered in women with severe disease.

They also reported the use of desmopressin which caused water intoxication.

Most persons with vonWillebrand disease are heterozygous and have only a mild bleeding disorder. When both parents have the disorder, their offspring may, if homozygous, develop a serious bleeding disorder. Chorionic villus biopsy with DNA analysis to detect the missing genes has been accomplished (see Chap. 32, p. 586). Some recommend cesarean delivery to avoid trauma to a possibly affected fetus if the mother has had severe disease.

OTHER INHERITED COAGULATION FACTOR DEFICIENCIES

Factor XI deficiency is probably the consequence of an autosomal trait which is manifested as severe disease in the homozygous individuals but a minor defect in the heterozygote. This deficiency state is most prevalent in persons of Jewish extraction. It is rarely encountered in pregnancy.

Inherited abnormalities of fibrinogen usually involve the formation of a functionally defective fibrinogen, commonly referred to as *dysfibrinogenemia*. Familial hypofibrinogenemia has been described very infrequently. Our experiences suggest that the condition represents a heterozygous autosomal dominant state with 50 percent of the affected mother's offspring affected. Typically thrombin-clottable protein has ranged from 80 to 110 mg per dL when nonpregnant and then increased by 40 or 50 percent as in normal pregnancy. Those pregnancy complications that give rise to acquired hypofibrinogenemia were more common in our cases, but the existence of such conditions provided the impetus for study at the outset. Reports of pregnancy experiences for women with congenital afibrinogenemia are rare. The potential for grave problems would undoubtedly exist.

A number of important regulatory proteins inhibit clotting. Examples include antithrombin III and protein C and its cofactor, protein S. Deficiencies of these inhibitory proteins may be associated with recurrent thromboembolism, and a few cases in which pregnancy was complicated by them have been reported. Nelson and colleagues (1985) described the pregnancy courses of two women with antithrombin III deficiency, and although these were uneventful, one woman had suffered numerous thrombotic episodes before pregnancy. Brenner and co-workers (1987) reported a woman with protein C deficiency who had placental infarctions and preeclampsia, as well as multiple episodes of venous thromboses. Continuous heparinization did not prevent preeclampsia and fetal growth retardation. According to Comp and colleagues (1986), total protein S plasma concentrations, as well as functional protein S activity, are substantively diminished during normal pregnancy. Since these levels are similar to those seen in nonpregnant patients with protein S deficiency, diagnosis during pregnancy may be difficult. Rose and associates (1986) reported the course of a woman with protein S deficiency who elected termination because of warfarin ingestion. Because of the thrombotic tendency, these investigators recommend that anticoagulation with heparin be given during pregnancy; however, many of these patients are already receiving warfarin when they conceive. Chronic warfarin ingestion is associated with several fetal anomalies (Chap. 32, p. 565).

CARDIOVASCULAR DISEASE

Heart disease probably complicates about 1 percent of pregnancies. Rheumatic heart disease formerly accounted for the great majority of cases, but this has changed remarkably as new cases of rheumatic fever have almost disappeared in this country (Land and Bisno, 1983). This is related to earlier treatment of streptococcal infection as well as observations that streptococci that are now prevalent appear to have less potential for inducing rheumatic disease or glomerulonephritis. At the same time, better medical management, together with a number of newer surgical techniques, has enabled more young girls with congenital heart disease to reach the childbearing age in reasonably good health and to conceive. Hypertensive heart disease contributes a few cases of organic heart disease in pregnancy, whereas other varieties, such as coronary, thyroid, syphilitic, and kyphoscoliotic cardiac disease, as well as cor pulmonale, constrictive pericarditis, various forms of heart block, and isolated myocarditis are even less common.

Heart disease may be a very serious complication of pregnancy leading to maternal death, but in the great majority of instances it need not be so.

PROGNOSIS

The likelihood of a favorable outcome for the mother with heart disease and her child-to-be depends upon (1) the functional capacity of her heart, (2) the likelihood of other complications that increase further the cardiac load during pregnancy and the puerperium, (3) the quality of medical care provided, and (4) the psychological and socioeconomical capabilities of the expectant mother, her family, and the community. The last item may assume great importance, since a favorable outcome for pregnancy is often achieved even in instances of markedly impaired cardiac function if the mother, her family, and the community will accept the need for, and provide an environment suitable for, a very sedentary life. For some women, these requirements may amount to hospitalization with essentially complete bed rest throughout pregnancy and the early puerperium.

The prognosis and recommended treatment of cardiac disease have been influenced inappropriately in some instances by certain physiological measurements, the imprecise or incorrect interpretation of which led the authors to conclude that there was a maternal hemodynamic burden that peaked some weeks before term and following which the risk of cardiac failure dropped dramatically. Considerable emphasis has been placed, for example, on an apparent reduction in cardiac output after the 32nd week of pregnancy (see Chap. 7, p. 144). The misconception that cardiac decompensation would seldom develop after this time is not supported by clinical observations. The decrease in maternal blood volume during the last weeks of pregnancy reported by some has been similarly considered to bring about a decrease in cardiac work. Most reported measurements, however, fail to identify a decrease in blood volume of any appreciable magnitude during the last several weeks. **It is important that the physician understand that cardiac failure is just as likely to develop during the last few weeks of preg-**

nancy, or during labor and the puerperium. Of 542 women whose pregnancies were complicated by heart disease reported by Etheridge and Pepperell (1977), there were 10 maternal deaths and 8 of these were during the puerperium.

CONGENITAL HEART DISEASE IN OFFSPRING

Many congenital heart lesions appear to be inherited as polygenic characteristics (see Chap. 32, p. 574). Thus it might be expected that some women with congenital lesions would give birth to similarly affected infants. According to Whittemore and associates (1982), who followed 233 such women through 482 pregnancies, 16 percent of their infants were found by 3 years of age to have congenital heart disease. Interestingly, about half of the lesions were concordant with the maternal cardiac defect. Conversely, Shime and colleagues (1987) found congenital cardiovascular lesions, including Marfan syndrome, in only 3 percent of 87 infants born to women with congenital heart lesions.

DIAGNOSIS

As discussed at some length in Chapter 7 (p. 144), many of the physiological changes of normal pregnancy tend to make the diagnosis of heart disease more difficult than it is in the nonpregnant state. For example, in normal pregnancy systolic heart murmurs that are functional are quite common. Moreover, as the uterus enlarges and the diaphragm is elevated, the heart is elevated and rotated so that the apex is moved laterally while the heart is somewhat closer to the anterior chest wall. Cardiac filling is increased, accounting for the augmented stroke volume during much of pregnancy. Respiratory effort in normal pregnancy is accentuated, at times suggesting dyspnea. Presumably, this change is brought about in large part by a stimulatory effect of progesterone on the respiratory center. Edema, a further source of confusion, is often prevalent especially in the lower extremities during the latter half of pregnancy. Therefore, systolic murmurs and edema, as well as changes that suggest cardiac enlargement and dyspnea, are commonplace in normal pregnancy. It becomes obvious that the physician must be quite careful not to diagnose heart disease during pregnancy when none exists, but not fail to detect and treat appropriately heart disease when it does exist.

Burwell and Metcalfe (1958) list the following criteria, any one of which confirms the diagnosis of heart disease in pregnancy: (1) a diastolic, presystolic, or continuous heart murmur, (2) unequivocal cardiac enlargement, (3) a loud, harsh systolic murmur, especially if associated with a thrill, or (4) serious arrhythmias. Pregnant women who have none of these findings rarely have serious heart disease. While failure to detect clinically significant heart disease is inappropriate, faint suspicion of dysfunction should not lead to diagnostic efforts so intense that procedural costs become great or that seeds of anxiety are firmly planted in the mind of the patient.

CLINICAL CLASSIFICATION

There is no clinically applicable test for accurately measuring functional capacity of the heart. A helpful clinical classification has been provided by the New York Heart Association, which is based on past and present disability and is uninfluenced by the presence or absence of physical signs:

- **Class I.** Uncompromised: Patients with cardiac disease and *no limitation of physical activity*. These patients do not have symptoms of cardiac insufficiency, nor do they experience anginal pain.
- **Class II.** Slightly compromised: Patients with cardiac disease and *slight limitation of physical activity*. These women are comfortable at rest, but if ordinary physical activity is undertaken, discomfort results in the form of excessive fatigue, palpitation, dyspnea, or anginal pain.
- **Class III.** Markedly compromised: Patients with cardiac disease and *marked limitation of physical activity*. These women are comfortable at rest, but less than ordinary activity causes discomfort in the form of excessive fatigue, palpitation, dyspnea, or anginal pain.
- **Class IV.** Patients with cardiac disease and *inability to perform any physical activity without discomfort*. Symptoms of cardiac insufficiency or of the anginal syndrome may develop even at rest, and if any physical activity is undertaken, discomfort is increased.

GENERAL MANAGEMENT

The treatment of heart disease in pregnancy is dictated by the functional capacity of the heart. In all pregnant women, but especially those with cardiac disease, excessive weight gain, *abnormal* fluid retention, and anemia should be prevented. Increased bodily bulk increases the cardiac work, and *anemia* with its compensatory rise in cardiac output also predisposes to cardiac failure. The development of *pregnancy-induced hypertension* is hazardous, for in this circumstance cardiac output can be maintained only by an increase in cardiac work commensurate with increased afterload. At the same time, hypotension is undesirable, especially in women with septal defects or patent ductus arteriosus that allow shunting of blood from the right to the left heart chambers and from the pulmonary artery to aorta. *Infection* increases cardiac workload appreciably, and should be prevented if possible, and treated vigorously if it develops.

MANAGEMENT OF CLASSES I AND II

With rare exceptions, women in class I and most in class II are allowed to go through pregnancy. Throughout pregnancy and the puerperium, special attention should be directed toward both prevention and early recognition of heart failure. As emphasized by Sugrue and associates (1981), a more favorable functional classification at the outset should not engender any relaxation in vigilance of management. In 39 percent of their patients who developed frank cardiac failure the functional classification had been class I early in pregnancy. According to Sullivan and Ramanathan (1985), maternal morbidity is 0.4 percent in classes I and II. McFaul and co-workers (1988) encountered no maternal deaths in 445 women in these two classes.

A specific routine that assures adequate rest should be outlined for each patient. The recommendations of Hamilton and Thomson (1941) are still pertinent: The pregnant woman must rest in bed 10 hours each night and, in addition, must lie down for half an hour after each meal. Light housework and walking without climbing stairs is permitted. She should do no heavy work. Items rich in sodium should be avoided. Weight gain should not exceed the 24 pounds or so that are accounted for by the physiological changes induced by normal pregnancy. In essence, the pregnant woman must learn to spare herself all unnecessary effort and must rest as much as possible.

Not infrequently, infection has proved to be an important factor in precipitating cardiac failure. Each woman should receive instructions to avoid contact with others who have respiratory infections, including the common cold, and to report at once any evidence of an infection. Pneumococcal and influenza vaccines are recommended.

The onset of congestive heart failure is often gradual and may be detected if attention is continually directed to specific signs. The first warning sign of cardiac failure is likely to be persistent rales at the base of the lungs, frequently with a cough. To be significant, the rales must persist after two or three deep breaths, for the rales that are sometimes heard in normally pregnant women disappear after one or two deep inspirations. A sudden diminution in the woman's ability to carry out her household duties, increasing dyspnea on exertion, attacks of smothering with cough, and hemoptysis, are other signals warning of serious heart failure, as are progressive edema and tachycardia.

Serial measurements of the vital capacity may be of value, for a sudden decrease may denote cardiac failure. Although the program outlined for the early detection of cardiac failure may seem scarcely applicable to patients in classes I or II, since they rarely decompensate during pregnancy, the interests of the mother and the fetus dictate that all cases of cardiac disease in pregnancy be regarded as at risk of possible decompensation.

Hospitalization

Admission remote from delivery of women with class II cardiac disease has become common practice. Delivery should be accomplished vaginally unless there are obstetrical indications for cesarean section. In spite of the physical effort inherent in labor and vaginal delivery, less morbidity and mortality have been recorded when such a delivery has been accomplished.

Labor and Delivery

Relief from pain and apprehension without undue depression of the infant or the mother is especially important during labor and delivery. For the multiparous woman with a soft, effaced, somewhat dilated cervix, in whom little soft-tissue resistance is offered by the vagina and perineum, analgesics in moderate doses usually provide satisfactory pain relief. For some women, especially nulliparas, in whom cervical dilatation, descent of the presenting part, and delivery will probably require greater force over a longer time, continuous epidural analgesia often proves valuable for reducing pain and apprehension. The major danger of conduction analgesia is maternal hypotension. This is especially dangerous in women with intracardiac shunts, in whom flow may be reversed with blood passing from the right to the left side of the heart or the aorta, thereby bypassing the lungs. For example, in women with pulmonary hypertension, aortic sterosis, or hypertrophic cardiomyopathy, general anesthesia is given if needed for delivery. Continuous conduction analgesia is considered further in Chapter 17.

For cesarean section, the combination of thiopental, succinylcholine, nitrous oxide, and at least 30 percent oxygen, with an endotracheal tube placed after previously neutralizing gastric juice, also has proved satisfactory.

During labor, the mother should be kept in a semirecumbent position. Measurements of the pulse and respiratory rates should be made at least four times every hour during the first stage of labor, and every 10 minutes during the second stage. Increases in the pulse rate much above 100 per minute or in the respiratory rate above 24, particularly when associated with dyspnea, suggest cardiac decompensation that may progress to overt ventricular failure. With any evidence of cardiac decompensation, intensive medical management must be instituted immediately. Only in the presence of the completely dilated cervix and an engaged presenting part may these changes be taken as an indication for immediate delivery. With the cervix only partially dilated and the mother showing obvious evidence of cardiac embarrassment, there is no method of delivery that will not first intensify rather than relieve heart failure.

Immediate medical treatment usually calls for the use of morphine, oxygen, intravenously administered furosemide, perhaps a rapidly acting digitalis preparation, and the Fowler position. Morphine should be given intravenously and titrated so as to allay apprehension and also provide relief from pain. It will serve not only to allay apprehension and reduce the elevated respiratory rate, but in the second stage of labor it will reduce reflex abdominal muscular activity associated with uterine contractions. In the presence of pulmonary edema, oxygen may best be given by intermittent positive-pressure breathing to promote adequate oxygenation and to help clear aveolar edema. Digitalis in the form of a rapidly acting glycoside should be given intravenously. Care must be exercised to avoid toxicity especially in the woman who is depleted of potassium as the consequence of previous diuretic therapy.

Furosemide, given intravenously in a dose of 50 to 100 mg, promptly stimulates diuresis, and it also relaxes the capacitance system, which, in turn, decreases preload by reducing venous return, lowers intrapulmonary and left atrial blood pressures, and thereby reduces pulmonary congestion. A common precipitating event of heart failure is pregnancy-induced hypertension, and if identified, hydralazine is given to reduce cardiac afterload.

Hypotension further reduces cardiac output, and its cause must be identified. If coincidental hemorrhage is the cause, as for example from severe placental abruption with concealed hemorrhage, then careful blood replacement and arrest of the hemorrhage are important to a successful outcome. Successful therapy should be reflected by satisfactory hematocrit and adequate urinary output. If the hypotension is the consequence of a severely impaired myocardium, treatment is more difficult. Specifically, if there is no improvement after instituting the treatment just outlined, invasive cardiac monitoring with a pulmonary artery catheter is begun in order to obtain serial hemodynamic measurements that are likely essential in decision-making involving further therapy.

Signs of cardiac embarrassment developing after complete dilatation of the cervix and engagement of the vertex are indications for prompt forceps delivery unless easy spontaneous birth is expected within a few minutes.

Puerperium

Women who have shown little or no evidence of cardiac distress during pregnancy, labor, or delivery sometimes decompensate after delivery. Therefore it is important that the same meticulous care provided during the antepartum and intrapartum periods be continued into the puerperium. Postpartum hemorrhage, infection, and thromboembolism are much more serious complications of pregnancy in the woman with heart disease. If there was no evidence of cardiac embarrassment during labor, delivery, and the early puerperium, breast feeding is usually not contraindicated. In general, if tubal sterilization is to be performed, it should be delayed for several days until it is obvious that the mother is afebrile, not anemic, and has demonstrated hat she can ambulate without evidence of distress. Women who do not undergo tubal sterilization should be given detailed contraceptive advice, as should all puerperal women.

MANAGEMENT OF CLASS III

Women whose cardiac function is so seriously diminished as to be placed in class III present difficult problems that demand expert medical care. Maternal mortality for classes III and IV has been reported to be 4 percent (McFaul and colleagues, 1988) to 6.8 percent (Sullivan and Ramanathan, 1985). The important question is whether they should become pregnant. The rational answer is no, but many women will risk much for a baby. They and their families must understand the risk and cooperate fully.

Bunim and Appel (1950) reported that about a third of class III cardiac patients will decompensate during pregnancy, unless preventive measures are taken. When such a woman is seen in the first trimester, a question of therapeutic abortion inevitably arises. Her desire for a child may be a determining factor, but class III cardiac disease should lead to strong consideration for therapeutic abortion unless the mother can be hospitalized for the duration of the pregnancy.

The experience of Gorenberg and Chesley (1958) at the Margaret Hague Maternity Hospital led them to conclude that any woman with heart disease seen early in gestation can be carried through pregnancy successfully if she and her family are willing to abide by certain strict rules. Their recommended regimen included bed rest in the hospital for the duration of the pregnancy in any patient with class III disease. The application of this basic principle, together with good medical and obstetrical care to well over 1,000 women, reduced the maternal death rate to not much more than that of the general obstetrical population. The extreme importance of rigid adherence to their rules is demonstrated clearly by the fact that cardiac disease was the leading cause of maternal death at the hospital, but those who died were not women attending their cardiac clinic.

The preferred method of delivery is vaginal, as in classes I and II, and cesarean section is limited to obstetrical indications. Any pregnant woman with a history of previous cardiac failure that was not associated with acute rheumatic carditis or whose cardiac lesion causing the failure has not been corrected surgically is best managed as class III, regardless of their current functional classification.

Even though the woman has recently been in failure or is in failure at the time of labor, vaginal delivery, in general, is safer than cesarean section. These very sick women withstand major surgical procedures poorly and heart disease itelf is a contraindication rather than an indication for cesarean section.

Whereas it is well established that the woman with cardiac disease who receives appropriate care rarely dies during pregnancy or the puerperium, the possibility has been raised that pregnancy causes obscure deleterious effects that ultimately shorten her life span. In other words, it has been suggested that pregnancy in some way might accelerate the rate of deterioration of cardiac function. The conclusions derived from the comprehensive studies by Chesley (1980) of a large number of pregnant women observed over a long period are consistent with the view that pregnancy has no deleterious remote effect on the course of rheumatic heart disease.

MANAGEMENT OF CLASS IV

The treatment of women with class IV heart disease is essentially that of cardiac failure in pregnancy, labor, and the puer-

perium. In the presence of cardiac failure, delivery by any known method carries a high maternal mortality rate. Accordingly, the treatment of heart failure in pregnancy is primarily medical rather than obstetrical. The prime objective is to correct the decompensation, for only then will delivery be safe.

EFFECTS ON FETUS AND NEWBORN

In general, any disease complicated by severe maternal hypoxia is likely to lead to abortion, preterm labor and delivery, or fetal death. A relationship of chronic hypoxia and the polycythemia it causes to the outcome of pregnancy has been demonstrated in studies on women with cyanotic heart disease. Whittemore and colleagues (1980) identified fetal wastage to be 36 percent in women with hypoxic congenital heart disease. **When hypoxia is so intense as to stimulate a rise in the hematocrit reading above 65, pregnancy wastage is virtually 100 percent.**

SURGICALLY CORRECTED HEART DISEASE

To improve cardiac function, several kinds of procedures have been performed on the heart and large vessels, with many cases requiring open heart surgery and bypass. With successful repair, many of these women now are likely to attempt pregnancy. In fact, Löwenstein and colleagues (1988) reported a successful pregnancy following heart transplantation! In unusual instances, surgical corrections of cardiac lesions have been performed even during pregnancy.

VALVE REPLACEMENT

A number of women of reproductive age have had a cardiac valvar prosthesis implanted to replace a severely damaged mitral or aortic valve. Reports of subsequent pregnancy outcomes in these circumstances include those of Chen and associates (1982) and O'Neill and co-workers (1982). In fact, pregnancies with successful outcomes have followed replacement of these heart valves by prostheses (Nagorney and Field, 1981).

Following replacement with a mechanical valvar prosthesis, these women must be maintained on anticoagulants, and at least when not pregnant, warfarin is recommended. Unfortunately, as discussed in Chapter 32 (p. 565), warfarin is teratogenic, especially when given during early pregnancy. The recent observations of Iturbe-Alessio and colleagues (1986) provide an estimate of risk for both mother and fetus. They studied prospectively 72 women with cardiac valve prostheses. In some women warfarin derivatives were given throughout pregnancy, while in others 5,000 U of heparin given subcutaneously twice daily was substituted for coumarin from the 6th through 12th week, after which coumarin therapy was again given. Three of 35 women taking the low-dose heparin suffered massive thromboses of a Björk-Shiley mitral prosthesis and two of them died. On the other hand, while the women taking warfarin had no thromboses, there was evidence for embryopathy in 28 percent of their fetuses. Although they did not study the effects of full anticoagulation with heparin, these investigators concluded that pregnancy was inadvisable in women with such prostheses.

Certainly, if these women choose to risk pregnancy, then full anticoagulation is recommended with either warfarin or heparin after the woman is appraised of the respective risks. We feel that heparin is the antepartum anticoagulant of choice. It does not cross the placenta and the pregnant woman can usually be instructed to inject heparin satisfactorily. Some complications associated with prolonged heparin administration are discussed in Chapter 28 (p. 480). Just before delivery, the heparin is stopped. If delivery supervenes while the anticoagulant is still effective and extensive bleeding is encountered, protamine sulfate is given. Anticoagulant therapy with warfarin or heparin may be restarted by the day after vaginal delivery, usually with no problems.

The likelihood that a young woman undergoing valve replacement might wish to procreate subsequently has led to the insertion by some of a tissue valve, typically porcine. Unfortunately, such valves are not proving to be as durable as mechanical prostheses. Deviri and colleagues (1985) observed no thrombi in 22 pregnancies in 11 unanticoagulated women with porcine xerografts.

It is not surprising that severe complications can arise during pregnancy when the mother has a prosthetic valve. Other than thromboembolism and hemorrhage from anticoagulation, there may be deterioration in cardiac function, and even maternal death. Spontaneous abortions, stillborns, low birthweight infants, and malformed fetuses are identified more often than in the normal population. Therefore, pregnancy is not advised and sterilization should be considered. Because of their possible thrombogenic action, oral contraceptives containing estrogen and a progestin are contraindicated.

Valve Replacement During Pregnancy

Although it is advisable to postpone open-heart surgery until after pregnancy, occasionally valve replacement during pregnancy may be lifesaving. Bernal and Miralles (1986) reviewed the outcomes of 21 pregnant women in whom open-heart surgery while using cardiopulmonary bypass had been performed since 1969. Almost half of these women had mitral or aortic valve prostheses placed. Surprisingly, the women tolerated these procedures well and there was only one stillborn infant and one instance of preterm labor and delivery. The fetal response to cardiopulmonary bypass is usually bradycardia, and it is recommended that high-flow, normothermic perfusion be used if possible so that any theoretical risk of fetal hypoxia is obviated.

Mitral Valvotomy

El-Maraghy and associates (1983) reported their experiences in 42 pregnant women who were in class IV from mitral stenosis and who underwent valvotomy during pregnancy. The 42 mothers did well and there was only one spontaneous abortion two days after surgery. Subsequent to surgery, 32 were in class I, 7 in class II, and only 3 were in class III. In our experiences at Parkland Hospital, mitral valvotomy is the most common open-heart surgery performed during pregnancy, and these women generally have done quite well.

SPECIFIC HEART DISEASE

RHEUMATIC HEART DISEASE

Despite its overall decline, rheumatic heart disease is still a common cause of cardiovascular morbidity during pregnancy. *Mitral stenosis* is the most common lesion as well as the most important hemodynamically. With tight stenosis, left atrial pressure is chronically elevated and may result in significant pulmonary hypertension if not surgically corrected. The increased preload of normal pregnancy, as well as other factors that stimulate increased cardiac output, may cause ventricular failure with pulmonary edema. In fact, 25 percent of women with mitral stenosis have cardiac failure for the first time during pregnancy (Sullivan and Ramanathan, 1985), and we have reported how this may be confused with idiopathic peripartum cardiomyopathy (Cunningham and colleagues, 1986). Another common and frightening sign is hemoptysis. Atrial fibrillation is common with mitral valve stenosis, and since rapid ventricular response may precipitate heart failure, digoxin prophylaxis is recommended. Atrial fibrillation also predisposes to mural thrombosis formation and aortic embolization. For women who develop intractable heart failure, mitral valvotomy as described above, frequently provides dramatic relief of heart failure. Epidural analgesia for labor, with strict attention to avoid intravenous fluid overload, is ideal unless preeclampsia supervenes. Intrapartum endocarditis prophylaxis should be given.

Mitral or aortic valve insufficiency, whether due to rheumatic disease or another cause, is usually well tolerated during pregnancy. Patients with symptomatic disease, however, tend to be quite ill even when not pregnant and should undergo valve replacement before attempting pregnancy.

Mild *aortic stenosis* is well tolerated; however, with severe disease there is fixed cardiac output and these women tolerate poorly decreased preload, such as encountered with spinal or epidural analgesia and hemorrhage at delivery. **Arias and Pineda (1978) reported 17 percent maternal mortality with severe aortic stenosis.**

PATENT DUCTUS ARTERIOSUS

Some patients with patent ductus arteriosus develop pulmonary hypertension and, particularly if the systemic blood pressure falls, may have a reversal of blood flow from the pulmonary artery into the aorta with consequent cyanosis. Sudden drops in blood pressure at delivery, as with conduction analgesia or hemorrhage, may lead to fatal collapse. Therefore, hypotension should be avoided whenever possible and treated vigorously if it develops. Burwell and Metcalfe (1958) suggested that the ductus should not be ligated during pregnancy. In our limited experience, however, the operation has proved to be relatively simple, and cardiac function improved dramatically.

CYANOTIC HEART DISEASE

These women do poorly during pregnancy. If the hematocrit is very high, spontaneous early abortion usually follows conception. With somewhat lesser degrees of polycythemia there is still an increased incidence of abortion and low birthweight infants. Shime and associates (1987) reported that 13 of 23 women with cyanotic heart disease developed functional deterioration during pregnancy, and seven had cardiac failure. Perinatal mortality was 3 of 23 (13 percent), and low birthweight infants were common.

Whereas uncorrected cyanotic heart disease carries a high risk for both the mother and the fetus, when surgical correction prior to pregnancy is satisfactory, the fetal environment is improved remarkably and maternal risks decreased dramatically. Singh and associates (1982), on the basis of 40 pregnancies in 27 patients with surgically corrected tetralogy of Fallot, state that a woman with no major residual defects after surgery may be reassured that pregnancy will be well tolerated and delivery can be accomplished in the normal manner.

Eisenmenger Syndrome

The prognosis for pregnancy complicated by these lesions is poor as it is whenever there is *pulmonary hypetension* from any cause. **Both maternal and perinatal mortality rates for Eisenmenger syndrome have been identified to be about 30 percent (Gleicher and colleagues, 1979).** Shime and colleagues (1987) reported 19 pregnancies in nine such women, and half were terminated by spontaneous or therapeutic abortion, and there were only four term births. Three women developed heart failure and one died. These women tolerate hypotension poorly, and the cause of death is usually right-ventricular failure and hypotension that causes cardiogenic shock.

PULMONARY HYPERTENSION

This is most commonly secondary to cardiac or pulmonary disease. *Primary pulmonary hypertension* is idiopathic but some previously unexplained cases may be due to the presence of antiphospholipid antibodies (p. 839). The abnormality is associated with medial hypertrophy and plexiform lesions. Pregnancy should be avoided since maternal mortality has been reported as high as 50 percent. These reports describe women with severe primary pulmonary hypertension, but milder degrees of secondary pulmonary hypertension probably go unnoticed. For example, with the more common use of pulmonary artery catheterization in women with heart disease, we have identified women with mild to moderate secondary pulmonary hypertension who tolerated pregnancy, labor, and delivery quite well.

CORONARY THROMBOSIS AND ISCHEMIC HEART DISEASE

These are rare complications of pregnancy but the treatment is quite similar to that for the nonpregnant patient. The advisability of a woman undertaking a pregnancy after a myocardial infarction is not clear, but since the underlying vascular disease is usually progressive, and since it frequently is associated with hypertension, pregnancy probably is contraindicated. Cortis and Gensini (1977) recommended coronary angiography and, if severe involvement is detected, pregnancy should be discouraged.

Myocardial infarction during pregnancy has been described, but fortunately, it is quite rare. Hankins and co-workers (1985) reported two cases of myocardial infarction during pregnancy with favorable outcomes for both mothers and infants. They presented in detail their management techniques, which included labor and vaginal delivery under very close hemodynamic monitoring. They also provided an extensive review of the literature.

In both instances vaginal delivery was planned for under carefully controlled conditions at or very near term. Spontaneous labor developed in one at 39 weeks, 3 weeks after myocardial infarction, and in the other it was induced with oxytocin at 38 weeks. Epidural or epidural plus caudal analgesia was used to minimize both the discomfort of labor and vigorous expulsive efforts that might otherwise have accompanied the second stage of labor. Rapid infusion of fluid before commencing the epidural analgesia was not done. Throughout labor, delivery, and the early puerperium maternal hemodynamic function was carefully monitored using pressure measurements made through a pulmonary artery catheter, blood pressure measurements through an arterial line, continuous EKG recording, and cardiac outputs determined repeatedly by the thermodilution technic. Uterine pressures were continuously monitored as was the fetal heart rate. The 39-year-old primigravida was delivered with low forceps and the other woman delivered spontaneously. Cardiac outputs increased 7 to 10 percent during the first stage of labor, 21 to 23 percent during the second stage, and 35 percent during delivery. During the first stage of labor, central venous and pulmonary capillary wedge pressures averaged 10 mm Hg between uterine contractions, but transiently reached levels as high as 25 mm Hg during a contraction.

One year later, both mothers were alive and the infants were thriving.

PERIPARTUM HEART FAILURE

The term *peripartum cardiomyopathy* is now widely used to describe women with peripartum heart failure with no readily apparent etiology, but it is doubtful that there is a cardiomyopathy unique to pregnancy. We reported our experiences with 28 women with peripartum heart failure of obscure etiology cared for at Parkland Hospital over a 12-year period (Cunningham and associates, 1986). Although initially these women were thought to have idiopathic cardiomyopathy, heart failure in 21 subsequently was attributed to underlying chronic hypertension, previously unrecognized mitral stenosis, obesity, or viral myocarditis. The following case illustrates this concept:

E.G., an obese (111 kg) 36-year-old Hispanic multipara presented at term in early labor having had no prenatal care. Her blood pressure was 210/130 mm Hg, urine protein was 2+, and there was clinically obvious pulmonary edema. A radiograph of the chest taken at admission confirmed pulmonary edema and cardiomegaly (Fig. 39–6). Cardiac afterload was soon reduced with 5 mg hydralazine doses given intravenously, diuresis was effected with 20 mg of furosemide given intravenously, and magnesium sulfate was administered intravenously and intramuscularly to prevent eclampsia. Her symptoms improved dramatically, labor progressed, and she was soon delivered of a healthy infant. The initial impression of cardiology consultants was peripartum cardiomyopathy. However, an electrocardiogram was suggestive of left ventricular hypertrophy, and echocardiography confirmed the presence of concentric left ventricular hypertrophy and global hypokinesis. The pulmonary edema cleared completely by the following day, and cardiomegaly resolved over the next five days. One month after discharge she remained hypertensive despite diuretic therapy.

Regardless of the underlying condition that causes cardiac dysfunction, women who develop peripartum heart failure often have superimposed preeclampsia, they are frequently obese, and they usually have coexisting obstetrical complications that either contribute to or precipitate heart failure. Factors commonly associated with heart failure include anemia and infection. Anemia, both chronic from iron deficiency and acute from hemorrhage at delivery, especially with cesarean section, likely magnifies compromised ventricular function. Similarly, infection and the accompanying fever increase cardiac output and oxygen utilization. While it is unlikely that any of these factors alone would cause overt cardiac failure, they are important contributors in the woman with underlying ventricular dysfunction. Thus, individual complications that are known to further increase cardiac work, acting in concert with hypertensive cardiac disease, or any other underlying cause, may result in congestive heart failure.

Idiopathic Cardiomyopathy

In some women in whom a thorough search for an underlying cause for heart failure is unsuccessful, idiopathic cardiomyopathy may be considered. At Parkland Hospital, we identified

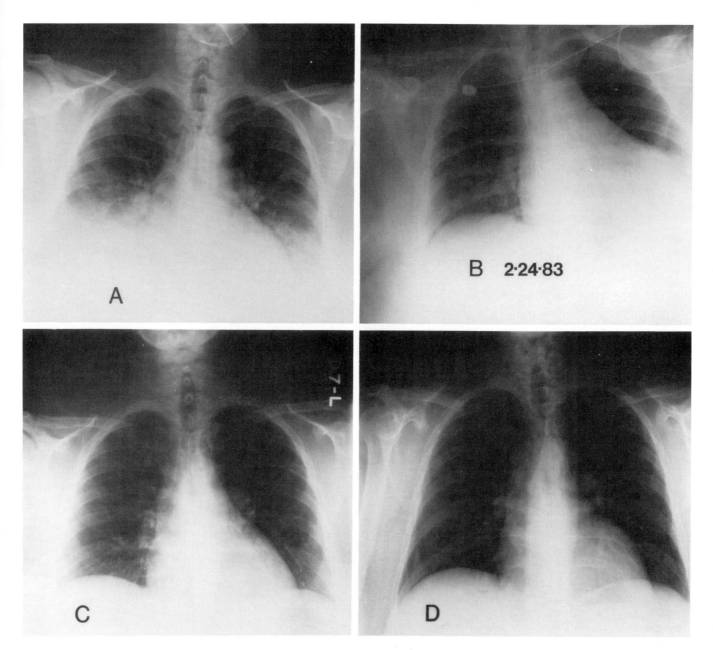

Figure 39–6. An obese 36-year-old Hispanic multipara with heart failure. **A.** She presented at term with severe preeclampsia, cardiomegaly, and pulmonary edema. **B.** One day later, pulmonary edema resolved but cardiomegaly persisted. Cardiomegaly improved in 2 days **(C)**, and almost completely resolved in 3 days **(D)**. (*From Cunningham and associates: Obstet Gynecol 67:157, 1986, with permission.*)

this in about 1 in 15,000 deliveries (Cunningham and colleagues, 1986). This syndrome does not appear to be different from idiopathic cardiomyopathy in nonpregnant young women, and is probably caused in most cases by clinically undetected myocarditis (James 1983; Sanderson and colleagues, 1988).

The distinction between peripartum heart failure from explicable causes versus idiopathic is important, as the prognosis for the latter is poor (Fig. 39–7). In nonpregnant patients, idiopathic cardiomyopathy results in death in over 75 percent from unrelenting cardiomegaly and failure (Johnson and Palacios, 1983; Homans, 1985). In contrast, in such as those discussed

above who have peripartum heart failure and who subsequently are identified to have underlying heart disease, the typical response is rapid reversal of heart failure with furosemide diuresis and correction of associated obstetrical complications. Within days their heart size returns to normal and their long-term prognosis is consonant with the underlying lesion.

INFECTIVE ENDOCARDITIS

Bacterial endocarditis, acute or subacute, is uncommon during pregnancy and the puerperium, but it has contributed appre-

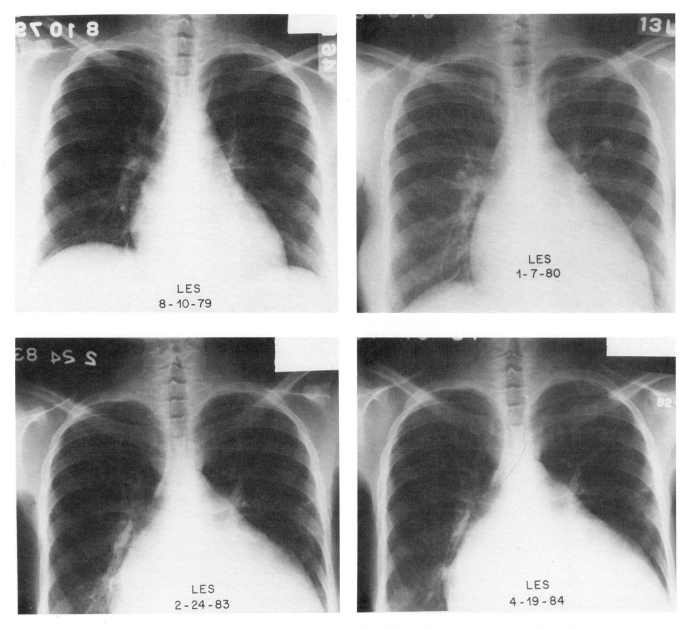

Figure 39–7. Idiopathic peripartum cardiomyopathy. Patient LES developed peripartum heart failure without any identifiable underlying cardiac disease and no associated preeclampsia. Despite an initially good symptomatic response and clearing of pulmonary edema, mild cardiomegaly persisted 3 months postpartum (8-10-79). Over the ensuing 5 years (1980–84) cardiomegaly worsened, and she died of end-stage heart failure at 23. (*From Cunningham and colleagues: Obstet Gynecol 67:156, 1986, with permission.*)

ciably to the relatively few maternal deaths at Parkland Hospital in recent years. Most often the pregnant women were taking illicit drugs intravenously, then developed bacterial endocarditis, and died from valvar incompetence or cerebral emboli. Cox and associates (1988a) reported these recent experiences, and over 7 years the incidence of endocarditis was about 1 in 16,000 deliveries at Parkland Hospital. Two of seven women died. Surgical intervention with prosthetic valve replacement of the destroyed valve along with antimicrobial therapy and meticulous supportive care may prevent a fatal outcome. Cavalieri and associates (1982) described a woman in whom a ruptured, abscessed aortic valve was replaced early in the puerperium and the mother discharged after 6 weeks of antibiotic therapy. Pastorek and

associates (1983) described in some detail their management of three women treated antepartum. Seaworth and Durack (1986) reviewed the literature and reported a 33 percent maternal death rate associated with infective endocarditis.

Antimicrobial Prophylaxis

Most recommend that antimicrobial agents be given prophylactically during labor in order to minimize the risk of bacterial endocarditis and infective arteritis in pregnant women with valvar prostheses, mitral valve prolapse, or with aortic abnormalities such as patent ductus arteriosus or coarctation. Even though there is meager evidence that a significant number of cases of bacterial endocarditis have been prevented with antimicrobial prophylaxis (McFaul and associates, 1988; Seaworth and Durack, 1986), the risk and costs of prophylaxis are not great. If prophylaxis is to be effective, however, administration should begin during labor and be continued for at least one more dose after delivery. The regimen currently recommended by the American Heart Association (Shulman and colleagues, 1984) calls for ampicillin 2 g intravenously or intramuscularly, plus gentamicin 1.5 mg per kg, followed by a second dose of both 8 hours later. Women allergic to penicillin are given vancomycin 1 g intravenously in place of ampicillin. For individuals with a history of rheumatic fever or rheumatic heart disease, the recommendation is that benzathine penicillin G 1.2 million U be given intramuscularly monthly.

MITRAL VALVE PROLAPSE

This condition has been identified in nearly 10 percent of all women. Nishimura and colleagues (1985) identified only those patients with redundant mitral valve leaflets to be at increased risk of sudden death, infective endocarditis, or cerebral embolism. Artal and colleagues (1988) described such a pregnant woman with transient cerebral ischemia. In our experience, mitral valve prolapse has not been deleterious to pregnancy; however, we manage these women as if not pregnant and prescribe β-blocker drugs if they are symptomatic. Mitral valve prolapse is considered by some, but certainly not all, to be a significant risk factor for development of bacterial endocarditis (Clemens and associates, 1982).

MARFAN SYNDROME

This syndrome is characterized by a generalized weakness of connective tissue which can result in dangerous cardiovascular complications. Women with Marfan syndrome have a seriously affected prognosis during pregnancy, and deaths due to dissecting aortic aneurysm are more common during pregnancy. Marfan syndrome is considered further on p. 841.

COARCTATION OF THE AORTA

This is a relatively rare lesion. The collateral circulation arising above the level of the coarctation expands, often to a striking extent, to cause localized erosion of margins of the ribs by the hypertrophied intercostal arteries. Frequently a bicuspid aortic valve is demonstrated by echocardiography. The typical findings on physical examination are hypertension in the upper extremities, but normal or reduced blood pressures in the lower extremities.

The major complications of coarctation are congestive heart failure when there has been long-standing severe hypertension, bacterial endocarditis of the biscupid aortic valve, and rupture of the aorta. Cerebral hemorrhage from aneurysms of the circle of Willis also may develop. Aortic rupture is more likely to occur late in pregnancy or early in the puerperium and may be associated with changes in the media that are histologically similar to those of Erdheim's idiopathic medial cystic necrosis.

Congestive heart failure demands vigorous efforts to improve cardiac function and usually warrants interruption of the pregnancy. It has been recommended by some that resection of the coarctation be undertaken during pregnancy to protect against the possibility of a dissecting aneurysm and rupture of the aorta. The operation, however, has significant risk, especially for the fetus, because all the collaterals must be clamped

for variable periods of time during the procedure, possibly leading to serious fetal hypoxia.

Some authorities recommend that the woman with coarctation of the aorta be delivered by cesarean section lest the transient elevation of arterial blood pressure that commonly accompanies labor lead to rupture of either the aorta or a coexisting cerebral aneurysm. The available evidence, however, is consistent with the conclusion that cesarean section should be limited to obstetrical indications.

HYPERTROPHIC CARDIOMYOPATHY

This condition is synonymous with *idiopathic hypertrophic subaortic stenosis.* It is an autosomally dominant disorder characterized by idiopathic left ventricular myocardial hypertrophy that may provide a pressure gradient to left ventricular outflow. Diagnosis is confirmed by echocardiography. The majority of affected women are asymptomatic, but dyspnea, anginal or atypical chest pain, and arrhythmias may develop. Complex arrhythmias may progress to sudden death. Symptoms are usually worsened by exercise.

Propranolol is given if symptoms develop. There is little published experience with this lesion complicating pregnancy, but limited reports suggest that pregnancy outcome is good (Oakley and colleagues, 1979). Epidural analgesia is avoided as in aortic stenosis (p. 800). Infants rarely demonstrate inherited lesions at the time of birth.

KYPHOSCOLIOTIC HEART DISEASE

During pregnancy, severe degrees of kyphoscoliosis commonly cause serious cardiopulmonary problems, sometimes referred to as *kyphoscoliotic heart disease.* In these circumstances, some regions of the lungs in the markedly deformed thoracic cage may be quite emphysematous, while others are atelectatic, with both lesions contributing to an inadequate ventilatory capacity. In these circumstances, *cor pulmonale* is a frequent complication.

The increased oxygen demands and the cardiac work imposed by pregnancy and delivery must be taken into account in reaching a decision whether to allow the pregnancy to continue or to perform a therapeutic abortion. If pulmonary function studies indicate that the vital capacity is not reduced appreciably, the outcome most often is favorable. In women with marked degrees of kyphoscoliosis and markedly impaired pulmonary function, therapeutic abortion is indicated.

Frequently the bony pelvis is so distorted that cesarean section is necessary. Kopenhager (1977) reported that 40 percent of 49 women had to be delivered by cesarean section because of cephalopelvic disproportion. The supine position during delivery may result in serious hypotension. The commonly used analgesics such as meperidine should be used carefully, since respiratory depression is very poorly tolerated. During and after delivery, meticulous care should be directed toward the prevention of further atelectasis, which could lead rapidly to severe hypoxia and death. Intermittent positive-pressure breathing using appropriate concentrations of oxygen with mucolytic agents is of value. Sterilization often is indicated. Kopenhager (1977) provided an analysis of the obstetrical and medical complications in 50 women with kyphoscoliosis.

ARRHYTHMIAS

Cardiac arrhythmias commonly are encountered during pregnancy, labor and delivery, or the puerperium. It is debated whether arrhythmias are more common during pregnancy, but in our experiences, their detection probably is increased because of closer observation, especially during the vigorous exercise of normal labor and delivery. Perhaps the normal but mild hypokalemia of pregnancy induces arrhythmias.

Bradyarrhythmias, including complete heart block, are compatible with a successful pregnancy outcome. Women with artificial pacemakers usually tolerate pregnancy well (Jaffe and associates, 1987). With fixed-rate devices, cardiac output is apparently increased by augmented stroke volume.

Tachyarrhythmias are more common. Supraventricular tachycardias and fibrillation can be treated with digoxin, β-blocker drugs, or calcium channel blocking drugs. Although these drugs cross the placenta, they do not appear to harm the fetus. Rotmensch and colleagues (1983) provided a review of their use. Cardioversion is not contraindicated by pregnancy per se.

Supraventricular tachycardia in association with Wolff-Parkinson-White syndrome complicating three pregnancies was described by Gleicher and associates (1981). Propranolol proved effective when used in two instances. Atrial fibrillation associated with mitral stenosis may cause pulmonary edema in late pregnancy if the ventricular rate is increased so that rate-related failure follows.

CARDIOPULMONARY RESUSCITATION

Cardiac arrest is fortunately rare during pregnancy and special considerations for resuscitation have been reviewed by Lee and colleagues (1986). After 25 weeks, when there is likelihood of fetal viability, these authors recommend emergency cesarean section if there is no response to cardiopulmonary resuscitation by 15 minutes. They emphasize that the hemodynamics of resuscitation in pregnant humans or animals have not been systematically evaluated.

PULMONARY DISORDERS

Pregnancy induces a number of changes in the respiratory system. Uterine enlargement causes the diaphragm to rise, the transverse thoracic diameter to increase, the vertical chest diameter to decrease, and the residual lung volume to be reduced. In reponse to the modest hyperventilation that is normal for pregnancy, the tidal volume is increased somewhat and the plasma carbon dioxide is lowered slightly. Of importance, during the latter part of pregnancy, oxygen consumption is increased 15 to 25 percent above that of normal nonpregnant women (Chap. 7, p. 147).

PNEUMONIA

Pneumonitis causing an appreciable loss of ventilatory capacity is tolerated less well by women during pregnancy. This generalization seems to hold true regardless of whether the cause of the pneumonia is bacterial, viral, or chemical. Moreover, as emphasized in the discussions of heart disease and of diabetes, hypoxia and acidosis are poorly tolerated by the fetus, and they frequently lead to preterm labor after midpregnancy. Therefore, it is important to the pregnant woman and her fetus that pneumonia be diagnosed as soon as possible and that she be promptly hospitalized so that the disease can be treated most effectively. **Any pregnant woman suspected of having pneumonia should undergo anteroposterior and lateral chest radiography.**

There are no extensive epidemiological studies concerning the incidence of various etiologies of pneumonias in young adults. Foy and colleagues (1973) reported 7 to 17 cases per 1,000 for all adults. In a review of six studies totalling nearly 700 adults, Luby (1987) found that 65 percent were bacterial with *S. pneumoniae* causing two thirds of these. About 20 percent were of nonbacterial origin and *Mycoplasma pneumoniae* and influenza A each caused 5 percent of all cases. The etiology was not determined in the remaining 20 percent. It is probably safe to say that the majority of community-acquired pneumonias in young adults are also caused by pneumococci. However, mycoplasmal pneumonias are much more common in pregnant women than in older patients, and *Legionella pneumophilia* occasionally causes outbreaks or sporadic cases of Legionnaire's disease. Influenza A is the most commonly encountered viral pneumonia. It is usually seen during winter epidemics, and many of these women will have bacterial suprainfection. Finally, the TWAR strain of *Chlamydia psittaci* was reported recently to cause 12 percent of pneumonias diagnosed in college students (Grayston and colleagues, 1986), and it is reasonable to believe that this organism may cause pneumonia during pregnancy.

In some cases these pneumonias may be distinguishable from one another, but generally, chest x-ray findings are not reliable predictors of etiology. During pregnancy at least, initially erythromycin is a good therapeutic choice since the most common agents that cause adult pneumonias usually are sensitive.

There are few recent reports that deal specifically with pneumonia complicating pregnancy. Benedetti and associates (1982) summarized their experiences with 39 cases caused by a variety of organisms, but most often *Streptococcus pneumoniae.* They used prompt hospitalization, antimicrobials, and arterial Po_2 measurement, and when low, oxygen therapy was given. All of the mothers survived. One fetus expired whose mother also had sickle cell anemia. These, for the most part favorable outcomes, should not serve to minimize the apparent severity of the problem of pneumonia complicating pregnancy but rather to emphasize the value of prompt diagnosis and effective treatment.

Pneumonia from *Mycoplasma pneumoniae* is relatively common during pregnancy. It is sometimes difficult to diagnose and to treat. High titers of anti-I, or cold, agglutinins are detectable in about half of the cases and eventually complement-fixing antibodies increase fourfold. Erythromycin is recommended for treatment during pregnancy. In the absence of hypoxia this form of pneumonitis probably does not affect pregnancy adversely.

Viral pneumonitis, especially that caused by varicella or influenza A, can prove devastating to the mother and, in turn, the hypoxic fetus. Although influenza A pneumonitis destroys respiratory tract epithelium and it can destroy pneumocytes, many women with severe pneumonitis have morbidity from suprainfections with *S. pneumoniae, Hemophilus pneumoniae,* or *Staphylococcus aureus.* Pregnant women at high risk because of underlying diseases should be given influenza vaccine annually. If not immunized, amantadine may be given for prophylaxis or treatment. Amantadine is a category C drug (see Chap. 32, p. 563).

Aspiration Pneumonitis

Aspiration of gastric contents during anesthesia for delivery can cause severe chemical pneumonitis, primarily as the consequence of the necrotizing effects of hydrochloric acid. Diagnosis and treatment are discussed in Chapter 17 (p. 331). The aspiration of gastric contents is not limited to anesthesia for delivery. For example, treatment of eclampsia with large doses of morphine or barbiturates, and inebriating the pregnant woman with ethanol to try to arrest labor sometimes has been followed by the aspiration of gastric contents and a bad outcome.

ASTHMA

This rather common respiratory illness is encountered relatively often in pregnant women. With active but otherwise uncomplicated asthma, indices of expiratory air flow are reduced while diffusing capacity is normal. A low PCO_2 indicates hyperventilation and an elevated PCO_2 is evidence of carbon dioxide retention and is ominous.

Pregnancy does not seem to exert any consistent predictable effect on bronchial asthma. In some women asthma appears to be less of a problem, but in others it becomes more troublesome, while in still others it remains unchanged from its nonpregnant status. Turner and colleagues (1980) reviewed nine studies of 1,054 pregnancies complicated by asthma and reported that in 22 percent asthma worsened, in 29 percent it improved, and in the remaining 49 percent it was unchanged. Schatz and associates (1988) described 366 pregnancies prospectively managed in 330 asthmatic women and reported 35, 28, and 33 percent respectively. The great majority of women with asthma can be carried safely through pregnancy, labor, and delivery. The pregnant woman in whom signs and symptoms of asthma previously have been mild is at low risk of serious asthmatic attacks during pregnancy. However, the woman who suffers severe attacks when not pregnant is likely to continue to do so when pregnant.

ACUTE ASTHMA

In general, therapeutic regimens which have been beneficial when the woman was not pregnant will continue to be effective during pregnancy. This applies both to agents used chronically to minimize bronchospasm and promote clearance of secretions as well as those used in vigorous treatment of a severe asthmatic attack causing hypoxia and hypercapnea. It is emphasized again that oxygen consumption increases during pregnancy by up to 25 percent and that the fetus tolerates severe hypoxia poorly. Asthma is a reactive airway disease that, unless complicated by other pulmonary disorders, for example pneumonia, is not associated early on with oxygen-diffusing abnormalities. Therefore, unless unusually severe, there is frequently little evidence for hypoxemia early in an attack. Alternatively, hypocapnea is the expected finding early since hyperventilation is characteristic of the disease. **It must be remembered that arterial PCO_2 normally falls during pregnancy, and levels considered normal for nonpregnant persons may reflect ominous carbon dioxide retention in a pregnant woman.** Measurement of the *1-second forced expiratory volume* (FEV_1) is important, and any decreases measured should improve with treatment.

Soon after assessment, treatment with β-adrenergic agents

such as epinephrine or terbutaline, corticosteroids such as hydrocortisone or methylprednisolone and, with caution, theophyllines such as aminophylline, should be given. Adequate hydration is often beneficial as is respiratory care to remove tenacious secretions. A search for a precipitating or aggravating factor, especially infection, is begun. It is difficult to provide written guidelines for admission, but during pregnancy it is better to be overly cautious. At Parkland Hospital, if the woman who presents to the obstetrical emergency room with asthma is not markedly improved quickly following bronchodilator therapy, then she is admitted for close observation and further therapy. Persistent tachycardia, labored respirations, hypertension, dyspnea while speaking full sentences, pulsus paradoxus, or use of accessory respiratory muscles should prompt consideration for admission (Greenberger, 1985). Cyanosis, hypoxemia (PO_2 less than 70 mm Hg), hypercarbia (PCO_2 greater than 38 mm Hg), severe dyspnea, or subcutaneous emphysema mandate immediate hospitalization. **The mortality of asthma is that of ventilatory fatigue from the work of breathing, and careful assessment must be made to determine if tracheal intubation and mechanical ventilation are indicated.**

Iodide-containing medications should be avoided, since iodide is transported across the placenta and concentrated in the fetal thyroid. When the mother ingests iodide chronically, the large amount reaching the fetus may induce a goiter.

Therapeutic abortion might be indicated in the uncommon woman who, as the consequence of long-standing asthma, has reduced cardiopulmonary function. Since asthma is a chronic disease that in the adult is likely to persist for many years after the pregnancy, sterilization should be considered.

TUBERCULOSIS

The considerable influx of women from Southeast Asia, Mexico, and Central America has been accompanied by an increased frequency of tuberculosis in pregnant women, especially those attending public clinics. In 1985, the tuberculosis rate for Hispanics in the United States was four times that of the non-Hispanic white population (Centers for Disease Control, 1987).

The prognosis has improved remarkably during the past 30 years for the woman with active pulmonary tuberculosis. Chemotherapy that has proved to be effective in the absence of pregnancy is also effective during pregnancy, and fortunately, several first-line tuberculostatic drugs do not appear to affect the fetus adversely. Active disease is always treated with at least two tuberculostatic drugs. In a review, Snider and colleagues (1980) found no increase in birth defects among children whose mothers during pregnancy had been treated with isoniazid, ethambutol, or rifampin. Mild auditory and vestibular abnormalities have been identified after streptomycin therapy. When isoniazid is used during pregnancy, supplemental pyridoxine probably should also be administered to minimize the potential for neurotoxicity in the fetus (Atkins, 1982).

Bowes (1975) recommended that all women registering for prenatal care be screened for tuberculosis by appropriate skin testing. If the intracutaneously applied purified protein derivative is negative, no further evaluation is needed. If positive, a thorough history is obtained and a complete physical examination and chest radiograph with the abdomen shielded are performed. If negative, no treatment is necessary until after delivery when generally isoniazid chemoprophylaxis is given for one year. Very few clinics routinely screen all prenatal patients in this way, and a reasonable alternative is to skin test women in high-risk groups. This is our practice at Parkland Hospital, however, in an asymptomatic tuberculin-positive woman who has a close contact with someone with active disease, we began isoniazid chemoprophylaxis during pregnancy.

Evaluation of the degree of activity of the pulmonary disease radiographically at times may be difficult. As pregnancy advances and the diaphragm rises, the lungs undergo some degree of compression, which may mask the extent of the tuberculosis lesion. In fact, this mechanical effect of pregnancy on the lung may conceal pulmonary cavitation. Therefore, treatment may have to be undertaken in the pregnant woman on less firm ground than if she were not pregnant.

In the absence of seriously impaired pulmonary infection, analgesia and anesthesia for labor and delivery usually can be accomplished with any of the techniques used for normal pregnancy. Tuberculosis is seldom an indication for therapeutic abortion unless there is disseminated tuberculosis or severely compromised cardiopulmonary function. Sterilization is warranted for women who desire no more children. Rifampin, which has been used usually in combination with isoniazid, may impair the efficacy of oral contraceptives.

Congenital tuberculosis is rare even when the mother has widespread disease, but it has been reported and can prove fatal (Myers and co-workers, 1981). The newborn is also quite susceptible to tuberculosis. Therefore, the infant should be isolated immediately from the mother suspected of having active disease. Because of the risk of active disease developing in the infant, either isoniazid chemoprophylaxis or BCG vaccination may be beneficial.

Pelvic tuberculosis usually causes sterility. When pregnancy does supervene, often it terminates ectopically or in abortion followed at times by activation of the pelvic infection. Treatment is given with a combination of multiple drug chemotherapy.

ADULT RESPIRATORY DISTRESS SYNDROME

Respiratory failure is either caused by or is associated with a growing number of illnesses or injuries, and it is now widely recognized that frequently these are nonpulmonic in origin. In 1967, Ashbaugh and colleagues provided the first clinical description of what is now termed the *adult respiratory distress syndrome* which is characterized by lung injury with increased capillary membrane permeability, pulmonary edema, and reduced lung compliance. The injury also causes loss of surfactant which is followed by alveolar collapse and worsening of hypoxia.

A number of conditions may lead to the syndrome, but in obstetrics, the most common predisposing causes are viral or bacterial pneumonias; severe acute hemorrhage with ectopic pregnancy (Chap. 30, p. 511), placenta previa or abruption (Chap. 36, p. 695); aspiration of gastric acid contents (Chap. 17, p. 331); or septicemia most commonly complicating acute pyelonephritis, septic abortion, or postpartum metritis (Chap. 27, p. 472). Moreover, if plasma colloid oncotic pressure is decreased further than in normal pregnancy, such as is common with severe preeclampsia (Chap. 35, p. 684), then pulmonary edema is made worse.

There is usually a lag phase before respiratory insufficiency is apparent, and at varying times following the initial injury, the woman becomes dyspneic and arterial blood gas analysis discloses progressive hypoxemia. Usually at first the chest is clear

to auscultation, but inspiratory rales may be heard. The chest x-ray often shows only minimal changes, and at this early stage, hypoxemia easily is corrected by administering oxygen by mask. With ultimate progression, these findings worsen and the chest radiograph shows extensive alveolar infiltrates and pleural effusions which become confluent and show up as "whited-out" lungs.

Treatment is aimed at eradication of the initiating cause, for example, infection and septicemia, and supportive care is given. In many cases, mechanical ventilation with increased oxygen concentration is needed to reverse dangerous hypoxemia. Positive end-expiratory pressure usually is necessary to increase lung volume and maintain alveoli open at end expiration to decrease shunting. Pulmonary artery catheter placement for central hemodynamic monitoring may be useful for management, especially if there are other complications.

The syndrome carries a high mortality rate, but the prognosis in an otherwise healthy young woman is good if ventilatory support can be maintained until the underlying disease is appropriately treated.

OTHER PULMONARY DISORDERS

SARCOIDOSIS

This multisystem granulomatous disorder of unknown etiology uncommonly complicates pregnancy and deRegt (1987) found only 14 cases over a 12-year period at Downstate Medical Center, during which time nearly 20,000 women were delivered. The available evidence is suggestive that sarcoidosis seldom affects pregnancy adversely unless there is severe preexisting disease, especially extensive pulmonary granulomas and fibrosis (O'Leary, 1968; deRegt, 1987). DeRegt reported two fatal cases due to extensive disease, and we have observed one maternal death in a woman in whom severe pulmonary sarcoidosis and extensive hilar adenopathy were further complicated by placenta previa, extreme obesity, and aspiration of gastric contents.

Pregnancy is not a contraindication to the use of corticosteroids to treat sarcoidosis and symptomatic women are given treatment.

CYSTIC FIBROSIS

This disease is transmitted as an autosomal recessive trait and its frequency is estimated to be in 1 per 1,500 white births and 1 per 17,000 black births. Because of improvements in diagnosis and treatment, more girls with cystic fibrosis are now surviving to adulthood. Although most are infertile because of delayed sexual development and perhaps abnormal cervical mucus production, pregnancy is not uncommon. Males who survive to adulthood often have aspermia.

Most clinical manifestations of cystic fibrosis are caused by abnormal mucus production, and the pulmonary involvement can prove very deleterious to a pregnancy. Chronic hypoxia and frequent pulmonary infections characterize the pregnancy state. Pancreatic dysfunction can contribute significantly to poor maternal nutrition. Cohen and associates (1980), in a survey of cystic fibrosis centers, obtained information on 129 pregnancies and reported that increased maternal and perinatal mortality were related to severe pulmonary infection.

THROMBOEMBOLISM AND PULMONARY INFARCTION

These may be encountered during pregnancy, but they develop more often during the puerperium. Diagnosis and treatment of these serious problems are discussed in Chapter 28 (p. 477).

PULMONARY RESECTION

The effect of pulmonary resection, usually for bronchiectasis or tuberculosis, will depend upon the functional capacity of the remaining pulmonary tissue. In general, if function is equivalent to one normal lung and active pulmonary disease does not persist, pregnancy is tolerated without undue risk to the mother and with a good likelihood of delivery of a healthy infant (Laros, 1980).

CARBON MONOXIDE POISONING

Pregnant women, and especially the fetus, tolerate poorly excessive carbon monoxide inhalation. The odorless, tasteless gas has a high affinity and binding for hemoglobin, thus displacing oxygen and impeding its transfer. Fetal carboxyhemoglobin levels are 10 to 15 percent higher than those in the mother (Longo, 1977). Symptoms usually appear when carboxyhemoglobin concentration is 20 percent, and concentrations over 50 percent may be fatal to the mother, and presumably lesser concentrations may be fatal for the fetus. Treatment is supportive along with administration of inspired 100 percent oxygen. Recently Hollander and colleagues (1987) reported the successful use of hyperbaric oxygen to treat an affected woman.

DISEASES OF THE KIDNEY AND URINARY TRACT

A few diseases of the urinary tract may be associated with pregnancy by chance and be little affected by it. Much more likely, pregnancy predisposes to the development or exacerbation of these disorders. An example of the former is pyelonephritis and of the latter lupus nephritis with hypertension. The remarkable changes—anatomical and functional—induced in the urinary tract by normal pregnancy are considered elsewhere, especially in Chapter 7 (p. 148).

URINARY TRACT INFECTIONS

Infections of the urinary tract are the most common bacterial infections encountered during pregnancy. Asymptomatic bacteriuria is more common, but symptomatic infection may involve the lower tract to cause *cystitis*, or it may involve the renal calyces, pelvis, and parenchyma to cause *pyelonephritis*. Most symptomatic urinary infections are acute and self-limited; however, they are characterized by a high frequency of recurrence, especially during pregnancy.

Organisms that cause urinary infections are those from the normal perineal flora, which in most cases have gained urinary tract access before pregnancy. There is now evidence that some strains of *Enterobacteriaceae*, especially *E. coli*, have pili that enhance their virulence (Svanborg-Eden, 1982). Also called *adhesins* or *P-fimbriae*, these appendages allow bacterial attachment to glycoprotein receptors on uroepithelial cell membranes. Thus, bacteria are not washed out normally by urine flow, and multiplication and invasion follow. Pregnancy does not seem to enhance these virulence factors, but urinary stasis and diminished ureteral tone and peristalsis caused by ureteral compression of the enlarging uterus, and to a lesser extent by the smooth muscle relaxant effects of progesterone (see Chap. 7, p. 149), predispose to symptomatic urinary infections.

In the early puerperium, bladder sensitivity to intravesical fluid tension is often decreased as the consequence of analgesia, especially epidural or spinal, and after the effects dissipate, sensations of bladder distension are likely diminished by discomfort caused by a large episiotomy, periurethral lacerations, or vaginal wall hematomas. Moreover, starting immediately after delivery, oxytocin is commonly infused with an appreciable volume of fluid at rates which cause antidiuresis. When the oxytocin is stopped, a diuresis often follows with copious urine production and bladder distension. Overdistension, coupled with catheterization to provide relief, commonly leads to urinary infection.

ASYMPTOMATIC BACTERIURIA

Asymptomatic bacteriuria refers to persistent actively multiplying bacteria within the urinary tract without symptoms. The reported prevalence of bacteriuria during pregnancy varies from 2 to 12 percent, and depends on parity, race, and socioeconomic status. The highest incidence has been reported in black multiparas with sickle cell trait, and the lowest incidence has been found in affluent white women of low parity.

Bacteriuria is typically present at the time of the first prenatal visit, and after an initial negative urine culture, only about 1 percent of women develop urinary infection (Whalley, 1967). Asymptomatic infection is identified when significant numbers of bacteria are demonstrated in the urine. In most instances, this can be accomplished by culturing clean-voided midstream specimens without resorting to catheterization. A clean-voided specimen containing more than 100,000 organisms of the same species per mL of urine is evidence for infection. Smaller numbers of bacteria may represent contamination during collection, although with dilute urine a lesser number of organisms of the same species likely represents infection.

If asymptomatic bacteriuria is not treated, about 25 percent of infected women subsequently develop an acute symptomatic infection during that pregnancy. Fortunately, eradication of bacteriuria with antimicrobial agents has been shown to prevent most of these clinically evident infections.

Bacteriuria has been thought by some investigators to cause preterm labor and, in turn, increased neonatal morbidity and mortality. In early studies by Kass (1962, 1965), the incidence of premature births, defined as a birthweight of 2,500 g or less, was 27 percent among 95 bacteriuric women given a placebo during pregnancy, whereas it was only 7 percent among 84 women treated with antimicrobial agents. The corresponding perinatal death rates were 14 and 0 percent, respectively. Kincaid-Smith and Bullen (1965) also reported a relatively high proportion of low birthweight infants among untreated bacteriuric women, but they were unable to reduce significantly this proportion with antimicrobial therapy (21 versus 17 percent).

They concluded that bacteriuria in pregnancy is commonly a manifestation of underlying chronic renal disease, which accounts for the higher incidence of low birthweight infants and perinatal loss. Other investigators have been unable to corroborate this possible relation between bacteriuria and low birthweight (Table 39–5). Although there may be a relation between bacteriuria and low birthweight and preterm infants, from the evidence currently available it is unlikely that bacteriuria is a prominent factor in their genesis.

Even though bacteriuria plays a pivotal role in the causation of acute pyelonephritis during pregnancy, nearly three fourths of women with bacteriuria remain asymptomatic throughout pregnancy. Some have bacteriuria limited to the bladder, but evidence has been presented in several studies that others have potentially serious renal disease. Bacteriuria persists after delivery in many of these women and there is also a significant number of women with pyelographic evidence of chronic infection, obstructive lesions, or congenital urinary abnormalities (Kincaid-Smith and Bullen, 1965; Whalley and associates, 1965, 1967).

During pregnancy bladder infection also is identified when there has been recent instrumentation of the urinary tract. Since bacteria are normally found in the outer portion of the urethra, single catheterization or the use of an indwelling catheter is likely to introduce bacteria into the bladder. Brumfitt and associates (1961) showed that routine bladder catheterization before delivery resulted in infection in 9 percent of puerperal women. It follows that the number of puerperal infections can be reduced appreciably by avoiding routine bladder catheterization at the time of delivery.

Treatment

Women with asymptomatic bacteriuria are given treatment as outpatients. Treatment for 10 days with nitrofurantoin macrocrystals (Macrodantin), 100 mg once daily, or with sulfisoxazole (Gantrisin), 1 g 4 times a day, has proved effective in the great majority of cases so treated at Parkland Hospital. Other regimens that are successful include ampicillin or a cephalosporin given four times daily for 10 days. The recurrence rate for all of these regimens is about 30 percent. Recurrence following short-term therapy, that is 10 to 14 days, is likely to be a *relapse*, whereas recurrence following a 3-week course are more likely *reinfections* (Leveno and colleagues, 1981).

Harris and co-workers (1982) evaluated single-dose treatment of asymptomatic bacteriuria during pregnancy. In 75 to 80 percent of cases a single dose of sulfisoxazole (2 g), nitrofurantoin macrocrystals (200 mg), or ampicillin (2 g) plus probenecid (1 g) eradicated the bacteria.

TABLE 39–5. INCIDENCE OF LOW BIRTHWEIGHT INFANTS BORN TO WOMEN WITH AND WITHOUT BACTERIURIA DURING PREGNANCY

Study	Bacteriuric Patients[a]	Nonbacteriuric Patients
Gilstrap and colleagues (1981b)	248 (12)	248 (13)
Little (1966)	141 (9)	4,735 (8)
Norden and Kilpatrick (1965)	114 (15)	109 (13)
Whalley (1967)	176 (15)	176 (12)
Wilson and associates (1966)	230 (11)	6,216 (10)

[a] Numbers in parenthesis indicate percent of low birthweight infants.

CYSTITIS AND URETHRITIS

There is evidence that bladder infection during pregnancy develops without antecedent covert bacteriuria (Harris and Gilstrap, 1981). Typically, cystitis is characterized by dysuria, particularly at the end of urination, as well as urgency and frequency. There are few associated systemic findings. Usually there is pyuria as well as bacteriuria. Erythrocytes also are found commonly in the urinary sediment, and occasionally there is gross hematuria. Although cystitis is usually uncomplicated, the upper urinary tract may soon be involved in an ascending infection. For example, 40 percent of pregnant women with acute pyelonephritis have preceding symptoms of lower-tract infection (Gilstrap and associates, 1981a).

Treatment

Women with bacterial cystitis respond readily to any of several regimens. Harris and Gilstrap (1981) reported a 97 percent cure rate with a 10-day ampicillin regimen. Sulfonamides, nitrofurantoin, or a cephalosporin also are effective when given for 10 days. Single-dose therapy as described above has been shown to be effective for both nonpregnant and pregnant women, but since 40 percent of women with early pyelonephritis initially have lower-tract symptoms, renal infection must be confidently excluded before one-dose therapy is given.

Frequency, urgency, dysuria, and pyuria accompanied by a "sterile" urine culture may be the consequence of urethritis caused by *Chlamydia trachomatis*, a common pathogen of the genitourinary tract. Erythromycin therapy is effective.

ACUTE PYELONEPHRITIS

Acute pyelonephritis is one of the most common serious medical complications of pregnancy. At Parkland Hospital, the incidence of acute pyelonephritis complicating pregnancy or the puerperium was nearly 3 percent before routine detection and treatment for bacteriuria was begun (Gilstrap and colleagues, 1981a). The incidence is now about 1 percent. Pyelonephritis is more common after mid-pregnancy, and is unilateral and right-sided in more than half of cases and bilateral in a fourth. In most cases, renal parenchymal infection is caused by bacteria that ascend from the lower tract. More than 90 percent of renal infections are caused by bacteria that have P-fimbriae adhesins (Väisänen and colleagues, 1981).

The onset of pyelonephritis is usually rather abrupt. The woman who has previously been well or has complained of dysuria or hematuria suddenly develops fever, shaking chills, and aching pain in one or both lumbar regions. There may be anorexia, nausea, and vomiting. The temperature most often is elevated, but the course of the disease may vary remarkably with fever to as high as 40°C or more and hypothermia to as low as 34°C. Tenderness can usually be elicited by firm palpation in one or both costovertebral angles. The urinary sediment contains many leucocytes, frequently in clumps, and numerous bacilli. During 1987 at Parkland Hospital, *Escherichia coli* was isolated from the urine in 81 percent of cases, *Klebsiella pneumoniae* and *Enterobacter* each in 6 percent, and *Proteus* in 2 percent (Cunningham, 1988). About 15 percent of these women also had bacteremia.

Pain in one or both lumbar regions, characteristic urinary findings, as well as fever and costovertebral tenderness, usually make the diagnosis apparent. The condition may be mistaken, however, for labor, appendicitis, placental abruption, or infarction of a myoma and, in the puerperium, for metritis with pelvic cellulitis.

Treatment

Pregnant women with acute pyelonephritis should be hospitalized for prompt treatment. **Intravenous hydration to insure adequate urinary output is essential.** During the first few days of therapy, these women should be watched carefully to detect symptoms of bacterial shock or its sequelae. Although this serious complication is quite uncommon, its gravity demands early recognition and prompt therapy. Urinary output should be recorded carefully and frequently and blood pressure and temperature observed closely. High fever should be treated, usually with a cooling blanket. A marked fall in body temperature is ominous in that it may precede somewhat or coincide with worrisome hypotension. Plasma creatinine should be measured early in the course of therapy. As shown in Figure 39–8, acute pyelonephritis in some pregnant women causes a considerable reduction in glomerular filtration rate that is reversed by effective treatment (Whalley and co-workers, 1975). More recently we have described the clinical courses of 15 women with severe antepartum pyelonephritis who developed varying degrees of respiratory insufficiency (Cunningham and associates, 1987). It appears that endotoxin-induced alveolar injury causes pulmonary edema, which is also termed the *adult respiratory distress syndrome* (see p. 807). Pulmonary injury may be severe and in some women tracheal intubation and mechanical ventilation is lifesaving (Fig. 39–9). Anemia commonly develops due to erythrocyte destruction by lipopolysaccharide (Cox and colleagues, 1988b).

These serious urinary infections usually respond quickly to intravenous hydration and antimicrobial therapy. The choice of drug is empirical, and ampicillin, a cephalosporin, or an extended-spectrum penicillin is satisfactory (Cox and Cunningham, 1988a). Antimicrobial resistance of *E. coli* to ampicillin is reported commonly, and many prefer to give gentamicin or tobramycin along with ampicillin. Serial determinations of serum creatinine are important if nephrotoxic drugs are given. Clinical symptoms for the most part resolve during the first two days of therapy, but even though the symptoms promptly abate, therapy is recommended for a total of 10 days. Cultures of urine usually become sterile within the first 24 hours. Changes in the urinary tract induced by pregnancy persist and reinfection is always possible. If subsequent cultures of the urine are positive remote from the time of therapy, prolonged treatment is indicated using a drug to which the organism appears sensitive.

If improvement is not obvious by 48 to 72 hours, then underlying urinary obstruction must be considered. The most common cause will be a *calculus,* and nearly 90 percent of these are visualized with a plain abdominal x-ray. A *perinephric phlegmon* or *perinephric abscess* also may cause prolonged fever (Cox and Cunningham, 1988b). Identification and surgical drainage of the latter, using one-shot intravenous pyelography or limited computed tomography, may be lifesaving.

Recurrent infection, both covert and symptomatic, are common and can be demonstrated in 30 to 40 percent of these women following completion of treatment (Cunningham and associates, 1973; Van Dorsten and colleagues, 1987). Unless assiduous attention is given to insure urine sterility, then Macrodantin, 100 mg nightly, is given through the remainder of the pregnancy. Van Dorsten and co-workers (1987) reported that this regimen reduces recurrence of bacteriuria to 8 percent.

CHRONIC PYELONEPHRITIS

Chronic interstitial nephritis from bacterial infection is termed *chronic pyelonephritis.* In contrast to acute pyelonephritis, chronic infection is usually not symptomatic, and in advanced cases, symptoms are those of renal insufficiency. There may or may not be a history of prior symptomatic urinary infection, and fewer than half of women with chronic pyelonephritis have a clear history of preceding cystitis or acute pyelonephritis. The pathogenesis of this disease is therefore obscure. As in all chronic progressive renal diseases, the maternal and fetal prognosis in a particular case depends on the extent of renal destruction. Women with hypertension or renal insufficiency have a poor prognosis, whereas those with adequate renal function and no hypertension usually tolerate pregnancy without serious complications. Regardless of the extent of renal destruction, chronic pyelonephritis complicated by bacteriuria during pregnancy is associated with an increased risk of superimposed acute pyelonephritis, which, in turn, may lead to further deterioration of renal function.

RENAL TUBERCULOSIS

Tuberculosis of the kidney is a serious, but rare, complication of pregnancy. Renal tuberculosis is believed by some to pursue a rapidly unfavorable course, particularly during the later months of pregnancy. Therefore, the advisability of allowing a pregnancy to continue in any case of proven renal tuberculosis is a therapeutic dilemma. A decision regarding termination of pregnancy should be based upon the individual findings in each case, however. With either choice, aggressive multidrug chemotherapy is initiated promptly.

Whether the women who has undergone nephrectomy for tuberculosis should be allowed to become pregnant is another question. The consensus is that pregnancy should be inter-

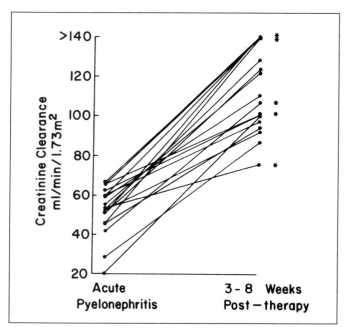

Figure 39–8. Endogenous creatinine clearance values in 18 pregnant women during and 3 to 8 weeks after an attack of acute pyelonephritis. Asterisk indicates patients reevaluated while still pregnant. (*From Whalley and colleagues: Obstet Gynecol 46:174, 1975.*)

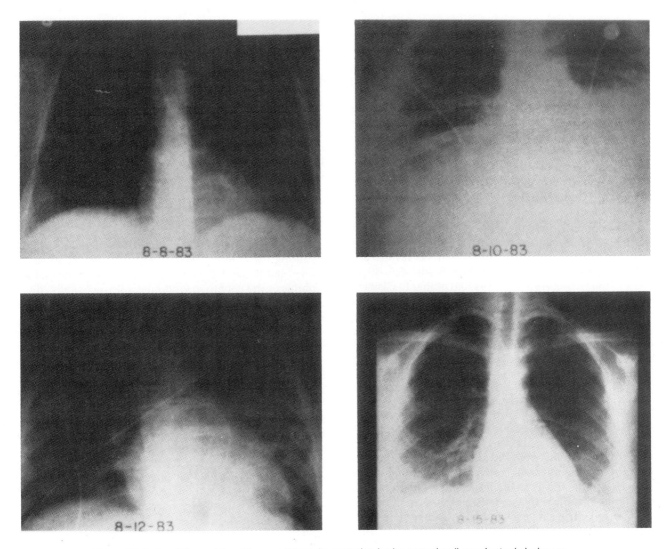

Figure 39–9. An 18-year-old multipara at 20 weeks gestation had a normal radiograph at admission on 8-8-83. Respiratory distress 20 hours later was accompanied by a left-sided pulmonary infiltrate which progressed to bilateral infiltrates by 8-10-83, despite normal cardiovascular function. The infiltrates improved, and she had a normal x-ray by 8-15-83. (*From Cunningham and colleagues: Am J Obstet Gynecol 156:797, 1987.*)

dicted for about two years until absence of infection and good function are demonstrated in the remaining kidney.

URINARY CALCULI

Renal and ureteral lithiasis are uncommon complications of pregnancy. Since in pregnant women there are some of the cardinal prerequisites for stone formation—urinary stasis and infection—the incidence might be expected to be higher were it not for the relatively short duration of pregnancy. Urinary tract dilatation also may predispose to fewer symptoms.

Women who have formed renal stones previously are generally at risk of doing so again; however, Coe and associates (1978) found no evidence that pregnancy increased that risk. Moreover, stone disease did not appear to have any prejudicial effect on pregnancy outcome except for an increased frequency of urinary infections. They concluded that a woman with nephrolithiasis need not forego pregnancy as long as renal function

is adequate. Calculi seldom cause severe symptomatic obstruction during pregnancy. **Persistent pyelonephritis despite adequate antimicrobial therapy should prompt a search for renal obstruction, which is most frequently due to nephrolithiasis.**

Sonography may help to confirm a suspected renal stone, but pregnancy hydronephrosis may obscure these findings. Stones may be identified in most women by carefully performed radiography, with or without contrast media. Treatment depends on the symptoms and the duration of pregnancy. In over half of the cases, the stone passes spontaneously, but about a third of pregnant women with symptomatic stones will need cystoscopy, percutaneous nephrostomy, basket extraction or surgical exploration (Maikranz and colleagues, 1987). Associated infection is treated vigorously. If symptoms persist, especially severe infection, then surgical removal may be mandatory. Loughlin and Bailey (1986) reported that ureteral double-J stents, placed via cystoscopy under local anesthesia, relieved persistent symptoms from ureteral calculi in eight pregnant women. We have used this method to successfully avoid the more invasive surgical procedures, including percutaneous nephrostomy, basket extraction, nephrolithotomy, and perhaps even nephrectomy. During the latter half of pregnancy, the blood vessels supplying the kidney and ureter are remarkably enlarged, and proper exposure of the lower ureter without emptying the uterus is often impossible.

Lattanzi and Cook (1980) and Maikranz and colleagues (1987) have reviewed much of the literature regarding these complications. When calculi are discovered, the possibility of hyperparathyroidism also should be considered.

GLOMERULOPATHIES

The kidney, and especially the glomerulus and its capillaries, are subject to a large number and variety of acute and chronic diseases, which may result from a single stimulus such as poststreptococcal glomerulonephritis, or from a multisystem disease such as systemic lupus erythematosus. According to Glasscock and Brenner (1987), there are five major glomerulopathic syndromes: acute and chronic glomerulonephritis, rapidly progressive glomerulonephritis, the nephrotic syndrome, and those caused by asymptomatic urinary abnormalities. The majority of these diseases are encountered in young women of childbearing age, and thus they may complicate pregnancy.

ACUTE GLOMERULONEPHRITIS

Like most glomerulopathies, acute glomerulonephritis may result from any of several causes, including those following infectious diseases, multisystem diseases, or primary disorders unique to the glomerulus. All are characterized by an abrupt onset of hematuria and proteinuria accompanied by varying degrees of renal insufficiency and salt and water retention causing edema, hypertension, and circulatory congestion. Acute poststreptococcal glomerulonephritis is prototypical of these syndromes.

Poststreptococcal glomerulonephritis rarely develops acutely during pregnancy. In reviewing the literature, Nadler and coworkers (1969) found reports of only 19 pregnant women with acute glomerulonephritis, and in only three of them was the diagnosis verified by biopsy. The diagnosis during pregnancy is easier if there is a history of pharyngeal or cutaneous streptococcal infection a few weeks before and supporting evidence is provided by red cell casts in urine and an elevated antistreptolysin titer. Acute glomerulonephritis that would arise during the second half of pregnancy especially is in most cases clinically indistinguishable from preeclampsia. Renal biopsy might be of value in unusual circumstances to try to exclude preeclampsia and identify the type of glomeruler disease (Madaio and Harrington, 1983).

In general, the treatment of glomerulonephritis is the same as in the nonpregnant woman. There are insufficient data to predict fetal or maternal prognosis. Some investigators have noted a high fetal loss from abortion, immaturity, or stillbirth, whereas others have documented otherwise uneventful pregnancies. Since the clinical syndrome usually subsides within two weeks, a course of expectant observation is warranted. In nonpregnant women the mortality rate is about 1 percent with death usually the result of heart failure or unrelenting renal failure. Some patients never completely recover, and *rapidly progressive glomerulonephritis* leads to end-stage renal failure. In some, chronic glomerulonephritis follows. Women with a his-

tory of acute glomerulonephritis that subsequently has healed may undergo additional pregnancies without any appreciable increase in the incidence of complications (Felding, 1968).

RAPIDLY PROGRESSIVE GLOMERULONEPHRITIS

In some cases, acute glomerulonephritis does not resolve, and rapidly progressive glomerulonephritis progresses to end-stage renal failure within weeks to months. Since extensive extracapillary or *crescenteric glomerulonephritis* is commonly identified, the two terms are often used interchangeably (Glasscock and Brenner, 1987).

CHRONIC GLOMERULONEPHRITIS

Chronic glomerulonephritis is characterized by progressive renal destruction over a period of years or decades, eventually producing the *end-stage kidney*. In many cases the cause is unknown, but it may follow almost any type of acute glomerulonephritis or the nephrotic syndrome. Microscopically, the renal lesions are categorized as proliferative, sclerosing, or membranous.

Chronic glomerulopathies may be detected in any of several ways: (1) Some patients may remain asymptomatic for years, and proteinuria or abnormal urinary sediment, or both, detected by screening are the only indicators of the disease. (2) It may be discovered in some women during the course of evaluation for chronic hypertension. (3) The disease may first manifest as the nephrotic syndrome. (4) It may exacerbate and the clinical presentation may be quite similar to acute glomerulonephritis. (5) Renal failure may be the first manifestation. (6) A woman with symptoms and signs of preeclampsia–eclampsia, but without their resolution, may be found to have chronic glomerulonephritis.

NEPHROTIC SYNDROME

The nephrotic syndrome, or *nephrosis*, is also a spectrum of renal disorders of many causes. It is characterized by proteinuria in excess of 3 to 4 g per day, hypoalbuminemia, hyperlipidemia, and edema. Most patients have microscopic renal abnormalities and many have accompanying evidence for renal dysfunction. The defects in the barriers of the glomerular capillary wall which allow excessive filtration of plasma proteins may follow immunological or toxic injury or metabolic or vascular diseases, or commonly it is a primary glomerular disease. Some causes of the first four include lupus nephritis, diabetic glomerulopathy, poststreptococcal glomerulonephritis, heavy metals, insect stings, and drug reactions. Examples of lesions that primarily affect the kidney to cause nephrosis are minimal change disease, mesangial proliferative glomerulonephritis, focal and segmental glomerulosclerosis, and membranous glomerulonephritis (Glasscock and Brenner, 1987).

When the nephrotic syndrome complicates pregnancy, the maternal and fetal prognosis and the treatment depend on the underlying cause of the disease and the extent of renal insufficiency. For example, we identified two women with antepartum syphilis that likely caused the nephrotic syndrome since after pencillin therapy, the nephrosis cleared and pregnancy outcomes were both satisfactory. Whenever possible, the specific cause should be ascertained and renal function assessed. In this regard, when the cause is not apparent, percutaneous renal biopsy, usually after pregnancy, may be of value. In our experiences, serial studies of renal function in women without appreciably diminished renal function will demonstrate some augmentation of renal function. This is related to blood volume expansion, which we have reported to be normal in these women if the serum creatinine is less than 3 mg per dL (Cox and colleagues, 1989).

A review of reported cases of nephrosis indicates that the majority of women who are not hypertensive and do not have severe renal insufficiency usually will have a successful pregnancy, particularly since adrenal glucocorticoids have been available (Weisman and colleagues, 1973). In certain cases, however, in which there is evidence for renal insufficiency or moderate to severe hypertension, or both, the prognosis for mother and fetus is poor.

PREGNANCY OUTCOME IN CHRONIC RENAL DISEASE

Chronic renal disease is a global term used to describe women with either underlying renal insufficiency or proteinuria, or in many cases, both. As described above, there are a number of primary renal disorders as well as multisystem diseases that affect the kidneys. In many cases, renal biopsy will be necessary to determine the cause of underlying renal disease; however, most defer this until pregnancy is completed. Packham and Fairley (1987) performed 111 percutaneous biopsies in 104 pregnant women before the third trimester and reported a 5 percent complication rate. Lindheimer and Davison (1987) emphasize that such good outcomes are unusual and attributable to the experience of the Australian group, and we agree with them that biopsy is usually best reserved until after pregnancy.

There is good evidence that the degree of renal insufficiency is more important than the type of lesion in determining pregnancy outcome. Importantly, accompanying preexisting hypertension also is predictive of pregnancy outcome. **However, even if renal function is normal and the woman normotensive, pregnancy outcome is still not always good.** Katz and associates (1980) reviewed 89 pregnancies in women with chronic renal disease, the exact diagnosis of which was established by renal biopsy. In none of the 38 women with diffuse or focal glomerulonephritis was there evidence before pregnancy of appreciable impairment of renal function. Plasma creatinine levels were 1.2 mg per dL or less and blood urea nitrogen levels were 17 mg per dL or less. Nonetheless, of 59 pregnancies in these 38 women, there were 10 perinatal deaths, 14 infants were delivered preterm, and 15 were small for gestational age. Superimposed preeclampsia was common and severe abruptio placentae developed in three instances.

Surian and colleagues (1984) described the clinical course of 123 pregnancies in 86 women with biopsy-proven glomerular disease. Some, but definitely not all of these women had renal dysfunction. In about 60 percent of these women pregnancy was uncomplicated. In the remaining 40 percent, about a third each had obstetrical or renal complications, or a combination of both. Hypertension developed in 20 percent and it persisted in half of these after pregnancy ended. In 8 percent of the women, renal function deteriorated, and this persisted in half. They concluded that in most women pregnancy does not alter the course of glomerular disease.

Hou and her colleagues (1985) reported the outcomes of 25 pregnancies in 23 women studied because of moderate renal insufficiency and whose baseline serum creatinine ranged from 1.2 to 1.7 mg per dL. Pregnancy-induced or -aggravated hypertension developed in slightly more than half of these women

and early delivery frequently was forced. Although 92 percent of the fetuses were liveborn and 84 percent survived, nearly 60 percent were preterm. Pregnancy was associated with accelerated renal dysfunction in about a third of women with moderate renal insufficiency. The effects of underlying severe hypertension which is made worse by pregnancy are considerable, and pregnancy-aggravated hypertension was identified in most women whose renal function worsened.

Our experiences at Parkland Hospital (Harstad and colleagues, 1989) with 37 pregnancies complicated by moderate to severe renal insufficiency are that perinatal outcomes were surprisingly good. Common complications included chronic hypertension (73 percent), anemia (76 percent), preeclampsia (57 percent), fetal growth retardation (30 percent) and preterm delivery (48 percent). Birthweight correlated inversely and significantly with serum creatinine concentration. We conclude that except for an increased risk of superimposed preeclampsia, women with relatively normal renal function and no hypertension before pregnancy are more likely, but not guaranteed, to have a relatively normal pregnancy. Because of the inevitable likelihood of long-term progression of the chronic disease, however, the ultimate maternal prognosis is guarded. Conversely, in women with extreme hypertension and/or renal insufficiency, the outcome is much more likely to be poor for them and for the pregnancy. Because of varying degrees and causes of renal destruction, it is difficult to evaluate the influence of pregnancy on progression of the disease. In most women, *in the absence of superimposed preeclampsia or severe placental abruption*, pregnancy does not appear to accelerate appreciably deterioration in renal function. In the absence of complications, affected kidneys may show the same pattern of response to pregnancy as do normal kidneys, with some increase in both glomerular filtration and renal plasma flow.

ACUTE RENAL FAILURE

Acute renal failure associated with pregnancy has become less common but it certainly has not been eliminated, as shown by the experiences of Grünfeld and associates (1980) which are summarized in Table 39–6. The most common causes of acute renal failure were abruptio placentae and eclampsia. A third of these 57 women had cortical necrosis, and 15 percent died.

Identification of acute renal failure and, in turn, its cause or

TABLE 39–6. PRINCIPAL CAUSES AND OUTCOME OF ACUTE RENAL FAILURE IN 57 PREGNANT WOMEN

Primary Cause	Number	Cortical Necrosis	Died
Abruptio placentae	13	7	2
Eclampsia	11	1	0
Preeclampsia	1	0	0
Prolonged fetal death	6	5	2
Uterine hemorrhage	4	2	0
Acute pyelonephritis	3	0	0
Other infections	5	0	0
Amnionic fluid embolism	1	1	1
Ectopic pregnancy	1	0	1
Miscellaneous unrelated	7	0	0
Postpartum idiopathic	5	3	2
Totals	57	19	8

From Grünfeld and associates: Kidney Int 18:179, 1980.

causes is important. Appropriate therapy initiated promptly will minimize the intensity and duration of functional impairment. Oliguria is an important sign of acutely impaired renal function. Unfortunately, potent diuretics such as furosemide can increase urine flow without correcting but rather intensifying some causes of oliguria. Moreover, their use may negate the value of various urinary indices that might be used to try to differentiate prerenal from intrarenal or postrenal causes of acute renal failure. A urine:plasma creatinine ratio of greater than 20 is strongly suggestive, at least, of prerenal azotemia as is an elevated urine:plasma osmolality ratio of more than 1.5. Also, with prerenal azotemia most filtered sodium is reabsorbed so that the urinary concentration typically is less than 20 mEq per L. In obstetrical cases, however, both prerenal and intrarenal factors commonly are operative. For example, with total placental abruption, severe hypovolemia is common from massive concealed hemorrhage. Moreover, chronic hypertension with superimposed preeclampsia is frequent, and these women may have diminished sodium resorption (Chap. 35, p. 666). Finally, intense consumptive coagulopathy commonly triggered by abruption might impede the intrarenal microcirculation, but causes even more blood loss from lacerations and surgical incisions.

ACUTE TUBULAR NECROSIS

This clinical entity may be prevented, most often, by the following means: (1) Prompt and vigorous replacement of blood in instances of massive hemorrhage, as in placental abruption, placental previa, uterine rupture, and postpartum uterine atony, following the guidelines described in Chapter 36 (p. 697); (2) termination of pregnancies complicated by severe preeclampsia and eclampsia with careful blood replacement if loss is excessive; (3) close observation for early signs of septic shock especially in women with pyelonephritis, septic abortion, amnionitis, or sepsis from other pelvic infections; (4) avoidance of potent diuretics to treat oliguria before initiating appropriate efforts to assure cardiac output adequate for renal perfusion; and (5) avoidance of vasoconstrictors to treat hypotension unless pathological vasodilation is unequivocally the cause of the hypotension.

When azotemia is evident and severe oliguria persists, hemodialysis should be initiated before marked deterioration of general well-being occurs. Early dialysis appears to reduce mortality appreciably and may enhance the extent of recovery of renal function. Acute tubular necrosis is not chronically progressive. In fact, after healing has taken place, renal function usually returns to normal or near normal. Future pregnancies therefore are not necessarily contraindicated.

RENAL CORTICAL NECROSIS

Compared to acute tubular necrosis, bilateral necrosis of the renal cortex is uncommon. When cortical necrosis has developed, however, it often has been associated with pregnancy. For example, among 38 cases studied by Kleinknecht and co-workers (1973), 26 were obstetrical. Most of the reported cases in pregnant women have followed such complications as placental abruption, preeclampsia–eclampsia, or endotoxin-induced shock. Histologically, the lesion appears to result from thrombosis of segments of the renal vascular system. The lesions may be focal, patchy, confluent, or gross. Clinically, renal cortical necrosis follows the course of acute renal failure with oliguria or anuria, uremia, and generally death within 2 to 3 weeks unless dialysis is initiated. Differentiation from acute

tubular necrosis during the early phase is not possible. The prognosis depends on the extent of the necrosis, since recovery is a function of the amount of renal tissue spared. When the lesion is confluent, the mortality rate approaches 100 percent unless chronic dialysis or renal transplantation is performed.

OBSTRUCTIVE RENAL FAILURE

Rarely, bilateral ureteral compression by a very large pregnant uterus is greatly exaggerated causing ureteral obstruction and, in turn, severe oliguria and azotemia. O'Shaughnessy and co-workers (1980), as well as others, have described this phenomenon as the consequence of a markedly overdistended gravid uterus. Homans and associates (1981) described a case in which massive hydramnios was associated with renal failure in a woman with a single left kidney. When placed in the right lateral recumbent position, diuresis was prompt and the plasma creatinine dropped from 6.0 to 2.0 mg per dL over the 60-hour period that she maintained that posture.

We have observed this phenomenon on several occasions. In one woman with massive hydramnios (9.4 L) and an anencephalic fetus, amniocentesis and removal of some of the amnionic fluid was followed promptly by a diuresis and a lowering of the plasma creatinine concentration. In another instance, progressive oliguria and azotemia were identified during two successive pregnancies early in the third trimester in a woman who as a child had been subjected to reimplantation of both ureters into the bladder to try to prevent reflux. During the second pregnancy, using cystoscopy, ureteral catheters were teased through the markedly narrowed ureteral lumens and provided significant relief from the obstructions (Laverson and colleagues, 1984).

THROMBOTIC MICROANGIOPATHIES

In 1968 Wagoner and Robson and their associates described what they believed to be a new syndrome of *acute irreversible renal failure* that developed within the first 6 weeks postpartum. Pregnancy and delivery appeared to have been normal in the seven cases reported and none of the known causes of renal failure was found. The pathological changes identified by renal biopsy were necrosis and endothelial proliferation in glomeruli, plus necrosis, thrombosis, and intimal thickening of the arterioles. No vascular abnormalities were demonstrated in the other visceral organs in the four cases in which autopsy was performed. Morphological changes in the erythrocytes consistent with microangiopathic hemolysis and thrombocytopenia were usually present. These findings are similar to those reported for the *postpartum hemolytic uremic syndrome*. Moreover, they are also similar to those in which renal failure is identified as part of the syndrome of *thrombotic thrombocytopenic purpura*. It is obvious that these disorders are not limited to the kidneys, and in most cases there is widespread arteriolar hyalinization and evidence for endothelial damage. Although these three syndromes may be due to different etiologies, it is difficult currently to separate them, at least clinically. They are discussed in detail on page 793.

PREGNANCY AFTER RENAL TRANSPLANTATION

Murray and associates in 1963 reported two successful pregnancies in a woman who had a kidney transplanted from her identical twin sister. Since that time many pregnancies have been reported in women who previously had received a kidney from immunologically nonidentical donors.

Davison (1987) recently reviewed the outcomes in 1,569 pregnancies in 1,009 women, 80 percent of whom had cadaveric transplants. The incidence of spontaneous abortion was 16 percent, or about the same as in the general population; however, therapeutic abortion was performed for another 22 percent. Of the pregnancies that continued beyond the first trimester, 92 percent had a successful outcome. Beginning early in pregnancy, glomerular filtration in these women usually increased. Preeclampsia developed in 30 percent and signs of kidney rejection were observed in 9 percent. Unfortunately, without renal biopsy, rejection may be difficult to distinguish from acute pyelonephritis, recurrent glomerulopathy, or severe preeclampsia. Serious infections, most likely related to immunosuppressive therapy, complicated some pregnancies. Urinary infections were diagnosed in 40 percent and viral infections were increased.

Almost half of infants who were liveborn were delivered preterm. Prematurely ruptured membranes and preterm labor were common. Growth-retarded infants averaged 20 percent in the series reviewed. Respiratory distress was common among the preterm infants but seldom was it fatal. Fetal malformations were identified in only 2 percent, and no specific type predominated. The newborns, as well as the mother, were at increased risk of infection because of maternal immunosuppressive therapy.

From these experiences, recommendations were formulated for factors requisite before pregnancy should be attempted, and these include good general health without severe hypertension for at least two years after transplantation, since graft rejection is more common in this period. There should be no evidence of graft rejection or persistent proteinuria. Even so, the effects of pregnancy are unpredictable and not necessarily related to previous rejection episodes, lack of problems in previous pregnancies, or human leucocyte antigen typing. If stable, prednisone intake should be maintained at 15 mg a day or less and azathioprine at 2 mg per kg or less. We and others have observed azathioprine hepatotoxicity with severe jaundice developing during pregnancy (Ware and co-workers, 1979). A reduction in dosage is likely to improve hepatic function.

Concern persists over the possibility of late effects in the offspring subjected to immunosuppressive therapy in utero, such as malignancy, germ cell dysfunction, and malformations in the offspring's children. Penn and colleagues (1980) reported that 58 of 60 babies sired by fathers who had undergone renal transplant were normal. One infant was born with a meningomyelocele, hip dislocation, and talipes equinovarus. The other infant with congenital anomalies, including microcephaly and polycystic kidneys, died at birth.

Pregnancy following renal transplantation has been reviewed in detail by Davison (1987), Davison and Lindheimer (1982), and Hadi (1986).

HEMODIALYSIS DURING PREGNANCY

Most often, significantly impaired renal function is accompanied by infertility. With chronic hemodialysis, however, fertility may be restored (Perez and colleagues, 1978). A few women on chronic hemodialysis have become pregnant and have been so managed throughout pregnancy, but with marginal success. For example, Hou (1987) reported the outcomes in 37 women in whom hemodialysis was used during pregnancy. Hypertension complicated half of the pregnancies and placental abruption occurred in four. Only a fourth of the pregnancies resulted in a liveborn infant and half of these were delivered before 36 weeks because of preterm labor, preeclampsia, abruptio placentae, ruptured membranes, fetal jeopardy, or growth retardation. Hou (1987), as well as others, reported that an increased frequency of dialysis was required during pregnancy, but even with such management it was unclear if this improved fetal survival.

In our experiences, the likelihood of salutary pregnancy outcome with a chronically dialysed woman is very low. If it is to be attempted, then vigorous dialysis treatments are recommended.

OTHER KIDNEY DISORDERS

POLYCYSTIC KIDNEY DISEASE

An in-depth study of the apparent effects of polycystic kidney disease on pregnancy and vice versa has been provided by Milutinovic and co-workers (1983). Of 137 women at risk of having inherited the autosomal dominant gene, 55 percent demonstrated multiple renal cysts. Fertility, spontaneous abortion, stillbirth, and symptomatic urinary tract infection were comparable in both groups. Hypertension was more common both when pregnant and nonpregnant in those with polycystic disease, but no evidence was obtained of an adverse effect from pregnancy on the disease. Hossack and colleagues (1988) studied 163 nonpregnant patients and reported substantivley increased cardiac valvar lesions detected by echocardiography. Mitral valve prolapse was 13-fold increased over that in the control group, and there was excessive mitral, aortic, and tricuspid incompetence.

PREGNANCY AFTER UNILATERAL NEPHRECTOMY

Because the excretory capacity of two kidneys is much in excess of ordinary needs, and because the surviving kidney usually undergoes hypertrophy with increased excretory capacity, women with one normal kidney most often have no difficulty in pregnancy. If the remaining kidney is chronically infected, however, further damage may result from the stasis induced by pregnancy, and its likelihood to lead to more intense infection. Accordingly, before advising a woman with one kidney about the risk of future pregnancy, a thorough functional evaluation of the remaining organ is essential. Should it be found impaired, childbearing is risky. Even asymptomatic women should be carefully monitored to make certain that the single kidney is functioning satisfactorily.

ORTHOSTATIC PROTEINURIA

Proteinuria is sometimes detectable in urine formed while the pregnant woman is ambulatory but not when recumbent. No other evidence for renal disease is apparent. The estimate of 5 percent in pregnant women appears too high in our experience. The pregnant woman with orthostatic proteinuria should be evaluated for bacteriuria, abnormal urinary sediment, reduced glomerular filtration rate, and hypertension. In the absence of these abnormalities the prognosis for pregnancy is good.

Intermittent proteinuria may be the consequence of a suburethral diverticulum that empties its proteinaceous contents into the voided urine from time to time, especially following examination of the anterior vaginal wall.

ENDOCRINE DISORDERS

It is quite evident from the following discussions that a variety of endocrine disorders can complicate pregnancy and vice versa. The most common, diabetes mellitus, is made more difficult to manage by pregnancy and also increases appreciably the risk of a number of pregnancy complications. With some other conditions, for example, thyrotoxicosis, pregnancy often only appears to worsen the endocrinopathy by increasing the concentration of circulating thyroxine but not necessarily the amount of free, or active, hormone.

DIABETES MELLITUS

Before insulin therapy many women with diabetes were too ill to conceive. For example, Williams (1915), after 13 years as Chief of Obstetrics at the Johns Hopkins Hospital, and with a large consulting practice, had encountered only one case of pregnancy complicated by recognized diabetes. The exact cause of infertility in diabetic women during the preinsulin era is not clear, but the incidence of anemorrhea has been placed as high as 50 percent. Of the infrequent pregnancies, about one fourth of the mothers and half of the fetuses and infants died.

PREVALENCE

The lack of agreement about the minimal requirements for the diagnosis of diabetes makes it difficult to acquire satisfactory figures for its prevalence. Even so, by diagnostic criteria acceptable to most, it is estimated that perhaps 1 percent of the general population of childbearing-age women now has overt diabetes, and about one-fourth of these have insulin-dependent disease (Foster, 1987). The cause or causes for the remarkable increase in recent years are not known, but environmental factors, as well as genetic predisposition, are implicated. The bases for incriminating environmental factors is provided principally by the observations that for most young persons with insulin-dependent diabetes there is no family history of diabetes. Moreover, the concordance rate for diabetes in monozygous twins, rather than being nearly 100 percent if diabetes were solely genetic in origin, is less than 50 percent (Foster, 1987).

The probability of interaction of environmental factors, especially viral, and of genetic predisposition, is supported by demonstrations of considerable variation in susceptibility to diabetes among different animal strains injected with the same virus. In human population studies an association has been found between the human leucocyte antigen (HLA) system and some, but not all, forms of diabetes.

CLASSIFICATION

Women whose pregnancies are complicated by diabetes can be separated into those who were known to have diabetes before pregnancy and those with gestational diabetes. Although White (1978) provided an update of her classification, its increasing complexity may have impaired its usefulness. Shown in Table 39–7 is the classification presented by the American College of Obstetricians and Gynecologists (1986). It follows the classification of White, and its salient features are that the duration of diabetes relates to the severity of end-organ derangement, especially the eyes, kidneys, and cardiovascular system.

DIAGNOSIS DURING PREGNANCY

The woman who presents with glucosuria, high plasma glucose levels, and ketonemia and ketonuria presents no problem in diagnosis. The woman at the opposite end of the spectrum, with only minimal metabolic derangement, may be difficult to identify. The likelihood of impaired carbohydrate metabolism and related metabolic stigmata of diabetes is increased appreciably in women who have a strong familial history of diabetes, have given birth to large infants, demonstrate persistent glucosuria or have unexplained fetal losses.

Reducing substances are commonly found in the urine of pregnant women, but their presence does not necessarily mean diabetes. Unless a method that is specific for glucose is used, often the material is lactose, which should not be a source of needless concern. The commercially available testing substances, Tes-Tape and Clinistix, may be used to identify glucosuria while avoiding a positive reaction from lactose. Even then, glucosuria most often does not reflect impaired glucose tolerance, but rather an increased glomerular filtration rate and an

TABLE 39–7. CLASSIFICATION OF DIABETES COMPLICATING PREGNANCY

		Pregestational Diabetes			
Class	Age Onset		Duration (Yr)	Vascular Disease	Therapy
A	Any		Any	None	A-1, diet only
B	Over 20		Less than 10	None	Insulin
C	10 to 19	or	10 to 19	None	Insulin
D	Before 10	or	More than 20	Benign retinopathy	Insulin
F	Any		Any	Nephropathy	Insulin
R	Any		Any	Proliferative retinopathy	Insulin
H	Any		Any	Heart disease	Insulin

	Gestational Diabetes		
Class	Fasting Plasma Glucose		Postprandial Plasma Glucose
A-1	Less than 105 mg per dL	and	Less than 120 mg per dL
A-2	More than 105 mg per dL	and/or	More than 120 mg per dL

From The American College of Obstetricians and Gynecologists: Technical Bulletin No. 92, May, 1986.

amount of filtered glucose which exceeds normal tubular reabsorption capacity (see Chap. 7, p. 149). Nonetheless, the detection of glucosuria during pregnancy warrants further testing.

EFFECT OF PREGNANCY ON DIABETES

The diabetogenic effects of pregnancy are borne out by the fact that some women who have no evidence of diabetes when not pregnant develop during pregnancy distinct abnormalities of glucose tolerance and, at times, clinically overt diabetes. Most often these changes are reversible. After delivery, evidence for either the induction of or a worsening of diabetes usually disappears rapidly, and the ability of the mother to metabolize carboyhdrate returns to the prepregnancy status. As discussed in Chapter 7 (p. 138), physiological pregnancy alterations impair peripheral insulin action. The insulin antagonism during pregnancy is the consequence probably of the actions of *placental lactogen*, which is secreted in enormous quantities, and to lesser degrees those actions of *estrogens* and *progesterone*. Also, *placental insulinase* may contribute to pregnancy-induced diabetogenicity by accelerating insulin degradation.

During pregnancy, diabetes control is usually made more difficult by a variety of complications. Nausea and vomiting, by precluding food intake to counteract exogenously administered insulin, may lead on one hand to insulin shock and, on the other, to insulin resistance if starvation is severe enough to cause ketosis. The pregnant woman, even in the absence of diabetes, is more prone to develop metabolic acidosis than when nonpregnant. Presumably, placental lactogen is responsible for this tendency by virtue of its carbohydrate-sparing and lipolytic actions. With diabetes, the likelihood of severe metabolic acidosis is increased appreciably. Infection during pregnancy commonly results in insulin resistance and ketoacidosis unless the infection is promptly recognized and both the infection and diabetes are effectively treated. The vigorous muscular exertion of labor accompanied by the ingestion of little or no carbohydrate may result in troublesome hypoglycemia unless the amount of insulin given is reduced appropriately or an intravenous infusion of glucose is provided.

After delivery, the need for exogenous insulin most often decreases at a rapid rate and to a considerable degree. Puerperal infection, however, may obtund this response or perhaps even increase insulin requirements. Presumably, the rapid decrease in insulin requirements that is usually seen in the absence of other complications stems from the rapid disappearance of those pregnancy factors cited above following delivery of the placenta, and at a time that levels of pituitary growth hormone remain low for several days.

It was once thought by some that the fetus ameliorates maternal diabetes by producing insulin which was supposedly transferred in significant amounts across the placenta to the mother. There is no evidence, however, that the fetal pancreas is capable of providing insulin to the mother.

EFFECTS OF DIABETES ON PREGNANCY

Diabetes may be deleterious to pregnancy in a number of ways. Adverse maternal effects include the following:

1. The likelihood of preeclampsia–eclampsia is increased about fourfold, and an increased incidence is noted even in the absence of demonstrated preexisting vascular or renal disease.

2. Some infections are common, and they are likely to be more severe in women with diabetes.
3. The fetus can be much larger and his size may lead to difficult delivery with injury to the birth canal.
4. Because of substantively increased perinatal jeopardy, as well as the possibility of dystocia, the rate of cesarean delivery is increased and the maternal risks that are imposed by surgery are increased.
5. Hydramnios is common, and at times the large volume of amnionic fluid, coupled with fetal macrosomia, may cause cardiorespiratory symptoms in the mother.
6. Postpartum hemorrhage is more common than in the general obstetrical population.

Maternal diabetes adversely affects the fetus and newborn infant in several ways:

1. In the absence of excellent diabetes and pregnancy management, the perinatal death rate is considerably elevated compared with that of the general population.
2. Major anomalies are increased threefold in the fetuses of women with overt diabetes.
3. Morbidity is common in the newborn. In some instances, the morbidity is direct and results from birth injury as the consequence of fetal macrosomia with disproportion between the size of the infant and the maternal pelvis. In other instances, it is indirect and takes the form of severe respiratory distress and metabolic derangement that include hypoglycemia and hypocalcemia.
4. The infant may inherit at least a predisposition to diabetes.

Except for the brain, most fetal organs are affected by macrosomia that commonly, but not always, characterizes the fetus of the diabetic woman. At the same time, body fat is increased (Fig. 39–10). The mechanisms responsible for the extra growth of the fetus are not well defined. In several studies, however, the degree of fetal macrosomia appeared to correlate well with the degree of maternal hyperglucemia and lack of maternal vascular disease. Both favor the transfer of excessive glucose across the placenta to the fetus. This stimulates fetal insulin secretion, which is a potent growth factor. Thus, hyperglucemia and hyperinsulinemia in concert enhance glycogen synthesis, lipogenesis, and protein synthesis (Hill, 1978). There is abundant experimental evidence to support this concept. Mintz and co-workers (1972) injected streptozotocin into the pregnant monkey to destroy the β-cells of the maternal islets of Langerhans and the subsequent maternal diabetes resulted in fetal macrosomia. Cheek (1968) injected streptozotocin into the circulation of the monkey fetus to destroy the capacity of the fetus to make insulin and, conversely, fetal size was reduced appreciably. Moreover, marked fetal growth retardation with very poor development of striated muscle and near absence of adipose tissue has been observed in a newborn infant whose plasma and vestigial pancreas contained no insulin (Hill, 1978).

A fairly common finding at autopsy in the newborn infant of a diabetic mother is hypertrophy and hyperplasia of the islets of Langerhans. Although the changes are not specific and also can be noted in erythroblastotic infants, they are sufficiently characteristic when found to suggest that the mother had impaired glucose metabolism. It has been suggested that maternal hyperglucemia and, in turn, fetal hyperglucemia are responsible for the striking increase in the size, and sometimes the number, of islets.

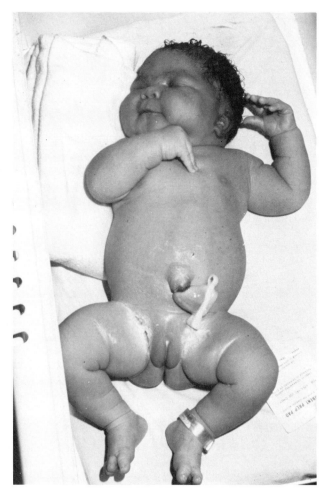

Figure 39–10. This macrosomic infant who weighed 6,050 g was born to a woman with gestational diabetes.

PRINCIPLES OF MANAGEMENT

Management which is based on a full appreciation of the following general principles will provide the best outcome for both the fetus-infant and his diabetic mother:

1. Abnormal carbohydrate metabolism should be detected and defined precisely.
2. The pregnant woman with overt diabetes should be cared for throughout her pregnancy by experienced individuals.
3. Control of maternal glucemia in overtly diabetic women is an important factor in determining fetal outcome.
4. The newborn of a mother with diabetes should be cared for from the time of birth by experienced individuals.

GESTATIONAL DIABETES

Gestational diabetes is carbohydrate intolerance induced by pregnancy. Because it is frequently a covert abnormality, its impact on maternal and perinatal morbidity have not been fully defined, and indeed Hunter and Milner (1985) have commented that *"gestational diabetes is a diagnosis still looking for a disease."*

In 1984 the Second Workshop-Conference on Gestational Diabetes was held in Chicago. Gestational diabetes was defined as carbohydrate intolerance of variable severity with onset or first recognition during the current pregnancy. This definition did not exclude the possibility that glucose intolerance may have antedated pregnancy. Use of the diagnostic term *gestational diabetes* was encouraged in order to communicate the need for high-risk surveillance to third-party payers or others responsible for the financing of health care delivery, and to convince women of the need for further testing postpartum. The conferees concluded that gestational diabetes is a heterogeneous disorder with varied worldwide prevalence. Indeed, in a 10-year survey, the reported prevalence of gestational diabetes varied from 0.15 to 12.3 percent, but there was no international agreement on the most appropriate diagnostic criteria. Obesity is a common cofactor and Johnson and her colleagues (1987) reported that 8 percent of 588 women who weighed more than 250 pounds had gestational diabetes compared to less than 1 percent of women who weighed less than 200 pounds.

It was concluded at the 1984 Workshop that obstetrical and perinatal risks were increased for women with undetected gestational diabetes. Also, more than half of women with gestational diabetes ultimately develop overt diabetes, and there is mounting evidence for long-range complications that include obesity and diabetes in offspring born to these women.

As shown in Table 39–7, the classification previously presented includes in class A_1 those women with postprandial glucose intolerance but fasting euglucemia.

SCREENING

Screening for gestational diabetes is controversial. For example, the 1984 Workshop-Conference recommended that *all* pregnant women should be screened using a 50-g oral glucose tolerance test between the 24th and 28th week of gestation without regard to time of day or last meal, and that a plasma value at 1 hour exceeding 140 mg per dL be used as the cutoff for performing a 100-g oral glucose tolerance test. Values used are the same as those originally recommended by O'Sullivan and Mahan (1964), and abnormal values for the 100-g test, administered after at least an 8-hour overnight fast, are shown in Table 39–8. In contrast, the American College of Obstetricians and Gynecologists (1986) recommends screening only for women considered at high risk, which includes age over 30; family history of diabetes; a prior macrosomic, malformed, or stillborn infant; obesity; hypertension; or glucosuria. β-mimetic drugs impair carbohydrate tolerance and Angel and colleagues (1988) reported a 12 percent incidence in 86 women receiving oral terbutaline for preterm labor.

ADVERSE EFFECTS

There has now been an important shift in focus concerning adverse fetal consequences of gestational diabetes. Fetal anom-

TABLE 39–8. CRITERIA FOR DIAGNOSIS OF GESTATIONAL DIABETES USING 100 G OF ORAL GLUCOSE

Timing of Glucose Measurement	Whole Venous Blood (mg per dL)	Plasma (mg per dL)
Fasting	90	105
1-hour	165	190
2-hour	145	165
3-hour	125	145

From the Second International Workshop-Conference on Gestational Diabetes: Diabetes 34s: 1, 1985.

alies are not increased (Reece and Hobbins, 1986). While women with fasting hyperglucemia are at greater risk for fetal death, this danger is not apparent for those with postprandial hyperglucemia only. Indeed, the perinatal focal point now is avoidance of difficult delivery due to macrosomia, with concomitant neonatal morbidity from birth trauma.

One supposed advantage of identifying gestational diabetes is increased awareness of potential shoulder dystocia. Unfortunately, precise identification of macrosomic infants is currently not possible (see Chap. 19, p. 365). Bochner and colleagues (1987) reported the outcomes of 201 gestational diabetics whose fasting and postprandial glucose values were normal with diet. Fetal abdominal circumference was measured ultrasonically between 30 and 33 weeks. If more than the 90th percentile, then 40 percent of those infants weighed more than 4,000 g at delivery and there was an increased incidence of cesarean section for failure to progress, shoulder dystocia, and birth trauma. Conversely, if the circumference was less than the 90th percentile, these complications were not increased compared to the normal population. Unfortunately, the predictive value of abdominal circumference greater than the 90th percentile was only 56 percent.

It is emphasized that the pregnant woman with a normal fasting glucose level but an abnormal glucose tolerance test early in pregnancy may occasionally develop overt diabetes late in pregnancy. The incidence is estimated to be about 15 percent, and thus fasting plasma glucose levels likely should be checked periodically.

MANAGEMENT

Pregnant women without persistent fasting hyperglucemia, but with an abnormal oral glucose tolerance test, are treated typically by diet alone. A liberal exercise program is encouraged. An acceptable diet is that recommended by the American Diabetes Association in amounts that provide 30 to 35 kilocalories per kg of ideal body weight each day. In general, for women with gestational diabetes who do not require insulin, there is seldom need for early delivery. Thus in the absence of other indications, these women are delivered at term. Labor induction at 40 weeks, while ideal, is not done unless the cervix is favorable.

It long has been debated whether prophylactic insulin will decrease complications related to macrosomia, and the participants of the 1984 Workshop-Conference concluded that data were insufficient to draw conclusions. Coustan and Imarah (1984) concluded from a nonrandomized study that routine insulin treatment given to women with gestational diabetes decreased the incidence of macrosomia, midforceps and cesarean deliveries, and birth trauma from shoulder dystocia. Persson and colleagues (1985) randomized insulin treatment to supplant diet in 202 women with gestational diabetes and reported no difference in mean birthweight, macrosomic infants, or neonatal hypoglyucemia and polycythemia. Finally, Leikin and co-workers (1987) reported that women with gestational diabetes and fasting euglucemia, when treated by diet alone, had the same incidence of macrosomia as a group of women at high risk for diabetes, but who had postprandial euglucemia. In this study, women with fasting hyperglucemia were given NPH insulin in addition to diet therapy, and macrosomia developed only in those who were obese. Importantly, half of these women with gestational diabetes and postprandial hyperglucemia were morbidly obese.

When carefully managed, perinatal mortality in infants of women with gestational diabetes is not greater than that for the general obstetrical population (Gabbe, 1978). However, if the diabetes worsens as pregnancy advances, the prognosis for the fetus-infant also worsens. Adverse outcome is also more likely if there was a prior stillbirth, or if pregnancy-induced hypertension develops (Gabbe, 1985). Therefore, throughout the remainder of pregnancy, periodic checks of fasting plasma glucose concentration are essential to detect the 10 to 15 percent of women who may possibly develop overt diabetes.

POSTPARTUM CONSEQUENCES

In about one-fourth of women with gestational diabetes without fasting hyperglucemia, diabetes will be found to persist at 1 year, and another 15 percent will have abnormal glucose tolerance (Metzger and colleagues, 1985). Moreover, according to the 1984 Workshop-Conference, if followed longer, about half of gestational diabetics ultimately will develop overt diabetes. According to Metzger and associates (1985), if fasting hyperglucemia is identified during pregnancy, diabetes is more likely to persist postpartum, and for women with fasting glucose levels of 105 to 130 mg per mL this figure is 43 percent. When fasting glucose exceeded 130 mg per dL during pregnancy, 86 percent of women remained overtly diabetic.

OVERT DIABETES

The likelihood of successful outcomes for the fetus-infant and the overtly diabetic mother parallels closely the degree of diabetes control as well as the intensity of any underlying maternal cardiovascular or renal disease. Therefore, as the letter classification shown in Table 39–7 advances the likelihood of a good pregnancy outcome lessens.

The criterion for diagnosis of diabetes during pregnancy is the identification of fasting hyperglucemia on two or more occasions. During pregnancy, this has been defined to be a *plasma* level of 105 mg per dL or higher, compared to 140 mg per dL or higher in nonpregnant individuals. The decision to establish a lower value during pregnancy was influenced, in part, by the fact that the plasma glucose level in women is lower during much of normal pregnancy than when nonpregnant (Gabbe, 1985).

MANAGEMENT BEFORE CONCEPTION

Overtly diabetic women have a threefold increased incidence of offspring with congenital malformations (Reece and Hobbins, 1986). It is now believed by most that the increased frequency of severe malformations is the consequence of poorly controlled diabetes both preconceptionally as well as early in pregnancy (Cousins, 1983; Miller and colleagues, 1981). Congenital heart defects are the most common lesions and their incidence is increased fivefold over the general population while neural tube defects are encountered in 20 per 1,000 pregnancies (Reece and Hobbins, 1986). The retrospective study from Miller and co-workers (1981) suggested that women with lower glycosylated hemoglobin values at the time of conception have a reduced incidence of anomalous fetuses compared to women with abnormally high values. Unfortunately, the recent report from the National Institutes of Health sponsored Diabetes in Early Pregnancy Study (Mills and colleagues, 1988) did not corroborate these findings. This investigation included over 600 diabetic women, and it was concluded that a normal glycosylated hemoglobin did not guarantee that diabetes-associated anomalies were absent. Conversely an elevated level did not necessarily indicate an increased risk for such anomalies. While it is hoped that normalization of maternal plasma glucose periconceptionally will influence favorably development of the embryo and fetus, this remains to be documented. Hopefully, the Diabetes in Early Pregnancy Study, as well as the Maine Diabetes in Pregnancy Project (Centers for Disease Control, 1987) may provide answers to this important question.

PERINATAL AND MATERNAL MORTALITY

In several reports of overtly diabetic pregnancies published in recent years, if substantively increased congenital malformations are disregarded, perinatal mortality rates have not been much higher than those for the general population. For example, the perinatal mortality rate was reported to be 4.6 percent by Gabbe and associates (1977), 3.6 percent by Kitzmiller and co-workers (1978), 4.5 percent by Leveno and co-workers (1979), 3.7 percent by Schneider and associates (1980), 4 percent by Coustan and associates (1980), and 3.9 percent by Martin and colleagues (1987). Severe congenital malformations accounted for much of the increase in perinatal mortality over those values observed in the general population.

Recently, the Vanderbilt University group (Diamond and colleagues, 1987) reported that Pederson's prognostically bad signs are still cogent for pregnant diabetics. Specifically, ketoacidosis, pregnancy-induced hypertension, pyelonephritis, or matenal neglect were associated with a perinatal mortality rate of 17 percent compared to only 7 percent in insulin-dependent diabetic women without any of these complications. Reece and associates (1988) reported that women with diabetic nephropathy, with good care, had pregnancy outcomes comparable to such women without renal disease.

Although it was generally felt that women with overt diabetes suffer disproportionate mortality, there were no maternal deaths reported in the above-cited studies of nearly 600 pregnancies. Still, as emphasized by Cousins (1987), maternal mortality is increased tenfold in diabetic women, most often as a result of ketoacidosis, underlying hypertension, preeclampsia, and pyelonephritis.

PRENATAL CARE

In all of the reports cited above regarding management of the pregnant diabetic, early diagnosis and meticulous management of diabetes and pregnancy was stressed. It was emphasized that, ideally, the maternal glucose level should be kept as close to normal as possible and the pregnancy should continue until the fetus is functionally mature unless the intrauterine environment is deteriorating. With evidence of deterioration, the fetus most often is better off being delivered even though preterm. The specific techniques emphasized by the several investigators to provide control of the diabetes and to monitor fetal well-being differed, yet the perinatal outcomes were nearly identical!

Important to a successful pregnancy outcome is precise knowledge of fetal age. A carefully obtained menstrual history and accurate measurements of uterine height during the second trimester provide useful information (see Chap. 38, p. 741). Ultrasonic confirmation of fetal age often will be of value. Although the value of ultrasonic examination performed before midpregnancy to try to identify fetal malformations has not been clearly established, it should be considered in conjunction with maternal serum α-fetoprotein screening at 16 to 18 weeks

(Gabbe, 1985). Sonographic evaluation later in pregnancy may serve to document either fetal macrosomia, a common phenomenon with less severe diabetes, or growth retardation, a complication seen especially when the mother has underlying vascular disease.

Effective maternal counseling is an extremely important function of prenatal care. She must not only be seen often but also be instructed carefully as to how to recognize and deal with problems that arise in the interim. She must be encouraged to report immediately any of a variety of events. For example, respiratory or urinary infection are rather common occurrences during pregnancy which can rapidly precipitate diabetic ketoacidosis that is poorly tolerated by the fetus. The common complication of pregnancy—nausea and vomiting—may, if the mother does not eat appropriately, lead to the characteristic reaction of hyperinsulinism, and when more severe and prolonged, the starvation may lead to both serious acidosis and insulin resistance much sooner than in the nonpregnant woman.

Similar to normal pregnancy, the woman is likely to develop glucosuria as the consequence of pregnancy-induced glomerular hyperfiltration of glucose without increased tubular reabsorption (see Chap. 7, p. 149). If she were to increase her insulin dosage to a level that avoids glucosuria, she likely would develop symptomatic hypoglycemia. In general, glucosuria is a signal to evaluate carefully the plasma glucose levels. Overt acetonuria should never be ignored and most often means that the insulin dosage should be increased.

The intelligent, well-coached, highly-motivated pregnant woman with relatively stable diabetes, who conscientiously follows her appropriate diet, which may have to be ingested in as many as five meals a day, and who takes multiple forms of insulin two or more times a day, has the best chance for achieving normoglucemia. In actuality, many women who attempt such rigid control commonly run the risk of hypoglycemia episodes that are dangerous not only to themselves but also to their fetuses. Frequent measurements of plasma glucose, especially before meals, and adjustment of insulin dosage and of diet on the basis of these measurements will help achieve the goal of avoiding both serious hyper- and hypoglucemia.

Within the past decade there has been an impetus to monitor the effects of insulin therapy by blood glucose levels determined several times daily at home by the pregnant woman. At her first evaluation, the woman is taught to use the glucose oxidase reagent strips, preferably with a reflectance meter (Landon and Gabbe, 1985). Blood is obtained by finger prick and glucose concentration is estimated upon arising in the morning, then again before each meal, and at bedtime. Combinations of intermediate-acting and regular insulin are then appropriately adjusted to achieve desired levels.

Schneider and co-workers (1980) formulated and evaluated a method of management which emphasized ambulatory care throughout pregnancy until actual delivery. The expectant mother was taught self-measurement of blood glucose using a reflectance meter and, depending upon the results, either the alterations to make in insulin dosage and diet, or how to obtain expert advice immediately. They emphasized that an expert especially knowledgeable in obstetrics and diabetes, and one who was intimately concerned with the mother's problem, always should be available through electronic paging to provide such advice and to direct appropriate action whenever needed. As pointed out above, their low perinatal mortality rate is meritorious.

Hemoglobin A$_{1c}$

Glycosylated hemoglobin A, commonly referred to as hemoglobin A$_{1c}$, is likely to be elevated in diabetes and the magnitude of the elevation generally correlates inversely with the degree of long-term control of plasma glucose concentration that has been achieved. Some investigators measure the total hemoglobin A$_1$ fraction, which includes A$_{1a}$, A$_{1b}$, and A$_{1c}$. Morris and colleagues (1985) also have shown a good correlation between glycosylated serum protein and blood glucose control over a 1-week period. Brans and colleagues (1982) found no correlation between maternal hemoglobin A$_{1c}$ levels measured at the time of delivery and either infant birthweight or neonatal hypoglycemia. Conversely, Hahm and associates (1983) reported a correlation between large infants and maternal hyperglucemia reflected by elevated hemoglobin A$_{1c}$ levels. Edidin and Menella (1983) also reported elevated glycosylated hemoglobin levels in both maternal and cord blood in cases of fetal macrosomia. It is emphasized that there are several pitfalls in the analysis of glycosylated hemoglobin (Garlick and co-workers, 1983).

Urine or Plasma Estriol Measurement

The daily measurement of 24-hour urinary estriol excretion, or of plasma unconjugated estriol concentration to monitor fetal well-being, in the past received considerable attention from many workers, including several whose reports are cited above. The majority of those cited no longer attempt serial measurements of estriol. Studies have been carried out at several centers to evaluate the benefits that might be achieved from monitoring estriol excretion at daily intervals during the latter half of the third trimester. As pointed out in Chapters 5 (p. 79) and 15 (p. 289), the bulk of evidence indicates that estriol measurements can be grossly misleading, often being "abnormally low" when the immature fetus is not otherwise compromised (Dooley and associates, 1984; Lavin and co-workers, 1983). The measurements are mentioned only for historical purposes.

Insulin Pump

Subcutaneous insulin infusion by a calibrated pump may be used during pregnancy. The pump has both advantages and disadvantages, and as emphasized by Kitzmiller and associates (1985) and Leveno and colleagues (1988), any salutary pregnancy effects have yet to be determined. If a distinct advantage to the mother and her fetus from its use can be documented, its use will undoubtedly become more popular during pregnancy.

Oral Hypoglycemia Agents

Tolbutamide and the other oral hypoglycemic agents are not used during pregnancy, but instead insulin is given. Tolbutamide in large doses is teratogenic in some animals, but there is no evidence that doses used clinically are teratogenic for humans. Serious hypoglycemia has been observed, however, in the newborn infants of mothers treated with tolbutamide.

Estrogen Treatment

For many years, White (1965) administered an estrogen and a progestin to diabetic mothers throughout much of pregnancy. Compounds used included estradiol or stilbestrol with either progesterone or ethisterone, or a mixture of estradiol valerate and 17-hydroxyprogesterone caproate. These hormones are no longer used by White (1978), and their elimination certainly has not adversely affected the improved pregnancy salvage witnessed in more recent years.

Hospitalization

Because of increased hospitalization costs, as well as reluctance of third-party payers for reimbursement, routine antepartum hospitalization for the overt diabetic woman is no longer commonly practiced. In our predominantly indigent population at Parkland Hospital, this practice was associated with a doubling of the perinatal mortality rate (Table 39–9). Specifically, for 266 insulin-dependent pregnant women routinely admitted to the High Risk Pregnancy Unit at 32 weeks from 1972 through 1982, the perinatal mortality was 4.5 percent. Bed space in this unit was then decreased, and from 1982 through 1985, diabetic women were not admitted routinely until 36 to 37 weeks, and for these 132 women, the perinatal mortality rate was 9 percent. This doubling of perinatal mortality was due solely to unexplained fetal death that typically occurred at about 36 weeks.

TIMING OF DELIVERY

Ideally, delivery of the overtly diabetic woman is accomplished close to term. At Parkland Hospital, because of experiences related above, currently these women are requested to enter the hospital at 34 weeks gestation and to stay until delivered. Typically the lecithin-spingomyelin ratio in amnionic fluid is measured at about 37 weeks and, if 2 or greater, delivery is effected during the 38th week. For women whose gestational age is known for certain, tests to determine fetal pulmonary maturation are not done and delivery is planned after 38 completed weeks. Until that time, the fetus is considered in no serious jeopardy as long as he is growing in utero and there are no other complications, especially overt maternal hypertension or gross hydramnios. If severe hypertension develops, delivery is carried out even though the L/S ratio is less than 2. Of 118 liveborn infants who were delivered according to this policy, all survived except one who had trisomy 18. Of the four stillbirths during the same period, one who died in utero at 34 weeks might have been salvaged if delivery had been performed even earlier (Leveno and co-workers, 1979). An L/S ratio of 2 or more as measured in our laboratory has served to exclude severe respiratory distress and its serious sequelae in infants of insulin-dependent diabetic mothers. It has become evident, however, from the experiences of others that in some circumstances identification of such a ratio does not always do so, especially in pregnancies complicated by gestational diabetes (Gabbe, 1985; Leveno and Whalley, 1982).

Others who report very favorable success rates have em-

TABLE 39–9. CHANGES IN PERINATAL MORTALITY IN 398 OVERTLY DIABETIC WOMEN RELATED TO THE TIME OF ROUTINE ADMISSION TO THE PARKLAND HOSPITAL HIGH-RISK PREGNANCY UNIT

Time	Policy	Percent		
		Stillbirths	Neonatal Deaths	Perinatal Mortality
1972–82 (n = 266)	Routine admission at 32 weeks	2.6	1.9	4.5
1982–85 (n = 132)	Routine admission at 36–37 weeks	7.6	1.6	9.0[a]

[a] Increase due to unexplained stillbirths.

Unpublished data courtesy of Drs. K. Leveno and P. Whalley.

phasized other plans of management in an effort to optimize the time selected for delivery. Most employ various tests of fetal well-being as described in Chapter 15 (p. 290). These tests are those biophysical techniques which include nonstress testing, the biophysical profile, and contraction stress testing. Golde and co-workers (1984) reported good perinatal results in diabetic pregnancies in which nonstress testing was used for screening and biophysical profiles and contraction stress testing performed for back-up. Nonstress testing twice weekly proved sufficient to assure fetal well-being in 90 percent of their patients. Gabbe (1985), as well as the American College of Obstetricians and Gynecologists (1986), recommend that serial nonstress tests be performed weekly beginning at 28 to 30 weeks. If nonreactive, then a contraction stress test is performed. At Parkland Hospital, for women hospitalized on the High Risk Unit, but not those followed as outpatients, assessment of fetal heart rate activity is done weekly. It is emphasized that acceleration with movement does not predict fetal health for seven days. Similarly, a reassuring test should not dissuade the physician to induce delivery in a woman whose clinical condition is deteriorating as in the case of severe preeclampsia.

METHOD OF DELIVERY

In the diabetic woman with an A or B White classification, cesarean section has been used commonly to avoid traumatic delivery of a large infant at or near term. In women with advanced classes of diabetes, especially those associated with vascular disease, the reduced likelihood of inducing labor safely remote from term also has contributed appreciably to an increased cesarean delivery rate. In the several reports cited above with low perinatal mortality, the cesarean section rates were more than 50 percent in Melbourne (Martin and colleagues, 1987), 55 percent in Los Angeles (Gabbe and colleagues, 1977), 69 percent in Boston (Kitzmiller and associates, 1978), 70 percent in a midwestern multicenter study (Schneider and co-workers, 1980), and 81 percent in Dallas (Leveno and associates, 1979). At Parkland Hospital, the cesarean delivery rate for overtly diabetic women has remained at about 80 percent for the past 15 years (K. Leveno, personal communication).

Labor induction may be attempted when the following criteria are met: (1) The fetus is not excessively large nor is the pelvis contracted. (2) Parity is not great. (3) The cervix is soft, appreciably effaced, and somewhat dilated. (4) The vertex is presenting and is fixed in the pelvis.

It is important to reduce considerably or delete the dose of long-acting insulin given on the day of delivery. Regular insulin should be utilized to meet most or all of the insulin needs of the mother at this time, since the insulin requirements typically drop markedly after delivery. We have found that constant insulin infusion by calibrated pump is most satisfactory. During and after either cesarean section or labor and delivery, the mother should be adequately hydrated intravenously as well as supplied with glucose in sufficient amounts to maintain normoglycemia. Plasma glucose levels should be checked frequently and regular insulin administered accordingly. The urine, or preferably the plasma, should be tested for ketones. It is not unusual for the woman to require virtually no insulin for the first 24 hours or so and then insulin requirments may fluctuate markedly during the next few days after delivery. Starvation with resistance to insulin must be avoided and infection must be quickly detected and promptly treated.

PERINATAL MORBIDITY

Even though perinatal mortality among infants of diabetic mothers has been reduced remarkably in recent years, troublesome morbidity persists. This is clearly evident in the reports just cited. The most serious morbidity is severe *congenital malformations*. Hopefully, more assiduous preconceptual metabolic control and its maintenance during embryogenesis will reduce the frequency and severity of these malformations.

Infants delivered at Parkland Hospital are taken to the Special Care Nursery for close observation. *Hypoglucemia* is commonplace in the newborn infant presumably due in part, at least, to persistent hyperstimulation of the fetal β-islet cells by chronic hyperglucemia. *Hypocalcemia* and *hyperbilirubinemia* are also common complications of the newborn period. Fortunately, these three are readily treatable. *Idiopathic respiratory distress* is likely to be somewhat more common among infants of diabetic mothers compared to other infants of the same gestational age, although Gabbe (1977) and Leveno (1979) and their co-workers did not find this to be a major problem.

It is extremely important that the large size and robust appearance of the newly-delivered infant not lead to inappropriate care. Although the infant may appear mature on the basis of his size, functionally he may be quite premature and must be so treated.

CONTRACEPTION

The two most common forms of reversible contraception, estrogen-progestin oral contraceptives and the intrauterine device, may be contraindicated in women who have overt diabetes when nonpregnant. Oral contraceptives are likely to intensify the diabetes. Moreover, the vascular disease that rather often is associated with diabetes may potentiate the variety of hazards from vascular disease that have been described following use of oral contraceptives in the absence of diabetes (see Chap. 42, p. 926). On the other hand, women with gestational diabetes are reported to have minimal adverse effects from triphasic preparations (Skouby and colleagues, 1985). The risk of pelvic infection from an intrauterine device is very likely increased in the diabetic woman. Therefore, barrier methods seem the best choice for reversible contraception followed by sterilization once it is certain that the woman wants no more children.

THYROID DISEASES

It is difficult at times to differentiate some of the usual findings of thyroid dysfunction, especially mild to moderate thyrotoxicosis, from several changes induced by normal pregnancy: (1) Cutaneous blood flow is increased appreciably and some degree of heat intolerance is common especially during warm weather. (2) Modest tachycardia is normal. (3) Plasma thyroxine concentration and thyroid radioiodine uptake are increased and both suggest hyperthyroidism. However, free thyroxine concentration is not increased and binding in vitro of triiodothyronine by resin is actually decreased, suggestive of thyroid hormone deficiency. These diverse changes in thyroxine and triiodothyronine are the consequence of estrogen-induced increases in binding proteins in plasma, especially thyroid binding globulin. In some studies, free thyroxine and triiodothyronine levels in clinically euthyroid pregnant women have been identified actually to be somewhat lower than in healthy nonpregnant women (Franklyn and co-workers, 1983).

HYPERTHYROIDISM

Helpful signs for identifying hyperthyroidism during pregnancy are (1) tachycardia which exceeds the increase caused by normal pregnancy, (2) abnormally elevated sleeping pulse rate, (3) thyromegaly, (4) exophthalmos, and (5) failure to gain weight despite normal or increased food intake. In the great majority of cases of thyrotoxicosis, the level of plasma thyroxine is markedly elevated even when compared to the elevated but normal values induced by pregnancy. At the same time, in vitro binding tests fail to demonstrate the appreciably decreased uptake of triiodothyronine that is characteristic of normal pregnancy. Rarely, hyperthyroidism may be associated with normal plasma thyroxine values, but instead, the triiodothyronine level is abnormally high, causing T_3 -*toxicosis*. Measurement of radioiodine uptake by the thyroid is usually contraindicated during pregnancy. **It is emphasized that careful clinical evaluation, using those signs described above, is most important to a successful pregnancy outcome.**

The vast majority of cases of thyrotoxicosis in pregnancy are caused by Graves' disease, and it is widely held that there is spontaneous remission in late pregnancy (Amino and colleagues, 1982; Burrow, 1985). As shown in Figure 39–11, exacerbation of disease was common at 10 to 15 weeks, then remission ensued in almost all, followed by postpartum exacerbation within 4 months in nearly 80 percent. Our clinical observations, discussed subsequently, do not support the concept of late pregnancy remission.

Treatment of thyrotoxicosis may be medical, or medical until such time as the mother is nearly euthyroid, and then surgical. Hyperthyroidism nearly always can be controlled by thioamide drugs, so that the disease need not be a serious threat to the mother. However, medical treatment has the potential for causing fetal complications. Propylthiouracil and methimazole readily cross the placenta and may induce fetal hypothyroidism and goiter. Therefore, it became a common, but unsound practice to give propylthiouracil in doses that effectively suppressed maternal thyroid activity while the mother was given thyroid hormone simultaneously to provide hormone to the fetus. Thyroxine so administered does not cross the placenta in significant amounts and it served only to increase the maternal requirements for propylthiouracil and thereby increase, rather than decrease, the risks to the fetus, including goiter. However, some persist in administering thyroxine in conjunction with antithyroid drugs (Ramsay and associates, 1983). A regimen employing propylthiouracil without thyroid hormone administration has been followed at Parkland Hospital for nearly three decades with very satisfactory pregnancy outcomes for women who become euthyroid (Davis and associates, 1988b).

The dose of propylthiouracil is empirical, and depending upon symptoms, the starting dose is 300 to 450 mg daily (Burrow, 1985). If necessary, this dose should be increased until the woman, by clinical assessment, appears to be only minimally thyrotoxic and the serum thyroxine level is reduced to the upper normal range for pregnancy. In our experiences, much higher doses than previously reported are needed for metabolic control (Davis and colleagues, 1988b). In more than 50 women with Graves' thyrotoxicosis given an initial mean propylthiouracil dose of 600 mg, in only a third did this induce remission. In another third, it was necessary to increase the dose, while in the other third, this dose was maintained. In only 10 percent of these women were we able to decrease the dose to 150 mg by the end of pregnancy as recommended by some (Burrow, 1985). Importantly, there was evidence for hypothyroidism in only

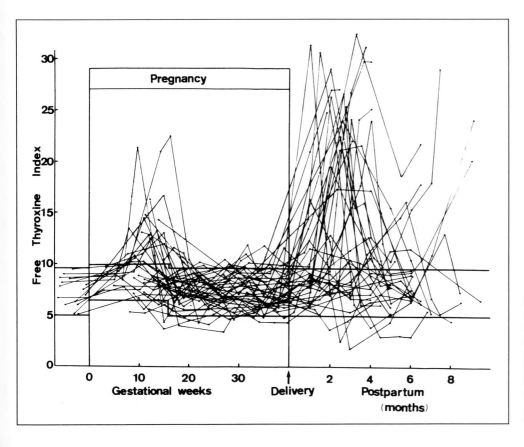

Figure 39–11. Early pregnancy and postpartum exacerbation of Graves' disease during 41 pregnancies in 35 untreated women considered to be in remission. Spontaneous sequential changes in free thyroxine index are plotted as a function of pregnancy duration. (*From Amino and colleagues: J Clin Endocrinol Metab 55:108, 1982.*)

one infant. Momotani and associates (1986) reported that cord serum thyroxine levels were lower in neonates born to thyrotoxic mothers who were taking propylthiouracil up until delivery when compared to mothers in whom the drug had been discontinued earlier. However, they found no dose-response relationship nor were any of these infants hypothyroid. In our experiences, principal morbidity and mortality are encountered in infants born to women who remain thyrotoxic despite therapy, or those who do not present for prenatal care (Table 39–10).

Thyroidectomy may be carried out after thyrotoxicosis has been brought under medical control. Opinions differ as to the wisdom of surgical treatment during the first trimester, a time when abortion is relatively common, or during the third trimester, when preterm labor may ensue. From the beginning of the second trimester until early in the third trimester, however, either for elective treatment, or for the woman who cannot adhere to medical treatment, or for women for whom drug therapy proves toxic, subtotal thyroidectomy may be the treatment of choice after appropriate pharmacological control.

Thyroid Storm or Heart Failure

In our experiences, thyroid storm is encountered rarely in untreated women during pregnancy and the puerperium (Davis and associates, 1989). Much more likely is heart failure apparently caused by long-term thyroxine effects on the myocardium, which are intensified by other pregnancy complications that include severe preeclampsia, infection, anemia, or combinations of these. Treatment consists of 1-g propylthiouracil plus 1-g potassium iodide given orally or through a nasogastric tube if the woman is unable to swallow. Propranolol may be given intravenously, but this must be done carefully if there is heart failure. A principal directive of therapy is aggressive treatment to treat serious hypertension, infection, and anemia.

Effects on the Neonate

Matsuura and colleagues (1988) presented evidence that neonatal thyrotoxicosis is caused by thyroid-stimulating antibodies transferred from the mother. Burrow and associates (1978) carried out a long-term study of the intellectual and physical development, including thyroid function, of children born to thyrotoxic mothers treated with propylthiouracil during pregnancy. Although the study was small, no adverse effects on

subsequent growth and development were identified. The prolonged administration of iodide to the mother along with propylthiouracil appears to increase appreciably the likelihood of obvious goiter in the fetus. Iodide should be used only preceding the time of thyroidectomy and *never* for long-term therapy.

Breast feeding has been considered by some to be contraindicated when the mother is taking antithyroid drugs, even though the concentrations of the antithyroid drugs in breast milk are low and therefore the amount of drug ingested by the infant is quite small. At least according to the American Academy of Pediatrics (1983), propylthiouracil is not contraindicated.

Even after being rendered euthyroid by surgery or radiation, women with Graves' disease may give birth to infants with manifestations of thyrotoxicosis, including goiter and exophthalmos. Thyroid-stimulating immunoglobulins, whose actions are similar to thyrotropin, are synthesized by the mother presumably as an autoimmune phenomenon, and these are transferred across the placenta and stimulate the fetal thyroid. The condition is suggested by a maternal history of thyrotoxicosis, identification of appreciable levels of a thyroid-stimulating immunoglobulin in maternal serum, a history of a previously affected fetus-infant, and by persistent fetal tachycardia. Cases have been reported in which the mother was given antithyroid medication to try to treat the fetus plus thyroxine to maintain maternal euthyroidism (Robinson and associates, 1979; Volpé and colleagues, 1984). The newborn may require antithyroid treatment for several weeks until these immunoglobulins are ultimately metabolized.

The infant recipient of thyroid-stimulating immunoglobulins and whose mother is treated up until the time of delivery with propylthiouracil may be euthyroid at birth but becomes hyperthyroid a few days later as the drug is cleared, but the thyrotoxic effect of the immunoglobulin persists.

HYPOTHYROIDISM

Hypothyroidism is diagnosed if the expected rise during pregnancy in the level of circulating thyroxine fails to take place and the level of thyrotropin is elevated. In most women, a history of surgical or radioiodine treatment, usually for Graves' thyrotoxicosis, will be elicited. Overt hypothyroidism complicating pregnancy is rare and is often associated with infertility. In our experiences from Parkland Hospital, those hypothyroid women who do become pregnant have a high incidence of preeclampsia and placental abruption with a correspondingly inordinate number of low birthweight and stillborn infants (Davis and colleagues, 1988). Heart failure also was encountered.

Perhaps much more common is *subclinical hypothyroidism*, which is characterized by elevated serum thyrotropin levels and normal serum thyroxine and triidothyronine levels unaccompanied by symptoms. Its effects on pregnancy outcome are unknown, but thyroxine replacement should be given. Jovanovic-Peterson and associates (1988) reported a high incidence of subclinical hypothyroidism in 26 of 51 pregnant women with type I diabetes. About a third of the 26 developed abnormally low serum thyroxine levels, and they usually also developed nephrotic-range proteinuria.

Effect on Fetus and Infant

In general, infants of hypothyroid mothers appear healthy without evidence of thyroid dysfunction (Montoro and co-workers, 1981). The infant of a mother with severe hypothyroidism may be a *cretin* if hypothyroidism followed maternal radioiodine therapy (not tracer doses) during pregnancy. Any infant whose

TABLE 39–10. PREGNANCY OUTCOME IN 60 WOMEN WITH OVERT THYROTOXICOSIS

Factor	Treated and Euthyroid (n = 36)	Thyrotoxic Despite Therapy (n = 16)	Untreated Thyrotoxicosis (n = 8)
Maternal Outcome			
Preeclampsia	2	3	2
Delivery (weeks)	38.6 ± 0.5	38.8 ± 1.1	33.1 ± 1.5
Heart failure	0	0	5
Neonatal Outcome			
Birthweight (g)	2,905 ± 97	2,665 ± 155	2,140 ± 164
Less than 2,000 g	1	1	2
Abortion	0	0	1
Stillbirth	0	2	4
Thyrotoxicosis	0	1	0
Hypothyroidism	1	0	0

From Davis and associates: Am J Obstet Gynecol, 160:63, 1989.

mother was so treated during pregnancy must be carefully evaluated and probably treated prophylactically for hypothyroidism. Abortion should be considered.

The clinical diagnosis of *congenital hypothyroidism* during the neonatal period is difficult to make and often is missed. This is unfortunate since if treatment is started early, mental retardation most often can be prevented. Such screening efforts are recommended by the American Academy of Pediatrics (1987), and in some states, including Texas, screening is mandatory. According to various reports based on mass screening of newborns, the frequency of congenital hypothyroidism detected is one in 4,000 to 7,000 infants. Most, but not all, infants with these conditions are detected and prompt treatment usually prevents mental retardation (Fisher, 1987).

OTHER THYROID DISEASES

Most other thyroid conditions encountered during pregnancy are rare and the woman is treated as if nonpregnant. *Hashimoto's thyroiditis* and *simple colloid goiter* are examples. *Thyroid nodules* pose a particular problem since radioiodine scanning is usually avoided during pregnancy. More recently, we have pursued a course of fine-needle aspiration to rule out malignancy, followed by attempts at suppression with thyroxine. Rosen and Walfish (1986) provided data from 30 pregnant women assessed for thyroid neoplasia because of a solitary nodule. Surprisingly, 43 percent of these women were found to have a malignancy and 37 percent had an adenoma. They recommend that surgery be performed for these women either during the middle trimester or to await until after delivery. With carcinoma, a delay in surgical therapy seems difficult to justify.

Postpartum hyperthyroidism is usually caused by painless lymphocytic thyroiditis that may be identified in 1 to 5 percent of women within about six months following delivery (Walfish and Chan, 1985). There is evidence that the condition is autoimmune mediated (Vargas and colleagues, 1988). It must be differentiated from an exacerbation of Graves' thyrotoxicosis as shown in Figure 39–11. The disease is usually self-limited, and it can be differentiated from the much more common Graves' disease by showing an abnormally low radioiodine uptake despite other evidence for mild thyrotoxicosis. Symptomatic treatment is usually given, but follow-up is important since some of these women will have Graves' disease and some will become hypothyroid.

PARATHYROID DISEASE

HYPERPARATHYROIDISM

Hyperparathyroidism is more common than once thought, and occurs more often in women with a peak incidence before the menopause. Despite this, only about 100 cases complicating pregnancy have been reported (Patterson, 1987; Pitkin, 1985). Whalley (1963) described four cases. One woman had parathyroid storm characterized by hypercalcemia and convulsions which were coexistent with chronic pyelonephritis and chronic hypertension. The combination of these might erroneously have been considered to be eclampsia.

The disease usually is caused by a parathyroid adenoma, but can be due to ectopic parathyroid hormone production, or rarely due to parathyroid carcinoma (Parham and Orr, 1987). Hyperparathyroidism causes hyperemesis, generalized weakness, renal calculi, pancreatitis, and psychiatric disorders and

adverse pregnancy outcomes are likely (Pitkin, 1985). Definitive treatment is surgical removal of the parathyroid adenoma.

Tetany has been noted occasionally in the newborn infants of mothers with hyperparathyroidism. At times, neonatal tetany alone has led to a search that identified a maternal parathyroid adenoma. Shangold and colleagues (1982) have reviewed much of the published experiences concerning hyperparathyroidism and pregnancy.

HYPOPARATHYROIDISM

Hypoparathyroidism is extremely uncommon. Treatment with 1-25-dihydroxyvitamin D_3 or large doses of vitamin D (50,000 to 150,000 U per day), together with calcium gluconate or calcium lactate (3 to 5 g daily), and a diet low in phosphates, usually prevents symptomatic hypocalcemia. The risk to the fetus from large doses of vitamin D has not been established. Whether these compounds cause cardiovascular and other anomalies is not clear.

DISEASES OF THE ADRENAL GLANDS

PHEOCHROMOCYTOMA

Pheochromocytoma is a rare but dangerous complication of pregnancy. Geelhoed (1983) reviewed a total of 89 cases in which 43 mothers died. Maternal death was much more common (58 versus 18 percent) if the tumor was not diagnosed antepartum. Using computed tomography and magnetic resonance imaging, tumor localization is now possible as shown in Figure 39–12. In some women, surgery may be performed during pregnancy, but in all cases, medical management with phenoxybenzamine or a similar drug is imperative. Favorable outcomes have been described more recently for women in whom the diagnosis was made late in pregnancy and the blood pressure controlled pharmacologically during cesarean section and tumor resection (Burgess, 1979; Schenker and Granat, 1982). In recent years, we have cared for three women in whom recurrent pheochromocytoma was identified during pregnancy. Pharmacological control of hypertension with phenoxybenzamine was successfully induced in all three. Two infants were healthy, but a third was stillborn in a mother with a massive tumor load who was receiving 100 mg daily of phenoxybenzamine. In all three women, resection of the tumor was carried out postpartum, one at the time of cesarean section and in the others at 2 and 6 months postpartum. The diagnosis, localization, and treatment of pheochromocytoma has been reviewed by Bravo and Gifford (1984).

ADDISON DISEASE

Before 1953, only 50 published cases of Addison disease in pregnancy had been identified, suggesting that untreated adrenal hypofunction caused sterility. With the advent of cortisone and related compounds, pregnancy has become much more common in women with adrenocortical hypofunction. It is important that a diagnosis made during pregnancy include the documentation of a lack of response to infused corticotropin (O'Shaughnessy and Hackett, 1984).

It is essential during pregnancy and the puerperium to observe the mother quite closely for evidence of either inadequate or excessive steroid replacement. Except at times of stress, replacement therapy need not be greater than in the nonpreg-

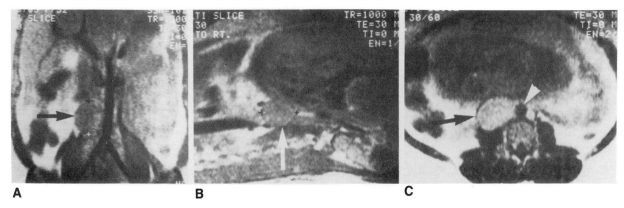

Figure 39–12. Magnetic resonance imaging of a nonadrenal pheochromocytoma in a woman 27-weeks pregnant. **A.** Coronal image obtained through the abdomen demonstrates a well-circumscribed, rounded mass (*arrow*) situated to the right of the aorta and approximately 2 cm above the bifurcation. **B.** Sagittal image obtained through the abdomen to the right of midline. The mass (*arrow*) can be seen just posterior to the fundus of the uterus and it compresses the inferior vena cava. **C.** Axial image demonstrates the relationship of the mass (*arrow*) to the aorta (arrow-head). The inferior vena cava is not visualized, probably as a result of compression. (*From Greenberg and co-workers: Radiology 161:475, 1986.*)

nant state. There may be little need during pregnancy for potent mineralocorticoid compounds. During and after labor and delivery or after a surgical procedure, the amount of steroid replacement should be increased appreciably to approximate the normal response in women with intact adrenal glands. It is important that shock from causes other than adrenocortical insufficiency be promptly recognized and treated, especially that caused by blood loss or bacterial septicemia.

CUSHING SYNDROME

Pregnancy associated with Cushing syndrome is rare and perhaps 35 cases have been reported (Geelhoed, 1983; Koerten and colleagues, 1986). Hypertension is inevitable, and preeclampsia and pulmonary edema are reported to be especially common if there is an adenoma. Liu and associates (1983) diagnosed Cushing syndrome in a woman who promptly thereafter conceived before given any treatment. The signs of Cushing syndrome increased appreciably during and after pregnancy. Spontaneous labor and delivery followed at 32 weeks and the infant survived. Three months postpartum, bilateral hyperplastic adrenal glands were resected. Abrahamson and colleagues (1986) reported successful resection at 17 weeks of a right-sided adrenal adenoma which had been localized by computed tomography.

PRIMARY ALDOSTERONISM

A few cases of primary aldosteronism in association with pregnancy have been reported. In view of the very high levels of aldosterone in normal pregnancies, it is not surprising that there may be amelioration of symptoms as well as of electrolyte disturbances during pregnancy (Biglieri and Slaton, 1967). Lotgering and colleagues (1986) reported a case in which a woman at midpregnancy presented with severe hypertension and hypokalemia. She was treated with aldosterone antagonists and antihypertensives and at 36 weeks was delivered by cesarean section of a severely growth-retarded but otherwise normal female infant without clitoromegaly. An adrenal adenoma was resected 2 months later.

DISEASES OF THE PITUITARY

PITUITARY MICROADENOMAS

Amenorrhea, galactorrhea, and hyperprolactinemia caused by pituitary microadenomas are amenable to therapy with bromocriptine. A relatively large number of pregnancies have now been observed in women so treated. Jewelewicz and Vande-Wiele (1980) concluded that the presence of a pituitary microadenoma without neurological or visual symptoms is not a contraindication to ovulation induction and pregnancy. Bromocriptine taken by the mother during pregnancy does not appear to affect the fetus adversely (Turkalj and associates, 1982).

The association of pregnancy and prolactin-secreting pituitary adenomas has been reviewed by Moltich (1985). In almost 250 women with previously untreated *microadenomas* who became pregnant, only four had symptoms during pregnancy and another 11 who were asymptomatic had radiographic evidence for enlargement. Symptomatic tumor enlargement was more common with *macroadenomas* and 15 percent of 45 such women developed headaches or visual field defects during pregnancy. Serial serum prolactin concentrations and visual field testing were not found to be effective, and Moltich recommends computed tomography during pregnancy only if symptoms develop. However, computed tomography was recommended for all women postpartum to assess pregnancy effects on the tumor. Symptomatic tumor enlargement during pregnancy is treated with bromocriptine and surgery is reserved for women with no response to this drug.

Development of *acromegaly* in a pregnant woman and in turn her fetus-infant has been described by Fisch and associates (1974). The mother was treated with x-irradiation to the pituitary fossa during the third trimester. The newborn infant presented a constellation of skeletal anomalies.

DIABETES INSIPIDUS

The condition is a rare complication of pregnancy. Only four cases have been cared for in the last 35 years at Parkland Hospital, during which time there were nearly 250,000 deliveries. This incidence is remarkably close to that cited by Hime and Richardson (1978). As long as the women took vasopressin appropriately for replacement therapy, their pregnancies progressed without serious complication. The specific agent of choice is the synthetic analogue of vasopressin, L-deamino-8d-arginine vasopressin. Most women with diabetes insipidus require increased doses during pregnancy, thought to be due to increased metabolic clearance, likely mediated through placental vasopressinase or oxytocinase (Dürr, 1987).

In a few instances of diabetes insipidus, there appeared to have been an impairment of labor, possibly caused by dimin-

ished or absent endogenous oxytocin (Hime and Richardson, 1978). Sende and associates (1975) were unable to detect oxytocin by radioimmunoassay in plasma of a pregnant woman with diabetes insipidus before labor, but during labor and puerperium there was a surge of oxytocin. A woman described by Chau and associates (1969) lactated normally, with measured milk ejection pressures comparable to those of normal lactating women.

Diabetes insipidus with or without anterior pituitary deficiency characteristic of *Sheehan syndrome* has been described following massive obstetrical hemorrhage and prolonged shock (Dürr, 1987).

DISEASES OF THE LIVER AND GALLBLADDER

Pregnancy normally induces appreciable change in many of the tests as well as some physical findings that usually are employed to assess liver function. Physiological alterations are considered in Chapter 7 and are summarized now: (1) serum albumin concentration is decreased about 25 percent, (2) serum urea nitrogen concentration is lowered, (3) serum alkaline phosphatase and leucine aminopeptidase activities are increased, (4) serum cholesterol and some lipids are increased, (5) excretion of sulfobromophthalein is delayed, and (6) palmar erythema and spider angiomata develop commonly.

Liver diseases complicating pregnancy more often than not are coincidental with pregnancy; however, there are some that are induced by pregnancy and, unless fatal, disappear following termination of gestation. Diseases induced by pregnancy include (1) intrahepatic cholestasis of pregnancy with or without icterus gravidarum, (2) acute fatty liver of pregnancy, (3) hepatocellular damage of varying intensity that is the direct consequence of severe preeclampsia and eclampsia, and (4) hepatic dysfunction associated with hyperemesis gravidarum.

INTRAHEPATIC CHOLESTASIS OF PREGNANCY

This syndrome also has been referred to as *recurrent jaundice of pregnancy, idiopathic cholestasis of pregnancy, cholestatic hepatosis, and icterus gravidarum*. The condition is characterized clinically by pruritus, icterus, or both. The major histological lesion is intrahepatic cholestasis with centrilobular bile staining without inflammatory cells or proliferation of mesenchymal cells. Its cause is unknown, but it appears to be stimulated in susceptible persons by high estrogen concentrations. For example, it has been identified as especially common among pregnant Scandinavian women and members of a tribe of Chilean Indians (Burroughs and colleagues, 1982; Steven, 1981). There is evidence that it may be an autosomal dominantly-inherited characteristic (Holzbach and colleagues, 1983).

Bile acids are incompletely cleared by the liver and accumulate in plasma of women with cholestasis. Levels typically are much greater than in normal pregnancy, and total bile acids may be elevated 30-fold and cholic acid 70-fold. Lunzer and associates (1986) studied serial serum levels of the glycine conjugate of cholic acid, cholylglycine, and observed that there was a threefold elevation during pregnancy in 297 normal women. About 10 percent of these women had an abrupt rise of cholylglycine beginning early in the third trimester, and half of these

had sustained pruritus until delivery. Other factors are involved since 20 percent of those with normally elevated cholylglycine levels had significant pruritus.

Modest hyperbilirubinemia results predominantly from retention of conjugated pigment. Sulfobromophthalein excretion is delayed appreciably and serum alkaline phosphatase may be elevated more so than is usual for pregnancy. Serum aspartate aminotransferase activity is usually mildly to moderately elevated. These changes disappear after delivery but often recur in subsequent pregnancies or when an oral contraceptive containing estrogen is taken.

Ultrasound examination often will serve to exclude bilary obstruction by gallstones, and if the serum aspartate aminotransferase is not appreciably elevated thereby excluding viral hepatitis, the likely diagnosis is cholestasis of pregnancy.

Pruitus associated with cholestasis is caused by elevated plasma bile salts and may be quite troublesome. Cholestyramine has been reported to provide relief; however, Shaw and associates (1982) did not find it to be effective. This too has been our experience at Parkland Hospital, and frequently there is only marginal clinical improvement despite 20 g of cholestyramine administered daily. Absorption of fat-soluble vitamins, already impaired, is magnified with cholestyramine. Thus, impaired coagulation as the consequence of vitamin K deficiency may develop, affecting both the mother and the fetus-neonate, unless supplemental vitamin K is provided.

Reid and associates (1976) reported appreciable pregnancy wastage among women with obstetric cholestasis. There were five stillbirths and one neonatal death among 56 pregnancies, intrapartum asphyxia was observed in five infants, 18 infants were delivered preterm, and five mothers had postpartum hemorrhage. Johnston and Baskett (1979) observed much lower pregnancy wastage but found an abnormally high incidence of preterm births and postpartum hemorrhage. Shaw and colleagues (1982) recommend close monitoring of fetal well-being with delivery once lung maturity has been achieved.

ACUTE FATTY LIVER OF PREGNANCY

Acute liver failure may occur with fulminant viral hepatitis, drug-induced hepatic toxicity, or acute fatty liver of pregnancy. The latter is fortunately a rare complication of pregnancy which often has proved to be fatal for both mother and fetus (Riely, 1987; Sherlock, 1983; Steven, 1981). The prominent histological

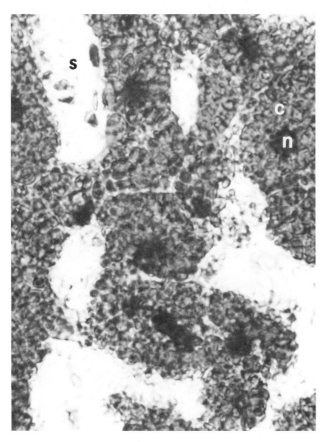

Figure 39–13. Fatty liver of pregnancy. High-magnification picture of liver plates and sinusoids **(s)** showing hepatocyte cytoplasm **(c)** filled with microvesicular fat globules. Note hepatocyte nucleus **(n)** remains centrally located in cell despite large amount of fat present. Oil red 0 fat stain. (*Courtesy of Dr. E. Eigenbrodt.*)

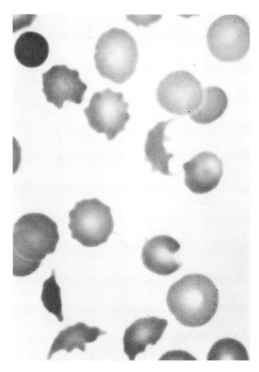

Figure 39–14. Schizocytes and echinocytes associated with microangiopathic (fragmentation) hemolysis in a woman with acute fatty liver of pregnancy. (*Courtesy of Ms. R. Mason.*)

abnormality consists of swollen hepatocytes in which the cytoplasm is filled with microvesicular fat with central nuclei and periportal sparing with minimal hepatocellular necrosis (Fig. 39–13). The mechanism by which pregnancy incites fatty liver changes is not known. Excessive doses of tetracycline, especially in women with impaired renal function, can cause these histological changes and clinical picture in nonpregnant individuals, as well as pregnant women. The histological changes in the liver with Reye's syndrome are also very similar to those of acute fatty liver of pregnancy, those sometimes induced by therapy with sodium valproate, or those seen with carnitine deficiency. Riely (1987) suggests that acquired abnormalities in mitochondria or intermediary metabolism of fatty acids, or both, may be the cause of fatty liver.

Acute fatty liver of pregnancy almost always develops in late pregnancy. It is probably more common with multifetal gestation. Typically, there is rapid onset of malaise, anorexia, nausea and vomiting, upper abdominal pain, and progressive jaundice. In many women there is also hypertension, proteinuria, and edema, all signs suggestive of preeclampsia. Often these signs have been detected shortly before or coincident with the development of clinical features of fatty liver of pregnancy. We have concluded that there is a spectrum of liver aberrations, and that liver failure is not universal, but rather it represents the most extensive involvement. Probably many milder cases of this syndrome go unnoticed, and are attributed to preeclampsia or mild hepatitis.

Fortunately, either the disease is self-limited or delivery arrests rapid deterioration of liver function. Recovery often follows as was the course in the case described now:

The 27-year-old gravida 2, para 2, white woman was transferred to Parkland Hospital 24 hours after vaginal delivery of an appropriately grown healthy infant at 38 weeks. About 5 days before delivery, malaise and anorexia developed and intensified. Epigastric pain developed and the color of the feces became light. She was admitted to active labor at which time jaundice was identified. She was not hypertensive at that time, but postpartum became so transiently. Vaginal bleeding persisted after delivery and she was given packed red cells, fresh-frozen plasma, and cryoprecipitate.

At the time of transfer coagulation was impaired as the consequence of severe hypofibrinogenemia, pathological elevation of fibrin degradation products, prolonged prothrombin time, and moderate thrombocytopenia. Vitamin K and fresh-frozen plasma were administered without dramatic effect clinically; however, ligation of a previously unrecognized bleeding vaginal artery helped to achieve hemostasis. Three days after delivery the intensity of the coagulopathy had diminished remarkably. Packed red cells were transfused to maintain the hematocrit near 30. Schizocytosis and echinocytosis, along with other evidence for microangiopathic hemolysis (Fig. 39–14), as well as bleeding from the vagina, were important in the genesis of anemia which developed postpartum and contributed to the hyperbilirubinemia.

Serum aspartate transferase activity was 200 units per L, and at no time was the activity elevated to the high levels that would be anticipated if the jaundice were the consequence of viral hepatitis. Liver function, as assessed by serial measurements of transaminases, alkaline phosphatase, bilirubin, and serum protein concentrations, was improved appreciably by 6 days after delivery. During that time, however, she had developed severe ascites which was treated by modest restriction of both sodium and fluids. During the illness she consumed a low-sodium general diet. She also received

150 g of glucose per day intravenously because of hypoglycemia. She ate little until late in the 1st week. Diuresis, beginning spontaneously on the 7th day, was vigorous, and resulted in a weight loss of 14 kg in less than a week.

Liver biopsy done on the 11th postpartum day confirmed the clinical diagnosis of acute fatty liver of pregnancy (Fig. 39–13). Renal function, which was impaired when she was first hospitalized (plasma creatinine 2.2 mg per dL), began to return to normal by the 5th day after delivery.

One year later, when evaluated for hepatic, renal, and hematological abnormalities, none persisted.

COAGULOPATHY

The pathogenesis of the coagulopathy that complicates fatty liver of pregnancy almost certainly results from increased consumption of procoagulants and their impaired production by the liver. Shown in Table 39–11 are laboratory data suggestive, at least, of consumptive coagulopathy in six women with idiopathic acute fatty liver of pregnancy cared for at Parkland Hospital. All had reduced plasma fibrinogen levels, and in some this was marked. The hypofibrinogenemia was accompanied by variable elevations of fibrin split products in serum. These observations are compatible with both decreased production and increased destruction of fibrinogen. Severe thrombocytopenia was not identified, but in some of these women, there was evidence for microangiopathic hemolysis. Echinocytes were the predominant red cell abnormality, presumably caused by impaired hepatic synthesis of various lipid components of the erythrocyte membrane, the lack of which renders red cells more susceptible to fragmentation hemolysis.

TREATMENT

Since spontaneous resolution usually follows delivery, many assume that delivery is essential for cure. Some authors recommend cesarean delivery to minimize the time until repair of hepatic function begins. In fact, immediate delivery also is likely to benefit the fetus who often is distressed. However, cesarean section in the presence of a severe coagulopathy may prove dangerous for the mother, as might an abdominal incision in circumstances in which severe hypoproteinemia and ascites are likely complications of the early puerperium. Because of severe maternal acidosis that develops from liver failure in severe cases, some fetuses are dead by the time the diagnosis is made, and many others tolerate poorly the stresses of even normal labor. Procrastination in effecting delivery can increase the risk

of coma and death from hyperammonemia usually further complicated by hypoglycemia, renal failure, acidosis, and severe hemorrhage.

Either coincidental with delivery, or with time, hepatic dysfunction resolves. In the interim, intensive medical support is required. Interestingly, subsequent pregnancies in an appreciable number of women who previously had severe acute fatty liver of pregnancy have proved to be totally benign.

Acute fatty liver of pregnancy has been reviewed extensively by Riely (1987) and Snyder and Hankins (1986).

PREECLAMPSIA–ECLAMPSIA

The liver may be involved in women with severe preeclampsia and eclampsia. Both the degree of dysfunction and the histological changes that develop can vary considerably. Typically, upper abdominal pain—epigastric or right upper quadrant—signals potentially dangerous liver involvement. Intrahepatic and subcapsular hemorrhage may develop and become so intense as to rupture the liver and produce extensive and even fatal hemorrhage. Hepatic dysfunction from preeclampsia and eclampsia is considered in Chapter 35 (p. 667).

HYPEREMESIS GRAVIDARUM

Nausea and vomiting of moderate intensity are especially common complaints from early pregnancy until about 16 weeks (see Chap. 14, p. 270). Fortunately, vomiting sufficiently pernicious to produce weight loss, dehydration, acidosis from starvation, alkalosis from loss of hydrochloric acid in vomitus, and hypokalemia, has become quite rare. Hyperemesis may lead to some elevation in serum transaminases, slight jaundice, and retention of sulfobromophthalein, all of which return to normal with hydration and feeding.

Treatment of pernicious vomiting of pregnancy comprises correction of fluid and electrolyte deficits and of acidosis or alkalosis. This requires appropriate amounts of sodium, potassium, chloride, lactate or bicarbonate, glucose, and water, which should be administered parenterally until the vomiting has been controlled. **Appropriate steps should be taken to detect other diseases, for example, gastroenteritis, cholecystitis, pancreatitis, hepatitis, peptic ulcer, and pyelonephritis.** In many instances, social and psychological factors contribute to the illness, as in the case of the young unwed mother who continues to live

TABLE 39–11. CONSUMPTIVE COAGULOPATHY AND ERYTHROCYTE CHANGES IN SIX WOMEN WITH ACUTE FATTY LIVER OF PREGNANCY

Patient	Plasma Fibrinogen[a] (mg per dL)	Serum FSP[b] (μg per mL)	Platelets[a] (per μL)	Reticulocytes (%)	Peripheral Erythrocytes (% Totals)		
					Abnormal	*Echinocytes*	*Schizocytes*
1	178	32	ND[c]	4.8	37	35	2
2	<20	128	73,000	2.6	ND	ND	ND
3	182	128	103,000	1.2	60	59	1
4	89	16	150,000	ND	10	9	1
5	95	16	189,000	ND	9	8	1
6	45	128	198,000	1.0	36	35	1

[a] Lowest value recorded
[b] FSP = Fibrin split products—highest value recorded
[c] ND = Not done

with her parents while they harass her because of her "sin." Commonly, in this circumstance, the woman improves remarkably while hospitalized, only to relapse after discharge. Positive assistance with psychological and social problems often proves quite beneficial. Only rarely is it necessary to interrupt the pregnancy. In some women with severe disease parenteral nutrition has been used as discussed on page 835.

VIRAL HEPATITIS

Hepatitis is the most common liver disease that afflicts pregnant women. There are at least five distinct types of viral hepatitis, and during their acute phases, they often are clinically quite similar. However, long-term complications in the mother and the risks to the fetus and infant are quite different.

The Centers for Disease Control has issued guidelines for patients when hospitalized with viral hepatitis. They recommend that feces, secretions, and bedpans and other articles in contact with the intestinal tract be handled with glove-protected hands. These precautions need not be continued once hepatitis A is excluded. Extra precautions such as double gloving during delivery may be wise in case of hepatitis B and non-A, non-B hepatitis. In these instances, instruments in contact with blood should be thoroughly cleaned and appropriately autoclaved.

VIRAL HEPATITIS A

Viral hepatitis A was previously referred to as *infectious hepatitis.* It is caused by an RNA picornavirus transmitted by the fecal-oral route. Individuals who are developing this disease shed the virus in their feces, and during the relatively brief period of viremia their blood is also infectious. The infection is usually spread by ingestion of contaminated blood or water, and the incubation period is about 2 to 7 weeks. The signs and symptoms are not very specific, and it may go undiagnosed or be considered an influenza-like illness unless jaundice is detected; however, the majority of cases are anicteric. Confirmation of the disease is made by detection of IgM antibody to hepatitis A, and although this may indicate acute infection, it also may persist for months (Snydman, 1985).

The effects of hepatitis A on pregnancy and vice versa are not dramatic in developed countries. However, at least in some underprivileged populations, both perinatal and maternal deaths are substantively increased. Treatment consists of a well-balanced diet and sedentary living. We have long followed the policy of hospitalizing all pregnant women with suspected hepatitis until it was clear that they were able to eat and drink and that liver function was improving, or at best not continuing to deteriorate.

There is no evidence that hepatitis A virus is teratogenic. Risk of transmission to the fetus appears to be nil and to the newborn infant quite small. The risk of preterm birth appears to be increased somewhat for pregnancies complicated by hepatitis A (Steven, 1981). The pregnant woman who has been recently exposed to hepatitis A should be given gamma globulin prophylactically as if she were not pregnant (see Chap. 14, p. 269).

VIRAL HEPATITIS B

Viral hepatitis B, once referred to as *serum hepatitis,* is found worldwide but is endemic in some regions, especially in Asia and in Africa. Hepatitis B is a DNA hepadnavirus and a variety of immunological markers to it have been identified in patients with acute or chronic disease, in those who have had the disease and now are immune, and in chronic carriers. The hepatitis B virus (Dane particle), core (c) antigen, and surface (s) antigen and their corresponding antibodies, and the e antigen and antibody are all detectable by various techniques.

The viral genome is incorporated into the hepatocyte nucleus where the viral core of DNA is produced, and the viral coat is produced in the cytoplasm. These viral components then are assembled and secreted from the cell as infectious virus. The e antigen correlates with infectivity and the presence of intact viral particles.

Hepatitis B disease is found most often among intravenous drug abusers, homosexuals, health care personnel, and individuals who have been treated often with blood products, for example, hemophiliacs. It is transmitted usually in infected blood or blood products, and in saliva, vaginal secretions, and semen; thus, a sexually transmitted disease.

The course of hepatitis B infection in the mother does not seem to be altered by pregnancy, at least in developed countries. Fulminant hepatitis may occasionally complicate hepatitis B infections, but does not seem to be more prevalent during pregnancy. As with hepatitis A, the likelihood for preterm delivery is increased. Treatment is supportive.

Transplacental transfer of the virus from the mother to the fetus except at delivery is thought to be rare (Goudeau and co-workers, 1983). Infection of the fetus-infant is by ingestion of infected material during delivery or exposure subsequent to birth. The infant may possibly obtain the virus through breast feeding. Some infected infants are asymptomatic, but others develop fulminant disease and succumb. The majority, nearly 85 percent, become chronic carriers who can infect others. They are also at appreciable risk for later development of hepatocellular carcinoma or cirrhosis or both.

The discovery of the e antigen of hepatitis B virus and its correlation with the number of circulating viral particles led to recognition that vertical transmission of hepatitis B correlates closely with the maternal e antigen status. Mothers with hepatitis B surface antigen and e antigen are very likely to transmit the disease to their infants, whereas those who are negative for e antigen but positive for anti-HBe antibody do not appear to transmit the infection.

Infection of the newborn infant whose mother chronically carries the virus usually can be prevented by the administration of hepatitis B immune globulin very soon after birth followed promptly by hepatitis B vaccine (Beasley and associates, 1983; Hsu and co-workers, 1988). For these reasons, the Centers for Disease Control (1988c) now recommends screening for all patients. If positive, and especially if e antigen is identified in the mother, the offspring should be given immune globulin and vaccine. Cruz and colleagues (1987), Kumar and associates (1987), and Wetzel and Kirz (1987) have provided data for the cost-effectiveness of such screening for inner-city lower socioeconomic women in Gainesville, Cleveland, and Chicago. Surface antigen positivity prevalence was about 1 percent, but risk factors were not predictive. Wetzel and Kirz emphasized that detection of one case of hepatitis B antigenemia costs only half as much as to detect one case of syphilis! Arevalo and Washington (1988) reviewed the literature and calculated that routine screening of all American women would result in net savings of $105 million annually.

DELTA HEPATITIS

Delta hepatitis, a recently described RNA virus, is a hybrid particle with a hepatitis B surface antigen coat and a delta core. The virus must coinfect with hepatitis B and cannot persist in serum longer than hepatitis B virus. Anti-delta antibody is produced only transiently unless chronic infection develops.

Transmission is similar to hepatitis B viral infection. Generally, simultaneous infection with B and delta hepatitis is not more virulent than B alone; however, particularly virulent epidemics in homosexuals and parenteral drug abusers have been associated with a case fatality rate of 5 to 10 percent (Dienstag and colleagues, 1987; Lettau and colleagues, 1987). Neonatal transmission has been reported, but it seems reasonable to assume that hepatitis B vaccination will prevent delta hepatitis.

NON-A, NON-B HEPATITIS

Nearly 90 percent of individuals who develop hepatitis after blood or blood products have non-A, non-B hepatitis. In one study, 18 of 842 cardiac surgery patients developed post-transfusion hepatitis and 14 were attributed to non-A, non-B hepatitis (Cossart and colleagues, 1982). Most cases are anicteric and are not diagnosed. After transfusion-related acute infections, about 50 percent of patients have an abnormal transaminase levels for a year, and most of these have histological evidence for chronic active hepatitis (Dienstag and associates, 1987). Unfortunately, 20 percent of these patients will develop cirrhosis by 10 years. The disease also may be contracted from an infected sexual partner, and the injection of some preparations of human immunoglobulin has been implicated in the causation of non-A, non-B hepatitis (Lane, 1983).

There are at least two variants, although current terminology would allow an unlimited number since most yet unidentified viruses that cause hepatitis would be classified as such. For example, hepatitis from *cytomegalovirus* or *Epstein-Barr* virus probably has been classified in the past as non-A, non-B, but now can be excluded by detecting cytomegalovirus titers and by tests for mononucleosis. Hepatitis from *herpesvirus* is frequently fatal (Wertheim and co-workers, 1983), and because of its rarity it will seldom be confused with non-A, non-B hepatitis.

Studies to evaluate immune serum globulin for prophylaxis against non-A, non-B hepatitis have been somewhat disappointing. Nonetheless, it probably should be given to the newborn of the mother with active disease since it may prevent acquisition of the disease by the offspring.

CHRONIC ACTIVE HEPATITIS

The effect of pregnancy on chronic active hepatitis and vice versa will depend in large part on the intensity of the disease process, which has a propensity to progress to cirrhosis, portal hypertension, hepatic failure, and shortened life span. When severe, anovulation is common. Adrenal glucocorticoid and immunosuppressive drugs have increased both fertility and survival in those with autoimmune chronic active hepatitis.

Chronic active hepatitis does not necessarily warrant therapeutic abortion. Steven and associates (1979) concluded that with chronic active hepatitis (1) fertility is reduced, but pregnancies which do occur can proceed without serious detriment to the mother if prednisolone treatment is maintained, (2) fetal loss will be increased, and (3) preterm delivery will be common

but malformations are not increased. The few women who we have managed have done well, but since their long-term prognosis is poor, sterilization should be considered.

CIRRHOSIS

Women with cirrhosis are very likely to be infertile. Cheng (1977) reviewed the clinical features of pregnancy in women with hepatic cirrhosis and concluded that perinatal loss is high and the maternal prognosis grave. Esophageal varices were prone to bleed with fatal hemorrhage as the consequence.

Schreyer and associates (1982) provided another review of hepatic cirrhosis complicating pregnancy. There were 69 pregnancies in 60 women without shunts and 28 pregnancies in 23 women who had undergone portal decompression. These authors also confirmed the high morbidity and appreciable mortality associated with cirrhosis. Severe gastrointestinal hemorrhage was increased sevenfold in nonshunted patients compared to those who had been shunted (24 versus 3.3 percent). The authors raised the possibility that the high incidence of esophageal hemorrhage and, in turn, the high mortality rate might be decreased by prophylactic portal-systemic shunting but hasten to emphasize that the procedure and its sequelae are not benign.

LIVER TRANSPLANT AND PREGNANCY

Walcott and associates (1978) described the delivery of a normal infant at term after an uncomplicated prenatal course even though the mother had undergone a liver transplant because of necrosis from hepatic vein thrombosis two years before. She was being treated continuously with azathioprine and prednisolone, and did not ovulate until treated with clomiphene citrate.

CHOLELITHIASIS AND CHOLECYSTITIS

There is a greater frequency—2 or 3 times as high—of cholelithiasis in women than in men. Gallbladder kinetics during pregnancy have been investigated by Braverman and associates (1980) using real-time sonography. After the first trimester, both gallbladder volume during fasting and residual volume after contracting in response to a test meal were twice as great as in nonpregnant subjects. Incomplete emptying may result in retention of cholesterol crystals, a prerequisite for cholesterol gallstones. These findings are supportive, at least, of the view that pregnancy increases the risk of gallstones. Presumably, the very high progesterone levels that characterize the second and third trimester of pregnancy are responsible for the diminished gallbladder motility. Singletary and colleagues (1986) documented that gallbladder tissue has both nuclear and cytosolic receptors for estrogens and progesterone. Progesterone has been shown to impair the gallbladder response to exogenously administered cholecystokinin in experimental animals.

Acute cholecystitis during pregnancy or the puerperium, in general, is managed in a similar manner as for nonpregnant women. About 75 percent of nonpregnant women with acute cholecystitis diagnosed for the first time will respond to medical therapy within 2 to 7 days. The other 25 percent develop complications that include gangrene and perforation, and surgical therapy is mandatory. About one-fourth of those whose symptoms undergo remission will have a recurrence within 1 year and more than half will do so within 5 years. While most now recommend cholecystectomy, optimal timing of surgery even in the nonpregnant woman is debated.

Landers and colleagues (1987) reported their experiences with 30 women with acute cholecystitis complicating pregnancy. The incidence was about 1 in 1,000 deliveries. Despite the fact that 21 of these women presented for care before the third trimester, these investigators elected medical therapy in 25 which was successful in 21. Four patients required cholecystectomy for persistent or worsening pain. In the other five women, cholecystectomy was done primarily. Gallstones were successfully visualized in 96 percent of women undergoing ultrasonic scanning.

If cholecystectomy is to be performed during pregnancy, the second trimester is the optimal time since the risk of spontaneous abortion or preterm labor and delivery is reduced and the uterus is not yet large enough to impinge on the field of operation. **Regardless, when surgery is thought to be indicated in the pregnant women, procrastination should be avoided.**

Delay can only place the woman and her fetus in greater jeopardy. At times, gallbladder drainage may be the procedure of choice. Recent surgery does not complicate labor except for the discomfort from the incision.

Hill and associates (1975) described 20 women undergoing cholecystectomy during pregnancy at the Mayo Clinic. There was one spontaneous abortion at 10 weeks gestation, almost 42 days after the operation. Maternal morbidity was low.

Asymptomatic Gallstones

Gallstones are not uncommon findings in asymptomatic women undergoing sonography during pregnancy or upon routine upper abdominal exploration at the time of cesarean section. Stauffer and colleagues (1982) and Chesson and co-workers (1985) found, respectively, an incidence of asymptomatic stones of 2.5 and 4.2 percent at the time of routine obstetrical ultrasonic evaluation in over 500 women. Although ideal treatment for silent stones is debated, pregnancy is not the appropriate time for surgical removal if they remain asymptomatic.

GASTROINTESTINAL DISORDERS

During normal pregnancy the gastrointestinal tract and its appendages undergo changes, both anatomical and functional, that can alter appreciably the criteria for diagnosis and treatment of several diseases to which they are susceptible. For example, heartburn has been said to occur in half of women at some time during pregnancy, and this has been attributed to reduced physiological tone in the lower esophageal sphincter caused by progesterone (Cohen, 1980). Importantly, during advanced pregnancy symptoms of gastrointestinal disease become difficult to assess and physical findings are greatly obtunded by the large uterus and its contents. A considerable degree of vigilance and a high index of suspicion are needed to diagnose many of these complications.

APPENDICITIS

Pregnancy does not predispose to appendicitis, but reflecting the general prevalence of the disease, its incidence is about 1 in 2,000 pregnancies, as shown in Black's extensive review (1960). Pregnancy often makes diagnosis more difficult: (1) Anorexia, nausea, and vomiting that accompany normal pregnancy are fairly common symptoms of appendicitis. (2) As the uterus enlarges, the appendix commonly moves upward and outward toward the flank, so that pain and tenderness may not be prominent in the right lower quadrant (Fig. 39–15). (3) Some degree of leucocytosis is the rule during normal pregnancy. (4) During pregnancy especially, other diseases may be readily confused with appendicitis, such as pyelonephritis, renal colic caused by a stone or kinking of a ureter, placental abruption, and red or carneous degeneration of a myoma.

Appendicitis increases the likelihood of abortion or preterm labor, especially if there is peritonitis. The fetal loss rate, therefore, in most series is about 15 percent. As the appendix is pushed progressively higher by the growing uterus, containment of the infection by the omentum becomes increasingly unlikely and appendiceal rupture causes generalized peritoni-

tis. The latter is more common if treatment is delayed and gangrene supervenes. Acute appendicitis in the last trimester, therefore, may carry a poor prognosis. Although antimicrobials have reduced the mortality rate from acute appendicitis in pregnancy, it remains a serious complication of gestation.

If appendicitis is suspected, then treatment, regardless of the stage of gestation, is immediate surgical exploration (Cunningham and McCubbin, 1975; Gomez and Wood, 1979). **Even though diagnostic errors sometimes lead to the removal of a normal appendix, it is better to operate unnecessarily than to postpone intervention until generalized peritonitis has developed.** In most reports, the diagnosis is verified in slightly less than half of women who undergo surgical exploration. According to DeVore (1980), the mortality with perforative appendicitis during pregnancy is 4 percent. This increased mortality rate in the obstetrical patient is due in most cases to surgical delay.

It is important that during surgery and the period of recovery both hypoxia and hypotension be avoided. Intravenous antimicrobials are given if there is gangrene, perforation, or a periappendiceal phlegmon. If this is done promptly, and generalized peritonitis does not develop, then the prognosis is quite good. Seldom, if ever, is cesarean section indicated at the time of appendectomy, and aside from local tenderness, a recent abdominal incision should present no problem during labor and vaginal delivery.

In some of these cases in our experiences at Parkland Hospital, undiagnosed appendicitis in all likelihood stimulated labor, and in many of these cases, it was before term. The large uterus helped to contain infection locally, but after delivery when the uterus rapidly empties, the walled-off infection was disrupted with spillage of free pus into the peritoneal cavity. In these cases, an acute surgical abdomen is encountered postpartum.

Simply because it is coincidental, appendicitis during the early puerperium is rare. In some cases, especially with early appendicitis, there is difficulty in diagnosis because of the normal robust leucocytosis as well as the frequency of other dis-

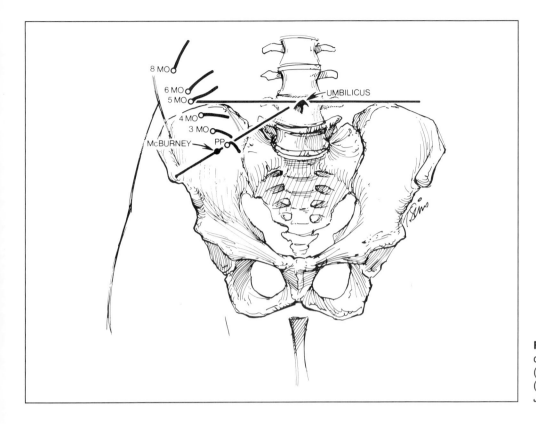

Figure 39–15. Changes in position of appendix as pregnancy advances (MO = month, PP = postpartum). (*Modified from Baer and associates: JAMA 92:1539, 1932.*)

eases with similar signs and symptoms. Anorexia with any evidence of peritoneal irritation such as distension and lack of bowel sounds should suggest appendicitis. **It is worth emphasizing that puerperal pelvic infections typically do not cause peritonitis (Chap. 27, p. 467).**

UPPER ABDOMINAL PAIN

Most obstetricians, but not most internists or gastroenterologists, are aware that upper abdominal pain—epigastric or right upper quadrant—can be an ominous sign of severe preeclampsia and act accordingly. An ultrasonic examination negative for gallstones, or a normal serum amylase value, or absence of free acid in gastric juice does not serve to exclude serious disease but rather supports the diagnosis of severe preeclampsia or eclampsia.

PEPTIC ULCER

An active peptic ulcer is extremely uncommon during pregnancy, and complications such as perforation or hemorrhage are even more rare. Conversely, women with a symptomatic peptic ulcer most often note considerable improvement during pregnancy. This has been attributed to the mucus-stimulating effects of progesterone as well as decreased gastric acid production.

Occasionally, especially during early pregnancy, nausea and vomiting may be accompanied by worrisome upper gastrointestinal bleeding. The obvious concern is that there is a bleeding peptic ulceration; however, in our experiences, most of these women have minute mucosal tears near the gastro-esophageal junction, or so-called *Mallory–Weiss* tears. These women usually respond promptly to conservative measures that include iced-saline irrigations, antacids and cimetidine. Rarely, blood transfusions are needed. **Endoscopy, if indicated, should not be withheld because of pregnancy.**

HIATAL HERNIA

Rigler and Eneboe (1935) performed upper gastrointestinal radiological examinations in 195 unselected women in the last trimester of pregnancy. Among 116 multiparas, 18 percent had hiatal hernias, and among 79 primigravidas, 5 percent had such hernias. When 10 of these women were reexamined 1 to 18 months postpartum, hernias were observed in only three. Hiatal hernias seen during pregnancy may be produced by intermittent but prolonged increase in intra-abdominal pressure. These hernias are an occasional cause of vomiting, epigastric pain, and even bleeding from ulceration.

ACHALASIA

Achalasia is a motor disorder of esophageal smooth muscle in which the lower sphincter does not relax properly with swallowing and there are abnormal esophageal contractions. The condition has received little attention as a pregnancy complication, but it has been said to be worsened by pregnancy. However, Mayberry and Atkinson (1987) described pregnancy outcomes in 20 such women and reported no excessive reflux esophagitis compared to nonpregnant women with achalasia. Of 16 women who became pregnant after symptoms developed, 11 had no change in symptomatology, two improved, and three worsened.

PANCREATITIS

Pancreatitis complicating pregnancy is uncommon. Unlike non-pregnant patients, these women seldom have associated alcoholism. In our experiences, associated cholelithiasis is common. The diagnosis of pancreatitis may be more difficult to confirm since some, but not all, have reported that normal pregnancy is associated with increased serum amylase concentrations. Kaiser and associates (1975) reported that serum amylase values were increased fourfold at midpregnancy compared to early pregnancy. However, Strickland and colleagues (1984) found no significant change in 413 women studied at various stages of gestation and again six weeks postpartum. If the diagnosis is uncertain, some advocate measuring the amylase:creatinine clearance ratio, but this has not gained widespread usage. Serial determinations of serum amylase and lipase activity remain the best methods to confirm the clinical diagnosis. Importantly, amylase values do not correlate with the severity of disease.

The principles of therapy are the same as for nonpregnant patients, and if the diagnosis is secure, then treament is medical. Ultrasonic or radiological examination, including *endoscopic retrograde cholangiopancreatography (ERCP)* may be necessary to visualize associated gallstones. Nasogastric suction is begun and intravenous fluids are given to ensure adequate blood volume as indicated by urine output. Careful monitoring for severely ill women is essential, and bad prognostic signs include respiratory insufficiency, hypotension, need for massive fluid replacement, and hypocalcemia. In most women, mild inflammation will subside in response to conservative therapy, but in some who remain ill, surgical exploration may be lifesaving. In these women, fetal loss is high because of associated hypovolemia, hypoxia, and acidosis.

After discharge, these women are followed closely for development of pancreatic pseudocysts, which may cause recurrent pain or pancreatitis, and they may even rupture. Sonographic evaluation of the pancreas will detect most of these complications, but limited computed tomography, or magnetic resonance imaging may be necessary. Corlett and Mishell (1972) and Wilkinson (1973) have reviewed pancreatitis and pregnancy and stress the necessity for prompt medical management.

INTESTINAL OBSTRUCTION

Intestinal obstruction is a grave complication of pregnancy and results most frequently from pressure of the growing uterus on intestinal adhesions that were formed after previous abdominal surgical procedures. The mortality rate can be very high, principally because of errors in diagnosis, late diagnosis, reluctance to operate on a pregnant woman, and inadequate preparation for surgery. Limited x-ray examinations, including plain abdominal films, and those following administation of soluble contrast medium, either orally or by enema, should be done if indicated.

Kohn and colleagues (1944) reported a remarkable case in which the same patient was operated upon for *volvulus* four times, three of the operations having been performed in the course of two pregnancies. In a review of the literature, they collected 79 cases of volvulus in pregnancy. In one third of the cases reported by Harer and Harer (1958), emptying the uterus by cesarean section was necessary to obtain proper exposure.

Volvulus, especially of the cecum, has been observed early in the puerperium after cesarean section (Pratt and colleagues, 1981).

INFLAMMATORY BOWEL DISEASE

Chronic inflammatory bowel disease, either ulcerative colitis or Crohn disease, is relatively common in women of childbearing age, and thus either may complicate pregnancy. Donaldson (1985) addressed four questions concerning these disorders and concluded the following: (1) Pregnancy does not increase the likelihood of an attack of inflammatory bowel disease. If the disease is quiescent in early pregnancy, then flares are uncommon, but if they develop, they may be severe. (2) Active disease at conception increases the likelihood of poor pregnancy outcome. (3) Diagnostic evaluations, including limited radiological studies, should not be postponed if their results are likely to affect management in a substantive way. (4) The usual treatment regimens, including corticosteroids, may be continued during pregnancy, and if indicated, surgery should be performed.

ULCERATIVE COLITIS

In an analysis of one of the largest series reported, Crohn and associates (1956) found that colitis that was quiescent at the beginning of gestation was reactivated during pregnancy, usually in the first trimester, in about half the cases. If the colitis was already active at the time of conception, it was materially aggravated in three-quarters of the cases. They emphasized also the excessive and prolonged severity of postpartum recurrences.

In an extensive review of more than 1,000 cases, Miller (1986) reported that ulcerative colitis quiescent at conception was worsened during pregnancy in about one third of cases. However, women with active disease at the time of conception had a worse prognosis (Table 39–12).

When ulcerative colitis becomes worse in gestation, the etiological factor may be psychogenic, rather than related to any intrinsic effect of pregnancy. The woman's fear that pregnancy will aggravate her disease, for example, may precipitate an exacerbation. Reassurance is therefore an important part of management. As indicated above, the disease is treated as if the woman were not pregnant. We occasionally have employed parenteral nutrition for women with severe exacerbations. In the very few cases in which emergency surgery for *toxic mega-*

TABLE 39–12. EFFECT OF PREGNANCY ON INFLAMMATORY BOWEL DISEASE

Condition	Percent		
	Improved	No Change	Worse
Inactive disease at conception			
Ulcerative colitis (n = 528)	—	66	34
Crohn disease (n = 186)	—	73	27
Active disease at conception			
Ulcerative colitis (n = 227)	27	24	45
Crohn disease (n = 93)	34	32	33

From Miller: J Royal Soc Med 79:221, 1986.

colon was performed, the results have been poor, and one woman died from sepsis.

REGIONAL ENTERITIS

There is no evidence that pregnancy exerts adverse effects on the course of Crohn's disease or that there is increased mortality (Fieldring and Cooke, 1970; Norton and Patterson, 1972). Miller (1986) reported findings very similar to those with ulcerative colitis, and disease quiescent at conception carries a good prognosis (Table 39–12). Homan and Thorbjarnarson (1976) observed relapses in one fourth of postpartum women with Crohn's disease. Abortion, preterm delivery, and stillbirths were not increased.

Parenteral hyperalimentation has been used successfully for women with severe recurrences of inflammatory bowel disease during pregnancy (Lee and colleagues, 1986). We also have had success with this at Parkland Hospital, and have used it for women with both types of inflammatory bowel disease.

Ostomy and Pregnancy

Women with a colostomy or an ileostomy are not prohibited from conception. Gopal and colleagues (1985) described 82 pregnancies in 66 women following ostomy, usually done for inflammatory bowel disease. Although stomal dysfunction was common, it responded to conservative management in all cases. Bowel obstruction developed in six women and in three surgery was necessary. Ileostomy prolapse was surgically corrected in three women during pregnancy or at cesarean section, and in a fourth postpartum. The cesarean section rate was 37 percent, and one third of these were done because of prior abdominoperineal resection.

PARENTERAL NUTRITION

For some of the gastrointestinal disorders discussed above, parenteral feeding or hyperalimentation, may be considered. Its purpose is to provide calories, essential amnio acids, vitamins, and minerals when the gastrointestinal tract must be kept quiescent. Peripheral venous access may be adequate for supplemental nutrition, however, jugular or subclavian venous catherization is necessary for total parenteral nutrition which is hyperosmolar.

Catanzarite and associates (1986) and Lee and colleagues (1986) have reviewed the relatively large number of women who have been given parenteral nutrition ranging from 1 to 37 weeks during pregnancy. In about half, nutritional supplementation was given for 4 weeks or less. Complications were identified in about one third, and one that is particularly worrisome is the reversible Wernicke–Karsakoff psychosis which complicated 10 percent of cases. Lee and colleagues (1986) emphasize that parenteral nutrition for the woman with diabetic gastroenteropathy is particularly hazardous and they reported one antepartum maternal death and four women with deteriorating renal function. Sepsis is also common. Nutritional support costs about $4,000 per week, and Catanzarite and colleagues (1986) rightly caution that careful informed consent with patient participation in decision making is important.

OBESITY

Marked obesity is a hazard to the pregnant woman and her fetus. Johnson and colleagues (1987) described the pregnancy outcomes of 588 women who weighed more than 250 pounds and who were cared for at the University of Iowa from 1961 to 1980. Complications were common and those found to be significantly different when compared to a group of control women who weighed less than 200 pounds are compared in Table 39–13. Hypertension, diabetes, and postterm pregnancy were substantively increased and this led to a higher oxytocin induction and augmentation rate, as well as a doubled primary cesarean rate. Our experiences at Parkland Hospital are similar, and we also have identified obesity, commonly further complicated by hypertension, to be a cause of peripartum heart failure (Cunningham and associates, 1986). Kliegman and Gross (1985) reported similar complications in their review.

Management of obesity during pregnancy is a challenge. A program of weight reduction utilizing a diet restricted in calories but providing all essential nutrients commonly has been recommended for obese pregnant women. It seems unrealistic that weight reduction will be substantive, but if such a regimen is chosen, it is mandatory that the quality of the diet be monitored closely and that ketosis be avoided.

SURGICAL PROCEDURES FOR OBESITY

Jejunoileal Bypass

Jejunoileal bypass has been followed by significant long-term morbidity and mortality, and the operation has been abandoned by most. In some cases, however, a small-intestinal bypass operation performed to treat obesity was followed by pregnancy. Knudsen and Källén (1986) reported results of the Danish-Swedish registry of 77 pregnancies after intestinal bypass. They described a lower mean birthweight, shorter gestations, and increased small for gestational age infants when compared to normal control women.

Eight pregnant women with a jejunoileal bypass have been cared for at Parkland Hospital. Seven of the pregnancies were quite benign. All of the women were given supplemental iron, folic acid, vitamin B_{12}, as well as a commercially available prenatal vitamin-mineral preparation. Seven infants were appropriately grown and in good health. In one woman who had previously undergone bypass operation which excluded nearly all of the small intestine and utilized an end-to-end anastomosis, pregnancy created myriad problems: She lost appreciable

TABLE 39–13. PERCENTAGE OF COMPLICATIONS THAT WERE SIGNIFICANTLY INCREASED IN 588 OBESE (MORE THAN 250 POUNDS) WOMEN COMPARED TO 588 NONOBESE (LESS THAN 200 POUNDS) CONTROLS

Complication	Obese	Nonobese
Diabetes		
All types	10	2
Gestational	8	0.7
Hypertension	28	3
Postterm pregnancy	15	4
Oxytocin induction	23	8
Oxytocin augmentation	17	8
Macrosomic infant	24	7
Shoulder dystocia	5	0.6
Primary cesarean section	13	6
Wound infection	38	10
Excessive blood loss	38	14

Modified from Johnson and colleagues: Surg Gynecol Obstet 164:431, 1987.

weight while consuming between 6,000 and 9,000 calories per day! A slightly growth-retarded infant was delivered by cesarean section which was necessitated by a prolapsed cord. He subsequently thrived. Postpartum, the mother developed severe hypoproteinemia, hypocalcemia with tetany, hypokalemia, hypomagnesemia, and vitamin K deficiency sufficiently intense to prolong appreciably the prothrombin time. She responded well to vitamin K, calcium gluconate, potassium chloride, magnesium sulfate (given parenterally), and to a generous high-protein diet.

Gastric Bypass

Gastroplasty, in which stomach volume is reduced by 90 percent using a variety of surgical techniques, is used currently to treat morbid obesity. Printen and Scott (1982) have described the experience during 51 pregnancies in 45 women who under-

went *gastric bypass* surgery because of morbid obesity. Of the 46 infants delivered, fetal growth retardation was not a problem, but one had a serious malformation. They concluded that neither the mother nor the developing fetus is endangered unduly by a pregnancy conceived subsequent to the period of rapid postoperative weight loss.

Richards and colleagues (1987) reported similar experiences from 57 pregnancies cared for at the University of Utah. These women weighed an average of 194 pounds before and 147 after surgery. Using pregnancies before gastroplasty as controls, they showed that the mean birthweight decreased from 3,600 g to 3,200 g, and that large for gestational age infants were delivered to 16 percent of the women after bypass surgery compared to 37 percent before. Importantly, the incidence of hypertension complicating pregnancy fell from 46 to 9 percent in women who had lost weight.

CONNECTIVE-TISSUE DISORDERS

Connective-tissue or collagen-vascular disorders are a group of diseases characterized principally by connective tissue abnormalities which are immunopathologically mediated as the consequence of a variety of autoantibodies. A review of the pathogenesis and clinical features of several of these disorders has been provided by Kohler and Vaughan (1982) and Mor-Yosef and colleagues (1984). Although the pathogenesis for all of these has not been elucidated, immunologically-mediated tissue destruction of various organ systems is the common denominator. Diseases in this category include systemic lupus erythematosus, rheumatoid arthritis, progressive systemic sclerosis (scleroderma), mixed connective tissue disease, Sjögren syndrome, ankylosing spondylitis, Reiter and Behcet syndromes, and a multitude of vasculitis syndromes.

SYSTEMIC LUPUS ERYTHEMATOSUS

Lupus is notoriously variable in its presentation, course, and outcome. The American Rheumatism Association has provided the following revised criteria for the identification of systemic lupus (Tan and associates, 1982). If any four or more of the 11 following criteria are present, serially or simultaneously, the diagnosis of lupus erythematosus is made: (1) malar rash, (2) discoid rash, (3) photosensitivity, (4) oral ulcers, (5) arthritis, (6) serositis, (7) renal disorder, (8) neurological disorder (seizures), (9) hematological disorder (hemolysis, leucopenia, or thrombocytopenia), (10) immunological disorder (positive LE preparation, anti-DNA, anti-Sm, or false-positive serological tests for syphilis), and (11) antinuclear antibody.

Clinical manifestations may be confined initially to one organ system, with other systems becoming involved as the disease progresses, or it may be manifest initially by multisystem involvement (Table 39–14). In addition, Galve and colleagues (1988) demonstrated clinically important cardiac valvar lesions in 18 percent of 74 patients with lupus.

It has been estimated that nearly a half million individuals in the United States have lupus, and the great majority of these are women. Even so, only recently have there been reports of lupus and pregnancy in which a large number of pregnancies provided the basis for the publication. Consequently, it is not

surprising that disagreements persist concerning systemic lupus and pregnancy, although opinions expressed in more recent reports seem much less divergent than in the past.

Fine and co-workers (1981) analyzed their experiences with one or more pregnancies in 39 women with systemic lupus erythematosus to provide answers to the following questions:

1. *Does pregnancy alter the natural history of systemic lupus erythematosus?* They concluded that pregnancy was not accompanied by an increased prevalence of major systemic nonrenal manifestations of lupus unless immunosuppressive therapy was stopped because of pregnancy.
2. *Are the effects of systemic lupus on renal function exaggerated by pregnancy?* They observed that for those women with no more than minimal prepregnancy renal impairment, renal function remained good in the great majority, deteriorated but recovered postpartum in about 10 percent, and in another 10 percent deteriorated and remained depressed. One such woman who also demonstrated florid extrarenal involvement died soon after hemodialysis was begun. It was difficult to distinguish clinically

TABLE 39–14. SOME CLINICAL MANIFESTATIONS OF SYSTEMIC LUPUS ERYTHEMATOSUS

Organ System	Percent
Systemic—fatigue, malaise, fever, weight loss	95
Musculoskeletal—arthralgias, myalgias, myopathy	95
Hematological—anemia, hemolysis, leucopenia, thrombocytopenia, lupus anticoagulant	85
Cutaneous—malar rash, discoid rash, photosensitivity, oral ulcers, alopecia, skin rashes	80
Neurological—organic brain syndromes, psychosis, seizures	60
Cardiopulmonary—pleuritis, pericarditis	60
Renal—proteinuria, casts	50
Gastrointestinal—anorexia, nausea, ascites, vaculitis	45
Thrombosis—arterial and venous	15
Ocular—conjunctivitis	15

From Hahn: Chapter 262. Systemic Lupus Erythematosus. In *Harrison's Principles of Internal Medicine. Eleventh Edition.* New York, McGraw-Hill, 1987.

between preeclampsia and lupus nephritis as the cause of the renal impairment as it was in the case summarized below. Induced abortions were not accompanied by any discernible deleterious effect on renal function.

3. *Should pharmacological treatment of systemic lupus be altered during pregnancy?* Their experiences led them to recommend the use of glucocorticoids and azathioprine antepartum in doses no different from those used when not pregnant. Moreover, they concluded that there probably is merit in increasing the dosage during labor and for up to two months thereafter to minimize the risk of exacerbation.

4. *How does systemic lupus affect the fetus and neonate?* Stillbirths were frequent (23 percent), as were preterm birth (33 percent) and fetal growth retardation (33 percent). Persistent proteinuria or reduced creatinine clearance were associated with a high prevalence of stillbirths and low birthweight infants even though the mothers were not overtly azotemic. When both proteinuria and appreciably reduced glomerular filtration coexisted, fetal wastage was very high. Talipes equinovarus was the only anomaly detected. Congenital heart block was not described.

Since this report, verification of most of these observations was made by several groups (Table 39–15). Varner and associates (1983) reported their experiences with pregnancies in women with systemic lupus erythematosus. One of the 36 mothers died 5 weeks postpartum with poorly controlled vascular disease. Perinatal mortality was increased but was not as great as reported by Fine and co-workers (1981). One fetus-infant demonstrated heart block. They too concluded that women whose disease is in remission and stays in remission can anticipate a favorable pregnancy outcome. They recommend that women taking immunosuppressive therapy at the onset of pregnancy continue therapy since its risk is less than the risk from the disease without treatment. This conclusion also was reached by Hayslett and Lynn (1980), who analyzed the pregnancy outcomes for a large group of women with lupus nephropathy. It is not clear at this time whether there is any advantage from increasing immunosuppressive dosage at delivery and during the puerperium. It often has been stated that this is the time that activation or exacerbation are most likely to develop, but evidence to support this is not striking.

Mor-Yosef and associates (1984) summarized their results with 159 pregnancies and concluded that lupus was not usually exacerbated. Nearly 80 percent of their patients had no appreciable clinical changes, while the remainder suffered some form of exacerbation. They confirmed that pregnancy following a period of quiesence, even with nephropathy, may be uneventful, or at least have a successful outcome in many cases. Of these 159 pregnancies, 10 percent each were terminated by spontaneous or induced abortion, 10 percent were stillborn, 10 percent were delivered preterm, and 60 percent had term, healthy infants.

Gimovsky and colleagues (1984) reported 77 pregnancy outcomes in 39 women with lupus, half of whom had renal involvement. They found an increased incidence of preterm, growth-retarded, and stillborn infants. These adverse outcomes were more likely if there was renal involvement. Although exacerbation during pregnancy was common, these were seldom encountered postpartum.

Mintz and co-workers (1986) provided data from a prospective study of 102 pregnancies in 75 women cared for from 1974 to 1983. They reported that exacerbations were common during pregnancy (60 percent), but that these were no more likely than in a group of nonpregnant control women taking progestational contraceptives. Their observations confirmed a high incidence of growth-retarded, preterm, and stillborn infants, especially in women with active disease.

Burkett (1985), in an excellent review, summarized maternal and fetal outcomes in systemic lupus erythematosus in 156 women with 242 pregnancies. He concluded that optimal pregnancy outcome was observed when clinical conditions included prepregnancy remission for at least 6 months, along with good renal function estimated by serum creatinine of 1.5 mg per dL or less, creatinine clearance of 60 mL per min or more, or proteinuria of less than 3 g per 24 hr.

LABORATORY EVALUATION

Various laboratory procedures have been recommended to monitor systemic lupus activity. The sedimentation test is widely used; however, an increase in this is uninterpretable during pregnancy since there is an appreciable rise induced by normal pregnancy. Serial measurements of C_3, C_4 and CH_{50} components of complement have been recommended, and while falling or low levels are more likely to be associated with active disease, unfortunately, higher levels provide no guarantee against significant disease activation. Varner and co-workers (1983), for example, found no correlation between clinical manifestations of disease and C_3 and C_4 complement levels in nearly half of their pregnant patients. Our experiences at Parkland Hospital have been similar.

Frequent hematological evaluation and measurements of renal and hepatic functions are essential to detect changes in the

TABLE 39–15. MATERNAL AND FETAL OUTCOMES IN PREGNANCIES COMPLICATED BY SYSTEMIC LUPUS ERYTHEMATOSUS

	Pregnancies	Exacerbations During Pregnancy (%)	Abortions[a] (%)	Perinatal Outcome (%)				
				Stillborn	Neonatal Death	Growth Retarded	Preterm	Term
Gimovsky (1984)	77	30	45	17	10	50	33	50
Mor-Yosef (1984)	159	20	25	about 8	N.S.[b]	N.S.	about 8	60
Fine (1981)	52	Not increased	27	24	N.S.	N.S.	33	43
Mintz (1986)	102	48	16	18	4	23	49	34

[a] Includes induced and spontaneous abortions.
[b] N.S. = Not stated

activity of the disease during pregnancy and the puerperium. Hemolysis is characterized by a positive Coombs' test, anemia, reticulocytosis, and usually unconjugated hyperbilirubinemia. Thrombocytopenia, leucopenia, or both, may develop. Increased serum transaminase activity reflects hepatic involvement as does a rise in serum bilirubin that is predominantly conjugated. At times azathioprine therapy will induce abnormalities in these tests of hepatic function. Overt and increasing proteinuria that persists is an ominous sign and is even more ominous if accompanied by other evidence for the nephrotic syndrome or an abnormal serum creatinine concentration. In general, the prognosis becomes worse as the number of abnormal findings increase, especially if immunosuppressive therapy provides no amelioration.

LUPUS VERSUS PREECLAMPSIA–ECLAMPSIA

Preeclampsia is common in all women with lupus, and superimposed preeclampsia is encountered even more often in those with lupus nephropathy. It may be difficult, if not impossible, sometimes to differentiate clinically lupus nephropathy from severe preeclampsia. Moreover, central nervous system involvement with systemic lupus may culminate in convulsions similar to those of eclampsia. Thrombocytopenia with or without hemolysis may further confuse the diagnosis. We have elected to manage such problem cases of systemic lupus as if they were the consequences of preeclampsia–eclampsia, utilizing magnesium sulfate, hydralazine intravenously, and delivery as described elsewhere (Chap. 35, p. 677). At the same time immunosuppressive therapy is continued. It should be emphasized that remote from pregnancy the most common causes of death are malignant hypertension with glomerulonephritis and neurological catastrophes such as seizures, strokes, and coma.

Some problems of differential diagnosis of preeclampsia–eclampsia from systemic lupus with vascular, renal, and central nervous system involvement during pregnancy and the puerperium are illustrated in the following woman cared for at Parkland Hospital.

A 21-year-old primigravida was observed throughout pregnancy. By term, her blood pressure had risen from its first trimester value of 100/60 to 130/80 mm Hg and intrapartum to 140/90. Edema was obvious, but proteinuria was not detected. She convulsed one hour after spontaneous delivery of a healthy infant who weighed 3,985 g. Transiently, her blood pressure was elevated to 160/108 mm Hg and proteinuria appeared. Hematocrit, platelet count, and plasma creatinine were normal. She was treated with magnesium sulfate parenterally for 24 hours and had no more convulsions. One week later she was discharged normotensive and asymptomatic.

Two weeks after delivery, she experienced bizarre neurological changes, which included tremors and transient loss of vision and consciousness. The cranial computed tomographic scan was normal, but an electroencephalogram was abnormal. The lupus erythematosus (LE) preparation was positive, antinuclear antibody titer was 1:640, and the serological test for syphilis was falsely positive. While hospitalized, she developed a malar (butterfly) rash. The diagnosis was systemic lupus erythematosus with central nervous system involvement. Did she have eclampsia 2 weeks before? We concluded that she did not, but rather that she had lupus.

EFFECTS ON FETUS AND INFANT

Most report substantively increased rates of fetal growth retardation, and this has been our experience. The fetus should therefore be observed closely for adverse effects imposed by a hostile intrauterine environment, which would warrant prompt delivery unless perhaps the fetus is very immature and then close monitoring until delivery is effected.

Neonatal lupus erythematosus is caused by transplacental passage of IgG anti-SS-A(Ro), anti-SS-B(La) and probably other antibodies (Cobbe, 1983; Vetter and Rashkind, 1983). Diffuse myocarditis causes fibrosis and *congenital heart block*, as the consequence especially of myocarditis and fibrosis in the region between the atrioventricular node and bundle of His. Heart block may be tolerated or may lead to Stokes-Adams attacks or heart failure in the fetus or infant. The neonate may require a pacemaker. Heart block also may develop in fetuses whose mothers appear normal but are destined subsequently to develop clinical lupus erythematosus or some other connective tissue disease. Mothers of infants with isolated complete heart block should be so evaluated. Cutaneous lupus, thrombocytopenia, and autoimmune hemolysis are transient and clear within a few months (Lee, 1984). McCune and colleagues (1987) recently described 24 children with congenital lupus: 12 had heart block, 10 cutaneous lesions, and two had both. Three died as neonates and 5 of 11 survivors had permanent pacemakers. Importantly, of 12 subsequent liveborns in these women, 3 were similarly affected.

Singsen and colleagues (1985) recommend maternal and newborn screening of women at risk. Certainly, if SS-A or SS-B antibodies are detected in maternal blood, careful ultrasound screening of the fetus should be conducted to detect any evidence of heart block so that plans can be made for delivery in an appropriately staffed and equipped center.

SUBSEQUENT REPRODUCTION

If systemic lupus has been induced by a drug, the disease most likely will ameliorate when the drug is stopped. Otherwise, it is a lifelong disease. If the disease has been characterized by prolonged remissions, pregnancy should be undertaken during such a remission.

In general, women with systemic lupus and chronic vascular or renal disease should limit their family size because of the poor prognosis for the fetus and also the mother. Wallace and associates (1981) made the following observations on 609 cases of systemic lupus erythematosus: The 10-year survival was 87 percent for those without nephritis but 65 percent for those with nephritis. The most common causes of death were renal disease and sepsis. No appreciable difference between whites and nonwhites was noted.

Tubal sterilization may be advantageous. It is performed with greatest safety when the disease is reasonably quiescent. We have not recommended oral contraceptives for women with systemic lupus since vascular disease is a relatively common component. There is some evidence which suggests that systemic lupus may be worsened by their use. Intrauterine devices should be prescribed with caution, especially if the woman is receiving immunosuppressive therapy.

Since vascular disease, especially of the microvasculature, is common in women with lupus, it is not surprising that vessels so involved during pregnancy can include those of the decidua. This may account for the prevalence of fetal growth retardation and pregnancy wastage associated with maternal systemic lupus. Additionally, the lupus anticoagulant and anticardiolipin antibody have been associated with high rates of fetal wastage.

ANTIPHOSPHOLIPID ANTIBODIES—LUPUS ANTICOAGULANT AND ANTICARDIOLIPIN ANTIBODY

The lupus anticoagulant is either an IgG or IgM immunoglobin that has been identified in some patients with systemic lupus erythematosus and in others with no apparent evidence of lupus. In vitro, the lupus anticoagulant is characterized by a prolonged kaolin partial thromboplastin time. The anticoagulant, paradoxically, can incite thrombosis. Interest in this entity by obstetricians has resulted from the association of the lupus anticoagulant with decidual vasculopathy, placental infarction, fetal growth retardation, and recurrent abortion and fetal death (Carreras and colleagues, 1981; DeWolf and associates, 1982). The anticoagulant also is associated with a high incidence of venous and arterial thromboses, hypertension, hemolytic anemia, and biologically false-positive tests for syphilis.

Diagnosis

The partial thromboplastin time is generally prolonged since the anticoagulant interferes with conversion of prothrombin to thrombin in vitro by adhering to the phospholipid surface, thereby inhibiting attachment and assembly of other clotting factors. Tests considered more specific are the *tissue thromboplastin-inhibition test* and the *platelet neutralization procedure*. There is currently disagreement as to which of these three is best for screening.

In a group of 68 women with lupus anticoagulant activity who had 264 pregnancies reported in the literature, about a third had no symptoms, a third had a history of thrombotic episodes, and another third had systemic lupus (Gant, 1986). In addition, about a fourth each had a false-positive serological test for syphilis and a positive Coombs' test.

Obstetrical Implications

Although there is no doubt that the lupus anticoagulant is associated with increased fetal wastage in some women, it is unclear as to the extent of these adverse sequelae in all women who have the anticoagulant. In most studies that report recurrent abortions and fetal deaths, women were usually chosen because of these repeated adverse pregnancy outcomes. The incidence of lupus anticoagulant in a general obstetrical population, and thus any adverse effects on reproduction, has not been carefully ascertained (Lockwood and colleagues, 1988).

There is now evidence that women who have suffered excessive reproductive losses associated with the lupus anticoagulant will have improved outcomes if given treatment consisting of *low-dose aspirin* (about 75 mg) along with 20 to 80 mg of prednisone daily (Branch and associates, 1985; Lubbe and co-workers, 1983). Gant (1986) reviewed treatment results and reported that the number of liveborn infants increased from 6 to 80 percent in women so treated by these and other investigators. The effects of therapy are measured by reversal of clotting abnormalities (Fig. 39–16). Despite improved outcome, Branch and associates (1985) caution that fetal growth retardation and preeclampsia are still common. They also state that low-dose aspirin and glucocorticosteroid therapy is not universally successful. On the other hand, women with lupus and the lupus anticoagulant have had normal pregnancy outcomes despite that they were not treated (Stafford-Bradley and colleagues, 1988). Moreover, women with the lupus anitcoagulant and prior bad pregnancy outcomes had liveborn infants subsequently despite no treatment (Trudinger and associates, 1988). Lubbe

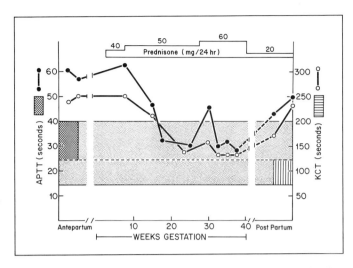

Figure 39–16. Activated partial thromboplastin time (APTT) and kaolin clotting time (KCT) in a single patient before, during and after pregnancy. Therapy during pregnancy consisted of aspirin, 75 mg daily plus prednisone as illustrated. (*Modified from Lubbe and associates: Lancet 1:1361, 1983.*)

(1985) recommends that treatment be given only to those women with a history of fetal death.

ANTICARDIOLIPIN ANTIBODY

Technically speaking, the lupus anticoagulant functions as an anticardiolipin antibody since the antibody reacts with a phospholipid antigen associated with normal coagulation. Lockshin and co-workers (1985) have developed an enzyme-linked immunosorbent assay (ELISA) for the anticardiolipin antibody, and with this technique, it is now apparent that a large number of patients with systemic lupus erythematosus have circulating antibodies directed against cardiolipin. For example, Harris and associates (1983) reported that 61 percent of serum samples obtained from a group of their patients with systemic lupus had such antibodies. Triplett and colleagues (1988) reported that 71 percent of 100 patients with evidence of lupus anticoagulant activity also had antiphospholipid antibody.

The presence of anticardiolipin antibodies is associated with clinical symptoms very similar to those caused by the lupus anticoagulant. Specifically, when they are present in high concentrations, arterial and venous thromboses, cerebral thrombosis, thrombocytopenia, pulmonary hypertension, and multiple abortions and fetal wastage have been observed (Derue and associates, 1985; Harris and colleagues, 1983; Lockshin and co-workers, 1985). Kochenour and colleagues (1987) recently described the clinical courses of three women who had lupus anticoagulant, antocardiolpin antibody, or both, who developed a postpartum syndrome of pleural effusion, pulmonary infiltrates, and fever. These women did not fulfill all requirements for the diagnosis of lupus erythematosus, and the authors suggest that this is a specific pleuropulmonary and cardiac disease.

RHEUMATOID ARTHRITIS

Although a number of humoral and cellular immunological abnormalities have been identified, the cause of rheumatoid arthritis, or rheumatoid disease, is unknown. Rheumatoid disease, like lupus, is more common in women than men.

In 1938, Hench reported marked improvement in the inflammatory component of rheumatoid arthritis during pregnancy. The pattern of improvement was the same as in spontaneous remission and involved gradual amelioration of the signs and symptoms of the rheumatoid process. Apparently on the basis that corticosteroid levels in plasma were considered to be markedly increased in pregnancy, Hench began to treat with cortisone individuals who had rheumatoid arthritis and there was a favorable effect. Smith and West (1960) demonstrated subsequently that increased secretion of cortisol did not readily account for all of the remissions rather commonly found in pregnancy.

Unger and associates (1983) studied a group of women with rheumatoid arthritis and in two-thirds disease activity diminished during pregnancy. In the group in which activity subsided, pregnancy-associated α_2-glycoprotein was considerably higher (mean 1,250 mg per L) than in those in whom the disease remained the same or worsened (mean 470 mg per L). Pregnancy-associated glycoprotein is known to have immunosuppressive properties in vitro, and therefore it is tempting to implicate the high level of this protein in the remission of rheumatoid arthritis in pregnancy, as Hench did for cortisol. Pope and associates (1983) reported that concentrations of immune complexes detected by the Clq-binding assay were decreased during pregnancy. They found no reproducible effect of pregnancy on IgM or IgG-rheumatoid factors.

Neely and Persellin (1977) similarly identified amelioration of activity of rheumatoid arthritis in 62 percent of 56 pregnancies, but in the other 38 percent there was either no change in activity or the arthritis actually became worse. In four women signs and symptoms of the disease first appeared during pregnancy. Thus in some women the course may occasionally worsen during pregnancy, and sometimes the disease may first appear at that time as illustrated by the case summarized below.

Ostensen and Husby (1983) reported prospective observations in women with either rheumatoid arthritis or ankylosing spondylitis. They confirmed the remarkable amelioration of symptoms even during early pregnancy in women with rheumatoid arthritis as well as exacerbations within 12 weeks postpartum in 11 of 12 women. Conversely, more than half of women with ankylosing spondylitis had active disease throughout pregnancy.

The drug most commonly used to treat rheumatoid arthritis remote from pregnancy has been aspirin in doses that, if used in pregnancy, might possibly affect the fetus and neonate adversely in one or more of the following ways; impaired hemostasis, prolonged gestation, and premature closure of the ductus arteriosus. Nonetheless, aspirin usually has been the drug of choice during pregnancy. Gold compounds have been used in pregnancy, but experiences are not sufficient to recommend their use. Prednisone and other adrenal corticosteroids have been used, usually without adverse side effects.

Intense involvement of certain joints may interfere with delivery. For example, severe deformities of the hip may preclude vaginal delivery.

We have observed the clinical onset of rheumatoid arthritis during the first trimester of pregnancy in a 22-year-old nullipara. Treatment with aspirin (600 mg every 4 hours) did not produce relief. Prednisolone 7.5 mg daily begun at 20 weeks gestation, plus enteric-coated aspirin, three tablets every 4 hours, provided considerable relief. Supplemental iron was provided during pregnancy and she never was anemic. Fetal growth retardation and oligohydramnios became evident during the third trimester. The mother was not hypertensive. The infant when delivered at 35 weeks gestation weighed 1,720 g but thrived subsequently. The placenta contained multiple infarcts.

Rheumatoid arthritis requiring vigorous treatment has persisted during the 2 years since delivery. Therapy has consisted primarily of gold by injection and indomethacin. She is contemplating another pregnancy.

PROGRESSIVE SYSTEMIC SCLEROSIS (SCLERODERMA)

Progressive systemic sclerosis is seen most commonly in women during the fourth decade, but its rarity prevents an accumulation of extensive data relative to its effect on pregnancy. Scleroderma was formerly considered to have a markedly deleterious effect upon pregnancy; however, Johnson and associates (1964) were more encouraging in their report of 36 pregnancies in a group of 337 women in whom scleroderma developed before the age of 45. They concluded that pregnancy had little or no effect on the course of the disease and that scleroderma had a minimal effect on the pregnancy. In our limited experience, dysphagia seems to be aggravated by pregnancy, and women with renal or cardiac involvement, hypertension or pulmonary fibrosis do poorly. Renal insufficiency and malignant hypertension are common causes of death in nonpregnant women, and whether preeclampsia enhances their onset and severity is not known. Almost certainly, preexisting vascular-renal disease increases the risk of preeclampsia–eclampsia. A fatal case of apparent eclampsia in a woman with scleroderma has been reported (Fear, 1968). The fetus also succumbed.

Vaginal delivery may be anticipated, unless the soft tissue changes wrought by scleroderma produce dystocia requiring abdominal delivery.

POLYARTERITIS NODOSA

Polyarteritis (periarteritis) nodosa is a rare disease with protean manifestations. The classic variety is one of the vasculitis syndromes and is progressive and characterized clinically by myalgia, neuropathy, gastrointestinal disorders, hypertension, and renal disease. Only a few documented cases of polyarteritis nodosa in association with pregnancy have been reported and the experience is too scant to draw any definitive conclusions other than that generally the combination is associated with an unfavorable maternal outcome (Siegler and Spain, 1965). Typically, the mother died postpartum with hypertension and renal involvement. Burkett and Richardson (1982) reported one case in which the disease was considered to be in remission throughout pregnancy and the puerperium. Although it was her fourth pregnancy, she developed hypertension (160/110 mm Hg), proteinuria, and edema which necessitated delivery at 37 weeks gestation. Interestingly, the surviving infant was not growth retarded. The mother continued taking antihypertensive therapy postpartum, but 18 months later died of progressive renal failure, uremia, and congestive heart failure.

DERMATOMYOSITIS

Dermatomyositis (polymyositis) is an uncommon acute, subacute, or chronic inflammatory disease of unknown cause involving especially skin and muscle. The disease may manifest as a severe generalized myositis with a cutaneous eruption, fever, and a fatal outcome within a few days or weeks. It also may assume a chronic form, characterized by the gradual development of paresis with little, if any, cutaneous or systemic involvement.

About 15 percent of adults developing dermatomyositis have an associated maligant tumor. The time of appearance of the two diseases, however, may be separated by several years. Extirpation of the malignant lesion is sometimes followed by a permanent remission of the dermatomyositis. The most common sites of the associated cancer are the breast, lung, stomach, and ovary. The uterus and cervix also have been reported as primary sites.

There are so few reports of dermatomyositis in pregnancy that it is difficult to draw any definite conclusions about the effect of one upon the other. Gutierrez and colleagues (1984) reported pregnancy outcomes in 10 pregnancies among seven women with active disease and there were three abortions, three perinatal deaths, and five preterm deliveries. We have cared for one woman disgnosed and treated with prednisone before pregnancy. During and after the pregnancy the mother actually improved and the infant thrived.

MARFAN SYNDROME

This disorder of connective tissue exhibits a Mendelian autosomal pattern of dominant inheritance. Both sexes are affected equally, and there appears to be no racial or ethnic basis for the syndrome. There are many mild cases in which the intrinsic lesion of the connective tissue affects neither well-being nor longevity and consequently escapes detection. Although the specific defect is still controversial, there is a degeneration of the elastic lamina in the media of the aorta. The cardiovascular lesion is the most serious abnormality, involving most of the ascending aorta, and predisposing to aortic dilatation or dissecting aneurysm. Early death in Marfan syndrome is thus ulti-

mately caused by either valvar insufficiency and congestive heart failure or by rupture of a dissecting aneurysm.

Pyeritz (1981) reviewed the literature and reported that 20 of 32 women with Marfan syndrome who became pregnant either died or had aortic dissection during or shortly after pregnancy. Since most of these were case reports, he concluded that there was significantly biased reporting of bad outcomes. Indeed, only one of his own 26 patients died postpartum from infective endocarditis, and this woman had severe preexisting cardiac disease. He concluded that women with significant aortic root dilatation (more than 40 mm in diameter) or mitral valve dysfunction are at high risk for life-threatening cardiovascular complications during pregnancy. Conversely, women with minimal or no dilatation, and those with normal cardiac function by echocardiography are counseled regarding the small but potential risk of aortic dissection.

Marfan syndrome alone is not an indication for abdominal delivery, for cesarean section does not protect against excessive stress on the aorta before the onset of labor. The role of cardiovascular surgery in Marfan disease is poorly defined.

EHLERS-DANLOS SYNDROME

This disorder of connective tissue is characterized by a variety of changes in connective tissue including hyperelasticity of the skin. In the more severe types there is a strong tendency for fatal rupture of any of several arteries. There are at least 10 reported varieties, some autosomal dominant, some recessive, and some X-linked (Peaceman and Cruikshank, 1987). There is an increased frequency of preterm rupture of membranes, antepartum and postpartum hemorrhage, and tissue fragility that makes episiotomy repair and cesarean section difficult. Case reports and literature reviews have been provided by Peaceman and Cruikshank (1987), Snyder and co-workers (1983), and Taylor and associates (1982b).

DISEASES OF THE SKIN

Most skin diseases are encountered with about the same frequency during pregnancy as in nonpregnant women. There are, however, a few dermatoses that appear to be unique to pregnancy. Moreover, episodes of pruritus are common during pregnancy, and in some instances, itching is not accompanied by a skin eruption but is due to *pruritus gravidarum* caused by intrahepatic cholestasis and bile salt retention. (p. 827).

ABNORMALITIES OF PIGMENTATION

During pregnancy, there is frequently an increased pigmentation called *chloasma*. This may be particularly marked along the linea nigra, the perineum, umbilicus, areola of the breasts, as well as freckles and nevi. Occasionally, unsightly, more or less symmetric, brownish splotches appear upon the face, and this *melasma gravidarum* or *mask of pregnancy*, most often involves the forehead and cheeks. After pregnancy, the hyperpigmentation usually disappears or at least recedes appreciably. Oral contraceptives may cause similar changes in pigmentation.

ALOPECIA

During pregnancy hair growth is stimulated; however, postpartum, hair reenters the resting phase and the numbers of hairs shed within 3 to 6 months may increase considerably. Thinning of the hair, or *telogen effluvium*, ceases gradually. The mother can be reassured that the phenomenon is temporary, it is not pathological, and that she can anticipate full recovery.

PRURITIC URTICARIAL PAPULES AND PLAQUES OF PREGNANCY

This is the most common pruritic dermatosis of pregnancy and is an intensely pruritic cutaneous eruption of late pregnancy. Erythematous urticarial papules and plaques (Fig. 39–17) first develop on the abdomen, usually in the periumbilical area, and spread to the thighs and extremities (Alcalay and associates, 1987; Yancey and colleagues, 1984). Typically, the face is spared

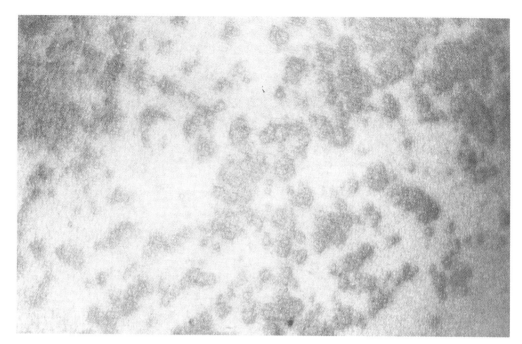

Figure 39–17. Pruritic urticarial papules and plaques of pregnancy. Numerous edematous and erythematous papular lesions are present on the lower trunk. (*From Yancey and colleagues: J Am Acad Dermatol 10:473, 1984.*)

and seldom is there excoriation. **The disease is more common in nulliparas and seldom recurs in subsequent pregnancies.** It may resemble herpes gestationis, but there are no vesicles or bullae. Furthermore, immunofluorescent staining of skin shows no immunoglobulin or complement deposition. Rather there is a mild nonspecific lymphohistiocytic perivasculitis. Alcalay and associates (1988) found no differences between serum concentrations of β-chorionic gonadotropin, estradiol, and cortisol or urinary estriol excretion in 11 women with this dermatosis compared to gestational-age matched controls.

Topical corticosteroid preparations usually provide relief, but occasionally oral prednisone is given for intense pruritus. There is no evidence that perinatal morbidity is increased (Yancey and associates, 1984).

HERPES GESTATIONIS

Herpes gestationis is a serious but rare dermatological disease peculiar to pregnancy. Unlike the name implies, it is not a viral-induced illness. This blistering disease of pregnancy usually presents as an extremely pruritic widespread eruption with lesions that vary from erythematous and edematous papules to large, tense bullae (Fig. 39–18). Common sites of involvement are the abdomen and the extremities. Although morphological changes may develop in the small intestinal mucosa similar to those of adult celiac disease, they do not appear to cause significant malabsorption.

Katz and co-workers (1976) described a herpes gestationis serum factor which is a thermostable IgG class protein. Immunofluorescent technics applied to a skin biopsy are of value for confirming the diagnosis and both IgG and C_3 complement are deposited along the basement membrane zone.

Prednisone in doses of 40 to 60 mg daily usually brings relief promptly and inhibits the formation of new lesions. Azathioprine is reserved for severe cases. Where the skin heals, the healed sites are not scarred but are usually hyperpigmented. The process may recur in subsequent pregnancies. Lawley and

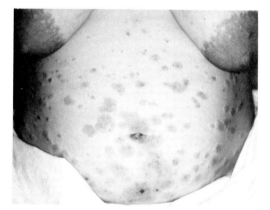

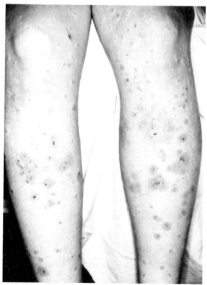

Figure 39–18. Herpes gestationis at 30 weeks gestation. Subsequently, remarkable relief from the intense pruritis, as well as considerable decrease in the intensity of the skin reaction, was provided by glucocorticoid treatment.

colleagues (1978) reported a high incidence of preterm birth and stillborn infants; however, Shornick and associates (1983) did not find such an association in 28 cases.

Lesions similar to those of the mother have been reported to develop in the neonate and to clear spontaneously within a few weeks (Chorzelski and colleagues, 1976). C_3 complement desposited at the basement membrane of the infant's skin and the herpes gestationis factor in cord serum have been described by Katz and associates (1976).

PAPULAR DERMATITIS OF PREGNANCY

This is an extremely rare dermatitis of late pregnancy described by Spangler and colleagues in 1962. It is characterized by a generalized pruritic eruption, the lesions of which consist of soft, red to violet to red-brown papules some of which have a centrally hemorrhagic crust. **Lesions clear spontaneously soon after pregnancy but can recur in subsequent pregnancies.** Corticosteroids orally may control this form of pregnancy-induced dermatitis. Perinatal mortality is increased especially if the mother is not treated with corticosteroids.

THERMAL INJURY

Although Parkland Hospital is a major burn center for the United States, we have not seen a large number of pregnant women with severe burns. It has become apparent, however, that pregnant women who suffer chemical pneumonitis from smoke inhalation tolerate this poorly, as they do most all forms of pneumonitis.

Mathews, on the basis of experience with 50 burned pregnant women (1982), recommended that women in the second or third trimester of pregnancy with burns over 50 percent or more of their body should be delivered immediately as maternal death is otherwise almost certain and the fetal survival rate is not improved by waiting. He emphasized that, if undelivered, the maternal prognosis is markedly worse than for a nonpregnant woman suffering otherwise comparable burns. Conversely, Amy and colleagues (1985) reported that pregnancy did not alter maternal outcome compared to nonpregnant women of similar age. Fetal survival usually parallels the percentage of burned surface area and survival of the mother (Amy and colleagues, 1985; Rayburn and co-workers, 1984). For severely burned women, the fetal prognosis is poor. Usually the woman enters labor spontaneously within a week, and often delivers a stillborn infant. Contributory factors are hypovolemia, pulmonary injury, septicemia, and the intensely catabolic state.

Skin contracture following serious abdominal burns may be painful during a subsequent pregnancy and may even necessitate surgical decompression and split skin autographs (Mathews, 1982). It has been our limited experience that the burn scar during pregnancy undergoes considerable softening and therefore can stretch appreciably.

Loss or distortion of nipples may cause problems in breast feeding. Daw and Mohandas (1983) described cases in which breast feeding was satisfactory from one breast without problems in the contralateral breast without a nipple.

ACNE

Some women, but certainly not all, note that their acne improves during pregnancy. **The retinoic acid, isoretinoin (Accutane), commonly has been prescribed to treat severe cystic acne, but unfortunately it has proven to be highly teratogenic.** Lammer and colleagues (1985) reported a 26-fold risk for craniofacial, cardiac, and central nervous system malformations in exposed fetuses (see Chap. 32, p. 562).

HIDRADENITIS SUPPURATIVA

This is a chronic, progressive inflammatory and suppurative disorder of skin and supporting structures characterized by apocrine gland plugging and infection that resembles acne vulgaris in many ways. In most cases, skin involvement is in multiple apocrine gland sites, but it may be seen only in the axillas, groin, perineum, perirectal area, or breasts.

The disease is hormonally responsive and thus not seen until puberty. In our experiences it is not worsened by pregnancy. Treatment is control of secondary infections with either systemic antimicrobials or clindamycin ointment. Definitive treatment is wide surgical excision, but this most often should be postponed during pregnancy.

NEUROLOGICAL DISORDERS

In general, most coincidental nervous system disorders are compatible with normal pregnancy outcome, and seldom does pregnancy appreciably exacerabate underlying neurological disease. There are however, exceptions to these generalizations as some of these diseases, or their treatment, may adversely affect pregnancy. Eclampsia, earlier in this century, was a common and serious disorder involving the nervous system, but is no longer the threat it once was. This complication, unique to pregnancy, is discussed in Chapter 35.

SEIZURE DISORDERS

More than 2 million people in the United States have some form of epilepsy. Seizures are caused by chronic, paroxysmal disorders of brain electrical activity, and if accompanied by motor manifestations, they are termed convulsive seizures. The new classification of seizure disorders is provided by Delgado-Escueta and co-workers (1983).

The effect of pregnancy on the frequency of epileptic seizures has been argued for more than 100 years. It appears that if seizures are well controlled before pregnancy there is little risk of an increased frequency during pregnancy. If seizures are poorly controlled before pregnancy, however, there is a likelihood that even further deterioration may occur during pregnancy (Schmidt and associates, 1983).

TREATMENT

The therapeutic goal for the treatment of epilepsy during pregnancy is to administer to the mother the least amount of a drug likely to affect her fetus adversely yet effectively control her convulsions. There is increasing evidence that the use of several of the most effective antiepileptic agents during pregnancy is accompanied by higher frequencies of fetal malformations as described below.

An increased likelihood of seizures during pregnancy may be the consequence of several often compounding factors. During early pregnancy, nausea and vomiting may interfere with the ingestion and absorption of anticonvulsant medications. Some women may reduce their dosage of medication or abstain completely because of fear of adverse effects on the fetus. During labor, delivery, and the early puerperium, medication may be withheld by the obstetrical staff deliberately or inadvertently, similarly increasing the likelihood of convulsions.

The effects of pregnancy on the metabolic clearance rate of some anticonvulsant drugs have been of interest for some years. Phenytoin has been used in the past very commonly during pregnancy. The drug is cleared more rapidly during pregnancy; and, as a consequence, with a constant dose of the medication, plasma levels are likely to be lower than when nonpregnant (Kochenour and co-workers, 1980; Lander and associates, 1977). While it seems that this should increase the risk of seizures, the amount of free or nonprotein-bound drug in plasma increases during pregnancy. This likely offsets to some degree the lower total concentration of phenytoin (Perucca and associates, 1981). The fall in plasma levels that accompanies pregnancy commonly has been interpreted by many as an indication for frequent measurements of plasma levels and, consequently an increase in dosage. This approach fails to take into account the enhanced therapeutic effect that results from decreased protein binding of the drug as pregnancy advances. Moreover, appropriate plasma levels for women throughout pregnancy, as yet, have not been established. Although some (Dalessio, 1985) recommend that plasma levels be determined routinely, this is not our practice at Parkland Hospital.

EFFECT OF ANTICONVULSANTS ON FETUS-INFANT

Women with epilepsy who take anticonvulsant medications have a two- to threefold increased risk for giving birth to infants with congenital anomalies. It is unclear whether epilepsy per se causes these increased malformations, or whether it is anticonvulsant drug teratogenicity, or a combination of these two (see Chap. 32, p. 566). In 1975, Hanson and Smith described a *fetal phenytoin syndrome* that included craniofacial anomalies, distal limb dysmorphosis, and mental deficiency. In this report, 11 percent of exposed infants studied were adversely affected. Use of phenytoin also has been accompanied by increased frequencies of cleft lip and palate and of congenital heart lesions. Kelly and associates (1984) subsequently reported that 30 percent of 468 infants exposed to phenytoin in utero had minor craniofacial and digital anomalies, but that there was no increased frequency of major malformations or mental retardation.

Maternal phenytoin ingestion alone or with phenobarbital has been implicated in the deficiency of four vitamin K-dependent clotting factors (II, VII, IX, and X) in the plasma of the neonate (Mountain and co-workers, 1970). *Hemorrhagic disease of the newborn* described in this circumstance usually can be prevented by the prompt parenteral administration of vitamin K to the newborn. It might be worthwhile, however, to give the mother vitamin K at least at the onset of labor, if not before, to minimize further the risk of hemorrhage in the fetus and infant (see Chap. 33, p. 611).

Other anticonvulsants have been implicated as having an increased risk for fetal malformations. *Phenobarbital* is difficult to assess as a teratogen since it was once commonly used in conjunction with phenytoin. *Trimethadione*, used principally for petit mal seizures, has been implicated in causing birth defects in excess of those associated with hydantoin, and this drug should be avoided in pregnancy (Briggs and colleagues, 1986). *Valproic acid* has been estimated to cause neural tube defects in 2 percent of exposed offspring, and it should not be given to pregnant women (Centers for Disease Control, 1983).

Carbamazepine is a tricyclic anticonvulsant that has been used widely since 1962, and because of the possible adverse effects reported for the drugs discussed above, it currently is used more frequently for convulsive disorders. Its teratogenic potential is unsettled, but there is evidence that it is associated with a lesser risk for fetal malformations than phenytoin. For these reasons, some recommend carbamazepine for new-onset epilepsy in pregnancy (Paulson and Paulson, 1981), and at Parkland Hospital, we have for several years used it as a first-line drug.

COUNSELING

Consideration should be given to stopping the anticonvulsant medication for the woman who wishes to conceive. The various conditions in which treatment may be stopped with little likelihood of recurrence have been described by Delgado-Escueta and associates (1983). Generally, if the woman has not convulsed for a long time on medication and does not do so while off medication before conception, she very likely will have no problem during pregnancy. Precautions to protect her and others must be taken during the trial period off medication. **However, if she does convulse, treatment during pregnancy is essential.**

Several of the anticonvulsant drugs in common use tend to precipitate or aggravate a deficiency of folic acid, and megaloblastic anemia has been described in these circumstances (Chanarin, 1969). At Parkland Hospital, maternal folate deficiency identified by low plasma folate levels is much more common in these women taking anticonvulsants than in the general obstetrical population. Interestingly, no cases of overt megaloblastic anemia have been identified among these women treated with anticonvulsant drugs even though they were not given supplemental folic acid (Pritchard and co-workers, 1969). Folic acid has been claimed by some to increase the likelihood of convulsions; however, Hiilesmaa and associates (1983) found no association between the number of seizures during pregnancy and serum folate concentrations. The benefits, if any, to be derived from folic acid supplementation in these circumstances are not clear and we do not prescribe supplemental folic acid.

At times, it may be difficult to differentiate between eclampsia and epilepsy in the hypertensive pregnant woman. Magnesium sulfate parenterally administered most often promptly controls the convulsions of epilepsy as well as those of eclampsia (Pritchard and Cunningham, unpublished).

CEREBROVASCULAR DISEASES

Cerebrovascular disease refers to disorders of one or more blood vessels of the brain, and the majority of lesions that arise from these are from arterial diseases. The resultant pathological lesion is a stroke, which is a neurological injury arising from ischemia, embolization, occlusion, or a ruptured vessel (Kistler and colleagues, 1987).

While distinctly uncommon in young women, disorders of the cerebral circulation have continued to be a prominent cause of maternal deaths in the United States. Kaunitz and colleagues (1985) reported that cerebrovascular accidents caused 5 percent of 2,067 nonabortion-related maternal deaths in the United States from 1974 to 1978. Sachs and colleagues (1987) showed that while the incidence of intracranial hemorrhage as a cause of maternal death decreased threefold over a 30-year period, it remained the third or fourth leading cause.

CEREBRAL THROMBOSIS

The vast majority of strokes are in older, nonpregnant individuals, and are caused by cerebral artery thrombosis as a result of atherosclerosis. Because of the low incidence of strokes in young women, the exact contribution of cerebral thrombosis as a cause of stroke during pregnancy is uncertain, but it probably is not more common than stroke from cerebral embolism or intracranial hemorrhage. In 29,099 consecutive births at the Mayo Clinic, Wiebers and Whisnant (1985) identified only one case each of cerebral thrombosis and intracranial hemorrhage. Unexplained cerebral thrombosis and other thrombotic complications may occur more frequently in women who have antiphospholipid antibodies (Gant, 1986). Therefore, with such a complication, a search for these antibodies should be made.

CEREBRAL EMBOLISM

Since infarction follows cerebral embolization, it is sometimes confused with cerebral thrombosis. Many cases of cerebral embolism in young women never are found to have an underlying cause, and the risk of recurrence is speculative. On the other hand, if an underlying cause is identified, recurrence is more common unless treatment can be given. Thus, it is important to pursue aggressively a source when these are identified during pregnancy. The most commonly found origin of emboli is the heart. Emboli may result from arrhythmias, especially atrial fibrillation associated with rheumatic valvar disease. They also may arise from a heart valve affected by old rheumatic disease or from infective endocarditis (Cox and associates, 1988).

INTRACRANIAL HEMORRHAGE

Several lesions may cause serious intracranial hemorrhage. *Intracerebral hemorrhage* from hypertension is uncommon during pregnancy, but may complicate chronic essential hypertension with superimposed preeclampsia (see Chap. 35, p. 669). Lesions that cause *subarachnoid hemorrhage* are more likely to be associated with otherwise normal pregnancy and include ruptured saccular aneurysms and bleeding arteriovenous malformations which complicate about 1 in 15,000 pregnancies (Noronha, 1985).

Ruptured Aneurysm
Subarachnoid hemorrhage from a *ruptured aneurysm* is said to be more common later in pregnancy. It usually can be recognized readily by computed tomography. If the diagnosis is uncertain, then cerebral angiography should be performed. Whether to attempt repair of a potentially accessible vascular lesion during pregnancy is debatable. The advantages achieved by reducing the risk of a subsequent intracranial hemorrhage are obvious; however, the potential for adverse effects on the fetus from maternal hypotension and hypothermia during the surgical procedure are real. Because of maternal danger, it is our general policy to favor repair; and if the woman is near term, cesarean delivery immediately followed by craniotomy has proven successful. Antifibrinolytic agents commonly are used to try to impede clot dissolution and in turn reduce perhaps the risk of further hemorrhage. Since fibrinolytic activity already is reduced as the consequence of the pregnancy per se, we have counseled against their use in pregnancy or the immediate puerperium and thus avoid the risks associated with their use.

Following surgical repair, vaginal delivery is not prohibited. The main obstetrical problem concerns the management of pregnancy and delivery in women who survive intracranial hemorrhage, but in whom repair is not done. Some, but certainly not all, authorities favor cesarean section for delivery, and in cases in which the cerebral hemorrhage occurred shortly before or very early in pregnancy, some believe that therapeutic abortion is indicated. On the basis of a review of 142 cases of intracranial aneurysms that ruptured before or during pregnancy, Hunt and co-workers (1974) concluded that there is little indication for elective cesarean section to replace vaginal delivery. Barrett and associates (1982) provided an extensive review of pregnancy-related rupture of arterial aneurysms, including cerebral artery aneurysms.

Arteriovenous Malformations
According to the review of Tuttelman and Gleicher (1981), *arteriovenous malformations* are encountered in younger women and most commonly bleed before 20 weeks or during labor and the early puerperium. These lesions commonly rebleed; therefore, the conduct of labor and delivery following such a bleeding episode during pregnancy from an inoperable lesion is more critical than for aneurysmal hemorrhage. Under these circumstances, we prefer cesarean delivery.

CEREBRAL VENOUS THROMBOSIS

Lateral or superior sagittal venous sinus thromboses are rare in the absence of infection or trauma, but pregnancy and especially the puerperium seem to be predisposing events (Donaldson, 1981). The prognosis is variable and coma and death may ensue rapidly or, conversely, full recovery may follow. Most authorities recommend that heparin not be given since bleeding frequently follows clot resolution, thus intensifying the size of the lesion. Our general method of management has been careful observation and supportive care, but this has not always been associated with a good outcome.

OTHER NEUROLOGICAL DISORDERS

VENTRICULOPERITONEAL SHUNTS

A few instances of pregnancy have been described in women with ventriculoperitoneal shunts for hydrocephalus (Howard and Herrick, 1981; Kleinman and co-workers, 1983). Pregnancy outcomes have usually been satisfactory. Antimicrobial prophylaxis probably is indicated if the peritoneal cavity is entered for cesarean delivery or tubal sterilization.

MATERNAL BRAIN DEATH

A few instances of maternal brain death during pregnancy have been described in which life support systems and parenteral alimentation were utilized for some time while the fetus hopefully achieved sufficient maturity not only to survive but also to enjoy good health (Dillon and associates, 1982; Field and colleagues, 1988). The ethical, financial, and legal implications, both civil and criminal, that may arise from attempting—or not attempting—such care are profound!

PSEUDOTUMOR CEREBRI

Benign intracranial hypertension, or pseudotumor cerebri, is characterized by headache, visual disturbances, and papilledema from increased intracranial pressure in an otherwise healthy individual. Criteria for diagnosis include elevated pressure of cerebrospinal fluid of normal composition along with normal cranial computed tomography. Interestingly, Bates and associates (1982) reported in men and nonpregnant women with this condition a significantly increased prolactin concentration in cerebrospinal fluid.

Usually, but not always, the disease is self-limited. Corticosteroids usually provide prompt relief. Infrequently, surgical shunting of cerebrospinal fluid is required. Kassam and colleagues (1983), Koontz and associates (1983), and Peterson and Kelly (1985) have provided a general review.

SPINAL CORD INJURY

Spinal cord lesions caused by trauma or tumor do not prevent conception. In women so affected, the pregnancy is likely to be complicated by urinary infections, pressure necrosis of the skin, and autonomic hyperreflexia. The latter is common with lesions above T5-6, and some stimuli, including cervical dilatation, may precipitate dangerous hypertension which should be treated immediately (Young and associates, 1983). Labor often is easy—even precipitous—and comparatively painless. The second stage may be prolonged due to diminished expulsive efforts. Trauma causing paraplegia also may cause pelvic deformity and, in turn, fetopelvic disproportion. Greenspoon and Paul (1986) provided a concise review of care for these women.

MULTIPLE SCLEROSIS

Multiple sclerosis is a neurological disease which rarely complicates pregnancy and there is no evidence that pregnancy precipitates the disease in women who were destined to develop it. In most cases, pregnancy has no deleterious effect on the course of multiple sclerosis; however, 20 to 40 percent of women have an exacerbation during the first few months postpartum (Birk and Rudick, 1986). Conversely, Frith and McLeod (1988) questioned 431 women with multiple sclerosis and reported that during 52 pregnancies the relapse rate was reduced significantly during the first two trimesters, but was not increased in the third trimester or postpartum up to 6 months. Perinatal outcome is not altered significantly, but the incidence of multiple sclerosis in the offspring is nearly 3 percent.

GUILLAIN-BARRÉ SYNDROME

Guillain-Barré syndrome, an acute demyelinating polyneuropathy, probably is mediated immunologically. Sudo and Weingold (1975) reported two pregnancies complicated by this syndrome and reviewed 25 others previously reported. After insidious onset, paresis and paralysis most often continue to ascend. Respiratory insufficiency is a common serious problem in both pregnant and nonpregnant patients, and about a fourth of patients need ventilatory assistance. Bravo and associates (1982) successfully ventilated a mother for 5 weeks before delivery of a healthy infant who did not appear to be affected neurologically.

Recently, there have been efforts to diminish the severity and duration of this illness by using plasmapheresis. The Guillain-Barré Syndrome Study Group (1985) reported the results of its randomized study of nearly 250 nonpregnant patients with this syndrome. Significant benefits of plasmapheresis included lessened severity and duration of paralysis. At least in pregnancy, our experiences are too preliminary to conclude that such treatment either shortens the course or improves outcome.

MYASTHENIA GRAVIS

Myasthenia gravis is a rare acquired autoimmune disorder that is caused by acetylcholine-receptor deficiency and involves the neuromuscular endplate. It is most common in women of reproductive age, and long-term therapy has consisted of anticholinesterase drugs, corticosteroids, immunosuppression, and thymectomy, alone or in combination. Clinical improvement of myasthenia gravis has been reported following intravenously administered immunoglobulin (Minnefor and Oleske, 1987) and may be life-saving in some cases. Cyclosporine also has been used with some success (Tindall and co-workers, 1987), but not during pregnancy. Most women respond well to pyridostigmine given every 3 to 4 hours. In severely ill women, short-term relief may be achieved with plasmapheresis. With occasional exceptions, women with myasthenia gravis go through pregnancy and labor without difficulty. During the second stage of labor some may demonstrate impairment of voluntary expulsive efforts. Any drug with a curare-like effect must be used with extreme caution. Such drugs include magnesium sulfate and aminoglycoside antibiotics. Apparently, even the quinine in tonic water may be harmful (Donaldson, 1978).

Acetylcholine-receptor antibodies have been detected in most myasthenic patients, and although these IgG antibodies are transferred from the mother to her fetus, only perhaps 10 percent of neonates have symptoms. This is more likely if neonatal antibody levels are high, according to Donaldson and associates (1981). Transient symptomatic myasthenia gravis in the affected infant typically is demonstrated by a feeble cry, poor suckling, and respiratory distress which are corrected by parenteral neostigmine. Neonatal myasthenia also responds to small doses of edrophonium or similar drugs and most often subsides completely within 4 to 6 weeks. Without prompt recognition and treatment, including good nursing care, the affected newborn infant may succumb to respiratory insufficiency caused by muscular weakness and the effects of aspiration. The fetus appears to be protected while in utero by a factor, perhaps α-fetoprotein, that inhibits the interaction between the receptors and antibody to the receptors (Noronha, 1985).

HUNTINGTON DISEASE

Huntington disease is a degenerative disease of the cerebral cortex and basal ganglia that is inherited as an autosomal dominant trait. With the description of a DNA probe localizing the gene to the short arm of chromosome 4, prenatal diagnosis is now possible and may be used soon to detect affected fetuses (Hayden and colleagues, 1987).

MIGRAINE HEADACHES

Nearly 25 percent of the population suffer from migraine headaches, and they are three times more common in women than in men. Such headaches especially are common in young women. The exact pathophysiology is uncertain, but there is general agreement that prodromal neurological symtoms are caused by cerebral artery vasoconstriction and decreased blood flow. Presumably, vasodilation follows and is responsible for the headache. *Common migraine* begins with a headache that is frequently accompanied by nausea and vomiting. *Classic migraine* implies neurological prodromata. *Complicated migraine* is accompanied by neurological symptoms which may include parasthesias, paresis, and even temporary paralysis that resembles a stroke, although full recovery is usually forthcoming.

There is said to be dramatic improvement of migraine during pregnancy (Noronha, 1985), and certainly, we infrequently encounter severe varieties during pregnancies cared for at Parkland Hospital. Fortunately, most of these headaches respond to simple analgesics, such as aspirin or acetaminophen, especially if given early in the course of symptoms. Ergotamine preparations are successful in preventing the headaches when taken during the prodrome. These drugs should be avoided if possible during pregnancy, although their effects on the pregnant uterus are not nearly so profound as ergonovine. For severe headaches not responsive to simple measures, then codeine or meperidine are given along with promethazine for antiemetic and sedative effects. For women with frequent attacks, propanolol, 40 mg three times daily has been used with success, and such a regimen should not be withheld during pregnancy in the woman with severe disease.

BELL PALSY

Isolated facial nerve palsy, or Bell palsy, is relatively common. Pregnancy seems to be complicated by a disparate number of these cases which develop typically in late gestation (McGregor and colleagues, 1987). Pregnancy does not seem to alter the overall good prognosis for spontaneous recovery, and nearly 90 percent of these women will recover function within a few weeks to months. Treatment with corticosteroids remains controversial, but the bulk of evidence suggests that these drugs do not hasten resolution (McGregor and associates, 1987). Surgical decompression is not recommended routinely. Supportive care includes prevention of injury to the constantly exposed cornea, facial muscle massage, and reassurance to the woman that she will in all likelihood regain total neurological function.

CARPAL TUNNEL SYNDROME

The median nerve is vulnerable to compression within the carpal tunnel at the wrist. Symptoms of nerve compression are common during pregnancy, and as many as 25 percent of women may complain of these symptoms (Voitk and colleagues, 1983). Typically, the woman awakens with burning, numbness, or tingling in the thenar half of one or both hands. The fingers otherwise feel numb and useless. A splint applied to the very slightly flexed wrist and worn during sleep usually provides relief. The signs and symptoms most often regress after delivery, and in our experiences at Parkland Hospital, surgical decompression and corticosteroid injections have not been necessary.

CHOREA GRAVIDARUM

Chorea gravidarum is a rare complication since rheumatic fever has become uncommon. Zegart and Schwarz (1968) identified only one case in the course of over 100,000 deliveries. Often the woman previously has suffered chorea which sooner or later abated spontaneously as it is likely to do during or after the pregnancy. Chloropromazine or haloperidol has been used to treat the disorder.

PSYCHIATRIC DISORDERS

Pregnancy and the puerperium are at times sufficiently stressful to induce psychosis. Postpartum depression is discussed in Chapter 28. In general, most psychiatric disorders are managed as if the woman were not pregnant, and the prognosis will be the same. Some of the fetal and maternal effects of major and minor tranquilizers, antidepressants, and other psychotropic drugs are considered in Chapter 32.

Electroshock therapy has been used often in the past during pregnancy. The risks, if any, to mother and fetus have not been carefully evaluated. One pregnant woman was transferred to Parkland Hospital when she convulsed spontaneously with eclampsia during the course of electroshock therapy. The mother and infant survived.

Lithium carbonate, when given in early pregnancy to treat manic-depressive women, appears to have teratogenic effects that are principally cardiovascular (see Chap. 32, p. 568). In addition, the neonate may suffer adverse effects (Briggs and colleagues, 1986). Thus, if used, the smallest effective dose should be administered and then only after 12 weeks gestation. The excretion of lithium by the kidney is increased in normal pregnancy but decreased by sodium-depleting diuretics and sodium-poor diets.

INFECTIONS DURING PREGNANCY

The pregnant woman is susceptible to many infections and infectious diseases. Some of these have a profound impact on pregnancy outcome by virtue of a high likelihood of teratogenesis and are discussed in Chapter 33. Considered now are some infections that pose unique problems created during a coexisting pregnancy, for example, chickenpox, or because of historical interest, for example, smallpox.

VIRAL INFECTIONS

VARICELLA

Most adults have acquired chickenpox during childhood and are immune. For adults who do become infected, varicella tends to be much more severe than in children. This is especially so during pregnancy, and Paryani and Arvin (1986) reported that 4 of 43, or about 10 percent of infected pregnant women, developed pneumonitis. Two of these women required ventilatory support and one died. Treatment has consisted of oxygenation, assisted ventilation when necessary, and control of bacterial suprainfection. Acyclovir given intravenously may be of value in preventing and treating varicella pneumonitis (Hirsch and Schooley, 1983; Landsberger and colleagues, 1986). We have observed severe thrombocytopenia plus prolonged prothrombin and partial thromboplastin times in pregnancies complicated by varicella pneumonia, especially in cases that proved fatal.

Maternal chickenpox during the first trimester has been implicated to cause congenital malformations as the consequence of transplacental infection. Paryani and Arvin (1986) reported that 10 percent of maternal infections resulted in clinical evidence for fetal infection, and this risk was the same for all trimesters. Another 12 percent of fetuses exposed during the second or third trimester had immunological evidence for infection. Infection early in pregnancy resulted in severe congenital malformations including chorioretinitis, cerebral cortical atrophy, hydronephrosis, and cutaneous and bony leg defects (Fig. 39–19). Fetal exposure later in pregnancy was associated with congenital varicella lesions, and zoster developed in one child at seven months of age.

Exposure of the fetus to the virus just before or during delivery, and therefore before he has received antibody from the mother, poses a serious threat to the newborn. In some instances the infant will develop disseminated visceral and central nervous system disease which in the past, at least, were likely to be fatal. Varicella-zoster (VZIG) or zoster immune globulin (ZIG) should be administered to the neonate whenever the onset of maternal clinical disease was within five days before delivery or two days postpartum.

Administration of varicella-zoster immune globulin will either prevent or attenuate varicella infection in exposed susceptible individuals. This is recommended by the Centers for Disease Control (1984) for immunocompromised susceptible adults who are exposed, but some recommend this routinely for pregnant women (McGregor and colleagues, 1987; Paryani and Arvin, 1986). Since 80 to 90 percent of adults are immune because of prior symptomatic or asymptomatic infection, antibody testing with enzyme-linked immunosorbent assay (ELISA) or fluorescent antibody to membrane antigen (FAMA) should be done if possible, prior to immune globulin therapy.

An experimental attenuated live-virus vaccine has been developed and if successful, will be of value for susceptible nonpregnant women.

INFLUENZA

Influenza is caused by an RNA myxovirus that is classified into A and B types which are futher subclassified by its hemagglu-

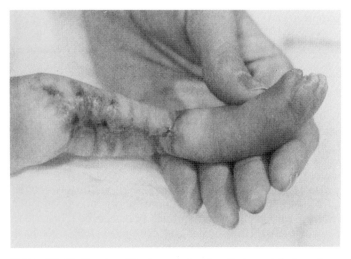

Figure 39–19. Atrophy of the lower extremity with bony defects and scarring in a fetus infected during the first trimester by varicella. (*From Paryani and Arvin: N Engl J Med 314:1542, 1986.*)

tinin (H) and neuraminidase (N) antigenic make-up. The viral strain is further characterized by its origin and the year of isolation. For example, one component in the 1988–89 vaccine was A/Taiwan/1/86 (H_1N_1), the first influenza A virus isolated from a patient in Taiwan in 1986 and having antigens of the H_1 hemagglutinin and N_1 neuraminidase subtypes. Influenza A is more serious than influenza B and usually develops during epidemics in winter months.

If pneumonia develops, the prognosis at once becomes serious. Although antibiotics are not effective against the influenza viruses, they are of value in the treatment of a secondary bacterial pneumonia. In the influenza pandemic of 1918, the disease, particularly the pneumonic type, was a grave complication of pregnancy. Harris (1919), in a statistical study based on 1,350 cases, found a gross maternal mortality rate of 27 percent, which increased to 50 percent when pneumonia developed. The 1957 pandemic, caused by A/Japan/305/57 (H_2N_2), also affected pregnant women with particular frequency and severity. In August and September 1957, for instance, 50 percent of childbearing-age women who died of influenza in Minnesota were pregnant (Freeman and Barno, 1959). In the same year in that state, the leading cause of maternal death was influenza. In New York City, the incidence of influenza in pregnant women was 50 percent higher than in nonpregnant controls and the mortality rate was also appreciably higher (Bass and Molloshok, 1960).

There is no firm evidence that influenza A virus causes congenital malformations (Larsen, 1982; Walker and McKee, 1959; Wilson and associates, 1959). However, McGregor and colleagues (1984) have demonstrated convincingly that the virus can infect the fetus, at least late in pregnancy. Vaccination against influenza is recommended by the Centers for Disease Control (1987) for pregnant women who have chronic underlying medical disorders and health-care workers who are likely to be exposed to high-risk patients.

MUMPS

This uncommon disease during pregnancy probably increases the risk of abortion and preterm labor. Pregnancy per se does not appear to increase the frequency or severity of complications associated with mumps. While parotid enlargement is a common feature, not all parotid enlargement is the consequence of mumps. For example, we have seen overtly enlarged parotid glands as the consequence of *pica* in the form of intense starch eating.

Manson and associates (1960) described 501 cases of mumps and reported that major fetal anomalies were not much more common than in the general population. Congenital mumps is very rare. Thus, whether intrauterine mumps infection endangers the health of the fetus and infant in any way is not clear.

RUBEOLA

Most adults are immune to measles, and thus it is a rare complication during pregnancy. An increased frequency of abortion and preterm delivery has been described if the mother develops measles. If she does so shortly before birth, there is considerable risk of measles developing in the neonate and, in turn, some risk of death, especially in preterm infants. The virus does not appear to be teratogenic. Passive immunization can be achieved by administering immune serum globulin intramuscularly. Vaccination should not be attempted during pregnancy since the vaccine contains live virus.

COMMON COLD

Rhinovirus, coronavirus, and adenovirus are major causes of the common cold. The first two are RNA viruses and usually produce a trivial, self-limited illness characterized by rhinorrhea, sneezing, and congestion. The DNA-containing adenovirus is more like to produce cough and lower respiratory tract involvement, including pneumonia. The pregnant woman is possibly slightly more susceptible to acute upper repiratory infections than the nonpregnant woman. Cases of pneumonia complicating pregnancy are often preceded by an acute upper respiratory viral infection. Puerperal infections from hemolytic streptococci may develop in patients who had acute respiratory infections at the time of delivery, and the incidence of hemolytic streptococci in the upper respiratory passages of such women is much higher than it is in healthy women.

ENTEROVIRUS INFECTIONS

Enteroviruses are RNA viruses that include poliovirus, Coxsackie virus, and echovirus. Even though they are trophic for intestinal epithelium, they can cause widespread infection that may include the central nervous system, heart, and lungs.

Coxsackievirus

These infections are usually clinically inapparent, but may cause aseptic meningitis, a polio-like illness, rashes, respiratory disease, or pleuritis, pericarditis, and myocarditis. The virus can be a serious complication of pregnancy, since it can be fatal to the fetus-infant, although causing only symptoms of a minor illness in the mother. Viremia in the fetus may cause hepatitis, myocarditis, and encephalomyelitis which can cause fetal death (Brady and Purdon, 1986). According to Amstey and colleagues (1988), there is clinical evidence that the Coxsackie virus seldom infects the fetus. However, it is certainly possible that maternal Coxsackie virus infection causes sublethal injuries of the embryo and fetus, thus producing congenital anomalies.

Poliomyelitis

The inactivated poliomyelitis vaccine (Salk) is recommended for adult vaccination, including immunization during pregnancy. With the widespread use of vaccination during childhood, polio has become rare in the United States. Siegel and Goldberg (1955), in a carefully controlled study in New York City, demonstrated that pregnant women not only are more susceptible to the disease, but have a higher death rate. Although the perinatal loss was about 33 percent, rarely was the fetus infected. Cesarean section was not necessarily required even in the presence of extensive paralysis and diminished expulsive efforts during the second stage of labor.

OTHER VIRUSES

Prior to the 13th edition of this book, the first disease discussed in this chapter was smallpox. In 1980 the World Health Organization declared that smallpox had been eradicated throughout the world!

Human *B19 parvovirus* causes erythema infectiosum, or fifth disease, and maternal infection has been linked in almost 40 percent of cases with adverse pregnancy outcomes, including abortion, fetal death, and congenital anomalies (Rodis and colleagues, 1988).

BACTERIAL INFECTIONS

STREPTOCOCCAL INFECTIONS

Although the causative organism of scarlet fever, *Streptococcus pyogenes*, is sensitive to certain antibiotics, the disease in the early months of pregnancy has a tendency to cause abortion, presumably because of the high fever in the mother. Regardless of treatment, rigid isolation must be instituted and maintained in the pregnant woman, parturient, or puerperal patient with scarlet fever. For no obvious reasons, scarlet fever has become very uncommon in recent years.

Erysipelas is an acute streptococcal skin infection and bacteremia is common. It is always a serious disease, but is particularly dangerous in pregnant women because of the potential hazard of puerperal infection. The hemolytic streptococci produce fetal infection and even death. For the protection of other patients, strict isolation of women with erysipelas is essential. Prompt treatment with penicillin G certainly has decreased the substantive mortality reported from the preantibiotic era.

LISTERIOSIS

Listeria monocytogenes is an uncommon but probably underdiagnosed cause of neonatal sepsis. From 1 to 5 percent of adults have listeria in their feces, and outbreaks of listeriosis have been reported from contaminated cabbage, pasteurized milk, and fresh Mexican-style cheese. Listeriosis during pregnancy may be asymptomatic or cause a febrile illness that is confused for influenza or pyelonephritis, and the diagnosis is not apparent until the blood culture is reported as positive. Maternal listeremia causes fetal infection that produces characteristically disseminated granulomatous lesions with microabscesses. There is evidence that maternal antimicrobial treatment may also be effective for fetal infection (Linnan and colleagues, 1988). Occult or clinical infection also may stimulate labor (Boucher and Yonekura, 1986). In these cases, early-onset neonatal sepsis is common, while late-onset listeriosis manifests as meningitis after 3 to 4 weeks of age. In this regard, these infections are very similar to those caused by group B β-hemolytic streptococci (see Chap. 33).

TYPHOID FEVER

Salmonella typhi is spread by oral ingestion of contaminated food, water, or milk. The disease is more likely to be encountered during epidemics (Duff and Engelsgjerd, 1983). According to Alimurung and Manahan (1952), pregnancy complicated by typhoid fever in former years resulted in abortion or preterm labor in 60 to 80 percent of cases, with a fetal mortality rate of 75 percent and a maternal mortality rate of 15 percent. However, the subsequent experiences of Riggall and co-workers (1974) are much more favorable. Chloramphenicol is the drug of choice, but ampicillin or trimethoprim-sulfamethoxazole may be given. Antityphoid vaccines appear to exert no harmful effects when administered to pregnant women and should be given in an epidemic or when otherwise indicated (see Chap. 14).

SHIGELLOSIS

Bacillary dysentery caused by *Shigella* species is a relatively common cause of watery diarrhea in adults. Since shigellosis is more common in children attending day-care centers, and since it is highly contagious, it is occasionally encountered in pregnant women. Clinical manifestations range from mild diarrhea to severe dysentery, abdominal cramping, tenesmus, fever, and systemic toxicity. Although shigellosis is self-limited, careful attention to treatment of dehydration is essential in severe cases. We have encountered women in whom secretory diarrhea exceeded 10 L per day! The treatment of choice is trimethoprim-sulfamethoxazole but ampicillin also may be given.

HANSEN DISEASE

According to Maurus (1978) and Duncan (1980), women with leprosy generally do well in pregnancy. Dapsone and clofazimine for treatment appear to be safe for use during pregnancy (Farb and associates, 1982). Duncan (1980) reported a high incidence of low-birthweight infants born to women infected with *Mycobacterium leprae*, and this was not explained by treatment given or maternal nutritional status. Fetal and placental infection must be rare since Duncan and associates (1984) were unable to demonstrate any morphological evidence of placental infection in 82 pregnant women infected with leprosy.

LYME DISEASE

This spirochetal disease, caused by *Borrelia burgdorferi,* is the most commonly reported tick-borne illness in the United States. It causes a distinctive skin lesion, *erythema chronicum migrans,* which may be followed by a flulike syndrome as well as rheumatic, cardiac, and neurological manifestions. In early infection, treatment is given with erythromycin, but in later infection with meningitis or carditis, intravenous penicillin G is recommended. There is concern that infection may be teratogenic, since other spirochetes, notably *Treponena pallidum* (see p. 851), cause congenital infection. Schlesinger and colleagues (1985) documented the persistence of spirochetes in fetal spleen, kidney, and bone marrow at 35 weeks in a woman who had Lyme disease during the first trimester. Markowitz and associates (1986) reviewed 19 cases of Lyme disease complicating pregnancy, and reported that 25 percent had preterm labor, fetal death, or rashlike illness in the newborn. They suggested further epidemiological surveillance to determine more conclusively if Borrelia causes abnormal pregnancy sequelae.

PROTOZOAL INFECTIONS

MALARIA

Nearly 200 million persons worldwide are infected with malaria at any given time. The incidence of abortion and preterm labor is increased with malaria, although the likelihood of either re-

lates to the severity of the disease and the promptness with which therapy is instituted. The increased fetal loss may be related to placental and fetal infections with malaria. The evidence for this is somewhat contradictory, however, since parasites rarely cross the placenta to infect the fetus. Covell (1950) studied this extensively in Africa and cited an incidence of neonatal malaria of 0.03 percent. According to Jones (1950), parasites have an affinity for the decidual vessels and may involve the placenta extensively without affecting the fetus. There is a marked tendency toward recrudescence of the disease during pregnancy and the puerperium, and after surgical operations. In women anemic from severe malarial infestation, fetal distress during labor is common (Looareesuwan and colleagues, 1985).

Commonly used antimalarial drugs are not contraindicated during pregnancy. Some of the newer antimalarial agents have antifolic acid activity, and theoretically may contribute to the development of megaloblastic anemia. In actual practice, this does not appear to be the case. Nonetheless, folic acid supplementation has been recommended (Bruce-Chwatt, 1983; Main and co-workers, 1983). For the woman with chloroquine-resistant falciparum infection, quinine is given orally. It may be given intravenously in severe infections, but careful attention must be given to the risk of hypoglycemia (Looareesuwan and colleagues, 1985).

Prophylaxis with chloroquine, 300 mg of base orally once a week, is initiated before an endemic area is entered and this is continued until 4 weeks after return to nonendemic areas (Centers for Disease Control, 1988b). Travel to areas endemic for chloroquine-resistant *P. falciparum* is discouraged.

AMEBIASIS

Dysentery caused by *Entamoeba histolytica,* especially if complicated by a hepatic abscess, may be a quite serious illness during pregnancy. Therapy is similar to that for the nonpregnant woman.

MYCOTIC INFECTIONS

In the past, disseminated *coccidiomycosis* during pregnancy commonly ended in maternal death. Powell and colleagues (1983) have presented data that are consistent with the view that *C. immitus* is stimulated in vitro by estrogen and progesterone through a specific cytosol protein-binding system. In more recent years treatment with amphotericin B has been employed successfully in a number of cases (Catanzaro, 1984; McCoy and associates, 1980). The drug must be administered carefully because of the risk of serious toxicity.

Disseminated infection during pregnancy is even less common with blastomycosis, cryptococcosis, or histoplasmosis, but their identification mandates prompt treatment with amphotericin B (McGregor and associates, 1986).

SEXUALLY TRANSMITTED DISEASES

There are more than 20 infectious diseases that may be transmitted by sexual contact, and pregnancy confers immunity to none of them. In fact, during a single act of intercourse a woman may become pregnant and acquire such a disease. Equally as important to the mother's health and well-being is the potential impact that some of these diseases may

have on her developing fetus. Many of these adverse fetal effects are considered also in Chapter 33.

In the following treatment protocols for sexually transmitted diseases, we attempt to adhere to the intensive, but frequently modified *Treatment Guidelines* provided by the Centers for Disease Control (1985b).

SYPHILIS

An unusually critical time to detect and treat syphilis is during pregnancy, not only to protect the mother and her sexual partner from the numerous complications of syphilis but, especially important, to protect the fetus from the extensive pathological changes that characterize congenital syphilis (see Chap. 33, p. 617). Fortunately, of the many congenital infections, syphilis is not only the most readily prevented, but it also is one of the most susceptible to therapy.

IDENTIFICATION

Following an incubation period of 10 to 90 days, but usually less than 6 weeks, primary syphilis appears. When infection is acquired during pregnancy, the primary lesion, or sometimes multiple lesions, involving the genital tract may be of such small size or be so located as to go unnoticed. For example, the lesion may be confined to the cervix. In some instances, however, the lesion may be somewhat larger than usual, presumably because of the increased vascularity of the genitalia. The primary lesion or chancre persists from 2 to 6 weeks and then heals spontaneously, but the chancre often is accompanied by the development of nontender, enlarged inguinal lymph nodes.

Approximately 6 to 8 weeks after healing of the chancre, secondary syphilis usually appears in the form of a highly variable skin rash. About 15 percent of women still have a chancre. The lesions of secondary syphilis may be mild and go unnoticed in 25 percent of patients. In some, lesions are limited to the genitalia, where they appear usually as elevated areas, or *condylomata lata*, which occasionally cause vulvar ulcerations. In many women no history of a local sore or rash can be elicited. At times the first suggestion of the disease is the delivery of an infant that may be either stillborn or liveborn but severely afflicted with congenital syphilis.

Syphilis of any stage during pregnancy can result in an infected and affected fetus. The more recent infections are more likely to be associated with fetal morbidity. Fetal syphylitic infection from maternal transmission is considered in Chapter 33, p. 617.

A suitable serological screening test such as the *Venereal Disease Research Laboratory (VDRL)* slide test or the *rapid plasma reagin (RPR)* test must be performed on blood obtained at the time of the first prenatal visit. Testing is required by law. Fortunately, serological tests for syphilis almost always will be positive by 4 to 6 weeks after contracting the disease. Because such reagin tests lack specificity, a treponemal test such as the *fluorescent treponemal antibody absorption test (FTA-ABS)* or the *microhemagglutination assay for antibodies to Treponema pallidum (MHA-TP)* is used to confirm a positive result. Especially for women at high risk for syphilis, a second nontreponemal test should be done during the third trimester, and the cord blood should be tested.

ANTIMICROBIAL TREATMENT FOR SYPHILIS

Penicillin remains the treatment of choice. The recommendations for treatment provided by the Centers for Disease Control (1985b) follow.

Incubating Syphilis

Patients exposed to infectious syphilis within the preceding 3 months, or those at high risk based on epidemiological grounds, should be treated as for early syphilis as outlined below. Where possible a diagnosis should be established. Women who are culture positive for gonorrhea with no lesion and a nonreactive serology also must be considered at high risk. The aqueous procaine penicillin G plus probenecid regimen for gonorrhea (p. 852) is also effective therapy for incubating syphilis. A reagin test for syphilis should be repeated 3 months after the initial therapy.

Syphilis of Less Than 1-Year Duration

This includes women with primary or secondary syphilis, as well as those known to be seronegative a year or less before becoming positive.

1. Benzathine penicillin G, 2.4 million units as a single dose intramuscularly, half in each buttock. This regimen has the advantage of single-visit treatment.
2. Penicillin-allergic patients:
   Erythromycin, 500 mg orally four times a day for 15 days.
   Tetracycline hydrochloride, 500 mg orally four times a day for 15 days.
   Tetracycline is not recommended during pregnancy.

If during the year following treatment, clinical signs recur or persist, a spinal fluid examination should be done and the patient retreated using the regimen described below for syphilis acquired more than one year previously. The same retreatment regimen is used if the initial nonspecific antibody titer of 1:8 or greater fails to decrease at least fourfold, or if it rises fourfold within a 12-month period.

Late Latent or Latent Syphilis of Uncertain Duration

This includes treatment of syphilis of indeterminate length but more than 1-year duration. Most women in this category are those found to be positive at routine screening, but they have no history of syphilitic infection.

1. Benzathine penicillin G, 2.4 million U intramuscularly weekly (1.2 million units in each buttock) for 3 successive weeks, a total of 7.2 million units.
2. Penicillin-allergic pregnant women are given erythromycin, 500 mg orally, four times daily for 30 days, for a total of 60 g. For nonpregnant patients a spinal fluid examination is performed prior to therapy and if abnormal, treatment is given as for neurosyphilis.

Treatment of Neurosyphilis

If the spinal fluid is positive, treatment is more intense. Since about 25 percent of patients with neurosyphilis have had recurrences following one dose of 2.4 million U of benzathine penicillin G, this regimen alone is not recommended for neurosyphilis.

1. Hospitalization is recommended to institute therapy with intravenous penicillin G, 2 to 4 million U every 4 hours for 10 days followed by benzathine penicillin G, 2.4 million U intramuscularly weekly for 3 doses.
2. Alternatively, aqueous procaine penicillin G, 2.4 million U intramuscularly daily plus probenecid 500 mg orally four times daily, both for 10 days, can be given, followed by benzathine penicillin G, 2.4 million U intramuscularly weekly for 3 doses.

3. For the penicillin-allergic nonpregnant patient, alternative treatment includes tetracycline, 500 mg daily for 30 days. Erythromycin is not recommended for neurosyphilis.

All patients with abnormal spinal fluid results should have spinal fluid testing at least every 6 months for 3 years.

Treatment of Syphilis in Pregnancy

For pregnant women not allergic to penicillin, treatment is the same as for the corresponding stage of syphilis in nonpregnant patients. For pregnant women who are allergic to penicillin, the only recommended therapy is erythromycin using the same guidelines as for nonpregnant women for the same stage of disease.

Unfortunately, erythromycin does not guarantee that fetal syphilis will be adequately treated. The drug crosses the placenta poorly, and it is our conclusion that other therapy should be given. One alternative is to desensitize these women to penicillin after which benzathine penicillin G is used as recommended (Wendel and colleagues, 1985). If this is not practical, then we agree with Fiumara (1984) that tetracycline should be given. Holmes (1987) suggests doxycycline, 200 mg orally twice daily for 15 days. Cephalosporins as yet have not been evaluated extensively and their use is not recommended.

The mother who has been treated successfully often remains susceptible to a subsequent syphilitic infection, as does her fetus. Therefore, it is important during pregnancy to treat her sexual partner, as well as to observe her closely for evidence of reinfection. When reinfection is detected, retreatment is necessary. Women who have been treated for syphilis during pregnancy should have monthly quantitative nontreponemal serological tests (VDRL or RPR) for the remainder of the pregnancy. Women who show a fourfold or greater rise in titer should be retreated.

Treatment of Congenital Syphilis

Every infant with suspected or proven congenital syphilis should have a cerebrospinal fluid examination prior to treatment, and should be followed at monthly intervals until the nontreponemal serological tests become negative or serofast. Symptomatic infants or those with abnormal spinal fluid examination should be treated with aqueous penicillin G, 50,000 U per kg intramuscularly or intravenously in two divided doses each day for at least 10 days, or aqueous procaine penicillin G, 50,000 U per kg intramuscularly each day for a minimum of 10 days.

Asymptomatic seropositive infants with a normal spinal fluid examination can be treated with a single dose of benzathine penicillin G, 50,000 U per kg intramuscularly.

Infants born of mothers treated with erythromycin for syphilis during pregnancy should be retreated as though they have congenital syphilis.

GONORRHEA

Female infection caused by *Neisseria gonorrhoeae* may be limited to the lower genital tract, including the cervix, urethra, and periurethral and Bartholin glands, or it may spread across the endometrium to infect the oviducts and the peritoneum. The organism also may enter the bloodstream to cause arthritis uncommonly and endocarditis rarely.

Acute gonococcal salpingitis is not a problem in pregnancy after about 12 weeks when the chorion laeve has fused with the decidua parietalis to obliterate the endometrial cavity between the cervix and oviducts. Rarely, a fallopian tube previously damaged by infection with *N. gonorrhoeae* may become reinfected during pregnancy with other organisms that apparently reach it through the bloodstream or lymphatics, or perhaps there is reactivation of a previously acquired but subclinical infection. Regardless, these infections are rarely seen during early pregnancy even at Parkland Hospital, where acute salpingitis is seen commonly in nonpregnant women.

The greatly increased prevalance of gonorrhea in recent years has not spared pregnant women, and many public obstetrical clinics have reported gonococcal infections of the lower genitourinary tract to be common. At Parkland Hospital, for example, the prevalence of asymptomatic cervical infection is about 3 percent (Dr. George Wendel, personal communciation).

The pregnant woman may have asymptomatic local infection involving singly, or in combination, the lower genital tract, lower urinary tract, rectum, or pharynx. The infection may antedate the pregnancy or the woman may have acquired the disease at the time of the insemination that resulted in pregnancy. Finally, she may have become infected after conception. In any event, without adequate treatment, persistence of the infection may allow her to infect her sexual partner, to suffer gonococcal arthritis or other disseminated disease, to infect her infant at the time of delivery, thereby causing gonorrheal ophthalmia (see Chap. 12, p. 241), or to develop an ascending genital infection postpartum. Consequently, even asymptomatic disease during pregnancy should be identified and eradicated. Ideally all pregnant women should have an endocervical culture made to detect gonorrhea at the time of their first visit. In high-risk women, an initial culture should be made at the first visit, followed by another culture obtained late in pregnancy (see Chap. 14, p. 259).

TREATMENT OF GONORRHEA

In recent years there has been an increasing frequency of infections caused by plasmid-mediated penicillinase-producing *Neisseria gonorrhoeae*. Chromosomally and plasmid-mediated tetracycline-resistant organisms also are becoming common. Recently, Boslego and colleagues (1987) reported a disturbingly high incidence of chromosomally-mediated resistance of gonococci to spectinomycin which is the drug previously recommended for penicillinase-producing strains. To further complicate therapy, chlamydial infections coexist commonly with gonococcal disease.

Sexual partners exposed to gonorrhea should be examined, cultured, and treated at once using one of the following regimes. Individuals treated for gonorrhea should be recultured 5 to 7 days after completion of the treatment.

Uncomplicated Infection in Adults

Several regimens are suitable.

1. Aqueous procaine penicillin G, 4.8 million U injected intramuscularly, half in each of two injection sites, plus 1 g of probenecid by mouth.
2. Ampicillin 3.5 g, or amoxicillin 3 g, plus probenecid 1 g, both by mouth. (This regimen is not effective against pharyngeal infection.)

3. For penicillin-allergic women, spectinomycin 2 g, intramuscularly, is recommended. (Incubating syphilis is not adequately treated by spectinomycin. A penicillin-resistant gonococcus has been identified that is also resistant to spectinomycin.)
4. Ceftriaxone, 250 mg intramuscularly, is given to high-risk patients in areas endemic for penicillinase-producing gonococci.
5. Tetracycline is not recommended during pregnancy; otherwise, the recommended dose is 500 mg orally four times a day for 7 days.

Coexistent Chlamydial Infection
All adults treated for gonorrhea should be treated for coexistent chlamydial infection. For pregnant women, the suggested treatment is the addition, to one of the above regimens, of erythromycin, 500 mg given orally four times a day for at least 7 days. Optimal dosage has not been established. In the absence of pregnancy, tetracycline 500 mg is given orally four times daily or doxycycline 100 mg is given orally twice daily, either regimen for 7 days.

Treatment Failures or Penicillinase-Producing Gonococci
Ceftriaxone, 250 mg intramuscularly, or spectinomycin, 2 g intramuscularly, may prove effective. Spectinomycin is not recommended for pharyngeal gonorrhea.

Disseminated Gonococcal Infections
There are several acceptable treatment schedules for arthritis and dermatitis including aqueous crystalline penicillin G intravenously at the outset, and either ampicillin or amoxicillin, 500 mg by mouth four times daily to complete 7 days of therapy. Tetracycline is recommended in case of penicillin allergy unless the woman is pregnant. Then erythromycin can be used as described above.

For gonococcal endocarditis and meningitis, long-term high-dose penicillin is given intravenously.

Infants of Mothers with Gonorrhea. Aqueous crystalline penicillin G, 50,000 U in a single injection is recommended (20,000 U is given to low birthweight infants).

Gonococcal Ophthalmia. The infant should be isolated until treated for 24 hours with intravenously administered penicillin G, 100,000 U per kg daily for 10 days. Local care of the eyes by an expert is also important. Topical antibiotic preparations are not appropriate. Both parents also should be treated for gonorrhea.

CHLAMYDIAL INFECTIONS

Chlamydia trachomatis is an obligate intracellular bacterium thought to be the most prevalent cause of sexually transmitted disease in the United States. The organism has several serotypes, and includes those that cause *lymphogranuloma venereum*, but the most commonly encountered are those that attach only to columnar or transitional cell epithelium and cause cervical, but not vulvar infection. The replication rate for chlamydiae is long compared to other bacteria, and this characteristic may explain the long latency period and frequent minimal symptomatology. Thus, chlamydial infections are characterized by their low-grade indolence, often associated with a paucity of clinical findings.

MATERNAL INFECTIONS
A profile of women at high risk for chlamydial infections, along with syndromes caused by chlamydiae, is given in Table 39–16.

Symptomatic Infection
Lower genital tract infections generally are minimally symptomatic. They are manifest most often by mucopurulent cervicitis characterized by cervical erythema and edema with cloudy or white "mucopus" which contains abundant polymorphonuclear leucocytes. It is difficult to distinguish normal cervical eversion and erythema of pregnancy from chlamydial cervicitis. Since the organism is incapable of attachment to stratified squamous epithelium, the vagina is not involved, which in part explains the lack of symptoms. Chlamydiae are, however, capable of attachment to and invasion of transitional cell epithelium, which may cause dysuria and frequency, and this may be attributed to conventional bacterial cystitis. Routine urine culture methods do not include techniques for chlamydia isolation, and women with the *acute urethral syndrome* caused by chlamydial infection have persistent dysuria, frequency, and pyuria with cultures reported as sterile (Stamm and colleagues, 1980).

Verification of these infections has been made easier by the use of a direct-slide fluorescence-tagged chlamydia monoclonal antibody test which is considered by many to be almost as accurate as culture. When these tests confirm maternal genital chlamydial infection, treatment is given with either erythromycin base 500 mg, or erythromycin ethylsuccinate 800 mg, four times daily for 7 days. In the absence of techniques to verify infection, and in the clinical settings described above, especially if the male sexual partner has nongonococcal urethritis, it is reasonable to treat the woman empirically with erythromycin. It is important that the male consort be treated with tetracycline or erythromycin.

Asymptomatic Infection
Depending upon epidemiological variables, the prevalence of asymptomatic *C. trachomatis* cervical carriage ranges from 3 to 26 percent (Eschenbach, 1985). Its incidence increases with the number of sexual contacts, and is higher in socioeconomically deprived women. Importantly, it frequently coexists with gonococcal infection, and the Centers for Disease Control recommends empirical therapy be given for chlamydiae whenever gonorrhea is treated (p. 852). It has been recommended by

TABLE 39–16. CHLAMYDIAL INFECTIONS

Women at High Risk	Symptomatic Syndromes
Less than 20 years of age	**Maternal**
Unmarried	Mucopurulent cervicitis
Lower socioeconomic status	Nongonococcal urethritis
Inner city population	Proctitis
Multiple sexual partners	Acute salpingitis
Other sexually transmitted diseases	Conjunctivitis
	Neonatal
	Conjunctivitis
	Pneumonia

From Centers for Disease Control: Chlamydia trachomatis *Infections. Policy Guidelines for prevention and control. Publication No. 00–4770, Atlanta, August, 1985.*

some that women at high risk for asymptomatic chlamydial infection (Table 39–16) undergo diagnostic testing and treatment during pregnancy, and indeed, Schachter and associates (1986) recently reported that such a practice reduces appreciably the incidence of neonatal chlamydial infections (see Chap. 33, p. 619).

PRETERM BIRTH AND LOW BIRTHWEIGHT INFANTS

It is unclear if cervical chlamydial infection causes preterm labor and delivery and low birthweight infants. Martin and colleagues (1982) reported a tenfold increased perinatal mortality and five-fold increased preterm birth rate in a small group of women identified to be chlamydia-positive early in pregnancy. Similarly, Gravett and co-workers (1986) found that chlamydial cervical infection was associated with a higher incidence of both preterm prematurely ruptured membranes and preterm labor. Harrison and associates (1983) studied a larger group with a similar prevalence of infection and found no such association. They did identify, however, a subgroup of women with serum IgM antibody who were at increased risk for low birthweight infants and prematurely ruptured membranes.

Sweet and colleagues (1987) studied prospectively 270 pregnant women with untreated cervical chlamydial infection and compared their pregnancy outcomes to chlamydia-negative controls. There were no differences in the incidences of preterm labor, prematurely ruptured membranes, chorioamnionitis, neonatal sepsis, or postpartum uterine infections. However, they found that women with evidence for recent infection characterized by IgM antibody to *C. trachomatis* were more likely to have preterm labor or prematurely ruptured membranes. Berman and colleagues (1987) also reported this association in 1,152 Navajo women whose cervical carriage rate for chlamydia was 22 percent.

If silent chlamydial cervical infection predisposes to poor pregnancy outcome, it will likely be from preterm labor caused by subclinical ascending chorioamnionitis or prematurely ruptured membranes. There is now substantial evidence that at least one third of women with preterm labor have occult chorioamnionitis (see Chap. 38, p. 749). The pathogens as yet have not been well elucidated, and it is possible that chlamydial co-pathogens also may contribute to perinatal morbidity. For example, genital mycoplasmas have been associated both with preterm labor and chorioamnionitis, and both *Ureaplasma urealyticum*, and *Mycoplasma hominis*, as well as *N. gonorrhoeae*, frequently co-exist with chlamydiae. To determine the impact of these asymptomatic cervical infections, as well as their treatment, large prospective investigations are necessary, and the National Institutes of Health is currently sponsoring such a study.

PUERPERAL INFECTION

The role of chlamydiae in most postpartum infections appears minimal; however, as many as one half of women with late infection manifested at 1 to 6 weeks postpartum will be culture-positive for *C. trachomatis* (Eschenbach, 1985; Wager and colleagues, 1980). Women whose infants have chlamydial conjunctivitis have a much higher incidence of these late infections when compared to mothers of uninfected infants. Clinically, they are mild, but may cause infertility if not treated, and tetracycline 500 mg four times daily for 7 days is the drug of choice.

LYMPHOGRANULOMA VENEREUM

The L serotypes of *Chlamydia trachomatis* cause lymphogranuloma venereum (lymphopathia venereum). The primary genital infection is transient and seldom recognized. Inguinal adenitis may follow and at times lead to suppuration. Utimately, the lymphatics of the lower genital tract and perirectal tissues may be involved with sclerosis and fibrosis, which can cause vulvar elephantiasis and especially severe rectal stricture.

Fistula formation involving the rectum, perineum, and vulva also may be quite troublesome. Sometimes attention is first drawn to the disease in pregnant women when rectal examination is attempted. In the absence of pregnancy, tetracycline 500 mg orally four times daily for at least 2 weeks is recommended. Otherwise erythromycin, in the same dosage, can be tried as can sulfamethoxazole, 1 g orally twice a day for at least 2 weeks. Stricture and fistula formation may necessitate surgical intervention. Some of these infections that we have encountered at Parkland Hospital have been long-standing, and there was little response to multiple antimicrobial regimens that in one case included erythromycin, sulfamethoxazole, tetracycline, and chloramphenicol.

HERPES SIMPLEX VIRUS INFECTIONS

Management of pregnancy complicated by maternal genital infection with herpesvirus remains a frustrating exercise for the obstetrician who often is expected to make intelligent management decisions during labor based on results from cervical and vulvar cultures often more than a week old and which seldom accurately reflect intrapartum conditions. There are no currently available rapid diagnostic tests that reliably document contemporary infection. Finally, there are minimal data to estimate risks for the neonate exposed to recurrent maternal infection.

VIROLOGY

Two types of herpesvirus have been distinguished based on immunological as well as clinical differences. Type 1 herpes simplex virus is responsible for most nongenital herpetic infections, but infrequently involves the genital tract. Type 2 virus is recovered almost exclusively from the genital tract and is transmitted in the great majority of instances by sexual contact (National Institutes of Health, 1985). The incidence of antibodies specific for type 2 herpes increases with age and varies considerably with the population studied, and it approaches 100 percent among prostitutes. In the absence of antibody, exposure to a sexual partner with active herpetic lesions will in the majority of instances result in clinical disease.

CLINICAL INFECTION

After primary mucocutaneous infection, viral particles infect contiguous nerve ganglia and establish a latent infection which appears to be lifelong. Latent infection is periodically interrupted by virus reactivation that results in either clinically silent (viral shedding) or apparent (recurrent) infections.

Primary Infection

Although frequently symptomatic, primary infection with herpesvirus may be asymptomatic, probably due to some immunity from cross-reacting antibody from childhood-acquired type 1 infection. The typical incubation period of 3 to 6 days is followed by a papular eruption with itching or tingling which then becomes painful and vesicular with multiple vulvar and perineal lesions that may coalesce. Inguinal adenopathy may be severe. Transient systemic influenza-like symptoms are common and are presumably caused by viremia. The vulvar and perineal vesicles are easily traumatized, eventually ulcerate, and can become secondarily infected. Vulvar lesions are likely to be extremely painful and may cause considerable debility. Urinary retention may occur because of the pain induced by micturition or because of sacral nerve involvement. In 2 to 4 weeks, all signs and symptoms of infection disappear, but later recurrences are common because of viral reactivation from the nerve ganglia. Cervical involvement is common with primary infection and may show inflammation, ulceration or be clinically inapparent.

There is no really effective treatment. Acyclovir used topically perhaps modifes the symptomatology. Oral or parenteral preparations have been shown to attenuate clinical infection as well as duration of viral shedding, but have not been used extensively during pregnancy and are not recommended routinely. Severe secondary bacterial infection should respond to broad-spectrum antimicrobial therapy. For intense discomfort, analgesics and topical anesthetics may provide some relief, and severe urinary retention is treated with an indwelling bladder catheter.

Recurrent Infection

During the latency period in which viral particles reside in nerve ganglia, reactivation is common and mediated through variable but poorly understood stimuli. Reactivation is termed recurrent infection and results in herpesvirus shedding with or without symptomatic lesions. These lesions are generally fewer in number, less tender, and shed virus for shorter periods (2 to 5 days) than those of primary infection, and they typically recur at the same sites. Although commonly involved in primary infection, cervical infection is less frequent with recurrent infections (Brown and colleagues, 1985; Yeager and Arvin, 1984).

While the episodic nature of asymptomatic viral shedding is well appreciated, its predictability is of particular concern in pregnant women who have recurrent genital infections. The reported prevalence rates for isolation of genital tract herpesvirus vary considerably, but may be as high as 4 to 5 percent in a high-risk population of women in whom the cervix is routinely cultured near term (Jacob and co-workers, 1984). While the rate of viral isolation in asymptomatic women varies considerably depending upon the population studied, equally important is whether or not women were included (or excluded) because of prior symptomatic infection. Prober and colleagues (1988) obtained specimens for culture from mothers and infants at the time of 6,904 deliveries without regard to the mothers' history of genital herpes. Only 14 (0.2 percent) were positive for herpesvirus, and 12 of these were recurrent infections.

Diagnosis of Herpesvirus Infection

Recovery of virus by tissue culture is most optimum for confirmation of clinically apparent infection and asymptomatic recurrences. The sensitivity of culture is nearly 95 percent before the lesions undergo crusting as long as specimens are properly obtained and handled. There are virtually no false-positives. With symptomatic recurrences, more than half of the cultures will be positive after 48 hours, but it may take longer to demonstrate cytopathic effects with asymptomatic recurrences, because of lower viral titers.

Cytologic examination after alcohol fixation and Papanicolaou staining is commonly used as a rapid means of diagnosis of clinical recurrences, and smears taken from scrapings of the base of lesions may show large multinucleated cells and eosinophilic viral inclusion bodies. This method is limited by its specificity and sensitivity. *Immunoperoxidase staining* and *enzyme-linked immunosorbent assay* (ELISA) techniques have been evaluated for rapid diagnosis of direct smears, but there is little experience with these tests during pregnancy.

HERPESVIRUS INFECTION DURING PREGNANCY

There is little evidence that herpesvirus causes early pregnancy wastage. However, Brown and associates (1987) presented preliminary data that primary infection, especially if acquired in the last trimester, may cause preterm labor and delivery or fetal growth retardation. Until appropriately studied, there is no justification for maternal systemic therapy with acyclovir to prevent fetal infection, or amniocentesis for culture to diagnose fetal infection.

Brown and colleagues (1985) have provided insight into the natural history of recurrent infection during pregnancy. They reported that in women whose initial infection was indentified prior to pregnancy, 84 percent had at least one recurrent infection during pregnancy, and these women had symptomatic recurrences on the average every 2 to 3 months. Asymptomatic viral shedding was identified at some time during pregnancy in 15 percent of these women. Although labial shedding was more common, almost 40 percent of these women with symptomless shedding had positive cervical cultures, and half were concomitant with a positive vulvar culture. Interestingly, recurrences were more common as pregnancy progressed, and this phenomenon has been attributed by some to suppressed cell-mediated immune responses (Weinberg, 1984). Brown and co-workers (1987) subsequently described the courses of women with a first episode of genital herpes during pregnancy. Following resolution of lesions, these women were then cultured weekly throughout pregnancy, and only 11 percent of cultures were positive.

NEONATAL DISEASE

Infection is transmitted only rarely across the placenta or an intact chorioamnion to the embryo or fetus. Almost always the fetus becomes infected by virus shed from the cervix or lower genital tract. The virus then either invades the uterus following rupture of the membranes or contacts the fetus at delivery. The incidence of neonatal herpesvirus infection has increased remarkably in some, and presumably most, areas of the United States. For example, Sullivan-Bolyai and associates (1983) reported an increase in King County, Washington, from 2.6 per 100,000 live births in 1969 to 12 per 100,000 in 1981.

Newborn infection takes on one of three forms: (1) disseminated, with involvement of major viscera (Fig. 39–20), (2) localized, with involvement confined to the central nervous system, eyes, skin, or mucosa, or (3) asymptomatic. Nearly half of the neonates infected with herpesvirus are preterm and their risk of infection correlates with whether there is primary or recurrent maternal infection. For example, Nahmias and colleagues (1971) reported a 50 percent risk of neonatal infection with primary maternal infection, but only 4 to 5 percent with recurrent infection. Prober and associates (1987) reported that none of 34 neonates exposed to recurrent viral shedding at delivery became infected. This is thought to be due to a smaller viral inoculum

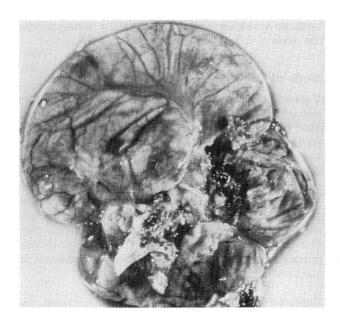

Figure 39–20. Cross-section showing necrotic brain tissue in a newborn infant who died from disseminated herpesvirus infection.

with recurrent infection, and as well as transplacentally acquired antibody which decreases the incidence, and severity of neonatal disease (Prober and colleagues, 1987; Yeager and Arvin, 1984).

Neonatal infection is associated with a mortality rate of at least 60 percent, and importantly, serious ophthalmic and central nervous system damage has been identified in at least half of survivors. In general, treatment of the neonate has been disappointing; therefore, considerable emphasis is placed upon prevention of contact between fetus and virus during delivery.

ANTEPARTUM MANAGEMENT

Because of the severity of neonatal herpesvirus infection, cesarean delivery has been used widely in instances when genital herpetic lesions are suspected or a recent culture or Pap smear has been positive for virus. For some, the unproven threat of asymptomatic viral shedding by women previously diagnosed as having genital herpes is considered sufficient grounds for cesarean section. While the latter approach seems overcautious, it is certainly prudent to choose cesarean delivery if there is *reasonable* chance that virus is being shed. In many cases, however, this is difficult to prove with currently available technology.

The premise that all neonatal infections can be avoided by carefully screening the obstetrical population is incorrect. A history consistent with a recurrent maternal genital infection is elicited in only one-fourth of mothers of infected infants (Yeager and Arvin, 1984). Many of the remaining women have peripartum primary infection, undiagnosed recurrent infection, or a sexual partner with recurrent genital infection. Another source of neonatal infection is oral lesions from the mother, family members, or even health personnel.

Several points should be emphasized with respect to women with a history of recurrent genital infection. The presence, absence, or frequency of recurrences does not predict asymptomatic shedding at delivery. Such shedding appears to be an entirely random event of short duration, usually less than

7 days (Wittek and associates, 1984). Indeed, according to some, there is greater than a 95 percent chance of a negative viral culture 7 days after an episode of asymptomatic shedding during pregnancy.

Many investigators have proposed protocols advocating the use of weekly cervicovaginal cultures to detect asymptomatic shedding, some beginning at 32 weeks, 36 weeks, or even a 38-week single culture. While 1 to 5 percent of randomly selected women have been shown to shed virus asymptomatically near term, cultures taken during labor are rarely positive. This may be due to antibody in cervical secretions, blood, or amnionic fluid (Hankins and colleagues, 1984). In addition to its unpredictability, detection of asymptomatic shedding during pregnancy in women with recurrent genital herpes also is expensive. The Centers for Disease Control estimated that $1.8 million would be spent yearly in the United States to prevent each case of neonatal herpes infection in women with recurrent infections (Binkin and associates, 1984). Moreover, only 11 neonatal deaths and 3.7 cases of severe mental retardation would be averted, but 3 to 4 women would die from complications of the cesarean sections performed because of positive viral cultures. Finally it is estimated that only one-fourth of women shedding virus at the time of delivery would be identified.

Arvin and colleagues (1986) recently provided data that are consistent with the view that serial genital cultures for herpesvirus are not predictive of the risk for neonatal infection. They studied 414 pregnant women with a history of recurrent genital herpes infections and found that in none of these women did antepartum cultures predict the 1.4 percent with positive cultures at delivery. This had been our experience at Parkland Hospital, and for some time our policy has been to use a management plan with the method of delivery based on the presence or absence of genital lesions. In this scheme, it is imperative that a diligent search in a well-motivated patient be carried out in early labor or with prematurely ruptured membranes. Cesarean delivery is performed if there are prodromal symptoms of a recurrence, or if primary or recurrent lesions are visualized near the time of labor or when the membranes are ruptured. This approach is now recommended by the American College of Obstetricians and Gynecologists (1988b), as well as the Infectious Disease Society for Obstetrics and Gynecology (Gibbs and colleagues, 1988).

Ruptured Membranes

With ruptured membranes, the "four-hour rule" has been commonly applied: If genital herpes is diagnosed or strongly suspected, and the membranes have been ruptured less than 4 hours, cesarean delivery is performed; otherwise, vaginal delivery is allowed. With recurrent perineal or vulvar lesions, this plan is not always justified since only about 20 to 40 percent of these women have concomitant cervical (and thus membrane-contiguous) infection. In the absence of previous examination or instrumentation, there is no evidence that these external lesions cause ascending membrane and fetal infection. We disregard the duration of membrane rupture in formulating a plan of delivery for women with perineal lesions, and unless there are other contradictory factors, for example, gross immaturity, we deliver these women with lesions by cesarean section.

CARE OF THE NEONATE

An exposed infant of a mother known or suspected of having genital herpes should be isolated and cultures taken for herpes.

Additionally, liver function and spinal fluid should be monitored serially along with close infant observation for up to 2 weeks. It has been considered impractical and unnecessary by some neonatologists, but certainly not all, to separate baby and mother when the mother has herpetic lesions. Instead, she may be instructed to wash her hands carefully and avoid any contact between her lesions, her hands, and the baby. Breast feeding has been allowed under these conditions; however, it should be pointed out that this was implicated in one case of disseminated neonatal infection. Some have recommended that parents and personnel with oral herpetic lesions be isolated from newborn infants, although Schriner and associates (1979) found that over 50 percent of 110 neonatal centers questioned did not do so.

ACQUIRED IMMUNODEFICIENCY SYNDROME

Acquired immunodeficiency syndrome (AIDS) was first described in 1981 when a cluster of patients was found to have defective cellular immunity and *Pneumocystis carinii* pneumonia. Within 4 years, another 10,000 cases were reported. In addition to its medical ramifications, the syndrome has had far-reaching psychological impact on medical workers and the general public.

The etiological agent of AIDS is the human immunodeficiency virus (HIV), an RNA-retrovirus capable of inducing severe immunological dysfunction in T-4 helper lymphocytes. Retroviruses have genomes which encode the enzyme, *reverse transcriptase*, which allows DNA to be transcribed from RNA. Thus the virus can make DNA copies of its own genome in host cells. Transmission is similar to hepatitis B virus, and sexual intercourse, especially amongst male homosexuals, is the major mode of transmission. It also is transmitted by blood or blood-contaminated products, and infected mothers may infect their infants.

The prevalence of asymptomatic infection in the United States in 1987 was estimated at 1 to 1.5 million persons, and by the end of 1988, the Centers for Disease Control (1988a) had reported more than 70,000 cases of AIDS. The exact incubation period is unknown; however, it may be as short as 2 months or as long as 5 years. The stimuli that cause progression from asymptomatic viremia to the immunodeficiency syndrome are presently unclear, but perhaps 10 percent of patients with serological evidence for infection will develop clinical illness within 3 years (Fauci and Lane, 1987). There may be less severe manifestations characterized by immune dysfunction and generalized lymphadenopathy associated with malaise, nausea and vomiting, and usually fever. When further complicated by Kaposi's sarcoma, and/or multiple opportunistic infections, including tuberculosis, cytomegalovirus, toxoplasmosis, and others, then AIDS is diagnosed. The mortality rate of AIDS is extremely high, and 60 to 80 percent who develop the syndrome die within 2 years.

SEROLOGICAL TESTING

In 1985, the Food and Drug Administration approved three test kits to determine the presence of antibodies to human immunodeficiency virus. Currently used tests are based on enzyme immunoassay (EIA), which has sensitivities and specificities of 99 percent when repeatedly positive. The Centers for Disease Control recommends that all positive tests be followed by ad-

ditional testing of the same serum sample using the *Western blot technique*, which establishes the specificity of the immunological reaction between the antibody and viral proteins. Although highly specific, this technique is less sensitive than immunoassay since more antibody is required for a positive result, and thus the Western blot test may have false-negative results.

There is disagreement as to who should be screened, and more importantly, what should be done with positive results. Certainly it is reasonable to test all blood products, and the American Red Cross found immunodeficiency virus antibody in 0.22 percent of the first 100,000 units screened (American Medical Association, 1985). Thus, if there are nearly 40,000 positive tests from 20 million blood units processed annually, even assuming false-positive test results of 95 percent, only a relatively small number of units are discarded. Of greater concern are the donors with incubating virus who test seronegative. Ward and colleagues (1988) estimate that 1 of 40,000 units from donors screened as negative will be infective.

Shown in Table 39–17 are prevalences of immunodeficiency viral antibody in heterosexual populations. The Centers for Disease Control (1987a) recommends that persons in the following categories be counseled and tested for immunodeficiency viral antibody: (1) persons who may have sexually transmitted disease, (2) intravenous illicit drug users, (3) persons who consider themselves at risk, (4) women of childbearing age with identifiable risk by virtue of intravenous drug use, prostitution, sexual partners who are bisexual or hemophiliac or intravenous drug users, or those living in communities or born in countries with a high prevalence rate, or who were given blood transfusions between 1978 and 1985, (5) persons planning marriage, (6) persons undergoing diagnostic testing that have evidence for AIDS, (7) persons of high risk admitted to hospitals, (8) persons in correctional institutions, and (9) prostitutes.

MATERNAL AND FETUS–INFANT INFECTION

There is insufficient experience to ascertain the risk of fetal infection from pregnant women with asymptomatic immunodeficiency virus infection, or those with clinical immunodeficiency syndromes. Of the 40,051 cases of AIDS reported through August, 1987, 558 were in children (Centers for Disease Control, 1987b). Half of these were less than one year of age and nearly three-fourths were born to mothers from groups with known increased prevalence of immunodeficiency viral infection such as listed in Table 39–17. Another 18

TABLE 39–17. PREVALENCE OF HUMAN IMMUNODEFICIENCY VIRUS (HIV) ANTIBODY IN UNITED STATES HETEROSEXUAL POPULATIONS

Population	Prevalence (%)
Intravenous drug users	9 to 59
Hemophiliacs	40 to 74
Female prostitutes	5 to 40
Female sex partners of males with AIDS or AIDS-related complex	47 to 71
Female sex partners of males with asymptomatic immunodeficiency viral infection	20
Haitians	4 to 8
Female blood donors	0.01

Adapted from MMWR 34:721, 1985a.

percent were attributed to blood or blood products, and 6 percent were inexplicable. Drug abuse (48 percent), Haitian origin (17 percent), and sex partners of male bisexuals or drug users (10 percent) were the most common risk factors.

Landesman and co-workers (1987) found a 2 percent seroprevalence rate for asymptomatic immunodeficiency virus infections in 602 cord blood specimens collected at Kings County Hospital in Brooklyn. Importantly, while all women were from an inner-city minority population, only about half were considered high risk by factors previously outlined. They recommended that serological testing and counseling be offered to all pregnant women in areas of increased seroprevalence in which there is poor identification of risk factors.

The rate of perinatal transmission of immunodeficiency virus is unknown but available data suggest that it is from 45 to 75 percent (Minkoff, 1987). Perinatal transmission is by transplacental infection, and almost all women who are delivered of infants who subsequently develop AIDS have been asymptomatic during pregnancy. Minkoff and associates (1987a) reported that only 4 of 32 such women were symptomatic; however, low birthweight infants (32 percent), prematurely ruptured membranes (29 percent), and cesarean delivery (29 percent) were common complications. Gloeb and colleagues (1988) reported that 35 percent of 50 seropositive women had preterm labor and delivery. However, according to the American College of Obstetricians and Gynecologists (1988), there is no evidence that preterm birth, low birthweight, or other pregnancy complications are increased in seropositive women.

The possibility exists that during pregnancy clinical illness is more likely to follow asymptomatic infection, presumably because of suppressed cell-mediated immunity. Sridama and colleagues (1982), as well as others, have reported during pregnancy diminished lymphocyte function and decreased helper T cells. In the report by Scott and colleagues (1985), of 16 asymptomatic infected mothers, one third had developed AIDS and another half AIDS-related complex within 30 months of delivery. Similarly, in the report by Minkoff and co-workers (1987b), almost half had one of these syndromes by 24 months following delivery. Progression of asymptomatic infection to clinical immunodeficiency syndromes is usually at a much slower rate in nonpregnant homosexuals and drug abusers. However, as emphasized by Minkoff (1987), there have been no controlled studies and women who transmit the virus perinatally may be at unique risk for disease progression. At least until fetal and maternal risks can be defined better, it is reasonable to advise that pregnancy be delayed in seropositive women.

PREVENTION OF TRANSMISSION

For the pregnant woman with symptomatic infection, or who is seropositive but asymptomatic, the same precautions as for nonpregnant individuals with these findings should be followed. Precautions for antepartum, peripartum and pediatric care of infected mothers and infants are similar to those for hepatitis B, with avoidance of exposure to blood and body fluids. Unfortunately, if heightened awareness of these precautions is reserved for women known to be seropositive, a large number of women with incubating infection or who are untreated will pose a larger threat to medical personnel. Eichberg and colleagues (1988) reported transplacental viral transfer in the chimpanzee, and at the present time there is no reason to think that cesarean delivery will decrease the chance of peripartum transmission (American College of Obstetricians and Gynecologists, 1988). The effects of maternal antiviral therapy on

the fetus are conjectural, however, Fortunato and associates (1989) found active transfer of zidovudine in the perfused cotyledon system.

The Centers for Disease Control (1987c) emphasizes that since medical history and examination cannot reliably identify all patients infected with immunodeficiency virus, or other blood-borne pathogens, blood and body-fluid precautions should be used consistently in all patients:

1. All health-care workers who participate in invasive procedures, including surgical procedures or obstetrical deliveries, must use appropriate barrier precautions to prevent skin and mucous-membrane contact with blood and other body fluids of all patients. Gloves, surgical masks, and protective eyewear must be worn for all invasive procedures that commonly result in the generation of droplets, splashing of blood or other body fluids, or the generation of bone chips. Gowns or aprons made of materials that provide an effective barrier should be worn during invasive procedures that are likely to result in the splashing of blood or other body fluids. All health-care workers who perform or assist in vaginal or cesarean deliveries should wear gloves and gowns when handling the placenta or the infant until blood and amnionic fluid have been removed from the infant's skin and should wear gloves during care of the cord.

2. If a glove is torn or there is a needlestick or other injury, the glove should be removed and a new glove used as promptly as patient safety permits. The needle or instrument involved in the incident also should be removed from the sterile field.

HUMAN PAPILLOMAVIRUS

Several types of human papillomaviruses cause mucocutaneous warts. *Condylomata acuminata* are also called genital warts or venereal warts and are usually caused by types 6 and 11. Viral types 16, 18, 31, 33, and 35 have been implicated in the cause of cervical intraepithelial neoplasia and possibly invasive cancer, as well as other female genital cancers. The virus also can cause laryngeal papillomatosis in children, and evidence is consistent that types 6 and 11 in some cases may be transmitted by aspiration of infected material at delivery.

CONDYLOMATA ACUMINATA

For unknown reasons, in some women the growth of genital warts is stimulated during pregnancy (Fig. 39–21). Certainly the constant mucorrhea throughout pregnancy offers ideal moist conditions for their growth. Treatment may be very unsatisfactory, but it is usual for these lesions to clear rapidly following delivery. During pregnancy, local washing of the external genitalia, plus cleansing of the vagina by gentle douching (see Chap. 14. p. 269) followed by thorough drying of the external genitalia, performed at least once daily, may inhibit proliferation of the warts, as well as minimize discomfort.

A 20 percent solution of podophyllin in tincture of benzoin applied to condylomata has long been used to try to eradicate these lesions. Its use during pregnancy is not likely to be highly effective, and considerable local discomfort may ensue. Rarely, topical application is toxic, and Slater and colleagues (1978) described intense systemic toxicity with coma following local application. Fortunately, it resolved after charcoal hemoperfu-

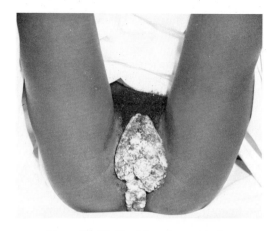

Figure 39–21. Condylomata acuminata.

sion. They also cited previously reported maternal and fetal deaths following topical application of podophyllin.

Occasionally, condylomata acuminata attain enormous size as shown in Figure 39–21, and these may even necessitate cesarean section. If the woman is seen several weeks before delivery, the large lesions sometimes can be removed by excision, electrocautery, cyrosurgery, or laser ablation. Matsunaga and colleagues (1987) reported successful results in 51 women with rather extensive cervical or labial lesions. Enthusiasm has been expressed for use of the carbon-dioxide laser during pregnancy to remove large lesions under anesthesia (Ferenczy, 1984). Calkins and associates (1982) have used laser therapy successfully on an outpatient basis. They noted, however, that a third of the pregnant women so treated had bleeding that was easily controlled with pressure.

NEONATAL INFECTION

An indeterminate, but probably small number of infants and children born to women with genital lesions caused by papillomavirus will become infected and develop laryngeal papillomatosis. These papillomas are usually found on the true vocal cords and HPV-6 or 11 were identified in 92 percent of 57 cases

(Abramson and colleagues, 1987). The question has been posed that cesarean section might avoid infection of the fetus-infant, but this is not recommended currently (Hallden and Majmudar, 1984).

CHANCROID

Hemophilus ducreyi can cause painful non-indurated genital ulcers, or soft chancre, at times accompanied by painful inguinal lymphadenopathy. Chancroid is common in some developing countries. While it has become rare in the United States, in 1986 its incidence was increased fourfold over the previous 5 years and prostitutes were shown to be an important reservoir of infection (Schmid and co-workers, 1987). Diagnosis should be confirmed by culture obtained from the ulcers or in aspirates from the enlarged nodes. Treatment consists of erythromycin, 500 mg orally four times daily for at least 10 days and until the ulcers and nodes have healed. Trimethoprim 160 mg-sulfamethoxazole 800 mg orally twice a day is efficacious. Single-dose 250 mg ceftriaxone given intramuscularly has been used.

GRANULOMA INGUINALE

In the pregnant woman the lesions of this now rare disorder tend to be multiple, large, quite foul-smelling ulcerations of the vulva, lower vagina, perineum, and cervix. The causative organism, *Donovania granulomatis*, at times disseminates to cause remote lesions, especially in bone. Diagnosis depends upon identification of Donovan bodies in large mononuclear cells in Giemsa-stained smears from the lesions. Antibiotic therapy is the same as described for lymphogranuloma venereum.

OTHER SEXUALLY TRANSMITTED DISEASES

There are many more infections and infestations that can be acquired as the consequence of sexual intercourse. Among others, these include *trichomonal vaginitis* (see Chap. 14, p. 273), *candida vulvovaginitis* (see Chap. 14, p. 273), *scabies*, and *pediculosis pubis*. Sexual partners at risk of fecal-oral transmission may acquire any of a number of enteric infections.

NEOPLASTIC DISEASES

Cancer during pregnancy is not rare. Donegan (1983) reviewed the literature and estimated that 1 in 1,000 women will be afflicted by cancer while pregnant. According to the Third National Cancer Survey (1975), about 13 percent of cancers in females develop during the childbearing years. The most frequent malignant tumors complicating pregnancy are those of the breast, cervix, ovary, hematopoietic and lymphatic systems, and colon. As discussed in regard to most other medical and surgical disorders complicating pregnancy, and as outlined by Donegan (1983), specific questions to be asked when confronted by the pregnant women with a neoplasm include: (1) Does pregnancy adversely influence maternal cancer? (2) What risk does cancer or its treatment pose to the fetus? (3) Is pregnancy advisable following cancer treatment? Doll and colleagues (1988) provided a review of therapeutic approaches, including radia-

tion, surgery, and chemotherapy, to a number of malignancies complicating pregnancy.

BREAST CARCINOMA

Breast cancer is the most common malignancy of women, and it is not surprising that it is encountered with some frequency during pregnancy. Its exact incidence is not known, but it has been estimated to be about 1 in 3,000 to 10,000 pregnancies (Donegan, 1983; Orr and Shingleton, 1983; Parente and associates, 1988). A large number of breast cancers have female sex hormone receptors and appear to be estrogen- or progesterone-dependent. Theoretically at least, they therefore should be more aggressive because of the hyperestrogenemia and hyperprogesteronemia that characterize normal pregnancy. However, there is no proof of this, and two observations may serve to explain this. Firstly, there is the widely held view that pregnancy is protective because the dominant estrogen is estriol that displaces the substantively more potent estradiol from tumor cell receptors. Secondly, Nugent and O'Connell (1985) reported that more than 70 percent of breast tumors in their pregnant patients were estrogen-receptor negative. Paradoxically, this latter characteristic is seen in many of the more aggressive neoplasms in young women.

Pregnancy does not appear to exert much influence on the course of mammary cancer, and therapeutic abortion does not improve its prognosis. In the extensive investigations of Westberg (1946), based on 224 cases of pregnant women and a control series of 3,000 nonpregnant women with mammary cancer, the difference in the survival rates was scarcely significant. Hochman and Schreiber (1953), and others since then, contended that the 5-year survival rate in breast cancer coexisting with pregnancy is primarily dependent on the state of the disease at the time of diagnosis, and that interruption of pregnancy has no influence on the course. Thus, results to be anticipated will be comparable to the survival rates expected with the same stage of the disease in nonpregnant women.

Unfortunately, pregnant women as a group have more advanced stages of cancer at diagnosis, and thus their prognosis is worse. King and colleagues (1985) described their experiences with 63 pregnant women treated for breast carcinoma at the Mayo Clinic and reported that 63 percent had axillary nodal metastases compared to only 38 percent of nonpregnant women of the same age who had been described by others. Similarly, Ribeiro and colleagues (1986) reported advanced stages of tumors diagnosed during pregnancy compared to nonpregnant women. Specifically, in their series 72 percent of pregnant women had nodal metastases compared to only 51 percent of those not pregnant. These results can best be explained by delayed diagnosis because of confusion between tumor growth with normal breast growth during pregnancy. It also has been hpothesized that increased breast vascularity may accelerate cancer spread. **Any suspicious breast mass found in the pregnant woman should prompt an aggressive plan to determine its cause, whether by fine-needle aspiration, mammography, or excisional biopsy.**

Surgical treatment should not be delayed because of pregnancy and termination is not necessary. In addition, several chemotherapeutic agents have been administered for metastatic disease during the second and third trimesters without apparent harm to the fetus-infant. Radiation therapy is not recommended during pregnancy since abdominal scatter is considerable, even with shielding (Orr and Shingleton, 1983).

No strong evidence has been provided that pregnancy after mastectomy for cancer of the breast has an adverse effect on survival (Donegan, 1983; Harvey and associates, 1981; Zinns, 1979).

LYMPHOMAS AND LEUKEMIAS

HODGKIN DISEASE

Reliable incidence figures are unavailable, but Hodgkin disease is the most common lymphoma encountered in childbearing-age women. There are no convincing data that pregnancy adversely affects Hodgkin lymphoma, nor does the disease cause pregnancy wastage. Holmes and Holmes (1978) have analyzed pregnancy outcomes when either the expectant mother or the father had the disease, and the great majority of the outcomes for 93 pregnancies were satisfactory. Jacobs and associates (1981) reported their experiences from Stanford University and found that neither chemotherapy during the second and third trimesters nor irradiation to the mediastinum and neck appeared to affect adversely the fetus or neonate.

The pregnant woman with Hodgkin disease presents special management considerations. Careful staging is essential before treatment, but pregnancy will limit the use of some x-ray studies of the abdomen and pelvis. Magnetic resonance imaging may prove to be a reasonable alternative to computed tomographic scanning for evaluating paraaortic lymph nodes. In some centers, staging laparotomy is done routinely, and while this may be reasonable in early pregnancy, especially if accompanied by pregnancy termination if disease is found, it is probably not advisable later. If the diagnosis is made before midpregnancy, termination should be considered so that appropriate staging can be done.

Treatment should be individualized depending upon the suspected stage and duration of pregnancy, and is given either by select radiotherapy or combination chemotherapy. Radiotherapy seems preferable for isolated cervical adenopathy, but with more advanced disease, chemotherapy should be started. **Pregnant women with Hodgkin disease are very susceptible to infections and sepsis, and radiotherapy or chemotherapy increases this susceptibility.**

Horning and co-workers (1981) evaluated the reproductive potential of women after treatment for Hodgkin disease. They reported that 55 percent of these women resumed normal menses after chemotherapy. In several instances, signs and symptoms of ovarian failure that developed soon after pelvic irradiation eventually receded and a successful pregnancy outcome followed. No birth defects nor developmental abnormalities were evident in the 24 infants studied. Chapman and associates (1979) observed ovarian failure, diagnosed clinically and by endocrinological studies, in 25 of 41 women following chemotherapy for Hodgkin disease.

The risk of second cancers is substantively increased in patients with Hodgkin disease. Tucker and colleagues (1988) reported this risk to be 18 percent within 15 years. The risk for leukemia, for example, was increased almost 100-fold if chemotherapy had been given. The risk for solid tumors was also increased.

LEUKEMIA

The incidence of acute leukemia complicating pregnancy is cited to be 1 in 75,000 (McLain, 1974; Orr and Shingleton, 1983). Associated with the overall improved survival rate with some of these malignancies, most women who develop acute leukemia during pregnancy usually can be successfully treated with chemotherapy to induce remission at least during pregnancy. For these reasons, the maternal and fetal outcomes have improved substantively (Catanzarite and Ferguson, 1984; Reynoso and colleagues, 1987). McLain (1974) reported that the maternal mortality rate was 100 percent and perinatal mortality rate was 34 percent in 256 women with acute leukemia treated before 1970. However, according to Lewis and Laros (1986), maternal mortality with acute leukemia since 1970 has become negligible, although many of these unfortunate women die months to years following pregnancy. As with other malignancies, infections are

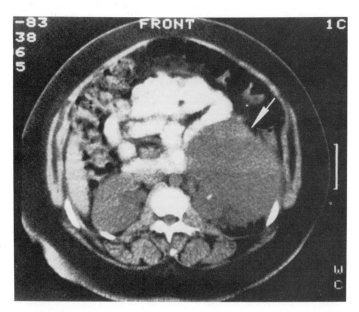

Figure 39–22. Renal cell carcinoma. Computed axial tomography scan of the abdomen shows a solid mass arising from the left kidney (*arrow*). Right kidney is normal. (*From Klein and colleagues: Obstet Gynecol 69:531, 1987.*)

associated with high mortality. Fetal outcome is especially poor if leukemia develops in the first two trimesters, and excluding abortions, Reynoso and associates (1987) reported that only 40 percent of these pregnancies resulted in liveborn infants.

The survival also has improved for chronic myelogenous and lymphocytic leukemias. Most of the cytotoxic drugs used in treatment cross the placenta, and therefore it was predicted generally that these agents would severely affect the fetus. To date this does not appear to be the case, at least during the latter two trimesters. Several cases of congenital leukemia in infants of nonleukemic mothers have been recorded, although no case of transmission of leukemia to the fetus has been authenticated.

Levine and Collea (1979) reviewed the problem of pregnancy complicated by chronic granulocytic leukemia and Lilleyman (1978) and Reynoso (1987) and their colleagues have done the same for acute leukemia.

MELANOMA

It has been said that pregnancy stimulates growth of malignant melanoma; however, this is not substantiated. Certainly, pregnancy is associated with increased melanocyte stimulating hormone (see Chap. 7, p. 136), and some of these tumors have sex steroid hormone receptors. In his review of 11 studies, Holly (1986) concluded that there was no adverse effect on survival if melanoma was first diagnosed during pregnancy, or if pregnancy developed in a woman with previously recognized melanoma. Prognosis is determined by staging of the lesion, and those with deep cutaneous invasion or regional node involvement, as expected, have a much poorer prognosis.

Melanoma is the malignancy most commonly identified to metastasize to the placenta, but as discussed in Chapter 31 (p. 553), this is unusual.

UTERINE LEIOMYOMAS

Benign uterine leiomyomas are common in older pregnant women, and especially in black women. Some of these tumors, presumably stimulated by estrogen, may undergo enormous growth during pregnancy and lead to pregnancy wastage; degeneration with pain, tenderness, and fever; or obstructed labor (see Chap. 21, p. 387). Not all of these benign tumors grow during pregnancy. Lev-Toaff and her associates (1987) performed serial ultrasonic measurements in 113 pregnant women with uterine leiomyoma and reported that half remained unchanged. Interestingly, tumors bigger than 6 cm often enlarged in the first trimester, but did so in only 10 to 15 percent of cases during the second and third trimesters.

LEIOMYOMATOSIS PERITONEALIS DISSEMINATA

Rarely at cesarean section or puerperal tubal ligation, numerous subperitoneal smooth muscle tumors are found that at first appear to be disseminated carcinomatosis. Leiomyomatosis peritonealis disseminata results from stimulation, probably by estrogen, of multicentric subcoelomic mesenchymal cells to become smooth muscle cells. Although surgery has been recommended, there is evidence that these tumors regress after pregnancy (Minassian and colleagues, 1986), and this has been our experience with the few women with this condition cared for at Parkland Hospital. Rubin and associates (1986), however, reported a malignant variety of this neoplasm.

OTHER NEOPLASTIC DISEASES

Renal cell carcinoma rarely complicates pregnancy and we have encountered only six pregnant women with this malignancy during the past 20 years at Parkland Hospital. These women either presented because of painless hematuria or the tumor was found by abdominal palpation done routinely in conjunction with cesarean section. If suspected antepartum, the diagnosis can be confirmed by intravenous pyelography, ultrasonicdirected needle biopsy, or limited computed tomography scanning as shown in Figure 39–22.

Cervical carcinoma complicating pregnancy is discussed in Chapter 37.

Colon carcinoma is rare during pregnancy. Tsukamoto and associates (1986) found 20 reported cases and added another. The most common symptoms were abdominal pain, nausea and vomiting, and constipation. Mortality was over 60 percent. Occasionally, intra-abdominal tumors may cause symptoms of intestinal obstruction (Yazigi and Driscoll, 1986). **It is emphasized that appropriate diagnostic studies to exclude neoplastic disease during pregnancy should not be avoided.**

REFERENCES

Abrahamson MJ, Miller JL, Alperstein AL, Barron J: Cushing's syndrome in pregnancy: A case report. S Afr Med J 69:834, 1986

Abramson AL, Steinberg BM, Winkler B: Laryngeal papillomatosis: Clinical histopathologic and molecular studies. Laryngoscope 87:678, 1987

Agre P, Orringer EP, Bennett V: Deficient red-cell spectrin in severe, recessively inherited spherocytosis. N Engl J Med 306:1155, 1982

Alcalay J, Ingber A, David M, Hazaz B, Sandbank M: Pruritic urticarial papules and plaques of pregnancy: A review of 21 cases. J Reprod Med 32:315, 1987

Alcalay J, Ingber A, Kafri B, Segal J, Kaufmann H, Hazaz B, Sandbank M: Hormonal evaluation and autoimmune background in pruritic urticarial papules and plaques of pregnancy. Am J Obstet Gynecol 158:417, 1988

Alger LS, Golbus MS, Laros RK Jr: Thalassemia and pregnancy: Results of an antenatal screening program. Am J Obstet Gynecol 134:662, 1979

Alimurung MM, Manahan CP: Typhoid in pregnancy: Report of a case treated with chloramphenicol and ACTH. J Philipp Med Assoc 28:388, 1952

Ambrose A, Welham RT, Cefalo RC: Thrombotic thrombocytopenic purpura in early pregnancy. Obstet Gynecol 66:267, 1985

American Academy of Pediatrics. Committee on drugs: The transfer of drugs and other chemicals into human breast milk. Pediatrics 72:375, 1983

American Academy of Pediatrics: Newborn screening for congenital hypothyroidism: Recommended guidelines. Pediatrics 80:745, 1987

American College of Obstetricians and Gynecologists: Human immune deficiency virus infections. Tech Bull No 123, December 1988a

American College of Obstetricians and Gynecologists: Management of diabetes mellitus in pregnancy. Tech Bull No 92, May 1986

American College of Obstetricians and Gynecologists: Perinatal herpes simplex virus infections. Tech Bull No 122, November 1988

American Medical Association Council on Scientific Affairs: Status report on the acquired immunodeficiency syndrome: Human T-cell lymphotrophic virus III testing. JAMA 254:1342, 1985

Amino N, Tanizawa O, Mori H, Iwatani Y, Yamada T, Kurachi K, Kumahara Y, Miyai K: Aggravation of thyrotoxicosis in early pregnancy and after delivery in Graves' disease. J Clin Endocrinol Metab 55:108, 1982

Amstey MS, Menegus MA, Miller RK, di Sant 'Agnese PA: Non-polio enterovirus infection in adults and pregnant women. Am J Obstet Gynecol (in press), 1988

Amy BW, McManus WF, Goodwin CW, Mason A Jr, Pruitt BA Jr: Thermal injury in the pregnant patient. Surg Gynecol Obstet 161:209, 1985

Angel JL, O'Brien WF, Knuppel RA, Morales WJ, Sims CJ: Carbohydrate intolerance in patients receiving oral tocolytics. Am J Obstet Gynecol 159:762, 1988

Arevalo JA, Washington E: Cost-effectiveness of prenatal screening and immunization for hepatitis B virus. JAMA 259:365, 1988

Arias F, Pineda J: Aortic stenosis and pregnancy. J Reprod Med 20:229, 1978

Artal R, Greenspoon JS, Rutherford S: Transient ischemic attack: A complication of mitral valve prolapse in pregnancy. Obstet Gynecol 71:1028, 1988

Arvin AM, Hensleigh PA, Prober CG, Au DS, Yasukawa LL, Wittek AE, Palumbo PE, Paryani SG, Yeager AS: Failure of antepartum maternal cultures to predict the infant's risk of exposure to herpes simplex virus at delivery. N Engl J Med 315:796, 1986

Ashbaugh DG, Bigelow DB, Petty TL, Levine BE: Acute respiratory distress in adults. Lancet 2:319, 1967

Atkins JN: Maternal plasma concentration of pyridoxal phosphate during pregnancy: Adequacy of vitamin B_6 supplementation during isoniazid therapy. Am Rev Respir Dis 126:714, 1982

Ball EW, Giles C: Folic acid and vitamin B_{12} levels in pregnancy and their relation to megaloblastic anemia. J Clin Pathol 17:165, 1964

Barnes PM, Hendrickse JP deV, Watson-Williams EJ: Low-molecular weight dextran in treatment of bone-pain crises in sickle-cell disease: A double blind trial. Lancet 2:1271, 1965

Barrett JM, Van Hooydonk JE, Boehm FH: Pregnancy-related rupture of arterial aneurysms. Obstet Gynecol Surv 37:557, 1982

Bass MH, Molloshok RE: In Guttmacher AF, Rovinsky JJ (eds): Medical, Surgical and Gynecological Complications of Pregnancy. Baltimore, Williams & Wilkins, 1960, p 526

Bates GW, Whitworth NS, Parker JL, Johnson MP: Elevated cerebrospinal fluid prolactin concentration in women with pseudotumor cerebri. South Med J 75:807, 1982

Bayever E, Champlin R, Ho W, Lenarsky C, Storch S, Ladisch S, Gale RP, Feig SA: Comparison between bone marrow transplantation and antithymocyte globulin in treatment of young patients with severe aplastic anemia. J Pediatr 105:920, 1984

Beasley RP, Lee G C-Y, Roan C-H, Hwang L-Y, Lan C-C, Huang FY: Prevention of perinatally transmitted hepatitis B virus infections with hepatitis B immune globulin and hepatitis B vaccine. Lancet 2:1099, 1983

Benedetti TJ, Valle R, Ledger WJ: Antepartum pneumonia in pregnancy. Am J Obstet Gynecol 144:413, 1982

Berman SM, Harrison HR, Boyce WT, Haffner WJJ, Lewis M, Arthur JB: Low birth weight, prematurity, and postpartum endometritis. JAMA 257:1189, 1987

Bernal JM, Miralles PJ: Cardiac surgery with cardiopulmonary bypass during pregnancy. Obstet Gynecol Surv 41:1, 1986

Bierling P, Farcet JP, Dveradi N, Rochant H, Mondor HH: Gamma globulin for idiopathic thrombocytopenic purpura. N Engl J Med 307:1150, 1982

Biglieri EG, Slaton PE Jr: Pregnancy and primary aldosteronism. J Clin Endocrinol Metab 27:1628, 1967

Binkin NJ, Koplan JP, Cates W: Preventing neonatal herpes: The value of weekly viral cultures in pregnant women with recurrent genital herpes. JAMA 251:2816, 1984

Birk K, Rudick R: Pregnancy and multiple sclerosis. Arch Neurol 43:719, 1986

Black WP: Acute appendicitis in pregnancy. Br Med J 1:1938, 1960

Blanchette V, Hogan V, Hsu E, Luke B, Rock G: Mechanism of action of high-dose intravenous gammaglobulin therapy in childhood immune thrombocytopenic purpura. Pediatr Res 17 [No 4, Part 2] [Abstract No 853], 1983

Bochner CJ, Medearis AL, Williams J III, Castro L, Hobel CJ, Wade ME: Early third-trimester ultrasound screening in gestational diabetes to determine the risk of macrosomia and labor dystocia at term. Am J Obstet Gynecol 157:703, 1987

Boehm CD, Antonarakis SE, Phillips JA III, Stetten G, Kazazian HH Jr: Prenatal diagnosis using DNA polymorphisms. N Engl J Med 308:1054, 1983

Boslego JW, Tramont EC, Takafuji ET, Diniega BM, Mitchell BS, Small JW, Khan WN, Stein DC: Effect of spectinomycin use of the prevalence of spectinomycin-resistant and of penicillinase-producing Neisseria gonorrhoeae. N Engl J Med 317:272, 1987

Boucher M, Yonekura ML: Perinatal listeriosis (early onset): Correlation of antenatal manifestations and neonatal outcome. Obstet Gynecol 68:593, 1986

Bowes WA Jr: Detection and treatment of tuberculosis. Contemp Ob/Gyn 6:43, 1975

Brady WK, Purdon A Jr: Intrauterine fetal demise associated with enterovirus infection. South Med J 79:770, 1986

Branch DW, Scott JR, Kochenour NK, Hershgold E: Obstetric complications associated with lupus anticoagulant. N Engl J Med 313:1322, 1985

Brans YW, Huff RW, Shannon DL, Hunter MA: Maternal diabetes and neonatal macrosomia. Pediatrics 70:576, 1982

Braverman DZ, Johnson ML, Kern F Jr: Effects of pregnancy and contraceptive steroids on gallbladder function. N Engl J Med 302:362, 1980

Bravo FI, Gifford RW Jr: Pheochromocytoma: Diagnosis, localization and management. N Engl J Med 311:1298, 1984

Bravo RH, Katz M, Inturisi M, Cohen NH: Obstetric management of Landry-Guillain-Barré syndrome. Am J Obstet Gynecol 142:714, 1982

Brenner B, Shapira A, Bahari C, Haimovich L, Seligsohn U: Hereditary protein C deficiency during pregnancy. Am J Obstet Gynecol 157:1160, 1987

Briggs GG, Freeman RK, Yaffee SJ: Drugs in Pregnancy and Lactation, 2nd ed. Baltimore, Williams & Wilkins, 1986

Brown ZA, Vontver LA, Benedetti J, Critchlow CW, Hickok DE, Sells CJ, Berry S, Corey L: Genital herpes in pregnancy: Risk factors associated with recurrences and asymptomatic shedding. Am J Obstet Gynecol 153:24, 1985

Brown ZA, Vontver LA, Benedetti J, Critchlow CW, Sells CJ, Berry S, Corey L: Effects on infants of a first episode of genital herpes during pregnancy. N Engl J Med 317:1246, 1987

Bruce-Chwatt LJ: Malaria and pregnancy. Br Med J 286:1457, 1983

Brumfitt W, Davies BI, Rosser E: Urethral catheter as a cause of urinary-tract infection in pregnancy and puerperium. Lancet 2:1059, 1961

Bunim JJ, Appel SB: A principle for determining prognosis of pregnancy in rheumatic heart disease. JAMA 142:90, 1950

Burgess GE: Alpha blockade and surgical intervention of pheochromocytoma in pregnancy. Obstet Gynecol 53:266, 1979

Burkett G: Lupus nephropathy and pregnancy. Clin Obstet Gynecol 28:310, 1985

Burkett G, Richardson R: Periarteritis nodosa and pregnancy. Obstet Gynecol 59:252, 1982

Burroughs AK, Seong NH, Dojcinov DM, Scheur PJ, Sherlock SVP: Idiopathic acute fatty liver of pregnancy in 12 patients. Q J Med, New Series LI:481, 1982

Burrow GN: The management of thyrotoxicosis in pregnancy. N Engl J Med 313:562, 1985

Burrow GN, Klatskin EH, Genel M: Intellectual development in children whose mothers received propylthiouracil during pregnancy. Yale J Biol Med 51:151, 1978

Burrows RF, Kelton JG: Incidentally detected thrombocytopenia in healthy mothers and their infants. N Engl J Med 319:142, 1988

Burwell CS, Metcalfe J: Heart Disease and Pregnancy. Boston, Little, Brown, 1958

Calkins JW, Masterson BJ, Magrina JF, Capen CV: Management of condylomata acuminata with carbon dioxide laser. Obstet Gynecol 59:105, 1982

Camitta BM, Storb R, Thomas ED: Aplastic anemia: Pathogenesis, diagnosis, treatment, and prognosis. N Engl J Med 306:645, 712, 1982

Carache S, Scott J, Niebyl J, Bonds D: Management of sickle cell disease in pregnant patients. Obstet Gynecol 55:407, 1980

Carreras LO, Vermylen J, Spitz B, Van Assche A: "Lupus" anticoagulation and inhibition of prostacyclin formation in patients with repeated abortion, intrauterine growth retardation and intrauterine death. Br J Obstet Gynaecol 88:890, 1981

Carroll RR, Noyes WD, Kitchens CS: High-dose intravenous immunoglobulin therapy in patients with immune thrombocytopenic purpura. JAMA 249:1748, 1983

Catanzarite VA, Arguright K, Mann BA, Brittain VL: Malnutrition during pregnancy: Consider parenteral feeding. Contemp Ob/Gyn 27:110, 1986

Catanzarite VA, Ferguson JE: Acute leukemia and pregnancy: A review of management and outcome, 1972–1982. Obstet Gynecol Surv 39:663, 1984

Catanzaro A: Pulmonary mycosis in pregnant women. Chest 86:14S, 1984

Cavalieri RL, Watkins L, Abraham RA, Berkay HS, Niebyl JR: Acute bacterial endocarditis with postpartum aortic valve replacement. Obstet Gynecol 59:124, 1982

Centers for Disease Control: Diabetes in pregnancy project—Maine, 1986–1987. MMWR 36:741, 1987

Centers for Disease Control: 1985 STD treatment guidelines. MMWR 34:75S, 1985b

Centers for Disease Control: Prevention and control of influenza. MMWR 36:373, 1987

Centers for Disease Control: Public Health Service guidelines for counseling and antibody testing to prevent HIV infection and AIDS. MMWR 36:509, 1987a

Centers for Disease Control: Quarterly report to the domestic policy council on the prevalence and rate of spread of HIV and AIDS—US. MMWR 37:551, 1988a

Centers for Disease Control: Recommendations for assisting in the prevention of perinatal transmission of human T-lymphotrophic virus type III/lymphadenopathy-associated virus and acquired immunodeficiency syndrome. MMWR 34:721, 1985a

Centers for Disease Control: Recommendations for prevention of HIV transmission in health-care settings. MMWR 36:3S, 1987c

Centers for Disease Control: Recommendations for the prevention of malaria in travelers. MMWR 37:17, 1988b

Centers for Disease Control: Recommendations of the Immunization Practices Advisory Committee: Prevention of perinatal transmission of hepatitis B virus: Prenatal screening of all pregnant women for hepatitis B surface antigen. MMWR 37:341, 1988c

Centers for Disease Control: Tuberculosis among Hispanics—United States, 1985. MMWR 36:568, 1987

Centers for Disease Control: Update: Acquired immunodeficiency syndrome—United States. MMWR 36:552, 1987b

Centers for Disease Control: Valproate: A new cause of birth defects—report from Italy and follow-up from France. MMWR 32:439, 1983

Centers for Disease Control: Varicella-zoster immune globulin for the prevention of chickenpox. MMWR 33:84, 1984

Chanarin I: The Megaloblastic Anaemias. Oxford and Edinburgh, Blackwell Scientific Publications, 1969

Chang JC, Kan YW: A sensitive new prenatal test for sickle cell anemia. N Engl J Med 307:30, 1982

Chapman RA, Sutcliffe SB, Malpas JS: Cytotoxic-induced ovarian failure in Hodgkin's disease: II. Effects on sexual function. JAMA 242:1882, 1979

Chasis JA, Agre P, Mohandas N: Decreased membrane mechanical stability and in vivo loss of surface area reflect spectrin deficiencies in hereditary spherocytosis. J Clin Invest 82:617, 1988

Chau SS, Fitzpatrick RJ, Jamieson B: Diabetes insipidus and parturition. Br J Obstet Gynaecol 76:444, 1969

Chediak JR, Alban GM, Maxey B: Von Willebrand's disease and pregnancy: Management during delivery and outcome of offspring. Am J Obstet Gynecol 155:618, 1986

Cheek DB (ed): Human Growth. Philadelphia, Lea & Febiger, 1968

Chen WCC, Chan CS, Lee PK, Wang RYC, Wong VCW: Pregnancy in patients with prosthetic valves: An experience with 45 pregnancies. Q J Med New Series LI:358, 1982

Cheng Y-S: Pregnancy in liver cirrhosis and/or portal hypertension. Am J Obstet Gynecol 128:812, 1977

Chesley LC: Severe rheumatic cardiac disease and pregnancy: The ultimate prognosis. Am J Obstet Gynecol 136:552, 1980

Chesson RR, Gallup DG, Gibbs RL, Jones BE, Thomas B: Ultrasonographic diagnosis of asymptomatic cholelithiasis in pregnancy. J Repro Med 30:921, 1985

Chorzelski TP, Jablonska S, Beutner EH, Maciejowska EWA, Jarzabek-Chorzelska M: Herpes gestationis with identical lesions in the newborn. Arch Dermatol 112:1129, 1976

Cines DB, Dusak B, Tomaski A, Mennuti M, Schreier AD: Immune thrombocytopenic purpura and pregnancy. N Engl J Med 306:826, 1982

Clemens JD, Horwitz RI, Jaffe CC, Feinstein AR, Stanton BF: A controlled evaluation of the risk of bacterial endocarditis in persons with mitral valve prolapse. N Engl J Med 307:776, 1982

Cobbe SM: Congenital complete heart block. Br Med J 286:1769, 1983

Coe FL, Parks JH, Lindheimer MD: Nephrolithiasis during pregnancy. N Engl J Med 298:324, 1978

Cohen LF, diSantAgnese PA, Friedlander J: Cystic fibrosis and pregnancy: A national survey. Lancet 2:842, 1980

Cohen S: The sluggish gallbladder of pregnancy. N Engl J Med 302:397, 1980

Committee on Drugs, American Academy of Pediatrics: Psychotropic drugs in pregnancy and lactation. Pediatrics 69:241, 1982

Comp PC, Thurnau GR, Welsh J, Esmon CT: Functional and immunologic protein S levels are decreased during pregnancy. Blood 68:881, 1986

Conti M, Mari D, Conti E, Muggiasca L, Mannucci PM: Pregnancy in women with different types of von Willebrand disease. Obstet Gynecol 68:282, 1986

Corlett RC Jr, Mishell DR Jr: Pancreatitis in pregnancy. Am J Obstet Gynecol 113:381, 1972

Cortis BS, Gensini GG: Can the risks of myocardial infarction in pregnancy be reduced? Bull Tex Heart Inst 4:49, 1977

Cossart YE, Kirsch S, Ismay SL: Post-transfusion hepatitis in Australia. Lancet 1:208, 1982

Cousins L: Congenital anomalies among infants of diabetic mothers. Am J Obstet Gynecol 147:333, 1983

Cousins L: Pregnancy complications among diabetic women: Review 1965–1985. Obstet Gynecol Surv 42:140, 1987

Coustan DR, Berkowitz RL, Hobbins JC: Tight metabolic control of overt diabetes in pregnancy. Am J Med 68:845, 1980

Coustan DR, Imarah J: Prophylactic insulin treatment of gestational diabetes reduces the incidence of macrosomia, operative delivery, and birth trauma. Am J Obstet Gynecol 150:836, 1984

Covell G: Congenital malaria. Trop Dis Bull 47:1174, 1950

Cox JV, Steane E, Cunningham G, Frenkel EP: Risk of alloimmunization and delayed hemolytic transfusion reactions in patients with sickle cell disease. Arch Intern Med 148:2485, 1988

Cox SM, Cunningham FG: Acute focal pyelonephritis (lobar nephronia) complicating pregnancy. Obstet Gynecol 71:510, 1988b

Cox SM, Cunningham FG: Ureidopenicillin therapy for acute antepartum pyelonephritis. Curr Ther Research 44:1029, 1988a

Cox SM, Hankins GDV, Leveno KJ, Cunningham FG: Bacterial endocarditis: A serious pregnancy complication. J Reprod Med 33:671, 1988a

Cox SM, Harstad TW, Mason RA, Cunningham FG, Pritchard JA: Blood volume changes during pregnancy complicated by chronic renal insufficiency: Society of Perinatal Obstetricians. [Abstract] New Orleans, Louisiana, February 1989

Cox SM, Shelburne P, Mason RA, Cunningham FG: Erythrocyte morphology in women with acute pyelonephritis: Infectious Disease Society for Obstetrics-Gynecology. [Abstract] Aspen, Colorado, August 1988b

Crohn BB, Yarnis H, Walter RI, Gabrilov JL, Crohn EB: Ulcerative colitis as affected by pregnancy. NY J Med 56:2651, 1956.

Cruz C, Frentzen M, Behnke M: Hepatitis B: A case for prenatal screening of all patients. Am J Obstet Gynecol 156:1180, 1987

Cunningham FG: Urinary tract infections complicating pregnancy. Clin Obstet Gynecol 1:891, 1988

Cunningham FG, Leveno KJ, Hankins GDV, Whalley PJ: Respiratory insufficiency associated with pyelonephritis during pregnancy. Obstet Gynecol 63:121, 1984

Cunningham FG, Lucas MJ, Hankins GDV: Pulmonary injury complicating antepartum pyelonephritis. Am J Obstet Gynecol 156:797, 1987

Cunningham FG, McCubbin JH: Appendicitis complicating pregnancy. Obstet Gynecol 45:415, 1975

Cunningham FG, Morris GB, Mickal A: Acute pyelonephritis of pregnancy: A clinical review. Obstet Gynecol 42:112, 1973

Cunningham FG, Pritchard JA: Prophylactic transfusions of normal red blood cells during pregnancies complicated by sickle cell hemoglobinopathies. Am J Obstet Gynecol 135:994, 1979

Cunningham FG, Pritchard JA, Hankins GDV, Anderson PL, Lucas MK, Armstrong KF: Idiopathic cardiomyopathy or compounding cardiovascular events. Obstet Gynecol 67:157, 1986

Cunningham FG, Pritchard JA, Mason R: Pregnancy and sickle hemoglobinopathy: Results with and without prophylactic transfusions. Obstet Gynecol 62:419, 1983

Daffos F, Capella-Pavlovsky M, Forestier F: Fetal blood sampling during pregnancy with use of a needle guided by ultrasound: A study of 606 consecutive cases. Am J Obstet Gynecol 153:655, 1985

Dalessio DJ: Seizure disorders and pregnancy. N Engl J Med 312:559, 1985

Davis LE, Leveno KL, Cunningham FG: Hypothyroidism complicating pregnancy. Obstet Gynecol 72:108, 1988

Davis LE, Lucas MJ, Hankins GDV, Roark ML, Cunningham FG: Thyrotoxicosis complicating pregnancy. Am J Obstet Gynecol 160:63, 1989

Davison JM: Renal transplantation and pregnancy. Am J Kidney Dis 9:374, 1987

Davison JM, Lindheimer MD: Pregnancy in renal transplant recipients. J Reprod Med 27:613, 1982

Daw E, Mohandas I: Pregnancy in patients after severe abdominal burns. Br J Obstet Gynaecol 90:69, 1983

Deaver JE, Leppert PC, Zaroulis CG: Neonatal alloimmune thrombocytopenic purpura. Am J Perinatol 3:127, 1986

Delgado-Escueta AV, Treiman DM, Walsh GO: The treatable epilepsies. N Engl J Med 308:1508, 1576, 1983

deRegt RH: Sarcoidosis and pregnancy. Obstet Gynecol 70:369, 1987

Derue GJ, Englert JH, Harris EN, Gharavi AE, Morgan SH, Hull RG: Fetal loss in systemic lupus: Association with anticardiolipin antibodies. J Obstet Gynaecol 5:207, 1985

Deviri E, Levinsky L, Yechezkel M, Levy MJ: Pregnancy after valve replacement with porcine xenograft prothesis. Surg Gynecol Obstet 160:437, 1985

DeVore GR: Acute abdominal pain in the pregnant patient due to pancreatitis, acute appendicitis, cholecystitis, or peptic ulcer disease. Clin Perinatol 7:349, 1980

DeWolf F, Carreras LO, Moerman P, Vermylen J, Van Assche A, Renaer M: Decidual vasculopathy and extensive placental infarction in a patient with repeated thromboembolic accidents, recurrent fetal loss, and lupus anticoagulant. Am J Obstet Gynecol 142:829, 1982

Diamond MP, Salyer SL, Vaughn WK, Cotton R, Boehm FH: Reassessment of White's classification and Pedersen's prognostically bad signs of diabetic pregnancies in insulin-dependent diabetic pregnancies. Am J Obstet Gynecol 156:599, 1987

Dienstag JL, Wands JR, Koff RS: Acute hepatitis. In Braunwald E, Isselbacher KJ, Petersford RG, Wilson JD, Martin JB, Fauci AS (eds): Harrison's Principles of Internal Medicine, 11th ed. New York, McGraw-Hill, 1987, p 1325

Dillon WP, Lee RV, Tronolone MJ, Buckwald S, Foote RJ: Life support and maternal death during pregnancy. JAMA 248:1089, 1982

Doll DC, Ringenberg S, Yarbro JW: Management of cancer during pregnancy. Arch Intern Med 148:2058, 1988

Donaldson JO: Neurology of Pregnancy. Philadelphia, Saunders, 1978

Donaldson JO: Stroke. Clin Obstet Gynecol 24:825, 1981

Donaldson JO, Penn AS, Lisak RP, Abramsky O, Brenner T, Schotland DL: Antiacetylcholine receptor antibody in neonatal myasthenia gravis. Am J Dis Child 135:222, 1981

Donaldson RM: Management of medical problems in pregnancy—inflammatory bowel disease. N Engl J Med 312:1618, 1985

Donegan WL: Cancer and pregnancy. CA 33:194, 1983

Dooley SL, Depp R, Socol ML, Tamura RK, Vaisrub N: Urinary estriols in diabetic pregnancy: A reappraisal. Obstet Gynecol 64:469, 1984

Duff P, Engelsgjerd B: Typhoid fever on an obstetrics-gynecology service. Am J Obstet Gynecol 145:113, 1983

Duncan ME: Babies of mothers with leprosy have small placentae, low birth weights and grow slowly. Br J Obstet Gynaecol 87:461, 1980

Duncan ME, Fox H, Harkness RA, Rees RJW: The placenta in leprosy. Placenta 5:189, 1984

Dürr JA: Diabetes insipidus in pregnancy. Am J Kidney Dis 9:276, 1987

Edidin DV, Menella J: Increased glycosylated hemoglobin in maternal and cord blood of macrosomic infants of diabetic mothers. Pediatr Res 17:288A [Abstract No 1211], 1983

Eichberg JW, Lee DR, Allan JS, Cobb KE, Barbosa LH, Nemo GJ, Prince AM: In utero infection of an infant chimpanzee with HIV. N Engl J Med 319:722, 1988

El-Maraghy M, Abou Senna I, El-Tehewy F, Bassiouni M, Ayoub A, El-Sayad H: Mitral valvotomy in pregnancy. Am J Obstet Gynecol 145:708, 1983

Eschenbach DA: Contending with the problem of chlamydial infection. Contemp Ob/Gyn 25:125, 1985

Etheridge MJ, Pepperell RJ: Heart disease and pregnancy at the Royal Women's Hospital. Med J Aust 2:277, 1977

Falk RH, Hood WB: The heart in sickle cell anemia. Arch Intern Med 142:1680, 1982

Farb H, West DP, Pedvis-Leftick A: Clofazimine in pregnancy complicated by leprosy. Obstet Gynecol 59:122, 1982

Fauci AS, Lane HC: The acquired immunodeficiency syndrome. In Braunwald E, Isselbacher KJ, Petersdorf RG, Wilson JD, Martin JB, Fauci AS (eds): Harrison's Principles of Internal Medicine, 11th ed. New York, McGraw-Hill, 1987, p 1392

Fear RE: Eclampsia superimposed on scleroderma. Obstet Gynecol 31:69, 1968

Fehr J, Hofman V, Kappeler U: Transient reversal of thrombocytopenia by high-dose intravenous gamma globulins. N Engl J Med 306:1254, 1982

Felding C: The obstetric prognosis in chronic renal disease. Acta Obstet Gynecol Scand 47:166, 1968

Ferenczy A: Treating genital condyloma during pregnancy with the carbon dioxide laser. Am J Obstet Gynecol 148:9, 1984

Ferguson JE II, O'Reilly RA: Hemoglobin E and pregnancy. Obstet Gynecol 66:136, 1985

Field DR, Gates EA, Creasy RK, Jonsen AR, Laros RK Jr: Maternal brain death during pregnancy. JAMA 260:816, 1988

Fieldring JF, Cooke WT: Pregnancy and Crohn's disease. Br Med J 2:76, 1970

Fine LG and several participants: UCLA Conference: Systemic lupus erythematosus in pregnancy. Ann Intern Med 94:667, 1981

Fisch RO, Prem KA, Feinberg SB, Gehrz RC: Acromegaly in a gravida and her infant. Obstet Gynecol 43:861, 1974

Fisher DA: Effectiveness of newborn screening programs for congenital hypothyroidism: Prevalence of missed cases. Clin North Am 34:881, 1987

Fiumara NJ: Letters to the editor. Sex Transm Dis 11:49, 1984

Fortunato SJ, Bawdon RE, Swan KF, Sobhi S: Transfer of azidothymidine (AZT) across the in vitro perfused human placenta: 36th Annual Meeting of the Society for Gynecological Investigation. [Abstract] San Diego, California, March 1989

Foster DW: Diabetes mellitus. In Braunwald E, Isselbacher KJ, Petersdorf RG, Wilson JD, Martin JB, Fauci AS (eds): Harrison's Principles of Internal Medicine, 11th ed. New York, McGraw-Hill, 1987, p 1778

Foy HM, Cooney MK, McMahan R, Grayston JT: Viral mycoplasmal pneumonia in a prepaid medical care group during an eight-year period. Am J Epidemiol 97:93, 1973

Franklyn JA, Sheppard MC, Ramsden DB: Serum free thyroxine and free triiodothyronine concentrations in pregnancy. Br Med J 287:394, 1983

Freedman WL: Alpha and beta thalassemia and pregnancy. Clin Obstet Gynecol 12:115, 1969

Freeman DW, Barno A: Deaths from Asian influenza associated with pregnancy. Am J Obstet Gynecol 78:1172, 1959

Friedland GH, Klein RS: Transmission of the human immunodeficiency virus. N Engl J Med 317:1125, 1987

Frith JA, McLeod JG: Pregnancy and multiple sclerosis. J Neurol Neurosurg Psychiatry 51:495, 1988

Gabbe SG: Application of scientific rationale to the management of the pregnant diabetic. Semin Perinat 2:361, 1978

Gabbe SG: Management of diabetes mellitus in pregnancy, Am J Obstet Gynecol 153:824, 1985

Gabbe SG, Mestman JH, Freeman RK, Goebelsmann UT, Lowensohn RI, Nochimson D, Cetrulo C, Quilligan EJ: Management and outcome of diabetes mellitus, classes B-R. Am J Obstet Gynecol 129:723, 1977

Galve E, Candell-Riera J, Pigrau C, Permanyer-Miralda G, Garcia-Del-Castillo H, Soler-Soler J: Prevalence, morphologic types, and evolution of cardiac valvular disease in systemic lupus erythematosus. N Engl J Med 319:817, 1988

Gant NF: Lupus erythematosus, the lupus anticoagulant, and the anticardiolipin antibody. Williams Obstetrics (suppl 6), May/June 1986

Garlick RL, Mazer JS, Higgins PJ, Bunn HF: Characterization of glycosylated hemoglobins. J Clin Invest 71:1062, 1983

Gasser C, Gautier E, Steck A, Siebenmann RE, Dechslin R: Hamolytisch-uramisch syndrome: Bilaterale Nierenrindennekrosen bie akuten erworbenin haemolytischen Anamien. Scweiz Med Wochenschr 85:905, 1955

Geelhoed GW: Surgery of the endocrine glands in pregnancy. Clin Obstet Gynecol 26:865, 1983

Gehlbach DL, Morgenstern LL: Antenatal screening for thalassemia minor. Obstet Gynecol 71:801, 1988

Gibbs RS, Amstey MS, Sweet RL, Mead PB, Sever JL: Management of genital herpes infection in pregnancy. Obstet Gynecol 71:779, 1988

Gilstrap LC III, Cunningham FG, Whalley PJ: Acute pyelonephritis in pregnancy: An anteroposterior study. Obstet Gynecol 57:409, 1981a

Gilstrap LC III, Leveno KJ, Cunningham FG, Whalley PJ, Roark ML: Renal infection and pregnancy outcome. Am J Obstet Gynecol 141:708, 1981b

Gimovsky ML, Montoro M, Paul RH: Pregnancy outcome in women with systemic lupus erythematosus. Obstet Gynecol 63:686, 1984

Glasscock RJ, Brenner BM: The major glomerulopathies. In Braunwald E, Isselbacher KJ, Petersdorf RG, Wilson JD, Martin JB, Fauci AS (eds): Harrison's Principles of Internal Medicine, 11th ed. New York, McGraw-Hill, 1987, p 1173

Gleicher N, Meller J, Sandler RZ, Sullum S: Wolff-Parkinson-White syndrome in pregnancy. Obstet Gynecol 58:748, 1981

Gleicher N, Midwall J, Hochberger D, Jaffin H: Eisenmenger's syndrome and pregnancy. Obstet Gynecol Surv 34:721, 1979

Gloeb DJ, O'Sullivan MJ, Efantis J: Human immunodeficiency virus infection in women. Am J Obstet Gynecol 159:756, 1988

Golde SH, Montoro M, Good-Anderson B, Broussard P, Jacobs N, Loesser C, Trujillo M, Walla C, Phelan J, Platt L: The role of nonstress tests, fetal biophysical profile, and contraction stress tests in the outpatient management of insulin-requiring diabetic pregnancies. Am J Obstet Gynecol 148:269, 1984

Gomez A, Wood M: Acute appendicitis in pregnancy. Am J Surg 137:180, 1979

Gopal KA, Amshel AL, Shonberg IL, Levinson BA, Vanwert M, Vanwert J: Ostomy and pregnancy. Dis Colon Rectum 28:912, 1985

Gorenberg H, Chesley LC: Rheumatic heart disease in pregnancy: The remote prognosis in patients with "functionally severe" disease. Ann Intern Med 49:278, 1958

Goudeau A, Yvonnet B, Lesage G, Barin F, Denis F, Coursaget P, Chiron JP: Lack of anti-HBc IgM in neonates with HBs Ag carrier mothers argues against transplacental transmission of hepatitis B virus infection. Lancet 2:1103, 1983

Gravett MG, Nelson HP, DeRouen T, Critchlow C, Eschenbach DA, Holmes KK: Independent associations of bacterial vaginosis and Chlamydia trachomatis infection with adverse pregnancy outcome. JAMA 256:1899, 1986

Grayston JT, Kuo CC, Wang SP, Altman J: A new Chlamydia psittaci strain, TWAR, isolated in acute respiratory tract infections. N Engl J Med 315:161, 1986

Greenberg M, Moawad AH, Wieties BM, Goldberg LI, Kaplan EI, Greenberg B, Lindheimer MD: Extraadrenal pheochromocytoma: Detection during pregnancy using MR imaging. Radiology 161:475, 1986

Greenberger PA: Asthma in pregnancy. Clin Perinatol 12:571, 1985

Greene MF, Frigoletto FD Jr, Claster S, Rosenthal D: Pregnancy and paroxysmal nocturnal hemoglobinuria: Report of a case and review of the literature. Obstet Gynecol Surv 38:591, 1983

Greenspoon JS, Paul RH: Paraplegia and quadriplegia: Special considerations during pregnancy and labor and delivery. Am J Obstet Gynecol 155:738, 1986

Grünfeld J-P, Ganeval D, Bournérias F: Acute renal failure in pregnancy. Kidney Int 18:179, 1980

Guillain-Barré Syndrome Study Group: Plasmapheresis and acute Guillain-Barré syndrome. Neurology 35:1096, 1985

Gutiérrez G, Dagnino R, Mintz G: Polymyositis/dermatomyositis and pregnancy. Arthritis Rheum 27:291, 1984

Hadi HA: Pregnancy in renal transplant recipients: A review. Obstet Gynecol Surv 41:264, 1986

Hahm S, Kaplan S, Nitowsky HM: Hemoglobin A_{1c} levels in mothers of large birth weight infants. Pediatr Res 17:315A [Abstract No 1370], 1983

Hallden C, Majmudar B: The relationship between juvenile laryngeal papillomatosis and maternal Condylomata acuminata. J Reprod Med 31:804, 1986

Hamilton BE, Thomson KJ: The Heart in Pregnancy and the Childbearing Age. Boston, Little, Brown, 1941

Hankins GD, Wendel GD Jr, Leveno KJ, Stoneham J: Myocardial infarction during pregnancy: A review. Obstet Gynecol 65:138, 1985

Hankins GVD, Cunningham FG, Luby JP, Butler SL, Stroud J, Roark M: Asymptomatic genital excretion of herpes simplex virus during early labor. Am J Obstet Gynecol 150:100, 1984

Hanson JW, Smith DW: The fetal hydantoin syndrome. So J Pediatr 87:285, 1975

Harer WB Jr, Harer WB Sr: Volvulus complicating pregnancy and the puerperium: A report of three cases and review of the literature (37 references cited). Obstet Gynecol 12:399, 1958

Harris EN, Boey ML, Mackworth-Young CG, Gharavi AE, Patel BM, Loizou S, Hughes GRV: Anticardiolipin antibodies: Detection by radioimmunoassay and association with thrombosis in systemic lupus erythematosus. Lancet 2:1211, 1983

Harris JW: Influenza occurring in pregnant women. JAMA 72:978, 1919

Harris RE, Gilstrap LC III: Cystitis during pregnancy: A distinct clinical entity. Obstet Gynecol 57:578, 1981

Harris RE, Gilstrap LC III, Pretty A: Single-dose antimicrobial therapy for asymptomatic bacteriuria during pregnancy. Obstet Gynecol 59:546, 1982

Harrison HR, Alexander ER, Weinstein L, Lewis M, Nash M, Sim DA: Cervical Chlamydia trachomatis and mycoplasmal infections in pregnancy. JAMA 250:1721, 1983

Harstad TW, Cox SM, Cunningham FG, Pritchard JA: Pregnancy outcome in chronic renal insufficiency: Society of Perinatal Obstetricians. [Abstract] New Orleans, Louisiana, February 1989

Harvey JC, Rosen PP, Ashikari R, Robbins GF, Kinne DW: The effect of pregnancy on the prognosis of carcinoma of the breast following radical mastectomy. Surg Gynecol Obstet 153:723, 1981

Hayden MR, Kastelein JJP, Wilson RD, Hilbert C, Hewitt J, Langlois S, Fox S, Bloch M: First-trimester prenatal diagnosis for Huntington's disease with DNA probes. Lancet 1:1284, 1987

Hayslett JP: Current concepts: Postpartum renal failure. N Engl J Med 312:1556, 1985

Hayslett JP, Lynn RI: Effect of pregnancy in patients with lupus nephropathy. Kidney Int 18:207, 1980

Hench PG: Ameliorating effect of pregnancy on chronic atrophic (infectious rheumatoid) arthritis, fibrositis and intermittent hydrarthrosis. Proc Mayo Clin 13:161, 1938

Hendrickse JP deV, Watson-Williams EJ: The influence of hemoglobinopathies on reproduction. Am J Obstet Gynecol 94:739, 1966

Herbert V, Cunneen N, Jaskiel L, Kopff C: Minimal daily adult folate requirement. Arch Intern Med 110:649, 1962

Hiilesmaa VK, Teramo K, Granström M-L, Bardy AH: Serum folate concentration during pregnancy in women with epilepsy: Relation to antiepileptic drug concentrations, number of seizures, and fetal outcome. Br Med J 287:577, 1983

Hill DE: Effect of insulin on fetal growth. Semin Perinatol 2:319, 1978

Hill LM, Johnson CE, Lee RA: Cholecystectomy in pregnancy. Obstet Gynecol 46:291, 1975

Hime MC, Richardson JA: Diabetes insipidus and pregnancy: Case report, incidence, and review of literature. Obstet Gynecol Surv 3:375, 1978

Hirsch MS, Schooley RT: Treatment of herpesvirus infections. N Engl J Med 309:963, 1983

Hobbins JC, Grannum PA, Romero R, Reece EA, Mahoney JM: Percutaneous umbilical blood sampling. Am J Obstet Gynecol 152:1, 1985

Hochman A, Schreiber H: Pregnancy and cancer of the breast. Obstet Gynecol 2:268, 1953

Hollander DI, Nagey DA, Welch R, Pupkin M: Hyperbaric oxygen therapy for the treatment of acute carbon monoxide poisoning in pregnancy. J Reprod Med 32:615, 1987

Holly EA: Melanoma and pregnancy. Recent Results Cancer Res 102:118, 1986

Holmes GE, Holmes FF: Pregnancy outcomes of patients treated for Hodgkin's disease: A controlled study. Cancer 41:1317, 1978

Holmes KK, Lukhart SA: Syphilis. In Braunwald E, Isselbacher KJ, Petersdorf RG, Wilson JD, Martin JB, Fauci AS (eds): Harrison's Principles of Internal Medicine, 11th ed. New York, McGraw-Hill, 1987, p 639

Holzbach RT, Sivak DA, Braun WE: Familial recurrent intrahepatic cholestasis of pregnancy: A genetic study providing evidence for transmission of a sex-limited, dominant trait. Gastroenterology 85:175, 1983

Homan WP, Thorbjarnarson B: Crohn disease and pregnancy. Arch Surg 111:545, 1976

Homans DC: Peripartum cardiomyopathy. N Engl J Med 312:1432, 1985

Homans DC, Blake GD, Harrington JT, Cetrulo CL: Acute renal failure caused by ureteral obstruction by a gravid uterus. JAMA 246:1230, 1981

Horning SJ, Hoppe RT, Kaplan HS, Rosenberg SA: Female reproductive potential after treatment for Hodgkin's disease. N Engl J Med 304:1377, 1981

Hossack KF, Leddy CL, Johnson AM, Schrier RW, Gabow PA: Echocardiographic findings in autosomal dominant polycystic kidney disease. N Engl J Med 319:907, 1988

Hou S: Pregnancy in women requiring dialysis for renal failure. Am J Kidney Dis 9:368, 1987

Hou SH, Grossman SD, Madias NE: Pregnancy in women with renal disease and moderate renal insufficiency. Am J Med 78:185, 1985

Howard TE, Herrick CN: Pregnancy in patients with ventriculoperitoneal shunts. Am J Obstet Gynecol 141:589, 1981

Hsu HM, Chen DS, Chuang CH, Lu JCF, Jwo DM, Lee CC, Lu HC, Cheng SH, Wang YF, Wang CC, Lo KJ, Shih CJ, Sung JL: Efficacy of a mass hepatitis B vaccination program in Taiwan: Studies on 3463 infants of hepatitis B surface antigen-carrier mothers. JAMA 260:2231, 1988

Hunt HB, Schifrin BS, Suzuki K: Ruptured berry aneurysms and pregnancy. Obstet Gynecol 43:827, 1974

Hunter DJ, Milner R: Gestational diabetes and birth trauma. Am J Obstet Gynecol 152:918, 1985

Hurd WW, Miodovnik M, Stys SJ: Pregnancy associated with paroxysmal nocturnal hemoglobinuria. Obstet Gynecol 60:742, 1982

Hurst D, Little B, Kleman KM, Emburg SH, Lubin GH: Anemia and hemoglobinopathies in Southeast Asian refugee children. J Pediatr 102:692, 1983

Iturbe-Alessio I, Fonseca MDC, Mutchinik O, Santos MA, Zajarias A, Salazar E: Risks of anticoagulant therapy in pregnant women with artificial heart valves. N Engl J Med 315:1390, 1986

Jacob AJ, Epstein J, Madden DL, Sever JL: Genital herpes infection in pregnant women near term. Obstet Gynecol 63:480, 1984

Jacobs C, Donaldson SS, Rosenberg SA, Kaplan HS: Management of the pregnant patient with Hodgkin's disease. Ann Intern Med 95:669, 1981

Jaffe R, Gruber A, Fejgin M, Altaras M, Ben-Aderet N: Pregnancy with an artificial pacemaker. Obstet Gynecol Surv 42:137, 1987

James TN: Myocarditis and cardiomyopathy. N Engl J Med 308:39, 1983

Jewelewicz R, VandeWiele RL: Clinical course and outcome of pregnancy in twenty-five patients with pituitary microadenomas. Am J Obstet Gynecol 136:339, 1980

Johnson RA, Palacios I: Dilated cardiomyopathies of the adult. N Engl J Med 307:1119, 1983

Johnson SR, Kolberg BH, Varner MW, Railsback LD: Maternal obesity and pregnancy. Surg Gynecol Obstet 164:431, 1987

Johnson TR, Banner EA, Winkelmann RK: Scleroderma and pregnancy. Obstet Gynecol 23:467, 1964

Johnston WG, Baskett TF: Obstetric cholestasis. Am J Obstet Gynecol 133:299, 1979

Jones BS: Congenital malaria: 3 cases. Br Med J 2:439, 1950

Jovanovic-Peterson L, Peterson CM: De novo clinical hypothyroidism in pregnancies complicated by type I diabetes, subclinical hypothyroidism, and proteinuria: A new syndrome. Am J Obstet Gynecol 159:442, 1988

Junzer M, Barnes P, Byth K, O'Halloran M: Serum bile acid concentrations during pregnancy and their relationship to obstetric cholestasis. Gastroenterology 91:825, 1986

Kaiser R, Berk JE, Fridhandler L: Serum amylase changes during pregnancy. Am J Obstet Gynecol 122:283, 1975

Karpatkin M, Porges RF, Karpatkin S: Platelet counts in infants of women with autoimmune thrombocytopenia. N Engl J Med 305:936, 1981

Kass EH: Progress in Pyelonephritis, Philadelphia, Davis, 1965. (Contains six articles by various authors on bacteriuria in pregnancy.)

Kass EH: Pyelonephritis and bacteriuria. Ann Intern Med 56:46, 1962

Kassam SH, Hadi HA, Fadel HE, Sims W, Joy WM: Benign intracranial hypertension in pregnancy: Current diagnostic and therapeutic approach. Obstet Gynecol Surv 38:314 1983

Katz AI, Davison JM, Hayslett JP, Singson E, Lindheimer MD: Pregnancy in women with kidney disease. Kidney Int 18:192, 1980

Katz M, Quagiorello J, Young BK: Severe polycystic kidney disease in pregnancy. Obstet Gynecol 53:119, 1979

Katz SI, Hertz KC, Yaoita H: Immunopathology and characterization of the HG factor. J Clin Invest 57:1434, 1976

Kaunitz AM, Hughes JM, Grimes DA, Smith JC, Rochat RW, Kafrissen ME: Causes of maternal mortality in the United States. Obstet Gynecol 65:605, 1985

Kazazian H Jr, Boehm C: Molecular basis and prenatal diagnosis of β-Thalassemia. Blood 72:1107, 1988

Kelly TE, Edwards P, Rein M, Miller JQ, Dreifuss FE: Teratogenicity of anticonvulsant drugs: II. A prospective study. Am J Med Genet 19:435, 1984

Kelton JG, Inwood MJ, Barr RM, Effer SB, Hunter D, Wilson WE, Ginsburg DA, Powers PJ: The prenatal prediction of thrombocytopenia in infants of mothers with clinically diagnosed immune thrombocytopenia. Am J Obstet Gynecol 144:449, 1982

Kincaid-Smith P, Bullen M: Bacteriuria in pregnancy. Lancet 1:395, 1965

King RM, Welch JS, Martin JK, Coulam CB: Carcinoma of the breast associated with pregnancy. Surg Gynecol Obstet 160:228, 1985

Kistler JP, Ropper AH, Martin JB: Cerebrovascular disease. In Braunwald E, Isselbacher KJ, Petersdorf RG, Wilson JD, Martin JB, Fauci AS (eds): Harrison's Principles of Internal Medicine. New York, McGraw-Hill, 1987, p 1930

Kitzmiller JL, Cloherty JP, Younger MD, Tabatabaii A, Rothchild SB, Sosenkol I, Epstein MF, Singh S, Neff RK: Diabetic pregnancy and perinatal outcome. Am J Obstet Gynecol 131:560, 1978

Kitzmiller JL, Younger MD, Hare JW, Phillippe M, Vignati L, Fargnoli B, Grause A: Continuous subcutaneous insulin therapy during early pregnancy. Obstet Gynecol 65:606, 1985

Kleigman RM, Gross T: Perinatal problems of the obese mother and her infant. Obstet Gynecol 66:299, 1985

Klein VR, Laifer S, Timoll EA, Repke JT: Renal cell carcinoma in pregnancy. Obstet Gynecol 69:531, 1987

Kleinknecht D, Grünfeld J-P, Gomez PC, Moreau J-F, Garcia-Torres R: Diagnostic procedures and long-term prognosis in bilateral renal cortical necrosis. Kidney Int 4:390, 1973

Kleinman G, Sutherling W, Martinez M, Tabsh K: Malfunction of ventriculoperitoneal shunts during pregnancy. Obstet Gynecol 61:753, 1983

Knudson LB, Källén B: Intestinal bypass operation and pregnancy outcome. Acta Obstet Gynecol Scand 65:831, 1986

Kochenour NK, Branch W, Rote NS, Scott JR: A new postpartum syndrome associated with antiphospholipid antibodies. Obstet Gynecol 69:460, 1987

Kochenour NK, Emery MG, Sawchuk RJ: Phenytoin metabolism in pregnancy. Obstet Gynecol 56:577, 1980

Koeffler HP, Goldwasser E: Erythropoietin radioimmunoassay in evaluating patients with polychythemia. Ann Intern Med 94:44, 1981

Koerten JM, Morales WJ, Washington Sr III, Castaldo TW: Cushing's syndrome in pregnancy: A case report and literature review. Am J Obstet Gynecol 154:626, 1986

Kohler PF, Vaughan J: The autoimmune diseases. JAMA 248:2646, 1982

Kohn SG, Briele HA, Douglass LH: Volvulus complicating pregnancy. Am J Obstet Gynecol 48:398, 1944

Koontz WL, Herbert WNP, Cefalo RC: Pseudotumor cerebri in pregnancy. Obstet Gynecol 62:325,1983

Kopenhager T: A review of 50 pregnant patients with kyphoscoliosis. Br J Obstet Gynaecol 84:585, 1977

Koshy M, Burd L, Wallace D, Moawad A, Baron J: Prophylactic red-cell transfusions in pregnant patients with sickle cell disease: A randomized cooperative study. N Engl J Med 319:1447, 1988

Kumar ML, Dawson NV, McCullough AJ, Radivoyevitch M, King KC, Hertz R, Kiefer H, Hampson M, Cassidy R, Tavill AS: Should all pregnant women be screened for hepatitis B? Ann Intern Med 107:273, 1987

Lammer EJ, Chen DT, Hoar RM, Agnish ND, Benke PJ, Braun JT, Curry CJ, Fernhoff PM, Grix AW, Lott IT, Richard JM, Sun SC: Retinoic acid embryopathy. N Engl J Med 313:837, 1985

Land MA, Bisno AL: Acute rheumatic fever: A vanishing disease in suburbia. JAMA 249:895, 1983

Lander CM, Edwards VE, Eadie MJ, Tyrer JH: Plasma anticonvulsant concentrations during pregnancy. Neurology 27:128, 1977

Landers D, Carmona R, Crombleholme W, Lim R: Acute cholecystitis in pregnancy. Obstet Gynecol 69:131, 1987

Landesberger EJ, Hager WD, Grossman JH III: Successful management of varicella pneumonia complicating pregnancy: A report of three cases. J Reprod Med 31:311, 1986

Landesman S, Minkoff H, Holman S, McCalla S, Sijin O: Serosurvey of human immunodeficiency virus infection in parturients: Implications for human immunodeficiency virus testing programs of pregnant women. JAMA 258:2701, 1987

Landon MB, Gabbe SG: Glucose monitoring and insulin administration in the pregnant diabetic patient. Clin Obstet Gynecol 3:496, 1985

Lane RS: Non A-non B hepatitis from intravenous immunoglobulins. Lancet 2:974, 1983

Larcos KD: The postpneumonectomy mother. Respiration 39:185, 1980

Larsen JW Jr: Influenza and pregnancy. Clin Obstet Gynecol 25:599, 1982

Lattanzi DR, Cook WA: Urinary calculi in pregnancy. Obstet Gynecol 56:462, 1980

Laverson PL, Hankins GD, Quirk JG Jr: Ureteral obstruction during pregnancy. J Urol 131:327, 1984

Lavin JP, Lovelace DR, Miodovnik M, Knowles HC, Barden TP: Clinical experience with 107 diabetic pregnancies. Am J Obstet Gynecol 147:742, 1983

Lawley TJ, Stingl G, Katz SI: Fetal and maternal risk factors in herpes gestationis. Arch Dermatol 114:552, 1978

Lee GR: The anemia of chronic disease. Semin Hematol 20:61, 1983

Lee LA, Weston WL: New findings in neonatal lupus syndrome. Am J Dis Child 138:233, 1984

Lee RV, Rodgers BD, White LM, Harvey RC: Cardiopulmonary resuscitation of pregnant women. Am J Med 81:311, 1986

Lee RV, Rodgers BD, Young C, Eddy E, Cardinal J: Total parenteral nutrition during pregnancy. Obstet Gynecol 68:563, 1986

Leiken M, Jenkins JH, Graves WL: Prophylactic insulin in gestational diabetes. Obstet Gynecol 70:587, 1987

Lettau LA, McCarthy JG, Smith MH, Hadler SC, Morse LJ, Ukena T, Bessette R, Gurwitz A, Irvine WG, Fields HA, Grady GF, Maynard JE: Outbreak of severe hepatitis due to delta and hepatitis B viruses in parenteral drug abusers and their contacts. N Engl J Med 317:1256, 1987

Leveno KJ, Fortunato SJ, Raskin P, Williams ML, Whalley PJ: Continuous subcutaneous insulin infusion during pregnancy. Diabetes Res Clin Pract 4:257, 1988

Leveno KJ, Harris RE, Gilstrap LC, Whalley PJ, Cunningham FG: Bladder versus renal bacteriuria during pregnancy: Recurrence after treatment. Am J Obstet Gynecol 139:403, 1981

Leveno KJ, Hauth JC, Gilstrap LC III, Whalley PJ: Appraisal of "rigid" blood glucose control during pregnancy in the overtly diabetic woman. Am J Obstet Gynecol 135:793, 1979

Leveno KJ, Whalley PJ: Dilemmas in the management of pregnancy complicated by diabetes. Med Clin North Am 66:1325, 1982

Levine AM, Collea JV: When pregnancy complicates chronic granulocytic leukemia. Contemp Ob/Gyn 13:47, 1979

Lev-Toaff AS, Coleman BG, Arger PH, Mintz MC, Arenson RL, Toaff ME: Leiomyomas in pregnancy: Sonographic study. Radiology 164:375, 1987

Lewis BJ, Laros RK Jr: Leukemia and lymphoma. In Laros RK Jr (ed): Blood Disorders in Pregnancy. Philadelphia, Lea & Febiger, 1986, pp 85–100

Lilleyman JS, Hill AS, Anderton KJ: Consequences of acute myelogenous leukemia in early pregnancy. Obstet Gynecol Surv 33:393, 1978

Lindheimer MD, Davison JM: Renal biopsy during pregnancy: "To b . . . or not to b . . .?" Br J Obstet Gynaecol 94:932, 1987

Linnan MJ, Mascola L, Lou XD, Goulet V, May S, Salminen C, Hird DW, Yonekura ML, Hayes P, Weaver R, Audurier A, Plikaytis BD, Fannin SL, Kleks A, Broome CV: Epidemic listeriosis associated with Mexican-style cheese. N Engl J Med 319:823, 1988

Liu L, Jaffe R, Borowski GD, Rose LI: Exacerbation of Cushing's disease during pregnancy. Am J Obstet Gynecol 145:110, 1983

Lockshin MD, Druzin ML, Goei S, Qamar T, Magid MS, Jovanovic L, Ferenc M: Antibody to cardiolipin as a predictor of fetal distress or death in pregnant patients with systemic lupus erythematosus. N Engl J Med 313:152, 1985

Lockwood C, Romero R, Costigan K, Hobbins J: The prevalence and the significance of lupus anticoagulant and anticardiolipin antibodies: Society of Perinatal Obstetricians eighth annual meeting. [Abstract 11], Las Vegas, Nevada, February 1988

Longo L: The biologic effects of carbon monoxide on the pregnant woman, fetus and newborn infant. Am J Obstet Gynecol 129:69, 1977

Looareesuwan S, White NJ, Karbwang J, Turner RC, Phillips RE, Kietinun S, Rackow C, Warrell DA: Quinine and severe falciparum malaria in late pregnancy. Lancet 2:4, 1985

Lotgering FK, Derkx FMH, Wallenburg HCS: Primary hyperaldosteronism in pregnancy. Am J Obstet Gynecol 155:986, 1986

Loughlin KKR, Bailey RB: Internal ureteral stents for conservative management of ureteral calculi during pregnancy. N Engl J Med 315:1647, 1986

Löwenstein BR, Vain NW, Perrone SV, Wright DR, Boullón FJ, Favaloro RG: Successful pregnancy and vaginal delivery after heart transplantation. Am J Obstet Gynecol 158:589, 1988

Lubbe WF, Buttler WS, Palmer SJ, Liggins GC: Fetal survival after prednisone suppression of maternal lupus-anticoagulant. Lancet 1:1361, 1983

Lubbe WF, Liggins GC: Lupus anticoagulant and pregnancy. Am J Obstet Gynecol 153:322, 1985

Luby JP: Pneumonias in adults due to mycoplasma, chlamydiae, and viruses: Presented at Medical Grand Rounds, University of Texas Southwestern Medical Center at Dallas, February 26, 1981

McCoy MJ, Ellenberg JF, Killam AP: Coccidioidomycosis complicating pregnancy. Am J Obstet Gynecol 137:739, 1980

McCune AB, Weston WL, Lee LA: Maternal and fetal outcome in neonatal lupus erythematosus. Ann Intern Med 106:520, 1987

McFaul PB, Dornan JC, Lamki H, Boyle D: Pregnancy complicated by maternal heart disease: A review of 519 women. Br J Obstet Gynaecol 95:861, 1988

McGregor JA, Burns JC, Levin MJ, Burlington B, Meiklejohn G: Transplacental passage of influenza A/Bangkok (H3N2) mimicking amniotic fluid infection syndrome. Am J Obstet Gynecol 149:856, 1984

McGregor JA, Guberman A, Goodlin R: Idiopathic facial nerve paralysis (Bell's palsy) in late pregnancy and the early puerperium. Obstet Gynecol 69:435, 1987

McGregor JA, Kleinschmidt-DeMasters BK, Ogle J: Meningoencephalitis caused by Histoplasma capsulatum complicating pregnancy. Am J Obstet Gynecol 154:925, 1986

McGregor JA, Mark S, Crawford GP, Levin MJ: Varicella zoster antibody testing in the case of pregnant women exposed to varicella. Am J Obstet Gynecol 157:281, 1987

McLain CR Jr: Leukemia in pregnancy. Clin Obstet Gynecol 17:185, 1974

Madaio MP, Harrington JT: The diagnosis of acute glomerulonephritis. N Engl J Med 309:1299, 1983

Maikranz P, Coe FL, Parks J, Lindheimer MD: Nephrolithiasis in pregnancy. Am J Kidney Dis 9:354, 1987

Main EK, Main DM, Krogstad DJ: Treatment of chloroquine-resistant malaria during pregnancy. JAMA 249:3207, 1983

Manson MM, Logan WPD, Loy RM: Rubella and Other Virus Infections during Pregnancy. London, Her Majesty's Stationery Office, 1960

Markowitz LE, Steere AC, Benach JL, Slade JD, Broome CV: Lyme disease during pregnancy. JAMA 255:3394, 1986

Martin DH, Koutsky L, Eschenbach DA, Daling JR, Alexander ER, Benedetti JK, Holmes KK: Prematurity and perinatal mortality in pregnancies complicated by maternal Chlamydia trachomatis infections. JAMA 247:1585, 1982

Martin FIR, Health P, Mountain KR: Pregnancy in women with diabetes mellitus: Fifteen years' experience: 1970–1985. Med J Aust 146:187, 1987

Martin JN, Morrison JC, Files JC: Autoimmune thrombocytopenic purpura: Current concepts and recommended practices. Am J Obstet Gynecol 160:86, 1984

Mathews RN: Old burns and pregnancy. Br J Obstet Gynecol 89:610, 1982

Matsunaga J, Bergman A, Bhatia NN: Genital condylomata acuminata in pregnancy: Effectiveness, safety and pregnancy outcome following cryotherapy. Br J Obstet Gynaecol 94:168, 1987

Matsuura N, Fujieda K, Iida Y, Fujimoto S, Konishi J, Kasagi K, Hagisawa M, Fukushi M, Takasugi N: TSH-receptor antibodies in mothers with Graves' disease and outcome in their offspring. Lancet 1:14, 1988

Maurus JN: Hansen's disease in pregnancy. Obstet Gynecol 52:22, 1978

Mayberry JF, Atkinson M: Achalasia and pregnancy. Br J Obstet Gynaecol 94:855, 1987

Metzger BE, Bybee DE, Freinkel N, Phelps RL, Radvany RM, Vaisrub N: Gestational diabetes mellitus: Correlations between the phenotypic and genotypic characteristics of the mother and abnormal glucose tolerance during the first year postpartum. Diabetes 34:111, 1985

Miller DM, Winslow RM, Klein HG, Wilson KC, Brown FL, Statham NJ: Improved exercise performance after exchange transfusion in subjects with sickle cell anemia. Blood 56:1127, 1980

Miller E, Hare JW, Cloherty JP, Dunn PJ, Gleason RE, Soeldner JS, Kitzmiller JL: Elevated maternal hemoglobin A_{1c} in early pregnancy and major congenital anomalies in infants of diabetic mothers. N Engl J Med 304:1331, 1981

Miller JP: Inflammatory bowel disease in pregnancy: A review. J R Soc Med 79:221, 1986

Mills JL, Knopp RH, Simpson JL, Jovanovic-Peterson L, Metzger BE, Holmes LB, Aarons JH, Brown Z, Reed GF, Bieber FR, Van Allan M, Holzman I, Ober C, Peterson CM, Withiam JM, Duckles A, Mueller-Heubach E, Polk BF, and the National Institute of Child Health and Human Development Diabetes in Early Pregnancy Study: Lack of relation of increased malformation rates in infants of diabetic mothers to glycemic control during organogenesis. N Engl J Med 318:671, 1988

Milner PF, Jones BR, Döbler J: Outcome of pregnancy in sickle cell anemia and sickle cell-hemoglobin C disease. Am J Obstet Gynecol 138:239, 1980

Milutinovic J, Fialkow P, Agodoa LY, Phillips LA, Bryant JI: Fertility and pregnancy complications in women with autosomal dominant polycystic kidney disease. Obstet Gynecol 61:566, 1983

Minassian SS, Frangipane W, Polin JI, Ellis M: Leiomyomatosis peritonealis disseminata: A case report and literature review. J Reprod Med 31:997, 1986

Minkoff H: Care of pregnant women infected with human immunodeficiency virus. JAMA 258:2714, 1987

Minkoff H, Nanda D, Menez R, Fikrig S: Pregnancies resulting in infants with acquired immunodeficiency syndrome or AIDS-related complex. Obstet Gynecol 69:285, 1987a

Minkoff H, Nanda D, Menez R, Fikrig S: Pregnancies resulting in infants with acquired immunodeficiency syndrome or AIDS-related complex: Follow-up of mothers, children, and subsequently born siblings. Obstet Gynecol 69:288, 1987

Minnefor AB, Oleske JM: Intravenous immune globulin: Efficacy and safety. Hosp Pract 22:171, 1987

Mint G, Niz J, Gutiérrez G, Garcia-Alonso A, Karchmar S: Prospective study of pregnancy in systemic lupus erythematosus: Results of a multidisciplinary approach. J Rheumatol 13:732, 1986

Mintz DH, Chez RA, Hutchinson DL: Subhuman primate pregnancy complicated by streptozotocin-induced diabetes mellitus. J Clin Invest 51:837, 1972

Moltch ME: Pregnancy and the hyperprolactinemic woman. N Engl J Med 312:1364, 1985

Momotani N, Noh J, Oyanagi H, Ishikawa N, Ito K: Antithyroid drug therapy for Graves' disease during pregnancy: Optimal regimen for fetal thyroid status. N Engl J Med 315:24, 1986

Monni G, Ibba RM, Olla G, Rosatelli C, Cao A: Chorionic villus sampling by rigid forceps: Experience with 300 cases at risk for thalassemia major. Am J Obstet Gynecol 156:921, 1987

Montoro M, Collea JV, Frasier SD: Successful outcome of pregnancy in women with hypothyroidism. Ann Intern Med 94:31, 1981

Morris MA, Grandis AS, Litton J: The correlations of glycosylated serum protein and glycosylated hemoglobin concentrations with blood glucose in diabetic pregnancy. Am J Obstet Gynecol 153:257, 1985

Morrison JC, Fort AT, Wiser WL, Fish SA: The modern management of pregnant sickle cell patients: A preliminary report. South Med J 65:533, 1972

Mor-Yosef S, Navot D, Rabinowitz R, Schenker JG: Collagen diseases in pregnancy. Obstet Gynecol Surv 39:67, 1984

Moschcowitz E: An acute febrile pleiochromic anemia with hyaline thrombosis of the terminal arterioles and capillaries. Arch Intern Med 31:89, 1925

Mountain KR, Hirsh J, Gallers AS: Neonatal coagulation defect due to anticonvulsant drug treatment in pregnancy. Lancet 1:265, 1970

Murphy JR, Wengard M, Brereton W: Rheological studies of Hb SS blood; influence of hematocrit, hypertonicity, separation of cells, deoxygenation, and mixture with normal cells. J Lab Clin Med 87:475, 1976

Murray JE, Reid DE, Harrison JH, Merrill JP: Successful pregnancies after human renal transplantation. N Engl J Med 269:341, 1963

Murray MJ, Murray AB, Murray NJ, Murray MB: The effect of iron status of Nigerian mothers on that of their infants at birth and 6 months, and on the concentration of Fe in breast milk. Br J Nutr 39:627, 1978

Myers JP, Peristein PH, Light IJ, Towbin RB, Dincsoy HP, Dincsoy MY: Tuberculosis in pregnancy with fatal congenital infection. Pediatrics 67:89, 1981

Nadler N, Salinas-Madrigal L, Charles AG, Pollak VE: Acute glomerulonephritis during late pregnancy. Obstet Gynecol 34:277, 1969

Nagorney DM, Field CS: Successful pregnancy 10 years after triple cardiac valve replacement. Obstet Gynecol 57:386, 1981

Natelson EA, White D: Recurrent thrombotic thrombocytopenic purpura in early pregnancy: Effect of uterine evacuation. Obstet Gynecol 66:54S, 1985

National Institutes of Health Conference: Herpes simplex virus infection: Biology, treatment and prevention. Ann Intern Med 103:404, 1985

Neely NT, Persellin RH: Activity of rheumatoid arthritis during pregnancy. Tex Med 73:59, 1977

Nehmias AJ, Josey WE, Naib ZM, Freeman MG, Fernandez RJ, Wheeler JH: Perinatal risk associated with maternal genital herpes simplex virus infection. Am J Obstet Gynecol 110:825, 1971

Nelson DM, Stempel LE, Brandt JT: Hereditary antithrombin III deficiency and pregnancy: Report of two cases and review of the literature. Obstet Gynecol 65:848, 1985

Nishurmura RA, McGoon MD, Shub C, Miller FA, Ilstrup DM, Tajik AJ: Echocardiographically documented mitral-valve prolapse: Long-term follow-up of 237 patients. N Engl J Med 313:1305, 1985

Noronha A: Neurologic disorders during pregnancy and the puerperium. Clin Perinatol 12:695, 1985

Norton RA, Patterson JF: Pregnancy and regional enteritis. Obstet Gynecol 40:711, 1972

Nugent P, O'Connell TX: Breast cancer and pregnancy. Arch Surg 120:1221, 1985

Nussbaum RL, Powell C, Graham HL, Caskey CT, Fernbach DJ: Newborn screening for sickle hemoglobinopathies: Houston, 1976 to 1980. Am J Dis Child 138:44, 1984

Oakley GDG, McGarry K, Limb DG, Oakley CM: Management of pregnancy in patients with hypertrophic cardiomyopathy. Br Med J 1:1749, 1979

O'Neill H, Blake S, Sugrue D, MacDonald D: Problems in the management of patients with artificial valves during pregnancy. Br J Obstet Gynaecol 89:940, 1982

Orkin SH, Little PFR, Kazazian HH Jr, Boehm CD: Improved detection of the sickle mutation by DNA analysis. N Engl J Med 307:32, 1982

Orr JW Jr, Shingleton HM: Cancer in pregnancy. In Hickey RC (ed): Current Problems in Cancer. Chicago, Year Book, 1983, pp 1–50

O'Shaughnessy R, Weprin SA, Zuspan FP: Obstructive renal failure by an overdistended pregnant uterus. Obstet Gynecol 55:247, 1980

O'Shaughnessy RW, Hackett KJ: Maternal Addison's disease and fetal growth retardation. J Reprod Med 29:752, 1984

Ostensen M, Husby G: A prospective clinical study of the effect of pregnancy on rheumatoid arthritis and ankylosing spondylitis. Arthritis Rheum 26:1155, 1983

O'Sullivan JB, Mahan CM: Criteria for the oral glucose tolerance test in pregnancy. Diabetes 13:278, 1964

Packham D, Fairley KF: Renal biopsy: Indications and complications in pregnancy. Br J Obstet Gynaecol 94:935, 1987

Parente JT, Amsel M, Lerner R, Chinea F: Breast cancer associated with pregnancy. Obstet Gynecol 71:861, 1988

Parham GP, Orr JW Jr: Hyperparathyroidism secondary to parathyroid carcinoma in pregnancy. J Reprod Med 32:123, 1987

Paryani SG, Arvin AM: Intrauterine infection with varicella-zoster virus after maternal varicella. N Engl J Med 314:1542, 1986

Pastorek JG III, Plauche WC, Faro S: Acute bacterial endocarditis. J Reprod Med 28:611, 1983

Patriarco M, Yeh S-Y: Immunological thrombocytopenia in pregnancy. Obstet Gynecol Surv 41:661, 1986

Patterson R: Hyperparathyroidism in pregnancy. Obstet Gynecol 70:457, 1987

Paulson GW, Paulson RB: Teratogenic effects of anticonvulsants. Arch Neurol 38:140, 1981

Peaceman AM, Cruikshank DP: Ehlers-Danlos syndrome and pregnancy: Association of type IV disease with maternal death. Obstet Gynecol 69:428, 1987

Penn I, Makowski EL, Harris P: Parenthood following renal transplant. Kidney Int 2:221, 1980

Perez RJ, Lipner H, Abdulla N, Cicotto S, Abrams M: Menstrual dysfunction of patients undergoing chronic hemodialysis. Obstet Gynecol 51:552, 1978

Persson B, Stangenberg M, Hansson U, Nordlander E: Gestational diabetes mellitus (GDM): Comparative evaluation of two treatment regimens, diet versus insulin and diet. Diabetes 34S:101, 1985

Perucca E, Ruprah M, Richens A: Altered drug binding to serum proteins in pregnant women: Therapeutic relevance. J R Soc Med 74:422, 1981

Peterson CM, Kelly JV: Pseudotumor cerebri in pregnancy: Case reports and review of literature. Obstet Gynecol Surv 40:323, 1985

Pitkin RM: Calcium metabolism in pregnancy and the perinatal period: A review. Am J Obstet Gynecol 151:99, 1985

Poddar D, Maude GH, Plant MJ, Scorer H, Serjeant GR: Pregnancy in Jamaican women with homozygous sickle cell disease: Fetal and maternal outcome. Br J Obstet Gynaecol 93:927, 1986

Poncz M, Colman N, Herbert V, Schwartz E, Cohen AR: Therapy of congenital folate malabsorption. J Pediatr 98:76, 1981

Pope RM, Yoshinoya S, Rutstein J, Persellin RH: Effect of pregnancy on immune complexes and rheumatoid factors in patients with rheumatoid arthritis. Am J Med 74:973, 1983

Powars DR, Sandhu M, Niland-Weiss J, Johnson C, Bruce S, Manning PR: Pregnancy in sickle cell disease. Obstet Gynecol 67:217, 1986

Powell BL, Drutz DJ, Huppert M, Sun SH: Relationship of progesterone- and estradiol-binding proteins in *Coccidioides immitis* to coccidioidal dissemination in pregnancy. Infect Immun 40:478, 1983

Pratt AT, Donaldson RC, Evertson LR, Yon JL Jr: Cecal volvulus in pregnancy. Obstet Gynecol (Suppl) 57:37, 1981

Printen KJ, Scott D: Pregnancy following gastric bypass for the treatment of morbid obesity. Am Surg 48:363, 1982

Pritchard JA: Hereditary hypochromic microcytic anemia in obstetrics and gynecology. Am J Obstet Gynecol 83:1193, 1962a

Pritchard JA, Cunningham FG, Mason RA: Coagulation changes in eclampsia: Their frequency and pathogenesis. Am J Obstet Gynecol 124:855, 1976

Pritchard JA, Mason RA: Iron stores of normal adults and replenishment with oral iron therapy. JAMA 190:897, 1964

Pritchard JA, Scott DE: Iron demands in pregnancy. In Hallberg L, Harwerth H-G, Vanotti A (eds): Iron Deficiency Pathogenesis, Clinical Aspects, Therapy. New York, Academic, 1970

Pritchard JA, Scott DE, Whalley PJ: Folic acid requirements in pregnancy-induced megaloblastic anemia. JAMA 208:1163, 1969

Pritchard JA, Scott DE, Whalley PJ, Cunningham FG, Mason RA: The effects of maternal sickle cell hemoglobinopathies and sickle cell trait on reproductive performance. Am J Obstet Gynecol 117:662, 1973

Prober CG, Hensleigh PA, Boucher FD, Yasukawa LL, Au DS, Arvin AM: Use of routine viral cultures at delivery to identify neonates exposed to herpes simplex virus. N Engl J Med 318:887, 1988

Prober CG, Sullender WM, Yasukawa LL, Au DS, Yeager AS, Arvin AM: Low risk of herpes simplex virus infections in neonates exposed to the virus at the time of vaginal delivery to mothers with recurrent genital herpes simplex virus infections. N Engl J Med 316: 240, 1987

Pyeritz RE: Maternal and fetal complications of pregnancy in the Marfan syndrome. Am J Med 71:784, 1981

Ramsay I, Kaur S, Krassas G: Thyrotoxicosis in pregnancy: Results of treatment by antithyroid drugs combined with T4. Clin Endocrinol 18:73, 1983

Rayburn W, Smith B, Feller I, Varner M, Cruikshank D: Major burns during pregnancy: Effects on fetal well-being. Obstet Gynecol 63:392, 1984

Reece EA, Coustan DR, Hayslett JP, Holford T, Coulehan J, O'Connor TZ, Hobbins JC: Diabetic nephropathy: Pregnancy performance and fetomaternal outcome. Am J Obstet Gynecol 159:56, 1988

Reece EA, Fox HE, Rapoport F: Factor VIII inhibitor: A cause of severe postpartum hemorrhage. Am J Obstet Gynecol 144:985, 1982

Reece EA, Hobbins JC: Diabetic embryopathy: Pathogenesis, prenatal diagnosis, and prevention. Obstet Gynecol Surv 41:325, 1986

Reid R, Ivey KJ, Rencoret RH, Storey B: Fetal complications of obstetric cholestasis. Br Med J 1:870, 1976

Reynoso EE, Shepherd FA, Messner HA, Farquharson HA, Garvey MB, Baker MA: Acute leukemia during pregnancy: The Toronto Leukemia Study Group experience with long-term follow-up of children exposed in utero to chemotherapeutic agents. J Clin Oncol 5:1098, 1987

Ribeiro G, Jones DA, Jones M: Carcinoma of the breast associated with pregnancy. Br J Surg 73:607, 1986

Richards DS, Miller DK, Goodman GN: Pregnancy after gastric bypass for morbid obesity. J Reprod Med 32:172, 1987

Riely CA: Acute fatty liver of pregnancy. Semin Liver Dis 7:47, 1987

Riggall F, Salkind G, Spellacy W: Typhoid fever complicating pregnancy. Obstet Gynecol 44:117, 1974

Rigler LG, Eneboe JB: Incidence of hiatus hernia in pregnant women and its significance. J Thorac Surg 4:262, 1935

Robson JS, Martin AM, Ruckley VA, MacDonald MK: Irreversible postpartum renal failure. Q J Med 37:423, 1968

Rodis JF, Hovick TJ, Quinn DL, Rosengren SS, Tattersall P: Human parvovirus infection in pregnancy. Obstet Gynecol 72:733, 1988

Rose PG, Essig GF, Vaccaro PS, Brandt JT: Protein S deficiency in pregnancy. Am J Obstet Gynecol 155:140, 1986

Rosen IB, Walfish PG: Pregnancy as a predisposing factor in thyroid neoplasia. Arch Surg 121:1287, 1986

Rotmensch HH, Elkayam U, Frishman W: Antiarrhythmic drug therapy during pregnancy. Ann Intern Med 98:487, 1983

Rubin SC, Wheeler JE, Mikuta JJ: Malignant leiomyomatosis peritonealis disseminata. Obstet Gynecol 68:126, 1986

Ruch WA, Klein RL: Polycythemia vera and pregnancy. Obstet Gynecol 23:107, 1964

Rust LA, Goodnight SH, Freeman RK, Johnson CS: Pregnancy and delivery in a woman with hemophilia B. Obstet Gynecol 46:483, 1975

Sachs BP, Brown DA, Driscoll SG, Schulman E, Acker D, Ransil BJ, Jewett JF: Maternal mortality in Massachusetts: Trends and prevention. N Engl J Med 316:667, 1987

Sanderson JE, Olsen EGJ, Gatei D: Peripartum heart disease: An endomyocardial biopsy study. Br Heart J 56:285, 1986

Schachter J, Sweet RL, Grossman M, Landers D, Robbie M, Bishop E: Experience with the routine use of erythromycin for chlamydial infections in pregnancy. N Engl J Med 314:276, 1986

Schatz M, Harden K, Forsythe A, Chilingar L, Hoffman C, Sperling W, Zeiger RS: The course of asthma during pregnancy, post partum, and with successive pregnancies: A prospective analysis. J Allergy Clin Immunol 81:509, 1988

Schenker JG, Granat M: Phaeochromocytoma and pregnancy—An updated appraisal. Aust NZ J Obstet Gynaecol 22:1, 1982

Schlesinger PA, Duray PH, Burke BA, Steere AC, Stillman MT: Maternal-fetal transmission of lyme disease spirochet, *Borrelia burgdorferi*. Ann Intern Med 103:67, 1985

Schmid GP, Sanders LL, Blount JH, Alexander ER: Chancroid in the United States: Reestablishment of an old disease. JAMA 258:3265, 1987

Schmidt D, Canger R, Avanzini G, Battino D, Cusi C, Beck-Mannagetta G, Koch S, Rating D, Janz D: Change of seizure frequency in pregnant epileptic women. J Neurol Neurosurg Psychiatry 46:751, 1983

Schneider JM, Curet LB, Olson RW, Shay G: Ambulatory care of the pregnant diabetic. Obstet Gynecol 56:144, 1980

Schneider RG, Hightower H, Hasty TS, Ryder H, Tomlin G, Atkins R, Brimhall B, Jones RT: Abnormal hemoglobins in a quarter million people. Blood 48:629, 1976

Schreyer P, Caspi E, El-Hindi JM, Eschar J: Cirrhosis—Pregnancy and delivery: A review. Obstet Gynecol Surv 37:304, 1982

Schriner RL, Kleiman MB, Gresham EL: Maternal oral herpes: Isolation policy. Pediatrics 63:247, 1979

Schwartz ML, Brenner W: Severe preeclampsia with persistent postpartum hemolysis and thrombocytopenia treated by plasmapheresis. Obstet Gynecol 65:53S, 1985

Scott DE, Pritchard JA: Iron deficiency in healthy young college women. JAMA 199:147, 1967

Scott GB, Fischl MA, Klimas N, Fletcher MF, Dickinson GM, Levine RS, Parks WP: Mothers of infants with the acquired immunodeficiency syndrome: Evidence for both symptomatic and asymptomatic carriers. JAMA 253:363, 1985

Scott JR, Rote NS, Cruikshank DP: Antiplatelet antibodies and platelet counts in pregnancies complicated by autoimmune thrombocytopenic purpura. Am J Obstet Gynecol 145:932, 1983

Seaworth BJ, Durack DT: Infective endocarditis in obstetric and gynecologic practice. Am J Obstet Gynecol 154:180, 1986

Second International Workshop-Conference: Gestational diabetes mellitus. Diabetes 34S:1, 1985

Sende P, Pantelakis N, Suzuki K, Bashore R: Plasma oxytocin level in pregnancy with diabetes insipidus. Clin Res 23:242A, 1975

Shangold MM, Dor N, Welt SI, Fleischman AR, Crenshaw MC Jr: Hyperparathyroidism and pregnancy: A review. Obstet Gynecol Surv 37:217, 1982

Shaw D, Frohlich J, Wittmann BAK, Willms M: A prospective study of 18 patients with cholestasis of pregnancy. Am J Obstet Gynecol 142:621, 1982

Sherlock S: Acute fatty liver of pregnancy and microvesicular fat diseases. Gut 24:265, 1983

Shime J, Mocarski EJM, Hastings D, Webb GD, McLaughlin PR: Congenital heart disease in pregnancy: Short- and long-term implications. Am J Obstet Gynecol 156:313, 1987

Shornick JK, Bangert JL, Freeman RG, Gilliam JN: Herpes gestationis: Clinical and histologic features of 28 cases. J Am Acad Dermatol 8:214, 1983

Shulman ST, Amren DP, Bisno AL, Dajani AS, Durack DT, Gerber MA, Kaplan EL, Millard HD, Sanders WE, Schwartz RH: Prevention of bacterial endocarditis: A statement for health professionals by the Committee on Rheumatic Fever and Infective Endocarditis of the Council on Cardiovascular Disease in the Young. Circulation 70:1123A, 1984

Siegel M, Goldberg M: Incidence of poliomyelitis in pregnancy. N Engl J Med 253:841, 1955

Siegler AM, Spain DM: Periarteritis nodosa in pregnancy. Clin Obstet Gynecol 8:280, 1965

Singh H, Bolton PJ, Oakley CM: Pregnancy after surgical correction of tetralogy of Fallot. Br Med J 285:168, 1982

Singletary BK, Van Thiel DH, Eagon PK: Estrogen and progesterone receptors in human gallbladder. Hepatology 6:574, 1986

Singsen BH, Akhter JE, Weinstein MM, Sharp GC: Congenital complete heart block and SSA antibodies: Obstetric implications. Am J Obstet Gynecol 152:655, 1985

Skouby SO, Kühl C, Milsted-Pedersen I, Petersen K, Christensen MS: Triphasic oral contraception: Metabolic effects in normal women and those with previous gestational diabetes. Am J Obstet Gynecol 153:495, 1985

Slater GE, Rumack RH, Peterson RG: Podophyllin poisoning. Obstet Gynecol 52:94, 1978

Smith EW, Krevans JR: Clinical manifestations of hemoglobin C disorders. Bull Johns Hopkins Hosp 104:17, 1959

Smith MB, Whiteside MG, DeGaris CN: An investigation of the complications and outcome of pregnancy in heterozygous beta-thalassaemia. Aust NZ J Obstet Gynecol 15:26, 1975

Smith WD, West HF: Pregnancy and rheumatoid arthritis. Acta Rheumat Scand 6:189, 1960

Snider DE Jr, Layde PM, Johnson MW, Lyle MA: Treatment of tuberculosis during pregnancy. Am Rev Respir Dis 122:65, 1980

Snyder RR, Gilstrap LC, Hauth JC: Ehlers-Danlos syndrome and pregnancy. Obstet Gynecol 61:649, 1983

Snyder RR, Hankins GDV: Etiology and treatment of acute fatty liver of pregnancy. Clin Perinatol 13:813, 1986

Snydman DR: Hepatitis in pregnancy. N Engl J Med 313:1398, 1985

Spangler AS, Reddy W, Bardawil WA, Roby CC, Emerson K: Papular dermatitis of pregnancy: A new clinical entity. JAMA 181:577, 1962

Sridama V, Pacini F, Yang SL, Moawad A, Reilly M, DeGroot LJ: Decreased levels of helper T cells: A possible cause of immunodeficiency in pregnancy. N Engl J Med 307:352, 1982

Stafford-Brady FJ, Gladman DD, Urowitz MB: Successful pregnancy in systemic lupus erythematosus with an untreated lupus anticoagulant. Arch Intern Med 148:1647, 1988

Stamm WE, Wagner KF, Amsel R, Alexander R, Turck M, Counts GW, Holmes KK: Causes of the acute urethral syndrome in women. N Engl J Med 303:409, 1980

Starksen NF, Bell WR, Kickler TS: Unexplained hemolytic anemia associated with pregnancy. Am J Obstet Gynecol 146:617, 1983

Stauffer RA, Adams A, Wygal J, Lavery JP: Gallbladder disease in pregnancy. Am J Obstet Gynecol 144:661, 1982

Steven MM: Progress report: Pregnancy and liver disease. Gut 22:592, 1981

Steven MM, Buckley JD, Mackay IR: Pregnancy in chronic active hepatitis. Q J Med 48:519, 1979

Strickland DM, Hauth JC, Widish J, Strickland K, Perez R: Amylase and isoamylase activities in serum of pregnant women. Obstet Gynecol 63:389, 1984

Sudo N, Weingold AB: Obstetric aspects of the Guillain-Barré syndrome. Obstet Gynecol 45:39, 1975

Sugrue D, Blake S, MacDonald D: Pregnancy complicated by maternal heart disease at the National Maternity Hospital, Dublin, Ireland, 1969 to 1978. Am J Obstet Gynecol 139:1, 1981

Sullivan JM, Ramanathan KB: Management of medical problems in pregnancy: Severe cardiac disease. N Engl J Med 313:304, 1985

Sullivan-Bolyai J, Hull HF, Wilson C, Corey L: Neonatal herpes simplex virus infection in King County, Washington. JAMA 250:3059, 1983

Surian M, Imbasciati E, Cosci P, Banfi G, di Belgiojoso B, Brancaccio D, Minetti L, Ponticelli C: Glomerular disease and pregnancy: A study of 123 pregnancies in patients with primary and secondary glomerular diseases. Nephron 36:101, 1984

Svanborg-Eden C, Hagberg L, Leffler H, Lonberg H: Recent progress in the understanding of the role of bacterial adhesion in the pathogenesis of urinary tract infection. Infection 10:327, 1982

Sweet RL, Landers CV, Walker C, Schachter J: *Chlamydia trachomatis* infection and pregnancy outcome. Am J Obstet Gynecol 156:824, 1987

Tan EM, Cohen AS, Fries JF, Masi AT, McShane DJ, Rothfield NF, Schaller JG, Talal N, Winchester RJ: The 1982 revised criteria for the classification of systemic lupus erythematosus. Arthritis Rheum 25:1271, 1982

Taylor DJ, Mallen C, McDougal N, Lind T: Effect of iron supplementation on serum ferritin levels during and after pregnancy. Br J Obstet Gynaecol 89:1011, 1982a

Taylor DJ, Wilcox I, Russell JK: Ehlers-Danlos syndrome during pregnancy: A case report and review of the literature. Obstet Gynecol Surv 36:277, 1982b

Third National Cancer Survey: Incidence data. Natl Cancer Inst Monogr 41:108, 1975

Tindall RS, Rollins JA, Phillips JT, Greenlee RG, Wells L, Belendiuk G: Preliminary results of a double-blind, randomized placebo-controlled trial of cyclosporine in myasthenia gravia. N Engl J Med 316:1987

Triplett DA, Brandt JT, Musgrave KA, Orr CA: The relationship between lupus anticoagulants and antibodies to phospholipid. JAMA 259:550, 1988

Trudinger BJ, Stewart GJ, Cook CM, Connelly A, Exner T: Monitoring lupus anticoagulant-positive pregnancies with umbilical artery flow velocity waveforms. Obstet Gynecol 72:215, 1988

Tsukamoto N, Uchino H, Matsukuma K, Kamura T: Carcinoma of the colon presenting as bilateral ovarian tumors during pregnancy. Gynecol Oncol 24:385, 1986

Tuck SM, Studd JWW, White JM: Pregnancy in women with sickle cell trait. Br J Obstet Gynaecol 90:108, 1983

Tucker MA, Coleman CN, Cox RS, Varghese A, Rosenberg SA: Risk of second cancers after treatment for Hodgkin's disease. N Engl J Med 318:76, 1988

Turkalj I, Braun P, Krupp P: Surveillance of bromocriptine in pregnancy. JAMA 247:1589, 1982

Turner ES, Greenberger PA, Patterson R: Management of the pregnant asthmatic patient. Ann Intern Med 6:905, 1980

Tuttleman RM, Gleicher N: Central nervous system hemorrhage complicating pregnancy. Obstet Gynecol 58:651, 1981

Unger A, Kay A, Griffin AJ, Panayi GS: Disease activity and pregnancy associated α_2-glycoprotein in rheumatoid arthritis. Br Med J 286:750, 1983

Väisänen V, Elo J, Tallgren LG, Siitonen A, Makela PH, Svanborg-Eden C, Kallenius G, Svenson SB, Hultbert H, Korhonen T: Mannose-resistant haemagglutination and P antigen recognition are characteristic of Escherichia coli causing primary pyelonephritis. Lancet 2:1366, 1981

Vandekerckhove F, Noems L, Coldardyn F, Thiery M, Delbarge W: Thrombotic thrombocytopenic purpura mimicking toxemia of pregnancy. Am J Obstet Gynecol 150:320, 1984

Van Dorsten JP, Lenke RR, Schifrin BS: Pyelonephritis in pregnancy: The role of in-hospital management and nitrofurantoin suppression. J Reprod Med 32:897, 1987

Vargas MT, Briones-Urbina R, Gladman D, Papsin FR, Walfish PG: Antithyroid microsomal autoantibodies and HLA-DR5 are associated with postpartum thyroid dysfunction: Evidence supporting an autoimmune pathogenesis. J Clin Endocrinol Metab 67:327, 1988

Varner MW, Meehan RT, Syrop CH, Strottman MP, Gopelrud CP: Pregnancy in patients with systemic lupus erythematosus. Am J Obstet Gynecol 145:1025, 1983

Ventura CS: Hereditary spherocytosis with haemolytic crisis during pregnancy. Aust NZ J Obstet Gynaecol 22:50, 1982

Vetter VL, Rashkind WJ: Congenital complete heart block and connective-tissue disorders. N Engl J Med 309:236, 1983

Vichinsky E, Hurst D, Earles A, Kleman K, Lubin B: Newborn screening for sickle cell disease: Effect on mortality. Pediatrics 81:749, 1988

Voitk AJ, Mueller JC, Farlinger DE, Johnston RU: Carpel tunnel syndrome in pregnancy. Can Med Assoc J 129:277, 1983

Volpé R, Ehrlech R, Steiner G, Row VV: Graves' disease in pregnancy years after hypothyroidism with recurrent passive-transfer neonatal Graves' disease in offspring. Am J Med 77:572, 1984

Wager GP, Martin DH, Koutsky L, Eschenbach DA, Daling JR, Chiang WT, Alexander FR, Holmes KK: Puerperal infectious morbidity: Relationship to route of delivery and to antepartum Chlamydia trachomatis infection. Am J Obstet Gynecol 138:1028, 1980

Wagoner RD, Holley KE, Johnson WJ: Accelerated nephrosclerosis and postpartum acute renal failure in normotensive patients. Ann Intern Med 69:237, 1968

Walcott WO, Derick DE, Jolley JJ, Synder DL, Schmid R: Successful pregnancy in a liver transplant patient. Am J Obstet Gynecol 132:340, 1978

Walfish PG, Chan JYC: Postpartum hyperthyroidism. J Clin Endocrinol Metab 14:417, 1985

Walker WM, McKee AP: Asian influenza in pregnancy: Relationship to fetal anomalies. Obstet Gynecol 13:394, 1959

Wallace DJ, Podell T, Weiner J, Klinenberg JR, Forouzesh S, Dubois EL: Systemic lupus erythematosus—Survival patterns. JAMA 245:934, 1981

Ward JW, Holmbert DS, Allen JR, Cohn DL, Critchley SE, Kleinman SH, Lenes BA, Ravenholt O, Davis JR, Quinn MG, Jaffee HW: Transmission of human immunodeficiency virus (HIV) by blood transfusions screened as negative for HIV antibody. N Engl J Med 318:473, 1988

Ware AJ, Luby JP, Hollinger B, Eigenbrodt EH, Cuthert JA, Atkins CR, Shorey J, Hull AR, Combs B: Etiology of liver disease in renal transplant patients. Ann Intern Med 91:364, 1979

Weatherall DJ, Pressley L, Wood WG, Higgs DR: Molecular basis for mild forms of homozygous beta-thalassemia. Lancet 1:527, 1981

Weinberg ED: Pregnancy-associated depression of cell-mediated immunity. Rev Infect Dis 6:814, 1984

Weisman SA, Simon NA, Herdson PB, Franklin WA: Nephrotic syndrome in pregnancy. Am J Obstet Gynecol 117:867, 1973

Wendel GD Jr, Stark RJ, Jamison RR, Molina RD, Sullivan TJ: Penicillin allergy and desensitization in serious infections during pregnancy. N Engl J Med 312:1229, 1985

Wertheim RA, Brooks BJ Jr, Rodriguez RH Jr, Lesesne HR, Jennette JC: Fatal herpetic hepatitis in pregnancy. Obstet Gynecol (Suppl) 62:38 1983

Westberg SV: Prognosis of breast cancer for pregnant and nursing women. Acta Obstet Gynecol Scand (Supl 4) 25:1, 1946

Wetzel AM, Kirz DS: Routine hepatitis screening in adolescent pregnancies: Is it cost effective? Am J Obstet Gynecol 156:166, 1987

Whalley PJ: Bacteriuria of pregnancy. Am J Obstet Gynecol 97:723, 1967

Whalley PJ: Hyperparathyroidism and pregnancy. Am J Obstet Gynecol 86:517, 1963

Whalley PJ, Cunningham FG, Martin FG: Transient renal dysfunction associated with acute pyelonephritis of pregnancy. Obstet Gynecol 46:174, 1975

Whalley PJ, Martin FG, Peters PC: Significance of asymptomatic bacteriuria detected during pregnancy. JAMA 198:879, 1965

White P: Classification of obstetric diabetes. Am J Obstet Gynecol 130:228, 1978

White P: Pregnancy and diabetes, medical aspects. Med Clin North Am 49:1015, 1965

Whittemore R, Hobbins JC, Engle MA: Pregnancy and its outcome in women with and without surgical treatment of congenital heart disease. Am J Cardiol 50:641, 1982

Whittemore R, Wright MR, Leonard MF, Johnson M: Results of pregnancy in women with congenital heart defects. Pediatr Res 14:452, 1980

Wiebers DO, Whisnant JP: The incidence of stroke among pregnant women in Rochester, Minn, 1955 through 1979. JAMA 253:3055, 1985

Wilkinson EJ: Acute pancreatitis in pregnancy: A review of 98 cases and a report of 8 new cases. Obstet Gynecol Surv 28:281, 1973

Williams JW: The limitations and possibilities of prenatal care. JAMA 64:95, 1915

Wilson MG, Heins HL, Imagawa DT, Adams JM: Teratogenic effects of Asian influenza. JAMA 171:638, 1959

Wittek AE, Yaeger AS, Au DS, Hensleigh PA: Asymtomatic shedding of herpes simplex virus from the cervix and lesion site during pregnancy. Am J Dis Child 138:439, 1984

Yancey KB, Hall RP, Lawley TJ: Pruritic urticarial papules and plaques of pregnancy: Clinical experience in 25 patients. J Am Acad Dermatol 10:473, 1984

Yazigi R, Driscoll SG: Sarcoma complicating pregnancy. Gynecol Oncol 25:125, 1986

Yeager AS, Arvin AM: Reasons for the absence of a history of recurrent genital infections in mothers of neonates infected with herpes simplex virus. Pediatrics 73:188, 1984

Young BK, Katz M, Klein SA: Pregnancy after spinal cord injury: Altered maternal and fetal response in labor. Obstet Gynecol 62:59, 1983

Zegart KN, Schwarz RH: Chorea gravidarum. Obstet Gynecol 32:24, 1968

Zinns JS: The association of pregnancy and breast cancer. J Reprod Med 22:297, 1979

Anatomy of the Reproductive Tract of Women

he organs of reproduction of women are classified according to hose that are external and those that are internal. The external rgans and the vagina serve for copulation; the internal organs rovide for ovulation, a site of ovum fertilization and blastocyst ansport, implantation, and thence development and birth of he fetus.

EXTERNAL GENERATIVE ORGANS

he *pudenda*, or the external organs of generation, are comnonly designated the *vulva*, which includes all structures visible xternally from the pubis to the perineum, that is, the mons ubis, the labia majora and minora, the clitoris, hymen, vestiule, urethral opening, and various glandular and vascular structures (Fig. 40–1).

MONS PUBIS

he mons pubis, or mons veneris, is the fat-filled cushion that es over the anterior surface of the symphysis pubis. After uberty, the skin of the mons pubis is covered by curly hair that orms the *escutcheon*. Generally, the distribution of pubic hair iffers in the two sexes. In women, it is distributed in a trianular area, the base of which is formed by the upper margin of he symphysis, and a few hairs are distributed downward over he outer surface of the labia majora. In men, the escutcheon is ot so well circumscribed, hairs from the pubic area grow in a gion that extends upward toward the umbilicus and downard and inward over the inner surface of the thighs.

LABIA MAJORA

here are two rounded folds of adipose tissue that are covered ith skin, and that extend downward and backward from the ons pubis; these are the labia majora. Among adult women, ese structures vary somewhat in appearance, principally acording to the amount of fat that is contained within these ssues. Embryologically, the labia majora are homologous with e scrotum of men. The round ligaments terminate at the uper borders of the labia majora. After repeated childbearing, the bia majora are less prominent, and in old age usually begin to rivel. Ordinarily, these structures are 7 to 8 cm in length, 2 to

3 cm in width, and 1 to 1.5 cm in thickness, and are somewhat tapered at the lower extremities. In children and nulliparous women, the labia majora usually lie in close apposition and thereby completely conceal the underlying tissues, whereas in multiparous women, the labia majora may gape widely (Fig. 40–2). The labia majora are continuous directly with the mons pubis above and merge into the perineum posteriorly, at a site where these structures are joined medially to form the *posterior commissure.*

Before puberty, the outer surface of each labium majus is similar to that of the adjacent skin, but after puberty each is covered with hair. In nulliparous women, the inner surface is moist and resembles a mucous membrane, whereas in multiparous women, the inner surface becomes more skinlike, but is not covered with hair. The labia majora are richly supplied with sebaceous glands. Beneath the skin, there is a layer of dense connective tissue that is rich in elastic fibers and adipose tissue, but is nearly void of muscular elements. Unlike the squamous epithelium of the vagina and cervix, in parts of the vulvar skin there are epithelial appendages. Beneath the skin, there is a mass of fat, which provides the bulk of the volume of the labium; this adipose tissue is supplied with a plexus of veins that, as the result of external injury, may rupture to create a hematoma.

LABIA MINORA

Two flat reddish folds of tissue are visible when the labia majora are separated; these structures are the labia minora, or nymphae, structures that join at the upper extremity of the vulva. Among women, the labia minora vary greatly in size and shape. In nulliparous women, the labia minora usually are not visible behind the nonseparated labia majora, whereas in multiparous women, it is common for the labia minora to project beyond the labia majora.

Each labium minus is a thin fold of tissue that, when projected, is moist and reddish in appearance and thus is similar to that of a mucous membrane. These structures, however, are covered by stratified squamous epithelium into which numerous papillae project. There are no hair follicles in the labia minora, but there are many sebaceous follicles and, occasionally, a few sweat glands. The interior of the labial folds is comprised of connective tissue in which there are many vessels and some

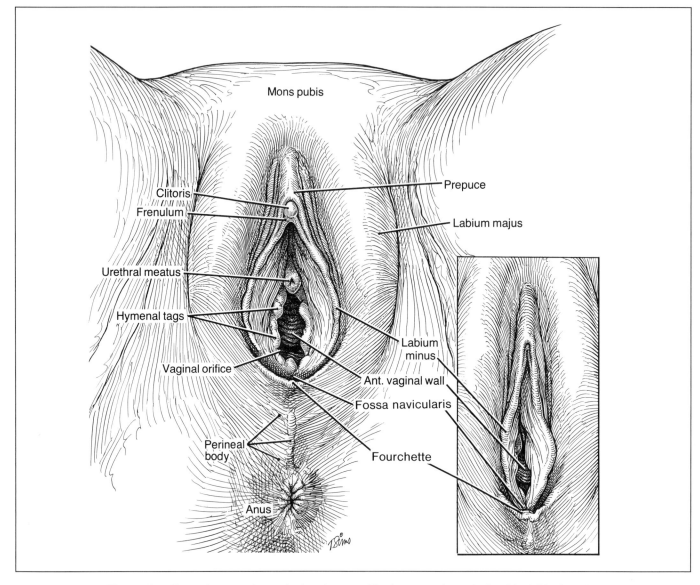

Figure 40–1. External organs of reproduction of women. The lower anterior vaginal wall is visible through the labia minora. In nulliparous women, the vaginal orifice is not so readily visible (*inset*) because of the close apposition of the labia minora.

smooth muscular fibers, as is the case in typical erectile structures. These structures are extremely sensitive and are supplied with a variety of nerve endings.

The tissues of the labia minora converge superiorly where each is divided into two lamellae, the lower pair of which fuse to form the *frenulum of the clitoris,* and the upper pair merges to form the *prepuce* of the clitoris. Inferiorly, the labia minora extend to approach the midline as low ridges of tissue that fuse to form the *fourchet* that is readily visible in nulliparous women; in multiparous women, however, the labia minora usually are imperceptibly contiguous with the labia majora.

CLITORIS

The clitoris, the homologue of the penis, is a small, cylindrical, erectile body that is located near the superior extremity of the vulva. This organ projects downward between the branched extremities of the labia minora, which, as stated, converge to form the prepuce and frenulum of the clitoris. The clitoris is comprised of a glans, a body (corpus), and two crura. The glans is made up of spindle-shaped cells, and in the body there are two corpora cavernosa, in the walls of which are smooth muscle fibers. The long, narrow crura arise from the inferior surface of the ischiopubic rami and fuse just below the middle of the pubic arch to form the body of the clitoris.

Rarely does the clitoris exceed 2 cm in length, even in a state of erection, and it is bent sharply by traction that is exerted by the labia minora. As a result, the free end of the clitoris is pointed downward and inward toward the vaginal opening. The glans, which rarely exceeds 0.5 cm in diameter, is covered by stratified squamous epithelium that is richly supplied with nerve endings and is, therefore, extremely sensitive to touch. The vessels of the erectile clitoris are connected with the vestibular bulbs; the clitoris is believed to be one, if not the principal, erogenous organ of women.

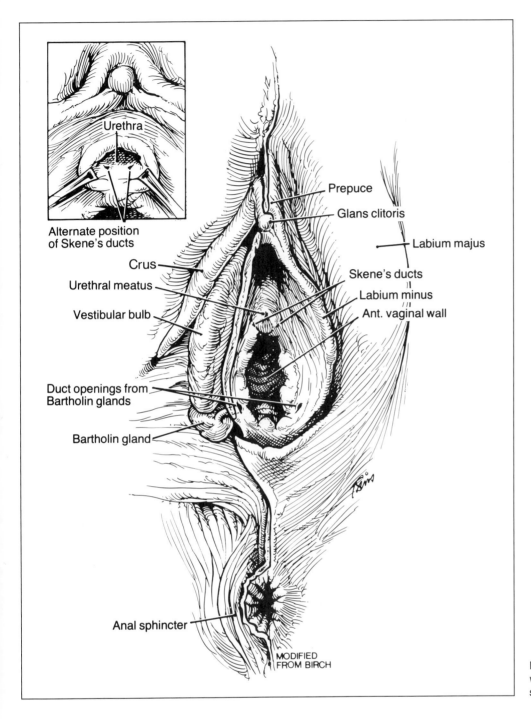

Figure 40–2. The external genitalia with the skin and subcutaneous tissue removed from the right side.

Krantz (1958) studied the nerve supply of the external genitalia; in the labia majora, as well as the labia minora and clitoris, he found that there is a delicate network of free nerve endings, the fibers of which terminate in small knoblike thickenings in or adjacent to the cells. These nerve endings are encountered more frequently in the papillae than elsewhere; moreover, tactile discs also are found in abundance in these areas. The number of genital corpuscles, which are considered the main structures that are mediators of erotic sensation, vary considerably. These structures are distributed sparsely and randomly in the labia majora deep in the corium, but in the labia minora there are a great number of these corpuscles, particularly in the prepuce and skin that overlies the glans clitoris.

VESTIBULE

The vestibule is an almond-shaped area that is enclosed by the labia minora laterally and extends from the clitoris above to the fourchet below. The vestibule is the functionally mature female structure of the urogenital sinus of the embryo; in the mature state it usually is perforated by six openings: the urethra, the vagina, the ducts of the Bartholin glands, and, at times, the ducts of the paraurethral glands, also called the Skene ducts and glands (Fig. 40–2). The posterior portion of the vestibule between the fourchet and the vaginal opening is called the *fossa navicularis*. Rarely is it observed except in nulliparous women, since usually it is obliterated as the result of childbirth.

Related to the vestibule are the *major vestibular glands,* i.e., the *Bartholin glands* (Fig. 40–2). These are a pair of small compound glands that are about 0.5 to 1 cm in diameter; each is situated beneath the vestibule on either side of the vaginal opening. The Bartholin glands lie under the constrictor muscle of the vagina and sometimes are found to be covered partially by the vestibular bulbs. The gland ducts are 1.5 to 2 cm long and open on the sides of the vestibule just outside the lateral margin of the vaginal orifice. The small lumina of the glands ordinarily admit only the finest of probes. At times of sexual arousal, mucoid material is secreted from these glands. The ducts sometimes harbor *Neisseria gonorrhoeae,* or other bacteria, that may gain access to the gland, and cause suppuration and a Bartholin gland abscess.

URETHRAL OPENING

The lower two thirds of the urethra lies immediately above the anterior vaginal wall and terminates externally in the urethral meatus. The urethral meatus is in the midline of the vestibule, 1 to 1.5 cm below the pubic arch, and a short distance above the vaginal opening; usually it is puckered in appearance. The orifice of the urethra appears as a vertical slit, which can be distended to 4 or 5 mm in diameter. Ordinarily, the *paraurethral ducts* open onto the vestibule on either side of the urethra, but occasionally open on the posterior wall of the urethra just inside the meatus (Fig. 40–2). These ducts are of small caliber, about 0.5 mm in diameter, and of variable length. In the United States, the paraurethral ducts generally are known as the Skene ducts.

VESTIBULAR BULBS

Beneath the mucous membrane of the vestibule on either side are the vestibular bulbs, which are almond-shaped aggregations of veins, 3 to 4 cm long, 1 to 2 cm wide, and 0.5 to 1 cm thick. These bulbs lie in close apposition to the ischiopubic rami and are partially covered by the ischiocavernosus and constrictor vaginae muscles. The lower terminations of the vestibular bulbs usually are at about the middle of the vaginal opening, and anteriorly, the vestibular bulbs extend upward toward the clitoris.

Embryologically, the vestibular bulbs correspond to the anlage of the corpus spongiosum of the penis. The vestibular bulbs of women, during childbirth, usually are pushed up beneath the pubic arch; since the posterior ends partially encircle the vagina, however, these structures are liable to injury and rupture, which may give rise to a hematoma of the vulva or else to profuse hemorrhage.

VAGINAL OPENING AND HYMEN

The vaginal opening is in the lower portion of the vestibule and varies considerably in size and shape among women. In virginal women, it most often is hidden entirely by the overlapping labia minora, and when exposed, it usually appears almost completely closed by the membranous hymen.

There are also marked differences in shape and consistency of the hymen. This tissue is comprised mainly of connective tissue, both elastic and collagenous. Both the outer and inner surfaces are covered by stratified squamous epithelium. Connective tissue papillae are more numerous on the vaginal surface and at the free edge. According to Mahran and Saleh (1964), there are no glandular or muscular elements in the hymen and it is not richly supplied with nerve fibers.

In the newborn, the hymen is very vascular and redundant; in pregnant women, the epithelium is thick and the tissue is rich in glycogen; after menopause, the epithelium of the hymen is thin and focal cornification may develop. In adult virginal women, the hymen is a membrane of various thickness that surrounds the vaginal opening more or less completely; among virginal women, the aperture of the hymen varies in diameter from that of a pinpoint to a caliber that admits the tip of one or even two fingers. The hymenal opening usually is crescentic or circular, but occasionally may be cribriform, septate, or fimbriated. As the fimbriated type of hymen in virginal women may be mistaken for one that has been penetrated during intercourse, it is wise to exercise caution when making definite statements with regard to "rupture" of the hymen.

As a rule, the hymen is torn at several sites during first coitus, usually in the posterior portion. The edges of the torn tissue soon cicatrize, and the hymen becomes divided permanently into two or more portions that are separated by narrow sulci that extend down to its base. The extent to which rupture occurs varies with the structure of the hymen and the extent to which it is distended. Although commonly it is believed that rupture of the hymen is accompanied by bleeding, this is not the case or else is not evident in all women. Occasionally with hymenal rupture, however, there my be profuse bleeding. Rarely, the hymenal membrane may be very resistant to penetration or perforation and surgical incision of the tissue may be necessary before coitus can be accomplished.

The changes in the hymen that are brought about by coitus are occasionally of medico-legal importance, especially in instances of alleged rape, in which the physician is called upon to examine the victim and to testify concerning the physical findings. In virgins who are examined a few hours after the alleged sexual attack, the finding of fresh hymenal lacerations or abrasions, or the finding of bleeding points on the hymen constitute corroborative evidence of recent vaginal penetration, possibly by intercourse. The absence of such findings is of no significance, however, since the hymen may not be lacerated even with repeated coitus in a short time period. In fact, many cases of pregnancy have been reported in women in whom the hymen did not appear to have been "ruptured."

As a rule, the changes produced in the hymen by childbirth are readily recognizable. After the puerperium, several cicatrized nodules of various sizes are formed, the tissue remnants of the hymen, the *myrtiform caruncles.*

Imperforate hymen, a rare lesion, is a condition in which the vaginal orifice is occluded completely, causing retention of the menstrual discharge.

VAGINA

The vagina is a tubular, musculomembranous structure that extends from the vulva to the uterus; the vagina is interposed anteriorly and posteriorly between the urinary bladder and the rectum (Fig. 40–3). The vagina is an organ of many functions: the excretory canal of the uterus, through which uterine secretions and menstrual flow escape; the female organ of copulation; and part of the birth canal at the time of childbirth. The upper portion of the vagina arises from the müllerian ducts; the lower portion is formed from the urogenital sinus. Anteriorly, the vagina is in contact with the bladder and urethra, from which it is separated by connective tissue that often is referred to as the vesicovaginal septum. Posteriorly, that is, between the lower portion of the vagina and the rectum, there are similar tissues that, together, form the rectovaginal septum. Usually, the up-

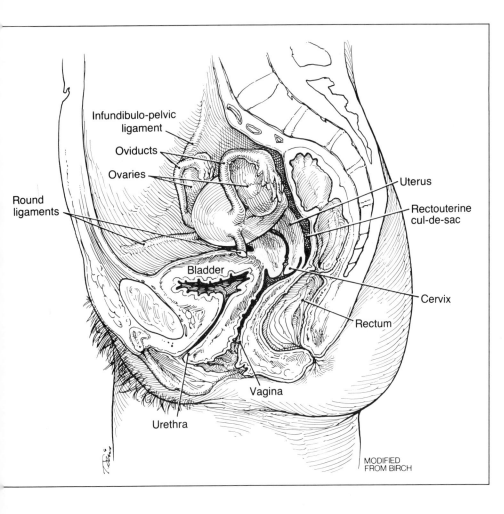

Figure 40–3. Sagittal section of the pelvis of an adult woman that is illustrative of relations of pelvic viscera.

MODIFIED
FROM BIRCH

er one fourth of the vagina is separated from the rectum by the ectouterine pouch, or, as it is sometimes called, the cul-de-sac f Douglas.

Normally, the anterior and posterior walls of the vagina lie n contact with only a slight space that intervenes between the ateral margins. Thus, when not distended, the vaginal canal on ansverse section is H-shaped (Fig. 40–4). The vagina can be istended markedly, a characteristic that is most evident during hildbirth.

The upper end of the vagina is the termination of a vault nto which the lower portion of the uterine cervix projects. The aginal vault is subdivided into the anterior, posterior, and two ateral fornices. Since the vagina is attached higher up on the osterior wall than on the anterior wall of the cervix, the depth f the posterior fornix is appreciably greater than the anterior. he lateral fornices are intermediate in depth. The fornices are f considerable clinical importance since the internal pelvic or- ans usually can be palpated through the thin walls of the ornices. Moreover, by way of the posterior fornix, there usually provided ready surgical access to the peritoneal cavity. mong women, the vagina varies considerably in length. Com- only, the anterior and posterior vaginal walls are, respec- vely, 6 to 8 cm, and 7 to 10 cm in length.

Prominent longitudinal ridges project into the vaginal lu- en from the midlines of both the anterior and posterior walls. nullparous women, these numerous transverse ridges, or gae, extend outward from, and almost at right angles to, the ongitudinal vaginal ridges. The rugae gradually recede as the

lateral walls are approached. The rugae are such as to form a corrugated surface, which is not present before menarche and is one that gradually becomes obliterated after repeated childbirth and after menopause. In elderly multiparous women, the vag- inal walls often are smooth.

The mucosa of the vagina (Fig. 40–5) is comprised of non- cornified stratified squamous epithelium. Beneath the epithe- lium there is a thin fibromuscular coat; usually, there is an inner circular layer and an outer longitudinal layer of smooth muscle that can be identified. There is a thin layer of connective tissue that overlies the mucosa and the muscularis, one that is rich in blood vessels, and one in which there are a few small lymphoid nodules. The mucosa and muscularis are attached very loosely to the underlying connective tissue, and, by surgical means, these tissues are easily dissected free. Some argument remains as to whether this connective tissue, which sometimes is re- ferred to as perivaginal endopelvic fascia, is a definite fascial plane in the strict anatomical sense.

Normally, glands are not present in the vagina. In parous women, however, fragments of stratified epithelium, which sometimes give rise to cysts, are occasionally embedded in the vaginal connective tissue. These vaginal inclusion cysts are not glands; rather, these are remnants of mucosal tags that were buried during the repair of vaginal lacerations after childbirth. Other cysts that are lined by columnar or cuboidal epithelium may be found; these are believed to be derived from embryonic remnants.

From early in infancy until after menopause, there is a

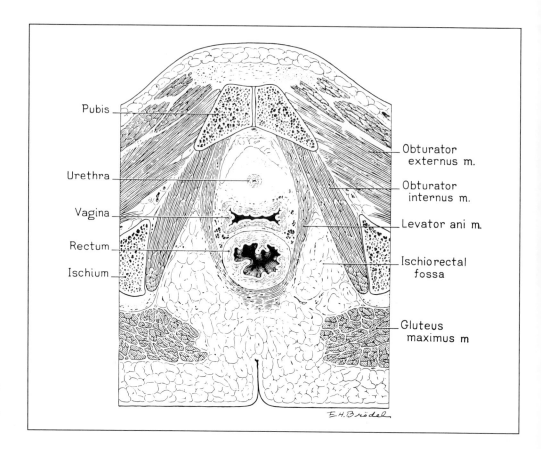

Figure 40–4. Cross-section of the pelvis of an adult woman; the H-shaped lumen of the vagina is apparent (m. = muscle).

considerable amount of glycogen in the cells of the superficial layer of the vaginal mucosa. By examination of cells that are exfoliated from the vaginal epithelium, one can identify the various hormonal events of the ovarian cycle.

In nonpregnant women, the vagina is kept moist by a small amount of secretion from the uterus. During pregnancy, there is copious vaginal secretion, which normally consists of a curd-like product of exfoliated epithelium and bacteria, which is markedly acidic. *Lactobacillus* species are recovered from most pregnant women, and in higher concentrations than in non-pregnant women (Larsen and Galask, 1980). These bacilli are the predominant bacteria of the vagina during pregnancy. The

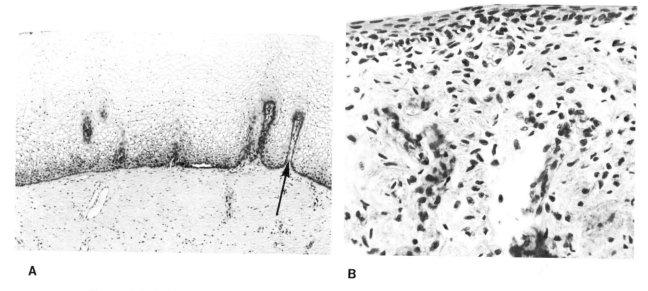

A   B

Figure 40–5. A. Photomicrograph of the vagina of an adult woman that is characterized by noncornified, thick, stratified squamous epithelium; note that epithelial appendages are not present. Arrow is pointed to a papilla. **B.** Photomicrograph of typical thin vaginal epithelium of a prepubertal girl.

acidic reaction is attributable to the presence of lactic acid, which arises from the metabolism of glycogen from the cells in the mucosa by lactobacilli. The pH of the vaginal secretion varies with the nature of the ovarian hormones that are secreted. Before puberty, the pH of the secretions of the vagina varies between 6.8 and 7.2, whereas in adult women it is well below this, and typically ranges from 4.0 to 5.0.

There appear to be both qualitative as well as quantitative changes in the microbial flora during pregnancy, but as Larsen and Galask (1980) emphasize, carefully done longitudinal studies are lacking. Most investigators report that *Lactobacillus* species are isolated more commonly during pregnancy, and probably in higher concentrations. There is also evidence that anaerobic organisms commonly isolated from nonpregnant women are not as numerous during pregnancy. Postpartum, this rapidly reverses and, probably related to lochial discharge, anaerobic bacteria increase dramatically and are the most common isolates causing infection in puerperal women (Chap. 27, p. 463).

There is an abundant vascular supply to the vagina; the upper third is supplied by the cervicovaginal branches of the uterine arteries, the middle third by the inferior vesical arteries, and the lower third by the middle hemorrhoidal and internal pudendal arteries. There is an extensive venous plexus that immediately surrounds the vagina, vessels which follow the course of the arteries; eventually, these veins empty into the hypogastric veins. For the most part, the lymphatics from the lower third of the vagina, along with those of the vulva, drain into the inguinal lymph nodes, those from the middle third into the hypogastric nodes, and those from the upper third into the iliac nodes. According to Krantz (1958), the vagina is devoid of any special nerve endings (genital corpuscles); occasionally, however, free nerve endings are found in the papillae.

THE PERINEUM

The many structures that make up the perineum are illustrated in Figure 40–6. Most of the support of the perineum is provided by the pelvic and urogenital diaphragms. The *pelvic diaphragm* consists of the levator ani muscles plus the coccygeus muscles posteriorly and the fascial coverings of these muscles. The levator ani muscles form a broad muscular sling that originates from the posterior surface of the superior rami of the pubis, from the inner surface of the ischial spine, and between these two sites, from the obturator fascia. The muscle fibers are inserted in several locations as follow: around the vagina and rectum to form efficient functional sphincters for each; into a raphe in the midline between the vagina and rectum; into a midline raphe below the rectum; and into the coccyx. The *urogenital diaphragm* is positioned external to the pelvic diaphragm, i.e., in the triangular area between the ischial tuberosities and the symphysis pubis. The urogenital diaphragm is comprised of the deep transverse perineal muscles, the constrictor of the urethra, and the internal and external fascial coverings.

PERINEAL BODY

The median raphe of the levator ani, which is positioned between the anus and the vagina, is reinforced by the central tendon of the perineum, on which converge the bulbocavernosus muscles, the superficial transverse perineal muscles, and the external anal sphincter. These structures, which contribute to the perineal body and provide much of the support for the perineum, often are lacerated during delivery unless an adequate episiotomy is made at an appropriate time (Chap. 16, p. 323).

INTERNAL GENERATIVE ORGANS

UTERUS

The uterus is a muscular organ that is covered, partially, by peritoneum, or serosa. The cavity of the uterus is lined by the endometrium. During pregnancy, the uterus serves for reception, implantation, retention, and nutrition of the conceptus, which it then expels during labor.

Anatomical Relationships

The uterus of the nonpregnant woman is situated in the pelvic cavity between the bladder anteriorly and the rectum posteriorly. The inferior portion, i.e., the cervix, projects into the vagina. Almost the entire posterior wall of the uterus is covered by serosa, or peritoneum, the lower portion of which forms the anterior boundary of the *rectouterine cul-de-sac*, or pouch of Douglas. Only the upper portion of the anterior wall of the uterus is so covered (Fig. 40–7). The lower portion is united to the posterior wall of the bladder by a well-defined but normally loose layer of connective tissue (Figs. 40–3, 40–8).

Size and Shape

The uterus is a structure that resembles a flattened pear in shape (Figs. 40–7, 40–8) and consists of two major but unequal parts: an upper triangular portion, the *body* (or *corpus*) and a lower, cylindrical, or fusiform portion, the *cervix*. The anterior surface of the body of the uterus is almost flat, whereas the posterior surface is distinctly convex. The oviducts, or fallopian tubes, emerge from the *cornua* of the uterus at the junction of the superior and lateral margins. The convex upper segment between the points of insertion of the fallopian tubes is called the *fundus*. The lateral margins extend from the cornua on either side to the pelvic floor. Laterally, the portion of the uterus below the insertion of the fallopian tubes is not covered directly by peritoneum, but it is the site of the attachments of the broad ligaments.

The uterus varies widely in size and shape, and the age and parity of the woman influence this tremendously. Before puberty, the organ varies in length from 2.5 to 3.5 cm. The uterus of adult nulliparous women is from 6 to 8 cm in length as compared with 9 to 10 cm in multiparous women (Fig. 40–8). Uteri of nonparous and parous women also differ considerably in weight; normally, the former weighs from 50 to 70 g, and the latter weighs 80 g or somewhat more (Langlois, 1970). The relationship between the length of the body of the uterus and that of the cervix likewise varies widely. In the young girl, the body of the uterus is only half as long as the cervix; in nulliparous women, the two are about equal in length; in multiparous women, the cervix is only a little more than one third of the total length of the organ (Fig. 40–8).

The great bulk of the body of the uterus, but not the cervix, is comprised of muscle. The inner surface of the anterior and posterior walls of the uterus lie almost in contact; the cavity between these walls forms a mere slit (Figs. 40–8, 40–9). The cervical canal is fusiform and is open at each end by small apertures, the *internal os* and the *external os*. On frontal section, the cavity of the body of the uterus is triangular, whereas that of the cervix is fusiform in shape. The margins of parous uteri

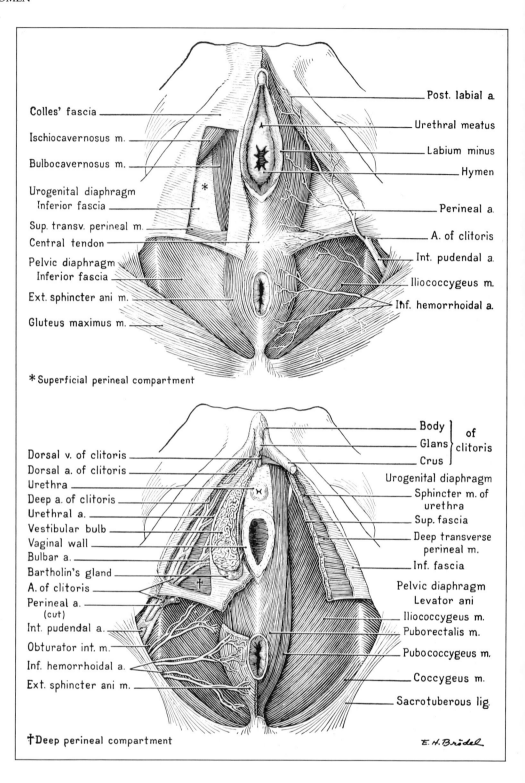

Figure 40–6. The perineum. The moresuperficial components are illustrated above and the deeper structures below (m. = muscle; a. = artery; lig. = ligament; Int. = internal; Ext. = external; Inf. = inferior).

become concave instead of convex, and hence the triangular appearance of the uterine cavity is less pronounced. After menopause, the size of the uterus decreases as a consequence of atrophy of the myometrium and the endometrium also is atrophic.

The *isthmus* (Fig. 40–8) is of special obstetrical significance because, in pregnancy, it is essential to the formation of the lower uterine segment (See Chap. 10, p. 214).

UTERINE CERVIX

The cervix is the specialized portion of the uterus that is below the isthmus. Anteriorly, the upper boundary of the cervix, the internal os, corresponds, approximately, to the level at which the peritoneum is reflected upon the bladder.

The cervix is divided by the attachment of the vagina into vaginal and supravaginal portions. The supravaginal segment

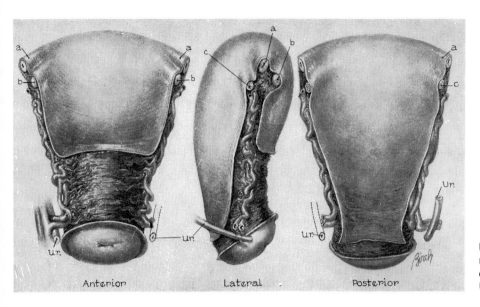

Figure 40–7. Anterior, right lateral, and posterior views of the uterus of an adult woman; a, oviduct; b, round ligament; c, ovarian ligament; Ur. = ureter.

on its posterior surface is covered by peritoneum. Laterally, it is attached to the cardinal ligaments; and, anteriorly, it is separated from the overlying bladder by loose connective tissue. The external os is located at the lower extremity of the vaginal portion of the cervix, the *portio vaginalis.*

The external os of the cervix varies greatly in appearance; before childbirth, it is a small, regular, oval opening; after childbirth, the orifice is converted into a transverse slit that is divided such that there are the so-called anterior and posterior lips of the cervix. If the cervix was torn deeply during delivery, it might heal in such a manner that it appears to be irregular, nodular, or stellate. These changes are sufficiently characteristic to permit an examiner to ascertain with some certainty whether a given woman has borne children by vaginal delivery (Figs. 40–10 and 40–11).

The cervix is composed of some smooth muscle fibers, but predominantly of collagenous tissue plus elastic tissue and blood vessels. The transition from the primarily collagenous tissue of the cervix to the primarily muscular tissue of the body of the uterus, although generally abrupt, may be gradual, and may extend over as much as 10 mm. The results of studies by Danforth and colleagues (1960) are suggestive that the physical properties of the cervix are determined, in large measure, by the state of the connective tissue, and that during pregnancy and labor the remarkable ability of the cervix to dilate is the result of dissociation of collagen. Buckingham and co-workers (1965) quantified the amount of muscle and collagen in the tissue of the cervix of women. In the normal cervix, the proportion of muscle is, on average, about 10 percent, whereas in women with an *incompetent cervix,* sometimes the proportion of muscle is appreciably greater.

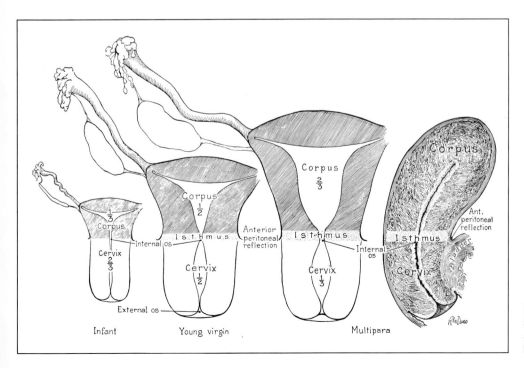

Figure 40–8. Comparison of the size of uteri of prepubertal girls and adult nonparous and parous women by frontal and sagittal sections.

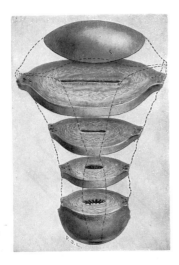

Figure 40–9. Reconstruction of the uterus to illustrate the shape of the uterine cavity.

formed by the peritoneum that covers the uterus, and to which it is firmly adherent except at sites just above the bladder and at the lateral margins where the peritoneum is deflected in a manner to form the broad ligaments.

Endometrium

The innermost portion of the uterus, or mucosal layer, that lines the uterine cavity in nonpregnant women, is the *endometrium*. It is a thin, pink, velvet-like membrane, which on close examination is found to be perforated by a large number of minute openings; these are the ostia of the uterine glands. Because of the repetitive cyclic changes that occur during the reproductive years of a woman's life, the endometrium normally varies greatly in thickness and measures from 0.5 mm to as much as 5 mm. The endometrium is comprised of surface epithelium, glands, and interglandular mesenchymal tissue in which there are numerous blood vessels.

The epithelium of the endometrial surface is comprised of a single layer of closely packed, high columnar, ciliated cells. During much of the endometrial cycle, the oval nuclei are situated in the lower portions of the cells but not so near the base as in the endocervix.

Cilia have been demonstrated in the cells of the endometria of many mammals; the ciliated cells are located in discrete patches, whereas secretory activity appears to be limited to nonciliated cells. The ciliary current in both the fallopian tubes and the uterus is in the same direction and extends downward from the fimbriated end of the tubes toward the external os.

The tubular *uterine glands* are invaginations of the epithelium, which, in the resting state, are reminiscent of the fingers of a glove. The glands extend through the entire thickness of the endometrium to the myometrium, which is occasionally penetrated for a short distance. Histologically, the inner glands resemble the epithelium of the surface and are lined by a single layer of columnar, partially ciliated epithelium that rests upon a thin basement membrane. The glands secrete a thin alkaline fluid that serves to keep the uterine cavity moist (see Figs. 3–3, and 3–4, pp. 29 and 30).

In the classic monograph of Hitschmann and Adler, published in 1908, it was reported that the endometrium undergoes constant, hormonally controlled changes during each ovarian cycle. These three fundamental phases—*menstrual, proliferative (follicular), and secretory (luteal)*—are discussed in detail in Chapter 3 in the section on menstruation. In brief, immediately after menstruation the endometrium is normally quite thin, and the tubular glands are well separated. Thereafter, the endometrium rapidly increases in thickness and, before the next menses, usually contains many convoluted or sacculated glands. After menopause, the endometrium is atrophic: the epithelium flattens, the glands gradually disappear, and the interglandular tissue becomes more fibrous.

Characteristically, the mucosa of the cervical canal, although embryologically a direct continuation of the endometrium, is differentiated in such a way that the appearance of sections through the canal are reminiscent of a honeycomb. The mucosa is composed of a single layer of very high, columnar epithelium that rests upon a thin basement membrane. The oval nuclei are situated near the base of the columnar cells, the upper portions of which appear to be rather clear because of content of mucus. These cells are supplied abundantly with cilia.

There are numerous cervical glands that extend from the surface of the endocervical mucosa directly into the subjacent connective tissue; since there is no submucosa as such, these glands furnish the thick, tenacious secretion of the cervical canal. If the ducts of the cervical glands are occluded, retention cysts may form, which are a few millimeters in diameter, the so-called *Nabothian follicles or Nabothian cysts.*

Normally, the squamous epithelium of the vaginal portion of the cervix and the columnar epithelium of the cervical canal form a sharp line of division very near the external os, i.e., the squamo-columnar junction. In response to inflammation or trauma, however, the stratified epithelium may extend gradually up the cervical canal and come to line the lower third, or occasionally even the lower half, of the canal. This change is more marked in the cervices of multiparous women, in whom the lips of the cervix often are everted. Uncommonly, the two varieties of epithelium abut on the vaginal portion outside the external os, as in *congenital ectropion.*

Changes in the characteristics of the cervical mucosa are dependent upon the variations in the hormonal patterns of the ovarian cycle, as discussed in Chapter 3 (p. 36).

BODY OF THE UTERUS

The wall of the body of the uterus is composed of three layers: the serosal, the muscular, and the mucosal. The serosal layer is

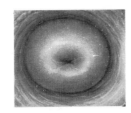

Figure 40–10. Cervical external os of a nonparous woman.

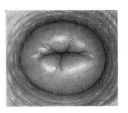

Figure 40–11. Cervical external os of a parous woman.

The connective tissue of the endometrium, between the surface epithelium and the myometrium, is a mesenchymal stroma. Immediately after menstruation, the stroma is comprised of closely packed cells with oval and spindle-shaped nuclei, around which there is very little cytoplasm. When separated by edema, the cells appear to be stellate, with cytoplasmic processes that branch to form anastomoses. These cells are packed more closely around the glands and blood vessels than elsewhere. Several days before menstruation, the stromal cells usually become larger and more vesicular, like decidual cells; and, at the same time, there is a diffuse leucocytic infiltration.

The vascular architecture of the endometrium is of signal importance in the phenomena of menstruation and pregnancy. Arterial blood is transported to the uterus by way of the uterine and ovarian arteries. As the arterial branches penetrate the uterine wall obliquely inward and reach its middle third, these vessels ramify in a plane that is parallel to the surface and thence these vessels are named the *arcuate arteries*. Radial branches extend from the arcuate arteries at right angles toward the endometrium. The endometrial arteries are comprised of *coiled* or *spiral arteries*, which are a continuation of the radial arteries, and *basal arteries*, which branch from the radial arteries at a sharp angle, as illustrated in Figures 40–12 and 40–13. The coiled arteries supply most of the midportion and all of the superficial third of the endometrium. It has been shown by several criteria that the walls of these vessels are responsive, i.e., sensitive, to the action of hormones, especially by vasoconstriction, and thus probably serve an important role in the mechanism(s) of menstruation as described in Chapter 3 (p. 28). The straight basal endometrial arteries are smaller in both caliber and length than are the coiled vessels. These vessels extend only into the basal layer of the endometrium, or at most a short distance into the middle layer, and are not responsive to hormonal action.

Myometrium

The tissue that makes up the major portion of the uterus, the myometrium, is comprised of bundles of smooth muscle that are united by connective tissue in which there are many elastic fibers. According to Schwalm and Dubrauszky (1966), the num-

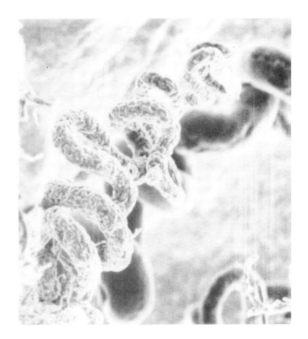

Figure 40–13. Corrosion cast of the complexly branching endometrial capillary network of the upper compact layer of a Rhesus monkey on the 25th day of the menstrual cycle × 400. (*From Ferenczy and Richart: Female Reproductive System: Dynamics of Scanning and Transmission Electron Microscopy. New York, Wiley, 1974.*)

ber of muscle fibers of the uterus progressively diminishes caudally such that in the cervix, muscle comprises only 10 percent of the tissue mass. In the inner wall of the body of the uterus, there is relatively more muscle than in the outer layers, and in the anterior and posterior walls, there is more muscle than in the lateral walls. During pregnancy, the myometrium, through hypertrophy primarily, increases greatly but there is no significant change in the muscle content of the cervix. The anatomical changes that occur in the myometrium during pregnancy are presented in detail in Chapter 7.

LIGAMENTS OF THE UTERUS

The broad, the round, and the uterosacral ligaments extend from either side of the uterus. The *broad ligaments* are comprised of two winglike structures that extend from the lateral margins of the uterus to the pelvic walls and thereby divide the pelvic cavity into anterior and posterior compartments. Each broad ligament consists of a fold of peritoneum in which there are enclosed various structures and of which there are superior, lateral, inferior, and medial margins. The inner two thirds of the superior margin form the *mesosalpinx*, to which the fallopian tubes are attached. The outer third of the superior margin of the broad ligament, which extends from the fimbriated end of the oviduct to the pelvic wall, forms the *infundibulopelvic ligament* (suspensory ligament of the ovary), through which the ovarian vessels traverse.

At the lateral margin of each broad ligament, the peritoneum is reflected onto the side of the pelvis. The base of the broad ligament, which is quite thick, is continuous with the connective tissue of the pelvic floor. The densest portion—referred to as the *cardinal ligament,* the transverse cervical ligament, or Mackenrodt ligament—is composed of connective

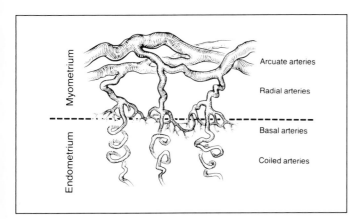

Figure 40–12. Stereographic representation of myometrial and endometrial arteries in the macaque. Above are shown parts of myometrial arcuate arteries from which myometrial radial arteries course toward the endometrium. Below are shown the larger endometrial coiled arteries and the smaller endometrial basal arteries. (*From Okkels and Engle: Acta Pathol Microbiol Scand 15:150, 1938.*)

tissue that medially is united firmly to the supravaginal portion of the cervix. In the base of the broad ligament, the uterine vessels and the lower portion of the ureter are enclosed.

A vertical section through the uterine end of the broad ligament is triangular; the uterine vessels are found within its broad base (Fig. 40–14). In its lower part, it is widely attached to the connective tissues that are adjacent to the cervix, i.e., the *parametrium*. The upper part is comprised of three folds that, in turn, nearly cover the oviduct, the utero-ovarian ligament, and the round ligament.

The *round ligaments* extend on either side from the lateral portion of the uterus; these ligaments arise somewhat below and anterior to that of the origin of the oviducts. Each round ligament is located in a fold of peritoneum that is continuous with the broad ligament and extends outward and downward to the inguinal canal, through which it passes to terminate in the upper portion of the labium majus. In nonpregnant women, the round ligament varies from 3 to 5 mm in diameter, and is comprised of smooth muscle cells that are continuous directly with those of the uterine wall and a certain amount of connective tissue. The round ligament corresponds, embryologically, to the gubernaculum testis of men. During pregnancy, the round ligaments undergo considerable hypertrophy and increase appreciably in both length and diameter.

Each *uterosacral ligament* extends from an attachment posterolaterally to the supravaginal portion of the cervix to encircle the rectum, and thence insert into the fascia over the second and third sacral vertebrae. The uterosacral ligaments are comprised of connective tissue and some smooth muscle and are covered by peritoneum. These ligaments form the lateral boundaries of the rectouterine cul-de-sac, or pouch of Douglas, and are of some importance in retaining the body of the uterus in its usual anterior position by traction that is exerted posteriorly upon the cervix.

Position

When a nonpregnant woman stands upright, the body of the uterus most often is almost horizontal and is flexed somewhat anteriorly and the fundus is resting upon the bladder, whereas the cervix is directed backward toward the tip of the sacrum with the external os approximately at the level of the ischial spines. The position of the body of the uterus is variable as a function of the degree of distension of the bladder or rectum or both.

Normally, the uterus is a partially mobile organ; whereas the cervix is anchored, the body of the uterus is free to move in the anteroposterior plane. Therefore, posture and gravity are factors that influence the position of the uterus.

Blood Vessels

The vascular supply of the uterus is derived principally from the uterine and ovarian arteries. The uterine artery, a main branch of the hypogastric artery (Fig. 40–15A through G), descends for a short distance, enters the base of the broad ligament, and

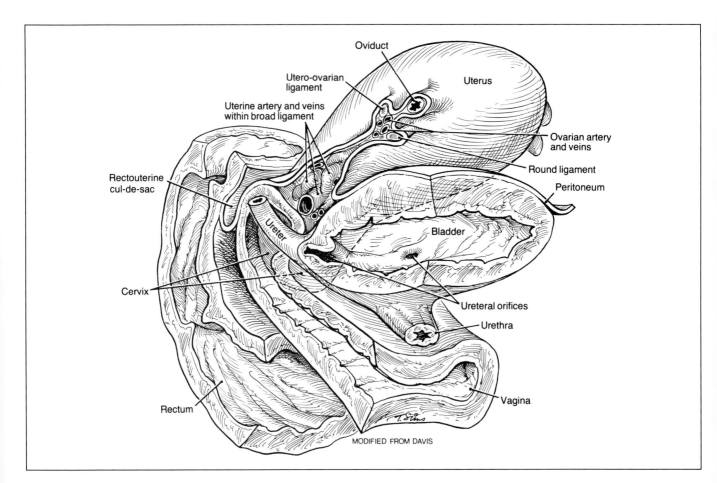

Figure 40–14. Vertical section through uterine end of right broad ligament.

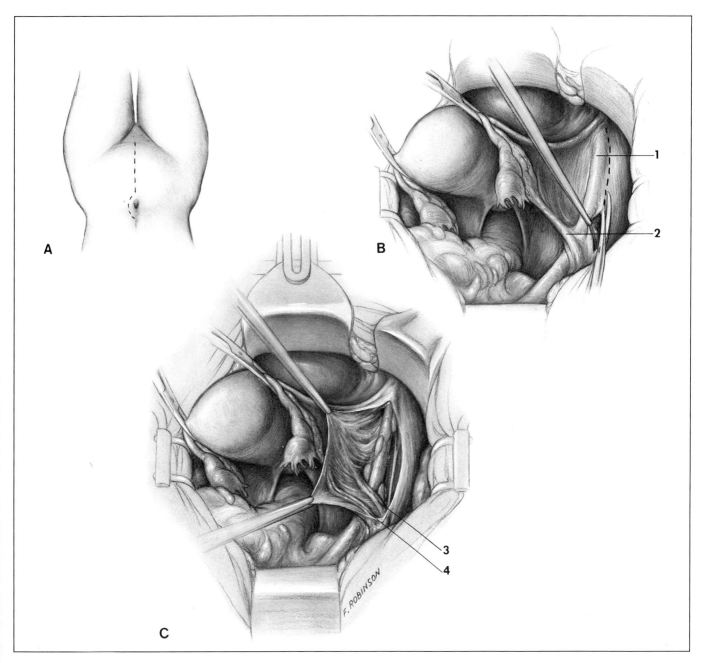

Figure 40–15 (A–C). Illustrated are the pelvic viscera as seen through a long midline incision **(A)** made in the lower abdomen. **B.** Retractors have been placed to spread the abdominal incision. The small intestine and omentum that overlie the pelvic contents have been displaced from the operative field. The oviducts, utero-ovarian ligaments, and round ligaments have been clamped bilaterally at their origin immediately adjacent to the uterus. Peritoneum just lateral to the right external iliac artery (1) is incised and the right infundibulopelvic ligament (2) is tensed by pulling the uterus to the left. **C.** The right broad ligament has been opened laterally. The right ureter (3) is now visible as it crosses the iliac vessels at the pelvic brim and courses medially and downward toward the cervix and bladder. The right ovarian artery and vein (4) are visible after dissection of the infundibulopelvic ligament. (*From Nelson JH Jr. Atlas of Radical Pelvic Surgery, 2nd ed. New York, Appleton, 1977, p. 131.*) **Note: D–G shown on page 884.**

makes its way medially to the side of the uterus. In so doing, it crosses anterior to the ureter, as described subsequently. Immediately adjacent to the supravaginal portion of the cervix, the uterine artery is divided into two main branches. The smaller cervicovaginal artery supplies blood to the lower portion of the cervix and the upper portion of the vagina. The main branch turns abruptly upward and extends thereafter as a highly con-

voluted vessel that traverses along the margin of the uterus; a branch of considerable size extends to the upper portion of the cervix and numerous other branches penetrate the body of the uterus. Just before the main branch of the uterine artery reaches the oviduct, it is divided into three terminal branches: fundal, tubal, and ovarian. The ovarian branch of the uterine artery anastomoses with the terminal branch of the ovarian artery; the

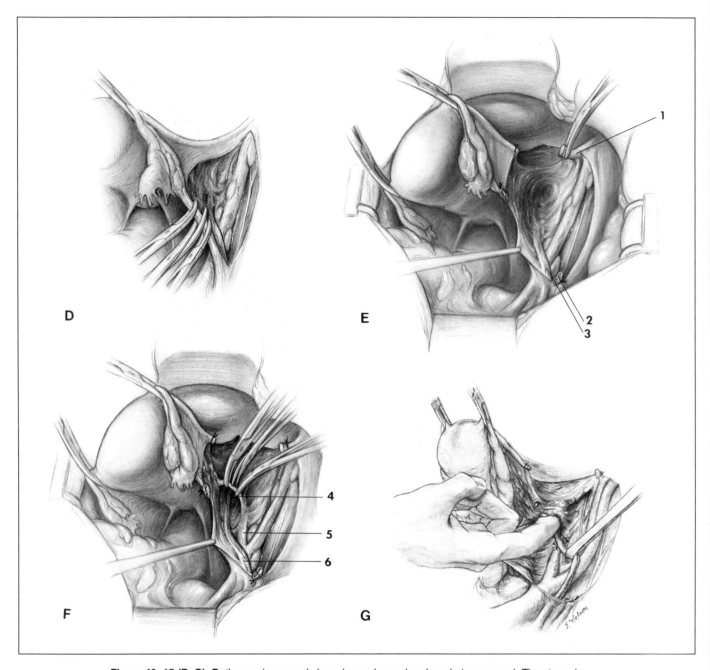

Figure 40–15 (D–G). D. the ovarian vessels have been clamped and are being severed. The uterus is retracted to the left and the external iliac artery is seen to the right. **E.** The round ligament (1) and the ovarian vessels (2) have been ligated and severed. More of the ureter is visible (3). **F.** The origin of the right uterine artery (4) from the right hypogastric artery (5) is illustrated. Note the ureter (6) coursing beneath the uterine artery (4) just lateral to the junction of the cervix and body of the uterus. **G.** The operator's finger is in the paracervical ureteral tunnel through the right cardinal ligament just lateral to supravaginal portion of the cervix. The ureter is being retracted laterally. (*From Nelson JH Jr. Atlas of Radical Pelvic Surgery, 2nd ed. New York, Appleton, 1977, p. 133.*)

tubal branch makes it way through the mesosalpinx and supplies part of the blood supply to the oviduct; the fundal branch is distributed to the uppermost portion of the uterus.

About 2 cm lateral to the cervix, the uterine artery crosses over the ureter, as shown in Figures 40–7, 40–15, and 40–16. The proximity of the uterine artery and uterine vein to the ureter at this point is of great surgical significance because, during hysterectomy, the ureter may be injured or ligated in the process of clamping and ligating the uterine vessels.

The *ovarian artery*, a direct branch of the aorta, enters the broad ligament through the infundibulopelvic ligament. At the ovarian hilum, it is divided into a number of smaller branches that enter the ovary, whereas the main stem of the ovarian artery traverses the entire length of the broad ligament very near the mesosalpinx and makes its way to the upper portion of the lateral margin of the uterus, where it anastomoses with the ovarian branch of the uterine artery. There are numerous additional communications among the arteries on both sides of the uterus.

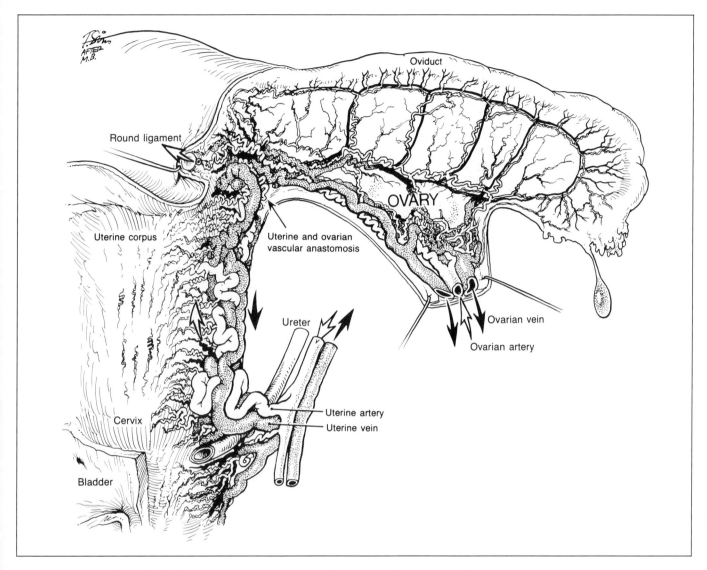

Figure 40–16. Blood supply to the left ovary, left oviduct, and the left side of the uterus. The ovarian and uterine vessels anastomose freely. Note the uterine artery and vein crossing over the ureter that lies immediately adjacent to the cervix.

When the uterus is in a contracted state, the lumina of its veins, which are in abundance, are collapsed; however, in injected specimens the greater part of the uterine wall appears to be occupied by dilated venous sinuses. On either side, the arcuate veins unite to form the *uterine vein,* which empties into the hypogastric vein and thence into the common iliac vein.

Some of the blood from the upper part of the uterus and blood from the ovary and upper part of the broad ligament is collected by several veins that, within the broad ligament, form the large *pampiniform plexus,* the vessels from which terminate in the ovarian vein. The right ovarian vein empties into the vena cava, whereas the left ovarian vein empties into the left renal vein.

Lymphatics

The endometrium is abundantly supplied with lymphatics, but true lymphatic vessels are confined largely to the basal layer. The lymphatics of the underlying myometrium are increased in number toward the serosal surface and form an abundant lymphatic plexus just beneath it, especially on the posterior wall of the uterus and, to a lesser extent, on the anterior wall.

The lymphatics from the various segments of the uterus drain into several sets of lymph nodes. Those from the cervix terminate mainly in the hypogastric nodes, which are situated near the bifurcation of the common iliac vessels between the external iliac and hypogastric arteries. The lymphatics from the body of the uterus are distributed to two groups of nodes. One set of vessels drains into the hypogastric nodes; the other set, after joining certain lymphatics from the ovarian region, terminates in the periaortic lymph nodes.

Innervation

The nerve supply is derived principally from the sympathetic nervous system, but also partly from the cerebrospinal and parasympathetic systems. The parasympathetic system is represented on either side by the pelvic nerve, which is comprised of a few fibers that are derived from the second, third, and fourth sacral nerves; it loses its identity in the cervical ganglion of Frankenhaüser. The sympathetic system enters the pelvis by way of the hypogastric plexus that arises from the aortic plexus just below the promontory of the sacrum. After descending on either side, it also enters the uterovaginal plexus of Frankenhaüser, which is comprised of ganglia of various sizes, but particularly of a large ganglionic plate that is situated on either side of the cervix and just above the posterior fornix in front of the rectum.

Branches from these plexuses supply the uterus, bladder, and upper part of the vagina and are comprised of both myelinated and nonmyelinated fibers. Some of these fibers terminate freely between the muscular fibers, whereas others accompany the arteries into the endometrium.

In the eleventh and twelfth thoracic nerve roots, there are sensory fibers from the uterus that transmit the painful stimuli of uterine contractions to the central nervous system of women. The sensory nerves from the cervix and upper part of the birth canal pass through the pelvic nerves to the second, third, and fourth sacral nerves, whereas those from the lower portion of the birth canal pass primarily through the pudendal nerve (Chapter 17).

OVIDUCTS

The oviducts, or fallopian tubes, extend from the uterine cornua to a site near the ovaries and provide access for the ova to the uterine cavity. The oviducts vary from 8 to 14 cm in length, are covered by peritoneum, and the lumen is lined by mucous membrane. Each fallopian tube is divided into an *interstitial portion, isthmus, ampulla,* and *infundibulum.* The interstitial portion is embodied within the muscular wall of the uterus. Its course is roughly obliquely upward and outward from the uterine cavity. The isthmus, or the narrow portion of the tube that adjoins the uterus, passes gradually into the wider, i.e., lateral portion, or *ampulla.* The *infundibulum,* or fimbriated extremity, is the funnel-shaped opening of the distal end of the fallopian tube (Fig. 40–17). The oviduct varies considerably in thickness; the nar-

rowest portion of the isthmus measures from 2 to 3 mm in diameter and the widest portion of the ampulla measures between 5 to 8 mm. The oviduct is surrounded completely by peritoneum except at the attachment of the mesosalpinx.

The fimbriated end of the infundibulum opens into the abdominal cavity. One projection, the *fimbria ovarica,* which is considerably longer than the other fimbriae, forms a shallow gutter that approaches or reaches the ovary.

The musculature of the fallopian tube is arranged, in general, in two layers, an inner circular and an outer longitudinal layer. In the distal portion of the oviduct, the two layers are less distinct and, near the fimbriated extremity, are replaced by an interlacing network of muscular fibers. The tubal musculature undergoes rhythmic contractions constantly, the rate of which varies with the hormonal changes of the ovarian cycle. The greatest frequency and intensity of contractions is reached during transport of ova and are slowest and weakest during pregnancy.

The fallopian tube is lined by a mucous membrane, the epithelium of which is composed of a single layer of columnar cells, some of them ciliated and others secretory. The ciliated cells are most abundant at the fimbriated extremity; elsewhere, these cells are found in discrete patches. There are differences in the proportions of these two types of cells in different phases of the ovarian cycle. Since there is no submucosa, the epithelium is in close contact with the underlying muscle. In the tubal mucosa, there are cyclic histological changes similar to, but much less striking than, those of the endometrium. The postmenstrual phase is characterized by a low epithelium that rapidly increases in height. During the follicular phase, the cells are taller, the ciliated elements are broad, with nuclei near the margin, and the nonciliated cells are narrow, with nuclei nearer the base. During the luteal phase, the secretory cells enlarge, project beyond the ciliated cells, and the nuclei are extruded. During the menstrual phase, these changes are even more marked. Changes in the fallopian tubes during late pregnancy and in the puerperium include the development of a low mucosa, plugging of the capillaries with leucocytes, and a decidual reaction.

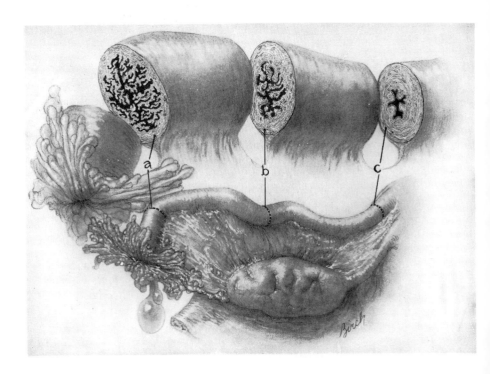

Figure 40–17. The oviduct of an adult woman with cross-sectioned illustrations of the gross structure of the epithelium in several portions: a, infundibulum; b, ampulla; c, isthmus.

The mucosa of the oviducts is arranged in longitudinal folds that are more complex toward the fimbriated end; consequently, the appearance of the lumen varies from one portion of the tube to another. On cross sections through the uterine portion, four simple folds are found that form a figure that resembles a Maltese cross. The isthmus is more complex; in the ampulla, the lumen is occupied almost completely by the arborescent mucosa, which consists of very complicated folds (Figs. 40–17 and 40–18).

The current produced by the tubal cilia is such that the direction of flow is toward the uterine cavity; indeed, minute foreign bodies that are introduced into the abdominal cavities of animals may eventually appear in the vagina after these are transported through the tubes and the cavity of the uterus. Tubal peristalsis also is believed to be an extraordinarily important factor in transport of the ovum.

The tubes are richly supplied with elastic tissue, blood vessels, and lymphatics. Sympathetic innervation of the tubes is extensive, in contrast to parasympathetic innervation. The role of these nerves in tubal function is poorly understood (Hodgson and Eddy, 1975).

Diverticula may extend occasionally from the lumen of the tube for a variable distance into the muscular wall and reach almost to the serosa. These diverticula may serve a role in the development of ectopic pregnancy (Chapter 30).

Pertinent gross anatomical, histological, and ultrastructural information about the human oviduct is well summarized by Woodruff and Pauerstein (1969).

Embryological Development of the Uterus and Oviducts

The uterus and the tubes arise from the müllerian ducts, which first appear near the upper pole of the urogenital ridge in the fifth week of development in embryos that are 10 to 11 mm long. This ridge is comprised of the mesonephros, the gonad, and associated ducts. The first indication of the development of the müllerian duct is a thickening of the coelomic epithelium at about the level of the fourth thoracic segment. This thickening becomes the fimbriated extremity (infundibulum) of the fallopian tube, which invaginates and grows caudally to form a slender tube at the lateral edge of the urogenital ridge. In the 6th week of embryonic life, the growing tips of the two müllerian ducts approach each other in the midline and reach the sinus 1 week later (embryos of 30 mm). At that time, a fusion of the two müllerian ducts is begun at the level of the inguinal crest, or gubernaculum (primordium of the round ligament), to form a single canal. Thus, the upper ends of the müllerian ducts produce the oviducts and the fused parts give rise to the uterus. The uterine lumen from the fundus to the vagina is completed during the 3rd month of fetal life. According to Koff (1933), the vaginal canal is not patent throughout its entire length until the 6th month of fetal life.

THE OVARIES

The ovaries are almond-shaped organs, the functions of which are the development and extrusion of ova and the synthesis and secretion of steroid hormones. Among women, the ovaries vary considerably in size. During the childbearing years, the ovaries are 2.5 to 5 cm in length, 1.5 to 3 cm in breadth, and 0.6 to 1.5 cm in thickness. After menopause, the size of the ovary is diminished remarkably.

Normally, the ovaries are situated in the upper part of the pelvic cavity and rest in a slight depression on the lateral wall of the pelvis between the divergent external iliac and hypogastric

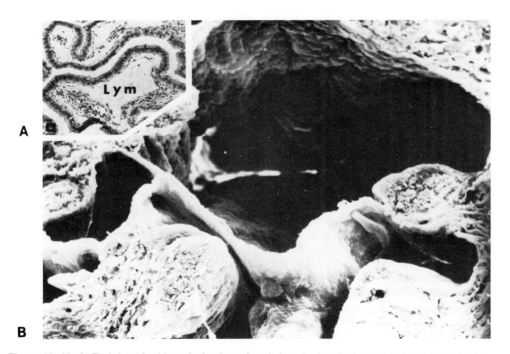

Figure 40–18. A. Fimbriae of oviduct. At the time of ovulation, the lymphatic vessels (Lym) in the lamina propria of the fimbria become greatly distended by the rapid accumulation of lymph. The dilatation of the lymphatic vasculature in the fimbriated end is believed to contribute to the fimbrial "erection" in grasping the ovary as follicles rupture at the time of ovulation (H & E stain, × 30). **B.** Fimbria of oviduct. Scanning electron micrograph of greatly dilated, labyrinthine lymphatic channels at the time of ovulation (× 200). (*From Ferenczy and Richart: Female Reproductive System: Dynamics of Scanning and Transmission Electron Microscopy. New York, Wiley, 1974.*).

vessels—the ovarian fossa of Waldeyer. When the woman stands, the long axes of the ovaries are almost vertical, but become horizontal when women are supine. The position of the ovaries, however, is subject to marked variation, and it is rare to find both ovaries at exactly the same level.

The lateral surface of the ovary is in contact with the ovarian fossa whereas the medial surface is facing the uterus. The margin of the ovary that is attached to the mesovarium is more or less straight and is designated as the hilum, whereas the free margin is convex and is directed backward and inward toward the rectum.

The ovary is attached to the broad ligament by the *mesovarium*. The *utero-ovarian ligament* extends from the lateral and posterior portion of the uterus, just beneath the tubal insertion, to the uterine, i.e., the lower pole, of the ovary. Usually, it is several centimeters long and 3 to 4 mm in diameter. It is covered by peritoneum and is made up of muscle and connective tissue fibers that are continuous with those of the uterus. The *infundibulopelvic* or *suspensory ligament of the ovary* extends from the upper, or tubal, pole to the pelvic wall (Fig. 40–15B); through it course the ovarian vessels and nerves.

The exterior surface of the ovary varies in appearance with age. In young women, the organ is smooth, with a dull white surface through which glisten several small, clear follicles. As the woman grows older, the ovaries become more corrugated; in elderly women, the exterior surfaces may be convoluted markedly.

The general structure of the ovary can be studied best in cross sections, in which two portions may be distinguished, the *cortex* and the *medulla*. The cortex, or outer layer, varies in thickness with age and becomes thinner with advancing years. It is in this layer that the ova and graafian follicles are located. The cortex of the ovary is composed of spindle-shaped connective tissue cells and fibers, among which there are scattered primordial and graafian follicles that are in various stages of development. As the woman grows older, the follicles become less numerous. The outermost portion of the cortex, which is dull and whitish, is designated as the *tunica albuginea;* on its surface, there is a single layer of cuboidal epithelium, the germinal epithelium of Waldeyer.

The medulla, or central portion, of the ovary is composed of loose connective tissue that is continuous with that of the mesovarium. There are a large number of arteries and veins in the medulla and a small number of smooth muscle fibers that are continuous with those in the suspensory ligament; the muscle fibers may be functional in movements of the ovary.

Both sympathetic and parasympathetic nerves are supplied to the ovaries. The sympathetic nerves are derived, in large part, from the ovarian plexus that accompanies the ovarian vessels; a few are derived from the plexus that surrounds the ovarian branch of the uterine artery. The ovary is richly supplied with nonmyelinated nerve fibers, which, for the most part, accompany the blood vessels. These are merely vascular nerves, whereas others form wreaths around normal and atretic follicles, and these give off many minute branches that have been traced up to, but not through, the membrana granulosa.

Development of the Ovary

The developmental changes in the human urogenital system have been described in ovaries from the third gestational week after conception to maturity. At first, the changes in the gonads are the same in both sexes. The earliest sign of a gonad is one that appears on the ventral surface of the embryonic kidney at a site between the 8th thoracic and 4th lumbar segments at about 4 weeks. As illustrated in Figure 40–19, the coelomic epithelium is thickened, and clumps of cells are seen to bud off into the underlying mesenchyme. This circumscribed area of the coelomic epithelium often is called the *germinal epithelium.* By the 4th to 6th week, however, there are many large ameboid cells in this region that have migrated into the body of the embryo from the yolk sac; these cells have been recognized in this region as early as the 3rd week. These *primordial germ cells* are distinguishable by a large size and certain morphological and cytochemical features. They react strongly in tests for alkaline phosphatase (McKay, Robinson, and Hertig, 1949), and are recognizable even after repeated divisions. Primordial germ cells have been studied in many animals. If they are destroyed before migration begins or prevented from reaching the genital area, a "gonad" that is lacking germ cells will develop.

When the primordial germ cells reach the genital area, some enter the germinal epithelium and others mingle with the groups of cells that proliferate from it or lie in the mesenchyme. By the end of the 5th week, rapid division of all these types of cells results in development of a prominent *genital ridge*. The ridge projects into the body cavity medially to a fold in which there are the mesonephric (wolffian) and the müllerian ducts (Fig. 40–20A through E). Since the growth of the gonad at the surface is more rapid, it enlarges centrifugally. By the seventh week (Figs. 40–19, 40–20), it is separated from the mesonephros except at the narrow central zone, the future hilum, where the blood vessels enter. At this time, the sexes can be distinguished since the testes can be recognized by well-defined radiating strands of cells (sex cords). These cords are separated from the germinal epithelium by mesenchyme that is to become the tunica albuginea. The sex cords, which consist of large germ cells and smaller epithelioid cells that are derived from the germinal epithelium, develop into the seminiferous tubules and tubuli rete. The rete, probably derived from mesonephric elements, establishes connection with the mesonephric tubules that develop into the epididymis (Fig. 40–20). The mesonephric ducts become the vas deferens.

In the female, the germinal epithelium continues to proliferate for a much longer time. The groups of cells thus formed lie at first in the region of the hilum. As connective tissue develops between them, these appear as sex cords. These give rise to the medullary cords and persist for variable times (Forbes, 1942). By the 3rd month, medulla and cortex are defined, as illustrated in Figure 40–20. The bulk of the organ is comprised of cortex, a mass of crowded germ and epithelioid cells that show some signs of grouping, but there are no distinct cords as in the testis. Strands of cells extend from the germinal epithelium into the cortical mass, and mitoses are numerous. The rapid succession of mitoses soon reduces the size of the germ cells to the extent that these no longer are differentiated clearly from the neighboring cells; now, these cells are called *oogonia*. Some of the oogonia in the medullary region soon are distinguishable by a series of peculiar nuclear changes. Large masses of nuclear chromatin appear, very different from the chromosomes of the oogonial divisions. This change marks the beginning of *synapsis*, which involves interactions between pairs of chromosomes that are derived originally from father and mother. Various stages of synapsis soon can be seen throughout the cortex; since similar changes occur in adjacent cells, groups (or "nests") appear. During one stage of synapsis, the chromatin is massed at one side of the nucleus, and the cytoplasm becomes highly fluid. Unless the in vitro preservation is prompt and perfect, these

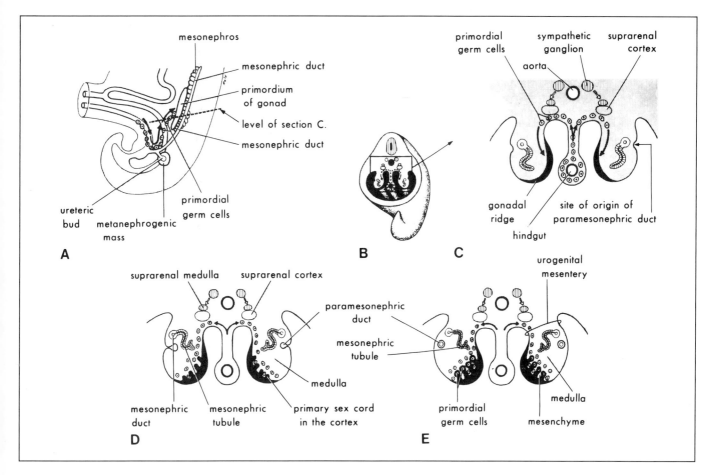

Figure 40–19 A. Sketch of 5-week embryo illustrating the migration of primordial germ cells. **B.** Three-dimensional sketch of the caudal region of a 5-week embryo showing the location and extent of the gonadal ridges on the medial aspect of the urogenital ridges. **C.** Transverse section showing the primordium of the adrenal glands, the gonadal ridges, and the migration of primordial germ cells. **D.** Transverse section through a 6-week embryo showing the primary sex cords and the developing paramesonephric ducts. **E.** Similar section at later stage showing the indifferent gonads and the mesonephric and paramesonephric ducts. (*From Moore K: The Developing Human, Philadelphia, Saunders, 1983.*).

cells appear to be degenerating. Such artifacts frequently have been misinterpreted as evidence of widespread degeneration among oogonia.

By the 4th month, some germ cells, again in the medullary region, having passed through synapsis, begin to enlarge. These are called *primary oocytes* (Fig. 40–21) at the beginning of the phase of growth that continues until maturity is reached. During this period of cell growth, many oocytes undergo degeneration, both before and after birth. The primary oocytes soon become surrounded by a single layer of flattened *follicle* cells that were derived originally from the germinal epithelium. These structures are now called *primordial follicles* and are first seen in the medulla and later in the cortex. Some follicles begin to grow even before birth and some are believed to persist in the cortex almost unchanged until menopause.

By 8 months of gestation, the ovary has become a long, narrow, lobulated structure that is attached to the body wall along the line of the hilum by the *mesovarium*, in which lies the *epoophoron*. At that stage of development, the germinal epithelium has been separated for the most part from the cortex by a band of connective tissue (tunica albuginea), which is absent in many small areas where strands of cells, usually referred to as

cords of Pflüger, are in contact with the germinal epithelium. Among these cords are cells believed by many investigators to be oogonia that have come to resemble the other epithelial cells as a result of repeated mitoses. In the underlying cortex, there are two distinct zones. Superficially, there are nests of germ cells in synapsis, interspersed with Pflüger cords and strands of connective tissue. In the deeper zone, there are many groups of germ cells in synapsis, as well as primary oocytes, prospective follicular cells, and a few primordial follicles. In addition, there are numerous, but scattered, degenerating cells, although this zone is well vascularized. Such cellular degeneration is present regularly at certain stages in various rapidly growing regions of normal embryos.

At term, the various types of ovarian cells in the human female fetus may still be found. In some cases, there are vesicular follicles in the medulla, which are all doomed to early degeneration.

Microscopic Structure of Ovary

From the first stages of its development until after the menopause, the ovary undergoes constant change. The number of oocytes at the onset of puberty has been estimated variously at

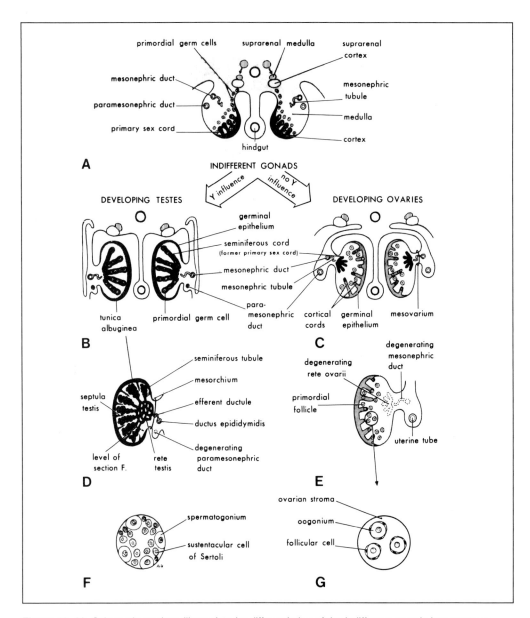

Figure 40–20. Schematic sections illustrating the differentiation of the indifferent gonads into testes or ovaries. **A.** Six weeks, showing the indifferent gonads that are comprised of an outer cortex and an inner medulla. **B.** Seven weeks, showing testes developing under the influence of a Y chromosome. Note that the primary sex cords have become seminiferous cords and that they are separated from the surface epithelium by the tunica albuginea. **C.** Twelve weeks, showing ovaries beginning to develop in the absence of Y chromosome influence. Cortical cords have extended from the surface epithelium, displacing the primary sex cords centrally into the mesovarium, where they form the rudimentary rete ovarii. **D.** Testis at 20 weeks, showing the rete testis and the seminiferous tubules derived from the seminiferous cords. An efferent ductule has developed from a mesonephric tubule, and the mesonephric duct has become the duct of the epididymis. **E.** Ovary at 20 weeks, showing the primordial follicles formed from the cortical cords. The rete ovarii derived from the primary sex cords and the mesonephric tubule and duct are regressing. **F.** Section of a seminiferous tubule from a 20-week fetus. Note that no lumen is present at this stage and that the seminiferous epithelium is comprised of two kinds of cells. **G.** Section from the ovarian cortex of a 20-week fetus showing three primordial follicles. (*From Moore K: The Developing Human, Philadelphia, Saunders, 1983.*)

200,000 to 400,000. Since only one ovum ordinarily is cast off during each ovarian cycle, it is evident that a few hundred ova suffice for purposes of reproduction. The mode by which the others disappear is discussed in the section dealing with the corpus luteum and follicular atresia.

Mossman and co-workers (1964), in an attempt to clarify the terminology of glandular elements of ovaries of adult women, distinguished interstitial, thecal, and luteal cells. The interstitial glandular elements are formed from cells of the theca interna of degenerating or atretic follicles; the thecal glandular

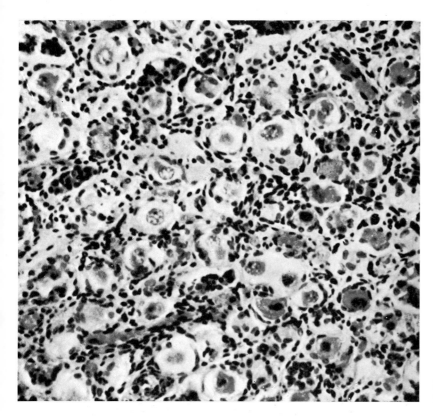

Figure 40–21. Ovary of newborn girl. Numerous primordial follicles are shown.

cells are formed from the theca interna of ripening follicles; and the true luteal cells are derived from the granulosa cells of ovulated follicles and from the undifferentiated stroma that surround them.

The huge store of primordial follicles at birth is exhausted gradually during the time of sexual maturation. Block (1952) found that there is a gradual decline from a mean of 439,000 oocytes in girls under 15 years to a mean of 34,000 in women over the age of 36. Öhler (1951) and others have refuted the concept of continued oogenesis after birth in higher mammals, which include women.

In the young girl, the greater portion of the ovary is comprised of the cortex, which is filled with large numbers of closely packed primordial follicles. Those nearest the central portion of the ovary are at the most advanced stages of development. In young women, the cortex is relatively thinner but still contains a large number of primordial follicles that are separated by bands of connective tissue cells in which there are spindle-shaped or oval nuclei. Each primordial follicle is comprised of an oocyte and its surrounding single layer of epithelial cells, which are small and flattened, spindle-shaped, and somewhat sharply differentiated from the still smaller and spindly cells of the surrounding stroma. (Fig. 40–21).

The oocyte is a large, spherical cell in which there is clear cytoplasm and a relatively large nucleus that is located near the center of the ovum. In the nucleus, there is one large and several smaller nucleoli, and numerous masses of chromatin. The diameter of the smallest oocytes in the ovaries of adult women averages 0.033 mm, and that of the nuclei, 0.020 mm.

EMBRYOLOGICAL REMNANTS

The *parovarium*, which can be found in the scant loose connective tissue within the broad ligament in the vicinity of the mesosalpinx, comprises a number of narrow vertical tubules that are lined by ciliated epithelium. These tubules connect at the upper ends with a longitudinal duct that extends just below the oviduct to the lateral margin of the uterus, where ordinarily it ends blindly near the internal os, but, infrequently, it may extend laterally down the vagina to the level of the hymen. This canal, the remnant of the wolffian (mesonephric) duct in women, is called *Gartner's duct*. The parovarium, also a remnant of the wolffian duct, is homologous, embryologically, with the caput epididymis in men. The cranial portion of the paraovarium is the *epoophoron*, or organ of Rosenmüller; the caudal portion, or *paroophoron*, is a group of vestigial mesonephric tubules that lie in or around the broad ligament. It is homologous, embryologically, with the paradidymis of men. Usually, the paroophoron in adult women disappear; but, on occasion, macroscopic cysts are formed from these remnants.

REFERENCES

Block E: Quantitative morphological investigation of the follicular system in women. Acta Anat 14:108, 1952

Buckingham JC, Buethe RA Jr, Danforth DN: Collagen-muscle ratio in clinically normal and clinically incompetent cervices. Am J Obstet Gynecol 91:232, 1965

Danforth DN, Buckingham JC, Roddick JW Jr: Connective tissue changes incident to cervical effacement. Am J Obstet Gynecol 80:939, 1960

Forbes TR: On the fate of the medullary cords of the human ovary. Contrib Embryol 30:9, 1942

Hitschmann F, Adler L: The structure of the endometrium of the sexually mature woman. Mschr Geburtsh Gynaek 27:1, 1908

Hodgson BJ, Eddy CA: The autonomic nervous system and its relationship to tubal ovum transport—A reappraisal. Gynecol Invest 6:161, 1975

Koff AK: Development of the vagina in the human fetus. Contrib Embryol 24:59, 1933

Krantz KE: Innervation of the human vulva and vagina. Obstet Gynecol 13:382, 1958

Langlois PL: The size of the normal uterus. J. Reprod Med 4:220, 1970

Larsen B, Galask RP: Vaginal microbial flora: Practical and theoretic relevance. Obstet Gynecol 55:100S, 1980

Mahran M, Saleh AM: The microscopic anatomy of the hymen. Anat Rec 149:313, 1964

McKay DG, Robinson D, Hertig AT: Histochemical observations on granulosa cell tumors, thecomas and fibromas of the ovary. Am J Obstet Gynecol 58:625, 1949

Mossman HW, Koering MJ, Ferry D Jr: Cyclic changes in interstitial gland tissue of the human ovary. Am J Anat 115:235, 1964

Öhler I: Contribution to the knowledge of the ovarian epithelium and its relationship to oogenesis. Acta Anat 12:1, 1951

Schwalm H, Dubrauszky V: The structure of the musculature of the human uterus-muscles and connective tissue. Am J Obstet Gynecol 94:391, 1966

Woodruff JD, Pauerstein CJ: The Fallopian Tube. Baltimore, Williams & Wilkins, 1969

Reproductive Success and Failure: Ovulation and Fertilization

OVERVIEW

The female of most species is the limiting resource with respect to reproduction. This clearly is the case in the human. But as Short (1976) observes, the human is the only mammal in which the female has forsaken the periodic behavioral phenomenon of estrus, when she is instinctively attractive and receptive to the male. In the human, this has been exchanged for a situation in which she is attractive and potentially receptive at any time from adolescence to old age. Humans are the only primate in which puberty is delayed until the second decade of life; and humans are the only primate in which full breast development occurs at puberty. In others, breast development occurs with first pregnancy (Milligan and associates, 1975). And, there is good evidence that breasts are regarded as erotic in primitive as well as modern societies (Ford and Beach, 1952). Because women at all times of the ovarian cycle are attractive to men and because women are potentially receptive at all times of the ovarian cycle, humans seem to be adapted for low levels of continuous sexual activity (Short, 1984).

This is an important consideration in devising predictions of successes and failures of human reproduction. Indeed as we will discuss, this situation seems to constitute a perplexing and unique problem for human reproduction. In other animals, the existence of an estrus state guarantees that spermatozoa are ready in the fallopian tube at the time of ovulation. But in the human, spermatozoa may arrive late—and the life span of the fertilizable ovum may exceed the time within which fertilization will lead to a normal, healthy fetus (Adams, 1972). It seems that the human may have accepted the advantages of family bonding that can result from continuous sexual activity in exchange for the risks that may obtain from late or absent fertilization of the ovum.

HUMAN REPRODUCTIVE SUCCESS IN THE EXTREME

From one vantage point, the success of reproduction in humans is the source of one of the greatest concerns of man, viz., a population explosion leading to overpopulation of the world. In an expression of worldwide interest in the rapid rate of population increase and in apprehension about the consequences of continued rapid growth, The United Nations designated 1974 as World Population Year. This fear, i.e., overpopulation of the world, is believed by many, and with considerable justification, potentially to be the greatest hazard to the health of man.

Until about 10,000 years ago, at least 35,000 years were required for the population of the earth to double. In the late 1970s, the doubling time of the world population was estimated to be 35 years. At this rate, 10 doublings (350 years) would produce a population of more than 4 trillion! (Coale, 1974). The population doubling time in some countries today is projected to be less than 20 years, perhaps as low as 15 years. The population of the world has just passed the 5 billion mark!

In the United States, one of the momentous social problems of the day is that of the high and continuing increase in the number of unwanted pregnancies among teenage girls.

The sexually-transmitted acquired immune deficiency syndrome (AIDS), caused by human immunodeficiency virus (HIV), threatens the world with a horrific, deadly epidemic. At the time of this writing, 1 in 60 babies born in New York City are HIV-antibody positive! (Centers for Disease Control, 1988).

Therefore, one view of the current status of human reproduction is that of a worldwide sexual orgy that is unencumbered by the use of contraceptive methods or protection against sexually-transmitted disease, a dilemma that will be reconciled by way of competition between overpopulation-induced starvation and AIDS-induced sure death.

HUMAN REPRODUCTIVE FAILURES

From another vantage point, the problem of human reproduction that haunts many obstetricians-gynecologists is the vision of a 25 percent incidence of absolute or relative infertility among married couples and a living newborn pregnancy success rate for in vitro fertilization and embryo transfer that seems currently to be paralyzed at just under 20 percent. At the same time, and in concert with this dilemma, pregnancy failure caused by embryonic or fetal wastage occurs at every possible step of human reproduction, commencing with failure of oocyte fertilization, and proceeding through failure of zygote cleavage and blastocyst implantation; and high fetal losses from spontaneous abortion, malformations, and preterm birth are a major concern.

From this perspective, it would be easy to reach the judgment that difficulty will be encountered in maintaining the human race, either quantitatively or qualitatively.

HUMAN REPRODUCTION IN PERSPECTIVE

For physicians, researchers, demographers, anthropologists, indeed all those interested in reproductive biology, it is important to be able to envision a theoretical norm, i.e., human reproduction uncluttered by social, religious, or pharmacological intervention. To gain such a vision, it would be essential to comprehend the natural history of human reproduction. But, such an understanding and such a vision is difficult to attain because of man's cunning. According to Short (1976), ordinarily, the reproductive variables that would lead to some sort of reproductive equilibrium would include (1) age of puberty, (2) extent of embryonic and fetal death, (3) neonatal (perinatal) mortality, and, (4) the duration of lactational amenorrhea (anovulation infertility). But man has been able to modify these constraints, albeit at times unwittingly.

Therefore, the natural history of reproduction in our species, the human, has been obscured by social overlay (Short, 1976). Nonetheless, it is worth remembering, as pointed out by Short, *"that genetically speaking we are still primitive hunter-gatherers; it is only 80 generations since the birth of Christ, and at most a few hundred since the dawn of civilization, hardly time for any meaningful genetic change to have occurred."*

Reproduction in Other Primates
One perspective of "natural human reproduction" may be gained from an examination of reproduction in closely related primates living in the wild. Among female chimpanzees in the jungle, the birth interval is almost 6 years; but, this interval is shortened by infant death, suggesting that the long interval between successive births normally is caused by lactation-induced infertility (anovulation). Chimpanzees in the wild suckle their young several times per hour, secrete a milk similar to humans, and sleep with the infant at their breast during the night (Short, 1984). Therefore, one factor in the social evolution of man's reproductive successes or failures may have been related to the duration of breast feeding of the newborn.

Reproduction in Primitive Societies
To remove some of the social overlay that obscures our view of uncluttered reproduction in the human, anthropologists from around the world also have studied a particular primitive tribe in South Africa. The !Kung hunter-gatherers of the Kalahari Desert of South Africa may be a people who provide useful clues as to the impact of demographic changes that have affected man's reproductive life. [The exclamation point in "!Kung" denotes an alveolar-palatal click. The tip of the tongue is pressed against the roof of the mouth and than drawn away sharply, producing a hollow popping sound (Kolata, 1974)]. The !Kung have lived as hunter-gatherers for at least 11,000 years; but recently, they have begun to live in agrarian villages near those of the Bantus.

Among nomadic !Kung women, who are hunters as well, the age of menarche is relatively late, 15½ years. This lateness of menarche has been attributed to the leaner body mass of the nomadic young !Kung women compared to the more sedentary women who now live in farming-like villages. The !Kung women marry in early puberty; but the nomadic women do not conceive until 19½ years of age on average, presumably because of post-menarchal anovulation. The !Kung do not practice any form of contraception, and the time interval between births is about 4.1 years. Because of the nomadic, hunter-gatherer life style of these !Kung women, there is very little soft food available to feed their infants. Probably for this reason, the !Kung women breast-feed their newborns for 4 to 5 years. And, they choose to breast-feed frequently, as many as four times per hour during the daytime, even if only for a minute or so at a time. Additionally, the !Kung women

sleep with their infants and small children who suckle the breasts during the night. This may account for the long birth interval. There seems to be a better relationship between the number of times per day that the infant suckles and anovulation and amenorrhea than between the duration of suckling or the amount of milk produced and the duration of lactation-induced infertility. During lactation-induced amenorrhea and anovulation, fertility is low, as reviewed by Kolata (1974) and Short (1976, 1984).

Among nomadic !Kung women, the average completed family size is 4.7 children; and, the population doubling time of the nomadic !Kung people is estimated to be 300 years.

In !Kung women who have adopted the agrarian lifestyle, menarche occurs earlier; first pregnancy occurs earlier; and the interval between births is diminished. Population explosion among the !Kung!

Possibly menarche in more sedentary women occurs earlier because of increased body fat. The time of menarche is related most closely to body weight (Chap. 3, p. 33). Lactation-induced amenorrhea intervals are shortened by the availability of soft food and alternate (animal) sources of milk for the babies, reducing the duration of breast feeding.

In the !Kung, therefore, "we may be witnessing in microcosm the transformation that occurred in human fertility as we changed from a nomadic to an agrarian way of life" (Short, 1976).

The North American Hutterites
The ethnic Hutterites of North America are an example of an agrarian group of people with an exceptionally high rate of fertility. This group is an anabaptist religious sect who live in hamlets, which they refer to as colonies. By anabaptist is meant that they reject the notion of baptism of infants. Baptism is conducted as a ritual of adulthood and is a prerequisite for marriage. The mean age of marriage for Hutterite women in 1950 was 22.0 years of age (Eaton and Mayer, 1953).

Reproduction among the Hutterites is encouraged; but premarital sex is forbidden, and very rarely practiced. In Hutterite women, age 25 to 29, the age-specific nuptial fertility rate is 498. In particular, around 1950, there were 498 births per year for each 1,000 married women between the ages of 25 and 29. Stated differently, there was one birth per woman every two years. The average completed family size of these women is 10.6 children.

The average maximum fecundity of the Hutterite population has been estimated based on the data presented and assuming an earlier marriage, e.g., 15 years of age. The average maximum fecundity computed was 12 to 14 children, or only about 1 to 3 children fewer than the actual number in the completed family. The largest number of children (live births) reported for Hutterite women is 16. This number is considerably less than the 32 infants (all but four of them liveborn) born to the wife of a Viennese linen-weaver (Pearl, 1929, cited by Eaton and Mayer, 1953). The incidence of sterility in Hutterites is very low, viz., 3.4 percent; but nonetheless, 33 percent of Hutterite women had three children or fewer.

Compared to the nomadic !Kung women, Hutterite women experience earlier puberty and ovulation, breast-feed their children on a rigid schedule, and supplement breast feeding with soft foods early in the infant's life. Based on the reproductive history of the Hutterite women, the population doubling time of this group was estimated to be 16 years, as reviewed by Eaton and Mayer (1953) and Short (1976, 1984).

MODERN WOMAN

As observed in Chapter 2, the physiological investments obliged in women (in the absence of pharmacological intervention) to achieve pregnancy are phenomenal. The depth of this investment is so great that Short comes to the view that "women are physiologically ill-adapted to spend the greater part of their reproductive lives in the nonpregnant state."

There appear to be two major factors that have impacted upon the natural course of human reproduction: nutrition and contraception. Nutritional advances have led to (1) earlier menarche (and ovulation), (2) artificial feeding of the newborn, resulting in decreased duration of lactation and associated amenorrhea and anovulation after childbirth, and (3) longer infant survival.

It seems reasonable to conclude that the sedentary, agrarian way of life of the past few centuries has contributed to a change in body composition and mass that favors earlier menarche and ovulation. Menarche in women in the United States today occurs at about 12½ years of age (Chap. 3, Fig. 3–6); and whereas anovulation is more common immediately after menarche than later in reproductive life, most young post-menarchal girls today are ovulatory and therefore potentially fertile. And today, of the women who choose to breast-feed their newborns, few will continue to do so for more than a few weeks or at most a few months. Most women who do breast-feed their infants choose to suckle the baby no more than eight times per 24 hours compared with 48 times per 12 hours of daylight for !Kung women (Short, 1984).

Modern Woman's Sexual Partner

From the vantage point of optimal reproductive success, men are relatively inefficient contributors to successful pregnancy. In the ejaculates of men, there are large numbers of abnormal spermatozoa, which is not true of other mammals. If ejaculation occurs more often than once every 48 to 72 hours in man, semen volume and sperm numbers decline. Therefore, in men, there are relatively small reserves of spermatozoa compared with some other primates, e.g., the male chimpanzee. The male chimpanzee has very large testes with an enormous sperm reserve and is able to copulate repeatedly with several female chimpanzees who come into estrus at the same time. The ejaculate of the chimpanzee contains 603 million sperm. And the testes produce 2,737 million sperm per day, sufficient for at least four ejaculates. In man, the ejaculate contains 253 million sperm but only 176 million are produced by the testes each day, fewer than the number in one ejaculate (Short, 1980). Indeed, it is reasoned that the large sperm reservoirs of the chimpanzee serve to permit genetic competition among the males. The male that deposits the greatest number of sperm in the vaginas of the estrus females is likely to be the one whose genetic material is transmitted by way of the winning sperm (Harcourt and colleagues, 1981).

PREDICTIONS OF SUCCESS AND FAILURE IN HUMAN REPRODUCTION

It is useful to predict the likelihood of success in human reproduction for many reasons. First, such predictions are necessary to understand the factors that contribute to the success of human reproduction. This is true if we are to devise optimal strategies for the prevention of pregnancy when the woman makes this choice. Second, it is imperative that we understand the natural limits of success of human reproduction to devise strategies for improving the likelihood of a liveborn infant in women desirous of pregnancy. Third, it is essential that we comprehend the likelihood of reproductive failure at each juncture of the reproductive process if we are to understand the cause of pregnancy failure in those who are infertile or else suffer pregnancy losses.

For this purpose, we have developed estimates of **the likelihood of pregnancy success and failure under optimal conditions.** In particular, we now present an analysis of the probable outcome of a given menstrual cycle in 1,000 young (20 to 29 years), healthy, fertile women in whom we assume there are normal viable spermatozoa in the fallopian tube at the time of ovulation (Fig. 41–1).

Whereas it may be that in young, healthy, fertile women, a fertilizable ovum enters the oviduct in the vast majority of ovarian cycles, the likelihood of viable spermatozoa being present at the time that the ovum enters the fallopian tube is decidedly less. To be able to estimate reproductive success and failure, it is important to recognize this limitation in human reproduction. In the long term, i.e., during the course of several or even many ovarian cycles, this limitation is diminished provided that sexual intercourse with a fertile male occurs at reasonable intervals. Nonetheless, late fertilization of the ovum, i.e., conception occurring in an ovum several hours after ovulation may portend an unfavorable outcome of the resulting zygote (Adams, 1972). And for the purpose of developing models to describe the natural course of human reproduction, which we are about to do, this is a consideration of substantial weight. Namely, **what are the probabilities of conception (fertilization of the ovum), implantation of the blastocyst, and birth of a normal living infant during each menstrual cycle in fertile women in whom the presence of living spermatozoa in the fallopian tube at ovulation is not limiting?**

Life Span of Spermatozoa and Ova

The life span of the liberated germ cells, both spermatozoa and ova, is short. Precise data still are not available for the longevity of spermatozoa in the female reproductive tract or the fertilizable life span of the ova. But, it is probable that few spermatozoa are capable of fertilization after more than 24 hours and it is likely that the optimum time for fertilization of the ovum is substantially shorter, perhaps no more than 1 to 2 hours, possibly less. But perhaps more importantly, as the liberated germ cells age, the likelihood of formation of an abnormal zygote increases. If these estimates are reasonable, it follows that viable spermatozoa must be present in the fallopian tube at the time of ovulation for optimal fertilization.

The timing of intercourse, therefore, becomes more crucial in establishing the likelihood of successful conception with any given ovulation. This is especially important recognizing that the semen volume and sperm density, even in normal men, declines when ejaculation occurs more often than every 48 hours.

Theoretical Basis for Predictions

For purposes of estimating *female fertility efficiency*, we assumed that fertilization in vivo takes place in the fallopian tube and we have assumed further that viable spermatozoa are in the fallopian tube at the time of ovulation. In particular, spermatozoa are not and must not be rate limiting in defining female fertility efficiency.

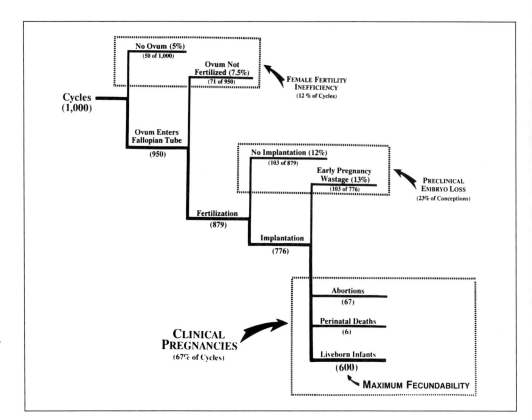

Figure 41–1. Predictions of reproductive success and failure: Estimates were made on the basis of two assumptions. First, the population of women is young, healthy, and fertile. Second, spermatozoa capable of ovum fertilization are present in the fallopian tube at the time of ovulation.

Based on these assumptions, can we estimate the reasonable likelihood of conception, pregnancy, early embryonic loss, and the number of liveborn infants as a function of the number of menstrual cycles in young, healthy, fertile women? We believe that reasonable estimates can be made. Such estimates are useful in (1) predicting pregnancy success, (2) defining the contribution of both male and female infertility to pregnancy failures, (3) determining at what stage of reproduction the greatest risk of failure exists, (4) ascertaining the theoretical limits of success for therapy of fertility, and (5) devising strategies for contraception.

To this end, a flow chart was developed to describe the estimates of important variables that affect human reproduction; and this chart is presented in diagrammatic form in Figure 41–1. By use of this approach, we have made estimates of human reproductive success and failure at each step of the process from ovulation to liveborn infant. The estimates were developed to describe the probability of the outcome of a given menstrual cycle in 1,000 young, healthy, fertile women.

To develop estimates for each step in the reproductive process, it was necessary to make use of the best sets of data available for some processes and thence to derive estimates of other processes by difference.

For example, we begin arbitrarily with 1,000 cycles by definition. We end with the prediction that theoretical maximum fecundability according to the assumptions made (young, fertile women, and spermatozoa not limiting) is 60 percent. Namely, in this theoretical circumstance, 60 percent of cycles would result in a living newborn infant. There is persuasive evidence in support of the validity of this assumption, which is presented in a later section. Nonetheless, this figure will come as a surprise to many, as it did to us.

Reproductive biologists are, and for the past few decades have been, extraordinarily concerned with high pregnancy losses that seem to occur at every stage of human reproduction, and for good reason. Perinatal mortality rates of 40 per 1,000 or more are not uncommon; yet among healthy, young women with appropriate prenatal care and optimum postnatal management of the newborn, many medical centers now experience perinatal mortality rates of less than 10 per 1,000. Spontaneous abortion rates upwards of 25 percent are reported frequently; but in healthy, fertile women, abortion of clinically recognized pregnancies in the first trimester of pregnancy is probably no more than 10 percent.

Some investigators have reported extraordinarily high preclinical embryonic losses, i.e., early pregnancy wastage, which occurs after implantation but before or at the time of the next expected menses (Chap. 29). But in some of these reports, definitive data were few or else estimates were made with essentially no data. In addition, many reports of high fetal wastage are based on studies of women who were acknowledged to be infertile; such data may not be relevant directly to estimates of reproductive success in normal, healthy, fertile women. We know that pregnancy failures are influenced by a number of factors, geographic, racial, ethnic, and environmental. For example, the incidence of hydatidiform mole in some areas of Southeast Asia is 1 per 100 pregnancies; in the United States, it is 1 per 2,500. The incidence of anencephaly in Ireland is 5 to 10 times greater than in other parts of the world.

To develop indices for deciphering the cause of fertility failure or loss of conceptuses, it first is helpful to attempt to estimate the ideal or the norm. The model presented is designed to address this goal.

FEMALE FERTILITY INEFFICIENCY

Given that spermatozoa are not limiting for conception, *female fertility inefficiency is* attributable to (1) failure of ovulation, (2) failure of entrance of ova into the fallopian tube, or (3) nonfertilizability of the ovum.

Ovum Availability

Provided that spermatozoa are not limiting, the first delimiting step in human conception is entry of an ovum into the oviduct. Anovulation among young, fertile women is relatively uncommon, but not absent. Most investigators agree that, on occasion, all women experience an anovulatory cycle. This has been estimated to occur as often as once a year or about once in 13 cycles. In our own experience, this estimate seems a bit too high. In a study designed to evaluate early pregnancy wastage, Edmonds and colleagues (1982) found, for example, that only 9 of 207 cycles (4.3 percent) seemed to be anovulatory.

In some cases, failure of ovulation may be associated with a luteinized follicle or "trapped ovum". Indeed, this may be one cause of the so-called short luteal phase.

There are very few data available to estimate the frequency of failure of the released ovum to enter the fallopian tube. Based on the findings of some studies involving the likelihood of transuterine migration of fertilized ova; however, this situation must exist. But in normal women, it probably is uncommon.

For these reasons, we estimate that in about 95 percent of menstrual cycles of young, fertile women, an ovum will actually enter the fallopian tube; or conversely, in only 5 percent of cycles of young, healthy, fertile women, there is no ovum to fertilize (Fig. 41–1).

Fertilizable Ova

Therefore, in 1,000 menstrual cycles in healthy, fertile, young women, 950 ova should be available for fertilization. The second delimiting step in female fertility efficiency is the fertilizability of the ovum. There must be some number, albeit probably small, of ova that cannot be fertilized even by a normal spermatozoa. To make this estimate, we assume that fertilization in vivo is at least as likely as that which can be attained in vitro. From the findings of in vitro fertilization, we surmise that, in vivo, the number of nonfertilizable ova is small, perhaps about 7 to 8 percent of those that enter the fallopian tube.

Based on these estimates, we deduce that of 1,000 menstrual cycles in young, fertile women, the maximum number of ova fertilized would be 879, or a female fertility efficiency of 88 percent. Stated conversely, minimal female fertility inefficiency is about 12 percent (Fig. 41–1). These estimates are similar to those made by Hertig and associates (1959) based on a study of the presence of a conceptus in the uteruses removed from women during the luteal phase of the ovarian cycle.

FECUNDABILITY

Natural Fecundability

To continue this analysis, it is convenient (and more data are available) to analyze next the likelihood of pregnancy success (living newborn) per menstrual cycle (fecundability). One approach to make such an estimate is to evaluate the number of living newborns that can be expected per menstrual cycle of young, healthy women desirous of pregnancy. This has been done in a number of studies, as reviewed by Short (1976). The results are expressed as the fecundability rate. We choose to refer to this value as the *natural fecundability rate,* because in these women, during some cycles, fertilization must have been precluded because of the absence of viable spermatozoa in the fallopian tube at the time of ovulation. In addition, absolute or relative infertility of the population under study may limit maximal natural fecundability. Nonetheless, the data available are very useful. In these studies, embryonic or fetal losses occurring at any time from conception are not considered, only living births are included in estimates of fecundability.

In rural French villages during the eighteenth century, the mean fecundability of women aged 20 to 29 was 23 percent. Several other studies have been conducted to ascertain how long it takes for a newlywed woman to conceive a pregnancy that results in a living newborn. In a study of 15,000 women who were contestants in a large-family competition in France after the First World War, the peak in fecundability (27 percent) was observed in women at age 25. Similar values were obtained in studies of North American Hutterites believed to be reproducing at close to the maximum natural rate. The mean postnuptial fecundability in these women was 28 percent.

In other studies, Tietze and Potter (1962) calculated the probability of pregnancy in a given menstrual cycle at different frequencies of intercourse. Their estimates ranged from a minimum probability of 28 percent at a coital frequency of six times per cycle to a maximum of 45 percent at a coital frequency of 12 times per cycle. Similar estimates were made by Lachenbruch (1967).

If we assume that absolute infertility affects 10 percent of married couples, and that relative infertility affects another 15 percent, it is obvious that even the estimates of 45 percent maximum natural fecundability are underestimates of the theoretical maximal fecundability in fertile women in whom spermatozoa are not limiting. Taking the 28 percent natural fecundability rate that is found most commonly in young, healthy women and correcting for absolute infertility (10 percent), the natural fecundability rate among fertile women is 31 percent. But, this value is not corrected for (1) relative infertility or (2) absence of spermatozoa in the fallopian tube at the time of ovulation. Correcting for relative infertility (assuming 15 percent), natural fecundability in fertile women becomes 37 percent. Even in Hutterite women with a 28 percent fecundability and an average of 10.6 children, 33 percent have three or fewer offspring. Eliminating this group of relatively infertile Hutterile women may give rise to greater than 40 percent natural fecundability in this group.

Hertig and colleagues (1959) estimated fecundability as 43 percent in a group of presumably fertile women who were somewhat older, on average (33 years), than those women believed to be maximally fertile. And even in women of the studies of Hertig and co-workers, intercourse may have occurred only on the day after ovulation, a time unlikely to result in optimal conception. Thus, the presence of spermatozoa in the fallopian tube at the time of ovulation is crucial in computing fecundability.

This same limitation exists for estimates of the corrected natural fecundability rate of 37 percent. These estimates were made from the findings of studies in which we cannot know how many ovulations occurred when viable spermatozoa were not present in the fallopian tube. It is likely that intercourse with a fertile male must occur within the 24 to 36 hours preceding ovulation for optimal fertilization and zygote outcome to occur in that particular cycle. Even in couples for whom intercourse is frequent, spermatozoa will not always be present at the critical time. Surely ovulation must have no preference for day of the week; and frequent intercourse for several days prior to the 36 hours preceding ovulation will no doubt limit sperm supplies. A conservative estimate, we believe, is that spermatozoa are present in the fallopian tubes at the time of three of five ovulations in the general population of young, fertile women desirous of pregnancy.

If this were correct, theoretical maximal fecundability in young, fertile women is 60 percent. Stated differently, of 1,000 menstrual cycles in young, healthy, fertile women, 600 liveborn infants should result if viable spermatozoa were present in the fallopian tube at the time of entry of the ovum into the oviduct.

This estimate also is consistent with the probability that sperm regeneration time (42 to 48 hours) is about twice as long as is the fertilizable life span of the spermatozoa in the female reproductive tract (24 hours). It is probable that sperm motility persists longer than does the fertilizing capacity of the spermatozoa. Therefore, we deduce that natural fecundability in a population of young women desirous of pregnancy (28 to 30 percent) is about one-half the theoretical maximum fecundability in young, healthy, fertile women if spermatozoa were not limiting.

SOURCE OF PREGNANCY LOSSES

Defining pregnancy as commencing at the time of implantation, we recognize that pregnancy wastage can take place at any time after implantation of the blastocyst. First, we know that fetal loss may occur after the time of expected viability for reasons of preterm labor, fetal anomalies, and intrauterine or neonatal death. Second, spontaneous abortion may occur, usually within the first trimester of pregnancy. Third, the products of conception may be sloughed before or at about the time of the next anticipated menstruation. In such cases, the pregnancy is not clinically recognized.

PERINATAL MORTALITY (LATE PREGNANCY WASTAGE)

For purposes of this model of menstrual cycle outcome in young, healthy women, we have assumed a perinatal mortality rate of 10 per 1,000 births, or 1 percent.

EARLY CLINICAL PREGNANCY WASTAGE (SPONTANEOUS FIRST TRIMESTER ABORTION)

We have accepted a relatively low incidence of spontaneous clinical (i.e., after the time of the first missed menses) abortion rate, viz., 10 percent. It is likely that the rate of spontaneous clinical abortion in young, healthy, fertile women is low compared with the rate of abortion in the general population of women (Chap. 29).

EARLY LOSS OF CONCEPTUS

Preimplantation
It is clear that some number, albeit not precisely defined, of human conceptuses are lost early after fertilization of the ovum. Some fertilized ova may never undergo cleavage; and yet other blastocysts may never implant. This naturally gives rise to fundamental inquiries as to the development and maturation of the ova as well as the genetics and environment of the zygote.

With the advent of new techniques for addressing successfully therapeutic remedies for infertility, it is imperative that we gain some insights into the long-range rate-limiting steps in the successful attainment of pregnancy by a given woman. It is becoming quite clear that *one of the limiting steps in the success of fertility*, including the use of in vitro fertilization, gamete intra-

fallopian transfer (GIFT), ovulation induction, and microsurgical correction of the obstructed fallopian tube, *is the quality of the fertilized ovum.*

Early Postimplantation (Preclinical) Embryonic Loss
Other blastocysts, after implantation, may be lost before or at the time of the next anticipated menstruation. Early fetal wastage also has been referred to as occult pregnancy. Namely, the implanted embryonic tissues are lost at or before the time of the next expected menses and therefore not interpreted by the woman (or by the physician) as a pregnancy episode.

Recognizing that chorionic gonadotropin (hCG) begins to enter the maternal circulation on the day of implantation, several studies have been conducted to evaluate early pregnancy wastage by monitoring the levels of hCG in blood or urine of women during the luteal phase of the ovarian cycle. The detection of hCG has been cited as evidence of "chemical" pregnancy. Other investigators have conducted similar investigations by use of pregnancy-specific proteins other than hCG, e.g., early pregnancy factor (EPF). EPF also may serve to identify the presence of a fertilized ovum before implantation.

In a prospective study of 226 ovulatory cycles in 91 healthy, young women, Whittaker and associates (1983) detected chemical evidence (β-hCG in serum) of pregnancy in 92 cycles. Of these, 74 (80 percent) ended in the delivery of normal, living babies. In the model presented in Figure 41–1, 77 percent would have been predicted. Eleven (11.9 percent) terminated in spontaneous clinical abortion. In the model presented (Fig. 41–1), 8.6 percent would have been predicted.

In seven cycles (8 percent), chemical evidence of pregnancy was obtained, but these ended with apparently normal menstruation. In the model presented, 14 percent preclinical pregnancy losses would have been predicted. The criticism of the study of Whittaker and colleagues has been that β-hCG levels were determined only at weekly intervals and thus some early postimplantation embryo losses may have been missed.

In other studies, appreciably higher percentages of preclinical pregnancy wastage were observed (Chap. 29). For example, Miller and associates (1980) in a study of β-hCG levels in urine during the luteal phase of the cycle, estimated a preclinical, postimplantation pregnancy loss of 33 percent (50 of 152 conceptions). They concluded that a small portion of their population sample was relatively infertile.

In the classic morphological study of Hertig and colleagues (1959), they concluded that 10 of 34 embryos (29 percent) found in the fallopian tube or uterus would have aborted at some time, before or after the next menses. In the model presented in Figure 41–1, the postconception pregnancy loss predicted is 31 percent.

Chartier and co-workers (1979) found a 21 percent postimplantation, preclinical pregnancy loss in infertile women, at least one-third of whom were treated to induce ovulation and at least 10 percent of whom were pregnant with multiple fetuses.

In a prospective, pilot study of recruited volunteers, Sweeney and associates (1988) found that early pregnancy loss (1 to 91 days after implantation) was 18 percent. The model (Fig. 41–1) predicts 22 percent. Wilcox and associates (1988), in a study of 221 healthy women attempting to conceive, found a 22 percent postimplantation preclinical pregnancy wastage and a total (including spontaneous abortion) of 31 percent.

In other studies, appreciably higher early fetal losses were estimated. For example, Edmonds and co-workers (1982) presented evidence for total postimplantation loss of 62 percent based on the finding of β-hCG in urine samples of 82 test subjects attempting to conceive.

PREDICTIONS OF PREGNANCY OUTCOME IN YOUNG, HEALTHY, FERTILE WOMEN

The data presented and the computations made were evaluated and collated into the flow chart presented in Figure 41–1 to estimate the likelihood of pregnancy outcome in young women. It is important to emphasize, however, that these predictions are based on the health, youth, and fertility of the women and upon the supposition that spermatozoa are present in the fallopian tube at the time of ovulation.

Conception

Based on these assumptions, we deduce that fertilization of the human ovum would occur in 88 percent of the menstrual cycles of fertile, young women.

Postconceptional, Preclinical Embryo Loss

We estimate that the fate of the 879 fertilized ova (of 1,000 cycles) will be as follows: 206 (23 percent) will be lost, either as a consequence of failure of cleavage or failure of implantation or else by abortion before or at the time of the next expected menstruation. This estimate is appreciably lower than that produced in many different studies. We arbitrarily elected to assign one-half of these losses to preimplantation failure and one-half to postimplantation failure. It is possible, indeed likely, that this arbitrary assignment is incorrect and that a greater proportion should be allocated to one category compared with the other. As yet, however, we can find no data that permit a more rational assignment.

There is no doubt that our low estimate of postconception loss is caused by our estimates of high fecundability among young, healthy, fertile women. On the other hand, it is probable that high estimates of early pregnancy wastage are derived from data assembled from the studies of relatively infertile women. No doubt, high embryonic and fetal wastage contributes to absolute or relative infertility.

Clinical Pregnancy

Of 1,000 cycles in young, healthy, fertile women, 673 clinically discernible pregnancies are predicted with an incidence of spontaneous clinical abortion of 10 percent and a perinatal mortality of 1 percent.

Summary and Conclusions

The important features of the estimates presented by way of the diagram illustrated in Figure 41–1 are that the optimal fecundability in young, healthy, fertile women may be twice that observed in a general population of women of the same age who are desirous of pregnancy. In the general population of young women, intercourse may occur frequently; but there is no doubt that in such women viable spermatozoa are not in the fallopian tubes of all of the women at every ovulation time. And, there is no doubt that in this general population of young women, absolute and relative infertility affects a sizable number of the couples.

Application of the Model

Some investigators have argued that because pregnancy rates with in vitro fertilization and embryo transfer are, in some clinics, not appreciably lower than natural fecundity (28 percent), early pregnancy losses occurring in either case must be similar. We reject this analysis completely! We suggest that natural fecundability is decreased equally or more by failure of ovum fertilization immediately after ovulation. And ordinarily, natural fecundability is based upon the entrance of one fertilized ovum into the uterine cavity, whereas in the case of in vitro fertilization, several embryos are transferred to achieve pregnancies that end with liveborn infants in the order of 20 percent.

In cattle, a single artificial insemination late on the day of estrus results in 75 percent fecundity. Importantly, estrus in cows lasts only a single day, ovulation taking place at the end of estrus. Therefore, the success of artificial insemination in cows likely resides in having fresh spermatozoa in the fallopian tube when the ovum enters the oviduct.

But ours is an optimistic appraisal; this obtains because if it were correct, it means that the next plateau that could be achieved by in vitro fertilization would approach 70 percent liveborn infants per embryo transfer: maximum fecundability (60 percent) divided by female fertility efficiency (88 percent).

THE FUTURE

We are rapidly approaching the time that the regulation of reproductive function to achieve or not to achieve pregnancy can be the choice of the woman. At that time, women can elect to control the destiny of their own reproductive function. Given the likelihood that we can approach this meritorious plateau in evolution and civilization, we as obstetricians are challenged as never before to contribute to the goal of guaranteeing that every newborn is well born. This meritorious goal is shared by all interested physicians and scientists. Indeed, the topic of the 1988 plenary session of the annual meeting of the Institute of Medicine was "Advances in Reproductive Biology: Implications for Research, Application, and Policy Development."

THE LIMITING RESOURCE IN HUMAN REPRODUCTION:OVARIAN FUNCTION

Notwithstanding the fact that many men are sterile or else subfertile (thus contributing to less than optimal fecundability), it still is clear that in the human, women are physiologically the limiting resource in reproduction.

One of the keys to the success of human development and reproduction is the postponement of puberty until the second decade of life—something unknown in other mammals (Short, 1984); and an acceptable definition of the completion of puberty is the periodic release of germ cells. Indeed, the cyclic release of a mature ovum by the ovaries of women or else the surgical retrieval of mature ova is limiting in human reproduction. To be sure, ideal reproduction involves the woman's choice of the male sperm donor, but this is not a limiting physiological factor. Accordingly, a comprehensive understanding of the development of the ovaries, including the maturation of the oocytes and ovulation, is fundamental to the role of the obstetrician-gynecologist as reproductive biologist.

OBSTETRICIAN-GYNECOLOGIST AS ENDOCRINOLOGIST

Whereas only a few of us will become students of the molecular events that serve to regulate ovarian function, ovum maturation, and cyclic ovulation, we all can become knowledgeable of the reproductive physiology and pathophysiology of women. For example, normality of the ovarian cycle—i.e., predictable alterations in hormone production and cyclic extrusion of a single ovum at approximately one month intervals—is the rule and not the exception. It is true that some women are, on occasion, anovulatory—and a few are permanently so—but this situation is rare compared with the reverse, i.e., the regular, predictable, cyclic repetition of the ovarian cycle and the morphological changes in reproductive tissues that accompany these events.

The obstetrician-gynecologist commonly must assume the role of endocrinologist, but as such has a significant advantage over his internist colleagues who are obliged to deal with endocrine abnormalities in men. This is so because knowledge of the physiological events that accompany the ovarian cycle and the clinical manifestations of abnormalities thereof serve as sensitive guides to the endocrine milieu of women.

Cyclic, Spontaneous, Predictable Menses

Specifically, the occurrence of spontaneous, predictable menses at reasonable intervals is strong evidence for the occurrence of ovulation. Moreover, if such menses are associated with some degree of discomfort, which may vary from only a prodroma of impending menstruation to that of severe dysmenorrhea, the likelihood of cyclic ovulation is even greater. This is probably true because progesterone withdrawal-induced menstruation (i.e., that which is characteristic of ovulation) is associated with endometrial formation of $PGF_{2\alpha}$, which causes endometrial ischemia and myometrial contractions, the parturition of fertility failure (Chap. 3).

Ovulation Equals Normal Sex Hormone Production

We do not accept the possibility that regular, predictable menses occur with any frequency in anovulatory women (excepting those that are artificially produced by exogenous steroid compounds). This being the case, two equations can be formulated: (1) cyclic, predictable, spontaneous menses = ovulation; (2) ovulation = normal sex hormone production.

In women who are ovulatory, therefore, it can be assumed with considerable confidence that the production of pituitary gonadotropins, both follicle-stimulating hormone (FSH) and luteinizing hormone (LH), as well as estrogens, androgens, and progesterone, is appropriate. One exception to this general rule may be found in women with so-called *luteal phase deficiency*. But ordinarily, the history of cyclic, predictable, spontaneous menstruation is more valuable than many hundreds of dollars worth of endocrine tests. For this reason, a thorough and carefully obtained menstrual history is of real as well as potential value. Consider the woman, for example, who experiences the regular, cyclic, predictable onset of menstruation, but who sustains abnormal bleeding thereafter. Such a woman almost invariably will have some organic disease of the uterus to account for the abnormal bleeding. At the same time, except in women over 40 years of age, the occurrence of unpredictable uterine bleeding, i.e., unpredictable in onset, amount, or duration of bleeding, which usually is painless, is most often the result of chronic anovulation or undiagnosed pregnancy rather than organic uterine disease.

OVERVIEW OF OVARIAN FUNCTION

The history of the study of the physiological regulation of the ovarian cycle and its hormones is not dissimilar to that of the investigations of many other reproductive processes. From a very simplistic, but at the same time quite sophisticated interpretation of events—i.e., that the pituitary served as the "master gland"—we have marched through a host of hypotheses. Many of these were meritorious and were supported by data that, while convincing at the time, were obviously incomplete. Perhaps, the pervading theory of the preceding few decades was one in which it was envisioned that the brain—and in particular specialized functions of the hypothalamus—served as the central processing site for receipt of and thence transmittal of signals that controlled the function of the anterior pituitary. The release of small peptides into hypophyseal-portal blood were and are now considered to be of signal importance in the hypothalamic regulation of anterior pituitary release of gonadotropins.

OVARIAN FAIL-SAFE SYSTEMS

In the past decade, however, many investigators have guided our thinking to a consideration of internal control mechanisms within the ovary that may constitute the fail-safe systems so important in the successful maintenance of cyclic ovarian function. We know that the levels of various hormones in blood at any given stage of the ovarian cycle vary widely among women and even in a given woman from one cycle to the next. Yet, the *sine qua non* of perfection in ovarian function, viz., ovulation, is accomplished. It is recognized that the nature of the molecular events that are controlled by these fail-safe systems are of such real and potential importance that new, descriptive, and even somewhat romantic terms now are used to describe some of the putative agents, e.g., inhibin and activin, cybernins, gonadocrinins and gonadostatins, cytokines and monokines.

THE OVARY, THE FOLLICLE AND OVULATION

George W. Corner (1943) provided a translation of the observations (in Latin) of the Dutch anatomist, Regner de Graaf (1641–73), for whom the graafian follicle is named, concerning the anatomy and function of the human ovaries, which, de Graaf initially referred to as the female testes:

> The testes of women differ much from those of the male as to position, form, size, substance, integuments, and function. . . . [They] are located in the interior cavity of the abdomen, in order that they may be nearer the uterus and serve the better and more easily their intended purpose.

In Chapter 2, we put forward the proposition that the physiological expenditures involuntarily obliged in women to achieve pregnancy are phenomenal. In the absence of pharmacological intervention, the function of the ovary is directed primarily toward the achievement of ovulation. Indeed, de Graaf, long before us, put forward a somewhat similar view:

> Thus, the general function of the female testicles is to generate the ova, to nourish them, and to bring them to maturity so that they serve the same purpose in women as the ovaries of birds. On this account, many have considered these bodies useless, but this is incorrect, because they are indispensable for reproduction. Hence, they should rather be called ovaries than testes because they show no similarity, either in form or contents, with the male testes properly so called.

EMBRYOLOGY

The morphological and physiological and anatomical parade of events that lead to the development of the mature graafian follicle and release of the mature ovum begins early in embryonic development. Baker (1978) states, with considerable conviction, that, "One of the most important concepts in reproductive physiology is that the definitive germ cells—the eggs and spermatozoa—are derived solely from the primitive sex cells (that are) found early in embryonic development." He goes on to say that there is "a continuity of the germ-cell line from embryo to adult." As Baker again emphasizes, "there is overwhelming evidence in support of the classical view of the continuity of the germ-cell line," but no evidence for "the transformation of epithelial (somatic) cells into those of the germinal line."

About 3 weeks after conception, the germ cells in the human fetus are localized in the epithelium of the yolk sac near the developing allantois (Baker, 1978; Fig. 41–2). Thereafter, these germ cells migrate to the connective tissue of the hindgut and thence move progressively to the gonadal primordia or ridges (Fig. 40–19). The number of germ cells is believed to increase by mitosis. There may be a substance (telopheron) that directs the anatomical migration of the germ cell to the genital ridge. The exact means by which germ cells migrate is not fully defined; ameboid activity, chemotactic substances, and lytic enzyme activities all may be involved. Even movement by way of blood with "hone-in" mechanisms to the gonad may be involved (Baker, 1978). Generally, the germ cells remain in the cortex

if the presumptive gonad is to be an ovary. The differentiation of the fetal female gonad is late when compared with that of the male. The number of germ cells in developing ovaries, by mitosis, changes rapidly during gestational development (Fig. 41–3).

After a definitive number of mitoses, the oogonia are transformed into oocytes—at this time, prophase is entered (Baker, 1978), which is the first of two meiotic divisions—thereafter, there are no new oocytes formed. Therefore, as oogonia are eliminated from the ovary—before birth primarily—the population of germ cells only can be reduced in number.

Prodigality—as Baker states—is the *keynote* in the early history of the germ cells—i.e., the oogonia. But if this were true of ova, consider the extraordinary extent of prodigality in the case of spermatogonia when more than a billion may be ejaculated in a single copulation.

The life-time history of germ cell maturation, loss, atresia, development, and ovulation is recapitulated in Figure 41–3, which is reproduced, in large measure, from data assembled by Baker.

There is no reliable evidence in support of the proposition that ova normally are formed in the human after birth. It has been estimated that there are 600,000 oogonia in the ovaries of female fetuses at 2 months gestation and 6,800,000 at 5 months gestation. Degeneration occurs thereafter and 2,000,000 are found at birth, but only 300,000 in prepubertal girls (Baker, 1978; Fig. 41–3). Before puberty, mature graafian follicles are found only in the deeper portions of the cortex. Later, however, mature follicles also develop in the superficial portions of the

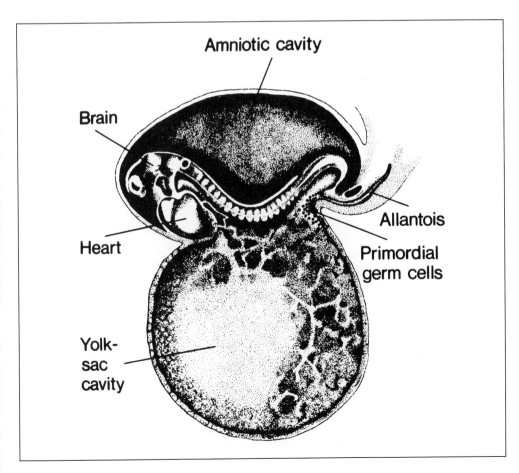

Figure 41–2. Reconstruction of 24-day human embryo in its amnion. The primordial germ cells (black dots) are grouped at the top of the yolk sac and in the ventral wall of the developing hindgut. (*From Baker. In Austin and Short (eds): Primordial Germ Cells in Germ Cells and Fertilization. Cambridge, Cambridge University Press, 1978.*)

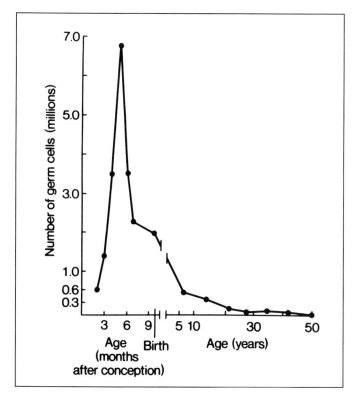

Figure 41–3. Changes in the total population of germ cells in the human ovary with increasing age. (*From Baker: Am J Obstet Gynecol 110:746, 1978.*)

ovary. During each cycle, one follicle makes its way to the surface, and there it appears as a transparent vesicle that may vary from only a few to 10 or 12 mm in diameter. As the follicle approaches the surface of the ovary, the wall becomes thinner and is supplied more abundantly with vessels (Fig. 41–4), ex-

cept in the most prominent projecting portion, which appears almost bloodless. This avascular locus is designated as the *stigma*, the site on the follicle where rupture is to occur.

FOLLICULOGENESIS

After formation of the oocytes in the early primordial follicles, these cells are surrounded by flattened epithelial-like cells (Fig. 41–5). As folliculogenesis progresses, the follicular cells proliferate and become cuboidal (Figs. 41–6 and 41–7) and then commence to secrete a fluid that accumulates, ultimately, into one large pool—and an antrum is formed. Ovarian stromal cells differentiate to form the theca externa and theca interna (Figs. 41–10 and 41–11). This stage of follicular development appears to proceed in a manner that is independent of gonadotropin action. Hereafter, an integrated set of metabolic events appears to be necessary for complete maturation of the follicle, viz., the choosing of the dominant follicle, which is destined to be the source of the ovum to be ovulated in a given cycle. Thereafter, as folliculogenesis proceeds, there is an orderly and progressive sequence of hormonally responsive and operative events that permit and facilitate the final stages in the maturation of the dominant follicle in preparation for ovulation.

During this time of folliculogenesis, two major functions emerge: (1) a gonadotropin hormone-receptor adenylate cyclase coupling system and (2) a cell-contact system for intercellular communication. It is recognized that not only do gonadotropins serve to stimulate and to activate the enzymatic processes of the cells of the follicles, but estradiol-17β, synthesized within the granulosa cells, also acts to alter gonadotropin receptor content and serves to stimulate growth and development of gap junctions in preantral follicles. The great majority of vesicular follicles, including all of those before puberty, undergo degeneration at various stages of formation (Baker, 1978; Fig. 41–3). As Roger Short (1980 puts it, "only a minute proportion of the total population of oocytes in the

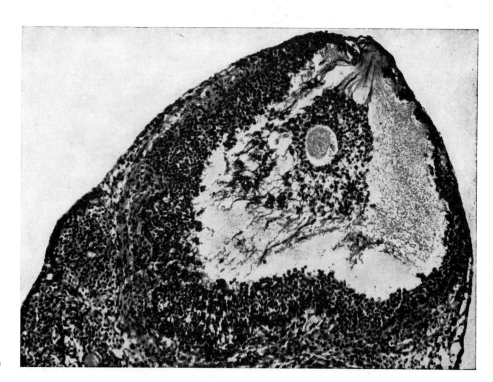

Figure 41–4. Rat ovary just prior to ovulation. (*Courtesty of Dr. Richard J. Blandau.*)

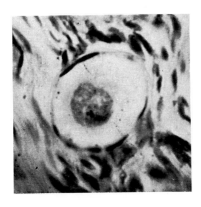

Figure 41–5. Primordial follicle from ovary of an adult woman.

From what has just been said, everyone will readily gather that it is the vesicles or their contents solely, which the nerves, arteries, veins, integuments, and the other structures normally observed in the [female] testes are designed to serve. These vesicles have been described under various names by Vesalius, Fallopius, Volcher Coiter, Laurentius, Castro, Riolan, Bartholin, Wharton, Marchettis, and others. Fallopius says: "I have seen in them indeed certain vesicles, as it were, swollen out with a watery humor, in some yellow, in other transparent." Castro also says: "The [female] testes have within them, besides the vessels, certain cavities full of a thin and watery humor which is like whey or white of egg." But the celebrated Dr. van Horne in his prodromum preferred to call them ova, a term which since it seems to me more convenient than the others, we shall in the future use, and we shall call these vesicles ova.

It seems, therefore, that de Graaf mistook the entire follicles as ova, but correctly deduced, nonetheless, that these were the structures from which the female germ cells were derived. The follicular cells, or granulosa cells, which immediately surround the ovum, constitute the *cumulus oophorus* or *discus proligerus*, a group of granulosa cells that project into the now abundant follicular fluid in the antrum of the mature follicle.

As the graafian follicle grows, the stromal cells that surround it enlarge and the capillary net about these cells becomes closer and forms the theca interna (Fig. 41–11), which is the cellular site of synthesis of C_{19}-steroids, and in particular androstenedione, which serves as the precursor for estradiol-17β formation in the granulosa cells. In the cells of the theca interna, lipid droplets develop; after ovulation, these cells persist and lie immediately adjacent to the enlarged follicular cells that are now called the granulosa lutein cells.

The results of measurements of diameters of ova in sections of a well-preserved ovary are indicative that although the ovum grows slowly during the development of the graafian follicle, the volume of the ovum increases about 40-fold before maturity is completed. The nucleus, however, increases in size only about 3-fold during this period. The large increase in cytoplasm is accompanied by the accumulation of nutrients such as yolk granules.

From the outside inward, the mature graafian follicle is

ovary at birth are ever ovulated; the majority perish through atresia."

As follicular maturation progresses, the order of events is as follows: (1) increase in size of the oocyte; (2) alteration in granulosa cells from flat to cuboidal, followed by replication; and (3) formation of the zona pellucida (Baker, 1978). The zona pellucida is a clear, mucoid band that envelops the ovum and persists until after the fertilized ovum reaches the uterus (Figs. 41–8 and 41–9). Thereafter, the theca interna is vascularized and is surrounded by the theca externa (Figs. 41–10 and 41–11). The follicle increases in size disproportionately to the ovum (Fig. 41–12).

During any ovarian cycle, 20 or more follicles may embark on the processes that appear to be on the road to ovulation. We know little, in fact nothing, of how these few of so many thousand are chosen, let alone how one of these 20 or so follicles becomes the dominant or **chosen one!**

MATURE GRAAFIAN FOLLICLE

The mature follicle is known as a *graafian follicle*; de Graaf described this structure in 1677. Referring to the developing follicles of the ovary, de Graaf said:

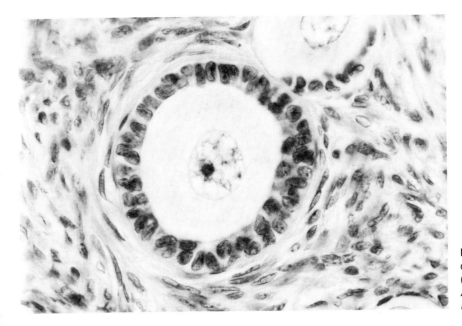

Figure 41–6. An early growing follicle in an ovary of a 4-year-old girl. A theca layer begins to form. (*From Peters: In Midgley and Sadler (eds): Some Aspects of Early Follicular Development. New York, Raven, 1979.*)

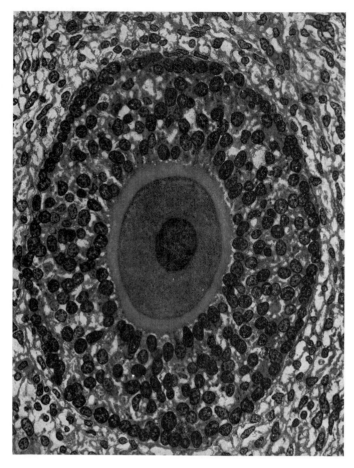

Figure 41–7. Developing follicle.

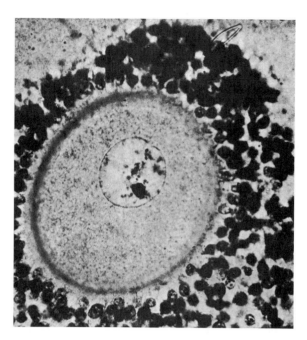

Figure 41–8. Human oocyte from a large graafian follicle. (*Courtesy of Carnegie Institution.*)

comprised of (1) a layer of specialized connective tissue, the theca folliculi; (2) an epithelial lining, the membrana granulosa; (3) the ovum; and (4) the liquor folliculi. The theca folliculi is comprised of an outer layer of cells, the theca externa and an inner layer, the theca interna. The theca externa is comprised of ordinary ovarian stroma that is arranged concentrically about the follicle, but the connective tissue cells of the theca interna are modified greatly.

Almost as soon as the primordial follicle begins to develop, mitotic figures appear in the cells of the surrounding stroma, considerable multiplication of cells occurs, and these cells become distinctly larger than those of the surrounding connective tissue. As the follicle increases in size, these cells, i.e., the *theca lutein cells,* accumulate lipid and a yellowish pigment, and this gives rise to a granular appearance. Simultaneously, a striking increase in the vascularity of and in the number of lymphatic spaces of the theca develops.

Before ovulation, the theca cells are separated from the granulosa cells by a highly polymerized membrane. It is possible that luteinizing hormone may act to depolymerize this membrane at about the time of ovulation and thus allow vascularization of the granulosa cells to take place.

The epithelial lining of the follicle, or membrana granulosa, is one that consists of several layers of small polygonal or cuboid cells in which there are round, darkly staining nuclei; the larger the follicle, the fewer the number of layers. At one time, the membrana granulosa is much thicker than elsewhere, and a

mound is formed in which the ovum is included, i.e., the cumulus oophorus (discus proligerus).

The follicle is filled with a clear, proteinaceous fluid, the *liquor folliculi,* i.e., the follicular fluid. The usual fat stains are not taken up by the granulosa cells until the stage of preovulatory swelling, a time of rapid growth that commences about 24 hours before ovulation and apparently is related to the onset of, or preparation for, the secretion of progesterone.

Ovarian follicles develop throughout childhood and occasionally attain considerable size, but normally do not rupture at this time, instead these undergo atresia in situ. The relative rates of increase in oocyte size and follicular size with matura-

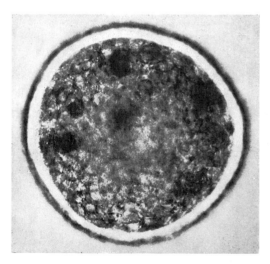

Figure 41–9. Human ovum washed from fallopian tube. Fresh specimen, surrounded by semitransparent zona pellucida, consists largely of lipoid masses. Ovum measured 0.136 mm in the living state. (*Carnegie Collection No. 6289, Dr. WH Lewis.*)

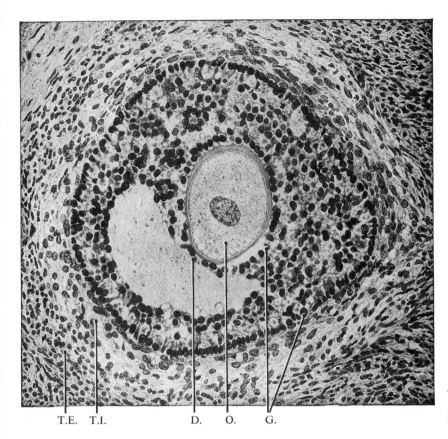

Figure 41–10. Graafian follicle approaching maturity. T.E.—theca externa,; T.I.—theca interna; D.— discus proligerus (cumulus oophorus); O.—ovum; G.—granulosa cell layer.

T.E. T.I.   D.   O.   G.

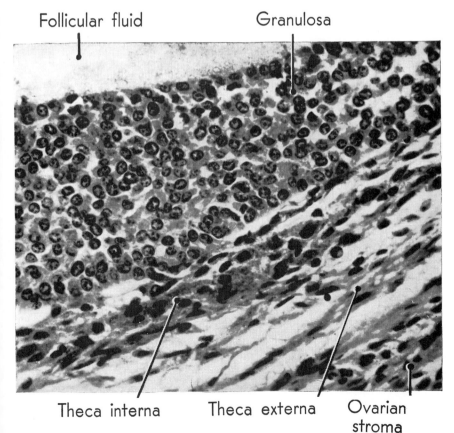

Follicular fluid   Granulosa

Theca interna   Theca externa   Ovarian stroma

Figure 41–11. Section through the wall of a mature graafian follicle.

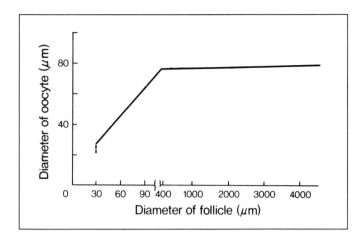

Figure. 41–12. Growth of the oocyte and follicle in the human ovary. First the oocyte alone enlarges, then both grow at a corresponding pace; finally, growth is restricted almost entirely to the follicle. (*From Baker: In Austin and Short (eds): Primordial Germ Cells and Fertilization. Cambridge, Cambridge University Press, 1978.*)

tion are considerably different (Fig. 41–12). Even in adult women, many follicles that reach a diameter of 5 mm or more undergo atresia. Usually, only one of a group of enlarging follicles continues to grow and to produce a normal mature egg that is extruded by ovulation. The mechanisms that normally limit maturation and ovulation to only one of the enlarging follicles has not been defined, and this phenomenon continues to constitute one of the major enigmas of ovarian physiology.

Concerning ovarian development, de Graaf wrote,

> Moreover, their size varies not a little with age, for in developing girls and [in women] in the flower of their life they weigh almost one and a half drachms, so that they attain a size about half that of the male testis, although in proportion they are wider and more succulent. In the old and decrepit, they are smaller, firmer, and more dried up, and slowly wither more and more, but never disappear completely; we have observed that the smallest testicles of old women weigh from five grains to half a scruple; and therefore are smaller in these than in the very old, although most anatomists say they are larger in infants and gradually diminish with the thymus gland.

THE MATURE OVUM

The human ovum, as it approaches maturity, is barely visible to the naked eye when brightly illuminated on a dark background. According to Hartman (1929) and Allen and co-workers (1930), the average diameter of the mature human ovum is 0.133 mm.

If the nearly mature ovum is examined in the follicular fluid or in physiological saline, the structures that can be distinguished in and about it are as follow: (1) a surrounding corona radiata; (2) a zona pellucida; (3) a perivitelline space; (4) a small clear zone of protoplasm; (5) a broad, finely granulated zone of protoplasm; (6) a central, deutoplasmic zone; (7) the nucleus, or germinal vesicle, within it a germinal spot; and, if appropriately stained, (8) many small spheroidal mitochondria. The ovum is free to rotate within the zona pellucida even though the outer vitelline membrane of the ovum appears to be applied closely to it. After fertilization, shrinkage of the ovum results in its complete separation from the zona pellucida as it floats in the perivitelline fluid. During growth, the oocyte accumulates

deutoplasm (yolk granules). Before ovulation, the ovum, in the living state, is transparent with a faint yellowish tinge. There also are larger lipoid granules, which in preserved material appear to surround the nucleus (germinal vesicle). Numerous mitochondria are distributed through the cytoplasm. The spherical nucleus is located near the center of the oocyte; and, in it, there is a large nucleolus and sparsely distributed chromatin. Shortly before ovulation, the nucleus migrates toward the periphery, and meiosis is reinitiated. At the completion of the first and second meiotic divisions, the number of chromosomes in the oocyte is halved, and two polar bodies are formed: the first before ovulation and the second after penetration of the oocyte by a spermatozoan. Both polar bodies are extruded into the perivitelline space.

OOGENESIS

For many decades, our most talented reproductive biologists, physiologists, cytogeneticists, and biochemists have labored diligently to define the molecular events that are essential to successful reproduction. Such fundamental information has provided great insight for the development of approaches to the correction of or at least the successful treatment of infertility due to anovulation caused by a variety of disorders. The results of these many studies of the mechanisms of control of the ovarian cycle also have provided means of addressing in a very meaningful way, effective and principally safe and acceptable means of population control. Many other examples could be given but those cited are obviously among the important issues that affect, directly or indirectly, every person of the world.

At the same time, generally, while investigations of the regulation of the processes of follicular maturation and ovulation were proceeding with great success, other investigators were pursuing, with equal vigor, dedication, and talent, a definition of the molecular events that serve to control the biochemistry of gametogenesis, fertilization, ovum and blastocyst transport, and implantation. Still others were evaluating the role of cervical mucus in sperm penetration and transport, the potential role of spermatozoa capacitation, and the difficult dilemma of antibody formation as a cause of infertility—or even as a means to induce infertility. But whereas these investigations were proceeding with success at a rate equal to that of the definition of the hormonal regulation of the reproductive processes, the clinical applicability of the knowledge so attained has lagged behind by two to three decades. We clinicians could not keep pace.

But at the time of this writing, a new era has emerged. In vitro fertilization of ova of women and embryo transfer with successful pregnancy and birth after reimplantation of the fertilized ovum is a reality. New tests are being developed to evaluate the nature of infertility in couples in whom previously no cause was found.

As customarily is the case, we still are far behind our veterinarian colleagues who for years have successfully frozen and preserved sperm from prize males, artificially inseminated many species, developed ova transport systems, succeeded with in vitro fertilization, effected superovulation—and on and on.

But again, at the time of this writing, the future is bright—in many cases, only further development and refinement of technical details appear to stand in front of a new era—one that may hold the promise for the solution of many problems of infertility not previously believed to be treatable—but perhaps (and possibly of greater socioeconomic significance for all the world) also the development of new means of population control, the delivery systems for which may be the answer to population control in underdeveloped nations. It is with this optimism that we now can address with renewed enthusiasm the issues of gametogenesis, fertilization, and development, and transport of the fertilized ovum. For it surely follows that the **absolute limiting step in successful pregnancy is the quality of the zygote.**

GAMETOGENESIS

Primitive germ cells are present in the human embryo by the end of the 3rd week of development. Both *oogenesis*, in the course of which mature ova are formed from primitive oogonia, and *spermatogenesis*, which results in the production of spermatids, share a basic biologic feature of maturation, i.e., reduction and division (Fig. 41–13). Such special cellular division, known as *meiosis*, is limited to germ cells. The process of meiosis is characterized by a long and unusual prophase, and involves a process that provides for the exchange of genetic material between homologous chromosomes and the reduction of the *diploid* number of chromosomes, i.e., 46, to the *haploid* number, i.e., 23. In man, the diploid number of chromosomes is comprised of 44 autosomes and 2 sex chromosomes; during meiosis, mature gametes are formed, in each of which there are 22 autosomes and 1 sex chromosome. The diploid number of chro-

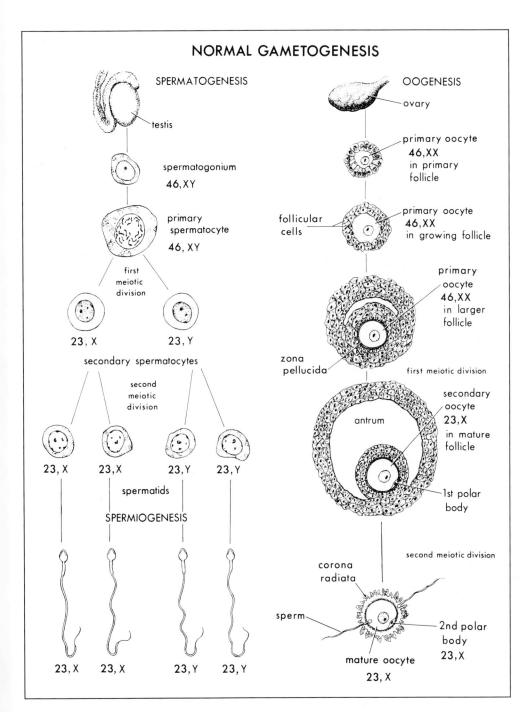

Figure 41–13. Drawings to compare spermatogenesis and oogenesis. The chromosome complement of the germ cells is shown at each stage. The number designates the total number of chromosomes, including the sex chromosome(s) shown after the comma. Note that (1) after the two meiotic divisions, the diploid number of chromosomes, 46, is reduced to the haploid number, 23; (2) four sperm form from one primary spermatocyte, whereas only one mature oocyte (ovum) results from maturation of a primary oocyte; and, (3) the cytoplasm is conserved during oogenesis to form one large cell, the mature oocyte (ovum). (*From Moore: The Developing Human, 2nd ed. Philadelphia, Saunders, 1977.*)

mosomes is not restored until fertilization with the union of the ovum and sperm. Spermatogenesis is the process that encompasses the final maturational events that lead to production of mature male gametes and is one that involves changes in the shape of the spermatids and the transformation of these cells to spermatozoa. The fact that the mature germ cells are derived directly from primitive cells that may have migrated from the yolk sac to the developing gonads as early as the 5th week of embryonic life, is one that underlies the concept of continuity of the germ plasm. In the case of human ova, some germ cells may remain dormant for as long as 40 years.

Meiosis

In all primitive germ cells, i.e., *oogonia* and *spermatogonia*, there are a diploid number of chromosomes (i.e., 46). When these stem cells divide to produce primary oocytes and spermatocytes, each chromosome undergoes replication by splitting longitudinally to form a double-stranded structure. During this typical *mitosis*, one strand of each chromosome enters each daughter cell, and in this manner, the identical chromosomal components of the parent cells are obtained.

When the primary oocytes and spermatocytes continue maturation to form secondary oocytes and spermatocytes, respectively, however, the meiotic division that ensues is quite different; this is the case in that each of the newly formed cells receives only 23, or the haploid number of chromosomes. The basic difference between meiosis and mitosis is the prolonged prophase in meiosis, in which there is, in meiosis, preliminary pairing of homologous chromosomes before division. During the *leptotene* stage of meiotic prophase, the 46 chromosomes appear as single slender threads; in the next stage, i.e., the *zygotene*, the homologous chromosomes are aligned in a parallel manner to one other in *synapsis*, with the formation of 23 bivalent components. Each chromosome then divides longitudinally, except at the *centromere*, and the ensuing *pachytene* stage is comprised of *tetrads* of four chromatids, the shape of which is dependent upon the position of the centromere. At this stage, the chromatids break and thence recombine with strands from the homologous chromosome to effect an exchange of genetic material. During the next, i.e., *diplotene*, stage, the homologous strands separate. During the metaphase of the first meiotic division, the bivalents (two chromatids that comprise each chromosome) become oriented on the spindle; when the cell divides, the members of each pair move toward opposite poles into the daughter cells, which then contain the haploid number of chromosomes, still as chromatid pairs. *The individual chromosomes now are no longer genetically identical with those of the parent cell.* Each secondary oocyte will thus receive 22 autosomes and an X chromosome, and each secondary spermatocyte will receive 22 autosomes and either an X or Y chromosome.

At the second meiotic division, the *diad* splits at the centromere to form two *monads,* one of which becomes associated with each daughter cell, probably having already undergone a typical mitotic longitudinal replication. The mature ovum (23,X), if fertilized by a spermatocyte with a Y chromosome (23,Y) will produce a male zygote (46, XY), whereas if the ovum was fertilized by a spermatocyte with an X chromosome (23,X), the result will be a female(46,XX).

Biochemistry of Cellular Division

During mitotic interphase, duplication of the chromosomes is accomplished by replication of DNA. The results of autoradiographic studies of the incorporation of tritium-labeled thymidine into chromosomes are indicative that duplication is accomplished by separation of the two original DNA strands of each chromosome and by subsequent synthesis of two new DNA strands. At the next cellular division, each chromatid receives one original and one newly synthesized strand.

Oogenesis

Pinkerton and colleagues (1961) were able to trace the development of the human ovum by use of histochemical technics that were dependent principally upon the high content of alkaline phosphatase that is characteristic of the germ cells. In the first phase (migration), the germ cells reach the medial slope of the mesonephric ridge where the gonads arise, divide rapidly, and become oogonia; in the second phase (division), the germ cells divide mitotically at a rate that is maximal during the 8th to 20th weeks, but slows thereafter, and finally ceases at birth. In the third phase (maturation), the cells enter the prophase of the first meiotic division, acquire a ring of granulosa cells, and become definitive oocytes within the primary follicles.

It is well to remember that all oocytes are derived from the primitive germ cells. Blandau and co-workers (1963) have recorded, cinematographically, in the mouse, the ameboid-like migration of primitive germ cells from the yolk sac to the germinal ridges. The primitive oogonia, furthermore, continue movements locally within the developing ovary even after the pachytene stage of meiosis is reached.

The primary oocytes increase in size and cuboidal follicular cells proliferate to form increasingly thick coverings around them (Fig. 41–14). The follicular cells, furthermore, deposit on the surface of the oocyte an *acellular* glycoprotein mantle that thickens gradually to form the *zona pellucida* (Figs. 41–14 and 41–15). Irregular fluid-filled spaces between the follicular cells then coalesce to form an antrum. The radially elongated follicular cells that surround the zona pellucida form the corona radiata (Fig. 41–14). A solid mass of follicular cells, the cumulus oophorus, surrounds the ovum in a developing vesicular ovarian follicle (Figs. 41–14 and 41–15). As the follicle nears maturity, the cumulus projects further into the antrum and as a consequence, the oocyte appears to be supported by this column of follicular cells. At this stage, the follicle may vary from 6 to 12 mm in diameter and lies immediately beneath the surface of the ovary.

The formation of the oocyte completes the first meiotic division, which was begun before birth, during the final stage of transformation of the primordial follicle into the mature graafian follicle. The important result is the formation of two daughter cells, each with 23 chromosomes but of greatly unequal size. One receives almost all of the cytoplasm of the mother cell and becomes a secondary oocyte; the other, the first polar body, receives very little cytoplasm. The polar body lies between the zona pellucida and the vitelline membrane of the secondary oocyte.

The Chosen Ovum

Not only is there a chosen follicle—or dominant follicle—there is a dominant oocyte because it is the only oocyte in the preovulatory follicle that matures; all others do not develop beyond the immature dictyotene state (Channing and associates, 1982). It is believed that a cybernin called *oocyte maturation inhibitor* (OMI) may serve an important role in oocyte maturation. Oocyte maturation inhibitor appears to be present in all follicles except preovulatory ones. From the results of a variety of experiments beginning with those of Chang (1955), it seems reasonably clear

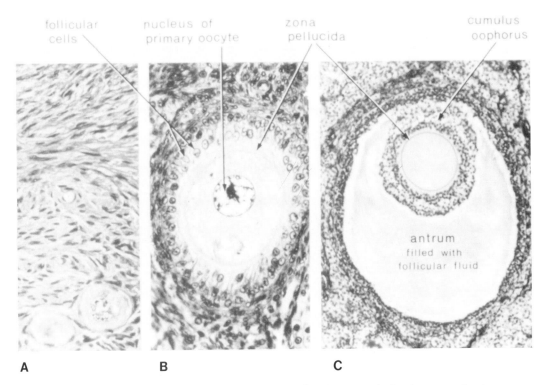

Figure 41–14. Photomicrographs of sections from ovaries of adult women. **A.** Ovarian cortex showing two primordial follicles that contain primary oocytes that have completed the prophase of the first meiotic division and have entered the dictyotene stage, a "resting" stage between prophase and metaphase (×250). **B.** Growing follicle that contains a primary oocyte, surrounded by the zona pellucida and a stratified layer of follicular cells (×250). **C.** An almost mature follicle with a large antrum. The oocyte, embedded in the cumulus oophorus, does not show a nucleus because it has been sectioned tangentially (×100). (*From Moore: The Developing Human. 3rd ed. Philadelphia, Saunders, 1982.*)

that a substance in follicular fluid that arises from granulosa cells inhibits oocyte maturation.

As summarized by Channing and Pomerantz (1981), there is in human (and other mammalian) follicular fluid an inhibitor of oocyte maturation—of molecular weight of less than 2,000—which is probably a polypeptide that is secreted by granulosa cells. The action of oocyte maturation inhibitor likely is mediated by cells of the cumulus. LH, in all likelihood, acts on the chosen follicle to block the action of the oocyte maturation inhibitor.

In studies of tubal ova, Hertig and Rock (1944) found that the first polar body is cast off while still in the ovary. A second division is consummated in the formation of the second polar body at about the moment that the sperm penetrates the egg.

A most interesting, but unsolved, riddle in this field is the mechanism(s) that prevents all follicles but one from undergoing simultaneous maturation and ovulation during the first, or any given, cycle. The factors that normally are believed to be responsible for allowing only one ovum to reach maturity each month are considered subsequently.

In ova of women, the second maturation division is completed only if the ovum is fertilized. If penetration by a spermatozoan does not occur within a few hours of ovulation, the ovum begins to degenerate. Although it is not certain that the first polar body always undergoes subsequent division, fertilized ova have been found that were accompanied by three polar bodies. During maturation, the diameter of the human ovum increases from 19 microns in the original oocyte to 135 microns in the fully mature ovum, a sevenfold increase in size.

TRANSPORT OF OVA AND SPERMATOZOA

Tubal Transport

Eddy and Pauerstein (1980) have presented an excellent review of the anatomy and physiology of the fallopian tube. In women, the ovaries normally lie free in the peritoneal cavity except for the supporting mesovarium and ovarian ligament. About the time of ovulation, however, the fimbriae of the oviduct, possibly as the consequence of appropriate hormonal and neural (doubtful) regulation, are believed to cover completely the ovary at the site of ovulation. Ovulation is not an explosive phenomenon; instead, as the stigma is digested by proteolytic enzymes, there is a gentle outpouring of the contents of the follicle, which include the egg that is surrounded by the zona pellucida and the cumulus oophorus. The cumulus cells appear to be important for uptake and transport of the ovum by the oviduct. In the oviduct of the monkey, ciliary action is believed to be the prominent force in the movement of the ovum in the tube, whereas peristalsis appears to be so in the rabbit. The relative contribution of each of these mechanisms in sperm and ovum transport in women is not known. Because, in mammals, fertilization usually occurs in the ampulla, whatever the roles of the tubal cilia and peristalsis may be, an adequate theory must be one whereby movement of ova and spermatozoa in opposite directions can be explained.

Migration of Fertilized Ovum

In most mammals, the fertilized ovum migrates through the oviduct and reaches the cavity of the uterus about 3 to 4 days

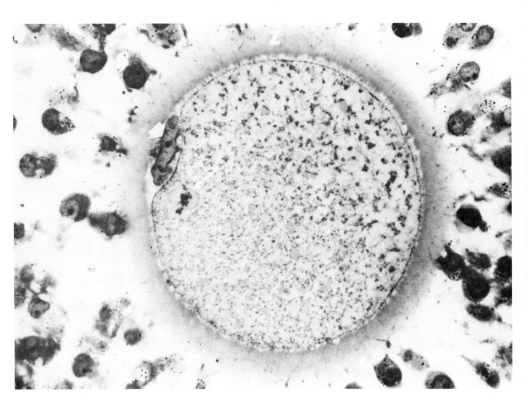

Figure 41–15. Light micrograph of a human follicular oocyte. The first polar body (short arrow) has been liberated and lies in the perivitelline space, which separates the oocyte from the zona pellucida (*Z*). The oocyte chromosomes are aligned on the equator of the meiotic spindle (long arrow). They will remain in this position until penetration of the fertilizing spermatozoan, when the second meiotic division will resume. The cells of the cumulus oophorus are more dispersed than in the previous stages. Some of them are undergoing regression, as shown by the presence of numerous fat droplets in the cytoplasm and pyknosis of nuclei. These features represent the onset of the denudation of the oocyte, a process that will be completed in the oviduct (× 1500). (*From Ferenczy and Richard (eds): The Female Reproductive System. Dynamics of Scan and Electron Microscopy. New York, Wiley, 1974.*)

after ovulation. In women, the ovum is believed to be able to wander across the pelvis and then to be taken up by the opposite tube (*external migration*) or else, theoretically, the ovum may cross inside the uterus and migrate up to the opposite tube (*internal migration*). Presumptive clinical evidence of migration of the ovum includes a successful intrauterine pregnancy in women who have only one tube and only the contralateral ovary. It is likely that the entire subject of migration of the ovum in women has received more attention than it deserves. In consideration of known normal anatomical relationships, as observed at laparotomy, both tubes usually are freely mobile, and the fimbriated extremities lie posterior to the uterus and in rather close approximation. In view of the recognized motility of the fallopian tubes, it is reasonable to presume that the ovum may be taken up directly by the opposite tube, without recourse to complicated explanations that involve mechanisms of internal or external migration.

Transport of Spermatozoa

During human coitus, there is in each ejaculate, on average, a volume of 2 to 5 mL in which there are approximately 70 million sperm per mL that are deposited in the vagina. Of these 100 million spermatozoa, or more, of which between 80 and 90 percent are presumed to be normal forms, perhaps fewer than 200 actually reach the site of fertilization, i.e., the ampulla of the tube. For successful fertilization, Eddy and Pauerstein (1980) asked the important question as to why "so many sperm are required in the ejaculate when so few arrive at the site of fertilization?" Only one spermatozoan must meet, in the upper portion of the fallopian tube, the single mature ovum that is released during each ovulatory cycle.

Sperm reach the site of fertilization in the ampulla of the oviduct shortly (often only 5 minutes) after ejaculation, a time that is much faster than can be explained by the flagellar action of spermatozoa. Eddy and Pauerstein are of the view that there are reservoirs (i.e., the ejaculate and the uterus may be considered as reservoirs for spermatozoa) whereas "the cervix, uterotubal junctions, and possibly the oviductal isthmus may be considered as barriers to the passage of sperm." An unbelievably sharp decrement occurs in the number of sperm between those deposited in the vagina and those that reach the ampulla of the fallopian tube (Eddy and Pauerstein, 1980).

It still remains a biological curiosity that spermatozoa can reach the ampulla of the fallopian tube with such rapidity from the time of insemination. Indeed, it has been reported that this transit time may be no more than 5 minutes, but on average, a time of 4 to 6 hours seems more reasonable. The loss of sperm in the ejaculate, however, is remarkable. In one study, it was estimated that for every 14 million sperm deposited in the vagina, only one could be recovered from the fallopian tubes within 15 to 45 minutes of insemination. It is clear, however, that there are mechanisms that are operative in the genital tract of women that provide for accelerated transport of sperm—at rates that are considerably greater than can be accounted for by sperm migration by flagellation. It is believed that movement of spermatozoa that is caused by flagellar action is necessary for maintenance of the sperm in suspension and in the facilitation of transport; moreover, such movement is believed to be necessary for transit of the spermatozoan through the cumulus oophorus and zona pellucida of the ovum.

It is believed that the spermatozoa must make their own way through the mucus that fills the cervical canal. The first spermatozoa appear to burrow through the mucus by chemical as well as mechanical means; the leaders among the spermatozoa very likely depolymerize the cervical mucus by releasing proteases that are contained in the acrosome, and thereby render the mucus more easily penetrable by the spermatozoa that follow and successfully enter the uterine cavity. The uterine cavity in vivo may well be nearly obliterated except for canals that extend from the internal os of the cervix to the uterotubal junctions; as the consequences of such canals, sperm are directed to the oviduct.

Fertilization

As soon as the sperm penetrates the zona pellucida and comes in contact with the vitelline membrane, a second polar body is formed and the female pronucleus, as well as the male pronucleus, are evident in the ovum. Ordinarily, the penetration of the zona pellucida and vitelline membrane by one sperm acts in a manner to inhibit entry by other sperm; but at times, more than one sperm does enter. The mechanism by which the sperm penetrates the zona pellucida is not defined clearly, but probably involves enzymatic action. Materials other than genetic material that are contained in the sperm degenerate within the ovum.

Zona Pellucida

Dickman and Noyes (1961) found that the zona pellucida in the rat is shed from the blastocyst during the 5th day after fertilization. The shedding, moreover, appears unrelated to a specific uterine environment, but rather is an intrinsic manifestation of growth and maturation of the blastocyst. The zona clearly is not necessary for implantation; on the contrary, its removal is a prerequisite for implantation, at least in the laboratory rodents studied thus far.

Presently, and even more so heretofore, the cause of involuntary infertility in a large number of infertile couples, i.e., 25 percent, was unknown. By conventional testing, both partners appeared to be normal and, yet, pregnancy was not achieved. These findings obviously were suggestive that a variety of undefined and, at that time, undetectable factors were important in the processes that lead to gametogenesis, gamete maturation, fertilization, transport of fertilized ova, implantation, and embryogenesis. For a variety of reasons, it was suspected that there was a "male" factor involved in a large proportion of instances of unexplained infertility. At that time, in the evaluation of male fertility, we were restricted to evaluation by history and by physical examination and by evaluation of ejaculates for semen volume, sperm density, morphology, and motility. Even then, it was reasonable to assume that these data gave us little insight into sperm survival, cervical penetration, migration, or capacity for ovum penetration and fertilization. And this is to say nothing of the potential—and perhaps the likelihood—that antibodies of either male or female origin can act to inhibit—in one manner or another—the capacity of sperm to reach and thence to fertilize a receptive ovum.

Possibly, the most obvious cause of unexplained infertility (other than pregnancy wastage) is that based upon an immunological disorder. The difficulty, to date, with this proposition is the development of immunological tests with sufficient specificity to permit conclusions to be drawn from the results obtained. Many reports appear to be anecdotal and others are replete with what appear to be the findings of false positives—i.e., antisperm antibodies in biological fluid(s) of women known to be fertile or even to be pregnant. As stated by Warren R. Jones (1980), "human semen is an antigenic nightmare."

A novel test was introduced in 1976 by Yanagimachi and colleagues to assess the capacity of human spermatozoa to fertilize. This test is dependent upon the capacity of the sperm of one species, man, to penetrate the ovum of another species, provided that the acellular, sperm-resistant (possibly specific antigen-containing) zona pellucida of such ova are removed. These investigators demonstrated that capacitated human spermatozoa could penetrate zona-free hamster eggs. Thereafter, there was decondensation of the sperm chromatin and pronucleus formation—events analogous to those of fertilization. In some clinics, this test is proving to be correlated reasonably well with male fertility. It also is of particular potential importance in that there appear to be zona pellucida–specific antigens. Such antibodies appear to react with eggs in such a manner that binding receptors for sperm are masked; thus, fertilization cannot take place. Indeed, there are reports of infertility due to the presence of circulating antizonal antibodies, but the status of this entity is as yet not clear. Nonetheless, the possibility is real of an antizonal-antibody to produce passive and even temporary infertility in this day of monoclonal antibody technology.

Aging of Gametes

The increased incidence of the trisomy 21 variety of Down syndrome late in reproductive life is well established. It may be related to an increased tendency toward nondisjunction in ova that have remained dormant in the ovary for 40 years or more. Although the incidence of this syndrome in the population as a whole is only 3 per 2,000 live births, the incidence rises to about 1 in 100 in women by age 40 (Chap. 32, p. 570).

Tesh and Glover (1969) noted that gametes of aging males also exerted deleterious effects on the embryo and fetus. They reported that aging of rabbit sperm in the male reproductive tract led to a decrease in the capacity for fertilization. Moreover, if eggs were fertilized by such sperm, an increase in embryonic anomalies resulted. Friedman (1981) found that the risk of new autosomal dominant mutations in children is increased many times among the offspring of fathers who are 40 years of age or older. Indeed, he found that such risk was similar to that of Down syndrome in infants of 35- to 40-year-old mothers.

Vickers (1969) observed that delayed fertilization also led to an increase in chromosomal anomalies of the embryo. In mice, in which fertilization was delayed (7 to 13 hours), triploidy, for example, was increased ninefold. Vickers postulated that the chromsomal aberrations may have resulted from errors in meiosis, fertilization, or cleavage.

THECA-GRANULOSA CELL COOPERATIVITY AND STEROIDOGENESIS

MOLECULAR EVENTS INVOLVED IN THE FINAL STAGES OF FOLLICULAR MATURATION AND OVULATION

It now is clear that a variety of molecular events in the theca and granulosa cells of the ovaries of women are subject to regulatory processes that involve the actions of gonadotropins and of steroids as well. It is recognized that follicular maturation can proceed in the absence of pituitary hormone stimulation to the preantral stage of development and even to replication of granulosa cells to a finite point, i.e., four-cell layer thickness. Beyond this stage, however, gonadotropin and most likely steroids produced in response to gonadotropin action are required for full expression of follicular maturation and responsiveness.

THE TWO-CELL HYPOTHESIS OF OVARIAN STEROIDOGENESIS

The characteristic cyclicity of secretion of estradiol-17β and progesterone, as well as the formation of the C_{19}-steroids, androstenedione, dehydroisoandrosterone, and testosterone, by the ovaries of young women is regulated by mechanisms that are considerably different with respect to C_{18}- and C_{21}-steroids (estrogen and progesterone) as compared with those of the C_{19}-steroids (androgen or androgen-like).

FSH acts to increase the enzymatic activity in granulosa cells that catalyzes the aromatization of C_{19}-steroids to produce estrogen. This activity is believed to be modulated by an increase in adenylate cyclase activity and by "androgens" that act in an, as yet, undefined manner to increase aromatase activity. But more than that, estradiol-17β synthesized by the dominant follicle also appears to act to increase the follicular cell actions of FSH to enhance LH responsiveness. The stimulation of aromatase activity by cyclic-AMP likely is mediated by cyclic-AMP-dependent phosphorylation of a number of cellular proteins, and by an increase in the rate of transcription of the specific gene that encodes for the aromatase protein. It is only after FSH-priming that cells become competent to LH action. This is believed to be the result of FSH-induced LH receptors and, perhaps, FSH-induced prolactin receptors. Thus, FSH appears to act to induce an increase in aromatase activity (by way of synthesis of new enzyme), as well as LH receptors.

Approximately three decades ago, a new, or revised, hypothesis, i.e., *the two-cell hypothesis*, was put forward and championed by Ryan and Smith (1959) with respect to the mechanism of steroid production in the ovary, and in particular, the maturing follicle. This postulate is to describe the cooperativity between theca and granulosa cells in steroid formation.

LH is known to act in theca cells to increase cholesterol side-chain cleavage enzyme activity (which is believed to be the rate-limiting step in steroidogenesis in many steroidogenic tissues) and to increase the activities of steroid 17α-hydroxylase/17,20-lyase, an enzyme important, indeed crucial, to the formation of C_{19}-steroids, i.e., androgen-like compounds such as dehydroisoandrosterone, androstenedione, and testosterone.

Androstenedione, formed in theca, diffuses into the follicular fluid and thereby becomes available to the granulosa cells for aromatization to form estrone and thence estradiol-17β (Fig. 41–16). Before ovulation, there is little or no de novo synthesis of steroids in granulosa cells because of limited capacity for the de novo synthesis of cholesterol. We will return to this issue.

STEROID PRODUCTION IN ISOLATED CELL TYPES

Granulosa cells can be isolated and maintained in culture. But strange, if not inexplicable, events accompany the maintenance of granulosa cells in vitro; importantly, spontaneous luteinization of such cells occurs in culture. Before ovulation, granulosa cells in vivo do not produce steroids de novo; rather, these cells are dependent upon preformed C_{19}-steroids (from theca cells) for estradiol-17β formation. This probably is true because human granulosa cells cannot form cholesterol de novo.

Source of Cholesterol for Steroidogenesis

We have known for many years that ultimately cholesterol must be the precursor of all steroid hormones. What we did not consider, until recently, was that the source of cholesterol for a given steroidogenic cell may differ. Together with the pioneering studies of Brown, Goldstein and colleagues (1979), who

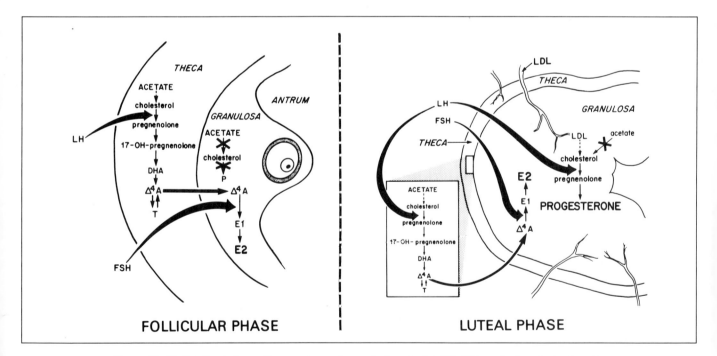

Figure 41–16. Relation between theca and granulosa cells in estradiol-17β (E2) production. Androstenedione (Δ⁴A) is synthesized by way of pregnenolone and dehydroisoandrosterone (DHA) formation in theca cells. Note that LH stimulates the formation of pregnenolone by increasing side-chain cleavage of cholesterol. Aromatization occurs in granulosa cells to give E2 by way of estrone (E1). The aromatization of androstenedione is stimulated by FSH. Progesterone synthesis from plasma low-density lipoprotein (LDL) occurs in luteinized granulosa cells. Testosterone (T) also is synthesized in the ovary.

demonstrated that many extrahepatic tissues assimilate cholesterol by uptake and processing of circulating lipoproteins, it was soon demonstrated that similar processes are applicable to the assimilation of cholesterol for steroidogenesis in endocrine glands and placenta (Chap. 5).

The specific form and source of cholesterol utilized by a given gland, however, varies widely among species and perhaps within a given cell type of a given gland in the same species. By way of example, the source of cholesterol for progesterone biosynthesis by the corpus luteum of various mammals is among the most diverse. Consider the following: In the rabbit, cholesterol is synthesized in the corpus luteum de novo, i.e., from 2-carbon fragments such as acetate. In the rat, however, circulating plasma high-density lipoprotein (HDL) is used as the cholesterol source. But in women, thre is little de novo synthesis of cholesterol in granulosa cells or in the corpus luteum. HDL is not assimilated by human granulosa cells; but rather, low-density lipoprotein (LDL) is the near exclusive form of cholesterol that can be used for progesterone biosynthesis. The molecular weight of LDL is approximately 3 million. Recall that follicular granulosa cells are not vascularized; it is apparent, therefore, that a precursor source of cholesterol becomes extraordinarily important in the mechanisms that provide for full luteinization and optimal progesterone biosynthesis.

LDL Utilization by Granulosa Cells

Let us consider the extremes. In women, there is very limited capacity for the de novo synthesis of cholesterol in granulosa cells and these cells do not utilize HDL as a source of cholesterol. In the follicular fluid that surrounds the avascular granulosa cells, there is little or no LDL. Thus, it is obvious that little or no steroidogenesis by way of the utilization of LDL-cholesterol could proceed in this unique environment. Therefore, before ovulation, there is little progesterone produced by the granulosa cells of women. The steroid produced, estradiol-17β, is synthesized from androstenedione provided by theca.

On the other hand, if granulosa cells obtained from the follicles of women are placed in culture, these cells luteinize and respond to appropriate trophic stimuli by producing progesterone in large amounts. It must be remembered, however, that the culture medium that bathes these cells usually contains serum—and thus LDL, a lipoprotein not present in follicular fluid, but the one known to be used specifically as a source of cholesterol in human granulosa cells. Thus, the "spontaneous" luteinization of granulosa cells and thence the biosynthesis of progesterone may be attributable, in part, to the addition of a utilizable source of cholesterol, viz., LDL to these cells.

Cholesterol Source for Steroidogenesis in Theca and Granulosa Cells

The cooperativity in the follicular, i.e., theca-granulosa cell production of estradiol-17β, is illustrated in Figure 41–16. But as stated, the corpus luteum of women is dependent upon plasma LDL for a source of cholesterol as precursor for progesterone biosynthesis.

As is the case in many studies of physiological events in the human, there is an entity, abetalipoproteinemia, that is particularly helpful in defining the origin of steroids produced in the ovaries of women. The steroid levels in a presumably ovulatory woman with abetalipoproteinemia are supportive of these deductions (Illingworth and colleagues, 1982). In such a woman, there is no LDL, hence the term, abetalipoproteinemia. As illustrated in Figure 41–17, there appeared to be cyclic ovarian function in this woman, i.e., a mid-cycle LH surge, appropriate levels of FSH and LH, *but no progesterone!* These findings are strongly supportive of the proposition that de novo cholesterol synthesis in theca can be sufficient to support the biosynthesis of C_{19}-steroids that enter follicular fluid to become available to the granulosa cells for estradiol-17β production that is characteristic of cyclic estrogen biosynthesis during the ovarian cycle. On the other hand, in this woman, there was no post-LH surge increase in progesterone secretion. We take this as evidence that the granulosa cells are dependent almost exclusively upon LDL as the source of cholesterol precursor for progesterone biosynthesis. This woman no doubt was ovulatory because she became pregnant and delivered a normal child at term (Chap. 10).

Thus, the *two-cell hypothesis* seems to be complete. We cannot disregard the potential of theca cells to utilize LDL-cholesterol; but, from the findings in the case of the woman with abetalipoproteinemia presented, it seems likely that sufficient de novo synthesis of cholesterol can proceed in theca to provide adequate quantities of androstenedione for granulosa cell estradiol-17β synthesis.

OVULATION

As the graafian follicle grows to a size of 10 to 12 mm in diameter, it gradually reaches the surface of the ovary and ultimately protrudes above it. Necrobiosis of the overlying tissues, rather than pressure within the follicle, is the principal factor that causes

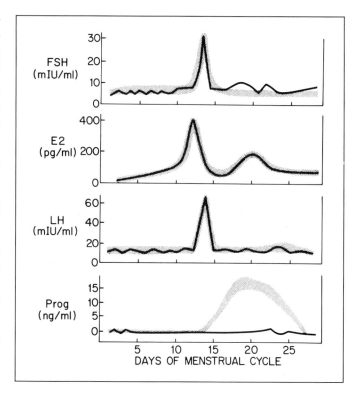

Figure 41–17. Hormones throughout the menstrual cycle. The shaded areas represent mean values noted in normal ovulatory women. The solid lines represent those values measured in a woman with abetalipoproteinemia. (*Adapted from Illingworth: Proc Natl Acad Sci USA 79:6685, 1982.*)

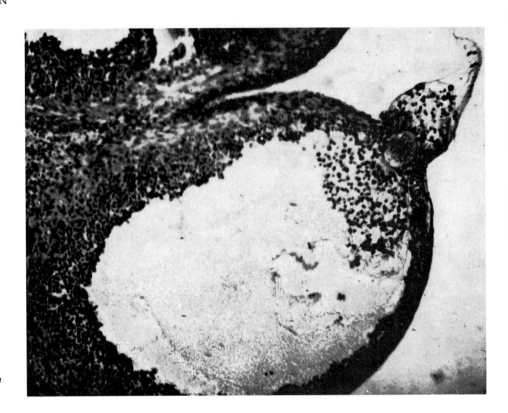

Figure 41–18. Moment of ovulation in the rat. (*Courtesy of Dr. Richard J. Blandau.*)

follicular rupture. The cells at the exposed tip of the follicle float away at the site of the pale stigma so that the region becomes transparent. The thinnest clear area then bursts, and the follicular liquid and the ovum surrounded by the zona pellucida and corona radiata are extruded at the time of ovulation. The actual rupture of the follicle is not explosive; the discharge of the ovum together with the zona pellucida and attached follicular cells takes not more than 2 to 3 minutes; and in the rabbit at least, it is expedited by the separation, just before rupture, of the ovum with the surrounding granulosa cells (corona radiata) from the follicular wall as the result of accumulation of fluid in the cumulus; hence, the ovum floats freely in the liquor.

Strickland and Beers (1979) demonstrated that granulosa cells produce plasminogen activator. The extracellular level of this enzyme is correlated closely with ovulation, and the activity of the enzyme, is modulated by the action of gonadotropins, cyclic nucleotides, and prostaglandins. Further, by the action of this enzyme on plasminogen, which is present in follicular fluid, plasmin is generated, a proteolytic enzyme that has been shown to weaken the follicular wall (Beers, 1975).

Excellent motion pictures of the process of ovulation in the rat have been obtained by Richard Blandau and others. In Figures 41–4 and 41–18, two frames from these movies are illustrated. The follicle is shown just before ovulation and the expulsion of the ovum also is shown. In the first (Fig. 41–4), the stigma is clearly visible, whereas in the second (Fig. 41–18) the actual expulsion of the ovum is illustrated. In Figure 41–19, a scanning electron micrograph of an oocyte and the follicle of a mouse at the time of ovulation is presented.

TIME OF OVULATION

The exact time of ovulation in the cycle is of the utmost importance for several reasons. First, since the life span of both the spermatozoa and the unfertilized ovum are limited, fertilization must take place within hours (preferably minutes) after ovulation if conception is to occur in that cycle. In some infertile couples, detection of the time of ovulation and appropriate adjustment of the time of coitus are important considerations in therapy. Importantly, for couples who use the "rhythm method" to avoid conception, coitus should be limited to that part of the cycle several days removed from the time of ovulation, or the "safe period." Ovulation usually marks approximately the midpoint of both the ovarian and menstrual cycles. The period from the first day of menstrual bleeding to ovulation is designated as the proliferative phase of the menstrual cycle. The proliferative phase encompasses roughly the first half of the menstrual cycle; the *postovulatory phase* is known as the secretory phase (Chap. 3).

Various methods have been used in attempts to determine the time of ovulation in women. Allen and colleagues (1930) recovered mature unfertilized ova from the fallopian tube on the 12th, 15th, and 16th days of the cycle, and concluded that ovulation occurs approximately on day 14 of a 28-day menstrual cycle. Other indirect methods by which to ascertain the time of ovulation are the examination of fertilized ova and evaluation of the changes that have taken place at the site of the ruptured follicle. By use of these techniques, it has been demonstrated that, although ovulation frequently occurs between the 12th and 16th days of the cycle, there is considerable variation in the timing of ovulation. It is not uncommon for ovulation to take place at any time between the 8th and 20th days, as illustrated in Figure 41–20. The time of ovulation bears a closer temporal relation to the onset of the next menstrual period than to the previous menses. Ovulation usually occurs approximately 14 days before the first day of the succeeding menstrual bleeding.

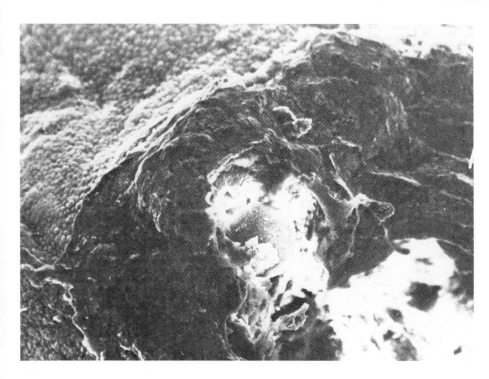

Figure 41–19. Scanning electron micrograph of an oocyte and the follicle of a mouse at the time of ovulation. (*From Motta and Hafez (eds): Biology of the Mouse Ovary. The Hague, Martinus Nijhoff, 1980.*)

SIGNS AND SYMPTOMS OF OVULATION

On or about the day of ovulation, as many as 25 percent of women experience lower abdominal discomfort on the involved side. This so-called *Mittelschmerz* is believed to be caused by peritoneal irritation by follicular fluid or blood that escapes from the ruptured follicle. The symptoms rarely occur during every cycle.

A useful means of detecting ovulation is by documentation of a shift in basal body temperature from a relatively constant lower level during the follicular or preovulatory phase to a somewhat higher level early in the luteal or postovulatory phase, as illustrated in Figure 41–21. Most likely, ovulation occurs just before or during the shift in temperature. The increase in the basal body temperature is believed to be caused by the thermogenic action of progesterone in the brain. Perhaps this is mediated by way of the progesterone-induced generation of the cytokine, interleukin-1β (Chap. 10, p. 201). A similar thermal response can be induced by the injection of progesterone into a castrated woman. The rise in basal body temperature,

therefore, may be evidence for the development of a corpus luteum and the secretion of progesterone. Extensive luteinization of the granulosa, however, may occur in a follicle that still contains an ovum (luteinized follicle or entrapped ovum). Such an event is believed to be one cause of a short luteal phase and thereby infertility.

CORPUS LUTEUM FORMATION

De Graaf also provided a clear description of the corpus luteum:

> Those structures, which thought normal, are only at certain times found in the testes of women, are globular bodies in the form of conglomerate glandulae which are composed of many particles, extending from the center to the circumference in straight rows, and are enveloped by a special membrane. We assert that these globules do not exist at all times in the testicles of females; on the contrary, they are only detected in them after coitus, [being] one or

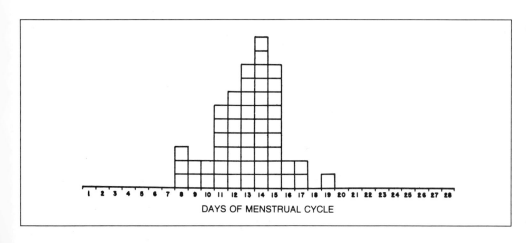

DAYS OF MENSTRUAL CYCLE

Figure 41–20. Day of ovulation in 54 women calculated from the apparent age of the corpus luteum. Each block represents an observation of one woman.

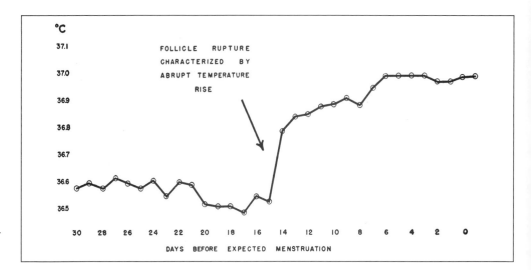

Figure 41–21. Basal temperature shift characteristic of rupture of follicle. (*From Palmer: Obstet Gynecol Survey 4:1, 1949.*)

more in number according as the animal brings forth one or more foetuses from that congress.

Probably, de Graaf concluded that coitus brought about the appearance of the corpus luteum because of comparisons he made with anatomical findings in animals that are induced-ovulators, such as the rabbit.

The corpus luteum forms in the ovary at the site of the ruptured follicle immediately after ovulation (Fig. 41–22). It is colored by a golden pigment, from which it derives its name, which means "yellow body." Microscopically, it has been observed that the corpus luteum undergoes four stages of development and demise: proliferation, vascularization, maturity, and regression.

When the mature graafian follicle ruptures, the ovum, follicular liquid, and a considerable portion of the surrounding granulosa are discharged. The collapsed walls of the empty follicle form convolutions about the blood-filled cavity (Fig. 41–23). The remaining granulosa cells appear polyhedral, with round, vesicular nuclei, and frothy cytoplasm. There are many large lacunae that contain extravasated blood but, initially, no blood vessels. The theca interna is invaginated, and its vascular channels are greatly dilated. Endothelial sprouts from the vessels penetrate the granulosa and the hemorrhagic cavity of the ruptured follicle. Hertig (1964) described the K cells (Fig. 41–24) that can be recognized in the mature graafian follicle as stellate cells in which there is deeply eosinophilic, homogenous cytoplasm. During the proliferative stage, strands of K cells, which

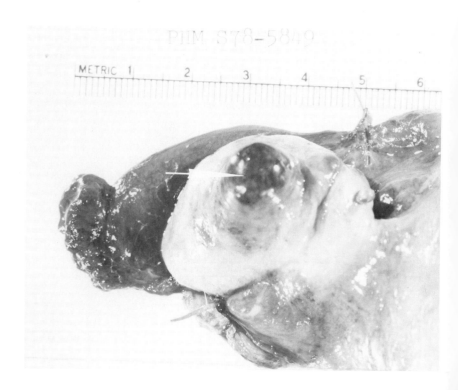

Figure 41–22. Arrow points to an intact corpus luteum of early pregnancy. (*Courtesy of Dr. R. Vogt.*)

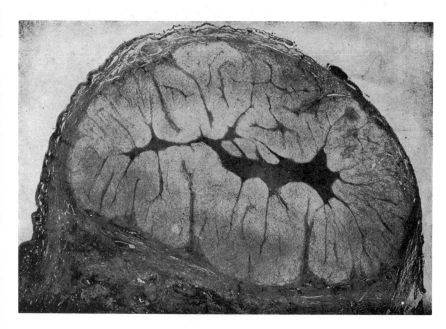

Figure 41–23. Corpus luteum of pregnancy. (Low power; see also Fig. 41–25.)

migrate from the theca, extend into the membrana granulosa to a position as far as the central coagulum.

In the stage of vascularization (which soon follows ovulation), the blood-filled cavity of the ruptured follicle undergoes rapid organization. Grossly, the central coagulum appears pale gray with only a few hemorrhagic foci. Microscopically, there are fibroblasts, but no capillaries, within the coagulum. Elsewhere in the granulosa layer, dilated capillaries are conspicu-

ous. As the stage of vascularization of the corpus luteum progresses to maturity, there is vacuolation in the periphery of the luteinized cells that originate from granulosa; this finding is suggestive that the luteinized cells are physiologically active. The theca interna cells also are vaculated; when stained for lipid, many more coarse droplets are present in the theca interna cells than in the granulosa lutein cells. The K cells continue to constitute a prominent portion of the corpus luteum cell

"K" cell   Theca lutein   Lutein cells

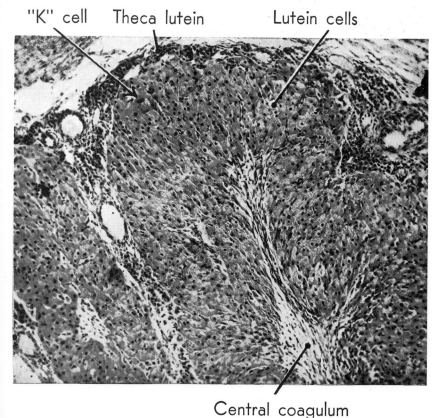

Central coagulum

Figure 41–24. Section through the wall of a mature corpus luteum of menstruation.

mass at that stage and also contain lipid, as well as alkaline phosphatase activity in great amounts. The mature corpus luteum is usually 1 to 3 cm in diameter but occasionally may occupy a third or more of the entire ovary. At this stage, the corpus luteum characteristically is bright yellow.

Regressive changes occur in the corpus luteum, occasionally as early as the 23rd day of the menstrual cycle. These changes become progressively more marked, up to the onset of menstruation, until the central coagulum has been obliterated by connective tissue, and blood pigment has been removed by leucocytes. There is no further capillary proliferation; the nuclei of the granulosa lutein cells become pale, and vacuolization of the peripheral cytoplasm decreases as coarse lipid droplets accumulate. The theca cells can be seen only in widely separated clumps. The K cells develop hyperchromatic nuclei, and the cellular outlines almost disappear. There is a progressive loss of lipid-staining material throughout the entire corpus luteum. Before menstruation, complete regression of the corpus luteum takes place. If fertilization does not take place, the corpus luteum is destined to be a *corpus luteum of menstruation*. If fertilization does take place, a *corpus luteum of pregnancy* is initiated, presumably by the action of chorionic gonadotropin, and the degenerative changes that otherwise would occur as postponed (Fig. 41–25).

Ultrastructure of the Corpus Luteum of Menstruation

Adams and Hertig (1969a) described the ultrastructure of human corpora lutea obtained approximately 2, 3, 5, 11, and 15 days after ovulation. The day 5 (menstrual cycle day 19) corpus luteum, compared with younger, differentiating and with older, regressing specimens, is one in which ultrastructural characteristics that are consistent with maximal secretion of progesterone are apparent. In the day 5 luteal cell, there is a peripheral mass

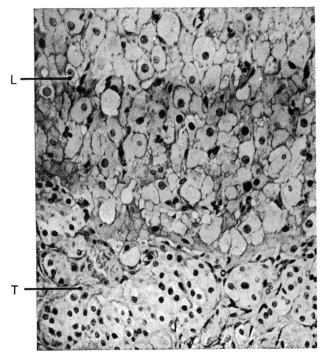

Figure 41–25. Corpus luteum of pregnancy. (High power; L = lutein cells; T = theca lutein cells.)

of agranular endoplasmic reticulum, which is merged with a large paranuclear Golgi area. Parallel cisternae of granular endoplasmic reticulum are present in the periphery. Lipid droplets and mitochondria with tubular cristae are numerous in the physiologically active cells, and the complex plasma membranes are suggestive of specialized activities.

CORPUS LUTEUM OF PREGNANCY

The duration and the function of the corpus luteum of pregnancy are the subjects of much speculation and investigation (Chaps. 5 and 10). The scientific validity of hormonal therapy in the prevention of early abortion after surgical removal of the corpus luteum is dependent on an understanding of the function of this structure.

Hertig (1964) enumerated the morphological criteria of a very early corpus luteum of pregnancy; these include (1) a surge of hyperplasia from the 23rd to 28th day after the last menstrual period, which results presumably, at least in part, from the stimulus of chorionic gonadotropin; (2) an increasing number of K cells; and (3) the absence of atrophic, ischemic, or regressive changes that are similar to those that appear when menstruation is imminent. The degenerative changes in the corpus luteum are delayed for a variable time but take place most frequently at about 6 months of gestation, although corpora lutea that appear to be normal have been found at term.

Ultrastructure of the Corpus Luteum of Pregnancy

Adams and Hertiz (1969b) compared the ultrastructure of human corpora lutea obtained during the 6th, 10th, 16th, and 35th weeks of pregnancy with that of those obtained during the menstrual cycle. In pregnancy, the luteal cell appears to be more highly compartmentalized with a peripheral mass of endoplasmic reticulum and a central area in which mitochondria and Golgi complexes are concentrated. The area that is rich in mitochondria and Golgi complexes extends to the cell surface where microvilli are found that face a vascular space. In certain luteal cells with irregular nuclear membranes, there are vesicular aggregates within the peripheral nucleoplasm or the perinuclear cytoplasm. These nuclear vesicular aggregates and certain spherical bodies may be reflective of prolonged endocrine stimulation and thence secretory exhaustion, which ultimately produce electron-dense cells in which there are pyknotic nuclei.

Crisp and co-workers (1970), in an ultrastructure study, compared the granulosa and theca lutein cells of human corpora lutea. In early pregnancy, granulosa lutein cells may be distinguished from theca lutein cells on the basis of more homogeneous, electronlucent matrix, enlarged pleomorphic mitochondria, abundant endoplasmic reticulum, and several other important ultrastructural features. Furthermore, granulosa lutein cells of early pregnancy may be distinguished from those of the progestational phase of the ovarian cycle by a well-developed endoplasmic reticulum, large spherical mitochondria, more numerous membrane-bound granules, and greater numbers of intercellular canaliculi. These investigators suggested that these differences are a result of the action of chorionic gonadotropin during early gestation. On the basis of morphological specializations, it seems likely that the corpus luteum secretes, in addition to steroids, proteinaceous products, i.e., relaxin and oxytocin (see Chap. 7, p. 134).

Function of the Corpus Luteum in Pregnancy

Numerous human pregnancies have succeeded despite early ablation of the corpus luteum. Pratt (1927) reported continuation of pregnancy after an operation was performed as early as the 20th day after the last menstrual period to remove the corpus luteum, or about the time of implantation. In a review of cases in which the corpus luteum had been removed early in pregnancy, Hall (1955) reported a rate of abortion of a little greater than 20 percent. He believed that such a rate was not higher than expected after any abdominal surgery that is conducted in the first trimester of pregnancy. In a well-designed study, Tulsky and Koff (1957) removed the corpora lutea from 14 women who requested sterilization and therapeutic abortion. Spontaneous abortion occurred in only two; in the remainder, the pregnancies were terminated by dilatation and curettage; 10 of the 14 women continued to excrete normal quantities of pregnanediol until the conceptus was removed.

The degenerative changes in the corpus luteum of an infertile cycle are delayed by the administration of chorionic gonadotropin. The corpus luteum, of course, secretes progesterone; soon after implantation, however, the human placenta apparently produces enough progesterone to maintain pregnancy. Thus, the corpus luteum, while necessary for implantation in the human, is not required for pregnancy in women beyond the earliest stages of pregnancy (Chap. 10).

Inevitably, however, the clinician must face certain therapeutic choices when obliged to remove the corpus luteum in early pregnancy from a woman who wishes to continue that pregnancy. Our choice is the use of a parenteral progestin, e.g., 17α-hydroxyprogesterone caproate (Delalutin, 150 mg) when the corpus luteum is removed prior to 10 weeks gestation. We choose 17α-hydroxyprogesterone caproate because of (1) the predictable duration of action; (2) rarely, if ever, does such treatment lead to virilization of a female fetus; and, (3) it can be given intramuscularly. Beyond 8 weeks gestation, we administer the progestin only at the time of surgery, if at all. Between 6 and 8 weeks, there may be some merit in a second injection 1 week after surgery.

CORPORA ALBICANTIA

In the absence of pregnancy, degenerated lutein cells are rapidly resorbed; and, in a short time, the corpus luteum is replaced by newly formed connective tissue that resembles closely that of the surrounding ovarian stroma. The structures formed,

called corpora albicantia, appear, on cut-section, to be dull and white, somewhat like scar tissue (Fig. 41–26); these are, however, invaded gradually by the surrounding stroma and are broken up into increasingly smaller hyaline masses, which eventually are completely resorbed. Ultimately, the site of the original follicle is indicated only by an area of slightly thickened connective tissue. In older women, this process may be slower and less complete. In women near the age of menopause, it is not uncommon to find that ovaries are almost filled by scars of various sizes.

ATRETIC FOLLICLES

Theca lutein cells are admixed somewhat with granulosa lutein cells, but, for the most part, the two cell types are distinctive in appearance. The granulosa lutein cells are larger, more highly vacuolated, and there is a smaller nucleus; the theca lutein cells are somewhat smaller, more deeply stained, and there is a relatively larger nucleus. The theca lutein cells serve a prominent role in the life history of follicles that degenerate without rupture. This process, i.e., *follicular atresia*, is particularly pronounced during pregnancy. In this circumstance, after the follicle has attained a certain size, the ovum undergoes cytolysis, while the membrana granulosa degenerates, is cast off into the liquor folliculi, and eventually is resorbed. While these changes are in progress, the theca lutein cells proliferate to form, about the follicle, a tunic many layers thick that frequently becomes yellowish. Eventually, as the follicular fluid disappears, the walls of the follicle collapse and in the theca cells that surround it, there are fatty and hyaline changes. Finally, an irregular hyaline body results that cannot be distinguished from a similar structure that was derived from a corpus luteum.

Artesia is the fate of the vast majority of follicles that develop beyond the primordial stage; the process begins during intrauterine life and continues until after the menopause. Corpora lutea, however, always develop only from the comparatively few follicles, usually one each ovarian cycle, that rupture after reaching maturity. Possibly, one of the functions of the corpus luteum is the obliteration of the spaces left by the ruptured follicles without the formation of cicatricial tissue; thus, the conversion of the entire ovary to scar tissue is prevented.

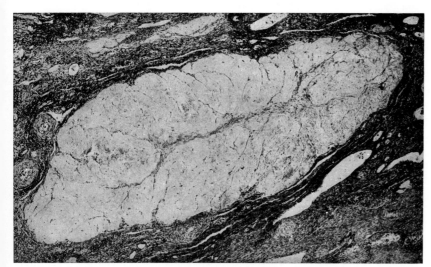

Figure 41–26. Corpus albicans.

INFERTILITY

Despite the remarkable success of pregnancy achievement in some women and despite the incredible investment of the female organism nominally in guaranteeing pregnancy, infertility (absolute or relative) probably affects no fewer than one of four married couples. Until relatively recently, obstetricians and gynecologists were obliged, for both diagnostic and therapeutic reasons, to consider only three causes of infertility: (1) anovulation; (2) obstruction of the fallopian tubes; and, (3) male infertility.

To be sure, these three causes of infertility remain as the major issues in the pathophysiology of fertility failure. But today, we recognize that infertility can be caused by (1) immunological phenomenon, (2) possibly by inadequacy of corpus luteum development or function, (3) genetic factors, and (4) for reasons not definable, but now treatable. Indeed, the therapeutics of infertility have been revolutionized in the past decade.

During this time, we have witnessed the birth of the first baby conceived by in vitro fertilization and embryo transfer. Reasonably reliable techniques for ovulation induction have been developed. Microsurgery to correct obstruction of the fallopian tubes has become commonplace and highly successful. Successful management of microadenomas of pituitary, permitting ovulation and pregnancy, is now commonplace.

Today, in cases of infertility, the greatest single challenge to successful pregnancy, i.e., the delivery of a normal, healthy baby, is to define the cause of pregnancy failure after fertilization. We have estimated that as many as 23 percent of fertilized ova are lost before clinical pregnancy is detected in normal, healthy, fertile women. Estimates conducted by others and the results of in vitro fertilization are indicative that this pregnancy loss may be much greater, especially in older women, infertile women, and in the case of late fertilization involving aging germ cells. Thus, the principal challenge of infertility is the challenge to define the nature and cause of conceptus wastage.

REFERENCES

Adams EC: Aging and reproduction. In Austin CR, Short RV (eds): Reproduction in Mammals: 4. Reproductive Patterns. Cambridge, Cambridge University Press, 1972, p 136

Adams EC, Hertig AT: Studies on the human corpus luteum: I. Observations on the ultrastructure of development and regression of the luteal cells during the menstrual cycle. J Cell Biol 41:696, 1969a

Adams EC, Hertig AT: Studies on the human corpus luteum: II. Observations on the ultrastructure of luteal cells during pregnancy. J Cell Biol 41:716, 1969b

Allen E, Pratt JP, Newell QU, Bland LJ: Human tubal ova: Related early corpora lutea and uterine tubes. Contrib Embryol 22:45, 1930

Baker TG: Oogenesis and ovulation. In Austin CR, Short RV (eds): Reproduction in Mammals: I. Germ Cells and Fertilization. Cambridge, Cambridge University Press, 1978

Beers WH: Follicular plasminogen and plasminogen activator and the effect of plasmin on ovarian follicle wall. Cell 6:379, 1975

Blandau RJ, White BJ, Rumery RE: Observations on the movements of the living primordial germ cells in the mouse. Fertil Steril 14:482, 1963

Brown MS, Kovanen PT, Goldstein JL: Receptor-mediated uptake of lipoprotein cholesterol and its utilization for steroid synthesis in the adrenal cortex. Recent Prog Horm Res 35:215, 1979

Centers for Disease Control: Human immunodeficiency virus infection in the United States. MMWR 37:4, 1988

Chang MC: The maturation of rabbit oocytes in culture and their maturation, activation, fertilization and subsequent development in the fallopian tubes. J Exp Zool 128:378, 1955

Channing CP, Anderson LD, Hoover DJ, Kolena J, Osteen KG, Pomerantz SH, Tanabe K: The role of nonsteroidal regulators in control of oocyte and follicular maturation. Recent Prog Horm Res 38:331, 1982

Channing CP, Pomerantz SH: Studies on an oocyte maturation inhibitor partially purified from porcine and human follicular fluids. In Franchimont P, Channing CP (eds): Intragonadal Regulation of Reproduction. New York, Academic, 1981, pp 81–96

Chartier M, Roger M, Barrat J, Michelon B: Measurement of plasma human chorionic gonadotropin (hCG) and β-hCG activities in the late luteal phase: Evidence of the occurrence of spontaneous menstrual abortions in infertile women. Fertil Steril 31:134, 1979

Coale AJ: The history of the human population. Sci Am 231:41, 1974

Corner GW: On the female testes or ovaries, by Regner de Graaf. In Farquar ST, Leake CD, Lyons WR, Simpson ME (eds): Essays in Biology. Los Angeles, University of California Press, 1943, p 123

Crisp TM, Dessouky DA, Denys FR: The fine structure of the human corpus luteum of early pregnancy and during the progestational phase of the menstrual cycle. Am J Anat 127:37, 1970

de Graaf R: De Mulierum organis generationi inservientibus. Lugd, Batav, 1677, p 161

Dickman Z, Noyes RW: Zona pellucida at the time of implantation: Fertil Steril 12:310, 1961

Eaton JW, Mayer AJ: The social biology of very high fertility among the Hutterites: The demography of a unique population. Hum Biol 25:206, 1953

Eddy CA, Pauerstein CJ: Anatomy and physiology of the fallopian tube. Clin Obstet Gynecol 23:1177, 1980

Edmonds DK, Linsay KS, Miller KF, Williamson E, Wood PJ: Early embryonic mortality in women. Fertil Steril 38:447, 1982

Ford CS, Beach FA: Patterns of Sexual Behavior. London, Eyre and Spottiswood, 1952

Friedman JM: Genetic disease in the offspring of older fathers. Obstet Gynecol 57:745, 1981

Hall RE: Removal of the corpus luteum in early pregnancy: A review of the literature and report of 2 cases. Bull Sloane Hosp Women 1:49, 1955

Harcourt AH, Harvey PH, Larson SG, Short RV: Testis weight, body weight and breeding system in primates. Nature 293:55, 1981

Hartman CG: How large is the mammalian egg? Q Rev Biol 4:581, 1929

Hertig AT: Gestational hyperplasia of endometrium: A morphologic correlation of ova, endometrium, and corpora lutea during early pregnancy. Lab Invest 13:1153, 1964

Hertig AT, Rock J: On the development of the early human ovum with special reference to the trophoblast of the previllous stage: A description of 7 normal and 5 pathologic human ova. Am J Obstet Gynecol 47:149, 1944

Hertig AT, Rock J, Adams EC, Menkin MC: Thirty-four fertilized human ova, good, bad and indifferent, recovered from 210 women of known fertility: A study of biologic wastage in early human pregnancy. Pediatrics (Suppl) 23:202, 1959

Illingworth DR, Corbin DK, Kemp ED, Keenan EJ: Hormone changes during the menstrual cycle in abetalipoproteinemia: Reduced luteal phase progesterone in a patient with homozygous hypobetalipoproteinemia. Proc Natl Acad Sci USA 79:6685, 1982

Jones WR: Immunologic infertility—Fact or fiction? Fertil Steril 33:577, 1980

Kolata GB: !Kung hunter-gathers: Feminism, diet and birth control. Science 185:932, 1974

Lachenbruch P: Frequency and timing of intercourse: Its relation to the probability of conception. Popul Stud 21:23, 1967

Miller JF, Williamson E, Glue J, Gordon YB, Grudzinskas JG, Sykes A: Fetal loss after implantation: A prospective study. Lancet 9:13, 1980

Milligan D, Drife JO, Short RV: Changes in breast volume during normal menstrual cycle and after oral contraceptives. Br Med J 4:494, 1975

Pinkerton JHM, McKay DG, Adams EC, Hertig AT: Development of the human ovary: Study using histochemical technics. Obstet Gynecol 18:152, 1961

Pratt JP: Corpus luteum in its relation to menstruation and pregnancy. Endocrinology 11:195, 1927

Ryan KJ, Smith OW: Biogenesis of estrogens by the human ovary: I. Conversion of acetate-1-C^{14} to estrone and estradiol. J Biol Chem 234:268, 1959

Short RV: Breast feeding. Sci Am 250:35, 1984

Short RV: The evolution of human reproduction. Proc R Soc Lond 195:3, 1976

Short RV: The origins of human sexuality. In Austin CR, Short RV (eds): Reproduction in Mammals: 8. Human Sexuality. Cambridge, Cambridge University Press, 1980, p 2

Strickland S, Beers WH: Studies of the enzymatic basis and hormonal control of ovulation. In Midgley AR, Sadler WA (eds): Ovarian Follicular Development. New York, Raven Press, 1979

Sweeney AM, Meyer MR, Aarons JH, Mills JL, LaPorte RE: Evaluation of methods for the prospective identification of early fetal losses in environmental epidemiology studies. AMJ Epidemiol 127:843, 1988

Tesh JM, Glover TD: Aging of rabbit spermatozoa in the male tract and its effect on fertility. J Reprod Fertil 20:287, 1969

Tietze C, Potter RG: Statistical evaluation of the rhythm method. Am J Obstet Gynecol 84:692, 1962

Tulsky AS, Koff AK: Some observations on the role of the corpus luteum in early human pregnancy. Fertil Steril 8:118, 1957

Vickers AD: Delayed fertilization and chromosomal anomalies in mouse embryos. J Reprod Fertil 20:69, 1969

Whittaker PG, Taylor A, Lind T: Unsuspected pregnancy loss in healthy women Lancet 1:1126, 1983

Wilcox AJ, Weinberg CR, O'Connor JF, Baird DD, Schlatterer JP, Canfield RE, Armstrong EG, Nisula BC: Incidence of early pregnancy loss. N Engl J Med 319:189, 1988

Yanagimachi R, Yanagimachi H, Rogers BJ: The use of zona-free animal ova as a test-system for the assessment of the fertilizing capacity of human spermatozoa. Biol Reprod 15:471, 1976

Family Planning

The practice of obstetrics in the United States has been influenced by forces from outside the medical community more than any other specialty to date. For in no other branch of medicine are social, religious, and political forces more obvious than in family planning. While clearly the majority of fertile American women would prefer to avoid pregnancy in any one given year, they and their physicians are continuously confronted by these forces. Thus, in spite of the recent withdrawal from the market of an efficient contraceptive technique, countless lawsuits alleging that contraception causes fetal malformations, and a variety of new formulations, the physician must continue to counsel and prescribe in an area in which confusion is common, change seems continual, and scientific evidence is often conflicting or even ignored by the legal and judicial communities.

WHO NEEDS CONTRACEPTION?

The sexually active couple, both of whom are fertile but do not desire pregnancy, needs to use effective contraception. **When no contraception is used by presumably fertile sex partners, about 90 percent of the women will conceive within 1 year.**

Young women who do not want to be pregnant are best advised to use contraception whenever they become sexually active, no matter how young. At least some girls, and perhaps the majority, ovulate before their first menstrual period.

A more difficult question to answer is, "How late in life does a woman remain capable of becoming pregnant?" Results of one study of women in the age range of 40 to 50 imply that ovulation is related more closely to the regularity of menstruation than to the age of the woman (Metcalf, 1979). *When menstruation remained regular, there was evidence of ovulation in almost every cycle.* A recent history of oligomenorrhea or of increasing cycle length was associated with a diminished frequency but not the complete absence of ovulation. Even the presence of hot flashes, amenorrhea, and elevated levels of follicle-stimulating hormone in plasma or urine do not absolutely guarantee against subsequent ovulation (Metcalf and Donald, 1979). Primordial follicles with apparently normal oocytes have been observed in ovaries removed from women over 50 years of age.

Even so, pregnancies are rare in women over 50, and extremely rare after the age of 52 (Francis, 1970). Therefore, older women are probably best advised as follows: Regular menstrual periods imply recurrent ovulation irrespective of age; however, pregnancy is rare after the age of 50. A woman younger than this who has not menstruated for 2 years is very unlikely to ovulate spontaneously and to conceive, although there are reported instances in which conception occurred more than 2 years after the onset of documented hypergonadotropic, hypoestrogenic amenorrhea (Szlachter and co-workers, 1979).

COMMONLY EMPLOYED CONTRACEPTIVE TECHNIQUES

Methods of contraception of variable effectiveness currently employed include (1) oral steroidal contraceptives, (2) injected or implanted steroidal contraceptives, (3) intrauterine devices, (4) physical, chemical, or physicochemical barrier techniques, (5) withdrawal, (6) sexual abstinence around the time of ovulation, (7) breast feeding, and (8) permanent sterilization.

The results of a national survey of the contraceptive status and most of the methods used by women of reproductive age are presented in Figure 42–1. Estimates of the failure rate with each of these techniques *during the first year of use* are presented in Table 42–1. It is emphasized that failures from patient misuse of the method are included. Effective education, as well as motivation, undoubtedly would have reduced appreciably the failure rate cited in Table 42–1. The results of the Oxford Family Planning Association contraceptive study provide strong support for this view (Vessey and co-workers, 1982). Their failure rates for more than 17,000 women who have been observed for an average of 9½ years are among the lowest reported. Failure rates for various contraceptive techniques per 100 woman-years of use were as follows: estrogen plus progestin oral contraceptives, 0.16 to 0.32; various intrauterine devices, 0.4 to 2.4; diaphragm, 1.9; and condom, 3.6. The mature woman who continued to use one technique for a long time typically experienced a very low failure rate.

Elective abortion, strickly speaking, is not a contraceptive technique, although it serves at times as a less than ideal means for preventing the birth of unwanted children (see Chap. 29). The synthetic 19-norsteroid competitive progesterone antagonist, RU 486, has been reported to be an effective orally administered abortifacient (Couzinet and associates, 1986), and may at some time in the future provide an alternative to surgical techniques currently employed. Preliminary experience with epostane, a 3β-hydroxysteroid dehydrogenase inhibitor, induced early pregnancy termination in 84 percent of women given the drug orally (Crooij and colleagues, 1988). RU 486 competes with progesterone at the endometrial receptor level. Das and Catt (1987) also demonstrated receptor blockade in vitro on syncytiotrophoblast where RU 486 impaired production of human chorionic gonadotropin, human placental lactogen, and progesterone. Epostane prevents conversion of pregnenolone to progesterone.

Nieman and colleagues (1987) reported that the oral administration to women of a single dose of RU 486 during the midluteal phase will reliably induce menses. Menstruation began within 72 hours after RU 486 administration and was not prevented by augmented progesterone production induced by the

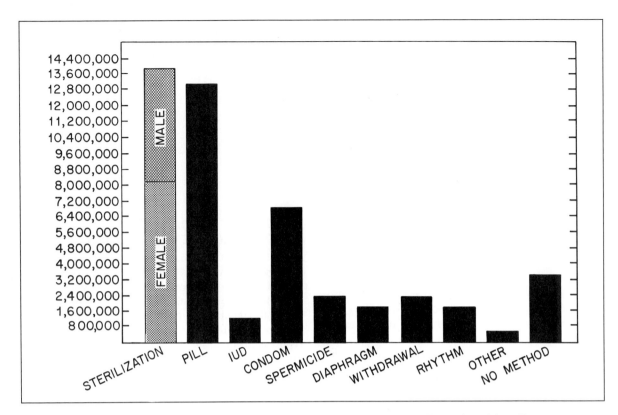

Figure 42–1. Contraceptive methods used in 1982 by women aged 15 to 44. (*Data adapted from Forrest JD, Fordyce RR: US women's contraceptive attitudes and practice: How have they changed in the 1980's? Fam Plann Perspect 20:112, 1988.*)

concomitant administration of chorionic gonadotropin. The potential usefulness of RU 486 as a once-a-month oral contraceptive is obvious, provided that long-term safety and appropriate dosage and timing can be established. Even then, the abortifacient action of the drug will preclude its being accepted by some women.

TABLE 42–1. FAILURE RATES DURING FIRST YEAR OF ATTEMPTED USE OF CONTRACEPTIVES

Methods	Lowest Observed Failure Rate (%)	Failure Rate in Typical Users (%)
Injectable progestin	0.25	0.25
Combination birth control pills	0.5	2
Progestin-only pill	1	2.5
Intrauterine device	1.5	5
Condom	2	10
Diaphragm (with spermicide)	2	19
Sponge (with spermicide)	9–11	10–20
Foams, creams, jellies, and vaginal suppositories	3–5	18
Withdrawal	16	23
Periodic rhythmic abstinence	2–20	24
Douche	—	40
Chance (no method)	90	90

Adapted from Williams NB: Contraceptive Technology 1986–1987. New York, Irvington, 1986.

HORMONAL CONTRACEPTIVES

Over 13 million women in the United States use one of the variety of hormonal contraceptives available for fertility control. Although hormonal contraceptives represented a dramatic departure from previous traditional methods, they also created a unique therapeutic dilemma. As stated in a report of an advisory committee to the Food and Drug Administration, "Never will so many people have taken such potent drugs voluntarily over such a protracted period for an objective other than for the control of disease." For some women, however, an unwanted pregnancy is in some ways a sexually transmitted disease.

ESTROGEN PLUS PROGESTIN CONTRACEPTIVES

The oral contraceptives most often employed now consist of a combination of an estrogen and a progestational agent taken daily for 3 weeks and omitted for 1 week, during which time withdrawal uterine bleeding normally occurs. In the United States the estrogen is ethinyl estradiol or its 3-methyl ether (mestranol), which is promptly metabolized to ethinyl estradiol. A greater variety of compounds with progestational activity is used, including norethindrone, norgestrel, ethynodiol diacetate, and norethindrone acetate.

MECHANISMS OF ACTION

The contraceptive actions of the combined estrogen-progestin steroidal medication are multiple. A most important effect is to prevent ovulation, almost certainly by suppression of hypothalamic releasing factors, which, in turn, leads to inappropriate secretion by the pituitary of follicle-stimulating and luteinizing hormones (Fig. 42–2). Other contraceptive effects induced by the combined steroids include altered maturation of the endometrium, rendering it inappropriate for successful implantation if a blastocyst were to develop, and the production of cervical mucus hostile to penetration by sperm. The possible role, if any, of altered tubal and uterine motility induced by the hormones is not clear. As the consequence of these actions, combined estrogen plus progestin oral contraceptives, *if taken daily for 3 weeks out of every 4,* provide virtually absolute protection against conception. An important exception, however, is the period of about a week immediately following initiation of use of an oral contraceptive. Indeed, in the woman with a maturing follicle who is soon to ovulate spontaneously, ovulation may actually be triggered by starting oral contraceptives in this circumstance.

DOSAGE AND ADMINISTRATION

To prevent induction of ovulation, as well as to help recognize preexisting early pregnancy, it is generally recommended that women begin the use of oral contraceptives on one of the first 7 days of the menstrual cycle. Many women, however, start their use after delivery or abortion, before the return of spontaneous menses. If their use is initiated at any time other than during or immediately after a normal menstrual cycle, or within 3 weeks of delivery, another means of birth control should be used throughout the first week to avoid the risk of induced ovulation.

To help achieve regular administration of the combined oral contraceptive, and thereby obtain maximum protection, several suppliers offer dispensers that provide sequentially 21 individually wrapped, color-coded tablets that contain hormones, followed by seven inert tablets of another color (Fig. 42–3). Many of these dispensers come with the day of the week imprinted next to each tablet or with a variable calendar that may be affixed to the dispenser.

It is important for maximum contraceptive efficiency and for peace of mind that the woman adopt an effective scheme for assuring daily (or nightly) self-administration. One technique is to keep her pill supply and toothbrush close to each other and to swallow a pill at the time of brushing the teeth. If one dose is missed, nothing serious will happen; it may be desirable to double the next dose to minimize breakthrough bleeding and to "stay on schedule." If several doses are missed, another form of effective contraception (a barrier technique) should be used whenever intercourse is contemplated. The pill can be started after withdrawal bleeding. Without any bleeding, the possibility of pregnancy must be considered.

Since oral contraceptives have come into use, the amounts of estrogen and progestational agent contained in each tablet have been reduced considerably. It is now known that effective contraception can be achieved with doses of the steroids that are quite small compared to those originally used. This is of considerable importance, since adverse effects are to a degree dose-related. The lowest acceptable limit of dosage is set by the ability of the medication to prevent unacceptable breakthrough bleeding from the endometrium (Edelman and associates, 1983). The amount of estrogen most commonly administered daily is 30 to 50 µg of either ethinyl estradiol or mestranol. Oral contraceptive tablets that contain as little as 20 µg of ethinyl estradiol per tablet are commercially available. No tablet sold in the United

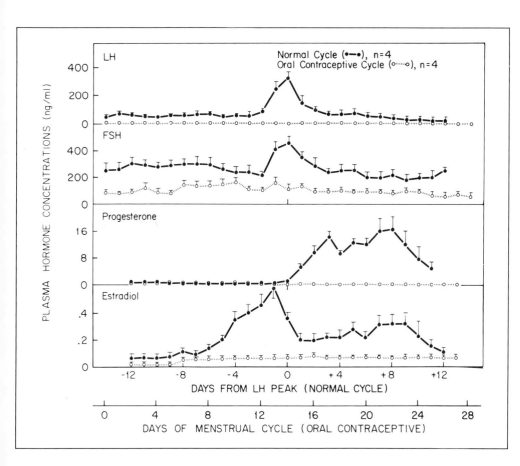

Figure 42–2. Plasma levels of luteinizing hormone (LH), follicle-stimulating hormone (FSH), progesterone, and 17-β estradiol in four ovulatory women and in four women who were ingesting one tablet daily of an oral contraceptive that contained 80 µg of mestranol and 1 mg of norethindrone. Note the suppression of all four hormones in the women taking the oral contraceptives. (*From Carr and colleagues: J Clin Endocrinol Metab 49:346, 1979.*)

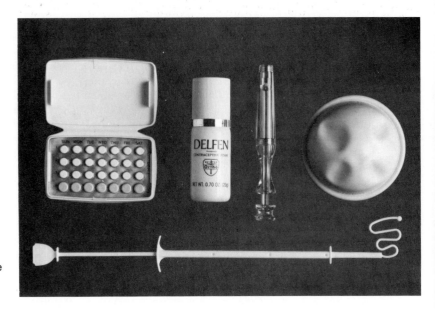

Figure 42–3. Shown left to right are oral contraceptive tablets in a container, a tube of vaginal contraceptive cream plus applicator, a diaphragm, and, below, a Lippes Loop intrauterine device and inserter. Just before insertion, the rod is withdrawn until all of the device is pulled into the inserter tube.

States contains more than 50 μg (FDA Drug Bulletin, 1988). The amount of progestin varies in two ways: (1) Among older, now well-evaluated formulations the progestational activity will vary depending upon the compound used but the daily dosage of the compound ingested throughout the cycle is constant, for example, 1 mg of norethindrone daily. (2) In some more recent preparations the dosage of the progestin varies throughout the cycle.

Phasic Pills

These preparations were developed in an effort to reduce the amount of total progestin ingested in a single cycle without sacrificing contraceptive efficacy or cycle control. This reduction of progestin dose is achieved by beginning the contraceptive cycle with a low dose of progestin and increasing this later in the cycle. They have been shown to be highly effective to prevent pregnancy (Ellis, 1987; Toews and colleagues, 1987). The theoretical advantage of a reduction in dose is a reduction in those metabolic changes which are attributable to the progestin, and thereby a reduction in those adverse effects from such metabolic changes. Any beneficial effects of oral contraceptives which may be the consequence of progestins, may also be reduced. The triphasic oral contraceptives initially marketed in 1984 in the United States have achieved great popularity and now account for the majority of new oral contraceptive prescriptions. Estrogen dose may be kept constant, or it is increased temporarily later in the cycle, but in all preparations it is kept low with only 30 to 40 μg of ethinyl estradiol.

Investigational Contraceptive Steroids

Three new potent progestins—desogestrel, norgestimate, and gestodene—are currently undergoing extensive study in both the United States and Europe for possible use in oral contraceptives. Preliminary reports suggest that oral contraceptives containing low doses of these new progestins may be associated with minimal metabolic changes but excellent cycle control (Runnebaum and Rabe, 1987). It is anticipated that these new progestins may be approved for commerical sale in both fixed dose and phasic pills within the next several years.

ADVERSE AND BENEFICIAL EFFECTS FROM ORAL CONTRACEPTIVES

The combined estrogen plus progestin pill taken 3 weeks out of every 4 is the most effective reversible form of contraception available. Failure rates of 0.32 per 100 woman-years or lower have been documented (Vessey and co-workers, 1982). Other reported beneficial effects include reduced menstrual blood loss; less dysmenorrhea, functional ovarian cysts and salpingitis; fewer premenstrual complaints; less endometrial and ovarian cancer; reduction in various benign breast diseases and possibly breast cancer; and less rheumatoid arthritis (Andersch and Hahn, 1981; Mishell, 1982; Centers for Disease Control, 1983).

At the outset, concern was rightfully raised for the safety of users of oral contraceptives. Fortunately, no major disasters have occurred, and, in general, the use of oral contraceptives, when appropriately monitored as outlined below, has proved to be safe for the great majority of women.

The possibility of adverse effects from oral contraceptives has received so much attention for so long that the major adverse effect among their users may be the anxiety that has been created by the almost incessant publicity so generated. It would seem that among the data banks of several centers the slightest suggestion of variation in the apparent health status of pill users automatically triggers an outflow of statistical probabilities to word processors for manuscript production, followed soon thereafter by publication and instant dissemination by the lay press, radio, and television. Physicians and public alike are frequently confused by the many and often conflicting reports with which they continue to be bombarded.

Metabolic Changes

A variety of metabolic changes, often qualitatively similar to those of pregnancy, has been identified in women taking oral contraceptives. For example, plasma thyroxine and thyroid binding proteins are elevated appreciably whereas triiodothyronine uptake by resin is lowered. Another change similar to that induced by normal pregnancy is elevation of plasma cortisol concentration with a nearly comparable increase in transcortin. It is extremely important, therefore, that evaluation of results of these laboratory tests and others be considered in light of whether or not the woman is using an estrogen-containing oral contraceptive. The estrogen in a combined pill appears to decrease the serum concentration of low-density lipoprotein cholesterol and to increase high-density lipoprotein cholesterol, but some progestins, at least, cause the reverse (Stadel, 1981). The importance of such changes in the genesis of *arterial vascular disease* such as myocardial infarctions or stroke in users of oral contraceptives is not clear but, nonetheless, is cause for concern. (Knopp, 1988; Meade, 1988; Mishell, 1988).

The contraceptive steroids may intensify preexisting *diabetes* or may prove sufficiently diabetogenic to induce clinically apparent disease in women prone to develop diabetes. However, the risk of the latter appears slight since in the great majority of women the effect on carbohydrate metabolism is slight. Phillips and Duffy (1973), for example, identified serum glucose levels 1 hour after administration of 75 g of glucose orally to average 11 mg per dL more in users of oral contraceptives than in nonusers. As with pregnancy, diabetogenic effects most often appear to be reversible when use of the oral contraceptive is terminated (Wingrave and associates, 1979).

The use of estrogen-progestin oral contraceptives in women who had *gestational diabetes* has been discouraged by some for many years. Initially concern centered around the possible acceleration of the appearance of permanent diabetes by the mild carbohydrate intolerance occasionally encountered in women who take oral contraceptives. In his brief review of this subject, Kalkhoff (1980) suggests that while the incidence of diabetes among normal women taking estrogen-progestin oral contraceptives is essentially identical to the incidence in a general population of women, the incidence of diabetes among women with previous gestational diabetes taking oral contraceptives is increased tenfold. Since the number of women with previous gestational diabetes studied while taking oral contraceptives is very small and the proportion of gestational diabetics who are expected to become permanent diabetics later in life is very large, the ability of oral contraceptives to hasten the appearance of permanent diabetes in gestational diabetics is still an important but largely unanswered question.

More recently, concern about the use of oral contraceptives in women with previous gestational diabetes has centered around the possible association between mild hyperglycemia and/or hyperinsulinemia and an increased risk for cardiovascular disease. In this context, a recent report by Skouby and associates (1985) is encouraging. These investigators described a small group of women with previous gestational diabetes who were using a triphasic oral contraceptive pill, and reported that glucose, insulin, and glucagon response, as well as serum cholesterol, high-density lipoproteins and low-density lipoproteins were unchanged compared to pretreatment values.

Argument persists as to whether women with *overt* diabetes should use oral contraceptives. A general policy established early in the development of the Greater Dallas Family Planning Program operated by the Department of Obstetrics and Gynecology of the University of Texas Southwestern Medical Center would preclude their use in this circumstance. The policy is as follows: **No women with systemic chronic disease shall be given an oral contraceptive except in circumstances where it can be verified that the merits from its use undoubtedly outweigh any risks.**

Cholestasis and *cholestatic jaundice* are uncommon complications in users of oral contraceptives; the signs and symptoms clear when the medication is stopped. A somewhat increased risk of surgically identified gallstones and *gallbladder disease* was reported for users of oral contraceptives. However, results of a more recent study by the Royal College of General Practitioners (1982) suggest that oral contraceptives may only accelerate the development of gallbladder disease in women who are susceptible and that there is no overall increased long-term risk. There appears to be no reason to withhold oral contraceptives from women fully recovered from viral hepatitis.

Neoplasia

The possible role of hormonal contraception in the causation of neoplasia is not clear. There are reports that suggest that the risk of malignant and premalignant change in the cervix and breast is increased, or decreased, or unchanged. If there is an increased risk, it most likely is slight (Vessey and co-workers, 1983a, 1983b; Pike and co-workers, 1983; McPherson and associates, 1983; Wiseman, 1983; Food and Drug Administration Advisory Committee, 1984).

Recent data from the Cancer and Steroid Hormone Study (1987 a,b) provide evidence that oral contraceptive use protects women from developing *endometrial and ovarian cancers*. In this case-controlled study, the relative risk for steroidal contraceptive users developing either type of cancer was 0.6 compared to nonusers. These protective effects were seen with use for as little as 3 to 12 months, and persisted for 15 years after use ended.

Use of estrogen plus progestin contraceptives has been linked circumstantially with the development of *hepatic focal nodular hyperplasia* and actual tumor formation that most often, but not necessarily always, is benign. In fact, Neuberger and associates (1986) reported an association between prolonged oral contraceptive use and *hepatocellular carcinoma* in women under the age of 50. A prominent feature of the benign tumor nodules is increased vascularity with extensive proliferation of large and small thin-walled blood vessels. Therefore, the lesions, upon rupture, can be complicated by bleeding, hemoperitoneum, and shock, which in 8 of 24 cases cited by Antoniades (1975) proved fatal. The liver may become enlarged to palpation, and by means of computed tomography, magnetic resonance imaging, sonography, liver scans, and angiography, a space-occupying lesion or lesions can be visualized. If identified before rupture, resection of the lesion, along with stopping the use of oral contraceptives, has been recommended. Some liver lesions appear to have disappeared after merely stopping the use of oral contraceptives. Increased growth and vascularity during pregnancy or the puerperium, leading to rupture, and causing death of the mother, have been described (Kent and co-workers, 1978). Fortunately, such liver lesions associated with the use of oral contraceptives are rare and steroid-dose related.

It is not clear at this time whether oral contraceptives contribute to the development of *breast cancer*. Three recently published studies fail to clarify this issue. In the Cancer and Steroid Hormone Study (1986), the largest study to date, no increased risk for breast cancer among oral contraceptive users was demonstrated. Moreover, the risk did not vary according to preparation or duration of use. While a New Zealand study (Paul and colleagues, 1986) confirmed these findings, a Swedish study (Meirik and associates, 1986) published on the same date contained evidence of a slightly increased risk of breast cancer among women who used oral contraceptives for 12 or more years. If there is an increased risk of breast malignancy from use of estrogen plus progestin oral contraceptives, the risk must be small.

Although it has been suggested that oral contraceptives might increase the risk of pituitary *prolactinomas*, the Pituitary Adenoma Study Group (1983) provided evidence that this is not the case. The awareness in recent years that these neoplasms may cause menstrual irregularities, along with the technology to visualize them radiographically, has resulted in the diagnosis of these adenomas even before steroidal contraceptives are given.

Nutrition

Aberrations in the levels of several *nutrients* have been described for women who use oral contraceptives and typically are similar to changes induced by normal pregnancy. Lower plasma levels in users compared to nonusers have been described by some investigators, but not all, for ascorbic acid, folic acid, vitamin B_{12}, niacin, riboflavin, and zinc. Moreover, biochemical changes compatible with, but not necessarily proof of, vitamin B_6 deficiency have been documented repeatedly but do not differ from those that accompany normal pregnancy (Theur, 1972; Wynn, 1975).

The possibilities of folate deficiency and of vitamin B_6 deficiency as the consequence of oral contraceptives have received considerable attention. *Folate deficiency* developing from use of oral contraceptives was suggested by Streiff (1970), who described in a few women who were using oral contraceptives severe megaloblastic anemia that responded to pteroylmonoglutamic acid but not to pteroylpolyglutamic acid unless the ingestion of the contraceptive was stopped. He believed that the estrogen of the contraceptive blocked intestinal conjugase (pteroylpolyglutamate hydrolase) and thereby prevented the cleavage of pteroylglutamate to an absorbable active form, a view not supported by the studies of Stephens and co-workers (1972). Shojania and associates (1968) reported serum folate levels of women who used oral contraceptives to be somewhat lower than those who did not. This triggered a chain reaction of reports that about equally confirmed and denied the findings of Shojania.

The observations of Pritchard and associates (1971) may provide an explanation for the discrepancies. In their initial study, they compared plasma folate levels of socioeconomically somewhat privileged users and nonusers of oral contraceptives who were employed by the hospital or medical school or were wives of employees. No difference in serum folate levels was found. They subsequently carried out similar studies of socioeconomically less privileged women who attended the free family planning clinics. Again they found no difference in plasma folate levels between users and nonusers, but their plasma folate levels were lower than those of the more affluent groups first studied. In other words, less affluent users and nonusers of oral contraceptives had lower folate levels than more affluent users.

Prasad and associates (1978) appear to have utilized about all of the possible permutations for apparent effects of oral contraceptives on blood folate levels when they reported the following: For nonusers of oral contraceptives blood folate levels were higher in women of upper socioeconomic class. With the use of oral contraceptives by women of upper socioeconomic class blood folate levels were lower than for nonusers in that class. In women of lower socioeconomic class, however, the blood folate levels were no lower in users than in nonusers.

A number of women with overt megaloblastic anemia resulting from folate deficiency during pregnancy have subsequently been followed, some of whom used an oral contraceptive beginning shortly after delivery (Scott and Pritchard, 1975). One relapsed remote from pregnancy while using an oral contraceptive, as did one who did not use an oral contraceptive. In both instances, relapse occurred while the women were consuming atrocious diets essentially devoid of any folate. We are therefore of the opinion that use of the typical estrogen-progestin oral contraceptive is rarely by itself a cause of clinically significant folate deficiency. This opinion is not shared by all.

Pyridoxine deficiency in women who use oral contraceptives has been implicated as a cause of mental depression, a phenomenon that is not a frequent complication of oral contraceptive use. Estrogens induce in the liver the rate-limiting enzyme, tryptophan oxygenase, that enhances tryptophan metabolism in a way that suggests pyridoxine deficiency (Wynn, 1975). To abolish these biochemical variations suggestive of pyridoxine deficiency, as much as 20 to 30 mg of pyridoxine, or 10 times the usual intake, need be ingested! Since altered tryptophan metabolism persists in contraceptive users even when other indices of vitamin B_6 nutrition are normal, Leklem and co-workers (1975) believe that oral contraceptives specifically affect tryptophan metabolism by some means other than through vitamin B_6 deficiency.

It also has been suggested that altered tryptophan metabolism, as the consequence of oral contraceptives, may have a diabetogenic effect. For example, tryptophan has been reported to bind to insulin (Larrson-Cohn, 1975). Moreover, Spellacy and associates (1972) claimed that women who were taking oral contraceptives and who experienced deterioration of glucose tolerance showed partial improvement in glucose tolerance after administration of pyridoxine. These observations have not been confirmed.

The similarity of changes in tryptophan and pyridoxine metabolism to those of normal pregnancy strongly implies that estrogen-progestin contraceptives do not induce significant pathologic changes as the consequence of pyridoxine deficiency any more than does normal pregnancy.

Combined estrogen-progestin oral contraceptives conserve *iron* by reducing blood loss from menstruation. Nilsson and Sölvell (1967) compared hemoglobin shed by apparently normal women during spontaneous menses with hemoglobin shed by withdrawal bleeding following estrogen-progestin contraceptives, and they noted that the contraceptives reduced the amount of hemoglobin shed by one half. By quantitative measurements, Pritchard (unpublished) has demonstrated blood loss from spontaneous menses to decrease from as much as 400 mL per cycle to less than 30 mL when 100 µg of mestranol plus 2 mg of norethindrone was ingested daily by two young women with cyclic menorrhagia of unknown cause. The menorrhagia recurred when the oral contraceptive was stopped. It is apparent, therefore, that women who typically lose more than the average amount of blood with their periods may benefit from oral contraceptives by becoming iron sufficient. Moreover, women with *dysmenorrhea* from endometriosis or from idiopathic causes are likely to enjoy appreciable relief from pain while using combined oral contraceptives.

At times, while using the combined medication, the amount of blood and endometrium shed is so scant that the woman believes she is amenorrheic and concludes that she is pregnant, especially if she has missed a tablet or two. She then stops taking the medication and, unfortunately, soon thereafter does conceive. Increasing the estrogen dose particularly for the first 7 days of a contraceptive cycle usually will alleviate the amenorrhea. Women who can recognize early pregnancy symptoms can be maintained on low estrogen doses and reassured that the amenorrhea is not harmful.

Cardiovascular Effects

The risk of *deep vein thrombosis* and *pulmonary embolism* has been estimated to be 3 to 11 times greater in women who used oral contraceptives than in otherwise apparently similar women who did not (Realini and Goldzieher, 1985; Stadel, 1981). Moreover, the use of oral contraceptives during the month before an operative procedure appears to increase the risk of postoperative thromboembolism significantly. Pills that contain less estrogen appear to be associated with a smaller increase in risk of venous thrombosis and thromboembolism. In 1988, all manufacturers of oral contraceptives stopped production of preparations containing more than 50 μg of estrogen.

The mechanism by which estrogen-progestin contraceptives enhance the risk of venous thrombosis and thromboembolism is not altogether clear. The development of distinctive vascular intimal and medial lesions with associated occlusive thrombi have been described (Irey and co-workers, 1970). Moreover, platelet aggregation may be accelerated and both plasma antithrombin III activity and endothelial plasminogen activator are likely to be reduced somewhat while using estrogen plus progestin oral contraceptives (Stadel, 1981).

The enhanced risk of thromboembolism appears to decrease rapidly once the oral contraceptive is stopped. The woman who developed thromboembolism while taking estrogen-containing contraceptives, however, appears also to be at increased risk of thromboembolism during pregnancy and the early puerperium (Badaracco and Vessey, 1974).

Arterial thrombosis has also been attributed to the use of estrogen plus progestin contraceptives. The relative risk of a stroke seems to be about four times greater than in women who do not use oral contraceptives and appears to be confined largely to women about 35 years old or older (Stadel, 1981).

An association between oral contraceptives and *hypertension* became apparent in the late 1960s, when several reports appeared of the occasional woman who, while using an estrogen-progestin contraceptive, became overtly hypertensive. Usually, but not always, she became normotensive when the medication was stopped. The oral contraceptives, presumably in response chiefly to the estrogen contained, were shown to increase markedly the plasma level of renin substrate and, to a lesser degree, renin, to near the levels found in normal pregnancy. The great majority of women using oral contraceptives demonstrate these changes, as in pregnancy, yet do not become hypertensive. The progestin appears to contribute to the hypertension that develops in some women. Weir (1982) observed that women who had developed hypertension while taking estrogen-progestin oral contraceptives and who had become normotensive after stopping the contraceptive became hypertensive again when oral contraception was reinstituted, even if the contraceptive employed contained no estrogen. Fisch and Frank (1977) evaluated blood pressures of a large number of women who were using oral contraceptives and identified the mean systolic and diastolic blood pressures to be only 5 to 6 and 1 to 2 mm Hg higher, respectively, than in the age-adjusted control group. Not surprisingly, the risk of hypertension attributable to oral contraceptives has been observed to increase with age (Stadel, 1981).

Unfortunately, normotensive women who are destined to become hypertensive in response to oral contraceptives usually cannot be identified in advance. The development of hypertension during pregnancy does not preclude subsequent use of oral contraceptives. Pritchard and Pritchard (1977) evaluated the pressor response to oral contraceptives in young black women who had developed overt pregnancy-induced hypertension but postpartum had diastolic blood pressures of 90 mm Hg or less when oral contraceptives were started. The contraceptive dose provided 50 μg of mestranol and 1 mg of norethindrone daily. Over an average of 1½ years, only 6 percent demonstrated a rise in diastolic pressure above 90 mm Hg, a frequency not remarkably different from that observed in initially normotensive young nulligravid black women who used the same kind of oral contraceptive. Moreover, Fisch and Frank (1977) found no significant association between hypertension from use of oral contraceptives and previous hypertension during pregnancy.

In keeping with the policy of not giving estrogen plus progestin contraceptives to women who demonstrate systemic chronic disease, we do not give them to hypertensive women. Moreover, every woman's blood pressure is rechecked when contraceptive refills are provided 3 months after starting the medication, and every 9 to 12 months thereafter. At each visit, usually a nurse or, at times, a physician performs a brief but pertinent interrogation designed to uncover other possibly adverse effects from the use of oral contraceptives. Smoking is discouraged. Physical examination is repeated annually, or more often if an abnormality is suspected. Whenever hypertension is detected, the oral contraceptive is stopped and another form of contraception is substituted.

Several epidemiolgoical studies very strongly imply, at least, that use of estrogen plus progestin oral contraceptives increases the risk of *myocardial infarction*. Mann and Inman (1975) noted a significant association, which became stronger with increasing age. Use of oral contraceptives by women who were heavy smokers, were obese, were being treated for hypertension and diabetes, or had type II hyperlipoproteinemia increased the risk of myocardial infarction remarkably, the effects being synergistic rather than merely additive.

The frequency and intensity of attacks of *migraine headaches* may be enhanced appreciably by estrogen plus progestin contraceptives. We prefer to avoid these contraceptives for a woman with migraine, not only because they are likely to be unacceptable to her, but also because some migraine symptoms and signs are indistinguishable from mild or impending stroke.

Realini and Goldzieher (1985) appropriately identified methodological flaws in essentially every published study associating oral contraceptive use with an increased risk of cardiovascular disease including venous thromboembolism, stroke, and myocardial infarction. They correctly warn physicians to interpret these studies with care and to continue to question the reported relationships. Nevertheless, from a medicolegal standpoint it seems foolhardy to ignore these studies. At the very least, women should be informed of the *possible* association between cardiovascular disease and the use of oral contraceptives. Fortuantely, Stampfer and colleagues (1988) showed from prospective data that use of steroidal contraceptives in the past does not increase the risk of subsequent cardiovascular disease.

Risk of Death

A number of adverse effects have been identified for users of oral contraceptives. As borne out by the data in Table 42–2, the risk of death from the use of an oral contraceptive is very low if the woman is under 35, has no systemic illness, and does not smoke. Porter and associates (1987) reported their experiences with nearly 55,000 woman-years of oral contraceptive use in the Group Health Cooperative of Puget Sound, and attributed only one death to their use. The risk of dying as the consequence of using an oral contraceptive is certainly less than that of pregnancy, even though the risk with the latter is actually quite low. Moreover, serious morbidity, as well as mortality, almost certainly would be minimized by avoiding the use of the estrogen plus progestin pill in those circumstances listed in Table 42–3.

Effects on Reproduction

When the estrogen-progestin contraceptive is discontinued, ovulation usually, but not always, promptly resumes. Similar to

TABLE 42–2. ESTIMATES OF MORTALITY RATES (PER 100,000) ASSOCIATED WITH PREGNANCY AND CHILDBIRTH, FIRST TRIMESTER LEGAL ABORTION, ORAL CONTRACEPTIVES, AND INTRAUTERINE DEVICES

| Age Group (Yr) | Pregnancy and Childbirth | First Trimester Legal Abortion | Oral Contraceptives | | Intrauterine Devices |
			Nonsmokers	Smokers	
15–19	11.1	1.2	1.2	1.4	0.8
20–24	10.0	1.2	1.2	1.4	0.8
25–29	12.5	1.4	1.2	1.4	1.0
30–34	24.9	1.4	1.8	10.4	1.0
35–39	44.0	1.8	3.9	12.8	1.4
40–44	71.4	1.8	6.6	58.4	1.4

Adapted from Tietze: Fam Plan Perspect 9:74, 1977.

the postpartum period, within 3 months after discontinuance at least 90 percent of women who previously ovulated regularly will have done so again. *Post-pill amenorrhea* poses no long-term threat to fertility (Hull and associates, 1981; Linn and colleagues, 1982). In the rare instance in which *anovulation* persists and is not caused by unrecognized early pregnancy or pituitary adenoma or by premature menopause, ovulation may be induced successfully.

Whether very recent use of oral contraceptives before a pregnancy or continued use during early unrecognized pregnancy might adversely affect the fetus has been the source of much concern. The report by Linn and co-workers (1983) provides some assurance that they do not. They did not show an increased risk of major fetal malformations among users of oral contraceptives (or for users of diaphragm or foam barrier techniques).

Even though an association between *congenital defects* and the use of oral contraceptives during early pregnancy has not been established, the woman who thinks that she may be pregnant is best advised to stop the oral contraceptive (*but use another contraceptive technique!*) until it can be established whether or not she is pregnant.

Harlap and Eldor (1980) and others reported a slight increase in both major and minor fetal malformations when the mother had recently used combined oral contraceptives. They

also noted a preponderance of male offspring and significantly increased frequency of twinning. Teratogenic effects in pregnancies conceived while taking or soon after taking the pill reported to date have included fetal limb-reduction deformities (Janevich and co-workers, 1974; Nora and Nora, 1975). Rothman and Louik (1978) and Savolainen (1981), however, found little difference for major malformations between infants whose mothers had very recently used oral contraceptives and those whose mothers had not. Lammer and Cordero (1986) found no association between any major malformation and oral contraceptive exposure in early pregnancy (see Chap. 32, p. 569).

Use of contraceptive hormones by nursing mothers tends to reduce the amount of *breast milk*; however, only very small quantities of the hormones are excreted in the milk.

Other Effects

Cervical mucorrhea is fairly common in response to the estrogen contained, and the mucus at times may be irritating to the vagina and vulva. *Vaginitis* or *vulvovaginitis,* especially that caused by *Candida,* may develop. Antibiotic therapy in pill users increases the frequency of such an infection.

Hyperpigmentation of the face and forehead (*chloasma*) is more likely to occur in women who demonstrate such a change during pregnancy. *Acne* may improve or, at times, be aggravated.

Uterine *myomas* may increase in size more rapidly in response to the estrogen of oral contraceptives than they would otherwise but this is not a consistent phenomenon.

Weight gain has been a troublesome complaint from women who use oral contraceptives, although an increase in weight is far from a uniform phenomenon. Some of the weight may be caused by fluid retention, but it is likely to be a consequence of increased dietary intake.

Oral contraceptives often ameliorate the *dysmenorrhea* associated with endometriosis. Their use may even reduce the risk of a woman developing severe endometriosis.

TABLE 42–3. SOME IMPORTANT CONTRAINDICATIONS TO USE OF ESTROGEN PLUS PROGESTIN CONTRACEPTIVES

1. Thromboembolism, current or past
2. Cerebrovascular accident, current or past
3. Coronary artery disease
4. Impaired liver function
5. Liver adenoma, current or past
6. Breast cancer
7. Hypertension
8. Diabetes
9. Gallbladder disease
10. Cholestatic jaundice during pregnancy
11. Sickle cell hemoglobinopathy
12. Surgery contemplated within 4 weeks
13. Major surgery on or immobilization of lower extremity
14. Over 40 years of age
15. Smoke heavily
16. Familial hyperlipidemia
17. Antiphospholipid antibodies

Postpartum Use

Recently pregnant women who do not nurse their children, and especially those who have undergone abortions, may ovulate before 6 to 7 weeks after pregnancy termination (Chap. 13, p. 254). The administration of bromocriptine for lactation suppression in puerperal women may hasten ovulation by 1 to 2 weeks. There is an advantage, therefore, to starting oral contraceptives before the traditional "6 weeks postpartum check." On the other hand, increased risks of adverse effects, especially venous thromboembolism, might be anticipated from use of estrogen-progestin contraceptives earlier in the puerperium. So far, in our now extensive experience in which oral contraceptives have been started typically during the third week postpartum, there has been no evidence of increased morbidity.

Cost

Unfortunately, the cost of oral contraceptives has increased remarkably in recent years perhaps as the consequence of extensive and expensive litigation arising from lawsuits filed by some users. Their price cannot accurately reflect the cost of the ingredients.

In January, 1987, fixed dose estrogen-progestin contraceptives containing norethindrone and either 35 μg or 50 μg of estrogen were first marketed as *generic products* in the United States. Because United States regulation allows a 25 percent variance in bioavailability, poor cycle control might follow their use in women as they change from one generic manufacturer to another. It is too early to tell whether this problem will develop at all or with sufficient frequency to offset the advantage of the modest cost reduction that certainly will be associated with the generic product.

PROGESTATIONAL AGENTS ALONE

ORAL PROGESTINS ALONE

The so-called mini-pill, consisting solely of 0.5 mg or less of a progestational agent daily, has not achieved widespread popularity because of a much higher incidence of irregular bleeding and a higher pregnancy rate. The progestational agent alone presumably impairs fertility, without necessarily inhibiting ovulation, by causing formation of cervical mucus that impedes sperm penetration and by altering endometrial maturation sufficiently to thwart successful implantation of a blastocyst.

INJECTABLE HORMONAL CONTRACEPTIVES

The advantages of injected medroxyprogesterone acetate (Depo-Provera) are a contraceptive effectiveness comparable to the combined oral contraceptives, long-lasting action with injections required only two to four times a year, and lactation not likely to be impaired. The mechanisms of action appear to be multiple, and include inhibition of ovulation, increased viscosity of cervical mucus, and an endometrium unfavorable to ovum implantation.

The disadvantages are prolonged amenorrhea, or uterine bleeding, or both, during and after its use, and prolonged anovulation after discontinuation (Cheng and associates, 1974). The risk of venous thrombosis and thromboembolism appears to be increased, as with estrogen plus progestin oral contraceptives (Schwallie, 1974). The potentially adverse effects of the unopposed progestin on serum lipoprotein concentrations are also of serious concern (Bradley, 1978). Obviously, these adverse effects must be explained to the woman and her consent obtained to use such a preparation for contraception. Unfortunately, the woman who may be best served by such a contraceptive agent may not be able to comprehend these potential problems.

Injected medroxyprogesterone acetate (Depo-Provera) has been widely used for contraception in several countries but not in the United States. It has been estimated that one million women throughout the world depend on an injectable progestin for contraception. Food and Drug Administration hearings are held periodically, with great public awareness through television, radio, newspapers, and magazines, but medroxyprogesterone acetate is still not marketed in the United States for contraceptive use, presumably because of the possibility that the compound may cause cancer (Williams, 1986). Interestingly, it is approved for use in this country to treat metastatic endometrial cancer. Moreover, studies on a large number of women users have not identified an increased risk of cancer (Liang and co-workers, 1983).

Hormonal Implants

These are being studied currently in several countries. The Norplant system, which provides the progestin levonorgestrel in a silastic container which is implanted subdermally, has been approved for use in Finland, Sweden, Thailand, Indonesia, and the Dominican Republic. The system is also being evaluated in 31 additional countries, including the United States (Segal, 1987). Some, but not all, ovulatory cycles are prevented by the progestin which works presumably by altering the endometrium and cervical mucus. Lopez and associates (1985) recently reported no pregnancies and a high patient acceptance with the use of Norplant in Columbia.

POSTCOITAL CONTRACEPTION

Stilbestrol administered after intercourse to prevent unwanted pregnancy has come to be known as the "morning-after pill." Kuchara (1971) reported no pregnancies in 1,000 women who had inadequate contraceptive protection at the time of intercourse but within 3 days began to take stilbestrol, 25 mg twice daily for the next 5 days. The mechanism of action is not fully understood but very likely implantation is interfered with in some way. Nausea and vomiting are common side effects. The possible teratogenic effect of the drug must be kept in mind if pregnancy does occur (Chap. 32, p. 562). Prevention of pregnancy has also been reported using either ethinyl estradiol or conjugated equine estrogens (Premarin) when taken in large doses for several days.

Yuzpe and colleagues (1982) devised an estrogen plus progestin regimen in which the combination was taken in two doses 12 hours apart starting within 72 hours of exposure. In a multicenter trial involving 692 women the pregnancy rate observed by them was 1.6 percent.

Luteinizing Hormone–Releasing Hormone

The natural hormone agonists and antagonists of luteinizing hormone–releasing hormone (LHRH) are being evaluated for contraceptive properties. Continuous administration of an LHRH agonist will reliably inhibit ovulation but the inhibition of follicular activity is variable. Thus a major drawback to use of LHRH agonists as contraceptives is the high incidence of irregular bleeding or amenorrhea. Recently, Lemay and Faure (1986) suggested combining intermittent intranasal LHRH agonist administration with oral progestin to achieve cycle control. At present LHRH agonists seem to offer no distinct advantage over combination oral contraceptives.

INTRAUTERINE CONTRACEPTIVE DEVICES

Since early in this century, attempts have been made, sporadic at the outset but very intense since 1960 to design a device that when inserted into the uterus would prevent pregnancy without causing adverse effects. One intriguing but unconfirmed story describes the first successful experience with an intrauterine device to have been the insertion of small stones into the uteri of camels to prevent pregnancy during long caravans.

At one time, it was estimated that in the United States 6 to 7 percent of sexually active women of reproductive age used an intrauterine device for contraception. Some of the devices used are demonstrated in Figures 42–3 and 42–4. The pregnancy rates in larger studies generally vary from 0.5 to 5 per 100 woman-years (Population Reports, 1982).

By 1986, the two most popular intrauterine devices used by American women were voluntarily withdrawn from the market by their manufacturers. The announced reason for the withdrawal of the Lippes loop and Cu 7 was the financial burden of defense in liability cases. Nearly 2 million women (Fig. 42–1) were suddenly left with doubts as to their ability to continue to employ this effective, generally safe contraceptive method of their preference which was approved by the Food and Drug Administration. At that time, about half of the women wearing intrauterine devices in the United States in 1986 were acceptable candidates for oral contraceptive therapy. Some of the remaining women continued to wear inert plastic devices, as these may be left in place indefinitely. Many women, however, would have been obliged to choose between alternative, albeit less effective, contraceptive measures and permanent sterilization. Fortunately, the Progestasert (Fig. 42–4) continued to be marketed in the United States in limited quantities and at a very high cost to the consumer. Although developed much earlier by the nonprofit Population Council, the copper-T model 380 A (Fig. 42–4) did not become commercially available in the United States until 1988. It too is very expensive.

THEORETICAL ADVANTAGES

Ideally, an intrauterine device would need to be inserted but once, would provide complete protection against pregnancy, would neither be expelled spontaneously nor have to be removed for adverse effects, and, after removal to allow a planned pregnancy, would have in no way induced changes detrimental to pregnancy. These objectives have not been fully achieved by any device so far.

TYPES OF INTRAUTERINE DEVICES

In general, devices are of two varieties: (1) those that appear to be chemically inert, in that they are made of a nonabsorbable material, most often polyethylene impregnated with barium sulfate for radiopacity; and (2) those in which there is more or less continuous elution from the device of a chemically active substance, such as copper or a progestational agent.

Of the chemically inert devices, the *Lippes loop* had been quite popular before it was withdrawn from the market in 1985. Even so, many American women continue to wear these devices that were inserted before that time.

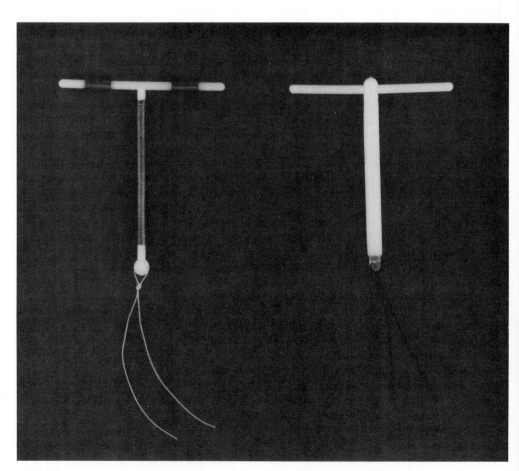

Figure 42–4. Intrauterine contraceptive devices available in 1989. At left is a Copper T 380A (*Courtesy of GynoPharma, Inc., Somerville, New Jersey*) and to the right is a Progestasert. (*Courtesy of ALZA Corp., Palo Alto, California.*)

Through 1987, the only continuing production device was the T-shaped *Progestasert* that releases approximately 65 μg of progesterone per day through the wall of the vertical shaft made of vinyl acetate copolymer. Of the copper-containing devices, the Cu7 was withdrawn in 1986, and the Copper T 380A introduced in 1988.

MECHANISMS OF ACTION

The mechanisms of action of the chemically inert device have not been defined precisely. Interference with successful implantation of the fertilized ovum in the endometrium seems to be the most prominent contraceptive action. The interference may result from induction of a local inflammatory response that, in turn, leads to lysosomal action on the blastocyst and perhaps phagocytosis of spermatozoa (Population Reports, 1982). Providing support for such a mechanism of action are the observations of Buhler and Papiernik (1983), who described two successive pregnancies in each of four women who had been fitted with intrauterine devices but were chronically taking antiinflammatory drugs. For the chemically inert devices, contraceptive effectiveness generally increases with size and extent of contact with the endometrium.

Certain metals, especially copper, greatly enhance the contraceptive action of inert devices. For example, one small T-shaped polyethylene device allowed a pregnancy rate of about 18 per 100 woman-years until the addition of fine copper ribbon with a surface area of 200 mm^2. Then the pregnancy rate dropped to about 2 per 100 woman-years. A local, rather than systemic, action from copper must be of major importance, since metallic copper placed in one uterine horn of a rabbit prevents blastocyst implantation there but not in the adjacent horn (Zipper and co-workers, 1971). The experiences of Lippes and co-workers (1978) that insertion of a Copper T or Cu7 device up to 7 days after coitus effectively prevents pregnancy strongly support the concept that the copper-bearing device compromises the blastocyst. Alvarez and associates (1988) suggested that some devices prevent fertilization.

ADVERSE EFFECTS

A great variety of complications has been described during the use of various intrauterine devices, but, for the most part, the common side effects have not been serious while the serious side effects have not been common. The earliest adverse effects are those associated with insertion. They include clinically apparent or silent *perforation of the uterus*, either while sounding the uterus or during insertion of the device, and *interruption of an unsuspected pregnancy*. The frequency of these will depend upon the skill of the operator and the precautions taken to avoid interrupting a pregnancy. Although devices may migrate spontaneously into and through the uterine wall at any time, most perforations occur, or at least begin, at the time of insertion.

Uterine *cramping* and some *bleeding* are likely to develop soon after insertion of an intrauterine device and to persist for variable periods of time. Considering unmedicated devices only, the smaller the device, the less the likelihood of cramping and bleeding but the greater the likelihood of a pregnancy with the device in situ or especially after spontaneous expulsion. Conversely, the larger and more rigid the device, the lower the probability of expulsion and pregnancy but the greater the likelihood of troublesome cramping and bleeding.

Blood loss with menstruation is commonly increased by a factor of about two but may be so great as to cause severe iron deficiency anemia (Guttorm, 1971). Therefore, it is wise to make an annual check of the hemoglobin level or hematocrit of women with intrauterine devices as well as any time they complain of heavy menstruation. Antifibrinolytic agents such as epsilon–aminocaproic acid and tranexamic acid have been used by some to reduce excessive uterine bleeding from intrauterine devices, the rationale being that plasminogen activation is inhibited by such agents. Unfortunately, these drugs may prove thrombogenic as well as antifibrinolytic and fatal cerebral thrombosis during the course of such treatment has been reported (Agnelli and associates, 1982).

As an aid for ascertaining appropriate placement in the uterine cavity, most devices have an attached synthetic filament, or tail, which protrudes through the external os and is cut off so that 2 cm or so are visible through the vagina. There has been concern from the outset that the tail might act as a wick and promote invasion of the uterine cavity by pathogenic bacteria. Purrier and co-workers (1979) identified potentially pathogenic bacteria colonizing the mucus that coated the tails of more than half of intrauterine devices.

Pelvic infections, including septic abortion, have developed following the use of a variety of intrauterine devices. Tuboovarian abscesses, which may be unilateral, have been described by W. Taylor and associates (1973), E. S. Taylor and co-workers (1975), Dawood and Birnbaum (1975), and several others. When infection is suspected, the device should be removed and the woman treated with effective antibiotics. She must be observed closely because there have been deaths from sepsis associated with the use of an intrauterine device. Even so, mortality attributable to such devices is probably lower than that attributed to estrogen plus progestin oral contraceptives or to pregnancy. Nonetheless, because of the risk of salpingitis, pelvic peritonitis, and pelvic abscess, and, as a consequence, sterility, use of an intrauterine device is usually discouraged for women under the age of 25 of no or very low parity as well as in women who appear to be at increased risk of developing an infection of the pelvic viscera. Vessey and associates (1983) have provided data that reinforce their earlier observations that parous women having an intrauterine device removed to try to achieve pregnancy have no prolonged impairment of fertility. They conclude that pelvic infection sufficient to impair fertility must be very uncommon, at least in parous users of such devices.

Subsequently, Daling (1985) and Cramer (1985) and their many associates provided data that were consistent with the view that intrauterine device use is associated with increased tubal infertility. These effects were negligible with copper-bearing devices, but more apparent in nulliparous women, especially if they were polygamous and used the Dalkon shield.

Actinomyces-like structures identified in Papanicolaou smears and the prolonged use of an intrauterine device have been linked, but the clinical importance of this finding is not clear but worrisome. In most studies an increased prevalence of *Actinomyces israelii* or actinomyces-like organisms was apparent only after several years of use of the device. Furthermore, the organisms were much less frequent when a copper-bearing device was used rather than an inert one, possibly because the former was changed more frequently. Of importance, the percentage of women reporting gynecological symptoms did not differ significantly between users with and without actinomyces-like organisms on smear (Petitti and associates, 1983). Keebler and co-workers (1983) identified actinomyces in 12.6 percent of device users. Once the smear became positive for actinomyces bodies, all subsequent smears remained positive until the intrauterine device was removed. Authorities agree that, if signs or symptoms of infection develop in women who harbor actinomyces bodies, the device should be removed and antibiotic therapy instituted. However, in the absence of signs or symptoms of pelvic infection there is considerable disagreement as to whether uniform removal of the device or simply close observation is the correct approach.

LOCATING A LOST DEVICE

When the tail cannot be visualized protruding from the cervical canal, the possibilities of expulsion or of extrauterine location must be considered. In either event, pregnancy is likely to occur. The tail may, however, simply be in the uterine cavity along with a normally positioned device. Often, gentle probing of the uterine cavity using a rod with a terminal hook or with a Randall stone clamp will retrieve the device. The simple assumption that the device has been expelled and thus another should be inserted can be carried to extremes. For example, we have observed a woman in whom two Dalkon shields and one Lippes loop were found adherent to the placenta at delivery at term! Almost certainly, each tail has been drawn into the uterine cavity by the rapidly growing pregnant uterus. The pregnancy was otherwise uncomplicated.

When the tail is not visible, and gentle probing of the uterine cavity fails to confirm the presence of the device and allow its removal, sonography is done to ascertain if the device is within the uterine cavity. If these findings are negative or inconclusive then a plain x-ray film of the abdomen and pelvis is performed with a radio-opaque probe (uterine sound) within the uterine cavity. Instillation of radiocontrast for hysterography may be done and hysteroscopy is yet another alternative. Obviously none of these maneuvers except sonography should be performed during early pregnancy.

An open device of inert material, such as the Lippes Loop, located outside the uterus may or may not do harm. Perforations of large and small bowel and bowel fistulas, with attendant morbidity, have developed remote from the time of insertion of the so-called inert devices. Closed devices, such as the Birnberg Bow, can cause *bowel obstruction* and for this reason are no longer used. A copper-bearing device in an extrauterine location is prone to induce an intense local inflammatory reaction and adhere to the inflamed structure. Although chemically inert devices have been readily removed from the peritoneal cavity by laparoscopy or through a posterior colpotomy, the copper-bearing device is likely to be too firmly adherent for successful removal by these techniques.

A device may penetrate the uterine wall in varying degrees. At times part of the device may extend into the peritoneal cavity while the remainder is firmly fixed in the myometrium. In one case, at the time of repeat cesarean delivery, part of a Lippes Loop that was inserted 3 years before was found protruding from the fundus posteriorly. Omentum was firmly adherent to the uterus around the protruding loop. Oozing from the tract left after the loop was extracted was controlled with a deep mattress suture.

The intrauterine device can also penetrate into the cervix and actually protrude into the vagina. This is more common with the Cu7 and Copper-T device than with the Lippes Loop. A more likely cause for pregnancy with a device in situ is displacement of the device into the uterine isthmus and cervix, although successful nidation may occur with the device in the fundus of the uterus.

PREGNANCY WITH A DEVICE IN UTERO

As emphasized in Chapter 14, it is important to identify all pregnant women who might be harboring an intrauterine device, whether it be within the uterine cavity or elsewhere. A device within the uterus and co-existing pregnancy is risky for mother and fetus. A device residing beyond the uterus may be risky for the mother. Appropriate steps are taken at delivery to identify and assure removal of the device.

When pregnancy is recognized and the tail of the device is visible through the cervix, the device should be removed. This will help reduce subsequent complications in the form of late abortion, sepsis, and preterm birth. Tatum and co-workers (1976) observed the abortion rate to be 54 percent with the device left in compared to 25 percent if promptly removed. Moreover, with the device remaining in situ, the frequency of low birthweight, chiefly from preterm delivery, was 20 percent, compared to about 5 percent if the device was removed early. Vessey and associates (1979) confirmed these observations. If the tail is not visible, attempts to locate and remove the device from the uterus by instrumentation may lead to abortion.

Not only is the likelihood of abortion during the second trimester much increased if an intrauterine device remains in a pregnant uterus, but, very importantly, the abortion is likely to be septic, with the sepsis, at times, being fulminant and fatal to the mother. Women pregnant with a device in utero and who demonstrate any evidence of uterine infection must have the products of conception and the device removed promptly as well as intensive antibiotic therapy. The following case illustrates the dangers of a device co-existing with a pregnancy:

A woman conceived with a Lippes Loop in place and attempts to visualize the strings and remove it were unsuccessful. She elected to continue the pregnancy, and did well until 20 weeks when she was admitted to a community hospital because of chills and fever. The membranes were intact, the cervix was closed and there were no contractions, and no pelvic or uterine tenderness was elicited. Blood cultures were obtained and broad-spectrum antimicrobials begun. She felt better initially, but in 24 hours she had another chill accompanied by temperature of 40° C. The initial blood cultures were sterile, however, others done at this time were subsequently positive for *Escherichia coli*. Also at this time she began to develop clinical and x-ray evidence for alveolar capillary leakage caused by injury from endotoxin (see Chap. 27, p. 472; Chap. 39, p. 807). Labor began spontaneously and the 20-week fetus was delivered shortly thereafter and the Loop was laying on his chest and not embedded in the placenta.

Although her pulmonary injury improved slowly over the next few days, and despite continued intravenous antimicrobial therapy, consumptive coagulopathy developed 7 days later and this was assumed to be due to continued sepsis. A computed tomographic scan (Fig. 42–5) disclosed evidence for uterine necrosis and at laparotomy the uterus and both adnexae were found to be necrotic and there was septic ovarian vein thrombophlebitis. Hysterectomy and bilateral adnexectomy were performed. After an extremely complicated and prolonged postoperative course, which included renal failure that required hemodialysis, she ultimately survived.

An increased incidence of fetal malformations has not been noted with pregnancies complicated by the presence of an intrauterine device.

EXTRAUTERINE PREGNANCIES

Although most intrauterine pregnancies are prevented, the device provides less protection against nidation in other locations.

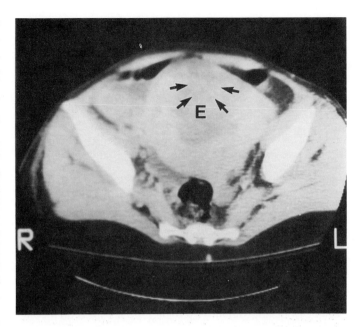

Figure 42–5. Computed tomographic scan showing uterine necrosis from an intrauterine device-related infection at 20 weeks gestation. Arrows surround areas of hypodensity indicating necrosis. E = endometrial cavity. (*Courtesy of Drs. K. Waldrep and L. Swygert.*)

There has been concern that use of an intrauterine device inordinately increases the risk of *ectopic pregnancy*, but Vessey and co-workers (1979) found that the risk remains rather constant with duration of use at 1.2 per 1,000 women per year. However, since the device does not prevent extrauterine pregnancy reliably, women already at high risk of an ectopic pregnancy (previous salpingitis, ectopic pregnancy, or tubal surgery) are poor candidates for an intrauterine contraceptive device.

PROCEDURES FOR INSERTION

The Food and Drug Administration requires that before an intrauterine device is inserted physicians must give women who request a device a detailed brochure detailing the side effects and apparent risks from use of such a device.

Most devices have a special inserter, usually a sterile graduated plastic tube into which the device is withdrawn just before insertion (Fig. 42–3). Timing of insertion of the device influences the ease of placement as well as the pregnancy and expulsion rates. Insertion near the end of a normal menstrual period when the cervix is usually softer and the canal somewhat more dilated may facilitate insertion and at the same time exclude an early pregnancy. However, insertion need not be limited only to this period. For the woman who is reasonably sure that she is not pregnant and she does not want to be pregnant, insertion may be carried out anytime during the menstrual cycle. Even though she engaged in coitus during the previous week, she is unlikely to conceive if a Copper T or Cu7 device is used (Lippes and associates, 1978).

Insertion at the time of delivery or very soon thereafter is followed by an unsatisfactorily high expulsion rate. The recommendation has been made, therefore, to withhold insertion for at least 8 weeks to reduce expulsion as well as to minimize the risk of perforation. The experience of the Greater Dallas Family Planning Program, however, has been that earlier insertion has not led to perforation or expulsion rates significantly higher than for insertion remote from pregnancy. In the absence of infection, the device may be inserted immediately after early abortion.

A satisfactory technique for insertion and plan for follow-up are outlined below:

1. Obtain a careful gynecological history. Contraindications to the use of an intrauterine device include the following: Untreated gonorrhea even though asymptomatic, a recent pelvic infection or a history of recurrent pelvic infections, severe dysmenorrhea, cervical stenosis, abnormalities of the uterine cavity, heavy menses, overt anemia, and abnormalities of blood coagulation. The woman who has had a previous ectopic pregnancy should be counseled against the use of an intrauterine device because she is already at considerable risk of another ectopic pregnancy and an intrauterine device does not prevent ectopic pregnancy efficiently.
2. Describe the various problems associated with use of an intrauterine device and obtain informed consent.
3. Perform a thorough pelvic examination to identify especially the position and size of the uterus and adnexa. If abnormalities are found, an intrauterine device often is contraindicated.
4. Visualize the cervix and grasp it with a tenaculum. Use sterile instruments and sterile intrauterine device. Wipe the cervix and the vaginal walls with an antiseptic solution. It is commonly recommended that the uterus first be sounded to help identify the direction and depth of the uterine cavity. Before identifying the depth of the uterine cavity with a sound, the cervical canal and uterine cavity are first straightened by applying gentle traction on the tenaculum. A device of appropriate size is selected based on the length of the uterine cavity. The inserter (Fig. 42–3), with the device contained within its most distal portion, is gently inserted to the fundus of the uterus. After rotating the inserter so that the device is positioned high in the transverse plane of the uterus, the inserter is removed while the device is held in place in the fundus by the plastic rod within the inserter behind the device. Thus, the device is not pushed out of the tube, but rather it is held in place by the rod while the inserter tube is withdrawn.
5. Cut the marker tail 2 cm from the external os, remove the tenaculum, observe for bleeding from the tenaculum puncture sites, and if there is no bleeding, remove the speculum.
6. Provide analgesia with aspirin or codeine to allay cramps. Advise the woman to report promptly any apparent adverse effects.

Expulsion

Loss of the device from the uterus is most common during the first month of use. The recipient should be instructed on how to palpate the strings protruding from the cervix by either sitting on the edge of a chair or squatting down and then advancing the middle finger into the vagina until the cervix is reached. The woman should be checked in 1 month, usually after menses, for appropriate placement of the device by identifying the tail protruding appropriately from the cervix. Barrier contraception may be desirable during this time, especially if a device has been expelled previously.

Replacement

The chemically inert device may be left in the uterus indefinitely. In some cases, the polyethylene compound becomes encrusted with calcium salts and endometrial erosion causes bleeding that prompts removal and insertion of another device. The copper-bearing devices will have to be replaced periodically. For the Cu7 and some Copper T devices, replacement every three years is recommended even though the device may remain effective for 6 to 8 years. The new copper-bearing device, Copper T-380 A is approved in the United States for 4 years of continuous use. The progesterone-bearing intrauterine device, Progestasert, should be replaced annually.

LOCAL BARRIER METHODS

Condoms, vaginal diaphragms, and spermicidal agents placed in the vagina have long been used for contraception with variable success.

CONDOMS

To date, the condom represents in the United States the only reversible, effective, "male method" of contraception except for *coitus interruptus*. Condoms can provide effective contraception. Their failure rate with experienced and strongly motivated couples has been as low as 3 or 4 per 100 couple-years of exposure. Generally, and during the first year of use especially, the failure rate is much higher (Table 42–1). Perhaps the recent availability in the United States of a condom with a spermicidal lubricant (Ramses Extra) will lower the failure rate.

When used properly, condoms provide considerable but not absolute protection against a broad range of sexually transmitted diseases, including gonorrhea, syphilis, herpes, chlamydia, and trichomoniasis; they possibly prevent and ameliorate premalignant changes in the cervix (Population Reports, 1982). Feldblum and Fortney (1988) reviewed the few published studies and concluded that there is some evidence that use of condoms provides protection, although not absolute, from infection with the *human immunodeficiency virus* (see Chap. 39, p. 857). The Centers for Disease Control recommends their use for patients at risk for infection with the virus, and this includes those women with multiple sex partners. Consequently, the use of condoms has escalated exponentially in the past few years, but not necessarily for contraception. It is estimated that 40 million couples in the world use condoms for birth control, and in Japan, 50 percent of married couples do so.

> Historically, the original condoms were made of intestine and other material, but with the introduction of rubber, the condom became much more effective, less expensive, and more widely available.
> The origin of the word "condom" is unknown. It has been stated, probably incorrectly, that is refers to Dr. Condom, a physician who provided King Charles II with a means of preventing more illegitimate offspring. Casanova (1725–98) is said to have mentioned condoms several times in his exhaustive memoirs.
> In Texas, and elsewhere, the earliest father–son discussion of sex and reproduction often was stimulated by the presence of condom-dispensing machines in the men's room of service stations. It is of interest that condoms were widely available at a time when attempts to make other family planning techniques more readily available were discouraged by much of society lest they promote sexual promiscuity or offend someone's religious beliefs. The condoms, or "prophylactics," in the gasoline stations, allegedly were

provided only to prevent sexually tansmitted diseases—a use that now has certainly become popular.

INTRAVAGINAL CONTRACEPTIVES

Such contraceptive agents are variously marketed as creams, jellies, suppositories, film, and foam in aerosol containers (Fig. 42–3), as well as sponges, and are widely used in this country, especially by women who find the oral contraceptive or an intrauterine device unacceptable, or who need temporary protection, for example, during the first week after starting oral contraceptives or while nursing.

Most such agents can be purchased over-the-counter, that is, a prescription is not needed. Typically, such preparations work by providing a physical barrier to sperm penetration as well as chemical spermicidal action. The active ingredient is nonoxynol-9. **To be highly effective, the spermicides must, shortly before intercourse, be deposited high in the vagina in contact with the cervix.** Their duration of maximal spermicidal effectiveness is usually no more than 1 hour and therefore they must be reinserted into the vagina before intercourse is repeated. Douching should be avoided for at least 6 hours after intercourse.

High pregnancy rates are attributable chiefly to inconsistent use rather than to failure of the method during use. If inserted regularly and correctly, use of the foam preparations for contraception probably results in no more than 5 pregnancies per 100 woman-years of use (Population Reports, 1984).

The spermicides in current use appear to provide some protection against some sexually transmitted disease, including gonorrhea and probably papillomavirus and human immunodeficiency virus (Feldblum and Fortney, 1988).

Malformations

One study suggested that the use of vaginal spermicides during the year before conception might be associated with an increased frequency of malformations. However, a well-defined syndrome of congenital disorders was not identified, and the investigators considered their results to be tentative (Jick and associates, 1981). Importantly, in studies by both Mills and coworkers (1982) and Shapiro and associates (1982) no association was identified between congenital malformations and maternal spermicide exposure before or after the last menstrual period.

In 1986, the Food and Drug Administration concluded that the evidence *does not* support an association between spermicide use and congenital malformations. In spite of the scientific evidence to the contrary, a recent court decision (*Wells* v. *Ortho Pharmaceutical*) was rendered in favor of the plaintiff in a suit alleging that congenital malformations were caused by maternal spermicide exposure. The decision was upheld by an appellate court. Subsequently, Louik and colleagues (1987) reported results from their case-controlled surveillance system, in which they examined specifically for possible effects of periconceptual use of spermicides on specific fetal malformations. They found no association with spermicide use and Down syndrome, hypospadias, limb-reduction defects, neoplasms, or neural tube defects. Concurrently, Warburton and associates (1987) reported no increased risk of trisomies with spermicide use. Similarly, Strobino and colleagues (1988) did not find increased congenital malformations in a cohort study.

DIAPHRAGM PLUS SPERMICIDAL AGENT

The vaginal diaphragm (Fig. 42–3), consisting of circular rubber dome of various diameters supported by a circumferentially placed metal spring, has long been used for contraception, in combination with a spermicidal jelly or cream. The spermicidal agent is applied to the superior surface both along the rim and centrally. The device is then placed in the vagina so that the cervix, vaginal fornices, and anterior vaginal wall are effectively partitioned from the rest of the vagina and the penis. At the same time, the centrally placed spermicidal agent is held against the cervix by the diaphragm. When appropriately positioned in the vagina, the rim of the diaphragm is lodged superiorly deep in the posterior vaginal fornix and inferiorly the rim lies in close promixity to the inner surface of the symphysis immediately below the urethra (Fig. 42–6). If the diaphragm is too small, it will not remain in place. If too large, it will be uncomfortable when it is forced into position. A cystocele or uterine prolapse is very likely to result in instability and therefore expulsion. Because the variables of size and spring flexibility must be specified, the diaphragm is available only by prescription.

The diaphragm and spermicidal agent can be inserted even hours before intercourse, but if more than 2 hours elapse, additional spermicide should be placed in the upper vagina for maximum protection and be reapplied before subsequent exposure. The diaphragm should be left for a least 6 hours after intercourse before removal.

The so-called toxic-shock syndrome following use of a diaphragm has been described in a few reports (Alcid and associates, 1982). For this reason, it may be worthwhile to remove the diaphragm at the end of 6 hours or so (or the next morning) to minimize this very uncommon event.

The diaphragm requires a high level of motivation for proper use that, when expended, is accompanied by a low pregnancy rate. Vessey and Wiggins (1974) reported a pregnancy rate of only 2.4 per 100 woman-years for already established users of the diaphragm. They rightfully emphasized that established users need not be encouraged to change to a "more modern" method of birth control.

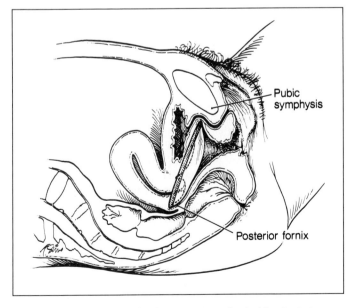

Figure 42–6. A diaphragm in place creates a physical barrier between the vagina and cervix and importantly provides for intimate contact between the contraceptive jelly or cream and the cervix. (The woman is lying supine.)

SPONGE OR CERVICAL CAP

Contraceptive sponges to be placed in the upper vagina continue to undergo extensive evaluation. One polyurethane sponge soaked with a spermicide has been approved by the Food and Drug Administration and is marketed under the trade name "Today." It has been claimed to be about as effective as other vaginal methods, although studies to date are not really adequate to define precisely its efficacy (Population Reports, 1984). In a randomized clinical trial conducted in Yugoslavia the sponge had a failure rate of 10 percent in one year (Borko and associates, 1985).

After falling into disuse in the United States for several decades, the *cervical cap* was approved for use (FDA Drug Bulletin, 1988). The flexible, cup-like device, made of natural rubber, is fitted around the base of the cervix. It can be self-inserted, is allowed to remain in place 48 hours, and is used with spermicide applied once at insertion. According to trials conducted by the National Institutes of Health, the cap is comparable in effectiveness to the diaphragm.

BREAST FEEDING

Breast feeding is important to infant health and to child-spacing. For mothers who are fully nursing their infants, ovulation during the first 10 weeks after delivery is very unlikely according to Pérez (1981). However, it is not a very reliable method of family planning for women whose infants are on a 3- to 4-hour, daytime-only feeding schedule and are receiving other food (see Chap. 13, p. 254). Waiting for first menses involves a risk of pregnancy because ovulation may antedate menstruation. Certainly, after the first menses contraception is essential unless the woman desires another pregnancy so soon after her last one.

Combined estrogen-progestin contraceptives have been thought by some to reduce somewhat both the rate and the duration of milk production. The benefits from prevention of pregnancy by the use of combined oral contraceptives would appear to outweigh the risks in selected patients.

Intrauterine devices have been recommended for the lactating but potentially ovulating, sexually active woman. An increased rate of uterine perforation has been identified in lactating women with an intrauterine device, perhaps as the consequence of vigorous myometrial contractions and involution brought about by the release of oxytocin in response to the stimulation from suckling (Heartwell and Schlesselman, 1983). However, the risk is not so great that intrauterine devices should not be used.

PERIODIC (RHYTHMIC) ABSTINENCE

The pregnancy rate with the various methods for application of periodic abstinence (rhythm methods, "natural" family planning) has been placed at from 5 to 40 per 100 woman-years (Population Reports, 1981). Ovulation most often occurs about 14 days before the onset of the next menstrual period, but, unfortunately, not necessarily 14 days after the onset of the last menstrual period. Therefore, *calendar rhythm* is not always reliable. In 1982, the International Planned Parenthood Federation concluded that "couples electing to use periodic abstinence should, however, be clearly informed that the method is not considered an effective method of family planning."

The human ovum probably is susceptible to successful fertilization only for about 12 to no more than 24 hours after ovulation. Motile sperm have been identified in cervical mucus as many as 7 days after coitus or artificial insemination and in oviducts of women undergoing laparotomy as long as 85 hours after coitus (Ahlgren, 1975). However, it is unlikely that sperm retain the capability for successful fertilization for this long a period.

Temperature rhythm relies on *slight* changes in basal body temperature that may occur just before ovulation. The temperature rhythm method is much more likely to be successful if during each menstrual cycle intercourse is avoided until well after the ovulatory temperature rise.

> A bedside clock, the Rite Time, is now marketed. Promotional literature claims that accuracy of the temperature rhythm method is greatly enhanced by the combination of a preprogrammed computer, a digital clock, and a very precise oral thermometer. (Another reason to ask "What time is it?")

Cervical mucus rhythm ("Billings method") depends upon awareness of "dryness" and "wetness" in the vagina as the consequence of changes in the amount and kind of cervical mucus formed at different times in the menstrual cycle. This approach has not achieved popularity. A small, hand-held device which detects small variations in electrolyte concentrations in vaginal or oral secretions is claimed to be capable of predicting ovulation 5 to 7 days in advance. The applicability of this technology to contraception is being studied. However, Roumen and Dieben (1988) found it to be of no use in predicting the day of ovulation.

An extensive review of "natural family planning" has been provided by Klaus (1982).

SURGICAL CONTRACEPTION

PREVALENCE

Surgical sterilization of one or both sexual partners is the most popular form of contraception among couples of reproductive age (Fig. 42–1). In 1981, according to the Association for Voluntary Sterilization, nearly 900,000 sterilization procedures were performed in the United States; 52 percent were performed on women.

Until recently, sterilization of women as a technique for effective family planning has been frowned upon by important segments of society, including not only some churches, but also medical groups and a variety of political bodies. For example, until 1969, the American College of Obstetricians and Gynecologists recommended that a woman 30 years of age should have four living children before qualifying for sterilization! Even now, multiple restrictions imposed by the federal government serve to discourage voluntary sterilization among financially underprivileged women by threatening to sever federal funding to the organization that provides the service.

Methods used for surgical sterilization, as well as counseling, recently were reviewed by the American College of Obstetricians and Gynecologists (1988).

TUBAL STERILIZATION

Over 5 million women underwent tubal sterilization in the United States during the 1970s. Medically speaking, the operation can be performed at any time. Many are done at cesarean section. For women who deliver vaginally the early puerperium

is a particularly convenient time. Because the fundus is near the umbilicus and the oviducts are readily accessible directly beneath the abdominal wall for several days after delivery, the operation is technically simple and hospitalization need not be prolonged.

Sterilization immediately following vaginal delivery has some disadvantages. Most often the mother is multiparous and has delivered without receiving anesthesia appropriate for entering the peritoneal cavity. The likelihood of postpartum hemorrhage in multiparous women subsides remarkably during the first 10 hours after delivery. Of particular importance, the status of the newborn infant can be determined much more precisely several hours after birth.

It was recommended previously that puerperal sterilization by partial resection of the oviducts be accomplished before 72 hours postpartum so as to minimize infection from ascending bacterial invasion of the fallopian tubes. However, in several studies no correlation was apparent between time interval and postoperative morbidity. At Parkland Hospital, the operation is performed in the obstetrical surgical suite, most often the morning after delivery, in order to minimize hospital stay.

TYPES OF TUBAL STERILIZATION

The first tubal sterilization reported in the United States more than 100 years ago consisted of ligating the oviducts with a strong silk ligature about 1 inch from their uterine attachment following the woman's second cesarean delivery (Lungren, 1881). Literally, the woman had her tubes tied. Subsequently, it became apparent that an unacceptably high failure rate followed ligation without some form of tubal resection to create discontinuity of the tubal lumen. A variety of techniques are now employed to try to disrupt tubal patency and thereby thwart union of sperm and egg, several of which are considered below.

Irving Procedure

This operation is least likely to fail. Briefly, the procedure, as illustrated in Figure 42–7A, involves severing the oviduct and separating it from the mesosalpinx sufficiently to create a medial segment of tube, the end of which is buried within a tunnel into the myometrium posteriorly, and a short lateral segment of tube, the proximal end of which is then buried within the mesosalpinx. The procedure requires considerably more exposure than do most other techniques and the likelihood of hemorrhage is much greater.

Pomeroy Procedure

Of all the techniques that divide the tube, the simplest, reasonably effective method of performing abdominal sterilization is the so-called Pomeroy procedure (Fig. 42–7B). It has generally been considered important that plain catgut be used to ligate the knuckle of tube, since the rationale of this procedure is based on prompt absorption of the ligature and subsequent separation of the severed tubal ends, which most often become sealed over by fibrosis.

Parkland Procedure

This was designed to avoid the initial intimate approximation of the cut ends of the oviduct that is inherent in the Pomeroy procedure (Fig. 42–7C). Through an infraumbilical abdominal wall incision, typically just long enough to allow a small Richardson retractor to be inserted, the oviduct is positively identified by grasping the midportion in a Babcock clamp and

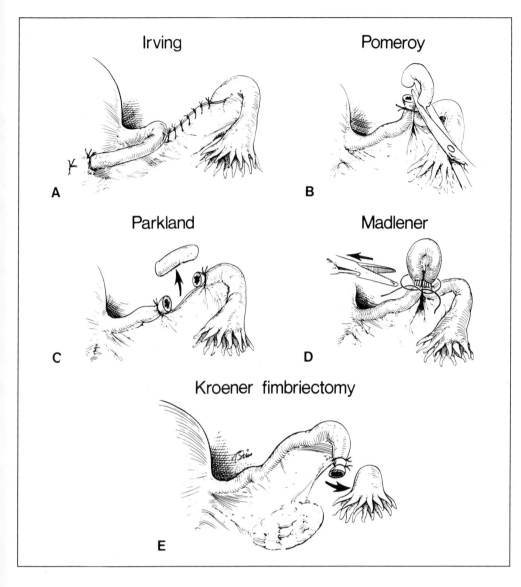

Irving

Pomeroy

A

B

Parkland

Madlener

C

D

Kroener fimbriectomy

E

Figure 42–7. Various techniques for tubal sterilization. **A.** Irving procedure: The medial cut end of the oviduct is buried in the myometrium posteriorly and the distal cut end is buried in the mesosalpinx. **B.** Pomeroy procedure: A loop of oviduct is ligated and the knuckle of tube above the ligature is excised. **C.** Parkland procedure: A midsegment of tube is separated from the mesosalpinx at an avascular site, the separated tubal segment is ligated proximally and distally and then excised. **D.** Madlener procedure: A knuckle of oviduct is crushed and then ligated without resection. **E.** Kroener procedure: The tube is ligated across the ampulla and the distal portion of the ampulla, including all of the fimbriae, is resected.

confirming by direct observation that indeed fimbriae are present on the distal end of the structure so held. Otherwise, it is easy to confuse the round ligament with the midportion of the oviduct. **Whenever the oviduct is inadvertently dropped, it is mandatory to repeat in toto the identification procedure just described!**

An avascular site (Fig. 42–8A) in the mesosalpinx adjacent to the oviduct is then perforated with a small hemostat and the jaws are opened to separate the oviduct from the adjacent mesosalpinx for about 2.5 cm (Fig. 42–8B). The freed oviduct is ligated proximally and distally (Fig. 42–8C) with 0 chromic suture and the intervening segment of about 2 cm is excised with sharp scissors (Fig. 42–8D). After inspecting for hemostasis, the now discontinuous oviduct is dropped in place and the procedure is repeated on the other side. Both resected segments of oviduct are labeled and submitted for histological confirmation. Excluding the rare instance in which the operator failed to resect the fallopian tube, which can be confirmed promptly in the surgical pathology laboratory, the subsequent failure rate has been approximately 1 in 400 procedures.

Madlener Procedure
A knuckle of tube is crushed and ligated with nonabsorbable suture but not resected (Fig. 42–7D). This procedure is men-

tioned only to discourage its use. Early experiences at Parkland Memorial Hospital indicated a failure rate of about 7 percent.

Fimbriectomy
Removal of all of the fimbriae to effect sterilization has been recommended by Kroener (1969) and by others. Kroener doubly ligated the oviduct with silk suture and then excised the fimbriated end (Fig. 42–7E). Although Kroener reported no failures, others have, and in some instances the rate has been unacceptable. Taylor (1972), for example, observed 6 pregnancies among about 200 women who were subjected to fimbriectomy; when the oviducts were subsequently examined, usually a small amount of fimbrial tissue had been left. Metz (1977) identified 7 failures among 388 women upon whom bilateral fimbriectomy was performed. Catgut suture had been used and the resected surface had been lightly electrocoagulated. In the cases that failed, tuboperitoneal fistulas lined with tubal epithelium were found in the remaining ampullary portion.

POSTOPERATIVE CARE

After puerperal sterilization, analgesia should be provided for abdominal soreness, which at times is aggravated in multip-

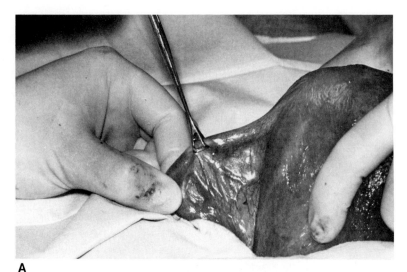

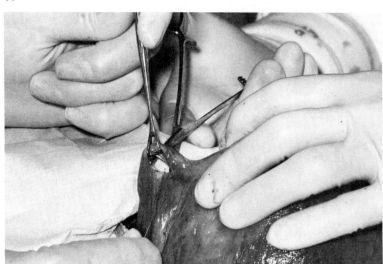

Figure 42–8 (A–B). Sterilization at cesarean section. **A.** An avascular site in the mesosalpinx adjacent to the midportion of the oviduct is identified. **B.** A small hemostat has been inserted through the avascular site and the jaws of the clamp opened to separate mesosalpinx from tube for about 2.5 cm. A ligature is being inserted.

arous women by uterine "afterbirth pains." Meperidine, 50 to 75 mg intramuscularly, given intermittently as needed during the first 24 hours, provides excellent analgesia. Within 8 hours, most women can ambulate, eat a regular diet, and care for and nurse their babies. We have found discharge from the hospital the day after the procedure to be satisfactory in most instances.

NONPUERPERAL TUBAL STERILIZATION

The techniques, including modifications that have been recommended to accomplish sterilization through tubal occlusion, are almost bewildering in number. Basically, they consist of (1) ligation and resection as described above for puerperal sterilization, (2) the permanent application of a variety of rings or clips to the fallopian tubes, and (3) electrocoagulation of a segment of the oviducts.

Laparotomy to perform sterilization can be a much more formidable procedure once the uterus has completely involuted and returned to the true pelvis. However, much of the difficulty of obtaining exposure is removed if the uterus and adnexa are pushed out of the true pelvis to beneath the abdominal wall above the symphysis using a manipulator previously inserted into the uterus with the handle protruding from the vagina. Utilizing this technique, "minilaparotomies" are being performed through a 3-cm incision made suprapubically and tubal sterilization effected.

Vaginal tubal sterilization can usually be performed on women who have delivered vaginally once the uterus has involuted and pregnancy-induced hyperemia has subsided. The peritoneal cavity is entered through the posterior vaginal fornix (colpotomy, culdotomy), the oviducts are grasped and drawn into view, and then, most often, either a Pomeroy type resection or fimbriectomy is performed. As expected, since the operation is performed through the vagina which is "contaminated" with normal bacterial flora, this approach has a higher infection rate.

Enthusiasm was generated for interval as well as post-abortal sterilizations using *laparoscopy* by an article in *Life* magazine (July 28, 1972) that referred to the technique as "Band-Aid" surgery. Commonly, the woman is cared for in an ambulatory surgical setting. Anesthesia, either general, usually with endotracheal intubation, or local, is induced, and after producing pneumoperitoneum with carbon dioxide, the sterilization procedure is accomplished. Most often the woman can be discharged several hours later.

HAZARDS FROM TUBAL STERILIZATION

The principal hazards associated with tubal sterilization are anesthetic complications, inadvertent coagulation of vital structures, the rare occurrence of pulmonary embolism, and failure to produce sterility with an unrecognized and therefore inappropriately treated ectopic pregnancy as the result (see Chap.

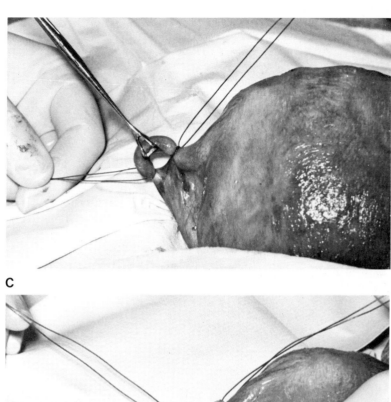

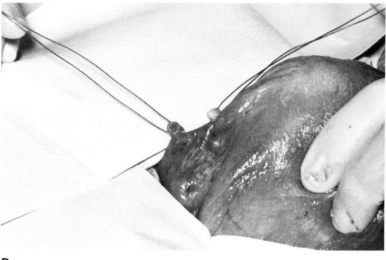

Figure 42–8 (C–D). C. The segment of oviduct separated from mesosalpinx has been ligated. **D.** The ligated segment of oviduct has been resected.

30, p. 511). Peterson and co-workers (1982, 1983) considered all deaths temporally associated with tubal sterilization and estimated the case-fatality frequency to be 8 per 100,000 procedures. When only deaths directly attributable to the procedure per se were considered, the case-fatality rate was at least 4 per 100,000. The leading cause of death, general anesthesia without endotracheal intubation, almost certainly could have been avoided in most cases by use of an endotracheal tube or another form of anesthesia.

Results of a multicenter, multinational randomized study of minilaparotomy with tubal ligation plus a midsegment resection procedure compared to laparoscopy with tubal electrocoagulation have been provided by the World Health Organization Task Force on Female Sterilization (1982). Significant complications were identified in 1.5 percent of the former and 0.9 percent of the latter. They concluded, however, that minilaparotomy is the preferred approach for such a service when provided away from a major institution.

DeStefano and co-workers (1983) identified intraoperative or postoperative complications in 1.7 percent of a large number of women who, remote from pregnancy, underwent laparoscopic tubal electrocoagulation for sterilization. Factors identi-fied to increase morbidity were previous abdominal or pelvic surgery, a history of previous pelvic infection, obesity, diabetes, and general anesthesia rather than local analgesia. These same factors would, undoubtedly, increase the risk of morbidity with minilaparotomy.

TUBAL STERILIZATION FAILURES

No method mentioned above is without failure, and subsequent pregnancy, both uterine as well as ectopic, may result from failure of the method itself or from improper performance of surgical sterilization. Soderstrom (1985) reviewed in detail causes of failures in 47 women referred because of failed sterilization procedures and concluded the following: (1) Resection method failures most often followed spontaneous reanastomosis or fistula formation. Fimbriectomy was particularly vulnerable to reanastomosis because the fimbria was not always removed. (2) Mechanical devices failed when the device was defective or placed improperly. (3) Tissue damage was evident but incomplete with failures following bipolar electrocoagulation, whereas failures following unipolar electrocoagulation were caused by fistula formation. He further concluded that most sterilization failures are not preventable.

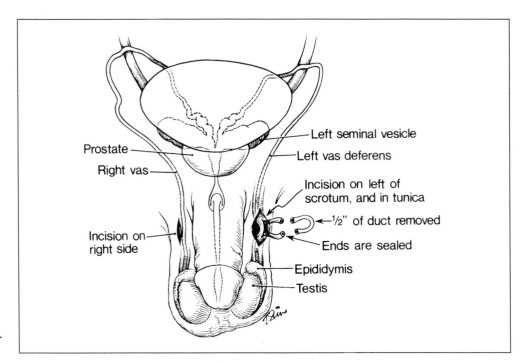

Figure 42–9. Male reproductive system showing the site of vasectomy.

"Post–Tubal Ligation Syndrome"

The possibility has been raised of a "post–tubal ligation syndrome" variably characterized by pelvic discomfort, ovarian cyst formation, and especially menorrhagia. That tubal ligation induces any of these changes remains to be established. Kasonde and Bonnar (1976) actually measured menstrual blood loss before and for 6 to 12 months after tubal sterilization and found that the operation made no significant difference in menstrual blood loss. They also noted that women who presented with menorrhagia soon after sterilization usually had had the problem beforehand or had been using oral contraceptives, which reduced blood loss, and then reverted to spontaneous heavier periods when their use was stopped after sterilization. More recently, DeStefano and co-workers (1983) followed 2,456 women for 2 years after tubal sterilization surgery and noted that, except for menstrual pain among women who underwent unipolar electrocoagulation procedures, there was no increase in the prevalence of adverse menstrual function. In fact, 50 percent or more of women with adverse menstrual function before sterilization had an improvement over the 2 years following the procedure. DeStefano and colleagues (1985) amplified their work by including a control group of women whose partners had undergone vasectomy, and they reported that abnormal menstrual bleeding seldom developed unless it was reported before sterilization. Interestingly, women with menstrual irregularities before sterilization were less likely than the controls to revert spontaneously to normal cyclic menses later. Vessey and associates (1983) compared the frequency of gynecologic and psychiatric disorders among women who had undergone tubal sterilization with the frequencies in women who had not, but their husbands had undergone vasectomy, and found little difference between the two groups.

Some women who had undergone tubal sterilization were reported by Hargrove and Abraham (1981) to have high serum estradiol and low serum progesterone levels compared to normal controls. Ladehoff and co-workers (1980), however, identified no change in ovarian endocrine function following tubal sterilization. Other investigators have failed to identify luteal phase dysfunction after tubal sterilization, except possibly after techniques that can cause obstruction of the uteroovarian artery (Donnez and associates, 1981).

Although complete transection of the oviduct is mandatory, at the same time preservation of blood supply through the adjacent mesosalpinx is desirable to minimize the possibility of "postligation" abnormalities that have been attributed by some to tubal sterilization. The Parkland technique (Fig. 42–7C) should not compromise blood supply to the ovary. Interestingly, El-Minawi and associates (1983), by means of venography, identified uterovaginal and ovarian varicosities commonly after the Pomeroy and some other procedures but not following the Parkland technique.

RESTORATION OF FERTILITY

Despite the recent enthusiasm for performing "microsurgery" on oviducts previously rendered nonpatent surgically, no woman should undergo tubal sterilization believing that her fertility can be restored by such means. Sterilization reversal is costly, difficult, and uncertain. Restoration of tubal continuity and function is technically feasible. The success rate, however, varies with the extent of tubal destruction or removal at the time of sterilization and the overall success rate is probably no more than 50 percent. If any doubt exists in the mind of the recipient, the sterilization should not be done.

HYSTERECTOMY

For the woman who desires no more children, hysterectomy has many theoretical advantages. The only known potential of the uterus, other than to house products of conception, is to harbor disease. However, in the absence of uterine or other pelvic disease, hysterectomy for sterilization at the time of cesarean section, early in the puerperium, or remote from pregnancy is difficult to justify (Barclay and associates, 1976; Laros and Work, 1975). Unfortunately, morbidity, mortality, and cost compared to tubal sterilization, usually preclude hysterectomy. With cesarean hysterectomy, blood loss is nearly always greater than with cesarean section plus tubal sterilization, leading to much more frequent use of blood transfusions and its sequelae. Injury to the urinary tract is also appreciably more common.

For reasons that are hard to identify, an increased failure rate for sterilization at the time of cesarean section has been reported by some. However, with the technique for tubal sterilization used at Parkland Hospital and described above, no difference was identified (Husbands and co-workers, 1970).

HYSTEROSCOPY

Sterilization utilizing *hysteroscopy* to visualize the tubal ostia and somehow obliterate them is a worthy goal and has received considerable attention. To date, the failure rate and other problems limit the clinical utility of this approach.

VASECTOMY

Sterilization of the male has emerged as a popular form of family planning. It has been estimated that one-half million men undergo vasectomy annually in the United States. Through a small incision in the scrotum, the lumen of the vas deferens is disrupted to block the passage of sperm from the testes (Fig. 42–9). The procedure is usually performed in 20 minutes or so on an outpatient basis under local analgesia. The procedure has less morbidity and mortality and is less expensive than female sterilization. The cost of vasectomy has been estimated to be only about one fifth that of tubal sterilization. In Dallas in 1989, the cost of vasectomy was $500 compared to $2,000 for outpatient tubal ligation (J. Pospahala, personal communication).

A disadvantage of vasectomy is that sterility is not immediate. Complete expulsion of sperm stored in the reproductive tract beyond the interrupted vas deferens may take a week to several months. The time appears to depend in part on the frequency of ejaculation. Semen should be checked until two consecutive sperm counts are zero. During this period, another form of contraception must be used. The failure rate for vasectomy is estimated to be about 1 in 100 (Population Reports, 1975).

Restoration of fertility after a successful vasectomy does not always succeed. A review of several reports suggests that odds for success are about 50–50, with somewhat higher success rates following microsurgical reanastomosis. As with women, the risks of regret after sterilization appear to relate primarily to immaturity at the time of sterilization (Howard, 1982). Three factors that appear to be important in restoration of fertility after previous vasectomy are (1) the application of meticulous microsurgical techniques for reanastomosis, (2) the length of time after vasectomy, since chronic obstruction of the vas and possibly the development of sperm antibodies reduce progressively the capacity for spermatogenesis, and (3) the presence of absence of sperm granulomas.

Long-term storage of semen collected before vasectomy remains an experimental procedure. The cost of storing frozen semen is high, the availability of facilities is limited, and the results remain uncertain (Beck, 1978).

Sperm antibodies can be identified rather often after vasectomy. Concern was raised over the possibility that the immune response may cause systemic changes of a harmful nature. Moreover, in some preliminary studies on previously vasectomized monkeys, atherosclerosis appeared to be increased. However, observations carefully made on a very large number of males who had undergone vasectomy several years before have not identified an increase in cardiovascular disease, circulating immune complexes, or damage to blood vessels of the retina (Linnet and co-workers, 1982; Petitti, 1982; Walker and associates, 1981; Goldacre and colleagues, 1983).

REVERSIBLE SYSTEMICALLY ACTING CONTRACEPTIVES FOR MEN

A safe, practical, consistently reliable, and reversible contraceptive for men that does not impair sexual function has not yet been developed.

In China, gossypol, extracted from cottonseed, has been widely used. The compound was discovered after an outbreak of illness and impaired fertility among Chinese farmers exposed to raw cottonseed oil after a change in processing techniques. Gossypol directly affects the testes to inhibit spermatogenesis. Toxic side effects limit its use.

The administration of some analogues of luteinizing hormone-releasing hormone has produced a decline in sperm density, a fall in sperm motility, and a decrease in testosterone production (Linde and co-workers, 1981). The loss of libido makes such a regimen unacceptable.

REFERENCES

Agnelli G, Gresele P, DeCunto M, Nenci GG: Tranexamic acid, intrauterine contraceptive devices and fatal cerebral arterial thrombosis. Br J Obstet Gynaecol 89:681, 1982

Ahlgren M: Sperm transport to and survival in the human fallopian tube. Gynecol Invest 6:206, 1975

Alcid DV, Kothari N, Quinn EP, Geismar L, Glowinsky LZ: Toxic-shock syndrome associated with diaphragm use for only nine hours, Lancet 1:1363 1982

Alvarez F, Brache V, Fernandez E, Guerrero B, Builoff E, Hess R, Salvatierra AM, Zacharias S: New insights on the mode of action of intrauterine contraceptive devices in women. Fertil Steril 49:768, 1988

American College of Obstetricians and Gynecologists: Sterilization. Tech Bull No 113, February 1988

Andersch B, Hahn L: Premenstrual complaints: II. Influence of oral contraceptives. Acta Obstet Gynecol Scand 60:579, 1981

Antoniades K, Campbell WN, Hecksher RH, Kessler WB, McCarthy GE Jr: Liver cell adenoma and oral contraceptives. JAMA 234:628, 1975

Badaracco MA, Vessey MP: Recurrence of venous thromboembolic disease and use of oral contraceptives. Br Med J 1:215, 1974

Barclay DL, Hawks BL, Frueh DM, Power JD, Struble RH: Elective cesarean hysterectomy: A five year comparison with cesarean section. Am J Obstet Gynecol 124:900, 1976

Beck WW Jr: Artificial insemination and preservation of semen. Urol Clin N Am 5:593, 1978

Bradley DD, Wingerd V, Petitti DB, Krauss RM, Rancharan S: Serum high-density-lipoprotein cholesterol in women using oral contraceptives, estrogens and progestins. N Engl J Med 299:17, 1978,

Buhler M, Papiernik E: Successive pregnancies in women fitted with intrauterine devices who take anti-inflammatory drugs. Lancet 1:483, 1983

Cancer and Steroid Hormone Study of the Centers for Disease Control and the National Institute of Child Health and Development: Combination oral contraceptive use and the risk of endometrial cancer. JAMA 257:796, 1987a

Cancer and Steroid Hormone Study of the Centers for Disease Control and the National Institute of Child Health and Development: The reduction in risk associated with oral-contraceptive use. N Engl J Med 316:650, 1987b

Cancer and Steroid Hormone Study of the Centers for Disease Control and the National Institute of Child Health and Development: Oral-contraceptive use and the risk of breast cancer. N Engl J Med 315:405, 1986

Centers for Disease Control: Oral contraceptive use and the risk of breast cancer. JAMA 249:1591, 1983

Centers for Disease Control: Oral contraceptive use and the risk of ovarian cancer. JAMA 249:1596, 1983

Centers for Disease Control: Oral contraceptive use and the risk of endometrial cancer. JAMA 249:1600, 1983

Cheng MCE, Lim YC, Ng AYH, Ratnam SS: Six-monthly Depo-Provera injection as a contraceptive agent: Its acceptability in Singapore. Aust NZ J Obstet Gynaecol 14:231, 1974

Couzinet B, Le Strat N, Ulmann A, Baulieu EE, Schaison G: Termination of early pregnancy by the progesterone antagonist RU 486 (mifepristone). N Engl J Med 315:1555, 1986

Cramer DW, Schiff I, Schoenbaum SC, Gibson M, Belisle S, Albrecht A, Stillman RJ, Berger MJ, Wilson E, Stadel BV, Seibel M: Tubal infertility and the intrauterine device. N Engl J Med 312:941, 1985

Crooij MJ, De Nooyer CCA, Rao BR, Berends GT, Gooren LJG, Janssens J: Termination of early pregnancy by the 3β-Hydroxysteroid dehydrogenase inhibitor epostane. N Engl J Med 319:813, 1988

Daling JR, Weiss NS, Metch BJ, Chow WH, Soderstrom RM, Moore DE, Spadoni LR, Stadel BV: Primary tubal infertility in relation to the use of an intrauterine device. N Engl J Med 312:937, 1985

Das C, Catt KJ: Antifertility actions of the progesterone antagonist RU 486 include direct inhibition of placental hormone secretion. Lancet 2:599, 1987

Dawood MY, Birnbaum SJ: Unilateral tubo-ovarian abscess and intrauterine contraceptive device. Obstet Gynecol 46:429, 1975

DeStefano F, Greenspan JR, Dicker RC, Peterson HB, Strauss LT, Rubin GL: Complications of interval laparoscopic tubal sterilization. Obstet Gynecol 61:153, 1983

DeStefano F, Perlman JA, Peterson HB, Diamond EL: Long-term risk of menstrual disturbances after tubal sterilization. Am J Obstet Gynecol 152:835, 1985

Donnez J, Wauters M, Thomas K: Luteal function after tubal sterilization. Obstet Gynecol 57:65, 1981

Edelman DA, Kothenbeutel R, Levinski MJ, Kelly SE: Comparative trials of low-dose combined oral contraceptives. J Reprod Med 28:195, 1983

Ellis JW: Multiphasic oral contraceptives: Efficacy and metabolic impact. J Reprod Med 32:38, 1987

El-Minawi MF, Masor N, Reda MS: Pelvic venous changes after tubal sterilization. J Reprod Med 28:641, 1983

FDA: Drug Bull 16:2, 1986

Feldblum PJ, Fortney JA: Condoms, spermicides and the transmission of human immunodeficiency virus: A review of the literature. Am J Public Health 78:52, 1988

Fisch IR, Frank J: Oral contraceptives and blood pressure. JAMA 237:2499, 1977

Forrest JD, Fordyce RR: US women's contraceptive attitude and practice; How have they changed in the 1980's? Fam Plann Perspect 20:112, 1988

Francis WJA: Reproduction at menarche and menopause in women. J Reprod Fertil (Suppl) 12:89, 1970

Goldacre JM, Holford TR, Vessey MP: Cardiovascular disease and vasectomy. N Engl J Med 308:805, 1983

Grimes DA: Reversible contraception for the 1980s. JAMA 255:69, 1986

Guttorm E: Menstrual bleeding with intrauterine contraceptive devices. Acta Obstet Gynecol Scand 50:9, 1971

Hargrove JT, Abraham GE: Endocrine profile of patients with post-tubal ligation syndrome. J Reprod Med 26:359, 1981

Harlap S, Eldor J: Births following oral contraceptive failures. Obstet Gynecol 55:447, 1980

Heartwell SF, Schlesselman S: Risk of uterine perforation among users of intrauterine devices. Obstet Gynecol 61:31, 1983

Howard G: Who asks for vasectomy reversal and why? Br Med J 285:490, 1982

Hull MGR, Savage PE, Bromham DR, Jackson JAM: Normal fertility in women with post-pill amenorrhea. Lancet 1:1329, 1981

Husbands, ME Jr, Pritchard JA, Pritchard SA: Failure of tubal sterilization accompanying cesarean section. Am J Obstet Gynecol 107:966, 1970

International Planned Parenthood Federation, International Medical Advisory Panel: Statement on periodic abstinence for family planning. IPPF Med Bull 18:2, 1982

Irey NS, Nanion WC, Taylor HB: Vascular lesions in women taking oral contraceptives. Arch Pathol 89:1, 1970

Janevich DT, Piper JM, Glebatis DM: Oral contraceptives and congenital limb reduction defects. N Engl J Med 291:697, 1974

Jick H, Walker AM, Rothman KJ, Hunter JR, Holmes LB, Watkins RN, D'Ewart DC, Danford A, Madsen S: Vaginal spermicides and congenital disorders. JAMA 245:1329, 1981

Kalkhoff RK: Relative sensitivity of postpartum gestational diabetic women to oral contraceptive agents and other metabolic stress. Diabetes Care 3:421, 1980

Kasonde JM, Bonnar J: Effect of sterilization on menstrual blood loss. Br J Obstet Gynaecol 83:572, 1976

Keebler C, Chatwani A, Schwartz R: Actinomyces infection associated with intrauterine contraceptive devices. Am J Obstet Gynecol 145:596, 1983

Kent DR, Nissen ED, Nissen SE, Ziehm DJ: Effect of pregnancy on liver tumor associated with oral contraceptives. Obstet Gynecol 51:148, 1978

Klaus H: Natural family planning: A review. Obstet Gynecol Surv 37:128, 1982

Knopp RH: Cardiovascular effects of endogenous and exogenous sex hormones over a woman's lifetime. Am J Obstet Gynecol 158:1630, 1988

Kroener WF Jr: Surgical sterilization by fimbriectomy. Am J Obstet Gynecol 104:247, 1969

Kuchara LK: Postcoital contraception with diethylstilbestrol. JAMA 218:562, 1971

Ladehoff P, Lindholm P, Qvist K, Sorenson T: Gonadotropins and estrogens before and after laparoscopic sterilization. Acta Obstet Gynecol Scand (Suppl) 93:77, 1980

Lammer EJ, Cordero JF: Exogenous sex hormone exposure and the risk for major malformations. JAMA 255:3128–3132, 1986

Laros RK Jr, Work BA Jr: Female sterilization: III. Vaginal hysterectomy. Am J Obstet Gynecol 122:693, 1975

Larrson-Cohn U: Oral contraceptives and vitamins: A review. Am J Obstet Gynecol 121:84, 1975

Leklem JE, Brown RR, Rose DP, Linkswiler HM: Vitamin B₆ requirements of women using oral contraceptives. Am J Clin Nutr 28:535, 1975

Lemay A, Faure N: Fourteen-day versus twenty-one-day regimens of intermittent intranasal luteinizing hormone-releasing agonist combined with an oral progestogen as antivulatory contraceptive approach. J Clin Endocrinol Metab 63:1379, 1986

Liang AP, Levenson AG, Layde PM, Shelton UD, Hatcher RA, Potts M, Michelson MJ: Risk of breast, uterine corpus, and ovarian cancer in women receiving medroxyprogesterone injections. JAMA 249:2909, 1983

Linde R, Doelle GC, Alexander N, Kirchner F, Vale W, Rivier J, Rabin D: Reversible inhibition of testicular steroidogenesis and spermatogenesis by a potent gonadotropin-releasing hormone agonist in normal men. N Engl J Med 305:663, 1981

Linn S, Schoenbaum SC, Monson RR, Rosner B, Ryan KJ: Delay in conception for former "pill" users. JAMA 247:629, 1982

Linn S, Schoenbaum SC, Monson RR, Rosner B, Stubblefield PG, Ryan KJ: Lack of association between contraceptive usage and congenital malformations in offspring. Am J Obstet Gynecol 147:923, 1983

Linnet L, Moller NPH, Bernth-Perersen P, Ehlers N, Brandslund I, Svehag S–E: No increase in arteriosclerotic retinopathy or activity in tests for circulating immune complexes 5 years after vasectomy. Fertil Steril 37:798, 1982

Lippes J, Tatum HJ, Maulid D, Zielezny M: A continuation of the study of postcoital IUDs. Presented at the annual meeting of the Association of Planned Parenthood Physicians, San Diego, October 25, 1978

Lopez G, Rodrigues A, Rengifo J, Sivin I: Two-year prospective study in Colombia of Norplant implants. Obstet Gynecol 68:204, 1985

Louik C, Mitchell AA, Werler MM, Hanson JW, Shapiro S: Maternal exposure to spermicides in relation to certain birth defects. N Engl J Med 317:474, 1987

Lungren SS: A case of cesarean twice. Am J Obstet Dis Women Child 14:78, 1881

Mann JI, Inman WHW: Oral contraceptives and death from myocardial infarction. Br Med J 2:245, 1975

McPherson K, Neil A, Vessey MP, Doll R: Oral contraceptives and breast cancer. Lancet 2:1414 1983

Meade TW: Risks and mechanisms of cardiovascular events in users of oral contraceptives. Am J Obstet Gynecol 158:1646, 1988

Meirik O, Lund E, Adami H, Bergstrom R, Christoffersen T, Bergsö P: Oral contraceptive use and breast cancer in young women: A joint national case-control study in Sweden and Norway. Lancet 1:650, 1986

Metcalf MG: Incidence of ovulatory cycles in women approaching the menopause. J Biosoc Sci 11:39, 1979

Metcalf MG, Donald RA: Fluctuating ovarian function in a perimenopausal woman. Aust NZ Med J 89:45, 1979

Metz KGP: Failures following fimbriectomy. Fertil Steril 28:66, 1977

Mills JL, Harley EE, Reed GF, Berendes HW: Are spermicides teratogenic? JAMA 248:2148, 1982

Mishell DR Jr: Noncontraceptive health benefits of oral contraceptives. Am J Obstet Gynecol 142:809, 1982

Mishell DR Jr: Use of oral contraceptives in women of older reproductive age. Am J Obstet Gynecol 158:1652, 1988

Neiman LK, Choate TM, Chrousos GP, Healy DL, Morin M, Renquist D, Merriam GR, Spitz IM, Bardin CW, Baulieu EE, Loriaux DL: The progesterone antagonist RU 486: A potential new contraceptive agent. N Engl J Med 316:187, 1987

Neuberger J, Forman D, Doll R, Williams R: Oral contraceptives and hepatocellular carcinoma. Br Med J 292:1355, 1986

Nilsson L, Sölvell L: Clinical studies on oral contraceptives. Acta Obstet Gynecol Scand (Suppl) 8:46, 1967

Nora AH, Nora JJ: A syndrome of multiple congenital anomalies associated with teratogenic exposure. Arch Environ Health 30:17, 1975

Paul C, Skegg DCG, Spears GFS, Kaldor JM: Oral contraceptives and breast cancer: A national study. Br Med J 293:723, 1986

Perez A: Natural family planning: Postpartum period. Int J Fertil 26:219, 1981

Peterson HB, DeStefano F, Greenspan JR, Ory HW: Mortality risk associated with tubal sterilization in United States hospitals. Am J Obstet Gynecol 143:125, 1982

Peterson HB, DeStefano F, Rubin GL, Greenspan JR, Lee NC, Ory HW: Deaths attributed to tubal sterilization in the United States, 1977 to 1981. Am J Obstet Gynecol 146:131, 1983

Petitti DB: Atherosclerotic disease in men 10 or more years after vasectomy. Presented at the annual meeting of the Association of Planned Parenthood Professionals, Baltimore, November 19, 1982

Petitti DB, Yamamoto D, Morgenstern N: Factors associated with actinomyces-like organisms on Papanicolaou smear in users of intrauterine contraceptive devices. Am J Obstet Gynecol 145:339, 1983

Phillips N, Duffy T: One-hour glucose tolerance in relation to the use of oral contraceptive drugs. Am J Obstet Gynecol 116:91, 1973

Pike MC, Henderson BE, Krailo MD, Duke A, Roy S: Breast cancer in young women and use of oral contraceptives: Possible modifying effect of formulation and age at use. Lancet 2:926, 1983

Pituitary Adenoma Study Group: Pituitary adenomas and oral contraceptives: A multi-center case controlled study. Fertil Steril 39:753, 1983

Population Reports: Vasectomy—What are the problems? Series D, No 1, January 1975, pp. 41–60

Population Reports: OC's—Update on usage, safety, and side effects. January 1979, p A-133

Population Reports: Periodic abstinence: How well do new approaches work? Series L, No 3, September 1981, pp. 33–71

Population Reports: IUDs: An appropriate contraception for many women. Series B, No 4, July 1982, pp. 101–135

Population Reports: Update on condoms—Products, protection, promotion. Series H, No 6, September–October 1982, pp. 121–156

Population Reports: Barrier Method—New developments in vaginal contraception. Series H, No 7, January–February 1984, pp. 157–190

Porter JB, Jick H, Walker AM: Mortality among oral contraceptive users. Obstet Gynecol 70:29, 1987

Prasad AS, Lei KY, Moghissi KS: The effect of oral contraceptives on micronutrients. In Mosely WH (ed): Nutrition and Human Reproduction. New York, Plenum Press, 1978

Pritchard JA, Pritchard SA: Blood pressure response to estrogen-progestin oral contraceptive after pregnancy-induced hypertension. Am J Obstet Gynecol 129:733, 1977

Pritchard JA, Scott DE, Whalley PJ: Maternal folate deficiency and pregnancy wastage: IV. Effects of folic acid supplements, anticonvulsants, and oral contraceptives. Am J Obstet Gynecol 109:341, 1971

Purrier BGA, Sparks RA, Watt PJ, Elstein M: In vitro study of the possible role of the intrauterine contraceptive device tail in ascending infection of the genital tract. Br J Obstet Gynaecol 86:374, 1979

Realini JP, Goldzieher JW: Oral contraceptives and cardiovascular disease: A critique of the epidemiologic studies. Am J Obstet Gynecol 152:729, 1985

Rothman KJ, Louik C: Oral contraceptives and birth defects. N Engl J Med 299:522, 1978

Roumen FJME, Dieben TOM: Ovulation prediction by monitoring salivary electrical resistance with the Cue fertility monitor. Obstet Gynecol 71:49, 1988

Royal College of General Practitioners' Oral Contraceptive Study: Oral contraceptives and gallbladder disease. Lancet 2:957, 1982

Runnebaum B, Rabe T: New progestogens in oral contraceptives Am J Obstet Gynecol 157:1059, 1987

Savolainen E, Saksela E, Saxen L: Teratogenic hazards of oral contraceptives analyzed in a national malformation register. Am J Obstet Gynecol 140:521, 1981

Schwallie PC: Experience with Depo-Provera as an injectable contraceptive. J Reprod Med 13:113, 1974

Scott DE, Pritchard JA: Hematologic effects of oral contraceptives after megaloblastic anemia in pregnancy: Gynecol Invest 6:40, 1975

Segal S: A new delivery system for contraceptive steroids. Am J Obstet Gynecol 157:1090, 1987

Shapiro S, Slone D, Heinonin OP, Kaufman DW, Rosenberg L, Mitchell AA, Helmrich SP: Birth defects and vaginal spermicides. JAMA 247:2381, 1982

Shojania AM, Hornaday G, Barnes PH: Oral contraceptives and serum-folate levels. Lancet 1:1376, 1968

Skouby SO, Kühl C, Mølsted-Pedersen L, Petersen K, Christensen MS: Triphasic oral contraception: Metabolic effects in normal women and those with previous gestational diabetes. Am J Obstet Gynecol 153:495, 1985

Soderstrom RM: Sterilization failures and their causes. Am J Obstet Gynecol 152:395, 1985

Spellacy WN, Buhi WC, Birk SA: The effects of vitamin B$_6$ on carbohydrate metabolism in women taking steroid contraceptives: Preliminary report. Contraception 6:265, 1972

Stadel BV: Oral contraceptives and cardiovascular disease. N Engl J Med 305:612, 672, 1981

Stampfer MJ, Willett WC, Colditz GA, Speizer FE, Hennekens CH: A prospective study of past use of oral contraceptive agents and risk of cardiovascular diseases. N Engl J Med 319:1313, 1988

Stephens MEM, Craft I, Peters TJ, Hoffbrand AV: Oral contraceptives and folate metabolism. Clin Sci 42:405, 1972

Streiff RR: Folate deficiency and oral contraceptives. JAMA 214:105, 1970

Strobino B, Kline J, Warburton D: Spermicide use and pregnancy outcome. Am J Public Health 78:260, 1988

Szlachter BN, Nachtigall LE, Epstein J, Young BK, Weiss G: Premature menopause: A reversible entity? Obstet Gynecol 54:396, 1979

Tatum HJ: Copper-bearing intrauterine devices. Clin Obstet Gynecol 17:93, 1974

Tatum HJ, Schmidt FH, Jain AK: Management and outcome of pregnancies associated with Copper-T intrauterine contraceptive device. Am J Obstet Gynecol 126:869, 1976

Taylor ES, McMillan JH, Greer BE, Droegemueller W, Thompson HE: The intrauterine device and tubo-ovarian abscess. Am J Obstet Gynecol 123:338, 1975

Taylor TS: Editorial comment. Obstet Gynecol Surv 27:168, 1972

Taylor WW, Martin FG, Pritchard SA, Pritchard JA: Complications from Majzlin spring intrauterine device. Obstet Gynecol 14:404, 1973

Theur RC: The effect of oral contraceptive agents on vitamin and mineral needs: A review. J Reprod Med 3:13, 1972

Toews M, Boone S, Watson M, Whillans J: A multicenter phase IV study of Ortho 7/7/7 tablets in previous users of oral contraceptives. Curr Ther Res 41:509, 1987

Vessey MP: Thromboembolism, cancer, and oral contraceptives. Clin Obstet Gynecol 17:65, 1974

Vessey MP, Baron J, Doll R, McPherson K, Yeates D: Oral contraceptives and breast cancer: Final report of an epidemiological study. Br J Cancer 47:455, 1983b

Vessey MP, Doll R, Jones K: Oral contraceptives and breast cancer. Lancet 1:941, 1975

Vessey MP, Doll R, Jones K, McPherson K, Yeates D: An epidemiological study of oral contraceptives and breast cancer. Br Med J 1:1757, 1979

Vessey MP, Huggins G, Lawless M, Yeates D: Tubal sterilization: Findings in a large prospective study. Br J Obstet Gynaecol 90:203, 1983

Vessey MP, Lawless M, McPherson K, Yeates D: Fertility after stopping use of intrauterine contraceptive device. Br Med J 286:106, 1983

Vessey MP, Lawless M, Yeates D: Efficacy of different contraceptive methods. Lancet 1:841, 1982

Vessey MP, McPherson K, Lawless M, Yeates D: Neoplasia of the cervix uteri and contraception: A possible adverse effect of the pill. Lancet 2:930, 1983a

Vessey MP, Meisler L, Flavel R, Yeates D: Outcome of pregnancy in women using different methods of contraception. Br J Obstet Gynaecol 86:548, 1979

Vessey MP, Wiggins P: Use-effectiveness of the diaphragm in a selected family planning clinic population in the United Kingdom. Contraception 9:15, 1974

Vessey MP, Yeates D, Flavel R: Risk of ectopic pregnancy and duration of use of an intrauterine device. Lancet 2:501, 1979

Walker AM, Hunter JR, Watkins RN, Jick H, Danford A, Alhadeff L, Rothman KF: Vasectomy and non-fatal myocardial infarction. Lancet 1:13, 1981

Warburton D, Neugut RH, Lustenberger A, Nicholas AG, Kline J: Lack of association between spermicide use and trisomy. N Engl J Med 317:478, 1987

Weir RJ: Effect on blood pressure or changing from high to low dose steroid preparations in women with oral contraceptive induced hypertension. Scott Med J 27:212, 1982

Williams NB: Contraceptive Technology 1986–1987. New York, Irvington, 1986, p 183

Wingrave AJ, Kay CR, Vessey MP: Oral contraceptives and diabetes mellitus. Br Med J 1:23, 1979

Wiseman RA: Oral contraceptives and breast cancer rates. Lancet 2:1415, 1983

World Health Organization Task Force on Female Sterilization: Minilaparotomy or laparoscopy for sterilization: A multicenter, multinational randomized study. Am J Obstet Gynecol 143:645, 1982

Wynn V: Vitamins and oral contraceptive use. Lancet 1:561, 1975

Yuzpe AA, Smith RP, Rademaker AE: A multicenter clinical investigation employing ethinyl estradiol combined with dl-norgestrel as a postcoital contraceptive agent. Fertil Steril 37:508, 1982

Zipper JA, Tatum JH, Medel M, Pastene L, Rivera M: Contraception through the use of intrauterine metals: I Copper as an adjunct to the T device. Am J Obstet Gynecol 109:771, 1971

Appendix: Système International (S.I.)

SYSTEME INTERNATIONAL (SI) CONVERSION FACTORS FOR SOME FREQUENTLY USED LABORATORY COMPONENTS

System[a]	Component	Present Reference Interval and Units (Examples)[b]	Conversion Factor	SI Reference Interval and Units	Significant Digits[c]	Suggested Minimum Increment
Hematology						
B	Hematocrit					
	Female	33–43%	0.01	0.33–0.43	0.XX	
	Male	39–49%	0.01	0.39–0.49	0.XX	
B	Hemoglobin concentration					
	Female	12.0–15.0 g/dL	10	120–150 g/L	XXX	
	Male	13.6–17.2 g/dL	10	136–172 g/L	XXX	
(B) Ercs	Mean corpuscular hemoglobin / *Mass concentration*	27–33 pg	1	27–33 pg	XX	
(B) Ercs	Mean corpuscular hemoglobin concentration	33–37 g/dL	10	330–337 g/L	XX0	
(B) Ercs	Mean corpuscular volume	76–100 cu µm	1	76–100 fL	XXX	
B	Erythrocytes (*Female*)	$3.5-5.0\ 10^6$/cu mm	1	$3.5-5.0\ 10^{12}$/L	XX	
B	Thrombocytes (platelets)	$150-450\ 10^3$/cu mm	1	$150-450\ 10^9$/L	XXX	
B Lkcs	White blood count	3,200–9,800/cu mm	0.001	$3.2-9.8\ 10^9$/L	XX.X	
Clinical Chemistry						
S	Aspartate aminotransferase (ASAT)	0–35 Units/L	1.00	0–35 U/L	XX	1 U/L
		0–35 Karmen units/mL	0.482	... U/L	XX	1 U/L
S	Albumin	4.0–6.0 g/dL	0.01	40–60 g/L	XX	1 g/L
S	Amylase, enzymatic	0–130 (37°C) Units/L	1.00	0–130 U/L	XXX	1 U/L
	(Somogyi/Caraway)	50–150 Somogyi units/dL	1.850	100–300 U/L	XX0	10 U/L
S	Bilirubin					
	Total	0.1–1.0 mg/dL	17.10	2–18 µmol/L	XX	2 µmol/L
	Conjugated	0–0.2 mg/dL	17.10	0–4 µmol/L	XX	2 µmol/L
S	Calcium	8.8–10.0 mg/dL	0.2495	2.20–2.50 mmol/L	X.XX	0.02 mmol/L
	Female<50 yr old					
B,P,S	Carbon dioxide content (bicarbonate + CO_2)	22–28 mEq/L	1.00	22–28 mmol/L	XX	1 mmol/L
S	Creatinine	0.6–1.2 mg/dL	88.40	50–110 µmol/L	XX0	10 µmol/L
S,U	Creatinine clearance	75–125 mL/min	0.01667	1.24–2.08 mL/s	X.XX	0.02 mL/s
P	Fibrinogen	200–400 mg/dL	0.01	2.0–4.0 g/L	X.X	0.1 g/L
P	Follicle-stimulating hormone (FSH)					
	Female	2.0–15.0 mIU/mL	1.00	2–15 IU/L	XX	1 IU/L
	Peak production	20–50 mIU/mL	1.00	20–50 IU/L	XX	1 IU/L
P	Glucose	70–110 mg/dL	0.05551	3.9–6.1 mmol/L	XX.X	0.1 mmol/L
S	Iron (*Female*)	60–160 µg/dL	0.1791	11–29 µmol/L	XX	1 µmol/L
S	Iron-binding capacity	250–460 µg/dL	0.1791	45–82 µmol/L	XX	1 µmol/L
S	Magnesium	1.8–3.0 mg/dL	0.4114	0.80–1.20 mmol/L	X.XX	.02 mmol/L
S	Phosphate (as phosporus)	2.5–5.0 mg/dL	0.3229	0.80–1.60 mmol/L	X.XX	.05 mmol/L
S	Potassium	3.5–5.0 mEq/L	1.00	3.5–5.0 mmol/L	X.X	0.1 mmol/L
S	Protein (*Total*)	6–8 g/dL	10.0	60–80 g/L	XX	1 g/L
S	Sodium	135–147 mEq/L	1.00	135–147 mmol/L	XXX	1 mmol/L
P	Testosterone (*Female*)	<0.6 ng/mL	3.467	<2.0 nmol/L	XX.X	0.5 nmol/L
S	Triiodothyronine (T_3)	75–220 ng/dL	0.01536	1.2–3.4 nmol/L	X.X	0.1 nmol/L

[a] P represents plasma; B, blood; S, serum; U, urine; Ercs, erythrocytes; and Lkcs, leukocytes.

[b] These reference values are not intended to be definitive since each laboratory determines its own values. These values are for males and nonpregnant females and many of these values are substantially altered by pregnancy.

[c] Number of digits used to describe reported results. XX implies that results expressed to the nearest whole number are meaningful; XX0 that results are meaningful when rounded to the nearest 10, and that results reported to lower number are beyond the sensitivity of the procedure.

Adapted from JAMA 260:73, 1988

Index

Page numbers followed by *f* refer to illustrations.
Page numbers followed by *t* refer to tables.

949

Cerebral blood flow, fetal, Doppler velocimetry of, 288

Cerebral embolism, in pregnancy, 845

Cerebral palsy, 597
  factors contributing to, 597

Cerebral-placental ratio, 770

Cerebral venous thrombosis, in pregnancy, 844, 845

Cerebrovascular accident. *See* Stroke

Cerebrovascular disease, complicating pregnancy, 844–845

Ceruloplasmin
  maternal, in pregnancy, 138
  plasma levels, in pregnancy, 140

Cervical anomalies. *See also* Cervix
  classification of, 730, 730*t*
    with DES exposure in utero, 736
  obstetrical significance of, 731

Cervical cancer
  carcinoma in situ, during pregnancy, 728
  dystocia and, 386
  invasive, during pregnancy, 728–729
  papillomaviruses and, 728
  screening for, 728
  therapeutic abortion with, 501

Cervical cytology, abnormal, 728

Cervical dilatation
  abnormalities of, with pelvic inlet contraction, 378
  after midpregnancy, risk of preterm birth with, 753
  evaluation of, at admittance, 308
  incomplete, delivery through, postpartum hemorrhage with, 415
  in labor, 341
  manual, 438
  mechanism of, 217–218, 218*f*–220*f*
  pattern of, 218–219, 220*f*
  protracted, 346
  secondary arrest of, 341–342, 342*t*, 346

Cervical dysplasia, 728

Cervical effacement, 218*f*
  evaluation of, at admittance, 308
  mechanism of, 217

Cervical erosions
  postpartum, 481–482
  in pregnancy, 133

Cervical eversions, postpartum, 481–482

Cervical incisions. *See* Dührssen incisions

Cervical mucorrhea, with oral contraceptives, 928

Cervical myoma, dystocia and, 388*f*, 389

Cervical neoplasia
  intraepithelial, with DES exposure in utero, 736
  management of, during pregnancy, 728–729

Cervical os, conglutination of, dystocia and, 386

Cervical pregnancy, 530–531, 531*f*

Cervix. *See also* Cervical; Engagement
  abnormalities of, dystocia and, 386
  acute edema of, 738
  adaptation to pregnancy, 133, 134*f*
  anatomy of, 877, 878–880
  annular (circular) detachment of, 405
  anterior and posterior lips, 879
  appearance of
    in multipara versus nullipara, 20
    in pregnancy, 258
  atresia of, dystocia and, 386
  biopsy, during pregnancy, 728
  changes in
    during labor, 341
    as symptom of pregnancy, 14
  cyclical changes in, 36
  double, 730
  examination of, at admittance, 308
  external os, 877, 879
    appearance, in parous woman, 879, 880*f*
  glands of, 880
  incompetent, 879
    preterm labor and, 749

Cervix (*cont.*)
  injuries to, in delivery, 405–406
  internal os, 877, 878
  in labor, 217, 217*f*
  mucosa, 880
  in parturition, 212
  portio vaginalis, 878
  position of
    in abdominal pregnancy, 528*f*, 529
    evaluation of, at admittance, 308
  puerperal infection in, 464–465
  in puerperium, 246–247
  ripening of, 212
    regulatory factors in, 212–213
  septate, 730
  squamo-columnar junction, 880
  stenosis of, dystocia and, 386
  supravaginal portion, 878

Cesarean hysterectomy, 453–455
  appendectomy at, 455
  for cervical neoplasia, 728
  indications for, 453–454
  oophorectomy at, 455
  technique, 454–455

Cesarean section, 441–447. *See also* Vaginal delivery, after cesarean section
  abdominal closure in, 452*f*, 452–453
  abdominal incisions in, 447–448
  active management of labor and, 313
  ambulation after, 456
  amnionic fluid volume and, 762
  anesthesia and analgesia for, 329, 330, 335, 447
    postoperative, 455
  bladder and bowel function after, 456
  blood loss in, 142
  breast care after, 456
  with breech presentation, 350, 352, 353, 355, 357, 399–400, 441–443
  classical, 447, 453
  coarctation of aorta and, 804
  contraindications, 445
  definition of, 441
  delivery of infant in, 450–451, 450*f*–451*f*
  diabetes and, 817, 822
  emergency
    after CPR, 805
    for entrapment of fetal head, with breech presentation, 399–400
  extraperitoneal, 453
  with fetal growth retardation, 772–773
  fluid therapy and diet with, postoperative, 455–456
  frequency of, 441–443
  gas pains after, 456
  heart disease and, 798
  in hemolytic disease, 608
  historical perspective on, 457–458
  hospital discharge after, 456
  in hypotonic uterine dysfunction, 344
  hysterectomy at, 940
  in immune thrombocytopenia, 791, 792–793
  incisional infection after, 465
  indications for, 441, 442*t*
  intravenous fluid administration in, 455
  with kyphoscoliosis, 804
  laboratory tests after, 456
  maternal morbidity and, 444
  maternal mortality and, 443–444
  versus midforceps delivery, 436
  in multifetal pregnancy, 648–649
  perinatal morbidity and mortality and, 442, 443*f*
  perinatal morbidity and mortality in, 444
  in placental abruption, 708
  placental delivery in, 451, 451*f*
  with placenta previa, 715–716
  postmortem, 453
    historical perspective on, 457
  postpartum infections in, 465–468, 472–474
  in postterm pregnancy, 759, 760, 763
  preoperative care, 455

Cesarean section (*cont.*)
  of preterm infant, 755
    with breech presentation, 353–354
  preterm rupture of membranes and, 750, 751
  prophylactic antimicrobial therapy with, 456–457, 457*f*
  recovery suite care, 455
  recurrent indications for, 445–446
  repair of uterus in, 451–452, 452*f*
  repeat, 441, 442
    timing of, 444
  scar
    classical versus lower-segment, 407–408
    dehiscence of, 407
    healing of, 408, 409*f*
    rupture of, 406–407, 408, 408*f*, 409*f*
  spinal analgesia for, 335
  sterilization at, 940
  technique of, 447–453
  with transverse lie, 362
  tubal sterilization in, 452, 936–937, 937*f*, 938*f*–939*f*
  with uterine anomalies, 731–736
  uterine incisional infection, 469
  uterine incision in, 447, 448*f*–449*f*, 448–450
  vital signs with, postoperative monitoring of, 455
  volvulus and, 834
  in von Willebrand disease, 796
  wound care for, 456

c-fms proto-oncogene, 201

Chadwick's sign, 13, 135

Chamberlen forceps, 438–439, 439*f*

Chancroid, in pregnancy, 859

Chiari-Frommel syndrome, 486

Chickenpox, complicating pregnancy, 847–848. *See also* Varicella

Chimerism, 63, 636

Chlamydial conjunctivitis, in newborn, 242

Chlamydial infections
  asymptomatic, 853–854
  coexistent in gonorrhea, 853
  complicating pregnancy, 853–854
  low birthweight and, 854
  neonatal, 619
    treatment of, 619
  preterm birth and, 854
  puerperal, 463, 463*t*, 854
  symptomatic, 853
  uterine, postpartum, 481

Chlamydia psittaci, pneumonia, 805

Chlamydia trachomatis, 853
  in pathogenesis of preterm labor, 750
  spontaneous abortion and, 493
  testing for, prenatal, 261
  UTI, 809

Chloasma, 136, 841
  oral contraceptives and, 928

Chloramphenicol, for puerperal infection, 464

Chlorodiazepoxide, teratogenic risks of, 568

Chloroprocaine, 333*t*
  for local anesthesia, 333*t*
  for paracervical block, 335

Chloroquine, teratogenic risks of, 565

Chlorothiazide, therapy, teratogenic risks of, 565

Chlorpromazine, teratogenic risks of, 568

Cholecalciferol. *See* Vitamin D

Cholecystectomy, 831–832

Cholecystitis, complicating pregnancy, 831–832

Cholelithiasis
  complicating pregnancy, 831–832
  in pregnancy, 834

Cholestasis
  intrahepatic, of pregnancy, 827
  oral contraceptives and, 925

Cholestatic hepatosis of pregnancy, 827

Cholestatic jaundice, oral contraceptives and, 925

Cholesterol. *See also* Low-density lipoprotein
  fetal levels of, regulation of, 76–77, 78*f*
  as precursor for progesterone biosynthesis, 82
  for steroidogenesis, 912–913

Cholesteryl ester storage disease, prenatal diagnosis of, 582*t*

Page numbers followed by f refer to illustrations.
Page numbers followed by t refer to tables.

Page numbers followed by f refer to illustrations.
Page numbers followed by t refer to tables.